Contents

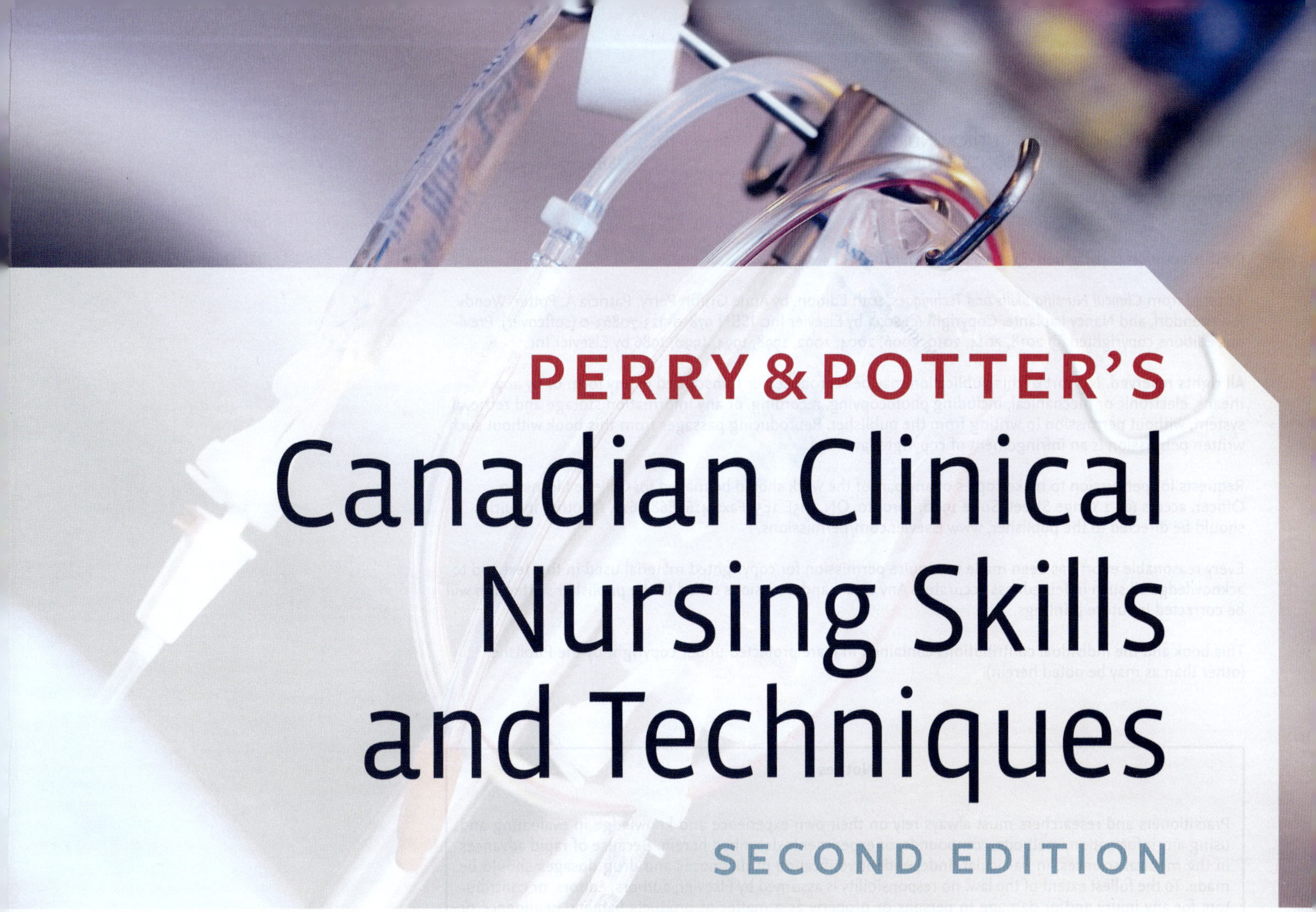

PERRY & POTTER'S

Canadian Clinical Nursing Skills and Techniques

SECOND EDITION

Shelley L. Cobbett, RN, BN, GnT, MN, EdD

Assistant Professor, Nursing and BScN Site Administrator
School of Nursing–Yarmouth Campus
Dalhousie University
Yarmouth, Nova Scotia

US TENTH EDITION EDITORS

Anne Griffin Perry, RN, MSN, EdD, FAAN
Professor Emerita
School of Nursing
Southern Illinois University—Edwardsville
Edwardsville, Illinois

Patricia A. Potter, RN, MSN, PhD, FAAN
Formerly, Director of Research
Patient Care Services
Barnes-Jewish Hospital
St. Louis, Missouri

Wendy R. Ostendorf, RN, MS, EdD, CNE
Contributing Faculty
Master of Science in Nursing Program
Walden University
Minneapolis, Minnesota

Nancy Laplante, PhD, RN, AHN-BC
Associate Professor of Nursing
School of Nursing
Widener University
Chester, Pennsylvania

ELSEVIER

PERRY & POTTER's CANADIAN CLINICAL NURSING SKILLS AND TECHNIQUES, SECOND EDITION

ISBN: 978-0-323-82744-7

Notices

Practitioners and researchers must always rely on their own experience and knowledge in evaluating and using any information, methods, compounds, or experiments described herein. Because of rapid advances in the medical sciences, in particular, independent verification of diagnoses and drug dosages should be made. To the fullest extent of the law, no responsibility is assumed by Elsevier, authors, editors, or contributors for any injury and/or damage to persons or property as a matter of products liability, negligence or otherwise, or from any use or operation of any methods, products, instructions, or ideas contained in the material herein.

Senior Content Strategist (Acquisitions, Canada): Roberta A. Spinosa-Millman
Content Development Manager: Lenore Gray Spence
Content Development Specialist: Martina van de Velde
Publishing Services Manager: Deepthi Unni
Senior Project Manager: Manchu Mohan
Cover Design and Design Direction: Brian Salisbury

Printed in India

Last digit is the print number: 9 8 7 6 5 4 3

Collaborating with expert professional nurses across Canada to ensure that the Second Edition of this textbook continues to be based on evidence-informed best practices, while remaining cognizant of jurisdictional differences, has been a deeply rewarding and enlightening experience. Nursing is not only a profession but a lifestyle, a way of being and interacting with people, and a profession that I am forever grateful to be a part of. As the seasons change each year, so too do our lives and our families.

I would like to dedicate this text to the first man I loved, the man that could see no wrong in my choices throughout life, the man that supported my life aspirations and goals without question or hesitation, the man that was proud to have his daughter become a nurse: my dad, Patrick William Gallagher (March 17, 1940–October 11, 2019). May he be resting in peace now that his work on this earth is done. Love you forever, love you always, Dad. XO

Shelley L. Cobbett

As always, this book is dedicated to my children. To be their mother brings more joy, honour, and sense of pride than I could have ever imagined. They and their loved ones are truly my shining stars. As they grow, things change, and I now also dedicate this book to:

My daughter, Rebecca Lacey Perry Bryan; her husband, Robert Donald Bryan; their three daughters, Cora Elizabeth Bryan, Amalie Mary Bryan, and Noelle Anne Bryan; and their son, Shepherd Charles Bryan.

And to my son, Mitch Perry-Cox, and his husband, Samuel Perry-Cox.

Anne Griffin Perry

Registered nurses, licensed practical nurses, and assistive personnel have sacrificed a great deal since the beginning of the pandemic while continuing to show compassion and strength in caring for COVID-19 patients. I salute you all for your dedication and resolve. This dedication is a small way of thanking you.

Patricia A. Potter

For Toba and Harris, who never saw this achievement but would be proud of its influence on today's and tomorrow's nurses. And, as always, for my ever-supportive and patient husband, who inspires me daily.

Wendy R. Ostendorf

I dedicate this textbook to my family. First, to my husband, Phil, who is my greatest support system and a wonderful partner to share this life with. And second, to my children, Chris and Charlotte, who have grown into adults that I respect and love more each and every day.

I am blessed to have this family.

Nancy Laplante

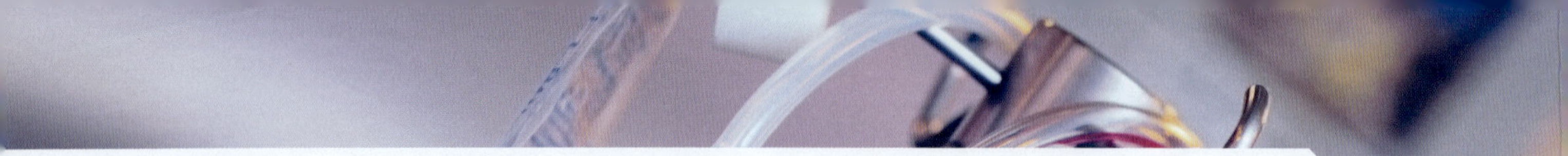

About the Authors

SHELLEY L. COBBETT, RN, BN GNT, MN, EdD

Dr. Shelley Cobbett received her Post-RN BN and her MN from Dalhousie University and her EdD from Charles Sturt University. Her clinical practice background is maternal-child nursing and she has been a nurse educator for over 33 years. Her main area of research during the last 15 years has focused on the scholarship of learning and teaching and led to more than 60 peer-reviewed publications, invited speaker engagements, and oral conference presentations. She is the co-editor of *Lewis's Medical-Surgical Nursing in Canada: Assessment and Management of Clinical Problems*, Fifth Edition. Dr. Cobbett is President of the Atlantic Region–Canadian Association of Schools of Nursing. She also serves as a member of the Education Advisory Committee of the Nova Scotia College of Nursing. She is currently Assistant Professor and Site Administrator at Dalhousie University School of Nursing, Yarmouth Campus.

ANNE GRIFFIN PERRY, RN, MSN, EdD, FAAN

Dr. Anne G. Perry, Professor Emerita at Southern Illinois University–Edwardsville, is a Fellow of the American Academy of Nursing. She received her BSN from the University of Michigan, her MSN from Saint Louis University, and her EdD from Southern Illinois University–Edwardsville. Dr. Perry is a prolific and influential author and speaker. As an author for over 40 years, her work includes four major textbooks (*Essentials for Nursing Practice*, *Fundamentals of Nursing*, *Nursing Interventions & Clinical Skills*, and *Clinical Nursing Skills & Techniques*) and dozens of journal articles, abstracts, and nursing research and education grants. She has presented numerous papers at conferences across the United States and internationally. Dr. Perry was one of a few key consultants on *Mosby's Nursing Video Skills* and *Mosby's Nursing Skills Online*.

Dr. Perry's passion for nursing education led her to become an instructor in 1973, after which she achieved the rank of Professor and assumed various leadership roles at Saint Louis University School of Nursing. She was a Professor and Associate Dean and Interim Dean at Southern Illinois University–Edwardsville. As a clinician and researcher, Dr. Perry's contributions to pulmonary nursing and nursing language development involve both research and policy-making. She has investigated and published findings on topics that include weaning from mechanical ventilation, use of the therapeutic intervention scoring system, critical care, and validation of nursing diagnoses.

PATRICIA A. POTTER, RN, MSN, PhD, FAAN

Dr. Patricia Potter received her BSN at the University of Washington in Seattle and her MSN and PhD at Saint Louis University in St. Louis, Missouri. A groundbreaking author for more than 30 years, her work includes four major textbooks (*Essentials for Nursing Practice*, *Fundamentals of Nursing*, *Nursing Interventions & Clinical Skills*, and *Clinical Nursing Skills & Techniques*) and publications in numerous professional journals. She has been an unceasing advocate of evidence-based practice and quality improvement in her roles as an administrator, educator, and, more recently, director of research.

Dr. Potter has devoted a lifetime to nursing education, practice, and research. She spent a decade teaching at Barnes Hospital School of Nursing and Saint Louis University. She held a variety of managerial and administrative positions, ultimately becoming the director of nursing practice at Barnes-Jewish Hospital. In that capacity, she sharpened her interest in the development of nursing practice standards and the measurement of patient outcomes in defining nursing practice. Her most recently developed passion is nursing research, specifically cancer family caregiving, the cancer patient symptom experience, fall prevention, and the effects of compassion fatigue on nurses. Recently, Dr. Potter worked with colleagues to develop an inpatient Innovation Unit, which is designed to incorporate current evidence into the selection and development of a unique work team and the creation of a care delivery model and innovative care practices. Dr. Potter was Director of Research for Patient Care Services at Barnes-Jewish Hospital in St. Louis, Missouri, until her retirement in 2017.

WENDY R. OSTENDORF, RN, MS, EdD, CNE

Dr. Wendy R. Ostendorf received her BSN from Villanova University, her MS from the University of Delaware, and her EdD from the University of Sarasota. She currently serves as a contributing faculty in the Master of Science in Nursing at Walden University. She has contributed more than 30 chapters to numerous nursing textbooks and served as author for two major textbooks: *Nursing Interventions & Clinical Skills* and *Clinical Nursing Skills & Techniques*. She has presented more than 25 papers at local, national, and international conferences.

Dr. Ostendorf has a diverse background in pediatric and adult critical care. She has taught at the undergraduate and graduate levels for 35 years. With decades of practice as a clinician, her educational experiences have influenced her teaching philosophy and perceptions of the nursing profession.

NANCY LAPLANTE, PhD, RN, AHN-BC

Dr. Nancy Laplante received her BSN from William Paterson University, Wayne, New Jersey; her MSN in Community Health from West Chester University, West Chester, Pennsylvania; and her PhD from Widener University, Chester, Pennsylvania. Dr. Laplante is also a board-certified advanced holistic nurse.

Dr. Laplante is Associate Professor of Nursing at Widener University and also serves as Director of the Accelerated RN to BSN to MSN program and Director of the RN to MSN bridge program. She teaches undergraduate courses in self-care, health policy, and gerontology and teaches graduate courses in technology, health policy, assessment and evaluation, population health, and epidemiology. Dr. Laplante teaches primarily in online formats and enjoys being able to connect with a diverse group of students both nationally and internationally.

Dr. Laplante strives to engage all students in respectful dialogue. She believes that teaching is a collaborative process between students and faculty and that reciprocal relationships form as we learn from one another. As an advanced holistic nurse, she incorporates self-care, self-responsibility, spirituality, and reflection in her teaching and seeks to be a role model for her students.

Dr. Laplante's research interests include creating a presence in online learning environments, health care applications of the Internet of Things (IoT), the image of nursing, and self-care practices for students and peers. Dr. Laplante has presented at local, national, and international conferences and has published recently in the areas of IoT and holistic nursing practice. In addition to her teaching and Director responsibilities, Dr. Laplante serves as a committee member and reader for doctoral nursing students. She believes this role is important for mentoring and supporting the next generation of nursing scientists.

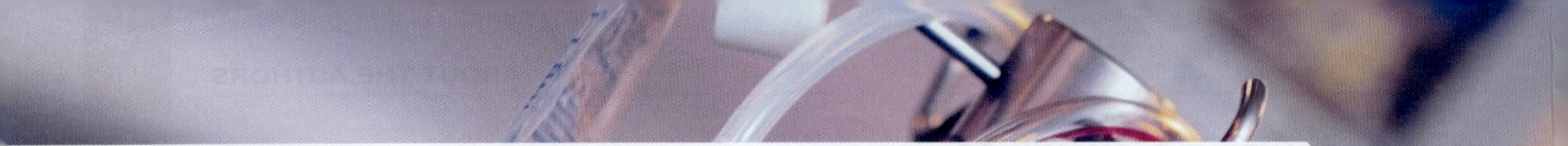

Contributors

Chantal Backman, RN, MHA, PhD
Associate Professor
School of Nursing
University of Ottawa
Ottawa, ON

Margie Burns, RN, MN, PhD
Assistant Professor
Faculty of Nursing
University of Prince Edward Island
Charlottetown, PEI

Danielle Byrne, RN, MN, CCSNE
Adjunct Lecturer and Clinical Instructor
School of Nursing
Dalhousie University
Halifax, NS

Paula D'Eon, RN, MN, CCSNE
Adjunct Lecturer and Clinical Instructor
School of Nursing
Dalhousie University
Yarmouth, NS

Adele deRosenroll, RN, CVAA(c), VA-BC
Clinical Resource Nurse, Vascular Access
Island Health
Vancouver, BC

Keri Durocher, RN, MN, PhD(c)
Graduate Teaching Assistant
Arthur Labatt Family School of Nursing
Western University
London, ON;
Nursing Professor
Lambton College
Sarnia, ON

Leslie Graham, RN, MN, PhD(c), CNCC, CHSE, CCSNE
Professor, Nursing
School of Health and Community Studies
Durham College;
Adjunct Professor
Faculty of Health Sciences
Ontario Tech University
Oshawa, ON

Giuliana Harvey, RN, PhD
Associate Professor
School of Nursing and Midwifery
Mount Royal University
Calgary, AB

Selena Hebig, RN, BSN, BScKin
Nurse Educator
School of Health and Human Services
Camosun College (Lansdowne)
Victoria, BC

Chen Jin, RN, MN, CMSN(C)
Instructor
College of Nursing
University of Manitoba
Winnipeg, Manitoba

Darlaine Jantzen, RN, MA, PhD
Associate Professor
School of Nursing
Trinity Western University
Langley, BC

Erika Kinney, RN, BN, MN, CNCC(c)
Assistant Teaching Professor
Department of Nursing and Health Sciences
University of New Brunswick
Saint John, NB

Holly Knight, RN, MN, CCN(c)
Assistant Teaching Professor
Department of Nursing and Health Sciences
University of New Brunswick
Saint John, NB

Rosemary Kohr, RN, BA (Arts Plastiques), BScN, MScN, PhD, Tertiary Care Nurse Practitioner Certificate
Program Director
Health Leadership and Learning Network
Faculty of Health
York University
Toronto, ON;
Adjunct Associate Professor
Faculty of Health Sciences
Western University
London, ON

Nicole Lewis-Power, RN, MN, PhD
Assistant Professor
School of Nursing
Memorial University
St. John's, NL

Maureen Loft, NP, MScN, PhD
Nurse Practitioner/Clinical Nurse Specialist
Middlesex Hospital Alliance
Strathroy, ON;
Adjunct Assistant Professor
Arthur Labatt Family School of Nursing
Western University
London, ON

Heather MacLean, RN, MN, CHSE
Associate Professor
School of Nursing and Midwifery
Mount Royal University
Calgary, AB

Lisa MacNaughton-Doucet, RN, BTHM, MN
Adjunct Assistant Professor
School of Nursing
Dalhousie University
Yarmouth, NS

Megan MacNeil, RN, MN, CEBN
Graduate Student
Arthur Labatt Family School of Nursing
Western University
London, ON

Rose McCloskey, RN, PhD, GNC(c)
Professor
Department of Nursing and Health Sciences
University of New Brunswick
Saint John, NB

Kateryna Metersky, RN, PhD
Assistant Professor
Daphne Cockwell School of Nursing
Toronto Metropolitan University
Toronto, ON

Joanne Newell, RN, MN
Adjunct Assistant Professor
School of Nursing
Dalhousie University
Yarmouth, NS

Stephanie Nunes, RN, MN
Instructor
College of Nursing
University of Manitoba
Winnipeg, Manitoba

Rachel Ollivier, RN, PhD
Women's and Newborn Health Services
IWK Health Centre
Halifax, NS

Noelle Ozog, RN, MSN
Staff Nurse, Emergency
Queen Elizabeth II Health Sciences Centre
Halifax, NS

Sayedeh Haddis Razeghi, RN, BScN
Clinical Instructor
Arthur Labatt Family School of Nursing
Western University
London, ON

Holly Richardson, RN, MA, PhD
Associate Professor
Rankin School of Nursing
St. Francis Xavier University
Antigonish, NS

Shawna Ryan, RN, COHN, MN
Nursing Faculty
Bachelor of Science in Nursing Program
Health and Human Services
College of the Rockies
Cranbrook, BC

Monakshi Sawhney, RN(EC), NP(Adult), MN, PhD
Associate Professor
School of Nursing & Department of Anesthesiology and Peri-operative Medicine
Queen's University
Kingston, ON

Catherine Sheffer, RN, PhD, PNC(c)
Associate Director
Undergraduate Studies
School of Nursing
Dalhousie University
Halifax, NS;
Coordinator
BScN Arctic Nursing Program
Dalhousie University/Nunavut Arctic College
Halifax, NS;
President
Canadian Association of Perinatal and Women's Health Nurses
Ottawa, ON

Chantal Singh, RN, MScN
Nursing Professional Practice Consultant
Interprofessional Practice and Academic Relations
London Health Sciences Centre & LHSC Children's Hospital
London, ON;
Lecturer
Arthur Labatt Family School of Nursing
Western University
London, ON

Alexis Smith, RN, MScN
Clinical Practice Faculty Lead
Arthur Labatt Family School of Nursing
Western University
London, ON

Crystal Thibodeau, RN, BScN, MN-NP
Adjunct Lecturer
School of Nursing
Dalhousie University
Yarmouth, NS

Jennifer Thorney, RN, MN
Arthur Labatt Family School of Nursing
Western University
London, ON

Debbie Turner, MSc(HQ), RN, HCM, ENC(c)
Director
Quality and Professional Practice
St. Thomas Elgin General Hospital
St. Thomas, ON

Kathryn Weaver, RN, MN, PhD
Honorary Research Professor
Department of Nursing and Health Sciences
University of New Brunswick
Fredericton, NB;
Mental Health Professional
Eating Disorder Care and Services
Fredericton, NB;
Adjunct Professor
Faculty of Nursing
Brandon University
Brandon, MB

CONTRIBUTORS TO THE US 10TH EDITION

Tim Buchanan, MSN
Safe Patient Handling and Mobility Facility Coordinator and Nurse Instructor
Nursing Education
Saint Louis University
St. Louis, Missouri

Hope Bussenius, DNP, APRN, FNP-BC, FAANP
Associate Professor, Clinical
Nell Hodgson Woodruff School of Nursing
Emory University
Atlanta, Georgia;
Owner/Provider
Health Connection Inc.
Jefferson, Georgia

Janice Colwell, MS, CWOCN, FAAN
Advanced Practice Nurse
General Surgery
University of Chicago Medicine
Chicago, Illinois

Christine Durbin, PhD, JD, RN
Professor Emerita
School of Nursing
Southern Illinois University–Edwardsville
Edwardsville, Illinois

Jane Fellows, MSN, CWOCN-AP
Wound/Ostomy CNS
Advanced Clinical Practice
Duke University Health System
Durham, North Carolina

Susan Fetzer, BA, BSN, MSN, MBA, PhD
Professor Emerita
College of Health and Human Services
University of New Hampshire
Durham, New Hampshire
Director of Research
Patient Care Services
Southern New Hampshire Medical Center
Nashua, New Hampshire

Lorri A. Graham, DNP-L, MSN, RN
Visiting Professor
Nursing
Chamberlain University
Downers Grove, Illinois

Kathleen Hudson, MSN, BSN, RN, CWOCN
Clinical Nurse Educator, Wound and Ostomy Care
Center for Nursing Professional Practice and Research
University of Chicago
Chicago, Illinois

Nelda Martin, MSN
Clinical Nurse Specialist, Heart and Vascular
Barnes-Jewish Hospital
St. Louis, Missouri

Karen A. May, PhD
Assistant Professor
School of Nursing
Widener University
Chester, Pennsylvania

Angela McConachie, FNP, DNP
Associate Professor
Goldfarb School of Nursing
Barnes-Jewish College
St. Louis, Missouri

Theresa Miller, PhD, MSN, MHA, RN
Associate Professor
Nursing
Saint Francis Medical Center College of Nursing
Peoria, Illinois

Nancy Mirarchi, MSN, RN, CNOR
Clinical Instructor
Nursing
West Chester University
West Chester, Pennsylvania;
Charge Nurse
Operating Room
Penn Medicine Chester County Hospital
West Chester, Pennsylvania

Jill Parsons, PhD, RN
Associate Professor
Nursing
MacMurray College
Jacksonville, Illinois

William Pezzotti, DNP, CRNP, AGACNP-BC
Critical Care Nurse Practitioner
Critical Care Medicine
Penn Medicine Chester County Hospital
West Chester, Pennsylvania

Theresa Pietsch, PhD, RN, CRRN, CNE
Associate Professor
Division of Nursing and Health Sciences
Neumann University
Aston, Pennsylvania;
Associate Dean
Undergraduate Nursing Program
Division of Nursing and Health Sciences
Neumann University
Aston, Pennsylvania

Carolyn J. Wright-Boon, MSN, BSN
Assistant Professor
Nursing
Saint Francis Medical Center College of Nursing
Peoria, Illinois

Rita Wunderlich, MSN, PhD
Associate Professor
Nursing
Maryville University
St. Louis, Missouri

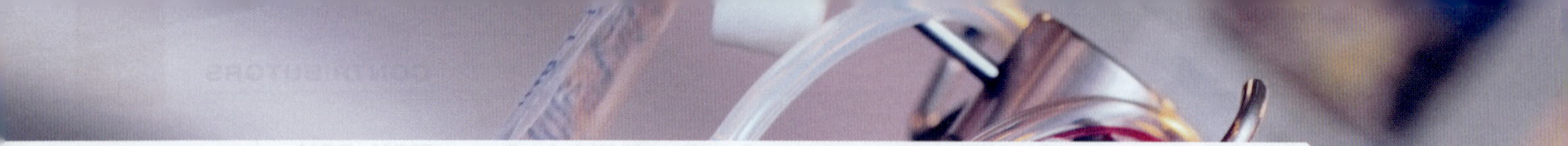

Reviewers

Joanne Gullison, RN, BScN
Coordinating Instructor
School of Health and Wellness
New Brunswick Community College–Fredericton
Fredericton, NB

Shauna Houk, RN, BScN, MN
Assistant Professor
Faculty of Nursing
Dalhousie University
Halifax, NS

Stephanie Janveaux, RN, BScN, MN
Professor
Health and Community Studies
Algonquin College/University of Ottawa
Ottawa, ON

Ruth Klann, RN, BScN, MLE, PIDP
Nursing Educator
Bachelor of Science in Nursing Program
Vancouver Community College
Vancouver, BC

Melissa Parker, RN, MScN, BScN, BSc
Professor
Bachelor of Science in Nursing Collaborative Program
Canadore College/Nipissing University
North Bay, ON

Kimberley Pinel, MEd, RN, CCSNE
Nursing Instructor
School of Health Sciences and Community Services
Red River College Polytechnic
Winnipeg, MB

Katie Pitt, RN, MN
Instructor
Practical Nursing Program
School of Health and Human Services
Nova Scotia Community College
Middleton, NS

Trina Propp, RN, BSN
Nursing Instructor
School of Health Sciences
Vancouver Community College
Vancouver, BC

Suzee Rocque, RN, BScN, MScN/Ed, CRFN, CPMHN(c)
Nursing Professor and Coordinator (Years 3 and 4)
School of Baccalaureate Nursing
St. Lawrence College
Cornwall, ON

Preface to the Student

Numerous features are built into this text to help you identif pieces of information and study more efficiently. Additional tools and review questions may be found on the companion E site: http://evolve.elsevier.com/Canada/Perry/clinicalskills/

Objectives highlight the primary aims of chapter content.

Evolve media resources are available for every chapter.

Standards of Care sections summarize the most recent evidence-informed practice standards or professional clinical standards recommended for skills within each chapter

Principles for Practice sections highlight key nursing principles that apply to all skills within a chapter.

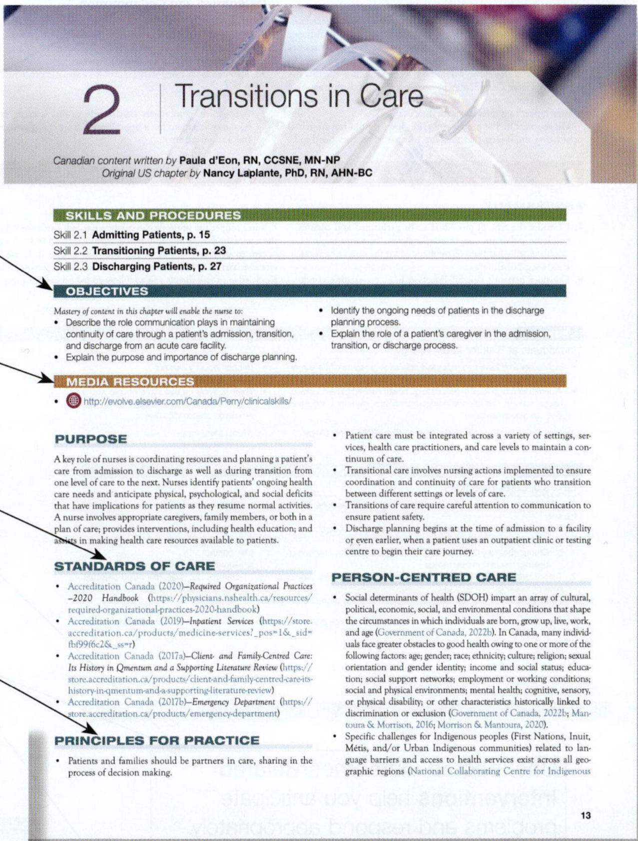

2 | Transitions in Care

Canadian content written by **Paula d'Eon, RN, CCSNE, MN-NP**
Original US chapter by **Nancy Laplante, PhD, RN, AHN-BC**

SKILLS AND PROCEDURES

Skill 2.1 **Admitting Patients, p. 15**
Skill 2.2 **Transitioning Patients, p. 23**
Skill 2.3 **Discharging Patients, p. 27**

OBJECTIVES

Mastery of content in this chapter will enable the nurse to:

- Describe the role communication plays in maintaining continuity of care through a patient's admission, transition, and discharge from an acute care facility.
- Explain the purpose and importance of discharge planning.
- Identify the ongoing needs of patients in the discharge planning process.
- Explain the role of a patient's caregiver in the admission, transition, or discharge process.

MEDIA RESOURCES

- http://evolve.elsevier.com/Canada/Perry/clinicalskills/

PURPOSE

A key role of nurses is coordinating resources and planning a patient's care from admission to discharge as well as during transition from one level of care to the next. Nurses identify patients' ongoing health care needs and anticipate physical, psychological, and social deficits that have implications for patients as they resume normal activities. A nurse involves appropriate caregivers, family members, or both in a plan of care; provides interventions, including health education; and assists in making health care resources available to patients.

STANDARDS OF CARE

- Accreditation Canada (2020)—*Required Organizational Practices –2020 Handbook* (https://physicians.nshealth.ca/resources/required-organizational-practices-2020-handbook)
- Accreditation Canada (2019)—*Inpatient Services* (https://store.accreditation.ca/products/medicine-services?_pos=1&_sid=fbf99f6c2&_ss=r)
- Accreditation Canada (2017a)—*Client- and Family-Centred Care: Its History in Qmentum and a Supporting Literature Review* (https://store.accreditation.ca/products/client-and-family-centred-care-its-history-in-qmentum-and-a-supporting-literature-review)
- Accreditation Canada (2017b)—*Emergency Department* (https://store.accreditation.ca/products/emergency-department)

PRINCIPLES FOR PRACTICE

- Patients and families should be partners in care, sharing in the process of decision making.
- Patient care must be integrated across a variety of settings, services, health care practitioners, and care levels to maintain a continuum of care.
- Transitional care involves nursing actions implemented to ensure coordination and continuity of care for patients who transition between different settings or levels of care.
- Transitions of care require careful attention to communication to ensure patient safety.
- Discharge planning begins at the time of admission to a facility or even earlier, when a patient uses an outpatient clinic or testing centre to begin their care journey.

PERSON-CENTRED CARE

- Social determinants of health (SDOH) impart an array of cultural, political, economic, social, and environmental conditions that shape the circumstances in which individuals are born, grow up, live, work, and age (Government of Canada, 2022b). In Canada, many individuals face greater obstacles to good health owing to one or more of the following factors: age; gender; race; ethnicity; culture; religion; sexual orientation and gender identity; income and social status; education; social support networks; employment or working conditions; social and physical environments; mental health; cognitive, sensory, or physical disability; or other characteristics historically linked to discrimination or exclusion (Government of Canada, 2022b; Mantoura & Morrison, 2016; Morrison & Mantoura, 2020).
- Specific challenges for Indigenous peoples (First Nations, Inuit, Métis, and/or Urban Indigenous communities) related to language barriers and access to health services exist across all geographic regions (National Collaborating Centre for Indigenous

13

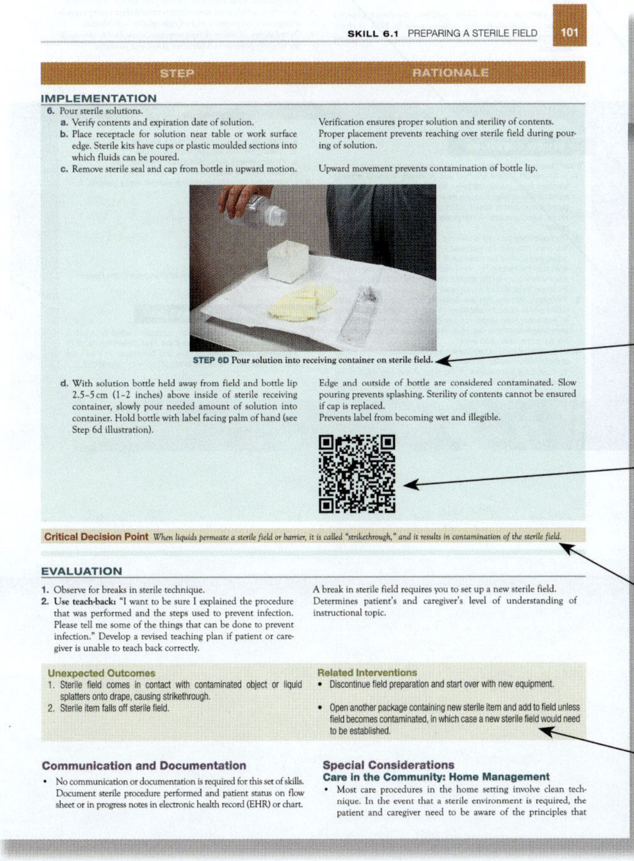

SKILL 6.1 PREPARING A STERILE FIELD 101

STEP	RATIONALE
IMPLEMENTATION	
6. Pour sterile solutions.	
a. Verify contents and expiration date of solution.	Verification ensures proper solution and sterility of contents.
b. Place receptacle for solution near table or work surface edge. Sterile kits have cups or plastic moulded sections into which fluids can be poured.	Proper placement prevents reaching over sterile field during pouring of solution.
c. Remove sterile seal and cap from bottle in upward motion.	Upward movement prevents contamination of bottle lip.
d. With solution bottle held away from field and bottle lip 2.5–5 cm (1–2 inches) above inside of sterile receiving container, slowly pour needed amount of solution into container. Hold bottle with label facing palm of hand (see Step 6d illustration).	Edge and outside of bottle are considered contaminated. Slow pouring prevents splashing. Sterility of contents cannot be ensured if cap is replaced. Prevents label from becoming wet and illegible.

STEP 6D Pour solution into receiving container on sterile field.

Critical Decision Point *When liquids permeate a sterile field or barrier, it is called "strikethrough," and it results in contamination of the sterile field.*

EVALUATION

1. Observe for breaks in sterile technique.	A break in sterile field requires you to set up a new sterile field.
2. Use teach-back: "I want to be sure I explained the procedure that was performed and the steps used to prevent infection. Please tell me some of the things that can be done to prevent infection." Develop a revised teaching plan if patient or caregiver is unable to teach back correctly.	Determines patient's and caregiver's level of understanding of instructional topic.

Unexpected Outcomes	Related Interventions
1. Sterile field comes in contact with contaminated object or liquid splatters onto drape, causing strikethrough.	• Discontinue field preparation and start over with new equipment.
2. Sterile item falls off sterile field.	• Open another package containing new sterile item and add to field unless field becomes contaminated, in which case a new sterile field would need to be established.

Communication and Documentation

- No communication or documentation is required for this set of skills. Document sterile procedure performed and patient status on flow sheet or in progress notes in electronic health record (EHR) or chart.

Special Considerations
Care in the Community: Home Management

- Most care procedures in the home setting involve clean technique. In the event that a sterile environment is required, the patient and caregiver need to be aware of the principles that

Extensive illustrations demonstrate step-by-step procedures for more thorough understanding.

Quick Response codes may be scanned to link to video clips directly from the text page

Clinical Decision Points highlight points to consider when performing skills, to ensure effective outcomes and promote safety.

Rationales for steps within skills help you learn the why as well as the how of each skill.

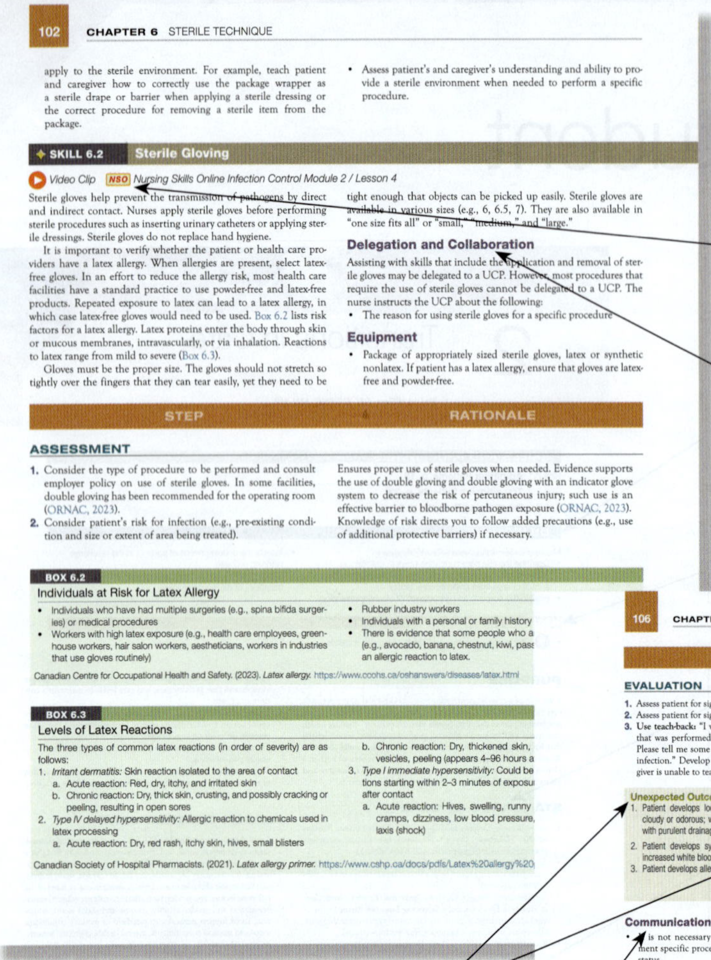

102 CHAPTER 6 STERILE TECHNIQUE

apply to the sterile environment. For example, teach patient and caregiver how to correctly use the package wrapper as a sterile drape or barrier when applying a sterile dressing or the correct procedure for removing a sterile item from the package.

- Assess patient's and caregiver's understanding and ability to provide a sterile environment when needed to perform a specific procedure.

SKILL 6.2 Sterile Gloving

Video Clip NSO Nursing Skills Online Infection Control Module 2 / Lesson 4

Sterile gloves help prevent the transmission of pathogens by direct and indirect contact. Nurses apply sterile gloves before performing sterile procedures such as inserting urinary catheters or applying sterile dressings. Sterile gloves do not replace hand hygiene.

It is important to verify whether the patient or health care providers have a latex allergy. When allergies are present, select latex-free gloves. In an effort to reduce the allergy risk, most health care facilities have a standard practice to use powder-free and latex-free products. Repeated exposure to latex can lead to a latex allergy, in which case latex-free gloves would need to be used. Box 6.2 lists risk factors for a latex allergy. Latex proteins enter the body through skin or mucous membranes, intravascularly, or via inhalation. Reactions to latex range from mild to severe (Box 6.3).

Gloves must be the proper size. The gloves should not stretch so tightly over the fingers that they can tear easily, yet they need to be tight enough that objects can be picked up easily. Sterile gloves are available in various sizes (e.g., 6, 6.5, 7). They are also available in "one size fits all" or "small," "medium," and "large."

Delegation and Collaboration

Assisting with skills that include the application and removal of sterile gloves may be delegated to a UCP. However, most procedures that require the use of sterile gloves cannot be delegated to a UCP. The nurse instructs the UCP about the following:

- The reason for using sterile gloves for a specific procedure

Equipment

- Package of appropriately sized sterile gloves, latex or synthetic nonlatex. If patient has a latex allergy, ensure that gloves are latex-free and powder-free.

STEP	RATIONALE
ASSESSMENT	
1. Consider the type of procedure to be performed and consult employer policy on use of sterile gloves. In some facilities, double gloving has been recommended for the operating room (ORNAC, 2023). 2. Consider patient's risk for infection (e.g., pre-existing condition and size or extent of area being treated).	Ensures proper use of sterile gloves when needed. Evidence supports the use of double gloving and double gloving with an indicator glove system to decrease the risk of percutaneous injury; such use is an effective barrier to bloodborne pathogen exposure (ORNAC, 2023). Knowledge of risk directs you to follow added precautions (e.g., use of additional protective barriers) if necessary.

BOX 6.2 Individuals at Risk for Latex Allergy

- Individuals who have had multiple surgeries (e.g., spina bifida surgeries) or medical procedures
- Workers with high latex exposure (e.g., health care employees, greenhouse workers, hair salon workers, aestheticians, workers in industries that use gloves routinely)
- Rubber industry workers
- Individuals with a personal or family history
- There is evidence that some people who a (e.g., avocado, banana, chestnut, kiwi, pass an allergic reaction to latex.

Canadian Centre for Occupational Health and Safety. (2023). Latex allergy. https://www.ccohs.ca/oshanswers/diseases/latex.html

BOX 6.3 Levels of Latex Reactions

The three types of common latex reactions (in order of severity) are as follows:

1. Irritant dermatitis: Skin reaction isolated to the area of contact
   a. Acute reaction: Red, dry, itchy, and irritated skin
   b. Chronic reaction: Dry, thick skin, crusting, and possibly cracking or peeling, resulting in open sores
2. Type IV delayed hypersensitivity: Allergic reaction to chemicals used in latex processing
   a. Acute reaction: Dry, red rash, itchy skin, hives, small blisters
   b. Chronic reaction: Dry, thickened skin, vesicles, peeling (appears 4–96 hours a
3. Type I immediate hypersensitivity: Could be tions starting within 2–3 minutes of exposu after contact
   a. Acute reaction: Hives, swelling, runny cramps, dizziness, low blood pressure, laxis (shock)

Canadian Society of Hospital Pharmacists. (2021). Latex allergy primer. https://www.cshp.ca/docs/pdfs/Latex%20allergy%20

NSO icon links to online course lessons

Delegation and Collaboration sections define communication within the patient care team and your responsibility when delegating to unregulated care providers.

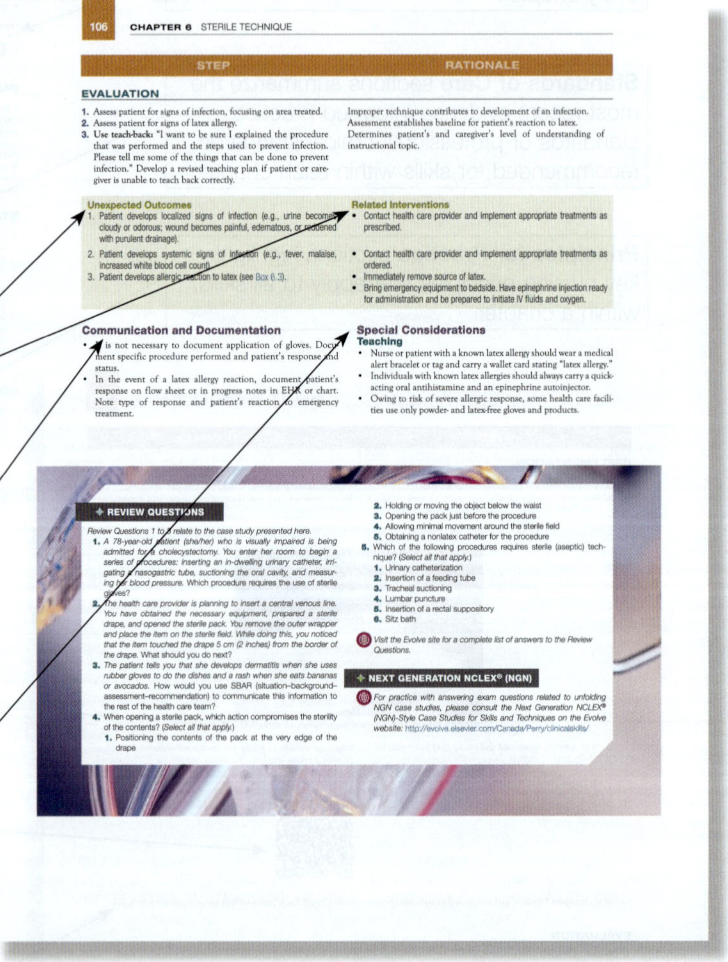

106 CHAPTER 6 STERILE TECHNIQUE

STEP	RATIONALE
EVALUATION	
1. Assess patient for signs of infection, focusing on area treated. 2. Assess patient for signs of latex allergy. 3. Use teach-back: "I want to be sure I explained the procedure that was performed and the steps used to prevent infection. Please tell me some of the things that can be done to prevent infection." Develop a revised teaching plan if patient or caregiver is unable to teach back correctly.	Improper technique contributes to development of an infection. Assessment establishes baseline for patient's reaction to latex. Determines patient's and caregiver's level of understanding of instructional topic.

Unexpected Outcomes	Related Interventions
1. Patient develops localized signs of infection (e.g., urine becomes cloudy or odorous; wound becomes painful, edematous, or reddened with purulent drainage).	• Contact health care provider and implement appropriate treatments as prescribed.
2. Patient develops systemic signs of infection (e.g., fever, malaise, increased white blood cell count).	• Contact health care provider and implement appropriate treatments as ordered.
3. Patient develops allergic reaction to latex (see Box 6.3).	• Immediately remove source of latex. • Bring emergency equipment to bedside. Have epinephrine injection ready for administration and be prepared to initiate IV fluids and oxygen.

Communication and Documentation

- It is not necessary to document application of gloves. Document specific procedure performed and patient's response and status.
- In the event of a latex allergy reaction, document patient's response on flow sheet or in progress notes in EHR or chart. Note type of response and patient's reaction to emergency treatment.

Special Considerations

Teaching

- Nurse or patient with a known latex allergy should wear a medical alert bracelet or tag and carry a wallet card stating "latex allergy."
- Individuals with known latex allergies should always carry a quick-acting oral antihistamine and an epinephrine autoinjector.
- Owing to risk of severe allergic response, some health care facilities use only powder- and latex-free gloves and products.

REVIEW QUESTIONS

Review Questions 1 to 4 relate to the case study presented here.

1. A 78-year-old patient (she/her) who is visually impaired is being admitted for a cholecystectomy. You enter her room to begin a series of procedures: inserting an in-dwelling urinary catheter, irrigating a nasogastric tube, suctioning the oral cavity, and measuring her blood pressure. Which procedure requires the use of sterile gloves?
2. The health care provider is planning to insert a central venous line. You have obtained the necessary equipment, prepared a sterile drape, and opened the sterile pack. You remove the outer wrapper and place the item on the sterile field. While doing this, you noticed that the item touched the drape 5 cm (2 inches) from the border of the drape. What should you do next?
3. The patient tells you that she develops dermatitis when she uses rubber gloves to do the dishes and a rash when she eats bananas or avocados. How would you use SBAR (situation-background-assessment-recommendation) to communicate this information to the rest of the health care team?
4. When opening a sterile pack, which action compromises the sterility of the contents? (Select all that apply.)
   1. Positioning the contents of the pack at the very edge of the drape
   2. Holding or moving the object below the waist
   3. Opening the pack just before the procedure
   4. Allowing minimal movement around the sterile field
   5. Obtaining a nonlatex catheter for the procedure
5. Which of the following procedures requires sterile (aseptic) technique? (Select all that apply.)
   1. Urinary catheterization
   2. Insertion of a feeding tube
   3. Tracheal suctioning
   4. Lumbar puncture
   5. Insertion of a rectal suppository
   6. Sitz bath

Visit the Evolve site for a complete list of answers to the Review Questions.

NEXT GENERATION NCLEX® (NGN)

For practice with answering exam questions related to unfolding NGN case studies, please consult the Next Generation NCLEX® (NGN)-Style Case Studies for Skills and Techniques on the Evolve website: http://evolve.elsevier.com/Canada/Perry/clinicalskills/

Unexpected Outcomes/Related Interventions help you anticipate problems and respond appropriately.

Communication and Documentation guidelines for each skill detail what to document and report.

Special Considerations indicate special teaching considerations, as well as procedure modifications needed for pediatric, gerontological, and self-care teaching in community populations.

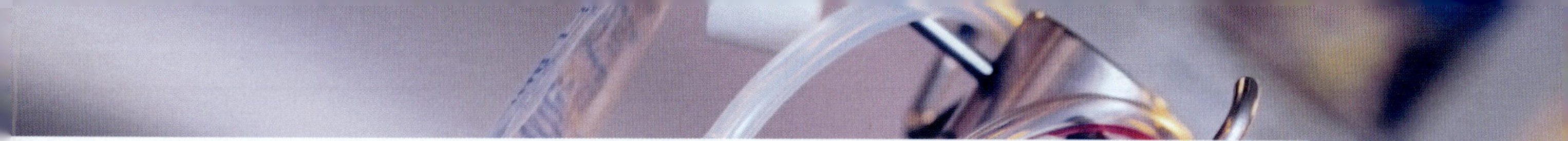

Preface to the Instructor

Though technological advances and knowledge expansion have without a doubt introduced many changes in nursing over the years, from the way we teach clinical skills to nursing students to how we improve the quality of care and enhance patient safety, the foundation for excellence in performing nursing skills remains the same: a competent, evidence-informed nurse who thinks critically, asks the right questions at the right time, and makes accurate and timely clinical judgements.

In this Second Edition of *Perry & Potter's Canadian Clinical Nursing Skills and Techniques*, we have consulted with nurses across Canada, including contributors from almost every province and territory. Each chapter opens by introducing students to key concepts: Standards of Practice, Principles for Practice, Person-Centred Care, Evidence-Informed Practice, and Safety Guidelines. We have streamlined these sections into a quick and easy-to-read bulleted format to emphasize, yet simplify, these important concepts.

The importance of interprofessional collaboration has been highlighted and threaded throughout the key concepts. Chapter 1, Evidence-Informed Nursing Practice, prepares students to understand and use the evidence-informed practice information included in every chapter.

All topics and skills, along with documentation examples, have been updated to meet the most recent Canadian standards in nursing practice.

Your students will find that the Second Edition of *Perry & Potter's Canadian Clinical Nursing Skills and Techniques* provides a comprehensive resource that will serve them well throughout their nursing education and well into their clinical practice careers.

CLASSIC FEATURES

- **Over 200 basic, intermediate, and advanced nursing skills and procedures** are covered.
- **Five-step nursing process format** provides a consistent presentation that helps students apply the process while learning each skill.
- **Skills and Procedures** list and **Objectives** open each chapter.
- **Over 1 200 full-colour photos and illustrations** help students master the material covered.
- **Standards of Care** sections summarize the most recent evidence-informed standards and the professional clinical standards recommended for the skills within each chapter.
- **Principles for Practice** sections highlight the key nursing principles that apply to skills within a chapter.
- **Evidence-Informed Practice** sections present students with the most recent evidence for the procedures presented. Recent research findings are discussed, and their implications for patient care are explored.
- **Person-Centred Care** sections prepare students to collaborate with patients when performing skills in a compassionate and coordinated way that is based on respect for a patient's cultural preferences, values, beliefs, and needs. "Person" in this context means the patient, their family, their caregivers (both formal and informal), and their identified support person(s).
- **Safety Guidelines** sections cover global and Healthcare Excellence Canada recommendations on the safe execution of the particular skill set covered in each chapter.
- **NSO icon** links text content with the latest edition of *Nursing Skills Online*, which has been simultaneously revised with the textbook to provide completely coordinated information.
- **Rationales** are given for steps within each skill so that students learn the *why* as well as the *how* of each step. Rationales include up-to-date citations from the literature.
- **Collaboration and Delegation** sections define communication within interprofessional teams and the nurse's responsibility when delegating to unregulated care providers.
- **Critical Decision Points** alert students to key steps that affect patient outcomes and help them modify care as needed to implement person-centred care.
- **Evaluation** sections highlight steps students must take to evaluate the outcomes of the skills performed.
- **Teach-back** is included in each evaluation section to demonstrate to students how to phrase a teach-back question appropriately.
- **Communication and Documentation** sections follow the evaluation discussion and alert students to what information should be documented in each situation. New in this edition are actual documentation examples provided with many of the skills.
- **Unexpected Outcomes and Related Interventions** sections inform students to be alert for potential problems and help them determine appropriate nursing interventions.
- **Special Considerations** sections include additional considerations to keep in mind when performing the skill for specific populations of patients or in specific settings and may include:
  - Teaching Considerations
  - Pediatric Considerations
  - Gerontological Considerations
  - Care in the Community Considerations
  - Patients With Physical and Cognitive Challenges Considerations
- **Quick Response (QR) codes** (scannable using the camera on a smartphone or tablet) on the text pages link to video clips of the appropriate skill or procedure, allowing students to view the video immediately after reading the implementation section of the skill.
- **Review Questions** at the end of each chapter include new case studies, opportunities to practise SBAR (situation–background–assessment–recommendation) communication, and other unique questions reviewing the chapter content.
- **Glossary** (on Evolve) contains a primer on medical terminology and combing forms as well as lists of common prefixes and suffixes.
- **Answers to Review Questions** (on Evolve) contain a complete list of detailed answers to the Review Questions found in each chapter.
- **TEACH for Nursing Lesson Plans** help you capitalize on the new clinical material in the text, skills video series, and online course. Additional discussion questions and activities unique to the TEACH manual expand the in-class material available to you.
- An **Image Collection** is available with *Perry & Potter's Clinical Nursing Skills and Techniques*.

FEATURES OF THE CANADIAN SECOND EDITION

This Second Canadian Edition highlights the importance of interprofessional collaboration and patient safety, referencing standards and recommendations from Healthcare Excellence Canada. We used the most current best practice standards; while some standards are over 5 years old, they are still current in practice. When referencing best practices, we have weighed the strength of the evidence as well as its currency to choose the most pertinent reference citation. There are also some best practice standards in use in Canada that refer to US standards or practices; this distinction is noted when applicable.

With continued changes in medication preparation and unit supply, for example, unit-dose systems, the third check for accuracy in medication preparation–which historically is when the nurse returns the stock medication to the cabinet/drawer–may not always be possible. In some instances, there may be no medication container to return to. In these circumstances, the third check for accuracy is done with the patient's MAR at the bedside, prior to administration, as part of following the 10 rights of medication administration. Throughout the text, we have included the three medication preparation checks for accuracy: the first check, before removing the medication vial/container from the drawer; the second check, when the prescribed amount of the medication is prepared (e.g., poured, drawn up); and the third check, before returning the medication container to storage or disposing of the single-use vial or ampoule.

Throughout each skill and procedure, we have emphasized the "4 moments for hand hygiene," prompting the nurse to assess when those moments ought to occur while they are performing a psychomotor skill. The 4 moments for hand hygiene are to be implemented before initial patient (or patient environment) contact, before an aseptic procedure, after body fluid exposure risk, and after patient (or patient environment) contact. Additional hand hygiene should be performed when hands are visibly soiled. As such, we have added a hand hygiene icon as a prompt for students to make the assessment at that step of the skill as to whether any of those 4 moments have occurred and thus whether hand hygiene is required. Each skill includes the 4 moments and the hand hygiene icon ( ) students/instructors know what we are referring to here whenever it is anticipated that 1 of the 4 moments will occur or has occurred.

Within the Canadian health care context, registered nurses (RNs) may "assign" skills to licensed practical nurses (LPNs) or registered practical nurses (RPNs), but there are very few skills that may be delegated. In order for a skill to be eligible for delegation from an RN to an RPN/LPN, the skill must fall outside of the RPN/LPN's scope of practice. Throughout this text, when a skill is specific to the role of the RN, we have used "registered nurse" or "RN"; in all other instances, we use the term "nurse" to refer to an RN and/or an RPN/LPN, depending on jurisdictional regulations. Using this terminology aligns the text with the changing membership of the Canadian Nurses Association, which, in June 2018, passed a motion that its membership would include all RNs and RPNs/LPNs and that all members would be termed "nurses."

As health care continues to change at a fast pace, many employers are developing policies to enable the delegation of tasks to unregulated care providers (UCPs), provided that specific criteria are met related to knowledge, skills, and abilities. It is important for the nurse to be informed of their employer's policy specific to the delegation of tasks. For example, historically, the skill of catheterization could not be delegated to a UCP; however, currently, in some jurisdictions (e.g., Ontario), this skill may be delegated provided that certain guidelines have been met. Throughout the text, the student/reader is always cautioned to check their employer's policy pertaining to delegation of skills to a UCP.

The authors and contributors recognize and acknowledge the diverse histories of the First Peoples of the lands now referred to as Canada. We recognize that individual communities identify themselves in various ways. Within this text, the term "Indigenous" is used to collectively refer to all First Nations, Inuit, Métis, and non-status peoples within Canada, unless research findings are cited for a particular population.

Specific terminology used within this text is grounded in the Canadian health care context to ensure consistency from one chapter to the next:

- "Health care provider" can include a physician, nurse practitioner, or an RN who has prescribing of medications and/or treatments within their scope of practice.
- Family member was changed to "caregiver" to be more inclusive; caregivers can be family or friends as well as formal or informal caregivers.
- Knowledge and language concerning sex, gender, and identity are fluid and continually evolving. The language and terminology presented in this text endeavours to be inclusive of all people and reflects what is, to the best of our knowledge, current at the time of writing. Gendered pronouns were removed whenever possible and replaced with the gender-neutral terms "they" and "them" as acceptable singular references (see https://www.oed.com/discover/a-brief-history-of-singular-they/), and preferred pronouns have been indicated in the case scenarios.
- "Prescriptions" was used to replace "order" and "medication order," and "prescribing" replaces "ordering."
- "Interprofessional collaboration" is used to refer to any collaboration among health care team members and others (e.g., spiritual caregivers).

LEARNING SUPPLEMENTS FOR STUDENTS

- The **Evolve Student Resources** are available online at http://evolve.elsevier.com/Canada/Perry/clinicalskills/ and include the following valuable learning aids, organized by asset:
- Animations
- Answers to Textbook Review Questions
- Glossary
- Calculation Tutorial
- Fluids and Electrolytes Tutorial
- Printable versions of Chapter Key Points
- Review Questions
- Skills Performance Checklists for each skill in the text
- Video Clips from the *Canadian Clinical Skills: Essentials Collection* highlighting common nursing skills

TEACHING SUPPLEMENTS FOR INSTRUCTORS

- The **Evolve Instructor Resources** (available online at http://evolve.elsevier.com/Canada/Perry/clinicalskills/) are a comprehensive collection of the most important tools instructors need, including the following:
- **TEACH for Nurses** ties together every chapter resource you need for the most effective class presentations, with sections dedicated to objectives, clinical judgement classroom tools, instructor chapter resources, teaching strategies, nursing curriculum standards, nursing concepts, and reference to the Canadian Interprofessional Health Collaborative (CIHC) framework. Teaching strategies include content highlights, student activities, online activities, and large group activities.

- The revised **Test Bank** contains more than 1 100 multiple-choice questions with textbook references and answers coded for NCLEX competencies and cognitive level for RN students. Educators can administer Elsevier's textbook Test Banks and Review Questions online using Evolve Course Tools. Test Banks, available for every chapter of the textbook, feature examination format test questions with rationales and answers for all chapters. Provided at no cost to faculty, these Test Banks can be administered to students in Evolve's convenient online test player. Student results can be automatically recorded to the Evolve gradebook, and analysis is available for each item. Evolve gradebooks are customizable and can be easily exported for import into most common Learning Management Systems.
- **PowerPoint Presentations** include over 1 500 slides for use in lectures.
- The **Image Collection** contains more than 1 200 illustrations from the text for use in lectures.
- **Simulation Learning System** is an online toolkit that helps instructors and facilitators effectively incorporate medium- to high-fidelity simulation into their nursing curriculum. Detailed patient scenarios promote and enhance the clinical decision-making skills of students at all levels. The system provides detailed instructions for preparation and implementation of the simulation experience, debriefing questions that encourage critical thinking, and learning resources to reinforce student comprehension. Each scenario in the Simulation Learning System complements the textbook content and helps bridge the gap between lectures and clinicals. This system provides the perfect environment for students to practise what they are learning in the text for a true-to-life, hands-on learning experience.

Next Generation NCLEX®

The National Council of State Boards of Nursing (NCSBN) is a not-for-profit organization whose members include nursing regulatory bodies. In empowering and supporting nursing regulators in their mandate to protect the public, the NCSBN is involved in the development of nursing licensure examinations, such as the NCLEX-RN®. In Canada, the NCLEX-RN® was introduced in 2015 and is, as of the writing of this text, the recognized licensure exam required for practising RNs in Canada.

The NCLEX-RN® has, as of 2023, changed to ensure that its item types adequately measure clinical judgement, critical thinking, and problem-solving skills on a consistent basis. The NCSBN also incorporates into the examination what they call the Clinical Judgement Measurement Model (CJMM), a framework that the NCSBN has created to measure a novice nurse's ability to apply clinical judgement in practice.

These changes to the examination come as a result of research findings indicating that novice nurses have a much higher-than-desirable error rate with patients (i.e., errors that cause patient harm) and, upon NCSBN's investigation, the discovery that the overwhelming majority of these errors were caused by failures in clinical judgement.

Clinical judgement has been a foundation underlying nursing education for decades and is based on the work of a number of nursing theorists. The theory of clinical judgement that most closely aligns with what the NCSBN has based their CJMM on is the work of Christine A. Tanner.

The new version of the NCLEX-RN® is referred to as the "Next Generation NCLEX" or "NGN," and features the following:

- Six key skills in the CJMM: Recognizing Cues, Analyzing Cues, Prioritizing Hypotheses, Generating Solutions, Taking Actions, and Evaluating Outcomes.
- Item types: multiple response, extended drag-and-drop, cloze (drop-down), enhanced hot-spot (highlight), matrix/grid, bow-tie, and trend.
- Item types are accompanied by case studies containing comprehensive patient information—some of it relevant to the question, and some of it not.
- Case information may be presented as a single, unchanging moment in time (a "single episode" case study) or multiple moments in time as a patient's condition changes (an "unfolding" case study).
- Single-episode case studies may be accompanied by one to six questions; unfolding case studies are accompanied by six questions that correspond to the six levels of the CJMM.

For more information regarding the NCLEX-RN® and the changes made to the exam, visit the NCSBN website: https://www.nclex.com/faqs.page and https://www.nclex.com/clinical-judgment-measurement-model.page.

For further NCLEX-RN® examination preparation resources, see *Elsevier's Canadian Comprehensive Review for the NCLEX-RN® Examination*, Third Edition, ISBN 9780323810333.

Prior to preparing for any nursing licensure examination, please refer to your provincial or territorial nursing regulatory body to determine which licensure examination is required in order for you to practise in your chosen jurisdiction.

MULTIMEDIA SUPPLEMENTS FOR INSTRUCTORS AND STUDENTS

- **Nursing Skills Online 5.0** contains 19 modules rich with animations, videos, interactive activities, and exercises to help students prepare for their clinical lab experience. The instructionally designed lessons focus on topics that are difficult to master and pose a high risk to the patient if done incorrectly. Lesson quizzes allow students to check their learning curve and review as needed, and the module exams feed out to an instructor grade book. Modules cover Airway Management, Blood Therapy, Bowel Elimination/Ostomy Care, Cardiac Care, Closed Chest Drainage Systems, Enteral Nutrition, Infection Control, Injections, Intravenous Fluid Administration, Intravenous Fluid Therapy Maintenance, Parenteral Medication Administration, Nonparenteral Medication Administration, Safe Medication Administration, Safety, Specimen Collection, Urinary Catheterization, Vascular Access, Vital Signs, and Wound Care. It is available alone or packaged with the text.
- **NEW *Canadian Clinical Skills: Essentials Collection*** provides videos covering more than 160 essential nursing skills. Each skill in the collection uses a seven-part framework to walk you through every aspect of the skill, including interactive learning tools; an overview of the purpose of the skill; safety alerts; patient and family education; delegation guides; equipment lists; preparation procedures; documentation guidelines; demonstration videos and animations; images and illustrations; additional reading suggestions; printable evaluation checklists; and interactive review questions and competency tests with rationales. It is available online.

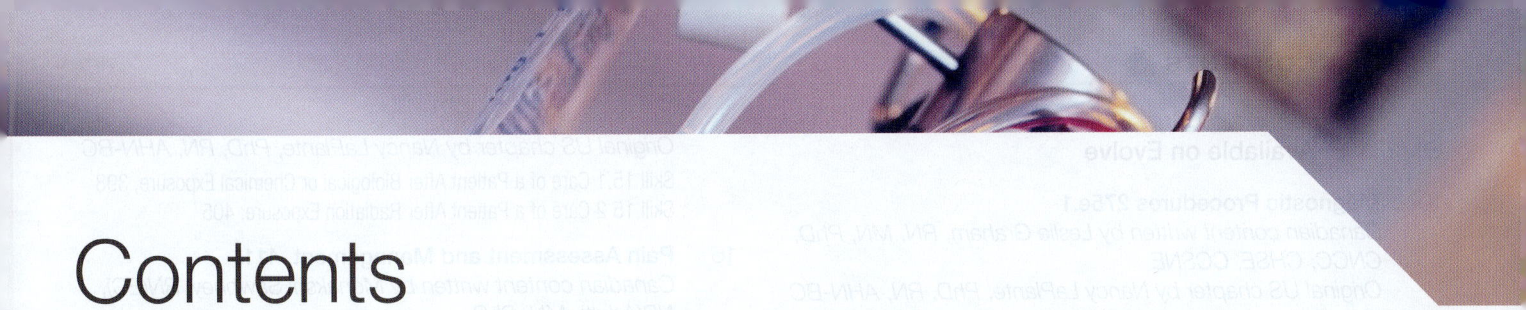

Contents

UNIT 15

Nursing in the Community

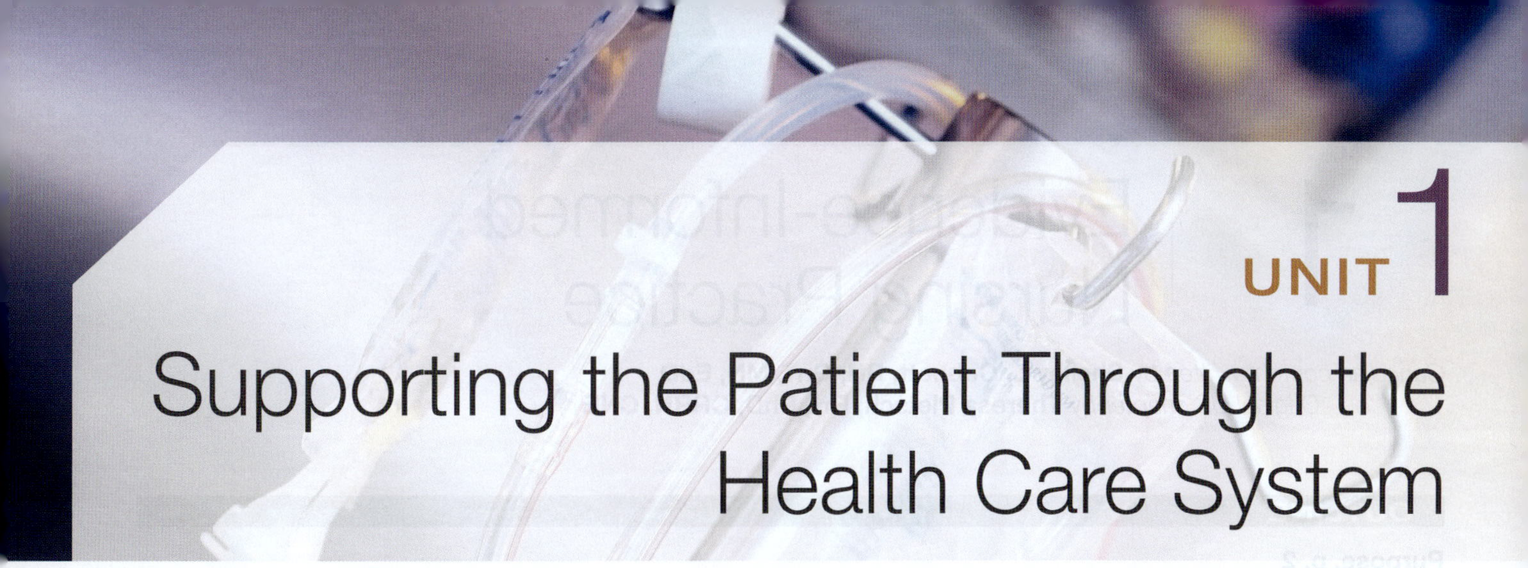

UNIT 1

Supporting the Patient Through the Health Care System

The skills in Unit 1 include evidence-informed practice and communication—both essential knowledge elements that enable you to think critically in the selection and performance of skills. Patients enter the health care system through a variety of settings and in various states of health. When nurses apply therapeutic communication principles, they are better able to perform the nursing process and make the clinical judgements needed to help patients transition through all health care settings. For example, a nurse applies therapeutic communication during assessment to gather data that give the whole picture of a patient being admitted to a health care setting, during a transition period, and prior to discharge.

Scientific evidence informs us and provides a scope of knowledge that directs us in the type of assessment information we need to learn when communicating with patients and families. For example, the newest scientific evidence enables a nurse to make recommendations about the frequency of various types of health screenings. In an outpatient centre, during an initial admission, such evidence-informed knowledge directs how a nurse interacts with patients to learn what they know about a particular screening and their own screening habits. The screening guidelines direct the type of questions a nurse poses to a patient (e.g., "What do you know about the frequency of screening and its purpose?").

Sound clinical judgements cannot be made without applying evidence and using excellent communication skills with patients, families, and health care team members. Therapeutic and collaborative communication enables us to become recipients of the type and depth of information we need to make informed clinical decisions. Effective communication is also a part of professional documentation—the conveying of relevant and accurate information that describes a patient's clinical course and response to nursing care.

The transition of patients through admission, transfer, and discharge, regardless of setting, requires an organized approach and emphasis on having accurate assessment information about patients. The methods we use to support patients in these phases of care depend in part on what we have learned from patients by using therapeutic communication. The same applies to our ability to collaborate effectively with colleagues and the interprofessional health care team. When a patient enters a hospital, the nurse becomes responsible for gathering as thorough a health history as possible to form a meaningful patient database. That database changes over time. During transfers within or between health care settings, the information pertinent to a patient's clinical care must be communicated and documented for other health care providers to use. Discharge is a critical time, requiring nurses to fully understand a patient's and caregiver's willingness and ability to follow the health care guidelines and restrictions needed for successful recovery.

When a patient enters the hospital setting, a nurse will also be mindful of the stress involved. Patients may feel uncertainty about their health conditions, the procedures to be performed, and the competence of health care staff, to name a few. Therapeutic communication can defuse some of that stress, enabling a nurse to establish trust and then obtain a thorough history. Therapeutic communication techniques are essential to help patients who have difficulty coping or understanding the hospital experience. The information exchanged about patients with other health care providers then becomes important for continuity of care and maintenance of quality care standards.

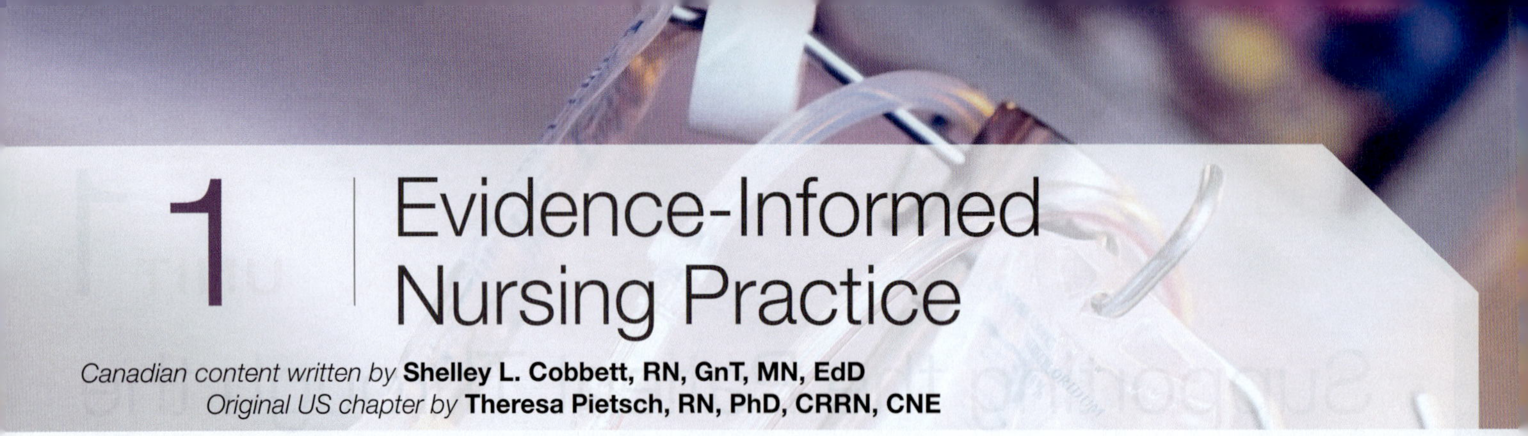

1 Evidence-Informed Nursing Practice

Canadian content written by **Shelley L. Cobbett, RN, GnT, MN, EdD**
Original US chapter by **Theresa Pietsch, RN, PhD, CRRN, CNE**

OUTLINE

OBJECTIVES

Mastery of content in this chapter will enable the nurse to:

- Describe how scientific evidence improves the relevance and efficacy of nursing skills.
- Explain the differences between research- and non–research-based evidence.
- Describe evidence-informed practice.
- Describe critical thinking, clinical reasoning, decision making, and clinical judgement.
- Explain the components of a PICO(TS) question.
- Describe the process for critiquing evidence in the literature.
- Identify the elements to review when critiquing a scientific article.
- Describe the seven steps of the action cycle of the Knowledge-to-Action Framework.
- Describe ways to apply evidence in nursing practice.
- Explain the importance of identifying outcomes in the evaluation of an evidence-informed practice change.

MEDIA RESOURCES

- http://evolve.elsevier.com/Canada/Perry/clinicalskills/

PURPOSE

Nurses must maintain and continuously update the knowledge, skills, attitude, and judgements required to meet patient needs in an ever-changing health care system. Evidence is a critical part of quality care in nursing practice and is fundamental to improving the health care system (Canadian Nurses Association [CNA], 2018). The foundation of *evidence-informed practice (EIP)* is research, embracing the principles of safety, effectiveness, and person-centredness; clinical expertise; and patient values, beliefs, and attitudes (White et al., 2021). Nurses advocate for evidence-informed decision making as part of their professional nursing practice (CNA, 2017). The CNA (2018) indicates that in evidence-informed decision making, the many factors that influence decision making—for example, available resources, cultural and religious norms, patient values, and legislation—are taken into account. The process of searching, selecting, appraising, and summarizing evidence is used in partnership with clinical expertise, patient preferences, and values, while remaining grounded in the local context, to implement person-centred, evidence-informed nursing practice.

There are various ways of knowing that are fundamental to nurses' ability to make competent and confident decisions. A seminal work (Carper, 1978) has outlined four ways of knowing: empirics (the science of nursing), esthetics (the art of nursing), personal knowledge in nursing, and ethics (moral knowledge in nursing). In 2010, Chinn and Kramer proposed a fifth type of knowing, emancipatory knowing, which advocates for social justice and human rights on behalf of patients and change on a societal level. Nursing is positioned to lead change and advance health through the use of EIP. Using many different levels and types of evidence, nurses ensure that the skills and procedures performed on patients incorporate best practices for efficiency, patient safety, and clinical effectiveness.

STANDARDS OF CARE

The CNA represents the family of nursing in Canada: registered nurses (RNs) (including nurse practitioners [NPs]), registered psychiatric nurses, and licensed (registered) practical nurses, with a membership of approximately 439 975 nurses in total (Almost, 2021).

Nursing registration and licensure is a provincial/territorial responsibility, and each jurisdiction has unique legislation that governs the practice of nursing. Entry-level competencies for the provinces and territories can be found on the website of each professional nursing association for RNs and licensed (registered) practical nurses:

- Canadian Council of Practical Nurse Regulators (2013)—*Code of Ethics for Licensed Practical Nurses in Canada* (https://ccpnr.ca/wp-content/uploads/2021/03/IJLPN-CE-Final.pdf)
- Canadian Council of Practical Nurse Regulators (2019)—*Entry-Level Competencies for Licensed Practical Nurses* (https://ccpnr.ca/wp-content/uploads/2021/03/CCPNR-ELCs_2019E.pdf)
- Canadian Council of Registered Nurse Regulators (2019)—*Entry-Level Competencies (ELCs) for the Practice of Registered Nurses* (https://www.ccrnr.ca/assets/ccrnr-rn-entry-level-competencies--2019.pdf)

- Canadian Nurses Association (2015a)—*Framework for the Practice of Registered Nurses in Canada* (https://www.cna-aiic.ca/en/nursing/regulated-nursing-in-canada/rn-practice-framework2)
- Canadian Nurses Association (2015b)—*Framework for Registered Nurse Prescribing in Canada* (https://www.cna-aiic.ca/en/nursing/regulated-nursing-in-canada/rn-prescribing-framework)
- Canadian Nurses Association (2017)—*Code of Ethics for Registered Nurses* (https://www.cna-aiic.ca/en/nursing/regulated-nursing-in-canada/nursing-ethics)
- Choosing Wisely Canada (2020)—*Nine Tests and Treatments to Question in Nursing* (https://choosingwiselycanada.org/recommendation/nursing/)
- Registered Nurses' Association of Ontario (2022)—*Best Practice Guidelines Program Published Resource List* (https://rnao.ca/bpg/resources/best-practice-guidelines-program-published-resource-list-2021)

PRINCIPLES FOR PRACTICE

This clinical case study highlights how professional nurses address problems in their practice.

Mary (she/her) works on a surgical intensive care unit (SICU) where patients recover from thoracic surgery, surgical oncology, and emergency surgery. Older persons are at higher risk for developing delirium postoperatively. Delirium usually develops abruptly in older surgical patients and manifests as a fluctuating change in attention, cognition, and consciousness. This change results in patient confusion and reduced awareness of the environment. Mary recently cared for an older patient who abruptly became confused and inattentive, then fell when they attempted to climb out of bed, resulting in a fracture of their hip. Mary discusses the situation with two nurse colleagues and asks, "How can we identify delirium sooner to prevent injuries to our patients on the SICU?" The nurse specialist for the unit tells Mary, "I know that there are different evidence-informed assessment scales available other than our current scale to help identify delirium. There may be more reliable and valid assessment scales to detect delirium in older persons who are intensive care patients. Let us ask this question: "For older intensive care patients, which assessment scale for delirium, compared with the current scale in use, will be most reliable and valid for detecting delirium during an ICU stay?" Feeling frustrated that their patient sustained a serious injury because the delirium was not identified prior to the fall, the group agrees that the question is the right one to search in the literature.

EIP is a process of making informed decisions about the way nurses care for patients. It begins with asking clinical questions to acquire an evidence base of knowledge. Clinical questions lead nurses such as Mary and her colleagues to find evidence from the research literature, clinical papers, quality improvement data, risk management trends, and the opinions of nurse experts. In addition to this evidence base, the nurse considers the context of the patient or population, along with their preferences and values, to implement EIP. This process guides the nurse in knowledge translation to make relevant and informed changes in practice, such as early identification of delirium in the case study.

In order to assist nurses in implementing EIP, there are evidence-informed elements of all nursing procedures presented throughout this textbook. For example, the length of time necessary to wash hands, the application and removal of gloves, the technique for determining the position of a feeding tube in the stomach, and the technique for giving an intramuscular injection are all based on evidence. Clinical research has answered the question of how these nursing procedures should be performed. The use of such evidence in practice enables clinicians to provide the highest quality of care to patients and their families.

Quality Health Care and Patient Safety

According to the CNA (2017), integrated care is based on six key principles: person-centred care, quality services, health promotion and illness prevention, equitable access to quality care, sustainability, and accountability. The Quadruple Aim Framework includes improved patient experience, improved population health, reduced costs, and improved work life of providers as a way to enhance health care system performance and nurture health care system sustainability (FPT Committee on Health Workforce, 2020). Implementing health care processes or practices that are evidence informed in a reliable and consistent manner is a feature of quality care that maximizes patient safety. Globally, patient harm is thought to be the fourteenth leading cause of morbidity and mortality (World Health Organization, 2019), with 1 in 17 patients in Canadian hospitals experiencing a preventable incident of patient harm (Canadian Institute for Health Information [CIHI], 2021). There are four categories of harmful events: health care and medications (e.g., bedsores or receiving the wrong medication, 46%); infections (e.g., surgical site infections, 30%); procedure-related events (e.g., bleeding after surgery, 20%); and patient accidents (e.g., falls, 4%) (CIHI, 2021). Implementing new knowledge into practice requires a systematic approach that applies the best available evidence to clinical, educational, and administrative practices. Clinical practice guidelines rely on the best evidence to decide which interventions produce the best outcomes, enhancing patient safety. Nurses play a key role in all areas of health care in questioning outdated, illogical, or unsafe practices, and then adopting evidence-informed practices that will alter patients' health status, maximize safety, and achieve desired outcomes.

Critical Thinking, Clinical Reasoning, Decision Making, and Clinical Judgement

The terms *critical thinking, clinical reasoning, decision making,* and *clinical judgement* are often used interchangeably. But within nursing, these terms have slightly different meanings. Critical thinking is complex and based on context and has no single "right" definition. Critical thinking is a broad term that refers to purposeful, informed, outcome-focused thinking and includes clinical reasoning, decision making, and clinical judgement (Alfaro-LeFevre, 2019). *Critical thinking* involves analysis and discrimination of evidence-informed research to guide practices and is essential for sound clinical judgement, identifying nursing diagnoses, planning patient care, and safely and effectively practising person-centred care. *Clinical reasoning* is a more specific term that refers to ways of thinking about patient care issues, whereas *clinical judgement* refers to the outcome of critical thinking, clinical reasoning, and decision making. It is helpful to think about critical thinking and clinical reasoning as the processes that lead to clinical judgement, the outcome or result (e.g., conclusion, decision, or opinion) (Alfaro-LeFevre, 2019). Critical thinking occurs in both clinical settings (e.g., identifying person-centred diagnoses) and nonclinical settings (e.g., test taking), whereas decision making, clinical reasoning, and clinical judgement usually occur in the clinical setting. As critical thinkers, you will use many skills, knowledge sources, and attitudes; as you progress in your nursing career, your critical thinking skills will continue to improve.

A Case for Evidence

EIP helps the nurse make accurate, timely, and appropriate clinical decisions. It is an interprofessional process of applying the newest knowledge available in health care sciences to the patient's bedside. Using a sliding board to transfer a patient from bed to stretcher instead of lifting and using the research-based Braden Scale to routinely assess a patient's risk for skin breakdown are examples of using evidence at the bedside. This textbook demonstrates how to use evidence in nursing procedures or skills and provides the scientific guidelines to perform skills more effectively, improve patient outcomes, and maximize patient safety.

As a professional nurse, you need to stay informed and be aware of the most current evidence. Typically, new students diligently read their textbooks and assigned scientific articles. A good textbook incorporates current evidence into the practice guidelines and nursing skills at the time it is published. However, because a textbook relies on the scientific literature, some information can become outdated by the time the book is published. Articles from the nursing and health care literature are available on almost any topic involving nursing practice. New research is reported every day. Although the scientific basis of nursing practice has grown, there are practices that are still not "research based" (based on findings from well-designed research studies) because the findings are inconclusive or because researchers have not yet studied the practices.

For example, in the past, nurses changed intravenous (IV) site dressings daily and applied antibiotic ointment to reduce the incidence of infection at a site. However, there was no evidence at the time to support this practice. IV care was based on tradition. Subsequent research demonstrated that topical antibiotics offer no benefit, and daily dressing changes are not beneficial unless a dressing becomes soiled or compromised. Today, the standard of care is to cleanse an adult's IV site with chlorhexidine antiseptic solution and not use antibiotic ointment on the IV site (Infusion Nurses Society [INS], 2021). A transparent semipermeable membrane (TSM) dressing change should be performed at least every 7 days, and gauze dressings every 2 days or when loose, wet, or visibly soiled, or when integrity is compromised (INS, 2021). The challenge is to obtain the best, most current information at the right time, when you need it for patient care.

The best evidence comes from well-designed, systematically conducted research studies that are reported in peer-reviewed scientific journals. Widespread access to online research articles has enhanced the availability of best-practice information in the health care setting, empowering nurses to move away from practices based on tradition, preference, or convenience. It is important for nursing leaders to provide a supportive environment and adequate facilitation of required changes. Researchers have found that leadership within health care institutions is vital for the process of implementing EIP in nursing (Välimäki et al., 2018). Strengths-based nurse leaders are agents of change (Waddell & Walton, 2020), and they empower nurses to fully engage in critiquing practice and in the translation of knowledge for ongoing efficiency and effectiveness. Information is widely portable, and as such, current practice is continuously evolving and changing based on the best available evidence. The acceptability of up-to-date information at the point of care is quickly becoming the norm.

EIP requires nurses to consider many different types and levels of evidence to become informed about practice issues (e.g., fall or infection rates). But remember, as a nurse it is important that you *not* rely on one type of evidence alone. When you face a clinical issue or problem, seek out all sources of evidence, including research, patient preferences, and patient values, to find the best solution in caring for patients in an evidence-informed, person-centred manner. When there is no research evidence for a practice question or issue, nurses have a range of non–research-based evidence available to them (Singh et al., 2022). Examples of non–research-based evidence include consensus or position statements, general literature reviews, quality improvement and risk management data, retrospective or concurrent chart review, and clinicians' expertise.

Even when you use the best evidence available, application and outcomes will differ based on patients' values, preferences, concerns, and expectations and the local context. You need to apply critical thinking and clinical reasoning competencies to determine whether evidence is relevant and appropriate to your patients to aid you in making sound decisions and clinical judgements. For example, some research suggests that spirituality positively affects and enhances older patients' psychological health and health promotion behaviours (Heidari et al., 2019). However, if a patient is reluctant to discuss their spirituality and you are unsure of their beliefs, an attempt to use spiritual health interventions is inappropriate. Using your clinical expertise and considering patients' cultures, values, and preferences ensures that you apply new evidence in practice both ethically and appropriately. EIP requires good nursing judgement; it does not entail finding research evidence and applying it blindly, but rather applying the best evidence from a variety of sources from a person-centred perspective.

Ask a Clinical Question

Asking a clinical question is the initial important step of the process, as the question will direct the search for the most relevant and best evidence. Every day, nurses perform interventions (e.g., providing comfort measures, caring for patients with wounds, and offering grief support to a family) that stimulate questions such as "Why do we use this approach?" and "Is there a better way?" or "This step causes patients distress. What other options are available?" Always think about your practice when caring for patients. Question what does not make sense to you and what you think needs clarification. Interprofessional collaboration involves various perspectives and might help to clarify or examine the clinical problem or issue. As practised in the previous case study, think about a patient care problem or an area of interest that is time consuming, costly, or not logical.

Clinical questions often arise because of either a problem- or knowledge-focused trigger. A problem-focused trigger occurs as the nurse cares for a patient or notices a trend on a nursing unit. For example, the following problem-focused trigger might arise while caring for an unconscious patient: "Which is the best anti-infective solution to use when giving oral care to patients on a ventilator?" Examples of problem-focused trends include the increase in the number of pressure injuries to patients' skin or tissues or the incidence of urinary tract infections on a nursing unit. A knowledge-focused trigger arises when the nurse asks a question regarding new information about a topic. For example, "What is the current evidence to reduce the incidence of postoperative delirium in patients over the age of 70 years?" Important knowledge sources often include standards and practice guidelines available from national and provincial/territorial agencies, for example, the Registered Nurses' Association of Ontario (RNAO; https://rnao.ca/bpg), Canadian Stroke Best Practices (https://www.strokebestpractices.ca/), and the Canadian Clinical Practice Guidelines InfoBase (https://www.cma.ca/).

There are two basic types of questions: background and foreground (Dang et al., 2022; Melnyk et al., 2018). Think of a forest and the trees. A *background question* gives us a view of a forest. It is broad and general about a condition or idea—for example, "Which interventions reduce falls in oncology patients?" The answer to the question provides general knowledge about the problem, concepts, or topic of interest (e.g., falls, fall occurrence among oncology patients, reasons oncology patients fall). In contrast, a *foreground question* gives us a closer look at the trees in a forest. It is used to find out specific information for making clinical decisions (Dang et al., 2022). A foreground question asks which of two interventions is likely to be more effective in addressing a practice issue. For example, "Does hourly rounding compared with a standard fall prevention protocol affect the incidence of falls?" A background question allows you to explore a vast array of options in the literature, whereas a foreground question produces a refined and limited body of evidence specific to your area of interest. In day-to-day clinical practice,

BOX 1.1

Developing a PICO(TS) Question

P Patient, population, or problem

- Be as specific as possible to identify the patient, population, or problem

I Intervention (quantitative studies) or issue of interest (qualitative studies)

- Can be an assessment, intervention, therapy, or evaluation

C Comparison (quantitative studies) or context (qualitative studies)

- Standard care versus the intervention or issue of interest; context of the question

O Outcomes (quantitative studies) or findings (qualitative studies)

- Which result do you wish to achieve or observe as a result of an intervention or issue of interest?

T Time (optional component for a clinical question)

S Search strategy (optional component using search limiters)

Adapted from Davies, B., & Logan, J. (2021). *Reading research: A user-friendly guide for health professionals* (7th ed., p. 34). Elsevier/Mosby; Brown, S. (2018). *Evidence-based nursing* (4th ed., p. 253). Jones & Bartlett Learning.

it helps to be able to identify foreground questions to reduce the extent of the literature to review.

A well-stated foreground question is clearly worded when you use a PICO(TS) format. Box 1.1 summarizes the elements of a PICO(TS) question. Using keywords in a PICO(TS) strategy makes it easier to search for evidence in the scientific literature because it restricts a search to only articles pertinent to the PICO(TS) terms (Brown, 2018). The use of "(TS)" denotes that T (time) and S (search strategy) are not required elements of every PICO(TS) question. The words used in the PICO(T) question are the key terms for a literature search, and the (S) limits the search strategy; for example, you may limit a search to only randomized controlled trials (RCTs). Examples of PICO(TS) questions are as follows: "For patients in intensive care units (P), does the Intensive Care Delirium Screening Checklist (ICDSC) (I) compared with the Nursing Delirium Scale (C) detect incidences of delirium (O) earlier during the ICU stay (T)?" "In medical patients (P) does the use of teach-back (I) compared with teach-back and a follow-up call-back system (C) improve patient medication adherence (O) during the first 60 days after discharge (T)?"

Well-designed PICO(TS) questions do not have to include all six elements. For example, a comparison intervention is not pertinent when a PICO(TS) question is about meaning, such as, "Do family caregivers (P) of hospice patients feel anxiety (O) when providing hands-on care (I)?" Also, if there is no comparison intervention, only the standard of care, a (C) is not required; nor does the time (T) or the search strategy (S) need to be included. For example, one such question could be, "Do family caregivers (P) of patients with dementia feel sadness (O) when providing hands-on care (I)?" The elements of Population, an Intervention or issue of interest, and Outcome are essential for a well-designed PICO(TS) question involving an intervention.

A clearly stated PICO(TS) question helps to identify knowledge gaps for a specific clinical, educational, or managerial problem or situation. When you form well-thought-out questions, the type of evidence you lack for clinical judgement and decision making becomes clearer when you search the literature. Examples of different knowledge gaps include the following:

- *Diagnosis:* Questions about the selection and interpretation of diagnostic tests. *Example:* Does the use of a smartphone app-assisted blood pressure (BP) monitoring system compared with a standard home BP monitoring system measure BP more accurately for a patient at home?
- *Prognosis:* Questions about a patient's likely clinical outcome. *Example:* Is there a difference in the level of functional decline in hospitalized older persons who are admitted to an acute care gerontological unit compared with those who are admitted to a general medical-surgical unit?
- *Therapy:* Questions about the selection of the most beneficial treatments. *Example:* Which bowel regimen is most effective in relieving constipation caused by the administration of opioid therapy in oncology patients with chronic pain (or persistent pain)?
- *Prevention:* Questions about screening and prevention methods to reduce the risk of disease. *Example:* Does the use of social media with educational messages compared with informational brochures reduce the incidence of vaping in adolescents?
- *Education:* Questions about the best teaching strategies for colleagues, patients, or family members. *Example:* Is there a difference in colon emptying from a bowel preparation regimen in preoperative patients who receive paper directions and follow-up text messages compared with those who receive paper directions only?
- *Meaning:* Questions that seek to understand a phenomenon. *Example:* How do nurses perceive the expression of pain in patients with opioid misuse?

Search for the Best Evidence

Once you have a clear and concise PICO(TS) question, you are ready to search for evidence. Numerous research and nonresearch resources are available to aid you in your search, including government and professional websites, employer procedure manuals, performance improvement reports, and computerized bibliographical databases. Do not hesitate to ask for help to find appropriate evidence. A reference librarian is an excellent resource with whom to collaborate on a literature search. If one is not available, go to your faculty member or an advanced practice nurse within the health care institution.

A reference librarian knows the relevant databases available to you for a literature search about your PICO(TS) question (Box 1.2). The databases are repositories of published scientific studies, including peer-reviewed research. A peer-reviewed article is preferable for retrieval because it has been evaluated by a panel of experts who are familiar with the topic or subject matter of the article. Working with the librarian, translate the elements of your PICO(TS) question into the language or keywords that will yield the best articles for your evidence search. For example, consider the following PICO(TS) question: "Does motivational interviewing (I) compared with teach-back (C) improve heart failure patients' (P) adherence to cardiac medications (O) over a 6-month period (T)?" The keywords include *heart failure patient, motivational interviewing, teach-back, cardiac medications,* and *adherence.* A good librarian will recommend using the indexing language or controlled vocabulary of the database that you are searching. The controlled vocabulary known as Medical Subject Headings (MeSH) is used in Canada and is updated annually from the US National Library of Medicine (2021). Proper use of MeSH terms facilitates a more thorough and focused literature search than one you might get from simply trying to search combinations of keywords on Google or Bing. In the previous example, the word *cardiac medications* might be entered instead of *cardiovascular medications* to fit the database language, whereas *adherence* might also be entered as *compliance.*

When working with a database, you need to enter keywords to search for articles. Because the vocabulary in published articles is often vague, the words you select sometimes have one meaning to one author and a very different meaning to another. Each keyword generates a set of articles. Boolean is a set of words or commands that can be used in most search engines and databases to help limit

BOX 1.2

Searchable Scientific Literature Databases and Sources

CINAHL	Cumulative Index of Nursing and Allied Health Literature; database for EBSCO nursing resources; includes studies in nursing, allied health, and biomedicine https://www.ebsco.com/products/research-databases/cinahl-complete
MEDLINE	US National Library of Medicine; bibliographical database that contains more than 29 million references to journal articles in life sciences with a concentration on biomedicine https://www.nlm.nih.gov/medline/medline_overview.html
Embase	Biomedical and pharmaceutical studies as well as abstracts and articles from biomedical, drug, and medical device conferences https://www.elsevier.com/solutions/embase-biomedical-research
APA PsycInfo	Interprofessional bibliographical resources in psychology and the behavioural and social sciences https://www.apa.org/pubs/databases/psycinfo/index
Cochrane Database of Systematic Reviews	Full text of regularly updated systematic reviews prepared by the Cochrane Collaboration; includes completed reviews and protocols https://www.cochranelibrary.com/
National Guideline Clearinghouse	Public resource for evidence-informed clinical practice guidelines. Available through the Agency for Healthcare Research and Quality; contains structured abstracts (summaries) about clinical guidelines and their development; also includes condensed version of guidelines for viewing https://www.ahrq.gov/gam/index.html
PubMed	Health science library at the US National Library of Medicine; free access to more than 34 million citations for biomedical literature from MEDLINE, life science journals, and online books https://pubmed.ncbi.nlm.nih.gov/
ERIC (Educational Resources Information Center)	Consists of resources in education and covers published literature from over 775 periodicals in the discipline of education https://eric.ed.gov/
JBI EBP Database	Includes full systematic reviews, protocols, evidence summaries, best practice recommendations, and consumer information https://www.wolterskluwer.com/en/know/jbi-resources
CPS (Compendium of Pharmaceuticals and Specialties)	Compendium of pharmaceuticals and specialties, drug information, and patient information https://joulecma.ca/clinical-tools/cps
Trip Medical Database	A clinical search engine that allows hundreds of evidence-informed resources to be searched simultaneously. https://www.tripdatabase.com/

your results to those that are most applicable to your clinical topic. The most common Boolean operators are AND, OR, and NOT; they should be keyed as all capital letters because some databases recognize them only in this format. Using Boolean operators or the function of Search Limits enables you to narrow the results of the search by combining key terms from your PICO(TS) question using the Boolean connector AND. For example, by entering the combination of "heart failure patient AND cardiovascular medications AND adherence" into the literature database, you will obtain a listing of only those articles that contain all three terms. A librarian can show you how to use the Search Limits function. Your search can be further narrowed by limiting it to certain categories, such as the time frame during which the article was written, types of studies, English-language publications, or age of patients. Use of Boolean connectors and Search Limits reduces the number of articles to a manageable number to review for a PICO(TS) question.

The pyramid in Fig. 1.1 represents a hierarchy for rating available scientific evidence obtained in your search. It is important to learn about the types of studies to help you know which ones provide the best scientific evidence to guide you in choosing which articles to review. The strongest level of evidence is at the top of the pyramid; the weakest is at the bottom. You can use the rating scale of I to VIII when you later critique each article that you obtain in your search of the literature. Table 1.1 describes types of studies with examples in the evidence hierarchy, beginning with the study at the top of the hierarchy, a systematic review.

If your PICO(TS) question leads you to an article that is a systematic review, celebrate! A systematic review is the perfect answer to a PICO(TS) question. Basically, a researcher has asked the same

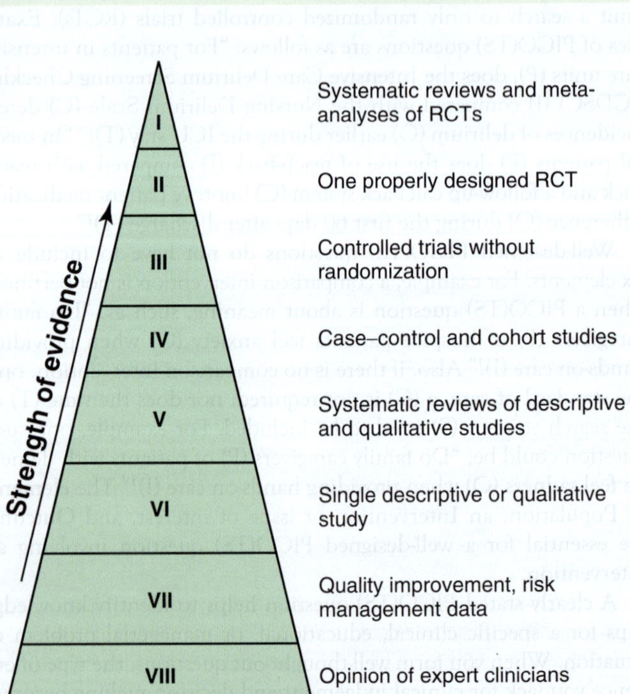

FIG 1.1 The evidence pyramid. *RCT,* Randomized controlled trial.

PICO(TS) question you have asked and then examined all the well-designed relevant research studies that ask the same question. The researcher creates a detailed and comprehensive plan and uses explicit methods to locate, appraise, and synthesize research on the

TABLE 1.1

Types of Studies in the Evidence Hierarchy

Study Type	Description	Example
Systematic review or meta-analysis	An author or panel of experts reviews the evidence from randomized controlled trials (RCTs) (and other defined types of research studies) about a specific clinical question and summarizes the state of the science. In a meta-analysis, there is the addition of a statistical analysis that combines data from all studies.	A study summarized and synthesized the current state of evidence-informed competencies adopted in clinical practice by health care professionals. Eleven systematic reviews were eligible for critical appraisal from the 3947 publications found in four databases. Evidence-informed practice (EIP) was not fully implemented in clinical practice, even though health care professionals' self-report of knowledge, skills, attitudes, and beliefs toward EIP was rated at a moderate to high level. Health care professionals' competencies were difficult to compare across studies because there were a variety of measurement tools to measure competencies. Practice changes to improve processes or patient care outcomes were minimally discussed in the 11 studies reviewed. The use of interdisciplinary evidence-informed competencies and common outcome measures can strengthen the implementation of EIP (Saunders et al., 2019).
Randomized controlled trial (RCT)	A researcher tests an intervention against the usual standard of care. Participants are randomly assigned to either a control group (receives standard care) or a treatment group (receives the experimental intervention), with both measured on the same outcomes to determine whether there is a difference.	This study, focusing on female incontinence in 12 nursing homes, evaluated the impact of implementing evidence-informed interventions for the treatment of incontinence. The nursing homes were randomly assigned to one of two groups. A control group received the current standard of care; the second group had nursing staff participate in incontinence education, and then these individuals were given handouts with urinary incontinence evidence-informed interventions. Supplemental content for their patients included posters with the interventions, bladder diaries, and questionnaires about quality of life with incontinence. Outcome measurements included number of urinary incontinence events, urinary incontinence diagnoses, and the number of nursing interventions for urinary incontinence. The 218 patients receiving care from the intervention group had significantly less use of incontinence pads and lower risk for episodes of urinary incontinence when compared with the control group of 165 patients (Hödl et al., 2019).
Quasi-experimental study	This research approach tries to show that an intervention causes a particular outcome. This type of study is done when one of the three elements of an RCT is not feasible, most commonly randomization (Davies & Logan, 2021).	In a quasi-experimental study (*N* = 103), the authors investigated the effectiveness of eye masks and earplugs on quality of sleep among patients in intensive care units (ICUs). The intervention group received eye masks and earplugs for sleep; the control group received routine sleep care, such as noise reduction. Subjects were not randomized to the groups. The researchers hypothesized that the intervention group (*n* = 52) would report better quality of sleep when compared with the control group (*n* = 51). All subjects received routine sleep care on day 1 followed by a pretest sleep questionnaire. On day 2, the intervention group used the eye masks and earplugs, and the control group received routine sleep care followed by a post-test questionnaire for all subjects. The findings suggest that the implementation of eye masks and earplugs may improve sleep among patients in the ICU, but that the quality of sleep still remains low. Further research is needed (Bani Younis et al., 2019).
Case–control or cohort study	Researchers study one group of subjects with a certain health condition (e.g., obesity) at the same time as another group of subjects who do not have the condition to determine whether there is an association between the health condition and the predictor variables (e.g., exercise pattern, family history, history of depression).	The objective of this descriptive cohort design was to validate the Cultural Capability Measurement Tool with a cohort of health professional students to better provide care to Indigenous peoples. The tool was tested for reliability, content, and construct validity using confirmatory factor analysis, and concurrent validity using the Cultural Understanding Self-Assessment Tool. Cronbach's alpha coefficient of 0.86 was obtained and a five-factor solution was confirmed. Measuring nursing students' cultural capabilities can inform their development of a culturally safe nursing workforce (West et al., 2018).
Descriptive study	Study describes a concept or topic of interest. It sometimes examines the prevalence, magnitude, or characteristics of a concept.	This study assessed oncology nurses' adherence to personal protective equipment (PPE) guidelines when handling and administering hazardous chemotherapy drugs. Data were collected using a valid and reliable research instrument tool—the Hazardous Drug Handling Questionnaire. Nurses' adherence to recommended guidelines for hazardous chemotherapy drugs was assessed during administration, disposal, and handling of excreta. Findings from this descriptive study indicate that nurses are not completely adhering to recommended hazardous drug administration guidelines for PPE with chemotherapy drugs (Menonna-Quinn et al., 2019).

Continued

TABLE 1.1
Types of Studies in the Evidence Hierarchy—cont'd

Study Type	Description	Example
Qualitative study	Study examines individuals' perceptions of experiences with health problems or life events and the contexts in which the experiences occur. A qualitative study provides narrative data from extensive interviews with subjects. A qualitative researcher encourages subjects to tell their story about an event or condition to obtain a full and rich description.	Researchers interviewed two oncology nurse focus groups to understand nurses' perceptions about using e-health content from the Oncology Interactive Navigator (OIN) to improve patient outcomes. The researchers of this descriptive qualitative study interviewed eight nurses prior to exposure to OIN content and then seven nurses 4 weeks after exposure. Three themes emerged about the nurses' experiences using the OIN: (1) it is an evolving and dynamic process; (2) it supports clinical practice and patient care; and (3) it provides a platform for professional development and networking (Lau & Loiselle, 2018).
Clinical experts	Accessing clinical experts on a nursing unit is an excellent way to learn about current evidence. Clinical experts often write clinical articles on topics that require application of evidence in the literature.	Telehealth nursing is a growing specialty in the nursing profession. The authors discuss the value of telehealth nursing for communities, education and credentialling for nurses, and specific competencies expected in telehealth nursing (Mataxen & Webb, 2019).

topic (Davies & Logan, 2021). The researcher sets criteria for the type of studies to review in the search. A systematic review explains whether the evidence for which you are searching about a specific question exists and whether it supports a change in practice. A systematic review of well-designed research studies provides the best evidence for the effectiveness of different interventions. A meta-analysis involves using statistical techniques to analyze the data from the studies in a systematic review to determine statistically the strength of the evidence.

An RCT is a formal experiment for testing therapies and establishing cause and effect. A researcher tests an intervention (e.g., a mobility program or a new type of wound covering) against the usual standard of care. Researchers randomly assign subjects in an RCT to either a control group or a treatment group. In other words, all the subjects in the study have an equal chance of being assigned to either group. In that way, it is unlikely that the two groups will be highly different. The treatment group receives the experimental intervention at the same time the control group receives the usual standard of care. Both groups are measured for the same outcomes to determine whether the experimental intervention made a difference. Following the completion of an RCT, the researcher knows whether the intervention leads to better outcomes than the standard of care.

More often you will find articles in the nursing literature that involve controlled trials without randomization (i.e., quasi-experimental studies) or descriptive studies. Regardless of the level of evidence, a study with relevant results helps you decide whether your PICO(TS) question can be answered. For example, if a quasi-experimental study resulted in a positive clinical improvement, even though it was not a statistically significant change, the clinical change might be worth strong consideration based on its clinical significance.

The use of clinical experts is located at the bottom of the evidence pyramid, but do not consider clinical experts to be a poor source of evidence. Expert clinicians frequently use evidence as they build their own practice, and they are rich sources of information for clinical problems as a result of their clinical experience.

Critique the Evidence

Continuing with the case study presented earlier, the nurses on the SICU conduct their unit practice committee (UPC) meeting. During the meeting, Mary and her colleagues decide that it is important to include key members of their interprofessional team (health care provider, respiratory therapist, and pharmacist). The UPC then reviews the articles carefully using a rapid-appraisal checklist, which includes criteria for evaluating the strength of an article. After the group evaluates the articles for the strength of evidence and synthesizes the findings, they decide that there is evidence for considering a different assessment scale for delirium: the Intensive Care Delirium Screening Checklist (ICDSC). The staff note that one of the articles recommends other considerations, such as the importance of staff education, to ensure an understanding of the assessment criteria and that the clinicians are applying the criteria to patients in the same way. Another article summarizes the risk factors for patients developing delirium during a hospitalization and highlights criteria to flag in a nursing assessment, such as decreased mobility or visual or hearing impairment. Yet another article suggests increasing the frequency of the delirium assessment. Critically reviewing and analyzing the available evidence requires a systematic approach. Each source of evidence (e.g., journal article, clinical guideline, expert summary) must be reviewed to determine its value, feasibility, and utility of evidence for making a practice change.

When you conduct a review, it should enable you to determine whether the research contains evidence that answers your question. It is important to use an approach that does not bog you down by requiring you to review every single element of each article. The Critical Appraisal Skills Programme (CASP), an international collaboration that supports the education of critical appraisal skills and provides several free appraisal tools, advocates answering three important questions when critically appraising evidence (CASP, 2021):

1. *Is the study valid?* Evaluate the study's methodological quality.
2. *What are the results?* Consider whether the study is statistically significant, clinically significant, or both.
3. *Are the results useful?* Consider how the information applies to your question.

Many organizations use appraisal checklists for recording article reviews; these can be helpful in your own article appraisal. Once you have decided that the article is relevant to your PICO(TS) question, you need to assess the validity of the study. This requires identifying the type of study using the evidence pyramid. For example, if you have an article on an RCT to review, were subjects randomized in the study? Was the sample of subjects large enough to test the intervention effectively? What approach was used in delivering the intervention and measuring the effects? Were all subjects measured for the same outcomes? In contrast, if you read a qualitative study, did the researcher study a sufficient number and representation of subjects, and did the approach allow for a thorough and objective review of findings? Studies that are not well designed cannot provide definitive support for the evidence they aim to produce.

As you read each article, ask the next question: What are the results? Do the findings apply to your patients and practice setting? If you have an RCT, you will want to know whether or not an intervention worked to help you decide whether it potentially makes sense to use it in your practice. Your analysis of statistics will help. For example, if an intervention was shown to be "statistically significant," the intervention shows benefit. If instead there was no statistically significant difference, you may reject the value of the intervention. However, if the intervention led to an improvement, though not a statistically significant one, you might still consider it to have clinical value. If you have a descriptive study, you will need to decide whether the information is relevant to your PICO(TS) question. For example, were characteristics of the patients in the study similar to those of your own patients?

You might also choose to review a clinical article that explains a clinical practice topic relevant to your PICO(TS) question. A clinical article is not rated for its level of evidence, but it can offer useful information, especially if you decide to implement a change related to the practice topic. To learn how to read research and clinical articles, you first need to understand each of the common elements. This will help you decide whether an article is complete and well explained. Articles should include the following elements:

- *Abstract:* A brief summary of the article that tells you whether the article is research or clinically based. An abstract summarizes the purpose of the study or clinical topic, the major themes or findings, and the implications for practice.
- *Introduction:* Contains information about the purpose of the article and the importance of the topic for the audience that reads it. There is usually a brief discussion of supporting evidence about why the topic is important from the author's point of view.

  After reading the abstract and introduction, decide whether you want to continue reading the entire article. At this stage, you will know whether the topic of the article is similar to your PICO(TS) question or related closely enough to provide you with useful information. Remember that the research question does not need to be the same as yours but close enough to offer useful information. If this is the case, continue to read the next elements of the article:
- *Literature review or background:* A good author offers a detailed background of the level of scientific or clinical information that exists about the topic of the article. The review explains what led the author to conduct the study or report on the clinical topic. Perhaps the article itself does not address your PICO(TS) question the way you desire, but it could possibly lead you to other more useful articles. The literature review gives you a good idea of how past research led to the researcher's question.
- *Article narrative:* The "middle section," or narrative, of an article differs depending on whether it is an empirical (research) or conceptual article. A conceptual article describes something—for example, a clinical topic—which often includes a description of a patient population, the nature of a certain disease or health problem and how it affects patients, and implications for nursing care or how to use a therapy or new technology. A research article describes the key elements of a research study, including its purpose, how the study was designed or the methods used, and the results and implications. The narrative of a research article contains several standard subsections:
  - *Purpose statement:* Explains the focus or intent of a study. It identifies which concepts or variables will be researched.
  - *Methods or design:* Explains how a research study was organized and conducted to answer the research question(s). This is where you learn the type of study (e.g., RCT, case-control, or qualitative). You will also learn how many subjects or people are in a study. In health care studies, subjects sometimes include patients, family members, or health care staff. The language in the methods section is sometimes confusing if it explains details about how the researcher designed the study to minimize bias so as to obtain the most accurate results possible. Use your faculty member as a resource to help interpret this section.
  - *Results (or findings) and discussion:* Both conceptual and research articles have a summary section. In a conceptual article, the author explains the clinical implications for the topic. In a research article, the author explains the results and how the research question was answered. For example, in a qualitative study there is a thorough summary of subject narratives, which provides a description of themes and ideas that arise from the researcher's analysis of the data. There is no statistical analysis of the data collected. By comparison, a quantitative study includes a full description of the study subjects and a statistical analysis of the findings. It is important to learn some of the common statistical terms used by researchers (Box 1.3). A good author also discusses the implications and limitations of a study in the discussion section.
  - *Clinical implications:* A research article includes a section that explains whether the findings from the study have clinical implications. The researcher explains how to apply the findings in a practice setting for the type of subjects studied.
  - *Limitations:* Limitations are the identified weaknesses of a study. The researcher suggests possible issues with the study, such as bias or missed procedural steps. The information on limitations will help you decide whether you want to use the evidence presented in the article in your own nursing practice.

As you critique each article, complete your critical appraisal checklist. You may choose to rate each article by its level and strength of evidence, using the scale of I to VIII from the evidence pyramid (see Fig. 1.1). It also helps to review multiple articles with a group of colleagues involved in the EIP process. Each person can review a single article; then you can come together as a group to review your total findings. Once all evidence has been reviewed, it is time to discuss the third important question: Are the results useful?

Use critical thinking to consider the scientific rigour of the evidence and how well it addresses your area of interest. Scientific rigour

BOX 1.3

Common Statistical Terms

Sample Size: Number (*n*) of individuals in a study.

Significance: A measure of the likelihood that a finding or a result of a study is caused by the intervention being tested and is not simply due to chance alone. Most researchers set the level of significance at a p value of 0.05 or 0.01. For example, if the effects of an intervention (e.g., use of the Intensive Care Delirium Screening Checklist) are significant at $p < 0.05$, it means that the likelihood of the effect (earlier identification of delirium) occurring by chance is less than 5%; thus, it is more than 95% likely that the intervention truly had an effect on the early identification of patients with delirium. When a study result has a p value (e.g., 0.61) greater than that originally set by the researcher (e.g., p value of 0.05), the researcher must conclude that the results were possibly due to chance and the intervention had no effect.

Confidence Interval (CI): The CI tells you the precision of a study finding, meaning the range (e.g., range of a mean score) in which clinicians judge the confidence of a finding. A 95% CI means that clinicians can be 95% confident that their findings will be within the range given in the study.

Effect Size: When the effect of an intervention is statistically significant, it does not necessarily mean that it is big, important, or helpful in decision making. It simply means that the researcher can be confident that there is a difference. An effect size greater than 0.5 is considered a large effect.

is the extent to which the findings of a study are valid, reliable, and relevant to a given patient population. Consider the evidence in light of your patients' concerns, preferences, and values. Your review of articles offers a snapshot conclusion based on combined evidence about one focused topical area. Ethically, always consider evidence that will benefit patients and do no harm. Decide whether the evidence is relevant, is easily applicable in your setting of practice, and has the potential to improve patient outcomes.

There will be times when you find that there is insufficient or no evidence to answer a PICO(TS) question. This finding warrants no change in practice because the evidence is weak and inconsistent or absent.

KNOWLEDGE-TO-ACTION FRAMEWORK

If a literature review and critique yields evidence that answers your PICO(TS) question and offers evidence that can be applied to practice, the next step is to translate that knowledge into practice. A common conceptual framework, the Knowledge-to-Action (KTA) Framework, includes two components: knowledge creation and an action cycle (Graham et al., 2006). This framework has been adopted by many professional organizations to guide the process of knowledge translation (e.g., RNAO, 2022). The framework utilizes a systems perspective that is responsive and adaptive and acknowledges the unpredictability of the environment when moving from evidence into action (RNAO, 2022). The action cycle provides a useful framework for knowledge translation and includes the following seven steps:

1. *Identifying the knowledge-to-action gaps:* Identify a situation or problem that needs to be addressed. Compare the evidence and current practice—is there a gap? Involve multiple sources of evidence and engage relevant partners. Critique the evidence that you collected when doing your PICO(TS) search.
2. *Adapting knowledge to local context:* It is critical that the evidence be adapted to fit local circumstances to make it relevant and promote successful implementation of person-centred care. The assimilation of the collected evidence with professional judgement within the local context provides a comprehensive and rational basis for decision making in patient care.
3. *Assessing barriers/facilitators to knowledge use:* Assess issues related to who will be using the evidence and in what context, as well as the evidence in and of itself, for factors that could potentially enhance or hinder knowledge use. If the barriers to practice change are excessive, adopting a practice change can be difficult, if not impossible. For example, if use of the Intensive Care Delirium Screening Checklist (ICDSC) is too difficult for staff to complete, or if all staff are not able to attend the educational sessions, the practice change may not be successful.
4. *Selecting, tailoring, and implementing interventions:* It is important to select and tailor the interventions to address the identified barriers to knowledge use and to enhance implementation while being mindful of the stakeholders involved (e.g., health care providers, patients, and community groups). A practice change should involve applying evidence in a manner that integrates well with existing practice for all interprofessional health team members. It is important to understand change theory and to lobby for early adopters of the practice change to act as champions while maintaining a focus on communicating the rationale for the change and the anticipated positive outcomes. When practice changes involve other health care team members, interprofessional collaboration related to planning, implementing, and evaluating the change is crucial for optimal success.

   Returning to the case study, the SICU UPC has identified evidence from multiple sources and assessed the barriers and facilitators to knowledge use. The evidence is considered in the context of the committee members' experiences, a review of the unit delirium rate and outcome reports, and knowledge of their patients' risk factors, enabling the UPC to base the knowledge in the local context of the unit and the patients. The UPC recommends use of the Intensive Care Delirium Screening Checklist (ICDSC). The nurses and patients are the stakeholders; the UPC will provide the nurses with professional development sessions related to the new screening tool during scheduled work time. Patients will be informed of the new program, along with the rationale for implementation. The nurses will complete the screening tool and conduct the focused assessments of patients for other risk factors identified from the literature, such as hearing or visual impairment and decreased mobility. The UPC works with the manager to create a staff education schedule and sets a date for the start of the use of the ICDSC. Before the start date, the UPC collects baseline measures of delirium rate data and number of patients with delirium who experienced injuries in the last 3 months.
5. *Monitoring knowledge use:* Once the type of knowledge (conceptual, instrumental, or persuasive) has been identified (RNAO, 2022), its use needs to be monitored. There are several ways to monitor knowledge use, such as recording the frequency of behaviour, observing for a change in attitude, or conducting a chart audit.
6. *Evaluating outcomes:* Evaluative measures must be rigorous, valid, and reliable and should consider both quantitative and qualitative information. Evaluations can be structural, process, or outcome measures (RNAO, 2022). It is important to plan how to collect baseline data on the outcomes that will be used to evaluate the effect of practice change. (For example, in the case study presented, the UPC will be able to use the unit's monthly quality performance report, which includes delirium rate and number of patients with delirium who experience injuries. The UPC collects data for 3 months before implementing the program, and will continue collecting this data each month once the new screening tool is implemented.) Collection of outcome measures is critical, and their selection should consider the following criteria:
   - Know which outcomes to measure and how to collect the measures consistently (e.g., to measure pain acuity, use a self-report pain scale; to measure ambulation, determine the distance a patient walks each time).
   - Be sure that the outcomes are measurable (Box 1.4). Use scales (e.g., pain and Braden Scales), physiological measures (e.g., temperature, blood pressure, pulse oximetry), survey tools, and performance improvement reports.
   - Choose outcomes that are inexpensive to collect. Use existing equipment if possible.
   - Educate team members on how to collect and record outcomes.

BOX 1.4

Patient Outcome Measurements

Patient Outcome	Outcome Measure
Fall occurrence	Fall index, falls with injuries
Functional abilities	Performance of daily activities, including bathing, dressing, toileting, transferring, and feeding
Medication adherence	Pill counts, patient self-report, number of filled prescriptions
Learning discharge instructions (topic specific)	Patient surveys, including questions on topic; nurse observations of patients performing skills (using a rating scale); patient self-report during a follow-up phone call or visit
Infection occurrence	Monthly infection control reports of laboratory tests on infection incidence

- Limit the number of staff who collect data to ensure greater accuracy and consistency in measurement. Be sure that each person collects data the same way, at the same time or frequency, and accurately.
- Establish a way to record all data.

Evaluation of outcomes tells you whether the practice change has improved conditions, created no change, or worsened conditions. It is important to include all members of the health care team and the stakeholders involved or affected by the practice change, including patients and their families, when applicable.

In the case study, the UPC on the SICU made sure that outcome measures were in place before implementing the ICDSC education program. The delirium rate and associated injuries were collected from monthly quality performance reports and included data for each of the 6 months before implementation as well as data for 6 months after the program began. The UPC designated three staff members to also collect surveys from staff at 1 month, 3 months, and 6 months after implementation began to see how their colleagues were reacting to the education and using the ICDSC with patients.

7. *Sustaining knowledge use:* Sustainability needs to be considered in relation to financial and human resources within the health care system or community to maximize continued knowledge translation. Consider not only whether the outcomes were met but also whether patients, families, and health care team members were affected by the change in other ways.

In the case study, 6 months after implementing the program, the SICU staff were cautiously optimistic. The interrater reliability with the ICDSC was 96% after education, and the injury rate associated with delirium had dropped to 1 after the education program. Based on the evidence that staff were consistently using the ICDSC as intended, the accuracy of detecting delirium improved. Although it was not an outcome measure, the nurses observed an interprofessional commitment to the project. The nursing staff surveys revealed that the majority were enthused and agreed that the additional education and verifying their use of the scale needed to be a routine part of their annual education. The nursing staff were able to see that the education program and validation process to use the scale improved patient outcomes and gave them more time to coordinate safe care because of earlier detection of delirium. Mary submits the protocol for an abstract in the hospital publication, Nursing Practice. *The SICU UPC's methodical and well-designed knowledge-to-action project leads to several outcomes: the development of hospital-wide delirium screening protocols; a review of the literature by other nursing units to customize the nursing assessment to their particular patient needs; and the establishment of an evidence-informed standard for other nursing units in the hospital.*

After applying the evidence, it is important to engage in interprofessional collaboration to communicate the change in practice and the results. As a professional, you are responsible for communicating important information about nursing practice. Sharing evidence and the effects of any practice change motivates others within a health care setting and makes them excited about potential practice improvements on their work units. When you successfully adopt an EIP way of thinking, it becomes very natural to talk about available evidence and continue seeking solutions for problems in patient care.

Implementing EIP changes in a health care setting takes time and the commitment to doing it well. Competency in EIP requires a commitment to learning new knowledge, adapting it to fit the local context, interprofessional collaboration to appropriately apply and evaluate new interventions in practice, and finding ways to maintain and continue interventions that are consistently effective. Patients expect nursing professionals to be informed and to use the safest and most appropriate interventions. Use of the action cycle to translate evidence can enhance nursing practice and improve patient outcomes.

✦ REVIEW QUESTIONS

An oncology interdisciplinary team composed of staff nurses, a physiotherapist, a social worker, and a health care provider discussed the increased incidence of falls for patients on the inpatient oncology unit. The staff nurses and social worker believe more nursing staff are needed to decrease the incidence of falls. They currently have a standard fall protocol, but falls continue to occur. The physiotherapist proposes that it could be helpful to use a different scale to determine patients' risk for falling, in addition to encouraging early supervised ambulation. The interdisciplinary team decides to use an evidence-informed approach to improve care for these patients.

1. What initial step is important for the oncology team to address for their evidence-informed approach to improve patient care?
2. Which of the following questions describes a comprehensive PICO(T) question for the interdisciplinary team to use?
   1. For patients on an inpatient oncology unit, which fall prevention intervention strategies are most effective to reduce the incidence of falls during hospitalization?
   2. Does the use of increased fall risk screening compared with the use of a standard fall prevention protocol reduce the incidence of falls?
   3. On an inpatient oncology unit, which fall prevention strategies are most effective to change the incidence of falls?
   4. Which scale best predicts the incidence of falls for hospitalized patients?
3. The chair of the UPC contacts the hospital librarian to collaborate on a literature search to find articles pertinent to the clinical question. The nurse tells the librarian that the team wants to see whether there is evidence supporting their approach to reducing falls in their patients diagnosed with cancer. Which of the alternative MeSH terms will capture key concepts from your PICO(T) question?
   1. Patients and oncology
   2. Chronic care and patient safety
   3. Fall risk and injuries
   4. Cancer patients and fall prevention
4. The committee meets to review the articles obtained from the literature review. Which type of article is likely to be the most useful to the committee?
   1. Clinical article discussing an evidence-informed project on fall prevention
   2. Systematic review of studies testing the effects of early ambulation on falls
   3. Qualitative study exploring patients' perceptions of their own fall risk
   4. Quasi-experimental study comparing the use of two different fall screening tools
5. What are the elements of a successful EIP project? (*Select all that apply.*)
   1. Baseline data collected before implementation
   2. Timeline for the project
   3. Orientation plan for staff involved in the project
   4. Measurement decision after implementation
   5. Sponsor with expertise and commitment to the project
   6. Adequate resources to address all steps of the project
   7. Identification of outcome measurement prior to initiating project

Visit the Evolve site for a complete list of answers to the Review Questions.

✦ NEXT GENERATION NCLEX® (NGN)

For practice with answering exam questions related to unfolding NGN case studies, please consult the Next Generation NCLEX® (NGN)-Style Case Studies for Skills and Techniques on the Evolve website: http://evolve.elsevier.com/Canada/Perry/clinicalskills/

REFERENCES

Alfaro-LeFevre, R. (2019). *Critical thinking, clinical reasoning, and clinical judgment: A practical approach* (7th ed.). Elsevier.

Almost, J. (2021). *Regulated nursing in Canada: The landscape in 2021*. Canadian Nurses Association. https://www.cna-aiic.ca/en/nursing/regulated-nursing-in-canada

Bani Younis, M, K., Hayajneh, F. A., & Alduraidi, H. (2019). Effectiveness of using eye mask and earplugs on sleep length and quality among intensive care patients: A quasi-experimental study. *International Journal of Nursing Practice*, *25*(3), e12740. https://doi.org/10.1111/ijn.12740

Brown, S. (2018). *Evidence-based nursing* (4th ed.). Jones & Bartlett Learning.

Canadian Council of Practical Nurse Regulators. (2013). *Code of ethics for licensed practical nurses in Canada*. https://ccpnr.ca/wp-content/uploads/2021/03/IJLPN-CE-Final.pdf [Seminal Reference]

Canadian Council of Practical Nurse Regulators. (2019). *Entry-level competencies for licensed practical nurses*. https://ccpnr.ca/wp-content/uploads/2021/03/CCPNR-ELCs_2019E.pdf

Canadian Council of Registered Nurse Regulators. (2019). *Entry-level competencies for the practice of registered nurses*. https://www.ccrnr.ca/assets/ccrnr-rn-entry-level-competencies--2019.pdf

Canadian Institute for Health Information. (2021). *Patient harm in Canadian hospitals? It does happen*. https://www.cihi.ca/en/patient-harm-in-canadian-hospitals-it-does-happen

Canadian Nurses Association. (2015a). *Framework for the practice of registered nurses in Canada*. https://www.cna-aiic.ca/en/nursing/regulated-nursing-in-canada/rn-practice-framework2 [Seminal Reference]

Canadian Nurses Association. (2015b). *Framework for registered nurse prescribing in Canada*. https://www.cna-aiic.ca/en/nursing/regulated-nursing-in-canada/rn-prescribing-framework [Seminal Reference]

Canadian Nurses Association. (2017). *Code of ethics for registered nurses*. https://www.cna-aiic.ca/en/nursing/regulated-nursing-in-canada/nursing-ethics

Canadian Nurses Association. (2018). *Position statement: Evidence-informed decision-making and nursing practice*. https://hl-prod-ca-oc-download.s3-ca-central-1.amazonaws.com/CNA/2f975e7e-4a40-45ca-863c-5ebf0a138d5e/UploadedImages/documents/Evidence_informed_Decision_making_and_Nursing_Practice_position_statement_Dec_2018.pdf

Carper, B. (1978). Fundamental patterns of knowing in nursing. *Advances in Nursing Science*, *1*, 13–24. [Seminal Reference]

Chinn, P. L., & Kramer, M. K. (2010). Nursing's fundamental patterns of knowing. In P. L Chinn, & M. K. Kramer (Eds.), *Integrated theory and knowledge development in nursing* (8th ed., pp. 1–23). Elsevier. [Seminal Reference]

Choosing Wisely Canada. (2020). *Nine tests and treatments to question in nursing*. https://choosingwiselycanada.org/recommendation/nursing/

Critical Appraisal Skills Programme. (2021). *Critical appraisal skills programme*. https://casp-uk.net/

Dang, D., Dearholt, S. L., Bissett, K., et al. (2022). *Johns Hopkins evidence-based practice for nurses and healthcare professionals: Model and guidelines* (4th ed.). Sigma Theta Tau International.

Davies, B., & Logan, J. (2021). *Reading research: A user-friendly guide for health professionals* (7th ed.). Elsevier/Mosby.

FPT Committee on Health Workforce. (2020). *A vision for the future of nursing in Canada*. https://www.nnpbc.com/pdfs/media/news/2020/Vision-for-the-Future-of-Nursing-in-Canada.pdf

Graham, I. D., Logan, J., Harrison, M. B., et al. (2006). Lost in knowledge translation: Time for a map? *Journal of Continuing Education in the Health Professions*, *26*(1), 13–24. https://doi.org/10.1002/chp.47

Heidari, M., Ghodusi Borujeni, M., Kabirian Abyaneh, S., et al. (2019). The effect of spiritual care on perceived stress and mental health among the elderlies living in nursing home. *Journal of Religion & Health*, *58*(4), 1328. https://doi.org/10.1007/s10943-019-00782-1

Hödl, M., Halfens, R. J. G., & Lohrmann, C. (2019). Effectiveness of conservative urinary incontinence management among female nursing home residents: A cluster RCT. *Archives of Gerontology and Geriatrics*, *81*, 245–251. https://doi.org/10.1016/j.archger.2019.01.003

Infusion Nurses Society. (2021). Infusion therapy standards of practice (8th ed.). *Journal of Infusion Nursing*, *44*(1S), S1–S224.

Lau, G. J., & Loiselle, C. G. (2018). E-health tools in oncology nursing: Perceptions of nurses and contributions to patient care and advanced practice. *Canadian Oncology Nursing Journal*, *28*(2), 118–124. https://doi.org/10.5737/23688076282118124

Mataxen, P. A., & Webb, L. D. (2019). Telehealth nursing: More than just a phone call. *Nursing*, *49*(4), 11–13. https://doi.org/10.1097/01.nurse.0000553272.16933.4b

Melnyk, B. M., Gallagher-Ford, L., Zellefrow, C., et al. (2018). Outcomes from the first Helene Fuld Health Trust National Institute for Evidence-Based Practice in Nursing and Healthcare Invitational Expert Forum. *Worldviews on Evidence-Based Nursing*, *15*(1), 5–15. https://doi.org/10.1111/wvn.12272

Menonna-Quinn, D., Polovich, M., & Marshall, B. (2019). Personal protective equipment: Evaluating usage among inpatient and outpatient oncology nurses. *Clinical Journal of Oncology Nursing*, *23*(3), 260–265. https://doi.org/10.1188/19.CJON.260-265

Registered Nurses' Association of Ontario (RNAO). (2022). *Knowledge-to-Action Framework*. https://rnao.ca/leading-change-toolkit/knowledge-to-action

Saunders, H., Gallagher-Ford, L., Kvist, T., et al. (2019). Practicing healthcare professionals' evidence-based practice competencies: An overview of systematic review. *Worldviews on Evidence-Based Nursing*, *16*(3), 176–185. https://doi.org/10.1111/wvn.12363

Singh, M., Thirsk, L., Stahlke, S., et al. (2022). *Lobiondo-Wood and Haber's nursing research in Canada: Methods, critical appraisal, and utilization* (5th ed.). Elsevier.

US National Library of Medicine. (2021). *Welcome to Medical Subject Headings*. https://www.nlm.nih.gov/mesh/meshhome.html

Välimäki, T., Partanen, P., & Häggman-Laitila, A. (2018). An integrative review of interventions for enhancing leadership in the implementation of evidence-based nursing. *Worldviews on Evidence-Based Nursing*, *15*(6), 424–431. https://doi.org/10.1111/wvn.12331

Waddell, J., & Walton, N. (2020). *Yoder-Wise's leading and managing in Canadian nursing* (2nd ed.). Elsevier.

West, R., Mills, K., Rowland, D., et al. (2018). Validation of the First peoples' cultural capability measurement tool with undergraduate health students: A descriptive cohort study. *Nurse Education Today*, *64*, 166–171. https://doi.org/10.1016/j.nedt.2018.02.022

White, J., Grant, K., Sarkies, M., et al. (2021). Translating evidence into practice: A longitudinal qualitative exploration of allied health decision-making. *Health Research Policy and Systems*, *19*(38). https://doi.org/10.1186/s12961-020-00662-1

World Health Organization. (2019). *Patient safety*. https://www.who.int/news-room/facts-in-pictures/detail/patient-safety

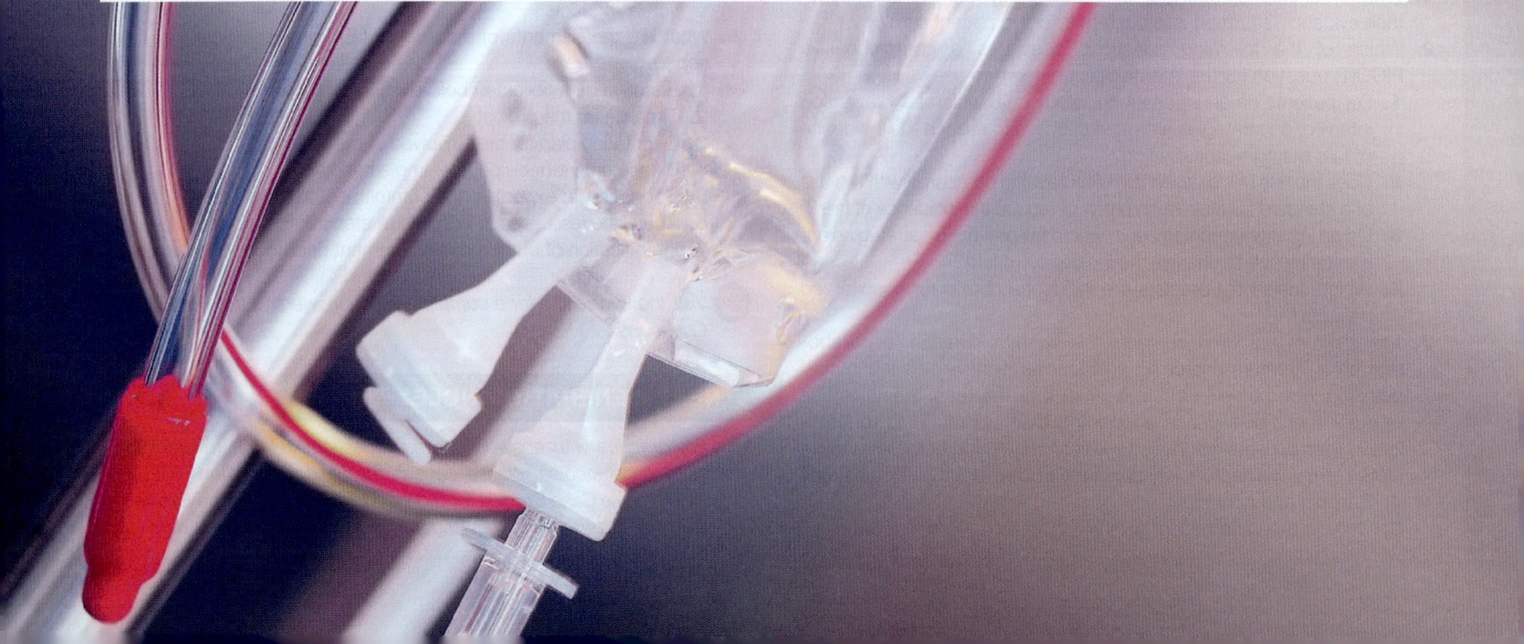

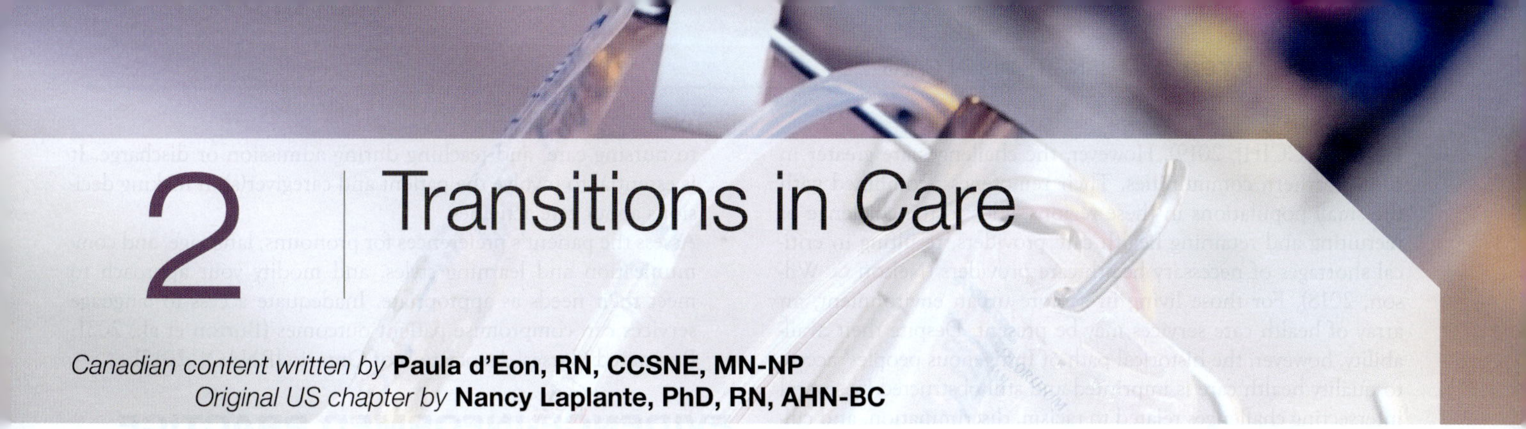

2 Transitions in Care

Canadian content written by **Paula d'Eon, RN, CCSNE, MN-NP**
Original US chapter by **Nancy Laplante, PhD, RN, AHN-BC**

SKILLS AND PROCEDURES

OBJECTIVES

Mastery of content in this chapter will enable the nurse to:

- Describe the role communication plays in maintaining continuity of care through a patient's admission, transition, and discharge from an acute care facility.
- Explain the purpose and importance of discharge planning.
- Identify the ongoing needs of patients in the discharge planning process.
- Explain the role of a patient's caregiver in the admission, transition, or discharge process.

MEDIA RESOURCES

- http://evolve.elsevier.com/Canada/Perry/clinicalskills/

PURPOSE

A key role of nurses is coordinating resources and planning a patient's care from admission to discharge as well as during transition from one level of care to the next. Nurses identify patients' ongoing health care needs and anticipate physical, psychological, and social deficits that have implications for patients as they resume normal activities. A nurse involves appropriate caregivers, family members, or both in a plan of care; provides interventions, including health education; and assists in making health care resources available to patients.

STANDARDS OF CARE

- Accreditation Canada (2020)—*Required Organizational Practices –2020 Handbook* (https://physicians.nshealth.ca/resources/required-organizational-practices-2020-handbook)
- Accreditation Canada (2019)—*Inpatient Services* (https://store.accreditation.ca/products/medicine-services?_pos=1&_sid=fbf99f6c2&_ss=r)
- Accreditation Canada (2017a)—*Client- and Family-Centred Care: Its History in Qmentum and a Supporting Literature Review* (https://store.accreditation.ca/products/client-and-family-centred-care-its-history-in-qmentum-and-a-supporting-literature-review)
- Accreditation Canada (2017b)—*Emergency Department* (https://store.accreditation.ca/products/emergency-department)

PRINCIPLES FOR PRACTICE

- Patients and families should be partners in care, sharing in the process of decision making.
- Patient care must be integrated across a variety of settings, services, health care practitioners, and care levels to maintain a continuum of care.
- Transitional care involves nursing actions implemented to ensure coordination and continuity of care for patients who transition between different settings or levels of care.
- Transitions of care require careful attention to communication to ensure patient safety.
- Discharge planning begins at the time of admission to a facility or even earlier, when a patient uses an outpatient clinic or testing centre to begin their care journey.

PERSON-CENTRED CARE

- Social determinants of health (SDOH) impart an array of cultural, political, economic, social, and environmental conditions that shape the circumstances in which individuals are born, grow up, live, work, and age (Government of Canada, 2022b). In Canada, many individuals face greater obstacles to good health owing to one or more of the following factors: age; gender; race; ethnicity; culture; religion; sexual orientation and gender identity; income and social status; education; social support networks; employment or working conditions; social and physical environments; mental health; cognitive, sensory, or physical disability; or other characteristics historically linked to discrimination or exclusion (Government of Canada, 2022b; Mantoura & Morrison, 2016; Morrison & Mantoura, 2020).
- Specific challenges for Indigenous peoples (First Nations, Inuit, Métis, and/or Urban Indigenous communities) related to language barriers and access to health services exist across all geographic regions (National Collaborating Centre for Indigenous

Health [NCCIH], 2019). However, the challenges are greater in rural northern communities. Their remoteness, combined with the small populations in these regions, adds to the challenge of recruiting and retaining health care providers, resulting in critical shortages of necessary health care providers (Nelson & Wilson, 2018). For those living in a more urban environment, an array of health care services may be present. Despite their availability, however, the historical path of Indigenous peoples' access to quality health care is imprinted and still obstructed by several intersecting challenges related to racism, discrimination, and culturally unsafe encounters with health care providers (NCCIH, 2019; Nelson & Wilson, 2018). By engaging with Indigenous peoples to understand and create health care practices that have meaning to them, including taking the time to understand and incorporate their cultural beliefs, traditional health practices, and medicines, nurses can help improve Indigenous peoples' access to health care services. Employing a nonjudgemental approach and culturally appropriate communication strategies, such as the use of Indigenous translators, patient navigators, and Indigenous health workers, are some of the essential first steps in creating a safe and welcoming care environment (NCCIH, 2019; Nelson & Wilson, 2018).

- Individuals who identify as members of the 2SLGBTQI+ (Two-Spirit, lesbian, gay, bisexual, transgender, queer, intersex, and additional sexual orientations and gender identities) community represent a broad range of people from all ethnicities, religions, and socioeconomic backgrounds. Despite the increased societal awareness and attention to gender diversity over the past few decades, members of the 2SLGBTQI+ community continue to remain at great risk of experiencing significant health disparities and adverse health outcomes (Burton et al., 2021). Sexual- and gender-diverse individuals are subject to discrimination from health care providers, may be reluctant to disclose their health information, and report a significant lack of trust in their care providers and in the health care system (Burton et al., 2021; Vermeir et al., 2018). Not only may this lack of trust prevent individuals from disclosing health information that can have an impact on their health outcomes, but in many instances it may also delay or prevent them from seeking necessary and sometimes urgent medical care (Vermeir et al., 2018).
- Nurses have an opportunity to improve health outcomes by practising gender-affirming care (Burton et al., 2021). This includes practising nursing care that conveys compassionate curiosity and nonjudgement within a paradigm of trauma-informed care. There are several ways nurses can contribute to creating a safe environment that welcomes members of the 2SLGBTQI+ community into health care settings. Advocating for the use of gender-inclusive assessment forms and ensuring the display of appropriate symbols or posters that represent and convey acceptance of the 2SLGBTQI+ community can contribute to creating a safe environment (Burton et al., 2021; Vermeir et al., 2018). Communicate in a respectful way by first introducing yourself with your own preferred pronouns and then asking for, and acknowledging, the patient's chosen pronouns (Burton et al., 2021; Vermeir et al., 2018).
- The nursing admission assessment should identify relevant SDOH and must incorporate patients' cultural beliefs and practices (see Chapter 4). When nurses identify gaps in their own understanding and enhance their own skills that will contribute to diverse, safe, and inclusive care environments, they are better able to provide person-centred care for all populations they encounter.
- Be aware of how SDOH and cultural variables, including gender diversity, will affect your patient and family assessment, approach to nursing care, and teaching during admission or discharge. It is essential to involve the patient and caregiver(s) in making decisions about care activities.
- Assess the patient's preferences for pronouns, language, and communication and learning styles, and modify your approach to meet their needs as appropriate. Inadequate access to language services can compromise patient outcomes (Burton et al., 2021; Registered Nurses' Association of Ontario [RNAO], 2015).

EVIDENCE-INFORMED PRACTICE

Many of today's patients have complex health needs that often call for more than one discipline to address those needs (Karam et al., 2018). These circumstances have led to the concept of shared care across teams, which requires interprofessional collaboration along with safe and effective transitions in care. Interprofessional collaboration can take on many forms, such as scheduled caregiver and patient meetings to discuss discharge arrangements; formal patient rounds to further explore the effectiveness of intervention; and frequent brief team huddles to provide team members with patient progress updates, to name just a few (Healthcare Excellence Canada, 2020).

Regardless of the form it takes, interprofessional collaboration involves the formation of a team or partnership between the patient, the caregiver, or both and at least two or more health care providers whose aim is to collaboratively address common goals such as patient safety, patient satisfaction, provider satisfaction, and improved care outcomes (Karam et al., 2018; Sowko et al., 2019). Additionally, transitions in care involve not only exchanging knowledge and information about the patient's health condition, but also identifying clear patient goals and management plans, including who will do what and by when; clarifying health care provider roles and relationships; identifying who is taking leadership of the patient's care; and clarifying how and to whom the patient and care team can reach out for support when things do not proceed as expected (Healthcare Excellence Canada, 2020).

Nurses have several opportunities to engage in interprofessional collaboration. Because of their close relationships with their patients, nurses are ideally positioned to be advocates for patients and can offer valuable insights related to patients' health circumstances and their individual and caregiver strengths and challenges (Karam et al., 2018). During care transitions, the nurse works as part of the interprofessional team to provide quality patient care. Through their leadership and communication skills, nurses play a key role in cultivating an environment in which the skills, abilities, and knowledge of all members of the care team are respected and recognized in the shared decision-making process (Karam et al., 2018).

The care team utilizes standardized information exchange processes during care transitions that support safe and efficient patient care (Accreditation Canada, 2019). Documentation tools and communication strategies that adhere to standardized organization of information conveyed during care transitions have been demonstrated to decrease the risk of communication errors and ambiguity, which can threaten patient safety. These standardized methods of communication have also been shown to improve the continuity of patient care. The necessary exchange or handover of information (including verbal) that occurs between care team members—be it during patient admission, patient relocation, a change in the team members providing patient care, or patient discharge to home—needs to be clearly defined and documented.

During care transitions, patients and families must also be given the information they require to make informed decisions (Healthcare Excellence Canada, 2020; Müller et al., 2018).

Lastly, evaluation mechanisms must be in place to assess care team members' compliance with the standardized information exchange processes and the quality of the information being shared in order to identify areas for improvement. Such evaluation methods may include audit tools for direct observation, chart review, and patient/care provider surveys to determine whether patients received the information they needed during the care transition (Accreditation Canada, 2019).

When nurse-to-nurse hand-offs (see Procedural Guideline 4.1) are performed effectively during care transitions (e.g., from shift to shift or transitions to different levels of care settings or different facilities), they can enhance patient safety by reducing risk of injury in multiple aspects of patient care, including falls (Müller et al., 2018; RNAO, 2015) and medication errors (Sowko et al., 2019).

- The implementation of standardized hand-off tools and processes (e.g., medication reconciliation; checklists; SBAR [situation-background-assessment-recommendation; see Chapter 3]; or I-START-END [introductions-story-tasks-assignment-resources-timely-exiting-next-documentation-debriefing; see Chapter 3]) should be built into the care transition process. Tools such as these need to be utilized in the same way each time a care transition occurs in order to reduce hand-off-related errors, and to ensure that critical information is communicated in a timely and effective matter. Some of the principles of care transition processes include the following: communication is always person to person; distractions are minimized; a structured framework is used during communication and documentation; contingency plans are discussed for what's next; and a close-the-loop strategy—such as read-back—is used (Accreditation Canada, 2021a; Healthcare Excellence Canada, 2020; Usher et al., 2018).
- Verbal hand-offs at the bedside serve important functions beyond the exchange of information. They have been shown to improve nurse-to-nurse communication and satisfaction and thus should be retained in practice. Transitions in care are recognized as vulnerable times for patients. Good communication with patients and caregivers is essential for safe and effective care transitions. For this reason, patients and their families should be encouraged to participate in the bedside hand-off process. Patients who are engaged in the process have reported being better informed, feeling part of the decision-making process, and feeling reassured that the health care team had the correct information and skill necessary to support their well-being (Bucknall et al., 2020).
- Medication reconciliation involves the process of creating the best possible medication history (BPMH) of the medications a patient is taking, including medication name, dosage, frequency, and route, then comparing that list with the health care provider's prescriptions with the goal of providing correct medications to the patient at all care transition points (Accreditation Canada, 2020; Healthcare Excellence Canada, 2020; Levesque et al., 2021).
- Medication reconciliation prevents medication errors such as omissions, duplications, incorrect medication, or medication interactions (Accreditation Canada, 2021b; Levesque et al., 2021).
- Protocols and processes for medication reconciliation must be in place. Medications need to be reviewed by either the nursing staff or pharmacy with the patient at the following transition points: on admission, during transitions between levels of care, when creating new medication administration records (MARs), and at discharge (Accreditation Canada, 2021b; Buck & Picinbono-Larose, 2018). When medications are reviewed at discharge, the nurse should emphasize to the patient the importance of keeping an updated list of medications and taking it along for future visits to hospital or their health care provider (Accreditation Canada, 2021b; Buck & Picinbono-Larose, 2018; Levesque et al., 2021; RNAO, 2014).

SAFETY GUIDELINES

- Identify whether a patient has a sensory or communication need (e.g., hearing aid, glasses, need for an interpreter).
- Identify whether a patient uses any assistive devices, and be sure that each is provided and deemed safe to use.
- Screen all patients on admission to a health care setting for possible discharge needs to ensure that appropriate teaching is completed to ensure a safe discharge.
- Include the patient, caregiver, and relevant health care providers early in planning care to promote successful transition through the health care system.
- Consider a patient's educational background, health literacy level, and ability to understand instructions.
- Use interprofessional collaboration (e.g., dietitian, social worker, pharmacist, physiotherapist) to assess appropriate resources needed as patients transition through the health care system.
- Use interprofessional collaboration to develop a plan of care for discharge to ensure a safe transition to home or an alternate care facility.

✦ SKILL 2.1 Admitting Patients

Patients enter the health care system in a variety of ways (e.g., hospital, clinic, presurgical screening visits, or health care provider's offices). The admission process is typically the first experience a patient has with a health care facility. There are common procedures for admitting patients to these settings (Box 2.1). Most patients enter the health care system through a standardized admission process that often requires an extensive registration process. However, some patients require emergency admission. A patient admitted through the emergency department (ED) is often not able to undergo the same registration process that takes place in a hospital admission office. Level of consciousness, pain, or other symptoms may prevent the patient from being a reliable resource. Caregivers or family members usually provide pertinent information for the facility records while the health care team cares for the patient. By comparison, an older person with self-care limitations undergoes extensive screening before being admitted into a long-term care facility.

Hospital registration staff and technicians are often the personnel involved in the preliminary admission process, such as interviewing patients and reviewing information related to provincial/territorial health insurance coverage (e.g., health care card number), demographic data, and facility regulations. A nurse performs the nursing admission assessment (see Chapter 8).

Admission Process

When admitted to hospital, patients should receive information about their safety, patient rights and responsibilities, and privacy (Accreditation Canada, 2019; RNAO, 2014). A private interview area should be used to provide patients and caregivers a place to reveal important identifying information, including a patient's full legal name, age, date of birth, address, next of kin, health care provider, religious preference, occupation, provincial/territorial health care insurance coverage, and any private insurance coverage. When a

BOX 2.1

Common Procedures for Admission to a Health Care System

- Placement of patient in appropriate receiving area
- Explanation of patients' rights (Accreditation Canada, 2020; RNAO, 2014) and elements of advance directives
- Orientation to relevant health care employer policies and procedures and room environment
- Assessment of patient's health care problems and needs (e.g., risk for falls, pressure injuries, and allergies)
- Preliminary testing and screening (specific to each facility and patient's condition)
- Development of a person-centred plan of care
- Determination of patient's payment source for facility fees (e.g., ward, semiprivate or private room) or health care for nonresidents of Canada

patient has a severe hearing impairment, the caregiver or a speech-language pathologist may assist. If a patient is not able to communicate because of a language barrier, a professional interpreter may be available, depending on the facility resources, to help during the admission procedure.

An identification (ID) bracelet that legibly states a patient's full legal name, address, acute care facility or provincial/territorial health card number, health care provider, and date of birth is secured to the patient's wrist. Health care providers use information from the ID band to identify a patient when administering medications and performing treatments or procedures. In many health care settings, an ID band contains a patient's unique bar code that then makes it easy to identify a patient for all prescribed procedures. Bar-code wristbands are typically created at the point of admission, and specific patient information is continually updated on the basis of the patient's needs (Accreditation Canada, 2017b). If a patient is unconscious, the nurse cannot ID them until a caregiver or family member arrives. When there is no family available, hospital staff provide an individualized ID band for the patient until the person can be identified. A patient who has been a victim of crime is given an anonymous name on their ID band under the facility's "blackout" or "do not publish" procedure.

Canada's Health Care System

It is essential for the nurse to have a comprehensive understanding of how Canada's health care system and financial governance work. This knowledge will facilitate identification of actual and potential issues that can have an impact on patient care transitions at the individual, organizational, and system levels. *Medicare* is a term that refers to Canada's publicly funded national health care system. Instead of having a single national plan, Canada has 13 provincial and territorial health care insurance plans (Martin et al., 2018). This system ensures that all Canadian residents have reasonable access to medically necessary acute care facility and health care provider services without having to pay out of pocket (Government of Canada, 2019a). The provincial and territorial governments are responsible for the management, organization, and delivery of health care services for their residents. The federal government is responsible for the following:

- Setting and administering national standards for the health care system through the *Canada Health Act* (Box 2.2)
- Providing funding support for provincial and territorial health care services
- Supporting the delivery of health care services to specific groups (Indigenous peoples living on reserves, Inuit, serving members of the Canadian Armed Forces, eligible veterans, inmates in federal penitentiaries, and some groups of refugee claimants)
- Providing other health-related functions, such as the regulation of consumer products (e.g., food, pharmaceuticals, cosmetics, chemical, pesticides, and medical devices)
- Supporting health research, health promotion and protection, and disease monitoring and prevention
- Providing tax support for health-related costs, such as tax credits and rebates and deductions for those with a disability, caregivers, and dependents living with a disability (Anthony & Krahn, 2019; Martin et al., 2018).

BOX 2.2

The Five Pillars of the *Canada Health Act*

Standard 1: Public Administration

- The provincial and territorial plans must be administered and operated on a nonprofit basis by a public authority.

Standard 2: Comprehensiveness

- The provincial and territorial plans must insure all medically necessary services provided by acute care facilities, physicians, and dentists (when the service must be performed in an acute care facility).
- Medically necessary services are not defined by the *Canada Health Act*. The provincial and territorial health care insurance plans consult with their respective physician colleges or groups. Together, they decide which services are medically necessary for health care insurance purposes.
- If a service is considered medically necessary, the full cost must be covered by the public health care insurance plan.

Standard 3: Universality

- The provincial and territorial plans must cover all residents.

Standard 4: Portability

- The provincial and territorial plans must cover all residents when they travel within Canada. Limited coverage is also required for travel outside the country.
- When a person relocates to another province, they can continue to use their original health care insurance card for 3 months, giving them time to register for the new plan and receive their new health insurance card.

Standard 5: Accessibility

- The provincial and territorial plans must provide all residents reasonable access to medically necessary services. Access must be based on medical need and not the ability to pay.

Adapted from Anthony S. E., & Krahn, M. (2019). Healthcare in Canada and issues of health-care reform. In D. Gregory, C. Raymond-Seniuk, L. Patrick, et al. (Eds.), *Fundamentals: Perspectives on the art and science of Canadian nursing* (2nd ed., pp. 28–31). Wolters Kluwer Health.

Adopted in 1984, the *Canada Health Act* is federal legislation that defines the conditions and criteria to which the provincial and territorial health insurance programs must conform in order to receive federal transfer payments under the Canada Health Transfer. This financial funding to the provinces and territories assists them with the sustainability of programs and services. There are four main transfers of funds: the Canada Health Transfer (CHT), the Canada Social Transfer (CST), Equalization, and Territorial Formula Financing (TFF). The CHT and CST are transfers that support specific policy areas such as health care, postsecondary education, social assistance and social services, early childhood development, and child care. The equalization and TFF programs provide unconditional transfer funds to the provinces and territories. Equalization enables less prosperous provincial governments to provide their residents with public services that are reasonably comparable to those of other provinces; TFF provides territorial governments with funding to support public services, in recognition of the higher cost of providing programs and services in the North (Government of Canada, 2019b; Martin et al., 2018). In 2020–2021, provinces and territories received $41.8 billion through the CHT (Government of Canada, 2022a).

Patients and families also have responsibilities, including providing truthful information, observing the rules and regulations of the facility, reporting any safety concerns, and treating others with respect (Accreditation Canada, 2019). During admission to a facility, a resuscitation care plan should be established outlining what measures the patient would like the health care team to take in the event they stop breathing or their heart stops (e.g., do not resuscitate [DNR], allow natural death [AND]; see Chapter 28). Patients should also receive information about advance care planning (e.g., advance directives) and be referred to appropriate resources if they want to discuss or receive help in completing an advance directive document (see Chapter 17).

Privacy is a deeply rooted core value in the nursing profession and a fundamental right of all individuals (Canadian Nurses Association [CNA], 2017). Privacy has become a matter of increasing concern in health care. With the growing adoption of electronic medical records, there are increasing demands for the use of electronic health care data in health research (CNA, 2018). Federal privacy laws include the *Privacy Act*, which came into force on July 1, 1983, and the *Personal Information Protection and Electronic Documents Act* (PIPEDA), which came into effect January 1, 2004. The *Privacy Act* governs the personal-information handling practices of federal government departments and agencies, while PIPEDA governs the collection, use, and disclosure of personal information in connection with commercial activities, including personal health information. Under PIPEDA, organizations need to obtain consent from individuals before collecting, using, or disclosing their personal information. They must also have appropriate security safeguards in place to protect personal information. In instances where there may be a privacy breach or complaint, PIPEDA outlines an ombudsman model in which complaints are directed to the Office of the Privacy Commissioner of Canada (Office of the Privacy Commissioner of Canada, 2019). Individuals have the right to withhold consent, to access personal information about themselves held by an organization, to have their personal information corrected if necessary, and to have recourse for a suspected information breach (Box 2.3). Several provinces and territories have their own privacy legislation. The Government of Canada requires all provinces and territories to comply with PIPEDA. Provinces whose legislation is deemed "substantially similar" to PIPEDA are exempt, whereas provinces whose legislation is not deemed similar to PIPEDA are not exempt (Office of the Privacy Commissioner of Canada, 2019). The CNA's *Code of Ethics for Registered Nurses* (2017) helps guide nurses through the decision-making process for ethical dilemmas involving privacy issues.

BOX 2.3

Patients' Rights

Health care laws and regulations vary slightly by province or territory, but generally Canadians share the following rights:

- The right to informed consent
- The right to recognition of a substitute decision maker
- The right to recognition of an advance care plan
- The right to a second opinion
- The right to confidentiality and privacy of personal health information
- The right to pain and symptom management
- The right to refuse treatment
- The right to request an assisted death
- The right to end-of-life care
- The right to advance directives
- The right to organ procurement

Adapted from Accreditation Canada. (2021a). *Standards: Long-term care services.* https://store.accreditation.ca/products/long-term-care-services; Dying With Dignity Canada. (2022). *Patient rights booklet.* https://www.dyingwithdignity.ca/education-resources/patient-rights-guide/; Registered Nurses' Association of Ontario. (2014). *Clinical best practice guidelines: Care transitions.* https://rnao.ca/bpg/guidelines/care-transitions

Role of the Nurse

On admission to a patient care area, nurses complete a thorough nursing assessment, review any advance directives, and ensure that necessary diagnostic testing is completed. If patients were receiving health care before admission (e.g., home health care, long-term care), a nurse from the sending care area provides appropriate information to the receiving nurse for continuity of care. In this situation, the nurse from the sending care area or facility should explain to the nurse receiving the hand-off report information about the patient's condition and why the patient is being admitted or transitioned to the particular health care setting (White-Trevino & Dearmon, 2018). A communication framework such as SBAR provides the nurse initiating the exchange of information (*the sender*) with clear expectations about what information is most important. SBAR has also gained attention as a focus for the nurse receiving report (*the receiver*) in that the same acronym is used to identify their responsibility as well. In the latter situation, SBAR stands for set aside assumptions–be attentive–ask questions–respond (White-Trevino & Dearmon, 2018) (see Chapter 3).

Nursing staff should ensure that a patient's room assignment is based on the patient's condition, health care needs, developmental level, activity level, expected length of stay, and personal preferences. For example, the best room for an older person who is acutely ill, at risk for falls, and receiving multiple treatments is one close to the nurses' station. The nurse identifies whether a patient has any known allergies; if any exist, the nurses places an allergy band on the patient and properly documents the known allergies in the medical record.

When a patient is admitted through the ED, the ED nurse provides a verbal report over the phone to the unit nurse receiving the patient. The ED nurse provides details on the patient's admission information, including their name; admitting health care provider; chief complaint; and any treatments or testing completed and the outcome, diagnosis, and pertinent information related to the patient's condition (e.g., initial vital signs, allergies, level of consciousness, and intravenous [IV] therapy). A physical hand-off report is seldom given, as most often the patient is brought to the care area by an escort (usually a facility porter or unregulated care provider [UCP]), who takes the patient and caregiver to the nursing unit and introduces them to the nurse assuming the patient's care. The ED nurse shares pertinent observations about the patient's behaviour (e.g., anxiety, fear, or level of knowledge regarding need for health care) with the nursing staff to foster continuity of care and help the patient and caregiver adjust to a new health care environment.

Many patients go to an acute care facility in advance for necessary preoperative diagnostic testing. In some cases, these patients and their caregivers also attend preoperative education classes. Other patients have contact with health care providers for the first time when they arrive at an acute care facility. Patients admitted on the morning of a surgical procedure or treatment are "same-day" admissions. A nurse provides basic instructions about the purpose of the surgery or treatment, preparatory procedures, and postsurgical or post-treatment care. Admission and consent forms, diagnostic tests, preoperative patient teaching (see Chapter 37), and instructions are usually completed before the actual day of surgery. When nurses are able to see patients several days in advance, they use a variety of resources, such as Internet sites, classes, videos, information booklets, and telephone calls, for patient teaching.

Nurses actively coordinate the initial admission process for all patients. A patient's condition influences the extent and type of admission activities. The nurse must always note the patient's level of fatigue and comfort. For example, when a critically ill patient reaches a critical care nursing unit, they undergo extensive examination and treatment procedures immediately. There may be little time available for the nurse to orient the patient and caregiver to the unit or learn of the patient's fears or concerns. When a patient enters an acute care facility for elective treatment, the nurse has more time to prepare the person psychologically for the stay and optimize patient outcomes with preadmission planning.

Delegation and Collaboration

The skill of completing the nursing assessment of a patient during admission to a health care facility cannot be delegated to an unregulated care provider (UCP). The nurse directs the UCP to do the following:

- Prepare the patient's room with the equipment needed before admission
- Gather and secure the patient's personal care items
- Escort and orient the patient and caregiver to the nursing unit

Equipment

- Hospital gown
- Bedpan and urinal (if needed)
- Washbasin, bath towel, and washcloth
- Toiletry items (e.g., soap, toothpaste, hand lotion; *optional in some facilities*)
- Facial tissues
- Water pitcher and drinking cup
- Kidney or emesis basin
- Disposable thermometer (see employer policy)
- Sphygmomanometer
- Stethoscope
- Clean gloves
- Pulse oximeter (*optional*)
- Safety equipment checked and available as needed (e.g., suction machine, oxygen equipment)
- Computer and documentation forms (see employer policy)

STEP	RATIONALE
ROOM PREPARATION	
1. Prepare room equipment and furniture. Prepare bed by adjusting it to the lowest horizontal position if patient is ambulatory. Place bed in high position if patient is arriving by stretcher. Turn down top sheet and bedspread. Arrange room furniture for easy access to bed. Adjust lights, temperature, and ventilation.	Promotes patient's comfort by preventing delays during admission. Proper position of bed lessens likelihood of a patient fall during transfer and also reduces risk of back injuries to staff helping patient into bed.
2. Be sure that equipment is in working order. Assemble any special equipment (e.g., suction, oxygen supplies, or intravenous [IV] pole) in patient's room.	Prevents delays in delivering immediate treatment and provides for smooth transition between caregivers.
ASSESSMENT	
1. Identify patient using at least two person-specific identifiers (e.g., name and date of birth, or name and medical record number) according to employer policy.	Ensures correct patient. Complies with Accreditation Canada's standards and improves patient safety (Accreditation Canada, 2020).
2. Throughout the procedure, the 4 moments for hand hygiene are to be implemented; hand hygiene should occur before initial patient (or patient environment) contact, before an aseptic procedure, after body fluid exposure risk, and after patient (or patient environment) contact. Additional hand hygiene should be performed when hands are visibly soiled.	Proper hand hygiene helps the prevent spread of infectious agents to health care providers.
3. Greet patient and caregiver cordially by name. Introduce yourself by full name (unless directed by employer policy to use first name only) and job title; explain your responsibilities in patient's care.	Providing personalized care reduces anxiety about admission, clarifies staff roles, and expedites patient requests.
4. Document findings while completing the patient admission assessment.	Real-time documentation saves valuable time and decreases the gap in time between collecting the data and documentation.
5. If the patient's preferred language differs from the nurse's, consider making arrangements for a professional translator to help with the nursing assessment. Use telephone or electronic device interpreter services as a supplemental system when an interpreter is needed instantly or when services are needed for an unusual or infrequently encountered language (Accreditation Canada, 2021a).	Translation services are preferable to using caregiver or family members to promote effective communication.
6. Use interprofessional collaboration (e.g., speech-language pathologist) when a patient has a severe hearing impairment.	A speech-language pathologist may have augmented hearing devices or resources to facilitate communication of assessment data.

STEP	RATIONALE

ASSESSMENT

STEP	RATIONALE
7. Assess patient's general appearance. Note signs or symptoms of physical distress (see Chapter 8).	Provides baseline assessment.

Critical Decision Point If patient is having acute physical problems, postpone routine admission procedures and taking of nursing history until their needs are met. Complete a focused assessment at this point.

STEP	RATIONALE
8. Assess patient's ability to understand and implement health information by asking a health literacy question, such as "How comfortable are you filling out medical forms by yourself?" The Rapid Estimate of Adult Literacy in Medicine–Short Form (REALM-SF) is a reliable and valid tool consisting of a list of seven words that the nurse asks the patient to read to determine their level of health literacy on a grade scale. For every correct word, the patient receives 1 point. Patients who score 7 points are considered to have a high school reading level and will be able to read most patient education materials. The tool is available at https://www.ahrq.gov/health-literacy/research/tools/index.html#rapid.	The REALM-SF is a simple, quick, and valid tool that helps the nurse determine at what reading level a patient can read, allowing the selection of appropriate educational material and teaching methods, such as teach-back (Nowak, 2019).
9. Assess patient's and caregiver's psychological status by noting verbal and nonverbal behaviours and responses to greetings and explanations.	Anxiety influences how well a patient adapts to a health care environment and retains instruction.
10. Assess vital signs (see Chapter 7), height and weight (see Chapter 8), and patient's level of discomfort (using an appropriate pain rating scale (see Chapter 16).	Provides baseline measurement to compare future findings. Determines alterations from normal range.
11. Assess for fall risk using an appropriate assessment tool (see employer policy). Ask patient to walk at end of bed and note gait and movement. Consider patient's risk factors (e.g., individual intrinsic factors: comorbidities [neurological disorders], muscle weakness, unsteady gait, and urinary incontinence [Buck, 2018]; transient factors: postural hypotension, polypharmacy, and use of high-risk medications [e.g., analgesics, antihypertensives] [Buck, 2018]). Provide patient who is at risk of falling with a fall risk band or bracelet.	Having a patient walk allows the nurse to more objectively assess the patient's gait and level of strength than asking the patient whether they have walking limitations. Provides data to determine patient's risk for injury and whether they need to be placed on fall precautions. For acute care facility inpatients, the maximum time frame for completing fall risk admission assessments is 24 hours (Accreditation Canada, 2017b; Buck, 2018). Promotes and enhances awareness of patient risk to all members of the care team.
12. Have caregivers leave room unless patient wishes to have them help with changing into a hospital gown or pyjamas. Close door and curtains. Help patient undress and get into comfortable position.	Demonstrates person-centred care because it provides for privacy and prepares patient for examination.
13. Obtain nursing history as soon as possible after patient's arrival to the nursing unit. Apply standards of nursing care adopted by facility (e.g., functional health patterns). Data include the following:	Each patient is to have an admission assessment prepared by a registered nurse (RN) (Accreditation Canada, 2021b). Each facility sets a time frame for completion of admission assessment (maximum time 24 hours).
a. Patient's perception of illness and health care needs	Establishes a baseline of patient's clinical status and enhances the nurse's understanding of the patient's perspective.
b. Past medical history	
c. Presenting signs and symptoms and reason for admission or transition in care	Identifies signs and symptoms in case patient's condition deteriorates.
d. Completion of a review of health status based on standards such as elimination, respiration, nutrition and metabolism, activity and exercise, self-concept, values and beliefs, cultural factors, social support, and cognitive function	Provides a holistic view of patient's health issues and response to those issues.
e. Risk factors for illness	Allows the nurse to institute preventive care measures and educate patient about health promotion behaviours.
f. History of allergies, including type of substance and a description of the reaction that patient has previously experienced	Patients often have sensitivity to a medication or substance rather than a true allergy; this needs to be clarified. Specify all allergens to prevent accidental exposure.

Critical Decision Point Provide patient with allergy arm band listing allergies to foods, medications, latex, or other substances; document allergies according to employer policy.

STEP	RATIONALE
ASSESSMENT	
g. Detailed medication history, including prescribed, over-the-counter (OTC), and alternative therapies such as herbs, hormones, and natural health products	Assesses potential for medication interactions; information often explains patient's presenting signs and symptoms.
h. Patient's knowledge of health problems and expectations of care	Enables the nurse to recognize and meet patient expectations when possible.
14. Apply clean gloves as appropriate. Conduct physical assessment of appropriate body systems (see Chapter 8). Inform patient of any necessary or additional specimens that need to be collected.	Provides objective data for identifying health problems. Unannounced procedures can make patients anxious. Preparation of patient relieves anxiety.
a. A priority is to assess a patient's skin integrity and any current skin breakdown at admission. Use a risk for pressure injury development scale (e.g., Braden Scale, Norton Scale [see Chapter 39]) to assess risk for potential skin breakdown. After assessment is complete, remove and dispose of gloves.	Provides baseline data for pressure injury prevention and identifies the presence of any previously acquired pressure injuries when patient is admitted. Existing pressure injuries must be documented within 24 hours of admission (Accreditation Canada, 2021a; RNAO, 2017). Pressure injuries that develop while patient is at an acute care facility are considered an adverse event or incident and become the financial responsibility of the facility responsible for their care.
b. Some facilities are now requiring assessment of risk for obstructive sleep apnea (OSA) in surgical patients (see Chapter 37). See employer policy. The STOP-Bang questionnaire has been specifically developed to meet the need for a reliable, concise, and easy-to-use screening tool. It consists of eight (yes/no) items related to the clinical features of sleep apnea (snoring, tiredness, observed apnea, high blood pressure, body mass index [BMI], age, neck circumference, and male gender). The total score ranges from 0 to 8. Patients can be classified for their OSA risk based on their respective scores (http://stopbang.ca/translation/pdf/caeng.pdf).	Allows the nurse to institute appropriate postoperative observations. OSA is a potentially serious sleep disorder in which breathing repeatedly stops and starts during sleep. Surgical patients with OSA are considered at risk for relaxation of their throat muscles and blockage of the airway during recovery from anaesthesia and sedation (Tyerman & Buchanan, 2023).
15. Check health care providers' prescriptions for treatment measures to initiate immediately.	Delay can cause deterioration of patient's condition.
16. Ask patient to identify their values regarding health care and needs or expectations of care: "To what extent do you believe being in the hospital will help you?" "Tell me what you hope will happen during your hospital stay?" "Tell me what is important to you for your care here to be satisfactory?" Note: Incorporate these questions during the physical examination.	Patient-centred care requires incorporation of patient needs, preferences, and values (Accreditation Canada, 2017b; RNAO, 2014).
17. Orient patient to the patient care unit.	
a. Introduce staff members who enter room. Always introduce patient by last name unless patient indicates otherwise.	Helps patient recognize caregivers. Demonstrates person-centred care by showing respect for patient.
b. Tell patient and caregiver the name of the nurse in charge of the unit/division and explain that person's role and responsibilities.	Provides means for patient and caregiver to understand unit/division communication structure.
c. If whiteboards are available within the hospital room, place names of assigned staff members for the patient and caregiver's reference. This may also be used to write reminders to the patient.	Promotes understanding of who team members are, as well as their roles, and aids in communication.
d. Explain visiting hours and their purpose (i.e., to provide time to administer needed procedures and give patient time to rest).	Provides knowledge and increases willingness to observe policy for visiting hours.
e. Discuss smoking policy and identify smoking areas (if available) for patient and caregiver.	A facility-wide smoking policy that prohibits the use of smoking materials throughout the facility is required. Some facilities may have a designated smoking area.
f. Demonstrate use of equipment (e.g., bed, over-bed table, lighting).	Patient's safety depends on patient understanding correct use of equipment.
g. Show patient how to use call light and position it in a convenient place. Have patient demonstrate use of light. Discuss with patient their specific fall risks and encourage the patient to ask for help when getting out of bed.	Ensures that patient knows why and how to call for assistance.

STEP	RATIONALE

ASSESSMENT

STEP	RATIONALE
h. Escort patient to bathroom (if able to ambulate).	Patient's safety depends in part on understanding how to use toilet facilities.

Critical Decision Point Ensure that patient knows how to call for help while in bathroom. (An emergency call light is usually installed in bathrooms.)

STEP	RATIONALE
i. Explain hours for mealtime and nourishments to patient and caregiver.	Caregiver often wishes to visit during evening to help with meals.
j. Describe services available (e.g., chaplain, beauty shop, activity therapy).	Offers patient options for making decisions.

NURSING DIAGNOSES

- Acute pain
- Chronic pain
- Anxiety
- Fear
- Insufficient knowledge regarding hospital procedures and planned therapies
- Inadequate coping, individual or caregiver
- Powerlessness
- Potential for injury
- Potential for falls

Related factors and risk factors are individualized on the basis of patient's condition or needs.

PLANNING

1. Expected outcomes following completion of procedure:

STEP	RATIONALE
• Patient is able to explain purpose and schedule of planned treatments and procedures.	Understanding treatment plan gives patient a better sense of control and reduces anxiety about the unknown.
• Patient demonstrates how to call for nurse when help is needed.	Falls commonly occur when patients attempt to get out of bed without help.
• Patient is able to ambulate (if condition permits) in room free of obstacles.	Ensures patient safety and mobility in room.
• Patient can safely and efficiently use equipment in room.	Equipment used in care of patient frequently poses hazards; helps to reduce anxiety.
• Patient verbalizes understanding of smoking policy, visiting hours, mealtimes, and services available.	Knowledge of facility policies helps patient adapt to health care environment.
• Patient self-reports improved comfort.	Basic pain and comfort measures are effective.

IMPLEMENTATION

STEP	RATIONALE
1. Complete patient medication reconciliation by checking home medication list for duplication, omission, or potential medication interactions with newly prescribed medications. Update medication list based on health care provider's prescriptions for treatment. Follow employer policy.	Medication reconciliation on admission helps ensure that patient is taking the correct medications and prevent medication errors (Accreditation Canada, 2021b).
2. Inform patient about procedures or treatments scheduled for the next shift or day (e.g., visits by health care provider or dietitian). These vary based on the nature of patient's condition.	Patient has right to be informed of any scheduled procedures or treatments. Being able to anticipate planned therapies reduces anxiety.
3. Perform basic comfort measures (positioning, temperature of room) and administer analgesic (if prescribed). Remove and dispose of gloves.	Enables patient to participate in planned therapies and education.
4. Complete learning readiness and learning needs assessment for patient and caregiver.	Identifies patient's and caregiver's educational needs and learning preferences.
5. Give patient and caregiver a chance to ask questions about procedures or therapies and to share their personal goals of care. (If patient is unresponsive or unable to understand, review with caregiver.)	Provides opportunity to clarify expectations and misconceptions. Provides for shared decision making.
6. Collect valuables that patient chooses to keep at bedside. Complete clothing and valuables listing sheet (see employer policy); have patient sign. Place valuables in facility safe or send home with caregiver. Document the location of valuables in the patient chart.	Accounts for placement of valuables and prevents loss.

STEP	RATIONALE
IMPLEMENTATION	
7. Ensure that patient and caregiver have time together alone if desired.	Admission is often stressful and fatiguing. Allows time for decision making.
8. Be sure that call light is within easy reach and bed is in low position.	Provides for patient safety.
EVALUATION	
1. Have patient explain own fall risks, facility policies, tests, and procedures through discussion and questions.	Patient demonstrates learning and understanding through feedback.
2. Ask patient to describe characteristics and severity of pain using an appropriate pain rating scale.	Determines whether pain severity has decreased.
3. Have patient demonstrate use of call light.	Return demonstration confirms learning.
4. Monitor patient's ability to ambulate independently.	Provides data to assess patient's safety in ambulating without injury.
5. Check patient's room setup regularly.	Determines whether care area is free of obstacles.
6. **Use teach-back:** After providing the patient with education on how to activate the call light system and discussing the importance of preventing falls by calling for assistance before getting out of bed, the nurse uses teach-back to ensure the patient has understood the instructions: "I want to be sure you understand how to use your call bell when you need help from the nurses. Can you show me how to use it and tell me when you should use it?" Develop a revised teaching plan if the patient or caregiver is unable to teach-back correctly.	Determines patient's and caregiver's level of understanding of instructional topic.

Unexpected Outcomes	Related Interventions
1. Patient is unable to explain facility policies (e.g., visitation, smoking) or does not know purpose or schedule for tests and procedures.	• Schedule follow-up session with patient. • Keep information focused and specific to patient's situation. Include caregiver if appropriate.
2. Patient becomes restless, expresses concerns, or displays tension in body movements.	• Give patient time to discuss fears and concerns. • Reassess comfort level or change in health status. • Demonstrate person-centred care with active listening skills and compassion to enhance open and honest communication.
3. Patient falls or is injured.	• Attend to patient's immediate physical needs. • Inform health care provider of fall and any injuries. • Follow the facility falls protocol (e.g., patient must have nursing assessment completed before moving and should have ongoing neurological vital signs monitored as appropriate). • Reassess patient's environment, alter care plan as needed, and ensure environment is free of safety hazards. • Complete adverse event/incident report.

Communication and Documentation

- Document history and assessment findings in appropriate forms or screens of electronic health record (EHR) or chart. Begin to develop nursing plan of care.
- Document your evaluation of patient and caregiver learning.
- If patient has an advance directive, place copy in the medical record. In the absence of a formal advance directive, document the essence of the directive in the medical record (Accreditation Canada, 2021a; RNAO, 2014).
- Notify health care provider of patient's arrival; report any unusual findings. Secure admission prescriptions if not previously provided.
- Most health care facilities will have standardized admission forms that will need to be completed as part of the admission process. Some of these forms may be multidisciplinary and can be filled in by a variety of health care providers.

DOCUMENTATION EXAMPLE

A 69-year-old patient (she/her) with no known drug allergies admitted from the ED to room 202 Bed B @ 0905 with a diagnosis of LCVA. T 36.7, HR 100, Resp 24. SpO_2 97% on room air. Patient transferred from bed to stretcher requiring assistance of 2 people. Pt alert and oriented ×3 and responding appropriately to verbal stimuli. Eyes PERRLA 3–4 mm. No slurring of speech. No JVD. Hand grips unequal, R strong, L diminished with limited L mobility due to weakness secondary to CVA. IV NS infusing @ 100 mL/hr in R forearm, no redness or erythema noted at insertion site. Lung sounds clear and equal bilaterally in all fields. S1 and S2 noted, no murmurs or additional sounds detected. BS present in all 4 quads and nontender to palpation. Last BM 2 days ago soft and formed, usual BM pattern for patient. Old scarring from previous surgery noted over R upper abdomen, patient identifies as scar from gallbladder removal over 30 years ago. Limited mobility L leg, and weakness due to CVA. Area over L hip noted to be warm, reddened, and tender to touch, size approx. 7 cm × 9 cm. Pt denies any other pain and does not require pain med at this time. #12 Fr Foley catheter draining clear amber urine approx. 200 mL noted in drainage bag. Lower legs cool, dry, cap refill <2 sec. with palpable pedal pulses bilaterally. Home medications reviewed with patient and sister who is also present. Pt and family member oriented to hospital room, call bell, and family presence policy. Encouraged to share care goals and questions and concerns as necessary. Pt admission ID band and Fall Risk bracelet applied. Side rails up ×4, call bell in reach, and patient aware to ring for assistance with repositioning and ambulating. For complete assessment refer to nursing health history and admission form. Referral sent to interprofessional stroke team.

Special Considerations

- Language barriers between patients and their care team members can contribute to negative health outcomes. Potential strategies to enhance communication include enlisting the assistance of a health care provider who speaks the same language as the patient or accessing hospital interpretation services.

Teaching

- Explain to patient that a different nurse provides care on each shift. Explain time frame for how assignments are made.
- Teaching occurs throughout the admission process. Provide information regarding physical assessment findings, risks for falling, purpose of allergy alert and fall risk bracelets, nature of patient's illness, planned diagnostic and treatment procedures, medications, goals of care, and acute care facility routines.
- In an emergency or if patient is unable to perform aspects of own care, teach caregivers about the rationale for any procedures and routines to be used in patient's care.

Pediatric

- Hospitalization is a major crisis for children, who feel stress from separation, loss of control, bodily injury, and pain. Separation anxiety is most common from middle infancy through the toddler years, especially at 16 to 30 months of age. Preschoolers are better able to tolerate brief periods of separation, but their protest behaviours are more subtle than those of younger children (e.g., refusal to eat, difficulty sleeping, withdrawing from others). School-age children can cope with separation but have an increased need for parental security and guidance (Keenan-Lindsay et al., 2022). Incorporating developmentally appropriate therapeutic play interventions before and during hospitalization enables children to have an autonomous and informed role in their health care. Therapeutic play has been shown to alleviate children's stress by reducing anxiety and improving pediatric confidence, attitudes, and care satisfaction.
- Explain the rooming-in and visiting policies of the facility. Allow and encourage familiar items from home—such as a stuffed toy or blanket—that may provide the child with a sense of comfort and normalcy in the unfamiliar hospital environment.
- Parental input during admission assessment can provide vital information on the child's normal behaviour and deviations caused by illness.
- Parents should be encouraged to be involved in as much of their child's care as possible, provided with the necessary supports to do so, and recognized as essential members of the care team.

Gerontological

- Hospitalized older persons experience functional declines such as new-onset incontinence, malnutrition, deconditioning, pressure injuries, and falls. Use interprofessional collaboration (e.g., physiotherapist, dietitian) to plan interventions that retain functional status (Buck, 2018).
- Patients who tend to fall in the acute care facility are typically those who have been admitted recently and are unfamiliar with surroundings, have acute illness, take four or more medications, or have been relocated recently. Visual changes that occur with aging often lead to falls in hospitalized older persons (Buck, 2018).
- Delirium, the most common complication in this population of patients, is linked to cognitive and functional decline and extended hospital stays. Nurses should remain alert to the risk factors and clinical signs of delirium.

✦ SKILL 2.2 Transitioning Patients

Patients transition to different points of care in order to receive alternate forms and levels of treatment and services and to continue receiving essential care closer to home. Evidence suggests that interprofessional collaboration and standardized tools increase the likelihood of positive patient outcomes and patient-centred care (White-Trevino & Dearmon, 2018). When a patient transitions to a different care level, the nurse often assumes the leadership role in ensuring the continuity of care. Nurses interact with patients and caregivers at their most vulnerable times and are often the ones who acquire information critical to successful transition planning. They play a key role in promoting successful transitions by developing, implementing, and evaluating the transition plan and identifying barriers to the plan (White-Trevino & Dearmon, 2018). Studies have shown that when nurses invite patients to participate during the information exchange, the nurse–patient relationship is strengthened. Nurses can accomplish this by encouraging the patient to listen and actively participate during the hand-off event. Patients who have had this opportunity report a high level of nursing competence and satisfaction with their care (White-Trevino & Dearmon, 2018).

When patients move between different points of care or health care facilities for diagnosis, treatment, and ongoing care, there is a safety risk at each interval. The hand-over (or hand-off) communication that occurs between staff on different units and between and among interprofessional teams might not include all the essential information, or information may be misunderstood. Hand-offs serve many functions, from coaching and teaching to team building, but their most important function is information processing–making sure that essential data are transferred for patient safety (Lavoie et al., 2021; Müller et al., 2018). Substandard or variable hand-offs have contributed to errors, care omissions, treatment delays, inefficiencies from repeated work, inappropriate treatment, adverse events with minor or major harm, increased length of stay, avoidable readmissions, and increased costs (White-Trevino & Dearmon, 2018).

When providing the hand-off of a patient to another unit, it is essential to clearly communicate information about the patient's care, treatment, services, and current condition and any recent or anticipated changes in prescriptions in order to meet patient safety goals (Accreditation Canada, 2021a). Nurses should also document in the patient chart details of what was shared in the hand-off and who the hand-off was provided to. Policies and procedures are usually similar throughout a facility.

Mnemonics such as SBAR, "I PASS THE BATON" (introduction–patient–assessment–situation–safety concerns–background–actions–timing–ownership–next), and I-START-END are examples of formats to use during communication of patient transitions in care that can be tailored for different clinical areas or purposes. These tools have demonstrated increased confidence for both the sender and receiver during a hand-off report (Healthcare Excellence Canada, 2018; Müller et al., 2018).

In the ED, when a patient is transferred from one facility to another, a nurse establishes the pertinent information to be included in the hand-off report. Patient circumstances will carry the most significance; however, at a minimum, details typically include the patient's full name and other person-specific identifiers, diagnoses, test results, procedures, contact information for the responsible providers, reason for the transition, and information about allergies, medications, and any advance directives (Accreditation Canada, 2017b; RNAO, 2014). Patient transitions at different points of care must be person centred (i.e., the patient agrees to the transition) and should also consider the following principles:

- Responsibility for the patient's care continues until service has ended or the patient has been transitioned to another care team, service, or facility or organization.
- Use interprofessional collaboration for shared decision making, and include the patient and caregiver or substitute decision maker.
- The patient's capacity and ability to make decisions needs to be considered.
- There is open and honest discussion of any risks associated with the transition.
- Risk of readmission is assessed, and if applicable, appropriate follow-up appointment and/or community referrals are made (Accreditation Canada, 2017b; RNAO, 2014).

Delegation and Collaboration

The task of assessment and decision making conducted during transitions cannot be delegated to a UCP. The nurse directs the UCP to do the following:

- Help the patient with dressing
- Gather and secure the patient's personal belongings and any equipment that goes with the patient
- Escort the patient to the nursing unit or transport area

Equipment

- Transfer forms
- Copies of documents such as medical records, radiology films, and laboratory test results (as appropriate)
- Special equipment as needed: wheelchair or stretcher, emesis basin, bedpan and urinal, oxygen tank and tubing, IV pole, cardiac monitor, and emergency medications

STEP	RATIONALE
ASSESSMENT	
1. Identify patient using at least two person-specific identifiers (e.g., name and date of birth, or name and medical record number) according to employer policy.	Ensures correct patient. Complies with Accreditation Canada's standards and improves patient safety (Accreditation Canada, 2020).
2. Throughout the procedure, the 4 moments for hand hygiene are to be implemented; hand hygiene should occur before initial patient (or patient environment) contact, before an aseptic procedure, after body fluid exposure risk, and after patient (or patient environment) contact. Additional hand hygiene should be performed when hands are visibly soiled.	Proper hand hygiene helps prevent the spread of infectious agents to health care providers.
3. Obtain and review transfer prescription from sending health care provider. Prescription includes name of the receiving facility (when applicable), receiving health care provider's name, and statement of patient's stability for transfer.	Health care provider is legally responsible for releasing patient from medical care and arranging for receiving health care provider. Patient has legal right to refuse transfer against medical advice.
4. In collaboration with health care provider and members of the interdisciplinary team, assess reason for patient's transfer (e.g., change in condition, services available at the facility, patient or caregiver preferences regarding patient's location).	Patient needs to have access to facility with best resources to meet health care needs. Health care provider determines patient's physical stability for transfer.
5. Assess individuals at high risk for transitional care problems (e.g., older persons with multiple health issues, patients with depression, non-English speakers, patients with sensory impairments, and low-income patients).	Identifying patients at risk for transitional care problems enables better continuity of care and improved patient outcomes (Müller et al., 2018). Patients may require consultation with needed resources (e.g., care manager, psychologist) when arriving at destination.

STEP	RATIONALE

ASSESSMENT

6. Explain purpose of transfer at care transitions thoroughly, and provide time to discuss patient's and caregiver's feelings about the change in care setting. As necessary, obtain patient's written consent to transfer. If patient is unable to consent, caregiver or substitute decision maker provides this consent.	Patients need to be informed of transfer plans in a timely manner (Accreditation Canada, 2020; RNAO, 2014). A patient requires adequate psychological preparation. In the event of a clinical emergency in which patient and caregiver are unable to consent, this consent is waived, and patient is transferred to a higher level of care on the basis of the clinical judgement of the health care provider requesting the transfer.
7. Assess patient's current physical condition and determine method of transport. When transferring to a new facility, assess method of transport to transferring vehicle (e.g., wheelchair or stretcher; consult employer policy).	Determines level of patient stability. Patient's condition often changes quickly and influences stability for transfer and type of support needed during transport.

Critical Decision Point Determine whether patient's status and safety require life-support equipment. Staff assisting with transfer need training in life-support measures. When transporting patient to new facility, a vehicle equipped with life-support equipment is necessary.

8. Assess whether patient requires pain relief or other medications for symptom management.	Ensures patient's comfort during transfer.
9. Ensure that staff have notified patient's caregiver or significant others of transfer as desired by patient.	Provides adequate communication with caregiver or significant others to help with patient's emotional and psychological adjustment to the transfer (Accreditation Canada, 2020; RNAO, 2014).

NURSING DIAGNOSES

- Anxiety
- Insufficient knowledge regarding transfer procedure
- Fear
- Powerlessness
- Relocation stress syndrome

Related factors are individualized on the basis of patient's condition or needs.

PLANNING

1. Expected outcomes following completion of procedure:	
• Patient's vital signs and physiological status remain the same following transfer.	Treatments are planned so as not to interrupt physical support of patient during transfer.
• Patient incurs no injury during transport procedures.	Safety measures are successful in transferring patient from wheelchair or stretcher to transport vehicle.
• Patient or caregiver explains purpose of transfer and procedure for transport.	Understanding provides patient with sense of control.
• Receiving nursing staff acquire and confirm written plan of care.	Ensures continuity of care.
2. Use interprofessional collaboration (e.g., social worker) to arrange for patient's transfer to the facility.	Transfer needs to occur without delays so that patient has access to all needed resources at all times.
3. When transfer is to a new facility, contact the facility and arrange for bed in appropriate setting. Confirm willingness of the facility to accept patient (usually social worker or discharge coordinator completes confirmation).	Prevents delays when patient arrives at destination. Receiving facility ensures that space and qualified personnel are available to treat patients and provides confirmation in advance to accept the transferred patient.

IMPLEMENTATION

1. Ensure that documentation in patient's record is complete and that care plan contains individualized nursing care measures.	Accurate information is necessary for receiving facility to assume patient's care.
2. Complete nursing care transfer form according to employer policy. (When transfer is to a different nursing unit, entire medical record accompanies patient.)	Form summarizes patient's pertinent nursing care needs to ensure continuity of care and prevent unnecessary duplication of services.
3. Complete medication reconciliation per employer policy. Check patient's current prescriptions for transfer against the most recent medication administration record and the original home medication list. Communicate updated medication list to next provider of care, including last medications given, with times and doses for ongoing consistency in care (e.g., last pain medication, antipyretics, insulin).	The new medication regimen prescribed at the time of transfer may omit needed medications, unnecessarily duplicate existing therapies, or contain incorrect dosages. Medication reconciliation ensures that patient receives correct medications at new facility and decreases medication errors (Accreditation Canada, 2020).

STEP	RATIONALE
IMPLEMENTATION	
4. Have UCPs gather patient's personal care items, clothing, and valuables. Check the entire room and all storage areas. Secure in suitcase or container.	Prevents loss of articles during transfer.
5. Anticipate problems that patient frequently develops just before or during transfer. Perform necessary nursing therapies such as suctioning or changing a dressing.	Ensures patient's comfort and safety during transport.
6. Help to transfer patient to stretcher or wheelchair using safe patient-handling techniques (see Chapter 11).	It is easier to move a patient being transported to outside facility by stretcher into transport vehicle.
7. Perform and document final assessment of patient's physical stability.	Minimizes risk of patient developing complications during transfer.

Critical Decision Point Priority assessment includes vital signs, clear airway, patency of IV tubing and accuracy of infusion rate, and patient's level of consciousness.

STEP	RATIONALE
8. When a patient is physically transferred to an outside facility, accompany patient to transport vehicle.	Ensures that medically qualified personnel are in attendance until patient leaves facility/unit.
9. Call receiving facility/unit and notify of impending transfer and patient's status (check employer policy).	Notification of nurse in charge or nurse assuming care of patient ensures better continuity of care at time of patient's arrival.
EVALUATION	
1. During the final assessment, compare data with the previous findings.	Determines whether patient's condition is changing.
2. Inspect patient's alignment and positioning on stretcher or in wheelchair.	Proper alignment and positioning reduce risk of injury occurring during transport.
3. Ensure that equipment needed for transfer is functioning.	Equipment such as oxygen must last through transport for patient safety.
4. Confirm that patient understands transfer and procedures through discussion and questions.	Feedback helps to ensure learning.
5. Determine whether receiving facility/nurse has questions about patient's care.	Provides for clear communication during hand-off and continuity of care.
6. **Use teach-back:** "I want to be sure you understand why you are being transferred to your new unit. Can you tell me why you are being transferred and what the name of your new unit is?" Develop a revised teaching plan if patient or caregiver is unable to teach-back correctly.	Determines patient's and caregiver's level of understanding of instructional topic.

Unexpected Outcomes	Related Interventions
1. Patient's physical status deteriorates during preparation.	• Call health care provider immediately. • Initiate interventions to stabilize patient's condition.
2. Patient is confused or uncertain about transfer.	• Provide clarification or additional explanation.
3. Receiving staff misinterpret directions for patient's care.	• Sending facility has nurse or health care provider call to confirm that there are no questions regarding patient's care.

Communication and Documentation

- The nurse sending the patient documents patient's status, including vital signs and other assessment findings regarding patient's condition, nursing plan of care, date and time of transfer, and method of transport, on appropriate transfer form.
- Document your evaluation of patient and caregiver learning.
- The nurse receiving the patient documents patient's arrival at facility by documenting date and time of arrival, reason for transfer, method of transport, patient's condition, and care provided at time of arrival.
- Most facilities have standardized transfer of care forms that will need to be completed as part of the patient care transition process. Some of these forms may be multidisciplinary and can be filled in by a variety of health care providers.

DOCUMENTATION EXAMPLE

A 69-year-old patient (she/her) with no known drug allergies with a diagnosis of LCVA. Transferred to 3rd floor Restorative Care Unit for intensive rehabilitative services via wheelchair. Patient condition stable last VS @0930, T 37, HR 75, Resp 20. SpO_2 98% on room air. IV in R forearm saline locked as prescribed. Patient has regained some mobility of L leg and L arm and is anticipating benefit from intensive rehabilitation service. Patient is able to communicate needs clearly and is excited to be going to the unit. Presently requires 1 person assist to complete ADLs. Pt hand-off report including review of patient transfer form given to P. Smith, RN.

Special Considerations

Teaching

- A transfer frequently creates anxiety for patients and caregivers. Carefully repeat instructions about the transfer when patient and caregiver are better able to understand your explanation. In this situation, be sure to have patient or caregiver restate any critical information.

Pediatric

- Children need their parents' comfort and security; thus, make sure that parents are well informed. Involve older children in any discussion regarding transfers. Allow a parent to accompany the child during the transfer.

Gerontological

- Relocation can be stressful for an older person being transferred to a new facility. Ensure that significant support people are still accessible and that patient and caregivers are thoroughly oriented to new surroundings. Practice person-centred care—ensure that the patient's and caregiver's opinions and sensitivities are included when establishing care needs (Accreditation Canada, 2021b; RNAO, 2014).

Long-Term Care

- It is important that patients receive the level of services appropriate to their physical and mental health needs. Use interprofessional collaboration (e.g., continuing care coordinator, social worker, discharge planner) in the transition process to ensure that placement at a long-term care facility is appropriate.
- Essential components of successful transfer to a long-term care facility are accurate communication of medication lists and advance directives (Accreditation Canada, 2021a; RNAO, 2014).

✦ SKILL 2.3 Discharging Patients

Early and comprehensive discharge planning facilitates the transition of a patient or resident from a health care facility to the most independent level of care, whether that is home or another facility. The overall goal of discharge planning is to provide the most appropriate level and quality of care throughout all stages of a patient's illness. Rates of hospital readmission and or return visits to the ED are common outcome measures of effective discharge planning (Luther et al., 2019). Evidence suggests that patients who receive an interprofessional collaborative approach to discharge planning are less likely to experience a readmission or visit to the ED (Luther et al., 2019). Preparation for discharge begins at the time of admission, and patient and caregiver perceptions of their physical and psychosocial readiness for the transition to discharge should be considered throughout the process (Accreditation Canada, 2021b). Favourable interventions must include an interprofessional approach that employs good communication between clinicians, patients, and care settings; areas of education and resources to support patient and caregiver knowledge of self-care management; and medication reconciliation and seamless transition to community resources, including primary care follow-up (Accreditation Canada, 2020; Luther et al., 2019).

The discharge planning process must be comprehensive and interdisciplinary, including all caregivers who are involved in the care of the patient. Every hospitalized patient requires patient-centred discharge planning, and it is equally essential for any patient permanently moving to a different health care facility. The trend toward shorter lengths of stay in acute care settings makes discharge planning increasingly difficult but all the more essential (Luther et al., 2019).

It is essential to develop a discharge plan whose outcomes are mutually accepted by patients and health care providers (Accreditation Canada, 2021b; Luther et al., 2019). Effective discharge planning prepares patients to assume self-care or prepares caregivers to provide needed support and thus can decrease hospital readmission and promote optimal patient outcomes (Luther et al., 2019). The discharge process may be simple or complex and occurs in three phases: acute, transitional, and continuing care. In the acute phase, medical attention dominates discharge planning efforts. During the transitional phase, the need for acute care is still present but its urgency declines, and patients begin to address and plan for their future health care needs. In the continuing care phase, patients are able to participate in planning and implementing the continuing care activities needed after discharge. In acute care facilities, these phases can occur very quickly, even within hours.

The greatest challenge in effective discharge planning is communication. Patients and families should be full partners in the discharge planning process and thus should be engaged in discussing what will be needed to make the transition in care safe and effective (Accreditation Canada, 2021b; Luther et al., 2019). When team members communicate during end-of-shift hand-offs, consultations, or huddle sessions, a patient's discharge readiness should be a central topic. Communication is enhanced if a facility has a discharge coordinator or case manager. Staff members in these roles thoroughly assess what each patient's needs will be at discharge, identify available and needed resources, and link patients and caregivers to these resources (e.g., community supports, Meals on Wheels, rehabilitation services). The coordination of necessary services (e.g., home health care) and appropriate follow-up on patients' progress after discharge should also occur.

Discharge from a facility can be stressful for a patient and caregiver. Before a patient is discharged, the patient and caregiver need to be prepared with the knowledge and skills to manage care in the home. They also need to know what to expect in regard to any continuing physical problems. Without the necessary equipment and professional resources, a patient risks loss of rehabilitation gains made before discharge. Failure to understand restrictions or the implications of health problems often causes a patient to develop complications. Poor discharge planning ignores a patient's needs within the home and increases the chance of the patient needing to re-enter the health care system prematurely.

Delegation and Collaboration

The tasks of assessment, care planning, and instruction included in discharging patients cannot be delegated to a UCP. The nurse directs the UCP to do the following:

- Gather and secure personal items and any supplies that the patient will take home or to the new setting
- Transport the patient to the discharge transport vehicle

Equipment

- Wheelchair or stretcher
- Discharge documentation forms (see employer policy)
- Patient instruction sheets
- Plastic bag for personal belongings

STEP	RATIONALE
ASSESSMENT	
1. Identify patient using at least two person-specific identifiers (e.g., name and date of birth, or name and medical record number) according to employer policy.	Ensures correct patient. Complies with Accreditation Canada's standards and improves patient safety (Accreditation Canada, 2020).
2. Throughout the procedure, the 4 moments for hand hygiene are to be implemented; hand hygiene should occur before initial patient (or patient environment) contact, before an aseptic procedure, after body fluid exposure risk, and after patient (or patient environment) contact. Additional hand hygiene should be performed when hands are visibly soiled.	Proper hand hygiene helps prevent the spread of infectious agents to health care providers.
3. From time of admission, assess patient's discharge needs using nursing history data, including assessments of patient's physical health, functional status, identified gender differences and preferences, psychosocial support system, financial resources, health values, cultural and ethnic background, level of education, and barriers to care, as needed. Also review ongoing assessment data during your shift of care (e.g., physical examinations and discussions with patient and health care provider). Make sure that the discharge plan is person centred and culturally appropriate (e.g., learn the patient's preferences and values about continuing health care after discharge).	Planning for discharge begins at admission and continues throughout patient's stay in a facility to help patient achieve maximum functioning. The discharge planning assessment determines patient's continuing care needs after they leave the acute care setting (Accreditation Canada, 2021b; RNAO, 2014).
4. Identify risk factors that may increase patient's chance of being readmitted after discharge (Accreditation Canada, 2021b; Luther et al., 2019; RNAO, 2014): diagnoses associated with high readmissions (e.g., heart failure, chronic lung disease); comorbidities; the need for numerous medications; a history of readmissions; psychosocial and emotional factors such as issues relating to mental health, interpersonal relationships, or family matters; the lack of a caregiver who could provide support or help with care; older age; financial distress; deficient living environment (e.g., water supply, heating).	Allows you to better prioritize care interventions that manage these risk factors during patient stay in facility. Conditions affect either patient's ability to become physically or psychologically ready for discharge or ability and readiness of caregiver to assume patient's care in the home.
5. If patient's destination at discharge is home, assess patient's and caregiver's learning needs as soon as possible (e.g., psychomotor skills, medication management, symptom recognition). Engage patient and caregiver as partners in the discharge teaching plan by having them identify their concerns about discharge.	Improves understanding of health care needs and ability to achieve self-care at home. Inclusion of caregiver in teaching sessions provides patient with available resource. Engaging patient and caregiver in the assessment supports person-centred nursing care (Accreditation Canada, 2020; Luther et al., 2019; RNAO, 2014).
6. Assess for current barriers to learning (e.g., age, fatigue, pain, lack of motivation). Assess patient's health literacy (see Skill 2.1, Assessment, Step 8).	Determines timing and approach to instruction. Different types of educational materials are effective with different individual learning styles. If printed material is to be used, be sure that material is written at proper reading level.
7. Ask patient, caregiver, or both to describe the home environment and assess for environmental factors that may interfere with self-care (e.g., size of rooms, doorway clearances for wheelchair, steps, lighting, bathroom facilities). (A community-based nurse is usually available on referral to help with assessment.)	Environmental factors within patient's home may pose safety risks or problems for self-care (see Chapter 42). Early identification of these factors allows you to arrange for home health referral.
8. Use interprofessional collaboration to assess patient's anticipated needs after discharge and their eligibility for care services in the community. Ask the following questions: "Does the patient have an injury or illness that makes it difficult to leave home (e.g., requires the aid of supportive devices such as a wheelchair or walker; requires the use of special transportation; needs the assistance of a caregiver)?" "Does the patient have a 'skilled need' that requires skills from a specific health care provider?"	These conditions are needed to meet eligibility criteria (which may vary) for reimbursement of home health care services in several provinces/territories. Generally, the patient must have a "skilled need" that requires the skills of a nurse, speech therapist, or physical therapist in order for the patient to perform the task. A health care provider's prescription is needed for nursing services.
9. Assess patient's and caregiver's perceptions of continued health care needs outside the facility. Assess caregivers' perceived ability to provide care to patient, including their level of social and community support and their ability to manage multiple medications with which the patient is discharged.	Caregiving can be a highly stressful experience. Caregivers may or may not be family members, and they may not be properly prepared for caregiving, as many are frequently overwhelmed by a patient's needs, which can lead to unnecessary facility readmissions.

STEP	RATIONALE

ASSESSMENT

10. Provide patient with copy of any written discharge instructions. Return original copy of any advance directives provided by the patient, provincial/territorial health card, and personal belongings, including home medications.	Evidence confirms that discharge instructions can achieve the following: • Reduce readmission rates for the same condition • Improve quality of patient care • Improve patient satisfaction • Support patient adherence to patient care plan

Critical Decision Point It is often necessary to talk with the patient and caregiver separately to learn about true concerns or doubts; in such instances, the nurse must ensure they maintain patient confidentiality.

11. Assess patient's acceptance of health problems and related restrictions.	Affects willingness to follow therapies and restrictions.

NURSING DIAGNOSES

- Anxiety
- Caregiver role strain
- Insufficient knowledge regarding home care restrictions
- Inadequate health management
- Interrupted family processes
- Openness to improving health management
- Relocation stress syndrome
- Reduced self-care: feeding, toileting, dressing/grooming, bathing/hygiene

Related factors are individualized on the basis of patient's condition or needs.

PLANNING

1. Expected outcomes following completion of procedure:	
• Patient or caregiver explains how health care is to continue in home (or other facility), which problems to observe and what to do, which treatments or medications patient needs, and when to go to next medical appointment.	Increases likelihood of care not being interrupted in home (or other facility) and reduces chance of unplanned readmission to the acute care facility.
• Patient can demonstrate self-care activities (or caregiver is able to administer care measures).	Feedback ensures learning.
• Obstacles to patient's mobility and hazards to ambulation in home setting are removed.	Patient is often physically weakened or has physical changes resulting from illness that predispose to injury.

IMPLEMENTATION

1. Preparation before day of discharge:	
a. Partner with patient and caregiver in identifying ways to change physical arrangement of home that will be required to meet patient's needs (see Chapter 42).	Maintains patient's level of independence and ability to retain function within safe environment.
b. Provide patient and caregiver with information about community health care resources (e.g., Health Link, medical equipment companies, Meals on Wheels, adult day care). Referrals are usually made while patient is in the facility.	Community resources offer services that patient or caregiver cannot provide.
c. Conduct teaching sessions with patient and caregiver as soon as possible during hospitalization. Cover these topics: description of what life at home will be like; review of medications and dosing schedules; warning signs of possible health problems; explanation of test results; explanation of how to provide therapies or use home medical equipment; assess knowledge and understanding of applicable community resources; review of restrictions resulting from health alterations; and when to make follow-up appointment. Use appropriate materials such as pamphlets, books, or multimedia resources. Refer patient to reliable and current resources on the Internet.	Gives patient opportunities to practise new skills, ask questions, and obtain necessary feedback to ensure learning. A combination of written and verbal information is effective in improving patient satisfaction and knowledge (Accreditation Canada, 2021b; RNAO, 2014). In some settings, electronic programs are available that allow the nurse to tailor patient-specific media instructions.
d. Communicate patient's and caregiver's response to teaching and proposed discharge plan to other health care team members.	Facilitates continuity and achievement of a person-centred individualized discharge plan.

STEP	RATIONALE
IMPLEMENTATION	
2. Procedure on day of discharge:	
a. Encourage patient and caregiver to ask questions or discuss issues related to home care. A final opportunity to demonstrate learned skills is helpful.	Allows for final clarification of information previously discussed. Helps relieve anxiety.
b. Check health care provider's discharge prescriptions, change in treatments, or need for special medical equipment. (Make sure that prescriptions are written as early as possible.) Arrange for delivery and setup of equipment (e.g., hospital bed, oxygen) before patient arrives home.	Only a health care provider is able to authorize a discharge. Early check of prescriptions permits the nurse to attend to any last-minute treatments or procedures well before discharge.
c. Determine whether patient or caregiver has arranged for transportation.	Patient's condition at discharge determines method of transport.
d. Provide privacy and assistance as patient dresses and packs all personal belongings. Check closets and drawers for belongings. Obtain copy of list of valuables signed by patient and have security or appropriate administrator deliver valuables to patient.	Prevents loss of personal items. Patient's signature verifies receipt of items and relieves nursing department of liability for losses.
e. Complete medication reconciliation per employer policy. Check discharge medication prescriptions against the medication administration record and home medication list. Provide patient with prescriptions or pharmacy-dispensed medications prescribed by health care provider. Offer a final review of information needed to facilitate safe medication self-administration.	Decreases risk of medication errors and ensures that patient is receiving correct medication at home (Accreditation Canada, 2020; RNAO, 2014). The new medication regimen prescribed at the time of discharge may inadvertently omit needed medications, unnecessarily duplicate existing therapies, or contain incorrect dosages (Holbrook et al., 2019). Review provides feedback to determine patient's success in learning about medications.
f. Provide information on follow-up appointments to health care provider's office.	Provides patient with contact for questions that arise after discharge. Ensures continuity of care to prevent rehospitalization.
g. Acquire utility cart to move patient's belongings. Obtain wheelchair for patient. Transport patient leaving by ambulance on an ambulance stretcher.	Provides for safe transport.
h. Help patient to wheelchair or stretcher using safe patient handling and transfer techniques (see Chapter 11). Escort patient to entrance of facility where source of transportation is waiting (see employer policy) (see Step 2h illustrations). Lock wheelchair wheels. Help patient transfer into transport vehicle. Help place personal belongings in vehicle.	Prevents injury to nurse and patient. Employer policy requires escort to ensure patient's safe exit. Facility's liability ends once patient is safely in vehicle.
i. Return to unit/division. Notify admitting or appropriate department of time of discharge. Notify housekeeping of need to clean patient's room.	Allows facility to prepare for admission of next patient.

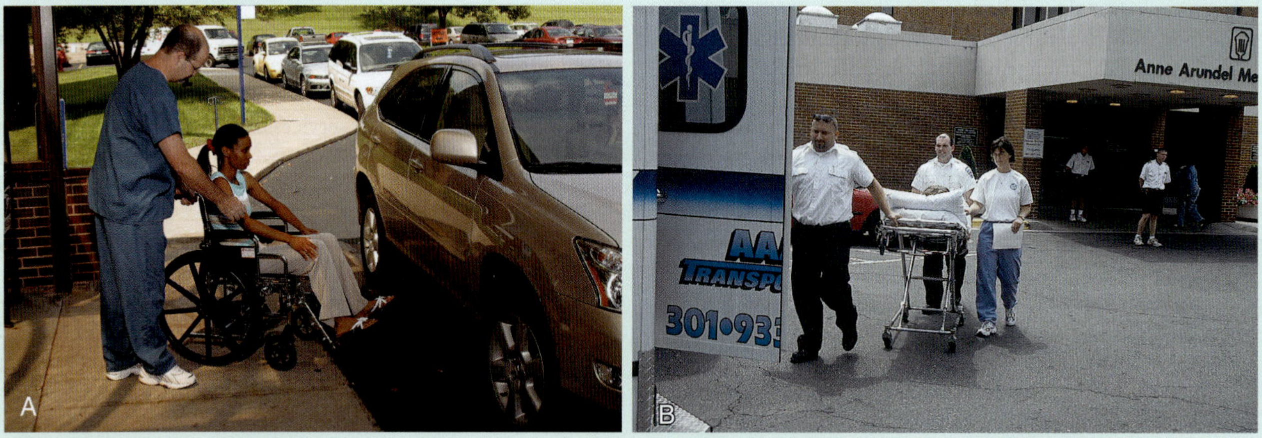

STEP 2h A, Nurse escorts patient to transport vehicle at time of discharge via a wheelchair. B, Many patients are discharged via stretcher.

STEP	RATIONALE
EVALUATION	
1. Ask patient or caregiver to describe nature of illness, treatment and medication regimens, and physical signs or symptoms to be reported to a health care provider.	Measures patient's or caregiver's learning.
2. Have patient or caregiver perform any treatments that will continue in the home.	Return demonstrations allow you to evaluate level of learning.

STEP	RATIONALE
EVALUATION	
3. Community-based nurse inspects home, identifies obstacles that pose risks for patient, and recommends revisions.	Provides continuity of care.
4. Use **teach-back:** "I want to be sure you understand when your follow-up appointment is. Can you tell me when you require a check-up?" Develop a revised teaching plan if patient or caregiver is unable to teach-back correctly.	Determines patient's and caregiver's level of understanding of instructional topic.

Unexpected Outcomes	Related Interventions
1. Patient or caregiver is unable to explain or demonstrate self-care measures.	• Provide immediate clarification or additional instruction. • Plan additional time to demonstrate treatment measures. • Ask patient to explain which aspect of procedure is difficult to perform and why. • If patient or caregiver continues to be unable to correctly demonstrate treatment measures, request referral for home care services.
2. Environmental risks are still present in home.	• Reassess reason why changes have not been implemented. • Community-based nurse will problem solve and seek appropriate solution.
3. Patient or caregiver resists discharge plans and refuses assimilation of new roles needed for home care.	• Use interprofessional collaboration (e.g., social work, home care, pastoral care) to provide additional resources.

Communication and Documentation

- Complete documentation of patient's discharge on discharge summary form (Box 2.4). Give patient a signed copy of form.
- Document unresolved problems and description of arrangements made for resolution in progress notes in EHR or chart.
- Document patient's vital signs and status of health problems at time of discharge in progress notes in EHR or chart.
- Document your evaluation of patient and caregiver learning.
- Most facilities will have standardized discharge forms or summaries that will need to be completed as part of the discharge process. Some of these forms may be multidisciplinary and can be filled in by a variety of health care providers.

BOX 2.4

Nursing Discharge and Referral Summaries

- Description of the patient's status at discharge (e.g., physical, mental, emotional)
- Discharge destination and mode of discharge (e.g., ambulatory, wheelchair, stretcher)
- Issues that have been resolved and those that still remain
- Functional and self-care abilities in terms of vision, hearing, speech, mobility (with or without aids), meal preparation and eating, and medication preparation and administration
- Instructions for continuing self-care needs: activity, diet, medications, special treatments such as wound care, insulin injections, self-catheterization, tracheostomy care
- Reconciled list of current medications with dose, frequency, and route
- Identified restrictions that relate to activity, diet, or personal care
- Patient's and caregiver's comfort level with discharge
- Signs and symptoms of complications or medication reactions to watch for
- Signs and symptoms that patient should consider normal
- Referral services (e.g., home health care, occupational therapy, social work)
- Patient support networks, including caregivers, significant other or family members, community self-help groups, home care, and spiritual advisor or other community agencies
- Scheduled follow-up appointment at health care provider's office, clinic
- Name and contact information of health care provider, nursing unit, or both
- Explanation of pertinent emergency procedures
- Patient's signature, showing understanding of instructions

Adapted from Foley, V. (2018). Documenting and reporting. In B. Kozier, G. Erb, A. Berman, et al. (Eds.), *Fundamentals of Canadian nursing: Concepts, process, and practice* (4th ed., p. 471). Pearson Canada Inc.

DOCUMENTATION EXAMPLE

Patient vital signs stable—B/P 124/76, T 37, HR 72, Resp 18, O_2 98% on room air. Right hip dsg is clean, dry, and intact and covered with a dry 4×8 sterile dressing. Patient is 1 assist with a walker and is being discharged home today with her sister for 1 month while continuing to rehab as an outpatient. Community-based nursing service referral completed for continued wound management, and family is aware nursing home care visits will begin tomorrow am. Discharge instructions and prescriptions explained to patient and sister, who were both able to repeat back key points related to mobility safety concerns at home and rationale for medication changes. Pt has follow-up appointments in place with outpatient rehab services and with their primary care provider in 1 week.

Special Considerations

Teaching

- Assess patient's fatigue and pain levels before beginning any instruction. Keep focused on the important teaching topics to cover.

Pediatric

- Once caregivers have learned how to perform any necessary caregiver skills, have them assume care before child returns home. Many facilities incorporate a trial period requiring caregivers to manage care before child's discharge home (Keenan-Lindsay et al., 2022).
- The nurse is a leader in the interprofessional process of discharge planning in partnership with other health care providers, children, and their parents. Throughout hospitalization, the nurse assesses factors that will affect the caregiver's ability to manage care at home (Keenan-Lindsay et al., 2022).

Gerontological

- Older persons and their caregivers often overestimate their ability to manage care after discharge. They may also disagree about what postdischarge care includes. Make referrals to home care to address needs associated with functional decline and help prevent readmission to the acute care facility.

Care in the Community: Home Management

- Assess availability and skill of primary caregiver (e.g., family member or friend): assess time availability, ability, and willingness to give care, emotional and physical stamina, knowledge of caregiving requirements, and type of relationship held with patient. Assess additional resources, including friends or neighbours who are available to help. Ensure that patient and caregiver are aware of how to access additional home care support if needs arise.
- Inform community care services and the patient's health care provider about whether the patient or caregiver will receive home support upon discharge.

✦ REVIEW QUESTIONS

A 69-year-old widow (she/her) has been admitted to the acute care unit with a left-sided stroke. The patient has a history of diabetes mellitus and arthritis. She is able to help with many care activities but requires help with eating. She has a sibling who will be her caregiver. On admission, her assessment shows an area of skin breakdown on her left hip, assessed as a stage 1 pressure injury. The patient's medications on admission were metformin, lisinopril, and St. John's wort. After 3 days, she is transferred to the rehabilitation unit. Her medications on transfer are metformin, lisinopril, and warfarin. She has left-sided weakness from her stroke and will likely require a walker.

Review Questions 1 to 3 and 6 relate to the case study presented here.

1. During the patient's admission assessment, which physical assessment findings are a priority to document and why?

2. During the patient's care transition, which key piece of information, reflecting a potential risk, should be shared during the hand-off with the nurse on the rehabilitation unit?

3. At the time the patient is admitted to rehabilitation, the nurse conducts an assessment in an effort to plan for discharge in 2 weeks. The patient will be going home and staying with a sibling for at least a month. During the assessment, the nurse learns that the sibling is concerned about being able to manage the patient. The patient's sibling has heart failure and limited exercise tolerance. Assessment also reveals that the patient's skin has cleared over the left hip. The patient will be trained to use the walker safely in rehabilitation. Write an SBAR to communicate this situation.

4. The nurse is admitting a patient from the emergency department. Which of the following steps should the nurse take to ensure that the patient is safely admitted? (*Select all that apply.*)
 1. Obtain a list of the patient's medications from the patient.
 2. Ask the family to provide interpreter services.
 3. Determine patient's level of health literacy.
 4. Obtain the patient's history as soon as possible.
 5. Wait 24 hours before assessing skin integrity.

5. The nurse is orienting a student nurse who asks when medication reconciliation is done. The nurse tells her that it is done: (*Select all that apply.*)
 1. On admission
 2. On transition to another level of care
 3. At the change of every shift
 4. On discharge
 5. Once every 24 hours

6. The nurse is preparing the patient on the day of discharge. Which of the following elements are important to address? (*Select all that apply.*)
 1. Reviewing health care providers' prescriptions
 2. Arranging for transportation
 3. Completing medication reconciliation
 4. Reviewing discharge instructions
 5. Beginning discharge planning

Visit the Evolve site for a complete list of answers to the Review Questions.

✦ NEXT GENERATION NCLEX® (NGN)

For practice with answering exam questions related to unfolding NGN case studies, please consult the Next Generation NCLEX® (NGN)-Style Case Studies for Skills and Techniques on the Evolve website: http://evolve.elsevier.com/Canada/Perry/clinicalskills/

REFERENCES

Accreditation Canada. (2017a). *Client- and family-centred care: Its history in Qmentum and a supporting literature review.* https://store.accreditation.ca/products/client-and-family-centred-care-its-history-in-qmentum-and-a-supporting-literature-review

Accreditation Canada. (2017b). *Emergency department.* https://store.accreditation.ca/collections/emergency/products/emergency-department

Accreditation Canada. (2019). *Inpatient services.* https://store.accreditation.ca/products/medicine-services

Accreditation Canada. (2020). *Required organizational practices handbook.* https://physicians.nshealth.ca/resources/required-organizational-practices-2020-handbook

Accreditation Canada. (2021a). *Standards: Long-term care services.* https://store.accreditation.ca/products/long-term-care-services

Accreditation Canada. (2021b). *Standards: Medication management.* https://store.accreditation.ca/collections/medication-management/products/medication-management-standards

Anthony, S. E., & Krahn, M. (2019). Healthcare in Canada and issues of health-care reform. In D. Gregory, C. Raymond-Seniuk, L. Patrick, et al. (Eds.), *Fundamentals: Perspectives on the art and science of Canadian nursing* (2nd ed., pp. 28–31). Wolters Kluwer Health.

Buck, M. (2018). Safety. In B. Kozier, G. Erb, A. Berman, et al. (Eds.), *Fundamentals of Canadian nursing: Concepts, process, and practice* (4th ed., pp. 761–792). Pearson Canada.

Buck, M., & Picinbono-Larose, G. (2018). Medications. In B. Kozier, G. Erb, A. Berman, et al. (Eds.), *Fundamentals of Canadian nursing: Concepts, process, and practice* (4th ed., pp. 792–874). Pearson Canada.

Bucknall, T. K., Hutchinson, A. M., Botti, M., et al. (2020). Engaging patients and families in communication across transitions of care: An integrative review. *Patient Education & Counselling, 103*(6), 1104–1117. https://doi.org/10.1016/j.pec.2020.01.017

Burton, C. W., Nolasco, K., & Holmes, D. (2021). Queering nursing curricula: Understanding and increasing attention to LGBTQIA+ health needs. *Journal of Professional Nursing, 37*(1), 101–107. https://doi.org/10.1016/j.profnurs.2020.07.003

Canadian Nurses Association (CNA). (2017). *Code of ethics for registered nurses.* https://www.cna-aiic.ca/en/nursing/regulated-nursing-in-canada/nursing-ethics

Canadian Nurses Association (CNA). (2018). *Protection of personal information.* https://www.cna-aiic.ca/en/protection-of-personal-information

Dying With Dignity Canada. (2022). *Patient rights booklet.* https://www.dyingwithdignity.ca/education-resources/patient-rights-guide/

Foley, V. (2018). Documenting and reporting. In B. Kozier, G. Erb, A. Berman, et al. (Eds.), *Fundamentals of Canadian nursing: Concepts, process, and practice* (4th ed., pp. 460–481.). Pearson Canada.

Government of Canada. (2019a). *Canada's healthcare system.* https://www.canada.ca/en/health-canada/services/health-care-system/reports-publications/health-care-system/canada.html

Government of Canada. (2019b). *Federal transfers to provinces and territories.* https://www.canada.ca/en/department-finance/programs/federal-transfers.html

Government of Canada. (2022a). *Canada Health Act annual report 2020–2021.* https://www.canada.ca/en/health-canada/services/publications/health-system-services/canada-health-act-annual-report-2020-2021.html

Government of Canada. (2022b). *Social determinants of health and health inequalities.* https://www.canada.ca/en/public-health/services/health-promotion/population-health/what-determines-health.html

Healthcare Excellence Canada. (2018). *Communications during transitions in care: Is there room for improvement?* https://www.patientsafetyinstitute.ca/en/toolsResources/Documents/Webcasts/2018-02-21%20-%20Human%20Factors%20Transitions%20in%20Care/Human%20Factors%20-%202018-02-21%20-%20Transitions%20in%20Care.pdf

Healthcare Excellence Canada. (2020). *The safety competencies: Enhancing patient safety across the health professions* (2nd ed.). https://www.patientsafetyinstitute.ca/en/toolsResources/safetyCompetencies/Documents/CPSI-SafetyCompetencies_EN_Digital.pdf

Holbrook, A., Bannerman, H., Ahmed, A., et al. (2019). Evaluation of a novel audit tool for medication reconciliation at hospital discharge. *Canadian Journal of Hospital Pharmacy*, *72*(6), 421–427. https://www.ncbi.nlm.nih.gov/pmc/articles/PMC6910843/

Karam, M., Brault, I., Van Durme, T., et al. (2018). Comparing interprofessional and interorganizational collaboration in healthcare: A systematic review of the qualitative research. *International Journal of Nursing Studies*, *79*, 70–83. https://doi.org/10.1016/j.ijnurstu.2017.11.002

Keenan-Lindsay, L., Sams, C., & O'Connor, C. L. (2022). *Perry's maternal child nursing care in Canada* (3rd ed.). Elsevier.

Lavoie, P., Clausen, C., Purden, M., et al. (2021). Nurses' experience of handoffs on four Canadian medical and surgical units: A shared accountability for knowing and safeguarding the patient. *Journal of Advance Nursing*, *77*(10), 4156–4169. https://doi.org/10.1111/jan.14997

Levesque, T., Abdelaziz, H., Smith, A., et al. (2021). Medication reconciliation at hospital admission: Proactive versus retroactive models. *Drugs & Therapy Perspectives*, *37*(11), 545–551. https://doi.org/10.1007/s40267-021-00872-9

Luther, B., Wilson, R. D., Kranz, C., et al. (2019). Discharge processes: What evidences tells us is most effective. *Orthopedic Nursing*, *38*(5), 328–333. https://doi.org/10.1097/NOR.0000000000000601

Mantoura, P., & Morrison, V. (2016). *Policy approaches to reducing health inequalities.* National Collaborating Centre for Healthy Public Policy. http://www.ncchpp.ca/docs/2016_Ineg_Ineq_ApprochesPPInegalites_En.pdf

Martin, D., Miller, A., Quesnel-Vallée, A., et al. (2018). Canada's universal health-care system: Achieving its potential. *Lancet*, *391*(10131), 1718–1735. https://doi.org/10.1016/S0140-6736(18)30181-8

Morrison, V., & Mantoura, P. (2020). *Approaches to reducing health inequalities: A practical exercise using the example of food insecurity.* National Collaborating Centre for Healthy Public Policy. https://ccnpps-ncchpp.ca/docs/2020-inequalities-policy-approaches-example-food-insecurity.pdf

Müller, M., Jürgens, J., Redaèlli, M., et al. (2018). Impact of the communication and patient hand-off tool SBAR on patient safety: A systematic review. *BMJ Open*, *8*(8). https://doi.org/10.1136/bmjopen-2018-022202

National Collaborating Centre for Indigenous Health (NCCIH). (2019). *Access to health services as a social determinant of First Nations, Inuit and Métis health.* https://www.nccih.ca/docs/determinants/FS-AccessHealthServicesSDOH-2019-EN.pdf

Nelson, S. E., & Wilson, K. (2018). Understanding barriers to health care access through cultural safety and ethical space: Indigenous people's experiences in Prince George, Canada. *Social Science & Medicine*, *218*, 21–27. https://doi.org/10.1016/j.socscimed.2018.09.017

Nowak, T. J. (2019). Implementation of a health literacy universal toolkit to improve postdischarge care at an urban trauma center. *Journal of Trauma Nursing*, *3*(4), 180–185. https://doi.org/10.1097/JTN.0000000000000446

Office of the Privacy Commissioner of Canada. (2019). *PIPEDA in brief.* https://www.priv.gc.ca/en/privacy-topics/privacy-laws-in-canada/the-personal-information-protection-and-electronic-documents-act-pipeda/pipeda_brief/

Registered Nurses' Association of Ontario (RNAO). (2014). *Care transitions.* https://rnao.ca/sites/rnao-ca/files/Care_Transitions_BPG.pdf [Seminal Reference]

Registered Nurses' Association of Ontario (RNAO). (2015). *Person- and family-centered care.* https://rnao.ca/sites/rnao-ca/files/FINAL_Web_Version_0.pdf [Seminal Reference]

Registered Nurses' Association of Ontario (RNAO). (2017). *Risk assessment and prevention of pressure ulcers.* https://rnao.ca/sites/rnao-ca/files/Risk_Assessment_and_Prevention_of_Pressure_Ulcers.pdf

Sowko, L. A., Fennimore, L. A., & Drahnak, D. M. (2019). Teaching workplace interprofessional communication to undergraduate nursing students. *Journal of Nursing Education*, *58*(9), 538–542. https://doi.org/10.3928/01484834-20190819-08

Tyerman, J., & Buchanan, D. T. (2023). Sleep and sleep disorders. In J. Tyerman, & S. L. Cobbett (Eds.), *Lewis's medical-surgical nursing in Canada: Assessment and management of clinical problems* (5th ed., pp. 120–134). Elsevier.

Usher, R., Cronin, S. N., & York, N. L. (2018). Evaluating the influence of a standardized bedside handoff process in a medical-surgical unit. *The Journal of Continuing Education in Nursing*, *49*(4), 157–163. https://doi.org/10.3928/00220124-20180320-05

Vermeir, E., Jackson, L. A., & Marshall, E. G. (2018). Barriers to primary and emergency healthcare for trans adults. *Culture, Health and Sexuality*, *20*(2), 232–246. https://doi.org/10.1080/13691058.2017.1338757

White-Trevino, K., & Dearmon, V. (2018). Transitioning nurse handoff to the bedside: Engaging staff and patients. *Nursing Administration Quarterly*, *42*(3), 261–268. https://doi.org/10.1097/NAQ.0000000000000298

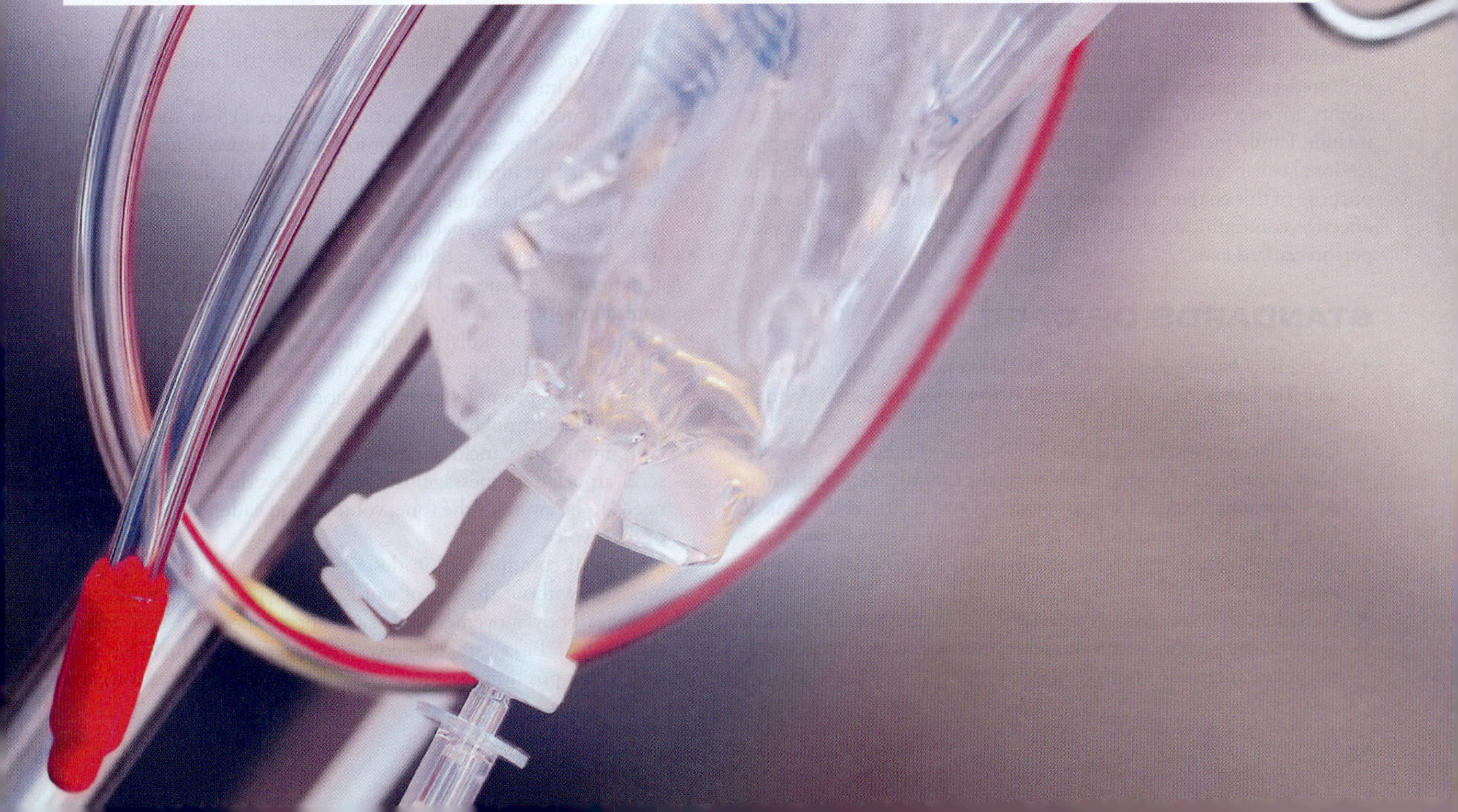

3 Communication and Collaboration

Canadian content written by **Crystal Thibodeau, RN, MN-NP**
Original US chapter by **Nancy Laplante, PhD, RN, AHN-BC**

SKILLS AND PROCEDURES

OBJECTIVES

Mastery of content in this chapter will enable the nurse to:

- Identify guidelines to use in therapeutic communication.
- Explain the communication process.
- Identify the purposes of therapeutic communication and communication in various phases of the nurse–patient relationship.
- Develop skills for therapeutic communication in various phases of the nurse–patient relationship.
- Develop therapeutic communication skills for communicating with patients who have difficulty coping because of feelings such as anxiety, anger, and depression.
- Develop therapeutic communication skills for communication with cognitively impaired patients.
- Develop skills for effective communication with colleagues.

MEDIA RESOURCES

- http://evolve.elsevier.com/Canada/Perry/clinicalskills/

PURPOSE

Communication is the interaction between two or more people. Effective communication positively influences how nursing care is delivered and patient satisfaction with that care. A nurse's responsibility to effectively communicate extends beyond the patient to include family members and significant others along with interprofessional collaboration with all members of the health care team. The purpose of this chapter is to provide you with a framework to develop effective communication skills that are essential to the delivery of person-centred care.

STANDARDS OF CARE

- Canadian Nurses Association (2021)—*Regulated Nursing in Canada: The Landscape in 2021* (https://www.cna-aiic.ca/en/nursing/regulated-nursing-in-canada)
- Canadian Nurses Association (2017)—*Code of Ethics for Registered Nurses—Part 1. Nursing Values and Ethical Responsibilities: A. Providing Safe, Compassionate, Competent, and Ethical Care: Ethical Responsibilities 1, 2, 3* (p. 8) (https://www.cna-aiic.ca/en/nursing/regulated-nursing-in-canada/nursing-ethics)
- Canadian Nurses Association (2022)—*Interprofessional Collaboration* (https://www.cna-aiic.ca/en/nursing/nursing-tools-and-resources/interprofessional-collaboration)

PRINCIPLES FOR PRACTICE

- Nurses must have the ability to express and receive written, verbal, and nonverbal information in a respectful and professional manner (Almost, 2021).
- Communication is an interaction between two or more people that involves the exchange of information between a sender and a receiver. This information can be expressed in the form of emotions, ideas, and thoughts, through both verbal (words or written language) and nonverbal (behaviours) exchanges (Fig. 3.1).
- It is important to establish and understand the purpose of a patient interaction. This is an essential quality of effective communication.
- Communication skills provide information and comfort, promote understanding, clarify misinformation, help to develop plans of care, promote interprofessional collaboration, and facilitate wellness through patient teaching.
- Communication includes both spoken and written words. To send an accurate message, the sender of verbal communication needs to be aware of the tone, volume, and cadence (pace or rate) of their voice.
- Nonverbal communication describes all behaviours that convey messages without the use of words. This type of communication includes body movement, physical appearance, personal space, and touch. Be aware of body language, which includes posture, body position, gestures, eye contact, facial expression, and

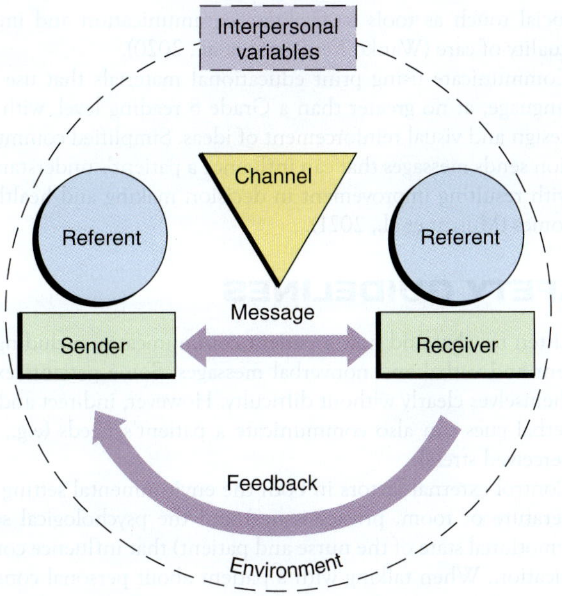

FIG 3.1 Communication is a two-way process.

movement. Nonverbal communication must be consistent with the spoken word.

- Nurse–patient relationships require special consideration in the use of self-disclosure. Nurses need to identify and recognize actions or behaviours that have the potential for crossing or violating professional boundaries (e.g., providing personal information such as an address or phone number, participating in social networking, or sharing information about past or current relationships) (Nova Scotia College of Nursing [NSCN], 2020). You need to use clinical judgement related to the amount of personal information revealed to patients, and ensure that anything you communicate about yourself is disclosed for the benefit of the patient as the focus of the relationship.

PERSON-CENTRED CARE

- Therapeutic communication enables nurses to deliver care that is respectful of and responsive to individual patient preferences, needs, and values, but is also in the best interest of the patient (Almost, 2021; Ellis-Smith et al., 2021). It also contributes to and promotes measures that optimize positive patient health outcomes at the individual, organizational, and system levels (Almost, 2021).
- Include patients and the people within their full social circle in collaboration with health care providers to make decisions related to wellness and illness care. Benefits include improved satisfaction with care, self-efficacy, quality of life, and empowerment to engage in self-care (Ellis-Smith et al., 2021; Giusti et al., 2020).
- Use appropriate communication strategies to create a safe and therapeutic environment for patient care (Almost, 2021).
- Understand how culture affects patients and their knowledge and values about health. Nurses need to recognize their own attitudes about working with patients from different backgrounds (Schill & Caxaj, 2019).
- It is essential to understand the impact that the residential school system and colonization have had on the overall wellness of Indigenous peoples in Canada (Crosschild & Varcoe, 2021). Through knowledge and understanding, nurses can work toward eliminating the significant power imbalance that still exists between non-Indigenous health care providers and Indigenous peoples

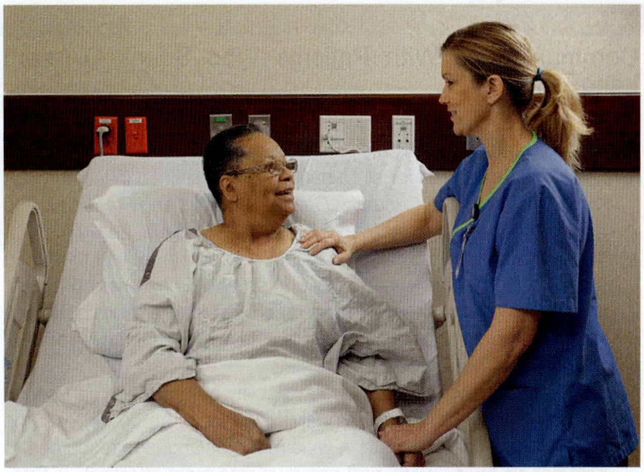

FIG 3.2 An open, relaxed posture conveys interest.

and that continues to create adverse experiences for Indigenous peoples within the health care system (Pepin & Myrick, 2021).
- Be mindful of cultural differences (e.g., when considering the use of touch), and of religious and ethnic practices because these influence methods of communication (Fig. 3.2).
- To avoid misinterpretation of nonverbal cues, be aware of any cultural norms or values (e.g., eye contact) that patients may have (see Skill 3.1).
- Adopt a flexible, respectful attitude that also communicates interest in a patient to bridge any communication barriers that exist because of cultural differences between patient and caregiver.
- When using language assistance:
  - Provide easy-to-understand print and multimedia materials and bedside communication tools that feature pictures and symbols (Gerchow et al., 2021).
  - Address the patient and family directly when using an interpreter; do not direct questions or comments to the interpreter. Take care to determine whether the patient understood (Box 3.1).

EVIDENCE-INFORMED PRACTICE

Recent studies have examined specific interventions or adjustments used to effectively communicate with people of varying developmental levels as well as people who may have difficulty communicating with others because of a physical or mental illness (Bingham & O'Brien, 2018; Heslop et al., 2019; Moloney et al., 2021).

- Methods that incorporate music, video, and hand gestures are often used to help people with disordered states of consciousness to communicate (Papadimitriou et al., 2022).
- Telemedicine technology, including the use of telephones, computers, and handheld devices that have been adapted to the health needs and capabilities of those with intellectual challenges, promotes social engagement and independence by enhancing communication (Krysta et al., 2021). The use of modern technologies can also help to optimize access to quality care for those with mental illness who may have limited access, such as during the COVID-19 pandemic (Krysta et al., 2021).
- Effective communication and support from health care providers often reduces psychological distress in patients and families in a variety of settings—for example, those undergoing cancer treatment. Health care providers benefit from communication skills training to interact more therapeutically with their patients who have cancer (Wittenberg et al., 2020).

BOX 3.1

Communicating With Patients Who Speak Different Languages

- Linguistic services for patients with limited English proficiency (LEP) may vary among health care settings across Canada. This is because ". . . language rights for all Canadians are enshrined in law through the Constitution, the *Canadian Charter of Rights and Freedoms* and the *Official Languages Act*." (Government of Canada, 2018, p. 8).
- In Canada, health care organizations that receive federal funds are required to offer services in both English and French, which means they must inform the public that such services are available and include bilingual greetings and signs (Office of the Commissioner of Official Languages, 2022).
- There are no laws enforcing the availability of translation services in Canada, but the Language Portal of Canada is an online resource that provides free access to a wide range of language resources to help people study, work, and communicate more effectively in English or French (Government of Canada, 2022).
- Professional interpreters improve communication, promote appropriate use of resources, and significantly increase patient and clinician satisfaction.
- When choosing an in-person, telephonic, or video interpreter, it is important to consider the resources available and the needs for your specific clinical situation. Select same-age and same-gender interpreters if possible.
- If there is no interpreter available:
  - Talk in short units, and pause frequently to promote accuracy of interpretation.
  - Remember that nonverbal communication is as important as verbal communication.
- Pantomime simple words and actions:
  - Keep messages simple and repeat them frequently.
  - Avoid using medical terms that a patient may not understand.

From Office of the Commissioner of Official Languages. (2022). *Understanding your language rights*. https://www.clo-ocol.gc.ca/en/language_rights/act; Government of Canada. (2018). *Action plan for official languages 2018–2023: Investing in our future*. https://www.canada.ca/en/canadian-heritage/services/official-languages-bilingualism/official-languages-action-plan/2018-2023.html; Government of Canada. (2022). *Resources of the language portal of Canada*. https://www.noslangues-ourlanguages.gc.ca/en/index; Balzer-Riley, J. (2020). *Communication in nursing* (9th ed., pp. 56–58). Elsevier.

- Health care providers need to consider the needs of older persons in order for person-centred communication to occur. Specific strategies include the use of environmental objects, eye contact, nonverbal communication matching verbal communication, and social touch as tools to facilitate communication and improve quality of care (Wanko Keutchafo et al., 2020).
- Communicate using print educational materials that use plain language, at no greater than a Grade 8 reading level, with basic design and visual reinforcement of ideas. Simplified communication sends messages that can influence a patient's understanding, with resulting improvement in decision making and health outcomes (Muscat et al., 2021).

SAFETY GUIDELINES

- Listen to what and how a patient communicates, including content and verbal and nonverbal messages. Some patients express themselves clearly without difficulty. However, indirect and nonverbal cues can also communicate a patient's needs (e.g., pain, perceived stress).
- Control external factors in both the environmental setting (temperature of room, privacy issues) and the psychological setting (emotional state of the nurse and patient) that influence communication. When talking with a patient about personal concerns, privacy is important.
- When teaching, try to have a caregiver present who can reinforce the content of the instruction. Use language-appropriate print and multimedia materials. This is necessary for caregivers to provide needed support when patients return home.
- Controlling background noise level is also important to limit errors in speech perception and recognition when communicating with patients (Karaminis et al., 2022).
- Establish and understand the purpose of the interaction. This is an essential quality of effective communication.
- Guide an interaction according to the patient's condition and response. For example, the purpose of an interaction may be patient teaching; however, the patient has just learned about the death of a loved one and expresses the need to talk about the death. Help the grieving patient by remaining flexible in the interaction. Or, if the patient indicates increased pain, provide relief measures.
- When communicating with colleagues, it is important to communicate clearly and to avoid indirect communication. A greater awareness of body language and positioning may increase the effectiveness of communication (Crist et al., 2022).
- Effective communication is the groundwork for efficient interprofessional collaboration.

✦ SKILL 3.1 Establishing the Nurse–Patient Relationship

A therapeutic nurse–patient relationship is the foundation of nursing care and involves using a variety of person-centred therapeutic communication skills (Box 3.2). Communication is essential in nursing, as effective communication among patients, families, and health care providers is an important part of patient-centred care (Cusatis et al., 2020; Sanders et al., 2018). The primary goal of therapeutic communication for a nurse is to promote patients' wellness and personal growth. Therapeutic communication empowers patients to make decisions but differs from social communication in that it is person centred and goal directed with limited disclosure from the professional.

Social communication provides an opportunity for personal needs to be met, but nurses do not routinely share intimate details of their personal lives with patients (NSCN, 2020). However, in their role as communicators, nurses use a variety of strategies and relevant technologies to create and maintain professional relationships, share information, and foster therapeutic environments (Almost, 2021). There are times when empathy is essential to establishing and maintaining the nurse–patient relationship. *Empathy* is being warm and genuine; it conveys an understanding of a patient's or family's feelings and communicating this understanding to them. Empathetic communication requires an accurate verbal reflection of what the patient said, accompanied by genuine caring (e.g., "You seem to be very upset" expressed with a concerned facial expression or gentle touch on the shoulder, if appropriate). Empathy differs from sympathy, because sympathy often shifts the emphasis to the nurse's feelings, which may prevent the patient from expressing feelings and inhibit the nurse's ability to view the patient's needs objectively. Barriers to therapeutic communication include giving an opinion, offering false reassurance, making insincere comments, being defensive, showing

BOX 3.2

Therapeutic Communication Techniques

Technique: Active Listening

Definition: An active process of receiving information and examining one's reaction to the messages received.

Example: Consider the cultural practices of your patient, maintain appropriate eye contact, and be receptive to nonverbal communication.

Therapeutic value: Nonverbally communicates your interest and acceptance to a patient.

Technique: Broad Openings

Definition: Encouraging patient to select topics for discussion.

Example: "Can you tell me what you are thinking about?"

Therapeutic value: Indicates your acceptance and valuing of patient's initiative.

Technique: Restating

Definition: Repeating main thought that patient has expressed.

Example: "You say that your mother left you when you were 5 years old."

Therapeutic value: Indicates that you are listening, and validates, reinforces, or calls attention to something important that has been said.

Technique: Clarification

Definition: Attempting to improve your understanding of words, vague ideas, or patient's unclear thoughts, or asking patient to explain what they mean.

Example: "I'm not sure what you mean. Could you tell me again?"

Therapeutic value: Helps to clarify patient's feelings, ideas, and perceptions and provides an explicit correlation between them and patient's actions.

Technique: Reflection

Definition: Directing back to patient ideas, feelings, questions, or content.

Example: "You're feeling tense and anxious, and it's related to a conversation you had with your sister last night?"

Therapeutic value: Validates your understanding of what patient is saying and signifies empathy, interest, and respect for patient.

Technique: Informing

Definition: Demonstrating skills or giving information.

Example: "I think it would be helpful for you to know more about how your medication works."

Therapeutic value: Helpful for patient education about relevant aspects of patient's well-being and self-care.

Technique: Focusing

Definition: Asking questions or making statements that help patient expand on a topic of importance.

Example: "I think it would be helpful if we talk more about your relationship with your father."

Therapeutic value: Allows patient to discuss central issues related to problem and keeps communication process goal directed.

Technique: Silence

Definition: Using silence or nonverbal communication for a therapeutic reason.

Example: Sitting with patient and nonverbally communicating interest and involvement.

Therapeutic value: Allows patient time to think and gain insights, slows the pace of the interaction, and encourages patient to initiate conversation while you convey support, understanding, and acceptance.

Adapted from Townsend, M. C., & Morgan, K. I. (2018). *Psychiatric mental health nursing: Concepts of care in evidence-based practice* (9th ed., pp. 152–154). F. A. Davis Company.

approval or disapproval, stereotyping, and asking, "Why?" The use of "why" questions causes increased defensiveness in patients and hinders communication. The therapeutic nurse–patient relationship is goal directed, with a patient moving toward productive modes of interpersonal functioning.

The therapeutic relationship between nurse and patient is supported through the interrelated phases of pre-interaction, orientation, working, and termination. The pre-interaction phase occurs prior to meeting the patient. The nurse uses self-reflection to become aware of personal feelings, values, and beliefs. This self-awareness allows a nurse to practise using a person-centred approach to develop the relationship and meet the patient's needs. The orientation phase is important in developing a foundation for the therapeutic relationship. The working phase of the helping relationship has two main components: exploring thoughts and feelings and facilitating and taking action (Kennedy, 2018). The final phase is the termination phase, which may occur at the end of shift, patient transfer, discharge, or death. Skills such as summarizing or reviewing what has been accomplished can assist in the termination process.

Delegation and Collaboration

All health care providers must practise effective communication. The nurse serves as a role model for effective communication for members of the interprofessional health care team.

The skill of establishing therapeutic communication cannot be delegated to an unregulated care provider (UCP). The nurse instructs the UCP about the following:

- The proper way to interact verbally and nonverbally with select patients
- The need to keep all patient communication confidential
- Ways to arrange the environment to ensure privacy and confidentiality
- Special considerations pertaining to communication with patients who are cognitively or sensorially impaired, older, children, or anxious, and with potentially violent patients

STEP	RATIONALE
ASSESSMENT	
1. Identify patient using at least two person-specific identifiers (e.g., name and date of birth, or name and medical record number) according to employer policy.	Ensures correct patient. Complies with Accreditation Canada's standards and improves patient safety (Accreditation Canada, 2020).
2. Prepare for orientation phase of therapeutic communication. Formulate individualized patient goals, consider time allocation (e.g., patient acuity and medical priorities), formulate initial questions, and mentally prepare to keep your mind clear of other concerns or distractions. Select the assessment questions most relevant to the clinical situation.	Preparation is part of a planned communication process that facilitates interaction. Planning for the orientation phase helps identify actual or potential problems, current health status, and experience. Without preparation, a risk exists for casual, non-goal-oriented communication.

STEP	RATIONALE
3. Address patient by preferred name and introduce yourself and your role on health care team ("Hello, my name is Jane Smith, and I am the registered nurse assigned to take care of you today . . . ") Use clear, specific communication, including verbal and nonverbal techniques (e.g., good eye contact, relaxed, comfortable position) to provide information and clarify concerns (see Fig. 3.2). Create a climate of warmth and acceptance.	Refer to provincial/territorial standards of nursing practice and employer policy related to relaying your full name. Professional presence "includes a registered nurse's verbal and nonverbal communications and the ability to articulate a positive role and professional image, including the use of full name and title" (NSCN, 2018, p. 2). However, some employers recommend the use of a first name only, for personal safety and security reasons. Ensure that when you are introducing yourself to a member or members of the interprofessional team that you include your full name and title. Congruent verbal and nonverbal communication expresses warmth and respect and helps establish rapport. The quality of communication in interactions between nurse and patient has important influences on patient outcomes (Ellis-Smith et al., 2021).
4. Assess the following during initial interaction: patient's needs, coping strategies, defences, and adaptation styles.	Recognizing recurrent themes in patient's responses helps identify problem areas related to health status (e.g., avoidance of questions, request for information, expression of a loss).
5. Determine patient's need to communicate (e.g., constant use of call light, crying, patient who does not understand an illness or who has just been admitted).	Patients in need of support, comfort, knowledge, or encouragement benefit from individualized meaningful communication.
6. Assess reason that patient needs health care. Ask patient about health status, lifestyle, support systems, patterns of health and illness, and strengths and limitations.	The nature of the illness affects a patient's coping ability and effectiveness in communicating needs and concerns. For example, patients who are fearful of a cancer diagnosis and patients who are having joint replacement surgeries probably have differing needs and concerns.
7. Assess for factors about yourself and the patient that normally influence communication. Examples of factors include perceptions, values, and beliefs; emotions; sociocultural background; severity of illness; knowledge; age; verbal ability; roles and relationships; environmental setting; physical comfort or discomfort (see Step 7 illustration).	Communication is a dynamic process influenced by interpersonal and intrapersonal processes. By assessing factors that influence communication, you can make the best use of opportunities to interact with patients. This will not only improve the patient's level of satisfaction, but also facilitate further development of the nurse–patient relationship and decrease the level of stress associated with future interventions (Lam et al., 2020).

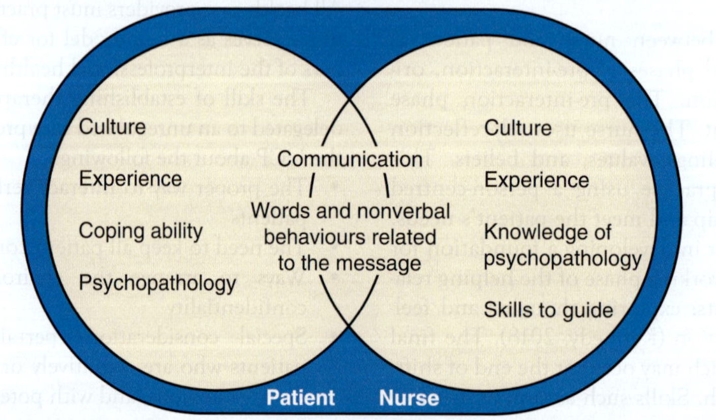

STEP 7 Essential and influencing variables of the therapeutic communication environment. *(Adapted from Keltner, N., & Steele, D. [2019]. Psychiatric nursing [8th ed.]. Mosby.)*

STEP	RATIONALE
8. Assess personal barriers to communicating with patient (e.g., bias toward patient's condition, anxiety from inexperience).	Barriers prevent you from conveying empathy and caring and from obtaining relevant assessment information.
9. Assess patient's language and ability to speak. Does patient have difficulty finding words or associating ideas with accurate word symbols? Does patient have difficulty with expression of language, reception of messages, or both? What is the patient's primary language?	Assessment determines the need for special techniques to address the communication needs of patients with limited English proficiency, hearing impairments, or literacy levels (Gerchow et al., 2021). Examples include picture boards, computers, sign language, or an interpreter (see Step 9 illustration).

STEP	RATIONALE

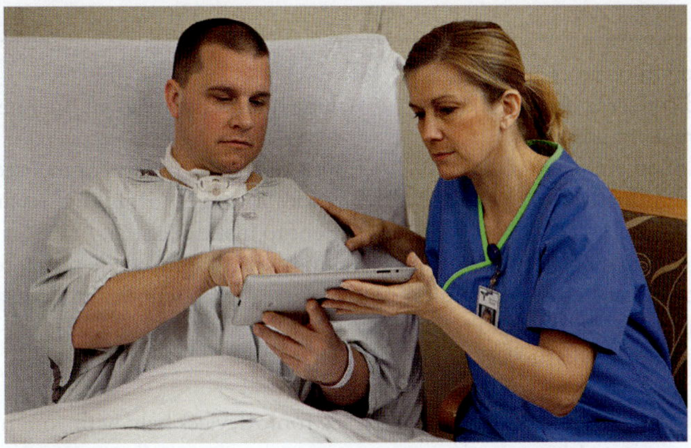

STEP 9 Communication tools for patients who cannot speak.

STEP	RATIONALE
10. Assess patient's literacy level. Does the patient skip over uncommon or hard words, avoid asking questions, or have difficulty discussing concepts about illness? *Option*: Use health literacy resources such as the Newest Vital Sign (NVS) or Test of Functional Health Literacy (Mock & Sethares, 2019).	Health literacy has a direct effect on health outcomes. Assessing a patient's level of health literacy allows you to design more effective communication and patient teaching approaches (Ellis-Smith et al., 2021; Gerchow et al., 2021). Patients with limited health literacy may avoid questions, show signs of nervousness, or make excuses (Wittenberg et al., 2018).
11. Assess patient's ability to hear. Be sure that hearing aid is functional if worn. Be sure that patient hears and understands words (see Chapter 19).	Patients with hearing deficits require techniques to enhance hearing reception (e.g., speaking in normal tone, speaking so patient can see your face).
12. Observe patient's pattern of communication and verbal or nonverbal behaviour (e.g., gestures, tone of voice, eye contact).	Observation determines type and manner of communication that you will use.
13. Assess resources available in selecting communication methods:	
a. Review information in medical record and reflect on your past patient communication experiences.	Relying totally on information from patient restricts the quality of interaction. Additional resources provide insight into best methods of communicating.
b. Consult with family, health care provider, and other interprofessional health care team members concerning patient's condition, problems, and impressions.	Effective interprofessional collaboration centres on effective communication among team members and facilitates your response to patients, based on integration of knowledge. A framework such as SBAR (situation–background–assessment–recommendation) requires that nurses use concise communication when relaying pertinent patient information, thus improving interprofessional collaboration, communication, and patient safety (Müller et al., 2018). Seek information from family after receiving patient approval. Patient privacy must be maintained (Phillips et al., 2020).
14. Before initiating the working phase of the nurse–patient relationship, assess patient's readiness to work toward goal attainment: "We want to work together with you to improve your health. Tell me your goals or what it is that you feel is important for you to recover."	Patient's goals are identified and agreed on by using effective communication skills such as restating and clarifying.
15. Consider when patient is due to be discharged or transferred from health care facility. Share that information with patient and caregiver.	Allows you to anticipate the amount of time available to work with the patient and when termination of relationship will occur.

NURSING DIAGNOSES

- Anxiety
- Fear
- Inadequate coping
- Altered verbal communication
- Deficient knowledge regarding communication skills
- Altered social interaction
- Deficient knowledge regarding communication skills
- Nonadherence
- Readiness for enhanced decision making

Related factors are individualized on the basis of patient's condition or needs.

STEP	RATIONALE
PLANNING	
1. Expected outcomes following completion of procedure:	
• Patient expresses ideas, fears, and concerns clearly, asks questions, and openly expresses relief of anxiety.	Asking questions shows an openness to communication.
• Patient health care goals are identified and achieved.	Interaction remains patient focused.
• Patient verbalizes understanding of information communicated by nurse.	Provides a means to build trust and develop a knowledge base for patient to make decisions.
2. Before engaging in the working phase, prepare patient physically (e.g., deliver pain relief measures, provide for hygiene or elimination), provide a quiet environment, maintain privacy, and reduce distractions or interruptions before beginning discussion.	Taking care of basic needs promotes an environment for interaction and decreases patient distractions and interruptions.
3. Working phase:	
a. Use appropriate communication tools such as iPads or other electronic devices for patients whose initial language is not English.	Electronic devices help with communication and provide translation resources.
b. Prepare open-ended questions to identify strategies for developing a realistic plan to meet identified health goals of patients (e.g., "Let's talk more about the goals you shared earlier for this hospitalization/visit").	Open-ended questions promote goal attainment and avoid risk of misinterpretation.
IMPLEMENTATION	
1. Working phase: Observe patient's nonverbal behaviours, including body language. If verbal behaviours do not match nonverbal behaviours, seek clarification from patient.	Congruence between patient's verbal and nonverbal behaviours ensures that you receive the correct message.
2. Explain purpose of interaction when information is to be shared.	Information and explanation can decrease anxiety about the unknown.
3. Continue to use therapeutic communication skills (see Box 3.2).	Fosters open, interactive communication with patient as a participant and the focus of the discussion.
4. Identify patient's expectations in seeking health care.	Identifying expectations conveys a level of interest in patient's needs.
5. Encourage patient to ask for clarification at any time during the communication.	Gives patient a sense of control and keeps channels of communication open.
6. Set mutual goals.	
a. Use therapeutic communication skills such as restating, reflection, and restating to identify and clarify strategies for attainment of mutual goals.	For communication between nurse and patient to be effective, both need to possess the skills and knowledge required for participation within the communicative interaction.
b. Discuss and prioritize problem areas.	A patient, nonjudgemental, supportive approach minimizes patient anxiety.
c. Provide information to patient and help them express needs and feelings.	Patient can respond to help, develop workable solutions based on goals, and fully participate in a realistic plan for their well-being.
d. Use questions carefully and appropriately. Ask one question at a time and allow sufficient time to answer. Use direct questions. Use open-ended statements as much as possible, such as "Tell me about how you're feeling today."	Strategy helps patient express self and allows for thorough collection of information about needs and concerns.

Critical Decision Point *Avoid asking questions about information that may not yet have been disclosed to the patient (e.g., human immunodeficiency virus [HIV] status, diagnostic test results). Avoid asking "why" questions, which can cause increased defensiveness in the patient that prevents communication.*

STEP	RATIONALE
e. Avoid communication barriers.	Barriers result in a message not being received, being distorted, or not being understood.
7. Termination phase: Communicate with the patient.	
a. Prepare by identifying methods of summarizing and synthesizing information pertinent to patient's aftercare (e.g., "Once you return home, what are your plans for follow-up to maintain your health status?").	Effective communication in the form of summarizing and synthesizing information reinforces behavioural change.

STEP	RATIONALE
b. Use therapeutic communication skills to discuss discharge or termination issues, and guide discussion related to specific patient changes in thoughts and behaviours.	Reinforces behaviours and skills learned during working phase of relationship.
c. Summarize with patient what you discussed during interaction, including goal achievement.	Termination phase consists of evaluation and summary of progress toward prescribed goals. Provides a sense of closure and mutual understanding.

EVALUATION

1. Observe patient's verbal and nonverbal responses to your communication, noting their willingness to share information and concerns during orientation phase.	Verbal and nonverbal feedback reveals patient's interest and willingness to communicate and reflects ability to form a therapeutic relationship.
2. Note your response to patient and patient's response to you. Reflect on effectiveness of therapeutic techniques used in establishing rapport with patient.	Sensitivity to one's ability to use therapeutic communication skills helps improve ability to adjust techniques when necessary.
3. During working phase, evaluate patient's ability to work toward identified goals. Elicit feedback (verbal and nonverbal) to determine success of goal attainment. Evaluate patient's health status in relation to identified goals. Re-evaluate and identify barriers if patient goals are not met.	Feedback is an essential step in evaluating new behaviours. Modifications are necessary if goals cannot be met.
4. During termination phase, summarize and restate. Reinforce patient's strengths, outline issues still requiring work, and develop an action plan.	Evaluates patient progress in terms of attainment of mutual goals.
5. **Use teach-back:** "I want to make sure that I explained things clearly. Show me how you would take your blood pressure." Revise the teaching plan if patient or caregiver is unable to teach back correctly.	Determines patient's and caregiver's level of understanding of teaching.

Unexpected Outcomes	Related Interventions
1. Patient continues to verbally and nonverbally express feelings of anxiety, fear, anger, confusion, distrust, and helplessness. Patient often responds to internal and external factors and cues.	• Reassess patient's level of anxiety, fear, and distrust. Attempt to determine the cause of anxiety or fear. • Repeat message to patient later. • Determine influence affecting clear communication (e.g., cultural, language, or literacy issues; physical limitations).
2. Feedback between you and patient reveals lack of understanding and ineffective communication.	• Assess for and remove barriers to communication such as literacy level or language issues (Wittenberg et al., 2018). • Repeat message using another approach, if possible. • Consider cultural norms associated with eye contact, use of touch, personal space, and nonverbal behaviours (Gasiorek & van de Poel, 2018). • Avoid using medical terms that patient does not understand.
3. You are unable to acquire information about patient's ideas, fears, and concerns. Communication techniques do not promote patient's willingness to communicate openly. Trust is not established. Goals are not identified and therefore cannot be achieved.	• Use alternative communication techniques to promote patient's willingness to communicate openly. • Offer another professional with whom patient can talk to obtain necessary information.
4. Caregiver answers for patient even when patient can answer.	• Direct question to patient, using patient's name. • Acknowledge answer given by caregiver; then state that you are interested in patient's response. • Resume interaction after caregiver has left or encourage caregiver to take a break for coffee or a meal.

Communication and Documentation

- Document in progress notes in electronic health record (EHR) or chart the communication pertinent to patient's health, response to illness or therapies, and responses that demonstrate understanding or lack of understanding (include verbal and nonverbal cues).
- Report any relevant information obtained through patient's verbal and nonverbal behaviours to members of interprofessional team.
- Document teach-back and any changes to teaching plan.

DOCUMENTATION EXAMPLE

Patient received sitting upright on stretcher with relaxed posture. Patient made eye contact with this writer and smiled when greeted. Patient stated, "I am feeling much better now that I know what was causing my headache." Patient stated that they were "so glad" they came to the emergency department when the headache seemed to worsen more than usual and that they are "very relieved" now that they know it was likely caused by elevated blood pressure. Patient able to accurately explain the purpose of ramipril and the importance of taking this medication as prescribed. Patient left department ambulatory with plan to have prescription filled at community pharmacy.

Patient accurately able to demonstrate application of blood pressure cuff following explanation and demonstration by this writer. Patient demonstrated uncertainty regarding which button to press on home BP monitor to obtain reading, as evidenced by hesitancy when asked which button to press. Key information written down by this writer to help patient remember instructions at home. Patient then demonstrated correct choice of button to obtain BP reading. Patient left ambulatory with plan to return on September 29, 2024, at 1000h for blood pressure recheck and review of recorded daily home readings.

Special Considerations

Teaching

- Use gestures, pictures, and role playing to help patient understand. Be alert to literacy status; determine whether patient can access health information adequately. Be alert to words that patient seems to understand and use them frequently.
- Individualize patient teaching to meet patient needs. Always conduct teaching with the purpose of meeting patient's learning needs with consideration for their preferred methods of learning.

Mental Health

- Communicating with patients who are experiencing anxiety, sadness, fear, and worry requires clear communication in order to ensure high quality of care.
- Focus on developing trust with the patient by providing support and empathy to encourage the patient to feel safe in expressing anxieties and symptoms.
- Use simple words in a calm and clear manner in order to understand the reason for the patient's distress.
- Teach the patient signs and symptoms of increasing anxiety and ways to control its progression (calming/relaxation skills) and how to apply these skills during periods of distress (Townsend & Morgan, 2018).

Pediatric

- Communicating with children requires an understanding of feelings and thought processes from the child's perspective (McKinney et al., 2022).
- Use vocabulary that is familiar to the child, based on their level of understanding (age and developmental level). Try to be on same eye level as the patient.
- Understand the child's cognitive, developmental, and functional level to select the most appropriate communication techniques. Some age-appropriate communication techniques include storytelling and drawing (McKinney et al., 2022).
- Nurses need to use effective communication skills to ensure that parents have been provided with education about the child's acute or preventive care and rationales to facilitate transition from the hospital to home setting (McKinney et al., 2022).

Gerontological

- Be aware of any cognitive or sensory impairment. Assess each patient individually, and avoid stereotyping older persons who have cognitive or sensory impairments (Ondrejka, 2018).
- Understand the crucial importance of effective communication skills, medical history, and personality in terms of providing both human and therapeutic responses to older persons.
- Ensure that older persons with visual or hearing impairment use assistive devices such as eyeglasses, large-print reading material, or hearing aids to facilitate communication (Ondrejka, 2018).

Care in the Community: Home Management

- Identify primary caregiver for patient, and adapt techniques to assess level of understanding regarding patient's condition.
- Incorporate communication into patient's daily activities (e.g., bathing and dressing).

✦ SKILL 3.2 Communicating With Patients Who Have Difficulty Coping

Patients in the health care setting may have difficulty coping for a variety of reasons and may therefore experience anxiety, anger, depression, or a combination of these feelings. The nurse can help the patient decrease or manage their feelings and ineffective coping behaviours through effective communication. Examples of factors that cause anxiety are a newly diagnosed illness, separation from loved ones, threat associated with diagnostic tests or surgical procedures, and expectations of life changes. How successfully a patient copes with anxiety depends in part on previous experiences, the presence of other stressors, the significance of the event causing anxiety, and the availability of supportive resources. There are four stages of anxiety with corresponding behavioural manifestations: mild, moderate, severe, and panic (Box 3.3).

Anger is a common factor underlying abusive and violent behaviour. Patients become angry for a variety of reasons. Anger is often directly related to a patient's experience with illness, or it can be associated with previous problems. In the health care setting, the nurse has frequent contact with a patient and thus often becomes the target of this unresolved anger. Understanding how to use de-escalation skills is a useful strategy to manage an angry or violent patient and help ensure a safe health care environment for other patients and health care personnel.

Depression is a state of feelings that is more than just sadness. It is a common mood disorder that affects a person's ability to function in day-to-day activities. Major depression is the fourth leading cause of years lived with disability (YLD) (Hancock, 2018). Approximately 9% of Canadians aged 12 years and older reported a diagnosis of a mood disorder in 2020 (Statistics Canada, 2021). There are many symptoms of depression, with the most common being apathy, feelings of sadness, fatigue, guilt, poor concentration, sleep disturbances, and suicidal thoughts. Depression results in both subjective and objective behaviours and patient reports of increased physical complaints (Box 3.4). Some patients report feeling anxious when depressed.

Delegation and Collaboration

The skill of communicating with a patient who has difficulty coping cannot be delegated to a UCP. The nurse instructs the UCP about the following:

- Basic communication skills needed to interact verbally and nonverbally with anxious, angry, or depressed patients
- Their support role as the nurse uses de-escalation techniques
- Appropriate safety measures for themselves and other patients
- How the nurse collaborates with the health care team to identify effective coping mechanisms

BOX 3.3

Behavioural Manifestations of Anxiety: Stages of Anxiety

Mild Anxiety
- Increased auditory and visual perception
- Increased awareness of relationships
- Increased alertness
- Able to problem solve

Moderate Anxiety
- Selective inattention
- Decreased perceptual field
- Focus only on relevant information
- Muscle tension; diaphoresis

Severe Anxiety
- Focus on fragmented details
- Headache, nausea, dizziness
- Unable to see connections between details
- Poor recall

Panic State of Anxiety
- Does not notice surroundings
- Feeling of terror
- Unable to cope with any problem

BOX 3.4

Symptoms of Depression

Common Symptoms
- Apathy
- Decreased socialization
- Sadness
- Sleep disturbances
- Hopelessness
- Helplessness
- Powerlessness
- Low self-esteem
- Difficulty experiencing pleasure in activities

Other Symptoms
- Fatigue
- Decreased performance of activities of daily living
- Thoughts of death
- Decreased libido
- Anorexia or overeating

From Townsend, M. C., & Morgan, K. I. (2018). *Psychiatric mental health nursing: Concepts of care in evidence-based practice* (9th ed., pp. 511–512). F. A. Davis Company.

STEP	RATIONALE
ASSESSMENT	
1. Identify patient using at least two person-specific identifiers (e.g., name and date of birth, or name and medical record number) according to employer policy.	Ensures correct patient. Complies with Accreditation Canada's standards and improves patient safety (Accreditation Canada, 2020).
2. Provide a brief, simple introduction; introduce yourself and explain purpose of interaction.	Ineffective coping behaviours may limit amount of information patient can understand.
3. Assess factors influencing communication with patient (e.g., environment, timing, presence of others, values, experiences, need for personal space because of heightened anxiety).	Identifies effective communication strategies.
4. Assess for possible factors causing patient anxiety (e.g., hospitalization, unknown diagnosis, fatigue).	Understanding the source of anxiety helps in patient support and communication.
5. Discuss possible causes of patient's anxiety, anger, or depression with family members, including past history of the illness, if necessary.	Gathering information about patient from a family perspective is useful because family members may provide new information or understanding of the situation (Ondrejka, 2018).
6. Observe for physical, behavioural, and verbal cues that indicate patient is anxious, such as dry mouth, sweaty palms, tone of voice, frequent use of call light, difficulty concentrating, wringing of hands, and statements such as "I'm scared."	Anxiety interferes with the usual manner of communication and thus with patient's care and treatment. Extreme anxiety interferes with comprehension, attention, and problem-solving abilities.
7. Assess for physical, behavioural, and verbal cues that indicate patient is depressed, such as feelings of sadness, tearfulness, difficulty concentrating, increase in reports of physical complaints, and statements such as "I'm sad/depressed."	Depression interferes with the usual manner of communication and thus with patient's care and treatment. If depression is severe, it interferes with comprehension, attention, and problem-solving abilities.
8. Assess for possible factors causing patient's depression (e.g., acute or persistent illness, personal vulnerability, recent loss).	Patient's depressive state is sometimes unknown. Understanding the possible cause of depression helps in patient support and communication.
9. Observe for behaviours that indicate the patient is angry (e.g., pacing, clenched fist, loud voice, throwing objects) and expressions that indicate anger (e.g., repeated questioning of nurse, not following requests, aggressive outbursts, threats).	Anger is a normal expression of frustration or response to feeling threatened. However, its expression often interferes with or blocks effective communication and interactions.
10. Assess factors that influence the angry patient's communication, such as refusal to adhere to treatment goals, use of sarcasm or hostile behaviour, having a low frustration level, or being emotionally immature.	Allows you to accurately evaluate the situation or patient experiences that block or facilitate effective communication.

STEP	RATIONALE
11. Assess for resources (e.g., social worker, pastoral care, or family) available to help in communicating with a potentially violent patient.	This helps to clarify cause and intervention required to deal with patient's anger.
12. Assess for underlying medical conditions that may potentially lead to violent behaviour.	Patients with medical conditions such as traumatic brain injury, dementia, or substance or alcohol withdrawal may exhibit hostile, aggressive behaviours.

Critical Decision Point *With some violent behaviours (e.g., physical aggression) you may not be able to de-escalate the situation. When this potential situation exists, know whom to call for assistance (e.g., Code White). Personal safety is essential.*

NURSING DIAGNOSES

- Anxiety
- Hopelessness
- Decisional conflict
- Defensive coping
- Inadequate coping
- Altered verbal communication
- Altered role performance
- Potential for other-directed violence
- Potential for self-directed violence

Related factors and risk factors are individualized on the basis of patient's condition or needs.

PLANNING

STEP	RATIONALE
1. Expected outcomes following completion of procedure:	
• Patient discusses factors causing anxiety, anger, or depression.	Reflects success in ability to communicate openly and build trust.
• Patient can discuss methods to cope with anxiety, anger, or depression.	Gains resources (e.g., use of breathing exercises, guided imagery) to cope with situations that cause anxiety, anger, or depression.
• Patient states that sensations of anxiety or depression are reduced.	Eases symptoms associated with anxiety and depression and allows patient to focus on problem.

Critical Decision Point *First acknowledge and address the anxious patient's physical and emotional discomfort. Focus on understanding the patient, providing feedback, helping them problem solve, and creating an atmosphere of warmth and acceptance.*

STEP	RATIONALE
• Patient no longer exhibits verbal and nonverbal expressions of anger.	De-escalation techniques successfully allow patient to express anger in a constructive way.
2. Prepare for therapeutic intervention by considering patient goals, time allocation, and resources.	Allows patient to establish rapport, achieve a sense of calm, and begin to analyze source of anxiety.
3. Recognize personal level of anxiety and consciously try to remain calm (breathe slowly and deeply) when communicating with an anxious, angry, or depressed patient. Be aware of nonverbal cues that indicate your own anxiety (e.g., body language, posture, cadence of speech). Remain nonjudgemental.	Your anxiety increases patient's anxiety. Your personal feelings and values may negatively affect interaction with patient.
4. Prepare a quiet, calm area, allowing personal space.	Decreasing stimuli has a calming effect. Invasion of personal space increases anxiety, anger, or depression.

Critical Decision Point *First acknowledge and address the depressed patient's physical and emotional discomfort. Focus on understanding patient, providing feedback, and helping them problem solve.*

STEP	RATIONALE
5. Prepare to de-escalate an angry patient.	
a. Pause to collect own thoughts, feelings, and reactions.	Awareness and control of your reaction and responses facilitates more constructive interaction.
b. Determine what patient is saying.	Clarification of patient needs or concerns may help de-escalate situation.
c. Prepare the environment to de-escalate a potentially violent patient.	Potentially violent patient needs to be in an environment with decreased stimuli and have protection from injury of self or others. Encourages patient's expression of anger rather than provoking it.
(1) Encourage other people, particularly those who provoke anger, to leave room or area.	Avoids pressuring patient; helps prevent injury if anger becomes out of control.
(2) Maintain an adequate distance and open exit. Position yourself closest to door to facilitate escape from a potentially violent situation. Do not block exit so that patient feels escape is unattainable.	Prevents feeling of being trapped for both you and patient. Feeling trapped may cause a violent outburst. Safety of both parties is essential.

STEP	RATIONALE
(3) When anger begins to disturb others, close door. This is particularly important when patient becomes agitated.	Agitation and anxiety can spread to others. Some hospital rooms are equipped with security windows and cameras to allow for observation of patients.

Critical Decision Point *Some patients are disruptive to one another, especially those who are hyperactive, intrusive, or threatening/exhibiting bizarre behaviours. For these patients, first try the least restrictive measures before using more restrictive measures such as seclusion.*

STEP	RATIONALE
(4) Reduce disturbing factors in room (e.g., noise, drafts, inadequate lighting).	Reduces irritants that may heighten anger.

IMPLEMENTATION

STEP	RATIONALE
1. Use appropriate nonverbal behaviours and active listening skills such as staying with patient at bedside and having a relaxed posture. Focus on understanding the patient's issues.	Patients experiencing an emotionally charged situation may not comprehend a verbally delivered message. Nonverbal messages to patient express interest and help alleviate anxiety.
2. Use appropriate verbal techniques that are clear and concise to respond to anxious patient. Use brief statements that acknowledge current state of feelings and provide direction to patient, such as "It seems to me that you're anxious" or "I notice that you seem to want to be alone. Would you like to go to your room to rest?"	Promotes effective communication so that patient can explore reasons for anxiety, anger, or depression. Appropriate techniques and statements provide reassurance.
3. Help patient develop alternative coping strategies such as progressive relaxation, breathing exercises, and visual imagery (see Chapter 16).	Coping strategies help patient reduce anxiety and depression and, in some cases, reduce anger.
4. Provide necessary comfort measures such as analgesics, positioning, or hygiene.	Pain heightens patient's anxiety or depression and can contribute to their anger.
5. Use open-ended questions, such as "Tell me about how you're feeling" or "You seem sad. Tell me about your sadness."	Encourages patient to continue talking, facilitating an in-depth discussion of symptoms.
6. Encourage and reward small decisions and independent actions. When necessary, make decisions that patients are not ready to make. Present situations that require no decision making.	Depressed patients are often overly dependent and indecisive.
7. Accept patient and focus on positive aspects. Provide positive feedback.	Depressed patients often have low self-esteem. This approach helps to focus on their strengths.
8. Be honest and empathetic.	Honesty and empathy facilitate the development of trust.

Critical Decision Point *If the patient seems depressed, ask the person about suicidal ideation. Ask, "Have you thought about hurting yourself? Tell me how you would do it. Do you have the means to carry out your plan?" The risk of suicide is greatly increased if the patient has developed a plan, has strong intentions, and has the means to complete the plan. Listen actively and encourage expression of feelings, including anger, in a nonjudgemental way. It is critical to be direct with the patient and to communicate openly and matter-of-factly about suicide. Refer to an appropriate mental health care provider (if available)* (Townsend & Morgan, 2018).

STEP	RATIONALE
9. De-escalation for an angry patient:	
a. Maintain personal space. It may be necessary to have someone with you and to keep the room door open. Position yourself between the patient and the exit.	Use of personal space may help to de-escalate patient's anger. Positioning promotes health care provider's safety if patient's anger continues to escalate and patient becomes violent.
b. Maintain nonthreatening verbal and nonverbal approach using a calm, reassuring tone of voice. Use open body language with a concerned, nonthreatening facial expression, open, unfolded arms, relaxed posture, and a safe distance. Use gestures that are slow and deliberate rather than sudden and abrupt.	Decreases chance of misinterpretation of message and is less threatening. A relaxed atmosphere prevents further escalation. Creates climate of acceptance for patient.
c. Use therapeutic silence and allow patient to vent feelings. Use active listening for understanding. Do not argue with patient.	Often de-escalates anger. Anger expends emotional and physical energy; patient runs out of momentum and energy to maintain anger at high level. Arguing escalates anger.
d. Respond to anger therapeutically; avoid becoming defensive or angry and encourage verbal expression of anger.	Some depressed patients are angry; understand that anger is a symptom of their depression. Verbal expression often reduces tension.

STEP	RATIONALE
e. Answer questions calmly and honestly as appropriate. If patient asks power-struggle type of question (challenging or confrontational type) (e.g., "Who said you were in charge?"), redirect and set limits by giving clear, concise expectations. Inform patient of potential consequences without sounding threatening and follow through with consequences if patient does not change behaviours.	Remaining calm and encouraging the patient to express concerns helps to set limits on power-struggle types of situations and helps resolve conflict (College of Nurses of Ontario [CNO], 2018).
f. If patient is making verbal threats to harm others, remain calm yet professional and continue to set limits on inappropriate behaviour.	Angry patient loses ability to process information rationally and therefore may impulsively express anger through intimidation.

Critical Decision Point *If imminent harm to another is present on discharge, notify proper authorities (e.g., nurse manager, security). A potentially violent patient can be impulsive and explosive; therefore, you need to keep personal safety skills in mind. In this case, avoid touch.*

STEP	RATIONALE
g. If patient appears to be calm and anger is defused, explore alternatives to situation or feelings of anger.	Processing with patient can prevent future explosive outbursts and teach patient effective ways of dealing with anger.

EVALUATION

STEP	RATIONALE
1. Observe for continuing presence of physical signs and symptoms or behaviours reflecting anxiety, anger, or depression.	Observation determines extent to which planned interaction relieved patient's emotions.
2. Ask patient to describe ways to cope with anxiety, depression, or anger in the future and make decisions about own care.	Measures patient's ability to assume more health-promoting behaviour.
3. Evaluate patient's ability to discuss factors causing anxiety, depression, or anger.	Measures patient's ability to attend to or focus on area of concern.
4. Note patient's ability to answer questions and problem solve.	Determines whether anger has lessened so that patient is able to focus on alternative coping skills.
5. Have patient discuss ways to cope in the future and make decisions about own care.	Allows evaluation of patient's ability to assume more health-promoting behaviour.
6. **Use teach-back:** "I want to be sure you understand what we went over today. We talked about different ways to help you manage your anxiety along with taking your medication. Tell me about the other methods you are going to use." Develop a revised teaching plan if patient or caregiver is unable to teach back correctly.	Determines patient's and caregiver's level of understanding of teaching.

Unexpected Outcomes	Related Interventions
1. Physical signs and symptoms of anxiety/anger continue. Your interaction has increased patient's anxiety/anger; source of anxiety/anger is not resolved.	• Use refocusing or distraction skills such as relaxation or guided imagery to reduce anxiety (Townsend & Morgan, 2018). • Reassess factors and remove or alter factors contributing to anxiety/anger. • Take charge with calm, firm directions. Give as-needed (prn) medications as prescribed for anxiety/agitation or escalating behaviours. • Ensure that health care team members are available to help if necessary.
2. Patient displays difficulty making decisions by avoiding your efforts to focus discussion or is unable to discuss real concerns. Anxiety/anger/depression continues to prevent problem solving.	• Be clear and direct when communicating with patient to avoid misunderstanding. • When used appropriately, touch helps control feelings of panic.
3. Depressive behaviours continue; interaction has been ineffective at relieving depressive symptoms or patient reports suicidal ideation, with or without plan.	• Continue to use therapeutic communication skills but try different techniques. • Refer patient to mental health provider for consultation regarding use of pharmacological medications, formal psychotherapy to treat depression, or both. • Refer patient to mental health provider for evaluation and possible admission to an inpatient psychiatric treatment facility.

Communication and Documentation

- Document cause of patient's anxiety/anger/depression and any exhibited signs and symptoms of behaviours on flow sheet or in progress notes in EHR or chart.
- Document de-escalation technique used and patient's response to de-escalation efforts on flow sheet or in progress notes in EHR or chart.
- Report methods used to relieve anxiety/anger/depression and patient's response to ensure continuity of care between nurses.
- Report technique used to de-escalate and patient's response to nurse in charge.
- Document your evaluation of patient and caregiver learning.

DOCUMENTATION EXAMPLE

Patient informed by this writer that their patience is appreciated while the emergency department is experiencing long wait times. Patient permitted to vent. Through use of calm, reassuring tone of voice and relaxed posture while providing 3 metres physical distancing, patient relaxed and seated self with relaxed posture into chair. Once patient anger de-escalated, patient educated regarding strategies such as decreasing stimuli to help reduce agitation. Patient demonstrated understanding by reporting to this writer their plans to pause and collect their thoughts when becoming angry and to try to move to a quiet, calm space, which will also provide personal space. Positive feedback provided.

Special Considerations

Teaching

- Teaching patient and caregiver to identify possible sources of anxiety such as illness, hospitalization, knowledge deficits, or other known stressors gives patient knowledge of anxiety and increases sense of control.
- Patients experiencing emotionally charged situations do not always comprehend instruction. Focus on understanding patient; provide feedback and help to problem solve, and provide an atmosphere of safety, warmth, and acceptance.
- Teaching patient and caregiver to identify possible factors that contribute to angry outbursts, such as inadequate coping skills, low frustration levels, illness, hospitalization, knowledge deficits, or other known stressors, may give patient a sense of control.
- Once anger has been de-escalated, teach patient new adaptive methods of coping with anger.
- Teach patient and caregiver to identify possible sources of depression. Knowledge of depression increases patient's sense of control over feelings of depression.

Pediatric

- Children often demonstrate anxiety through physical and behavioural signs but are unable to express anxiety verbally. Some children express anxiety through restless behaviour, physical complaints, or behavioural regression. Note any changes in child's behaviour that occur during illness or hospitalization (McKinney et al., 2022).
- Set limits for inappropriate behaviours exhibited by child such as using a time-out. Apply such limits immediately because children tend to have less internal control over their own behaviour (McKinney et al., 2022).
- Children's symptoms of depression often differ from those exhibited by adults. They manifest depression through physical (increased somatic complaints) and behavioural (poor school performance, social isolation) signs and are often unable to express it verbally. Some children express depression through restless behaviour or behavioural regression. It is important to note any changes in a child's behaviour that occur during illness or hospitalization (McKinney et al., 2022).

Gerontological

- Anxiety is one of the most common symptoms seen in older persons. Anxiety develops because of a specific event or a general pattern of change (e.g., decline in health) (Byrd & Luther, 2018).
- Psychosocial factors such as anxiety and confusion, lack of mobility, and spatial organization of a long-term or complex care facility are factors that decrease social contacts, thus hindering communication with peers and health care providers. This leads to further feelings of isolation, boredom, and increased anxiety.
- Older persons who are socially isolated often have multiple health problems and are more likely to have anxious or depressive symptoms. In addition, they are less likely to seek care for these symptoms.
- Depression among older persons is a major health concern. It is important to differentiate between depression and any underlying medical illness, such as cognitive impairment (Byrd & Luther, 2018).
- Suicide risk is increased in older persons because of loss of life partner, health status, independence, and social support system or financial losses (Byrd & Luther, 2018).

Patients With Cognitive or Physical Challenges

- A change in needs or a negative life event, such as loss of a support animal, loved one, or special caregiver, can lead to crisis. Assess and monitor patient and caregivers for stress and advocate for respite care as needed (Sullivan et al., 2018).

Care in the Community: Home Management

- Anticipation of a home care visit may increase a patient's anxiety (Dellosso, 2021). Personal safety for the nurse against a potentially violent patient or caregiver extends to all health care settings, including the patient's home. Assess patient's home and physical surroundings, including possible exits. You may be in a potentially dangerous situation while giving care to a patient at home because you are without support from other team members. Do not enter the home if you feel unsafe; call for help.
- Depression is often present in home care settings. Educate caregivers about how to identify symptoms. Manage depression based on patient's presenting behaviours with consideration of any cognitive or physical impairment.

✦ SKILL 3.3 Communicating With a Patient Who Is Cognitively Impaired

The act of communicating and expressing oneself is affected by a person's ability. Patients with cognitive impairments pose a challenge for nurses because these patients may have disabilities that negatively affect communication (Mendes & Palmer, 2018; van Manen et al., 2021). Acute cognitive impairment or delirium is largely reversible and may be caused by conditions such as infection, polypharmacy, and metabolic changes. Once the cause is identified and treated, the patient's mental status returns to a baseline condition. Persistent types of cognitive impairments are irreversible and progressive. These include dementia (Alzheimer's disease, vascular dementia, frontotemporal dementia), traumatic brain injury (TBI), and human immunodeficiency virus (HIV)–related cognitive dysfunction.

Cognitive impairments accompanied by communication deficits hinder a patient's ability to initiate conversation and participate in self-care. Since it is time consuming to interact with these patients, they may be deprived of human contact, which then leads to depression, detachment, and isolation. Patients with cognitive impairments may also be at risk for physical status changes such as infection, falls and injury, and poor nutrition. In these circumstances, a lack of quality nurse–patient interaction and communication is a possibility, which negatively affects patient outcomes. A person-centred approach stresses the individuality of each patient when assessing the patient's ability to communicate.

Delegation and Collaboration

The skill of communicating effectively with a cognitively impaired patient cannot be delegated to a UCP. The nurse instructs the UCP about the following:

- The proper communication skills needed to interact verbally and nonverbally with the cognitively impaired patient
- The possible causes and signs and symptoms of the patient's cognitive impairment
- The negative impact that lack of a high-quality relationship with the patient and family can have on patient outcomes
- Collaborate with interprofessional team members to communicate effectively.

STEP	RATIONALE
ASSESSMENT	
1. Identify patient using at least two person-specific identifiers (e.g., name and date of birth, or name and medical record number) according to the employer policy.	Ensures correct patient. Complies with Accreditation Canada's standards and improves patient safety (Accreditation Canada, 2020).
2. When you first meet a patient, approach from the front. Assess for physical, behavioural, and verbal cues that indicate a patient is cognitively impaired. Assess orientation status of patient (person, place, time). A mental health examination (see Chapter 8) may be used to assess for the presence of cognitive impairment in a person with suspected dementia or following a head injury.	You may startle and upset a patient if you touch the person unexpectedly or approach from behind. If the patient is unable to think, speak, or understand, adjust your communication strategies to communicate effectively.
3. Assess for possible factors causing patient's cognitive impairment (e.g., acute or persistent illness, fever, medications, fluid and electrolyte imbalance).	Understanding the possible cause of mental decline helps in conferring with the health care team on appropriate therapy and has implications for short-term and long-term communication strategies.
4. Assess factors influencing communication with patient (e.g., environment, timing, presence of others, values, experiences, prior sensory loss, poor concentration).	Understanding factors that influence communication helps you to identify effective communication strategies (Sanders et al., 2018).
5. Discuss possible causes of patient's cognitive impairment with family members or caregivers, including current illness, duration, treatment regimen, and past medical history.	Gathering information about the patient from a family perspective is useful because family members may provide new information or understanding of the situation. It is important to establish patient's baseline mental status.
6. Discuss with family or caregivers how patient typically communicates with them. Consider these questions: Does the patient lose their train of thought, struggle to organize words logically, need more time to understand what you're saying, or curse or use offensive language? (Mayo Clinic, 2021)	Allows you to anticipate pattern of patient's communication so you can use effective communication strategies.
7. Ascertain the most effective means of communication with patient (e.g., verbal or written communication, picture board). Ensure that this information is communicated and shared with all members of the interprofessional team.	Knowing how best to communicate and using alternative communication methods can help identify a patient's needs. It is essential that all team members are aware of the strategies that work best for the patient to enhance interprofessional collaboration and improve patient health outcomes.

NURSING DIAGNOSES

- Acute confusion
- Hopelessness
- Inadequate coping
- Decisional conflict
- Altered social interaction
- Altered verbal communication
- Altered role performance

Related factors are individualized on the basis of patient's condition or needs.

STEP	RATIONALE
PLANNING	
1. Expected outcomes following completion of procedure: • Patient can communicate physical and emotional discomfort needs to nurse.	Use of relevant communication techniques enables patient to express needs (e.g., physical and emotional discomfort) effectively given the limitations related to cognitive impairment.
2. Prepare for communication by considering type of cognitive and communication impairments, time allocation, and resources.	Effective communication allows you to establish rapport with patient and have a quality nurse–patient interaction.

STEP	RATIONALE
3. Be aware of your nonverbal cues that affect communication with the cognitively impaired patient (e.g., body language, posture, cadence of speech). Remain nonjudgemental.	Frustration in communication with patients with cognitive impairment may negatively affect interaction with patient.
4. Prepare environment physically by providing a quiet, calm area. Reduce distractions such as external noises.	Decreasing stimuli has a calming effect. Ensuring that the environment is quiet and free from distractions enhances the communication experience.

IMPLEMENTATION

STEP	RATIONALE
1. Approach patient from the front and face them when speaking.	This strategy avoids startling the patient and helps ensure that the patient both sees you and hears you.
2. Provide a brief, simple introduction. Introduce yourself, show respect, and explain purpose of interaction.	Symptoms associated with cognitive impairment limit amount of information that patient can understand.
3. Use appropriate nonverbal behaviours and active listening skills such as staying with patient at bedside or using touch appropriately.	Nonverbal messages to patient express your interest and convey empathy. Use of touch may help with concentration and reassurance.
4. Use clear and concise verbal techniques to respond to patient (Mayo Clinic, 2021). Use simple language and speak slowly; use short and simple sentences. Ask yes or no questions.	Appropriate techniques and statements provide reassurance to cognitively impaired patient.
5. Ask one question at a time and allow time for response. Avoid rushing patient. Do not interrupt patient.	Gives patient time to process the information and respond.
6. Repeat sentences using a steady voice, and avoid raising your voice or being too quick to guess what patient is trying to express.	Repetition allows time for patient to respond; it can be frustrating for patient if you misinterpret their message or pressure them to respond.
7. Use augmentative and assistive communication (AAC) devices such as pictogram grid, talking mats, objects, and iPads to facilitate communication.	Talking mats are communication aids that use picture symbols to enable patient to place relevant images below a visual scale to indicate feelings (Hagelskjær et al., 2019).
8. Make sure that patient is wearing eyeglasses or hearing aids to help with communication.	Some patients with cognitive impairments forget about eyeglasses or hearing aids and need to be reminded to use these to improve clarity of communication.
9. Do not argue with patient or correct them if mistakes are made.	Arguing can lead to increased frustration and agitation.
10. Maintain meaningful interactions with patients and use creative modes of communication based on patient's comfort level and abilities.	Meaningful interactions help patient engage with family or community and surroundings and help reduce sense of isolation and detachment.
11. Use individualized coping strategies such as progressive relaxation, breathing exercises, or guided imagery.	Helps reduce anxiety associated with confusion and difficulties in communication.

EVALUATION

STEP	RATIONALE
1. Observe patient's response for clarity and understanding of messages sent and received.	Observation determines extent to which cognitively impaired patient is able to express self.
2. Observe verbal and nonverbal behaviours.	Observation reveals whether patient is comfortable and needs have been met.
3. **Use teach-back:** "I want to be sure I explained how this picture board will help you communicate with your family. Tell me how to use the picture board to show your spouse that you want to take a shower or take a walk together." Develop a revised teaching plan if patient or caregiver is unable to teach back correctly.	Determines patient's and caregiver's level of understanding of teaching.

Unexpected Outcomes	Related Interventions
1. Messages that are sent and received are not understood.	• Continue to use therapeutic communication skills when interacting with cognitively impaired patient. Be creative in using alternative strategies (e.g., involving family members).
2. Patient becomes frustrated, and communication with nurse becomes more challenging.	• Remain patient and calm and speak in a soft voice (Twigg & Schwartzkopf, 2018). • Give patient time to respond and distract if possible. • Avoid touching; wait until patient is calmer. • Identify and address unmet needs (hunger, pain, toileting). • Allow for periods of adequate rest; make frequent attempts to interact to minimize social isolation.

Communication and Documentation

- Document both objective and subjective behaviours (associated with cognitive impairment) that patient is displaying on flow sheet or in progress notes in EHR or chart.
- Document and report the methods used to communicate with patient and patient's response.
- Document your evaluation of patient and caregiver learning.

DOCUMENTATION EXAMPLE

Patient frequently lost train of thought and struggled to organize words logically throughout encounter. Patient reported an inability to "find words" when they tried to tell their spouse what they wanted and implied frustration when being misunderstood. Patient was assisted to use picture board to show spouse that they wanted to go for a walk. Demonstrated understanding by pointing to the picture of people walking on communication board. Patient appeared pleased with ability to communicate as evidenced by smiling and relaxed posture. Patient and spouse demonstrated use of communication board. Plan made for patient and spouse to return on September 27, 2024, at 1000h for reassessment.

Special Considerations

Teaching

- Teach patient and caregiver how to use various methods to communicate, such as pictorial board or communication aids.
- Make teaching modifications with consideration of impaired concentration and memory related to patient's cognitive status (e.g., present a small amount of material at a time; use simple and short phrases; repeat information as needed).

Pediatric

- Children may exhibit cognitive impairments because of acute or persistent metabolic or neurological conditions. Communication strategies with children should take into consideration their developmental level. Use pictures and drawings for patients who are unable to read.

Gerontological

- Many older persons have cognitive impairments that pose serious barriers to the reliability of your assessment; therefore, it is important to use effective verbal and nonverbal communication strategies. Poor communication can compromise care, leading to increased anxiety and frustration.
- Patients who have cognitive impairments may exhibit tantrum-like behaviours in response to real or perceived frustration. Use distraction techniques to remove a cognitively impaired older person from disturbing stimuli or redirect patient to activity that is pleasurable (Twigg & Schwartzkopf, 2018).

Care in the Community: Home Management

- Manage care based on patient's presenting behaviours with consideration of any cognitive or physical impairment. Include the caregiver, family, and friends in using effective communication strategies.

✦ SKILL 3.4 Communicating With Colleagues

In health care settings communicating is a key part of everyday practice. As a nurse, you communicate with patients, members of the interprofessional health care team, and external colleagues. This communication occurs face to face, over the phone, and in writing. The quality of these interactions is a key component of error prevention; clarity and comprehension of treatment plans and adherence to them; and patient outcomes. Nevertheless, communication problems are common in health care settings, and failures in communication can have serious consequences (Müller et al., 2018). Interprofessional collaboration increases team members' awareness of each other's type of knowledge and skills, leading to continued improvement in decision making and patient outcomes. Moreover, teamwork and interprofessional collaboration are essential to quality patient care. Be aware of the differences in communication styles among members of the interprofessional team and adapt your style of communicating to effectively interact with team members (Kayser & Kaplan, 2020).

Conflict can arise when colleagues view issues or situations from different perspectives. Conflict that remains unresolved can have far-reaching effects that ultimately influence every aspect of patient care (CNO, 2018, p. 3; Kayser & Kaplan, 2020). If conflicts are not resolved, they can escalate into *workplace bullying*, which is abusive conduct that is threatening, humiliating, or intimidating and interferes with a productive work environment (Clark, 2019). Effective communication is necessary to resolve conflict among members of the health care team. Good communication in the form of conflict resolution skills can decrease the risk of conflict and its negative effects. Health care facilities need to be proactive in order to create healthy work environments, encouraging a shared philosophy of civility and respect (Clark, 2019).

Standardized communication using SBAR is structured to optimize effective communication among members of the health care team. Using SBAR, nurses are better prepared before calling a health care provider and when formulating a recommendation based on solid assessment. Nurses are more confident in their clinical judgement, resulting in better patient outcomes (Campbell & Dontje, 2019). Improved communication using structured communication techniques, including bedside reporting with the SBAR framework, streamlines information exchanges and promotes patient safety (e.g., important patient information does not get missed) (Campbell & Dontje, 2019). The evidence suggests that bedside reporting gives the oncoming nurse a chance for direct observation of a patient and a chance to ask questions related to the patient's status. This type of interaction promotes accountability between shifts. Bedside reporting and effective communication with the use of SBAR help to decrease adverse events and increase opportunities for units to move toward patient- and family-centred care (Campbell & Dontje, 2019). SBAR is one example of a simple interprofessional communication technique that can improve the culture of safety.

I-START-END (introductions–story–tasks–assignment–resources–timely–exiting–next–documentation–debriefing) is a communication tool that was created to improve the ability of health care providers to communicate in dynamic and often unpredictable settings. This tool provides a framework for interprofessional health care teams to work together effectively with patients, families, and one another, and to enhance communication. I-START-END is most commonly used during handover and team/family conferences.

Delegation and Collaboration

The skill of communicating effectively with colleagues can be delegated to a UCP. The nurse instructs the UCP about the following:

- The proper communication skills needed to effectively interact verbally and nonverbally with colleagues.

- The expectation that all members of the interprofessional health care team practise effective and respectful communication. Self-care workshops can be a means to enhance resilience and well-being and to create healing and healthy work environments (Barrett, 2019).

STEP	RATIONALE

ASSESSMENT

1. Identify purpose of interaction with colleague.	Sets the stage for the interaction; all members of the communication exchange are aware of purpose of the conversation.
2. Assess factors influencing communication with others (e.g., environment, timing, others' cultural beliefs and values, prior experiences).	Assessment allows you to accurately evaluate any barriers to communication or issues that may need to be considered to maintain open, clear channels of communication.
3. Consider level of stress in the situation; do you feel threatened?	Feeling threatened results in a sympathetic stress response that can impair judgement, emotional control, and ability to communicate clearly.

NURSING DIAGNOSES

- Decisional conflict
- Fear
- Altered coping
- Inadequate knowledge regarding communication skills
- Inadequate role performance
- Reduced social interaction
- Altered verbal communication

Related factors are individualized on the basis of patient's condition or needs.

PLANNING

1. Prepare for communication with members of the health care team who may have differing needs or concerns. Example: If you feel stressed, try to relax and use breathing exercises.	Effective communication allows members of the health care team to establish rapport and have a quality interaction. Adapt own style of communicating (e.g., relaxation) to meet the needs of the health care team.
2. Be aware of your nonverbal cues that affect communication with others. Remain nonjudgemental.	Frustration in communication may negatively affect interaction with others.
3. Prepare environment physically; go to a quiet, calm area. Reduce distractions such as external noises.	Factors to consider include privacy, noise control, seating space, and convenience to help ensure the space needed for effective teamwork.
4. Be aware that hierarchical differences among members of the health care team pose a common barrier to effective communication and collaboration.	Intimidating behaviour by individuals at the top of a hierarchy can hinder open communication.

IMPLEMENTATION

1. Approach colleague from the front and face directly when speaking. Maintain appropriate eye contact.	Strategy ensures that colleague both sees you and hears you and conveys an attitude of respect.
2. Provide a brief, simple introduction; introduce yourself and explain purpose of interaction.	Strategy ensures that colleague understands purpose of interaction.
3. Be aware of your own body language and tone. Assume an open stance; do not fold arms across your chest.	Nonverbal messages convey empathy. Be aware of how your nonverbal communication style may impact others.
4. Acknowledge and respond to a range of views. Allow equal time for all members to participate in expressing opinions.	Understand the perspectives of others and support the value of collaboration and teamwork.
5. Use effective verbal communication skills: ask open-ended questions, do not assume, do not interrupt, and do not blame others. Provide feedback. Use active listening and recognize nonverbal triggers. Ask for clarification when necessary.	Effective communication skills should be used for communicating and for resolving conflict.
6. Use a range of workplace written communication methods (e.g., verbal, written notes, memos, letters, charts, diagrams).	Standardized communication methods such as SBAR and I-START-END can help streamline information exchanges and promote patient safety.
7. Encourage discussion of both positive and negative feelings to increase opportunities for members to express all their concerns.	Discussion fosters active listening and understanding. All members of the exchange are valued and their contributions recognized.
8. Summarize key themes in the discussion and help develop alternative solutions to the issue.	Conflict resolution involves examining alternative solutions to an issue. It values the influence of system solutions in achieving effective functioning among colleagues (Kayser & Kaplan, 2020).

STEP	RATIONALE
EVALUATION	
1. Confirm clarity and understanding of messages sent and received.	Determines extent to which members of the exchange understand.
2. Observe verbal and nonverbal behaviours.	Observation reveals whether there are any negative emotions or further concerns that contradict a message.

Unexpected Outcomes	Related Interventions
1. Messages that are sent and received are not understood.	• Continue to use therapeutic communication skills when interacting with others. Be creative in using alternative strategies.
2. Frustration among colleagues persists, and communication becomes more challenging.	• Conflict among colleagues can have a direct impact on the nurse–patient relationship, affecting delivery of care (CNO, 2018). • Nurses should address conflict directly (CNO, 2018). Talk to colleague first; if that is not effective, consult your manager/director as appropriate for resolution, following employer policy. Continue to have empathy and use active listening to better understand colleagues.
3. Occurrence of bullying behaviours (verbal attacks, threats, spreading rumours and gossip, public ridicule, purposefully withholding vital information) (Clark, 2019).	• Follow employer policy to report behaviours immediately and seek assistance of security personnel if required.

✦ REVIEW QUESTIONS

You are assigned to care for an older patient (she/her) who was admitted to the hospital 2 days ago after falling at a family member's home. She recently moved in with her only child following the sudden death of her partner. Her partner (he/him) had been the primary caregiver since the patient's diagnosis with Alzheimer's disease 3 years ago. Neither her husband nor her son wanted to put her into a long-term or complex care facility. She had emergency surgery to repair a fractured wrist. During shift report on a medical-surgical unit, the nurse tells you that the patient is withdrawn and confused. In addition, she has difficulty understanding verbal direction from the interprofessional team members.

When you approach the patient to perform an initial assessment, she is looking out the window and seems disoriented. She appears dishevelled, and her lunch tray is untouched. You ask her whether she needs help with bathing, dressing, and feeding, but you get a response that you cannot understand. Her impaired communication is making the patient increasingly anxious, which is further hindering her communication with others and her ability to follow directions.

Review Questions 1 to 4 relate to the case study presented here.

1. Which steps are necessary to effectively communicate with a cognitively impaired patient?
2. Which strategies would you use to manage or decrease the patient's anxiety level? Explain your choice or choices.
3. Using the SBAR (situation–background–assessment–recommendation) format, describe strategies to communicate with the interprofessional team regarding the treatment plan for this patient.
4. The nurse is learning about barriers to effective nurse–patient communication. Which of the following approaches would be considered a barrier? (*Select all that apply.*)
   1. Discussing fears about a patient with members of the health care team
   2. Interrupting patient when the patient does not answer the question posed
   3. Obtaining information about a critically ill patient from their family
   4. Admitting a mistake to a patient's family
   5. Giving advice to the patient's health care provider
   6. Minimizing patient's concerns and issues
5. The nurse is caring for a patient recovering from a bilateral mastectomy for breast cancer who tearfully states that she is feeling depressed and worthless as a woman. Which of the following responses are therapeutic statements for the nurse to make? (*Select all that apply.*)
   1. "Many women have body image concerns after undergoing this surgery."
   2. "You will feel better soon."
   3. "Tell me more about how you feel."
   4. "Why do you feel depressed and worthless?"
   5. "How long have you been feeling this way?"
   6. "I am sure your husband will still love you no matter what you look like."
6. The nurse is caring for a patient with a cognitive impairment who is upset about not being able to describe what he wants to eat. The patient is talking loudly, which is annoying other patients. Which of the following actions would be **most** appropriate for the nurse to take? (*Select all that apply.*)
   1. Approach the patient from the front and make eye contact.
   2. Explain to the patient that he will benefit from acting calmer and not talking loudly.
   3. Ask the patient one question at a time about what he would like to eat.
   4. Use nonverbal communication methods.
   5. Ask family members which communication measures are successful at home.

Visit the Evolve site for a complete list of answers to the Review Questions.

✦ NEXT GENERATION NCLEX® (NGN)

For practice with answering exam questions related to unfolding NGN case studies, please consult the Next Generation NCLEX® (NGN)-Style Case Studies for Skills and Techniques on the Evolve website: http://evolve.elsevier.com/Canada/Perry/clinicalskills/

REFERENCES

Accreditation Canada. (2020). *Required organizational practices handbook*. https://physicians.nshealth.ca/resources/required-organizational-practices-2020-handbook

Almost, J. (2021). *Regulated nursing in Canada: The landscape in 2021*. Canadian Nurses Association. https://www.cna-aiic.ca/en/nursing/regulated-nursing-in-canada

Barrett, C. A. (2019). Self-care: A holistic nurse imperative. *AHNA Beginnings, 39*(3), 14.

Bingham, H., & O'Brien, A. J. (2018). Educational intervention to decrease stigmatizing attitudes of undergraduate nurses towards people with mental illness. *International Journal of Mental Health Nursing, 27*(1), 311–319. https://doi.org/10.1111/inm.12322

Byrd, L., & Luther, C. (2018). Anxiety and depression in the older adult. In K. Mauk (Ed.), *Gerontological nursing: Competencies for care* (4th ed., pp. 1362–1430). Jones & Bartlett Learning.

Campbell, D., & Dontje, K. (2019). Implementing bedside handoff in the emergency department: A practice improvement project. *Journal of Emergency Nursing, 45*(2), 149–154. https://doi.org/10.1016/j.jen.2018.09.007

Canadian Nurses Association. (2017). *Code of ethics for registered nurses*. https://www.cna-aiic.ca/en/nursing/regulated-nursing-in-canada/nursing-ethics

Canadian Nurses Association. (2021). *Regulated nursing in Canada: The landscape in 2021*. https://www.cna-aiic.ca/en/nursing/regulated-nursing-in-canada

Canadian Nurses Association. (2022). *Interprofessional collaboration*. https://www.cna-aiic.ca/en/nursing/nursing-tools-and-resources/interprofessional-collaboration

Clark, C. M. (2019). Accused of workplace bullying: What happens next? *American Nurse Today, 14*(3), 24–27. https://www.myamericannurse.com/accused-workplace-bullying/

College of Nurses of Ontario (CNO). (2018). *Practice guideline: Conflict prevention and management*. https://www.cno.org/globalassets/docs/prac/47004_conflict_prev.pdf

Crist, K., Laffery, M., Umberfield, E., et al. (2022). Which factors promote shared understanding between physicians and nurses in inpatient oncology care settings? A qualitative exploration. *Cancer Nursing, 45*(2), E338–E344. https://doi.org/10.1097/NCC.0000000000000959

Crosschild, C., & Varcoe, C. (2021). Piinaat'stikaanookiinan: A call to action for nursing leaders to decolonize nursing. *Nursing Leadership, 34*(4), 144–150. https://doi.org/10.12927/cjnl.2021.26677

Cusatis, R., Holt, J. M., Williams, J., et al. (2020). The impact of patient-generated contextual data on communication in clinical practice: A qualitative assessment of patient and clinician perspectives. *Patient Education and Counseling, 103*(4), 734–740. https://doi.org/10.1016/j.pec.2019.10.020

Dellosso, M. (2021). Anxiety: Every patient's silent enemy. *Home Healthcare Now, 39*(2), 118–119. https://doi.org/10.1097/NHH.0000000000000931

Ellis-Smith, C., Tunnard, I., Dawkins, M., et al. (2021). Managing clinical uncertainty in older people towards the end of life: A systematic review of person-centred tools. *BMC Palliative Care, 20*(1), 168. https://doi.org/10.1186/s12904-021-00845-9

Gasiorek, J., & van de Poel, K. (2018). Language-specific skills in intercultural healthcare communication: Comparing perceived preparedness and skills in nurses' first and second languages. *Nurse Education Today, 61*, 54–59. https://doi.org/10.1016/j.nedt.2017.11.008

Gerchow, L., Burka, L. R., Miner, S., et al. (2021). Language barriers between nurses and patients: A scoping review. *Patient Education and Counseling, 104*(3), 534–553. https://doi.org/10.1016/j.pec.2020.09.017

Giusti, A., Nkhoma, K., Petrus, R., et al. (2020). The empirical evidence underpinning the concept and practice of person-centred care for serious illness: A systematic review. *BMJ Global Health, 5*(12), Article e003330.

Hagelskjær, V., Krohn, M., Christensen, P. S., et al. (2019). Canadian occupational performance measure supported by talking mats: An evaluation of the clinical utility. *Occupational Therapy International, 2019*, Article 9367315. https://doi.org/10.1155/2019/9367315

Hancock, T. (2018). Mental health promotion must be a priority. *Canadian Medical Association Journal, 190*(16), ES22. https://doi.org/10.1503/cmaj.180464

Heslop, P., Turner, S., Read, S., et al. (2019). Implementing reasonable adjustments for disabled people in healthcare services. *Nursing Standard, 34*(8), 29–34. https://doi.org/10.7748/ns.2019.e11172

Karaminis, T., Hintz, F., & Scharenborg, O. (2022). The presence of background noise extends the competitor space in native and non-native spoken-word recognition: Insights from computational modeling. *Cognitive Science, 46*, Article e.13110. https://doi.org/10.1111/cogs.13110

Kayser, J., & Kaplan, L. (2020). Conflict management in the ICU. *Critical Care Medicine, 48*(9), 1349–1357. https://doi.org/10.1097/CCM.0000000000004440

Kennedy, E. (2018). Caring and communicating. In B. Kozier, G. Erb, A. Berman, et al. (Eds.), *Fundamentals of Canadian nursing: Concepts, process and practice* (4th ed., pp. 381–410). Pearson Canada.

Krysta, K., Romańczyk, M., Diefenbacher, A., et al. (2021). Telemedicine treatment and care for patients with intellectual disability. *International Journal of Environmental Research and Public Health, 18*(4), 1746. https://doi.org/10.3390/ijerph18041746

Lam, W., Wong, F. Y., & Chan, A. E. (2020). Factors affecting the levels of satisfaction with nurse-patient communication among oncology patients. *Cancer Nursing, 43*(4), 186–196. https://doi.org/10.1097/NCC.0000000000000672

Mayo Clinic. (2021). *Alzheimer's and dementia: Tips for effective communication*. https://www.mayoclinic.org/healthy-lifestyle/caregivers/in-depth/alzheimers/art-20047540

McKinney, E. S., James, S. R., Murray, S. S., et al. (2022). *Maternal-child nursing* (6th ed.). Elsevier.

Mendes, A., & Palmer, S. (2018). Communicating effectively with a person living with dementia. *British Journal of Nursing, 27*(2), 101. https://doi.org/10.12968/bjon.2018.27.2.101

Mock, M. S., & Sethares, K. A. (2019). Concurrent validity and acceptability of health literacy measures of adults hospitalized with heart failure. *Applied Nursing Research, 46*, 50–56. https://doi.org/10.1016/j.apnr.2019.02.007

Moloney, M., Hennessy, T., & Doody, O. (2021). Reasonable adjustments for people with intellectual disability in acute care: A scoping review of the evidence. *BMJ Open, 11*(2), Article e039647. https://doi.org/10.1136/bmjopen-2020-039647

Müller, M., Jürgens, J., Redaèlli, M., et al. (2018). Impact of the communication and patient hand-off tool SBAR on patient safety: A systematic review. *BMJ Open, 8*(8), Article e022202. https://doi.org/10.1136/bmjopen-2018-022202

Muscat, D. M., Smith, J., Mac, O., et al. (2021). Addressing health literacy in patient decision aids: An update from the International Patient Decision Aid Standards. *Medical Decision Making, 41*(7), 848–869. https://doi.org/10.1177/0272989X211011101

Nova Scotia College of Nursing (NSCN). (2018). *A guideline for nurses: Professional presence*. https://cdn3.nscn.ca/sites/default/files/documents/resources/ProfessionalPresence.pdf

Nova Scotia College of Nursing (NSCN). (2020). *Professional boundaries and the nurse–client relationship*. https://cdn3.nscn.ca/sites/default/files/documents/resources/ProfessionalBoundaries.pdf

Ondrejka, O. (2018). Teaching and communication with older adults and their families. In K. Mauk (Ed.), *Gerontological nursing: Competencies for care* (4th ed., pp. 524–619). Jones & Bartlett Learning.

Papadimitriou, C., Weaver, J. A., Guernon, A., et al. (2022). "Fluctuation is the norm": Rehabilitation practitioner perspectives on ambiguity and uncertainty in their work with persons in disordered states of consciousness after traumatic brain injury. *PLOS ONE, 17*(4), Article e0267194. https://doi.org/10.1371/journal.pone.0267194

Pepin, J. I., & Myrick, F. (2021). Critical consciousness in nursing education. *Quality Advancement in Nursing Education, 7*(2), 1–5. https://doi.org/10.17483/2368-6669.1327

Phillips, A., Niemiec, E., Howard, H. C., et al. (2020). Communicating genetic information to family members: Analysis of consent forms for diagnostic genomic sequencing. *European Journal of Human Genetics, 28*(9), 1160–1167. https://doi.org/10.1038/s41431-020-0627-7

Sanders, J. J., Curtis, J. R., & Tulsky, J. A. (2018). Achieving goal-concordant care: A conceptual model and approach to measuring serious illness communication and its impact. *Journal of Palliative Medicine, 21*(S2), S17–S27. https://doi.org/10.1089/jpm.2017.0459

Schill, K., & Caxaj, S. (2019). Cultural safety strategies for rural indigenous palliative care: A scoping review. *BMC Palliative Care, 18*(1), 21. https://doi.org/10.1186/s12904-019-0404-y

Statistics Canada. (2021). *Health characteristics, annual estimates–mood disorders by age group*. https://doi.org/10.25318/1310009601-eng

Sullivan, W. F., Diepstra, H., Heng, J., et al. (2018). Primary care of adults with intellectual and developmental disabilities: 2018 Canadian consensus guidelines. *Canadian Family Physician, 64*, 254–279. https://pubmed.ncbi.nlm.nih.gov/29650602/

Townsend, M. C., & Morgan, K. I. (2018). *Psychiatric mental health nursing: Concepts of care in evidence-based practice* (9th ed.). F. A. Davis Company.

Twigg, P., & Schwartzkopf, C. E. (2018). Nursing management of dementia. In K. Mauk (Ed.), *Gerontological nursing: Competencies for care* (4th ed., pp. 1091–1180). Jones & Bartlett Learning.

van Manen, A. S., Aarts, S., Metzelthin, S. F., et al. (2021). A communication model for nursing staff working in dementia care: Results of a scoping review. *International Journal of Nursing Studies, 113*, Article 103776. https://doi.org/10.1016/j.ijnurstu.2020.103776

Wanko Keutchafo, E. L., Kerr, J., & Jarvis, M. A. (2020). Evidence of nonverbal communication between nurses and older adults: A scoping review. *BMC Nursing, 19*, Article 53. https://doi.org/10.1186/s12912-020-00443-9

Wittenberg, E., Ferrell, B., Kanter, E., et al. (2018). Health literacy: Exploring nursing challenges to provide support and understanding. *Clinical Journal of Oncology Nursing, 22*(1), 53–61. https://doi.org/10.1188/18.CJON.53-61

Wittenberg, E., Goldsmith, J. V., Williams, Y., et al. (2020). Caring for family caregivers: A pilot test of an online COMFORT™ communication training module for undergraduate nursing students. *Journal of Cancer Education, 35*(1), 138–143. https://doi.org/10.1007/s13187-018-1452-3

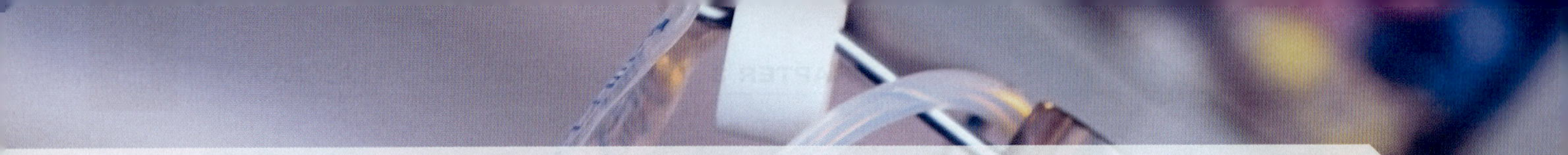

4 Documentation and Informatics

Canadian content written by **Joanne Newell, RN, MN**
Original US chapter by **Christine Durbin, PhD, JD, RN**

SKILLS AND PROCEDURES

Procedural Guideline 4.1 **Giving a Hand-Off Report, p. 62**

Procedural Guideline 4.2 **Documenting Progress Notes, p. 65**

Procedural Guideline 4.3 **Adverse Event/Incident Reporting, p. 66**

Procedural Guideline 4.4 **Guidelines for Meaningful Use of an Interoperable Electronic Health Record, p. 69**

OBJECTIVES

Mastery of content in this chapter will enable the nurse to:

- List guidelines for effective communication and reporting.
- Describe measures to maintain confidentiality of patient information.
- Identify the purpose of the patient record.
- Describe the elements of a hand-off report and when it would be used.
- Describe the role of digital technology in documentation and patient care.
- Explain the features and benefits of an electronic documentation system.
- Describe the elements of an SBAR hand-off report and when it would be used.
- Write a nurse's progress note using problem-oriented charting formats.
- Describe information found in a patient care profile, nursing kardex/patient care summary.
- Accurately complete a nursing flow sheet.
- Explain the guidelines used for documentation in long-term care and care in the community.
- Describe the role of critical pathways in interdisciplinary documentation.
- Complete an adverse event/incident report accurately.
- Describe the importance of medication reconciliation.

MEDIA RESOURCES

- http://evolve.elsevier.com/Canada/Perry/clinicalskills/

PURPOSE

Documentation is any information entered into a patient's electronic health record (EHR) or written in a patient record. The EHR (Fig. 4.1) is a longitudinal electronic record of patient health information generated by one or more encounters in a care delivery setting (Canada Health Infoway [CHI], 2018). The EHR includes information from multiple electronic medical records and health care providers (Accreditation Canada, 2020). Nursing documentation ensures continuity of care, provides legal evidence, and evaluates patient outcomes. The nurse's documentation provides a detailed account of a patient's plan of care, assessment, and treatment, which must be an accurate and timely evaluation of information. Electronic tools such as computers support documentation and patient care. Nursing informatics focuses on best practices with information and communication technology (Canadian Nurses Association [CNA], 2022).

STANDARDS OF CARE

- Accreditation Canada (2020)—*Required Organizational Practices Handbook* (https://physicians.nshealth.ca/resources/required-organizational-practices-2020-handbook)
- Canada Health Infoway (2021)—*Nursing Data Standards* (https://infocentral.infoway-inforoute.ca/en/standards/other-canadian/nursing-data-standards)
- Canadian Nurses Association (2017)—*Code of Ethics for Registered Nurses* (https://www.cna-aiic.ca/en/nursing/regulated-nursing-in-canada/nursing-ethics)
- Canadian Nurses Association (2022)—*Nursing Informatics* (https://www.cna-aiic.ca/en/nursing/nursing-tools-and-resources/nursing-informatics)
- Nova Scotia College of Nursing (2022)—*Documentation Guidelines for Nurses* (https://www.nscn.ca/professional-practice/practice-support/practice-support-tools/documentation/documentation-guidelines-nurses)

PRINCIPLES FOR PRACTICE

- All members of the health care team are legally and ethically obligated to keep patient information confidential and to adhere to

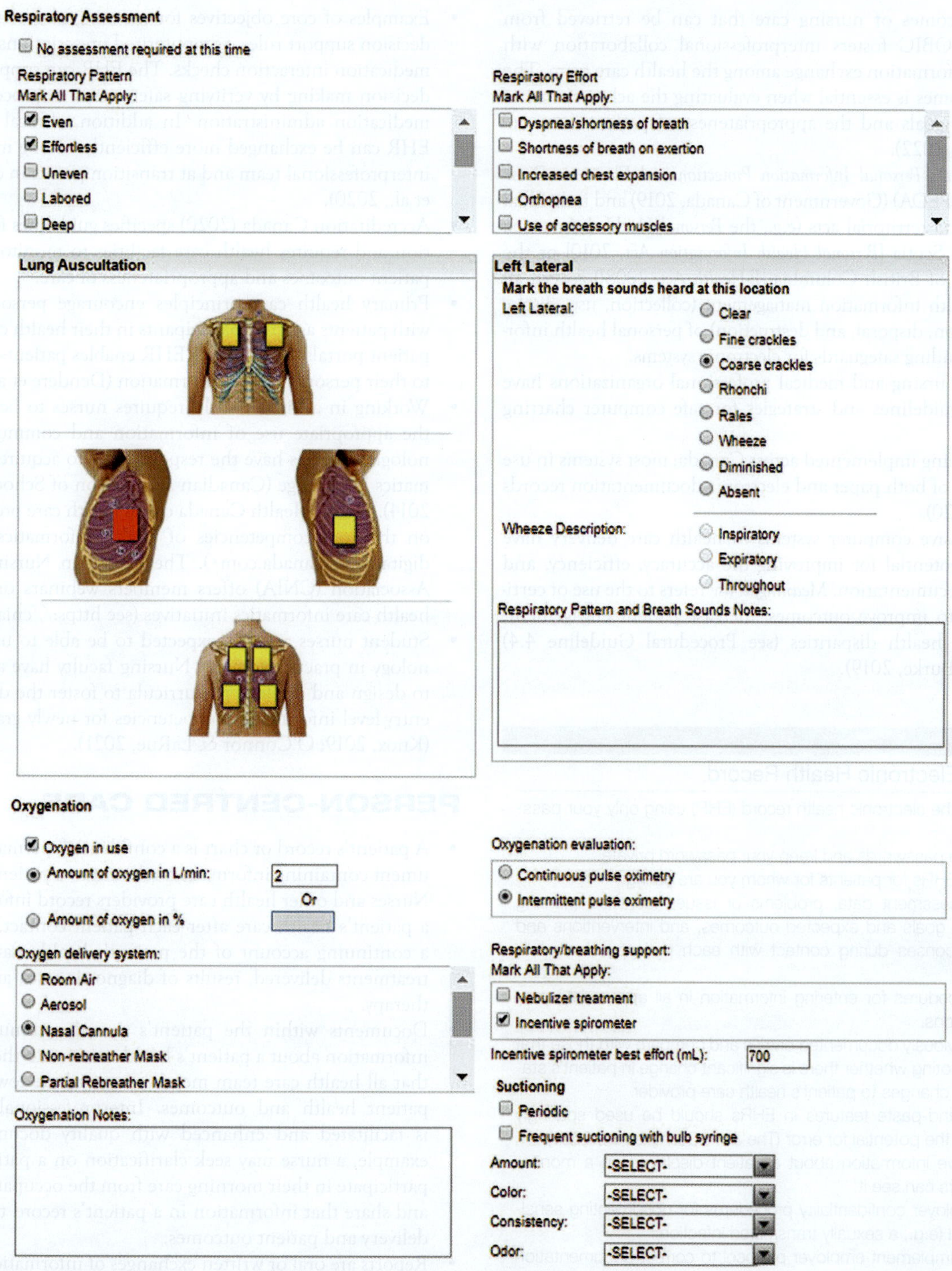

FIG 4.1 Computerized documentation provides many benefits. (*Williams, P. A. [2018]. deWit's fundamental concepts and skills for nursing [5th ed.]. Elsevier.*)

documentation standards (CNA, 2017; Canadian Nurses Protective Society [CNPS], 2020).

- Documentation occurs within the context of the nursing process, including documenting evidence of patient and family teaching and discharge planning (Nova Scotia College of Nursing [NSCN], 2022). Employer standards or policies often state the frequency of assessment; thus, it is essential to know the standards of your health care employer.
- Nursing diagnoses are part of the nursing care plan. They can be standardized (e.g., North American Nursing Diagnosis Association International [NANDA-I]; Olatubi et al., 2019) or employer or unit specific.
- The Nursing Interventions Classification (NIC) provides a list of nursing actions that are recognized internationally (Olatubi et al., 2019).
- Nursing Order Sets (NOS) provide a standardized list of evidence-informed interventions to address clinical conditions (Olatubi et al., 2019).
- The Canadian Health Outcomes for Better Information and Care (C-HOBIC) data set includes a list of measurable standardized

clinical outcomes of nursing care that can be retrieved from EHRs. C-HOBIC fosters interprofessional collaboration with improved information exchange among the health care team. The use of outcomes is essential when evaluating the achievement of patient care goals and the appropriateness of patient interventions (CNA, 2022).

- The Canadian *Personal Information Protection and Electronic Documents Act* (PIPEDA) (Government of Canada, 2019) and individual provincial and territorial acts (e.g., the *Personal Health Information Act* of Nova Scotia [*Personal Health Information Act*, 2010] or the *E-Health Act* of British Columbia [*E-Health Act*, 2008]) govern all areas of health information management (collection, use, disclosure, retention, disposal, and destruction) of personal health information, including safeguards for electronic systems.
- Numerous nursing and medical professional organizations have developed guidelines and strategies for safe computer charting (Box 4.1).
- EHRs are being implemented across Canada; most systems in use are a hybrid of both paper and electronic documentation records (Boothe, 2020).
- Comprehensive computer systems in health care delivery have unlimited potential for improving the accuracy, efficiency, and quality of documentation. *Meaningful use* refers to the use of certified EHRs to improve outcomes, increase patient engagement, and reduce health disparities (see Procedural Guideline 4.4) (Joneidy & Burke, 2019).

BOX 4.1

Use of the Electronic Health Record

- Sign on to the electronic health record (EHR) using only your password.
- Never share passwords and keep your password private.
- Only open EHRs for patients for whom you are caring.
- Review assessment data, problems or issues identified (nursing diagnoses), goals and expected outcomes, and interventions and patient responses during contact with each patient before data entry.
- Follow procedures for entering information in all appropriate program functions.
- Review previously documented entries and compare with those that you enter, noting whether there is significant change in patient's status. Report changes to patient's health care provider.
- The copy-and-paste features in EHRs should be used sparingly because of the potential for error (The Joint Commission, 2021).
- Do not leave information about a patient displayed on a monitor where others can see it.
- Follow employer confidentiality procedures for documenting sensitive material (e.g., a sexually transmitted infection).
- Know and implement employer protocol to correct documentation errors.
- Never create, change, or delete records unless your employer provides you with this authority.
- Software programs have a system for backup files. If you inadvertently delete part of the permanent record, follow employer policy. You must type an explanation into the computer file with the date, time, and your initials and submit an explanation in writing to your supervisor.
- Save information as documentation is completed.
- Protect printouts from computerized records. Shredding printouts and logging in the number of copies generated by each caregiver minimizes duplicate records and protects the confidentiality of patient information.
- Sign off when you leave the computer.

- Examples of core objectives for meaningful use include clinical decision support rules, computerized prescriptions, and real-time medication interaction checks. The EHR can support the nurse's decision making by verifying safety steps in procedures such as medication administration. In addition, clinical data from an EHR can be exchanged more efficiently among members of the interprofessional team and at transition points in care (Adamson et al., 2020).
- Accreditation Canada (2020) specifies guidelines for documentation and requires health care facilities to monitor and evaluate patient outcomes and appropriateness of care.
- Primary health care principles encourage person-centred care with patients as active participants in their health care. The use of patient portals to access the EHR enables patients to have access to their personal health information (Dendere et al., 2019).
- Working in a digital world requires nurses to be competent in the appropriate use of information and communication technologies. Nurses have the responsibility to acquire nursing informatics knowledge (Canadian Association of Schools of Nursing, 2014). Digital Health Canada offers health care providers courses on the core competencies of health informatics (see https://digitalhealthcanada.com/). The Canadian Nursing Informatics Association (CNIA) offers members webinars on nursing and health care informatics initiatives (see https://cnia.ca/).
- Student nurses are also expected to be able to use digital technology in practice settings. Nursing faculty have a responsibility to design and implement curricula to foster the development of entry-level informatics competencies for newly graduated nurses (Knox, 2019; O'Connor & LaRue, 2021).

PERSON-CENTRED CARE

- A patient's record or chart is a confidential, permanent legal document containing information relevant to a patient's health care. Nurses and other health care providers record information about a patient's health care after each patient contact. The record is a continuing account of the patient's health status and needs, treatments delivered, results of diagnostic tests, and response to therapy.
- Documents within the patient's record communicate specific information about a patient's health status and the interventions that all health care team members contribute toward improving patient health and outcomes. Interprofessional collaboration is facilitated and enhanced with quality documentation. For example, a nurse may seek clarification on a patient's ability to participate in their morning care from the occupational therapist and share that information in a patient's record to improve care delivery and patient outcomes.
- Reports are oral or written exchanges of information among caregivers (Fig. 4.2). Reports include information about a patient's clinical status, observations made about their behaviour, data pertaining to diagnostic tests, and directions for changes in therapy. Common reports given by nurses include telephone reports, transfer reports, and adverse event/incident reports (see Procedural Guideline 4.3).
- When a nurse receives a verbal prescription or critical test result, the nurse writes down the prescription or critical test result as it is given and then reads it back to the individual who has given the prescription. By stating the information back (called the *read-back*) to the individual giving the prescription or test result, the nurse verifies that the complete prescription or test result has been received and understood (NSCN, 2022).

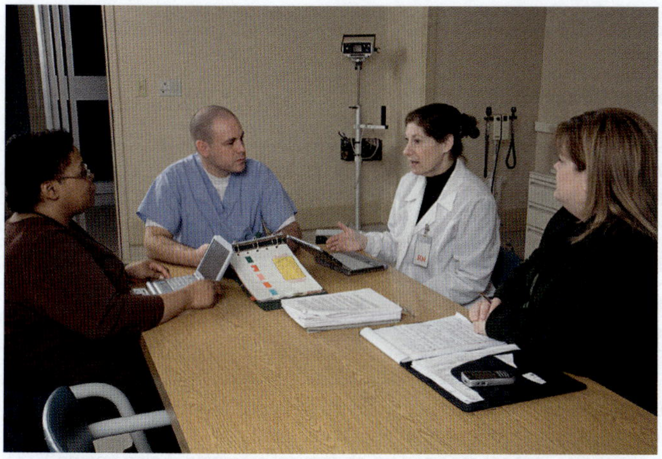

FIG 4.2 Communication among members of the health care team.

- Patient hand-off reports (see Procedural Guideline 4.1), a standardized approach to communication of patient information among caregivers, are being used by many health care facilities.
- A nurse should avoid using gender-specific pronouns when documenting, to respect gender diversity.

EVIDENCE-INFORMED PRACTICE

EHRs and digital technology have major implications for person-centred care, patient engagement, and evidence-informed practice. Basic nursing care interventions can be documented to provide meaningful data to the health care team.

- Use of EHRs improves patient outcomes, interprofessional communication, and collaboration for patients admitted to the critical care unit (Anderson, 2022).
- Quality EHRs allow retrieval of data to improve patient outcomes. For example, data are retrieved from EHRs when patients are identified and matched to their active medication lists. The bar coding of medications can reduce errors because the data retrieved match the right patients to the right medications (Strudwick et al., 2018).
- Nursing outcomes can be measured efficiently with EHRs. Incorporating an EHR promoted decision making and was connected with positive outcomes in the practice setting (Ardic & Turan, 2021).
- Nursing management of chronic diseases such as asthma can be done more effectively with EHRs. The EHR supports the sharing of data between health care settings and throughout the continuum of care. The access to data is more timely and the extraction of data is more efficient because of the standardization of language found in EHRs (Lougheed et al., 2018).
- Use of EHRs by nurses in clinical practice has been correlated with nurse satisfaction. Nurses who use fully electronic health records report a higher degree of satisfaction compared with nurses using a hybrid of paper and electronic systems (CHI, 2020).
- Use of digital technology, such as patient portals, has been associated with improved patient satisfaction, improved communication with health care providers, and increased patient engagement (Dendere et al., 2019; Stewart et al., 2020).
- Hands-free wireless devices (e.g., the Smartbadge developed by Vocera Communications [https://vocera.com]) have been effective in fostering interprofessional communication and workflow efficiency (Carreon & Dutra, 2020).

SAFETY GUIDELINES

- Quality documentation and reporting must be factual, accurate, complete, concise, current, and organized. Quality documentation must follow standardized safety, legal, and best practice guidelines.

Factual

- Factual data contain descriptive, objective information about what a nurse sees, hears, feels, and smells. Subjective data included in a record consists of statements that the patient actually verbalizes. Write subjective information with quotation marks, using the patient's exact words whenever possible. For example, record, "Patients states, 'My stomach hurts.'"

Accurate

- Data should be charted in measurable terms. The use of exact measurements in documentation establishes accuracy. For example, charting that an abdominal wound is "5 cm in length without redness, edema, or drainage" is more descriptive than "large wound healing well." Documenting that wound drainage is the "size of a quarter" versus "a lot of blood" provides more accurate information to inform clinical decisions.

Complete

- The information within a recorded entry or a report must be complete and contain appropriate and essential information. There are criteria for reporting and documenting information for health problems or nursing activities (Table 4.1).
- All entries in medical records must be dated and a method established to identify the authors of the entries. Each entry in a patient's record ends with the caregiver's full name or initials and status. A nursing student enters their full name, student nurse abbreviation (e.g., SN, NS), and educational institution, such as "David Jones, DalSN" (Dalhousie University [Dal] student nurse). An EHR generates the nurse's name and initials when the entry is submitted.

Concise

- Data need to be clear, to the point, and easy to understand. Avoid using unnecessary words and irrelevant detail. A concise statement provides a succinct description of the patient's situation and includes the most important information. For example, inclusion of the fact that a patient is watching television is only necessary when this activity is significant to the patient's status and plan.

Current

- Current documentation includes making timely entries in a patient's record, which avoids omissions and delays in patient care (CNPS, 2020; NSCN, 2022). To increase accuracy and decrease unnecessary duplication, many health care facilities locate medical records near a patient's bedside, which facilitates immediate documentation of care activities. The following activities or findings should be documented at the time of occurrence:
  - Vital signs
  - Pain assessment and evaluation
  - Administration of medications and treatments
  - Preparation for diagnostic tests or surgery
  - Change in patient's status and who was notified
  - Treatment for a sudden change in patient's status
  - Patient response to intervention
  - Admission, transfer, discharge, or death of patient

TABLE 4.1

Examples of Criteria for Communicating and Documenting

Topic	Criteria to Communicate or Document
Assessment	
Subjective data	Description of episode/event in patient's words in quotation marks. Clarify onset, location, description of condition (severity; duration; frequency; precipitating, aggravating, and relieving factors)
Patient behaviour (e.g., anxiety, confusion, hostility)	Onset, behaviours exhibited, precipitating factors
Objective data (e.g., rash, tenderness, breath sounds)	Onset, location, size, description of condition (severity; duration; frequency; precipitating, aggravating, and relieving factors)
Nursing Interventions and Evaluation	
Treatments (e.g., enema, bath, dressing change)	Time administered, equipment used (if appropriate), patient's response (objective and subjective changes) compared with previous treatment (e.g., rated pain 2 on a scale of 0–10 during dressing change or "patient reported no abdominal cramping during enema")
Medication administration	Immediately after administration, document the following: time medication given, dose, route, any preliminary assessment (e.g., pain level, vital signs), patient response or effect of medication. For example: "1200: Patient reports pain level 7 (scale 0 being no pain and 10 being worst pain ever). 12:30: Acetaminophen 650 mg given PO. 1330: Patient reports pain level 2 (scale 0–10)."
Patient teaching	Information presented; method of instruction (e.g., discussion, demonstration, videos, booklet); patient response, including questions and evidence of understanding such as return demonstration or change in behaviour
Discharge planning	Measurable patient goals or expected outcomes, progress toward goals, need for referrals

- Military time, a 24-hour system that prevents misinterpretation of morning and evening hours, is recommended to record the time of events. The military clock ends with midnight at 2400 and begins 1 minute after midnight at 0001. For example, 1:00 p.m. is 1300 military time, and 10:22 a.m. is 1022 military time. Fig. 4.3 compares military and civilian time. An EHR generates the time of entry when the nurse submits the entry.

Organized

- Information in the health record should be documented in a logical order following the steps of the nursing process. Application of the nursing process will assist in the documentation of pertinent information in a clear, comprehensive, and logical order. For example, an organized entry would describe a patient's pain, your assessment, resultant interventions, and the patient's response to the treatment provided.

Safety Principles

- Healthcare Excellence Canada (2020) (formerly the Canadian Patient Safety Institute) requires that health care facilities standardize abbreviations, symbols, acronyms, and dose designations and establish a list of abbreviations in accordance with the Institute for Safe Medication Practices (ISMP)'s *List of Error-Prone Abbreviations, Symbols, and Dose Designations* (ISMP, 2021). It is essential to know your employer abbreviation list and to use only the accepted abbreviations, symbols, and measures (e.g., metric) so that all documentation is accurate and in compliance with standards. For example, the abbreviation for *every day (qd)* **is no longer used** (Box 4.2). If a treatment or medication is needed daily, the written prescription or care plan should write out "daily" or "every day." The abbreviation *qd (every day)* can be misinterpreted to mean *O.D. (right eye)*. Neither abbreviation (i.e., qd, OD) is acceptable for use.

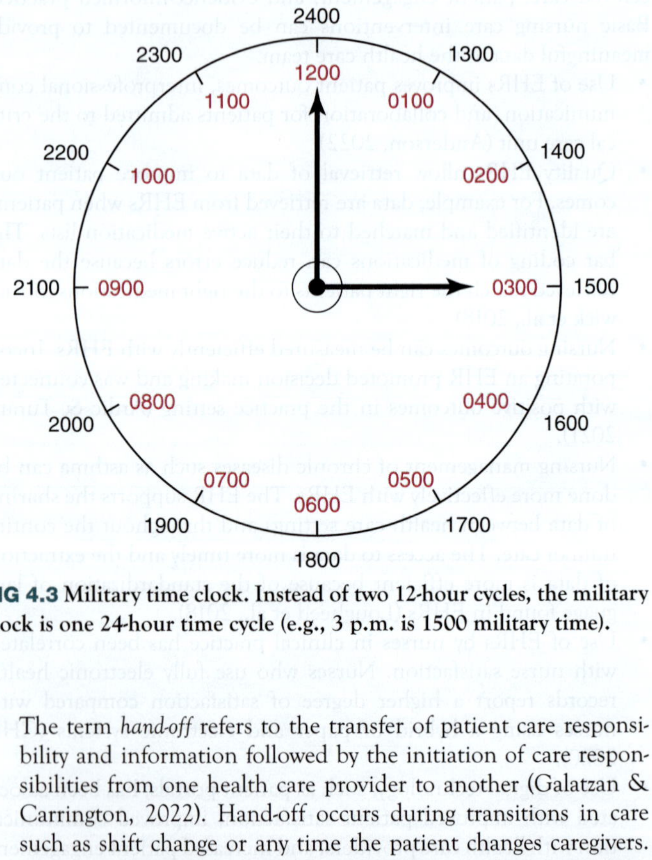

FIG 4.3 Military time clock. Instead of two 12-hour cycles, the military clock is one 24-hour time cycle (e.g., 3 p.m. is 1500 military time).

- The term *hand-off* refers to the transfer of patient care responsibility and information followed by the initiation of care responsibilities from one health care provider to another (Galatzan & Carrington, 2022). Hand-off occurs during transitions in care such as shift change or any time the patient changes caregivers. Key transition times include shift changes, rounds, moving from one organization to another or to another community provider, or even at the end of service (Accreditation Canada, 2020). Effective hand-off allows for face-to-face communication when available, which gives the care provider the opportunity to ask questions.

BOX 4.2

Official "Do Not Use" Abbreviations

Do Not Use	Potential Problem	Use Instead
U, u (unit)	Mistaken for "0" (zero), the number "4" (four), or "cc"	Use "unit"
IU (International Unit)	Mistaken for "IV" (intravenous) or the number "10" (ten)	Use "International Unit"
Q.D., QD, q.d., qd (daily)	Mistaken for one another	Use "daily"
Q.O.D., QOD, q.o.d, qod (every other day)	Period after the Q mistaken for "I" and the "O" mistaken for "I"	Use "every other day"
Trailing zero (X.0 mg)	Decimal point is missed	Use X mg
Lack of leading zero (.X mg)		Use 0.X mg
MS	Can mean morphine sulphate or magnesium sulphate	Use "morphine sulphate"
MSO_4 and $MgSO_4$	Confused for one another	Use "magnesium sulphate"

Adapted from Institute of Safe Medication Practices. (2018). *Do not use: Dangerous abbreviations, symbols, and dose designations*. https://www.ismp-canada.org/download/ISMPCanadaListOfDangerousAbbreviations.pdf

- During hand-off, the sender of the patient information initially presents the patient name, room number, age, gender, resuscitation status, diagnosis, medical history, and discharge planning. This is followed by patient vital signs and clinical assessments, changes in clinical condition, medication review, fluid balance, and patient safety risk assessment factors. Once hand-off is completed, the receiver of the information is given an opportunity to ask questions and confirm understanding. Incomplete or incomprehensible information can negatively affect a patient's safety. A comprehensive hand-off involves not only information sharing but also the acceptance and effective transfer of all patient authority and responsibility (Galatzan & Carrington, 2022).
- Common communication and documentation errors include (1) failing to document the correct time of events, (2) failing to record verbal prescriptions or have them signed, (3) charting actions in advance to save time, (4) documenting incorrect data, and (5) failing to give a report or giving an incomplete report to an oncoming shift. Nurses must be aware of the legal guidelines for documentation and reporting (Table 4.2).

COMMON RECORD-KEEPING FORMS OR SCREENS

The patient chart or medical record contains evidence of a patient's health status. The chart includes a variety of forms or screens (as in the case of EHRs) to facilitate quick and comprehensive documentation. Use of these forms or screens helps avoid duplication of information within the record.

Admission Nursing History Forms or Screens

A nurse completes a comprehensive nursing history form or screen to gather baseline assessment data when a patient is admitted to a nursing care unit. The nurse uses the admission data to form a plan of care and compare it with any changes in a patient's condition. The nursing history guides the admitting nurse through a complete assessment to identify relevant nursing issues or problems for the patient's care plan. Examples of information included in the nursing history are patient allergies, primary spoken/written language, advance directives, disabilities, mobility and fall risk, and medication reconciliation.

Flow Sheets and Graphic Records

Flow sheets and graphic records, which are used in both EHRs and paper charts, enable concise documentation of nursing information and patient data over time. They are especially useful for the documentation of routine observations or repeated specific measurements for a patient, such as vital signs (see Chapter 7), intake and output, hygiene measures, medication administration (see Chapter 20), and pain assessment. Flow sheets have a format or system for the entry of information, usually every 24 hours (Fig. 4.4). When you are documenting a significant change that you recognize on a flow sheet, describe the change in the progress notes, including the patient's response to nursing interventions. For example, if a patient's blood pressure becomes dangerously low, record in the progress notes the blood pressure, relevant assessment such as pallor or dizziness, and any interventions to raise the blood pressure. Also include an evaluation of the interventions, such as repeated blood pressures and relief of dizziness. Other health care providers may have the responsibility to document on nursing flow sheets or screens.

Patient Education Record

Many employers have an education record that identifies a patient's knowledge base about their diagnosis, treatment, and medications. The goal of patient and family education is to promote person-centred care by involving the patient, family, or both in self-care and decisions, which improves health outcomes. Standards for patient education include assessment of needs, functional abilities, learning styles, and readiness to learn (Flanders, 2018). The nurse should base patient education needs on the assessment and then teach patients about topics such as safe and effective use of medications, nutrition and dietary modifications, safe use of medical equipment, pain control, rehabilitative methods to promote and improve functional abilities, and self-care activities. When documenting on a patient teaching record, it is important to be specific about the information and skills taught, the patient's learning response, and information given to the patient.

Patient Care Summary or Kardex

Many health care facilities have computerized systems that provide a concise record of patient information in the form of a patient care summary or computer-generated kardex. This summary prints out for each patient during each shift. Data are updated automatically as new prescriptions and nursing decisions enter the system.

In some health care settings, a written kardex produced on a "cardboard flip-over" file is kept at the nurses' station. Parts of the kardex have information recorded in pencil, allowing changes to be made to patient information, which prevents it from being considered a legal document. The updated information in the patient summary or kardex eliminates the need for repeated referral to the chart for routine information throughout the day. The effectiveness of these forms as a communication tool is contingent on timely updates to patient information and transfer of prescriptions. Failure of the nurse to transfer a prescription to the kardex could result in an adverse event/incident and the nurse being liable. The patient care summary or kardex does not always become part of the permanent record (check employer policy). Information commonly found on the patient care summary or kardex includes the following:

- Basic demographic data (e.g., age, religion)
- Primary medical diagnosis

TABLE 4.2

Legal Guidelines for Documentation and Reporting

Guideline	Rationale	Correct Action
Use only your unique user identification and password to log onto the EHR.	An electronic signature is associated with each user identification and password login.	Protect the security of your user identification and password. Once logged on to the computer, do not leave the computer screen unattended.
Do not erase, apply correction fluid, or scratch out errors made while recording in a paper record.	The reason and content of the correction is understood (NSCN, 2022). Prevents accusations of defacing patient records and maintains legibility of the erroneous entry.	Draw single line through error, write word *error* or *mistaken entry* above it, and sign your name or initials. Then document note correctly. Check employer policy (NSCN, 2022).
Do not write retaliatory or critical comments about patient or care by other health care providers.	Statements can be used as evidence for nonprofessional behaviour or poor quality of care.	Enter only objective descriptions of patient's behaviour; use quotation marks for patient's comments.
Need to add patient information.	New information is acquired.	If additional information is to be added to an existing entry, write the date and time of the new entry in the next available space and mark it as an addendum (date and time of prior note).
	Forgot to chart during a shift.	Write the current date and time in the next available space and mark it as a late entry (date and time/shift missed).
Correct all errors promptly.	Errors in recording can lead to errors in treatment.	Avoid rushing to complete charting; be sure that information is accurate.
Document all facts.	Record must be accurate and reliable.	Be certain that entry is factual; do not speculate or guess.
Document all entries legibly and follow employer policy regarding colour of permanent ink for paper records (NSCN, 2022).	Illegible entries can be misinterpreted, causing errors and lawsuits; permanent ink cannot be erased and is more legible when records are photocopied or scanned.	**Never** erase entries, and **never** use correction fluid/tape or pencil. Use enough pressure so the ink will be dark in colour.
If prescription is questioned, record that you sought clarification.	If you perform an incorrect prescription, you are just as liable for prosecution as the health care provider that prescribed it.	Do not document "physician made error." Instead, chart that "Dr. Smith was called to clarify prescription for analgesic."
Chart only for yourself.	You are accountable for information that you document on the chart.	Never document for someone else. **Exception:** If caregiver has left unit for day and calls with information that needs to be documented, include the name of the source of information in the entry and that the information was provided via telephone.
Avoid using generalized, empty phrases such as "status unchanged" or "had good day."	Specific information about patient's condition or case can be deleted accidentally if information is too generalized.	Use complete, concise descriptions of care.
Begin each entry with time, and end each entry with your signature and title.	This guideline ensures that correct sequence of events is documented; signature indicates who is accountable for care delivered.	Do not wait until end of shift to document important changes that occurred several hours earlier; be sure to sign each entry.

EHR, Electronic health record.

- Current health care provider's prescriptions (e.g., diet, activity, dressing changes)
- Plan of care
- Nursing orders or interventions (e.g., intake and output, comfort measures, teaching)
- Scheduled tests and procedures
- Safety precautions used in the patient's care
- Factors related to activities of daily living
- Nearest relative or guardian or person to contact in an emergency
- Resuscitative care plan information (e.g., do not resuscitate [DNR], allow natural death [AND])
- Allergies

Acuity Records

Many health care facilities use a patient acuity system as a method of determining the intensity of nursing care required for a group of patients. Acuity measurements for patients on a unit serve as a guide for determining staffing needs. An acuity recording system determines the hours of nursing care and number of staff required for a nursing unit.

Typically, nurses enter acuity data into a computerized system in the morning. The administrative staff collect the acuity data electronically and use them to make appropriate staffing decisions. Acuity levels allow the nursing staff to compare patients with one another. For example, an acuity system might rate bathing patients from 1 to 5 (1 is totally dependent, 5 is independent); a patient returning from surgery who requires frequent monitoring and extensive care has an acuity level of 1. On the same continuum, another patient awaiting discharge after a successful recovery from surgery has an acuity level of 5. Accurate acuity ratings justify the number and qualifications of staff needed to safely care for patients on a particular unit.

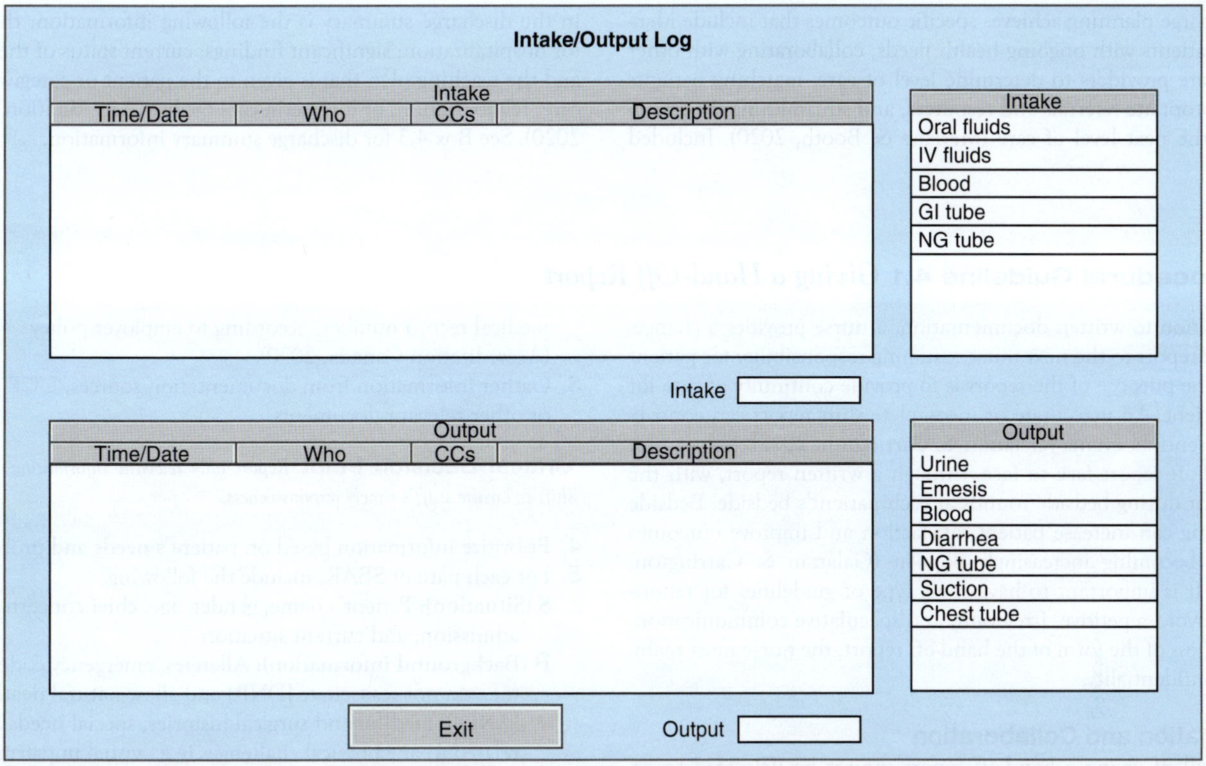

FIG 4.4 **Graphic and intake–output record, electronic version.** (*Courtesy ER Choice, Irving, TX.*)

Standardized Care Plans

The trend among many health care facilities is to computerize care plans. These systems provide daily computer-generated care plans, which incorporate several nursing diagnoses or problems in a single nursing or interprofessional plan of care. These systems improve documentation and facilitate high-quality care that is based on scientific evidence and past experiences (CHI, 2018). Standardized care plans are based on standards of clinical practice and established guidelines used to care for patients with similar health problems. Standardized care plans are often used with postoperative patients–for example, a care plan for a patient having bowel surgery. As the nurse, after completing a nursing assessment, identify the patient's nursing diagnosis or health problem and select an appropriate standardized care plan for the patient medical record. Always individualize it for each patient. Most standardized care plans allow for the addition of patient-specific outcomes and target dates for achieving these outcomes.

One advantage of standardized care plans is the establishment of evidence-informed standards of care. By using standardized plans, nurses learn to recognize the accepted requirements of care for patients. Implementation of digital standardized plans improves continuity of care among professional nurses (Østensen et al., 2020).

One disadvantage of standardized care plans is an increased risk that the unique, individualized therapies needed by patients will go unrecognized. Standardized care plans do not replace clinical judgement, critical thinking, and clinical reasoning. In addition, care plans need to be updated on a regular basis to ensure that content is current and appropriate.

Discharge Summaries

The discharge summary includes essential information for the patient, caregiver, and health care facility (Box 4.3) and is based on data obtained from the discharge planning process. Discharge planning is a comprehensive process with emphasis placed on preparing a patient for discharge. Nurses enhance discharge planning when they are responsive to changes in a patient's condition and involve the patient and caregiver in the planning process (Schjødt et al., 2022).

There must be evidence of the patient's and caregiver's involvement in the discharge planning process so that they have the necessary information and resources to return home (Schjødt et al., 2022). Accreditation Canada (2020) has standards for patient education required for effective discharge planning. When a patient is discharged from a health care facility, the members of the health care team prepare a discharge summary. It provides important information relating to the patient's ongoing health problems and need for health care after discharge.

BOX 4.3

Discharge Summary Information

- Use clear, concise descriptions in patient's own language.
- Provide step-by-step description of how to perform a procedure (e.g., home medication administration). Reinforce explanation with printed instructions for patient to take home.
- Provide a detailed list of all prescribed medications.
- Identify precautions to follow when performing self-care or administering medications.
- Review any restrictions that may relate to activities of daily living (e.g., bathing, ambulating, and driving).
- Review signs and symptoms of complications to report to health care provider.
- List names and phone numbers of health care providers and community resources for patient to contact.
- Identify any unresolved problems, including plans for follow-up and continuous treatment.
- List actual time of discharge, mode of transportation, and who accompanied patient.

Discharge planning achieves specific outcomes that include identifying patients with ongoing health needs, collaborating with other health care providers to determine level of care, matching patients with appropriate referrals and resources, and streamlining the transition to the next level of care (Merlane & Booth, 2020). Included in the discharge summary is the following information: the reason for hospitalization; significant findings; current status of the patient; and the teaching plan that is given to the patient or caregiver, home care, rehabilitation, or long-term care facility (Accreditation Canada, 2020). See Box 4.3 for discharge summary information.

Procedural Guideline 4.1 *Giving a Hand-Off Report*

In addition to written documentation, a nurse provides a change-of-shift report to the next nurse assuming responsibility for patient care. The purpose of the report is to provide continuity of care for the patient. An inaccurate or incomplete shift report can contribute to sentinel events (Galatzan & Carrington, 2022). Nurses give a hand-off report face to face, through a written report, with the EHR, or during bedside rounds at each patient's bedside. Bedside reporting can increase patient satisfaction and improve outcomes and is becoming increasingly popular (Galatzan & Carrington, 2021). It is important to have some type of guidelines for reporting to avoid repetitive, irrelevant, and speculative communication. Regardless of the form of the hand-off report, the nurse must maintain confidentiality.

Delegation and Collaboration

The skill of giving a hand-off report cannot be delegated to an unregulated care provider (UCP). The nurse directs the UCP to do the following:

- Report to the nurse (e.g., increased pain, changes in vital signs) so the nurse can reassess, validate, and report any changes in the hand-off report

Equipment

- Worksheets, patient care summary or nursing kardex, plan of care, critical pathway, or interprofessional treatment plan
- EHR (if implemented by employer)

Procedural Steps

1. Use an organized format for delivering report that provides a description of patient needs and problems. SBAR (situation–background–assessment–recommendation) can be used to organize and streamline reporting (Shahid & Thomas, 2018).
2. Identify the electronic patient record using at least two identifiers (e.g., name and date of birth, or name and medical record number) according to employer policy (Accreditation Canada, 2020).
3. Gather information from documentation sources, UCP report, or other relevant documents.

Critical Decision Point *Report only relevant information to next shift to ensure staff's timely responsiveness.*

4. Prioritize information based on patient's needs and problems.
5. For each patient SBAR, include the following:
   S (Situation): Patient's name, gender, age, chief concern on admission, and current situation
   B (Background information): Allergies, emergency code status (i.e., do not resuscitate [DNR] and allow natural death [AND]), medical and surgical histories, special needs as related to any physical challenges (e.g., visual impairment, hearing deficit, amputee), and immunizations
   A (Assessment data): Objective observations and measurements made by the nurse during the shift; emphasis on any recent changes
   Include any relevant information reported by patient, caregiver, or health care team members such as laboratory data and diagnostic test results. Include therapies or treatments administered during shift and expected outcomes (e.g., medication changes, use of oxygen, referral visits). Describe education given in the teaching plan and caregiver's ability to demonstrate learning. Report on evaluation by explaining patient's response and whether outcomes are met. Review patient's progress toward discharge during each change-of-shift report.
   R (Recommendation): Explanation of the priorities to which the oncoming nurse must attend, including referrals, nursing orders, and core measures
   Ask staff from the oncoming shift whether they have any questions regarding the information provided.

CHARTING SYSTEMS

A variety of documentation systems (computerized and written) exist for recording patient information and progress (Box 4.4). The documentation system selected by nursing reflects the philosophy of the health care facility. The same documentation system is used throughout a specific facility, but there are several acceptable methods for recording health care data.

Narrative Documentation

Narrative charting uses a story-like format to document specific information about a patient's conditions and nursing care, usually presented in chronological order. It is useful in emergency situations when the time and order of events are important. A narrative should be organized in a clear, concise way (e.g., by using the nursing process to order the data).

Problem-Oriented Medical Records

A problem-oriented medical record (POMR) is a structured method of documenting narratives that emphasizes a patient's problems. This method organizes data using the nursing process, which facilitates communication about patient needs. Data are organized by problem or diagnosis. Ideally, interprofessional collaboration should occur so that all members of the health care team can contribute to the list of identified patient issues. This approach helps to coordinate an individualized plan of care with the following sections: database, problem list, care plan, and progress notes.

Patient Database

A database contains all available information pertaining to a patient. This section is the foundation for identifying patient issues and problems and for planning care. The database remains active and current for each patient and is revised as new data become available.

BOX 4.4

Formats for Recording Progress Notes

Narrative Note

Describes patient data in a narrative paragraph

Example

Patient states, "I'm dreading this surgery because last time I had a terrible reaction to the anaesthesia and such terrible pain when they made me get out of bed." Noted muscle tension and loud, agitated voice. Notified anaesthesiologist of patient's prior experience. Discussed alternatives for anaesthesia and pain control options. Stressed importance of activity for circulation and healing. Encouraged patient to keep nurses informed of pain level and need for medication and that pain may be present but manageable.

SBAR (Situation–Background–Assessment–Recommendation)

System of structured communication used to share information about a patient's condition

Example

S (Situation): Patient verbalized preoperative fears. Nurse noted muscle tension and loud, agitated voice.

B (Background): Patient fearful of surgery because of past experiences with anaesthesia and pain.

A (Assessment): BP: 160/84, T: 37°C (98.6°F); P: 86; RR: 18. O_2 saturation: 96%. Skin warm and dry to touch. Respirations even and unlaboured.

R (Recommendation): Encourage patient to discuss preoperative fears. Assess pain level at least every 4 hours after surgery. Provide nonpharmacological pain management techniques and administer prescribed medication as needed.

SOAP (Subjective Data–Objective Data–Assessment–Plan)

Usually based on a numbered list of problems or nursing diagnoses

Example

S (Subjective data—patient's statements regarding the problem): Patient states, "I'm dreading this surgery because last time I had a terrible reaction to the anaesthesia and such terrible pain when they made me get out of bed."

O (Objective data—observations that support or are related to subjective data): Noted muscle tension and loud, agitated voice.

A (Assessment/Analysis—conclusions reached on basis of data): Fear related to pain/anaesthesia.

P (Plan—plan for dealing with the situation): Notified anaesthesiologist, Dr. Martin, of patient's prior experience. Discussed alternatives for anaesthesia and pain control options. Stressed importance of activity for circulation and healing. Encouraged patient to keep nurses informed of pain level and need for medication and that pain may be present but manageable.

PIE (Problem–Intervention–Evaluation)

Problem-oriented system in which progress notes are written on the basis of a list of identified problems; detailed data may be entered by any member of the health care team

Example

P (Problem): Patient states, "I'm dreading this surgery because last time I had a terrible reaction to the anaesthesia and such terrible pain when they made me get out of bed." Noted muscle tension and loud, agitated voice.

I (Intervention): Notified anaesthesiologist, Dr. Martin, of patient's prior experience. Discussed alternatives for anaesthesia and pain control options. Stressed importance of activity for circulation and healing. Encouraged patient to keep nurses informed of pain level and need for medication and that pain may be present but manageable.

E (Evaluation): Patient stated that they were "very relieved." Stated that they would tell the nurses about pain.

Focus or DAR Charting (Data–Action–Response)

A way to organize progress notes to make them clearer and organized

Example

D (Data): Patient states, "I'm dreading this surgery because last time I had a terrible reaction to the anaesthesia and such terrible pain when they made me get out of bed." Noted muscle tension and loud, agitated voice.

A (Nursing Action): Notified anaesthesiologist of patient's prior experience. Discussed alternatives for anaesthesia and pain control options. Stressed importance of activity for circulation and healing. Encouraged patient to keep nurses informed of pain level and need for medication and that pain may be present but manageable.

R (Patient Response): Patient stated that they were "very relieved." Stated understanding of the importance of informing the nurses about pain.

Note: Some facilities add **P (Plan)** and refer to this as DARP charting.

Example

P (Plan): Assess pain level at least every 4 hours after surgery. Provide nonpharmacological pain management techniques and administer medication as needed.

Problem List

The problem list includes the patient's physiological, psychological, sociocultural, spiritual, developmental, and environmental needs. To develop a patient's problem list, first analyze the assessment data. Identify and list priority problems in chronological order to serve as an organizing guide for the patient's care. Add new problems as they are identified during the ongoing nursing assessment. When a problem is resolved, record the date and draw a line through the problem and its number. In an electronic system, the problem is marked as resolved.

Plan of Care

Interprofessional collaboration is used to ensure that all health team members involved in a patient's care contribute to the development of an interprofessional plan of care. For example, for a patient experiencing a nutritional deficit, a nurse recommends feeding approaches, and a dietitian recommends types of dietary supplements. Some provincial legislation, such as the *Nursing Act* of Nova Scotia, and care plan standards require that a plan of care be developed for all patients on admission to a health care facility (Health Quality Ontario, 2018; NSCN, 2019). Generally, these plans include nursing diagnoses, expected outcomes, interventions, and evaluations.

Progress Notes

Health care team members use progress notes to monitor and record the progress of a patient's problem (see Box 4.4). Narrative notes, flow sheets, and discharge summaries are formats used to document patient progress (see Procedural Guideline 4.2).

SBAR Documentation. SBAR (situation-background-assessment-recommendation) is a concrete approach for framing conversations, especially critical ones that require a nurse's immediate attention and action. It allows for an easy and focused way to set expectations for what the team will communicate. SBAR promotes the provision of safe, efficient, timely, and person-centred communication (Shahid & Thomas, 2018). This method is used for written and verbal communication when a patient's condition changes, for a brief targeted report (e.g., a preprocedure or postprocedure report), or as a change-of-shift report (Shahid &Thomas, 2018).

SOAP Documentation. One way to structure narrative notes to document patient progress is the SOAP (subjective data–objective data–assessment–plan) format. Some facilities add an "I" and an "E" (i.e., SOAPIE). The *I* stands for *intervention,* and the *E* represents *evaluation.* The logic for SOAP(IE) notes is like that of the nursing process: collect data about a patient's problems, draw conclusions, and develop a plan of care. Number each SOAP note, and title it according to the problem on the list.

PIE Documentation. The PIE (problem–intervention–evaluation) note format of documentation is like that of SOAP charting in its problem-oriented nature. However, it differs from the SOAP method in that PIE charting has a nursing origin, whereas SOAP originated from a medical model.

The PIE format simplifies documentation by combining the care plan and progress note into one record. It differs from that of SOAP because there are no assessment data in the narrative note. Assessment data are included in documentation on the flow sheets of each shift. The nurse numbers or labels the PIE notes according to a patient's problems. Resolved problems are dropped from daily documentation after the nurse's review. Continuing problems are documented daily.

Focus Charting. Another narrative format is focus charting, or DAR (data–action–response). One distinction of focus charting is that it places less importance on patient problems and instead focuses on patient concerns such as a sign or symptom, condition, nursing diagnosis, behaviour, significant event, or change in condition. Each entry includes data (subjective and objective), actions or nursing interventions, and patient response (e.g., evaluation of effectiveness). Focus charting saves time because it is easy for caregivers to understand, is adaptable to most health care settings, and enables all caregivers to track a patient's condition and progress.

Source Records

In a source record, a patient's chart is organized so that each profession (e.g., nursing, medicine, respiratory therapy) has a separate section in which to record data. The advantage of a source record is that it is easy for each health care provider to locate the proper section of the record in which to make entries.

A disadvantage of the source record is that information about a specific problem may be distributed throughout the record. For example, the nurse describes the character of a patient's fractured femur pain and the use of repositioning and analgesia in the progress notes and EHR. The health care provider notes in a separate section of the record the patient's bone healing and the plan for casting or surgery. The results of radiographic examinations that show bone healing are in the radiology section of the record. This method makes it difficult to find chronological information about patient care or how the team is coordinating care to meet all the patient's needs.

Interprofessional Documentation

Interprofessional documentation involves members of the health care team charting in the same record and sharing documentation tools. When interprofessional teams collaborate, they develop and modify the plan of care for the patient together. This method eliminates duplication and improves patient outcomes (Adamson et al., 2020).

Charting by Exception

Charting by exception (CBE) is a system of documentation that aims to eliminate redundancy, makes documentation of routine care more concise, emphasizes abnormal findings, and identifies trends in clinical care. CBE is a shorthand method for documenting based on clearly defined standards of practice and predetermined criteria for nursing assessments and interventions (Fig. 4.5). This system involves completing a flow sheet that incorporates standard assessment and intervention criteria by placing a check mark in the appropriate standard box on the flow sheet to indicate normal findings and routine interventions. The nurse writes a narrative nurse's note *only* when there is an exception to the established standard or abnormal data are present (e.g., presence of pain, change in oral intake and physical activity, emotional distress, and actions the nurse took to address these concerns).

2200	Pt states that she feels nauseated. Vomited 100 mL of clear fluid.
	Sally Smith, RN
2205	Gravol 50 mg IV administered.
	Sally Smith, RN
2235	Pt states no longer feels nauseated.
	Sally Smith, RN

FIG 4.5 Charting by exception. Change in patient's condition requiring a narrative note.

The presumption with CBE is that the nurse assessed the patient and all standards are met unless otherwise documented. Nurses must be careful to not leave fields blank and assume that documentation was not required because a finding was normal. The nurse needs to initial or indicate "within defined limits" in charting templates to communicate that the assessment was completed (Elliott et al., 2018).

Changes in a patient's condition require thorough and precise descriptions of what happened, actions taken, and patient response to treatment. Legal risks in using CBE include difficulty in proving safe care if nurses are not disciplined in documenting exceptions. Nurses need to chart more frequently and thoroughly when patients have complex health needs, are acutely ill, or are deemed high risk (CNPS, 2020).

Critical Pathways

Critical pathways are a system of documentation that states the goals and important treatment interventions on the basis of best practice and patient expectations by documenting, monitoring, and evaluating variances. Key interventions and expected outcomes are established within an expected time frame for specific diseases (Fig. 4.6). Variances are unexpected occurrences, unmet goals, and interventions not specified within the critical pathway time frame and reflect a positive or negative change. A positive variance occurs when a patient progresses more rapidly than the pathway expected (e.g., use of a Foley catheter is discontinued a day early). A negative variance occurs when the activities on the critical pathway do not happen as predicted or outcomes are unmet (e.g., oxygen therapy is necessary for a new-onset breathing problem). The nurse documents the variance and includes causative factors, actions taken, patient response, and outcomes. Over time, the recurrence of similar variances leads the health care team to revise a critical pathway, particularly if it affects quality of care or length of stay.

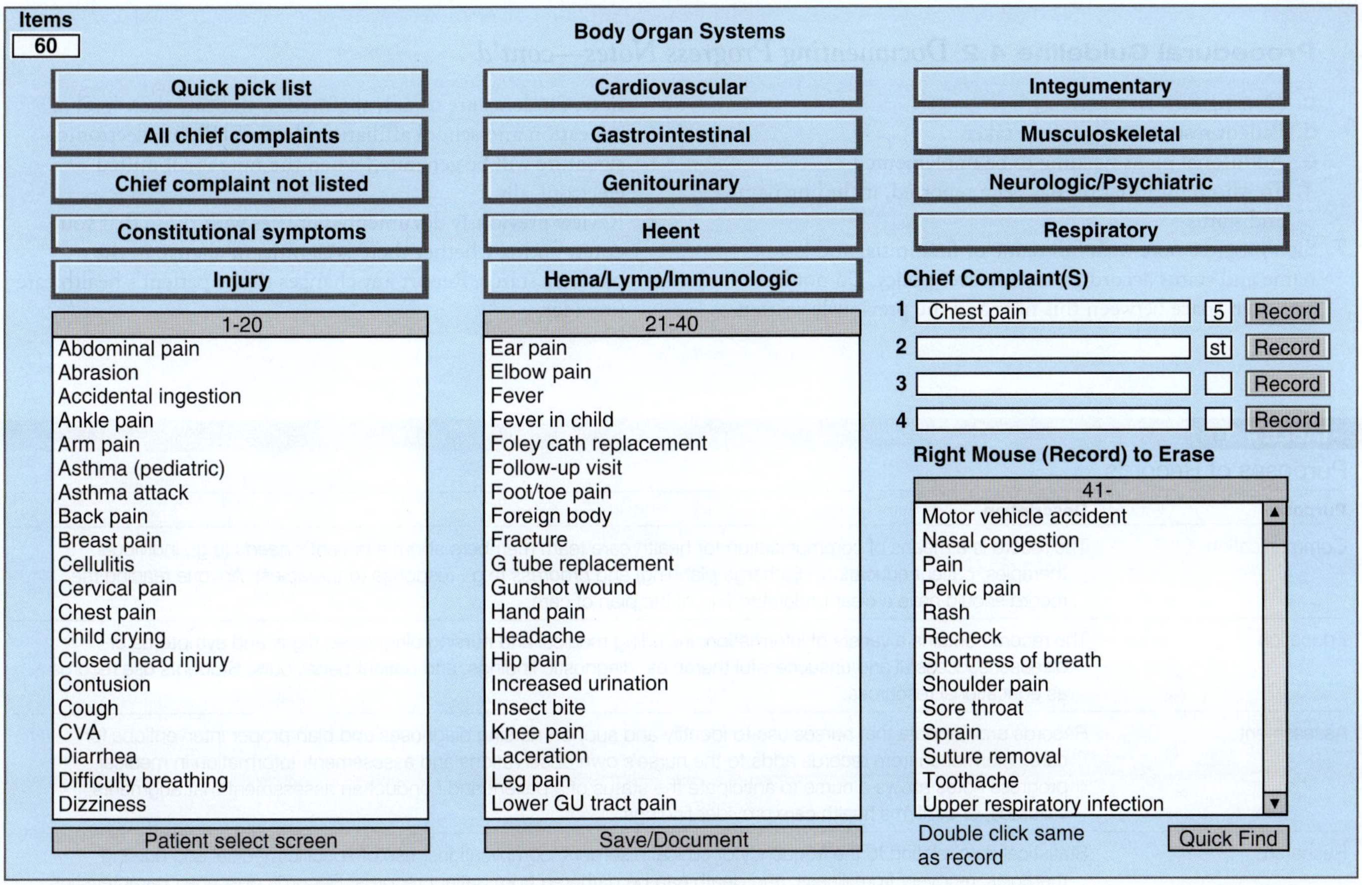

FIG 4.6 Electronic documentation, nursing record. (*Courtesy ER Choice, Irving, TX.*)

Procedural Guideline 4.2 *Documenting Progress Notes*

Accurate documentation reflects the quality of care and provides evidence of each health care team member's accountability in giving care. The purpose of a patient's record is to provide information for communication, education, assessment, research, financial billing, auditing, and legal documentation (Table 4.3).

Because the nursing process directs a nurse's approach to patient care, documentation needs to reflect this process. Nurses record assessment data, changes in a patient's condition, nursing interventions, and an evaluation of the patient's progress toward established outcomes. Prompt documentation of these data increases accuracy and promotes effective communication to all health care team members. The nurse caring for the patient is responsible for writing and signing each progress note, which includes the nurse's full name and title. All caregivers need to be able to read the progress note and have a clear picture of the problem, level of care required, and results of interventions.

Delegation and Collaboration

The skill of documenting progress notes cannot be delegated to a UCP. The nurse instructs the UCP about the following:

- Which repetitive care activities to document on flow sheets (e.g., vital signs, intake and output [I&O], routine care)
- What to report to the nurse (e.g., increased pain, changes in vital signs) so the nurse can reassess, validate, and document any changes in the progress note

Equipment

- Progress note form (written or electronic)
- Black pen or EHR

Procedural Steps

1. Identify the electronic patient record using at least two person-specific identifiers (e.g., name and date of birth, or name and medical record number) according to employer policy (Accreditation Canada, 2020).
2. Review assessment data, problems identified, goals and expected outcomes, nursing interventions, and patient response during contact with each patient and before documentation.
3. Document patient information in the format indicated by employer policy for charting to ensure quality documentation.
4. After each patient contact, identify information that needs to be documented. Consider the following:
   a. Abnormal findings
   b. Changes in status
   c. New problems identified
5. Document in a timely fashion without leaving open spaces between notes and include date and time. In an EHR, the date and time are entered automatically by the system.
6. Using employer format, document in chronological order the following:
   a. Pertinent, factual, objective data
   b. Selected subjective data that validate or clarify

Continued

Procedural Guideline 4.2 *Documenting Progress Notes—cont'd*

c. Nursing actions taken
d. Patient responses to actions taken
e. Additional plans needing to be implemented
f. To whom information has been reported, including name and status

7. Sign progress note with full name or first initial and last name and status according to employer policy. Do not leave any open space between this note and the previously written note. Students are usually required to indicate their level of education and school affiliation. In an EHR, an electronic signature will be generated when the note is submitted electronically.
8. Review previously documented entries with those that you enter, noting whether there is significant change in the patient's status. Report any changes to the patient's health care provider.

TABLE 4.3

Purposes of Records

Purpose	Description
Communication	The record is a means of communication for health care team members about a patient's *needs* (e.g., individual therapies, patient education, discharge planning) and *progress* (e.g., response to therapies). Anyone reading the record should have a clear understanding of the plan of care.
Education	The record contains a variety of information, including medical and nursing diagnoses, signs and symptoms of disease, successful and unsuccessful therapies, diagnostic findings, and patient behaviours. Students use records as educational resources.
Assessment	Records provide data that nurses use to identify and support nursing diagnoses and plan proper interventions for care. Information from records adds to the nurse's own observations and assessment. Information in medical progress notes allows a nurse to anticipate the status of a patient and conduct an assessment that augments, validates, or confirms health care provider findings.
Research	Statistical data relating to the frequency of clinical disorders, complications, use of specific medical and nursing therapies, recovery from illness, and death can be gathered from patient records. Records describe characteristics of patient populations in a health care facility.
Funding and billing	Information gathered from the patient record supports the allocation of human and physical resources required for safe, competent care. It serves as a resource for billing of nonfunded health care services.
Auditing and monitoring	A regular review of information in patient records gives a basis for evaluation of the quality and appropriateness of care provided in a facility. Accreditation Canada (2020) requires health care facilities to establish quality improvement programs to conduct objective, ongoing reviews of patient care. Review of records reveals information about the processes and outcomes of care.
Legal documentation	A medical record must be accurate because it is a legal document. In case of a lawsuit, the medical record, not the nursing care, is on trial. Nursing care may have been excellent; however, care not documented is care not done as far as a court of law is concerned.

Procedural Guideline 4.3 *Adverse Event/Incident Reporting*

An adverse event/incident is any event not consistent with the routine operation of a health care unit or routine care of a patient. Examples include patient falls, needle-stick injuries, medication errors, or a visitor becoming ill. Patient safety events are events that harm the patient, reach the patient but do not harm the patient, or did not reach the patient (known as a "near miss"), such as a medication error. Healthcare Excellence Canada and Health Quality Ontario (2015) have identified a standardized list of preventable *never events*, a subset of patient safety events, that facilitate the reporting of such events (Box 4.5). Completion of a report occurs when there is actual or potential patient injury (a "near miss"). The process involves documentation first in the patient health record and in an adverse event/incident report as per employer policy (also referred to as a "serious event report" or an "occurrence report"). Document in the patient's record an objective description of what you observed and follow-up actions taken without reference to the adverse/incident report. The actual report does not become part of the health record. Nurses are accountable to help develop quality practice environments. Reporting helps identify high-risk trends in nursing care or daily unit operations that warrant correction. You need to complete the report even if an injury does not occur or is not apparent. This information helps nursing staff find solutions to prevent repeated incidents. The reports are an important part of the quality improvement program of a unit.

Healthcare Excellence Canada (2022) provides guidance and strategies to health care agencies in the development of adverse event reporting systems. Adverse event/incident reports are important sources of data for enhancing understanding of underlying causes of events that, when analyzed, can improve patient safety (Healthcare Excellence Canada, 2022). Nurses are active participants in examining the causes of errors and redesigning systems to minimize repeated errors. By focusing on systems rather than on individual failures,

Procedural Guideline 4.3 *Adverse Event/Incident Reporting—cont'd*

there is greater opportunity to improve patient safety (Lee et al., 2018). For example, a patient is administered the wrong medication by a nurse. A review of the event focuses primarily on the medication process instead of placing blame. Interprofessional examination of adverse event cases, using reflective inquiry, allows those involved to share feelings, which contributes to a culture of support. This process of reflective inquiry creates a blame-free environment that contributes to a positive work environment and improvements in teamwork and patient safety (Hellyar et al., 2019).

Health care systems across Canada have adopted electronic reporting systems to document and track adverse events. While there is variation in the systems used (e.g., British Columbia Patient Safety and Learning System [BCPSLS], the Regional Occurrence System Enhanced [ROSE] adopted by Newfoundland), they all facilitate the tracking of events, help health care providers understand the reasons why events occurred, and inform organizational practices (Gregory, 2018).

Nurses are ethically responsible for reporting near misses and taking immediate action to prevent harm to persons receiving care (CNA, 2017). Accreditation Canada (2020) disclosure guidelines indicate that communication of near misses should take place immediately following the event in order to prevent further harm to others. Such disclosure allows the patients and families involved to heal and promotes patient safety practices.

Delegation and Collaboration

- Ensure that documentation is completed by the person who performed the action or witnessed the event (CNPS, 2020).

Equipment

- Adverse event/incident report form or screen
- Pen or digital technology

Procedural Steps

1. Identify the electronic patient record using at least two person-specific identifiers (e.g., name and date of birth, or name and medical record number) according to employer policy (Accreditation Canada, 2020).
2. Use clinical reasoning skills to systematically and carefully determine what was involved in the event. The person who witnessed the event is the person who documents the event. Document the exact sequence of events involved, including time and type of event; injury to patient, nurse, visitor, or other staff; and observation of factors that possibly contributed to the event (e.g., wet floor discovered in area of patient fall). Notify risk management per employer policy.

Critical Decision Point *Prepare the report on any questionable event. A just culture in health care values the reporting of errors without fear of punitive actions. This approach ensures that all contributing factors involved in the error are examined and processes are put in place to prevent future errors.*

3. Assess extent of any injury to patient or others, including patient's subjective report and objective physical examination findings.
4. If the adverse event/incident involves an injury, take steps to restore individual's safety, such as stabilizing patient's position after a fall and assessing for further injuries.
5. When patient sustains an injury, notify health care provider immediately.
6. When visitor or staff member sustains an injury, refer to emergency department or appropriate treatment setting.
7. Complete adverse event/incident report form.

Critical Decision Point *Document adverse event/incident on report form as quickly as possible. The closer in time to the event it is documented, the more accurate the recording.*

   a. Record time of event and describe exactly what occurred or was observed, using objective findings and observations. Use language that does not allow for subjective interpretation. Do not include personal opinions or feelings. Document person's interpretation of event by using quotes.
   b. Objectively describe person's condition when event was discovered or observed.
   c. Describe measures taken by any caregivers at time of event.
   d. Submit report as per employer policy.
8. When patient is involved, document events of incident in patient's chart.
   a. Only enter objective description of what happened.
   b. Record any assessment and intervention activities initiated because of event.
   c. Do not duplicate all information from report.
   d. Do not document that report was completed.
9. Submit the report properly to the risk management department or designated people.

BOX 4.5

15 Never Events for Hospital Care in Canada

- Surgery on the wrong body part or the wrong patient, or conducting the wrong procedure
- Wrong tissue, biological implant, or blood product given to patient
- Unintended foreign object left in patient following a procedure
- Patient death or serious harm arising from the use of improperly sterilized instruments or equipment provided by the health care facility
- Patient death or serious harm due to a failure to inquire whether patient has a known allergy to medication, or due to administration of a medication to patient whose allergy had been identified
- Patient death or serious harm due to administration of the wrong inhalation or insufflation gas
- Patient death or serious harm due to one of five pharmaceutical events:
  - Wrong route used for chemotherapy
  - Intravenous (IV) administration of a concentrated potassium solution
  - Injecting epinephrine intended for topical use
  - Overdose of hydromorphone by administering a higher concentration of solution

Continued

BOX 4.5

15 Never Events for Hospital Care in Canada—*cont'd*

- Neuromuscular blockade without sedation, airway control, and ventilation capability
- Patient death or serious harm as a result of failure to identify and treat metabolic disturbances (e.g., hypoglycemia or hyperbilirubinemia)
- Any stage III or stage IV pressure ulcer acquired after admission to hospital
- Patient death or serious harm due to uncontrolled movement of a ferromagnetic object in a magnetic resonance imaging (MRI) area
- Patient death or serious harm due to an accidental burn
- Patient under the highest level of observation leaves a secured facility or ward without the knowledge of staff (e.g., patient with dementia or suicide risk)
- Patient suicide, or attempted suicide that resulted in serious harm, in instances where suicide prevention protocols were to be applied to patients under the highest level of observation
- Infant abducted or discharged to the wrong person
- Patient death or serious harm due to transport of a frail patient, or patient with dementia, when protocols were not followed to ensure the patient was left in a safe environment

Adapted from Healthcare Excellence Canada & Health Quality Ontario (HQO). (2015). *Never events for hospital care in Canada: Safer care for patients.* https://www.patientsafetyinstitute.ca/en/toolsResources/NeverEvents/Documents/Never%20Events%20for%20Hospital%20Care%20in%20Canada.pdf

Mobile Communication Devices

Mobile devices have become a popular means by which to access clinical decision-making tools, deliver virtual care to patients, and monitor health conditions through medical apps. Technological advances enable patient data to be collected on mobile phones and transmitted to health care providers and EHRs through wearable sensors. Despite their global use, concerns remain about the security and privacy of the information stored on these devices. Mobile devices can store and retain personal health information (PHI) and—given their small size—they can also be easily lost or stolen. Encryption of devices and the use of strong passwords are essential to reducing the risk of unauthorized access to or disclosure of PHI (Yang et al., 2020).

Hands-free wireless devices have been adopted by many hospitals to improve health care communication. These devices are lightweight, are worn by health care providers, and are used to deliver real-time awareness of patient situations. These mobile devices enable health care providers to receive and deliver messages to individuals or groups, to produce audio reminders, and to receive urgent alerts (Carreon & Dutra, 2020).

Text and email communication has also gained popularity in health care systems and among health care providers. Health care systems should have policies and procedures in place for health care teams to interact with each other and with patients, and to access patient records, using mobile devices (NSCN, 2022). Consent and security measures are always required.

Liability Issues Related to Documentation

Failure to secure patient information that has been documented may result in a breach of information, liability for a wrongful act, and professional misconduct. Any changes made to a health record must follow employer policies to protect the integrity of the record. Changing another person's entry in the health record can result in an accusation of falsification of a record and professional misconduct (NSCN, 2022).

Students are accountable for their actions and should document the care they provide in the health record. Student documentation notes should not be co-signed (unless required by certain employer policies), as this may result in accountability issues for the co-signer (NSCN, 2022). However, students must be aware of practices that require supervision and confirming signature of a witnessed event (e.g., high-alert medications such as insulin, potassium, anticoagulants) (ISMP, 2018). In such events, a third nurse may be involved as a witness and co-signer in addition to the student nurse and instructor/preceptor. Employer policies provide guidance to nurses regarding documentation requirements for student nurses.

Poor documentation can affect the integrity of the health record. Lawyers rely on charting to show whether a nurse met the standard of care and did not cause harm to the patient that resulted in the legal act of negligence (CNPS, 2020). Working notes should become part of the health record in a timely manner and should be shredded following transcription into the health record. The use of notes outside of the patient chart should be avoided (CNPS, 2020).

BOX 4.6

Forms for Documentation of Care in the Community

The usual forms used to document care in the community include the following:

- Patient assessment
- Referral source information/intake form
- Discipline-specific care plans
- Health care provider's plan of treatment
- Medication sheet
- Clinical progress notes
- Miscellaneous (conference notes, verbal prescription forms, telephone calls)
- Discharge summary
- Reports to third-party payers

Privacy and Ethics Around Digital Health Information

Patients have the right to the confidentiality and security of their health information. Every effort should be made to ensure that those who are not involved in the care of the patient do not have access to patients' digital information. Nurses must follow professional standards, provincial/territorial privacy legislation, and employer policies on documentation and protection of PHI.

Patients have the right to access their PHI, and nurses should advocate and assist patients with the retrieval process in accordance with provincial/territorial legislation and employer policies.

DOCUMENTATION OF CARE IN THE COMMUNITY

Care in the community setting continues to grow as a result of shorter hospitalizations and an increasing numbers of persons requiring care in the home. Documentation when caring for a patient at home has different implications than in other areas of nursing. One primary difference is that it is the patient and family, rather than the nurse, who witness the majority of care. In addition, documentation systems need to provide the entire health care team with the necessary information to maximize the efficiency of interprofessional collaboration (Box 4.6).

Computerized patient records are evolving in the community setting. The EHR facilitates clarity, continuity of care, and comprehensiveness because of increased standardization of language (CHI, 2021). PHI stored electronically should be encrypted to prevent privacy breaches. Users need to make every effort to keep PHI secure by avoiding use of public wireless networks and free email services when accessing patient health information from an EHR.

LONG-TERM HEALTH CARE DOCUMENTATION

In Canada, a growing number of older persons and persons with disabilities require care in long-term care facilities. Nursing personnel in long-term care face documentation challenges much different from those in the acute care setting. EHRs in long-term care facilities improve documentation management, clinical decision making, and health outcomes (Hämäläinen & Hirvonen, 2020).

A nurse is responsible for coordinating the plan of care. Documentation supports the assessment and planning process for patients using an interprofessional approach. Communication among all health care team members is essential in the documentation process. The overall goal is a system of clinical documentation that identifies potential or actual problems and provides improved actions for each problem, resulting in improved care for residents (Hämäläinen & Hirvonen, 2020).

Procedural Guideline 4.4 *Guidelines for Meaningful Use of an Interoperable Electronic Health Record*

A CHI (2018) goal is to improve the health and health care experiences of Canadians by connecting health care information through an interoperable EHR (iEHR). In addition, health care facilities across the country are connecting health care information through technology to facilitate patient transitions across the continuum of care. Meaningful use means that health care providers effectively use iEHRs to improve patient care (Joneidy & Burke, 2019).

When health care facilities participate in meaningful use initiatives, health care providers use iEHRs to record universal patient data, practise person-centred care, and transmit critical patient data at care transition points (Rangachari et al., 2019). An example of a care transition is a patient discharge from a hospital to a long-term care facility. During transitions, there is a transfer of specific patient data collected from the sending facility to the new provider. Examples of the data sent include history of allergies, cognitive status, functional status, immunizations, medications, and smoking history.

An important component of care transitions is the process of medication reconciliation. *Medication reconciliation* is the process of comparing the patient's current medications against the medications actually prescribed at a care transition point. This process minimizes medication errors and adverse events (ISMP, 2018). The EHR provides efficiencies for all health care providers performing medication reconciliation. Medication reconciliation is one of the World Health Organization's top five mandated core objectives for reducing medication errors globally (ISMP, 2018). Medication reconciliation, which is a complex process requiring interprofessional collaboration, is also a national patient safety goal and a required organizational practice standard (Accreditation Canada, 2020). By using a standardized process to assess a patient's medications at a care transition point, medication discrepancies such as omissions, duplications, contraindications, and vague information can be reduced (Accreditation Canada, 2020). Although some facilities may assign other disciplines as the accountable discipline for medication reconciliation, the nurse plays an active collaborative role in the process (Mardani et al., 2020).

Delegation and Collaboration

The skill of using an iEHR for medication reconciliation cannot be delegated to a UCP. The nurse instructs the UCP to do the following:

- Report to the nurse any pertinent information the patient or caregiver reports about their medications

Equipment

- Admission medication list
- Current medication list
- Discharge medication list
- Medication reconciliation work screen or worksheet (follow employer policy)
- iEHR

Procedural Steps

1. Use an organized format for medication reconciliation. Gathering the best possible medication history (BPMH) is the first step in medication reconciliation and provides an important tool to refer to during care transitions (Accreditation Canada, 2020). Medication reconciliation reduces medication errors for patients transitioning across points of care (ISMP, 2018).
2. Identify the electronic patient record using at least two person-specific identifiers (e.g., name and date of birth, or name and medical record number) according to employer policy (Accreditation Canada, 2020).
3. Gather information from electronic documentation sources such as admission medications, active medications, or discharge medications.
4. Arrange for two nurses to complete the medication reconciliation at time of care transition. Assess the current medications prescribed to the medications prescribed for the care transition. If the patient is being discharged from a facility, assess the medications on admission and current medications to the discharge medications (Accreditation Canada, 2020).
5. Have the two nurses assess discrepancies.

Critical Decision Point *If discrepancies still exist after nurse review, a nurse-to-health care provider reconciliation occurs.*

6. If the patient is being discharged from a facility, reconcile the medication list before giving information to the patient. Provide the patient with the written reconciled list of medications.
7. Teach the patient how to keep their medication list current.
8. Educate the patient about the medications and the importance of sharing the current medication list at every health care visit. **Use teach-back:** "It is important to keep your medication list up to date. Tell me how you plan on doing this." Develop a revised teaching plan if the patient or caregiver is not able to teach back correctly.

✦ REVIEW QUESTIONS

A 55-year-old retired teacher (he/him) will be discharged this evening from the ambulatory care unit following his surgical hernia repair. The patient's admission medication list includes hydrochlorothiazide 12.5-mg tablet orally once per day and fluoxetine 40-mg tablet orally once daily in the morning. Immediately after surgery he rates his pain as 10 on a scale of 0 to 10 (0 = no pain, 10 = the worst pain ever), and he is medicated with hydromorphone 1 mg IV at 0930.

1. Based on the patient's admission medication list, which medications should you expect to find on the discharge medication list?
2. At 1400 hours, the patient rates his surgical pain as 9 on a scale of 0–10 (0 being no pain, 10 being worst pain ever). He receives two oxycodone 10 mg tablets orally for his pain at 1410. Thirty minutes later, he rates his pain as 2 on a scale of 0–10. At discharge, the medication list reads as follows: hydrochlorothiazide 12.5-mg tablet orally once per day and fluoxetine 40-mg tablet orally once daily in the morning. What are your nursing actions?
3. Using SBAR (situation–background–assessment–recommendation), show how you would communicate with the health care provider about the medication omission.
4. The patient falls on the unit. Which actions should the nurse perform? (*Select all that apply.*)
   1. Assess extent of any injury to the patient.
   2. Document the adverse event report in the EHR.
   3. Identify the patient using at least two person-specific identifiers.
   4. Complete an adverse event report on the basis of the nurse's initial reaction.
   5. Document the nurse's clinical assessment in the EHR.
5. During a hand-off report, the nurse will do which of the following? (*Select all that apply.*)
   1. Use the patient's first and last name as the two person-specific identifiers.
   2. Provide background information about the patient.
   3. Recommend the priority of care for the next shift.
   4. Include in the assessment the patient's response to pain medications.
   5. Exclude the patient from the hand-off report.
6. The patient is being transitioned from the hospital to a long-term care facility. Place the following criteria in the correct order for an SBAR report:
   1. Medical history, allergies, code status, isolation, significant interventions, pain management, responses to interventions, report of abnormal studies, who was notified, any interventions, intravenous (IV) access
   2. Admission date, chief complaint, and diagnosis
   3. Review of systems: neurological, respiratory, cardiac, gastrointestinal, genitourinary, musculoskeletal, peripheral vascular, skin, hematological, endocrine, and psychosocial
   4. Patient's daily goals, consultations, planned treatments, upcoming tests or surgery, discharge planning, and patient education

Visit the Evolve site for a complete list of answers to the Review Questions.

✦ NEXT GENERATION NCLEX® (NGN)

For practice with answering exam questions related to unfolding NGN case studies, please consult the Next Generation NCLEX® (NGN)-Style Case Studies for Skills and Techniques on the Evolve website: http://evolve.elsevier.com/Canada/Perry/clinicalskills/

REFERENCES

Accreditation Canada. (2020). *Required organizational practices handbook*. https://physicians.nshealth.ca/resources/required-organizational-practices-2020-handbook

Adamson, K., Maxwell, J., & Forbes, J. (2020). Interprofessional guide to documentation in electronic health records. *Journal of Interprofessional Education & Practice, 21*, 100387. https://doi.org/10.1016/j.xjep.2020.100387

Anderson, R. (2022). Effects of an electronic health record tool on team communication and patient mobility: A 2-year follow-up study. *Critical Care Nurse, 42*(2), 23–31. https://doi.org/10.4037/ccn2022385

Ardic, A., & Turan, E. (2021). Nursing care management based on the Omaha system for inpatients diagnosed with COVID–19: An electronic health record study. *Journal of Advanced Nursing, 77*(6), 2709–2717. https://doi.org/10.1111/jan.14793

Boothe, C. (2020). The history of technology in nursing: The implementation of electronic health records in Canadian healthcare settings. *Canadian Journal of Nursing Informatics, 15*(2). https://cjni.net/journal/?p=7192

Canada Health Infoway (CHI). (2018). *Connected health information in Canada: A benefits evaluation study*. https://www.infoway-inforoute.ca/en/component/edocman/3510-connected-health-information-in-canada-a-benefits-evaluation-study-document/view-document

Canada Health Infoway (CHI). (2020). *2020 National survey of Canadian nurses: Use of digital health technology in practice, final executive report*. https://www.infoway-inforoute.ca/en/component/edocman/3812-2020-national-survey-of-canadian-nurses-use-of-digital-health-technology-in-practice/view-document

Canada Health Infoway (CHI). (2021). *Nursing data standards*. https://infocentral.infoway-inforoute.ca/en/standards/other-canadian/nursing-data-standards

Canadian Association of Schools of Nursing. (2014). *Nursing informatics: Entry-to-practice competencies for registered nurses*. https://www.casn.ca/wp-content/uploads/2014/12/Nursing-Informatics-Entry-to-Practice-Competencies-for-RNs_updated-June-4-2015.pdf

Canadian Nurses Association (CNA). (2017). *Code of ethics for registered nurses*. https://www.cna-aiic.ca/en/nursing/regulated-nursing-in-canada/nursing-ethics

Canadian Nurses Association (CNA). (2022). *Nursing informatics*. https://www.cna-aiic.ca/en/nursing/nursing-tools-and-resources/nursing-informatics

Canadian Nurses Protective Society (CNPS). (2020). *InfoLaw: Quality documentation: Your best defense*. https://cnps.ca/article/infolaw-qualitydocumentation/

Carreon, H., & Dutra, D. (2020). Inpatient outcomes of a hands-free, wireless communication device implementation. *CIN: Computers, Informatics, Nursing, 38*(7), 323–328. https://doi.org/10.1097/CIN.0000000000000653

Dendere, R., Slade, C., Burton-Jones, A., et al. (2019). Patient portals facilitating engagement with inpatient electronic medical records: A systematic review. *Journal of Medical Internet Research, 21*(4), Article E12779. https://doi.org/10.2196/12779

E-Health Act, (2008). *SBC*, c 38. https://www.bclaws.gov.bc.ca/civix/document/id/complete/statreg/08038_01

Elliott, L., Weil, J., Dykstra, E., et al. (2018). Standardizing documentation: A place for everything (continuous quality improvement). *Medsurg Nursing, 27*(1), 32–37.

Flanders, S. A. (2018). Nurses as educators. Effective patient education: Evidence and common sense. *Medsurg Nursing, 27*(1), 55–58.

Galatzan, B., & Carrington, J. (2021). Examining the meaning of the language used to communicate the nursing hand–off. *Research in Nursing & Health, 44*(5), 833–843. https://doi.org/10.1002/nur.22175

Galatzan, B., & Carrington, J. (2022). Communicating data, information, and knowledge in the nursing handoff. *CIN: Computers, Informatics, Nursing, 40*(1), 21–27. https://doi.org/10.1097/CIN.0000000000000806

Government of Canada. (2019). *PIPEDA in brief*. https://www.priv.gc.ca/en/privacy-topics/privacy-laws-in-canada/the-personal-information-protection-and-electronic-documents-act-pipeda/pipeda_brief/

Gregory, D. (2018). *Adverse health event management: International and Canadian practices*. https://www.gov.nl.ca/ahe/additions/05_AdverseHealthEventManagementInternationalandCanadianPractices.pdf

Hämäläinen, A., & Hirvonen, H. (2020). Electronic health records reshaping the socio-technical practices in long-term care of older persons. *Technology in Society, 62*, 101316. https://doi.org/10.1016/j.techsoc.2020.101316

Healthcare Excellence Canada. (2020). *The safety competencies: Enhancing patient safety across the health professions* (2nd ed.). https://www.patientsafetyinstitute.ca/en/toolsResources/safetyCompetencies/Documents/CPSI-SafetyCompetencies_EN_Digital.pdf

Healthcare Excellence Canada. (2022). *Patient safety and incident management toolkit*. https://www.healthcareexcellence.ca/en/resources/patient-safety-and-incident-management-toolkit/

Healthcare Excellence Canada & Health Quality Ontario. (2015). *Never events for hospital care in Canada: Safer care for patients*. https://www.patientsafetyinstitute.ca/en/toolsResources/NeverEvents/Documents/Never%20Events%20for%20Hospital%20Care%20in%20Canada.pdf

Health Quality Ontario. (2018). *Adopting a common approach to transitional care planning: Helping health links improve transitions and coordination of care. Queen's Printer for Ontario.* http://www.hqontario.ca/Portals/0/documents/qi/health-links/bp-improve-package-traditional-care-planning-en.pdf

Hellyar, M., Madani, C., Yeaman, S., et al. (2019). Case study investigation decreases burnout while improving interprofessional teamwork, nurse satisfaction, and patient safety. *Critical Care Nursing Quarterly*, *42*(1), 96–105. https://doi.org/10.1097/CNQ.0000000000000243

Institute for Safe Medication Practices (ISMP). (2018). *Do not use: Dangerous abbreviations, symbols, and dose calculations.* https://www.ismp-canada.org/download/ISMPCanadaListOfDangerousAbbreviations.pdf

Institute for Safe Medication Practices (ISMP). (2021). *ISMP's list of error-prone abbreviations, symbols, and dose designations.* https://www.ismp.org/recommendations/error-prone-abbreviations-list

The Joint Commission. (2021). Preventing copy-and-paste errors in EHRs. *Quick Safety* (Issue 10). https://www.jointcommission.org/-/media/tjc/newsletters/quick-safety-10-update-7-19-21.pdf

Joneidy, S., & Burke, M. (2019). Towards a deeper understanding of meaningful use in electronic health records. *Health Information and Libraries Journal*, *36*(2), 134–152. https://doi.org/10.1111/hir.12233

Knox, A. (2019). Informatics in nursing education: What do we do next? *Canadian Journal of Nursing Informatics*, *14*(4). https://cjni.net/journal/?p=6351

Lee, S. E., Vincent, C., Dahinten, V. S., et al. (2018). Effects of individual nurse and hospital characteristics on patient adverse events and quality of care: A multilevel analysis. *Journal of Nursing Scholarship*, *50*(4), 432–440. https://doi.org/10.1111/jnu.12396

Lougheed, M. D., Thomas, N. J., Wasilewski, N. V., et al. (2018). Use of SNOMED CT® and LOINC® to standardize terminology for primary care asthma electronic health records. *Journal of Asthma*, *55*(6), 629–639. https://doi.org/10.1080/02770903.2017.1362424

Mardani, A., Griffiths, P., & Vaismoradi, M. (2020). The role of the nurse in the management of medicines during transitional care: A systematic review. *Journal of Multidisciplinary Healthcare*, *13*, 1347–1361. https://doi.org/10.2147/JMDH.S276061

Merlane, H., & Booth, Z. (2020). Discharge planning in end-of-life care. *British Journal of Nursing*, *29*(4), 202–203. https://doi.org/10.12968/bjon.2020.29.4.202

Nova Scotia College of Nursing (NSCN). (2019). *Nursing care plan guidelines for nurses.* https://cdn3.nscn.ca/sites/default/files/documents/resources/NursingCarePlan.pdf

Nova Scotia College of Nursing (NSCN). (2022). *Documentation guidelines for nurses.* https://www.nscn.ca/professional-practice/practice-support/practice-support-tools/documentation/documentation-guidelines-nurses

O'Connor, S., & LaRue, E. (2021). Integrating informatics into undergraduate nursing education: A case study using a spiral learning approach. *Nurse Education in Practice*, *50*, 102934. https://doi.org/10.1016/j.nepr.2020.102934

Olatubi, M., Oyediran, O. O., Faremi, F. A., et al. (2019). Knowledge, perception, and utilization of standardized nursing language (SNL) (NNN) among nurses in three selected hospitals in Ondo State, Nigeria. *International Journal of Nursing Knowledge*, *30*(1), 43–48. https://doi.org/10.1111/2047-3095.12197

Østensen, E., Hardiker, N. R., Bragstad, L. K., et al. (2020). Introducing standardised care plans as a new recording tool in municipal health care. *Journal of Clinical Nursing*, *29*(17–18), 3286–3297. https://doi.org/10.1111/jocn.15355

Personal Health Information Act, SNS 2010, c 41. https://nslegislature.ca/legc/bills/61st_2nd/3rd_read/b089.htm

Rangachari, P., Dellsperger, K. C., & Rethemeyer, R. K. (2019). A qualitative study of interprofessional learning related to electronic health record (EHR) medication reconciliation within a social knowledge networking (SKN) system. *Journal of Healthcare Leadership*, *11*, 23–41. https://doi.org/10.2147/JHL.S198951

Schjødt, K., Erlang, A. S., Starup-Linde, J., et al. (2022). Older hospitalized patients' experience of involvement in discharge planning. *Scandinavian Journal of Caring Sciences*, *36*(1), 192–202. https://doi.org/10.1111/scs.12977

Shahid, S., & Thomas, S. (2018). Situation, background, assessment, recommendation (SBAR) communication tool for handoff in health care—A narrative review. *Safety & Health*, *4*(1). https://0-doi-org.brum.beds.ac.uk/10.1186/s40886-018-0073-1

Stewart, M. T., Hogan, T. P., Nicklas, J., et al. (2020). The promise of patient portals for individuals living with chronic illness: Qualitative study identifying pathways of patient engagement. *Journal of Medical Internet Research*, *22*(7), Article E17744. https://doi.org/10.2196/17744

Strudwick, G., Reisdorfer, E., Warnock, C., et al. (2018). Factors associated with barcode medication administration technology that contribute to patient safety: An integrative review. *Journal of Nursing Care Quality*, *33*(1), 79–85. https://doi.org/10.1097/NCQ.0000000000000270

Yang, Y., Liu, X., Deng, R. H., et al. (2020). Lightweight sharable and traceable secure mobile health system. *IEEE Transactions on Dependable and Secure Computing*, *17*(1), 78–91. https://doi.org/10.1109/TDSC.2017.2729556

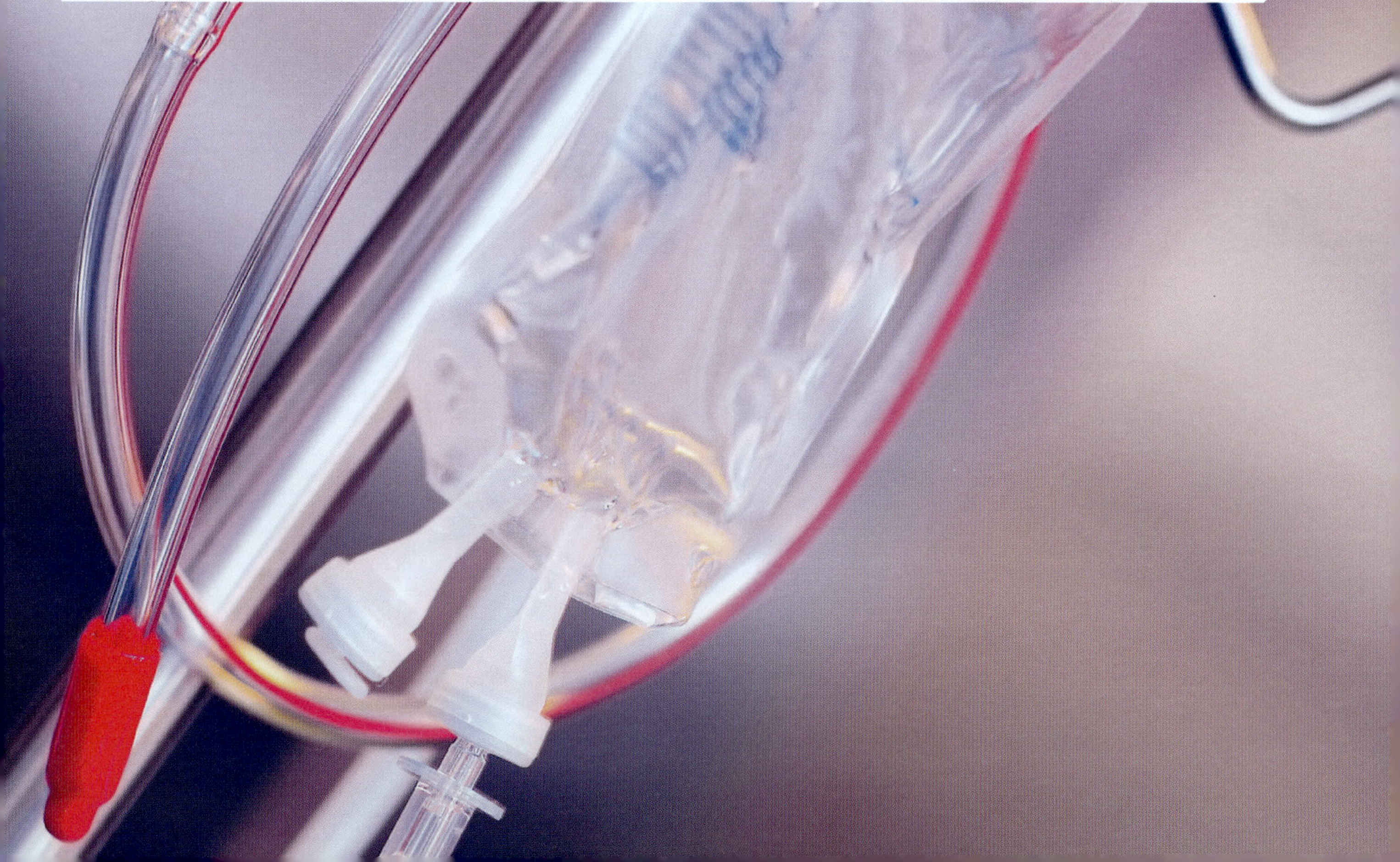

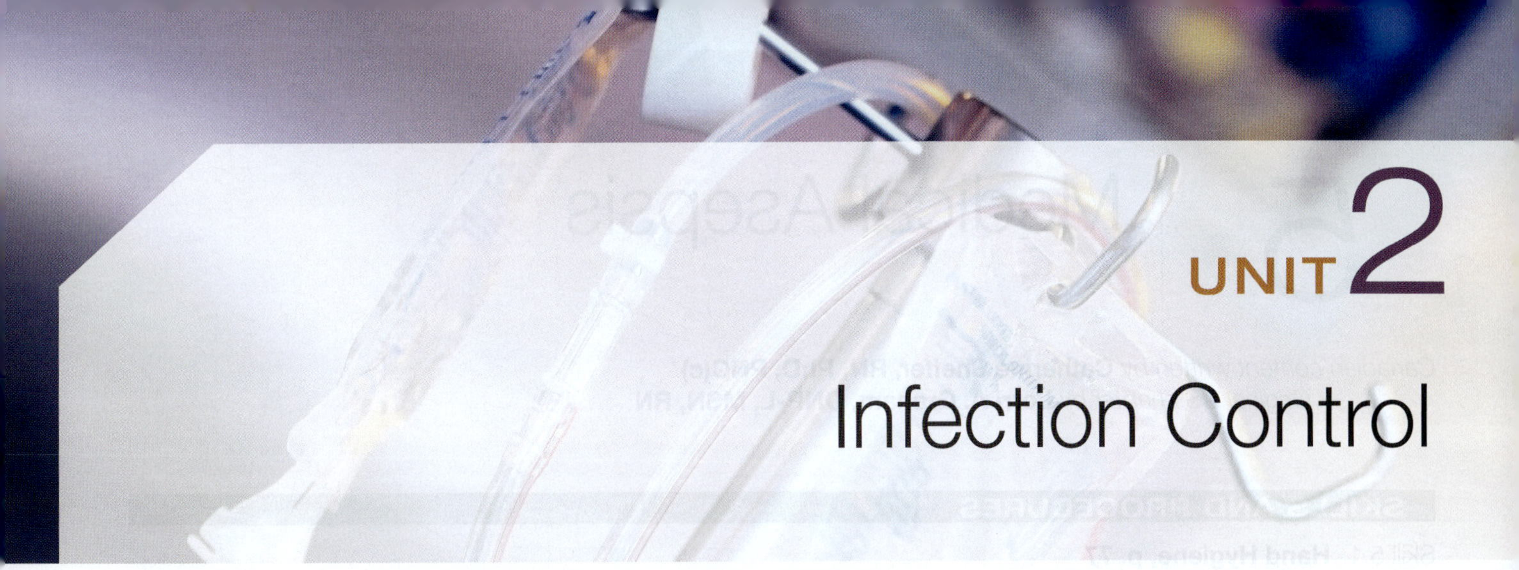

UNIT 2 Infection Control

Using clinical judgement to make accurate decisions about the appropriate skills to use for infection control requires the application of knowledge about the nature of infection, the pathology of different types of infection, and a patient's susceptibility and risks for infection. Knowing a patient's susceptibility and risks requires a thorough and focused assessment of the patient's clinical condition and common risk factors. A nurse needs to develop an infection control conscience when caring for patients. Basic infection control techniques, also known as routine practices or standard precautions, are the evidence-informed approaches that apply in the care of all patients. These techniques reduce the transmission of infection from nurses to patients and, conversely, the transfer of infection directly from patients to nurses. It is important to follow medically aseptic routine practices regardless of the health care setting because sources of infection are everywhere, including work surfaces in patient rooms and common work areas, patients' bodily fluids, and visitors' and health care workers' hands. Having an infection control conscience is the highest form of patient advocacy. It means anticipating sources of infection, understanding the risks to you and to patients, and carrying out the procedures necessary to reduce infection transmission.

Hand hygiene and clean gloving are two of the most common medically aseptic skills. The 4 moments for hand hygiene are to always be implemented; hand hygiene should occur (1) before initial patient (or patient environment) contact, (2) before an aseptic procedure, (3) after body fluid exposure risk, and (4) after patient (or patient environment) contact. Additional hand hygiene should be performed when hands are visibly soiled. Clinical judgement is necessary to perform these skills correctly during patient care. A nurse must always anticipate what the gloves have touched and what the next care activity involves. For example, a nurse will perform hand hygiene and then apply a pair of clean gloves before bathing a patient. During the bath, the nurse cleans the patient's perineal area. The gloves should immediately be removed, followed by handwashing and reapplication of clean gloves to complete the bath. The gloves used during perineal care should never be used to touch clean areas of the patient's body.

Sterile aseptic techniques are necessary when a nurse works in environments in which invasive procedures are performed. This is the norm in areas such as the operating room, interventional procedure areas, and special treatment rooms. The use of skills such as sterile gloving or creating a sterile field reduces infection transmission when foreign sterile objects such as a urinary catheter, intravenous catheter, or nasotracheal suction catheter are introduced into the body. Sterile objects must remain sterile, and proper aseptic technique achieves this goal. When you do not work in special procedure areas but a procedure is planned to be performed at a patient's bedside, anticipate how to use sterile aseptic technique in that situation. The risks for accidental contamination of a sterile work field at the bedside are higher than when you work in a more controlled procedure room.

Clinical judgement plays a role in deciding when to use medical versus sterile aseptic techniques. Consider the example of caring for a patient with leukemia, a cancer of the blood. Your scientific knowledge informs you that the patient is at increased risk for reduced immune function because of the nature of the disease. In addition, you know that the chemotherapy the patient receives can further lower immunity. The combination of reduced immunity and chemotherapy makes the patient highly susceptible to infection. The use of routine practices limits transmission of organisms that are normally transmitted through routine patient contact. However, when your assessment reveals additional patient risks such as a skin tear or pressure injury, you must decide whether more aggressive infection control techniques are needed, such as the use of sterile gloves during a dressing change. Depending on the degree to which the patient's immune system is depressed, consultation with infection control professionals could be necessary to implement additional precautions (contact, droplet, and airborne) to protect the patient from microorganism exposure.

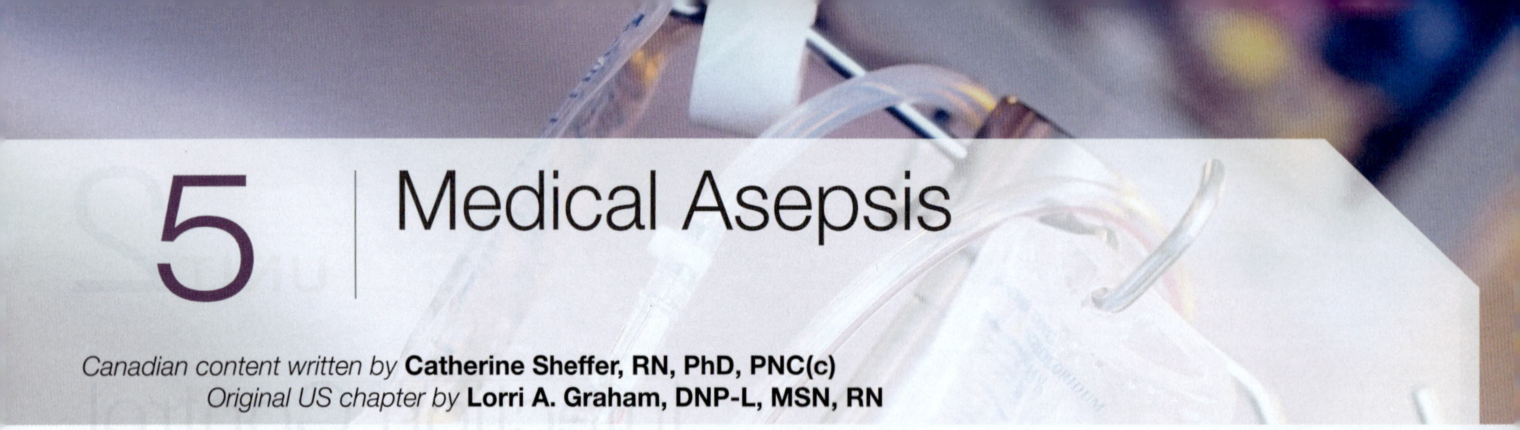

5 | Medical Asepsis

Canadian content written by **Catherine Sheffer, RN, PhD, PNC(c)**
Original US chapter by **Lorri A. Graham, DNP-L, MSN, RN**

SKILLS AND PROCEDURES

OBJECTIVES

Mastery of content in this chapter will enable the nurse to:

- Describe how to apply critical thinking in the prevention of the transmission of infection.
- Explain how and when to apply the principles of medical asepsis in patient care.
- Identify nursing care measures intended to break the chain of infection.
- Describe how each element of the infection chain contributes to infection.
- Describe the factors that influence nursing staff adherence to hand hygiene.
- Demonstrate proper procedures for hand hygiene.
- Apply and remove a cap, mask and protective eyewear correctly.
- Demonstrate correct routine practices and additional precautions in preventing the transmission of infection.

MEDIA RESOURCES

- http://evolve.elsevier.com/Canada/Perry/clinicalskills/

PURPOSE

Infection prevention and control practices reduce or eliminate sources and transmission of infection. These prevention and control practices are designed to protect patients and health care providers from disease. Medical asepsis, or clean technique, includes the procedures used for reducing the number of organisms and preventing their transfer. Surgical asepsis, or sterile technique (see Chapter 6), refers to the procedures used to eliminate all organisms from an area. Nurses play a critical role in the prevention of infection in all health care settings.

STANDARDS OF CARE

- Accreditation Canada (2020)—*Required Organizational Practices Handbook: Hand Hygiene Education and Training* (p.53)(https://physicians.nshealth.ca/resources/required-organizational-practices-2020-handbook)
- Infection Prevention and Control Canada (IPAC Canada, 2022)—*IPAC Canada Practice Recommendations: Hand Hygiene in Health Care Settings* (https://ipac-canada.org/photos/custom/Members/pdf/22Nov11_Hand%20Hygiene_Practice%20Recommendation.pdf)
- Ontario Agency for Health Protection and Promotion (Public Health Ontario [PHO]), Provincial Infectious Diseases Advisory Committee (PIDAC) (PHO-PIDAC, 2014)—*Best Practices for Hand Hygiene in All Health Care Settings*, 4th edition (https://www.publichealthontario.ca/-/media/documents/B/2014/bp-hand-hygiene.pdf)
- Public Health Agency of Canada (PHAC, 2017)—*Routine Practices and Additional Precautions for Preventing the Transmission of Infection in Healthcare Settings* (https://www.canada.ca/en/public-health/services/publications/diseases-conditions/routine-practices-precautions-healthcare-associated-infections.html)

PRINCIPLES FOR PRACTICE

- Hand hygiene practices are major principles of infection control and are essential to safe patient care (IPAC Canada, 2022; PHAC, 2021; World Health Organization [WHO], 2017).
- Patients in all health care settings are at risk of becoming colonized or infected because of an impaired immune response, exposure to an increased number of pathogenic organisms, and performance of invasive procedures (Shang et al., 2020).
- Patients have varying levels of susceptibility to infection and should be assessed. Age, nutritional status, stress, disease processes, and forms of medical therapy can place patients at risk (Bajpal & Nahrendorf, 2021).
- Health care–associated infections (HAIs), which are infections not present at the time of admission, result from direct contact with health care workers during provision of health services in a health care setting. A hospital is one of the most likely settings in which an HAI is acquired because staff, patients, and

environmental factors support a high population of pathogens that are resistant to antibiotics (Tan et al., 2021).

- Using interprofessional collaboration optimizes the prevention and control of infection and enhances patient safety (Saraswathy et al., 2021).
- The presence of a pathogen does not mean that an infection will occur. Infection occurs in a cycle, often referred to as the *chain of infection* (Cole, 2012). An infection develops if this chain remains intact (Fig. 5.1). By recognizing elements of the chain of infection and initiating measures to prevent the onset and spread of infection, it is possible to break an element in the chain so as not to transmit infection (Table 5.1). The six elements in the chain of infection are as follows:
    - An infectious agent or pathogen
    - A reservoir or source of pathogen growth

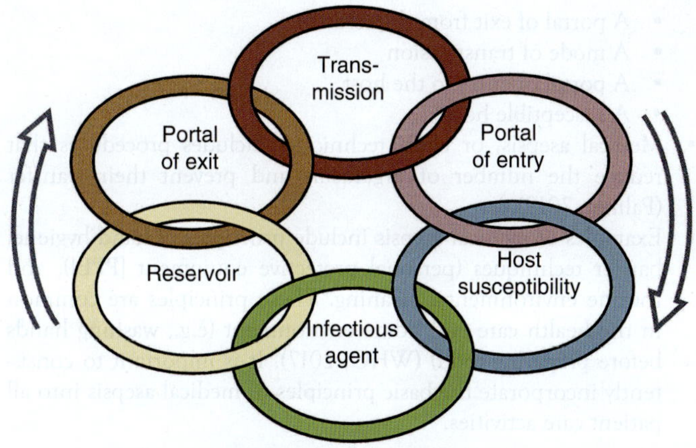

FIG 5.1 Chain of infection.

TABLE 5.1

Breaking the Chain of Infection

Element in the Chain of Infection	Medical Asepsis Practices
Infectious agent (pathogenic organism capable of causing disease)	Clean contaminated objects. Clean, disinfect, and sterilize.
Reservoir (site or source of microorganism survival and growth)	Perform hand hygiene before and after patient contact with appropriate antiseptic (e.g., alcohol-based hand rub) or soap and water. Control sources of body fluids and drainage. Bathe patient with soap and water or use disposable bath. If a patient is critically ill, chlorhexidine baths are more effective for infection prevention (Huang et al., 2019). Change soiled dressings. Dispose of soiled tissues, dressings, or linen in moisture-resistant bags. Place syringes, uncapped hypodermic needles, and intravenous needles in designated puncture-proof containers. Keep table surfaces clean and dry. Do not leave bottled solutions open for prolonged periods. Keep solutions tightly capped. Keep surgical wound drainage tubes and collection bags patent. Empty and dispose of drainage suction bottles according to employer policy.
Portal of exit (means by which microorganisms leave a site)	Respiratory • Avoid talking, sneezing, or coughing directly over wound or sterile dressing field. • Cover nose and mouth when sneezing or coughing. • Wear mask if suffering respiratory tract infection. Urine, feces, emesis, and blood • Wear clean gloves when handling blood and body fluids. • Wear gowns and eyewear if there is a chance of splashing fluids. • Handle all laboratory specimens as if infectious.
Mode of transmission (means of spread)	Reduce microorganism spread: • Perform hand hygiene according to the 4 moments for hand hygiene (Accreditation Canada, 2020) (Fig. 5.2). • Use personal set of care items for each patient. • Avoid shaking bed linen or clothes; dust with damp cloth. • Avoid contact of soiled item with uniform. • Discard any item that touches the floor. • Follow routine practices or additional precautions as indicated (e.g., transmission-based precautions).
Portal of entry (site through which microorganisms enter a host)	Skin and mucosa • Maintain skin and mucous membrane integrity; lubricate skin, offer frequent hygiene, turn and position. • Cover wounds as needed. • Clean wound sites thoroughly. • Dispose of used needles in puncture-proof container. Urinary • Keep all drainage systems closed and intact, maintaining downward flow.
Vulnerable host (patient)	Reduce susceptibility to infection. Provide adequate nutrition. Ensure adequate rest. Promote body defences against infection. Provide immunizations.

- A portal of exit from the reservoir
- A mode of transmission
- A portal of entry to the host
- A susceptible host
- Medical asepsis, or clean technique, includes procedures that reduce the number of organisms and prevent their transfer (Palmer, 2019).
- Examples of medical asepsis include principles of hand hygiene, barrier techniques (personal protective equipment [PPE]), and routine environmental cleaning. These principles are common in the health care and home environment (e.g., washing hands before preparing food) (WHO, 2017). It is important to consistently incorporate the basic principles of medical asepsis into all patient care activities.

PERSON-CENTRED CARE

- Nurses are responsible for educating patients and their families about infection control, including information concerning signs and symptoms of infection, modes of transmission, methods of prevention, knowledge of the infectious process, disease transmission, and critical thinking skills associated with the use of aseptic techniques and barrier protection.
- Some infections require transmission-based precautions, leading to isolation of the patient, which may negatively affect mental health and self-concept or body image (Hossain et al., 2020).
- It is important to know the cultural views and preferences of your patients. Patients who choose to incorporate alternative health care practices may require education on medical asepsis (Evgin & Muz, 2021).
- When a patient from another culture requires transmission-based precautions that include isolation, use caution to ensure that the patient and caregiver understand the therapeutic purpose (Gammon et al., 2019).

EVIDENCE-INFORMED PRACTICE

- Multimodal interventions such as ongoing education, reminders (e.g., posters), administrative support, wall-mounted alcohol dispensers, and pocket-size bottles improve hand hygiene practices (WHO, 2017).
- Handwashing with plain soap sometimes results in paradoxical increases in bacterial counts on the skin (WHO, 2009). A systematic review supports the WHO's "5 moments for hand hygiene" (refined to "4 moments for hand hygiene" in Canada; see Fig. 5.2), and adherence to hand hygiene practices among health care providers is increased through goal setting, incentives, and accountability (Assefa et al., 2021; PHO-PIDAC, 2014; WHO, 2017).
- Alcohol-based products are more effective for standard handwashing or hand antisepsis than soap or antiseptic soaps (WHO, 2022). Moreover, brisk alcohol-based rinses or gels containing emollients cause substantially less skin irritation and dryness than plain or antimicrobial soaps (Peters et al., 2022).
- Soap and water are still necessary for hand hygiene if hands are visibly soiled or when caring for patients infected with *Clostridioides difficile (C. difficile)* (Kiersnowska et al., 2021).

SAFETY GUIDELINES

- Hand hygiene with an appropriate alcohol-based hand antiseptic or soap and water is an essential part of patient care and infection prevention and is fundamental to patient safety (PHAC, 2021).
- Always assess a patient's susceptibility to infection. Age, nutritional status, stress, disease processes, and forms of medical therapy can place patients at risk.
- Recognize the elements of the chain of infection, and initiate measures to prevent the onset and spread of infection.
- Health care workers should not wear artificial nails or nail enhancements because of bacterial buildup (Alberta Health Services, 2021; IPAC Canada, 2022).
- Fingernails should not be longer than 0.625 cm (0.25 inches) in length, with evidence suggesting that nail polish should not be worn (Wu & Lipner, 2020).
- Consistently incorporate the basic principles of medical asepsis into patient care.
- Ensure that patients, caregivers, and health care workers follow "cough hygiene practices"—cover the mouth and nose with arm when coughing or sneezing, use tissues to contain respiratory secretions, dispose of tissues in the waste receptacle, and wash hands (Alberta Health Services, 2020).
- Use clean gloves when you anticipate contact with body fluids, nonintact skin, or mucous membranes when there is a risk of drainage.
- Use barrier protection (e.g., gown, mask, and eye protection) when there is a splash risk.

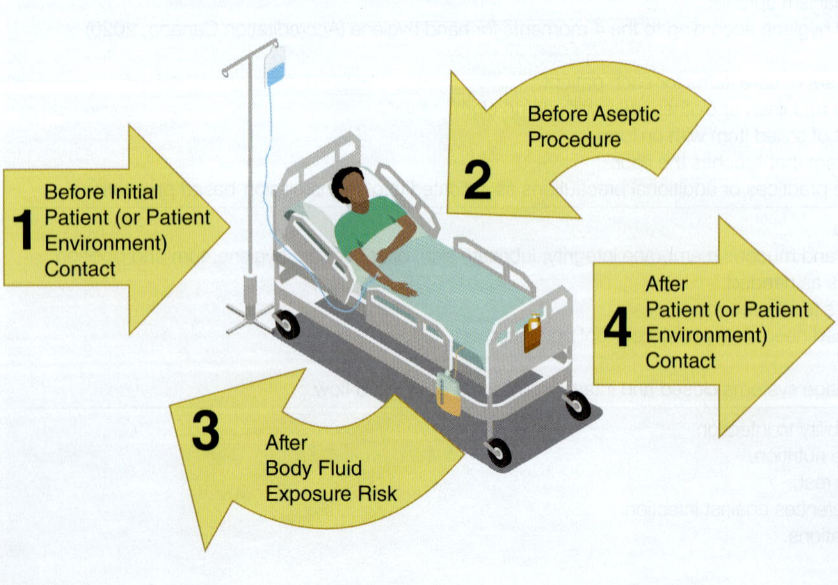

FIG 5.2 **The 4 moments for hand hygiene.** (*Adapted from Nova Scotia Department of Health and Wellness. [2021]. Hand hygiene. https://novascotia.ca/dhw/hsq/public-reporting/hand-hygiene-data.asp*)

- Protect other health care workers from exposure to infectious agents through proper use and disposal of equipment in appropriate receptacles.
- Be aware of body sites where HAIs are most likely to develop (e.g., urinary or respiratory tract). This enables you to direct preventive measures (Henderson et al., 2021).

SKILL 5.1 Hand Hygiene

Video Clip NSO Nursing Skills Online Infection Control Module 2 / Lessons 1 and 2

The most important and basic technique in preventing and controlling transmission of infection is hand hygiene (Hillier, 2020). *Hand hygiene* is a general term that applies to handwashing, antiseptic hand wash, antiseptic hand rub, or surgical hand antisepsis. *Handwashing* refers to washing hands with plain soap and water. An *antiseptic hand wash* is defined as washing hands with water and soap or other detergents containing an antiseptic agent. An *antiseptic hand rub* means applying an antiseptic hand rub product to all surfaces of the hands to reduce the number of microorganisms present. *Surgical hand antisepsis* is the use of an antiseptic hand wash or antiseptic hand rub before surgery by surgical personnel to eliminate transient microorganisms and reduce resident hand microorganisms (see Chapter 38, Skill 38.1).

Hand hygiene is performed at these junctures of clinical care (called the 4 moments for hand hygiene): (1) before initial patient (or patient environment) contact, (2) before any aseptic procedure, (3) after any blood or body fluid exposure risk, and (4) after patient (or patient environment) contact (Accreditation Canada, 2020; Hillier, 2020; PHO-PIDAC, 2014). It is a critical responsibility for all health care workers to follow these guidelines for hand hygiene (Lotfinejad et al., 2021):

- Wash hands with either plain soap and water or an antibacterial soap and water when they are visibly dirty or soiled with blood or other body fluids, before eating, and after using the toilet.
- Wash hands if exposed to spore-forming organisms such as *C. difficile* (Kiersnowska et al., 2021).
- If hands are not visibly soiled, use an alcohol-based hand rub for routinely decontaminating hands in the following clinical situations:
  - Before and after having direct contact with patients
  - Before applying sterile gloves and inserting an invasive device such as in-dwelling urinary catheters and intravenous peripheral vascular catheters
  - After contact with body fluids or excretions, mucous membranes, and nonintact skin
  - After contact with wound dressings (if hands are not visibly soiled)
  - When moving from a contaminated body site to a clean body site during patient care
  - After contact with inanimate objects (e.g., medical equipment) in the immediate vicinity of a patient
  - After removing gloves

Delegation and Collaboration

The skill of hand hygiene is performed by all caregivers. Hand hygiene is not optional (Lotfinejad et al., 2021). Members of the health care team should serve as role models for one another and provide reminders when hand hygiene is missed or incomplete.

Equipment

- Antiseptic hand rub
  - Alcohol-based waterless antiseptic containing emollients
- Handwashing
  - Easy-to-reach sink with warm running water
  - Antimicrobial or regular soap
  - Paper towels or air dryer
  - Disposable nail cleaner (*optional*)

STEP	RATIONALE
ASSESSMENT	
1. Inspect surface of hands for breaks or cuts in skin or cuticles. Cover any skin lesions with a waterproof dressing before providing care. If lesions are too large to cover, you may be restricted from direct patient care.	Open cuts or wounds can harbour high concentrations of microorganisms. Employer policy may prevent nurses from caring for high-risk patients if open lesions are present on hands (WHO, 2009).
2. Inspect hands for visible soiling.	Visible soiling requires handwashing with soap and water.
3. Inspect condition of nails. Natural tips should be no longer than 0.625 cm (0.25 inches) long. Be sure that fingernails are short, filed, and smooth.	Subungual areas of hands harbour high concentrations of bacteria. Long nails and chipped or old polish increase the number of bacteria residing on hands (IPAC Canada, 2022). Artificial nail applications increase microbial load on hands (Alberta Health Services, 2021).
NURSING DIAGNOSES	
This skill is required for all patients with a variety of nursing diagnoses. *Related factors are individualized on the basis of patient's condition or needs.*	
PLANNING	
1. Expected outcomes following completion of procedure:	
• Hands and areas under fingernails are clean and free of debris.	Transient bacteria have been removed.
• Skin of hands is without irritation or breakdown.	Proper hand hygiene technique used.
• Patient and caregivers perform hand hygiene appropriately in health care or home setting.	Reduces infection transmission.

STEP	RATIONALE
IMPLEMENTATION	
1. Throughout the procedure, the 4 moments for hand hygiene are to be implemented; hand hygiene should occur before initial patient (or patient environment) contact, before an aseptic procedure, after body fluid exposure risk, and after patient (or patient environment) contact. Additional hand hygiene should be performed when hands are visibly soiled.	Proper hand hygiene helps prevent the spread of infectious agents to health care providers.
Push wristwatch and long uniform sleeves above wrists. Avoid wearing rings; if worn, remove during hand hygiene.	Provides complete access to fingers, hands, and wrists. The skin underneath rings carries a higher bacterial count; bacteria include Gram-negative bacilli, enterobacteria, and *Staphylococcus aureus* (Wu & Lipner, 2020).
2. Antiseptic hand rub:	
a. According to manufacturer directions, dispense ample amount of product into palm of one hand (see Step 2a illustration).	Use enough product to cover hands thoroughly.
b. Rub hands together, covering all surfaces of hands and fingers with antiseptic (see Step 2b illustration).	Provides enough time for product to work.

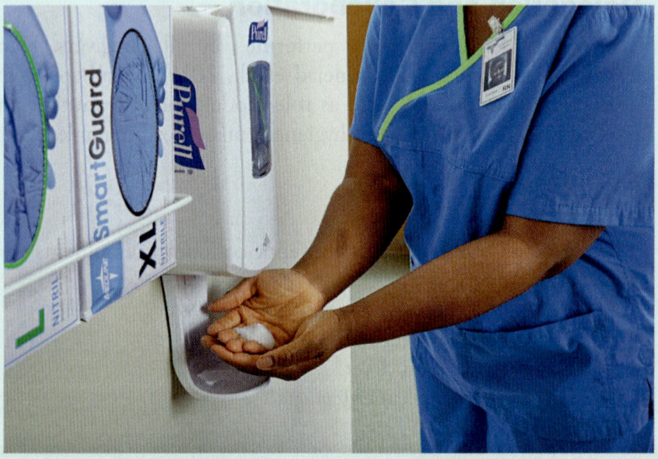

STEP 2A Apply waterless antiseptic to hands.

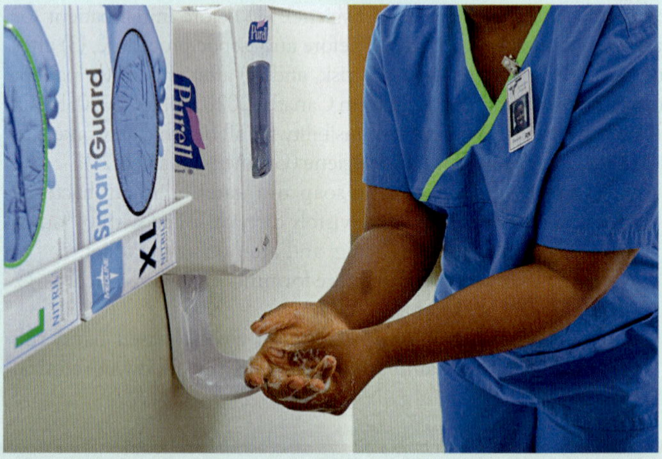

STEP 2B Rub hands thoroughly.

STEP	RATIONALE
c. Rub hands together until alcohol is dry. Allow hands to dry completely before applying gloves.	Ensures complete antimicrobial action.
3. Handwashing using regular or antimicrobial soap:	
a. Stand in front of sink, keeping hands and uniform away from sink surface. (If hands touch sink during handwashing, repeat sequence.)	Inside of sink is contaminated area. Reaching over sink increases risk of touching edge, which is contaminated.
b. Turn on water. Turn on faucet (see Step 3b illustration) or push knee pedals laterally or press pedals with foot to regulate flow and temperature.	Knee pads within operating room and treatment areas are preferred, to prevent hand contact with faucet. Faucet handles are likely to be contaminated with organic debris and microorganisms and should be manipulated using paper towel (Spruce, 2021).
c. Avoid splashing water against uniform.	Microorganisms travel and grow in moisture.
d. Regulate flow of water so temperature is warm.	Warm water removes less of protective oils from hands than hot water.
e. Wet hands and wrists thoroughly under running water. Keep hands and forearms lower than elbows during washing.	Hands are the most contaminated parts to wash. Water flows from least to most contaminated area, rinsing microorganisms into sink.

STEP	RATIONALE

IMPLEMENTATION

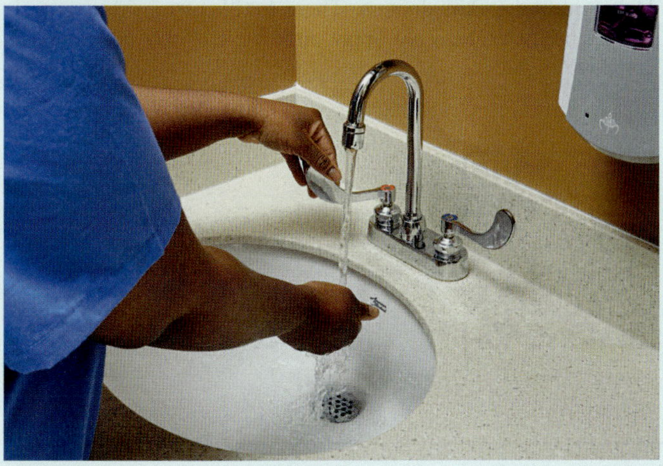

STEP 3B Turn on water.

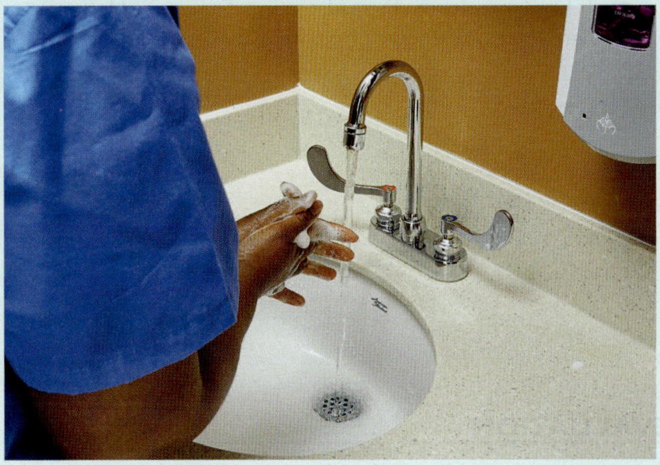

STEP 3F Lather hands thoroughly.

STEP	RATIONALE
f. Apply 3–5 mL of antiseptic soap and rub hands together (see Step 3f illustration).	Ensure that all surfaces of hands and fingers are cleaned.
g. Perform hand hygiene using plenty of lather and friction for at least 15 seconds. Interlace fingers and rub palms and back of hands with circular motion at least five times each. Keep fingertips down to facilitate removal of microorganisms.	Soap cleans by emulsifying fat and oil and lowering surface tension. Friction and rubbing mechanically loosen and remove dirt and transient bacteria. Interlacing fingers and thumbs ensures that all surfaces are cleaned. Adequate time is needed to expose skin surfaces to antimicrobial agent.
h. Areas underlying fingernails are often soiled. Clean them with fingernails of other hand and additional soap or with disposable nail cleaner.	Area under nails can be highly contaminated, which increases risk for transmission of infection from nurse to patient.
i. Rinse hands and wrists thoroughly, keeping hands down and elbows up (see Step 3i illustration).	Rinsing mechanically washes away dirt and microorganisms.
j. Dry hands thoroughly from fingers to wrists with paper towel, single-use cloth, or warm air dryer.	Drying from cleanest (fingertips) to least clean (wrist) avoids contamination. Drying hands prevents chapping and roughened skin. Do not tear or cut skin under or around nail.
k. If used, discard paper towel in proper receptacle.	Prevents transfer of microorganisms.
l. To turn off hand faucet, use clean, dry paper towel; avoid touching handles with hands (see Step 3l illustration). Turn off water with foot or knee pedals (if applicable).	Wet towel and hands allow transfer of pathogens from faucet by capillary action.

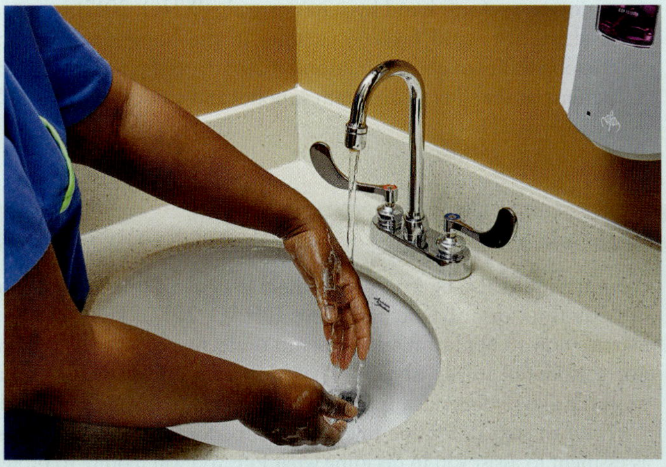

STEP 3I Rinse hands.

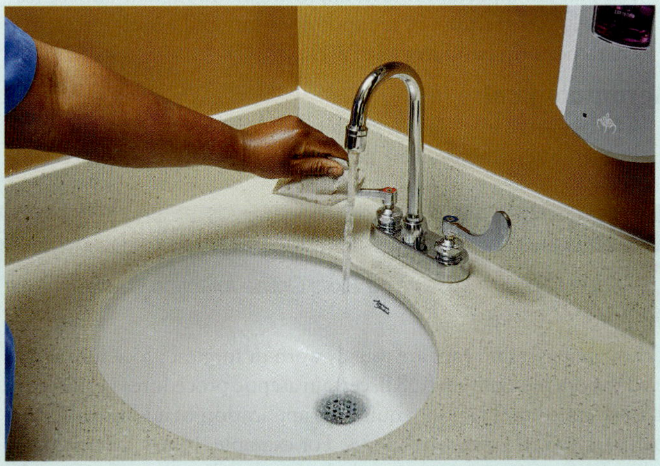

STEP 3L Turn off faucet.

STEP	RATIONALE
IMPLEMENTATION	
m. If hands are dry or chapped, use small amount of lotion or barrier cream dispensed from individual-use container.	Helps minimize skin dryness. There is risk of organism growth in lotion; therefore, only apply after patient care activities are complete.
EVALUATION	
1. Inspect surface of hands for obvious signs of dirt or other contaminants.	Determines whether hand hygiene is adequate.
2. Inspect hands for dermatitis or cracked skin.	Breaks in skin integrity increase risk for transmission of microorganisms.
3. Use teach-back: "Can you tell me when you or your caregiver would wash your hands and the different ways you can wash your hands?" Develop a revised teaching plan if patient or caregiver is unable to teach back correctly.	Determines patient's and caregiver's level of understanding of instructional topic (Fries et al., 2020).

Unexpected Outcomes	Related Interventions
1. Hands or areas under fingernails remain soiled.	• Repeat handwashing with soap and water.
2. Repeated use of soaps or antiseptics causes dermatitis or cracked skin.	• Rinse and dry hands thoroughly after using soap and water; avoid excessive amounts of soap or antiseptic; try various products. • Use approved hand lotions or barrier creams. Small individual-use containers are preferred because large containers have been found to harbour pathogens.

Special Considerations

Teaching

- Instruct patient and caregiver in proper techniques and situations for hand hygiene.
- When patients are educated about the risks for infections, they can play an important role in improving hand hygiene adherence in health care settings by reminding visitors and health care workers to perform hand hygiene (WHO, 2017).

Gerontological

- The impact of infections is greater in older persons. Hand hygiene by staff attending to older persons is of utmost importance and should be an ongoing continuing education requirement (Hillier, 2020).

Care in the Community: Home Management

- Evaluate patient and caregiver to determine their understanding of the transmission of microorganisms and their ability and motivation to perform hand hygiene correctly (WHO, 2017).
- Evaluate the hand hygiene facilities in the home to determine the possibility of contamination, proximity of the facilities to the patient, and ability to maintain supplies and equipment (Payne & Peache, 2021).

✦ SKILL 5.2 Applying and Removing Cap, Mask, and Protective Eyewear

Video Clip *NSO Nursing Skills Online Infection Control Module 2 / Lesson 1*

Although masks and caps are usually worn in surgical procedure areas (e.g., the operating room [OR]), certain aseptic procedures performed at a patient's bedside also require the application of additional PPE, such as eyewear, gown, and gloves. For example, it may be employer policy for a nurse to wear a mask during the changing of a central-line dressing or insertion of a peripherally inserted central catheter (PICC). Other policies might require that a nurse wear a mask and cap to secure hair during dressing changes on a patient with extensive burns or a central line (Infusion Nurses Society, 2021). Protective eyewear should also be worn when there is a risk of splattering blood or body fluid or airborne pathogens (PHAC, 2017). This skill summarizes how to apply a mask, cap, and protective eyewear, which are not considered sterile objects. The additional application of clean or sterile gloves depends on the type of procedure being performed.

The first step in routine practices is to perform a point-of-care risk assessment to assist you in deciding what PPE you will require to protect yourself, patients, and other members of the interprofessional health care team (Box 5.1). Assess a patient's potential for acquiring an infection and the splash risk before deciding whether to apply a mask (e.g., Does the patient have a large open wound? Is the person immunosuppressed?

Is there a splash risk from the wound?). If you wear a mask, change it when it becomes moist or soiled (e.g., splattered with blood). Wear eyewear when there is a risk of body fluids splashing into your eyes.

Delegation and Collaboration

The skill of applying and removing cap, mask, and protective eyewear is required of all caregivers working in areas in which sterile procedures are performed. However, the *procedures* performed at a patient's bedside that require cap, mask, gown, or eyewear generally cannot be delegated to an unregulated care provider (UCP). The skill of applying PPE can be delegated to a UCP. The nurse instructs the UCP to do the following:

- Be available to hand off equipment or help with patient positioning during a sterile procedure. If the procedure is to use sterile technique, the nurse must educate the UCP regarding the sterile field.

Members of the interprofessional health care team should collaborate to serve as role models for one another and provide reminders when sterile technique is missed or incomplete.

Equipment

- Surgical mask (different types are available for people with different skin sensitivities)
- Surgical cap (**Note:** Use in OR, or if employer policy requires. Use to secure hair if there is a possibility of contamination of a sterile field.)
- Hairpins, elastic bands, or both
- Protective eyewear (e.g., goggles or glasses with appropriate side shields). *Option:* Clean or sterile gloves (applied after cap, mask, or eyewear is applied). See Skill 5.3.

BOX 5.1

Point-of-Care Risk Assessment for Use of Personal Protective Equipment

Assess the task, the patient, and the environment prior to every patient encounter to determine the correct personal protective equipment (PPE) to use. Ask yourself the following questions:

- Will my hands be exposed to blood, body fluids, or contaminated items?
  - If yes, wear nonsterile gloves.
- Will my clothing or skin become contaminated from splashes/sprays or contact with items contaminated with blood or body fluids?
  - If yes, wear a gown.
- Will my eyes, face, or mucous membranes be splashed or sprayed with blood or body fluids or be within 2 metres of a coughing or vomiting patient?
  - If yes, wear facial protection (mask and eye).
- Is the patient suspected or confirmed to have COVID-19?
  - If yes, wear COVID-19–related PPE (including fit-tested N95 respirator).

Adapted from Alberta Health Services. (2022). *Point of care risk assessment (PCRA).* https://www.albertahealthservices.ca/assets/healthinfo/ipc/hi-ipc-acute-care-pcra.pdf

STEP	RATIONALE
ASSESSMENT	
1. Review type of sterile procedure to be performed and consult employer policy for use of mask, cap, gown, or protective eyewear.	Not all sterile procedures require mask, cap, gown, or protective eyewear. Ensures that nurse and patient are properly protected.
2. If you or other health care providers have symptoms of a respiratory infection, either avoid participating in procedure or apply a mask.	A greater number of pathogenic microorganisms reside within the respiratory tract when infection is present.
3. Assess patient's risk for infection (e.g., older person, neonate, or immunocompromised patient).	Some patients are at greater risk of acquiring an infection; therefore, use additional protective barriers.
NURSING DIAGNOSES	
• Insufficient protection • Potential for infection *Related factors and risk factors are individualized on the basis of patient's condition or needs.*	
PLANNING	
1. Expected outcome following completion of procedure: • Patient does not develop signs of localized infection (e.g., redness, tenderness, edema, drainage) or systemic infection (e.g., fever, change in white blood cell [WBC] count) 24 hours after procedure.	Indicates lack of microorganism transfer to patient and sterile field.
2. Prepare equipment and inspect packaging for integrity and exposure to sterilization.	Ensures availability of equipment and sterility of supplies before procedure begins.
IMPLEMENTATION	
1. Throughout the procedure, the 4 moments for hand hygiene are to be implemented; hand hygiene should occur before initial patient (or patient environment) contact, before an aseptic procedure, after body fluid exposure risk, and after patient (or patient environment) contact. Additional hand hygiene should be performed when hands are visibly soiled.	Proper hand hygiene helps prevent the spread of infectious agents to health care providers.
2. *Option:* In cases in which you are performing or assisting with a procedure at a patient's bedside, apply a clean gown if there is a risk of splatter or soiling. Apply the gown with opening to the back. Be sure that it covers all outer garments. Pull sleeves down to wrist. Tie securely at neck and wrist.	Proper gowning prevents transmission of infections when patient has excessive drainage or discharges.

STEP	RATIONALE

IMPLEMENTATION

3. Apply a cap:
   a. If hair is long, comb back behind ears and secure. — Cap must cover all hair entirely.
   b. Secure hair in place with pins. — Long hair should not fall down or cause cap to slip and expose hair.
   c. Apply cap over head as you would apply a hairnet. Be sure that all hair fits under edges of cap (see Step 3c illustration). — Loose hair hanging over sterile field or falling dander contaminates objects on sterile field.

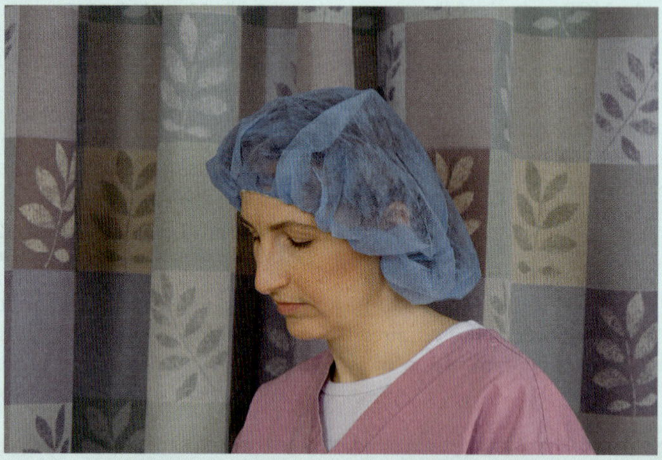

STEP 3C Apply cap over head, covering all hair.

4. Apply a mask:
   a. Find top edge of mask, which usually has a thin metal strip along edge. — Pliable metal fits snugly against bridge of nose.
   b. Hold mask by top two strings or loops, keeping top edge above bridge of nose. — Position prevents contact of hands with clean facial part of mask. Mask covers all of nose.
   c. Tie two top strings at top of back of head, over cap (if worn), with strings above ears (see Step 4c illustration). Alternatively, place loops over ears. — Position of ties at top of head provides tight fit. Strings over ears may cause irritation.
   d. Tie two lower ties snugly around neck with mask well under chin (see Step 4d illustration). — Tying prevents escape of microorganisms through sides of mask as you talk and breathe.

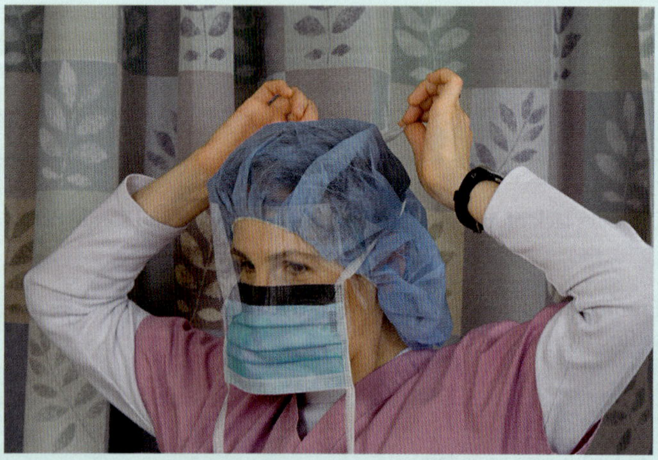

STEP 4C Tie top strings of mask.

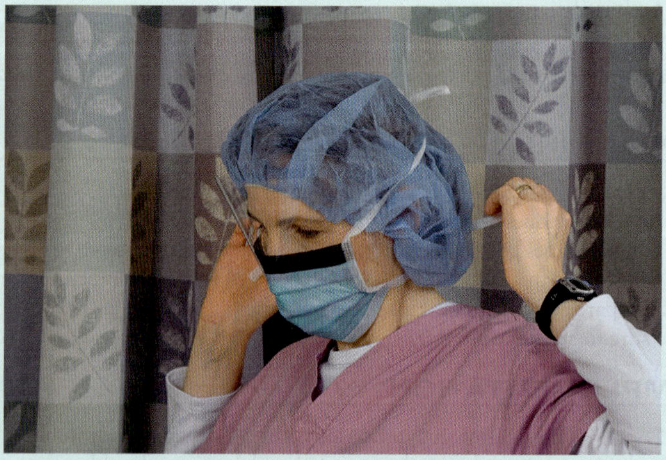

STEP 4D Tie bottom strings of mask.

   e. Gently pinch upper metal band around bridge of nose. — Pinching prevents microorganisms from escaping around nose and eyeglasses from steaming up.

5. Apply protective eyewear:
   a. Apply protective glasses, goggles, or face shield comfortably over eyes and check that vision is clear (see Step 5a illustration). — Positioning affects clarity of vision.
   b. Be sure that face shield fits snugly around forehead and face. — Snug fitting ensures that eyes are fully protected.

STEP	RATIONALE

IMPLEMENTATION

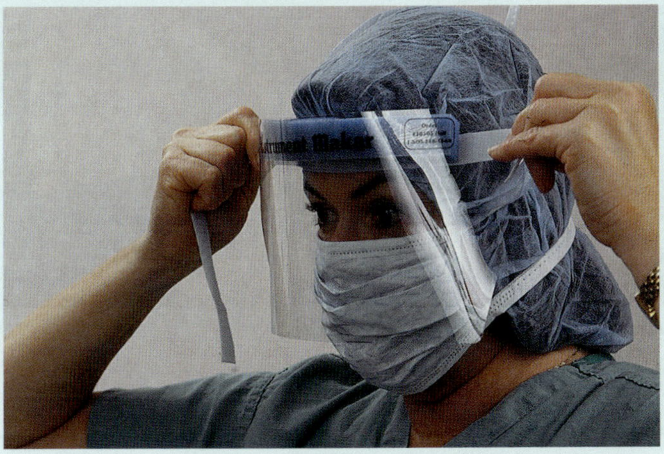

STEP 5A Apply face shield over cap.

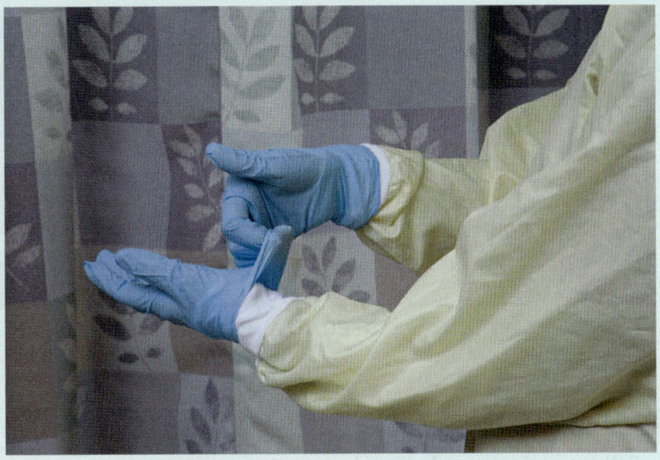

STEP 6 Apply gloves over gown sleeves.

Step	Rationale
6. If performing a sterile procedure, apply sterile gown (see Skill 5.3) at this time. After applying cap, mask, and eyewear, apply clean gloves for nonsterile procedures and sterile gloves (see Skill 6.2) for sterile procedures. Pull up clean gloves to cover each wrist (see Step 6 illustration). NOTE: Provide a latex-free environment if patient or nurse has a latex allergy.	Reduces transmission of microorganisms.
7. Remove protective barriers:	
a. Remove gloves first if worn (see Skill 6.2). Remove gloves by grasping cuff and pulling glove inside out over hand. Hold removed glove in other gloved hand. Slide fingers of ungloved hand under remaining glove at wrist (see Step 7a illustration). Peel glove off over first glove. Discard gloves in proper container.	Proper removal prevents contamination of hair, neck, and facial area.
b. Remove gown by unfastening neck ties and pulling away from neck and shoulders. Touching only inside of gown, turn gown inside out, roll, or fold into a bundle and discard.	Front and sleeves of gown are contaminated. This method of disposal prevents transmission of infection.
c. Remove eyewear. Avoid placing hands over soiled lens. NOTE: If wearing a face shield, remove it before removing mask.	Proper removal prevents transmission of microorganisms.
d. Untie bottom strings of mask. First, hold strings, untie top strings, and pull mask away from face while holding strings. Then remove mask from face and discard in proper receptacle (see Step 7d illustrations).	Proper removal prevents top part of mask from falling down over uniform. If mask falls and touches uniform, uniform will be contaminated.
e. Grasp outer surface of cap and lift from hair.	Proper removal minimizes contact of hands with hair.
f. Discard cap in proper receptacle.	Routine reduces transmission of infection.

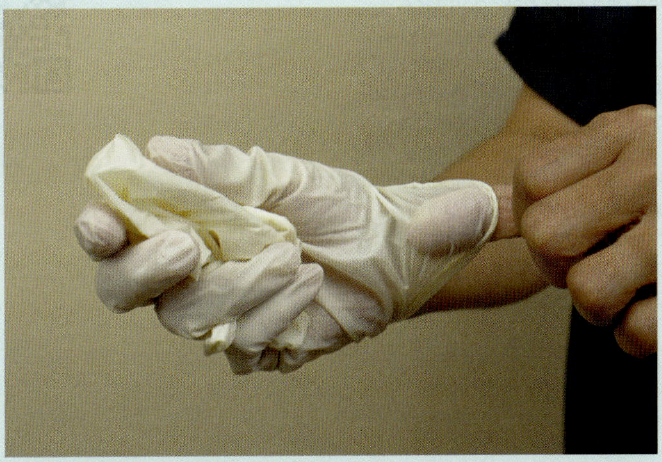

STEP 7A Remove second glove while holding soiled glove.

STEP	RATIONALE

IMPLEMENTATION

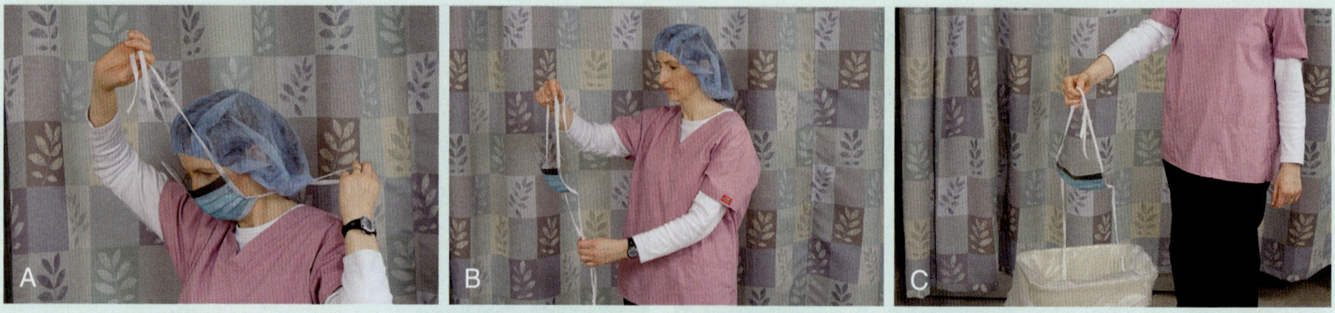

STEP 7D A, Untie top mask strings. B, Remove mask from face. C, Discard mask.

EVALUATION

STEP	RATIONALE
1. Following the procedure and as part of ongoing assessment, assess patient for signs of systemic infections or local area of body treated for drainage, tenderness, edema, or redness.	Assessment rules out presence of localized infection.
2. Use teach-back: "I want to be sure I explained why personal protective equipment is used. Please explain to me why you and your caregiver need to wear personal protective equipment and show me how you will put it on." Develop a revised teaching plan if patient or caregiver is unable to teach back correctly.	Determines patient's and caregiver's level of understanding of instructional topic.

Unexpected Outcomes	Related Interventions
1. Redness, heat, edema, pain, or purulent drainage develops at wound or treatment site, indicating possible infection.	• Notify health care provider of change in condition of affected area and initiate appropriate treatments as prescribed.

Communication and Documentation

- It is unnecessary to document use of PPE.
- Communicate required use of PPE to patients, families, caregivers and all interprofessional team members. Document patient and caregiver learning.

DOCUMENTATION EXAMPLE

Provided demonstration of donning and doffing of personal protective equipment (PPE) to one family member with permission to visit patient; family member demonstrated understanding by stating reasons for requiring PPE (to decrease spread of microorganisms to self, patient, and HCPs); was able to successfully don PPE (perform hand hygiene before donning PPE; put on gown first, then cap over hair; don face mask by fitting metal strip to nose, then tie upper strings above ears, lower strings around neck, then pinch metal band around nose; put on face shield) and doff PPE (remove gown and place in laundry bag, touching only the inside of the gown; perform hand hygiene; remove face shield; untie bottom strings, hold and untie top strings and pull mask away from face; discard in garbage bin; remove cap and discard in garbage bin) during practice session; family member stated they felt comfortable with this process; was encouraged to ask for help if required; correctly donned PPE; and entered room to visit patient.

Special Considerations

Care in the Community: Home Management

- Instruct family, caregiver, or both about specifics of when to use PPE and how to dispose of PPE properly.
- Determine ability of family, caregiver, or both to use equipment safely.
- Teach patient and caregiver to observe for signs and symptoms of infection.

✦ SKILL 5.3 Caring for Patients Under Transmission-Based Precautions

When a patient has a known or suspected source of colonization or infection, health care workers follow specific infection prevention and control practices to reduce the risk of cross-contamination to other patients. Certain procedures performed at a patient's bedside require the application of PPE such as a mask, cap, eyewear, gown, or gloves. Routine practices require the nurse to wear clean gloves before coming in contact with mucous membranes, nonintact skin, blood, body fluids, or other infectious material. Clean gloves are worn routinely when performing a variety of procedures (e.g., nasogastric tube insertion). Masks are worn when there is the risk of splashing during a procedure or when certain sterile procedures such as changing a central-line dressing are performed. Protective eyewear and masks become important when there is a risk of splashing of blood or other body fluids to the eyes or mouth (Woolley et al., 2020).

Assess the need for PPE for each task you plan and for all patients, regardless of their diagnoses. Because of increased attention to the prevention of bloodborne pathogens and tuberculosis (TB) (Box 5.2), the Public Health Agency of Canada (PHAC, 2017, 2021) has stressed the importance of barrier protection. The PHAC (2017, 2021) has published guidelines for infection control and prevention, including the use of PPE.

Routine practices apply to the care of all patients, regardless of risk or presumed infection status (Box 5.3). Routine practices are the primary strategies for prevention of infection transmission and apply to all patient interaction in all health care and community settings.

Additional precautions (Table 5.2) include precautions designed for the care of patients who are known or suspected to be infected, or colonized, with microorganisms transmitted by the contact, droplet, or airborne route (PHAC, 2021) or by contact with contaminated surfaces (see Table 5.2). The three types of transmission-based precautions—airborne, droplet, and contact—may be combined for diseases that have multiple routes of transmission (e.g., chickenpox). Whether used singly or in combination, use these precautions in addition to routine practices.

Delegation and Collaboration

The skill of caring for patients on transmission-based precautions can be delegated to a UCP. However, the nurse must assess the patient's status and transmission-based precaution indications. The nurse instructs the UCP about the following:

- Reason patient is on transmission-based precautions
- Precautions for bringing equipment into the patient's room
- Special precautions regarding individual patient needs such as transportation to diagnostic tests

When a patient develops an infection and the causative organism is unclear, collaborate with infection control personnel to determine proper transmission control procedures. Communication of transmission-based precautions is key among members of the interprofessional health care team who come into contact with the patient so that there is no breach in precautions.

Equipment

- PPE determined by type of transmission-based precautions required: clean gloves, mask, eyewear or goggles, face shield, and gown (gowns may be disposable or reusable, depending on employer policy)

BOX 5.2

Special Tuberculosis Precautions

The Public Health Agency of Canada (PHAC, 2014) has published guidelines to prevent tuberculosis (TB) transmission in health care facilities. The overall number of cases of TB remains virtually unchanged, and TB is most common among Indigenous and foreign-born individuals (LaFreniere et al., 2019).

- Current PHAC (2014) guidelines for preventing and controlling TB focus on early detection of infection, preventing close contact with patients with active TB disease, and applying effective infection control measures in health care settings.
- Suspect TB in any patient with respiratory symptoms lasting longer than 3 weeks accompanied by other suspicious symptoms such as unexplained weight loss, night sweats, fever, and a productive cough often streaked with blood.
- Consider the potential for infectious pulmonary or laryngeal TB from documented positive acid-fast bacilli (AFB) smear or culture, cavitation on chest X-ray film, or history of recent TB exposure.
- Transmission-based precautions for patients with suspected or confirmed TB include placing the patient on airborne precautions in a single-patient negative-pressure room.
- Health care workers who care for patients with suspected or confirmed TB must wear special respirators (e.g., N95 or P100) (Locke et al., 2021). These respirators are high-efficiency particulate masks that have the ability to filter particles at a 95% or better efficiency (Bartoszko et al., 2020).
- The PHAC (2014) recommends that diagnosis of active TB be made with chest radiography and microbiological testing, including sputum smear microscopy, mycobacterial culture, phenotypic drug sensitivity testing, and nucleic acid amplification testing. The use of blood testing may be appropriate in specific circumstances.
- Health Canada (2016) has developed a monitoring and performance framework for TB programs for Indigenous peoples to guide continuous quality improvement and help decrease the incidence of TB.

BOX 5.3

Provincial Infectious Diseases Advisory Committee (PIDAC) Isolation Guidelines

Routine Practices for Use With All Patients

- Perform hand hygiene using alcohol-based hand rub or soap and water: before and after patient contact; before and after providing direct care; before handling food; before donning gloves and personal protective equipment (PPE) and after removing PPE; when contact with secretions, excretions, blood, or body fluid may occur; after personal body functions; and after contact with items in the patient environment (Hillier, 2020; PHO-PIDAC, 2014).
- Use a mask and eye protection (goggles) or face shield based on point-of-care risk assessment (see Box 5.1).
- Wear a long-sleeved gown if contamination of skin or clothing is anticipated.
- Wear gloves if there is a risk of contact with blood, body fluids, nonintact skin or mucous membranes, or contaminated surfaces or objects. Glove use is not a substitute for hand hygiene.
- All equipment that is being used by more than one patient must be cleaned between patients.
- Handle soiled linen and waste appropriately to prevent personal contamination and transfer to other patients.
- A private room is unnecessary unless the patient's hygiene is unacceptable (e.g., uncontained secretions, excretions, or wound drainage). Perform hand hygiene on exiting the room.
- Never recap used needles. Discard all contaminated sharp instruments and needles in a puncture-resistant sharps container. Where possible, use safety-engineered medical devices.

Adapted from Public Health Agency of Canada. (2017). *Routine practices and additional precautions for preventing the transmission of infection in healthcare settings.* https://www.canada.ca/en/public-health/services/publications/diseases-conditions/routine-practices-precautions-healthcare-associated-infections.html

TABLE 5.2

Provincial Infectious Diseases Advisory Committee (PIDAC): Routine Practices and Additional Precautions in All Health Care Settings for Use With Specific Types of Patients

Transmission-Based Precaution	Indication for Use	Barrier Protection
Contact precautions	When contamination of the environment or intact skin is of consideration, such as: • Contamination of the patient environment • Infectious agents of very low infective dose (e.g., norovirus, rotavirus) • Patients who are infected or colonized with epidemiologically important microorganisms that may be transmitted by contact with intact skin or with contaminated environmental surfaces (e.g., methicillin-resistant *Staphylococcus aureus* (MRSA), vancomycin-resistant Enterococcus (VRE), *C. difficile*)	Private-room or cohort patients with dedicated sink and toilet (see employer policy), gloves, gowns. Patient may leave their room for procedures or therapy if infectious material is contained or covered, patient is placed in a clean gown, and patient's hands are cleaned.
Droplet precautions (droplet within 1 metre [3 feet] of patient)	When droplets carrying an infectious agent exit the respiratory tract of a person, such as: • Respiratory tract viruses (e.g., adenovirus, influenza and parainfluenza viruses, rhinovirus, human metapneumovirus, respiratory syncytial virus [RSV]) • Rubella, mumps, and *Bordetella pertussis*	Private room with a dedicated toilet and patient sink; door may remain open or there may be cohort patients. Mask or respirator (refer to employer policy).
Airborne precautions	When airborne particles remain suspended in the air, travel on air currents, and are then inhaled by others, such as: • Microorganisms transmitted by the airborne route (e.g., *Mycobacterium tuberculosis* [TB], varicella virus [chickenpox virus], and measles virus)	Private room with own toileting facilities. Room with negative-pressure ventilation, with room air exhausted outside through HEPA filter. Door must remain closed; monitor negative pressure daily while in use. N95 respirator; patient to wear mask during transport.

Adapted from Public Health Agency of Canada. (2017). *Routine practices and additional precautions for preventing the transmission of infection in healthcare settings*. https://www.canada.ca/en/public-health/services/publications/diseases-conditions/routine-practices-precautions-healthcare-associated-infections.html

- Other patient care equipment (as appropriate) (e.g., hygiene items, medications, dressing supplies, sharps container, disposable blood pressure [BP] cuff)
- Soiled linen bag and garbage receptacle
- Sign for door indicating type of transmission-based precaution and for visitors to come to the nurses' station before entering room (signs can be text, colour coded, or both)
- TB transmission-based precautions
  - Room with negative airflow
  - N95 or P100 respirator

STEP	RATIONALE
ASSESSMENT	
1. Assess patient's medical history for possible indications for transmission-based precautions (e.g., risk factors for TB, major draining wound, or purulent productive cough). Review specific transmission-based precautions system, including appropriate barriers to apply for each type (e.g., airborne, contact, droplet) (see Table 5.2).	Mode of transmission for infectious microorganism determines type and degree of precautions followed. Ensures adequate protection.
2. Review laboratory test results (e.g., wound culture, acid-fast bacillus [AFB] smears, changes in WBC count).	Reveals type of microorganism for which patient is being isolated, body fluid in which it was identified, and whether patient is immunosuppressed.
3. Review employer policy for transmission-based precautions necessary for patient circumstance, and consider types of care measures that you will perform while in patient's room (e.g., medication administration or dressing change).	Allows you to organize care items for procedures and time spent in patient's room.
4. Review nursing care plan notes or confer with colleagues regarding patient's emotional state and reaction or adjustment to transmission-based precautions. Also assess patient's understanding of purpose of transmission-based precautions.	Provides opportunity to plan for patient's need for emotional support and teaching.
5. Assess whether patient has known latex allergy. If allergy is present, refer to employer policy and resources available to provide full latex-free care.	Protects patient from serious allergic response.

STEP	RATIONALE

NURSING DIAGNOSES

- Insufficient knowledge regarding purpose of transmission-based precautions
- Reduced social interaction
- Inadequate protection
- Potential for infection

Related factors and risk factors are individualized on the basis of patient's condition or needs.

PLANNING

STEP	RATIONALE
1. Expected outcomes following completion of procedure:	
• Patient asks for information about disease transmission.	Active interaction reveals patient's willingness and ability to communicate and be taught and understand information.
• Patient explains purpose of transmission-based precautions.	Instruction about precautions improves patient's ability to cooperate in care.

IMPLEMENTATION

STEP	RATIONALE
1. Identify patient using at least two person-specific identifiers (e.g., name and date of birth, or name and medical record number) according to employer policy.	Ensures correct patient. Complies with Accreditation Canada's standards and improves patient safety (Accreditation Canada, 2020).
2. Throughout the procedure, the 4 moments for hand hygiene are to be implemented; hand hygiene should occur before initial patient (or patient environment) contact, before an aseptic procedure, after body fluid exposure risk, and after patient (or patient environment) contact. Additional hand hygiene should be performed when hands are visibly soiled.	Proper hand hygiene helps prevent the spread of infectious agents to health care providers.
3. Prepare all equipment to be taken into patient's room. In many cases dedicated equipment such as stethoscopes, BP equipment, and thermometers should remain in room until patient is discharged. If patient is infected or colonized with resistant organism (e.g., vancomycin-resistant *Enterococcus* [VRE], methicillin-resistant *Staphylococcus aureus* [MRSA]), equipment remains in room and is thoroughly disinfected before removal (see employer policy).	Prevents you from making more than one trip into room. The PHAC (2017) recommends use of dedicated noncritical patient care equipment.
4. Prepare for entrance into patient room according to appropriate transmission-based precautions. Ideally, before applying PPE, step into patient's room and stay by door. Introduce yourself and explain care that you are providing. If this is not possible, apply PPE outside of the room.	Proper preparation ensures protection from microorganism exposure. Allows patient to see you without PPE and without exposing yourself to risk of infection transmission.
a. Apply gown, being sure that it covers all outer garments. Pull sleeves down to wrist. Tie securely at neck and waist (see Step 4a illustration).	Prevents transmission of infection; protects you when patient has excessive drainage or discharges.
b. Apply either surgical mask or fitted respirator around mouth and nose (type and fit-testing depend on type of transmission-based precaution and employer policy). You must have a medical evaluation and be fit-tested before using a respirator.	Prevents exposure to airborne microorganisms or to microorganisms from splashing of fluids.
c. If needed, apply eyewear or goggles snugly around face and eyes. If you wear prescription glasses, side shields may be used.	Protects you from exposure to microorganisms that may occur during splashing of fluids.
d. Apply clean gloves. (NOTE: Wear unpowdered, latex-free gloves if you, patient, or another health care worker has latex allergy.) Bring glove cuffs over edge of gown sleeves (see Step 4d illustration).	Reduces transmission of microorganisms.

STEP	RATIONALE

IMPLEMENTATION

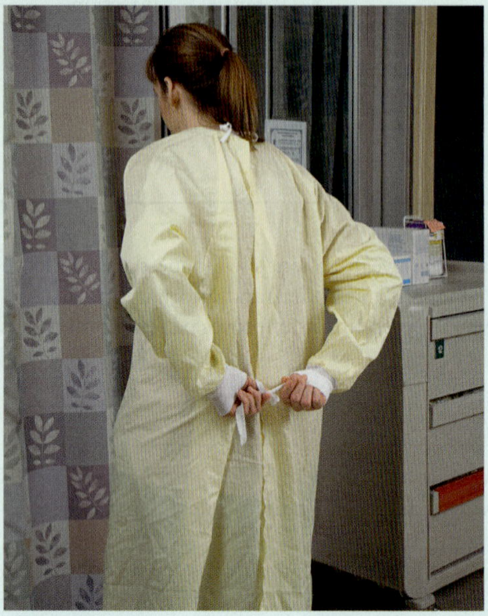

STEP 4A Tie isolation gown at waist.

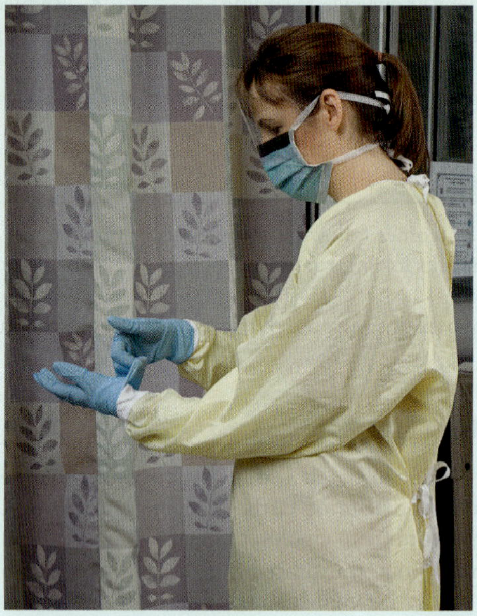

STEP 4D Apply gloves over gown sleeves.

STEP	RATIONALE
5. Enter patient's room. Arrange supplies and equipment. (NOTE: If equipment will be reused, place on clean paper towel.)	Prevents extra trips entering and leaving room. Minimizes contamination of care items.
6. Explain purpose of transmission-based precautions for patient and caregiver to take. Offer opportunity to ask questions. If patient is on TB precautions, instruct to cover mouth with tissue when coughing and to wear disposable surgical mask when leaving room.	Improves patient's and caregiver's ability to participate in care and minimizes anxiety. Identifies opportunity for planning social interaction and diversional activities. Reduces TB microorganism transmission.
7. Assess vital signs (see Chapter 7):	
a. If patient is infected or colonized with resistant organism (e.g., VRE, MRSA), equipment remains in room, including stethoscope and BP cuff (PHAC, 2017).	Decreases risk of infection being transmitted to another patient.
b. If stethoscope is to be reused, clean earpieces and diaphragm or bell with 70% alcohol or employer-approved germicide. Set aside on clean surface.	Systematic disinfection of stethoscopes with alcohol or approved germicide minimizes chance of spreading infectious agents between patients (Napolitani et al., 2020).
c. Use individual or disposable thermometers and BP cuffs when available.	Prevents cross-contamination.

Critical Decision Point *If disposable thermometer indicates a fever, assess for other signs and symptoms. Confirm fever using an alternative thermometer. Do not use electronic thermometer if patient has suspected or confirmed* C. difficile (McDonald et al., 2018).

STEP	RATIONALE
8. Administer medications (see Chapters 20, 21, and 22):	
a. Give oral medication in wrapper or cup.	Handle and discard supplies to minimize transfer of microorganisms.
b. Dispose of wrapper or cup in plastic-lined receptacle.	
c. Wear gloves when administering an injection.	Reduces risk of exposure to blood.
d. Discard needleless syringe or safety-sheathed needle into designated sharps container.	Needleless devices should be used to reduce risk of needle-sticks and sharps injuries to health care workers.
9. Administer hygiene, encouraging patient to ask any questions or express concerns about transmission-based precautions. Provide informal teaching at this time.	Hygiene practices further minimize transfer of microorganisms. Quality time should be spent with patient when in room.
a. Avoid allowing isolation gown to become wet; carry washbasin outward, away from gown; avoid leaning against wet tabletop.	Moisture allows organisms to travel through gown to uniform.

STEP	RATIONALE

IMPLEMENTATION

Critical Decision Point *When there is a risk for excess soiling, wear a gown impervious to moisture.*

STEP	RATIONALE
b. Help patient remove own gown; discard in leak-proof linen bag.	Reduces transfer of microorganisms.
c. Remove linen from bed; avoid contact with isolation gown. Place in leak-proof linen bag.	Handle linen soiled by patient's body fluids to prevent contact with clean items.
d. Provide clean bed linen.	
e. If gloves become excessively soiled and further care is necessary, remove gloves. Reglove.	
10. Collect specimens (see Chapter 9):	
a. Place specimen container on clean paper towel in patient's bathroom and follow procedure for collecting specimen of body fluids.	Container will be taken out of patient's room; prevents contamination of outer surface.
b. Follow employer procedure for collecting specimen of body fluids (see Chapter 9).	
c. Transfer specimen to container without soiling outside of container. Place container in plastic bag and place label on outside of bag or per employer policy. Label specimen in front of patient (PHAC, 2017). Perform hand hygiene and don gloves if additional procedures are needed.	Specimens of blood and body fluids are placed in well-constructed containers with secure lids to prevent leaks during transport. Proper labelling prevents diagnostic error.
d. Check label on specimen for accuracy. Send to laboratory (warning labels are often used, depending on employer policy). Label containers of blood or body fluids with biohazard sticker (see Step 10d illustration).	Ensures that health care providers who transport or handle containers are aware of infectious contents.

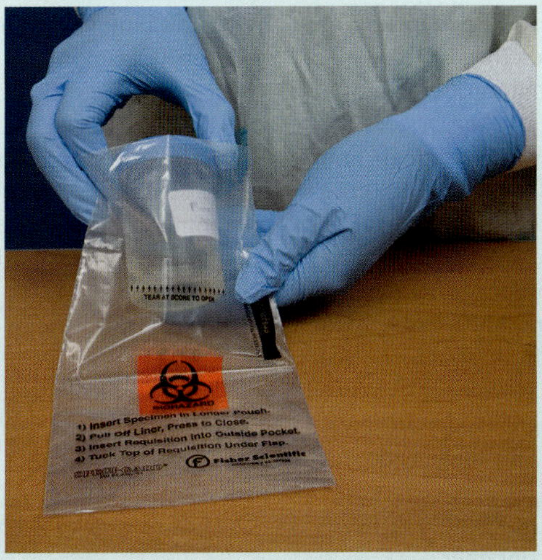

STEP 10D Place specimen container in biohazard bag.

STEP	RATIONALE
11. Dispose of linen, garbage, and disposable items:	
a. Use sturdy moisture-impervious bags to contain soiled articles. Use double bag if necessary for heavily soiled linen or heavy wet garbage.	Linen or refuse should be contained totally to prevent exposure of personnel to infectious material.
b. Tie bags securely at top in knot (see Step 11b illustration).	

STEP	RATIONALE

IMPLEMENTATION

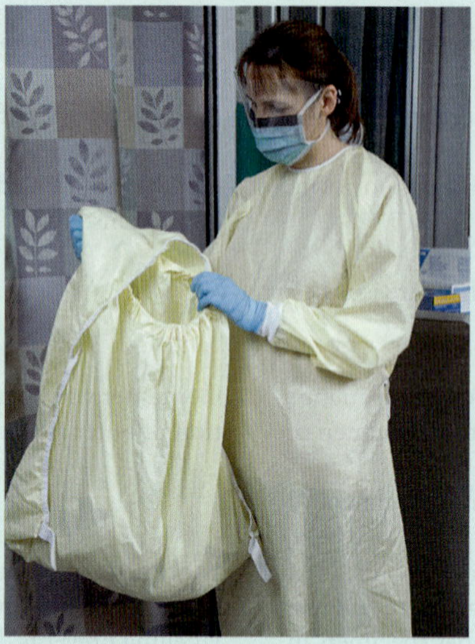

STEP 11B Tie bag securely.

12. Remove all reusable pieces of equipment. Clean and disinfect any contaminated surfaces according to employer policy.	All items must be properly cleaned, disinfected, or sterilized for reuse.
13. Resupply room as needed. Have colleague hand new supplies to you.	Limiting trips of personnel into and out of room reduces your and patient's exposure to microorganisms.
14. Leave patient room. Order of removal of PPE depends on what you wear in room. This sequence describes steps to take if all barriers were worn. PPE worn in room must be removed before leaving room:	Order of removal minimizes exposure to any infectious material on barriers (Osei-Bonsu et al., 2019).
a. Remove gloves. Remove one glove by grasping cuff and pulling glove inside out over hand. Hold removed glove in gloved hand (see Step 14a illustration). Slide fingers of ungloved hand under remaining glove at wrist. Peel glove off over first glove. Discard gloves in proper container.	Technique prevents contact with outer contaminated surface of glove. Change gloves between exposures to body sites and patient equipment. Inadequate glove changes and hand hygiene can lead to contamination, increasing the risk of HAIs (Lotfinejad et al., 2021).
b. Remove gown. Untie neck strings and then untie back strings of gown. Allow gown to fall from shoulders (see Step 14b illustration); touch inside of gown only. Remove hands from sleeves without touching outside of gown. Hold gown inside at shoulder seams and fold inside out into bundle; discard in laundry bag.	Hands do not come in contact with soiled front of gown.
c. Remove eyewear, face shield, or goggles. Handle by headband or earpieces. Discard in proper container.	Outside of goggles is contaminated. Hands have not been soiled.
d. Remove mask. If mask secured over ears, remove elastic from ears and pull mask away from face. For tie-on mask, untie *bottom* mask string and then top strings, pull mask away from face (see Step 14d, illustration *A*), and drop into garbage receptacle (see Step 14d, illustration *B*). (Do not touch outer surface of mask.)	Prevents contamination of ungloved hands by touching only elastic or mask strings. Prevents top part of mask from falling down over uniform.

STEP	RATIONALE

IMPLEMENTATION

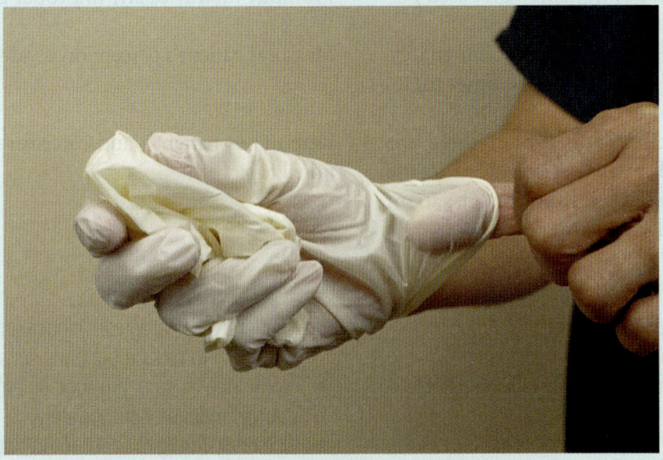

STEP 14A Remove gloves.

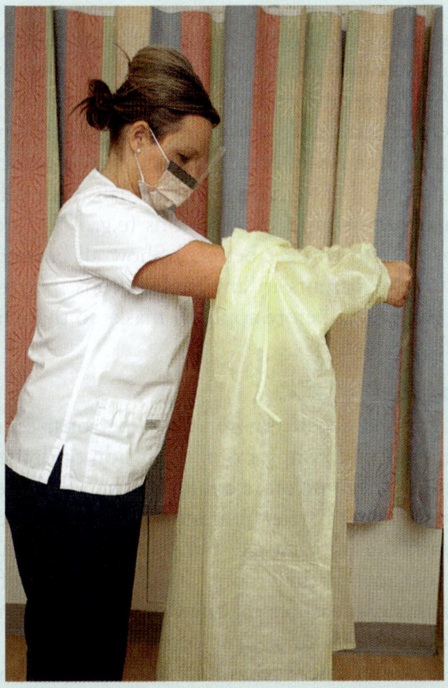

STEP 14B Remove gown by allowing it to fall from shoulders.

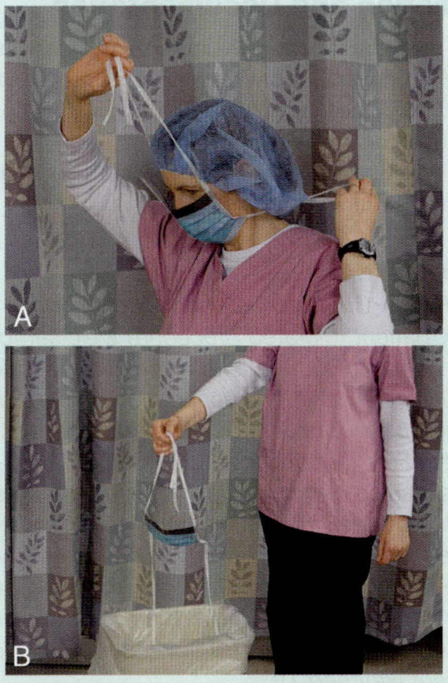

STEP 14D A, Pull mask away from face. B, Drop into trash receptacle.

Critical Decision Point *If patient is on TB precautions, place reusable mask in labelled paper bag for storage, being careful not to crush mask (check employer policy for number of times reusable masks can be used).*

STEP	RATIONALE
e. Retrieve wristwatch and stethoscope (unless items must remain in room).	
f. Explain to patient when you plan to return to room. Ask whether patient requires any personal care items. Offer books, magazines, and electronic devices.	Diversions can help minimize boredom and feeling of social isolation.
g. Dispose of all contaminated supplies and equipment in manner that prevents spread of microorganisms to other people (see employer policy).	
h. Leave room and close door if necessary. Close door if patient is on airborne precautions or in negative-airflow room.	Maintains negative-airflow environment and reduces transmission of microorganisms.

STEP	RATIONALE

EVALUATION

STEP	RATIONALE
1. Observe patient's and caregiver's use of transmission-based precautions when visiting.	Promptly identifies any improper use of precaution.
2. While in room, ask whether patient has had sufficient chance to discuss health problems, course of treatment, or other topics important to them.	Measures patient's perception of adequacy of discussions with caregivers.
3. Use teach-back: "I want to be sure I explained when these precautions are needed. Can you tell me when you need to use these precautions?" Develop a revised teaching plan if patient or caregiver is unable to teach back correctly.	Determines patient's and caregiver's level of understanding of instructional topic.

Unexpected Outcomes	Related Interventions
1. Patient avoids social and therapeutic discussions.	• Confer with caregiver, significant other, or both and determine best approach to reduce patient's sense of loneliness and depression.
2. Patient or health care worker may have an allergy to latex gloves.	• Notify health care provider or employee health, and treat sensitivity or allergic reaction appropriately. • Use latex-free gloves for future care activities.

Communication and Documentation

- Document procedures performed and patient's response to social isolation. Also document any patient or family education performed and reinforced on flow sheet or in progress notes in electronic health record (EHR) or chart.
- Document type of transmission-based precautions in use and the microorganisms (if known).

DOCUMENTATION EXAMPLE

Wearing full PPE, PCR test was performed without complication; patient tolerated procedure well; sample labelled and validated with patient; discussed need for isolation until COVID-19 status confirmed; discussed needs during isolation period; patient ably restated reasons for isolation at this time (unconfirmed COVID-19 status, need to prevent transmission of microorganism); patient stated, "I am doing okay. I don't feel much like entertaining my family right now because I am so tired. If I want to speak with them, I can FaceTime using my phone and I can keep my mask off when they aren't here"; reiterated availability of nursing staff if patient requires any help; wiped down surfaces and left room as patient watched TV.

Special Considerations

Teaching

- Teach visitors and caregivers how to follow the recommended transmission-based precautions when visiting a patient.

Pediatric

- Patient isolation is inherent in many transmission-based precautions, which creates a sense of separation from family and loss of control. A strange environment adds to the confusion that a child feels when experiencing isolation. Preschoolers are unable to understand the cause–effect relationship for being isolated. Older children may be able to understand the cause but still fantasize.
- Children require simple explanations (e.g., "You need to be in this room to help you get better.") Show all barriers to a child. Actively involve parents in any explanations. Nurses should let child see their faces before applying masks so that child does not become frightened.

Gerontological

- Isolation can be a concern for older persons, especially those who have signs and symptoms of confusion or depression. Many times, patients become more confused when they are confronted with a nurse using barrier precautions or when they are left in a room with the door closed. Nurses must assess need for closing door (negative-airflow room) along with safety of patient and additional safety measures that may need to be taken.
- Assess older persons for signs of depression, such as loss of appetite or decrease in verbal communications. If necessary, report to the health care team for appropriate interventions.

Care in the Community: Home Management

- Although transmission-based precautions followed in the hospital are not directly applicable to care in the community, caregivers should be aware of potential sources of contamination in the home (see Box 5.3) and practise good hand hygiene at all times.

Procedural Guideline 5.1 *Caring for Patients With Multidrug-Resistant Organisms and Clostridioides Difficile*

Multidrug-resistant organisms (MDROs) such as methicillin-resistant *Staphylococcus aureus* (MRSA) and vancomycin-resistant *Enterococcus* (VRE) have become increasingly common as a cause of colonization and health care–associated infections (HAIs). MRSA is a frequently identified pathogen associated with increased mortality. *Clostridioides difficile* infection is one of the most common and costly HAIs (Xia et al., 2019). In most instances, patient susceptibility to *C. difficile* infection requires prior treatment with antibiotics. There is no treatment for MRSA or VRE; prevention is key (Mehershahi et al., 2021). Unlike MRSA and VRE, *C. difficile* is more difficult to eliminate from the environment because it is a spore-forming organism, meaning that it can remain on surfaces in its dormant state for long periods of time. No matter which MDRO is involved, the most common means of transmission is by way of a health care worker's hands. To reduce the risk of cross-contamination among patients, transmission-based precautions (contact) should be used in addition to routine practices when caring for these patients (Edgeworth et al., 2020).

Delegation and Collaboration

Assessment of a patient's status and type of care required cannot be delegated to a UCP. Basic care procedures performed using transmission-based precautions can be delegated to a UCP. The nurse instructs the UCP to do the following:

- Clarify personal precautions used under transmission-based precautions (e.g., contact)
- Explain the type of changes in patient status to report to the nurse.

Equipment

- Clean gloves, gown, protective eyewear, surgical mask (based on patient's clinical condition)
- Basic care items (e.g., medication equipment, hygiene items)

Procedural Steps

1. Throughout the procedure, the 4 moments for hand hygiene are to be implemented.
2. Prepare all equipment needed in patient's room.
3. Before entering room, apply gown, being sure that it covers all outer garments. Pull sleeves down to wrists. Tie securely at neck and waist.
4. Apply clean gloves.
5. Explain purpose of contact precautions to patient and caregivers.
6. Provide personal care and treatments.
7. Leave room after telling patient when you will return and asking whether they have questions concerning their care.
8. Remove gloves and discard per employer policy.
9. Untie neck and waist ties on gown. Remove gown, allowing it to fall from shoulders. Discard in appropriate receptacle per employer policy.
10. If patient is being treated for *C. difficile* infection, clean hands with soap and water. Alcohol-based hand rubs are not effective against the spores of *C. difficile*.

✦ REVIEW QUESTIONS

Review Questions 1 to 3 relate to the case study presented here.

1. *A 78-year-old patient is admitted from a long-term care facility to an acute care hospital. The patient is confused and has a fever and decreased urinary output. After greeting the patient, the nurse begins to conduct a physical assessment. As the nurse turns the patient to check the condition of his skin, the nurse notices moisture on the skin. Assessing more closely, the nurse realizes that the moisture is from an open, oozing lesion measuring 2 cm × 2 cm on the patient's sacral area.* What should the nurse do next?
2. *A few hours later the nurse prepares to enter the patient's room. Wearing gloves, the nurse assesses the wound and quickly checks the position and function of the in-dwelling urinary catheter and then performs hand hygiene before leaving the patient's room.* Critique the nurse's approach. Was the correct technique used?
3. *Two days later, the patient is indicating increased pain at the wound site. On further assessment, the nurse sees that the wound now measures 3 cm × 3 cm; is red; and has thick, yellow drainage.* Use SBAR (situation–background–assessment–recommendation) to communicate this finding to the interprofessional health care team.
4. Which of the following are true statements regarding hand hygiene? (*Select all that apply.*)
   1. The percentage of health care workers using hand hygiene has been decreasing over the last few years.
   2. The incidence of health care–associated infections has decreased because of hand hygiene.
   3. There must be a mode of transmission for an infection to occur.
   4. Soap and water must be used when hands are visibly soiled.
   5. Hand hygiene can be antiseptic hand wash, antiseptic hand rub, or handwashing.
5. A nurse is taking care of a patient on airborne precautions for tuberculosis. Which interventions are appropriate for this patient? (*Select all that apply.*)
   1. Place patient in a private room.
   2. Explain why the patient across the hall is not on precautions.
   3. Wear gloves when giving an intramuscular injection.
   4. Educate patient regarding their specific transmission-based precautions.
   5. Wear a surgical mask into the room to take vital signs.
6. The nurse is having a complication of dermatitis related to repeated handwashing. Which interventions could be used to help the nurse with the situation? (*Select all that apply.*)
   1. Use personal hypoallergenic soap instead of the soap provided.
   2. Use only approved hand lotions or barrier creams.
   3. Rinse and dry hands thoroughly after every handwashing.
   4. Quickly wash hands when needed to avoid excess damage to skin.
   5. Wear gloves and change them frequently instead of washing hands.

Visit the Evolve site for a complete list of answers to the Review Questions.

✦ NEXT GENERATION NCLEX® (NGN)

For practice with answering exam questions related to unfolding NGN case studies, please consult the Next Generation NCLEX® (NGN)-Style Case Studies for Skills and Techniques on the Evolve website: http://evolve.elsevier.com/Canada/Perry/clinicalskills/

REFERENCES

Accreditation Canada. (2020). *Required organizational practices handbook*. https://physicians.nshealth.ca/resources/required-organizational-practices-2020-handbook

Alberta Health Services. (2020). *Routine practices: Infection prevention and control*. https://www.albertahealthservices.ca/assets/healthinfo/ipc/hi-ipc-routine-practices-info.pdf

Alberta Health Services. (2021). *Artificial nails in the healthcare environment: Why we care: Infection prevention and control*. https://www.albertahealthservices.ca/assets/info/hp/hh/if-hp-hh-artificial-nails-in-healthcare.pdf

Alberta Health Services. (2022). *Point of care risk assessment (PCRA)*. https://www.albertahealthservices.ca/assets/healthinfo/ipc/hi-ipc-acute-care-pcra.pdf.

Assefa, D., Melaku, T., Bayisa, B., et al. (2021). Knowledge, attitude and self-reported performance and challenges of hand hygiene using alcohol-based hand sanitizers among healthcare workers during COVID-19 pandemic at a tertiary hospital: A cross-sectional study. *Infection and Drug Resistance*, *14*, 303–313. https://doi.org/10.2147/IDR.S291690

Bajpal, G., & Nahrendorf, M. (2021). Infectious and lifestyle modifiers of immunity and host resilience. *Immunity*, *54*(6), 1110–1122. https://doi.org/10.1016/j.immuni.2021.05.011

Bartoszko, J., Farooqi, M. A. M., Alhazzani, W., et al. (2020). Medical masks vs N95 respirators for preventing COVID-19 in healthcare workers: A systematic review and meta-analysis of randomized trials. *Influenza and Other Respiratory Viruses*, *14*(4), 365–373. https://doi.org/10.1111/irv.12745

Cole, M. (2012). Breaking the chain of infection. *Nursing and Residential Care*, *14*(6), 288–291.

Edgeworth, J., Batra, R., Wulff, J., et al. (2020). Reductions in methicillin-resistant *Staphylococcus aureus*, *Clostridium difficile* infection and intensive care unit-acquired bloodstream infection across the United Kingdom following implementation of a national infection control campaign. *Clinical Infectious Diseases*, *70*(12), 2530–2540. https://doi.org/10.1093/cid/ciz720

Evgin, D., & Muz, G. (2021). Nursing students learning to care for refugee patients: A qualitative study. *International Nursing Review*, *68*(3), 341–348. https://doi.org/10.1111/inr.12641

Fries, K., Figueroa, A. M., Pickering, H., et al. (2020). Use of World Health Organization guidelines to improve hand washing efficacy. *The Journal of Continuing Education in Nursing*, *51*(10), 453–456. https://doi.org/10.3928/00220124-20200914-06

Gammon, J., Hunt, J., Williams, S., et al. (2019). Infection prevention control and organizational patient safety culture within the context of isolation: Study protocol. *BMC Health Services Research*, *19*, Article 296. http://dx.doi.org/10.1186/s12913-019-4126-x

Health Canada. (2016). *Health Canada's monitoring and performance framework for tuberculosis programs for First Nations on-reserve*. https://www.canada.ca/en/health-canada/services/publications/science-research-data/monitoring-performance-framework-tuberculosis-programs-first-nations-reserve-2015.html [Seminal Reference]

Henderson, J., Willis, E., Blackman, I., et al. (2021). Comparing infection control and ward nurses' views of the omission of infection control activities using the Missed Nursing Care Infection Prevention and Control (MNCIPC) Survey. *Journal of Nursing Management*, *29*(5), 1228–1238. https://doi.org/10.1111/jonm.13261

Hillier, M. (2020). Using effective hand hygiene practice to prevent and control infection. *Nursing Standard*, *35*(5), 45–50. https://doi.org/10.7748/ns.2020.e11552

Hossain, M., Sultana, A., & Purohit, N. (2020). Mental health outcomes of quarantine and isolation for infection prevention: A systematic umbrella review of the global evidence. *Epidemiology and Health*, *42*, Article e2020038. https://doi.org/10.4178/epih.e2020038

Huang, S., Septimus, E., Kleinman, K., et al. (2019). Chlorhexidine versus routine bathing to prevent multidrug-resistant organisms and all-cause bloodstream infections in general medical and surgical units (ABATE infection trial): A cluster-randomised trial. *The Lancet*, *393*(10177), 23–29. https://doi.org/10.1016/S0140-6736(18)32593-5

Infection Prevention and Control Canada (IPAC Canada). (2022). *IPAC Canada practice recommendations for hand hygiene in health care settings*. https://ipac-canada.org/photos/custom/Members/pdf/17JulHand%20Hygiene%20Practice%20Recommendations_final.pdf

Infusion Nurses Society. (2021). *Infusion therapy standards of practice* (8th ed.). https://www.ins1.org/publications/infusion-therapy-standards-of-practice/

Kiersnowska, Z. M., Lemiech-Mirowska, E., & Michałkiewicz, M. (2021). Hand hygiene as the basic method of reducing *Clostridium difficile* infections (CDI) in a hospital environment. *Annals of Agricultural and Environmental Medicine*, *28*(4), 535–540. https://doi.org/10.26444/aaem/131121

LaFreniere, M., Hussain, H., He, N., et al. (2019). Tuberculosis in Canada: 2017. *Canadian Communicable Disease Reports*, *45*(2/3), 68–74. https://doi.org/10.14745/ccdr.v45i23a04

Locke, L., Dada, O., & Shedd, J. S. (2021). Aerosol transmission of infectious disease and the efficacy of personal protective equipment (PPE): A systematic review. *Journal of Occupational and Environmental Medicine*, *63*(11), e783–e791. https://doi.org/10.1097/JOM.0000000000002366

Lotfinejad, N., Peters, A., Tartari, E., et al. (2021). Hand hygiene in health care: 20 years of ongoing advances and perspectives. *The Lancet Infectious Diseases*, *21*(8), e209–e221. https://doi.org/10.1016/S1473-3099(21)00383-2

McDonald, L. C., Gerding, D. N., Johnson, S., et al. (2018). Clinical practice guidelines for *Clostridium difficile* infection in adults and children: 2017 update by the infectious diseases society of America (IDSA) and Society for Healthcare Epidemiology of America (SHEA). *Clinical Infectious Diseases*, *66*(7), e1–e48. https://doi.org/10.1093/cid/cix1085

Mehershahi, S., Ghazanfar, H., Ashraf, S., et al. (2021). Concomitant vancomycin-resistant *Enterococcus faecium* and *Clostridium difficile* colitis. *Case Reports in Gastroenterology*, *15*(1), 372–378. https://doi.org/10.1159/000513165

Napolitani, M., Bezzini, D., Moirano, F., et al. (2020). Methods of disinfecting stethoscopes: Systematic review. *International Journal of Environmental Research and Public Health*, *17*(6), Article 1856. https://doi.org/10.3390/ijerph17061856

Ontario Agency for Health Protection and Promotion (Public Health Ontario [PHO]), Provincial Infectious Diseases Advisory Committee (PIDAC) (PHO-PIDAC). (2014). Best practices for hand hygiene in all health care settings (4th ed.). Queen's Printer for Ontario. https://www.publichealthontario.ca/-/media/documents/B/2014/ bp-hand-hygiene.pdf.

Osei-Bonsu, K., Masroor, N., Cooper, K., et al. (2019). Alternative doffing strategies of personal protective equipment to prevent self-contamination in the health care setting. *American Journal of Infection Control*, *47*(5), 534–539. https://doi.org/10.1016/j.ajic.2018.11.003

Palmer, S. J. (2019). Practising asepsis during dressing changes in community settings. *British Journal of Community Nursing*, *24*(12), 600–603. https://doi.org/10.12968/bjcn.2019.24.12.600

Payne, D., & Peache, M. (2021). The challenge of infection control in patients' homes. *British Journal of Community Nursing*, *26*(4), 168–174. https://doi.org/10.12968/bjcn.2021.26.4.168

Peters, A., Cave, C., Carry, J., et al. (2022). Tolerability and acceptability of three alcohol-based hand-rub gel formulations: A randomized crossover study. *Journal of Hospital Infection*, *123*, 112–118. https://doi.org/10.1016/j.jhin.2022.01.019

Public Health Agency of Canada (PHAC). (2014). *Canadian tuberculosis standards* (7th ed.). https://www.phac-aspc.gc.ca/tbpc-latb/pubs/tb-canada-7/assets/pdf/tb-standards-tb-normes-ch15-eng.pdf [Seminal Reference]

Public Health Agency of Canada (PHAC). (2017). *Routine practices and additional precautions for preventing the transmission of infection in healthcare settings* (Cat. No. HP40-83/2013E-PDF). https://www.canada.ca/en/public-health/services/publications/diseases-conditions/routine-practices-precautions-healthcare-associated-infections.html [Seminal Reference]

Public Health Agency of Canada (PHAC). (2021). *Infection prevention and control for COVID-19: Interim guidance for acute healthcare settings*. https://www.canada.ca/en/public-health/services/diseases/2019-novel-coronavirus-infection/health-professionals/infection-prevention-control-covid-19-second-interim-guidance.html

Saraswathy, T., Nalliah, S., Rosliza, A. M., et al. (2021). Applying interprofessional simulation to improve knowledge, attitude and practice in hospital-acquired infection control among health professionals. *BMC Medical Education*, *21*(482), 1–11. https://doi.org/10.1186/s12909-021-02907-1

Shang, J., Wang, J., Adams, V., et al. (2020). Risk factors for infection in home health care: Analysis of national outcome and assessment information set data. *Research in Nursing & Health*, *43*(4), 373–386. https://doi.org/10.1002/nur.22053

Spruce, L. (2021). Hand hygiene. *AORN Journal*, *113*(3), 286–294. https://doi.org/10.1002/aorn.13340

Tan, D., Wiseman, T., Betihavas, V., et al. (2021). Patient, provider, and system factors that contribute to health care-associated infection and sepsis development in patients after a traumatic injury: An integrative review. *Australian Critical Care*, 34(3), 269–277. https://doi.org/10.1016/j.aucc.2020.08.004

Woolley, K., Smith, R., & Arumugam, S. (2020). Personal protective equipment (PPE) guidelines, adaptations and lessons during the COVID-19 pandemic. *Ethics, Medicine and Public Health*, *14*, Article 100546. https://doi.org/10.1016/j.jemep.2020.100546

World Health Organization (WHO). (2009). *WHO guidelines on hand hygiene in health care*. https://www.who.int/publications/i/item/9789241597906 [Seminal Reference]

World Health Organization (WHO). (2017). *Evidence of hand hygiene as the building block for infection prevention and control*. https://apps.who.int/iris/handle/10665/330079 [Seminal Reference]

World Health Organization (WHO). (2022). *World hand hygiene day 2022–My 5 moments for hand hygiene*. https://www.who.int/campaigns/world-hand-hygiene-day/2022

Wu, A., & Lipner, S. (2020). A potential hidden reservoir: The role of nail hygiene in preventing transmission of COVID-19. *Journal of the American Academy of Dermatology*, *83*(3), e245–e246. https://doi.org/10.1016/j.jaad.2020.05.119

Xia, Y., Tunis, M. C., Frenette, C., et al. (2019). Epidemiology of *Clostridioides difficile* infection in Canada: A six-year review to support vaccine decision-making. *Canadian Communicable Disease Report*, *45*(7/8), 191–211. https://doi.org/10.14745/ccdr.v45i78a04

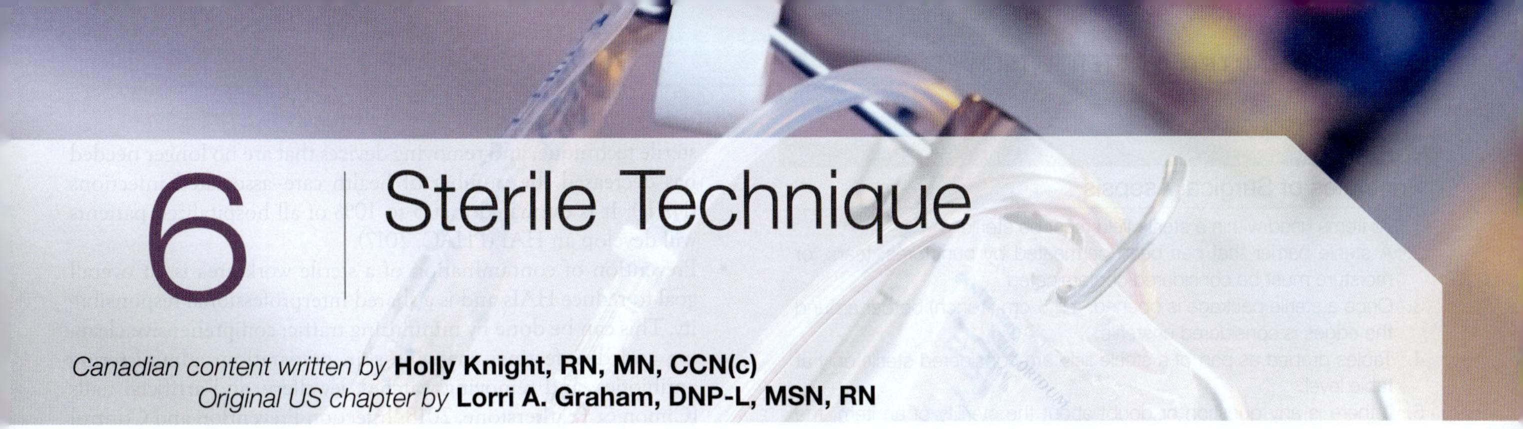

6 Sterile Technique

Canadian content written by **Holly Knight, RN, MN, CCN(c)**

Original US chapter by **Lorri A. Graham, DNP-L, MSN, RN**

SKILLS AND PROCEDURES

Skill 6.1 **Preparing a Sterile Field, p. 96**

Skill 6.2 **Sterile Gloving, p. 102**

OBJECTIVES

Mastery of content in this chapter will enable the nurse to:

- Describe settings where surgical aseptic techniques are necessary.
- Describe conditions when surgical asepsis is necessary.
- Identify the principles of surgical asepsis.
- Explain the importance of organization and caution when using surgical aseptic techniques.
- Identify individuals at risk for a latex allergy.
- Perform the following skills: preparing a sterile field, applying sterile gloves using the open-glove method, and applying a sterile drape correctly.
- Maintain a sterile field.

MEDIA RESOURCES

- http://evolve.elsevier.com/Canada/Perry/clinicalskills/

PURPOSE

Sterile technique and aseptic practices maintain an area that is free from pathogenic organisms, serve to isolate an operative area from the unsterile environment, and maintain a sterile field for surgery and invasive procedures. Proper sterile asepsis minimizes patient exposure to infection-causing agents, thereby reducing the patient's risk for infection. These techniques are common in the operating room (OR), labour and delivery area, and major diagnostic areas, but they are also used at the bedside (e.g., when inserting an intravenous [IV] or urinary catheter).

STANDARDS OF CARE

- Ontario Agency for Health Protection and Promotion (Public Health Ontario [PHO]), Provincial Infectious Diseases Advisory Committee (PIDAC) (PHO-PIDAC, 2012)—*Routine Practices and Additional Precautions in All Health Care Settings*, 3th edition (https://www.publichealthontario.ca/en/health-topics/infection-prevention-control/routine-practices-additional-precautions)
- Operating Room Nurses Association of Canada (ORNAC, 2023)—*ORNAC Standards, Guidelines, and Position Statements for Perioperative Registered Nurses*, 16th edition (http://www.ornac.ca/en/standards)
- Public Health Agency of Canada (PHAC, 2017)—*Routine Practices and Additional Precautions for Preventing the Transmission of Infection in Healthcare Settings* (https://www.canada.ca/en/public-health/services/publications/diseases-conditions/routine-practices-precautions-healthcare-associated-infections/part-b.html)

PRINCIPLES FOR PRACTICE

- The majority of sterile technique practices are used in the OR or in diagnostic procedure areas. These practices include using personal protective equipment (PPE) (e.g., applying a mask, protective eyewear, a gown, and a cap); performing a surgical hand scrub; applying a sterile gown; and applying sterile gloves.
- As with medical asepsis (see Chapter 5), proper hand hygiene, using the 4 moments for hand hygiene (Accreditation Canada, 2020) with an appropriate cleaner or antiseptic, is required before initiating any sterile procedure.
- Surgical aseptic technique is also used at the bedside in the following situations: during procedures that require intentional puncture of the skin or insertion of devices into an area of the body that is normally sterile (e.g., sterile dressing change) or in a situation in which skin integrity is compromised because of an incision or burn (Box 6.1).
- When sterile procedures are carried out in the OR or procedure area, health care providers must follow a series of steps to maintain sterile asepsis: applying a mask, protective eyewear, and cap (see Skill 5.2); performing a surgical hand scrub; and applying sterile gown and gloves. (See Chapter 38 for pandemic information related to surgical suites.)
- When sterile procedures such as a sterile dressing change are carried out at the bedside, the health care provider must perform hand hygiene and apply sterile gloves. When the risk of splashing is present, other PPE is required.
- When preparing to complete a sterile procedure at the bedside, ensure adequate preparation of the environment/surface to be used (i.e., remove flowers, cards, and gifts; close windows; use

BOX 6.1

Principles of Surgical Asepsis

1. All items used within a sterile field must be sterile.
2. A sterile barrier that has been permeated by punctures, tears, or moisture must be considered contaminated.
3. Once a sterile package is opened, a 2.5-cm (1-inch) border around the edges is considered unsterile.
4. Tables draped as part of a sterile field are considered sterile only at table level.
5. If there is any question or doubt about the sterility of an item, the item is considered to be unsterile.
6. Sterile contacting sterile equals sterile; sterile contacting unsterile equals unsterile. Movement around and in the sterile field must not compromise or contaminate the field.
7. A sterile object or field out of the range of vision or an object held below a person's waist is contaminated.
8. A sterile object or field becomes contaminated by prolonged exposure to air; stay organized and complete any procedure as soon as possible.

privacy curtains) and clean the surface with approved disinfectants before opening sterile supplies.

- When completing a sterile procedure at the bedside, communicate with the patient about what steps are being taken to prevent infection, including which actions the patient should avoid in order to keep the field sterile. These actions include avoiding sudden body movements, refraining from touching sterile supplies, and avoiding coughing or talking over the sterile area.

PERSON-CENTRED CARE

- Regardless of where invasive procedures such as starting an IV line or inserting a urinary catheter are performed—be it in a hospital, an ambulatory care setting, the patient's home, or a health care provider's office—they pose a risk for infection. As a nurse, it is your responsibility to protect patients from infection by adhering strictly to the principles of surgical asepsis when performing invasive procedures or when helping with such a procedure and to intervene to stop it when a break in sterile technique occurs. Maintaining surgical asepsis is a shared responsibility for those providing care to the patient (ORNAC, 2023).
- Take into consideration the patient's cultural background and beliefs when sterile asepsis is required. Provide individualized person-centred education for patients and families before starting any aseptic procedure to reduce fears and misconceptions about sterile asepsis attire. This also provides an opportunity for patients, caregivers, and family members to ask questions and express their concerns regarding surgical attire.

EVIDENCE-INFORMED PRACTICE

- Implementation of recommendations such as providing person-centred education, inserting devices only when necessary, using sterile technique, and removing devices that are no longer needed has decreased the number of health care–associated infections (HAIs). It is estimated that 5 to 10% of all hospitalized patients will develop an HAI (PHAC, 2017).
- Prevention of contamination of a sterile work area is an overall goal to reduce HAIs and is a shared interprofessional responsibility. This can be done by minimizing traffic; comprehensive cleaning and disinfecting; changing skin preparation; administering antibiotics; and removing watches, jewellery, and artificial nails (Cimon & Featherstone, 2018; Infection Prevention and Control Canada, 2022; ORNAC, 2023).
- Use of additional antiseptics such as chlorhexidine reduces bacterial count on the patient's skin (ORNAC, 2023).
- Most health care facilities have policies against artificial nails, including extensions or tips, gels and acrylic overlays, and resin wraps (Hewlett et al., 2018; ORNAC, 2023). The subungual area (under a fingernail) of the hand and the area exposed by the "lifting" of the product from the nail bed contain a high concentration of bacteria, more specifically coagulase-negative staphylococci, Gram-negative rods, and fungal growth (Cimon & Featherstone, 2018). These organisms are not removed effectively after hand hygiene.
- Preoperative prevention measures support using a dual agent (e.g., alcohol plus iodine or chlorhexidine) skin preparation. Intraoperative measures include using wound edge protectors for abdominal procedures and using triclosan-coated antibacterial sutures. Evidence supports use of postoperative prevention measures, including negative-pressure wound therapy for high-risk procedures such as abdominal and vascular cases (ORNAC, 2023).

SAFETY GUIDELINES

- Follow routine practices with all patients (PHAC, 2017).
- Complete a point-of-care risk assessment (see Chapter 5, Box 5.1) prior to every patient interaction as the initial step in routine practices.
- Review employer policies before conducting a sterile procedure.
- Assess the potential for splash and/or transmission of infection before choosing the PPE to be used (i.e., masks or protective eyewear).
- Use barrier techniques to decrease the transmission of microorganisms from health care personnel and the environment to a patient.
- Remain organized while performing any sterile procedure; keep bedside surfaces clean and free of clutter.
- Remember that hand hygiene is essential before and after initiating any sterile procedure to reduce HAIs (PHAC, 2017; World Health Organization, 2018).
- Apply the principles of surgical asepsis when conducting any sterile procedure.

✦ SKILL 6.1 Preparing a Sterile Field

Video Clip *NSO Nursing Skills Online Infection Control Module 2 / Lesson 3*

When performing sterile aseptic procedures, it is necessary to have a sterile work area in which objects can be handled with minimal risk for contamination. A sterile field provides a sterile surface for placement of sterile equipment. Sterile drapes establish a sterile field around a treatment site such as a surgical incision, venipuncture site, or site for introduction of an in-dwelling urinary catheter. Sterile drapes also provide a work surface for placing sterile supplies and manipulating items with sterile gloves. After a sterile kit is opened, the inside surface of the cover can be used as a sterile field. Prior to establishing the sterile field, the nurse should gather the equipment and supplies necessary to perform the procedure. Once a sterile field is created, the interprofessional team is responsible for performing the procedure and making sure that the field is not contaminated.

Delegation and Collaboration

Interprofessional collaboration may be a part of sterile field preparation. Surgical technicians may prepare a sterile field (see employer policy); however, an unregulated care provider (UCP) cannot prepare a sterile field. The nurse can direct the UCP to do the following:

- Help with patient positioning and obtain any necessary supplies

Equipment

- Sterile pack (commercial or institution wrapped)
- Sterile drape or kit that is to be used as a sterile field
- Sterile gloves (*optional*)
- Sterile solution and equipment specific to a procedure
- Waist-high table or countertop surface
- Appropriate PPE: gown, mask, cap, protective eyewear (see employer policy)

STEP	RATIONALE
ASSESSMENT	
1. Identify patient using at least two person-specific identifiers (e.g., name and date of birth, or name and medical record number) according to employer policy.	Ensures correct patient. Complies with Accreditation Canada's standards and improves patient safety (Accreditation Canada, 2020).
2. Throughout the procedure, the 4 moments for hand hygiene are to be implemented; hand hygiene should occur before initial patient (or patient environment) contact, before an aseptic procedure, after body fluid exposure risk, and after patient (or patient environment) contact. Additional hand hygiene should be performed when hands are visibly soiled.	Proper hand hygiene helps prevent the spread of infectious agents to health care providers.
3. Verify with employer policy that procedure requires surgical aseptic technique.	Some procedures require medical rather than surgical aseptic technique.
4. Assess patient's comfort, positioning, oxygen requirements, and elimination needs before preparing for procedure.	Certain procedures that require a sterile field may last a long time. Anticipates patient's needs so patient can relax and avoid any unnecessary movement that might disrupt procedure.
5. Instruct patient (and caregiver if present) not to touch work surface or equipment during procedure.	Instruction prevents contamination of sterile field.
6. Assess for latex allergies.	A review may reveal latex allergies and determine the need to use latex-free supplies.
7. Check sterile package integrity for punctures, tears, discoloration, moisture, or any other signs of contamination. If using commercially packaged supplies or those prepared by employer, check for sterilization indicator (e.g., marker that changes colour when exposed to heat or steam).	Inspection of packaging ensures that only sterile items are presented to sterile field (ORNAC, 2023).
8. Anticipate number and variety of supplies needed for procedure.	Not all sterile kits contain sufficient amounts or types of supplies. Failure to have necessary supplies can cause you to leave the sterile field, increasing risk for contamination.

NURSING DIAGNOSES

- Insufficient protection
- Potential for infection

Related factors and risk factors are individualized on the basis of patient's condition or needs.

STEP	RATIONALE
PLANNING	
1. Expected outcomes following completion of procedure:	
• Sterile field is not contaminated.	Correct surgical aseptic practice is performed.
• Patient is not exposed to microorganisms.	Lack of exposure prevents likelihood of infection transmission.
2. Complete all other nursing interventions (e.g., medication administration, suctioning patient) before beginning procedure.	Prepare sterile fields as close as possible to time of use to reduce potential for contamination (ORNAC, 2023).
3. Ask visitors to step out briefly during procedure. Instruct staff helping with procedure not to move.	Traffic or movement can increase potential for contamination through spread of microorganisms by air currents.
4. Arrange equipment at bedside.	Ensures availability before procedure and prevents break in sterile technique. (NOTE: Povidone–iodine and chlorhexidine are not considered sterile solutions and require separate work surfaces for preparation.)
5. Provide privacy. Position patient comfortably for specific procedure to be performed. If a body part is to be examined or treated, position patient so area is accessible. Have UCP help with positioning as needed.	Patient should be able to lie still in one position comfortably during procedure. Movement can contaminate sterile field.
6. Explain to patient purpose of procedure and importance of sterile technique.	Explanation ensures patient's ability to cooperate with procedure. Performing patient teaching before procedure reduces need to talk during procedure, which can cause air-droplet contamination of sterile area.

STEP	RATIONALE
IMPLEMENTATION	
1. Perform hand hygiene.	Proper hand hygiene helps prevent the spread of infectious agents to health care providers.
2. Apply PPE as needed (see employer policy) (see Skills 5.2 and 6.2).	PPE controls spread of airborne microorganisms.
3. Select a clean, flat, dry work surface above waist level.	A dry work surface is needed for a sterile field. A sterile object placed below a person's waist is considered contaminated.
4. Prepare sterile work surface.	
a. Use sterile commercial kit or pack containing sterile items.	
(1) Place sterile kit or pack on the prepared work surface.	Sterile object placed above waist level is considered sterile.
(2) Open outside cover (see Step 4a[2] illustration) and remove package from dust cover. Place on work surface.	Inner kit remains sterile.
(3) Grasp outer surface of tip of outermost flap.	Outer surface of package is considered unsterile. There is a 2.5-cm (1-inch) border around any sterile drape or wrap that is considered contaminated and can be touched with clean fingers.
(4) Open outermost flap away from body, keeping arm outstretched and away from sterile field (see Step 4a[4] illustration).	Reaching over sterile field contaminates it.
(5) Grasp outside surface of edge of first side flap.	Outer border is considered unsterile.
(6) Open side flap, pulling it to side and allowing it to lie flat on table surface. Keep arm to side and not over sterile surface (see Step 4a[6] illustration).	Drape or wrapper should lie flat so it does not accidentally rise up and contaminate inner surface or sterile contents.
(7) Repeat Step 4a(6) for second side flap (see Step 4a[7] illustration).	
(8) Grasp outside border of last and innermost flap (see Step 4a[8] illustration). Stand away from sterile package and pull flap back, allowing it to fall flat on table. Kit is ready to be used.	Outer border is considered unsterile. Never reach over a sterile field.

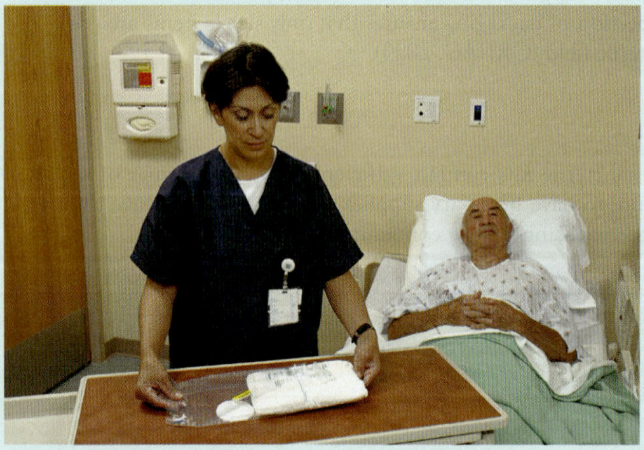

STEP 4A(2) Open outside cover of sterile kit.

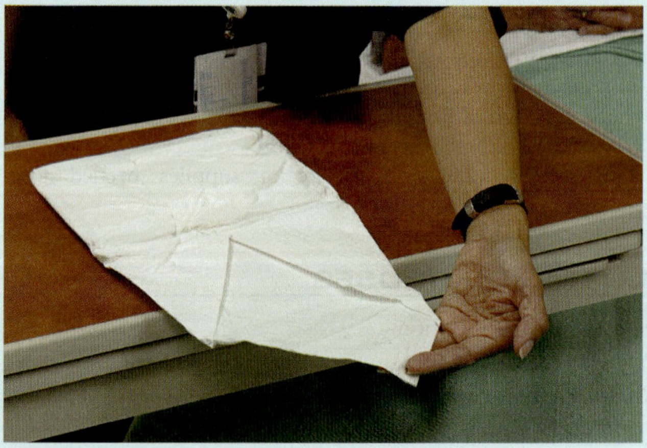

STEP 4A(4) Open outermost flap of sterile kit away from body.

STEP	RATIONALE

IMPLEMENTATION

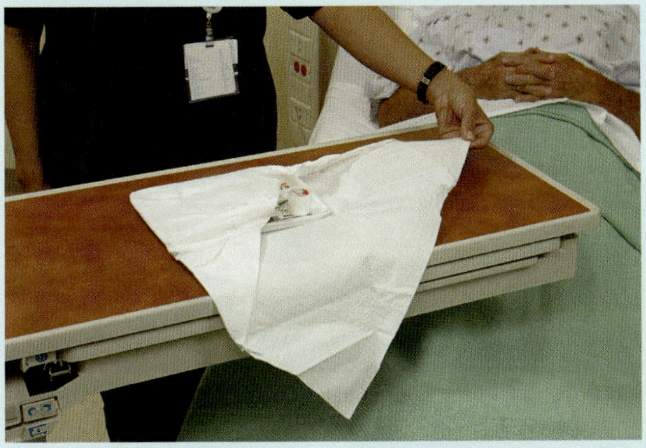

STEP 4A(6) Open first side flap, pulling to side.

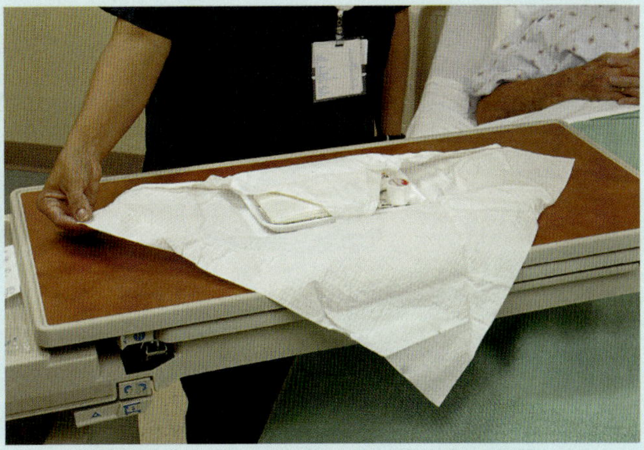

STEP 4A(7) Open second side flap, pulling to side.

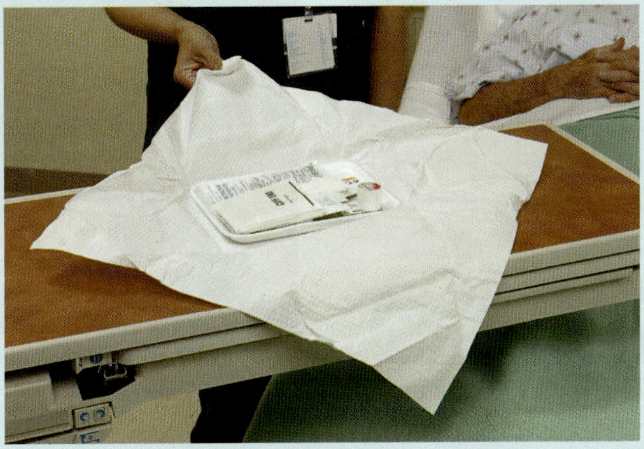

STEP 4A(8) Open last and innermost flap.

STEP	RATIONALE
b. Open sterile linen-wrapped package.	
(1) Place package on clean, dry, flat work surface above waist level.	Sterile items placed below waist level are considered contaminated.
(2) Remove sterilization tape seal and unwrap both layers following same steps (see Steps 4a[2] through 4a[8]) as for sterile kit.	Linen-wrapped items have two layers. The first is a dust cover. The second layer must be opened to view chemical indicator that verifies the sterility of the item.
(3) Use opened package wrapper as sterile field.	Inner surface of wrapper is considered sterile.
c. Prepare sterile drape.	
(1) Place pack containing sterile drape on flat, dry surface and open as described (see Steps 4a[2] through 4a[8]) for sterile package (see Step 4c[1] illustration).	Packaged drape remains sterile.
(2) Apply sterile gloves (*optional*; see employer policy). You may touch outer 2.5-cm (1-inch) border of drape without wearing gloves.	Sterile object remains sterile only when touched by another sterile object. Gloves are not necessary as long as fingers grasp the 2.5-cm (1-inch) unsterile border of the drape.
(3) Using fingertips of one hand, pick up folded top edge of drape along 2.5-cm (1-inch) border. Gently lift drape up from its wrapper without touching any object. Discard wrapper with other hand.	If sterile object touches any nonsterile object, it becomes contaminated.
(4) With other hand, grasp an adjacent corner of drape and hold it straight up and away from body. Allow drape to unfold, keeping it above waist and work surface and away from body (see Step 4c[4] illustration). (Carefully discard wrapper with other hand.)	An object held below a person's waist or above chest height is contaminated. Drape can now be placed properly with two hands.
(5) Holding drape, position bottom half over top half of intended work surface (see Step 4c[5] illustration).	Proper positioning prevents nurse from reaching over sterile field.
(6) Allow top half of drape to be placed over bottom half of work surface (see Step 4c[6] illustration).	Proper positioning creates flat, sterile work surface for placement of sterile supplies.

STEP	RATIONALE

IMPLEMENTATION

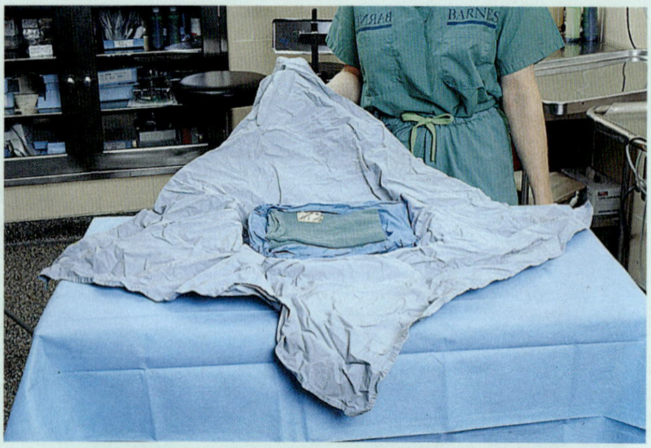

STEP 4C(1) Open sterile linen-wrapped package.

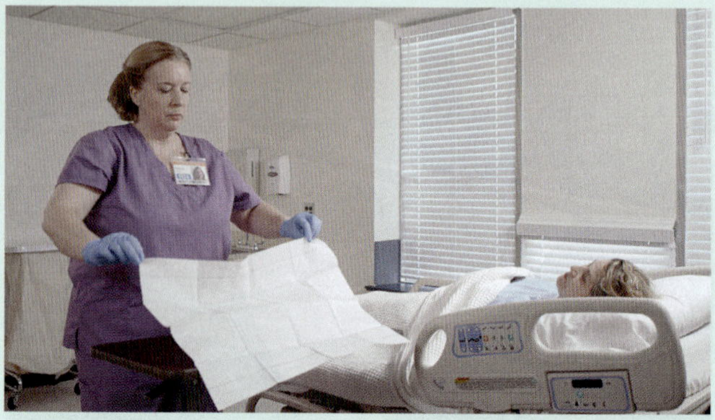

STEP 4C(5) Position bottom half of sterile drape over top half of work space.

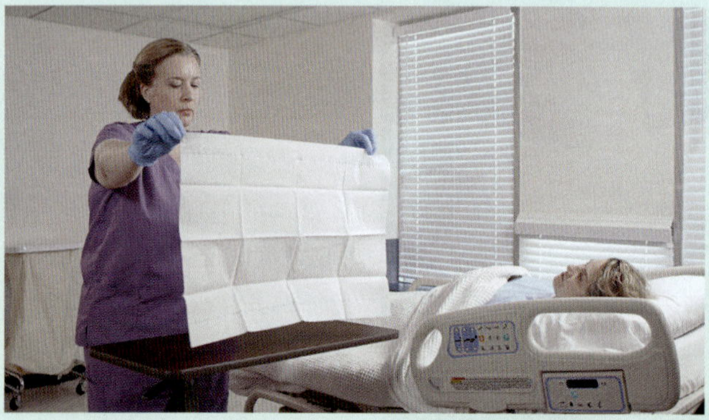

STEP 4C(4) Grasp corners of sterile drape, then hold up and away from body.

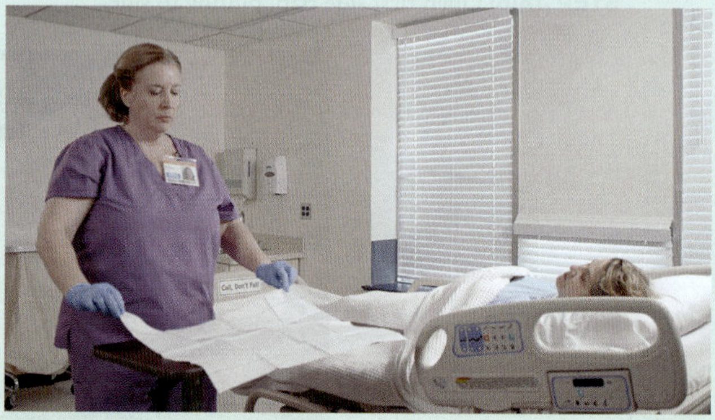

STEP 4C(6) Allow top half of drape to be placed over bottom half of work surface.

STEP	RATIONALE
5. Add sterile items to sterile field.	
a. Open sterile item (following package directions) while holding outside wrapper in nondominant hand.	Use of nondominant hand frees dominant hand for unwrapping outer wrapper.
b. Carefully peel wrapper over nondominant hand.	Item remains sterile. Inner surface of wrapper covers hand, making it sterile.
c. Be sure that the wrapper does not fall down onto the sterile field. Place the item onto the field at an angle (see Step 5c illustration). *Do not hold arms over sterile field.*	Secured wrapper edges prevent flipping of wrapper and contamination of contents of sterile field (ORNAC, 2023).

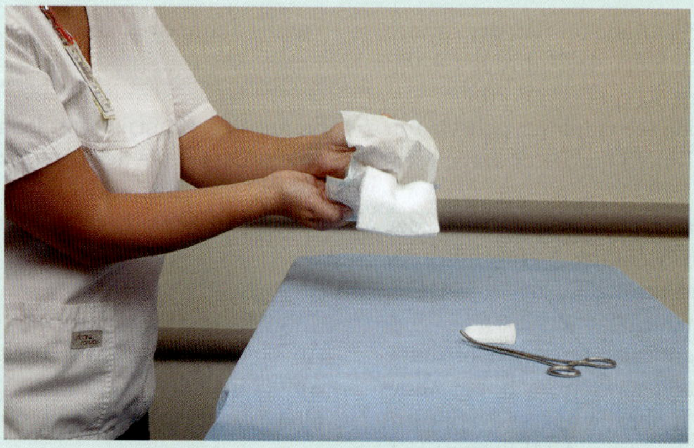

STEP 5C Add items to sterile field.

Critical Decision Point *Do not flip or toss objects onto sterile field.*

STEP	RATIONALE
d. Dispose of outer wrapper.	Disposal prevents accidental contamination of sterile field.

STEP	RATIONALE
IMPLEMENTATION	
6. Pour sterile solutions.	
a. Verify contents and expiration date of solution.	Verification ensures proper solution and sterility of contents.
b. Place receptacle for solution near table or work surface edge. Sterile kits have cups or plastic moulded sections into which fluids can be poured.	Proper placement prevents reaching over sterile field during pouring of solution.
c. Remove sterile seal and cap from bottle in upward motion.	Upward movement prevents contamination of bottle lip.

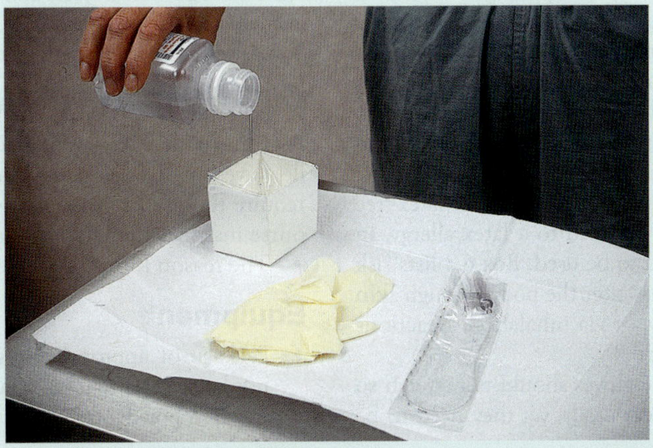

STEP 6D Pour solution into receiving container on sterile field.

STEP	RATIONALE
d. With solution bottle held away from field and bottle lip 2.5–5 cm (1–2 inches) above inside of sterile receiving container, slowly pour needed amount of solution into container. Hold bottle with label facing palm of hand (see Step 6d illustration).	Edge and outside of bottle are considered contaminated. Slow pouring prevents splashing. Sterility of contents cannot be ensured if cap is replaced. Prevents label from becoming wet and illegible.

Critical Decision Point *When liquids permeate a sterile field or barrier, it is called "strikethrough," and it results in contamination of the sterile field.*

EVALUATION	
1. Observe for breaks in sterile technique.	A break in sterile field requires you to set up a new sterile field.
2. Use teach-back: "I want to be sure I explained the procedure that was performed and the steps used to prevent infection. Please tell me some of the things that can be done to prevent infection." Develop a revised teaching plan if patient or caregiver is unable to teach back correctly.	Determines patient's and caregiver's level of understanding of instructional topic.

Unexpected Outcomes	Related Interventions
1. Sterile field comes in contact with contaminated object or liquid splatters onto drape, causing strikethrough.	• Discontinue field preparation and start over with new equipment.
2. Sterile item falls off sterile field.	• Open another package containing new sterile item and add to field unless field becomes contaminated, in which case a new sterile field would need to be established.

Communication and Documentation

- No communication or documentation is required for this set of skills. Document sterile procedure performed and patient status on flow sheet or in progress notes in electronic health record (EHR) or chart.

Special Considerations

Care in the Community: Home Management

- Most care procedures in the home setting involve clean technique. In the event that a sterile environment is required, the patient and caregiver need to be aware of the principles that apply to the sterile environment. For example, teach patient and caregiver how to correctly use the package wrapper as a sterile drape or barrier when applying a sterile dressing or the correct procedure for removing a sterile item from the package.

- Assess patient's and caregiver's understanding and ability to provide a sterile environment when needed to perform a specific procedure.

✦ SKILL 6.2 Sterile Gloving

Video Clip **NSO** *Nursing Skills Online Infection Control Module 2 / Lesson 4*

Sterile gloves help prevent the transmission of pathogens by direct and indirect contact. Nurses apply sterile gloves before performing sterile procedures such as inserting urinary catheters or applying sterile dressings. Sterile gloves do not replace hand hygiene.

It is important to verify whether the patient or health care providers have a latex allergy. When allergies are present, select latex-free gloves. In an effort to reduce the allergy risk, most health care facilities have a standard practice to use powder-free and latex-free products. Repeated exposure to latex can lead to a latex allergy, in which case latex-free gloves would need to be used. Box 6.2 lists risk factors for a latex allergy. Latex proteins enter the body through skin or mucous membranes, intravascularly, or via inhalation. Reactions to latex range from mild to severe (Box 6.3).

Gloves must be the proper size. The gloves should not stretch so tightly over the fingers that they can tear easily, yet they need to be tight enough that objects can be picked up easily. Sterile gloves are available in various sizes (e.g., 6, 6.5, 7). They are also available in "one size fits all" or "small," "medium," and "large."

Delegation and Collaboration

Assisting with skills that include the application and removal of sterile gloves may be delegated to a UCP. However, most procedures that require the use of sterile gloves cannot be delegated to a UCP. The nurse instructs the UCP about the following:

- The reason for using sterile gloves for a specific procedure

Equipment

- Package of appropriately sized sterile gloves, latex or synthetic nonlatex. If patient has a latex allergy, ensure that gloves are latex-free and powder-free.

STEP	RATIONALE
ASSESSMENT	
1. Consider the type of procedure to be performed and consult employer policy on use of sterile gloves. In some facilities, double gloving has been recommended for the operating room (ORNAC, 2023).	Ensures proper use of sterile gloves when needed. Evidence supports the use of double gloving and double gloving with an indicator glove system to decrease the risk of percutaneous injury; such use is an effective barrier to bloodborne pathogen exposure (ORNAC, 2023).
2. Consider patient's risk for infection (e.g., pre-existing condition and size or extent of area being treated).	Knowledge of risk directs you to follow added precautions (e.g., use of additional protective barriers) if necessary.

BOX 6.2

Individuals at Risk for Latex Allergy

- Individuals who have had multiple surgeries (e.g., spina bifida surgeries) or medical procedures
- Workers with high latex exposure (e.g., health care employees, greenhouse workers, hair salon workers, aestheticians, workers in industries that use gloves routinely)
- Rubber industry workers
- Individuals with a personal or family history of allergies
- There is evidence that some people who are allergic to certain foods (e.g., avocado, banana, chestnut, kiwi, passion fruit) may also develop an allergic reaction to latex.

Canadian Centre for Occupational Health and Safety. (2023). *Latex allergy.* https://www.ccohs.ca/oshanswers/diseases/latex.html

BOX 6.3

Levels of Latex Reactions

The three types of common latex reactions (in order of severity) are as follows:

1. *Irritant dermatitis:* Skin reaction isolated to the area of contact
   a. Acute reaction: Red, dry, itchy, and irritated skin
   b. Chronic reaction: Dry, thick skin, crusting, and possibly cracking or peeling, resulting in open sores
2. *Type IV delayed hypersensitivity:* Allergic reaction to chemicals used in latex processing
   a. Acute reaction: Dry, red rash, itchy skin, hives, small blisters
   b. Chronic reaction: Dry, thickened skin, crusting, scabbing sores, vesicles, peeling (appears 4–96 hours after exposure)
3. *Type I immediate hypersensitivity:* Could be life threatening, with reactions starting within 2–3 minutes of exposure and up to several hours after contact
   a. Acute reaction: Hives, swelling, runny nose, nausea, abdominal cramps, dizziness, low blood pressure, bronchospasm, anaphylaxis (shock)

Canadian Society of Hospital Pharmacists. (2021). *Latex allergy primer.* https://www.cshp.ca/docs/pdfs/Latex%20allergy%20primer.pdf

STEP	RATIONALE
ASSESSMENT	
3. Select correct size and type of gloves and examine glove package to determine whether it is dry and intact with no water stains.	Torn or wet package is considered contaminated. Signs of water stains on package indicate previous contamination by water.
4. Inspect condition of hands for cuts, hangnails, open lesions, or abrasions. In some settings, you can cover any open lesion with a sterile, impervious transparent dressing (check employer policy). In some cases, presence of such lesions may prevent you from participating in a procedure.	Cuts, abrasions, and hangnails tend to ooze serum, which possibly contains pathogens. Breaks in skin integrity permit microorganisms to enter and increase the risk for infection for both patient and nurse (ORNAC, 2023).
5. Assess patient for the following risk factors before applying latex gloves:	Risk factors determine level of patient's risk for latex allergy.
a. Previous reaction to the following items within hours of exposure: adhesive tape, dental or face mask, golf club grip, ostomy bag, rubber band, balloon, bandage, elastic underwear, IV tubing, rubber gloves, condom	Items are known to lead to latex allergy.
b. Personal history of asthma, contact dermatitis, eczema, urticaria, rhinitis	Patients with a history of these conditions are at higher risk of having a reaction.
c. History of food allergies, especially avocado, banana, peach, chestnut, passionfruit, raw potato, kiwi, tomato, papaya	Patients with a history of food allergies are at higher risk of developing a reaction.
d. Previous history of adverse reactions during surgery or dental procedure	Previous history suggests allergic response.
e. Previous reaction to latex product	Previous reaction suggests allergic response.

NURSING DIAGNOSES

- Insufficient protection
- Potential for infection
- Potential for injury

Related factors and risk factors are individualized on the basis of patient's condition or needs.

PLANNING

STEP	RATIONALE
1. Expected outcomes following completion of procedure:	
• Patient does not develop signs or symptoms of infection after procedure.	Lack of signs of infection indicates that microorganisms are not introduced into sterile body cavities or sites (such as skin or urinary tract).
• Patient does not develop latex sensitivity or latex allergy reaction.	Patient at risk for latex allergy is not exposed to latex proteins.

Critical Decision Point *Nonlatex gloves (latex-free/powder-free) must be used when patients are at risk for latex allergy or if nurse has sensitivity or allergy to latex.*

IMPLEMENTATION

STEP	RATIONALE
1. Apply sterile gloves:	
a. Throughout the procedure, the 4 moments for hand hygiene are to be implemented; hand hygiene should occur before initial patient (or patient environment) contact, before an aseptic procedure, after body fluid exposure risk, and after patient (or patient environment) contact. Additional hand hygiene should be performed when hands are visibly soiled.	Proper hand hygiene helps prevent the spread of infectious agents to health care providers.
b. Place glove package near work area.	Hand hygiene reduces number of bacteria on skin surfaces and transmission of infection. Proximity to work area ensures availability before procedure.
c. Remove outer glove package wrapper by carefully separating and peeling apart sides (see Step 1c illustration).	Proper removal prevents inner glove package from accidentally opening and touching contaminated objects.
d. Grasp inner package and lay on clean, dry, flat surface at waist level. Open package, keeping gloves on inside surface of wrapper (see Step 1d illustration).	Sterile object held below waist is contaminated. Inner surface of glove package is sterile.

STEP	RATIONALE

IMPLEMENTATION

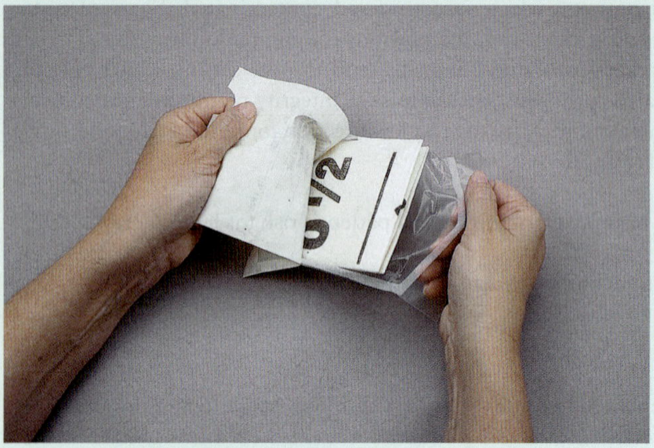

STEP 1C Open outer glove package wrapper.

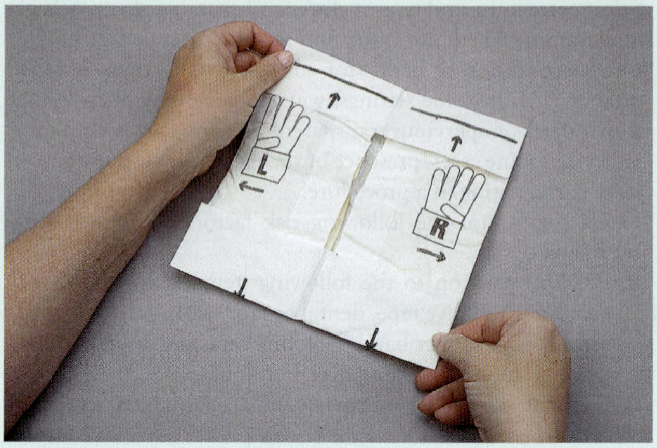

STEP 1D Open inner glove package on work surface.

STEP	RATIONALE
e. Identify right and left glove. Each glove has a cuff approximately 5 cm (2 inches) wide. Glove dominant hand first.	Proper identification of gloves prevents contamination by improper fit. Gloving of dominant hand first improves dexterity.
f. With thumb and first two fingers of nondominant hand, grasp glove for dominant hand by touching only inside surface of cuff.	Inner edge of cuff will lie against skin and thus is not sterile.
g. Carefully pull glove over dominant hand, leaving a cuff and being sure that cuff does not roll up wrist. Be sure that thumb and fingers are in proper spaces (see Step 1g illustration).	If outer surface of glove touches hand or wrist, it is contaminated.
h. With gloved dominant hand, slip fingers underneath cuff of second glove (see Step 1h illustration).	Cuff protects gloved fingers. Sterile touching prevents glove contamination.
i. Carefully pull second glove over fingers of nondominant hand (see Step 1i illustration).	Contact of gloved hand with exposed hand results in contamination.

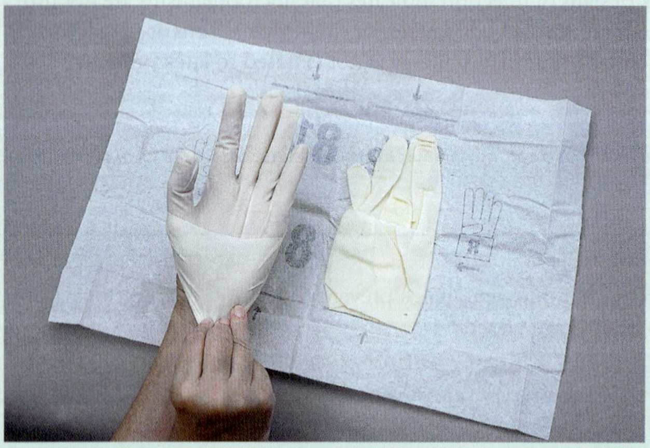

STEP 1G Pick up glove at cuff of dominant hand and insert fingers. Pull glove completely over dominant hand (example is for left-handed person).

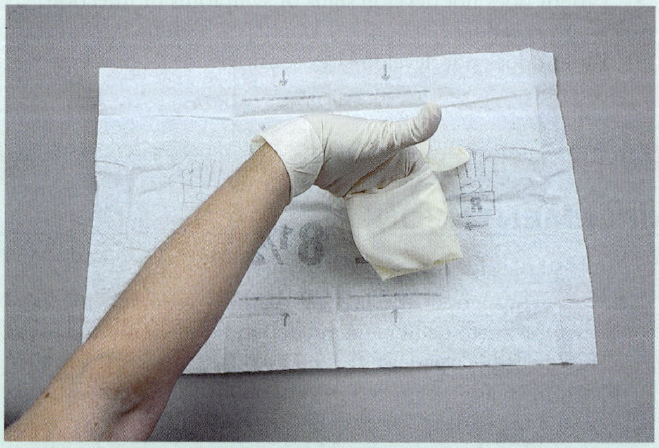

STEP 1H Pick up glove for nondominant hand.

STEP	RATIONALE

IMPLEMENTATION

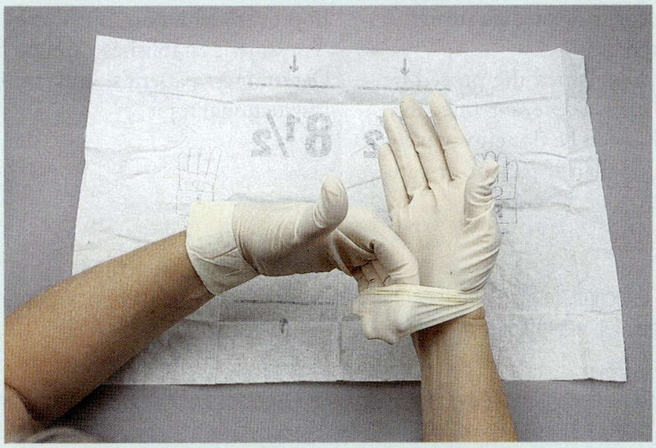

STEP 1I Pull second glove over nondominant hand.

Critical Decision Point *Do not allow fingers and thumb of gloved dominant hand to touch any part of exposed nondominant hand. Keep thumb of dominant hand abducted back.*

STEP	RATIONALE
j. After second glove is on, interlock hands together and hold away from body above waist level until beginning procedure (see Step 1j illustration).	Ensures smooth fit over fingers and prevents contamination.
2. Perform procedure.	
3. Remove gloves:	
a. Grasp outside of one cuff with other gloved hand; avoid touching wrist.	Procedure minimizes contamination of underlying skin.
b. Pull glove off, turning it inside out, and place it in gloved hand.	Outside of glove does not touch skin surface.
c. Take fingers of bare hand and tuck inside remaining glove cuff (see Step 3c illustration). Peel glove off inside out and over previously removed glove. Discard both gloves in receptacle.	Fingers do not touch contaminated glove surface. Hand hygiene protects health care worker from contamination resulting from any unseen tears or pinholes in gloves; also removes powder from hands to prevent skin irritation.

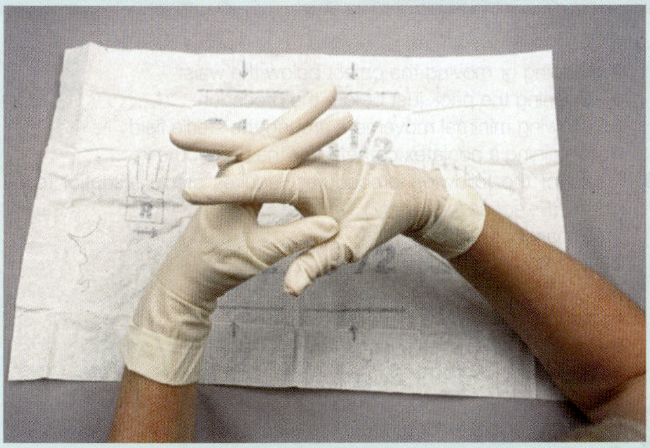

STEP 1J Interlock gloved hands.

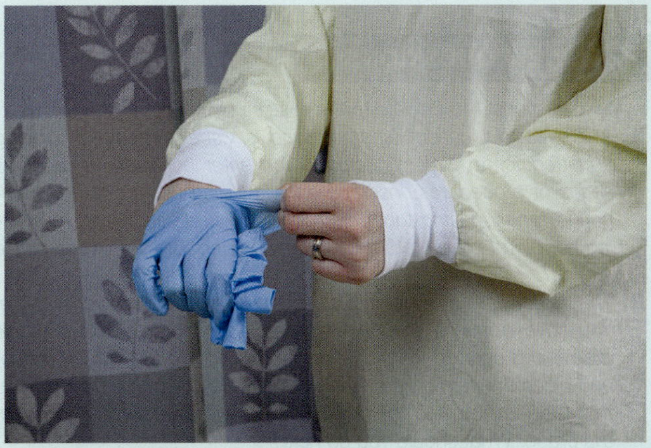

STEP 3C Remove second glove by turning it inside out.

STEP	RATIONALE

EVALUATION

1. Assess patient for signs of infection, focusing on area treated.	Improper technique contributes to development of an infection.
2. Assess patient for signs of latex allergy.	Assessment establishes baseline for patient's reaction to latex.
3. Use teach-back: "I want to be sure I explained the procedure that was performed and the steps used to prevent infection. Please tell me some of the things that can be done to prevent infection." Develop a revised teaching plan if patient or caregiver is unable to teach back correctly.	Determines patient's and caregiver's level of understanding of instructional topic.

Unexpected Outcomes	Related Interventions
1. Patient develops localized signs of infection (e.g., urine becomes cloudy or odorous; wound becomes painful, edematous, or reddened with purulent drainage).	• Contact health care provider and implement appropriate treatments as prescribed.
2. Patient develops systemic signs of infection (e.g., fever, malaise, increased white blood cell count).	• Contact health care provider and implement appropriate treatments as ordered.
3. Patient develops allergic reaction to latex (see Box 6.3).	• Immediately remove source of latex. • Bring emergency equipment to bedside. Have epinephrine injection ready for administration and be prepared to initiate IV fluids and oxygen.

Communication and Documentation

- It is not necessary to document application of gloves. Document specific procedure performed and patient's response and status.
- In the event of a latex allergy reaction, document patient's response on flow sheet or in progress notes in EHR or chart. Note type of response and patient's reaction to emergency treatment.

Special Considerations

Teaching

- Nurse or patient with a known latex allergy should wear a medical alert bracelet or tag and carry a wallet card stating "latex allergy."
- Individuals with known latex allergies should always carry a quick-acting oral antihistamine and an epinephrine autoinjector.
- Owing to risk of severe allergic response, some health care facilities use only powder- and latex-free gloves and products.

✦ REVIEW QUESTIONS

Review Questions 1 to 3 relate to the case study presented here.

1. *A 78-year-old patient (she/her) who is visually impaired is being admitted for a cholecystectomy. You enter her room to begin a series of procedures: inserting an in-dwelling urinary catheter, irrigating a nasogastric tube, suctioning the oral cavity, and measuring her blood pressure.* Which procedure requires the use of sterile gloves?

2. *The health care provider is planning to insert a central venous line. You have obtained the necessary equipment, prepared a sterile drape, and opened the sterile pack. You remove the outer wrapper and place the item on the sterile field. While doing this, you noticed that the item touched the drape 5 cm (2 inches) from the border of the drape.* What should you do next?

3. *The patient tells you that she develops dermatitis when she uses rubber gloves to do the dishes and a rash when she eats bananas or avocados.* How would you use SBAR (situation–background–assessment–recommendation) to communicate this information to the rest of the health care team?

4. When opening a sterile pack, which action compromises the sterility of the contents? (*Select all that apply.*)
   1. Positioning the contents of the pack at the very edge of the drape
   2. Holding or moving the object below the waist
   3. Opening the pack just before the procedure
   4. Allowing minimal movement around the sterile field
   5. Obtaining a nonlatex catheter for the procedure

5. Which of the following procedures requires sterile (aseptic) technique? (*Select all that apply.*)
   1. Urinary catheterization
   2. Insertion of a feeding tube
   3. Tracheal suctioning
   4. Lumbar puncture
   5. Insertion of a rectal suppository
   6. Sitz bath

Visit the Evolve site for a complete list of answers to the Review Questions.

✦ NEXT GENERATION NCLEX® (NGN)

For practice with answering exam questions related to unfolding NGN case studies, please consult the Next Generation NCLEX® (NGN)-Style Case Studies for Skills and Techniques on the Evolve website: http://evolve.elsevier.com/Canada/Perry/clinicalskills/

REFERENCES

Accreditation Canada. (2020). *Required organizational practices handbook*. https://physicians.nshealth.ca/resources/required-organizational-practices-2020-handbook

Canadian Centre for Occupational Health and Safety. (2023). *Latex allergy*. https://www.ccohs.ca/oshanswers/diseases/latex.html

Canadian Society of Hospital Pharmacists. (2021). *Latex allergy primer*. https://www.cshp.ca/docs/pdfs/Latex%20allergy%20primer.pdf.

Cimon, K., & Featherstone, R. (2018). *Jewellery and nail polish worn by health care workers and the risk of infection transmission: A review of clinical evidence and guidelines*. Canadian Agency for Drugs and Technologies in Health. https://europepmc.org/article/NBK/nbk487444

Hewlett, A. L., Hohenberger, H., Murphy, C. N., et al. (2018). Evaluation of the bacterial burden of gel nails, standard nail polish, and natural nails on the hands of health care workers. *American Journal of Infection Control*, *46*(12), 1356–1359. https://doi.org/10.1016/j.ajic.2018.05.022

Infection Prevention and Control Canada. (2022). *IPAC Canada practice recommendations: Hand hygiene in health care settings*. https://ipac-canada.org/photos/custom/Members/pdf/17JulHand%20Hygiene%20Practice%20Recommendations_final.pdf

Ontario Agency for Health Protection and Promotion (Public Health Ontario [PHO]), Provincial Infectious Diseases Advisory Committee (PIDAC) (PHO-PIDAC). (2012). *Routine practices and additional precautions in all health care settings* (3rd ed.). https://www.publichealthontario.ca/en/health-topics/infection-prevention-control/routine-practices-additional-precautions

Operating Room Nurses Association of Canada. (2023). *ORNAC standards, guidelines, and position statements for perioperative registered nurses* (16th ed.). http://www.ornac.ca/en/standards

Public Health Agency of Canada. (2017). *Routine practices and additional precautions for preventing the transmission of infection in healthcare settings* (Cat. No. HP40-83/2013E-PDF). https://www.canada.ca/en/public-health/services/publications/diseases-conditions/routine-practices-precautions-healthcare-associated-infections.html

World Health Organization. (2018). *Global guidelines on the prevention of surgical site infection* (2nd ed.). https://apps.who.int/iris/bitstream/handle/10665/277399/9789241550475-eng.pdf

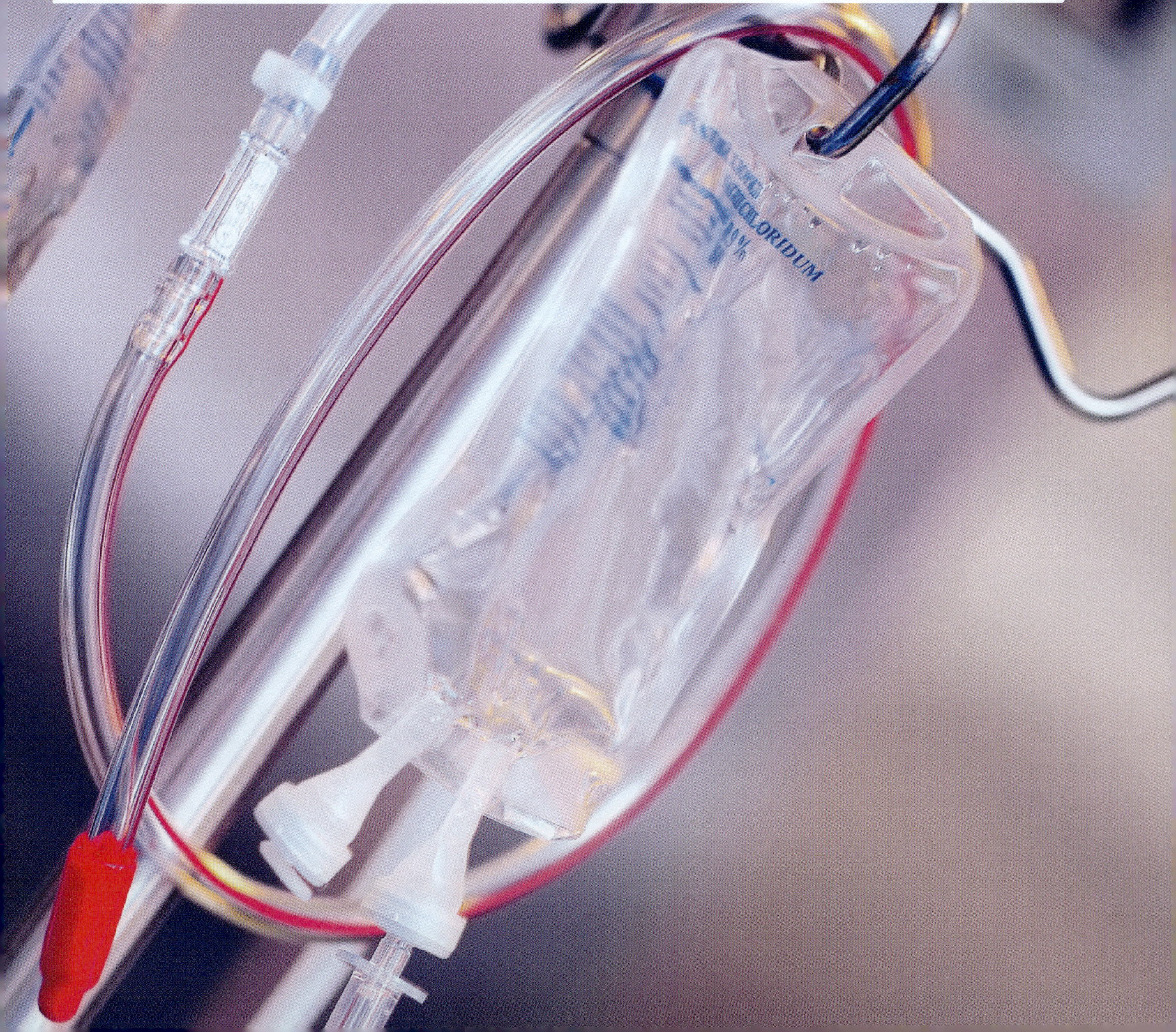

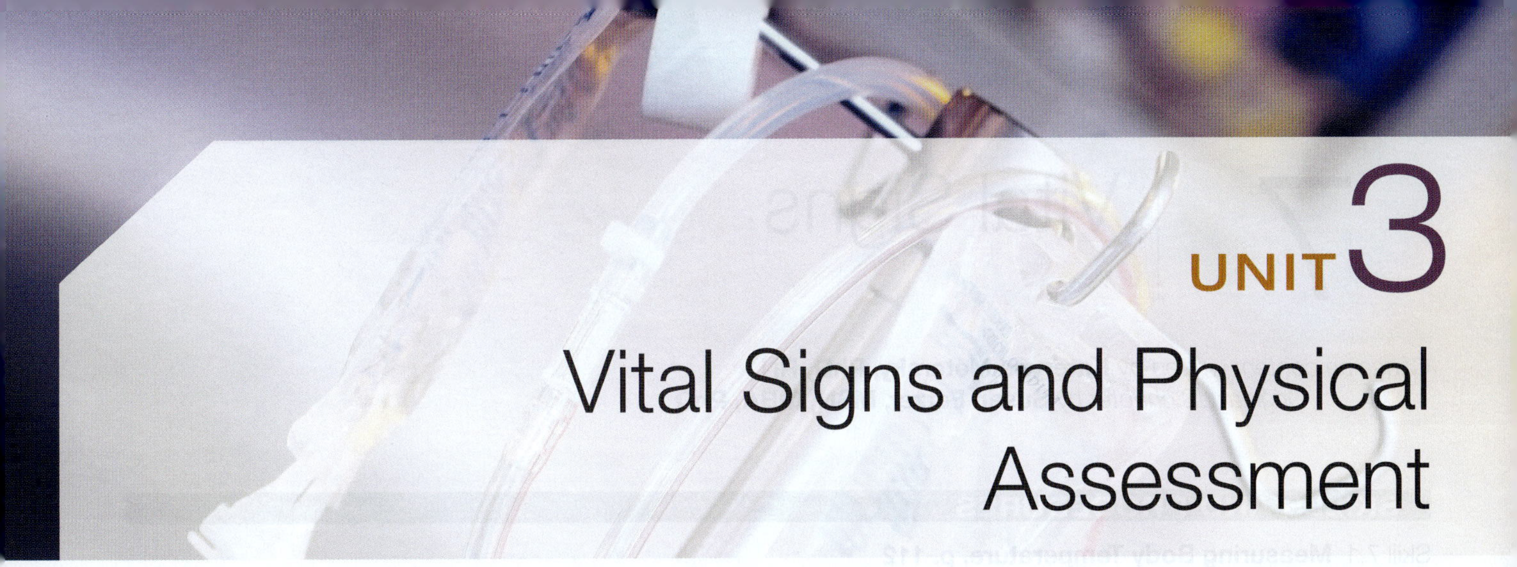

UNIT 3 Vital Signs and Physical Assessment

Any clinical decision about a patient is complex, requiring a nurse to gather sufficient assessment data that will reveal the cues pointing to the patient's health problems. In order to recognize cues, a nurse gathers significant data from many sources. Whether a patient presents with common symptoms of a back sprain or symptoms of an upper respiratory infection, a clinical decision cannot be made without sufficient data. A thorough assessment yields common sets of cues that form patterns. When analyzed critically, these patterns indicate patient problems and nursing diagnoses. A thorough assessment is comprehensive and patient centred.

Patient assessment includes a *health assessment* that incorporates the use of physical examination skills and direct patient questioning to uncover subjective and objective data about a patient's health status. Chapter 8 presents the comprehensive categories a nurse may choose to include when performing a health assessment. However, the amount of data that a nurse gathers in any clinical situation during a health assessment depends on the time spent with patients and the complexity and urgency of their problems. In addition, a nurse must make clinical judgements as to what should be further assessed when certain signs are discovered. For example, if a nurse notices swelling of a patient's ankle (edema), this observation should trigger further examination, including palpation of pulses in the patient's feet. The nurse then asks, Does the edema impair circulation? If a nurse observes the patient walking with an unsteady gait, that cue alone will prompt the nurse to examine whether the source of impairment is neurological or musculoskeletal.

Patient assessment also includes measurement of *vital signs*. At times, vital signs will be the primary reason a nurse assesses a patient, as in the case of a routine check following a procedure. Vital signs reveal the stability of a patient's vital functions. When a vital sign is found to be abnormal or significantly different from a patient's baseline findings, a nurse will then conduct appropriate health assessments to determine whether other cues exist. If a patient registers a fever on a thermometer, the nurse will palpate the skin for warmth and note whether the skin is diaphoretic. At other times, a physical finding such as a patient expressing chest pain will prompt a nurse to assess vital signs, specifically heart rate and blood pressure.

As a nurse analyzes the various cues available from a health assessment, including vital signs, there may be additional data available in the form of relevant *laboratory* and *diagnostic* test results. These data can help confirm the findings from the health assessment. When a patient presents with pallor and a thready pulse, a low hematocrit offers a cue to the problem of poor oxygenation.

A nurse decides whether assessment is complete for a specific clinical situation after connecting the available data with a patient's presentation. Anticipating the type of data to be expected, based on a patient's self-reported problem or a health care provider's medical diagnosis, prompts a nurse to be thorough. In addition, anticipating what to assess aids in the analysis of the meaning of assessment findings. When the data reveal unexpected findings, any potential problems need to be explored further. Patient assessment is central to providing the data needed for nurses to make clinical judgements regarding identification of patient problems and nursing diagnoses.

7 | Vital Signs

Canadian content written by **Kateryna Metersky, PhD, RN**
Original US chapter by **Susan Fetzer, MSN, MBA, PhD**

SKILLS AND PROCEDURES

OBJECTIVES

Mastery of content in this chapter will enable the nurse to:

- Identify when it is appropriate to assess each vital sign.
- Accurately assess a patient's oral, rectal, axillary, tympanic membrane, and temporal artery temperatures.
- Describe factors that cause variations in body temperature, pulse, respirations, blood pressure, and oxygen saturation.
- Describe factors influencing the selection of temperature measurement sites.
- Accurately assess a patient's radial and apical pulses.
- Explain implications of a pulse deficit.
- Accurately assess a patient's respirations.
- Accurately measure a patient's blood pressure using the techniques of auscultation and palpation.
- Describe benefits and disadvantages of using an electronic blood pressure machine.
- Describe factors influencing the selection of an extremity in which to measure blood pressure.
- Accurately assess a patient's oxygenation status using pulse oximetry.
- Identify ranges of acceptable vital sign values for infants, children, and adults.
- Correctly document vital signs.
- Appropriately delegate vital sign measurements to unregulated care providers.

MEDIA RESOURCES

- http://evolve.elsevier.com/Canada/Perry/clinicalskills/

PURPOSE

Vital signs, which include temperature, pulse, blood pressure, respirations, and oxygen saturation, reflect the physiological status of the body and its response to physical, environmental, and psychological stressors. Pain, a subjective symptom, is often referred to as the sixth vital sign. As a nurse, you will frequently perform an assessment of a patient's level of comfort and pain during vital sign measurements (see Chapter 16).

Vital signs reveal both sudden changes in a patient's condition and changes that occur progressively over time. Any difference between a patient's normal baseline measurement and present vital signs may indicate the need for interprofessional collaboration with other health care team members, nursing therapies, and medical interventions. Vital signs are also important in evaluating a patient's response to therapy—for example, how a patient with a fever responds to antipyretics, or how a patient with hypertension responds to medication.

STANDARDS OF CARE

- Canadian Agency for Drugs and Technologies in Health (2017)—*The Assessment of Postoperative Vital Signs: Clinical Effectiveness and Guidelines* (https://www.cadth.ca/assessment-postoperative-vital-signs-clinical-effectiveness-and-guidelines)
- Canadian Paediatric Society (CPS, 2022)—*Fever and Temperature Taking* (https://caringforkids.cps.ca/handouts/health-conditions-and-treatments/fever_and_temperature_taking)
- Hypertension Canada (2020a)—*Accurate Measurement of Blood Pressure* (https://guidelines.hypertension.ca/diagnosis-assessment/measuring-blood-pressure/)

PRINCIPLES FOR PRACTICE

- Vital signs are included in a routine health assessment (see Chapter 8). When vital signs are performed outside of a routine health assessment, a quick priority assessment (QPA) should be done.
- The nurse can perform a QPA each time the nurse interacts with the patient and in emergency situations. QPA is intended to be a guide for the nurse to gather information in a quick, concise manner to determine priorities of care (Box 7.1).
- Always obtain a baseline measurement of vital signs on first contact with a patient to provide a means for comparison with later vital sign measurements. Frequency of vital sign measurements depends on the specific patient's condition (Box 7.2).
- Use interprofessional collaboration and apply clinical reasoning and judgement to decide which vital sign to measure, when to obtain measurements, and the frequency of assessments.

PERSON-CENTRED CARE

- Interprofessional collaboration and patient involvement regarding vital signs and every other area of a patient's health are important in optimizing patient health and wellness and practising person-centred care. Patients should be actively engaged in the prevention, promotion, and management of their health (Canadian Nurses Association, 2011).
- Vital sign measurements can require the removal of clothing or exposure of areas considered inappropriate or offensive to patients from some cultures. Nurses must be sensitive to each patient's need for privacy and observation of cultural norms (i.e., providing privacy as part of person-centred care when performing apical pulse assessment).
- Always inform patients about their vital sign measurements. Many patients monitor their own vital signs at home and can be valuable partners in letting the nurse know which values are normal for them.
- Procedures that are normally noninvasive sometimes produce anxiety because of cultural variables of touch, privacy, and gender.
- When reporting findings, patients from some cultures rely on a male elder to receive information on their behalf.
- Provide culturally competent nursing care and assess patient preference related to decision making (e.g., independent or interdependent in health-related issues). Nurses must be aware that patients may make a decision based on what they think is best for their family, not necessarily themselves, and be prepared to advocate for and support the patient (Tyerman & Cobbett, 2023).

BOX 7.1

Quick Priority Assessment: ABC I&O PS

A Airway (Is the airway patent?)
B Breathing (What is the quality of breathing? Signs of compromised breathing?)
C Circulation (What is the patient's colour? Temperature of extremities?)
I In (What is going in? Identify all solutions, follow all tubes. Are volumes adequate? Rates accurate? Any evidence of complications?)
O Out (What is coming out? Are dressings dry and intact? Any drainage tubes present? If yes, what is the nature of the drainage? Are tubes patent? Any evidence of complications?)
P Pain (Is the patient in pain? Are analgesics given previously still effective? Is patient comfortable? Do they need to use the bathroom?)
S Safety (Is oxygen and suction equipment available? Are side rails up? Is patient call bell within reach? Are the bed/wheelchair brakes applied? Is the area clutter free? Always ask, "Is there anything you need from me at this time?")

Adapted from Anderson, R. (2018). 2.13 Quick priority assessment (QPA). In *Clinical procedures for safer patient care—Thompson Rivers University Edition*. BCcampus. https://pressbooks.bccampus.ca/clinicalproceduresforsaferpatientcaretrubscn/chapter/2-13-quick-priority-assessment-qpa/

BOX 7.2

When to Take Vital Signs

- On admission to a health care facility
- In a hospital or care facility on a routine schedule according to a health care provider's prescription or employer policy
- When assessing a patient during care in the community visits
- Before, during, and after a surgical or invasive diagnostic procedure
- Before, during, and after the administration of medications or application of therapies that affect cardiovascular, respiratory, or temperature-control functions
- Before, during, and after a transfusion of any type of blood products
- Before, during, and after nursing interventions influencing a vital sign (e.g., before and after patient previously on bed rest ambulates, before and after range-of-motion exercises)
- When a patient reports specific symptoms of physical distress (e.g., feeling "funny" or "different")
- When a patient's general physical condition changes (e.g., loss of consciousness, increased intensity of pain)
- Before a patient is sent home on a day or weekend pass and upon their return to the facility

EVIDENCE-INFORMED PRACTICE

Obtaining an accurate and reliable measurement of blood pressure (BP) requires consideration of measurement conditions.

- Slow breathing decreases systolic blood pressure (SBP) measurement by about 5.62 mm Hg and diastolic blood pressure (DBP) measurement by 2.97 mm Hg (Chaddha et al., 2019).
- Talking with a health care provider can increase SBP by 9.1 mm Hg and DBP by 4.5 mm Hg (Qi et al., 2017).
- The BP cuff should be placed at heart level on a bare arm (Hypertension Canada, 2020a).
- Respiratory rate has a strong relationship with mortality; some experts believe it is a better predictor of patient deterioration than BP or pulse (Takayama et al., 2019). Assessment of respiratory rate is an accurate predictor of cardiac arrest and patient deterioration (Rolfe, 2019).
- Try to obtain a respiratory assessment when the patient is not aware that you are counting their breaths, because the patient may try to control their respiratory rate, which prevents a true assessment (Rolfe, 2019).

SAFETY GUIDELINES

- A nurse caring for a patient is responsible for measuring vital signs. Nurses analyze vital signs to interpret their significance and make decisions about appropriate interventions.
- Equipment must be clean, functional, properly calibrated, and appropriate for the patient's size, age, condition, and characteristics.
- Ensure that patients who have latex allergies are provided with latex-free equipment, including BP cuffs and pulse oximeter probes.
- As the nurse, it is your responsibility to know each patient's usual range of vital signs. A patient's usual values may differ from the acceptable range for that age or physical state. They serve as a baseline for comparison with later findings, enabling you to detect changes in the patient's condition over time.
- You are also responsible for knowing a patient's medical history, therapies, and prescribed medications. Some illnesses or treatments cause predictable vital sign changes. Most medications affect at least one of the vital signs.

- Control or minimize environmental factors that affect vital signs. For example, assessing a patient's temperature in a warm, humid room may yield a value that is not a true indicator of their condition.
- Use an organized, systematic (step-by-step) approach when taking vital signs to ensure accurate findings.
- Based on a patient's condition, use interprofessional collaboration to decide the minimum frequency of vital sign assessment for each patient. Following surgery or treatment intervention, measure vital signs more frequently to detect complications. In a clinic or outpatient setting, take vital signs before the health care provider examines the patient and after any invasive procedures. As a patient's physical condition worsens, it is important to monitor vital signs as often as every 5 to 15 minutes. Use your clinical reasoning and judgement to determine whether more frequent assessments are necessary.
- Analyze the results of vital sign measurements and incorporate all the clinical findings about a patient in determining nursing diagnoses. Do not interpret vital signs in isolation. You need to know related physical signs or symptoms and be aware of the patient's ongoing health status.
- Verify, communicate, and document significant changes in vital signs. Baseline measurements allow you to identify changes in vital signs. When vital signs appear abnormal, it helps to have another nurse repeat the measurement. Inform the health care provider when vital signs become abnormal and report any changes to the nurse in charge.
- Always practise infection control. Perform hand hygiene according to the 4 moments for hand hygiene (Accreditation Canada, 2020). Conduct a point-of-care risk assessment (see Chapter 5, Box 5.1) to determine the appropriate personal protective equipment (PPE) required for each patient interaction. If possible, use disposable or dedicated patient-care equipment (e.g., BP cuffs). If disposable or dedicated equipment is not available, clean and disinfect the equipment before use on another patient (Lapum et al., 2021).

✦ SKILL 7.1 Measuring Body Temperature

Video Clip NSO *Nursing Skills Online Vital Signs Module 4 / Lessons 1 and 2*

Body temperature is the difference between the amount of heat produced by body processes and the amount lost to the external environment. The core temperature, or temperature of the deep body tissues, is controlled by the hypothalamus and remains within a narrow range. The thermostat regulated in the hypothalamus maintains this homeostasis by balancing heat production (from metabolism, exercise, food digestion, external factors) with heat loss (through radiation, evaporation of sweat, convection, and conduction) (Jarvis et al., 2024). Skin or body surface temperature can also fluctuate dramatically as it rises and falls with the changing temperature of the surrounding environment.

The body tissues and cells function best within a relatively narrow temperature range, from 36 to 38°C (96.8–100.4°F), but no single temperature is normal for all people. For healthy young adults, the average oral temperature is 37°C (98.6°F). In clinical practice, nurses learn the temperature range of individual patients. An acceptable temperature range for adults depends on age, gender, range of physical activity, hydration status, and state of health (Fig. 7.1).

Many factors affect body temperature, but physiological and behavioural control mechanisms act to maintain a constant core temperature. For example, the mechanism of peripheral vasodilation increases blood flow to the skin, which increases the amount of heat radiated to the environment. Control mechanisms have failed when heat produced by the body is not equal to heat lost to the environment. For example, patients without sweat gland function are unable to tolerate warm temperatures because they cannot adequately cool themselves. Fever occurs when heat-loss mechanisms are unable to keep pace with excess heat production, resulting in an abnormal rise in body temperature. When an individual has a febrile condition (i.e., pyrexia), the nurse needs to initiate temperature-control measures, such as administering prescribed antipyretics; providing a tepid sponge bath; applying cool compresses to the patient's forehead, wrists, and other body sites; dressing the patient in lightweight clothing; or providing a cooling blanket in cases of a high fever. It is important to carefully monitor the patient for shivering when using these cooling interventions because shivering increases core body temperature (Schlader & Vargas, 2018).

The purpose of measuring body temperature is to obtain a representative average temperature of core body tissues. Average usual temperature varies depending on the measurement site used. Research findings from numerous studies are contradictory; however, it is generally accepted that rectal temperatures are usually 0.5°C (0.9°F) higher than oral temperatures. Axillary temperatures are usually 0.5°C (0.9°F) lower than oral temperatures. Sites reflecting core temperature are more reliable indicators of body temperature than sites reflecting surface temperatures (Kiekkas et al., 2019) (Box 7.3).

To ensure accurate temperature readings, each site needs to be measured correctly. Use the same site when repeated measurements are necessary or when comparing temperature measurements over time.

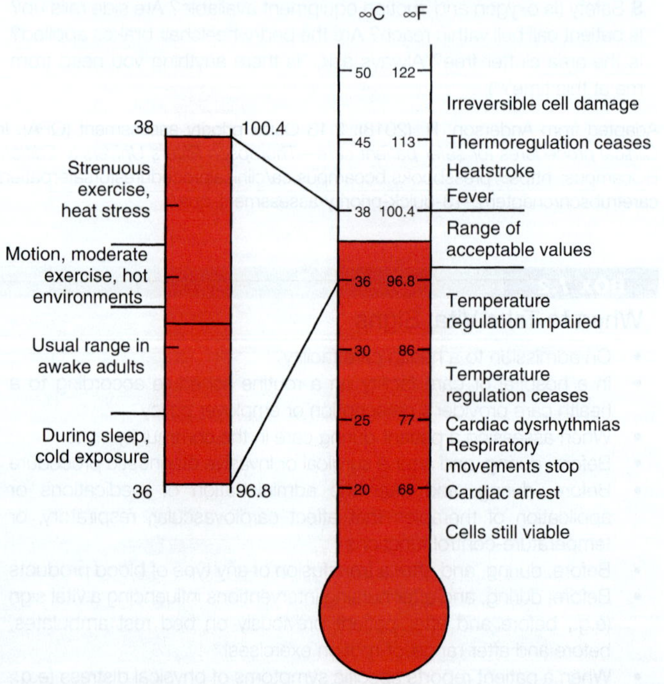

FIG 7.1 Ranges of normal temperature values and physiological consequences of abnormal body temperature. *(Adapted from Patton, K. T., & Thibodeau, G. A. [2018]. The human body in health and disease [7th ed.]. Elsevier.)*

BOX 7.3

Core and Surface Temperature Measurement Sites

Core Site
- Rectum
- Tympanic membrane
- Temporal artery
- Esophagus
- Pulmonary artery
- Urinary bladder

Surface Site
- Skin
- Oral cavity
- Axilla

Each site has advantages and disadvantages (Box 7.4). Determine the safest and most accurate site for a patient.

Several types of thermometers are commonly available to measure body temperature (Box 7.5). The mercury-in-glass thermometer, once the standard device found in the clinical setting, is now prohibited because of the potential hazards of mercury exposure. However, mercury-in-glass thermometers can still be found in patients' homes.

Delegation and Collaboration

The skill of temperature measurement can be delegated to an unregulated care provider (UCP). The nurse instructs the UCP by doing the following:

- Communicating the appropriate route, device, and frequency of temperature measurement

BOX 7.4

Advantages and Limitations of Selected Temperature Measurement Sites

Oral
Advantages
- Easily accessible—requires no position change
- Comfortable for patient
- Provides accurate surface temperature reading
- Reflects rapid change in core temperature
- Reliable route to measure temperature for intubated patients

Limitations
- Causes delay in measurement if patient recently ingested hot/cold fluids or foods, chewed gum, or smoked
- Not used with patients who have had oral surgery or facial trauma, are unable to position in mouth, or have shaking chills or history of seizures
- Not used with infants; small children; or confused, unconscious, or uncooperative patients (Sims et al., 2018)
- Not used with patients who are hypothermic (Sims et al., 2018)
- Risk for body fluid exposure

Tympanic Membrane
Advantages
- Easily accessible site
- Obtained without disturbing, waking, or repositioning patient
- No body fluid exposure
- Used for patients with tachypnea without affecting breathing
- Sensitive to core temperature changes
- Very rapid measurement (2–5 seconds)
- Unaffected by oral intake of food or fluids, smoking, or environmental temperatures

Limitations
- More variability of measurement than with other core temperature devices
- Requires removal of hearing aids before measurement
- Requires disposable sensor cover with only one size available
- Readings possibly distorted with otitis media and cerumen impaction (Sims et al., 2018)
- Not used with patients who have had surgery of the ear or tympanic membrane
- Environmental temperatures can affect the measurement reading, making it invalid
- Does not accurately measure core temperature changes during and after exercise
- Affected by ambient temperature devices such as incubators, radiant warmers, and facial fans
- Recent evidence indicates that tympanic temperature is a stable measurement only if the probe is directed at a specific site on the membrane and is influenced by head cooling (Foster et al., 2021).
- Anatomy of the ear canal makes it difficult to correctly position in neonates, infants, and children younger than 2 years of age. The thermometer probe is too large in relation to the size of the ear canal, so it will detect infrared emissions from both the tympanic membrane and the proximal meatus wall. The average of these two surface temperatures can produce an erroneously low reading. A slight tug of the pinna to straighten the ear canal can improve accuracy and consistency (Canadian Paediatric Society [CPS], 2022).
- Inaccuracies reported because of incorrect positioning of handheld unit

Rectal
Advantages
- Purported to be reliable when oral temperature is difficult or impossible to obtain
- Although controversial, it is still referred to as the gold standard for use in children under 3 years of age (CPS, 2022)

Limitations
- Lags behind core temperature during rapid temperature changes
- Not used for patients with diarrhea or those who have had rectal surgery, rectal disorders, bleeding tendencies, or neutropenia
- Requires positioning that can be a source of patient embarrassment and anxiety
- Risk for body fluid exposure and stoolborne pathogens (Kiekkas et al., 2019)
- Requires lubrication
- Not used for routine vital signs in newborns
- Readings influenced by impacted stool
- Should not be used with patients receiving chemotherapy because it increases the risk for infection

Axilla
Advantages
- Safe and inexpensive
- Reliable in stable neonates and those in the neonatal intensive care unit (NICU) (Sims et al., 2018)

Limitations
- Long measurement time
- Requires continuous positioning to ensure placement over axillary artery
- Poorly reflects core temperature (CPS, 2022)
- Not recommended for detecting fever in infants and young children
- Not used with patients who are hypothermic
- Requires exposure of thorax, which can result in temperature loss, especially in newborns
- Affected by exposure to the environment, including time it takes to place thermometer
- Underestimates core temperature in older persons and children (CPS, 2022; Fitzwater et al., 2019)

Skin
Advantages
- Inexpensive
- Provides continuous reading
- Safe and noninvasive
- Used for neonates

Continued

BOX 7.4

Advantages and Limitations of Selected Temperature Measurement Sites—cont'd

Limitations

- Measurement lags behind other sites during temperature changes, especially during hyperthermia
- Impaired adhesion from diaphoresis or sweat
- Affected by environmental temperature
- Cannot be used for patients with allergy to adhesives

Temporal Artery

Advantages

- Easy to access without position change
- Provides a considerable reduction in required nursing time to measure (Khan et al., 2021)
- Comfortable with no risk of injury to patient or nurse
- Eliminates need for patient to disrobe or unbundle
- Can be used for premature infants, newborns, and children (Kiekkas et al., 2019)
- Reflects rapid change in core temperature
- Sensor cover not required

Limitations

- Inaccurate with head covering or hair on forehead
- Affected by skin moisture such as diaphoresis or sweating
- Use not recommended when accurate measurement of body temperature is required to make informed clinical decisions (Brosinski et al., 2018)
- Considered inaccurate for children under 5 years of age (Mogensen et al., 2018)

BOX 7.5

Types of Thermometers

Electronic Thermometer (Fig. 7.2)

- The thermometer is a rechargeable battery-powered display unit with a thin wire cord and a temperature-processing probe covered by a disposable cover.
- Within 1 minute after placement, the thermometer displays a digital temperature reading.
- Separate probes are available for oral and axillary temperature measurement (blue tip) and rectal temperature measurement (red tip).

Tympanic Membrane Thermometer

- The probe consists of an otoscope-like speculum with an infrared sensor tip that detects heat radiated from the tympanic membrane of the ear (Fig. 7.3).
- Within seconds after placing probe in the ear canal and depressing the scan button, a digital reading appears on the display unit. A sound signals when the peak temperature has been measured.

Temporal Artery Thermometer

- An infrared scanner is swept across the forehead, lifted, and then placed behind the ear. If the patient is diaphoretic, a scan just behind the ear verifies the measurement accuracy (Fig. 7.4).
- Within seconds after scanning, a digital reading appears on the display unit.

Chemical Dot Single-Use or Reusable Thermometer

- The thermometer consists of thin strips of plastic with a temperature sensor at one end and chemically impregnated dots formulated to change colour at different temperatures, usually within 60 seconds (Fig. 7.5).
- It is useful for screening temperatures, especially in infants, during invasive procedures, for a patient on protective isolation, and in orally intubated critical care patients.
- It is not appropriate for monitoring fever in acutely ill patients or for temperature therapies.
- It can be used at axillary or rectal site if covered by a plastic sheath with a placement time of 3 minutes.
- Home disposable thermometers are useful for temperature screening but are not as accurate as nondisposable electronic thermometers.

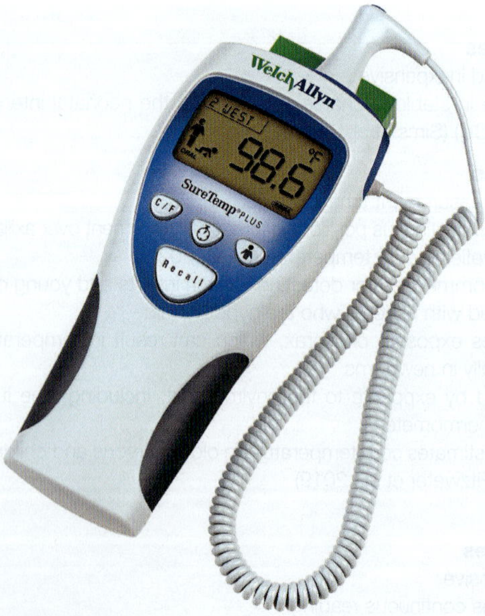

FIG 7.2 Electronic thermometer with disposable plastic probe cover. *(Photo courtesy Welch Allyn.)*

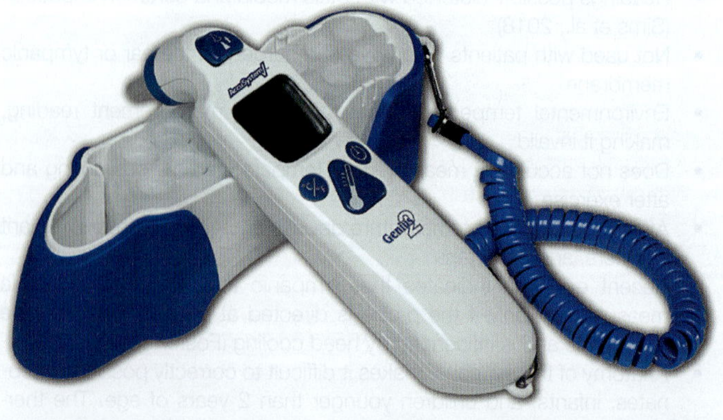

FIG 7.3 Tympanic membrane thermometer with disposable plastic probe cover. *(Copyright © Covidien. All rights reserved.)*

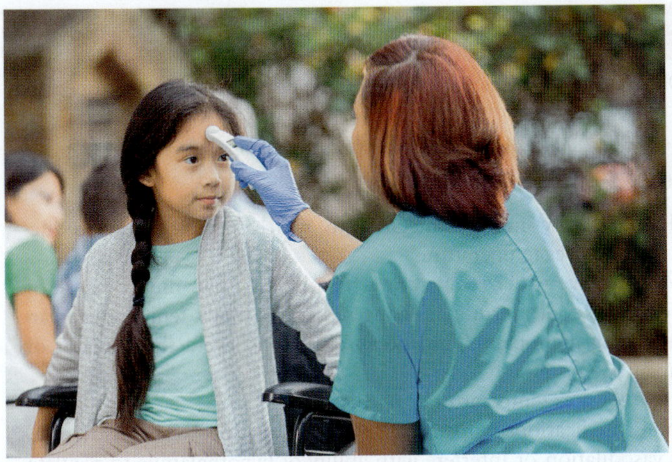

FIG 7.4 A temporal artery thermometer measures the heat from blood flowing through the superficial temporal artery. *(Steve Debenport/iStockphoto)*

- Explaining any precautions needed in positioning the patient (e.g., for rectal temperature measurement)
- Reviewing the usual temperature values and significant changes to report to the nurse

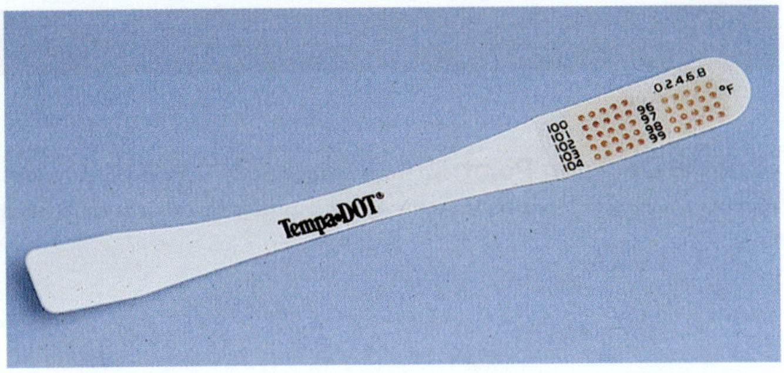

FIG 7.5 Chemical dot, disposable, single-use thermometer.

Equipment

- Thermometer (selected based on site used; see Box 7.4)
- Soft tissue or wipe
- Alcohol swab
- Water-soluble lubricant (for rectal measurements only)
- Pen and vital sign flow sheet, record form, or electronic health record (EHR)
- Clean gloves *(optional)*, plastic thermometer sleeve, disposable probe or sensor cover
- Towel

STEP	RATIONALE
ASSESSMENT	
1. Identify patient using at least two person-specific identifiers (e.g., name and date of birth, or name and medical record number) according to employer policy.	Ensures correct patient. Adheres to Accreditation Canada's standards and improves patient safety (Accreditation Canada, 2020).
2. Throughout the procedure, the 4 moments for hand hygiene are to be implemented; hand hygiene should occur before initial patient (or patient environment) contact, before an aseptic procedure, after body fluid exposure risk, and after patient (or patient environment) contact. Additional hand hygiene should be performed when hands are visibly soiled.	Proper hand hygiene helps prevent the spread of infectious agents to health care providers.
3. Determine need to measure patient's body temperature:	
a. Note patient's risks for temperature alterations: • Expected or diagnosed infection • Open wounds or burns • White blood cell count below 5–10 × 10^9/L or above 12 × 10^9/L • Immunosuppressive drug therapy • Injury to hypothalamus • Exposure to temperature extremes • Blood product infusion • Hypothermia or hyperthermia therapy • Postoperative status	Certain conditions place patients at risk for temperature alterations that require more frequent temperature measurement and nursing assessment.
b. Assess for other signs and symptoms that accompany temperature alteration: • *Hyperthermia:* Decreased skin turgor, dry mucous membranes; tachycardia; hypotension; decreased venous filling; concentrated urine • *Heatstroke:* Body temperature of 40°C (104°F) or more (Canada Safety Council, 2019); hot, dry skin; tachycardia; hypotension; excessive thirst; muscle cramps; visual disturbances; confusion or delirium • *Hypothermia:* Pale skin; skin cool or cold to touch; bradycardia and dysrhythmias; uncontrollable shivering; reduced level of consciousness; shallow respirations	Physical signs and symptoms alert you to alterations in body temperature.
c. Assess for factors that normally influence temperature:	Allows you to accurately assess for presence and significance of temperature alteration.

STEP	RATIONALE
• Age	Older persons have narrower range of temperature than younger persons.

Critical Decision Point *No single temperature is normal for all people. A temperature within an acceptable range in an adult may reflect a fever in an older person. Undeveloped temperature-control mechanisms in infants and children cause temperature to rise and fall rapidly.*

STEP	RATIONALE
• Exercise	Muscle activity increases metabolism, which increases heat production and raises temperature.
• Hormones	Women have wider temperature fluctuations than men because of menstrual cycle hormonal changes, because body temperature varies during menopause, and because women have a thicker layer of subcutaneous fat.
• Stress	Stress elevates temperature.
• Medications	Some medications impair or promote sweating, vasoconstriction, or vasodilation or interfere with ability of hypothalamus to regulate temperature.
• Daily fluctuations	Body temperature normally changes 0.5–1°C (0.9–1.8°F) during a 24-hour period. Temperature is lowest during early morning. Most patients have maximum temperature elevation between 5 and 7 p.m.; temperature falls gradually during the night.
• Damage to the hypothalamus	Damage to the hypothalamus caused by nervous system trauma, intracerebral bleeding, and increased intracranial pressure can cause a fever (sometimes called a *neurogenic fever*). This is a high-temperature fever where the patient does not sweat and is resistant to antipyretics (Tyerman & Cobbett, 2023).
• Environment	Environment influences body temperature. Infants, older persons, and those with spinal cord injuries are most likely to be affected, as their temperature-regulating mechanisms are less efficient. People with spinal cord injuries are often poikilothermic (body temperature adjusts to temperature of surrounding environment). The higher the level of injury, the greater the degree of poikilothermism, with high cervical injuries leading to greater loss of ability to regulate temperature (Tyerman & Cobbett, 2023).
4. Determine appropriate measurement site and device for patient (see Box 7.4). Use disposable thermometer for patient on isolation precautions.	Determines whether patient's status contraindicates selection of a specific method or site.
5. Determine previous baseline temperature and measurement site (if available) from patient's record.	Allows you to assess for change in condition. Provides comparison with future temperature measurements.
6. Assess patient's knowledge of procedure.	Encourages cooperation; minimizes risks and anxiety. Identifies teaching needs.

NURSING DIAGNOSES

- Hyperthermia
- Hypothermia
- Inadequate thermoregulation
- Potential for hyperthermia
- Potential for imbalanced body temperature
- Potential for perioperative hypothermia

Related factors and risk factors are individualized on the basis of patient's condition or needs.

PLANNING

STEP	RATIONALE
1. Expected outcomes following completion of procedure:	
• Body temperature is within acceptable range for patient's age group.	Thermoregulation is maintained.
• Body temperature returns to baseline range following therapies for abnormal temperature.	Environmental factors that alter temperature are controlled.
2. Explain to patient how you will measure temperature and the importance of maintaining proper position until reading is complete.	Promotes patient cooperation and increases adherence to procedure. Patients are often curious about their temperatures and should be cautioned against prematurely removing thermometer to read results.
3. Collect and bring appropriate supplies to patient's bedside.	Ensures an organized approach to measuring body temperature.
4. If patient is having oral temperature measured, verify that patient has not had anything to eat or drink in the last 20 minutes and has not chewed gum for 5 minutes or smoked within the past 2 minutes (Astle & Duggleby, 2024).	Food and fluids, smoking, and gum can alter oral temperature measurement (Astle & Duggleby, 2024).

STEP	RATIONALE
IMPLEMENTATION	
1.	Proper hand hygiene helps prevent the spread of infectious agents to health care providers.
2. Help patient to comfortable position that provides easy access to temperature measurement site.	Ensures patient's comfort and accuracy of temperature reading.
3. Obtain temperature reading.	
a. Oral temperature (electronic):	
(1) *Optional:* Apply clean gloves when there is risk for exposure to respiratory secretions or facial or mouth wound drainage.	Reduces transmission of microorganisms. An oral probe cover is removable without physical contact, thus gloves are not required.
(2) Remove thermometer pack from charging unit. Attach oral thermometer probe stem (blue tip) to thermometer unit. Grasp top of probe stem, being careful not to apply pressure on ejection button.	Charging provides battery power. Ejection button releases plastic cover from probe stem.
(3) Slide disposable plastic probe cover over thermometer probe stem until cover locks in place (see Step 3a[3] illustration).	Soft plastic cover will not break in patient's mouth and prevents transmission of microorganisms between patients.
(4) Ask patient to open mouth; gently place thermometer probe under tongue in posterior sublingual pocket lateral to centre of lower jaw (see Step 3a[4] illustration).	Heat from superficial blood vessels in sublingual pocket produces temperature reading. With electronic thermometer, temperatures in right and left posterior sublingual pocket are significantly higher than in area under front of tongue.
(5) Ask patient to hold thermometer probe with lips closed.	Maintains proper position of thermometer during recording.
(6) Leave thermometer probe in place until audible signal indicates completion and patient's temperature appears on digital display; remove thermometer probe from under patient's tongue.	Probe must stay in place until signal occurs to ensure accurate reading.
(7) Push ejection button on thermometer probe stem to discard plastic probe cover into appropriate receptacle.	Reduces transmission of microorganisms.
(8) If wearing gloves, remove and dispose in appropriate receptacle.	Reduces transmission of microorganisms.
(9) Return thermometer probe stem to storage position of thermometer unit.	Protects probe stem from damage. Returning thermometer probe stem automatically causes digital reading to disappear.
(10) Clean and disinfect the equipment that is not disposable before use on another patient.	Reduces transmission of microorganisms.

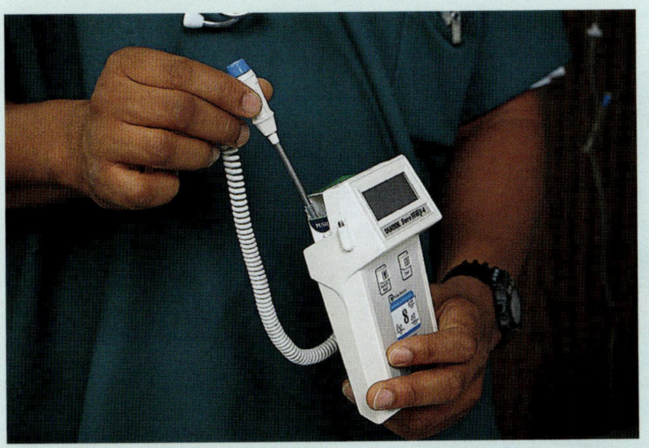

STEP 3A(3) **Nurse inserts electronic thermometer probe stem into probe cover. Cover snaps in place.**

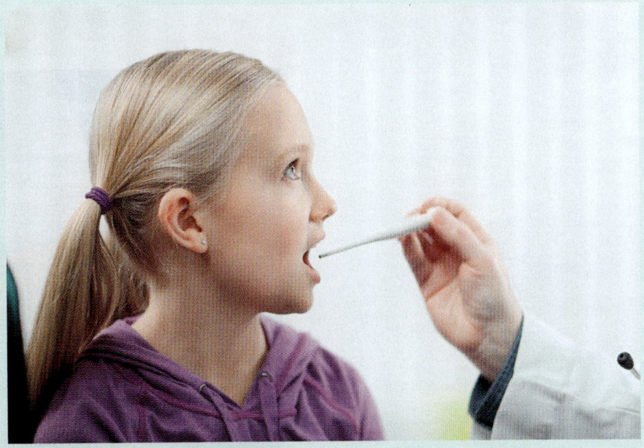

STEP 3A(4) **Probe placed under tongue in posterior sublingual pocket.** *(YinYang/iStockphoto)*

STEP	RATIONALE
b. Rectal temperature (electronic):	
(1) Draw curtain around bed and close room door. Help patient to side-lying position with upper leg flexed (modified left lateral recumbent position). Move aside bed linen to expose only anal area. Keep patient's upper body and lower extremities covered with sheet or blanket.	Maintains patient's privacy, minimizes embarrassment, and promotes person-centred care and comfort.
(2) Apply clean gloves. Cleanse anal region when feces or secretions are present. Remove soiled gloves and reapply clean gloves.	Reduces transmission of microorganisms. Maintains standard precautions when exposed to items soiled with body fluids (e.g., feces).
(3) Remove thermometer pack from charging unit. Attach rectal thermometer probe stem (red tip) to thermometer unit. Grasp top of probe stem, being careful not to apply pressure on ejection button.	Ejection button releases plastic cover from probe stem.
(4) Slide disposable plastic probe cover over thermometer probe stem until cover locks in place.	Soft plastic probe cover prevents transmission of microorganisms between patients.
(5) Using a single-use package, squeeze a liberal amount of lubricant on tissue. Dip probe cover of thermometer, blunt end, into lubricant, covering 2.5–3.5 cm (1–1.5 inches) for adult.	Lubrication minimizes trauma to rectal mucosa during insertion. Tissue avoids contamination of remaining lubricant in container.
(6) With nondominant hand, separate patient's buttocks to expose anus. Ask patient to breathe slowly and relax.	Fully exposes anus for thermometer insertion. Relaxes anal sphincter for easier thermometer insertion.
(7) Gently insert thermometer into anus in direction of umbilicus 3.5 cm (1.5 inches) for adult. Do not force thermometer.	Ensures adequate exposure against blood vessels in rectal wall.
(8) If you feel resistance during insertion, withdraw immediately. Never force thermometer.	Prevents trauma to mucosa.

Critical Decision Point *If you cannot adequately insert thermometer into rectum or resistance is felt during insertion, remove thermometer and consider alternative method for obtaining temperature. Never force thermometer.*

STEP	RATIONALE
(9) Once positioned, hold thermometer probe in place until audible signal indicates completion and patient's temperature appears on digital display; remove thermometer probe from anus (see Step 3b[9] illustration).	Probe must stay in place until signal occurs to ensure accurate reading.

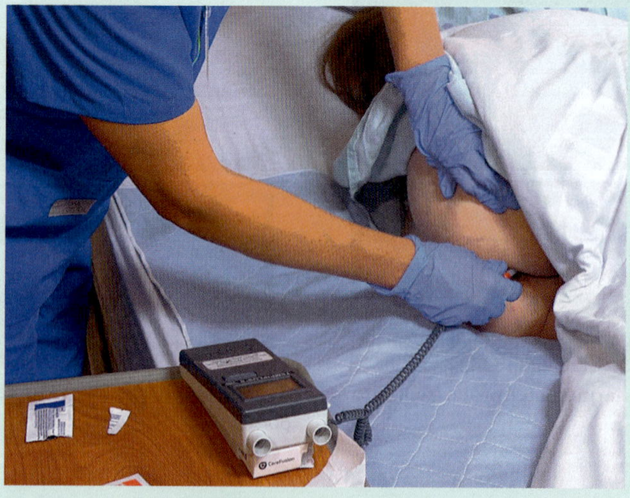

STEP 3B(9) Probe inserted into anus.

STEP	RATIONALE
(10) Push ejection button on thermometer stem to discard plastic probe cover into appropriate receptacle. Wipe probe stem with alcohol swab, paying particular attention to ridges where probe stem connects to probe, then remove and dispose of gloves in appropriate receptacle.	Reduces transmission of microorganisms.
(11) Return thermometer stem to storage position of recording unit. Don new gloves.	Protects probe stem from damage. Returning thermometer stem automatically causes digital reading to disappear.
(12) Wipe patient's anal area with soft tissue to remove lubricant or feces and discard tissue. Help patient to assume a comfortable position.	Provides for comfort and hygiene.
(13) Remove and dispose of gloves in appropriate receptacle.	Reduces transmission of microorganisms.
(14) Clean and disinfect the nondisposable parts of the equipment before use on another patient.	
c. Axillary temperature (electronic):	
(1) Draw curtain around bed and close room door. Help patient to supine or sitting position. Move clothing or gown away from shoulder and arm.	Maintains patient's privacy, minimizes embarrassment, and promotes comfort. Exposes axilla for correct thermometer probe placement.
(2) Remove thermometer pack from charging unit. Attach oral thermometer probe stem (blue tip) to thermometer unit. Grasp top of thermometer probe stem, being careful not to apply pressure on ejection button.	Charging provides battery power. Ejection button releases plastic cover from probe stem.
(3) Slide disposable plastic probe cover over thermometer stem until cover locks in place.	Soft plastic probe cover prevents transmission of microorganisms between patients.
(4) Raise patient's arm away from torso. Inspect for skin lesions and excessive perspiration; if needed, dry axilla or select alternative site. Insert thermometer probe into centre of axilla (see Step 3c[4] illustration), lower arm over probe, and place arm across patient's chest.	Maintains proper position of thermometer against blood vessels in axilla.
Critical Decision Point *Do not use axilla if skin lesions are present because local temperature is sometimes altered and area may be painful to touch.*	
(5) Once thermometer probe is positioned, hold it in place until audible signal indicates completion and patient's temperature appears on digital display; remove thermometer probe from axilla.	Thermometer probe must stay in place until signal occurs to ensure accurate reading.
(6) Push ejection button on thermometer stem to discard plastic probe cover into appropriate receptacle.	Reduces transmission of microorganisms.
(7) Return thermometer stem to storage position of recording unit.	Returning thermometer stem to storage position automatically causes digital reading to disappear. Protects stem from damage.
(8) Help patient to assume comfortable position, replacing linen or gown.	Restores comfort and sense of well-being.
(9) Clean and disinfect the nondisposable parts of the equipment before use on another patient.	Reduces transmission of microorganisms.
d. Tympanic membrane temperature:	
(1) Help patient to assume comfortable position with head turned toward side, away from you. If patient has been lying on one side, use other ear. Obtain temperature from patient's right ear if you are right-handed. Obtain temperature from patient's left ear if you are left-handed.	Ensures comfort and facilitates exposure of auditory canal for accurate temperature measurement. Heat trapped in ear facing down causes falsely high temperature reading. The less acute the angle of approach, the better the probe seal.
(2) Note whether there is an obvious presence of cerumen (earwax) in patient's ear canal.	Cerumen impedes lens cover of speculum. Switch to other ear or select alternative measurement site.
(3) Remove thermometer handheld unit from charging base, being careful not to apply pressure to ejection button.	Charging base provides battery power. Removal of handheld unit from base prepares it to measure temperature. Ejection button releases plastic probe cover from thermometer tip.
(4) Slide disposable speculum cover over otoscope-like lens tip until it locks in place. Be careful not to touch lens cover.	Soft plastic probe cover prevents transmission of microorganisms between patients. Lens cover should not have dust, fingerprints, or cerumen obstructing optical pathway.
(5) Insert speculum into ear canal following manufacturer instructions for tympanic probe positioning (see Step 3d[5] illustration):	Correct positioning of probe with respect to ear canal allows maximal exposure of tympanic membrane.

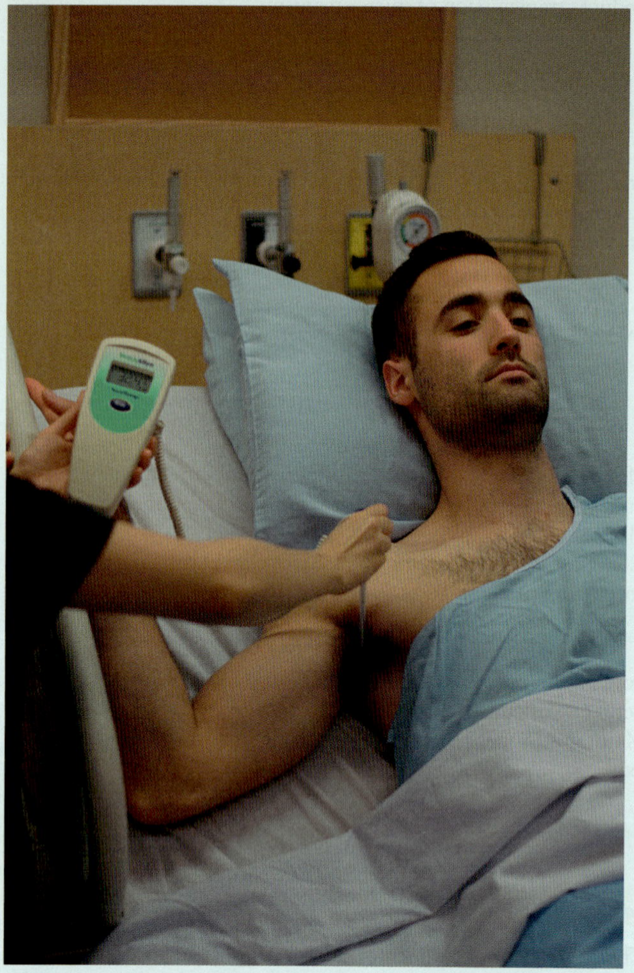

STEP 3C(4) **Insert thermometer probe into centre of axilla.** *(Courtesy Barbara J. Astle, RN, PhD.)*

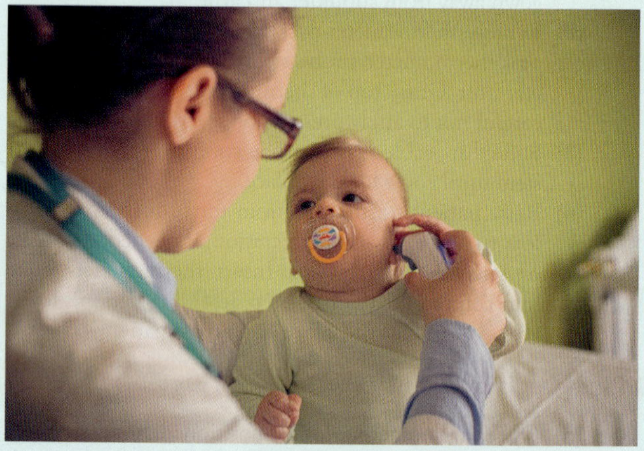

STEP 3D(5) **Tympanic membrane thermometer with probe cover placed in patient's ear.** *(aywan88/iStockphoto)*

STEP	RATIONALE
(a) Pull ear pinna backward, up, and out for an adult. For children less than 3 years of age, pull pinna down and back; point covered probe toward midpoint between eyebrow and sideburns. For children older than 3 years, pull pinna up and back (Hockenberry et al., 2024).	Ear tug straightens external auditory canal, allowing maximum exposure of tympanic membrane and therefore correctly positioning speculum (Hockenberry et al., 2024).
(b) Fit speculum tip snug in canal, pointing toward nose.	Gentle pressure seals ear canal from ambient air temperature, which alters readings by as much as 2.8°C (5°F).
(c) Move thermometer in figure-eight pattern.	Some manufacturers recommend movement of speculum tip in figure-eight pattern, which allows sensor to detect maximum tympanic membrane heat radiation.
(6) Once positioned, press scan button on handheld unit. Leave speculum in place until audible signal indicates completion and patient's temperature appears on digital display.	Pressing scan button causes detection of infrared energy. Speculum probe tip must stay in place until device has detected infrared energy noted by audible signal.
(7) Carefully remove speculum from auditory meatus. Push ejection button on handheld unit to discard speculum cover into appropriate receptacle.	Reduces transmission of microorganisms. Automatically causes digital reading to disappear.

STEP	RATIONALE
(8) If temperature is abnormal or second reading is necessary, replace probe cover and wait 2 minutes before repeating in same ear or repeat measurement in other ear. Consider an alternative temperature site or instrument.	Lens cover must be free of cerumen to maintain optical path. Time allows ear canal to regain usual temperature.
(9) Return handheld unit to thermometer base.	Protects sensor tip from damage.
(10) Help patient assume comfortable position.	Restores comfort and sense of well-being.
(11) Disinfect thermometer unit regularly when visibly soiled, after every use or once daily.	Reduces transmission of microorganisms.
e. Temporal artery temperature:	
(1) Ensure that forehead is dry; dry with towel if needed.	Moisture interferes with thermometer sensor.
(2) Place sensor firmly on patient's forehead.	Flush contact avoids measurement of ambient temperature.
(3) Press red scan button with your thumb. Slowly slide thermometer straight across forehead while keeping sensor flat and firmly on skin (see Fig. 7.4). Keeping scan button depressed, lift sensor after sweeping forehead and touch sensor on neck just behind earlobe. Read temperature when clicking sound during scanning stops. Release scan button.	Thermometer continuously scans for highest temperature when scan button is depressed. Area behind earlobe is less affected by diaphoresis and verifies temperature.
(4) Gently clean sensor with alcohol swab and return to storage unit.	Prevents transmission of microorganisms.
(5) If possible, use a disposable single-use sensor for patients on isolation precautions or disinfect before using it on another patient.	
4. Inform patient of temperature reading and record measurement.	Promotes patient's participation in care and understanding of health status.
5. Return thermometer to charger.	Maintains battery charge of thermometer unit.

EVALUATION

1. If you are assessing temperature for the first time, establish it as baseline if it is within acceptable range.	Used to compare future temperature measurements. A wider temperature range is acceptable in infants and young children, with temperature ranging from 35.5 to 37.7°C (95.9–99.8°F). In adults, the normal core body temperature is 36.5–37.5°C (97.7–99.5°F). Older persons tend to have lower body temperatures than other adults (Lapum et al., 2021).
2. Compare temperature reading with patient's previous baseline and acceptable temperature range for patient's age group.	Body temperature fluctuates within narrow range; comparison reveals presence of abnormality. Improper placement or movement of thermometer can cause inaccuracies. Second measurement confirms initial findings of abnormal body temperature (Kiekkas et al., 2019).
3. If patient has fever, take temperature approximately 30 minutes after administering antipyretics and every 4 hours until temperature stabilizes.	Determines whether temperature begins to fall in response to therapy.
4. Use **teach-back:** "I want to be sure I explained how to check your child's temperature at home. Show me how to swipe his forehead using the thermometer." Develop a revised teaching plan if caregiver is unable to teach back correctly.	Determines caregiver's level of understanding of instructional topic.

STEP	RATIONALE
Unexpected Outcomes	**Related Interventions**
1. Patient has temperature 1°C (1.8°F) or more above usual range.	• Initiate measures to lower body temperature: • Cool room environment. • Reduce external covering on patient's body to promote heat loss, but do not induce shivering. • Keep clothing and bed linen dry. • Apply hypothermia blanket as prescribed. • Limit physical activity and sources of emotional stress. • Administer antipyretics as prescribed. • Increase fluid intake to at least 3 L daily (unless contraindicated). • Initiate measures to stimulate appetite and provide nutrients to meet increased energy needs. • Prevent or control spread of infection.
2. Patient has temperature 1°C (1.8°F) or more below usual range.	• Initiate measures to raise body temperature: • Apply warm blankets and, unless contraindicated, offer warm liquids. • Apply hyperthermia blankets if prescribed. • Remove wet clothing or linen.
3. Unable to obtain temperature.	• Reassess correct placement of temperature probe or sensor. • Choose alternative temperature measurement site. • Obtain alternative temperature measurement device.

Communication and Documentation

- Document temperature, including unit of measurement, and route on vital sign flow sheet or in progress notes in EHR or chart.
- Report abnormal findings to nurse in charge or health care provider.
- Document your evaluation of patient and caregiver learning.

DOCUMENTATION EXAMPLE

Patient's vital signs stable. Patient's axillary temp is 37°C at 1100 hours. Pt is requesting a shower. Materials provided and patient assisted via commode to the shower with assistance by the UCP. Will reassess patient temp at 1600 hours.

Special Considerations

Teaching

- Identify patient's ability to initiate preventive health measures and recognize alteration in body temperature. Educate patient and caregiver about measures to prevent body temperature alterations.
- Educate patients about risk factors for hypothermia and frostbite: fatigue; malnutrition; hypoxemia; cold, wet clothing; alcohol intoxication.
- Educate patients about risk factors for heatstroke: strenuous exercise in hot, humid weather; tight-fitting clothing in hot environments; exercising in poorly ventilated areas; sudden exposures to hot climates; poor fluid intake before, during, and after exercise.
- Educate patients regarding importance of taking and continuing antibiotics as directed until course of treatment for infection is completed.

Pediatric

- Infants and young children may lose more heat to the environment because of their increased body surface area/volume ratios.
- Critically ill children sometimes have cool skin but high core temperature because of poor perfusion to the skin.
- Use axillary temperatures for screening purposes only; axillary temperature should not be relied on to detect a fever in children.
- Children may assume prone position for rectal temperature measurement.
- With children who cry or become restless, it is best to take temperature as the last vital sign.

Gerontological

- The temperature of older persons tends to be lower than the acceptable temperature range for an adult: 36°C (96.8°F).
- Temperatures considered within normal range often reflect a fever in an older person.
- Adults without teeth or older persons with poor muscle control may be unable to close their mouth tightly enough to obtain accurate oral temperature readings.
- Older persons are very sensitive to slight changes in environmental temperature because their thermoregulatory systems are not as efficient (Boscart et al., 2023).
- Oral temperature measurement is more reliable in older persons because cerumen tends to be drier and cilia become stiff, contributing to buildup of cerumen impaction, which interferes with accurate tympanic temperature measurement.
- A decrease in sweat gland activity in the older person results in a higher threshold for sweating at high temperatures, which can lead to hyperthermia.
- With aging, a loss of subcutaneous fat reduces the insulating capacity of the skin.
- Older persons are at high risk for hypothermia because of diminished sensation to cold, abnormal vasoconstrictor responses, and impaired shivering.

Care in the Community: Home Management

- Assess temperature and ventilation of patient's environment to determine existence of any environmental conditions that influence patient's temperature.
- In the home, some patients continue to use mercury-in-glass thermometers. Assess safe storage of these thermometers to protect from breakage and mercury spills. Educate patient and caregiver on proper use of the thermometer, mercury hazards, and proper disposal of any mercury-containing devices. Suggest alternative temperature measurement devices for home use.

✦ SKILL 7.2 Teaching Patients to Measure Body Temperature

An elevation in body temperature may be an early warning sign of serious health problems. Patients who are susceptible to temperature alterations (e.g., immunosuppressed patients) and their caregivers need to know how to measure temperature correctly so patients can seek medical attention earlier. Parents need to know how to measure their children's temperature because children can develop high fevers very quickly; older persons and their caregivers need to know the techniques for temperature measurement because older persons have impaired temperature-control mechanisms. Nurses need to teach patients and caregivers the skills of measuring body temperature and techniques to lower temperature when a fever occurs at home.

A variety of body temperature thermometers are currently available, including disposable single-use, electronic, noncontact, temporal, and tympanic thermometers. Mercury thermometers are not recommended for use; if a mercury thermometer breaks or is not disposed of properly, the mercury vapour gets into the air, posing a major health risk in the home and community (CPS, 2022). Nurses need to educate patients about the environmental hazards associated with mercury in the home and encourage them to purchase mercury-free thermometers. Patients should be encouraged to remove mercury thermometers from their homes and dispose of them at a toxic waste facility.

The nurse may help a patient choose the most appropriate thermometer to use in the home based on the patient's normal dexterity, vision, and financial resources. For example, a patient with visual impairment from glaucoma or retinopathy can read a thermometer with a large digital display more easily.

Delegation and Collaboration

The skill of teaching patients to measure body temperature cannot be delegated to a UCP. The nurse instructs the UCP to do the following:

- Inform the nurse of patient or caregiver concerns about measuring body temperature

Equipment

- Thermometer
- Disposable probe cover (if needed)
- Water-soluble lubricant (for rectal measurements)
- Paper and pencil or pen, or computer if frequent measurements are to be taken
- Disposable clean gloves (for rectal temperature taken by a caregiver)

STEP	RATIONALE
ASSESSMENT	
1. Identify patient using at least two person-specific identifiers during first visit (e.g., name and date of birth, or name and medical record number) according to employer policy. Facial recognition can be used as one of two identifiers for ongoing home visits.	Ensures correct patient. Complies with Accreditation Canada's standards and improves patient safety (Accreditation Canada, 2020).
2. Throughout the procedure, the 4 moments for hand hygiene are to be implemented; hand hygiene should occur before initial patient (or patient environment) contact, before an aseptic procedure, after body fluid exposure risk, and after patient (or patient environment) contact. Additional hand hygiene should be performed when hands are visibly soiled.	Proper hand hygiene helps prevent the spread of infectious agents to health care providers.
3. Assess patient's and caregiver's ability to manipulate and read thermometer. Have patient put on eyeglasses if necessary.	Physical restrictions in handling or reading a thermometer can prevent a patient from being able to read the thermometer and often require teaching the caregiver as well as the patient.
4. Assess patient's knowledge of normal temperature range, symptoms of fever and hypothermia, and patient's risk for body temperature alterations.	Identifies patient's ability to recognize alterations in body temperature and to initiate preventive health measures.
5. Assess patient's ability to determine appropriate type of thermometer to be used in varying situations.	Determines knowledge of age-related or medical conditions that determine selection of temperature.
6. Assess patient's learning readiness and ability to concentrate; consider presence of pain, nausea, or fatigue and patient interest in instruction.	Presence of significant illness, frailty, or confusion affects a patient's ability to attend to a teaching plan. Indicates need to rely on caregiver for learning and implementation (if available) on a short- or long-term basis.
7. Assess patient's and caregiver's previous knowledge of and experience in measuring temperature and maintaining a thermometer. Have the patient or caregiver perform a return demonstration if they indicate ability to measure temperature.	Allows assessment of patient's and caregiver's knowledge and use of safety precautions, aseptic technique, and time period for insertion.

NURSING DIAGNOSES

- Inadequate thermoregulation
- Insufficient knowledge regarding temperature measurement skill
- Potential for imbalanced body temperature
- Potential for infection

Related factors and risk factors are individualized on the basis of patient's condition or needs.

STEP	RATIONALE
PLANNING	
1. Expected outcomes following completion of procedure:	
• Patient or caregiver is able to correctly measure body temperature.	Indicates that skills are learned.
• Patient or caregiver demonstrates proper cleaning and storage of equipment.	Prevents transfer of microorganisms and maintains integrity of thermometer.
• Patient or caregiver states normal temperature range and factors that affect temperature, signs and symptoms of fever and hypothermia, and measures to take with abnormal temperatures.	Cognitive learning is achieved.
2. Select setting in the home where patient or caregiver is most likely to measure temperature.	Considers person-centred care.
3. Select setting in the home where patient is most likely to measure temperature and is a good location for teaching session:	Improves likelihood that patient and caregiver will be attentive to instruction.
a. Select a room that is well lit with comfortable seating.	
b. Be sure that the patient is close and can see the nurse clearly.	
c. Control sources of noise and distractions.	Room environment needs to minimize existing sensory alterations. A comfortable environment free of distractions increases patient's attention.
4. Discuss and demonstrate with patient and caregiver normal temperature ranges; instruct caregiver to remain with patient during measurement if age or physical status requires.	Learning by doing; active engagement is more effective than passive models.
IMPLEMENTATION	
1. Demonstrate steps of thermometer preparation, insertion, and reading. Provide rationale for steps to patient and caregiver.	Observing and evaluation of demonstration is cornerstone of person-centred care.
a. Instruct patient to take oral temperature 20–30 minutes after smoking or ingesting hot or cold liquids or foods and to wait at least an hour after a hot bath or vigorous exercise. Explain indications for selecting temperature site other than oral.	Waiting at least 15 minutes after drinking hot or cold liquids or foods improves accuracy of temperature reading (Vorvick, 2022).
b. Instruct caregiver to perform hand hygiene and wear clean, disposable gloves.	Patient and caregiver must be knowledgeable about infection prevention techniques.
c. Teach patient and caregiver the proper position of patient for temperature measurement.	Improves accuracy of readings.
d. Demonstrate temperature measurement technique and have patient or caregiver perform each step with guidance. Do not rush them.	Allows for correction of errors in technique as they occur and for discussion of potential consequences of errors.
e. Explain any special precautions in using thermometers: oral thermometer must be placed in the sublingual pocket; rectal thermometers must be lubricated with water-soluble lubricant; use rectal thermometer only for measuring rectal temperatures; never force a rectal thermometer into the rectum.	Ensures accurate reading and avoidance of injury to patient.
f. Discuss typical time frame needed for each type of temperature to register (based on thermometer type) and how to take reading.	Ensures accurate reading.
g. Teach proper method for removing, cleaning, and storing thermometer (when applicable) and select a suitable storage location.	Prevents transmission of infection. Thermometer is stored properly so it does not break or become inaccurate when not in use.
2. Discuss common symptoms of fever: warm, dry, flushed skin; feeling warm; chills; piloerection; malaise; and restlessness.	Patient or caregiver needs to recognize onset of fever for early detection and intervention.
3. Discuss common signs and symptoms of hypothermia: cool skin, uncontrolled shivering, loss of memory, and signs of poor judgement. Explain that people with inadequate home heating, older persons, or those unaware of the potential dangers of cold conditions are at risk.	Patient or caregiver needs to recognize onset of hypothermia for early detection and intervention.

STEP	RATIONALE
Critical Decision Point *Teach patient and caregiver to take temperature after chills or shivering subsides, to obtain an accurate temperature.*	
4. Discuss importance of notifying the health care provider when temperature elevations occur. Review common therapies for temperature reduction that are safe to perform at home, including when to use antipyretics; exposing skin to air; reducing room temperature; increasing air circulation; applying cool, moist compresses to skin (e.g., forehead); and drinking fluids. Patients receiving chemotherapy should be cautioned that any fever is a medical emergency and that they should immediately seek medical attention (Canadian Cancer Society, 2019).	Treating fever enhances patient comfort. Lowering the temperature can reduce risk of febrile seizures in children (Hockenberry et al., 2024).
5. Provide set of written guidelines for patient's reference at appropriate level of health literacy.	Patients prefer written materials that are clear and concise; bulleted lists are preferred to text blocks (National Institutes of Health, 2021).
6. Give patient or caregiver a paper or digital log to time and record temperature if frequent monitoring is required. Instruct patient and caregiver to use a written record to report temperatures to the health care provider.	Keeping an organized record of temperatures helps patient validate and report temperature fluctuations to the health care provider.

EVALUATION

1. Have patient or caregiver independently demonstrate technique for temperature measurement, including body placement and ability to read thermometer, three separate times.	When psychomotor skill is performed correctly, patient confidence is increased.
2. Ask patient or caregiver to identify the normal temperature range and the influence of smoking and hot and cold liquids or foods on oral readings; discuss safety implications for temperature measurement.	Measures cognitive learning and confirms understanding of information.
3. Have patient or caregiver describe common signs and symptoms of fever and hypothermia and methods for controlling these.	Measures cognitive learning.
4. Watch patient or caregiver clean and store equipment.	Proper cleaning prevents bacterial growth, and proper storage preserves accuracy of thermometer.
5. Watch patient or caregiver record temperature values and times in log. Review patient's log periodically to ensure that temperatures are being recorded correctly.	Health care providers make changes in patient care based on information provided by the patient. To ensure that changes are made appropriately, patient or caregiver needs to record accurate information.
6. Use **teach-back:** "I want to be sure I explained the importance of monitoring your temperature. Explain in your own words why it is important to know how to take your own temperature." Develop a revised teaching plan if patient or caregiver is unable to teach back correctly.	Determines patient's and caregiver's level of understanding of instructional topic.

Unexpected Outcomes	Related Interventions
1. Patient or caregiver is unable to measure temperature, clean and store thermometer correctly, or verbalize knowledge about fever and temperature measurement.	• Ask patient or caregiver to describe difficulties experienced while performing temperature measurement. • Use a different teaching strategy. • Plan for patient to perform another return demonstration during the next scheduled home care visit or plan to teach the caregiver.
2. Patient reports breaking mercury glass thermometer.	• Teach patient steps to dispose of thermometer safely (Box 7.6).

BOX 7.6

Steps to Take in the Event of a Mercury Spill

- If possible, close the room off from the rest of the house and increase ventilation in the affected room by opening windows or turning on a fan.
- Put on rubber, nitrile, or latex gloves. Do not touch the mercury. Do not allow children to help clean up the spill. Remove all pets from the area.
- Pick up glass pieces, place them in a folded paper towel, and place glass and towel into a plastic zip-lock bag.
- Use a squeegee or cardboard to gather mercury beads. Use an eyedropper to collect or draw up visible mercury beads. Slowly and carefully squeeze mercury onto a damp paper towel. Place the paper towel in a zip-lock bag and secure. Then put shaving cream on a small brush and "dot" the area or press duct tape in the area to pick up smaller beads.
- Place mercury, material used to pick up mercury, and broken glass in a plastic zip-lock bag. Triple bag the contaminated objects (place in a total of three sealed bags).
- Place gloves, mercury, and all other wastes into a garbage bag. Secure and label the bag.
- Call local health department to determine where to dispose of mercury safely.
- If possible, keep windows open and room well ventilated for at least 24 hours after cleanup.
- Instruct patient not to use a vacuum cleaner, a broom, or household cleaners when cleaning up mercury spill. Also instruct patient not to put mercury down the drain or place contaminated clothing into the washing machine.

Data from National Collaborating Centre for Environmental Health. (2015). *Cleanup instructions for small mercury spills.* https://ncceh.ca/sites/default/files/Small_Mercury_Spills_Clean-up_Oct_2015.pdf

Communication and Documentation

- Document information taught and patient's and caregiver's return demonstration in the home care record.
- Document temperature in home care record and home documentation system (e.g., log).
- Report high and low temperatures to health care provider.

DOCUMENTATION EXAMPLE

Patient's temp. is 38°C, tympanic. Patient is diaphoretic. Acetaminophen every 4 hours PRN 500 mg given PO at 1610 hours. Health care provider notified regarding elevated temp. Patient and caregiver were shown how to take patient temperature in the home. Patient and caregiver were able to return the demonstration without any reinforcement required. Both voiced being comfortable with the skill. Pamphlet with detailed instructions provided in case education gap present in future independent attempts.

Special Considerations

Teaching

- Instruct patient or caregiver to never force a thermometer into the rectum or to use a rectal thermometer after rectal surgery, when the patient has a rectal disorder such as a tumour or severe hemorrhoids, when the patient has a low platelet count, or when it is difficult to position the patient for proper thermometer placement.
- Use caution in recommending Aspirin or any other over-the-counter (OTC) or antipyretic medicine to patients whose conditions contraindicate their use (e.g., gastric ulcer, bleeding tendencies, allergic reactions, drug interactions, liver or kidney dysfunction). Encourage patient to contact the health care provider before using OTC antipyretics.
- Patients receiving chemotherapy who develop an increased temperature to seek immediate medical attention even if feeling well (Canadian Cancer Society, 2019).
- Instruct patient to never use sponging with isopropyl alcohol to lower a fever because of its neurotoxic effects (Hockenberry et al., 2024).
- Always leave a phone number and instructions on how to reach a home care nurse if needed.

Pediatric

- The stage of growth and development of a child will determine the site of measurement and type of equipment used.
- Different types of thermometers available for use with children (e.g., temporal artery, tympanic). Reliability of these different thermometers varies; ensure that parents know how to use the equipment correctly and detect the signs and symptoms of a fever (Hockenberry et al., 2024).
- Teach parents to take a child's temperature whenever the child feels warm to the touch, even if the temperature was recently normal (Hockenberry et al., 2024).
- Avoid using Aspirin in children under the age of 19 to prevent Reye's syndrome.

Gerontological

- Older persons' normal temperatures are often below 36.1°C (97°F); therefore, a normal temperature range for adults sometimes reflects a fever in the older person (Boscart et al., 2023).
- Older persons are more sensitive to temperature changes and tend to demonstrate symptoms of delirium or dementia with variations in body temperature.
- Altered internal temperature regulation or dehydration occurs frequently in frail, debilitated patients. Temperature measurement becomes very important to prevent severe states of hypothermia or hyperthermia.
- Consider common age-related sensory changes in the older person and direct teaching strategies to compensate for any alterations (e.g., a magnifying glass to read thermometer).

SKILL 7.3 Assessing Radial Pulse

Video Clip NSO *Nursing Skills Online Vital Signs Module 4 / Lesson 3*

The ejection of blood from the heart distends the walls of the aorta. Because of the force of the blood exiting the heart, aortic distension creates a pulse wave that travels rapidly toward the extremities. When the pulse wave reaches a peripheral artery, you can feel it by palpating the artery lightly against underlying bone or muscle. The pulse is the palpable bounding of the blood flow. The number of pulsing sensations occurring in 1 minute is the pulse rate.

Assessing a patient's peripheral pulses determines the integrity of the cardiovascular system. An abnormally slow, rapid, or irregular pulse indicates the inability of the heart to deliver adequate blood to the body; a pulse deficit may be present. The strength or amplitude of a pulse reflects the volume of blood ejected against the arterial wall with each heart contraction. If the volume decreases, the pulse often becomes weak and difficult to palpate. In contrast, a full bounding pulse is an indication of increased volume.

TABLE 7.1

Pulse Sites

Site	Location	Rationale for Selection
Temporal	Over temporal bone of head, above and lateral to eyebrow	Easily accessible site to assess pulse in children
Carotid	Along medial edge of sternocleidomastoid muscle in neck	Easily accessible site to assess character of peripheral pulse; used during physiological shock or cardiac arrest when other sites are not palpable
Apical	Fourth to fifth intercostal space at left midclavicular line	Site used to auscultate apical pulse
Brachial	Groove between biceps and triceps muscles at antecubital fossa	Site used to auscultate upper-extremity blood pressure; assesses status of circulation to lower arm
Radial	Radial or thumb side of forearm at wrist	Common site to assess character of peripheral pulse; assesses status of circulation to hand
Ulnar	Ulnar side of forearm at wrist	Site used to assess status of circulation to ulnar side of hand; used to perform Allen's test
Femoral	Below inguinal ligament, midway between symphysis pubis and anterior superior iliac spine	Site used to assess character of pulse during physiological shock or cardiac arrest when other pulses are not palpable; assesses status of circulation to leg
Popliteal	Behind knee in popliteal fossa	Site used to auscultate lower-extremity blood pressure; assesses status of circulation to lower leg
Posterior tibial	Inner side of each ankle, below medial malleolus	Site used to assess status of circulation to foot
Dorsalis pedis	Along top of foot between extension tendons of great and first toe	Site used to assess status of circulation to foot

The integrity of peripheral pulses indicates the status of blood perfusion to the area distributed by the pulse (Table 7.1). For example, assessment of the right femoral pulse determines whether blood flow to the right leg is adequate. If a peripheral pulse distal to an injured or treated area of an extremity feels weak on palpation, the volume of blood reaching tissues below the affected area may be inadequate, and surgical intervention may be necessary.

While any artery can be used to assess for pulse rate, the radial and carotid arteries are commonly used because they are easy to palpate (Fig. 7.6). When a patient's condition suddenly worsens, the carotid site is recommended for finding a pulse quickly. Assessment of other peripheral pulse sites, such as the brachial or femoral artery, is unnecessary when routinely obtaining vital signs. Other peripheral pulses are assessed when a complete physical examination (see Chapter 8) is conducted or when the radial artery is not available for assessment because of surgery, trauma, or impaired blood flow.

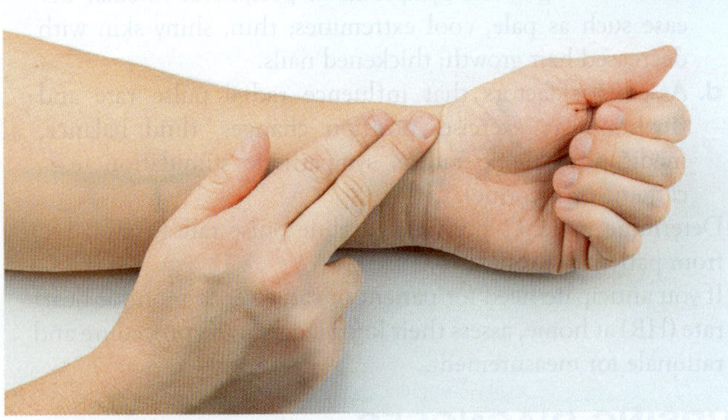

FIG 7.6 Palpating radial pulse. *(Maksim Sheliakin/iStockphoto)*

Delegation and Collaboration

The skill of radial pulse measurement can be delegated to a UCP if a patient's condition is stable. The skill cannot be delegated when a patient's condition is unstable (e.g., acute cardiac problem) or when the nurse is evaluating a patient's response to a treatment or medication. The nurse instructs the UCP by doing the following:

- Indicating the appropriate site for measuring pulse rate; frequency of measurement; and factors related to patient's history, such as risk for abnormally slow, rapid, or irregular pulse
- Reviewing patient's usual pulse rate and significant changes to report to the nurse for further assessment

Equipment

- Wristwatch with second hand or digital display
- Pen and vital sign flow sheet in chart or EHR

STEP	RATIONALE
ASSESSMENT	
1. Identify patient using at least two person-specific identifiers (e.g., name and date of birth, or name and medical record number) according to employer policy.	Ensures correct patient. Adheres to Accreditation Canada's standards and improves patient safety (Accreditation Canada, 2020).
2. Throughout the procedure, the 4 moments for hand hygiene are to be implemented; hand hygiene should occur before initial patient (or patient environment) contact, before an aseptic procedure, after body fluid exposure risk, and after patient (or patient environment) contact. Additional hand hygiene should be performed when hands are visibly soiled.	Proper hand hygiene helps prevent the spread of infectious agents to health care providers.
3. Determine need to assess radial pulse:	
a. Assess for any risk factors for pulse alterations: • History of heart disease • Cardiac dysrhythmia • Onset of sudden chest pain or acute pain from any site • Invasive cardiovascular diagnostic tests • Surgery • Sudden infusion of large volume of intravenous (IV) fluid • Internal or external hemorrhage • Administration of medications that alter cardiac function	Certain conditions place patients at risk for pulse alterations. A history of peripheral vascular disease often alters pulse rate and quality.
b. Assess for signs and symptoms of altered cardiac function such as presence of dyspnea, fatigue, chest pain, orthopnea, syncope, palpitations, edema of dependent body parts, cyanosis, or pallor of skin (see Chapter 8).	Physical signs and symptoms often indicate alteration in cardiac function, which affects radial pulse rate and rhythm.
c. Assess for signs and symptoms of peripheral vascular disease such as pale, cool extremities; thin, shiny skin with decreased hair growth; thickened nails.	Physical signs and symptoms indicate alteration in local arterial blood flow.
d. Assess for factors that influence radial pulse rate and rhythm: age, exercise, position changes, fluid balance, medications, temperature, sympathetic stimulation (e.g., caffeine or nicotine).	Anticipate factors that alter pulse, ensuring accurate interpretation. Dysrhythmics, cardiotonics, antihypertensives, vasodilators, and vasoconstrictors affect pulse rate and rhythm.
4. Determine patient's previous baseline pulse rate (if available) from patient's record.	Allows you to assess for change in condition. Provides comparison with future pulse measurements.
5. If you anticipate need for patient or caregiver to monitor heart rate (HR) at home, assess their knowledge of the procedure and rationale for measurement.	Determines need for patient or caregiver instruction.
NURSING DIAGNOSES	
• Reduced cardiac output • Reduced peripheral tissue perfusion • Reduced stamina • Potential for dehydration • Insufficient knowledge regarding pulse assessment *Related factors are individualized on the basis of patient's condition or needs.*	
PLANNING	
1. Expected outcomes following completion of procedure:	
• Radial pulse is palpable, within usual range for patient's age.	Usual range for adults is 60–100 beats/min.
• Rhythm is regular.	Cardiac status is stable.
• Radial pulse is strong, firm, and elastic.	Radial artery is patent.
2. Explain to patient that you will assess radial pulse rate (i.e., HR). Encourage patient to relax as much as possible. If patient has been active, wait 5–10 minutes before assessing pulse. If patient has been smoking or ingesting caffeine, wait 15 minutes before assessing pulse.	Anxiety, activity, caffeine, and smoking elevate HR. Assessing radial pulse rate at rest allows for objective comparison of values.
3. Collect appropriate equipment and bring to patient's bedside.	Ensures an organized approach to assessing a radial pulse.

STEP	RATIONALE
IMPLEMENTATION	
1.	Proper hand hygiene helps prevent the spread of infectious agents to health care providers.
2. If necessary, draw curtain around bed or close door.	Maintains privacy and minimizes embarrassment. Helps patient relax.
3. Help patient assume a supine or sitting position.	Provides easy access to pulse sites.
4. If patient is supine, place their forearm straight alongside or across lower chest or upper abdomen (see Step 4a illustration). If sitting, bend patient's elbow 90 degrees and support their lower arm on chair or on your arm. Place tips of first two or middle three fingers of hand over groove along radial or thumb side of patient's inner wrist (see Step 4b illustration). Slightly extend or flex wrist with palm down until you note strongest pulse.	Fingertips are most sensitive parts of hand to palpate arterial pulsation. Your thumb has pulsation that interferes with accuracy.
5. Lightly compress pulse against radius, losing pulse initially; relax pressure so pulse becomes easily palpable.	Pulse assessment is more accurate when using moderate pressure. Too much pressure occludes pulse and impairs blood flow.
6. Determine strength of pulse. Note whether thrust of vessel against fingertips is bounding (4+); full increased, strong (3+); expected (2+); barely palpable, diminished (1+); or absent, not palpable (0).	Strength reflects volume of blood ejected against arterial wall with each heart contraction. Decreased stroke volume (e.g., shock) is indicated by a "weak thready" pulse, while increased stroke volume (e.g., anxiety, exercise, and some abnormal conditions) is indicated by a "full bounding pulse" (Jarvis et al., 2024). Accurate description of strength improves communication, patient safety, and interprofessional collaboration.
7. After palpating a regular pulse, look at second hand of watch and begin to count rate. Count the first beat after the second hand hits the number on the dial; count as one, then two, and so on.	Rate is determined accurately only after pulse has been palpated. Timing begins with zero. Count of one is first beat palpated after timing begins.
8. If pulse is regular, count rate for 30 seconds and multiply total by 2.	A 30-second count is accurate for rapid, slow, or regular pulse rates.
9. If pulse is irregular, count rate for a full 60 seconds. Assess frequency and pattern of irregularity.	Inefficient contraction of heart fails to transmit pulse wave, resulting in irregular pulse. Longer time ensures accurate count.
10. When pulse is irregular, compare radial pulses bilaterally and assess apical pulse for a full 60 seconds.	A marked difference between pulses indicates that arterial flow is compromised to one extremity, and as a nurse you need to take action.
11. Help patient return to comfortable position.	Promotes comfort and sense of well-being.
12. Discuss findings with patient.	Promotes participation in care and understanding of health status. Reduces transmission of microorganisms.

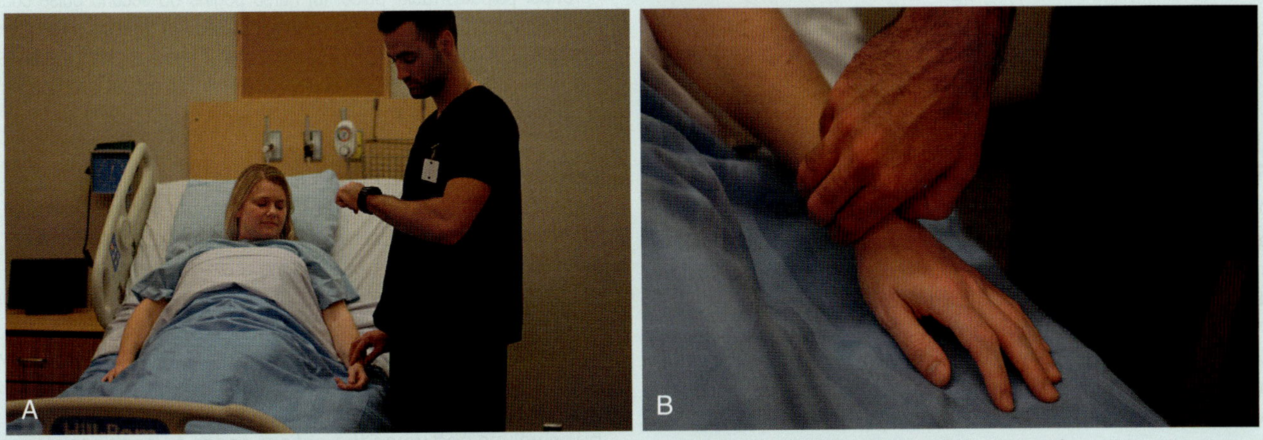

STEP 4 A, Pulse check with patient's forearm at side with wrist extended. **B,** Hand placement for pulse check. *(Courtesy Barbara J. Astle, RN, PhD.)*

STEP	RATIONALE
EVALUATION	
1. If assessing pulse for first time, establish radial pulse as baseline if it is within acceptable range.	Used to compare future pulse assessments. In newborns up to 1 month old, the typical HR range is 100–175 beats/min, while 1-month-olds to children 2 years of age have a HR range of 90–160 beats/min. Children aged 2 to 6 years have an HR range of 70–150 beats/min, and those aged 7 to 11 years have an HR range of 60–130 beats/min. In adolescents, the HR range is 50–110 beats/min, and in adults and older persons it is 60–100 beats/min (Lapum et al., 2021).
2. Compare pulse rate and character with patient's previous baseline and acceptable range for patient's age.	Allows for assessment of change in patient's condition and presence of cardiac alteration.
3. **Use teach-back:** "I want to be sure I explained why it is important to check your pulse at home. Tell me why it is important to check your pulse when you have a pacemaker." Develop a revised teaching plan if patient or caregiver is unable to teach back correctly.	Determines patient's and caregiver's level of understanding of instructional topic.

Unexpected Outcomes	Related Interventions
1. Patient has weak, thready, or difficult-to-palpate radial pulse.	• Assess both radial pulses and compare findings. • Observe for symptoms associated with ineffective tissue perfusion, including pallor and cool skin distal to weak pulse. • Assess for swelling in surrounding tissues or any encumbrance (e.g., dressing or cast) that may impede blood flow. • Obtain Doppler or ultrasonic stethoscope to detect low-velocity blood flow (see Chapter 8). • Have another nurse assess pulse.
2. An adult patient's pulse rate is less than 60 beats/min (bradycardia) or more than 100 beats/min (tachycardia).	• Assess the patient's baseline history of pulse rate to determine patient's "normal" and any medications the person is taking (e.g., beta blockers) that can affect pulse rate. • Identify related data, including fever, pain, fear or anxiety, recent exercise, low BP, blood loss, or inadequate oxygenation. • Observe for signs and symptoms associated with abnormal cardiac function, including dyspnea, fatigue, chest pain, orthopnea, syncope, palpitations, edema of body parts, cyanosis, or pallor of skin. • Auscultate apical pulse (see Skill 7.4). • Use interprofessional collaboration and prepare for possible electrocardiogram.
3. Patient has irregular pulse.	• Auscultate apical pulse (see Skill 7.4). • Assess for pulse deficit: (a) nurse auscultates apical pulse while second provider palpates radial pulse; (b) nurse begins 60-second pulse count by calling out loud when to begin counting pulses; (c) the two pulse rates are compared. If pulse count differs by more than 2 beats, a deficit exists; assess for other signs and symptoms of decreased cardiac output (see Chapter 8).

Communication and Documentation

- Document pulse rate (including pulse characteristics) and assessment site on vital sign flow sheet or in progress notes in EHR or chart. Document measurement of pulse rate after administration of specific therapies in progress notes EHR or chart.
- Document your evaluation of patient and caregiver learning.
- Check patient's baseline pulse and most recent pulse measurement and then report abnormal findings to nurse in charge or health care provider.

DOCUMENTATION EXAMPLE

Patient admitted to the unit at 1600 hours via stretcher with belongings from the ED, accompanied by partner. Patient admitting diagnosis is acute asthma exacerbation. Patient requires frequent pulse rate monitoring because patient is on an asthma protocol and receiving salbutamol at 4 puffs Q4min × 3. Current pulse rate is 110 bpm via 2nd digit pulse oximeter, while lying down; rhythm irregular. Will continue to monitor closely. Education provided to caregiver at bedside about normal pulse values and when the patient needs to seek assistance. Education reinforced with an information leaflet and all questions answered by writer. No further education is needed as patient was able to restate learned information accurately.

DOCUMENTATION EXAMPLE

Patient presented with a baseline pulse rate of 68 bpm at 0800 hours this morning. Current pulse rate is 115 bpm radially, while the patient is lying in bed; rhythm irregular, force: 4+, bounding, equal bilaterally. Page sent to health care provider re: findings. Will repeat page in 10 minutes if no response. Will continue to monitor patient. Charge nurse notified re: change in patient status.

Special Considerations

Teaching

- Patients taking certain prescribed cardiotonic or antidysrhythmic medications need to learn to assess their own pulse rates to detect adverse effects of medications.
- Patients undergoing cardiac rehabilitation need to learn to assess their own pulse rates to determine their response to exercise.
- Teach patients taking heart medications or starting a prescribed exercise regimen how to monitor carotid pulse rate.

Pediatric

- The radial artery is difficult to assess in an infant. Apical, femoral, or brachial pulse is the best site for assessing pediatric HR and rhythm until 2 years of age.
- Children often have a sinus dysrhythmia, which is an irregular heartbeat that speeds up with inspiration and slows down with expiration.
- Breath holding in a child temporarily lowers pulse rate.

Gerontological

- Older persons have a reduced HR with exercise because of a decreased responsiveness to catecholamines.
- It takes longer for the HR to rise in the older person to meet sudden increased demands that result from stress, illness, or excitement. Once elevated, the pulse rate of an older person takes longer to return to normal resting rate.
- Peripheral vascular disease is more common among older persons, making radial pulse assessment difficult.

Care in the Community: Home Management

- Patients taking certain prescribed cardiac medications should learn to assess their own pulse rates to detect adverse effects of medications (see Skill 7.7).

SKILL 7.4 Assessing Apical Pulse

Video Clip *NSO Nursing Skills Online Vital Signs Module 4 / Lesson 3*

The apical pulse is the most reliable noninvasive way to assess cardiac function. The apical pulse rate is the assessment of the number and quality of apical heart sounds in 1 minute. A single apical pulse is the combination of two heart sounds, S_1 and S_2. S_1 is the sound of the tricuspid and mitral valves closing at the end of ventricular filling, just before systolic contraction begins. S_2 is the sound of the pulmonic and aortic valves closing at the end of the systolic contraction. As you listen for sound waves with a stethoscope, you will hear the characteristic "lub-dub" as a single pulsation.

A stethoscope (Fig. 7.7) is a closed cylinder that amplifies sound waves as they reach the surface of the body. The five major parts of the stethoscope are the earpieces, binaurals, tubing, bell, and diaphragm. The plastic or rubber earpieces should fit snugly and comfortably in your ears. Binaurals should be angled and strong enough so the earpieces stay firmly in place without causing discomfort. The earpieces follow the contour of the ear canal, pointing toward the face when the stethoscope is in place.

The polyvinyl tubing should be flexible and 30 to 45 cm (12 to 18 inches) in length; longer tubing decreases sound transmission. Stethoscopes can have one or two tubes. At the end of the tubing is the chest piece, consisting of a bell and diaphragm that you rotate into position, depending on which part you choose to use.

The diaphragm is the larger, circular, flat-surfaced part of the chest piece. It transmits high-pitched sounds created by high-velocity movement of air and blood. Position the diaphragm to make a tight seal against a patient's skin. Exert enough pressure to complete the seal, leaving a temporary red ring on the patient's skin after you remove the diaphragm.

The bell is the cone-shaped part of the chest piece, usually surrounded by a rubber ring to avoid chilling the patient during placement. It transmits low-pitched sounds created by the low-velocity movement of blood. Hold the bell lightly against the skin for sound amplification.

Some stethoscopes have one chest piece that combines features of the bell and diaphragm. When you apply light pressure, the chest piece is a bell, whereas exerting more pressure converts the bell into a diaphragm. With the earpieces in your ears, tap lightly on the diaphragm and note which side you hear most clearly. This determines which side of the chest piece is functioning.

Delegation and Collaboration

The skill of apical pulse measurement cannot be delegated to a UCP. Often the apical pulse is measured when you suspect an irregularity in

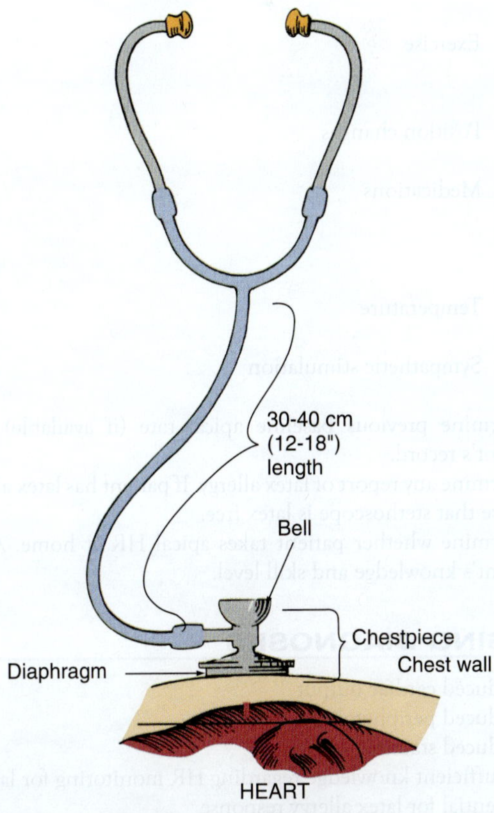

FIG 7.7 Acoustic stethoscope.

the radial pulse, before giving some medications, or when a patient's condition requires a more accurate assessment.

When apical pulse deficit is identified, collaborate with the interprofessional health care team (e.g., cardiac specialist, advanced practice nurse) to determine whether additional interventions such as medications are needed.

Equipment

- Stethoscope
- Wristwatch with second hand or digital display
- Pen and vital sign flow sheet in chart or EHR
- Alcohol swab

STEP	RATIONALE
ASSESSMENT	
1. Identify patient using at least two person-specific identifiers (e.g., name and date of birth, or name and medical record number) according to employer policy.	Ensures correct patient. Adheres to Accreditation Canada's standards and improves patient safety (Accreditation Canada, 2020).
2. Throughout the procedure, the 4 moments for hand hygiene are to be implemented; hand hygiene should occur before initial patient (or patient environment) contact, before an aseptic procedure, after body fluid exposure risk, and after patient (or patient environment) contact. Additional hand hygiene should be performed when hands are visibly soiled.	Proper hand hygiene helps prevent the spread of infectious agents to health care providers.
3. Determine need to assess apical pulse:	
a. Assess for any risk factors for apical pulse alteration: heart disease, onset of sudden chest pain or acute pain from any site, invasive cardiovascular diagnostic tests, surgery, sudden infusion of large volume of IV fluid, internal or external hemorrhage, administration of medications that alter heart function.	Certain conditions place patients at risk for pulse alterations.
b. Assess for signs and symptoms of altered cardiac function such as dyspnea, fatigue, chest pain, orthopnea, syncope, palpitations, edema of dependent body parts, cyanosis, or pallor of skin (see Chapter 8).	Physical signs and symptoms indicate alteration in cardiac output or stroke volume.
c. Assess for factors that normally influence apical pulse rate and rhythm:	Allows you to anticipate factors that alter apical pulse, ensuring an accurate interpretation.
• Age	Different age groups have different normal pulse ranges (see Skill 7.3, Evaluation).
• Exercise	Physical activity increases HR; a well-conditioned patient may have a slower-than-usual resting HR that returns more quickly to resting rate after exercise.
• Position changes	HR increases temporarily when changing from lying to sitting or standing position.
• Medications	Antidysrhythmics, sympathomimetics, and cardiotonics affect rate and rhythm of pulse; large doses of narcotic analgesics can slow HR; general anaesthetics slow HR; central nervous system stimulants such as caffeine can increase HR.
• Temperature	Fever or exposure to warm environments increases HR; HR declines with hypothermia.
• Sympathetic stimulation	Emotional stress, anxiety, or fear stimulates sympathetic nervous system, which increases HR.
4. Determine previous baseline apical rate (if available) from patient's record.	Allows nurse to assess for change in condition.
5. Determine any report of latex allergy. If patient has latex allergy, ensure that stethoscope is latex free.	Reduces risk of allergic reaction to stethoscope.
6. Determine whether patient takes apical HR at home. Assess patient's knowledge and skill level.	Determines level and type of instruction required by patient or caregiver.

NURSING DIAGNOSES

- Reduced cardiac output
- Reduced peripheral tissue perfusion
- Reduced stamina
- Insufficient knowledge regarding HR monitoring for latex allergy response
- Potential for latex allergy response

Related factors and risk factors are individualized on the basis of patient's condition or needs.

STEP	RATIONALE
PLANNING	
1. Expected outcomes following completion of procedure:	
• Apical HR is within acceptable range.	Average HR for adults is 60–100 beats/min.
• Rhythm is regular.	Cardiovascular status is stable.
2. Explain to patient that you will assess apical pulse rate. Encourage patient to relax and not speak. If patient has been active, wait 5–10 minutes before assessing pulse. If they have been smoking or ingesting caffeine, wait 15 minutes before assessing pulse.	Anxiety, activity, caffeine, and smoking elevate HR. Patient's voice interferes with nurse's ability to hear sound when measuring apical pulse. Assessing apical pulse rate at rest allows for objective comparison of values.
3. Collect and bring appropriate supplies to patient's bedside.	Ensures an organized approach to assessing radial pulse.
IMPLEMENTATION	
1.	Proper hand hygiene helps prevent the spread of infectious agents to health care providers.
2. If necessary, draw curtain around bed or close door.	Maintains privacy and minimizes embarrassment. Helps patient relax.
3. Help patient assume supine or sitting position. Move aside bed linen and gown to expose sternum and left side of chest.	Exposes part of chest wall for selection of auscultatory site. Stethoscope diaphragm must touch skin for best sounds.
4. Locate anatomical landmarks to identify point of maximal impulse (PMI), also called *apical impulse* (see Chapter 8). The heart is located behind and to the left of sternum, with base at top and apex at bottom. Find angle of Louis just below suprasternal notch between sternal body and manubrium; it feels like a bony prominence (see Step 4, illustration *A*). Slip fingers down each side of angle to find second intercostal space (ICS) (see Step 4, illustration *B*). Carefully move fingers down left side of sternum to fifth ICS and laterally to left midclavicular line (MCL) (see Step 4, illustration *C*). A light tap felt within area 1–2.5 cm (0.5 inches to 1 inch) of PMI is reflected from apex of heart (see Step 4, illustration *D*).	Use of anatomical landmarks allows correct placement of stethoscope over apex of heart. This position enhances ability to hear heart sounds clearly. If unable to palpate PMI, reposition patient on left side. In presence of serious heart disease, you may locate PMI to left of MCL or at sixth ICS. PMI may not be palpated in obese adults or patients in whom severe pulmonary disease has changed shape of thorax.

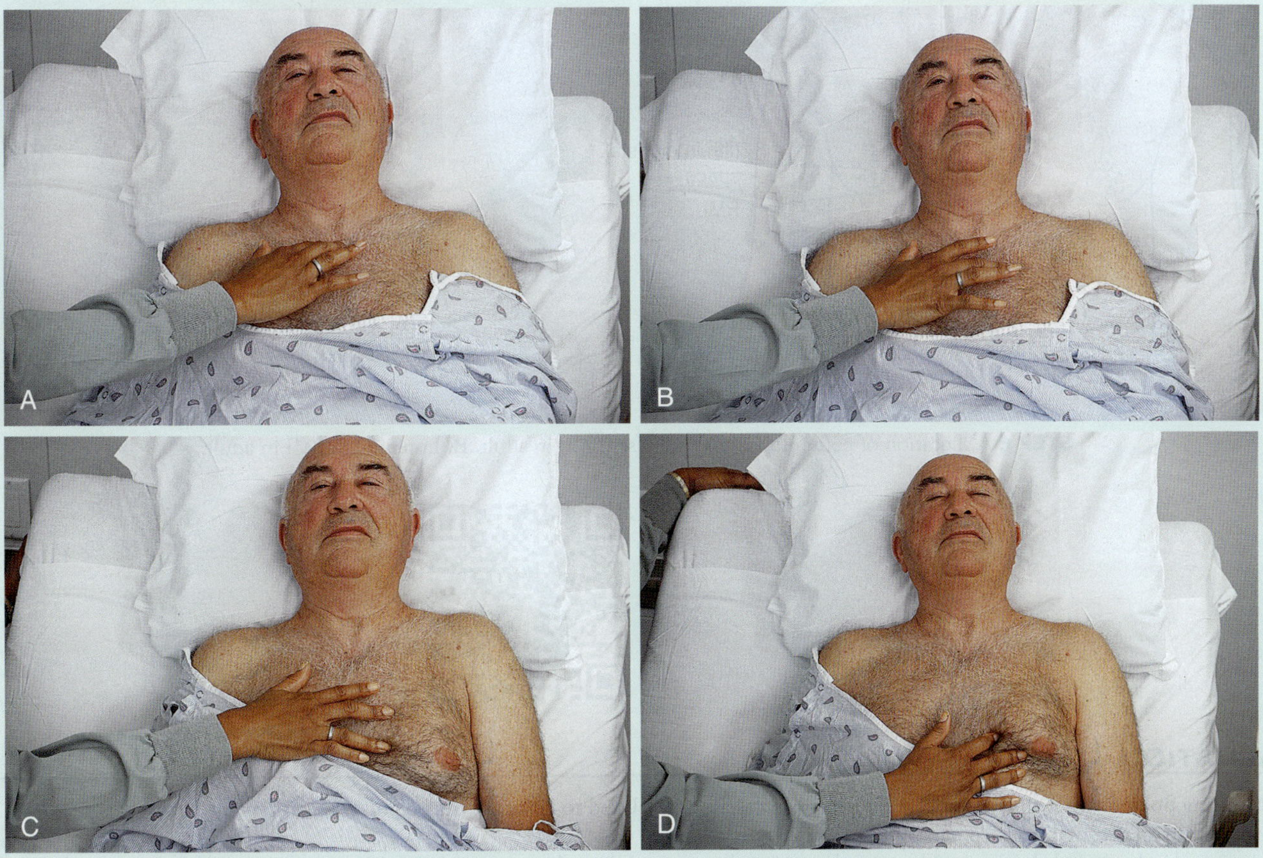

STEP 4 **A,** Nurse locates sternal notch. **B,** Nurse locates second intercostal space. **C,** Nurse locates fifth intercostal space. **D,** Nurse locates point of maximal impulse at fifth intercostal space at left midclavicular line.

STEP	RATIONALE
5. Place diaphragm of stethoscope in palm of hand for 5–10 seconds.	Warming of metal or plastic diaphragm prevents patient from being startled and promotes comfort.
6. Place diaphragm of stethoscope over PMI at fifth ICS, at left MCL, and auscultate for normal S_1 and S_2 heart sounds (heard as "lub-dub") (see Step 6 illustrations).	Allow stethoscope tubing to extend straight without kinks that would distort sound transmission. Normal S_1 and S_2 sounds are high pitched and best heard with diaphragm.
7. When you hear S_1 and S_2 with regularity, use second hand of watch and begin to count rate: when sweep hand hits number on dial, start counting with zero, then one, two, and so on.	Apical rate is determined accurately only after you are able to auscultate sounds clearly. Timing begins with zero. Count of one is first sound auscultated after timing begins.
8. If apical rate is regular, count for 30 seconds and multiply by 2.	You can assess regular apical rate within 30 seconds.
9. If HR is irregular or patient is receiving cardiovascular medication, count for 1 full minute (60 seconds).	Irregular rate is more accurately assessed when measured over longer interval.
10. Note regularity of any dysrhythmia (S_1 and S_2 occurring early or late after previous sequence of sounds) (e.g., every third or every fourth beat is skipped).	Regular occurrence of dysrhythmia within 1 minute indicates inefficient contraction of heart and potential alteration in cardiac output.
11. Replace patient's gown and bed linen; help them return to comfortable position.	Restores comfort and promotes sense of well-being.

Critical Decision Point *If apical rate is abnormal or irregular, repeat measurement or have another nurse conduct measurement. Original measurement may be incorrect. Second measurement confirms initial findings of an abnormal HR.*

STEP	RATIONALE
12. Discuss findings with patient.	Promotes person-centred care and understanding of health status.
	Reduces transmission of microorganisms.
13. Clean earpieces and diaphragm of stethoscope with alcohol swab routinely after each use.	Stethoscopes are frequently contaminated with microorganisms. Regular disinfection can control health care–associated infections (HAIs) (de Queiroz Junior et al., 2021).

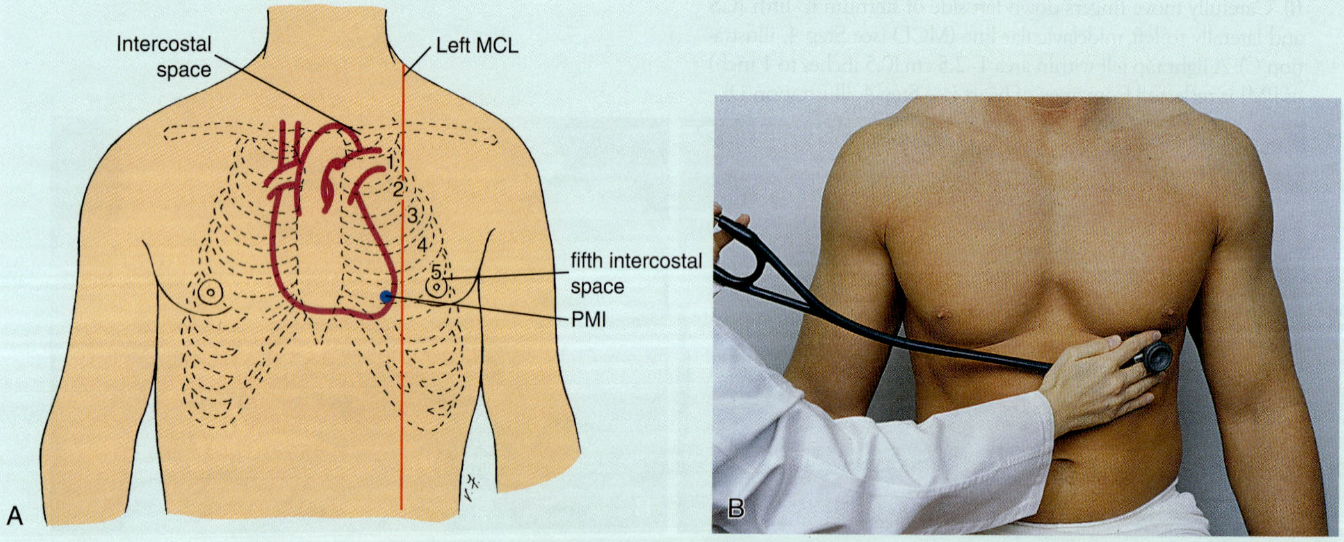

STEP 6 **A,** Location of point of maximal impulse (PMI) in adult. **B,** Listening to PMI in adult.

EVALUATION

1. If assessing pulse for first time, establish apical rate as baseline if it is within an acceptable range.	Used to compare future pulse assessments.
2. Compare apical rate and character with patient's previous baseline and acceptable range of HR for patient's age.	Allows for assessment of change in patient's condition and presence of cardiac alteration.

STEP	RATIONALE
3. Use **teach-back:** "I want to be sure I explained why it is important to check your heart rate at home. Tell me which medication you are taking that may decrease your heart rate." Develop a revised teaching plan if patient or caregiver is unable to teach back correctly.	Determines patient's and caregiver's level of understanding of instructional topic.

Unexpected Outcomes	Related Interventions
1. Adult patient's apical pulse is greater than 100 beats/min (tachycardia).	• Identify related data, including fever, pain, fear or anxiety, recent exercise, low BP, blood loss, or inadequate oxygenation. • Observe for signs and symptoms associated with abnormal cardiac function, including dyspnea, fatigue, chest pain, orthopnea, syncope, palpitations, edema of body parts, cyanosis, or dizziness.
2. Patient's apical pulse is less than 60 beats/min (bradycardia).	• Assess for factors that decrease HR, such as beta blockers and antiarrhythmic medications. • Observe for signs and symptoms associated with abnormal cardiac function, including dyspnea, fatigue, chest pain, orthopnea, syncope, palpitations, edema of body parts, cyanosis, or dizziness. • Have another nurse assess apical pulse. • Report findings to nurse in charge, health care provider, or both. It may be necessary to withhold prescribed medications that alter HR until health care provider can evaluate need to alter dosage.
3. Patient's apical rhythm is irregular.	• Assess for pulse deficit (see Skill 7.3): (a) nurse auscultates apical pulse while second provider palpates radial pulse; (b) nurse begins 60-second pulse count by calling out loud when to begin counting pulses; (c) if pulse count differs by more than 2 beats, assesses for other signs and symptoms of decreased cardiac output (see Chapter 8). • Report findings to nurse in charge and/or health care provider, who may prescribe an electrocardiogram to detect cardiac conduction alteration.

Communication and Documentation

- Document apical pulse rate and rhythm on vital sign flow sheet or in progress notes in EHR or chart. If apical pulse is not found at fifth ICS and left MCL, document location of PMI.
- Document measurement of apical pulse rate after administration of specific therapies in appropriate area in EHR per employer policy.
- Report abnormal findings to nurse in charge or health care provider.
- Document your evaluation of patient and caregiver learning.

DOCUMENTATION EXAMPLE

Patient apical pulse 125 bpm with a regularly irregular rhythm, confirmed by second RN. Findings reported to charge nurse and health care provider. Education provided to patient re: findings and symptoms patient needs to report to writer. Patient requires educational reinforcement.

Special Considerations

Teaching

- Teach caregivers of patients taking prescribed cardiotonic or antidysrhythmic medications how to assess apical pulse rates to detect adverse effects of medications.

Pediatric

- PMI of an infant is usually located at the third to fourth ICS near the left sternal border.
- In infants and children younger than 2 years, an apical pulse is more reliable and is counted for 1 full minute because of possible irregularities in rhythm (Hockenberry et al., 2024).
- Breath holding in an infant or child temporarily lowers apical pulse rate.

Gerontological

- PMI can be difficult to palpate in some older persons because the anterior–posterior diameter of the chest increases with age and the heart becomes repositioned because of left ventricular enlargement.
- When assessing older women, you may have to gently lift the breast tissue and place the stethoscope at the fifth ICS or the lower edge of the breast.
- Heart sounds are sometimes muffled or difficult to hear in older persons because of an increase in air space in the lungs.
- Older persons normally have a decreased HR at rest.

Care in the Community: Home Management

- Assess home environment and, if possible, use a room that affords a quiet, private environment for auscultation of apical rate.

✦ SKILL 7.5 Assessing Respirations

Video Clip NSO Nursing Skills Online Vital Signs Module 4 / Lesson 4

Respiration is the exchange of oxygen (O_2) and carbon dioxide (CO_2) between cells of the body and the atmosphere. The three processes of respiration are ventilation (i.e., mechanical movement of gases into and out of the lungs), diffusion (i.e., movement of oxygen and carbon dioxide between the alveoli and the red blood cells), and perfusion (i.e., distribution of red blood cells to and from the pulmonary capillaries). Ventilation is assessed by observing the rate, depth, and rhythm of respiratory movements. Accurate assessment of respirations depends on recognizing normal thoracic and abdominal movements. Normal breathing is both active and passive. On inspiration the diaphragm contracts, and the abdominal organs move down to increase the size of the chest cavity. At the same time, the ribs and sternum lift outward to promote lung expansion. On expiration the diaphragm relaxes upward, and the ribs and sternum return to their relaxed position (Fig. 7.8). During quiet breathing the chest wall gently rises and falls. The body uses more energy during inspiration than during expiration. Expiration is an active process only during exercise, voluntary hyperventilation, and certain disease states.

Delegation and Collaboration

The skill of counting respirations can be delegated to a UCP unless the patient is considered unstable (e.g., evidence of dyspnea). The nurse instructs the UCP by doing the following:

- Communicating the frequency of measurement and factors related to patient history or risk for increased or decreased respiratory rate or irregular respirations
- Reviewing any unusual respiratory values and significant changes to report to the nurse

If the patient has severe shortness of breath or persistent tachypnea, collaborate with the interprofessional health care team (e.g., advanced practice nurse or respiratory therapist) for additional interventions, such as medications or pulmonary chest physiotherapy.

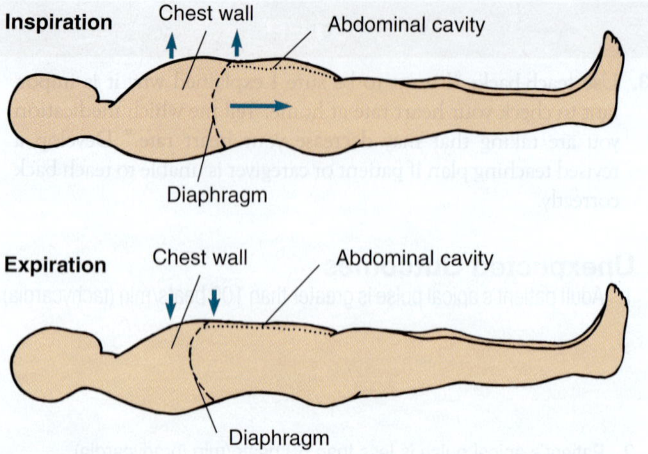

FIG 7.8 Diaphragmatic and chest wall movement during inspiration and expiration.

Equipment

- Wristwatch with second hand or digital display
- Pen and vital sign flow sheet in chart or EHR

STEP	RATIONALE
ASSESSMENT	
1. Identify patient using at least two person-specific identifiers (e.g., name and date of birth, or name and medical record number) according to employer policy.	Ensures correct patient. Adheres to Accreditation Canada's standards and improves patient safety (Accreditation Canada, 2020).
2. Throughout the procedure, the 4 moments for hand hygiene are to be implemented; hand hygiene should occur before initial patient (or patient environment) contact, before an aseptic procedure, after body fluid exposure risk, and after patient (or patient environment) contact. Additional hand hygiene should be performed when hands are visibly soiled.	Proper hand hygiene helps prevent the spread of infectious agents to health care providers.
3. Determine need to assess patient's respirations:	
a. Assess for risk factors of respiratory alterations: • Fever • Pain and anxiety • Diseases of chest wall or muscles • Constrictive chest or abdominal dressings • Presence of abdominal incisions • Gastric distension • Chronic pulmonary disease (emphysema, bronchitis, asthma) • Traumatic injury to chest wall with or without collapse of underlying lung tissue • Presence of chest tube • Respiratory infection (pneumonia, acute bronchitis) • Pulmonary edema and emboli • Head injury with damage to brainstem • Anemia	Certain conditions place patient at risk for ventilatory alterations, detected by changes in respiratory rate, depth, and rhythm.
b. Assess for signs and symptoms of respiratory alterations, such as: • Bluish or cyanotic appearance of nail beds, lips, mucous membranes, and skin • Restlessness, irritability, confusion, reduced level of consciousness • Pain during inspiration • Laboured or difficult breathing • Orthopnea • Use of accessory muscles • Adventitious breath sounds (see Chapter 8) • Inability to breathe spontaneously • Thick, frothy, blood-tinged, or copious sputum production	Physical signs and symptoms indicate alterations in respiratory status.

STEP	RATIONALE
c. Assess for factors that influence character of respirations:	Allows anticipation of factors that influence respirations, ensuring a more accurate interpretation.
• Exercise	Respirations increase in rate and depth to meet need for additional oxygen and rid body of carbon dioxide.
• Anxiety	Anxiety causes increase in respiration rate and depth because of sympathetic nervous system stimulation.
• Acute pain	Pain alters rate and rhythm of respirations; breathing becomes shallow. Patient inhibits or splints chest wall movement when pain is in area of chest or abdomen.
• Smoking	Chronic smoking changes pulmonary airways, resulting in increased respiratory rate at rest when not smoking.
• Medications	Opioids, analgesics, general anaesthetics, and sedative hypnotics depress rate and depth; amphetamines and cocaine increase rate and depth; bronchodilators cause dilation of airways, which ultimately slows respiratory rate.
• Body position	Standing or sitting erect promotes full ventilatory movement and lung expansion; stooped or slumped posture impairs ventilatory movement; lying flat prevents full chest expansion.
• Neurological injury	Damage to brainstem impairs respiratory centre and inhibits rate and rhythm.
• Hemoglobin function	Decreased hemoglobin levels lower amount of oxygen carried in blood, which results in increased respiratory rate to increase oxygen delivery. An increase in altitude lowers amount of saturated hemoglobin, which increases respiratory rate and depth.
4. Assess pertinent laboratory/clinical values:	
a. *Arterial blood gases (ABGs):* Normal ranges (values vary slightly among employers): • pH: 7.35–7.45 • $PaCO_2$: 35–45 mm Hg • HCO_3: 21–28 mmol/L • PaO_2: 80–100 mm Hg • SaO_2: 95–100%	ABG values measure arterial blood pH, partial pressure of oxygen (PaO_2) and carbon dioxide ($PaCO_2$), and arterial oxygen saturation (SaO_2), all of which reflect patient's ventilation and oxygenation status.
b. *Pulse oximetry (SpO_2):* Normal SpO_2 ≥95–100%; SpO_2 <90% may be a clinical emergency or may be due to a chronic condition (e.g., chronic obstructive pulmonary disease [COPD]) where a value in the upper 80s would not be considered an emergency (see Procedural Guideline 7.2).	SpO_2 <90% is often accompanied by changes in respiratory rate, depth, and rhythm.
• *Complete blood count (CBC):* Normal CBC for adults (values vary within employers): • *Hemoglobin:* 140–180 g/L in male patients; 120–160 g/L in female patients • *Hematocrit:* 0.42–0.52 in male patients; 0.37–0.47 in female patients • *Red blood cell count:* 4.6–6.2 × 10^{12}/L in male patients; 4.2–5.4 × 10^{12}/L in female patients	CBC measures red blood cell count, volume of red blood cells, and concentration of hemoglobin, all of which reflect patient's capacity to carry oxygen.
5. Determine previous baseline respiratory rate (if available) from patient's record.	Assesses for change in patient's condition. Provides comparison with future respiratory measurements.

NURSING DIAGNOSES

- Inadequate airway clearance
- Reduced spontaneous ventilation
- Inadequate breathing pattern
- Reduced gas exchange
- Reduced stamina

Related factors are individualized on the basis of patient's condition or needs.

STEP	RATIONALE
PLANNING	
1. Expected outcomes following completion of procedure:	
• Respiratory rate is within acceptable range.	Average respiratory rate in adults is 10–20 breaths/min.
• Respirations are regular and of normal depth.	Respiratory status is stable.
2. If patient has been active, wait 5–10 minutes before assessing respirations.	Exercise increases respiratory rate and depth. Assessing respirations while patient is at rest allows for objective comparison of values.
3. After taking the pulse measurement in an adult, immediately start counting respirations without informing the patient.	Assessing respirations immediately after the pulse without informing the patient prevents the patient from consciously or unintentionally altering rate and depth of breathing and provides a more accurate assessment.
4. Be sure that patient is in comfortable position, preferably sitting or lying with head of bed elevated 45–60 degrees.	Sitting erect promotes full ventilatory movement. Position of discomfort causes patient to breathe more rapidly.

Critical Decision Point *Assess patients who have difficulty breathing (dyspnea), such as those with heart failure or abdominal ascites or those in late stages of pregnancy, in the position of greatest comfort. Repositioning may increase the work of breathing, which increases respiratory rate.*

STEP	RATIONALE
IMPLEMENTATION	
1.	Proper hand hygiene helps prevent the spread of infectious agents to health care providers.
2. Draw curtain around bed or close door.	Maintains privacy.
3. Be sure that patient's chest is visible. If necessary, move bed linen or gown.	Ensures clear view of chest wall and abdominal movements.
4. Place patient's arm in relaxed position across abdomen or lower chest, or place your hand directly over patient's upper abdomen.	A similar position used during pulse assessment allows respiratory rate assessment to be inconspicuous. Patient's hand (or your hand) rises and falls during respiratory cycle.
5. Observe complete respiratory cycle (one inspiration and one expiration).	Rate is accurately determined only after viewing a complete respiratory cycle.
6. After observing a cycle, look at second hand of watch and begin to count rate: when sweep hand hits number on dial, begin time frame, counting one with first full respiratory cycle.	Timing begins with count of one. Respirations occur more slowly than pulse; thus, timing does not begin with zero.
7. If rhythm is regular, count number of respirations in 30 seconds and multiply by 2. If rhythm is irregular, less than 10, or greater than 20, count for 1 full minute.	Respiratory rate is equivalent to number of respirations per minute. Suspected irregularities require assessment for at least 1 minute (Box 7.7).
8. Note depth of respirations by observing degree of chest wall movement while counting rate. In addition, assess depth by palpating chest wall excursion or auscultating posterior thorax after you have counted rate (see Chapter 8). Describe depth as shallow, normal, or deep.	Character of ventilatory movement reveals specific disease states restricting volume of air from moving into and out of lungs.
9. Note rhythm of ventilatory cycle. Normal breathing is regular and uninterrupted. Do not confuse sighing with abnormal rhythm.	Character of ventilations reveals specific types of alterations. Periodically, people unconsciously take single deep breaths or sighs to expand small airways prone to collapse.

Critical Decision Point *Any irregular respiratory patterns or periods of apnea (cessation of respiration for several seconds) are symptoms of underlying disease in the adult, which you need to report to the health care provider or nurse in charge. Further assessment and immediate intervention are often necessary.*

STEP	RATIONALE
10. Replace bed linen and patient's gown.	Restores comfort and promotes sense of well-being.
11. Discuss findings with patient.	Promotes person-centred care and understanding of health status.

STEP	RATIONALE

EVALUATION

1. If assessing respirations for first time, establish rate, rhythm, and depth as baseline if within acceptable range.	Used to compare future respiratory assessment. Average respiratory rates are as follows: infants, 30–60 breaths/min; toddler (1–2 years), 22–37 breaths/min; and school age (6–11 years), 18–30 breaths/min (Lapum et al., 2021; PedsCases, 2018). In adults and older persons, average is 10–20 breaths/min (Lapum et al., 2021). In older persons, this range can also be higher (16–25 breaths/min) owing to changes in lung function (Wheatley, 2018).
2. Compare respirations with patient's previous baseline and usual rate, rhythm, and depth.	Allows for assessment of change in patient's condition and presence of respiratory alterations.
3. Correlate respiratory rate, depth, and rhythm with data obtained from pulse oximetry and ABG measurements if available.	Evaluations of ventilation, perfusion, and diffusion are interrelated.
4. Use teach-back: "I want to be sure I explained why you will be reminded to take deep breaths after surgery. Tell me why deep breathing is important." Develop a revised teaching plan if patient or caregiver is unable to teach back correctly.	Determines patient's and caregiver's level of understanding of instructional topic.

Unexpected Outcomes	Related Interventions
1. Adult patient's respiratory rate is below 10 breaths/min (bradypnea) or above 20 breaths/min (tachypnea). Breathing pattern is sometimes irregular (see Box 7.7). Depth of respirations is increased or decreased. Patient indicates dyspnea.	• Assess for related factors, including obstructed airway, abnormal breath sounds, productive cough, restlessness, anxiety, and confusion (see Chapter 8). • Help patient to supported sitting position (semi- or high Fowler's) unless contraindicated. • Provide oxygen as prescribed (see Chapter 23). • Assess for environmental factors that influence patient's respiratory rate, such as second-hand smoke, poor ventilation, or gas fumes. • Notify health care provider or nurse in charge if alteration continues.
2. Patient demonstrates Kussmaul's, Cheyne–Stokes, or Biot's respirations (see Box 7.7).	• Notify health care provider for additional evaluation and possible medical intervention.

BOX 7.7

Alterations in Breathing Pattern

Alteration	Description
Apnea	Respirations cease for several seconds. Persistent cessation results in respiratory arrest.
Biot's respiration	Irregular respirations varying in depth are followed by periods of apnea associated with central nervous system disorders.
Bradypnea	Rate of breathing is regular but abnormally slow (<10 breaths/min).
Cheyne–Stokes respiration	Respiratory rate and depth are irregular, characterized by alternating periods of apnea and hyperventilation. Respiratory cycle begins with slow, shallow breaths that gradually increase to abnormal rate and depth. The pattern reverses; breathing slows and becomes shallow, climaxing in apnea before respiration resumes.
Hyperpnea	Respirations are increased in depth and rate (>20 breaths/min); occurs normally during exercise.
Hyperventilation	Rate and depth of respirations increase. Hypocarbia, an abnormally low level of carbon dioxide in the blood, may occur.
Hypoventilation	Respiratory rate is abnormally low; depth of ventilation may be depressed. Hypercarbia, an abnormally elevated level of carbon dioxide in the blood, may occur.
Kussmaul's respiration	Respirations are abnormally rapid, deep, and laboured but regular; common with conditions that cause metabolic acidosis (e.g., diabetic ketoacidosis).
Tachypnea	Rate of breathing is regular but abnormally rapid (>20 breaths/min).

Communication and Documentation

- Document respiratory rate, depth, and rhythm on vital sign flow sheet or in progress notes in EHR or chart.
- Document measurement of respiratory rate after administration of specific therapies in progress notes in EHR or chart.
- Document your evaluation of patient and caregiver learning.
- Document type and amount of oxygen therapy, if used, in progress notes in EHR or chart.
- Review patient's baseline and previous respiratory measurement to report abnormal findings to nurse in charge or health care provider.

DOCUMENTATION EXAMPLE

Received patient lying in bed at 0730 hours for care. Pt alert and oriented × 3. Patient denies any pain. Pt temp, pulse, and BP within normal limits, but patient tachypneic with RR elevated at 25 bpm. No accessory muscle use present. No signs of respiratory distress. Oxygen saturation at 96% via 1 L nasal prongs. Cap refill at 1–2 seconds bilaterally. No signs of clubbing or colour changes noted. Education provided to caregiver at bedside re: patient's elevated RR. Pt reported being "mildly scared" about the upcoming procedure. Charge nurse notified re: increased RR. Will recheck vitals in 30 min.

Special Considerations

Teaching

- Patients who demonstrate decreased ventilation (e.g., after surgery) often benefit from learning deep breathing and coughing exercises (see Chapter 37).

- Instruct caregiver to contact community nurse or health care provider if unusual fluctuations in respiratory rate occur.

Pediatric

- Assess respiratory rates before other vital signs or assessments if you are able to view movement of chest wall or abdomen. This allows assessment of rate and rhythm before child becomes anxious because of stranger anxiety or fear of other assessment procedures.
- Average respiratory rate (breaths/min) for pediatric patients is dependent upon age (see Skill 7.5, Evaluation).
- Children up to age 7 breathe abdominally; thus, respirations are assessed by observing abdominal movement.
- An irregular respiratory rate and short apneic spells are normal for newborns.
- You can simply observe infant or young child while chest and abdomen are exposed.
- Use cardiorespiratory monitors for infants or newborns who are at risk for respiratory compromise or sustained apnea.

Gerontological

- Aging causes ossification of costal cartilage and downward slant of ribs, resulting in a more rigid rib cage, which reduces chest wall expansion. Kyphosis and scoliosis, frequent in older persons, may also restrict chest expansion.
- Depth of respirations tends to decrease with aging.
- Change in lung function with aging results in respiratory rates generally being higher in older persons, with a range of 16 to 25 breaths/min (Wheatley, 2018).
- Some older persons depend more on accessory abdominal muscles than weakened thoracic muscles during respiration.

Care in the Community: Home Management

- Assess for environmental factors in the home that influence patient's respiratory rate, such as second-hand smoke, poor ventilation, or gas fumes.

SKILL 7.6 Assessing Arterial Blood Pressure

Video Clip NSO Nursing Skills Online Vital Signs Module 4 / Lesson 5

Blood pressure (BP) is the force exerted by blood against the vessel walls. The peak pressure, or systolic blood pressure (SBP), occurs when the ventricular contraction of the heart forces blood under high pressure into the aorta. When the ventricles relax, the blood remaining in the arteries exerts a minimal or diastolic pressure against the arterial walls at all times.

The standard unit for measuring BP is millimetres of mercury (mm Hg). The most common technique for measuring BP is auscultation with a sphygmomanometer and stethoscope. As the sphygmomanometer cuff is deflated, the five different sounds heard over an artery are called *Korotkoff phases.* The sound in each phase has unique characteristics (Fig. 7.9). BP is recorded with the systolic reading (first sound) before the diastolic reading (beginning of the fifth sound). The difference between SBP and DBP is the pulse pressure. For a BP of 120/80 mm Hg, the pulse pressure is 40.

Hypertension

Hypertension is a major factor underlying death from heart attack and stroke in Canada. According to Hypertension Canada (2020b), a BP recording revealing a high SBP or DBP does not usually alone qualify as a diagnosis of hypertension. The non-automated office blood pressure (non-AOBP) mean or automated office blood pressure (AOBP) measurements are used to diagnose a patient with hypertension when they show a reading of SPB ≥180 mm Hg and/or DBP ≥110 mm Hg (Rabi et al., 2020). AOBP is performed using an automated device that can take a series of consecutive oscillometric measurements on the patient who is left unattended in a private area. Non-AOBP is performed using an electronic upper arm device with the provider in the room. The non-AOBP mean is calculated by discarding the first BP reading and then averaging the next two readings. If AOBP is used, the mean calculated and displayed by the device is used. If the mean of the AOBP from the first visit is an SBP of 135–179 mm Hg and/or DBP is 85–109 mm Hg or the mean of the non-AOBP SBP is 140–179 mm Hg and/or DBP is 90–109 mm Hg, out-of-office BP measurements should be performed before the second visit using ambulatory BP monitoring (Rabi et al., 2020) (Fig. 7.10). This is a validated oscillometric device that takes measurements at 20- to 30-minute intervals over a 24-hour period (Rabi et al., 2020). In patients with diabetes mellitus, diagnostic thresholds for AOBP, ambulatory BP monitoring, and home BP have yet to be established (and might be lower than 130/80 mm Hg). If it is thought that a patient has hypertension, a history and physical exam should be performed and diagnostic tests prescribed. Annual BP measurement is recommended for all adults in order to detect progression to hypertension (Rabi et al., 2020).

Hypotension

Hypotension occurs when SBP falls to 90 mm Hg or below. Although some adults normally have a low BP, for most people a low BP is an abnormal finding associated with illness (e.g., hemorrhage or myocardial infarction). Orthostatic hypotension is a sustained reduction in SBP by at least 20 mm Hg or a drop in DBP by at least 10 mm Hg

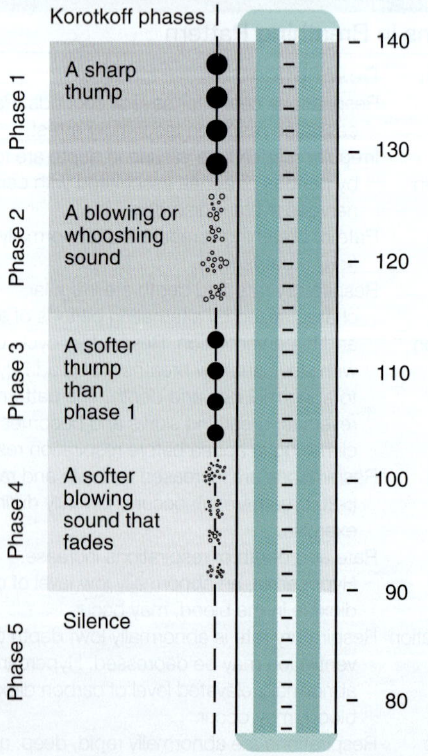

FIG 7.9 The sounds auscultated during blood pressure measurement can be differentiated into five phases. In this example, the blood pressure is 140/90 mm Hg.

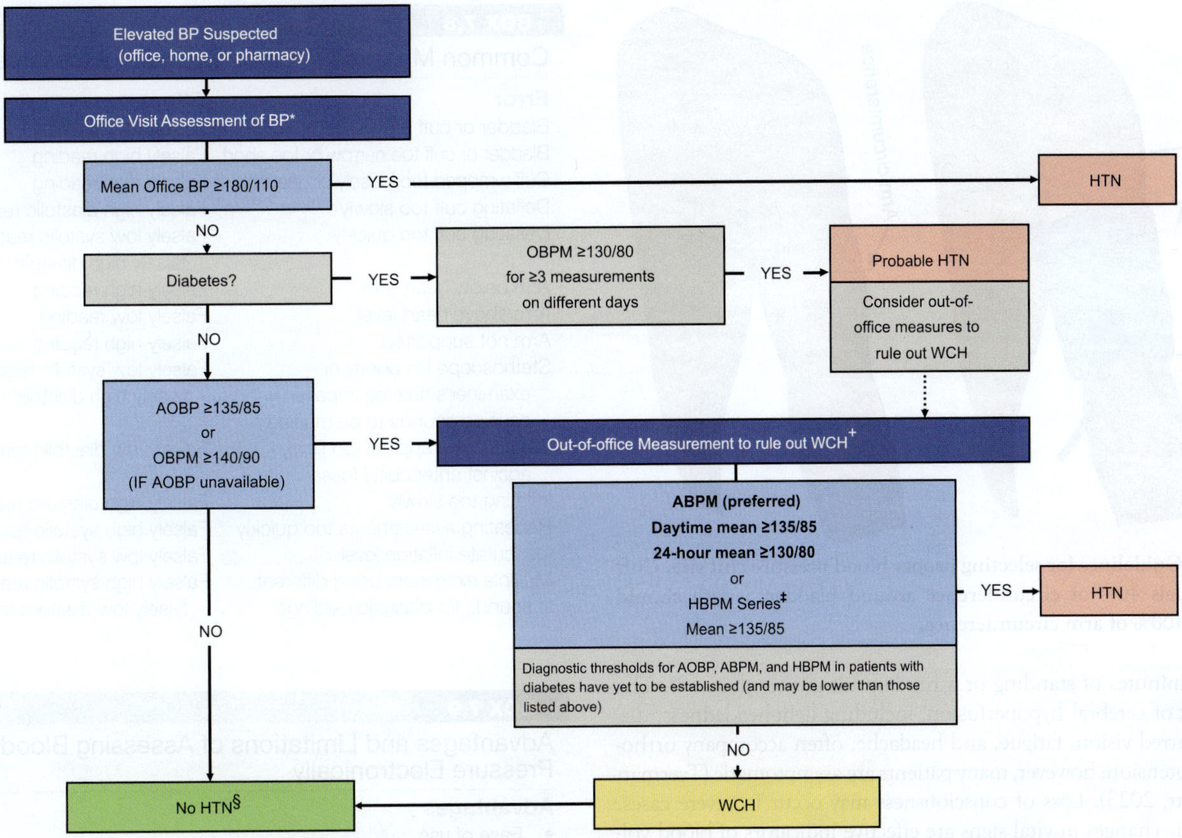

FIG 7.10 Hypertension diagnostic algorithm for adults. The diagnostic algorithm has been revised for the 2020 guidelines. In 2017 and 2018, diabetes was included in the diagnostic algorithm to provide a comprehensive overview of the diagnosis of hypertension. However, this change created several challenges: the OBPM diagnostic threshold is different in patients with diabetes; evidence for defining AOBP and out-of-office (ABPM and HBPM) diagnostic thresholds is lacking; and the potential prognostic value of out-of-office measurements in patients with diabetes, including the identification of white coat hypertension or masked hypertension, exists but definitions are not established. The committee elected to revise the 2018 algorithm to include the recommendation that a series of three to five office measurements can be used to establish a diagnosis of hypertension in diabetes. Although it is plausible that an AOBP threshold could be lower, there is currently no published evidence to guide a specific AOBP threshold. There are no studies to date that have established ABPM or HBPM thresholds in patients with diabetes. Other guideline bodies have elected to estimate corresponding values for HBPM and ABPM on the basis of the established thresholds for the general population; however, the evidence is not clear, and these are not validated for diabetes. With respect to identifying white coat hypertension in patients with diabetes, there are currently no evidence-based definitions. However, a comprehensive review of the published evidence is required to establish thresholds upon which diagnostic and treatment decisions can be based. *ABPM*, ambulatory blood pressure measurement; *AOBP*, automated office blood pressure (performed with the patient unattended in a private room); *BP*, blood pressure; *HBPM*, home blood pressure measurement; *HTN*, hypertension; *OBPM*, office blood pressure measurement (measurements are performed in the office using an electronic upper-arm device with a provider in the room); *WCH*, white coat hypertension.

*If AOBP is used, use the mean calculated and displayed by the device. If OBPM is used, take at least three readings, discard the first, and calculate the mean of the remaining measurements. A history and physical exam should be performed, and diagnostic tests ordered.

†Serial office measurements over three to five visits can be used if ABPM or HBPM is not available.

‡Home BP series: Two readings taken each morning and evening for 7 days (28 readings total). Discard first day's readings and average the readings from the last 6 days.

§In a patient with suspected masked hypertension, ABPM or HBPM could be considered to rule out masked hypertension.

(*From Rabi, D. M., McBrien, K. A., Sapir-Pichhadze, R., et al. [2020]. Hypertension Canada's 2020 comprehensive guidelines for the prevention, diagnosis, risk assessment, and treatment of hypertension in adults and children. Canadian Journal of Cardiology, 36*[5], *596–624.* https://doi.org/10.1016/j.cjca.2020.02.086)

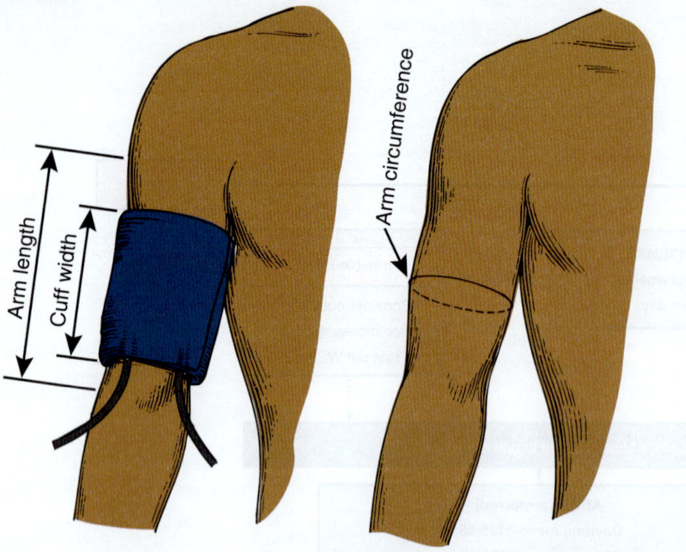

FIG 7.11 Guidelines for selecting proper blood pressure cuff size. Cuff width equals 40% of circumference around bladder, length should cover 80–100% of arm circumference.

BOX 7.8

Common Mistakes in Blood Pressure Assessment

Error	Effect
Bladder or cuff too wide	Falsely low reading
Bladder or cuff too narrow or too short	Falsely high reading
Cuff wrapped too loosely or unevenly	Falsely high reading
Deflating cuff too slowly	Falsely high diastolic reading
Deflating cuff too quickly	Falsely low systolic reading and falsely high diastolic reading
Arm below heart level	Falsely high reading
Arm above heart level	Falsely low reading
Arm not supported	Falsely high reading
Stethoscope fits poorly or examiner's hearing impaired, causing sounds to be muffled	Falsely low systolic reading and falsely high diastolic reading
Stethoscope applied too firmly against antecubital fossa	Falsely low diastolic reading
Inflating too slowly	Falsely high diastolic reading
Repeating assessments too quickly	Falsely high systolic reading
Inaccurate inflation level	Falsely low systolic reading
Multiple examiners using different sounds for diastolic readings	Falsely high systolic reading and falsely low diastolic reading

within 3 minutes of standing or a head-up tilt greater than 60°. The symptoms of cerebral hypoperfusion, including light-headedness, dizziness, blurred vision, fatigue, and headache, often accompany orthostatic hypotension; however, many patients are asymptomatic (Tyerman & Cobbett, 2023). Loss of consciousness may occur in severe cases. Orthostatic changes in vital signs are effective indicators of blood volume depletion. Some medications cause orthostatic hypotension, especially in young patients and older persons. Orthostatic hypotension occurs more frequently in older persons and can lead to an increased risk for falls and fall-related injuries (Tran et al., 2021).

Blood Pressure Equipment

Arterial BP is measured either directly (invasively) or indirectly (noninvasively). The direct method requires electronic monitoring equipment and the insertion of a thin catheter into an artery. The risks associated with invasive BP monitoring require a patient to be in a critical care setting.

Electronic or automatic BP machines consist of an electronic sensor positioned inside a BP cuff attached to an electronic processor (see Procedural Guideline 7.1). Cloth or disposable vinyl compression cuffs contain an inflatable bladder and come in several different sizes. The size selected is proportional to the circumference of the limb being assessed. Ideally, the bladder width should be close to 40% of arm circumference, and bladder length should cover 80 to 100% of arm circumference (Hypertension Canada, 2020a) (Fig. 7.11). Many adults require a large adult cuff. A regular-sized cuff holds a bladder the width of 12 to 13 cm (4.8 to 5.2 inches) and length of 22 to 23 cm (8.5 to 9 inches). An improperly fitting cuff produces inaccurate BP measurements (Box 7.8).

According to Hypertension Canada (2020a), measurement using validated electronic devices is preferred over auscultation because the former minimize errors (e.g., hearing deficits in the health care provider, rounding the reading to a 0 or 5, and rapid deflation) (Rabi et al., 2020) (Box 7.9). It is important that, unless specified otherwise, electronic measurement of BP be used; however, until manual BP is no longer being used, it is important for nurses to know proper technique.

Delegation and Collaboration

The skill of BP measurement can be delegated to a UCP unless the patient is considered unstable (e.g., hypotensive or hypertensive). The nurse instructs the UCP by doing the following:

- Explaining the appropriate limb to use for measurement, BP cuff size, and equipment (manual or electronic) to be used

BOX 7.9

Advantages and Limitations of Assessing Blood Pressure Electronically

Advantages

- Ease of use
- Efficient when frequent repeated measurements are indicated
- Stethoscope not required
- Allows blood pressure to be recorded more frequently, as often as every 15 seconds, with accuracy

Limitations

- Expensive
- Requires source of electricity
- Requires space to position machine
- Pressure from cuff on the arm may cause some patients discomfort and anxiety and lead to bruising of the arm, especially in older persons
- Sensitive to outside motion interference and therefore cannot be used in patients with seizures, tremors, or shivers or in patients unable to cooperate
- May not be accurate for patients with irregular heart rate or hypotension or in conditions with reduced blood flow (e.g., hypothermia)
- Accuracy standards for electronic blood pressure machine manufacturers are voluntary
- Vulnerable to error among older persons and obese patients

- Communicating the frequency of measurement and factors related to the patient's history, such as risk for orthostatic hypotension
- Reviewing the patient's usual BP values and significant changes or abnormalities to report to the nurse

When a patient has an abnormal BP that does not respond to treatment, collaborate with interprofessional health care team members (e.g., cardiac specialist) to determine whether additional interventions are needed.

Equipment

- Aneroid sphygmomanometer
- Cloth or disposable vinyl pressure cuff of appropriate size for patient's extremity
- Stethoscope
- Alcohol swab
- Pen and vital sign flow sheet in chart or EHR

STEP	RATIONALE
ASSESSMENT	
1. Identify patient using at least two person-specific identifiers (e.g., name and date of birth, or name and medical record number) according to employer policy.	Ensures correct patient. Adheres to Accreditation Canada's standards and improves patient safety (Accreditation Canada, 2020).
2. Throughout the procedure, the 4 moments for hand hygiene are to be implemented; hand hygiene should occur before initial patient (or patient environment) contact, before an aseptic procedure, after body fluid exposure risk, and after patient (or patient environment) contact. Additional hand hygiene should be performed when hands are visibly soiled.	Proper hand hygiene helps prevent the spread of infectious agents to health care providers.
3. Determine need to assess patient's BP:	
a. Assess risk factors for BP alterations: • History of cardiovascular disease • Renal disease • Diabetes mellitus • Circulatory shock (hypovolemic, septic, cardiogenic, or neurogenic) • Acute or persistent pain • Rapid IV infusion of fluids or blood products • Increased intracranial pressure • Postoperative status • Pregnancy-induced hypertension	Certain conditions place patients at risk for BP alterations.
b. Assess for signs and symptoms of BP alterations. In patients at risk for high BP, assess for headache (usually occipital), flushing of face, nosebleed, and fatigue in older persons. Hypotension is associated with dizziness; mental confusion; restlessness; pale, dusky, or cyanotic skin and mucous membranes; and cool, mottled skin over extremities.	Physical signs and symptoms indicate alterations in BP. Hypertension is often asymptomatic until pressure is very high.
c. Assess for factors that influence BP:	Allows you to anticipate factors that influence BP, ensuring a more accurate interpretation.
• Age	Acceptable values for BP vary throughout life (see Pediatric and Gerontological Considerations).
• Gender	During and after menopause, women often have higher BP than men of same age.
• Daily (diurnal) variation	BP varies throughout day; pressure is highest during the day between 1000 and 1800 hours and lowest in early morning.
• Position	BP falls as person moves from lying to sitting or standing position; normally, postural variations are minimal.
• Exercise	Increases in oxygen demand by body during activity increase BP.
• Weight	Obesity is an independent predictor of hypertension.
• Sympathetic stimulation	Pain, anxiety, and fear stimulate sympathetic nervous system, causing BP to rise.
• Medications	Antihypertensives, diuretics, beta-adrenergic blockers, vasodilators, calcium channel blockers, angiotensin-converting enzyme (ACE) inhibitors, angiotensin receptor blockers (ARBs), and antidysrhythmics lower BP; opioids and general anaesthetics also cause a drop in BP.
• Smoking	Nicotine in cigarettes smoke causes vasoconstriction, a narrowing of blood vessels, which raises BP. Smoking also makes BP medications less effective (Diabetes Canada, 2023).
• Ethnicity	Incidence of hypertension is higher among Indigenous, Black, and South Asian people (Heart and Stroke Foundation of Canada, 2018).
4. Determine best site for BP assessment. Avoid applying cuff to extremity when IV fluids are infusing or when breast or axillary surgery has been performed on that side. BP should also not be done on extremities that have dialysis access in the form of an arteriovenous graft (AVG) or arteriovenous fistula (AVF) (Tyerman & Cobbett, 2023). In addition, avoid applying cuff to traumatized or diseased extremity or one that has a cast or bulky bandage. After a stroke, BP should be measured in the unaffected arm (Maduagwu et al., 2018). Use lower extremities when brachial arteries are inaccessible.	Inappropriate site selection may result in poor amplification of sounds, leading to inaccurate readings. Application of pressure from inflated bladder temporarily impairs blood flow and can further compromise circulation in extremity that already has impaired blood flow. Studies have not directly determined the risk of lymphedema with BP measurement; however, BP cuffs on the affected arm of a person who has had a mastectomy *should be avoided*, as they use high-pressure focal compression that can lead to excessive constriction if not properly used (Tyerman & Cobbett, 2023). Avoiding BP measurement on extremities with AVG and AVF helps prevent possible infection and thrombosis in the vascular access (Tyerman & Cobbett, 2023). BP measurement in hemiplegic arm is often inaccurate owing to changes in muscle tone (Maduagwu et al., 2018).

STEP	RATIONALE
5. Determine previous baseline BP and site (if available) from patient's record. Determine any report of latex allergy.	Assesses for change in condition. Provides comparison with future BP measurements. If patient has latex allergy, verify that stethoscope and BP cuff are latex-free.
6. Assess patient's knowledge of procedure and any BP alterations that exist.	Encourages cooperation; minimizes risks and anxiety. Identifies teaching needs.

NURSING DIAGNOSES

- Reduced cardiac output
- Inadequate tissue perfusion
- Dehydration
- Fluid overload
- Potential for falls

Related factors and risk factors are individualized on the basis of patient's condition or needs.

PLANNING

STEP	RATIONALE
1. Expected outcome following completion of procedure: • BP is within acceptable range for patient's age.	Cardiovascular status is stable.
2. Explain to patient that you will assess BP. Have patient rest at least 5 minutes before measuring lying or sitting BP and 1 minute before measuring standing BP. Ask patient not to speak while you are measuring BP.	Reduces anxiety that can falsely elevate readings. Exercise causes false elevations in BP. Deep breathing lowers BP. Talking to a patient during assessment increases BP. A higher BP measurement occurs if the patient has not relaxed or rested (Mickley et al., 2018).
3. Be sure that patient has had no caffeine or tobacco 1 hour before BP measurement. Make sure patient has not exercised within past 30 minutes (Hypertension Canada, 2020a).	Smoking increases BP immediately, with increase lasting up to 15 minutes. Coffee or caffeine increase BP for up to 3 hours (Hypertension Canada, 2020a).
4. Select appropriate cuff size (see Fig. 7.11) and ensure that other equipment is in patient's room.	Use of improperly sized cuff causes falsely low or falsely high BP reading (see Box 7.8).

IMPLEMENTATION

STEP	RATIONALE
1.	Proper hand hygiene helps prevent the spread of infectious agents to health care providers.
2. Have patient assume sitting or lying position. Be sure that room is warm, quiet, and relaxing. Close room curtains.	Maintains patient's comfort during measurement. Patient's perceptions that physical or interpersonal environment is stressful affect BP.
3. Assess BP by auscultation:	
a. *Upper extremity:* With patient sitting or lying, position their forearm at heart level with palm turned up (see Step 3a illustration). If sitting, instruct patient to keep feet flat on floor without legs crossed. If supine, patient should not have legs crossed. If patient cannot be placed in prone position, position them supine with knee slightly bent.	If arm is extended and not supported, patient will perform isometric exercise that can increase DBP. Placement of arm above level of heart causes falsely low BP reading, 2 mm Hg for each 2.5 cm (1 inch) above heart level.
Lower extremity: With patient prone, position patient so knee is slightly flexed.	Leg crossing can falsely increase BP.
b. Expose extremity (arm or leg) fully by removing constricting clothing.	Ensures proper cuff application.

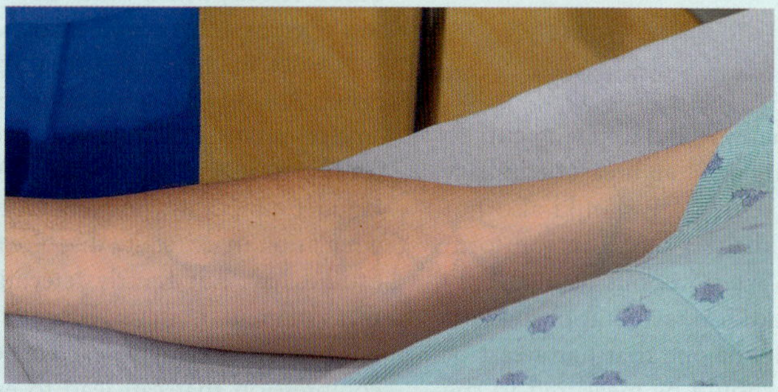

STEP 3A Patient's forearm supported on bed.

STEP	RATIONALE

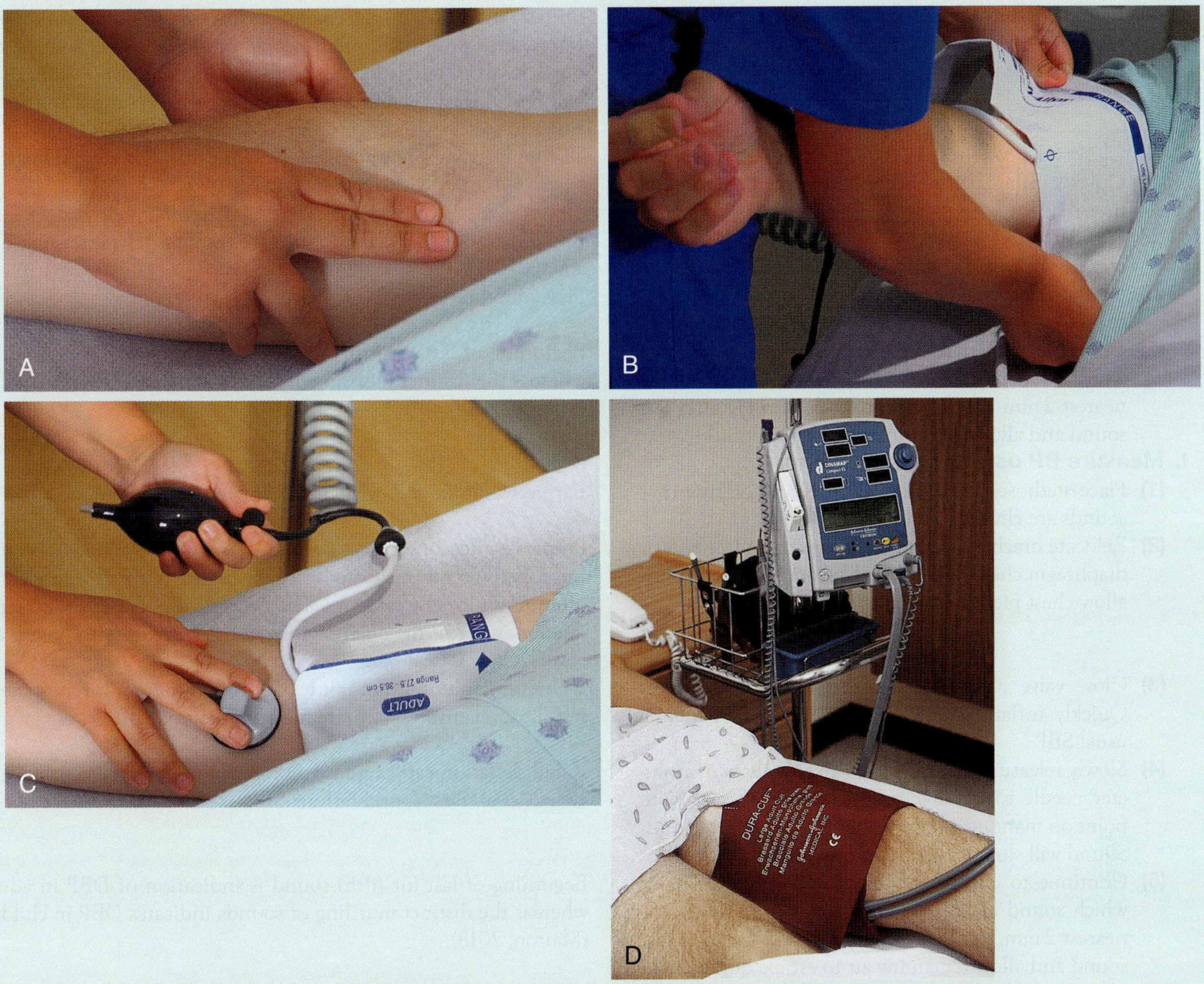

STEP 3C **A,** Palpating brachial artery. **B,** Aligning blood pressure cuff arrow with brachial artery. **C,** Blood pressure cuff wrapped around upper arm. **D,** Blood pressure cuff applied around thigh. *(D, Courtesy Barbara J. Astle, RN, PhD.)*

STEP	RATIONALE
c. Palpate brachial artery (arm, see illustration for Step 3c(*A*) or popliteal artery (leg). With cuff fully deflated, apply bladder of cuff above artery by centring arrows marked on cuff over artery (see illustration for Step 3c(*B*). If cuff does not have any centre arrows, estimate centre of bladder and place this centre over artery. Position cuff 2.5 cm (1 inch) above site of pulsation (antecubital or popliteal space). With cuff fully deflated, wrap it evenly and snugly around upper arm (see illustration for Step 3c[*C*] or leg (see illustration for Step 3c[*D*].	Brachial artery is along the groove between biceps and triceps muscles above elbow at antecubital fossa. Popliteal artery is just below patient's thigh, behind knee. Placing bladder directly over artery ensures that proper pressure is applied during inflation. A loose-fitting cuff causes falsely high BP readings.
d. Position manometer gauge vertically at eye level. You should be no farther than 1 metre (approximately 1 yard) away.	Looking up or down at scale can result in distorted readings.
e. Measure BP using two-step method:	
(1) Relocate brachial or popliteal pulse. Palpate artery distal to cuff with fingertips of nondominant hand while inflating cuff rapidly to pressure 30 mm Hg above point at which pulse disappears. Slowly deflate cuff and note point when pulse reappears. Deflate cuff fully and wait 30 seconds.	Estimating prevents falsely low BP readings. Determine maximal inflation point for accurate reading by palpation. If unable to palpate artery because of weakened pulse, use a Doppler ultrasonic stethoscope (see Chapter 8). Completely deflating cuff prevents venous congestion and falsely high BP readings.

STEP	RATIONALE
(2) Place stethoscope earpieces in ears and be sure that sounds are clear, not muffled.	Ensure that each earpiece follows angle of ear canal to facilitate hearing.
(3) Relocate artery and place bell or diaphragm chest piece of stethoscope over it. Do not allow chest piece to touch cuff or clothing.	Proper stethoscope placement ensures best sound reception. Improperly positioned stethoscope causes muffled sounds that often result in falsely low SBP and falsely high DBP readings. The bell provides better sound reproduction, whereas the diaphragm is easier to secure with fingers and covers a larger area.
(4) Close valve of pressure bulb clockwise until tight. Quickly inflate cuff to 30 mm Hg above patient's estimated SBP.	Tightening valve prevents air leak during inflation. Rapid inflation ensures accurate measurement of SBP.
(5) Slowly release pressure bulb valve and allow manometer needle to fall at rate of 2–3 mm Hg/sec.	Rapid deflation can cause inaccurate readings (Hypertension Canada, 2020a).
(6) Note point on manometer when you hear first clear sound. Sound will slowly increase in intensity.	First sound reflects SBP.
(7) Continue to deflate cuff gradually, noting point at which sound disappears in adults. Note pressure to nearest 2 mm Hg. Listen for 20–30 mm Hg after last sound and allow remaining air to escape quickly.	Beginning of last (or fifth) sound is indication of DBP in adults, whereas the distinct muffling of sounds indicates DBP in children (Mattoo, 2018).
f. Measure BP using one-step method:	
(1) Place stethoscope earpieces in ears and be sure that sounds are clear, not muffled.	Earpieces should follow angle of ear canal to facilitate hearing.
(2) Relocate brachial or popliteal artery and place bell or diaphragm chest piece of stethoscope over it. Do not allow chest piece to touch cuff or clothing.	Proper stethoscope placement ensures optimal sound reception. Improperly positioned stethoscope causes muffled sounds that often result in false readings. The bell provides better sound reproduction, whereas the diaphragm is easier to secure with fingers and covers a larger area.
(3) Close valve of pressure bulb clockwise until tight. Quickly inflate cuff to 30 mm Hg above patient's usual SBP.	Tightening valve prevents air leak during inflation. Inflation above systolic level ensures accurate measurement of SBP.
(4) Slowly release pressure bulb valve and allow manometer needle to fall at rate of 2–3 mm Hg/sec. Note point on manometer when you hear first clear sound. Sound will slowly increase in intensity.	Rapid deflation can cause inaccurate readings (Hypertension Canada, 2020a). First sound reflects SBP.
(5) Continue to deflate cuff gradually, noting point at which sound disappears in adults. Note pressure to nearest 2 mm Hg. Listen for 10–20 mm Hg after last sound and allow remaining air to escape quickly.	Beginning of last (or fifth) sound is indication of DBP in adults, whereas the distinct muffling of sounds indicates DBP in children (Mattoo, 2018).
(6) If non-AOBP is used to measure BP, the mean of at least three readings is used, discarding the first and calculating the remaining ones (Rabi et al., 2020).	Three sets of BP measurements help to prevent false-positive readings based on patient's sympathetic response (alert reaction). Averaging minimizes effect of anxiety, which often causes first reading to be higher than subsequent values (Basilie & Bloch, 2018).
4. Remove cuff from patient's arm or leg unless you need to repeat measurement.	Continuous cuff inflation causes arterial occlusion, resulting in numbness and tingling of patient's arm or leg.
5. If this is first assessment of patient, repeat procedure on other arm or leg.	Different BP readings in the right and left arms that vary by a few millimetres of mercury is not worrisome; however, a significant difference in pressure (>10 mm Hg) in the right and left arms can signal circulatory problems that may lead to stroke, peripheral artery disease, or other cardiovascular problems. Use arm with higher pressure for repeated measurements (Heshmat-Ghahdarijani et al., 2022).
6. Assess SBP by palpation:	
a. Follow Steps 3a through 3d of auscultation method.	
b. Locate and then continually palpate brachial, radial, or popliteal artery with fingertips of one hand. Inflate cuff to pressure 30 mm Hg above point at which you can no longer palpate pulse.	Ensures accurate detection of true SBP once pressure valve is released.

Critical Decision Point *If unable to palpate artery because of weakened pulse, use a Doppler ultrasonic stethoscope* (Fig. 7.12).

STEP	RATIONALE
c. Slowly release valve and deflate cuff, allowing manometer needle to fall at rate of 2 mm Hg/sec. Note point on manometer when pulse is again palpable.	Rapid deflation can cause inaccurate readings (Hypertension Canada, 2020a). Palpation helps identify SBP only.
d. Deflate cuff rapidly and completely. Remove cuff from patient's extremity unless you need to repeat measurement.	Continuous cuff inflation causes arterial occlusion, resulting in numbness and tingling of extremity.
7. Measure orthostatic hypotension:	
a. Have patient lie down for 5 minutes, then measure BP and pulse.	Gives baseline BP and pulse.
b. Have patient stand for 1 minute, then retake BP and pulse. **c.** Have patient continue to stand, and retake BP and pulse after 3 minutes. **d.** Always make sure patient has a safe place to sit or land while standing. If patient is too dizzy or weak to stand, have person sit at edge of the bed and dangle legs (Jarvis et al., 2024).	Rapid cardiovascular adaptations driven primarily by the autonomic nervous system maintain BP upon assumption of upright posture. A drop in BP upon standing can indicate failure of these compensatory mechanisms and can result in orthostatic hypotension (Tyerman & Cobbett, 2023).
8. Help patient return to comfortable position and cover upper arm or leg if previously clothed.	Restores comfort and provides sense of well-being.
9. Discuss findings with patient.	Promotes patient's participation in care and understanding of health status. Makes patient accountable for follow-up assessment. Systolic BP in leg is 10–40 mm Hg higher than in arm, but diastolic BP is same.
10. Clean earpieces and diaphragm of stethoscope with alcohol swab as needed. Wipe cuff with employer-approved disinfectant if used between patients.	Controls transmission of microorganisms when nurses share stethoscope. Reduces transmission of microorganisms.

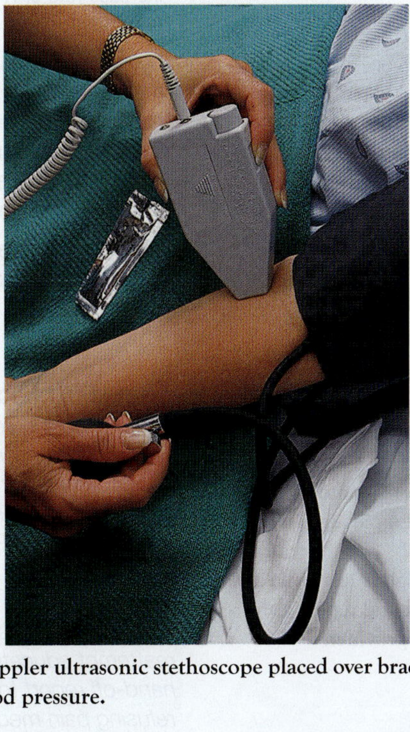

FIG 7.12 Doppler ultrasonic stethoscope placed over brachial artery to measure blood pressure.

EVALUATION

1. If assessing BP for first time, establish baseline BP if it is within acceptable range.
   Used to compare future BP measurements. See Table 7.2 for SBP and DBP ranges in patients based on age.
2. Compare BP reading with patient's previous baseline and usual BP for patient's age.
   Allows for assessment of change in patient's condition. Provides comparison with future BP measurements.
3. **Use teach-back:** "I want to be sure I explained why it is important to stand up slowly since you have high blood pressure. Tell me which of your medications might make you dizzy if you stand up too fast." Develop a revised teaching plan if patient or caregiver is unable to teach back correctly.
   Determines patient's and caregiver's level of understanding of instructional topic.

Unexpected Outcomes	Related Interventions
1. Patient's BP is above acceptable range.	• Repeat measurement in other extremity and compare findings. • Verify correct size and placement of BP cuff. • If BP was taken manually, have another nurse repeat measurement in 1–2 minutes to ensure it is not due to human error. • Observe for related symptoms that are not apparent unless BP is extremely high, including headache, facial flushing, nosebleed, and fatigue in older patients. • Report BP to nurse in charge or health care provider to initiate appropriate evaluation and treatment. • Administer antihypertensive medications as prescribed.
2. Patient's BP is not sufficient for adequate perfusion and oxygenation of tissues.	• Compare BP value to baseline. • Position patient in supine position to enhance circulation and restrict activity that further decreases BP. • Assess for signs and symptoms associated with hypotension, including tachycardia; weak, thready pulse; weakness; dizziness; confusion; and cool, pale, dusky, or cyanotic skin. • Assess for factors that contribute to low BP, including hemorrhage, dilation of blood vessels resulting from hyperthermia, anaesthesia, or medication adverse effects. • Report BP to nurse in charge or health care provider to initiate appropriate evaluation and treatment. • Increase rate of IV infusion or administer vasoconstriction medication if prescribed.
3. Unable to obtain BP reading.	• Determine that no immediate crisis is present by obtaining pulse and respiratory rate. • Assess for signs and symptoms of decreased cardiac output; if present, notify nurse in charge or health care provider immediately. • Use alternative sites or procedures to obtain BP: use Doppler ultrasonic instrument (see Chapter 8); palpate SBP.
4. Patient experiences orthostatic hypotension.	• Maintain patient safety. • Return patient to safe position in bed or chair.

Communication and Documentation

- Document BP and site assessed on vital sign flow sheet or in progress notes in EHR or chart.
- Document measurement of BP and any signs or symptoms of BP alterations after administration of specific therapies in progress notes in EHR or chart.
- Document your evaluation of patient and caregiver learning.
- Review baseline and previous BP measurement and report abnormal findings to nurse in charge or health care provider.

DOCUMENTATION EXAMPLE

Patient had a quiet afternoon. Ate 90% of supper. At 1800 hours patient reported a headache. Pain rated at 6/10 on rest and reported as pounding. Patient VS: T: 37.2°C; P: 94 beats/min; RR: 19 breaths/min; SpO_2 Sat: 98% on RA; BP: 154/87 mm Hg. Patient BP elevated from noon BP of 132/84. Amlodipine 5 mg q6h PRN given. Will recheck in 30 minutes. Clinical message sent to health care provider and charge nurse notified. Patient is not receptive to education at this time. Will reattempt education on BP reading in one hour or include in hand-off report to night RN to perform in evening. Pt is also refusing pain meds at this time. Will continue to monitor.

TABLE 7.2

Estimated Blood Pressure Ranges (mm Hg)

Age	Systolic Range	Diastolic Range
Newborn to 6 months	45–90	30–65
6 months to 2 years	80–100	40–70
Children (2–13 years)	80–120	40–80
Adolescent (14–18 years)	90–120	50–80
Adult (19–40 years)	95–135	60–80
Adult (41–60 years)	110–145	70–90
Older person (61 years and older)*	95–145	70–90

*The target blood pressure for adults less than 80 years of age is <140/90 mm Hg and those 80 years and older is <150/90 mm Hg (Rabi et al., 2020).

From Lapum, J. L., Verkuyl, M., Garcia, W., et al. (2021). *Vital sign measurement across the lifespan* (2nd ed., Table 5.1). BCcampus. https://opentextbc.ca/vitalsignmeasurement/

Special Considerations

Teaching

- Educate patient about risks for hypertension. People with family history of hypertension, premature heart disease, lipidemia, or renal disease are at significant risk. Obesity, cigarette smoking, heavy alcohol consumption, high serum lipids, high dietary sodium intake, sedentary lifestyle, and continued exposure to psychosocial stress are factors linked to hypertension (Rabi et al., 2020).
- Primary prevention and treatment of hypertension include health behaviour management: smoking cessation, physical exercise, weight reduction, decreased alcohol consumption, decreased sodium intake, stress management, and increased intake of dietary potassium in those who are not at risk for hyperkalemia (Rabi et al., 2020).
- Instruct primary caregiver to take BP at same time each day and after patient has had a brief rest. Take BP sitting or lying down; use same position and arm each time pressure is taken (see Skill 7.7).
- Instruct caregiver that if the BP is difficult to hear, it is probably caused by one of the following: cuff too loose, not large enough, or too narrow; stethoscope not over arterial pulse; cuff deflated too quickly or too slowly; or cuff not pumped high enough for systolic readings.

Pediatric

- BP measurement is not a routine part of assessment in children younger than 3 years.
- BP measurement can frighten children. Prepare child for squeezing feeling of inflated BP cuff by comparing sensation to elastic band on finger or a tight hug on the arm.
- Obtain BP in child before performing anxiety-producing tests or procedures.
- BP sounds are difficult to hear in children because of low frequency and amplitude. Using the bell of a pediatric stethoscope is often helpful.

Gerontological

- Older persons, especially frail older persons, have lost upper-arm mass, requiring special attention to selection of BP cuff size.
- Skin of older persons is more fragile and susceptible to cuff pressure when measurements are frequent. More frequent assessment of skin under cuff or rotation of measurement sites is recommended.
- Older persons commonly have pseudohypertension, which is an elevated SBP reading resulting from the inability of the BP cuff to adequately compress the arteries in those with arteriosclerosis (Spence, 2021) related to decreased vessel elasticity.
- Older persons often experience a fall in BP after eating.
- Instruct older persons to change position slowly and wait after each change to avoid postural hypotension and prevent injuries.

Care in the Community: Home Management

- Assess caregiver's financial ability to afford an electronic BP machine for performing BP evaluations on a regular basis. They should purchase and use only BP monitoring devices that have met the standards of the Association for the Advancement of Medical Instrumentation, the most recent requirements of the British Hypertension Society protocol, or the International Protocol for validation of automated BP-measuring devices. Patients should also be encouraged to use devices that can record the date or have automatic data transmission to increase the reliability of reported home BP monitoring (Rabi et al., 2020).
- Teach patient and caregiver on the correct way to measure BP in the home and, if necessary, repeat training (see Skill 7.7). Patient and caregiver should be observed to confirm that they can measure BP correctly and interpret the readings (Rabi et al., 2020).

✦ SKILL 7.7 Teaching Blood Pressure and Pulse Measurement

Patients with a variety of illnesses such as cardiac, kidney, or vascular diseases are susceptible to wide variations in their BP and pulse. They benefit from knowing how to assess their own BP and pulse because they are able to seek medical attention early when readings vary from their acceptable ranges. In addition, healthy people who exercise learn how their body responds to exercise and are able to determine appropriate exercise plans based on knowing what their pulse and BP are before, during, and after exercise.

Research related to home monitoring of BP has illustrated the importance of regular monitoring outside of acute care settings and medical offices so that the health care provider can treat patients with hypertension appropriately (Hypertension Canada, 2020c). If treatment is based on single readings during an office visit, health care providers do not have an accurate picture of a patient's health. To gather this essential information about patients living at home, nurses can teach them to measure their BP and pulse regularly and to interpret readings that are outside of their individualized normal values. For example, patients should be taught about factors that affect the accuracy of BP readings, such as cuff placement, movement of the tubing, speaking during measurement, and position and movement of the extremity or body.

Aneroid sphygmomanometers are available to measure BP in the home. Aneroid manometers are safe, lightweight, compact, and portable. In the home, many patients choose to use commercial automatic electronic BP devices. These devices may measure pulse rate and produce a BP measurement without needing to use a stethoscope. Measuring BP using these devices involves placing a cuff around the arm, the wrist, or a fingertip. A reading is displayed electronically for the patient. Electronic BP monitors are often easier to use, but their accuracy compared with manual BP monitoring is still a focus of debate. However, home monitoring of BP is still recommended because of the increased number of BP readings that can be obtained

(Hypertension Canada, 2020c). It is essential for patients to keep a record of all of their BP readings and to compare those obtained by a health care provider with those obtained using their electronic monitor to assess the accuracy of readings.

Additional factors that affect the accuracy of BP monitoring are cuff size and placement. Patients need to learn to place a cuff directly on their skin. BP cuffs that are too small tend to overestimate BP, whereas cuffs that are too large tend to underestimate it (Hypertension Canada, 2020c). Not all electronic home BP monitors come with interchangeable cuff sizes, which can complicate BP monitoring at home. Nurses need to help patients and caregivers determine cuff size, calibration, and accuracy of electronic equipment before they determine which type of BP monitor to purchase (see Fig. 7.11).

Delegation and Collaboration

The skill of teaching patients to measure BP and pulse cannot be delegated to a UCP. The nurse instructs the UCP as follows:

- Report concerns related to BP (e.g., episodes of suspected orthostatic hypotension) and measurements to the nurse

Equipment

For Blood Pressure

- Sphygmomanometer or electronic BP reading device. Cuff should be secure and fit snugly, encircling the arm (see Fig. 7.11 and Table 7.3). Most often, patients have an electronic BP machine in the home setting.

TABLE 7.3

Correct Blood Pressure Cuff Size for Electronic Monitor*

Cuff Size	Limb Circumference (cm)
Newborn	4–8
Infant	6–12
Older child	9–18
Small adult	17–25
Average adult	23–33
Large adult	31–40
Thigh	38–50

*A 3.7- to 7.3-metre (12- to 24-foot) cord is usually required for electronic adult blood pressure monitoring.

Data for pediatric sizes from Hockenberry, M. J., Duffy, E. A., & Gibbs, K. (2024). *Wong's nursing care of infants and children* (12th ed.). Elsevier.

- Stethoscope (two-headed teaching stethoscope is ideal) if using sphygmomanometer

For Pulse

- Wristwatch or clock with a second hand

For Both Blood Pressure and Pulse

- Paper or digital log

STEP	RATIONALE
ASSESSMENT	
1. Identify patient using at least two person-specific identifiers (e.g., name and date of birth, or name and medical record number, according to employer policy) during the first visit. Facial recognition can be used as one of two identifiers for ongoing subsequent visits.	Ensures correct patient. Complies with Accreditation Canada's standards and improves patient safety (Accreditation Canada, 2020).
2. Throughout the procedure, the 4 moments for hand hygiene are to be implemented; hand hygiene should occur before initial patient (or patient environment) contact, before an aseptic procedure, after body fluid exposure risk, and after patient (or patient environment) contact. Additional hand hygiene should be performed when hands are visibly soiled.	Proper hand hygiene helps prevent the spread of infectious agents to health care providers.
3. Assess patient's and caregiver's psychomotor function: visual (see dial and clock) and auditory (listen for Korotkoff sounds) acuity, ability to manipulate BP monitoring equipment, and ability to feel pulse.	Vision or hearing problems require use of equipment that has been adapted for these conditions (e.g., larger print). Other deficits may require the caregiver to perform skills.
4. Assess patient's and caregiver's knowledge of normal BP and pulse range for the patient and the symptoms of high or low readings. (Consult with health care provider regarding normal range desired.)	Identifies patient's and caregiver's ability to know when to initiate preventive health measures and recognize alterations in BP and pulse.
5. Assess patient's and caregiver's knowledge of what BP and pulse measure, specific medical issues that affect them, and why awareness of variations is important to the patient's health.	Identifies patient's and caregiver's understanding of potential cause-and-effect relationships between variations in BP and pulse and health status.
6. Assess patient's and caregiver's previous knowledge of and experience in measuring BP and pulse. Have patient or caregiver perform return demonstration if they indicate ability to measure BP or pulse.	Allows nurse to assess patient's and caregiver's knowledge and skill performance.
7. Assess patient's learning readiness and ability to concentrate; consider presence of pain, nausea, or fatigue and patient interest in instruction.	Presence of significant illness, frailty, or confusion affects a patient's ability to attend to a teaching plan. Indicates need to rely on caregiver for learning and implementation (if available) on a short- or long-term basis.

STEP	RATIONALE
8. Assess home environment for a favourable place to measure BP and pulse (e.g., quiet room with comfortable place to sit) along with quality of home BP equipment.	Ensures more accurate measurement.

NURSING DIAGNOSES

- Insufficient knowledge regarding pulse or BP measurement
- Inadequate health maintenance

Related factors and risk factors are individualized on the basis of patient's condition or needs.

PLANNING

STEP	RATIONALE
1. Expected outcomes following completion of procedure:	
• Patient or caregiver accurately measures BP and pulse.	Learning has occurred.
• BP and pulse are within range expected for patient's age and condition.	Cardiovascular status of patient is stable at level determined by health care provider.
• Patient or caregiver explains importance of measuring BP and pulse, common causes of changes, the best time for measurement, and when to communicate with the health care provider to evaluate changes in treatment regimen.	Measures cognitive learning.
2. Encourage patient or caregiver to perform measurements on a routine schedule for long-term monitoring plan.	Daily activities and many extrinsic and intrinsic factors affect measurement fluctuations. A routine schedule allows for daily comparisons.
3. Encourage patient to avoid exercise, caffeine, and smoking for 30 minutes before assessment to avoid inaccuracy.	These factors cause elevations in BP and pulse (Hypertension Canada, 2020a).
4. Have patient or caregiver perform measurement on patient in a comfortable position, with arm supported and feet flat on the floor and in a warm and quiet environment.	Maintains patient's comfort during measurement. Leg crossing can falsely increase BP.

IMPLEMENTATION

STEP	RATIONALE
1. BP measurement:	
a. Explain the importance of having patient sit quietly for 5 minutes with their back supported and feet on the floor before BP measurement. If patient cannot sit in this position, select a position that patient can maintain.	Reduces anxiety, which can falsely elevate BP readings. It is important for patient to maintain the same position for each reading.
b. Discuss with patient and caregiver the best sites for assessing BP. For self-measurement, the brachial artery is almost always used. If patient cannot sit in this position, select a position that patient can maintain. Instruct patient and caregiver to avoid applying cuff to an arm with: • IV catheter with or without fluids infusing • Arteriovenous shunt • Breast or axillary surgery • Trauma, inflammation, or disease	The most accessible sites are easiest to measure for accuracy of assessment. Appropriate site selection promotes accuracy in reading and minimizes potential for trauma. It is important for the patient to maintain the same position for each reading. Application of pressure from an inflated bladder temporarily impairs blood flow and compromises circulation in the extremity that already has impaired circulation.
c. Demonstrate steps for measuring BP (see Skill 7.6):	Eventual evaluation of psychomotor skill is measured through patient's performance and ability to follow instructions.
(1) *Use of sphygmomanometer and stethoscope:*	
(a) Teach palpation of artery, positioning cuff, wrapping cuff, placing stethoscope, inflating and releasing cuff, and listening for Korotkoff sounds.	Prepares patient or caregiver for measuring BP.
(b) Describe sounds of measurement and relationship to observation of gauge during BP reading. Caution patient and caregiver about level and length of time appropriate for cuff inflation.	Ensures accurate reading. Prolonged inflation of cuff impairs circulation to extremity.
(c) Teach patient and caregiver to routinely clean diaphragm and earpieces of stethoscope with rubbing alcohol or damp cloth.	Stethoscopes are frequently contaminated with microorganisms. Cleaning stethoscope routinely prevents transmission of microorganisms.

Critical Decision Point *If the patient or caregiver needs to use a stethoscope to take BP, use a double-headed teaching stethoscope to verify accuracy of the reading or read BP 1–2 minutes after the patient's attempt to verify accuracy. If the patient is having difficulty hearing Korotkoff sounds, ensure that they are applying the cuff appropriately and using the correct cuff size. Also determine correct use of equipment (e.g., cuff may have been deflated too quickly or too slowly; cuff may not have been pumped high enough for systolic readings).*

STEP	RATIONALE
(2) *Use of electronic BP monitor:*	
(a) Teach correct placement of cuff and use of electronic equipment for proper cuff inflation.	Using electronic equipment correctly helps ensure accurate BP readings.
2. Pulse measurement:	
a. Discuss with patient and caregiver the best sites for assessing pulse: radial and carotid.	Radial and carotid sites are accessible and usually easiest to palpate.

Critical Decision Point *If a carotid site is chosen, caution the patient against vigorously massaging their neck while attempting to locate pulse or attempting to locate both arteries at the same time. Stimulation of carotid sinus leads to reflex slowing of the heart rate from vagal stimulation. In addition, simultaneous occlusion of both carotid arteries decreases blood to the brain, resulting in fainting.*

STEP	RATIONALE
b. Demonstrate steps for palpating pulse (see Skills 7.2 and 7.3): position of artery on wrist or neck, how to locate artery, using fingertips for palpation, compressing artery, palpating pulse before counting, counting pulse, and calculating pulse rate (see Step 2b illustration).	Eventual evaluation of psychomotor skill is measured through patient's performance and ability to follow instructions.
(1) Instruct in use of gentle pressure; reinforce not to press hard over the pulse site.	Pressing too hard may occlude the artery.
(2) Instruct in use of watch or clock with second hand to count pulse.	Ensures correct timing of pulse.
(3) Instruct to count for a full 60 seconds, starting with the second hand at 1200 hours position.	Consistent timing of procedure reduces confusion or forgetfulness about time period or starting point used for pulse measurement. A full 60-second count increases accuracy of measure.
3. Educate patient and caregiver about normal desired BP and pulse ranges, the purposes of monitoring, and when to take measurements (e.g., before and after taking cardiac or antihypertensive medications; before, during, and after exercise).	Patient or caregiver needs to be able to determine when values are not in desired ranges and when measurements need to be taken.
4. Describe symptoms that indicate the need to perform BP and/or pulse measurement.	Promotes patient's understanding of health status alterations that need medical intervention.

Critical Decision Point *Discuss the importance of notifying the health care provider and withholding medications when abnormal values in BP or pulse occur (e.g., hypotension or bradycardia). The patient needs to understand preventive measures to take and to follow the health care provider's directions if alterations develop.*

STEP	RATIONALE
5. Have patient or caregiver attempt each step of skill on you or a family member.	Provides opportunity to correct any errors in technique as they occur.
6. Observe patient demonstrate techniques to measure pulse and BP on self. When patient is measuring BP, do not allow multiple repetitive BP attempts on any one limb.	After developing confidence in measuring values in others, the patient is ready to measure their own values. Making multiple repetitive BP attempts restricts circulation and alters measurement.
7. Teach patient and caregiver to monitor BP and pulse, even if they remain in normal range.	Continuous monitoring provides important information that evaluates the effectiveness of medications or other treatments.

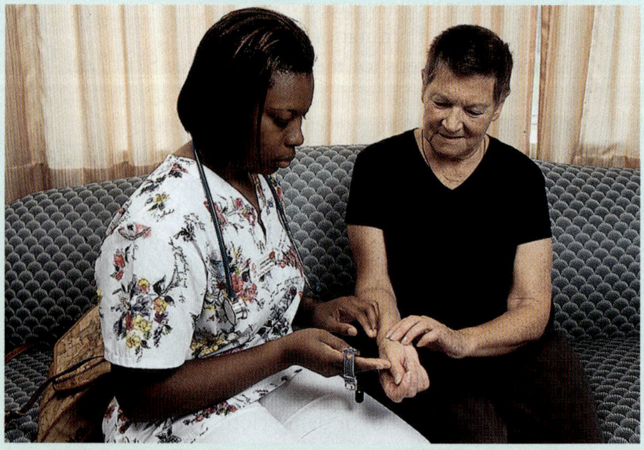

STEP 2B Nurse observes patient checking radial pulse.

STEP	RATIONALE
8. Provide patient and caregiver with printed instructions along with a written or pictorial guide or with a DVD or online demonstration of procedure if possible.	Printed and audiovisual teaching materials help stimulate patient's visual and auditory senses, which enhances learning.
9. Give patient or caregiver a paper or digital log to record BP and pulse and the time(s) they were taken. In addition, the patient must record whether or not medications that affect BP or pulse were taken. Instruct patient and caregiver to use a written record to report readings to the health care provider.	Keeping an organized record of BP and pulse readings and medications empowers the patient and provides accurate information to health care providers.
10. Instruct patient and caregiver in proper care of equipment (e.g., storage, cleaning, and battery care).	Improper care and storage of equipment affects accuracy of measurement.

EVALUATION

1. Observe patient or caregiver demonstrate technique for BP and pulse measurement on at least three different occasions and verify that patient or caregiver adds information to log correctly.	Feedback through return demonstration of psychomotor learning is the best means to evaluate learning.
2. Ask patient and caregiver whether readings are within the desired range and when to report abnormal readings to the health care provider.	Determines patient's and caregiver's ability to know when readings are within the proper range and what to do when abnormal readings are obtained.
3. Ask patient and caregiver to describe the reason for BP and pulse monitoring and any related medications (e.g., antihypertensives, antidysrhythmics) or treatment (e.g., diet and exercise).	Determines if patient understands monitoring and related therapies.
4. Have patient or caregiver demonstrate proper care of equipment.	Demonstrates learning.
5. **Use teach-back:** "I want to be sure I explained the importance of monitoring your BP. Explain to me how your medications can affect your BP readings." Develop a revised teaching plan if patient or caregiver is unable to teach back correctly.	Determines patient's and caregiver's level of understanding of instructional topic.

Unexpected Outcomes	Related Interventions
1. Patient or caregiver is unable to measure BP or pulse (e.g., inability to manipulate equipment, visualize numbers on equipment or clock, or hear BP sounds).	• Alter teaching plan to accommodate patient's or caregiver's problems (e.g., use other types of equipment that are easier to manipulate, see, or hear). • Reinforce information taught and continue return demonstrations until patient or caregiver can perform skill. • Teach skill to a different caregiver.
2. Patient or caregiver has difficulty explaining purposes of measurement or implications of therapy.	• Review and reinforce information that patient or caregiver does not understand.

Communication and Documentation

- Document teaching, patient and caregiver responses, and demonstration in the home care record.
- Document BP and pulse in home care record and home documentation system (e.g., logbook).
- Report BP and/or pulse findings that deviate from the patient's normal values to the health care provider.

DOCUMENTATION EXAMPLE

Education provided to patient and caregiver on proper technique for measuring pulse rate and BP at home. Patient was able to return demonstration accurately. Information leaflet reviewed re: normal values, documentation, and when to report values to health care provider. Patient and caregiver indicated reinforcement of information required. Will reinforce information on topic at next visit.

Special Considerations

Teaching

- Educate patient and caregiver about risks for hypertension, hypotension, or change in pulse rate.
- Ensure that patient or caregiver understands health care provider's recommendations for treatment regimen, including potential adverse effects and interactions of any medication therapies (e.g., patients taking thyroid medications might need to withhold them when BP is above normal range or pulse is above 100 beats/min). Confirm specific guidelines for BP and pulse with the health care provider; document information in home care record; and provide clear, written instructions for the patient and caregiver.
- Measurement should be performed before breakfast and 2 hours after dinner, before taking medication. Duplicate measurement should be taken in the morning and in the evening for 7 days (i.e., 28 measurements in total) (Hypertension Canada, 2020c).

- Average the results, excluding the first day's readings (Hypertension Canada, 2020c).
- Always leave a phone number and instructions about how to reach the home care nurse if needed.

Pediatric

- Readings (BP or pulse) are often inaccurate if an infant or child is anxious and uncooperative. BP is also inaccurate when the cuff size is inappropriate. Having others divert the child's attention or taking their BP or pulse while they are seated on the parent's lap usually helps calm the child (Hockenberry et al., 2024).
- Young children will be more likely to cooperate if allowed to touch or play with equipment before the procedure. Consider performing the procedure first on the parent or another person significant to child. This allows the child to observe that the procedure is safe.
- Use the radial pulse in children over 2 years of age. Femoral or brachial pulse is the best site for palpation of pulse for children under 2 years of age (Hockenberry et al., 2024). When the child is under 1 year, use a stethoscope to obtain the apical heart.

Gerontological

- Musculoskeletal changes such as arthritis or other joint conditions may impair a patient's ability to position a limb comfortably or perform the fine motor skills required to measure BP and pulse (Boscart et al., 2023).
- Older persons, especially those who are frail or who have lost upper-arm mass, require a smaller BP cuff.
- Home BP monitoring among older persons is not a replacement for BP monitoring by health care providers, but it can serve to provide more information to ensure the best treatment.

Procedural Guideline 7.1 *Noninvasive Electronic Blood Pressure Measurement*

NSO *Nursing Skills Online Vital Signs Module 4 / Lesson 5*

Many different styles of electronic BP machines are available to determine BP automatically (Fig. 7.13). Electronic machines rely on an electronic sensor to detect the vibrations caused by the rush of blood through an artery. They are easy to use and efficient and a stethoscope is not needed. The devices can be preprogrammed to take either single measurements or a series of measurements and then average the results. Hypertension Canada (2020a) strongly encourages the use of these validated electronic digital oscillometric devices as they can minimize or eliminate many auscultation-induced errors (Rabi et al., 2020).

Delegation and Collaboration

The skill of BP measurement using an electronic BP machine can be delegated to a UCP unless the patient is considered unstable (e.g., hypotensive). The nurse instructs the UCP by doing the following:

- Explaining the frequency and extremity to use for measurement
- Reviewing how to select an appropriately sized BP cuff for designated extremity and appropriate cuff for the machine
- Reviewing patient's usual BP and reporting significant changes or abnormalities to the nurse

Equipment

- Electronic BP machine
- BP cuff of appropriate size per manufacturer's recommendations
- Pen and vital sign flow sheet in chart or EHR

Procedural Steps

1. Identify patient using at least two person-specific identifiers (e.g., name and date of birth, or name and medical record number) according to employer policy (Accreditation Canada, 2020).
2. Assess need to measure BP (see Skill 7.6, Assessment, Step 2) and determine patient's baseline BP.
3. Throughout the procedure, the 4 moments for hand hygiene are to be implemented; hand hygiene should occur before initial patient (or patient environment) contact, before an aseptic procedure, after body fluid exposure risk, and after patient (or patient environment) contact. Additional hand hygiene should be performed when hands are visibly soiled. Determine best site for cuff placement; inspect condition of extremities.
4. Collect and bring appropriate equipment to patient's bedside. Select appropriately sized cuff for patient extremity (Table 7.3) and appropriate cuff for machine. Electronic BP cuff and machine must have same manufacturer and are not interchangeable.
5. Help patient to comfortable position, either lying or sitting. Plug device into electric outlet and place it near patient, ensuring that connector hose between cuff and machine reaches.
6. Locate on/off switch and turn on machine to enable device to self-test computer systems.
7. Remove constricting clothing to ensure proper cuff application.
8. Prepare BP cuff by manually squeezing all the air out of the cuff and connecting it to connector hose.
9. Wrap flattened cuff snugly around extremity, verifying that only one finger can fit between cuff and patient's skin. Make sure that "artery" arrow marked on outside of cuff is placed correctly (see Step 9 illustration).
10. Verify that connector hose between cuff and machine is not kinked. Kinking prevents proper inflation and deflation of cuff.
11. Following manufacturer directions, set frequency control for automatic or manual and press the start button. The first BP measurement pumps cuff to a peak pressure of approximately 180 mm Hg. After this pressure is reached, the machine begins a deflation sequence that determines the BP. The first reading determines peak pressure inflation for additional measurements.
12. When deflation is complete, the digital display shows the most recent values and flashes the time in minutes that have elapsed since the measurement occurred (see Step 12 illustration).

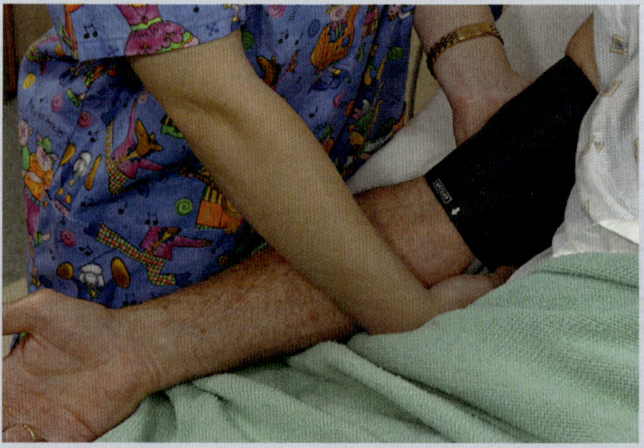

STEP 9 Aligning blood pressure cuff arrow with brachial artery.

Continued

Procedural Guideline 7.1 *Noninvasive Electronic Blood Pressure Measurement—cont'd*

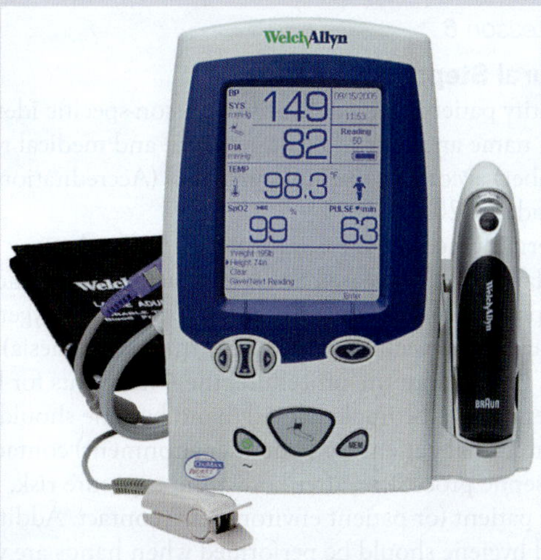

STEP 12 Digital electronic blood pressure display. *(Image courtesy Welch Allyn.)*

Critical Decision Point *If unable to obtain BP with electronic device, verify machine connections (e.g., plugged into working electrical outlet, hose–cuff connections tight, machine on, correct cuff). Repeat electronic BP measurement; if unable to obtain, use auscultatory technique (see Skill 7.6).*

13. Set frequency of measurements and upper and lower alarm limits for SBP, DBP, and mean BP readings. Intervals between measurements can be set from 1 to 90 minutes. A nurse determines frequency and alarm limits on the basis of patient's acceptable range of BP, nursing judgement, and health care provider prescription.
14. Obtain additional readings at any time by pressing the start button. Pressing the cancel button immediately deflates the cuff.
15. If frequent measurements are required, the cuff may be left in place. Remove it at least every 2 hours to assess underlying skin integrity and, if possible, alternate measurement sites. Patients with abnormal bleeding tendencies are at risk for microvascular rupture from repeated inflations. When patient no longer requires frequent BP monitoring, remove and clean cuff according to employer policy to reduce transmission of microorganisms. Disinfect electronic BP unit regularly when visibly soiled, after every use, or once daily. If possible, leave the machine in the room for patients on isolation precautions or disinfect before using it on another patient.
16. Discuss findings with patient.
17. Record BP and site assessed on vital sign flow sheet or in progress notes in EHR or chart; record any signs or symptoms of BP alterations in narrative form in progress notes; compare patient's baseline and most current previous BP findings to current readings; report abnormal findings to nurse in charge or health care provider.
18. **Use teach-back:** "I want to be sure I explained why you need to keep your arm straight while the machine is taking your blood pressure. Tell me why it is important to remain still." Develop a revised teaching plan if patient or caregiver is unable to teach back correctly.

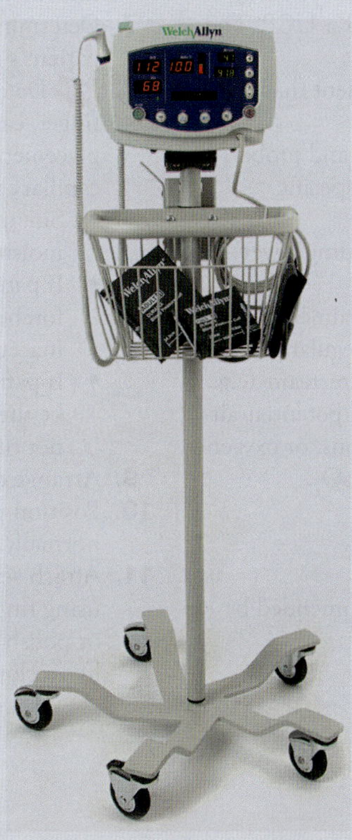

FIG 7.13 **Noninvasive electronic blood pressure machine.** (*Photo courtesy Welch Allyn.*)

Procedural Guideline 7.2 *Measuring Oxygen Saturation (Pulse Oximetry)*

Video Clip NSO *Nursing Skills Online Airway Management Module 9 / Lesson 6*

Pulse oximetry is the noninvasive measurement of arterial blood oxygen saturation, the percentage of hemoglobin saturated with oxygen. A pulse oximeter is a probe with a light-emitting diode (LED) connected by a cable to an oximeter. The LED emits light wavelengths that are absorbed differently by the oxygenated and deoxygenated hemoglobin molecules. The more hemoglobin saturated by oxygen, the higher the oxygen saturation (SpO_2). Normally, SpO_2 is greater than 95%; SpO_2 less than 90% is a clinical emergency in a patient without a chronic respiratory condition (World Health Organization, 2021).

Pulse oximetry measurement of SpO_2 is simple and painless and has few of the risks associated with more invasive measurements of oxygen saturation, such as arterial blood gas sampling. A vascular, pulsatile area is needed to detect the change in the transmitted light when making measurements with a finger or earlobe probe. Conditions that decrease arterial blood flow, including peripheral vascular disease, hypothermia, pharmacological vasoconstrictors, hypotension, or peripheral edema, affect accurate determination of oxygen saturation in these areas. For patients with decreased peripheral perfusion, you can apply a forehead sensor (Seifi et al., 2018). Factors that affect light transmission such as outside light sources or patient motion also affect the measurement of oxygen saturation. Carbon monoxide in the blood, jaundice, and intravascular dyes can influence the light reflected from hemoglobin molecules.

In adults, you can apply reusable and disposable oximeter probes to the earlobe, finger, toe, bridge of the nose, or forehead (Box 7.10). Pulse oximetry is indicated in patients who have an unstable oxygen status or are at risk for impaired gas exchange.

Delegation and Collaboration

The skill of SpO_2 measurement can be delegated to a UCP. The nurse instructs the UCP by doing the following:

- Communicating specific factors related to the patient that can falsely lower SpO_2
- Informing the UCP about appropriate sensor site and probe
- Notifying frequency of SpO_2 measurements for a specific patient
- Instructing to notify nurse immediately of any reading lower than SpO_2 of 95% or value for a specific patient
- Instructing the UCP to refrain from using pulse oximetry to obtain HR because oximeter will not detect an irregular pulse

Collaborate with the interprofessional health care team (e.g., respiratory therapy, pulmonary health specialist) for potential airway clearance measures, additional inhaled medications, or oxygen therapy when a patient has a persistent decrease in SpO_2.

Equipment

- Oximeter
- Oximeter probe appropriate for patient and recommended by oximeter manufacturer
- Acetone or nail polish remover if needed
- Pen and vital sign flow sheet in chart or EHR

Procedural Steps

1. Identify patient using at least two person-specific identifiers (e.g., name and date of birth, or name and medical record number) according to employer policy (Accreditation Canada, 2020).
2. Determine need to measure patient's SpO_2. Assess risk factors for decreased SpO_2 (e.g., acute or chronic compromised respiratory problems, change in oxygen therapy, chest wall injury, recovery from anaesthesia).
3. Throughout the procedure, the 4 moments for hand hygiene are to be implemented; hand hygiene should occur before initial patient (or patient environment) contact, before an aseptic procedure, after body fluid exposure risk, and after patient (or patient environment) contact. Additional hand hygiene should be performed when hands are visibly soiled. Assess for signs and symptoms of alterations in oxygen saturation (e.g., altered respiratory rate, depth, or rhythm; adventitious breath sounds [see Chapter 8]; cyanotic nails, lips, mucous membranes, or skin; restlessness; difficulty breathing).
4. Determine whether patient has a latex allergy; disposable adhesive sensors are made of latex.
5. Assess for factors that influence measurement of SpO_2 (e.g., oxygen therapy, respiratory therapy such as postural drainage and percussion; hemoglobin level, hypotension, temperature, nail polish [Luks & Swenson, 2020]; medications such as bronchodilators).
6. Review patient's medical record for health care provider's prescription and employer policy for standard of care for measurement of SpO_2.
7. Determine previous baseline SpO_2 (if available) from patient's record.
8. Determine most appropriate patient-specific site (e.g., finger, earlobe, bridge of nose, forehead) for sensor probe placement by measuring capillary refill (see Chapter 8). If capillary refill is greater than 2 seconds, select alternative site.
   - Site must have adequate local circulation and be free of moisture.
   - If patient has tremors or is likely to move, use earlobe or forehead. Motion artifact is the most common cause of inaccurate readings (Luks & Swenson, 2020).
   - If patient's finger is too large for the clip-on probe, as may be the case with obesity or edema, the clip-on probe may not fit properly; obtain a disposable (tape-on) probe.
9. Arrange equipment at the bedside.
10. Position patient comfortably. Instruct them to breathe normally.
11. Attach sensor to monitoring site (see Step 11 illustration). If using finger, remove fingernail polish from digit with acetone or polish remover. Instruct patient that clip-on probe will feel like a clothespin on the finger but will not hurt.

Continued

Procedural Guideline 7.2 *Measuring Oxygen Saturation (Pulse Oximetry)—cont'd*

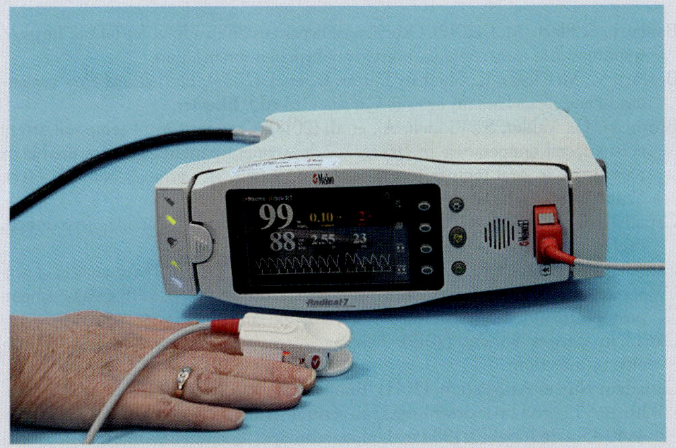

STEP 11 Oximeter sensor attached to finger.

Critical Decision Point *Do not attach probe to finger, ear, or bridge of nose if area is edematous or skin integrity is compromised. Do not use earlobe or bridge of nose sensors for infants and toddlers because of skin fragility. Do not attach sensor to fingers that are hypothermic. Select ear or bridge of nose if adult patient has a history of peripheral vascular disease. Do not use disposable adhesive sensors if patient has a latex allergy. Do not place sensor on same extremity as electronic BP cuff because blood flow to finger will be interrupted temporarily when cuff inflates and cause inaccurate reading that can trigger alarms* (Kitamoto et al., 2020).

12. Once sensor is in place, turn on oximeter by activating power. Observe pulse waveform/intensity display and audible beep. Correlate oximeter pulse rate with patient's radial pulse.
13. Leave sensor in place for 10–30 seconds or until oximeter readout reaches constant value and pulse display reaches full strength during each cardiac cycle. Inform patient that oximeter alarm will sound if sensor falls off or patient moves it. Read SpO_2 on digital display.
14. If you plan to monitor SpO_2 continuously, verify that SpO_2 alarm limits preset by manufacturer are at a low of 85% and a high of 100%. Determine limits for SpO_2 and pulse rate as indicated by patient's condition. For example, patients receiving oxygen because of an acute exacerbation of chronic obstructive pulmonary disease (COPD) should have their oxygen saturation levels maintained between 88 and 92% (Echevarria et al., 2021). Verify that alarms are on. Assess skin integrity under sensor probe every 2 hours; relocate sensor at least every 4 hours and more frequently if skin integrity is altered or tissue perfusion compromised.
15. If you plan intermittent or spot checking of SpO_2, remove probe and turn oximeter power off. Clean sensor and store sensor in appropriate location.
16. Discuss findings with patient.
17. Compare SpO_2 with patient's previous baseline and acceptable SpO_2. Compared with younger adults, older adults typically have lower SpO_2 levels within the normal limits (Lapum et al., 2021).
18. Record SpO_2 on vital sign flow sheet in chart or EHR; indicate type and amount of oxygen therapy used by patient during assessment; record any signs or symptoms of alterations in SpO_2 in narrative form in progress notes in EHR or chart.
19. Report abnormal findings to nurse in charge or health care provider.
20. **Use teach-back:** "I want to be sure I explained why you need to keep the probe on your finger. Tell me why this measurement is important and how moving your finger affects the reading." Develop a revised teaching plan if patient or caregiver is unable to teach back correctly.

BOX 7.10

Characteristics of Pulse Oximeter Sensor Probes and Sites

Finger Probe
- Easy to apply, conforms to various sizes

Earlobe Probe
- Clip-on is smaller and lighter, although more positional than finger probe
- Yields strong correlation with oxygen saturation
- Good when uncontrollable or rhythmic movements (e.g., hand tremors during exercise) are present
- Vascular bed least affected by decreased blood flow

Forehead Sensor
- Greater accuracy during decreased perfusion (Seifi et al., 2018)
- Reliable for patients on vasoactive medications
- Detects desaturation quicker than other sites (Seifi et al., 2018)
- Does not require a pulsatile vascular bed
- Good when uncontrollable or rhythmic movements (e.g., hand tremors) are present
- Requires headband to secure sensor

Disposable Sensor Pad
- Can be applied to a variety of sites: earlobe of adult; nose bridge; palm; or sole of infant
- Less restrictive for continuous oxygen saturation monitoring
- Expensive
- Contains latex
- Skin under adhesive may become moist and harbour pathogens
- Available in variety of sizes; pad can be matched to infant weight

✦ REVIEW QUESTIONS

The nurse is caring for a 56-year-old university professor who is admitted from the trauma unit following a motorcycle–automobile accident. The patient has a fractured left humerus and pelvis. Although the patient was wearing a helmet, they suffered a concussion. When doing the admission assessment, the nurse notes a cast on the patient's left arm and an intravenous (IV) line in the right antecubital fossa. The patient's sister is present and tells you that the patient is on a beta blocker for mild hypertension. The patient has received IV morphine sulphate 15 mg in the emergency department and is very sleepy. The patient awakens only to touch.

Review Questions 1 to 3 relate to the case study presented here.

1. Which admission vital signs can you assign to the unregulated care provider (UCP)? Which directions should the nurse provide the UCP regarding obtaining routine vital signs for this patient?
2. An hour after admission the patient has stabilized. One hour later, the UCP reports the radial pulse rate is 54 beats/min. The nurse notes that the emergency department nurse recorded a heart rate (HR) of 108. What might explain the change in HR? Which interventions should the nurse consider at this time?
3. Two hours after admission, the patient's respiratory rate is 12 breaths/min, oxygen saturation (SpO_2) is 90%, blood pressure (BP) is 112/60 mm Hg, and pulse is 92 beats/min. The nurse repeats and confirms these vital signs and notes that the patient is very difficult to rouse. Using SBAR (situation–background–assessment–recommendation), show how the nurse should communicate with the health care team about this patient.
4. Which of the following conditions should the nurse identify as possibly causing a falsely elevated BP measurement? (*Select all that apply.*)
   1. Arm positioned above heart level
   2. Deflating the cuff too slowly
   3. Inflating the cuff too fast
   4. Loose-fitting cuff
   5. Using an adult cuff on a toddler
5. Which of the following conditions should the nurse expect to cause an error in SpO_2 measurement? (*Select all that apply.*)
   1. Probe placed on finger with clear pink nail polish
   2. Finger probe on patient with a temperature of 35°C (95°F)
   3. Ear probe on patient with a temperature of 38.5°C (101.3°F)
   4. Foot probe on infant who is actively moving
   5. Forehead probe on patient who is perspiring

Visit the Evolve site for a complete list of answers to the Review Questions.

✦ NEXT GENERATION NCLEX® (NGN)

For practice with answering exam questions related to unfolding NGN case studies, please consult the Next Generation NCLEX® (NGN)-Style Case Studies for Skills and Techniques on the Evolve website: http://evolve.elsevier.com/Canada/Perry/clinicalskills/

REFERENCES

Accreditation Canada. (2020). *Required organizational practices handbook*. https://physicians.nshealth.ca/resources/required-organizational-practices-2020-handbook

Anderson, R. (2018). 2.13 Quick priority assessment (QPA). In *Clinical procedures for safer patient care–Thompson Rivers University Edition*. BCcampus. https://pressbooks.bccampus.ca/clinicalproceduresforsaferpatientcaretrubscn/chapter/2-13-quick-priority-assessment-qpa/

Astle, B. J., & Duggleby, W. (2024). *Canadian fundamentals of nursing* (7th ed.). Elsevier.

Basilie, J., & Bloch, M. J. (2018). Overview of hypertension in adults. *UpToDate*. https://www.uptodate.com/contents/overview-of-hypertension-in-adults

Boscart, V., McCleary, L., Sheiban Taucar, L., et al. (2023). *Ebersole and Hess' gerontological nursing and healthy aging in Canada* (3rd ed.). Elsevier.

Brosinski, C., Valdez, S., Riddell, A., et al. (2018). Comparison of temporal artery versus rectal temperature in emergency department patients who are unable to participate in oral temperature assessment. *Journal of Emergency Nursing, 44*(1), 57–63. https://doi.org/10.1016/j.jen.2017.04.015

Canada Safety Council. (2019). *Heat stroke is no joke*. https://canadasafetycouncil.org/heat-stroke-is-no-joke/

Canadian Agency for Drugs and Technologies in Health. (2017). *The assessment of postoperative vitals: Clinical effectiveness and guidelines*. https://www.cadth.ca/assessment-postoperative-vital-signs-clinical-effectiveness-and-guidelines

Canadian Cancer Society. (2019). *Infection*. https://cancer.ca/en/treatments/side-effects/infection

Canadian Nurses Association. (2011). *Position statement: Interprofessional collaboration*. https://hl-prod-ca-oc-download.s3-ca-central-1.amazonaws.com/CNA/2f975e7e-4a40-45ca-863c-5ebf0a138d5e/UploadedImages/documents/Interproffessional_Collaboration_position_statement.pdf [Seminal Reference].

Canadian Paediatric Society (CPS). (2022). *Fever and temperature taking*. https://caringforkids.cps.ca/handouts/health-conditions-and-treatments/fever_and_temperature_taking

Chaddha, A., Modaff, D., Hooper-Lane, C., et al. (2019). Device and non-device-guided slow breathing to reduce blood pressure: A systematic review and meta-analysis. *Complementary Therapies in Medicine, 45*, 179–184. https://doi.org/10.1016/j.ctim.2019.03.005

de Queiroz Junior, J. R. A., Melo, I. O., Calado, G. H. D. S., et al. (2021). Identification and resistance profile of bacteria isolated on stethoscopes by health care professionals: Systematic review. *American Journal of Infection Control, 49*(2), 229–237. https://doi.org/10.1016/j.ajic.2020.07.007

Diabetes Canada. (2023). *Hypertension*. https://www.diabetes.ca/diabetes-and-you/complications/high-blood-pressure

Echevarria, C., Steer, J., Watson, J., et al. (2021). Oxygen therapy and inpatient mortality in COPD exacerbation. *Emergency Medicine Journal, 38*(3), 170–177. https://dx.doi.org/10.1136/emermed-2019-209257

Fitzwater, J., Johnstone, C., Schippers, M., et al. (2019). A comparison of oral, axillary, and temporal artery temperature measuring devices in adult acute care. *Medsurg Nursing, 28*(1), 35–41. https://www.thefreelibrary.com/A+Comparison+of+Oral%2C+Axillary%2C+and+Temporal+Artery+Temperature...-a0577027472

Foster, J., Lloyd, A. B., & Havenith, G. (2021). Non-contact infrared assessment of human body temperature: The journal *Temperature* toolbox. *Temperature, 8*(4), 306–319. https://doi.org/10.1080/23328940.2021.1899546

Heart and Stroke Foundation of Canada. (2018). *Risk factors you cannot change*. https://www.heartandstroke.ca/heart/risk-and-prevention/risk-factors-you-cannot-change

Heshmat-Ghahdarijani, K., Ghasempour Dabaghi, G., Rabiee Rad, M., et al. (2022). The relation between inter arm blood pressure difference and presence of cardiovascular disease: A review of current findings. *Current Problems in Cardiology, 47*(11), 10187. https://doi.org/10.1016/j.cpcardiol.2021.101087

Hockenberry, M. J., Duffy, E. A., & Gibbs, K. (2024). *Wong's nursing care of infants and children* (12th ed.). Elsevier.

Hypertension Canada. (2020a). *Accurate measurement of blood pressure*. https://guidelines.hypertension.ca/diagnosis-assessment/measuring-blood-pressure/

Hypertension Canada. (2020b). *Hypertension Canada guidelines*. https://guidelines.hypertension.ca

Hypertension Canada. (2020c). *Recommended technique for home blood pressure measurement (HBPM)*. https://guidelines.hypertension.ca/diagnosis-assessment/supplementary-tables/#suptbl1d

Jarvis, C., Browne, J., MacDonald-Jenkins, J., & Luctkar-Flude, M. (2024). *Physical examination and health assessment* (4th ed.). Elsevier.

Khan, S., Saultry, B., Adams, S., et al. (2021). Comparative accuracy testing of non-contact infrared thermometers and temporal artery thermometers in an adult hospital setting. *American Journal of Infection Control, 49*(5), 597–602. https://doi.org/10.1016/j.ajic.2020.09.012

Kiekkas, P., Aretha, D., Almpani, E., et al. (2019). Temporal artery thermometry in pediatric patients: Systematic review and meta-analysis. *Journal of Pediatric Nursing, 46*, 89–99. https://doi.org/10.1016/j.pedn.2019.03.004

Kitamoto, N., Hitosugi, T., Kawakubo, Y., et al. (2020). The measurement of blood pressure by the linear method compared to the deflation methods differently modifies the pulse oximeter alarm frequency. *Blood Pressure Monitoring, 25*(1), 13–17. https://doi.org/10.1097/MBP.0000000000000408

Lapum, J. L., Verkuyl, M., Garcia, W., et al. (2021). *Vital sign measurement across the lifespan* (2nd ed.). BCcampus. https://opentextbc.ca/vitalsignmeasurement/

Luks, A. M., & Swenson, E. R. (2020). Pulse oximetry for monitoring patients with COVID-19 at home. Potential pitfalls and practical guidelines. *Annals of the American Thoracic Society, 17*(9), 1040–1046. https://doi.org/10.1513/AnnalsATS.202005-418FR

Maduagwu, S., Umeonwuka, C. I., Mohammad, H. W., et al. (2018). Reference arm for blood pressure measurement in stroke survivors. *Middle East Journal of Rehabilitation and Health Studies*, *5*(1), e62368. https://doi.org/10.5812/mejrh.62368

Mattoo, T. (2018). Definition and diagnosis of hypertension in children and adolescents. *UpToDate*. https://www.uptodate.com/contents/definition-and-diagnosis-of-hypertension-in-children-and-adolescents

Mickley, J. P., Evans, K. D., Tatarski, R. L., et al. (2018). Pilot application of varied equipment and procedural techniques to determine clinical blood pressure measurements. *Journal of Diagnostic Medical Sonography*, *36*(4), 446–458. https://doi.org/10.1177/8756479318800303

Mogensen, C. B., Wittenhoff, L., Fruerhøj, G., et al. (2018). Forehead or ear temperature measurement cannot replace rectal measurements, except for screening purposes. *BMC Pediatrics*, *18*(15), 1–6. https://doi.org/10.1186/s12887-018-0994-1

National Collaborating Centre for Environmental Health. (2015). *Cleanup instructions for small mercury spills*. https://ncceh.ca/sites/default/files/Small_Mercury_Spills_Clean-up_Oct_2015.pdf

National Institutes of Health. (2021). *Health literacy*. https://www.nih.gov/institutes-nih/nih-office-director/office-communications-public-liaison/clear-communication/health-literacy

PedsCases. (2018). *Pediatric vital signs reference chart*. https://www.pedscases.com/pediatric-vital-signs-reference-chart

Qi, W., Wu, Q., Wu, Y., et al. (2017). Talking with a doctor during a visit elicits increases in systolic and diastolic blood pressure. *Blood Pressure Monitoring*, *22*(5), 265–267. https://doi.org/10.1097/MBP.0000000000000270

Rabi, D. M., McBrien, K. A., Sapir-Pichhadze, R., et al. (2020). Hypertension Canada's 2020 comprehensive guidelines for the prevention, diagnosis, risk assessment, and treatment of hypertension in adults and children. *Canadian Journal of Cardiology*, *36*(5), 596–624. https://doi.org/10.1016/j.cjca.2020.02.086

Rolfe, S. (2019). The importance of respiratory rate monitoring. *British Journal of Nursing*, *228*(8), 504–508. https://doi.org/10.12968/bjon.2019.28.8.504

Schlader, Z. J., & Vargas, N. T. (2018). Regulation of body temperature by autonomic and behavioural thermoeffectors. *Exercise and Sports Sciences Reviews*, *47*(2), 116–126. https://doi.org/10.1249/JES.0000000000000180

Seifi, S., Khatony, A., Moradi, G., et al. (2018). Accuracy of pulse oximetry in detection of oxygen saturation in patients admitted to the intensive care unit of heart surgery: Comparison of finger, toe, forehead and earlobe probes. *BMC Nursing*, *17*(5), 15. https://doi.org/10.1186/s12912-018-0283-1

Sims, M. A., Patton, R. A., Williamson, J., et al. (2018). Selection of the most accurate thermometer devices for clinical practice. *Paediatric Nurse*, *44*(3), 134–154. https://www.thefreelibrary.com/Selection+of+the+Most+Accurate+Thermometer+Devices+for+Clinical...-a0546432762

Spence, J. D. (2021). Risk from low blood pressure in frail older adults: Diastolic pressure and pulse pressure are important. *Age and Ageing*, *50*(6), e5–e6. https://doi.org/10.1093/ageing/afaa084

Takayama, A., Takeshima, T., Nakashima, Y., et al. (2019). A comparison of methods to count breathing frequency. *Respiratory Care*, *64*(5), 555–563. https://doi.org/10.4187/respcare.06451

Tran, J., Hillebrand, S. L., Meskers, C. G. M., et al. (2021). Prevalence of initial orthostatic hypotension in older adults: A systematic review and meta-analysis. *Age and Ageing*, *50*(5), 1520–1528. https://doi.org/10.1093/ageing/afab090

Tyerman, J., & Cobbett, S. (Eds.) (2023). *Lewis's medical-surgical nursing in Canada: Assessment and management of clinical problems* (5th ed.). Elsevier Inc.

Vorvick, L. (2022). *Temperature measurement*. MedlinePlus. https://medlineplus.gov/ency/article/003400.htm

Wheatley, I. (2018). Respiratory rate 3: How to take an accurate measurement. *Nursing Times*, *114*(7), 21–22. https://www.nursingtimes.net/clinical-archive/respiratory-clinical-archive/respiratory-rate-3-how-to-take-an-accurate-measurement-25-06-2018/

World Health Organization. (2021). *Oxygen*. https://www.who.int/news-room/questions-and-answers/item/oxygen

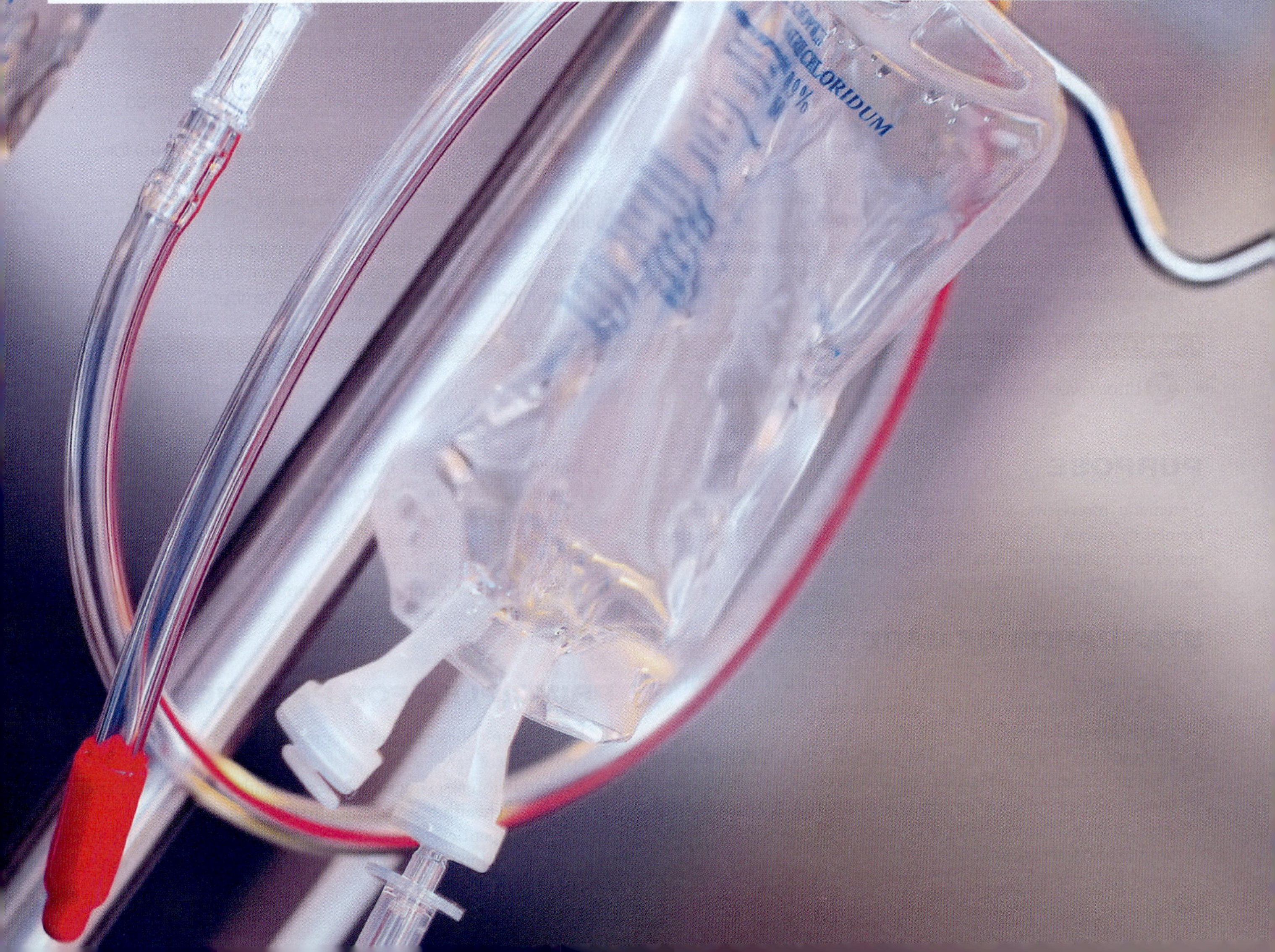

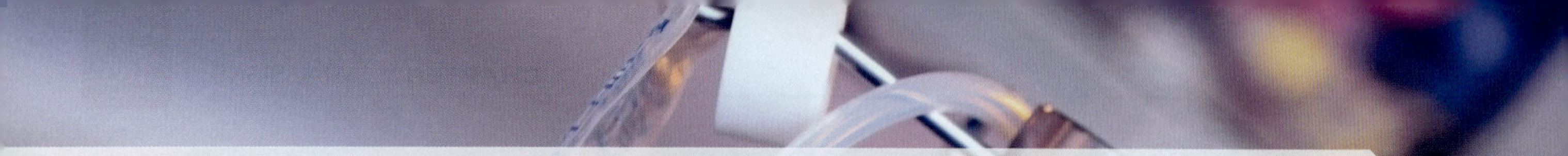

8 Health Assessment

Canadian content written by **Chantal Singh, RN, MScN**
Original US chapter by **Angela McConachie, FNP, DNP**

SKILLS AND PROCEDURES

OBJECTIVES

Mastery of content in this chapter will enable the nurse to:

- Explain the purposes of health assessment.
- Describe the techniques used with each physical assessment skill.
- Describe proper patient positioning during each phase of the examination.
- Describe how to conduct a physical examination on patients from different cultures.
- List techniques to promote a patient's physical and psychological comfort during an examination.
- Make environmental preparations before an assessment.
- Identify data to collect from the nursing history before an examination.
- Describe normal physical findings for patients across the lifespan.
- Describe ways to incorporate health promotion and health teaching into an assessment.
- Identify self-screening assessments commonly performed by patients.
- Identify preventive screenings and the appropriate age(s) for each screening.
- Apply physical assessment techniques and skills during routine nursing care.
- Document assessment findings on appropriate forms.
- Use interprofessional collaboration to communicate abnormal findings to appropriate team members.

MEDIA RESOURCES

- http://evolve.elsevier.com/Canada/Perry/clinicalskills/

PURPOSE

Systematic interviews and physical assessments are regularly performed by nurses to assess the status of a patient's health and their perception of their own health. The information gathered is documented in the patient's database.

STANDARDS OF CARE

- Canadian Task Force on Preventive Health Care (2019)—*Published Guidelines* (https://canadiantaskforce.ca/guidelines/published-guidelines/)
- College of Family Physicians of Canada (2013)—*Annual Physical Examination Practices by Province/Territory in Canada* (https://www.cfpc.ca/en/policy-innovation/health-policy-goverment-relations/cfpc-policy-papers-position-statements/annual-physical-examination)
- Indigenous Services Canada (2015)—*Clinical Practice Guidelines for Nurses in Primary Care* (https://www.canada.ca/en/indigenous-services-canada/services/first-nations-inuit-health/health-care-services/nursing/clinical-practice-guidelines-nurses-primary-care.html)
- Infection Prevention and Control Canada (2022)—*Guidelines and Standards* (https://ipac-canada.org/evidence-based-guidelines.php)

PRINCIPLES FOR PRACTICE

- Use ongoing objective and comprehensive assessment to promote continuity of care.
- An admission assessment involves a detailed review of a patient's condition, health history, and physical examination.
- Use therapeutic communication techniques, including open-ended questions, to encourage information sharing. For example,

as a patient is describing a symptom, you can say "go on" to probe further.

- Use critical thinking skills and clinical judgement for evaluation and interpretation of findings within the context of the individual patient.
- Initial assessment and examination provide a baseline for a patient's functional status and serve as a comparison for future assessment findings. In addition, the information is useful in making clinical decisions about the management of a patient's health problems.
- Use diagnostic or clinical reasoning to analyze health data and draw conclusions to identify actual or potential diagnoses and prioritize care.
- Immediately address any *first-level priority problems* encountered, such as life-threatening airway, breathing, or cardiac problems (Jarvis et al., 2024).
- Promptly intervene to address *second-level priority problems*, such as acute pain or mental status changes, to prevent further deterioration.
- Address *third-level priority problems*, such as knowledge deficits and health promotion, after more urgent health problems are resolved or stabilized.
- Use interprofessional collaboration to assess and manage patient health problems.
- Practise person-centred nursing care and ensure patient safety and confidentiality.

PERSON-CENTRED CARE

- Conduct a person-centred interview to learn about issues from the patient's perspective.
- The nurse should establish the therapeutic nurse–patient relationship by introducing themselves to the patient and caregiver(s). Show respect to patients, their families, and caregivers when seeking their involvement in the patient's plan of care.
- Have patients explain their symptoms by allowing them to offer details.
- After gathering data, group significant findings into patterns of data (clusters) that reveal actual or potential nursing diagnoses (Table 8.1).
- Be open to continually informing, communicating with, and educating patients and caregivers regarding relevant information or the plan of care.
- Integrate health promotion and education into physical assessment activities. It is an ideal time to offer individualized patient teaching and to encourage promotion of health practices such as breast (Box 8.1) and genital (see Box 8.6) self-examination.
- Ensure that the patient is comfortable and free from pain before beginning an examination and during your assessment.
- Acknowledge and respect patient's cultural diversity and beliefs when completing assessments; eye contact or physical touch may be considered inappropriate or offensive in some cultures (Ball et al., 2022).
- Communicate respect through proper use of distance, attention, eye contact, tone, loudness of voice, and other forms of body language.
- Use a professional interpreter familiar with a patient's culture and language if appropriate.
- Obtain information about health risks common to a cultural group (i.e., prevalence of certain diseases).
- Provide gender-affirming care by asking patients whether they have preferred pronouns or terms they would like used to address them (Rainbow Health Ontario, 2020).

TABLE 8.1

Development of Individualized Nursing Diagnoses

Assessment Method	Findings	Pattern	Nursing Diagnosis
Inspection of skin	Skin along sacral area is intact. There is a 3-cm area of redness around coccyx; skin blanches on palpation. No skin lesions are observed.	There is tissue injury area around coccyx.	Potential for impaired skin integrity
Palpation of skin	Skin is moist from diaphoresis. There is tenderness to palpation at sacral area. Skin turgor is elastic.	Skin moisture promotes maceration.	
Historical data	Patient suffered fractured left leg. Patient is immobilized because of left leg traction.	Continued pressure is exerted over sacrum.	

BOX 8.1

Breast Self-Examination

The updated Canadian Task Force on Preventive Health Care (2018) guidelines for breast cancer screening in average-risk cisgender women and nonoperative transgender men aged 40–74 years recommend not advising individuals to routinely practise breast self-examination (BSE) because neither clinical breast examination nor BSE has been shown to reduce mortality. Although research does not support a clear benefit of regular BSE, it is important for all persons to be aware of their breasts' normal appearance and feel, even if they get regular screening tests (Canadian Cancer Society [CCS], 2022b). To teach a patient to perform BSE, instruct them to disrobe to the waist and inspect their breasts in front of a mirror; to palpate their breasts while lying supine, which flattens the breast tissue; or to examine the breasts in the shower using soap and water, which assists with palpation (Jarvis et al., 2024). Patients should be told about the benefits and limitations of BSE and to report any breast changes to their health care provider right away. Reinforce that the great majority of breast lumps are benign.

- Drape the patient thoroughly, use the bedside curtains, and ask permission before touching the patient. This is an important part of person-centred care for patients from all cultures.

EVIDENCE-INFORMED PRACTICE

Organizations such as the Canadian Cancer Society support research and develop practice guidelines for the prevention and management of certain diseases such as skin cancer. The Canadian Cancer Society (CCS, 2022a) recommends that people practise the six principles of sun safety: (1) check the ultraviolet (UV) index every day; (2) seek shade; (3) cover up; (4) wear sunglasses; (5) use sunscreen properly; and (6) do not use indoor tanning beds. Risk factors for melanoma are as follows: exposure to UV radiation (from the sun or indoor tanning equipment); many moles or an atypical mole; familial atypical multiple mole melanoma (FAMMM) syndrome; light-coloured skin, eyes, and hair; personal or family history of skin cancer or *CDKN2A* gene mutation; history of blistering sunburn; and other inherited conditions such as xeroderma pigmentosum, Werner syndrome, and retinoblastoma (CCS, 2022k). The Canadian Cancer Society makes the following recommendations as part of prevention and early detection of skin cancer (CCS, 2022l):

- People should recognize symptoms of skin cancer and report symptoms or skin changes to their health care provider promptly.
- People should inform their health care provider promptly about any of the following: a sore that does not heal; areas of skin that are smooth and pearly, look waxy, and sometimes bleed; a firm spot or lump that may have a hard, rough, scaly, or crusted surface; a flat reddish patch of skin; any new moles; moles or spots that look different from other spots on the skin, or any change in the colour, size, and shape of existing skin lesions.
- People at higher-than-average risk should talk to their health care provider about a personal plan for testing that may include having regular skin exams by a health care provider.

SAFETY GUIDELINES

- Prioritize assessments based on the patient's presenting signs and symptoms or health needs. For example, when a patient develops sudden shortness of breath, first assess the lungs and thorax. If a patient is acutely ill, you may choose to assess only the involved body systems. Rule out urgent concerns utilizing critical thinking and clinical judgement, progressing to less urgent portions of the assessment.
- Organize an examination. Compare both sides of the body for symmetry. If a patient becomes fatigued, offer rest periods. Perform painful or intrusive procedures near the end of an examination.
- In a comprehensive assessment, use a head-to-toe approach following the sequence of inspection, palpation, percussion, and auscultation (except during abdominal assessment). This sequence facilitates an effective assessment.
- Encourage a patient's active participation. Patients usually know about their physical condition. Often a patient or caregiver can provide useful information regarding their baseline or changes.
- Follow routine practices for infection control with all patients and additional precautions when warranted. During an assessment, you may have contact with body fluids and discharge. Always wear clean gloves when there are breaks in the skin, lesions, or wounds or when having contact with mucous membranes. Complete a point-of-care risk assessment for use of personal protective equipment (PPE) before each patient encounter (see Chapter 5, Box 5.1).
- Consider the possibility of latex allergy. The incidence of serious allergic reaction to latex has increased dramatically (Ball et al., 2022).
- Record quick notes to facilitate accurate documentation. Inform the patient that you will be recording the data.
- Record a summary of the assessment using appropriate medical terminology and in the sequence that findings are gathered. Use only employer-approved documentation abbreviations. Be thorough and descriptive, especially for abnormal findings.

ASSESSMENT TECHNIQUES

Use assessment techniques during each patient contact, including activities such as bathing, administering medications, other therapies, or while talking with a patient. This practice will help you learn to become more observant and better able to identify changes quickly.

Inspection, palpation, percussion, auscultation, and olfaction are the five basic assessment techniques. Each skill allows you to collect a broad range of physical data about patients. Nurses need experience to recognize normal variations among patients and ranges of normal for an individual. Cultural diversity is one factor that influences both normal variations and potential alterations that you may find during an assessment. It is important to take the time needed to carefully assess each body part. Hurrying can cause you to overlook significant signs and make incorrect conclusions about a patient's condition.

Inspection

Inspection is the visual examination of body parts or areas. An experienced nurse learns to make multiple observations almost simultaneously while becoming very perceptive of any abnormalities. The secret is to always be observant—pay attention to patients. Watch all movements and look carefully at the body part you are inspecting. It is important to recognize normal physical characteristics of patients of all ages before trying to distinguish abnormal findings.

Inspection requires good lighting and full exposure of body parts. Inspect each area for size, shape, colour, symmetry, position, and the presence of abnormalities. If possible, inspect each area compared with the same area on the opposite side of the body. When necessary, use additional light such as a penlight to inspect body cavities such as the mouth and throat. *Do not hurry. Pay attention to detail.* Verify and clarify all abnormalities with subjective patient data. In other words, ask the patient for further information about each abnormality or change, such as whether the change is recent. Let patient data and your knowledge of anatomy, physiology, and pathophysiology guide your inspection.

Palpation

Palpation involves the sense of touch. Through palpation, the hands make delicate and sensitive measurements of specific physical signs. Palpation is used to detect resistance, resilience, roughness, texture, temperature, moisture, and mobility. Nurses often use it with or after visual inspection. Use different parts of the hand to detect specific characteristics. For example, the dorsum (back) of the hand is sensitive to temperature variations. The pads of the fingertips detect subtle changes in texture, shape, size, consistency, and pulsation of body parts. The palm of the hand is especially sensitive to vibration. Measure position, consistency, and turgor by lightly grasping a body part with the fingertips.

Help a patient relax and assume a comfortable position because muscle tension during palpation impairs the ability to palpate correctly. Asking the patient to take slow, deep breaths enhances muscle relaxation. Palpate tender areas last because they could cause the patient to become tense and impede the assessment. Ask the patient to point out areas that are more sensitive, and note any nonverbal signs of discomfort. Patients appreciate clean, warm hands; short fingernails; and a gentle approach. Palpation is either light or deep and is controlled by the amount of pressure applied with the fingers or hand. Light palpation precedes deep palpation. Consider a patient's condition, the area being palpated, and the reason for using palpation. For example, when a patient is admitted to the emergency department after an automobile accident, consider the factors surrounding the patient's injury and inspect the chest wall carefully before performing any palpation around the area of the ribs.

For light palpation, apply pressure slowly, gently, and deliberately, depressing approximately 1 cm (Fig. 8.1, *A*). Check tender areas further, using light, intermittent pressure. After light palpation, nurses in advanced practice roles may use deeper palpation to examine the condition of organs (Fig. 8.1, *B*). Depress the area you are examining by approximately 2 cm. Caution is the rule. Bimanual palpation involves one hand placed over the other while applying pressure. The upper hand exerts downward pressure as the other hand feels the subtle characteristics of underlying organs and masses. Seek the help of a qualified health care provider or nurse before attempting deep palpation.

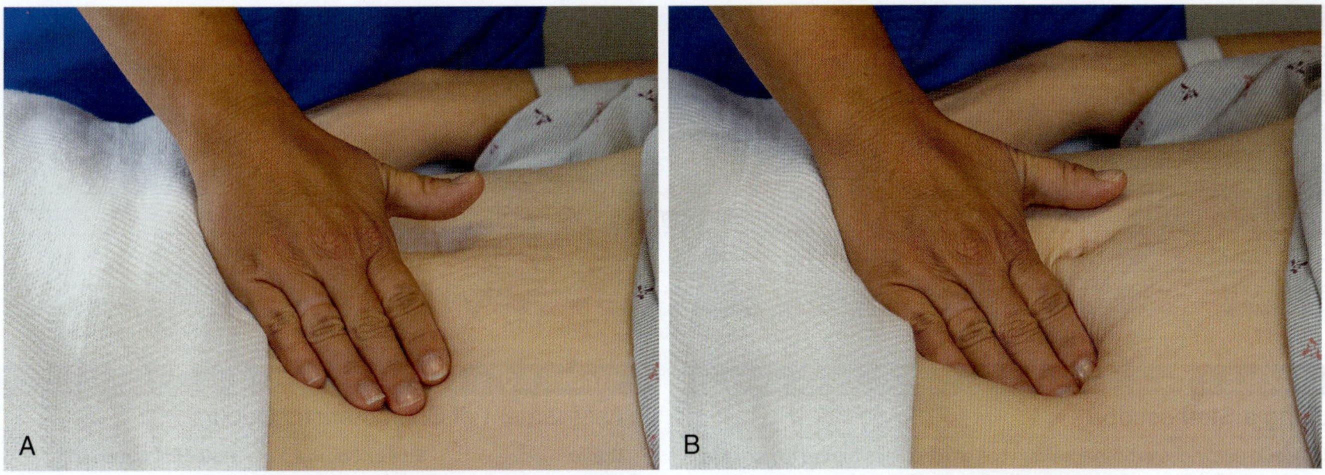

FIG 8.1 **A, During light palpation, use gentle pressure against underlying skin and tissues to detect areas of irregularity and tenderness. B, During deep palpation, depress tissue to assess condition of underlying organs.** *(From Ball, J. W., Dains, J. E., Flynn, J. A., et al. [2022]. Seidel's guide to physical examination: An interprofessional approach [10th ed.]. Elsevier.)*

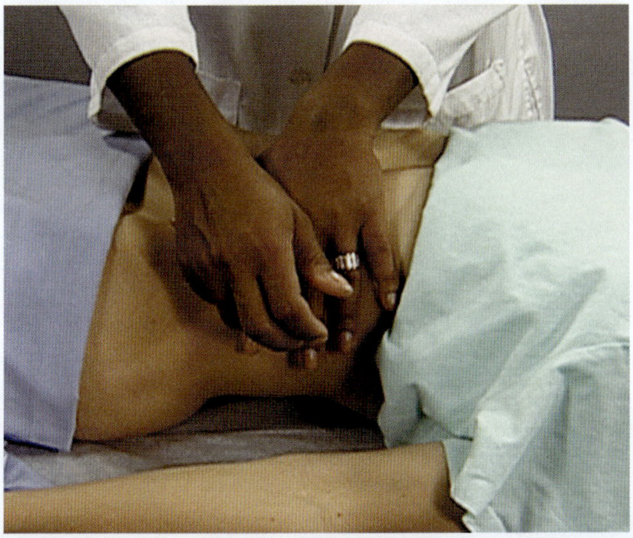

FIG 8.2 **Percussion technique: Tapping the interphalangeal joint.** *(From Ball, J. W., Dains, J. E., Flynn, J. A., et al. [2022]. Seidel's guide to physical examination: An interprofessional approach [10th ed.]. Elsevier.)*

Percussion

Percussion involves tapping the body with the fingertips to vibrate underlying tissues and organs. The vibration travels through body tissues, and the character of the resulting sound reflects the density of underlying tissue. The denser the tissue, the quieter the sound. By knowing various densities of organs and body parts, you learn how to locate organs or masses, map their edges, and determine their size. An abnormal sound suggests a mass or substance such as air or fluid in a body cavity.

The most commonly used percussion technique is the indirect technique. This is performed by placing the middle finger of the nondominant hand firmly against the body surface. With palm and fingers remaining off the skin, the tip of the middle finger of the dominant hand strikes the base of the distal joint of the finger (Fig. 8.2). Use a quick, sharp stroke, keeping the forearm stationary. Relax the wrist to deliver the proper blow. Once the finger has struck, the wrist snaps back. If the blow is not sharp, if the hand is held loosely, or if the palm rests on the body surface then the sound is softened, and you will not detect the presence of underlying structures. A light, quick blow produces the clearest sounds. Table 8.2 describes the five different percussive sounds.

Auscultation

Auscultation is listening with a stethoscope to sounds produced by the body. To auscultate correctly, listen in a quiet environment for both the presence of sound and its characteristics. To be successful in auscultation, you must first recognize normal sounds from each body structure, including the passage of blood through an artery, heart sounds, and movement of air through the lungs. These sounds vary according to the location in which they can be heard most easily. Likewise, you become familiar with areas that normally do not emit sounds. Practise listening to many normal sounds so you can recognize abnormal sounds when they arise.

To auscultate, the nurse needs good hearing acuity, a good stethoscope, and knowledge of how to use the stethoscope properly (Box 8.2). Nurses with hearing challenges may purchase stethoscopes with greater sound amplification. It is essential to place the stethoscope directly on a patient's skin because clothing obscures and changes sound. Through auscultation, the nurse will note that there are four characteristics of sound:

- *Frequency:* Number of sound wave cycles generated per second by a vibrating object. The higher the frequency, the higher the pitch of a sound and vice versa.
- *Loudness:* Amplitude of a sound wave. Auscultated sounds are described as loud or soft.
- *Quality:* Sounds of similar frequency and loudness from different sources. Terms such as *blowing* or *gurgling* describe the quality of sound.
- *Duration:* Length of time that sound vibrations last. Duration of sound is short, medium, or long. Layers of soft tissue dampen the duration of sounds from deep internal organs.

A nurse cannot be successful at auscultation without knowing how to use a stethoscope properly. Chapter 7 describes the parts of the acoustic stethoscope and use of the bell and diaphragm.

Olfaction

Olfaction uses the sense of smell to detect abnormalities that go unrecognized by any other means. Some alterations in body function and certain bacteria create characteristic odours (Table 8.3).

TABLE 8.2

Sounds Produced by Percussion

Sound	Intensity	Pitch	Duration	Quality	Common Location
Tympany	Loud	High	Moderate	Drumlike	Gastric air bubble, puffed-out cheek
Resonant	Loud	Low	Long	Hollow	Healthy lung
Hyperresonant	Very loud	Low	Longer than resonance	Booming	Emphysematous lung
Dull	Soft to moderate	Moderate to high	Moderate	Thudlike	Over liver
Flat	Soft	High	Short	Very dull	Over muscle

BOX 8.2

Using a Stethoscope

1. Place earpieces in both ears with tips of earpieces turned toward the face. *Lightly* blow against the diaphragm (flat side of chest piece). Now place the earpieces in both ears with the tips turned toward the back of the head and again blow against the diaphragm. Compare comfort in the ears and amplification of sounds with earpieces in both directions. After you have learned the right fit for the loudest amplification, wear the stethoscope the same way each time. Earpieces should fit snugly and comfortably.
2. If the stethoscope has both a diaphragm (flat side) and a bell (bowl-shaped with a rubber ring) (see Chapter 7, Fig. 7.7), put earpieces in ears and lightly blow against the diaphragm. The chest piece can be turned to allow sound to be carried through either side (bell or diaphragm). If sound is faint, lightly blow into the bell. Then turn the chest piece and blow again against both the diaphragm and the bell. The diaphragm is used for higher-pitched heart sounds, bowel sounds, and lung sounds. The bell is used for lower-pitched heart sounds and vascular sounds.
3. With earpieces in place and using the diaphragm, move the diaphragm lightly over the hair on your arm. The bristling sound mimics a sound heard in the lungs. When listening for significant sounds, hold the diaphragm still and firmly make a tight seal against the skin to eliminate extraneous sounds.
4. Place the diaphragm over the front of your chest directly on your skin and listen to your own breathing, comparing the bell and the diaphragm. Repeat the process while listening to your own heartbeat. Ask someone to speak in a conversational tone and note how the speech detracts from hearing clearly. When using a stethoscope, both you and the patient should remain quiet.
5. With the earpieces in your ears, gently tap the tubing. Note that it generates extraneous sounds. When listening to a patient, maintain a position that allows the tubing to extend straight and hang free. Movement may allow it to rub or bump objects, creating extraneous sounds. Kinked tubing muffles sounds.
6. *Care of a stethoscope:* Remove earpieces regularly and clean or remove cerumen (earwax). Keep the bell and diaphragm free of dust, lint, and body oils. Keep the tubing away from your body oils. To clean, wipe the entire stethoscope (e.g., diaphragm, tubing) with alcohol or soapy water. Be sure to dry all parts thoroughly. Follow manufacturer recommendations.
7. *Infection control:* Harmful bacteria, even antibiotic-resistant microorganisms, can be transferred from patient to patient when using portable equipment such as stethoscopes (Infection Prevention and Control Canada [IPCC], 2022). Follow employer infection control guidelines to decrease this risk. Clean the stethoscope between patients with isopropyl alcohol or ethanol-based cleaning products (IPCC, 2022).

TABLE 8.3

Assessment of Characteristic Odours

Odour	Site or Source	Potential Causes
Alcohol	Oral cavity	Ingestion of alcohol; diabetes mellitus
Ammonia	Urine	Urinary tract infection, renal failure
Body odour	Skin, particularly in areas where body parts rub together (e.g., under arms, beneath breasts, perineal area)	Poor hygiene, excessive perspiration (hyperhidrosis), foul-smelling perspiration (bromhidrosis)
	Wound site	Wound abscess; infection
	Vomitus	Abdominal irritation, contaminated food
Feces	Rectal area	Bowel incontinence; fistula
	Vomitus/oral cavity (fecal odour)	Bowel obstruction
Fetid, sweet odour	Tracheostomy or mucous secretions	Infection of bronchial tree (*Pseudomonas* bacteria)
Foul-smelling stools in infants	Stool	Malabsorption syndrome
Halitosis	Oral cavity	Poor dental or oral hygiene, gum disease; sinus infection
Musty odour	Casted body part	Infection inside cast
Stale urine	Skin	Uremic acidosis
Sweet, fruity ketones	Oral cavity	Diabetic acidosis
Sweet, heavy, thick odour	Draining wound	*Pseudomonas* (bacterial) infection

PREPARATION FOR ASSESSMENT

Preparation of the environment, equipment, and patient facilitates a smooth assessment. Ensure the environment is warm, quiet, private, and well lit (Jarvis et al., 2024). Practise person-centred care during the physical assessment by providing patient privacy. Position the bed or examination table at waist level to maintain safe body mechanics. During an examination, you must protect the patient from falls and injury and return the bed to a safe height at the completion of the assessment (Jarvis et al., 2024).

Preparing the Patient

Prepare patients both physically and psychologically for accurate assessments. A tense, anxious patient may have difficulty understanding, following directions, or cooperating with your instructions. To prepare a patient:

- Introduce yourself to the patient to begin establishing the therapeutic nurse–patient relationship.

- Ask the patient what their preferred name and/or pronouns are, to demonstrate respect.
- Implement comfort measures (e.g., positioning, hygiene) and provide the opportunity to empty the bowel or bladder (a good time to collect needed specimens).
- Minimize the patient's anxiety and fear by conveying an open, receptive, and professional approach. Using simple terms, thoroughly explain what will be done, what the patient should expect to feel, and how they can participate. Even if a patient appears unresponsive, or is nonverbal, it is still important to explain your actions.
- Provide access to body parts while draping areas that are not being examined.
- Help the patient assume positions during assessment so that body parts are accessible and the patient remains comfortable (Table 8.4). A patient's ability to assume positions depends on their physical strength and limitations. Some positions are

TABLE 8.4

Positions for Physical Assessment

Position	Areas Assessed	Rationale	Limitations
Sitting 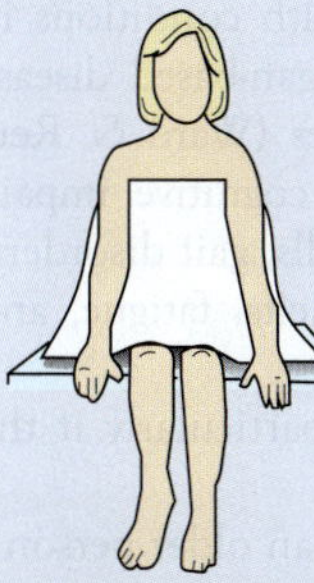	Head and neck, back, posterior thorax and lungs, anterior thorax and lungs, breasts, axillae, heart, vital signs, upper extremities	Sitting upright provides full expansion of lungs and better visualization of symmetry of upper body parts.	Physically weakened or developmentally challenged patient is sometimes unable to sit. Use supine position with head of bed elevated instead.
Supine 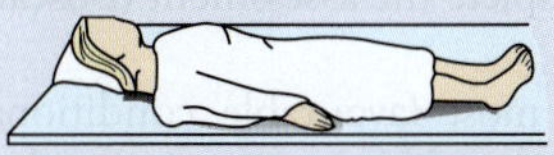	Head and neck, anterior thorax and lungs, breasts, axillae, heart, abdomen, extremities, pulses	This is normally the most relaxed position. It provides easy access to pulse sites.	If patient becomes short of breath easily, raise head of bed.
Dorsal recumbent 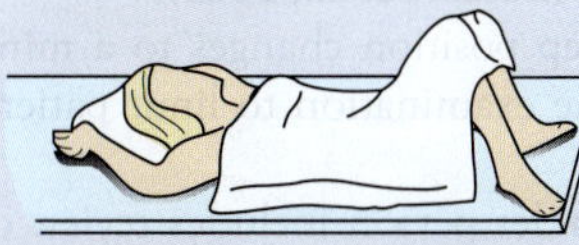	Head and neck, anterior thorax and lungs, breasts, axillae, heart, abdomen	Position is for abdominal assessment because it promotes relaxation of abdominal muscles.	Patients with painful disorders are more comfortable with knees flexed.
Lithotomy 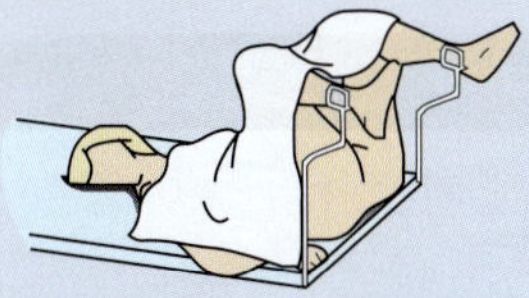	Female genitalia and genital tract	This position provides maximal exposure of genitalia and facilitates insertion of vaginal speculum.	Lithotomy position is embarrassing and uncomfortable; thus, examiner minimizes time that patient spends in it. Keep patient well draped. Patients with arthritis or other joint deformities may be unable to tolerate the position.
Modified left (or right) lateral recumbent position 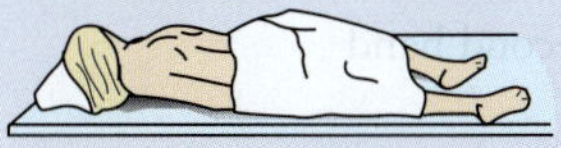	Rectum and vagina	Flexion of hip and knee improves exposure of rectal and genitourinary areas.	Joint deformities hinder patient's ability to bend hip and knee.
Prone 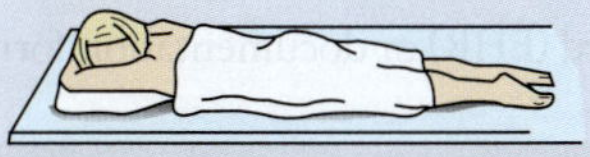	Musculoskeletal system	This position is for assessing extension of hip joint, skin, and buttocks.	Patients with respiratory difficulties do not tolerate this position well.
Lateral recumbent 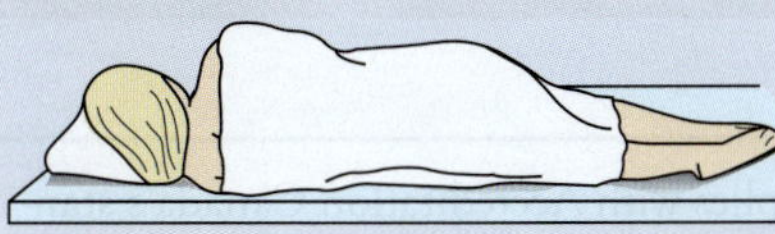	Heart	This position aids in detecting murmurs.	Patients with respiratory difficulties do not tolerate this position well.
Knee–chest 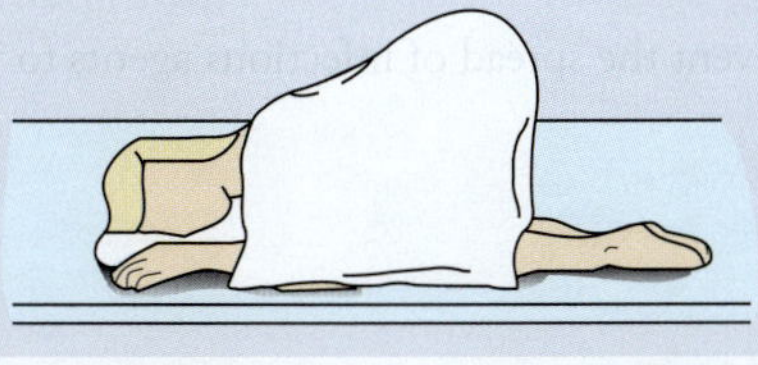	Rectum	This position provides maximal exposure of rectal area.	This position is embarrassing and uncomfortable. Patients with arthritis or other joint deformities may be unable to assume it.

uncomfortable or embarrassing; keep the patient in a given position no longer than necessary.

- Pace assessment according to an individual's physical and emotional tolerance.
- Use a relaxed tone of voice and facial expressions to put the patient at ease.
- Encourage the patient to ask questions and report discomfort felt during the examination.
- Given the potential for accusations of inappropriate conduct (e.g., during a genital exam), it is advisable to have a second health care provider assist in the examination room (see employer policy).
- Maintain a dialogue throughout the examination to explain your actions, ask and answer questions, and provide health teaching.
- At the conclusion of an assessment, ask the patient whether there are any concerns or questions.

PHYSICAL ASSESSMENT OF VARIOUS AGE GROUPS

Children and Adolescents

- Routine assessments of children focus on health promotion and illness prevention, particularly for care of well children with competent parenting and no serious health problems (Hockenberry et al., 2024). Focus on growth and development, sensory screening, dental examination, and behavioural assessment.
- Children who are living with chronic illness, physical or cognitive challenges, in foster care, or adopted internationally may require additional assessments because of unique health needs or risks.
- When obtaining histories of infants and children, gather information from parents or guardians.
- Parents may think that the examiner is testing or judging them. Explain the purpose of assessment, provide support during examination, and do not pass judgement.
- Call children and caregivers by their preferred names.
- Open-ended questions often allow parents to share more information and describe more of the child's problems.
- Older children and adolescents respond best when treated as adults and individuals and often can provide details about their health history and severity of symptoms.
- Older children also have a right to confidentiality. Some children may prefer caregivers to be present during the examination, while others may not. After talking with parents about historical information, arrange to be alone with adolescents to speak privately and perform the examination.

Older Persons

- Do not assume that aging is always accompanied by illness or disability. Older persons can adapt to change and maintain functional independence (Boscart et al., 2023).
- A thorough assessment of an older person provides critical information that can be used to maximize independence. *Geriatric syndrome* is a term that refers to common health conditions in older persons that do not fit into distinct organ-based disease categories and often have multifactorial causes (Ward & Reuben, 2020). Examples of conditions include cognitive impairment, delirium, incontinence, malnutrition, falls, gait disorders, pressure injuries, sleep disorders, sensory deficits, fatigue, and dizziness.
- Provide adequate space for an examination, particularly if the patient uses a mobility aid.
- Plan the history and examination, considering an older person's energy level, physical limitations, pace, and adaptability. You may need more than one session to complete the assessment (Boscart et al., 2023).
- Measure performance under the most favourable conditions. Take advantage of natural opportunities for assessment (e.g., during bathing, grooming, mealtime) (Boscart et al., 2023).
- Sequence the examination to keep position changes to a minimum. Be efficient throughout the examination to limit patient movement.
- Be sure that examination of an older person includes review of mental status.

✦ SKILL 8.1 General Survey

The general survey begins a review of a patient's primary health problems and includes assessment of vital signs, height and weight, general behaviour, and appearance. It provides information about the characteristics of an illness, a patient's hygiene, skin condition and body image, emotional state, recent changes in weight, and developmental status. The survey reveals important information about a patient's behaviour that influences how you communicate instructions and continue an assessment.

Equipment

- Stethoscope
- Sphygmomanometer and cuff
- Thermometer
- Digital watch or wristwatch with second hand
- Tape measure
- Clean gloves (use nonlatex if necessary)
- Tongue blade
- Appropriate electronic health record (EHR) or documentation form

STEP	RATIONALE
ASSESSMENT	
1. Identify patient using at least two person-specific identifiers (e.g., name and date of birth, or name and medical record number) according to employer policy.	Ensures correct patient. Complies with Accreditation Canada's standards and improves patient safety (Accreditation Canada, 2020).
2. Throughout the procedure, the 4 moments for hand hygiene are to be implemented; hand hygiene should occur before initial patient (or patient environment) contact, before an aseptic procedure, after body fluid exposure risk, and after patient (or patient environment) contact. Additional hand hygiene should be performed when hands are visibly soiled.	Proper hand hygiene helps prevent the spread of infectious agents to health care providers.

STEP	RATIONALE
3. Note whether patient has or has had any acute distress, namely difficulty breathing, pain, or anxiety. If such signs are present, defer general survey until later and focus immediately on affected body system.	Signs establish priorities regarding which part of examination to conduct first.
4. Review graphic sheet for previous vital signs and consider factors or conditions that may alter values (see Chapter 7).	Provides baseline and historical data about patient's vital signs.
5. Determine patient's primary language. If you identify the need for an interpreter, determine availability of a professional interpreter. It is best to have an interpreter of the same gender who is older and mature. Have interpreter translate verbatim if possible.	Facilitates patient understanding and promotes accuracy of information provided by patient.
6. After reviewing history, confirm primary reason patient has sought health care.	Keeps assessment focused on patient to ensure their expectations are addressed.
7. Identify patient's normal height, weight, and body mass index. If sudden gain or loss in weight has occurred, determine amount of weight change and period of time in which it occurred. Assess whether patient has recently been dieting or following an exercise program. Use growth chart for children under 18 years of age.	Generally, a body mass index of 25 to 29.9 kg/m^2 for men and women is overweight, whereas 30 kg/m^2 and over is obese (Ball et al., 2022). Fluid retention is one factor that must be ruled out. A person's weight can fluctuate daily because of fluid loss or retention (1 L of water weighs 1 kg [2.2 lbs]).
8. Ask if patient has noticed any changes in condition of skin (e.g., dryness, changes in colour or lack of pigment, changes in moles or new skin lesions).	Skin changes can indicate underlying illnesses (e.g., dry skin may be associated with hypothyroidism; changes in moles may indicate early signs of skin cancers) (Table 8.5).
9. Review patient's past fluid intake and output (I&O) records.	Fluid and electrolyte balance affects health and function in all body systems. Intake includes all liquids taken orally, by feeding tube, and parenterally. Liquid output includes urine, diarrhea stool, vomitus, drainage from fistulas and gastric suction, and drainage from postsurgical tubes such as chest tubes or Jackson–Pratt drains.
10. Identify patient's general perceptions about their personal health.	Assessment of patient's general appearance coupled with patient's own perceptions may reveal specific problem areas.

TABLE 8.5

Skin Colour Variations

Colour	Condition	Cause	Assessment Location
Bluish (cyanosis)	Increased amount of deoxygenated hemoglobin (associated with hypoxia and a late sign of decreased oxygen levels)	Heart or lung disease, cold environment	Nail beds, lips, base of tongue, skin (severe cases)
Pallor (decrease in colour from usual skin colour)	Reduced amount of oxyhemoglobin	Anemia Shock	Face, conjunctivae, nail beds, palms of hands
	Reduced visibility of oxyhemoglobin resulting from decreased blood flow		Skin, nail beds, conjunctivae, lips
Loss of pigmentation	Vitiligo	Congenital autoimmune condition causing lack of pigment	Patchy areas on skin over face, hands, arms
Yellow-orange (jaundice)	Increased deposit of bilirubin in tissues	Liver disease, destruction of red blood cells	Sclerae, mucous membranes, skin (may be more difficult to visualize in patients with increased melanin deposits—assess sclerae and alternate locations to rule out jaundice)
Red (erythema)	Increased visibility of oxyhemoglobin caused by dilation or increased blood flow	Fever, direct trauma, blushing, alcohol intake	Face; area of trauma; and areas at risk for pressure such as sacrum, shoulders, elbows, and heels
Tan-brown	Increased amount of melanin	Suntan, pregnancy	Areas exposed to sun: face, arms; areolae, nipples

STEP	RATIONALE
11. Assess for history of latex allergy, which may include contact dermatitis or systemic reactions. Ask if patient has risk factors such as food allergies (papaya, avocado, banana, peach, kiwi, or tomato); has high latex exposure (housekeepers, food handlers, health care workers); or must avoid products containing latex (rubber bands, adhesive tape, certain paints or carpets).	Gloves are worn during certain parts of the assessment. Repeated exposure to latex may result in more serious reactions, including asthma, itching, and anaphylaxis (Ball et al., 2022).

NURSING DIAGNOSES

- Inadequate breathing pattern
- Inadequate peripheral tissue perfusion
- Pain (acute, chronic)
- Inadequate fluid volume
- Excessive fluid volume
- Inadequate nutrition
- Reduced physical mobility
- Reduced skin integrity
- Anxiety
- Fear
- Decreased self-care: bathing
- Latex allergy response
- Obesity

Related factors are individualized on the basis of patient's condition or needs.

PLANNING

STEP	RATIONALE
1. Expected outcomes following completion of procedure:	
• Patient demonstrates alert, cooperative behaviour without evidence of physical or emotional distress during assessment.	Use calm and confident approach during assessment. Patient has no abnormal findings.
• Patient provides appropriate subjective data related to physical condition.	Patient able to cooperate with assessment.
2. *Prepare patient:* Tell patient that you will be using a routine process to check for areas of concern. Ask patient to tell you whether any area that you examine hurts when touched.	Understanding promotes patient's cooperation. Pain is an important finding during assessment.
3. Assemble necessary equipment.	Reduces transmission of infection. Promotes efficiency of examination.

IMPLEMENTATION

STEP	RATIONALE
1. Position patient initially, either sitting or lying supine with head of bed elevated. **2.** Throughout assessment note patient's verbal and nonverbal behaviours. Determine patient's level of consciousness (LOC) and orientation by observing and talking to patient (Box 8.3).	Behaviours may reflect specific physical abnormalities. Dementia and LOC influence ability to cooperate. Decreased LOC, such as lethargy or confusion, requires further investigation into causes such as fluid and electrolyte imbalance, oxygenation and circulation problems, and metabolic problems.
3. If patient's responses are inappropriate, ask short, to-the-point questions regarding information patient should know (e.g., "Tell me your name." "What is the name of this place?" "Tell me where you live." "What day is this?" "What month is this?" or "What season of the year is this?").	Measures patient's orientation to person, place, and time. Document exactly what the patient is oriented to. If disoriented in any way, include subjective and objective data rather than just documenting "disoriented."

BOX 8.3

Characteristics of Dementia

Cognition
- Memory impaired: trouble recalling recent conversations, events, and appointments
- Frequently misplaces objects

Speech/Language
- Struggles to find words
- Conversation possibly incoherent

Activity
- Unchanged from usual behaviour
- Difficulty performing tasks that require many steps

Mood and Affect
- Depressed
- Apathetic
- Uninterested

Delusions/Hallucinations
- Can be some delusions
- No hallucinations

Adapted from Ball, J. W., Dains, J. E., Flynn, J. A., et al. (2022). *Seidel's guide to physical examination: An interprofessional approach* (10th ed.). Elsevier.

STEP	RATIONALE
4. If patient is unable to respond to questions of orientation, offer simple commands (e.g., "Squeeze my fingers" or "Move your toes.").	LOC exists along a continuum, ranging from full responsiveness, to inability to consciously initiate meaningful behaviours, to unresponsiveness to stimuli.
5. Obtain temperature, pulse, respirations, and blood pressure (see Chapter 7). Inform patient of vital signs (where appropriate).	Vital signs provide important information regarding physiological changes related to oxygenation and circulation.
6. Ask patients about their preferred names and pronouns (he, she, they) rather than making assumptions based on their physical appearance or gender expression.	A person's chosen names and pronouns are common ways of expressing gender. As part of person-centred care, use respectful and gender-affirming language that aligns with how the patient self-identifies (Rainbow Health Ontario, 2020).
7. If uncertain whether patient understands a question, rephrase or ask a similar question.	Inappropriate response from a patient may be caused by language barriers or deterioration of mental status, preoccupation with illness, or decreased hearing acuity.
8. Assess affect and mood: Note whether verbal expressions match nonverbal behaviour and are appropriate to situation.	Reflects patient's mental and emotional status, consciousness, and feelings.
9. Watch patient interact with family members or caregiver. Be alert for indications of fear, hesitancy to report health status, or willingness to let caregiver control assessment interview. Does partner or caregiver have a history of violence, alcoholism, or substance misuse? Is person unemployed, ill, or frustrated with caring for the patient? Note whether patient has any obvious physical injuries.	Suspect abuse in patients who have suffered obvious physical injury or neglect, show signs of malnutrition, or have ecchymosis (bruises) on extremities or trunk. Health care providers are often the first to identify evidence of abuse because patients may not be able to tell family or friends. Partners or caregivers may have a history of abusive or addictive behaviours.

Critical Decision Point *Be discreet in how you conduct the interview. Ask direct questions about abuse in private. It is often necessary to delay assessment to a later time when the partner or caregiver is not present. Asking a partner or caregiver to leave during an assessment creates an awkward situation, but inquiring about possible abuse in front of an abuser puts a patient at risk for further abuse. Patients are more likely to reveal any problems when the suspected abuser is absent from the room.*

STEP	RATIONALE
10. Observe for signs of interpersonal violence (abuse):	
a. *Child:* Blood on underclothing, pain in genital area, difficulty sitting or walking, pain on urination, vaginal or penile discharge, itching or unusual colour in genital area,	Suggests child sexual abuse (Ball et al., 2022; Hockenberry et al., 2024).
physical injury inconsistent with parent's or caregiver's account of how injury occurred.	Suggests child physical abuse.
b. *Adult:* Injury or trauma inconsistent with reported cause or obvious injuries to head, face, neck, breasts, abdomen, and genitalia (e.g., black eyes, abrasions, bruises/welts, broken nose, lacerations, broken teeth, strangulation marks, burns, human bites, orbital fractures, fractured skull).	Suggests intimate partner violence (Ball et al., 2022).
c. *Older person:* Injury or trauma inconsistent with reported cause, injuries in unusual locations (e.g., neck or genitalia), pattern injuries (left when an object with which a person is struck leaves an imprint), parallel injuries (e.g., bilateral ecchymosis on upper arms suggesting that patient was held and shaken), burns (shaped like cigarette, iron, rope), fractures, poor hygiene, and poor nutrition.	Suggests elder abuse or neglect (Ball et al., 2022; Boscart et al., 2023). Prolonged interval between injury and time patient sought medical care also indicates elder abuse or neglect.

Critical Decision Point *Interpersonal violence includes intimate partner abuse, sexual assault, child abuse, and elder abuse or neglect. If abuse is suspected, ask the patient directly and in a nonjudgemental manner about the presence of interpersonal violence. A pattern of findings indicating abuse in children has mandatory reporting requirements in all Canadian provinces and territories, and some provinces/territories have reporting requirements for abuse of older persons or people with developmental challenges. Use immediate interprofessional collaboration to facilitate placement in a safer environment.*

STEP	RATIONALE
11. Assess posture and position, noting alignment of shoulders and hips while patient stands, sits, or both. Observe whether patient is slumped, stands erect, or has bent posture (see Step 10 illustration).	Reveals musculoskeletal problem, mood, or presence of pain.

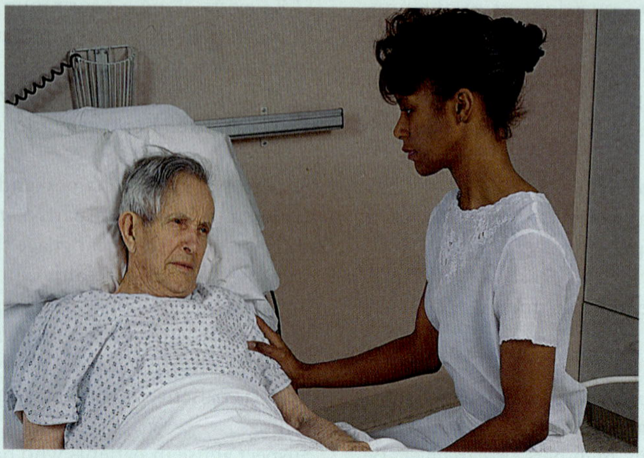

STEP 10 Observe patient's position and posture.

STEP	RATIONALE
12. Assess body movements. Are they purposeful? Are there tremors of extremities? Are any body parts immobile? Are movements coordinated or uncoordinated?	May indicate neurological or muscular problem or emotional stress (see Skill 8.7).
13. Assess speech. Is it understandable and moderately paced? Is there association with patient's thoughts?	Alterations reflect neurological impairment, injury or impairment of mouth, improperly fitting dentures, differences in dialect or language, and some mental illnesses.
14. Observe hygiene and grooming for presence or absence of makeup, type of clothes (hospital or personal), and cleanliness. Hair, teeth, and nails are good places to assess for hygiene status.	Grooming may reflect activity level before examination, resources available to purchase grooming supplies, patient's mood, and self-care practices. It may also reflect culture, lifestyle, economic status, and personal preferences.
a. Observe colour, distribution, quantity, thickness, texture, and lubrication of hair.	Changes in hair may reflect hormonal changes, changes from aging, poor nutrition, or hygiene.
b. Inspect condition of nails (hands and feet). Note colour, length, symmetry, cleanliness, and shape. Nails are normally transparent, smooth, and well rounded, with smooth, intact cuticle.	Changes indicate inadequate nutrition or grooming practices, nervous habits, or systemic diseases.
c. Assess presence or absence of body odour.	Body odour may result from physical exercise, deficient hygiene, or physical or mental abnormalities. Inadequate oral hygiene or unhealthy teeth cause bad breath.
15. Inspect exposed areas of skin and ask patient whether they have noted any changes, including the following:	Determines presence of abnormalities and cancerous lesions. Melanoma is an aggressive form of skin cancer; detection and prompt treatment are critical (Box 8.4).
a. Pruritus, oozing, bleeding	Itching could result from dry skin. Oozing could indicate infection, and bleeding may indicate a blood disorder.
b. Appearance of mole (nevus), bump, or nodule; change in sensation; itchiness, tenderness, or pain	These are key indicators that a lesion may be cancerous.
c. Petechiae (pinpoint-sized red or purple spots on skin caused by small hemorrhages in skin layers)	Petechiae may indicate serious blood clotting disorder, severe infection, medication reaction, or liver disease.
16. Inspect skin surfaces. Compare colour of symmetrical body parts, including areas unexposed to sun. Look for any patches or areas of skin colour variation.	Changes in colour can indicate pathological alterations (see Table 8.5).

Critical Decision Point *Be alert for basal cell carcinomas such as an open sore that does not heal, a shiny nodule, a pink or reddish growth, or a scar-like area. These are often seen in sun-exposed areas and frequently occur in sun-damaged skin.*

STEP	RATIONALE
17. Carefully inspect colour of face, oral mucosa, lips, conjunctiva, sclera, palms of hands, and nail beds.	Abnormalities are easier to identify in areas of body where melanin production is lowest.

STEP	RATIONALE

Critical Decision Point *When assessing the skin of a patient with bandages, a cast, restraints, or other restrictive devices, note report of pain or tingling and areas of pallor, decreased temperature, decreased movement, and impaired sensation, which may indicate impaired circulation. Immediate release of pressure from the restrictive device may be necessary.*

STEP	RATIONALE
18. Use ungloved fingertips to palpate skin surfaces to feel texture and moisture of intact skin.	Changes in texture may be first indication of skin rashes in dark-skinned patients. Hydration, body temperature, and environment may affect skin. Older persons are prone to xerosis, which presents as dry, scaly skin (Boscart et al., 2023).
a. Stroke skin surfaces lightly with fingertips to detect texture of surface of skin. Note whether skin is smooth or rough, thick or thin, or tight or supple and whether localized areas of hardness or lesions are present.	Localized texture changes result from trauma, surgical wounds, or lesions.
b. Palpate any areas that appear irregular in texture.	Allows detection of localized areas of hardness and/or tenderness within subcutaneous skin layers.
c. Using dorsum (back) of hand, palpate for temperature of skin surfaces. Compare symmetrical body parts. Compare upper and lower body parts. Note any distinct temperature differences and localized areas of warmth.	Skin on dorsum of hand is thin, which allows detection of subtle temperature changes. Cool skin temperature often indicates decreased blood flow. A stage 1 pressure injury may cause warmth and erythema (redness) of an area. Environmental temperature and anxiety may also affect skin temperature.

Critical Decision Point *In patients who receive routine injections (e.g., insulin, heparin), localized areas of hardness (lipodystrophy) may be palpated over injection sites; however, the use of human insulin reduces the risk for lipodystrophy. Rotation of insulin injection sites to different anatomical sites is no longer recommended as this causes variability in insulin absorption. Instead, advise patients to rotate injections within one particular site, such as the abdomen* (Tyerman & Cobbett, 2023).

STEP	RATIONALE
19. Apply clean gloves. Inspect character of any secretions; note colour, odour, amount, and consistency (e.g., thin and watery, thick and oily). Remove gloves.	Reduces transmission of microorganisms. Description of secretions helps to indicate type of lesion, presence of infection, or wound healing.
20. Assess skin turgor by grasping fold of skin on sternum, forearm, or abdomen with fingertips. Release skinfold and note ease and speed with which skin returns to place (see Step 19 illustration).	With reduced turgor, skin remains suspended, or "tented," for a few seconds before slowly returning to place, indicating decreased elasticity and possible dehydration. With altered turgor, provide education on prevention of pressure injuries (see Chapter 39). This may not be applicable to pediatric patients.
21. Assess condition of skin for pressure areas, paying particular attention to regions at risk for pressure injuries (e.g., sacrum, greater trochanter, heels, occipital area, clavicles). If you see areas of redness, place fingertip over area, apply gentle pressure, and release. Look at skin colour.	Normal reactive hyperemia (redness) is visible effect of localized vasodilation, the normal response of the body to lack of blood flow to underlying tissue. Affected area of skin normally blanches with fingertip pressure. If area does not blanch, suspect tissue injury.

BOX 8.4

Malignant Melanoma Mnemonics

The ABCDE Rule of Melanoma

Here is a simple way to remember the characteristics that should alert you to the possibility of malignant melanoma.

1. *A*symmetry of lesion: One side different from the other
2. *B*orders: Irregular (uneven, lumpy edges)
3. *C*olour: Blue–black or variegated; pigmentation not uniform; variations/multiple colours (tan, black) with areas of pink, white, grey, blue, or red
4. *D*iameter greater than 6 mm
5. *E*volving: Change in size, shape, colour; itching or bleeding

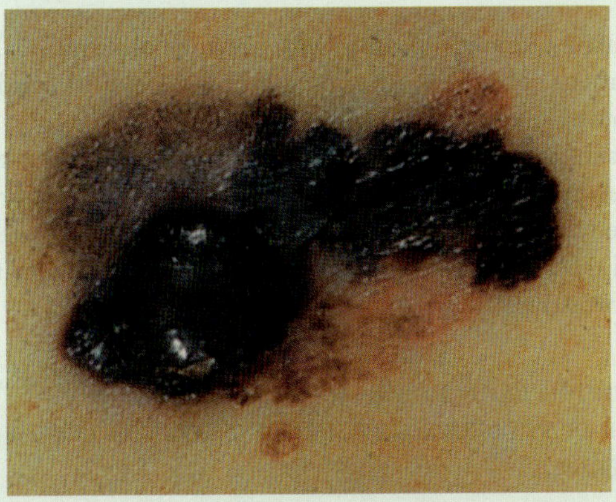

Figure from Ball, J. W., Dains, J. E., Flynn, J. A., et al. [2022]. *Seidel's guide to physical examination: An interprofessional approach* [10th ed.]. Elsevier.

STEP	RATIONALE

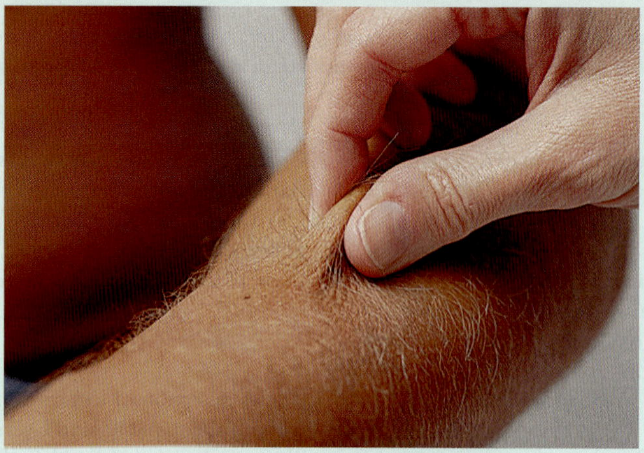

STEP 19 Checking skin turgor.

Critical Decision Point *When assessing darkly pigmented skin, visual inspection techniques to identify skin problems are ineffective. Skin inspection techniques for individuals with darkly pigmented skin must include assessment of temperature, edema, and changes in tissue consistency as compared with the surrounding skin* (Boyko et al., 2018).

Critical Decision Point *With evidence of normal reactive hyperemia, reposition patient and develop a turning schedule if the person is dependent.*

STEP	RATIONALE
22. When you detect a lesion, use adequate lighting to inspect colour, location, texture, size, shape, and type (Box 8.5). Also note grouping (e.g., clustered or linear) and distribution (e.g., localized or generalized).	Observation of skin lesions allows for accurate description and identification.
a. Apply gloves if lesion is moist or draining. Gently palpate any lesion to determine mobility, contour (e.g., flat, raised, or depressed), and consistency (e.g., soft or hard).	Gentle palpation prevents rupture of underlying cysts. Gloves reduce transmission of microorganisms.
b. Note whether patient reports tenderness with or without palpation.	Tenderness may indicate inflammation or pressure on body part.
c. Measure size of lesion (height, width, depth) with centimetre ruler.	Provides for baseline to assess changes in lesion over time.
23. Remove gloves. Dispose of all equipment in appropriate receptacles. Help patient to comfortable position.	Prevents transmission of infection.

EVALUATION

1. Observe throughout assessment for evidence of physical or emotional distress, which may alter assessment data.	Interaction during assessment reveals emotional problems. Manoeuvres used during physical examination reveal presence of physical problems.
2. Compare assessment findings with previous observations.	Determines whether change has occurred.
3. Ask patient if there is information about physical condition that you have not discussed.	Some patients think they are bothering you by asking questions unless opportunity for questions is provided.
4. Use teach-back: "I want to be sure I explained everything about the bleeding mole I found on your back during assessment. Tell me why it is important to see a dermatologist." Develop a revised teaching plan if patient or caregiver is unable to teach back correctly.	Determines patient's and caregiver's level of understanding of instructional topic.

Unexpected Outcomes	Related Interventions
1. Patient demonstrates acute distress (e.g., shortness of breath, acute pain, anxiety).	• Respond immediately to identified need (e.g., repositioning, oxygen, or medication as appropriate). • Obtain vital signs. • Notify health care provider.

BOX 8.5

Types of Skin Lesions

Macule: Flat, nonpalpable change in skin colour; smaller than 1 cm (e.g., freckle, petechia)

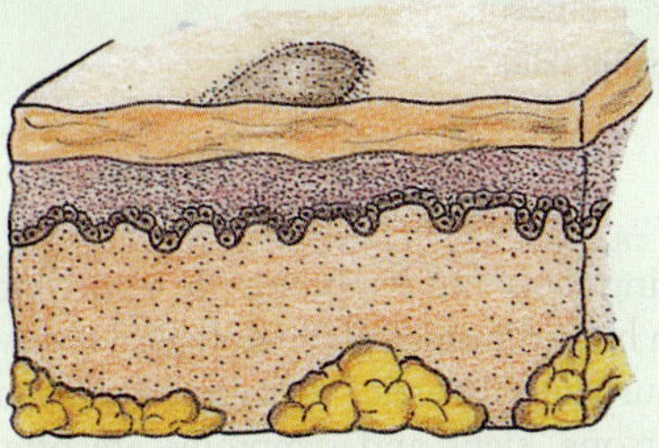

Vesicle: Circumscribed elevation of skin filled with serous fluid; smaller than 0.5 cm (e.g., herpes simplex, chicken pox)

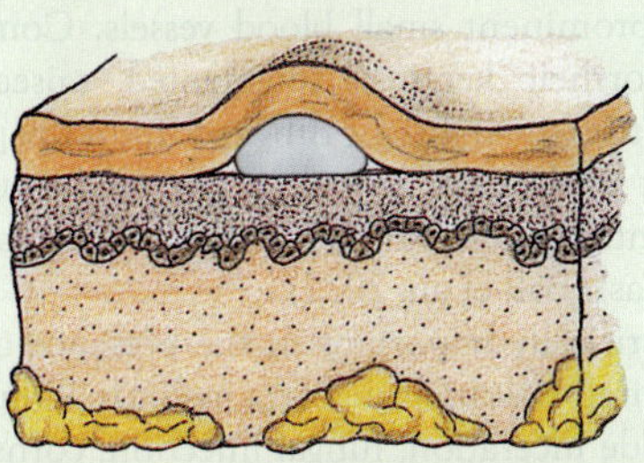

Papule: Palpable, circumscribed, solid elevation in skin; smaller than 0.5 cm (e.g., elevated nevus)

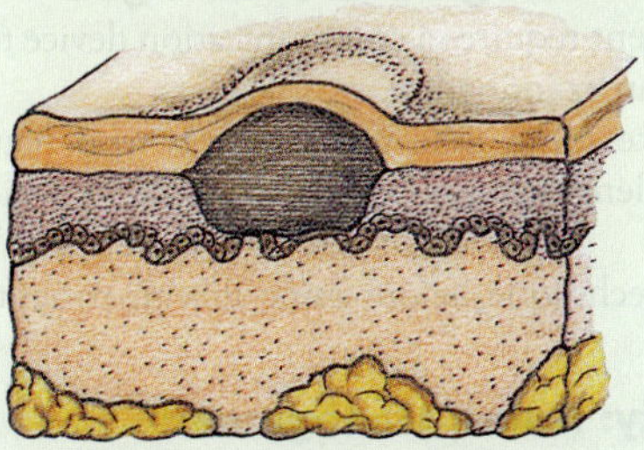

Pustule: Circumscribed elevation of skin similar to vesicle but filled with pus; varies in size (e.g., acne, staphylococcal infection)

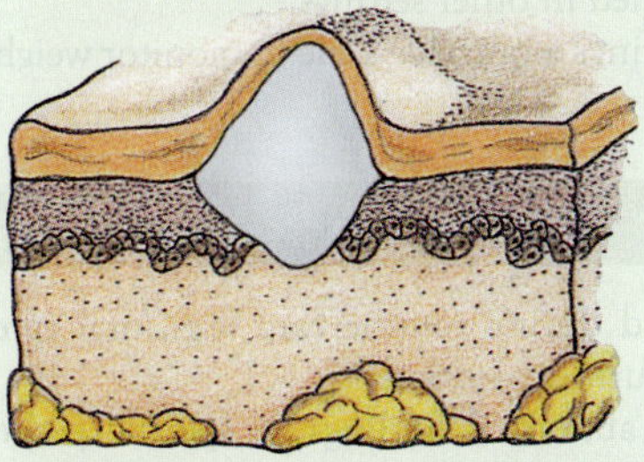

Nodule: Elevated solid mass, deeper and firmer than papule; 0.5–2 cm (e.g., wart)

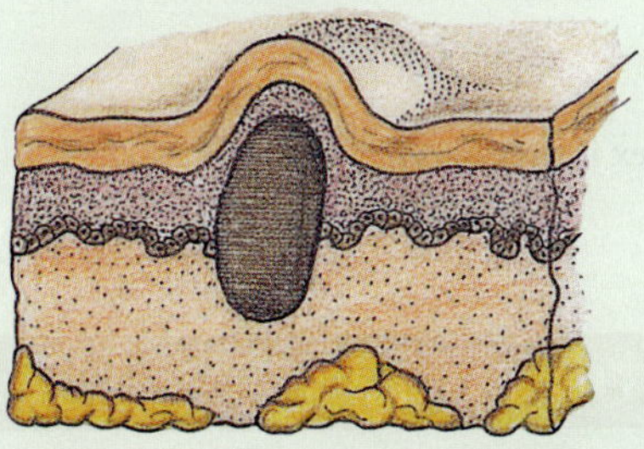

Ulcer: Deep loss of skin surface that may extend to dermis and frequently bleeds and scars; varies in size (e.g., venous stasis ulcer)

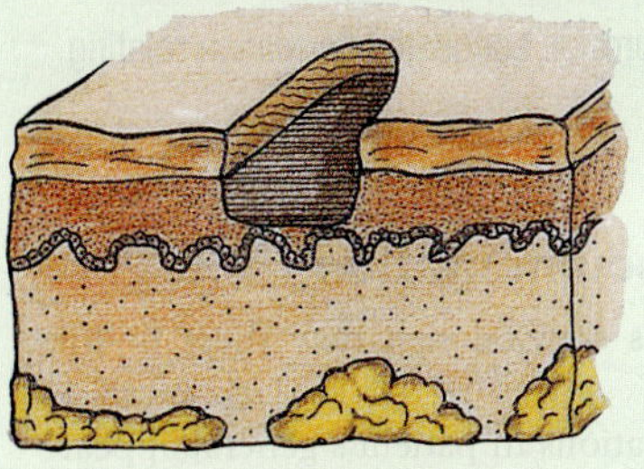

Tumour: Solid mass that may extend deep through subcutaneous tissue; larger than 1–2 cm (e.g., epithelioma)

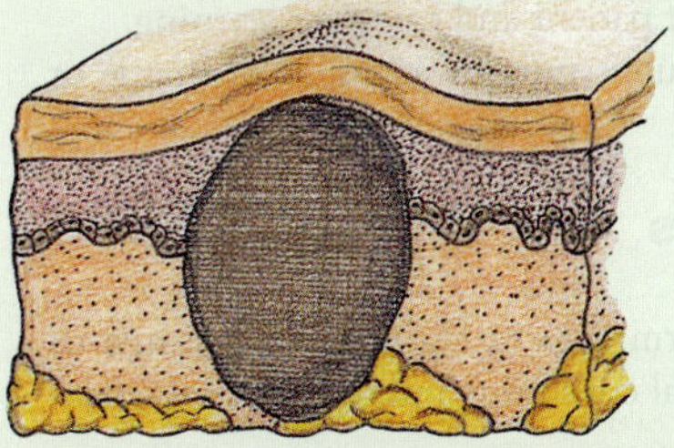

Atrophy: Thinning of skin with loss of normal skin furrow, with skin appearing shiny and translucent; varies in size (e.g., arterial insufficiency)

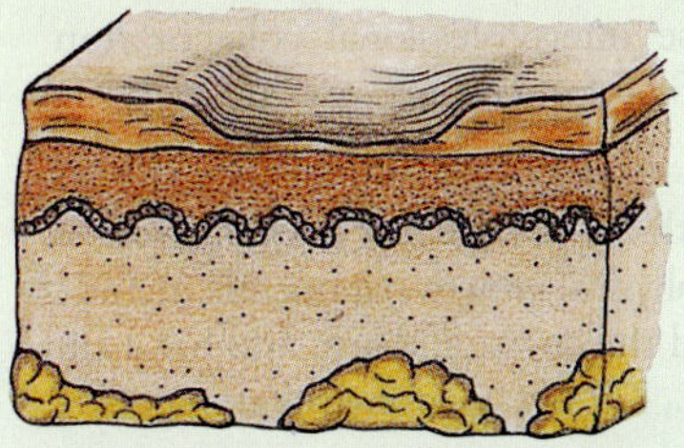

Wheal: Irregularly shaped, elevated area or superficial localized edema; varies in size (e.g., hive, mosquito bite)

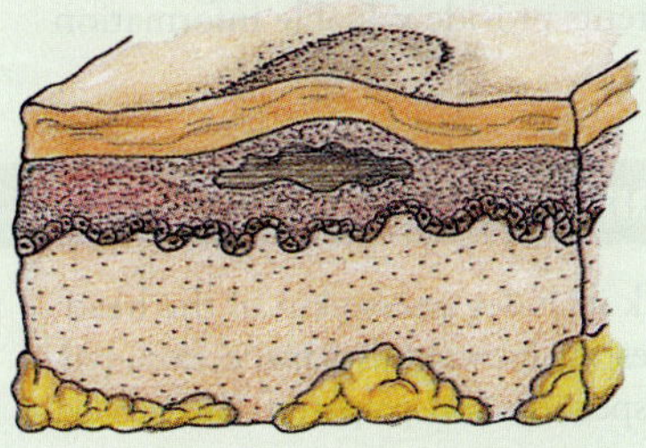

STEP	RATIONALE
Unexpected Outcomes	**Related Interventions**
2. Patient has abnormal skin condition (e.g., change in colour of a mole, dry texture, lesions, or erythema).	• Identify contributing factors and prevent continued irritation or damage as appropriate.
3. Patient is unwilling or unable to provide adequate information relating to identified concerns.	• Seek information from caregiver if present. • Review patient's record for baseline data.

Communication and Documentation

- Document patient's vital signs on vital sign flow sheet in the EHR or chart.
- Document description of alterations in patient's general appearance in the EHR or chart.
- Document patient's behaviours using objective terminology. Include patient's self-report of signs and symptoms.
- Document your evaluation of patient and caregiver learning.
- Report abnormalities and acute symptoms to nurse in charge or health care provider.

Special Considerations

Teaching

- During general survey, inform patient about normal range of vital signs for age and physical condition and normal body mass index.
- If patient is on therapeutic diet, discuss any problems that they have preparing or selecting food. The best form of weight reduction is to achieve gradual weight loss by increasing exercise and decreasing caloric intake. Use interprofessional collaboration (e.g., dietitian) to obtain specific information.

Pediatric

- Measurement of physical growth is a key element in evaluation of a child's health status. These physical growth parameters include height, length, weight, skinfold thickness, and arm and head circumference (Hockenberry et al., 2024). Use growth charts specific to child's age and condition.
- Weigh infants nude. Minimize length of time the infant is exposed. Weigh children in light underclothes or gown.
- A child's interactions with parents provide valuable information regarding the child's behaviour.

Gerontological

- An older person's presenting signs and symptoms are sometimes deceiving. An older person has a diminished physiological reserve that sometimes masks the usual, or "classic," signs and symptoms of a disease. In older persons, signs and symptoms are often blunted or atypical (Boscart et al., 2023).
- Common skin changes with aging include dryness, thinning, decreased elasticity, and prominent small blood vessels. Common lesions include seborrheic keratosis (pigmented, raised, warty lesion); cherry angioma (small, bright ruby-red, round papules); cutaneous tags (soft pinkish-tan to light-brown pedunculated lesions); and solar lentigines (grey-brown, irregular macular lesions on sun-exposed areas) (Ball et al., 2022).
- Inspection of the feet is critically important in the presence of impaired circulation, impaired vision, or diabetes mellitus. Common foot conditions include ulceration, fungal infection, corns, calluses, bunions, plantar warts, and hammertoe.

Patients With Physical or Cognitive Challenges

- Determine whether a patient requires a communication device to interact with you during an examination.
- An examination may take more time with patients who have physical or cognitive challenges, so schedule extra time to avoid being rushed.
- Demonstrate a physical technique before using it with patients who are nonverbal.

Care in the Community: Home Management

- In the home, the focus may be on the patient's ability to perform basic self-care tasks. Be sure that the home assessment builds on all health concerns identified in other settings.
- The home health nurse brings a portable scale to monitor weight changes.

✦ SKILL 8.2 Head and Neck Assessment

Examination of the head and neck includes assessment of the head, eyes, ears, nose, mouth, and sinuses. Assessment uses inspection, palpation, and auscultation, with inspection and palpation often used simultaneously.

Delegation and Collaboration

The skill of assessing the head and neck cannot be delegated to an unregulated care provider (UCP). The nurse directs the UCP to do the following:

- Observe for nasal discharge and nasal bleeding
- Report any findings found during routine care (e.g., oral care, bathing) to the nurse for further assessment

When assessment reveals abnormal findings or specific pathophysiological changes, collaborate with the interprofessional health care team (e.g., health care provider or audiologist).

Equipment

- Stethoscope
- Clean gloves (use nonlatex if necessary)
- Tongue blade
- Pen light

STEP	RATIONALE
ASSESSMENT	
1. Identify patient using at least two person-specific identifiers (e.g., name and date of birth, or name and medical record number) according to employer policy.	Ensures correct patient. Complies with Accreditation Canada's standards and improves patient safety (Accreditation Canada, 2020).

STEP	RATIONALE
2. Throughout the procedure, the 4 moments for hand hygiene are to be implemented; hand hygiene should occur before initial patient (or patient environment) contact, before an aseptic procedure, after body fluid exposure risk, and after patient (or patient environment) contact. Additional hand hygiene should be performed when hands are visibly soiled.	Proper hand hygiene helps prevent the spread of infectious agents to health care providers.
3. Assess for history of headache, dizziness, pain, or stiffness.	Headaches and dizziness are signs of stress, a symptom of another underlying problem such as high blood pressure, or a result of injury.
4. Determine whether patient has history of eye disease, diabetes mellitus, or hypertension.	Common conditions predispose patients to visual alterations requiring health care provider referral.
5. Ask if patient has experienced blurred vision, flashing lights, halos around lights, or reduced visual field.	These common symptoms indicate visual problems.
6. Ask if patient has experienced ear pain, itching, discharge, vertigo, tinnitus (ringing in the ears), or change in hearing.	These signs and symptoms indicate infection or hearing loss.
7. Review patient's occupational history.	Patient's occupation may create risk for injury, potential for eye fatigue, or prolonged noise exposure.
8. Ask if patient has history of allergies, nasal discharge, epistaxis (nosebleeds), or postnasal drip.	History is useful in determining source of nasal and sinus drainage.
9. Determine whether patient smokes or chews tobacco.	Tobacco users have greater risk for mouth and throat cancer.

NURSING DIAGNOSES

- Reduced health maintenance
- Insufficient knowledge regarding the need for head and neck assessment
- Inadequate oral mucous membranes
- Potential for injury

Related factors and risk factors are individualized on the basis of patient's condition or needs.

PLANNING

STEP	RATIONALE
1. Expected outcomes following completion of procedure:	
• Patient recognizes warning signs and symptoms of eye, ear, sinus, and mouth disease.	Awareness of warning signs improves adherence to reporting problems to health care provider.
• Patient takes appropriate safety precautions for occupational injury related to head and neck.	Awareness of safety precautions improves adherence to healthful behaviours.
• Patient exhibits good visual acuity, normal hearing, moist and intact oral mucosa, and head and neck without masses or lesions.	Patient has no abnormal findings.
2. Prepare patient. Tell them that you will be completing routine examination of the head and neck to check for areas of concerns.	Understanding promotes patient's cooperation.
3. Anticipate teaching topics so that during examination you can teach patient about common symptoms of eye, ear, sinus, and mouth problems and occupational health and safety.	Allows patient education to be incorporated into examination.
4. Assemble necessary equipment.	Reduces transmission of infection. Promotes efficiency of examination.

IMPLEMENTATION

STEP	RATIONALE
1. Position patient sitting upright if possible.	Proper hand hygiene helps prevent the spread of infectious agents to health care providers. Provides for more thorough examination of head and neck structures.
2. Inspect head. Note head position and facial features. Look for symmetry.	Head tilting to one side may indicate hearing or visual loss. Neurological disorders such as paralysis often affect facial symmetry.
3. Assess eyes (include discussion of signs and symptoms related to eye diseases).	
a. Inspect position of eyes, colour, condition of conjunctiva, and movement.	Asymmetrical positioning may reflect trauma or tumour growth. Differences in colour are sometimes congenital; changes in colour of conjunctiva may be result of local infection or symptomatic of another abnormality (e.g., pale conjunctiva is associated with anemia).

STEP	RATIONALE
b. Assess patient's near vision (ability to read newspaper or magazine) and far vision (ability to follow movement, read clock, watch television, or read signs at a distance).	Patient with visual acuity or visual field loss indicates need for supportive self-care measures (e.g., feeding, bathing, hygiene, dressing) and teaching.
c. Inspect pupils for size, shape, and equality (pupils equally round and reactive to light and accommodation [PERRLA]) (see Step 4c illustration).	Normal pupils are round, regular, and equal in size and shape, and have consensual response to light and accommodation.
d. Test pupillary reflexes. To test reaction to light, dim room lights. If you cannot dim lights, cup hand over eye to temporarily shield light. As patient looks straight ahead, move penlight from side of patient's face and direct light on pupil. Observe pupillary response of both eyes, noting briskness and equality of reflex (see Step 4d, illustrations A and B).	Darkened room normally ensures brisk response of pupils to light. Pupil that is illuminated constricts. Pupil in other eye should constrict equally (consensual light reflex).
(1) Test for accommodation by asking patient to focus on distant object, which dilates the pupil. Then have patient shift to near object about 7–8 cm (3–3.2 inches) from nose and observe for pupil constriction and convergence of eyes. **Note:** You can also ask patient to follow an object (e.g., finger, pen) with eyes from far to near point.	Absence of constriction, convergence, or an asymmetrical response requires further ophthalmological assessment (Ball et al., 2022).
4. Assess hearing. Note patient's response to questions and presence or use of hearing aid. If you suspect patient has hearing loss, ask them to repeat random words that you state. Use one- or two-syllable words. Repeat, gradually increasing voice intensity until patient correctly repeats the words.	Patients normally hear three to six sounds clearly when whispered (Ball et al., 2022). For patient with obvious hearing impairment, speak clearly and concisely, stand so patient can see your face, stand toward patient's good ear, use low pitch, and avoid yelling.

Critical Decision Point *If hearing deficit is present, have a qualified nurse inspect patient's ears. Impaired hearing may be the result of impacted cerumen, external otitis, or swelling in ear canal caused by allergic reactions to materials in hearing aids.*

STEP	RATIONALE
5. Inspect nose internally and externally for skin colour, drainage, and presence of deformity or inflammation. Additionally, inspect externally for shape and alignment. Note colour of mucosa and any lesions, discharge, swelling, or presence of bleeding. If drainage appears infectious, consult with health care provider about obtaining a specimen.	Character of discharge and inflammation indicates allergy or infection. Perforation and erosion of septum and puffiness and/or increased vascularity of mucosa indicate habitual substance misuse.
6. In patients with nasogastric (NG), nasointestinal (NI), or nasotracheal tube, inspect nares for excoriation, inflammation, or discharge. Using penlight, look up into each naris. Stabilize tube as needed.	Swallowing or coughing reflex causes movement of tubes against nares, and pressure against tissues and mucosa can result in tissue injury.

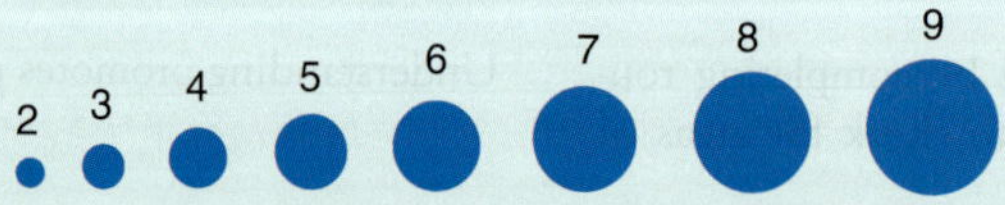

STEP 4C Pupil sizes in millimetres.

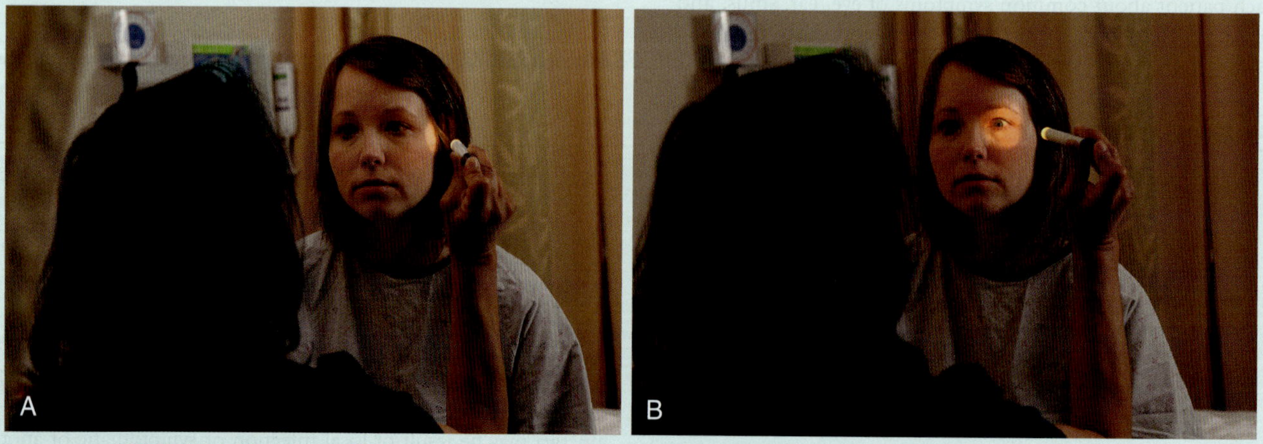

STEP 4D A, Holding penlight to side of patient's face. B, Illumination of pupil causes pupillary constriction.

STEP	RATIONALE
7. Inspect sinuses by palpating gently over frontal and maxillary areas. Use thumbs to apply pressure up and under eyebrows to assess frontal sinuses. Use thumbs to apply pressure over maxillary sinuses, about 0.4 cm (1 inch) below eyes.	Infection, allergy, or substance use sometimes causes tenderness.
8. Assess mouth (include discussion about signs and symptoms of oral cancer).	
a. Apply clean gloves. Inspect lips for colour, texture, hydration, and lesions. Patients wearing lipstick should remove it.	Reduces transmission of microorganisms. Normal lips are pink, moist, symmetrical, and smooth.
b. Inspect teeth and note position and alignment. Note colour of teeth and presence of dental caries, tartar, and extraction sites.	Reveals quality of hygiene and discoloration due to cola, coffee, and tobacco. Teeth are normally smooth, white, and shiny.
c. Inspect mucosa and gums. Determine whether patient wears dentures or retainers, and ask if they are comfortable. Remove dentures to visualize and palpate gums. Use tongue blade to lightly depress tongue and inspect oral cavity with penlight (see Step 9c illustration). Inspect oral mucosa, tongue, teeth, and gums for colour, hydration, texture, and obvious lesions.	Dentures and retainers can cause chronic irritation. Normal mucosa is glistening, pink, smooth, and moist. Precancerous lesions can go unnoticed and progress rapidly.
d. If oral lesions are present, palpate gently with gloved hand for tenderness, size, and consistency. Remove gloves.	Cancerous lesions tend to be hard and nontender.
9. Inspect and palpate the neck:	Assesses function of all neck structures, including neck muscles, lymph nodes, thyroid glands, and trachea.
a. Ask if patient has history of neck pain or difficulty moving neck.	May indicate muscle strain, head injury, local nerve injury, or swollen lymph nodes.
b. Neck muscles: Inspect neck for bilateral symmetry of muscles. Ask patient to flex and hyperextend neck and turn head from side to side.	Detects muscle weakness, strain, and range of motion (ROM).
c. Lymph nodes:	Lymph nodes are sometimes enlarged from infection or various diseases such as cancer.
(1) With patient's chin raised and head tilted slightly, inspect area where lymph nodes are distributed and compare both sides (see Step 10c[1] illustration).	
(2) To examine lymph nodes, have patient relax with neck flexed slightly forward. To palpate, face or stand to side of patient and use pads of middle three fingers of hand (see Step 10c[2] illustration). Palpate gently in rotary motion for superficial lymph nodes.	This position relaxes tissues and muscles.

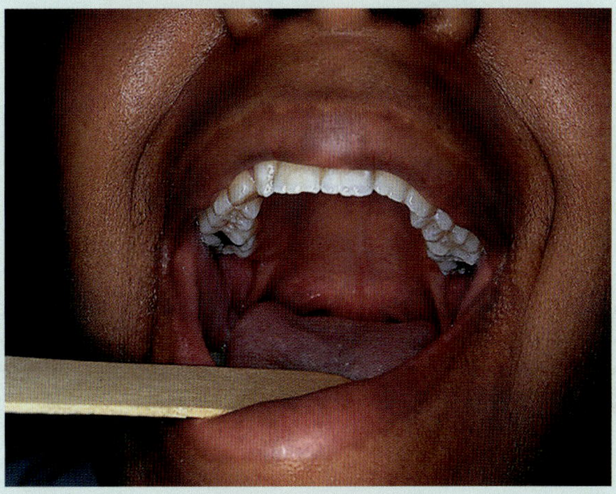

STEP 9C Inspect mouth.

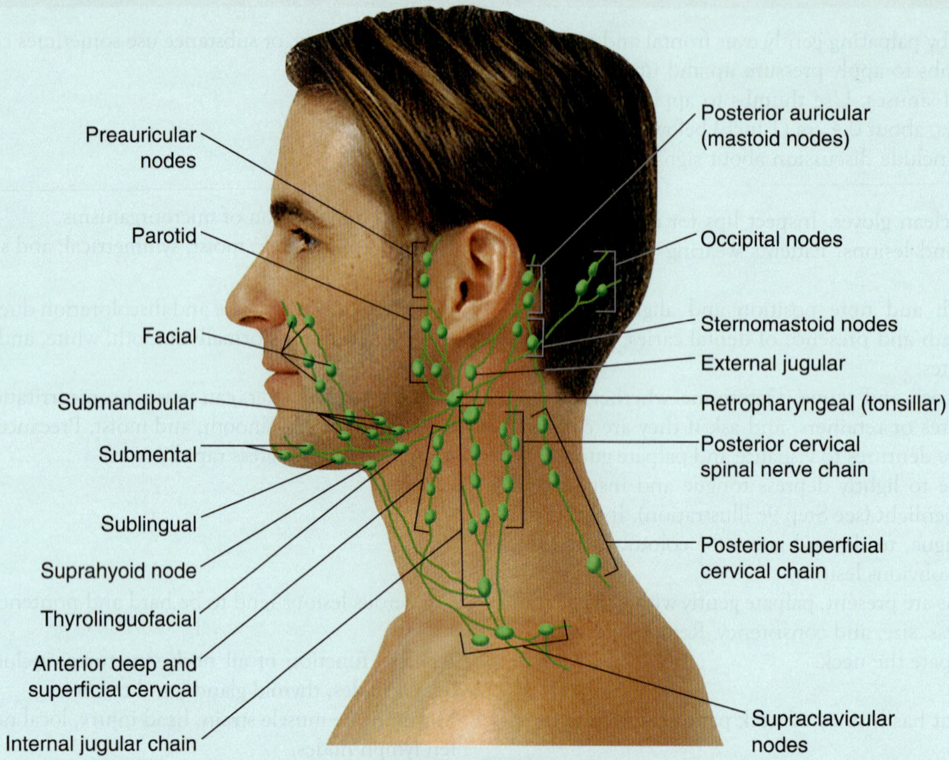

STEP 10C(1) **Palpable lymph nodes of head and neck.** (*From Ball, J. W., Dains, J. E., Flynn, J. A., et al. [2022]. Seidel's guide to physical examination: An interprofessional approach [10th ed.]. Elsevier.*)

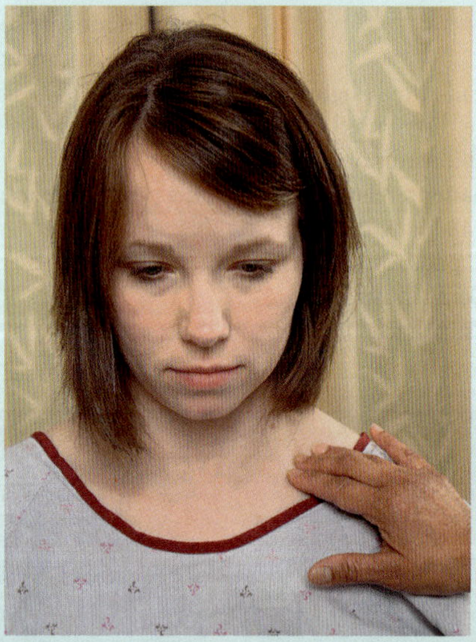

STEP 10C(2) **Palpation of cervical lymph nodes.**

(3) Note whether lymph nodes are large, fixed, inflamed, or tender.	Large, fixed, inflamed, or tender lymph nodes indicate local infection, systemic disease, or neoplasm.
10. Dispose of all equipment in appropriate receptacles. Help patient to comfortable position.	Reduces transmission of infection.

STEP	RATIONALE

EVALUATION

1. Compare assessment findings with previous observations.	Identifies changes in patient's condition.
2. Ask patient to describe common symptoms of eye, ear, sinus, or mouth disease.	Assesses patient's ability to recognize abnormalities.
3. Ask patient to list occupational safety precautions.	Knowledge allows patient to take safety precautions.
4. **Use teach-back:** "We've talked about some of the signs and symptoms of ear injuries that are related to your occupation. Tell me what you can do to reduce injury and potential hearing problems in your workplace." Develop a revised teaching plan if patient is unable to teach back correctly.	Determines patient's level of understanding of instructional topic.

Unexpected Outcomes	Related Interventions
1. Patient has yellow nasal discharge and sneezing, and indicates sinus pain.	• Reposition into semi-Fowler's or other comfortable position to relieve sinus pain. • Monitor temperature for fever. • Notify health care provider if these are new findings.
2. Patient indicates severe headache and dizziness when standing.	• Respond immediately by obtaining vital signs, especially blood pressure. • Return patient to bed in position of comfort to minimize dizziness and relieve headache. • Identify contributing factors (e.g., stress, pain, or elevated blood pressure). • Notify health care provider.
3. Patient has mouth sore that bleeds easily, lump or thickening in cheek, or white or red patch in mucosa.	• Notify health care provider.

Communication and Documentation

- Document all findings, including any abnormal findings such as hearing or visual loss, pain and its location, current infection, and character of drainage in progress notes in EHR or physical chart, as well as patient teaching and understanding of health information provided.
- Report any unexpected findings or changes to charge nurse or health care provider.

Special Considerations

Teaching

- Explain the common visual changes associated with aging, including reduced acuity (presbyopia), loss of or a reduction in peripheral vision, reduced tearing, and sensitivity to glare or bright lights. Inform patients when to seek help from an eye care professional.
- Educate patients and caregivers about strategies for preventing hearing loss (World Health Organization, 2019, 2021):
  - Immunizing children against childhood diseases, including measles, meningitis, rubella, and mumps
  - Immunizing people of reproductive age against rubella before pregnancy
  - Preventing cytomegalovirus infections in pregnant persons through good hygiene; screening for and treating syphilis and other infections in pregnant persons.

Pediatric

- Some infants resist eye examination by closing their eyes. Using distraction encourages eye opening (Hockenberry et al., 2024).
- Headaches in children are usually caused by loss of sleep, poor nutrition, eye fatigue, and allergies. Children as young as 3 years of age can develop severe migraine headaches, but the symptoms are vague and difficult to diagnose (Hockenberry et al., 2024).

Gerontological

- Older persons commonly experience loss of peripheral vision due to changes in the lens.
- Teach patients older than age 65 to have routine hearing checks.

Care in the Community: Home Management

- Teach the patient who is visually impaired and their caregivers how to adjust room arrangements at home to promote safer ambulation.
- Self-help aids are available to help patient function independently with daily activities.
- Measuring visual acuity helps determine level of assistance that patient requires with activities of daily living (ADLs) and ability of patient to safely ambulate and function independently within the home.
- Educate patients about proper techniques for maintaining glasses, contact lenses, and hearing aids (see Chapter 42).
- Encourage use of helmet during bike riding, motorcycling, and contact sports to prevent head injuries.

✦ SKILL 8.3 Thorax and Lung Assessment

Assessment of the thorax and lungs requires review of the ventilatory and respiratory functions of the lungs. It is a critical part of assessment because alterations can be life threatening. Changes in respiration can occur quickly as a result of immobility, infection, certain analgesic and sedative medications, and fluid overload. Use data from all body systems to determine the nature of pulmonary alterations. You will use inspection, palpation, and auscultation during the examination.

Before assessing the thorax and lungs, know the landmarks of the chest (Fig. 8.3, A–C). These landmarks help you identify findings and

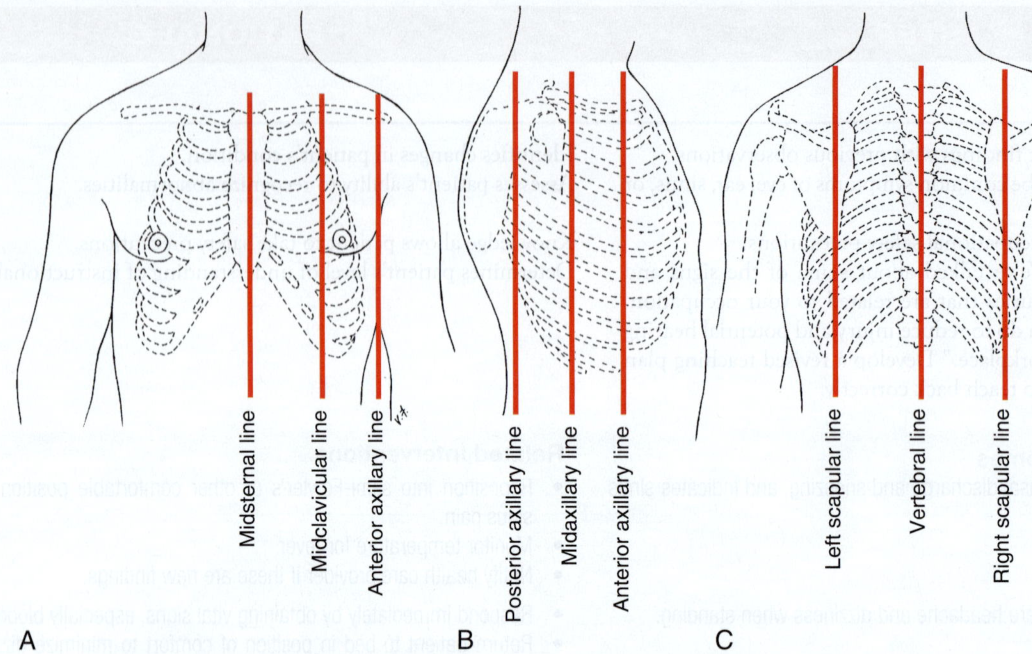

FIG 8.3 Anatomical landmarks and order of progression for examination of thorax. A, Anterior thorax. B, Lateral thorax. C, Posterior thorax.

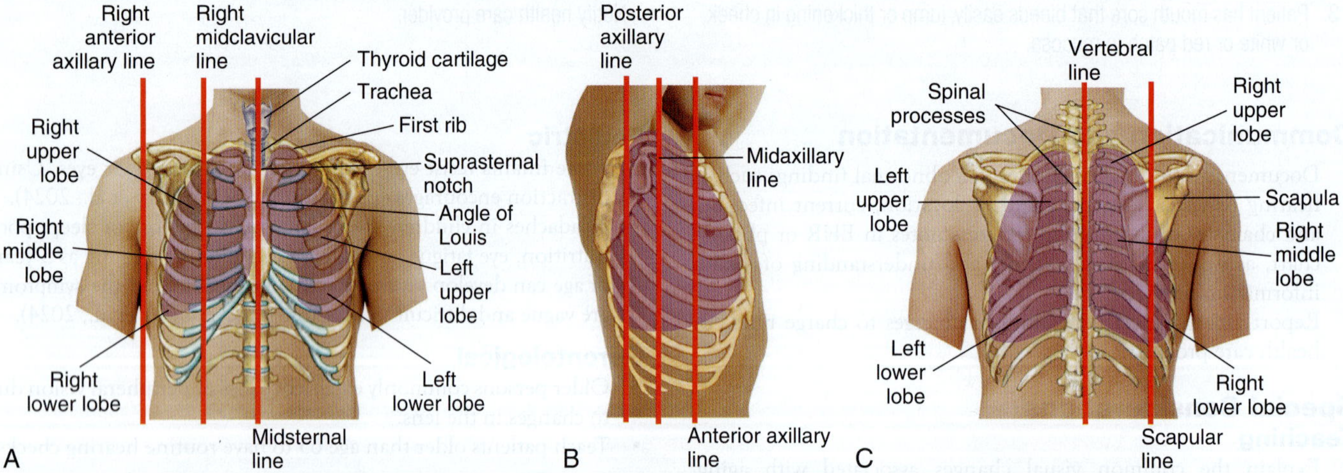

FIG 8.4 Position of lung lobes in relation to anatomical landmarks. A, Anterior position. B, Lateral position. C, Posterior position. *(From Ball, J. W., Dains, J. E., Flynn, J. A., et al. [2022]. Seidel's guide to physical examination: An interprofessional approach [10th ed.]. Elsevier.)*

use assessment skills correctly. A patient's nipples, angle of Louis at the sternum, suprasternal notch, costal angle, clavicles, and vertebrae are key landmarks. Keep a mental image of the location of the lobes of the lung and the position of each rib (Fig. 8.4, A–C).

Locating the position of each rib is critical to visualizing the lobe of the lung being assessed. To begin, locate the angle of Louis on the anterior chest by palpating the "speed bump" at the manubriosternal junction, where the second rib connects with the sternum. The angle is often visible and palpable. Count the ribs and intercostal spaces (between the ribs) from this point. The number of each intercostal space corresponds with that of the rib just above it. The spinous processes of the third thoracic vertebra and the fourth, fifth, and sixth ribs help to locate the lung lobes laterally. The lower lobes project laterally and anteriorly (see Fig. 8.4, *B*). Posteriorly, the tip (or inferior margin) of the scapula lies approximately at the level of the seventh rib (see Fig. 8.4, *C*).

During the examination, use auscultation to listen to breath sounds with a stethoscope. You can hear these sounds best when the person breathes deeply through the mouth. Adventitious sounds (abnormal sounds) result from air passing through fluid, mucus, or narrowed airways or from inflammation between the pleural linings. The four types of adventitious sounds are crackles, rhonchi, wheezes, and pleural friction rubs (Table 8.6). Additionally, stridor is a high-pitched inspiratory crowing sound originating in the larynx or trachea that is heard louder in the neck than over the chest wall; it results from an upper airway obstruction caused by swollen, inflamed tissues (e.g., croup or acute epiglottis in children) or foreign body inhalation (Jarvis et al., 2024). Note the location and characteristics of the sounds, diminished breath sounds, or absence of breath sounds. Determine where in the respiratory cycle the abnormal sounds are heard (inspiration versus expiration).

Delegation and Collaboration

The skill of assessing the lungs and thorax cannot be delegated to a UCP. The nurse directs the UCP to do the following:

TABLE 8.6

Adventitious Breath Sounds

Sound	Site Auscultated	Cause	Character
Crackles 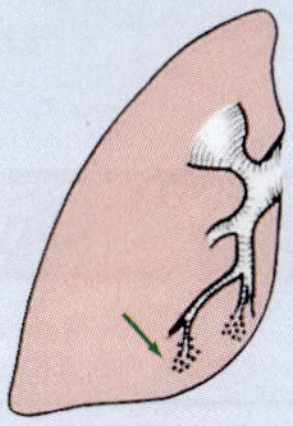	Most common in dependent lobes: right and left lung bases	Random, sudden reinflation of groups of alveoli; also related to increase in fluid in small airways	*Fine crackles:* Short, interrupted crackling sounds heard during end of inspiration, expiration, or both; may or may not change with coughing; sound like crushing cellophane *Medium crackles:* Lower, moister sounds heard during middle of inspiration; not cleared with coughing *Coarse crackles:* Loud bubbly sounds heard during inspiration; not cleared with coughing
Rhonchi (sonorous wheeze) 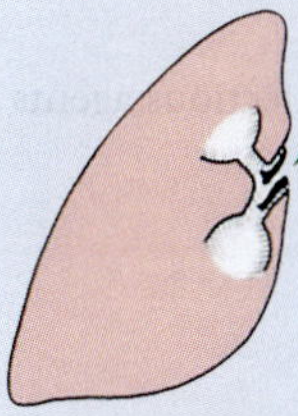	Heard primarily over trachea and bronchi; if loud enough, can be heard over most lung fields	Fluid or mucus in larger airways causing turbulence; muscular spasm	Loud, low-pitched, continuous sounds heard more during expiration; sometimes cleared by coughing Sound like blowing air through fluid with a straw
Wheezes (sibilant wheeze) 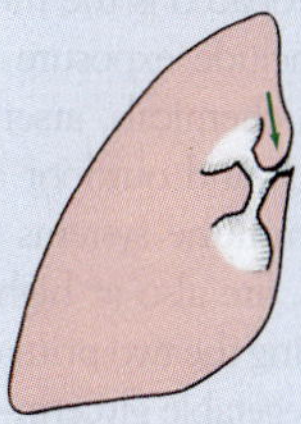	Heard over all lung fields but more distinct over posterior lung fields	High-velocity airflow through severely narrowed or obstructed bronchus	High-pitched, musical sounds such as a squeak heard continuously during inspiration or expiration; usually louder on expiration Not cleared with coughing
Pleural friction rub 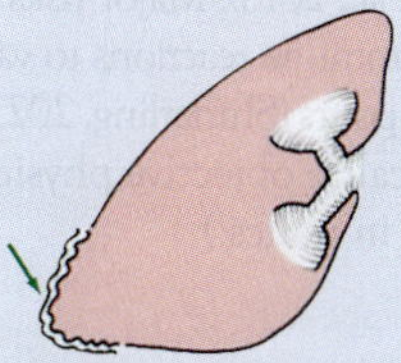	Heard over anterior lateral lung field (if patient is sitting upright)	Inflamed pleura, parietal pleura rubbing against visceral pleura	Has grating quality heard best during inspiration; does not clear with coughing; heard loudest over lower lateral anterior surface
Stridor	Heard loudest over the trachea but sounds may be transmitted to lung fields	Upper airway obstruction resulting from foreign body or inflamed, swollen tissues of the larynx or trachea	Loud, high-pitched crowing sound during inspiration, often heard without a stethoscope

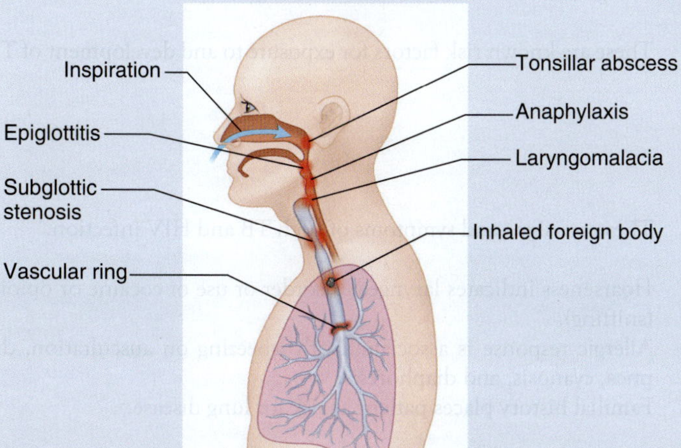

Data from Ball, J. W., Dains, J. E., Flynn, J. A., et al. (2022). *Seidel's guide to physical examination: An interprofessional approach* (10th ed.). Elsevier; Sarkar, M., Madabhavi, I., Niranjan, N., & Dogra, M. (2015). Auscultation of the respiratory system. *Annals of Thoracic Medicine, 10*(3), 158–168.

- Measure the patient's respirations after vital signs confirm that patient is stable
- Report respiratory distress, difficulty breathing, and changes in rate and depth
- Keep head of bed elevated for a patient who has respiratory difficulties

When assessment reveals changes in lung function or when assessments for specific pathophysiological changes reveal abnormal findings, collaborate with the interprofessional health care team (e.g., health care provider or respiratory therapist).

Equipment

- Stethoscope

STEP	RATIONALE
ASSESSMENT	
1. Identify patient using at least two person-specific identifiers (e.g., name and date of birth, or name and medical record number) according to employer policy.	Ensures correct patient. Complies with Accreditation Canada's standards and improves patient safety (Accreditation Canada, 2020).
2. Throughout the procedure, the 4 moments for hand hygiene are to be implemented; hand hygiene should occur before initial patient (or patient environment) contact, before an aseptic procedure, after body fluid exposure risk, and after patient (or patient environment) contact. Additional hand hygiene should be performed when hands are visibly soiled.	Proper hand hygiene helps prevent the spread of infectious agents to health care providers.
3. Assess history of tobacco use (cigarette, cigar, pipe, or vaping with e-cigarette [electronic nicotine delivery system]) or marijuana use, including type of tobacco, duration (number of years), and amount in pack-years. Pack-years equal number of years smoking times number of packs per day (e.g., 4 years × 0.5 packs/day = 2 pack-years). If patient has quit, determine length of time since smoking stopped. If patient vapes, determine device type and flavour preference, and identify the mix of tobacco products used (J. L. Pearson et al., 2018).	Smoking is a major cause of lung cancer, heart disease, and chronic lung disease (emphysema and chronic bronchitis). Smoking tobacco is the most important risk factor for lung cancer; other factors include exposure to second-hand smoke, radon, radiation, asbestos, certain chemicals, arsenic in drinking water, pollutants from cooking and heating, and outdoor air pollution (CCS, 2022e). Individuals with weakened immune systems or lupus, or smokers who take beta-carotene supplements, are also at higher risk of developing lung cancer. Even in small doses, inhaling the two primary ingredients found in e-cigarettes—propylene glycol and vegetable glycerin—is likely to expose users to a high level of toxins; and the more ingredients a user is inhaling, the greater the toxicity (Sassano et al., 2018). Major risks of vaping include chemical irritation and allergic or immune reactions to various chemicals or other substances in the inhaled vapours (Shmerling, 2022).
4. Ask if patient has experienced any of the following: *persistent cough* (productive or nonproductive), sputum production, *blood-streaked sputum*, *chest pain*, shortness of breath, orthopnea, dyspnea during exertion, activity intolerance, or *recurrent attacks of pneumonia or bronchitis*.	Symptoms of respiratory alterations help to localize objective physical findings. (Warning signals for lung cancer are in italics.)
5. Determine whether patient works in environment containing pollutants (e.g., asbestos, arsenic, coal dust, or chemical irritants) or requiring exposure to radiation. Does patient have exposure to second-hand cigarette smoke?	Patients with chronic respiratory disease, particularly asthma, have symptoms aggravated by changes in temperature and humidity, irritating fumes or smoke, emotional stress, and physical exertion.
6. Review history for known or suspected human immunodeficiency virus (HIV) infection, substance use, low income, residence or employment in a long-term care facility or shelter, homelessness, recent imprisonment, being a family member of patient with tuberculosis (TB), and immigration from a country where TB is prevalent. Ask when patient last had a TB test.	These are known risk factors for exposure to and development of TB.
7. Ask if patient has history of persistent cough, hemoptysis (bloody sputum), unexplained weight loss, fatigue, night sweats, or fever.	These are signs and symptoms of both TB and HIV infection.
8. Does patient have history of chronic hoarseness?	Hoarseness indicates laryngeal disorder or use of cocaine or opioids (sniffing).
9. Assess for history of allergies to pollen, dust, or other airborne irritants and to any foods, medications, or chemical substances.	Allergic response is associated with wheezing on auscultation, dyspnea, cyanosis, and diaphoresis.
10. Review family history for cancer, TB, allergies, asthma, or chronic obstructive pulmonary disease (COPD).	Familial history places patient at risk for lung disease.

NURSING DIAGNOSES

- Reduced airway clearance
- Inadequate breathing pattern
- Inadequate gas exchange
- Pain (acute, chronic)
- Fatigue
- Potential for infection

Related factors and risk factors are individualized on the basis of patient's condition or needs.

STEP	RATIONALE
PLANNING	
1. Expected outcomes following completion of procedure:	
• Respirations are passive, diaphragmatic or costal, and regular (10–20 breaths/min in adult) with symmetrical expansion.	Characteristics of normal respirations.
• Breath sounds are clear to auscultation and equal bilaterally.	Air flows without interference or obstruction. Corresponding sides should sound the same.
• Patient able to describe factors that predispose to lung disease.	Awareness of risks can improve patient adherence to healthy behaviour.
• Patient assumes appropriate posture for optimal breathing.	Patient can learn about benefits of good posture as examination manoeuvres are performed.
2. Anticipate teaching topics so that during the examination you can teach patient about any risk factors for lung disease.	Allows patient education to be incorporated into assessment process.
3. Assemble necessary equipment.	Reduces transmission of infection. Promotes efficiency of examination.
IMPLEMENTATION	
1. Position and prepare patient for examination:	Proper hand hygiene helps prevent the spread of infectious agents to health care providers.
a. Position patient sitting upright. For bedridden patient, elevate head of bed 45–90 degrees. If patient unable to tolerate sitting, use supine and side-lying positions.	Promotes full lung expansion during examination. Patients with chronic respiratory disease may need to sit up throughout examination because of shortness of breath. Help of another caregiver may be required to position unresponsive patients.
b. Remove gown or drape first from posterior chest, keeping front of chest and legs covered. As examination progresses, remove gown from area being examined.	Avoids unnecessary exposure and provides full visibility of thorax. Allows direct placement of diaphragm or bell on patient's skin, which enhances clarity of sounds.
c. Explain all steps of procedure, encouraging patient to relax and breathe normally through mouth.	Anxiety alters respiratory function. Breathing through mouth decreases extraneous sounds from air passing through nose.
2. Examine posterior thorax:	
a. If possible, stand behind patient. Inspect thorax for shape and symmetry. Note any deformities, position of spine, slope of ribs, retraction of intercostal spaces (ICS) during inspiration and bulging of ICS during expiration, and symmetrical expansion during inspiration. Note anteroposterior (AP) diameter.	Allows for identification of impairment in chest expansion and any symptoms of respiratory distress. Normal chest contour is symmetrical. In a child, the shape of chest is almost circular, with AP diameter in 1:1 ratio. In an adult, AP is one-third to one-half of side-to-side diameter. Chronic lung disease causes ribs to be more horizontal and increases AP diameter, resulting in "barrel chest." Patients with breathing problems assume postures that improve ventilation.

Critical Decision Point *When a patient holds the chest wall during breathing, it indicates localized chest pain. Assess the nature of pain, including onset, severity, precipitating factors, quality, region, and radiation.*

STEP	RATIONALE
b. Determine rate and rhythm of breathing (see Chapter 7). Examine thorax as a whole. Have patient relax.	This is a good time to count respirations, with patient relaxed and unaware of inspection. Awareness could alter respirations.

STEP	RATIONALE
c. Systematically palpate posterior chest wall, costal spaces, and ICS, noting any masses, pulsations, unusual movement, or areas of localized tenderness (see Step 3c illustration). If patient voices pain or tenderness, avoid deep palpation. If there is a suspicious mass, palpate lightly for shape, size, and qualities of lesion (see Skill 8.1). Do not palpate painful areas deeply.	Palpation is used to assess further characteristics and confirm or supplement findings from inspection. Localized swelling or tenderness indicates trauma to ribs or underlying cartilage. A fractured rib fragment could be displaced.
d. Assess chest expansion by standing behind patient and placing thumbs along spinal processes at tenth rib, with palms lightly contacting posterolateral surfaces (see Step 3d, illustration *A*). Keep thumbs about 5 cm (2 inches) apart, with thumbs pointing toward spine and fingers pointing laterally. Press hands toward patient's spine to form small skinfold between thumbs. After exhalation, have patient take deep breath. Note movement of thumbs (see Step 3d, illustration *B*) and symmetry of chest wall movement. Normally, symmetrical separation of thumbs occurs during chest excursion 3–5 cm (1.2–2 inches).	Palpation of chest expansion is used to assess depth of patient's breathing. This technique is a good measure to evaluate patient's ability to perform deep-breathing exercises. Limited movement on one side indicates that patient is voluntarily splinting during ventilation because of pain. Avoid allowing hands to slide over skin, which gives false measure of excursion.

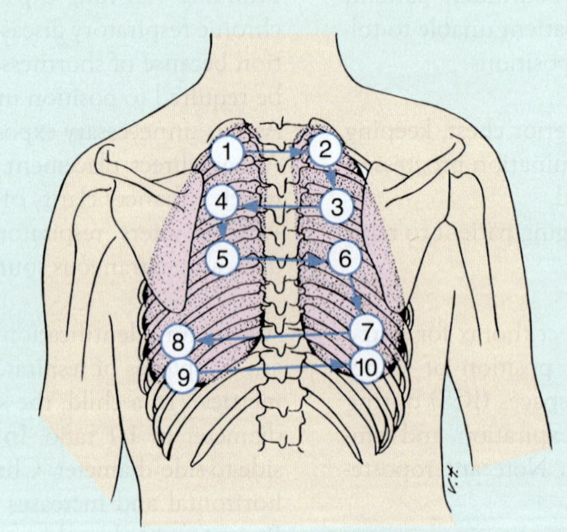

STEP 3C Pattern for assessment of posterior thorax.

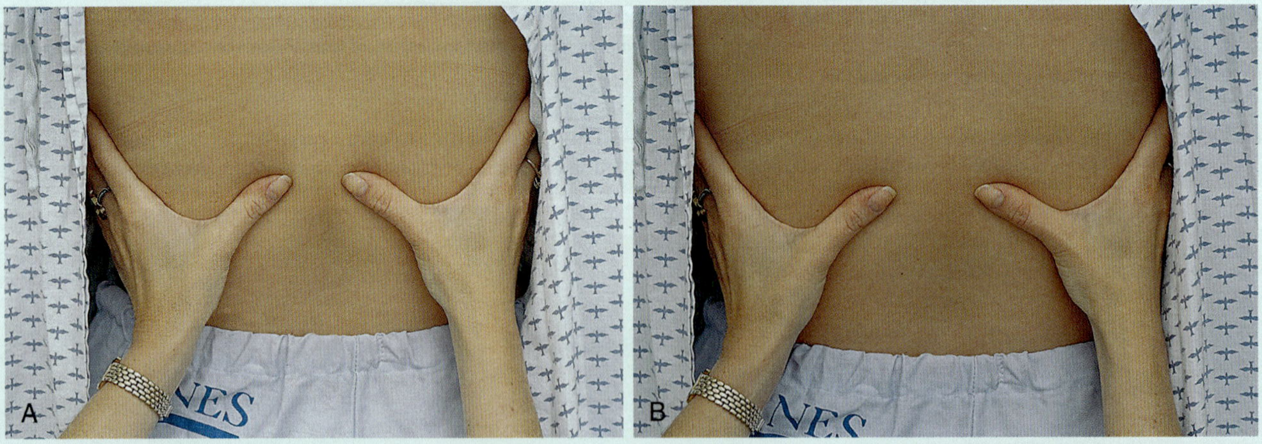

STEP 3D A, Position of hands for palpation of posterior thorax excursion. B, As patient inhales, movement of chest excursion separates nurse's thumbs.

STEP	RATIONALE
e. Auscultate breath sounds. Instruct patient to take slow, deep breaths with mouth slightly open. For an adult, place diaphragm of stethoscope firmly on chest wall over intercostal spaces (see Step 3e illustration). Listen to an entire inspiration and expiration at each stethoscope position (see pattern in Step 3c). If sounds are faint, as in obese patients, ask person to breathe harder and faster temporarily. Systematically compare breath sounds over right and left sides, listening for normal and adventitious sounds.	Assesses movement of air through tracheobronchial tree (Table 8.7). Recognition of normal airflow sounds allows detection of sounds caused by mucus or airway obstruction. Characterize sounds by length of inspiratory and expiratory phases.

Critical Decision Point *Use caution when asking patients to breathe harder or faster because inhaling and exhaling deeply or quickly can cause lightheadedness.*

STEP	RATIONALE
f. If you auscultate adventitious sounds, have patient cough. Listen again with stethoscope to determine whether sound has cleared with coughing. See Table 8.6 for a description of adventitious breath sounds.	Coughing may clear adventitious sounds. Rhonchi often are eliminated or altered by coughing. Crackles and wheezes are not.
3. Examine lateral thorax:	
a. Instruct patient to raise arms and inspect chest wall for same characteristics as reviewed for posterior chest.	Improves access to lateral thoracic structures.

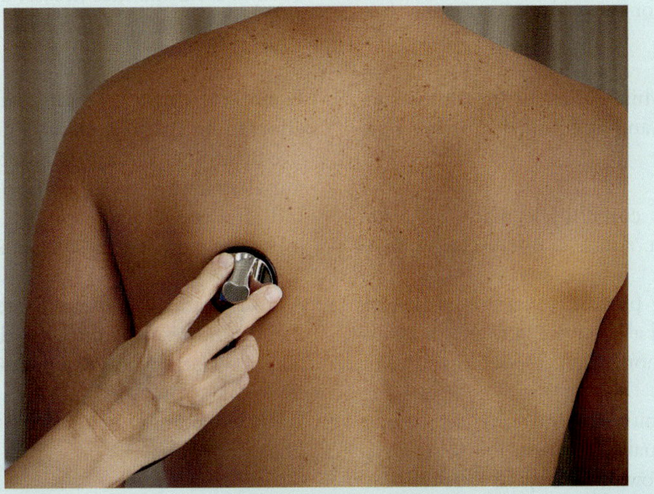

STEP 3E Auscultation with a stethoscope.

TABLE 8.7

Normal Breath Sounds

Type	Description	Location	Origin
Bronchial	Loud and high-pitched sounds with hollow quality Expiration lasts longer than inspiration (3:2 ratio)	Best heard over trachea	Created by air moving through trachea close to chest wall
Bronchovesicular	Medium-pitched and blowing sounds of medium intensity Inspiratory phase equal to expiratory phase	Best heard posteriorly between scapulae and anteriorly over bronchioles lateral to sternum at first and second intercostal spaces	Created by air moving through large airways
Vesicular	Soft, breezy, and low-pitched sounds Inspiratory phase 3 times longer than expiratory phase	Best heard over periphery of lung (except over scapula)	Created by air moving through smaller airways

STEP	RATIONALE

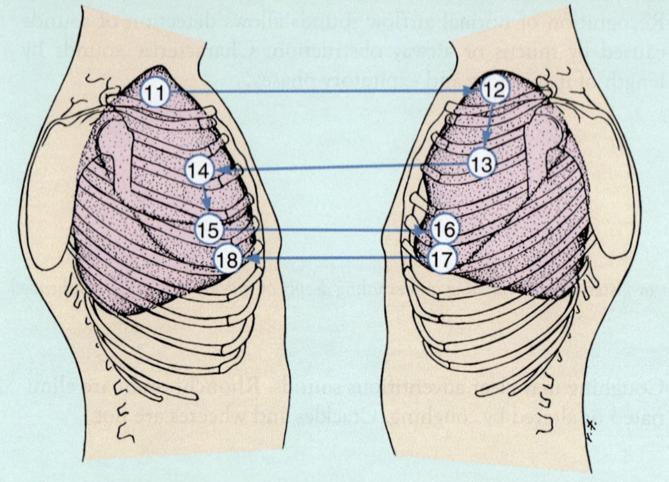

STEP 4B Pattern for assessment of lateral thorax.

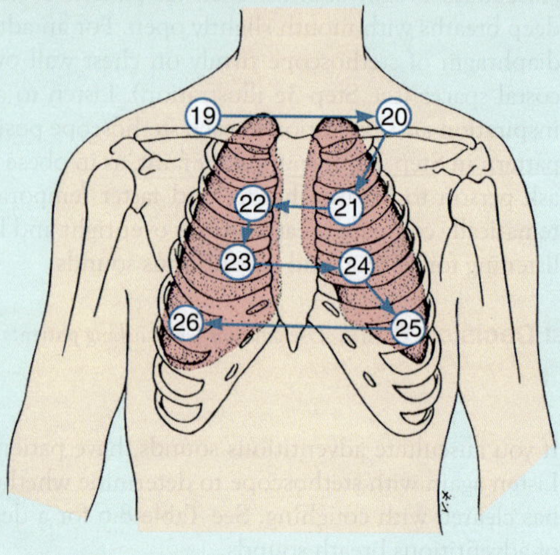

STEP 5D Pattern for assessment of anterior chest.

b. Extend palpation and auscultation of posterior thorax to lateral sides of chest, except for excursion measurement (see Step 4b illustration). — Locates abnormalities in lateral lung fields.

4. Examine anterior thorax:

a. Inspect accessory muscles while patient is breathing: sternocleidomastoid, trapezius, and abdominal muscles; note effort to breathe. — Extent to which accessory muscles are used reveals degree of effort to breathe. Accessory muscles move little with normal passive breathing. Patients who require great effort and rely on these muscles may produce a grunting sound.

b. Inspect width or spread of costal angle made by costal margins and tip of sternum. Angle is usually larger than 90 degrees between margins. — Indicates congenital, acquired, or traumatic alterations that may influence patient's chest expansion.

c. Observe patient's breathing pattern, observing symmetry and degree of chest wall and abdominal movement. Respiratory rate and rhythm are more often assessed on anterior chest wall. — Assesses patient's effort to breathe: symmetrical, passive movement indicates no respiratory distress. Male patients' breathing is diaphragmatic, whereas females patients' breathing is more costal.

d. Palpate anterior thoracic muscles and ribs for lumps, masses, tenderness, or unusual movement, following a systematic pattern across and down (see Step 5d illustration). — Localized swelling or tenderness indicates trauma to underlying ribs or cartilage.

e. Palpate anterior chest excursion. Place hands over each lateral rib cage, with thumbs approximately 5 cm apart and angled along each costal margin. As patient inhales deeply, thumbs should symmetrically move apart 3–5 cm (1.2–2 inches), with each side expanding equally. — Assesses depth of patient's breathing and ability to perform deep-breathing exercises. Certain abnormalities are evident if expansion is not symmetrical.

f. With patient sitting, auscultate anterior thorax following same pattern as in Step 5d. Begin above clavicles; move across and then down as during palpation. Compare right and left sides. Give special attention to lower lobes, where mucus commonly gathers. — A systematic pattern of assessment comparing sides helps to identify abnormal sounds.

5. Clean stethoscope. — Reduces transmission of infection.

EVALUATION

1. Compare respiratory findings with assessment characteristics for thorax and lungs. — Determines presence of abnormalities.
2. Have patient identify factors leading to lung disease. — Demonstrates learning.
3. **Use teach-back:** "We've talked about some of the risk factors your occupation poses for lung disease. Tell me what you can to do to reduce exposure in your workplace." Develop a revised teaching plan if patient is unable to teach back correctly. — Determines patient's level of understanding of instructional topic.

Unexpected Outcomes	Related Interventions
1. Patient has copious mucus production; audible inspiratory wheezing; or congested cough with thick mucus.	• Help patient cough by splinting chest; teach to inhale slowly through nose, exhale, and cough; encourage expectoration of mucus. • Auscultate breath sounds before and after cough to evaluate cough effectiveness. • Auscultate lungs for adventitious sounds. • Encourage increased oral intake (if permitted) to thin potential secretions. • If unable to clear airway by coughing, suctioning may be indicated. • Monitor vital signs. • Notify health care provider.
2. Respirations are rapid or slow and irregular (see Chapter 7) and bulging of intercostal spaces is present.	• Position patient more upright if appropriate. • Auscultate lungs for adventitious sounds. • Notify health care provider.
3. Chest excursion is reduced. Depth of breathing is reduced by pain, postural deformity, or fatigue.	• Reposition patient more comfortably. • Administer analgesic as prescribed if appropriate.

Communication and Documentation

- Document patient's respiratory rate and character; breath sounds, including type, location, and presence on inspiration, expiration, or both; changes noted after coughing; and other physical assessment findings in progress notes in EHR or chart.
- Report abnormalities immediately to the health care provider.
- Document your evaluation of patient learning.

Special Considerations

Teaching

- Educate patients about the risks of cigarette smoking. Smoking accounts for an estimated 30% of all cancer deaths in Canada and 85% of lung cancer cases (CCS, 2022b).
- Individuals who stop smoking have the potential to live longer than those who continue to smoke. The probability of these individuals dying from lung cancer or other related causes continues to decline with further abstinence.
- Explain to patients that exposure to radiation, radon, arsenic, and asbestos from occupational, medical, and environmental sources; air pollution; and second-hand smoke contribute significantly to lung cancer (CCS, 2022e).
- Discuss with patients the warning signs of lung cancer, such as a persistent cough, sputum streaked with blood, chest pains, and recurrent attacks of pneumonia or bronchitis.

Pediatric

- In children, observe for use of accessory muscles, which indicates respiratory distress. Retractions may involve intercostal, suprasternal, supraclavicular, or sternal muscles (Hockenberry et al., 2024).
- Use the bell of the stethoscope to auscultate lung sounds in children. Breath sounds are louder in children because of their thin chest walls.
- Children normally exhibit noticeable abdominal or diaphragmatic movement. Older children and adults exhibit more costal or thoracic movement.
- Head bobbing and nasal flaring in infants are signs of significant respiratory distress (Hockenberry et al., 2024).
- Pneumococcal vaccine is recommended for routine immunization of infants and children (Government of Canada, 2021).

Gerontological

- Older persons have a costal angle (anteriorly) of slightly less than 90 degrees. The AP diameter sometimes increases from kyphosis.
- In older persons, chest expansion is reduced because of calcification of rib cartilage and partial contraction of inspiratory muscles.
- Immunization with the pneumococcal vaccine is recommended for all adults 65 years of age and older. Individuals with chronic or immunosuppressed conditions, including asthma, or residents of long-term care facilities should receive the pneumococcal vaccine before age 64 (Government of Canada, 2021).

✦ SKILL 8.4 Cardiovascular Assessment

A patient who presents with signs or symptoms of heart (cardiac) problems such as chest pain may be suffering a life-threatening condition that requires immediate attention. In this situation, you need to act quickly and perform the parts of the examination that are absolutely necessary. This will reveal baseline heart function and any risks for heart disease. The heart, neck vessels, and peripheral circulation are assessed together because the systems work in unison. A more thorough assessment can be conducted once the patient is more stable.

Through your assessment you can determine the integrity of the circulatory system. Inadequate tissue perfusion results in an inadequate delivery of oxygen and nutrients to cells, a condition called *ischemia.* This condition is caused by constriction of vessels or occlusion (blockage) from clot formation. The effects of ischemia depend on the duration of the problem and the metabolic needs of the tissues. Ischemia results in pain. If lack of oxygen to tissues is unrelieved, tissue necrosis (death) occurs. An embolus is a blood clot that breaks loose and travels through the circulation. If the clot obstructs circulation to the lungs or brain, it can be life threatening.

Assessment of the heart begins after examination of the lungs because the patient is already in a suitable position with the chest exposed. Assessment then proceeds to the neck vessels and ends with evaluation of peripheral circulation. The skills of inspection, palpation, auscultation, and percussion are used during the examination.

Delegation and Collaboration

The skill of completing a comprehensive cardiovascular assessment cannot be delegated to a UCP. The nurse directs the UCP to do the following:

- Count peripheral pulses after vital signs confirm that the patient is stable
- Recognize skin temperature and colour changes of affected extremities and report any changes to the nurse
- Recognize changes in peripheral pulses and report any changes to the nurse
- Report any occurrence of chest pain to the nurse immediately

When assessment reveals changes in cardiovascular function or when assessments for specific pathophysiological changes reveal abnormal findings, collaborate with the interprofessional health care team (e.g., health care provider or cardiac specialist).

Equipment

- Stethoscope
- Doppler ultrasonic stethoscope *(optional)*
- Conducting gel (if a Doppler ultrasonic stethoscope is used)
- Clean gloves (use nonlatex if necessary)

STEP	RATIONALE
ASSESSMENT	
1. Identify patient using at least two person-specific identifiers (e.g., name and date of birth, or name and medical record number) according to employer policy.	Ensures correct patient. Complies with Accreditation Canada's standards and improves patient safety (Accreditation Canada, 2020).
2. Throughout the procedure, the 4 moments for hand hygiene are to be implemented; hand hygiene should occur before initial patient (or patient environment) contact, before an aseptic procedure, after body fluid exposure risk, and after patient (or patient environment) contact. Additional hand hygiene should be performed when hands are visibly soiled.	Proper hand hygiene helps prevent the spread of infectious agents to health care providers.
3. Assess patient for history of smoking, alcohol intake, caffeine intake (e.g., coffee, tea, soft drinks, energy drinks, and chocolate), and recreational substance use or misuse. Determine exercise habits and dietary patterns and intake.	These contribute to risk factors for cardiovascular disease. In addition, caffeine and alcohol cause tachycardia. Insufficient exercise and intake of fatty and salty foods increase risk for cardiovascular disease.
4. Ask if patient is taking medications for cardiovascular function (e.g., antiarrhythmics, antihypertensives, beta blockers, antianginals) and if they know their purpose, dosage, and adverse effects.	Allows you to assess patient's adherence to and understanding of medication therapies. Medications for cardiovascular function cannot be taken intermittently.
5. Ask if patient has experienced dyspnea, chest pain or discomfort, palpitations, excess fatigue, cough, leg pain or cramps, edema of the feet, cyanosis, fainting, or orthopnea. Ask if symptoms occur at rest or during exercise.	These are the cardinal symptoms of heart disease. Cardiovascular function is sometimes adequate during rest but not during exercise.
6. If patient reports chest pain, determine onset (sudden or gradual), precipitating factors, quality, region, and severity and whether it radiates. Anginal pain is usually a deep pressure or ache that is substernal and diffuse, radiating to one or both arms, neck, or jaw.	Symptoms reveal acute coronary syndrome or coronary artery disease.

Critical Decision Point *The most common heart attack symptom in women is the same as in men—some type of chest pain or pressure that lasts more than a few minutes or comes and goes. However, women are more likely than men to have symptoms unrelated to chest pain, including dyspnea, nausea/vomiting, indigestion, fatigue, sweating, and jaw, arm, or shoulder pain* (Fields, 2022).

STEP	RATIONALE
7. Assess family history for heart disease, diabetes mellitus, high cholesterol or lipid levels, hypertension, stroke, or rheumatic heart disease.	Family history of these conditions increases risk for heart and vascular disease.
8. Ask patient about history of any pre-existing heart conditions (e.g., heart failure, congenital heart disease, coronary artery disease, dysrhythmias, or murmurs), heart surgery, or vascular disease (e.g., hypertension, phlebitis, varicose veins).	Knowledge reveals patient's level of understanding of condition. Pre-existing condition influences which examination techniques to use and expected findings.
9. Ask if patient experiences leg cramps; numbness or tingling in extremities; sensation of cold hands or feet; pain in legs; or swelling or cyanosis of feet, ankles, or hands.	These are signs and symptoms of vascular disease.
10. If patient experiences leg pain or cramping in lower extremities, ask whether it is relieved by walking or standing for long periods or whether it occurs during sleep.	Relationship of symptoms to exercise clarifies if problem is vascular or musculoskeletal. Pain caused by vascular condition tends to increase with activity. Musculoskeletal pain is usually not relieved when exercise ends.
11. Ask patient if they wear tight-fitting underwear, hosiery, or tight-fitting trouser socks and if they sit or lie in bed with legs crossed.	Tight hosiery around lower extremities and crossing legs can impair venous return, promoting clot formation.

NURSING DIAGNOSES

- Reduced cardiac output
- Inadequate peripheral tissue perfusion
- Pain (acute, chronic)
- Reduced stamina
- Insufficient knowledge regarding the need for a cardiovascular assessment
- Potential for peripheral neurovascular dysfunction

Related factors and risk factors are individualized on the basis of patient's condition or needs.

STEP	RATIONALE
PLANNING	
1. Expected outcomes following completion of procedure:	
• Heart rate is 60–100 beats/min (adolescent through adult), without extra sounds or murmurs.	Indicates normal rate and sinus rhythm.
• Point of maximal impulse (PMI) is palpable at fifth intercostal space at left midclavicular line in children older than 7 years of age and in adults.	Indicates normal heart position.
• Patient describes changes in own behaviour that could improve cardiovascular function.	Instruction about cardiovascular disease risks may improve patient's health behaviour habits.
• Patient describes schedule, dosage, purpose, and benefits of medications being taken for cardiovascular function.	Information related to health benefits may improve adherence to therapy.
• Blood pressure is within normal limits for patient (see Chapter 7).	This is one indicator of normal cardiovascular function.
• Carotid pulse is localized, strong, elastic, and equal bilaterally. No change occurs during inspiration or expiration; without carotid bruit.	This indicates a patent vessel.
• Jugular veins distend when patient lies supine and flatten when patient is in sitting position.	Venous pressure is normal.
• Peripheral pulses are equal and strong (2+); extremities are warm and pink, with capillary refill <3 seconds; <1 second for infants.	Peripheral circulation is intact.
• There is no clubbing of fingernails.	
• There is no dependent edema.	
• Peripheral hair growth is symmetrical and evenly distributed, and skin is free of lesions.	
2. Anticipate teaching topics so that during the examination you can teach patient about risks for heart and vascular disease.	Allows patient education to be incorporated into examination.
3. Prepare necessary supplies.	Reduces transmission of infection. Promotes efficient examination.
IMPLEMENTATION	
1. Help patient be as relaxed and comfortable as possible.	Proper hand hygiene helps prevent the spread of infectious agents to health care providers. An anxious or uncomfortable patient can have mild tachycardia, which alters findings.
2. Have patient assume semi-Fowler's or supine position.	Provides adequate visibility and access to left thorax and mediastinum. Patient with heart disease often experiences shortness of breath while lying flat.
3. Explain procedure. Avoid facial gestures reflecting concern.	Patients with previously normal cardiac history may become anxious if you show concern.
4. Be sure that room is quiet.	Subtle, low-pitched heart sounds are difficult to hear.
5. Assess the heart:	
a. Form mental image of exact location of the heart (see Step 6a illustration). Base of heart is the upper part, and apex is the bottom tip. Surface of right ventricle constitutes most of the anterior surface of the heart.	Visualization improves ability to assess findings accurately and determines possible source of abnormalities.
b. Find angle of Louis, felt as ridge in sternum approximately 5 cm (2 inches) below suprasternal notch (between sternal body and manubrium). Slip fingers down each side of angle to feel adjacent ribs. Intercostal spaces (ICS) are just below each rib.	Provides you with landmarks to locate and assess heart sounds.
c. Find the following anatomical landmarks (see Step 6c illustration):	Familiarity with landmarks allows you to describe findings more clearly and ultimately may improve assessment.

STEP	RATIONALE

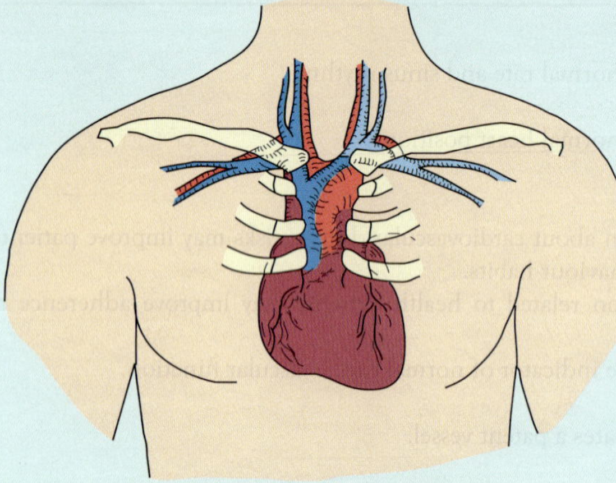

STEP 6A Anatomical position of heart.

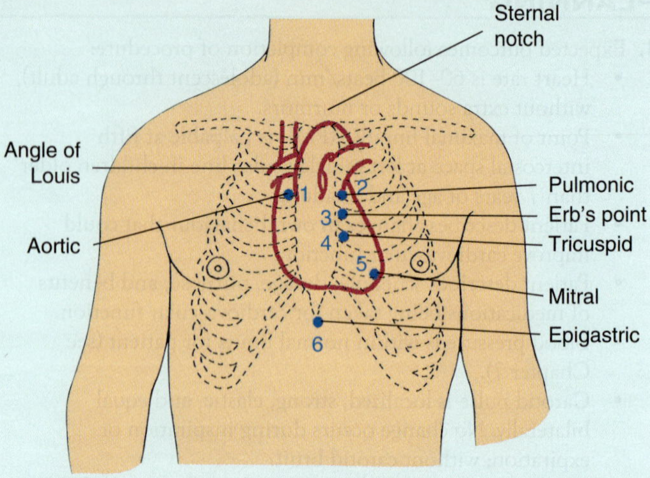

STEP 6C Anatomical sites for assessment of cardiac function.

(1) Aortic area is at second ICS, right of patient's sternum, close to sternal border *(1)*.

(2) Pulmonic area is at second ICS, left of patient's sternum, close to sternal border *(2)*.

(3) Second pulmonic area is found by moving down left side of sternum to third ICS, close to sternal border *(3)*, also referred to as *Erb's point*.

(4) Tricuspid area *(4)* is located at fourth left ICS along sternum, close to sternal border.

(5) Mitral area is found by moving fingers laterally to patient's left to locate fifth ICS at left midclavicular line *(5)*.

(6) Epigastric area *(6)* is at inferior tip of sternum.

Rationale: Listening to heart sounds from too far away from sternal border decreases the ability to hear them clearly.

d. Stand to patient's right to inspect and palpate precordium with patient supine. Note any visible pulsations and more exaggerated lifts. Closely inspect area of apex. Palpate for pulsations (placing proximal half of four fingers together and then alternating with ball of hand at all anatomical landmarks).

Rationale: Reveals size and symmetry of heart. Apical impulse may be visible at midclavicular line in fifth intercostal space. Apical impulse (PMI) may become visible only when patient sits up, bringing heart closer to anterior wall. Obesity obscures ability to visualize PMI. There should be no pulsations or vibrations. A thrill is a continuous palpable sensation, like purring of a cat. A thrust is the upward lift felt when palpating the chest wall.

e. Locate PMI by palpating with fingertips along the fifth ICS in midclavicular line (see Step 6e illustration). Note light, brief pulsation in area 1–2 cm (0.33–0.75 inches) in diameter at the apex.

Rationale: In presence of serious heart disease, PMI is located to left of midclavicular line, related to enlarged left ventricle. In chronic lung disease, PMI may be to right of midclavicular line as a result of right ventricular enlargement.

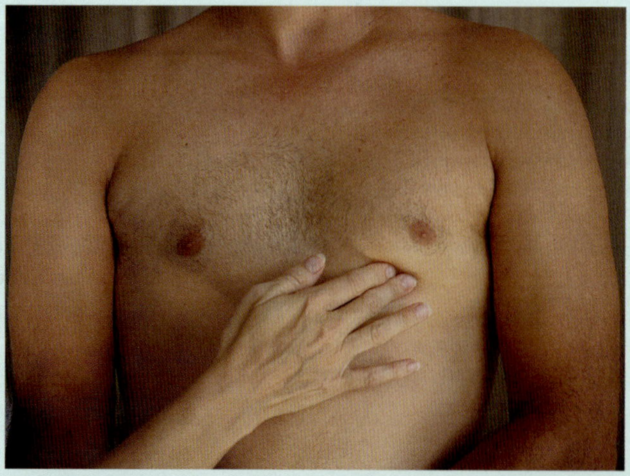

STEP 6E Palpation of point of maximal impulse (PMI).

STEP	RATIONALE

Critical Decision Point *Presence of a palpable thrill is not normal and indicates a disruption of blood flow caused by a defect in the closure of a heart valve or atrial septal defect. A stronger-than-expected impulse is a heave or lift, which indicates increased cardiac output or left ventricular hypertrophy. Report to health care provider.*

f. If palpating PMI is difficult, turn patient onto left side.

Manoeuvre moves heart closer to chest wall.

g. Inspect epigastric area and palpate abdominal aorta. **Note:** You should feel a localized strong beat.

Rules out reduced blood flow or diffuse pulse, which indicates abnormality.

h. Auscultate heart sounds:

(1) Have patient sit up and lean slightly forward; then have the person lie supine; end examination with patient in left lateral recumbent position (see Step 6h[1], illustrations A to C). In a patient with female genitalia, it may be necessary to lift left breast to hear heart sounds more effectively.

Different positions help to clarify type of sounds heard. Sitting position is best to hear high-pitched murmurs (if present). Supine is common position for hearing all sounds. Left lateral recumbent is best position to hear low-pitched sounds.

(2) While auscultating sounds at each anatomical landmark, ask patient not to speak but to breathe comfortably. Begin with diaphragm of stethoscope; alternate with bell. Use very light pressure for bell. Move stethoscope along slowly; avoid jumping from one area to another. Do not try to hear all heart sounds at once.

Auscultation requires you to isolate each heart sound at all auscultation sites, especially in patients with soft heart sounds.

(3) Begin at apex or PMI; move systematically to aortic area, pulmonic area, Erb's point, tricuspid area, and mitral area (see illustration in Step 6c). (**Note:** Some examiners use reverse sequence.) S_1 is loudest at apex and is simultaneous with carotid pulse. **Note:** Helpful mnemonic for remembering heart sound locations: **A P**ig **E**ats **T**oo **M**uch (**A**ortic, **P**ulmonic, **E**rb's point, **T**ricuspid, **M**itral).

At normal slow rates, S_1 is high pitched and dull in quality and sounds like a "lub." This sound precedes systolic phase of heart contraction.

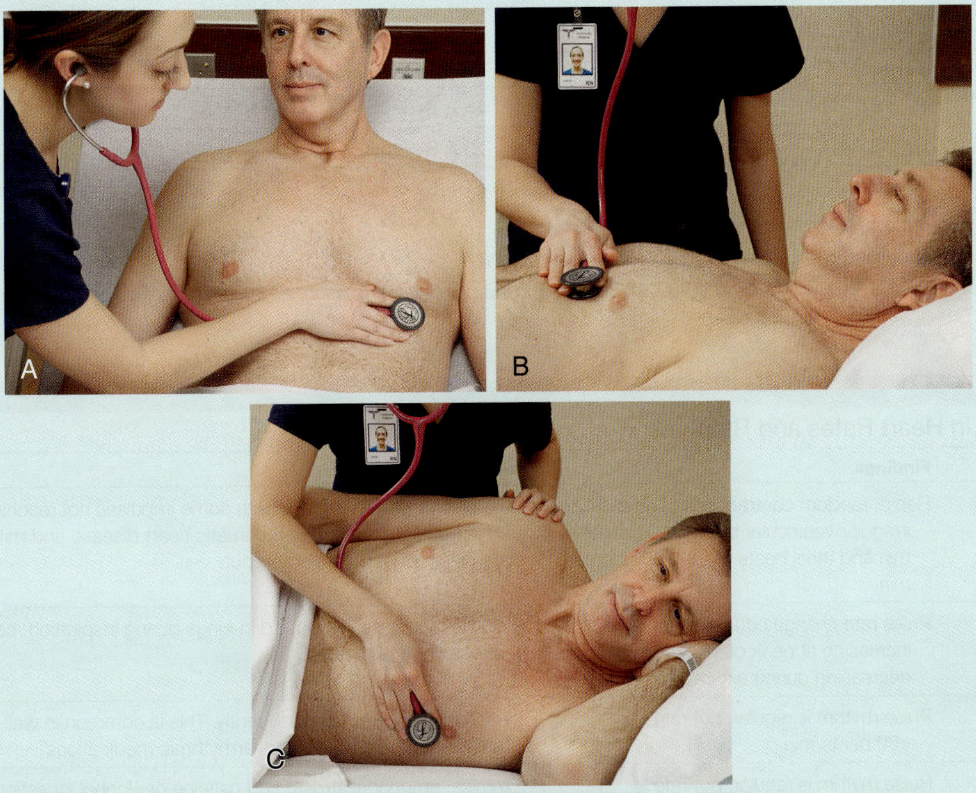

STEP 6H(1) Patient positions for auscultation of heart sounds. A, Sitting. B, Supine. C, Left lateral.

STEP	RATIONALE
(4) Listen for S_2 at each site. This sound is loudest at the aortic area. Heart sounds vary by pitch, loudness, and duration, depending on auscultatory site (Table 8.8).	Normal sounds of S_1 and S_2 are high pitched and best heard with diaphragm. S_2 precedes diastolic phase and sounds like "dub."
(5) After both sounds are heard clearly as "lub-dub," count each combination of S_1 and S_2 as one heartbeat. Count number of beats for 1 minute.	Determines apical pulse rate.
(6) Assess heart rhythm by noting time between S_1 and S_2 (systole) and then time between S_2 and the next S_1 (diastole). Listen to full cycle at each auscultation area. Note regular intervals between each sequence of beats. There should be a distinct pause between S_1 and S_2.	Failure of heart to beat at regular intervals is a dysrhythmia, which interferes with ability of heart to pump effectively.
(7) When heart rate is irregular, compare apical and radial pulses (Table 8.9). Auscultate apical pulse and then immediately palpate radial pulse. Also, you can ask a colleague to assess radial pulse while you simultaneously assess apical pulse.	Determines whether pulse deficit (radial pulse is slower than apical) exists. Deficit indicates that ineffective contractions of heart fail to send pulse waves to periphery.
i. Auscultate for extra heart sounds at each site. Note pitch, loudness, duration, timing, location on chest wall, and where it is heard in cardiac cycle.	Abnormal sounds include murmurs. Characteristics of murmurs help to identify contributing factors.
(1) Use stethoscope bell and listen for low-pitched extra heart sounds such as S_3 and S_4 gallops, clicks, and rubs. S_3, or a ventricular gallop, occurs just after S_2 at end of ventricular diastole. It sounds like "lub-dub-ee" or "Ken-tuc-ky." S_4, or an atrial gallop, occurs just before S_1 or ventricular systole. It sounds like "dee-lub-dub" or "Ten-nes-see."	Gallops are caused by premature rush of blood into a ventricle that is stiff or dilated or by an atrial contraction pushing against a ventricle that is not accepting blood.

TABLE 8.8

Heart Sounds According to Auscultatory Area

	Aortic	Pulmonic	Second Pulmonic	Mitral	Tricuspid
Pitch	$S_1 < S_2$	$S_1 < S_2$	$S_1 < S_2$	$S_1 > S_2$	$S_1 = S_2$
Loudness	$S_1 < S_2$	$S_1 < S_2$	$S_1 < S_2$*	$S_1 > S_2$†	$S_1 > S_2$
Duration	$S_1 > S_2$	$S_1 > S_2$	$S_1 > S_2$	$S_1 > S_2$	$S_1 > S_2$

*S_1 is relatively louder in second pulmonic area than in aortic area.

†S_1 may be louder in mitral area than in tricuspid area.

Adapted from Ball, J. W., Dains, J. E., Flynn, J. A., et al. (2022). *Seidel's guide to physical examination: An interprofessional approach* (10th ed.). Elsevier.

TABLE 8.9

Abnormalities in Heart Rates and Rhythms

Type	Findings	Description
Atrial fibrillation	Rapid, random contractions of atria cause irregular ventricular beats >100 beats/min and atrial beats at 200–350 beats/min.	Atria discharge very rapidly, with some impulses not reaching ventricles. This condition occurs in rheumatic heart disease and mitral stenosis. It causes reduced cardiac output.
Sinus arrhythmia	Pulse rate changes during respiration, increasing at peak of inspiration and decreasing during expiration.	Blood is momentarily trapped in lungs during inspiration, causing a fall in stroke volume of heart.
Sinus bradycardia	Pulse rhythm is regular, but rate is <60 beats/min.	Sinoatrial node fires less frequently. This is common in well-conditioned athletes and with use of antiarrhythmic medications.
Sinus tachycardia	Pulse rhythm is regular, but rate is accelerated to >100 beats/min.	Exercise, emotional stress, and caffeine or alcohol ingestion are common factors that cause increased firing of sinoatrial node.
Premature ventricular contraction	Premature beat occurs before regularly expected heart contraction. Underlying rhythm can be any rate.	Ventricle contracts prematurely because of electrical impulse bypassing normal conduction pathway. It may occur so early that it is difficult to detect as second beat. It may be followed by a pause.

STEP	RATIONALE
(2) With patient leaning forward or lying on left side, listen for friction rubs as "squeaky" or rubbing sounds.	Rubs result from lungs or inflamed visceral and parietal layers of the pericardium of the heart rubbing against one another.
j. Auscultate for heart murmurs over each auscultation site.	Murmurs are sustained swishing or blowing sounds heard at beginning, middle, or end of systole or diastole. Murmurs are caused by increased blood flow through a normal valve, forward flow through a stenotic valve or into a dilated vessel or chamber, or backward flow through a valve that fails to close.
(1) When you detect a murmur, listen carefully to note where you hear it best. Note intensity of the murmur.	Intensity is related to rate of blood flow through the heart or amount of blood regurgitated.
(2) Note whether murmur is low, medium, or high in pitch, using bell for low-pitched sounds.	Pitch depends on velocity of blood flow through the valves.
6. Assess neck vessels:	
a. To assess carotid arteries, have patient remain in sitting position.	Allows easier mobility of neck to expose artery for inspection and palpation.
b. Inspect neck on both sides for obvious arterial pulsations. Sometimes a pulse wave can be seen. Use a penlight to improve visibility if required.	Carotids are the only sites to assess quality of pulse wave (see Step 7b illustration). Experience is required to evaluate wave in relation to events of cardiac cycle.
c. Palpate each carotid artery separately with index and middle fingers around medial edge of sternocleidomastoid muscle. Ask patient to raise chin slightly, keeping head straight (see Step 7c illustration) or slightly away from artery. Note rate and rhythm, strength, and elasticity of artery. Also note whether pulse changes as patient inhales and exhales.	If both arteries were occluded simultaneously, patient could lose consciousness from reduced circulation to brain. Turning head improves access to artery. A change indicates a sinus arrhythmia.

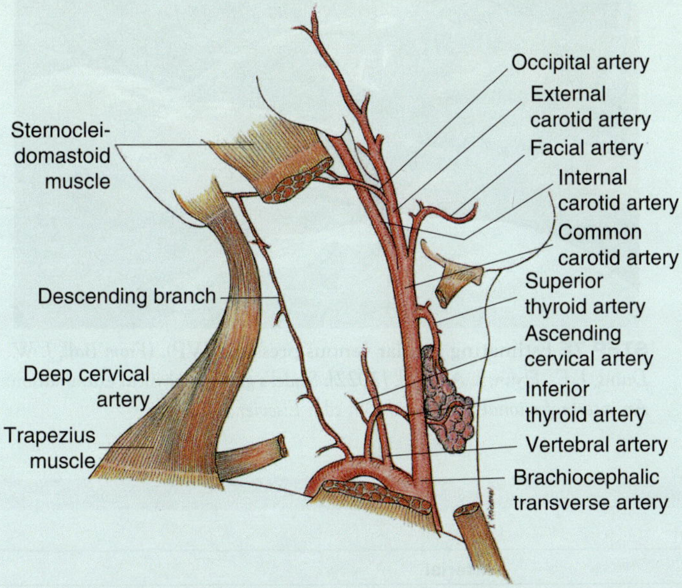

STEP 7B Anatomical position of carotid artery.

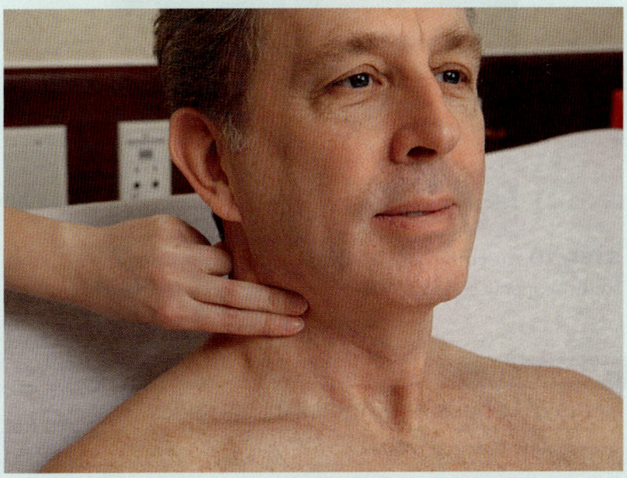

STEP 7C Palpate each carotid artery separately.

Critical Decision Point *Do not palpate or massage the carotid artery vigorously. Stimulation of carotid sinus causes a reflex drop in heart rate and blood pressure, which can result in cardiac arrest. Never palpate both arteries simultaneously because you could obstruct blood flow to the brain.*

STEP	RATIONALE
d. Place bell of stethoscope over each carotid artery, auscultating for blowing sound (bruit) (see Step 7d illustration). Ask patient to exhale and hold breath for a few heartbeats so respiratory sounds do not interfere with auscultation (Ball et al., 2022).	Narrowing of lumen of carotid artery by arteriosclerotic plaques causes disturbance in blood flow. Blood passing through narrowed section creates turbulence and emits blowing or swishing sound. Normally you do not hear a bruit.
e. To estimate the jugular venous pressure (JVP), hold a vertical ruler on the angle of Louis (sternal angle), align a straight edge on the ruler like a T-square, and adjust the level of the horizontal straight edge to the level of pulsation (Jarvis et al., 2024) (see Step 7e illustration). Read the level of intersection on the vertical ruler and state the patient's position, e.g., "JVP 3 cm above sternal angle when elevated 10 degrees." Changes in jugular venous distension (JVD) should also be noted, including pulsations or changes with patient position changes (i.e., from sitting to supine).	
7. Peripheral vascular assessment:	
a. Inspect lower extremities for changes in colour and condition of skin (Table 8.10). Note skin and nail texture, hair distribution, venous patterns, edema, and scars or impaired skin integrity. Compare skin colour with patient lying and standing.	Changes may reflect impaired peripheral circulation.

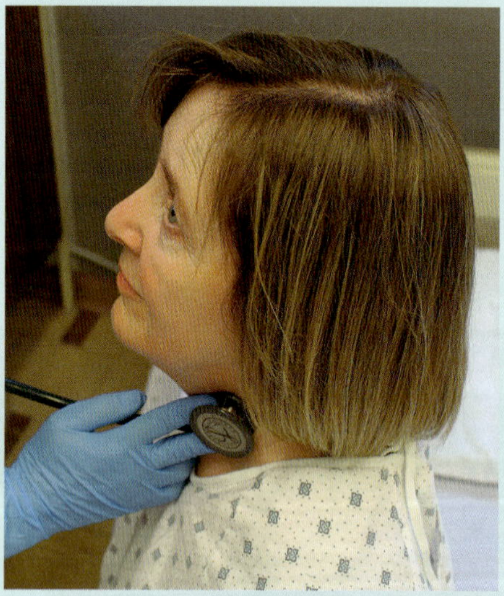

STEP 7D **Auscultation for carotid artery bruit using the bell of the stethoscope.** (*Courtesy Melanie Deveau and Jackie Hartigan-Rogers.*)

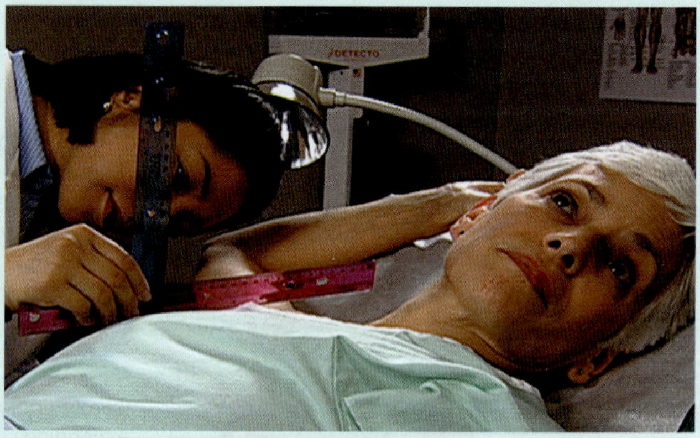

STEP 7E **Estimating jugular venous pressure (JVP).** (*From Ball, J. W., Dains, J. E., Flynn, J. A., et al. [2022]. Seidel's guide to physical examination: An interprofessional approach [10th ed.]. Elsevier.*)

TABLE 8.10

Signs of Venous and Arterial Insufficiency

Assessment Criterion	Venous	Arterial
Pain	Aching; increases in evening and with dependent position	Burning, throbbing, cramping; increases with exercise
Paresthesia	None	Numbness, tingling, decreased sensation
Temperature	Normal to touch	Cool to touch
Colour	Normal or cyanotic	Pale; worsened by elevation of extremity; dusky red when extremity is lowered
Capillary refill	Not applicable	>2 seconds
Pulse	Present	Decreased or absent
Skin changes	Brown pigmentation around ankles	Thin, shiny skin; decreased hair growth; thickened nails
Ulcerations	Shallow ulcers around ankles (chronic venous stasis); edema apparent	Deep, well defined at site of trauma or tips of toes

STEP	RATIONALE
b. Palpate edematous areas, noting mobility, consistency, and tenderness.	Helps to determine extent of edema.
c. Assess for pitting edema by pressing area firmly with one finger for 5 seconds and releasing. Depth of indentation determines severity (see Step 8c illustration): 2 mm 1+ edema 4 mm 2+ edema 6 mm 3+ edema 8 mm 4+ edema	Limb edema is a classic sign of deep vein thrombosis (DVT), although edema can also be seen in other conditions; therefore, if DVT is suspected, diagnostic tests must be performed. If DVT is diagnosed, emergency referral is needed owing to risk of pulmonary embolism (Jarvis et al., 2024).
d. Use tape measure to measure circumference of extremity.	Measuring circumference establishes baseline for future comparison.
e. Check capillary refill by grasping patient's fingernail or toenail and noting colour of nail bed. Apply gentle, firm pressure to nail bed. Release quickly, watching for colour change. Circulation is restored and normally returns to pink colour in less than 2 seconds.	Capillary refill is measured in seconds; less than 2 seconds is brisk, whereas greater than 4 seconds is sluggish. Cold environmental temperature with vasoconstriction and vascular disease can delay refill. Local pressure from cast or bandage also slows refill.
f. Inspect index fingers using the profile sign (viewing the finger from the side); the normal nail bed angle is 160 degrees.	Flattening of the nail bed angle suggests early clubbing, which may occur with chronic heart or lung diseases.
g. Ask if patient experiences pain or tenderness, and gently palpate for heat, firmness, or localized swelling of calf muscle, all of which are signs of phlebitis or DVT.	A frequent cause of DVT is prolonged immobility, such as in postoperative patients and in individuals after a long trip without adequate movement or exercise. Other factors that contribute to DVT include obesity, trauma, tobacco use, oral contraceptives, advanced age, malignancies, and stroke (Tyerman & Cobbett, 2023).

Critical Decision Point *Homans' sign (pain in calf on dorsiflexion of foot) is no longer considered a reliable indicator for the presence or absence of DVT* (Ball et al., 2022) *and should not be considered a reliable test. Trauma to a vein or muscle, reduced mobility, and increased blood clotting are reliable risk factors. If calf is swollen, tender, or red, notify patient's health care provider for further assessment and evaluation. If there is a strong suspicion of DVT, testing for Homans' sign is contraindicated. If a clot is present, it may become dislodged from its original site during this test, which could result in a pulmonary embolism.*

STEP	RATIONALE
h. Palpate peripheral arteries.	
(1) Start at most distal part of each extremity. Palpate each peripheral artery for equality, comparing side to side; elasticity of vessel wall (depress and release artery, noting ease with which it springs back to shape); and strength of pulse (force of blood against arterial wall) using the following rating scale (Ball et al., 2022): 0 Absent, not palpable 1+ Diminished, pulse barely palpable, weak and thready, easy to obliterate 2+ Normal pulse, easy to palpate 3+ Full, easy to palpate, increases 4+ Strong, bounding against fingertips, cannot be obliterated	Comparison of both arteries allows you to determine any localized obstruction or disturbance in blood flow. Pulses should be symmetrical side to side. If asymmetry is noted, look for other factors related to impaired circulation.
(2) Palpate radial pulse by lightly placing tips of first and second fingers in groove formed along radial side of forearm, lateral to flexor tendon of wrist (see Step 9h[2] illustration).	Pulse is relatively superficial and should not require deep palpation.
(3) Palpate ulnar pulse by placing fingertips along ulnar side of forearm (see Step 8h[3] illustration).	Palpated when arterial insufficiency to hand is expected or when you assess for radial occlusion (e.g., during arterial blood gas sampling), which may affect circulation to hand.

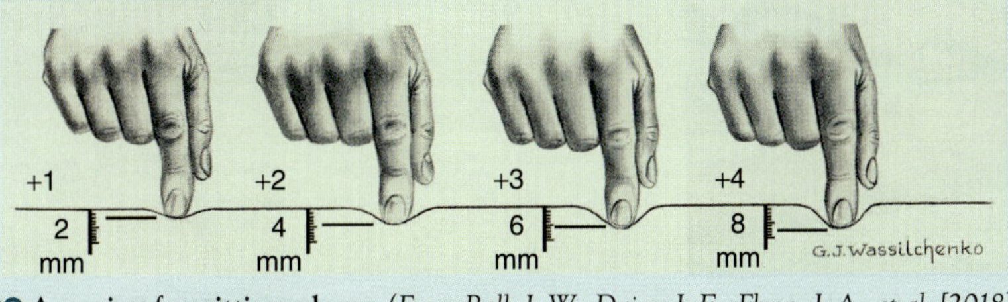

STEP 8C **Assessing for pitting edema.** (*From Ball, J. W., Dains, J. E., Flynn, J. A., et al. [2018]. Seidel's guide to physical examination [9th ed., Fig 15.12]. Mosby.*)

STEP	RATIONALE
(4) Palpate brachial pulse by locating groove between biceps and triceps muscles above elbow at antecubital fossa (see Step 8h[4] illustration). Place tips of first two fingers in muscle groove.	Artery runs along medial side of extended arm, requiring moderate palpation. If difficult to palpate, hyperextend arm to bring pulse site closer to the surface.
(5) Have patient lie supine with feet relaxed and palpate dorsalis pedis pulse. Gently place fingertips between great toe and first toe; slowly move fingers along groove between extensor tendons of great toe and first toe until pulse is palpable (see Step 8h[5] illustration).	Artery lies superficially and does not require deep palpation. Pulse may be congenitally absent.
(6) Palpate posterior tibial pulse by having patient relax and extend feet slightly. Place fingertips behind and below medial malleolus (ankle bone) (see Step 8h[6] illustration).	Artery is easily palpable with foot relaxed.
(7) Palpate popliteal pulse by having patient slightly flex knee with foot resting on table or bed. Instruct patient to keep leg muscles relaxed. Palpate deeply into popliteal fossa with fingers of both hands placed just lateral to midline. Patient may also lie prone to achieve exposure of artery (see Step 8h[7] illustration).	Flexion of knee and muscle relaxation improve accessibility of artery. Popliteal pulse is one of the more difficult pulses to palpate.
(8) Apply clean gloves. With patient supine, palpate femoral pulse by placing first two fingers over inguinal area below inguinal ligament, midway between pubic symphysis and anterosuperior iliac spine (see Step 8h[8] illustration).	Reduces transmission of microorganisms. Supine position prevents flexion in groin area, which interferes with artery access.

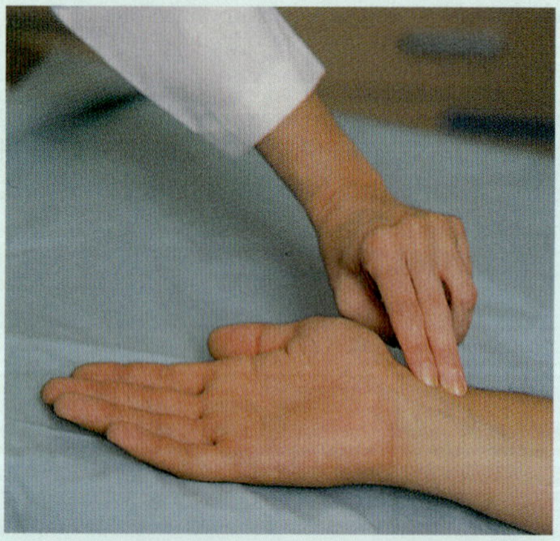

STEP 8H(2) Palpation of radial pulse.

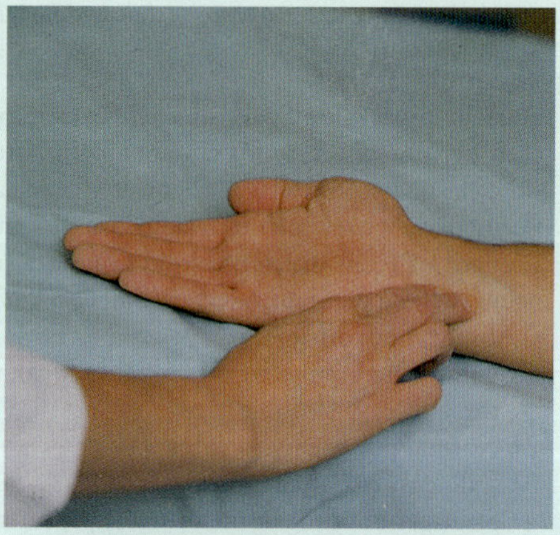

STEP 8H(3) Palpation of ulnar pulse.

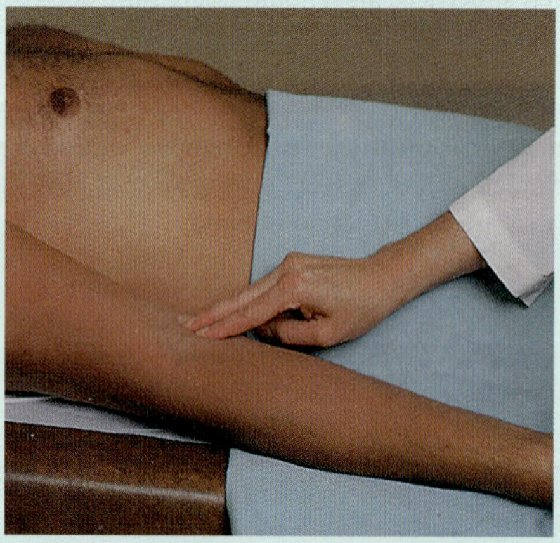

STEP 8H(4) Palpation of brachial pulse.

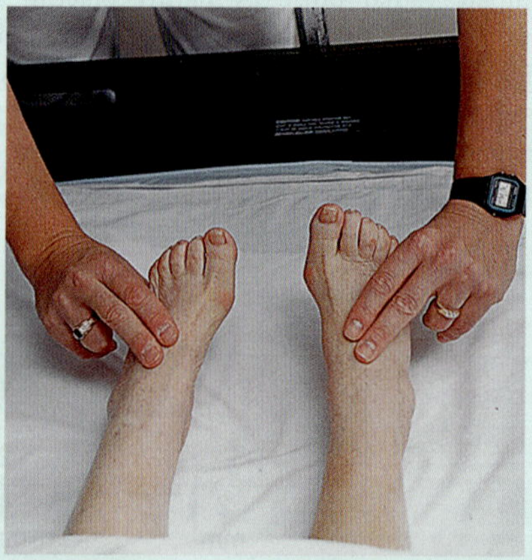

STEP 8H(5) Palpation of dorsalis pedis pulses.

STEP	RATIONALE
i. If pulses are difficult to palpate or are not palpable, use a Doppler ultrasonic instrument over pulse site: **(1)** Apply conducting gel to patient's skin over pulse site or onto transducer tip of probe. Turn Doppler on. **(2)** Gently apply ultrasound probe to skin, changing Doppler angle until pulsation is audible. Adjust volume as needed (see Step 8i[2] illustration). Wipe off gel from patient and Doppler.	Doppler amplifies sounds, allowing low-velocity blood flow through peripheral arteries to be heard.
8. Remove gloves and dispose of all equipment in appropriate receptacles. Help patient to comfortable position.	Reduces transmission of infection.

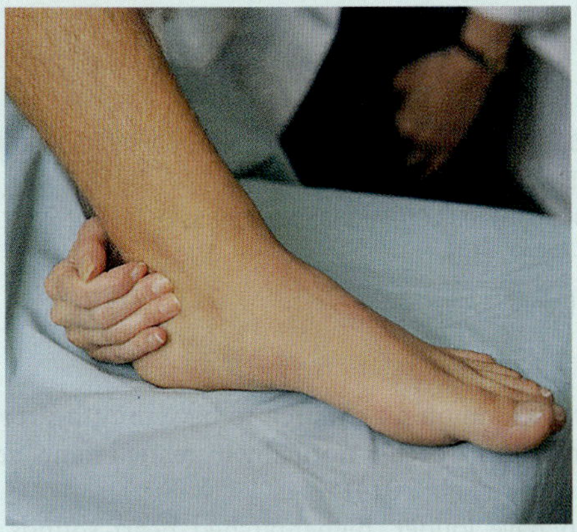

STEP 8H(6) Palpation of posterior tibial pulse.

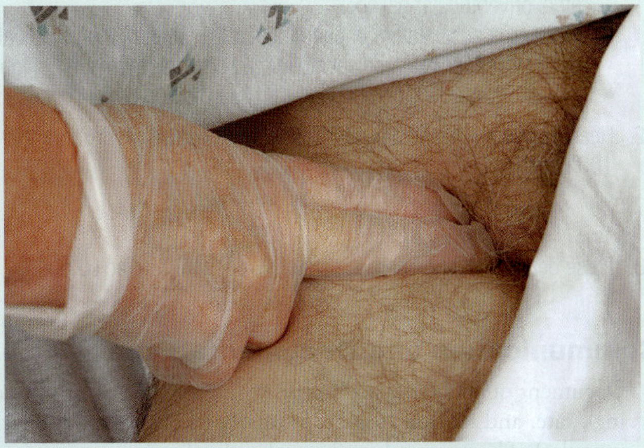

STEP 8H(8) Palpation of femoral pulse.

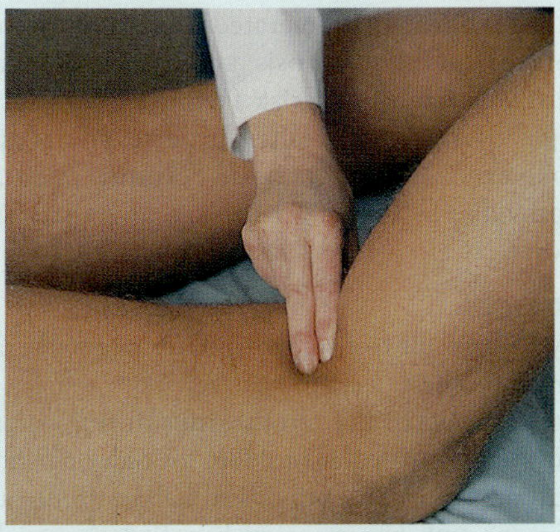

STEP 8H(7) Palpation of popliteal pulse with patient prone.

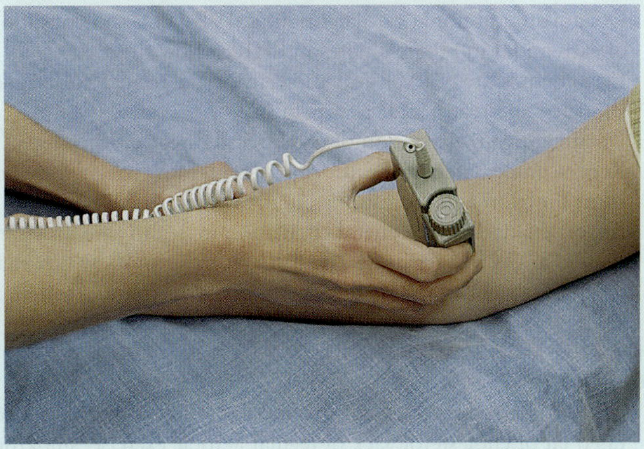

STEP 8I(2) Use of Doppler to assess brachial pulse.

EVALUATION

STEP	RATIONALE
1. Compare findings with normal assessment characteristics of heart and vascular system.	Determines presence of abnormalities.
2. If heart sounds are not audible or pulses are not palpable, ask another nurse to confirm assessment.	Validates abnormal assessment findings.
3. Ask patient to describe behaviours that increase risk for heart and vascular disease.	Demonstrates learning.
4. Compare pulses and capillary refill bilaterally with previous assessment.	Demonstrates change from baseline measures.

STEP	RATIONALE
5. Use teach-back: "I would like to make sure you understand some of the risks and behaviours that can lead to heart disease. Tell me how exercise affects your risk for heart disease." Develop a revised teaching plan if patient or caregiver is unable to teach back correctly.	Determines patient's and caregiver's level of understanding of instructional topic.

Unexpected Outcomes	Related Interventions
1. Findings differ from previous assessments, including the following: • Pulsations, vibrations, or both are palpable. These are the result of valvular problem, murmur, or both. • Extra heart sounds (S_3 or S_4) are auscultated. Extra sounds indicate atrial or ventricular gallop. • Murmur is auscultated. Impaired blood flow through heart indicates need for immediate medical attention. Some murmurs are benign. • JVP is elevated, a sign of right-sided heart failure or fluid overload.	• Prepare to obtain or help with electrocardiogram (ECG). • Use communication techniques to keep patient calm.
2. Heart rate is irregular, with rate less than 60 beats/min or more than 100 beats/min.	• Check blood pressure. If low, dysrhythmia is contributing to inadequate cardiac output. • Observe for sensations or reports of dizziness or feeling "faint." • Prepare to obtain ECG.
3. Pulse deficit is noted. There is risk for inadequate cardiac output.	• Obtain vital signs.

Communication and Documentation

- Document quality (clear or muffled), intensity (weak or pounding), rate, and rhythm (regular, regularly irregular, or irregularly irregular) of heart sounds and peripheral pulses in progress notes in EHR or physical chart.
- Document additional cardiac findings, JVP, JVD, and condition of extremities in progress notes in EHR or flow sheet.
- Document activity level and subjective data related to fatigue, shortness of breath, and chest pain.
- Document your evaluation of patient and caregiver learning.
- Report immediately to health care provider any irregularities in heart function and indications of impaired arterial blood flow.
- Report changes in peripheral circulation to health care provider; such changes may indicate circulatory compromise, which may result in permanent nerve damage or tissue death if untreated.

Special Considerations

Teaching

- Explain risk factors for heart disease: high dietary intake of saturated fat or cholesterol, lack of regular aerobic exercise, smoking, excess weight, stressful lifestyle, hypertension, and family history of heart disease.
- Refer patient (if appropriate) to available resources on controlling or reducing risks (e.g., nutrition counselling, exercise class, and stress reduction programs).
- Help patient find resources on how to quit smoking because this lowers the risk for cardiovascular disease (G. J. Pearson et al., 2021). Nicotine in cigarette smoke causes vasoconstriction.
- Use of daily low dose of Aspirin to prevent heart disease and DVT is no longer best practice. The Heart and Stroke Foundation of Canada (2021) indicates that daily Aspirin should not be used for prevention in patients who have not had a stroke or heart attack. Patients should consult their health care provider about therapy.

Pediatric

- PMI is at fourth intercostal space at left midclavicular line in children younger than 7 years of age (Hockenberry et al., 2024).
- Capillary refill in infants is usually less than 1 second.
- It is not uncommon for children to have third heart sounds (S_3). Sinus arrhythmia occurs normally in many infants and children (Hockenberry et al., 2024).
- Children have louder, higher-pitched heart sounds because of their thin chest walls.
- Atherosclerotic vascular changes can develop in childhood. Research has shown an accelerated burden of vascular changes and premature atherosclerosis among children and adolescents with well-established risk factors for cardiovascular disease (e.g., overweight/obesity, hypertension, dyslipidemia, and smoke exposure) (Hartz & de Ferranti, 2023). Caregivers should provide any child over the age of 2 years with a heart-healthy diet.

Gerontological

- PMI may be difficult to find in an older person because the AP diameter of the chest deepens.
- Accidental massage of the carotid sinus during palpation of the carotid artery is a particular problem for older persons, causing a sudden drop in heart rate from vagal nerve stimulation.
- Older persons with hypertension benefit from regular monitoring of blood pressure (daily, weekly, or monthly). Home monitoring kits are available. Teach patient how to use them correctly (see Chapter 7, Skill 7.7).

Care in the Community: Home Management

- The Heart and Stroke Foundation of Canada (2022) recommends the DASH eating plan to prevent cardiovascular disease. Help patients in the home to adapt food preferences and meal preparation resources. The DASH eating plan (or DASH diet) requires no special foods and instead provides daily and weekly nutritional goals. This plan recommends the following:
  - Eating vegetables, fruits, and whole grains
  - Including fat-free or low-fat dairy products, fish, poultry, beans, nuts, and vegetable oils
  - Limiting foods that are high in saturated fat, such as fatty meats, full-fat dairy products, and tropical oils such as coconut, palm kernel, and palm oils
  - Limiting sugar-sweetened beverages and sweets

✦ SKILL 8.5 Abdominal Assessment

Abdominal assessment is complex because of the multiple organs located within and near the abdominal cavity. This area of the body is associated with many health complaints; and many people are embarrassed by bowel or bladder dysfunction, reproductive problems, or urinary elimination problems. Abdominal pain is one of the most common symptoms that patients report when seeking medical care. It can be caused by alterations in organs such as the stomach, gallbladder, or intestines; or the pain may be the result of spinal or muscular injury. An accurate assessment requires matching the patient's history with a careful assessment of the location of physical symptoms (Table 8.11).

To perform an effective abdominal assessment, you need to know the location and function of the underlying structures involved, including the lower pelvis, kidneys, rectum, genitalia, liver, gallbladder, stomach, spleen, appendix, pancreas, intestines, and reproductive organs (Fig. 8.5). An abdominal assessment is routine after abdominal surgery, for any patient who has undergone invasive diagnostic tests of the gastrointestinal (GI) tract, and for patients with abnormalities affecting GI function. The order of an abdominal assessment differs from that of other assessments. You begin with inspection and follow with auscultation. It is important to auscultate before performing palpation and percussion because these manoeuvres alter the frequency and character of bowel sounds.

Delegation and Collaboration

The skill of abdominal assessment cannot be delegated to a UCP. The nurse directs the UCP to do the following:

- Report the development of abdominal pain and changes in the patient's bowel habits or dietary intake to the nurse

When assessment reveals changes in abdominal function or abnormal findings, communicate with the interprofessional health care team (e.g., health care provider, dietitian, urologist, ostomy nurse, or pain management team) for further follow-up.

Equipment

- Stethoscope
- Tape measure
- Examination light
- Water-based marking pen
- Drapes

TABLE 8.11

Common Causes of Abdominal Pain

Condition	Physical Alteration	Physical Signs and Symptoms
Appendicitis	Obstruction of appendix associated with inflammation, perforation, and peritonitis Patient often lies on back or side with knees flexed to decrease pain	Sharp pain directly over the irritated peritoneum 2–12 hours after onset. Often pain localizes in right lower quadrant between anterior iliac crest and umbilicus. Associated with rebound tenderness. Accompanied by anorexia, nausea, and vomiting.
Celiac disease	Damage to small intestine mucosa from ingestion of barley, rye, oats, and wheat	Foul-smelling diarrhea, abdominal distension, and symptoms of malnutrition may be present.
Cholecystitis	Obstruction of cystic duct causing inflammation or distension of gallbladder	*Murphy sign:* Apply gentle pressure below right subcostal arch and liver margin. Sharp pain and increased respiratory rate occur when patient takes a deep breath (Ball et al., 2022).
Crohn's disease	Chronic inflammatory disease of the ileum	Steady colicky pain in the right lower quadrant, with cramping, tenderness, flatulence, nausea, fever, and diarrhea. Often associated with bloody stools, weight loss, weakness, and fatigue. A tender mass of thickened intestine may be palpated in right lower quadrant.
Gastroenteritis	Inflammation of the stomach and intestinal tract	Generalized abdominal discomfort accompanied by anorexia, nausea, vomiting, diarrhea, and abdominal cramping.
Pancreatitis	Inflammation of the pancreas associated with alcoholism, medication reaction, and gallbladder disease	Steady severe epigastric pain close to umbilicus radiates to back. Associated with abdominal rigidity and vomiting. Pain is unrelieved by vomiting, worsens by lying supine.
Paralytic ileus	Obstruction of the small bowel that occurs after abdominal surgery, from abdominal radiation, or from use of anticholinergic medications	Generalized severe abdominal distension, nausea, and vomiting; decreased or absent bowel sounds.
Peptic ulcers (gastric and duodenal)	Damage of gastrointestinal (GI) mucosa at any area of the GI tract May be caused by bacterial infection (*Helicobacter pylori*) or nonsteroidal anti-inflammatory drugs (NSAIDs) Thought to be unrelated to stress Aggravated by smoking and excessive alcohol use	*Gastric ulcer:* Dull epigastric pain, localized midline. Early satiety; not usually relieved by food or antacids. *Duodenal ulcer:* Pain is episodic, lasting 30 minutes to 2 hours. It is located midline in epigastric region, may radiate around costal border to back; described as aching, burning, or gnawing. Typically occurs 1–3 hours after meals and at night (1200–0300 hours). Often relieved by food or antacid. *Both (dyspepsia syndrome):* Symptoms of fullness, epigastric discomfort, vague feeling of nausea, abdominal distension, and bloating; anorexia; weight loss.

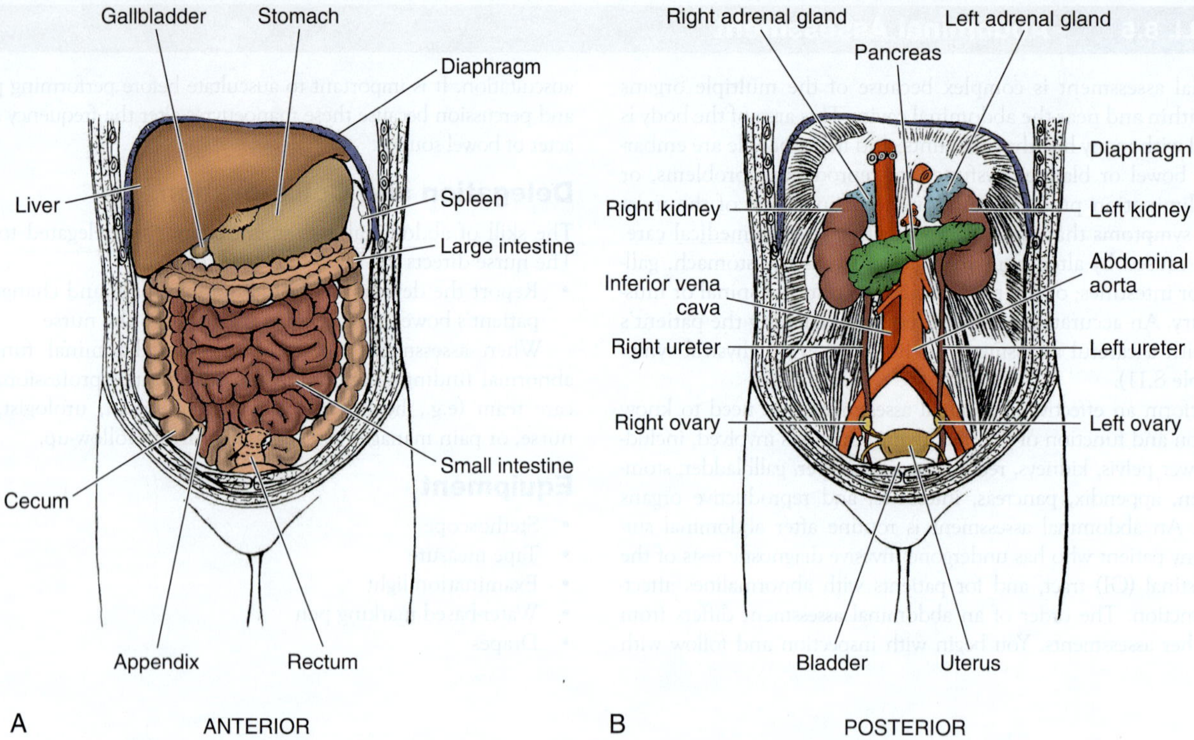

FIG 8.5 Location of organs in abdomen. A, Anterior. B, Posterior. *(Adapted from Monahan, F. D. [2008]. Mosby's expert physical exam handbook: Rapid inpatient and outpatient assessments [3rd ed.]. Mosby Elsevier.)*

STEP	RATIONALE
ASSESSMENT	
1. Identify patient using at least two person-specific identifiers (e.g., name and date of birth, or name and medical record number) according to employer policy.	Ensures correct patient. Complies with Accreditation Canada's standards and improves patient safety (Accreditation Canada, 2020).
2. Throughout the procedure, the 4 moments for hand hygiene are to be implemented; hand hygiene should occur before initial patient (or patient environment) contact, before an aseptic procedure, after body fluid exposure risk, and after patient (or patient environment) contact. Additional hand hygiene should be performed when hands are visibly soiled.	Proper hand hygiene helps prevent the spread of infectious agents to health care providers.
3. If patient has abdominal or low back pain, assess the character of pain in detail (location, onset, frequency, precipitating factors, aggravating factors, type of pain, severity, course).	Knowing pattern of characteristics of pain helps determine its source.
4. Carefully observe patient's movement and position, such as lying still with knees drawn up, moving restlessly to find a comfortable position, or lying on one side or sitting with knees drawn up to chest.	Positions assumed by patient reveal nature and source of pain (e.g., peritonitis, kidney stone, appendicitis). Patients with peritonitis lie still because movement aggravates pain. Supine position worsens acute pancreatitis pain; flexed knee with curved-back position brings relief. Patients with appendicitis lie on side or back with knees flexed in attempt to decrease muscle strain on abdominal wall.
5. Assess patient's normal bowel habits: frequency of stools; character of stools; recent changes in character of stools; measures used to promote elimination such as laxatives, enemas, and dietary intake; and eating and drinking habits.	Data compared with information from physical assessment may help identify cause and nature of elimination problems.
6. Ask if patient has had abdominal surgery, trauma, or diagnostic tests of GI tract.	Surgery or trauma to abdomen may result in altered position of underlying organs. Diagnostic tests may change character of stool.
7. Assess if patient has had recent weight changes or intolerance to diet (nausea, vomiting, cramping, especially in past 24 hours).	Changes may indicate alterations in upper GI tract (e.g., stomach or gallbladder) or lower colon.
8. Assess for difficulty in swallowing, belching, flatulence, bloody emesis (hematemesis), black or tarry stools (melena), heartburn, diarrhea, or constipation.	Indicative of GI alterations.

STEP	RATIONALE
9. Ask if patient takes anti-inflammatory medications (e.g., Aspirin, steroids, nonsteroidal anti-inflammatory drugs [NSAIDs]), or antibiotics.	These medications may cause GI upset or bleeding.
10. Review family history of cancer, kidney disease, alcoholism, hypertension, or heart disease.	Information may reveal risk for significant abdominal alterations. Chronic alcohol ingestion causes GI and liver problems.
11. Review patient's history for health care occupation, hemodialysis, intravenous medication use, household or sexual contact with hepatitis B virus (HBV) carrier, sexually active person (more than one sex partner in previous 6 months), or international traveller in an area of high HBV prevalence.	These are risk factors for HBV exposure. Abdominal findings for hepatitis include jaundice, hepatomegaly, anorexia, abdominal and gastric discomfort, tea-coloured urine, and clay-coloured stools (Tyerman & Cobbett, 2023).

NURSING DIAGNOSES

- Pain (acute, chronic)
- Constipation
- Diarrhea
- Inadequate nutrition
- Excessive nutrition
- Reduced health maintenance
- Nausea
- Insufficient knowledge regarding need for an abdominal assessment

Related factors are individualized on the basis of patient's condition or needs.

PLANNING

STEP	RATIONALE
1. Expected outcomes following completion of procedure:	
• Abdomen is soft and symmetrical, with smooth and even contour. No mass, distension, or tenderness is palpable. There are no forceful visible pulsations.	These are normal abdominal assessment findings.
• Bowel sounds are active and audible in all four quadrants.	Indicates normal peristaltic activity.
• No costovertebral angle (CVA) tenderness is present.	Indicates no inflammation of kidney.
• Patient denies discomfort or worsening of existing discomfort following examination.	Proper examination procedures have been implemented.
2. Anticipate teaching topics so that during the examination you can teach patient about warning signs of colorectal cancer.	Allows patient education to be incorporated into physical assessment.
3. Prepare necessary supplies.	Reduces transmission of infection. Ensures efficiency during examination.

IMPLEMENTATION

STEP	RATIONALE
1. Prepare patient for abdominal assessment:	Proper hand hygiene helps prevent the spread of infectious agents to health care providers.
a. Ask if patient needs to empty bladder or defecate.	Palpation of full bladder causes discomfort and feeling of urgency, making it difficult for patient to relax.
b. Keep upper chest and legs draped.	Maintains patient's comfort during examination, promoting relaxation.
c. Be sure that room is warm.	Promotes patient's comfort. Reduces risk of patient tensing abdominal muscles.
d. Have patient lie supine or in dorsal recumbent position with arms down at sides and knees slightly bent. Place small pillow under patient's knees.	Placing arms under head or keeping knees fully extended causes abdominal muscles to tighten. Tightening of muscles prevents adequate palpation.
e. Move sheet or blanket to expose area from just above xiphoid process down to symphysis pubis.	Provides full visualization of abdomen.
f. Maintain conversation during assessment except during auscultation. Explain steps calmly and slowly.	Patient's ability to relax during assessment improves accuracy of findings. Talking interferes with hearing bowel sounds.
g. Ask patient to point to tender areas.	Assess painful areas last. Manipulation of body part increases patient's pain and anxiety and makes remainder of assessment difficult to complete.
2. Abdominal assessment:	
a. Identify landmarks that divide abdominal region into quadrants. Boundary begins at tip of xiphoid process to symphysis pubis with line crossing and intersecting umbilicus, dividing abdomen into four equal sections (see Step 3a illustration).	Location of findings by common reference points helps successive examiners confirm findings and locate abnormalities.

STEP	RATIONALE
b. Inspect skin of surface of abdomen for colour, scars, venous patterns, rashes, lesions, silvery white striae (stretch marks), and artificial openings (stomas). Observe skin lesions for characteristics described in Skill 8.1.	Scars reveal evidence that patient has had past trauma or surgery. Striae indicate stretching of tissue from growth, obesity, pregnancy, ascites, or edema. Venous patterns reflect liver disease (portal hypertension). Artificial openings indicate bowel or urinary diversion (see Chapters 34 and 35).
c. If you note bruising, ask if patient self-administers injections (e.g., heparin or insulin).	Frequent injections may cause bruising and hardening of underlying tissues.

Critical Decision Point *Bruising may also indicate physical signs of abuse, accidental injury, or bleeding disorder. When bruising is noted, additional information may be needed from the patient.*

STEP	RATIONALE
d. Inspect contour, symmetry, and surface motion of abdomen. Note any masses, bulging, or distension. (Flat abdomen forms a horizontal plane from xiphoid process to symphysis pubis. Round abdomen protrudes in convex sphere from horizontal plane. Concave abdomen sinks into muscular wall. All are normal.)	Changes in symmetry or contour reveal underlying masses, fluid collection, or gaseous distension. Everted umbilicus (protruding outward) indicates distension. Hernia also causes umbilicus to protrude upward.
e. If abdomen appears distended, note whether distension is generalized. Look at flanks on each side.	Distension may be caused by the nine F's (*f*at, *f*latus, *f*eces, *f*luids, *f*ibroid, *f*ull bladder, *f*alse pregnancy, *f*atal tumour, and *f*etus) (Ball et al., 2022). If gas causes distension, flanks do not bulge. If fluid causes distension, flanks bulge. Tumour may cause more unilateral bulging or distension. Pregnancy causes symmetrical bulge in lower abdomen.
f. If you suspect distension, measure size of abdominal girth by placing tape measure under patient and around abdomen at level of umbilicus (see Step 3f illustration).	Consecutive measurements show any increase or decrease in abdominal distension. Make all subsequent measurements at same level of umbilicus to provide objective means to evaluate changes.
g. If patient has an NG or NI tube connected to suction, turn off momentarily.	Sound of suction obscures bowel sounds.
h. To auscultate bowel sounds, place diaphragm of stethoscope lightly over each of four abdominal quadrants. Ask patient not to talk. Listen until you hear repeated gurgling or bubbling sounds in each quadrant (minimum of once in 5–20 seconds). Describe sounds as normal, hyperactive, hypoactive, or absent. If initially there are no bowel sounds, listen for 5 minutes over each quadrant before deciding that bowel sounds are absent.	Normal bowel sounds occur irregularly every 5–15 seconds. Absence of sounds indicates cessation of gastric motility. Hyperactive bowel sounds not related to hunger or recent meal may indicate diarrhea or early intestinal obstruction. Hypoactive or absent bowel sounds indicate paralytic ileus or peritonitis. It is common for bowel sounds to be hypoactive after surgery for 24 hours or more, especially following abdominal surgery.

Critical Decision Point *Nausea and vomiting, increasing distension, and inability to pass flatus may accompany severe paralytic ileus.*

STEP	RATIONALE
i. Place bell of stethoscope over epigastric region of abdomen and each quadrant. Auscultate for vascular (whooshing) sounds.	Determines presence of turbulent blood flow (bruit) through thoracic or abdominal aorta, which may indicate an aneurysm.

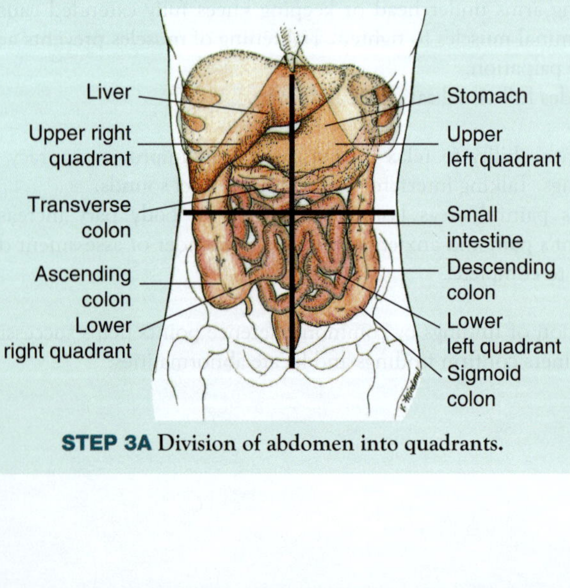

STEP 3A Division of abdomen into quadrants.

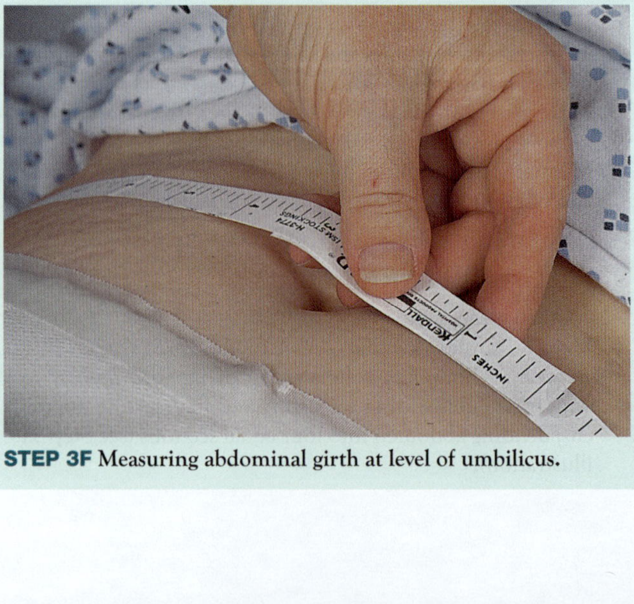

STEP 3F Measuring abdominal girth at level of umbilicus.

STEP	RATIONALE

Critical Decision Point *If aortic bruit is auscultated, suggesting presence of an aneurysm, stop assessment and notify health care provider immediately. Percussion or palpation over abdominal bruit could cause rupture of an already weakened vessel wall in the presence of an abdominal aneurysm.*

STEP	RATIONALE
j. With patient supine, gently percuss each of four abdominal quadrants systematically. Note areas of tympany and dullness.	Reveals presence of air or fluid in stomach and intestines. Normal percussion is tympanic because of swallowed air in GI tract. Presence of fluid or underlying masses is revealed by dull percussion.
k. Ask patient if abdomen feels unusually tight, and determine whether this is a recent development.	Continued sensation of fullness helps to detect distension. Feeling of fullness after heavy meal causes only temporary distension. Tightness is not felt with obesity.
l. With patient sitting, gently but firmly percuss over each CVA along scapular lines (see Step 3l, illustration A). Use ulnar surface of fist indirectly by placing nondominant hand flat against CVA and percussing with dominant hand or percuss directly against patient's skin (see Step 3l, illustration B). Note whether patient experiences pain.	Determines presence of kidney inflammation.

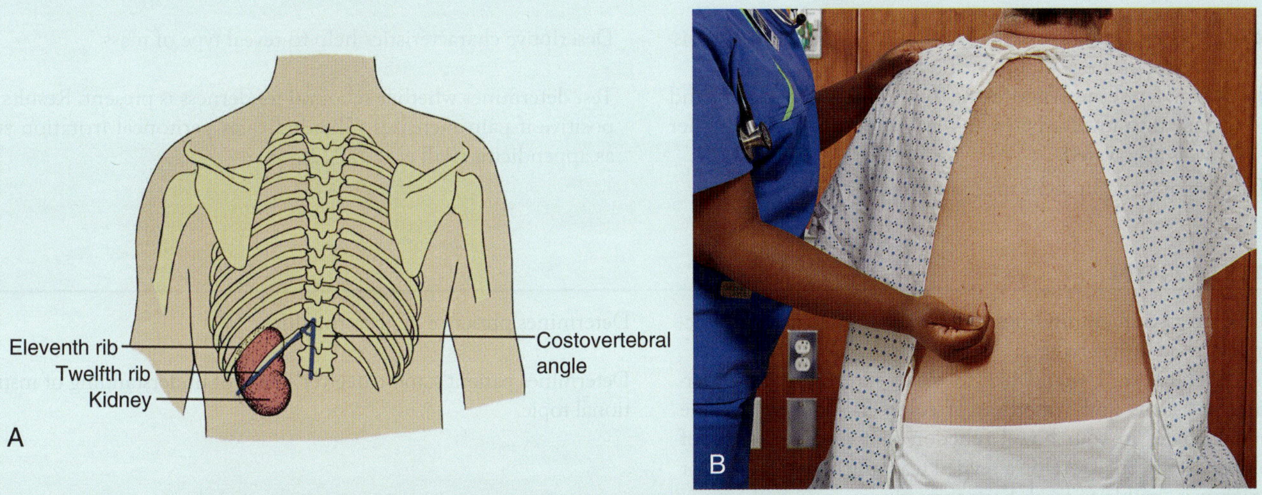

STEP 3L A, Position of kidney in relation to costovertebral angle (CVA). B, Direct percussion of kidney for CVA tenderness. (A *From Ball, J. W., Dains, J. E., Flynn, J. A., et al. [2018]. Seidel's guide to physical examination [9th ed.]. Mosby.*)

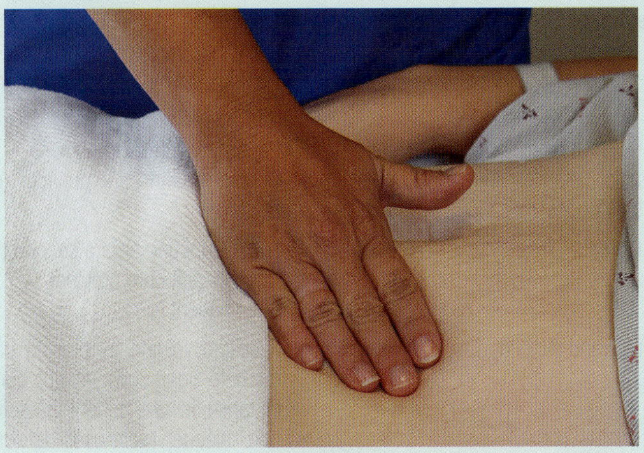

STEP 3M Light palpation of abdomen.

STEP	RATIONALE
m. Lightly palpate over each abdominal quadrant, laying palm of hand with fingers extended and approximated lightly on abdomen. Keep palm and forearm horizontal. Pads of fingertips depress skin no more than 1 cm (0.4 inches) in gentle dipping motion (see Step 3m illustration). Palpate painful areas last.	Detects areas of localized tenderness, degree of tenderness, and presence and character of underlying masses or fluid. Palpation of sensitive area causes guarding (voluntary tightening of underlying abdominal muscles).
(1) Note muscular resistance, distension, tenderness, and superficial masses or organs while observing patient's face for signs of discomfort.	Patient's verbal and nonverbal cues may indicate discomfort from tenderness. Firm abdomen indicates active obstruction with buildup of fluid or gas.
(2) Note whether abdomen is firm or soft to touch.	Soft abdomen is normal or reveals that obstruction is resolving.
n. Just below umbilicus and above symphysis pubis, palpate for smooth, rounded mass. While applying light pressure, ask if patient has sensation of need to void.	Detects presence of dome of distended bladder.

Critical Decision Point *Routinely check for distended bladder if patient has been unable to void, patient has been incontinent, or an in-dwelling Foley catheter is not draining well or has been removed recently.*

STEP	RATIONALE
o. If masses are palpated, note size, location, shape, consistency, tenderness, mobility, and texture.	Descriptive characteristics help to reveal type of mass.
p. When tenderness is present, press one hand slowly and deeply into involved area and let go quickly. Note whether pain is aggravated.	Test determines whether rebound tenderness is present. Results are positive if pain increases. This indicates peritoneal irritation such as appendicitis (Ball et al., 2022).
3. Dispose of all equipment in appropriate receptacles.	

EVALUATION

1. Compare assessment findings with previous assessment characteristics to identify changes.	Determines presence of abnormalities.
2. **Use teach-back:** "I would like to make sure that you understand the signs and symptoms of colorectal cancer. Tell me three changes in your bowel function that might be signs of colorectal cancer." Develop a revised teaching plan if patient or caregiver is unable to teach back correctly.	Determines patient's and caregiver's level of understanding of instructional topic.

Unexpected Outcomes	Related Interventions
1. Abdomen protrudes symmetrically with skin taut; patient complains of tightness and/or bowel sounds are absent. GI motility has ceased. Patient is vomiting. Signs suggest an obstruction.	• Keep patient on nothing by mouth (NPO) status and encourage ambulation. • Notify health care provider. • Gastric decompression following insertion of NG tube sometimes may be necessary.
2. Hyperactive bowel sounds are evident with GI motility. Commonly they result from anxiety, diarrhea, overuse of laxatives, inflammation of bowel, or reaction of intestines to certain foods.	• Patient may need to be NPO. • Contact health care provider to consider prescription for antidiarrheal medication.
3. Rebound abdominal tenderness is palpated.	• Avoid palpating area a second time. • Notify health care provider. • Keep patient NPO.
4. Bladder is palpable over symphysis pubis and distended.	• Facilitate voiding by placing patient in sitting position or encouraging them to bear down (if not contraindicated); run water within hearing distance or have patient place hand in basin of warm water. • Use bladder scan to determine extent of bladder fullness (see Chapter 34). • If unable to void, urinary catheterization is necessary (see Chapter 34).

Communication and Documentation

- Document appearance of abdomen, quality of bowel sounds, presence of distension, abdominal circumference, and presence and location of tenderness in progress notes in EHR or chart.
- Document evaluation of patient and caregiver learning.
- Document patient's ability to void and defecate, including description of output in the EHR or chart.
- Report serious abnormalities such as absent bowel sounds, presence of a mass, or acute pain to nurse in charge or health care provider.

Special Considerations

Teaching

- Explain that factors such as diet, regular exercise, limited use of over-the-counter medications causing constipation, establishment of regular elimination schedule, and adequate fluid intake promote normal bowel elimination.
- If patient is a health care worker or has contact with blood or body fluids of affected people, encourage them to receive series of three HBV vaccine doses.

Pediatric

- The most common palpable abdominal mass in a child is feces, usually palpated in right lower quadrant (Hockenberry et al., 2024).
- Have child stand erect and then lie supine during inspection of abdominal surface. Normal abdomen of infants and young children is cylindrical in erect position and flat in supine position. School-age children may have a rounded abdomen until 13 years of age when standing.
- In infants and children, skin of abdomen is usually taut and without wrinkles or creases.
- Infants and children until the age of 7 years are abdominal breathers.
- Some children perceive superficial palpation as tickling. Drawing attention to their laughter only causes it to increase. Have children help by placing their hand on top of yours or have them place their hand on their abdomen with their fingers separated and then palpate between their fingers.

Gerontological

- Older persons often lack abdominal tone; underlying organs are more easily palpable.
- Constipation along with nausea, flatulence, and heartburn is common.
- Stress to older persons the importance of adequate fluid intake, regular exercise, and a diet with at least four servings daily of fresh fruit, vegetables, and high-fibre food to promote normal defecation.

✦ SKILL 8.6 Genitalia and Rectum Assessment

The best time to examine a patient's external genitalia is while performing routine hygiene measures or preparing to insert or care for a urinary catheter. An examination of female and male external genitalia is part of preventive health screenings. Patients with male genitalia need to learn how to perform self-examinations of the genitalia to detect testicular cancer (Box 8.6). Adolescent and young adults are examined because of the growing incidence of sexually transmitted infections (STIs). The average age of menarche among individuals with female genitalia has declined, and most teenagers are sexually active by age 19 (Hockenberry et al., 2024). You can easily combine rectal and anal assessments with this examination because the patient assumes a lithotomy or dorsal recumbent position.

Examination of the genitalia of a transgender person must be done with sensitivity and must be relevant to the anatomy present, as sex organs and secondary sex characteristics will vary depending on whether the patient has had gender-confirming surgery (also known as *gender-affirming surgery* or *sex reassignment*) or hormone therapy (Jarvis et al., 2024).

Delegation and Collaboration

The skill of assessing the genitalia and rectum cannot be delegated to a UCP. The nurse directs the UCP to do the following:

- Report changes in patient's genitourinary function and presence of drainage in the perineal area

When assessment reveals changes in genitourinary function or abnormal findings, collaborate with the interprofessional health care team (e.g., health care provider, genitourinary advanced practice nurse) for further investigation

Equipment

- Examination light
- Clean gloves (use nonlatex if necessary)
- Drapes

> **BOX 8.6**
> **Genital Self-Examination**
>
> All persons with male genitalia aged 15 years and older should know what is normal for their testicles. The best time to feel the testicles is during or after a warm bath or shower, as the heat causes the testicles to descend and the scrotal sac to relax. It is normal to feel a soft cord or a small bump at the back of each testicle; this is the epididymis, a tube that collects and carries sperm. It is also normal for one testicle to be larger than the other. The patient should be encouraged to report any changes promptly to a health care provider.

STEP	RATIONALE
ASSESSMENT	
1. Identify patient using at least two person-specific identifiers (e.g., name and date of birth, or name and medical record number) according to employer policy.	Ensures correct patient. Complies with Accreditation Canada's standards and improves patient safety (Accreditation Canada, 2020).
2. Throughout the procedure, the 4 moments for hand hygiene are to be implemented; hand hygiene should occur before initial patient (or patient environment) contact, before an aseptic procedure, after body fluid exposure risk, and after patient (or patient environment) contact. Additional hand hygiene should be performed when hands are visibly soiled.	Proper hand hygiene helps prevent the spread of infectious agents to health care providers.

STEP	RATIONALE
3. Assessment of patient with female genitalia:	
a. Determine whether patient has signs and symptoms of vaginal discharge, painful or swollen perianal tissues, or genital lesions.	These signs and symptoms are consistent with an STI or other pathological condition.
b. Ask if patient has symptoms or history of genitourinary problems, including burning during urination (dysuria), frequency, urgency, nocturia, hematuria, or incontinence.	Urinary problems are associated with gynecological disorders, including STIs.
c. Ask if the patient has had signs of bleeding outside of normal menstrual cycle or after menopause or unusual vaginal discharge.	These are warning signs for cervical and endometrial cancer or vaginal infection.
d. Ask if patient has received human papillomavirus (HPV) vaccine.	To protect against cervical cancer, the National Advisory Committee on Immunization (NACI) recommends that healthy individuals with female genitalia aged 9–14 years receive a 2- or 3-dose schedule of the HPV4 (Gardasil), HPV2 (Cervarix), or HPV9 (Gardasil 9) vaccine, and healthy individuals with female genitalia aged 15 years or older receive a 3-dose schedule of one of the vaccines (Public Health Agency of Canada [PHAC], 2017). The Gardasil vaccine also protects against most genital warts and some cancers of the vulva, vagina, and anus. Gardasil or Gardasil 9 is recommended for individuals with male genitalia aged 9–14 years (2 or 3 doses) and individuals with male genitalia aged 15 or older (3 doses) (PHAC, 2017).
e. Ask if patient has history of HPV infection, smoking, giving birth many times, being sexually active, weakened immune system, has a low income, is the daughter of a woman who took diethylstilbestrol (DES) during pregnancy, or has taken oral contraceptives for a long time.	These are risk factors for cervical cancer (CCS, 2022c).
f. Ask if patient has a history of breast cancer, *BRCA* gene mutations, Lynch syndrome, hormone replacement therapy, smoking, asbestos exposure, or endometriosis; tall adult height; a family history of ovarian, colorectal, uterine, or pancreatic cancer; Ashkenazi Jewish ancestry; or has never been pregnant or given birth.	These are risk factors for ovarian cancer (CCS, 2022f).
g. Determine whether patient is overweight or obese; had early menarche or late menopause; has never given birth; has history of diabetes mellitus, polycystic ovarian syndrome, Lynch syndrome, or Cowden syndrome; or has a history of estrogen-related exposure (estrogen-only hormone replacement therapy, tamoxifen use), pelvic radiation, or low levels of physical activity.	These are risk factors for endometrial (uterine) cancer (CCS, 2022g).
h. Determine patient's knowledge of risk factors and signs of cervical and other gynecological cancers.	Provides baseline for patient education.
4. Assessment of patient with male genitalia:	
a. Review normal elimination pattern, including frequency of voiding; history of nocturia; character and volume of urine; daily fluid intake; symptoms of burning, urgency, and frequency; difficulty starting stream; and hematuria.	Urinary problems are directly associated with genitourinary problems because of anatomical structure of men's reproductive and urinary systems.
b. Ask if patient has noted penile pain or swelling, genital lesions, or urethral discharge.	These are signs and symptoms of STIs.
c. Determine whether patient has noted heaviness, painless enlargement, or irregular lumps of testis.	These signs and symptoms are early warning signs for testicular cancer.
d. Ask if patient has experienced any enlargement in inguinal area, and assess if intermittent or constant, associated with straining or lifting, and painful. Assess whether coughing, lifting, or straining at stool causes pain.	Signs and symptoms indicate potential inguinal hernia.
e. Ask if patient has experienced urinary frequency or urgency, difficulty starting urine flow, inability to empty the bladder completely, slow or interrupted urine stream, urinary or bowel incontinence, blood in the urine or semen, burning or pain during urination, painful ejaculation, erectile dysfunction, pain or stiffness in the bones of the hips, back, or chest, weakness or numbness in the legs or feet, shortness of breath, or a cough that does not go away.	These are warning signs and symptoms of prostate cancer (CCS, 2022j). Symptoms also may indicate infection or prostate enlargement.
f. Assess patient's knowledge of risk factors and signs of prostate and testicular cancer.	Provides baseline for patient education.

STEP	RATIONALE
5. Assessment of all patients:	
a. Determine whether patient has rectal bleeding, black or tarry stools (melena), rectal pain, change in bowel habits (constipation, diarrhea, or stool that looks narrower than usual), or weight loss.	These are warning signs of colorectal cancer (CCS, 2022i) or other GI alterations.
b. Determine whether patient has personal or family history of colorectal cancer, Ashkenazi Jewish ancestry, polyps, familial adenomatous polyposis, chronic inflammatory bowel disease, or personal history of breast, ovarian, or uterine cancer or Lynch syndrome. Determine whether patient is overweight or obese, smokes, drinks alcohol, has sedentary lifestyle, or eats a diet high in red and processed meats or low in fibre.	These are risk factors for colorectal cancer (CCS, 2022d).
c. Assess medication history for use of laxatives or cathartic medications.	Repeated use causes diarrhea and eventual loss of intestinal muscle tone.
d. Assess for use of opioids or iron preparations.	Opioids cause constipation. Iron turns stool black and tarry.
e. Assess patient's knowledge of risks and signs of colorectal cancer.	Provides baseline for patient education.

NURSING DIAGNOSES

- Pain (acute, chronic)
- Inadequate health maintenance
- Insufficient knowledge regarding need for a genital and rectal assessment
- Readiness for enhanced immunization status

Related factors are individualized on the basis of patient's condition or needs.

PLANNING

STEP	RATIONALE
1. Expected outcomes following completion of procedure:	
• Patient denies discomfort or worsening of existing discomfort following examination.	Proper examination procedures have been implemented.
• Patient able to list warning signs of colorectal cancer: patient with female genitalia (including cisgender woman or transgender man): cervical, endometrial, and ovarian cancer; patient with male genitalia (including cisgender man or transgender woman): testicular and prostate cancer.	Demonstrates learning.
• Patient able to discuss guidelines for HPV immunization.	Demonstrates learning.
2. Anticipate teaching topics so that during the examination you can teach patient about warning signs of colorectal cancer.	Prepares you to incorporate patient education into assessment activities.
3. Prepare necessary supplies.	Reduces transmission of infection.

IMPLEMENTATION

STEP	RATIONALE
1. Prepare patient for assessment:	Proper hand hygiene helps prevent the spread of infectious agents to health care providers.
a. Ask if patient needs to empty bladder or defecate.	Palpation of full bladder causes discomfort and feeling of urgency and makes it difficult for patient to relax.
b. Keep upper chest and legs draped and keep room warm.	Maintains patient's comfort during examination, promoting relaxation.
c. Position patient:	
(1) Patient with female genitalia should lie in dorsal recumbent position with arms down at sides and knees slightly bent. Place small pillow under the knees.	Placing arms under head or keeping knees fully extended causes tightening of abdominal muscles.
(2) Patient with male genitalia should lie supine with chest, abdomen, and lower legs draped; or have patient with male genitalia stand during examination.	

STEP	RATIONALE
(3) Transgender patient should be placed in a gender-affirming position. Physical examination should be relevant to the anatomy present.	
d. Apply clean gloves.	Reduces transmission of microorganisms.
2. Examine female genitalia (use this time to discuss patient's risk for STIs and the signs and symptoms of cervical, ovarian, and endometrial cancers):	
a. Expose perineal area, repositioning sheet as needed.	
b. Inspect surface characteristics of perineum and retract labia majora; observe for inflammation, edema, lesions, or lacerations. Note the presence of any vaginal discharge; discharge may indicate need for a culture.	Skin of perineum is smooth, clean, and slightly darker than other skin. Mucous membranes are dark pink and moist. Labia majora are symmetrical; may be dry or moist. Normally there is no vaginal discharge.
3. Examine male genitalia (use this time to discuss patient's risk for STIs and the signs and symptoms of testicular cancer):	
a. Expose perineal area. Observe genitalia for rashes, excoriations, or lesions.	Normally skin is clear without lesions.
b. Inspect and palpate penile surfaces (see also Box 8.6).	
(1) Inspect corona, prepuce (foreskin), glans, urethral meatus, and shaft. Retract foreskin in uncircumcised male genitalia. Observe for discharge, lesions, edema, and inflammation. Return foreskin to normal position.	Glans should be smooth and pink along all surfaces. Urethral meatus is slit-like and normally positioned at tip of glans. Foreskin should retract easily. Area between foreskin and glans is common site for venereal lesions.
c. Inspect and palpate testicular surfaces.	
(1) Inspect size, colour, shape, and symmetry; also gently palpate for lesions and edema.	Left testicle is normally lower than right. Scrotal skin is usually loose, surface is coarse, and skin colour is more deeply pigmented than body skin.
d. Palpate testes (see also Box 8.6).	
(1) Note size, shape, and consistency of tissue.	Testes are normally ovoid and approximately 2–4 cm (0.8–1.6 inches) in size, feel smooth and rubbery, and are free from nodules. Most common symptom of testicular cancer is irregular, nontender fixed mass.
(2) Ask if patient experiences tenderness with palpation.	Testes are normally sensitive but not tender.
4. Assess rectum:	
a. Patient with female genitalia remains in dorsal recumbent position or assumes side-lying position.	These positions allow for optimum visualization of the rectum.
b. Patient with male genitalia stands and bends forward with hips flexed and upper body resting across examination table; examine nonambulatory patient in side-lying position.	
c. View perianal and sacrococcygeal areas by gently retracting buttocks with your nondominant hand.	Perianal skin is smooth, more pigmented, and coarser than skin covering buttocks.
d. Inspect anal tissue for skin characteristics, lesions, external hemorrhoids (dilated veins that appear as reddened skin protrusion), inflammation, rashes, and excoriation.	Anal tissues are moist and hairless; voluntary sphincter holds anus closed.
5. Remove and discard gloves. Discard disposable supplies. Help patient to comfortable position.	Reduces transmission of infection.

EVALUATION

1. Compare assessment findings with previous assessment characteristics to identify changes.	Determines presence of abnormalities.
2. Ask patient to identify guidelines for HPV vaccination.	Demonstrates learning.
3. **Use teach-back:** "I would like to make sure that you understand the warning signs of different types of cancer. Tell me some of the signs and symptoms of the different types of cancer that we have discussed." Develop a revised teaching plan if patient is unable to teach back correctly.	Determines patient's level of understanding of instructional topic.

STEP	RATIONALE
Unexpected Outcomes	**Related Interventions**
1. Patient has vaginal/penile drainage and burning sensation during voiding. Patient with female genitalia may have vaginal bleeding between menstrual periods. Symptoms may suggest STI.	• Notify health care provider. • Prepare to collect a culture of the discharge. • Provide additional education.

Communication and Documentation

- Document results of assessment in progress notes in EHR or chart.
- Document patient's ability to void, including description of output, in EHR or chart.
- Document evaluation of patient learning.
- Report any abnormalities such as presence of a mass or acute pain to nurse in charge or health care provider.

Special Considerations

Teaching

- Discuss the screening guidelines of the Canadian Task Force on Preventive Health Care (2016) for early detection of colorectal cancer. The guidelines recommend that people aged 60–74 years (strong recommendation) and people aged 50–59 years (weak recommendation) should be screened every 2 years with a guaiac fecal occult blood test (gFOBT) or a fecal immunochemical test (FIT), or every 10 years by flexible sigmoidoscopy. These recommendations apply to adults aged 50 years and older who are not at high risk for colorectal cancer.
- Discuss warning signs of colorectal cancer, including long-term progressive weight loss, change in bowel habits, and blood in stools.
- Discuss dietary planning and healthy lifestyle choice to maintain or improve colon health.

Health Teaching for Cisgender Women and Nonoperative Trans Men.

- Teach patient about purpose and recommended frequency of Papanicolaou (Pap) tests, gynecological examinations, and HPV vaccines.
- Explain warning signs of STIs: pain or burning on urination, pain during sex, pain in pelvic area, bleeding between menstruation, itchy rash around vagina, and abnormal vaginal discharge.
- Teach measures to prevent STIs: use of condoms, restricting number of sexual partners, and avoiding sex with people who have multiple partners.
- Reinforce the importance of performing perineal hygiene (as appropriate).

Health Teaching for Cisgender Men and Nonoperative Trans Women

- Explain warning signs of STIs: pain on urination and during sex, abnormal penile discharge, swollen lymph nodes, or rash or ulcer on skin or genitalia.
- Teach measures to prevent STIs: use of condoms, HPV vaccines, avoiding sex with infected partner, avoiding sex with people who have multiple partners, and performing regular perineal hygiene.
- Tell patients with an STI to inform their sexual partners of the need to have an examination. Instruct patient to seek treatment as soon as possible if partner becomes infected with an STI.

Pediatric

- When examining the testes in an infant with male genitalia, avoid stimulating the cremasteric reflex, which causes the testes to pull higher into the pelvic cavity.

✦ SKILL 8.7 Musculoskeletal and Neurological Assessment

During the musculoskeletal and neurological assessment, you will use the skills of inspection and palpation. During the general survey, inspect gait, posture, and body position. A more thorough assessment of major bone, joint, and muscle groups and sensory, motor, and cranial nerve (CN) function is indicated in the presence of abnormalities. The assessment can be performed as you examine other body systems. For example, while assessing head and neck structures, assess neck ROM and examine selected CNs. Integrate assessment into routine activities of care (e.g., while bathing or positioning the patient). Assessment of these systems is important when a patient reports pain, loss of sensation, or impairment of muscle function. Prolonged illness or immobility may result in muscle weakness and atrophy. Neurological assessment is often conducted simultaneously because muscles may be weakened as a result of nerve involvement.

Delegation and Collaboration

The skill of assessing musculoskeletal and neurological function cannot be delegated to a UCP. The nurse directs the UCP to do the following:

- Report patient's problems with gait, balance, ROM, and muscle strength
- Be informed of patients at risk for falls (unsteady gait, foot dragging, weakness of lower extremities)
- Help patients with muscular weakness with transfer and ambulation

Equipment

- Cotton balls or cotton-tipped applicators
- Penlight
- Tape measure
- Tongue blade
- Tuning fork
- Reflex hammer

ASSESSMENT

STEP	RATIONALE
1. Identify patient using at least two person-specific identifiers (e.g., name and date of birth, or name and medical record number) according to employer policy.	Ensures correct patient. Complies with Accreditation Canada's standards and improves patient safety (Accreditation Canada, 2020).
2. Throughout the procedure, the 4 moments for hand hygiene are to be implemented; hand hygiene should occur before initial patient (or patient environment) contact, before an aseptic procedure, after body fluid exposure risk, and after patient (or patient environment) contact. Additional hand hygiene should be performed when hands are visibly soiled.	Proper hand hygiene helps prevent the spread of infectious agents to health care providers.
3. Review patient history for low calcium intake, low physical activity, smoking, consuming large amounts of alcohol, postmenopausal status.	These factors increase risk for osteoporosis (Jarvis et al., 2024).
4. Ask if patient has had a vertebral compression fracture, fragility fracture after age 40, either parent has had a hip fracture, more than 3 months' use of a glucocorticoid, or medical conditions or medications that inhibit absorption of nutrients or contribute to bone loss.	These are risk factors for fracture (Osteoporosis Canada, 2022b). Both women and men over the age of 50 should be assessed for risk factors for osteoporosis and fractures (Osteoporosis Canada, 2022a).
5. Determine whether patient has been screened for osteoporosis.	Both women and men aged 65 and older should be screened using bone mineral density (BMD) testing. Menopausal women, and men aged 50–64 years with clinical risk factors for fracture, should also be tested (Osteoporosis Canada, 2022a).
6. Ask patient to describe history of changes in bone, muscle, or joint function (e.g., recent fall, trauma, lifting heavy objects, bone or joint disease with sudden or gradual onset) and location of alteration.	History helps to assess nature of musculoskeletal problem. An estimated 2 million Canadians are affected by osteoporosis (Osteoporosis Canada, 2022b).
7. Assess height and weight (see Skill 8.1). Note whether there is a decrease in height among women aged 50 and older by subtracting current height from recall of maximum adult height.	Body mass index less than 22 kg/m^2 is a risk factor, and loss of height more than 7.5 cm is one of the first clinical signs of osteoporosis (Boscart et al., 2023).
8. Assess nature and extent of patient's musculoskeletal pain: location, duration, severity, predisposing and aggravating factors, relieving factors, and type of pain. If patient reports pain or cramping in lower extremities, ask if walking relieves or aggravates it. Assess distance walked and characteristics of pain before, during, and after activity.	Pain frequently accompanies alterations in bone, joints, or muscle. It has implications for comfort and also ability to perform ADLs. Pain caused by certain vascular conditions tends to increase with activity.
9. Ask if patient uses analgesics, antipsychotics, antidepressants, nervous system stimulants, or recreational substances.	These medications alter LOC or cause behavioural changes. Abuse sometimes causes tremors, ataxia, and changes in peripheral nerve function.
10. Ask if patient has recent history of seizures or convulsions: clarify sequence of events (aura, loss of muscle tone, falling, motor activity, loss of consciousness); character of any symptoms; and relationship to time of day, fatigue, or emotional stress.	Seizure activity often originates from central nervous system (CNS) alteration. Characteristics of seizure help determine its origin.
11. Screen patient for headache, tremors, dizziness, vertigo, numbness or tingling of body part; visual changes; weakness; pain; or changes in speech.	These symptoms commonly result from CNS dysfunction. Identifying patterns aids in diagnosis.
12. Discuss with partner, family member, or friends any recent changes in patient's behaviour (e.g., increased irritability, mood swings, memory loss, change in energy level).	Behavioural changes may result from intracranial pathology.
13. Ask if patient has noticed change in vision (CN II), hearing (CN VIII), smell (CN I), taste (CN VII), or touch.	Major sensory nerves originate from brainstem. These symptoms help to localize nature of problem during CN examination.
14. If patient displays sudden acute confusion (delirium), review history for medication toxicity (e.g., anticholinergics, digoxin, antihistamines, antipsychotics, benzodiazepines, opioid analgesics, sedative/hypnotics, steroids); serious infections; metabolic disturbances (e.g., diabetes mellitus); heart failure; and severe anemia.	Delirium is one of the most common mental health disorders in older people (Boscart et al., 2023), but it also occurs in children.
15. Review history for head or spinal cord injury, meningitis, congenital anomalies, neurological disease, or psychiatric counselling.	These neurological symptoms or behavioural changes help to focus assessment on possible cause.

STEP	RATIONALE

NURSING DIAGNOSES

- Inadequate peripheral tissue perfusion
- Pain (acute, chronic)
- Reduced physical mobility
- Decreased self-care abilities (bathing/hygiene, dressing/grooming, feeding, toileting)
- Reduced stamina
- Potential for injury
- Potential for peripheral neurovascular dysfunction
- Potential for trauma

Related factors and risk factors are individualized on the basis of patient's condition or needs.

PLANNING

STEP	RATIONALE
1. Expected outcomes following completion of procedure:	
• Patient demonstrates erect posture; strong grasp; steady gait, with arms swinging freely at side.	Indicates normal alignment, gait, and neuromuscular muscle strength.
• There is bilateral symmetry of extremities in length, circumference, alignment, position, and skinfolds.	
• Full active ROM is present in all joints, with good muscle tone and absence of contractures, spasticity, or muscular weakness.	Indicates normal ROM of joints.
• Patient is alert and oriented to person, place, and time. Behaviour and appearance appropriate for condition and situation.	Indicates normal cerebral function.
• Patient demonstrates normal pupil reaction to light and accommodation (see Skill 8.2); external ocular muscles (EOMs) intact; facial sensation intact; symmetrical facial expressions; soft palate and uvula midline and rise on phonation; gag reflex intact; speech clear without hoarseness; no difficulty swallowing.	Indicates normal functioning of CNs III, IV, V, VI, VII, IX, and X.
• Patient distinguishes between sharp and dull sensations and light touch on symmetrical areas of extremities. Position sense intact to lower extremities.	Indicates normal function of sensory nerves.
• Gait is coordinated and steady with appropriate stance and swing phases. Romberg test negative.	Indicates normal cerebellar and motor system functioning.
2. Prepare necessary supplies.	Reduces transmission of infection.

IMPLEMENTATION

STEP	RATIONALE
1. Prepare patient:	Proper hand hygiene helps prevent the spread of infectious agents to health care providers.
a. Integrate musculoskeletal and neurological assessments during other parts of physical assessment or during nursing care (e.g., when patient moves in bed, rises from chair, or walks).	You can conduct assessment as patient performs activities or goes through movements required during complete physical examination. Integration with care conserves patient's energy and allows patient to perform movements more naturally.
b. Plan time for short rest periods during assessment.	Movement of body parts and various manoeuvres may tire patient. Always plan rest periods with older person and very ill patients.
2. Assess musculoskeletal system. (Discuss any risks patient may have for falls or other injuries.)	
a. Observe ability to use arms and hands for grasping objects (e.g., pen, utensils).	Assesses coordination and muscle strength.
b. To assess hand grip strength, cross your hands and have patient grasp index and middle fingers of both of your hands and squeeze them as hard as possible (see Step 3b illustration).	It is common for patient's dominant hand to be slightly stronger than nondominant hand. By crossing your hands, patient's right hand grasps your right hand. This helps with recall of which is patient's right/left hand.

STEP	RATIONALE
c. To assess strength of lower arms or legs, first ask patient to contract the muscle you indicate by extending or flexing the joint. Then have patient resist as you apply force against that muscle contraction. Have patient maintain pressure until told to stop. Compare symmetrical muscle groups. Note weakness and compare right with left.	Compares strength of symmetrical muscle groups. Upper and lower extremities on dominant side are usually stronger. Rate muscle strength on scale of 0–5 as follows: 0 No voluntary contraction 1 Slight contractility, no movement 2 Full ROM, passive 3 Full ROM, active 4 Full ROM against gravity, some resistance 5 Full ROM against gravity, full resistance
d. Observe body alignment for sitting, supine, prone, and standing positions. Muscles and joints should be exposed and free to move to allow for accurate measurement.	Each joint or muscle group requires different position for measurement.
e. Inspect gait as patient walks. Have patient use their assistive device (e.g., cane, walker) if appropriate. Observe for foot dragging, shuffling, or limping, balance, presence of obvious deformity in lower extremities, and position of trunk in relation to legs.	Gait is more natural if patient is unaware of your observation. Assesses for neuromusculoskeletal disorder.
f. Perform timed up-and-go (TUG) test: Have adult wear regular footwear, sit back in comfortable chair, and use normal assist devices, if needed. Have a watch with a second hand. On the word "Go," begin timing as you have the patient stand from a sitting position without using chair arms for support, stand still momentarily, walk 3 m (10 feet) in a line, turn around and return to chair; and sit back in chair without using chair arms for support. Observe gait and ability to stand.	The TUG test is an assessment that should be conducted as part of routine evaluation of older persons. The test helps to detect a person's risk for falls. Normally, a person completes the task in less than 10 seconds; over 20 seconds is abnormal.

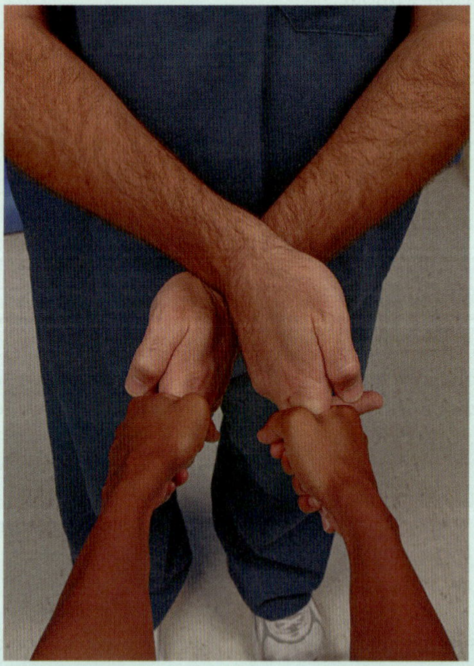

STEP 3B Assessing strength of hand grasps, comparing sides.

STEP	RATIONALE
g. Stand behind patient and observe postural alignment (position of hips relative to shoulders). Look sideways at cervical, thoracic, and lumbar curves (see Step 3g illustration).	Abnormal curves of posture include kyphosis (hunchback, exaggerated posterior curvature of thoracic spine), lordosis (swayback, increased lumbar curvature), and scoliosis (lateral spinal curvature). Postural changes indicate muscular, bone, or joint deformity; pain; or muscular fatigue. Head should be held erect.

STEP	RATIONALE
h. Make a general observation of extremities. Look at overall size, gross deformity, bony enlargement, alignment, and symmetry.	General review pinpoints areas requiring in-depth assessment.
i. Gently palpate bones, joints, and surrounding tissue in involved areas. Note any heat, tenderness, edema, or resistance to pressure.	Reveals changes resulting from trauma or chronic disease. Do not attempt to move joint when fracture is suspected or joint is apparently "frozen" by lack of movement over a long period of time.
j. Ask patient to put major joint through its full ROM (Table 8.12). Patients with deformities, reduced mobility, joint fixation, or weakness require passive ROM assessment. Observe equality of motion in same body parts:	Assessment of patient's normal ROM provides baseline for assessing later changes after surgery or inactivity.
(1) *Active motion:* (Patient needs no support or help and is able to move joint independently.) Teach patient to move each joint through its normal range. Sometimes it is necessary to demonstrate and then ask patient to mimic your movements.	Identifies muscle strength and detects limited ROM.
(2) *Passive motion:* (Joint has full ROM, but patient does not have strength to move it independently.) Have patient relax and move same joints passively until end of range is felt. Support extremity at joint. Do not force joint if there is pain or muscle spasm.	Determines ability to perform joint motion in presence of muscle weakness. Forcing joint causes injury and pain.
k. Palpate joint for swelling, stiffness, tenderness, and heat; note any redness.	Indicates acute or chronic inflammation. ROM causes pain or injury.
l. Assess muscle tone in major muscle groups. Normal tone causes mild, even resistance to movement through entire ROM.	If muscle has increased tone (hypertonicity), any sudden movement of joint is met with considerable resistance. Hypotonic muscle moves without resistance. Muscle feels flabby.
3. Neurological assessment:	
a. Assess LOC and orientation by asking patient to identify name, location, day of week, and year; note behaviour and appearance. This can be completed during general survey.	A fully conscious patient responds to questions spontaneously. As consciousness declines, patient may show irritability, shortened attention span, or unwillingness to cooperate. As consciousness continues to deteriorate, patient becomes disoriented to name, time, and place. Behaviour and appearance reveal information about patient's mental status.

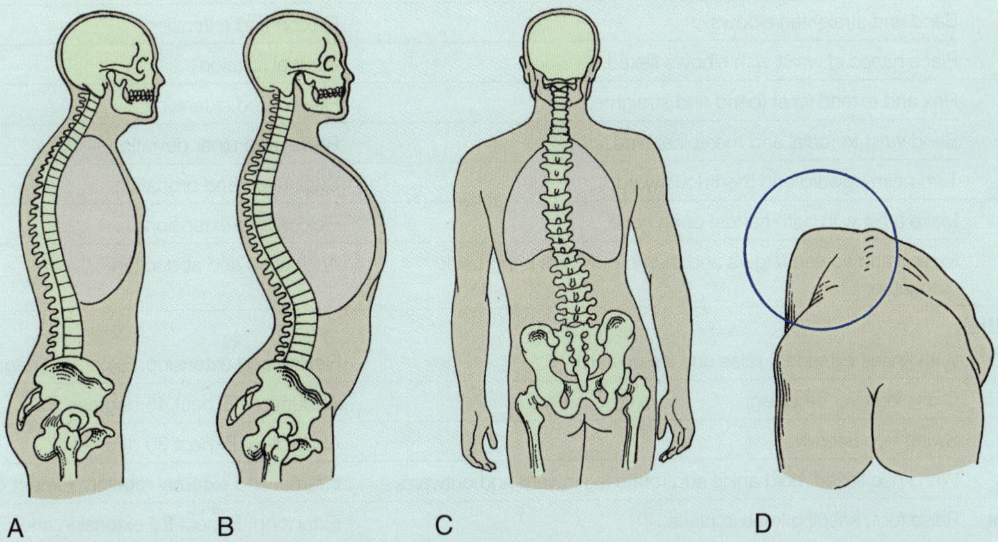

STEP 3G Observe spinal deformities. A, Kyphosis. B, Lordosis. C, Scoliosis. D, Scoliosis with patient bending forward.

STEP	RATIONALE
b. Assess cranial nerves (CNs):	
(1) For CN III (oculomotor), CN IV (trochlear), and CN VI (abducens), assess EOMs. Ask patient to look straight ahead without moving head and follow movement of your finger through six cardinal positions of gaze; measure pupillary reaction to light reflex and accommodation (see Skill 8.2) using penlight.	These CNs are those most likely to be affected by increasing intracranial pressure (ICP), which causes change in response or size of pupil; pupils may change shape (more oval) or react sluggishly. ICP impairs movements of EOMs. Accommodation is ability of eye to adjust vision from near to far.
(2) For CN V (trigeminal), apply light sensation with cotton ball to symmetrical areas of face.	Sensations should be symmetrical; unilateral decrease or loss of sensation may be caused by CN V lesion.
(3) For CN VII (facial), note facial symmetry. Have patient frown, smile, puff out cheeks, and raise eyebrows.	Expressions should be symmetrical; Bell's palsy causes drooping of upper and lower face; cerebrovascular accident causes asymmetry.
(4) For CN IX (glossopharyngeal) and CN X (vagus), have patient speak and swallow. Ask them to say "ah" while you use tongue blade and penlight. Check for midline uvula and symmetrical rise of uvula and soft palate. Use tongue blade and place on posterior tongue to elicit gag reflex.	Damage to CN IX causes impaired swallowing; damage to CN X causes loss of gag reflex, hoarseness, and nasal voice. When palate fails to rise and uvula pulls toward normal side, this indicates a unilateral paralysis.

TABLE 8.12

Assessing Range of Motion*

Body Part	Assessment Procedure	ROM
Upper Extremities		
Neck	Bend head forward and then backward. Bend neck side to side. Turn head to look over each shoulder.	Flexion, lateral flexion, rotation
Shoulders	Raise both arms to vertical position level at sides of head.	Flexion
	Bring arm across upper chest to touch opposite shoulder.	Adduction
	Place both hands behind neck, with elbows out to sides.	External rotation and abduction
	Place both hands behind small of back.	Internal rotation
	Have patient make small circles with hands, with arms extended at shoulder level.	Circumduction
Elbows	Bend and straighten elbows.	Flexion and extension
	Place hands at waist with elbows flexed.	Internal rotation
Wrists	Flex and extend wrist (bend and straighten).	Flexion and extension
	Bend wrist to radial and then ulnar side.	Radial and ulnar deviation
	Turn palm upward and then downward.	Supination and pronation
Hands	Make a fist with both hands; open hand.	Flexion and extension
	Extend and spread fingers and thumb outward; bring back together.	Adduction and abduction
Lower Extremities		
Hips (with patient supine)	With knees extended, raise one leg upward.	Flexion and extension: Expect 90 degrees flexion
	Cross leg over other leg.	Abduction: Expect 45 degrees
	Swing legs laterally.	Adduction: Expect 30 degrees
	With knee flexed, hold ankle and rotate leg inward and outward.	Internal and external rotation: Expect 40–45 degrees
Knees (with patient sitting)	Raise foot, keeping knee in place.	Extension: Expect full extension and up to 15 degrees hyperextension
Ankles	With foot held off floor, point toes downward and bring them back toward knee.	Plantar flexion: Expect 45 degrees Dorsiflexion: Expect 20 degrees
Toes	Turn foot (sole) inward and sole outward.	Inversion and eversion: Expect to reach 5 degrees
	Bend toes down and back.	Flexion and hyperextension: Expect to reach 40 degrees

AROM, Active range of motion; *PROM,* passive range of motion; *ROM,* range of motion.

*This may be done actively by the patient (AROM) or passively by the nurse (PROM).

STEP	RATIONALE
c. Assess extremities for sensation. Perform all sensory testing with patient's eyes closed so they are unable to see when or where a stimulus strikes skin. Use minimal stimulation initially, increasing gradually until patient is aware of it.	For all sensory stimulus testing, patient should note minimal differences side to side, correctly describe the sensation (sharp or dull, hot or cold), and recognize side of the body tested and location.
(1) *Pain:* Ask patient to indicate when sharp or dull sensation is felt as you alternately apply sharp and dull ends of a broken tongue blade to skin surface. Apply in symmetrical areas of extremities.	Patient should be able to distinguish sharp or dull sensations. Impaired sensations indicate disorders of spinal cord or peripheral nerve roots.
(2) *Light touch:* Apply light wisp of cotton to different points along surface of skin in symmetrical areas of extremities.	Patient should be able to distinguish when touched.
(3) *Position:* Grasp finger or toe, holding it by its sides with your thumb and index finger. Alternate moving patient's finger or toe up and down. Ask patient to state when finger is up or down. Repeat with toes.	Patient should be able to distinguish movements of a few millimetres. Decreased or absent position sense may occur in spinal anaesthesia, paralysis, or other neurological disorders.
d. Assess motor and cerebellar function:	
(1) *Gait:* Have patient walk across room, turn, and come back. Similarly note use of assistive devices. This is a good time to instruct in proper use of assistive devices.	Neurological and musculoskeletal disorders impair gait and balance.
(2) *Romberg's test:* Have patient stand with feet together, arms at sides, with eyes open and eyes closed (for 20–30 seconds). Protect patient's safety by standing at side; observe for swaying.	Romberg's test should be negative; slight swaying is considered normal.
e. Assess deep tendon reflexes (DTRs):	
(1) In patients with back pain or surgery, cerebrovascular accident, or spinal cord compression, it is appropriate to monitor DTRs (Ball et al., 2022). This requires an advanced level of skill. In most settings, this is not part of routine physical assessment.	Muscle spasticity and hyperactive reflexes may result from disorders such as stroke and paralysis. Diminished DTRs and muscle weakness may suggest electrolyte abnormalities or lower motor neuron disorders (e.g., amyotrophic lateral sclerosis [ALS] or Guillain-Barré syndrome).
(2) For each reflex tested, compare sides and assign a grade on the following scale: 0 No response 1+ Sluggish or diminished response 2+ Normal; active or expected response 3+ More brisk than expected; slightly hyperactive 4+ Very brisk; hyperactive, with clonus.	Grade indicates extent of neuron dysfunction. Clonus is described as repeated spasms of muscular contraction and relaxation.
(3) *Knee reflex:* Palpate patellar tendon just below patella. Tap pointed end of reflex hammer briskly on tendon (see Step 4e[3] illustration).	Knee reflex is the most common DTR assessment performed. The normal response is knee extension.
(4) *Plantar response (Babinski's reflex):* Using handle end of reflex hammer, stroke lateral aspect of sole from heel to ball of foot.	Toes should flex inward and downward (see Step 4e[4] illustration).

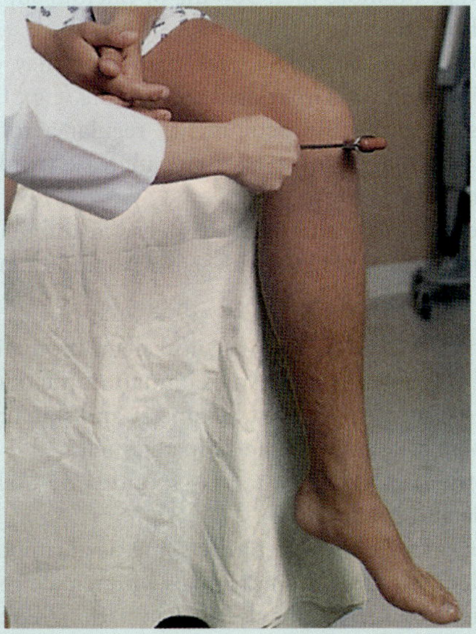

STEP 4E(3) Assessing knee reflex. Knee should extend.

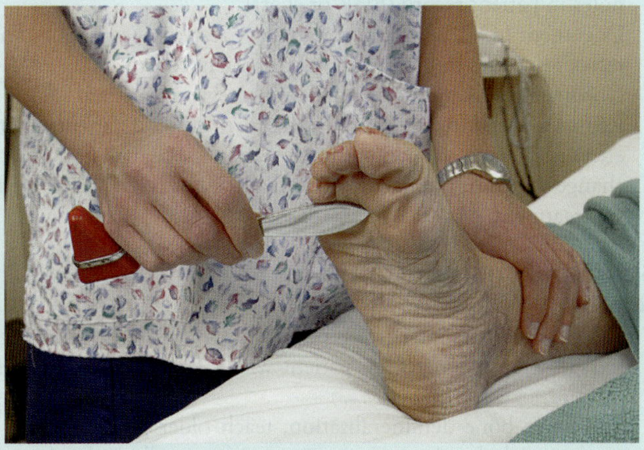

STEP 4E(4) Assessing plantar response. Toes should flex inward and downward.

STEP	RATIONALE
(5) After stroking soles of feet, if Babinski's reflex is present, great toe dorsiflexes, accompanied by fanning of the other toes.	Indicates CNS dysfunction. Dorsiflexion of great toe and fanning of the others are normal in children younger than age 2 (Hockenberry et al., 2024).
4. Dispose of all equipment in appropriate receptacles.	Reduces transmission of infection.

EVALUATION

1. Compare muscle strength and ROM with previous physical assessment.	Determines presence of abnormalities.
2. Compare neurological status with previous physical assessment.	Determines presence of abnormalities.
3. Evaluate level of patient's discomfort following procedure, using appropriate pain scale.	Determines whether manipulation of musculoskeletal structures intensifies patient's discomfort.
4. **Use teach-back:** "I want to be sure you understand the reasons why you are at risk of falling that we discussed during your exam. Tell me two reasons why you are at risk of falling." Develop a revised teaching plan if patient or caregiver is unable to teach back correctly.	Determines patient's and caregiver's level of understanding of instructional topic.

Unexpected Outcomes	Related Interventions
1. Joints are prominent, swollen, and tender with nodules or overgrowth of bone in distal joints, indicating signs of arthritis.	• Teach patient proper ROM. • Determine patient's knowledge regarding use of anti-inflammatory medications and nonpharmacological measures (see Chapter 16).
2. ROM is reduced in one or more major joints: shoulder, elbow, wrist, fingers, knee, hip.	• Assess further for pain during movement with joint unstable, stiff, painful, or swollen or with obvious deformity. • Notify health care provider. • Reduce mobility in extremity until cause of abnormal joint motion is determined.
3. Patient demonstrates weakness in one or more major muscle groups or has difficulty with gait or ability to walk and sit during TUG test, indicating a fall risk.	• Place patient on fall precautions. • Provide patient safety when ambulating (see Chapter 12). • Notify health care provider.
4. Patient has changes in mental status and pupillary response or other neurological deficits.	• Notify health care provider immediately. • Continue to assess patient's vital signs and LOC closely. • Place on fall precautions.

Communication and Documentation

- Document posture, gait, muscle strength, and ROM in progress notes in patient record (EHR or chart)
- Document LOC, orientation, pupillary response, sensation, and reflex responses in progress notes in patient record.
- Document evaluation of patient and caregiver learning.
- Report to nurse in charge or health care provider if patient experiences acute pain or sudden muscle weakness, change in LOC, or change in size or pupillary reaction, all of which require immediate treatment.

Special Considerations

Teaching

- Teach patient about correct postural alignment. Consult with physiotherapist to provide patient with exercises for improving posture.
- To reduce bone demineralization, teach older persons about a proper weight-bearing exercise program (e.g., walking, low-impact aerobics) to be followed three or more times a week.
- Encourage intake of calcium to meet the recommended daily allowance. Increased vitamin D aids calcium absorption (400 to 800 international units daily). Recommendation for daily calcium supplements for adults over age 50: 1 200 mg/day. Instruct patient to take no more than 500 mg of calcium supplements at one time (Boscart et al., 2023).
- Explain to patients with low back pain that they can benefit from modification of work-related risk factors (e.g., lifting heavy weights, use of protective equipment), regular aerobic exercise, exercises that strengthen the back and increase trunk flexibility, and learning how to lift properly.
- Explain measures to ensure safety (e.g., use of ambulation aids or safety equipment) for patients with sensory or motor impairments.

Pediatric

- Examine infants carefully for musculoskeletal anomalies resulting from genetic or fetal insults. An examination includes review of posture, generalized movement, symmetry and skin creases of the extremities, muscle strength, and hip alignment.
- Normally, the back of a newborn is rounded or C-shaped from the thoracic and pelvic curves.
- Scoliosis, or lateral curvature of the spine, is an important childhood problem, especially in individuals with female genitalia, usually identified at puberty. (For closer examination, have child stand

erect wearing only underclothes. Observe from behind, looking for asymmetry of shoulders and hips. Then observe from the back as child bends forward.) Uneven dress hems or trouser hems or uneven fit of clothing at the waist is an indication of scoliosis.
- Watching a child during play reveals information about musculoskeletal function.
- Children ages 13–19 years need 1 300 mg of calcium daily along with 400 international units of vitamin D (Hockenberry et al., 2024).

Gerontological

- Teach older persons about fall prevention. Make modifications in the home environment to reduce the risk for falls (see Chapter 42).
- Teach older persons and those with osteoporosis about proper body mechanics, ROM exercises, and moderate weight-bearing exercises (e.g., swimming, walking) to minimize trauma.
- Functional assessment is a measurement of an older person's ability to perform ADLs (Ball et al., 2022). When patient is unable to perform self-care easily, determine need for assistive devices (e.g., zippers on clothing instead of buttons, elevation of chairs to minimize bending of knees and hips).
- Older persons tend to assume a stooped, forward-bent posture, with hips and knees somewhat flexed, arms bent at the elbows, and level of arms raised.

Patients With Physical or Cognitive Challenges

- Research has shown high rates of osteoporosis documented among adults with intellectual and developmental challenges; earlier screening is recommended beginning at younger ages (age 40 if living in an institution, age 45 if community dwelling). Risk factors among women with intellectual and developmental disabilities include inactivity, long-term anticonvulsant use, and possible Down syndrome (Sullivan et al., 2018).

Procedural Guideline 8.1 *Monitoring Intake and Output*

Video Clip

Measuring and recording intake and output (I&O) during a 24-hour period is part of the assessment for fluid and electrolyte balance (Table 8.13). Nurses are responsible for the accurate recording of all intake (orally, by enteral feedings, and parenterally) and output (urine, diarrhea, vomitus, gastric suction, and drainage from surgical tubes). Accuracy is critical, as health care providers will use the findings to prescribe medications and IV fluids, and certain populations may be sensitive to even small fluid changes (i.e., neonatal and pediatric patients) (Hockenberry et al., 2024).

Monitor I&O for patients with a fever or edema or with a urinary catheter; receiving diuretic or intravenous therapy; or on restricted fluids as per employer policy or health care provider prescription. It is also important when a patient has electrolyte losses associated with vomiting, diarrhea, GI drainage, or extensive open wounds such as burns. Total and evaluate I&O at the end of each shift or at specified times such as every 8 hours. Significant alterations are apparent by comparing 24-hour totals over several days. Because fluid imbalance occurs at any time, be aware of I&O for all patients, even when documentation is not required. Certain disease processes (e.g., renal failure) and postoperative patients also require monitoring and documentation of I&O.

Delegation and Collaboration

The skills of assessing I&O totals at the end of each shift; comparing 24-hour totals over several days; and monitoring and recording intravenous therapy, wound or chest tube drainage, and tube feedings cannot be delegated to a UCP. The nurse needs to emphasize maintaining routine practices and additional precautions (e.g., transmission-based precautions) related to body fluids, accurately measuring and recording I&O, and using the metric system with standard containers. The nurse directs the UCP to do the following:

- Measure and record all sources of I&O
- Report changes in patient's condition such as alteration in intake or changes in colour, amount, or odour of output

Equipment

- Sign to alert personnel of I&O measurement
- Daily I&O record form or computer graphic
- Graduated measuring container
- Bedpan, urinal, bedside commode, or urine "hat" (a receptacle that fits under the toilet seat)
- Clean gloves
- Mask, eye protection, and gown (where appliable)

Procedural Steps

1. Identify patient using at least two person-specific identifiers (e.g., name and date of birth, or name and medical record number) according to employer policy (Accreditation Canada, 2020).
2. Throughout the procedure, the 4 moments for hand hygiene are to be implemented; hand hygiene should occur before initial patient (or patient environment) contact, before an aseptic procedure, after body fluid exposure risk, and after patient (patient environment) contact. Additional hand hygiene should be performed when hands are visibly soiled.
3. Identify patients with conditions that increase fluid loss (e.g., fever, diarrhea, vomiting, surgical wound drainage, chest tube drainage, gastric suction, major burns, or severe trauma).
4. Identify patients with impaired swallowing, unconscious patients, and patients with impaired mobility.
5. Identify patients on medications that influence fluid balance (e.g., diuretics and steroids).
6. Assess signs and symptoms of dehydration and fluid overload (e.g., bradycardia versus tachycardia, hypotension versus hypertension, and reduced skin turgor versus edema).
7. Weigh patients daily using the same scale, the same time of day, and with comparable clothing. (Rationale: Use of different scales, completing patient weight at different time of day, or different clothing weight may result in variable and inaccurate results of patient weight measurements).
8. Monitor laboratory reports:
   - Urine specific gravity (normal is 1.010–1.030)
   - Hematocrit (Hct) (normal range is 37–47% for female patients and 42–52% for male patients).

Continued

Procedural Guideline 8.1 *Monitoring Intake and Output—cont'd*

9. Assess patient's and caregiver's knowledge of purpose and process of I&O measurement.
10. Explain to patient and caregiver the reasons that I&O are important.
11. Measure and record all fluid intake:
    a. Liquids with meals, gelatin, custards, ice cream, popsicles, sherbets, ice chips (recorded as 50% of measured volume [e.g., 100 mL of ice chips equals 50 mL of water]). Convert household measures to the metric system: 1 oz equals 30 mL; therefore 12 oz (pop can) equals 360 mL.
    b. Count liquid medicines such as antacids and fluids with medications as fluid intake.
    c. Calculate fluid intake from tube feedings (see Chapter 32).
    d. Calculate fluid intake from parenteral fluids, blood components, and total parenteral nutrition solutions (see Chapters 29, 30 and 33).

Critical Decision Point *Record intake as soon as you measure it to maintain accuracy. If more than one patient is in the same room, each must have urine receptacles labelled with name and bed location.*

12. Instruct patient and caregiver to call you or the UCP to empty contents of urinal, urine hat, or commode each time patient uses it. Have patient and caregiver monitor incontinence, vomiting, and excessive perspiration and report it to the nurse.
13. Inform patient and caregiver that Foley catheter drainage bag and wound, gastric, or chest tube drainage are to be closely monitored, measured, and recorded and who is responsible for performing these tasks. Each patient must have a graduated container clearly marked with name and bed location and used only for the patient indicated.
14. Apply clean gloves. Measure drainage at the end of the shift or as indicated, using appropriate containers and noting colour and characteristics. If splashing is anticipated, wear mask, eye protection, and/or gown.
    a. Measure urine drainage using a "hat" into which patient voids or a graduated container (see Step 14a illustration).
    b. Observe colour and characteristics of urine in Foley tubing and drainage bag. Sometimes a measuring device is part of the drainage bag (see Step 14b illustration). Otherwise measure with a graduated container.
    c. Measure chest tube drainage by marking and recording the time on the collection chamber at specified intervals (see Step 14c illustration) (see Chapter 27). Chest tube collection devices are changed when they become full.
    d. Measure Jackson-Pratt/Hemovac drainage with a medicine cup (see Step 14d illustration) (see Chapter 39).
    e. Measure gastric drainage or larger drainage pouches by opening clamp and pouring into graduated cup with a 240-mL capacity (see Step 14e illustration).

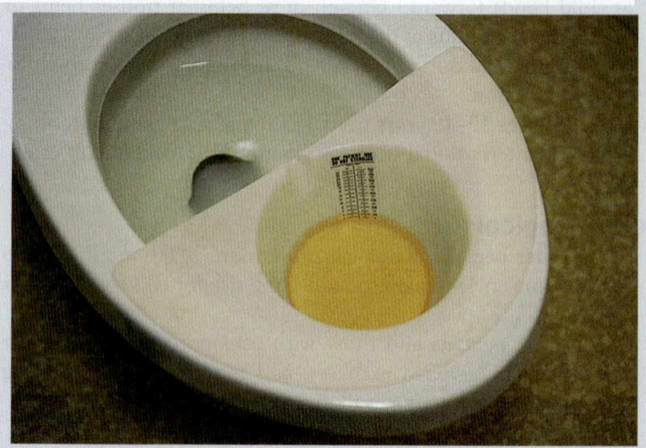

STEP 14A Urine "hat."

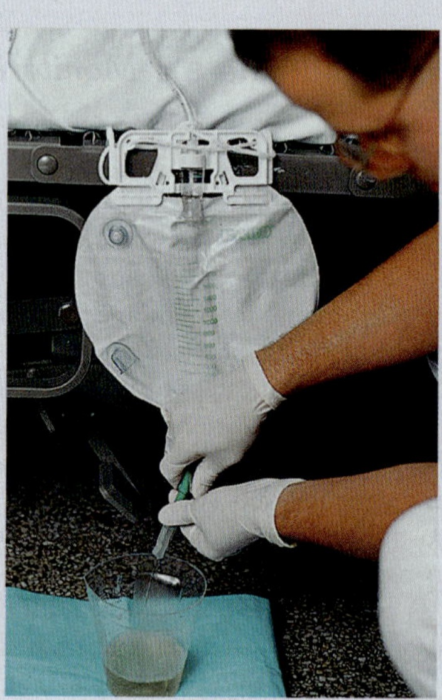

STEP 14B Device for monitoring hourly urine output.

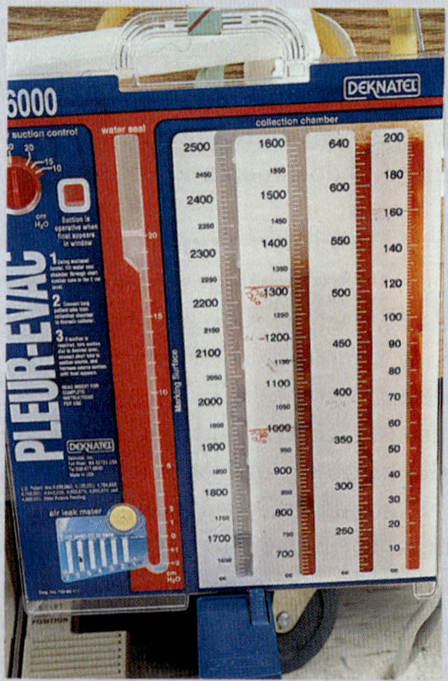

STEP 14C Collection chamber for measuring chest tube drainage.

Continued

Procedural Guideline 8.1 *Monitoring Intake and Output—cont'd*

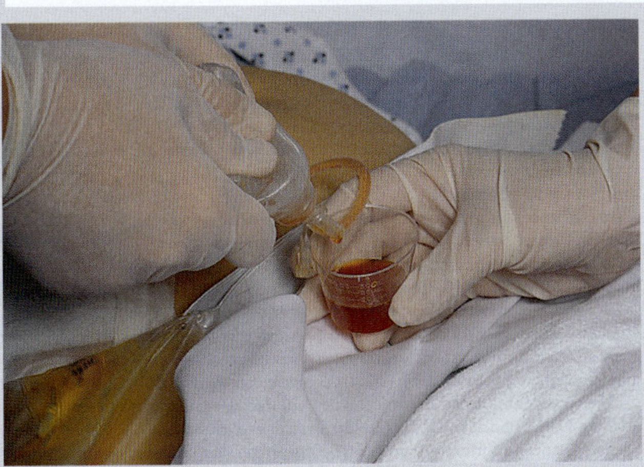

STEP 14D Measuring wound drainage through Jackson–Pratt drain.

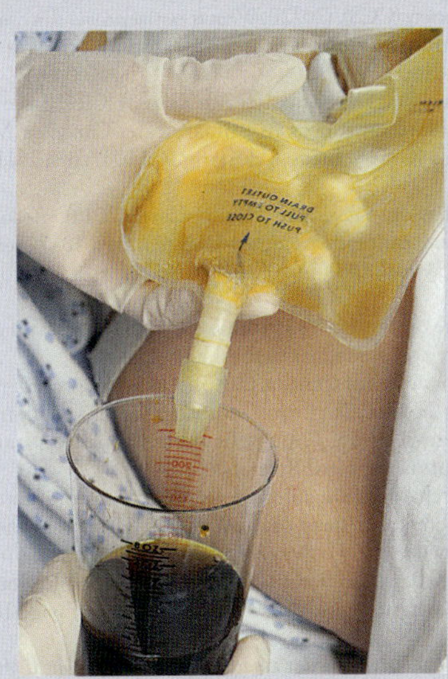

STEP 14E Measuring drainage from large drainage pouch.

TABLE 8.13

Adult Average Fluid Gains and Losses

Fluid Intake		**Fluid Output**	
Source	**Volume (mL)**	**Source**	**Volume (mL)**
Oral fluids	1 100–1 400	Kidneys	1 200–1 500
Solid foods	800–1 000	Skin	500–600
Oxidative metabolism	300	Lungs	400
		Gastrointestinal	100
Total Gains	2 200–2 700	**Total Losses**	2 200–2 700

From Hall, J. E., & Hall, M. (2020). *Guyton and Hall textbook of medical physiology* (14th ed.). Elsevier.

15. Remove gloves and dispose of them in appropriate receptacle.

16. Note I&O balance or imbalance and report to health care provider any urine output less than 30 mL/hr or significant changes in daily weight.

17. Document on I&O forms or EHR.

✦ REVIEW QUESTIONS

You are performing your morning assessment on a 69-year-old patient (he/him) 3 days post coronary artery bypass surgery (CABG). When asked about pain, the patient states, "My heart hurts. I feel short of breath and very hot."

Review Questions 1 to 4 relate to the case study presented here.

1. Which body systems should you assess on the patient and why?
2. You check the patient's last recorded temperature, which took place 1 hour ago, and it reads 37.7°C; you check it again and it is now 38.3°C. What could cause this change in temperature?
3. On auscultation of the patient's heart, you hear a "squeaky" or rubbing sound. Which cardiac abnormality should you suspect?
4. Your assessment of vital signs reveals the following: BP: 140/86 mm Hg; T: 38.3°C; HR: 90 beats/min; RR: 22 breaths/min; oxygen saturation, 91%. How should you document your assessment findings using SBAR (situation–background–assessment–recommendation), and what should your next step be?
5. Which of the following are characteristics of malignant melanoma? (*Select all that apply.*)
   1. An irregularly shaped lesion
   2. A lesion with lumpy edges
   3. A small papule with a dry, rough scale
   4. A pearly papule with a central crater and a waxy border
   5. A lesion with blue–black or variegated colour
   6. A lesion greater than 6 mm in size
6. In conducting a general survey of a patient, the nurse knows that the survey should include which of the following? (*Select all that apply.*)
   1. Appearance
   2. Obtaining peripheral pulses
   3. Measuring chest expansion
   4. Conducting a detailed history
   5. Behaviour
   6. Pupillary response
   7. Posture
7. You are about to begin an abdominal assessment on your patient. Place the following steps in the correct order:
   1. Auscultation
   2. Inspection
   3. Palpation
   4. Percussion

Visit the Evolve site for a complete list of answers to the Review Questions.

✦ NEXT GENERATION NCLEX® (NGN)

For practice with answering exam questions related to unfolding NGN case studies, please consult the Next Generation NCLEX® (NGN)-Style Case Studies for Skills and Techniques on the Evolve website: http://evolve.elsevier.com/Canada/Perry/clinicalskills/

REFERENCES

Accreditation Canada. (2020). *Required organizational practices–2020 handbook.* https://physicians.nshealth.ca/resources/required-organizational-practices-2020-handbook

Ball, J. W., Dains, J. E., Flynn, J. A., et al. (2022). *Seidel's guide to physical examination: An interprofessional approach* (10th ed.). Elsevier.

Boscart, V., McCleary, L., Sheiban Taucar, L., et al. (2023). *Ebersole and Hess' gerontological nursing and healthy aging in Canada* (3rd ed.). Elsevier.

Boyko, T. V., Longaker, M. T., & Yang, G. P. (2018). Review of the current management of pressure ulcers. *Advances in Wound Care*, 7(2), 57–67. https://doi.org/10.1089/wound.2016.0697

Canadian Cancer Society (CCS). (2022a). *Be sun safe.* https://cancer.ca/en/cancer-information/reduce-your-risk/be-sun-safe

Canadian Cancer Society (CCS). (2022b). *Live smoke-free.* https://cancer.ca/en/cancer-information/reduce-your-risk/live-smoke-free

Canadian Cancer Society (CCS). (2022c). *Risk factors for cervical cancer.* https://cancer.ca/en/cancer-information/cancer-types/cervical/risks

Canadian Cancer Society (CCS). (2022d). *Risk factors for colorectal cancer.* https://cancer.ca/en/cancer-information/cancer-types/colorectal/risks

Canadian Cancer Society (CCS). (2022e). *Risk factors for lung cancer.* https://cancer.ca/en/cancer-information/cancer-types/lung/risks

Canadian Cancer Society (CCS). (2022f). *Risk factors for ovarian cancer.* https://cancer.ca/en/cancer-information/cancer-types/ovarian/risks

Canadian Cancer Society (CCS). (2022g). *Risk factors for uterine cancer.* https://cancer.ca/en/cancer-information/cancer-types/uterine/risks

Canadian Cancer Society (CCS). (2022h). *Screening for breast cancer.* https://cancer.ca/en/cancer-information/cancer-types/breast/screening

Canadian Cancer Society (CCS). (2022i). *Symptoms of colorectal cancer.* https://cancer.ca/en/cancer-information/cancer-types/colorectal/signs-and-symptoms

Canadian Cancer Society (CCS). (2022j). *Symptoms of prostate cancer.* https://cancer.ca/en/cancer-information/cancer-types/prostate/signs-and-symptoms

Canadian Cancer Society (CCS). (2022k). *What is melanoma skin cancer?* https://cancer.ca/en/cancer-information/cancer-types/skin-melanoma/what-is-melanoma

Canadian Cancer Society (CCS). (2022l). *What is non-melanoma skin cancer?* https://cancer.ca/en/cancer-information/cancer-types/skin-non-melanoma/what-is-non-melanoma-skin-cancer

Canadian Task Force on Preventive Health Care. (2016). Recommendations on screening for colorectal cancer in primary care. *Canadian Medical Association Journal, 188*(5), 340–348. https://doi.org/10.1503/cmaj.151125 [Seminal Reference]

Canadian Task Force on Preventive Health Care. (2018). Recommendations on screening for breast cancer in average-risk women aged 40–74 years. *Canadian Medical Association Journal, 190*(49), E1441–E1451. https://doi.org/10.1503/cmaj.180463

Canadian Task Force on Preventive Health Care. (2019). *Published guidelines.* https://canadiantaskforce.ca/guidelines/published-guidelines/

College of Family Physicians of Canada. (2013). *Annual physical examination practices by province/territory in Canada.* https://www.cfpc.ca/en/policy-innovation/health-policy-goverment-relations/cfpc-policy-papers-position-statements/annual-physical-examination [Seminal Reference]

Fields, L. (2022, March 27). *Heart disease: 6 symptoms of women's heart attacks.* WebMD. https://www.webmd.com/heart-disease/features/womens-heart-attack-symptoms

Government of Canada. (2021). *Pneumococcal vaccine: Canadian immunization guide.* https://www.canada.ca/en/public-health/services/publications/healthy-living/canadian-immunization-guide-part-4-active-vaccines/page-16-pneumococcal-vaccine.html

Hall, J. E., & Hall, M. (2020). *Guyton and Hall textbook of medical physiology* (14th ed.). Elsevier.

Hartz, J. C., & de Ferranti, S. D. (2023). Overview of risk factors for development of atherosclerosis and early cardiovascular disease in childhood. *UpToDate.* https://www.uptodate.com/contents/overview-of-risk-factors-for-development-of-atherosclerosis-and-early-cardiovascular-disease-in-childhood

Heart and Stroke Foundation of Canada. (2021). *ASA for prevention: What you need to know.* https://www.heartandstroke.ca/articles/asa-for-prevention-what-you-need-to-know

Heart and Stroke Foundation of Canada. (2022). *The DASH diet to lower blood pressure.* https://www.heartandstroke.ca/healthy-living/healthy-eating/dash-diet

Hockenberry, J. N., Duffy, E. A., & Gibbs, K. (2024). *Wong's nursing care of infants and children* (12th ed.). Elsevier.

Indigenous Services Canada. (2015). *Clinical practice guidelines for nurses in primary care.* https://www.canada.ca/en/indigenous-services-canada/services/first-nations-inuit-health/health-care-services/nursing/clinical-practice-guidelines-nurses-primary-care.html [Seminal Reference]

Infection Prevention and Control Canada (IPCC). (2022). *Guidelines and standards.* https://ipac-canada.org/evidence-based-guidelines.php

Jarvis, C., Browne, J., MacDonald-Jenkins, J., & Luctkar-Flude, M. (2024). *Physical examination and health assessment* (4th ed.). Elsevier.

Osteoporosis Canada. (2022a). *Diagnosis: The importance of a comprehensive fracture risk assessment.* https://osteoporosis.ca/diagnosis/

Osteoporosis Canada. (2022b). *Facts and stats: Learn more about osteoporosis and related fractures.* https://osteoporosis.ca/facts-and-stats/

Pearson, G. J., Thanassoulis, G., Anderson, T. J., et al. (2021). 2021 Canadian Cardiovascular Society guidelines for the management of dyslipidemia for the prevention of cardiovascular disease in adults. *Canadian Journal of Cardiology*, 37(8), 1129–1150. https://doi.org/10.1016/j.cjca.2021.03.016

Pearson, J. L., Hitchman, S. C., Brose, L. S., et al. (2018). Recommended core items to assess e-cigarette use in population-based surveys. *Tobacco Control*, 27, 341–346. https://dx.doi.org/10.1136/tobaccocontrol-2016-053541

Public Health Agency of Canada (PHAC). (2017). *Updated recommendations on human papillomavirus (HPV) vaccines: 9-valent HPV vaccine 2-dose immunization schedule and the use of HPV vaccines in immunocompromised populations.* https://www.canada.ca/en/public-health/services/publications/healthy-living/updated-recommendations-human-papillomavirus-immunization-schedule-immunocompromised-populations.html

Rainbow Health Ontario. (2020). *Guidelines for gender-affirming primary care with trans and non-binary patients: A quick reference guide for primary care providers (PCPs).* https://www.rainbowhealthontario.ca/resource-library/qrg/

Sarkar, M., Madabhavi, I., Niranjan, N., et al. (2015). Auscultation of the respiratory system. *Annals of Thoracic Medicine, 10*(3), 158–168.

Sassano, M. F., Davis, E. S., Keating, J. E., et al. (2018). Evaluation of e-liquid toxicity using an open-source high-throughput screening assay. *PLOS Biology, 16*(3), Article e2003904. https://doi.org/10.1371/journal.pbio.2003904

Shmerling, R. H. (2022). *Can vaping damage your lungs? What we do (and don't) know.* Harvard Health Publishing. https://www.health.harvard.edu/blog/can-vaping-damage-your-lungs-what-we-do-and-dont-know-2019090417734

Sullivan, W., Diepstra, H., Heng, J., et al. (2018). Primary care of adults with intellectual and developmental disabilities: Clinical practice guidelines. *Canadian Family Physician, 64*(4), 254–279. https://www.cfp.ca/content/64/4/254.long

Tyerman, J., & Cobbett, S. (Eds.) (2023). *Lewis's medical-surgical nursing in Canada: Assessment and management of clinical problems* (5th ed.). Elsevier Inc.

Ward, K. T., & Reuben, D. B. (2020). Comprehensive geriatric assessment. *UpToDate* https://www.uptodate.com/contents/comprehensive-geriatric-assessment

World Health Organization. (2019). *Safe listening devices and systems: A WHO ITU standard.* https://apps.who.int/iris/bitstream/handle/10665/280085/9789241515276-eng.pdf

World Health Organization. (2021). *Deafness and hearing loss.* https://www.who.int/news-room/fact-sheets/detail/deafness-and-hearing-loss

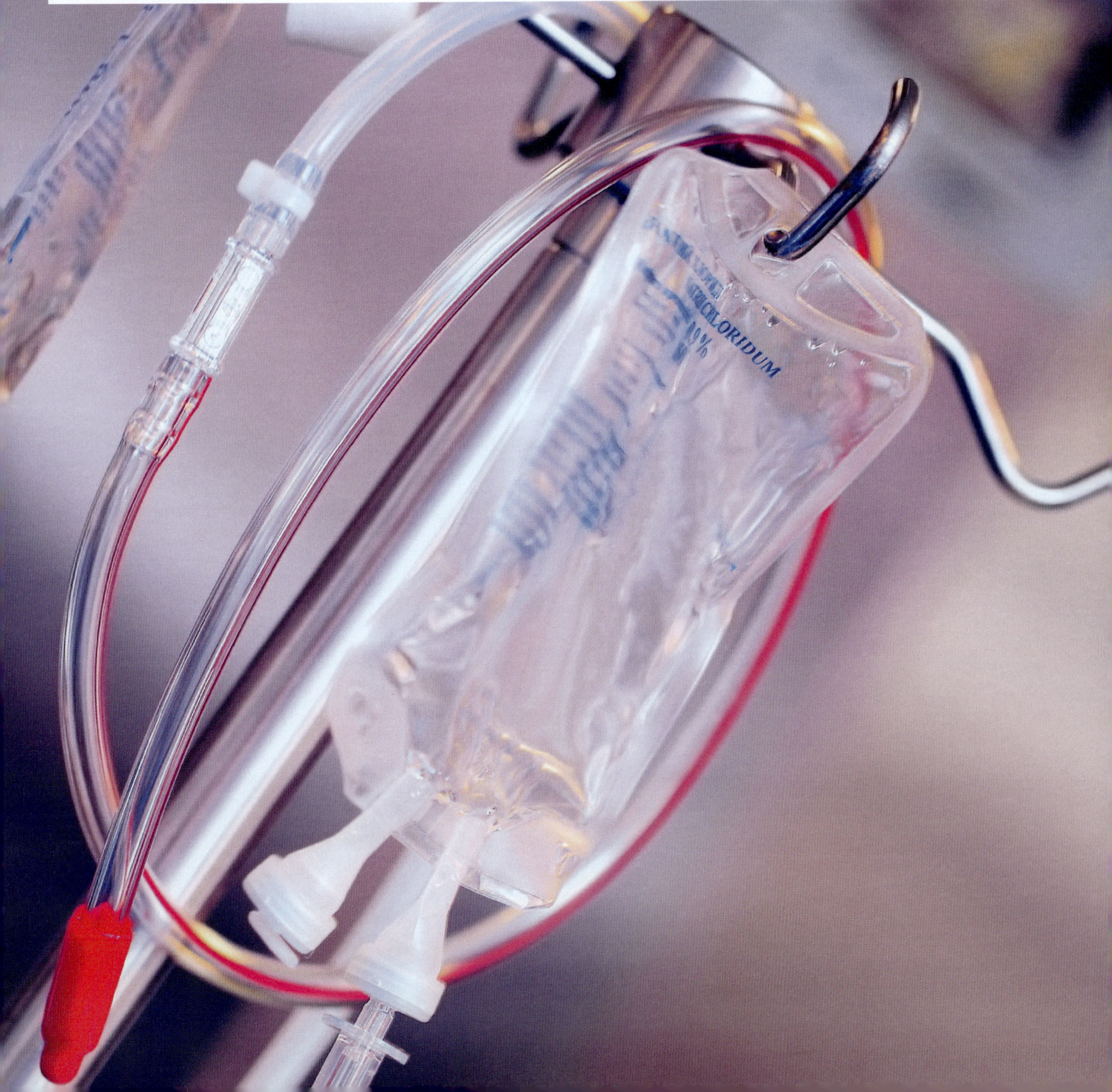

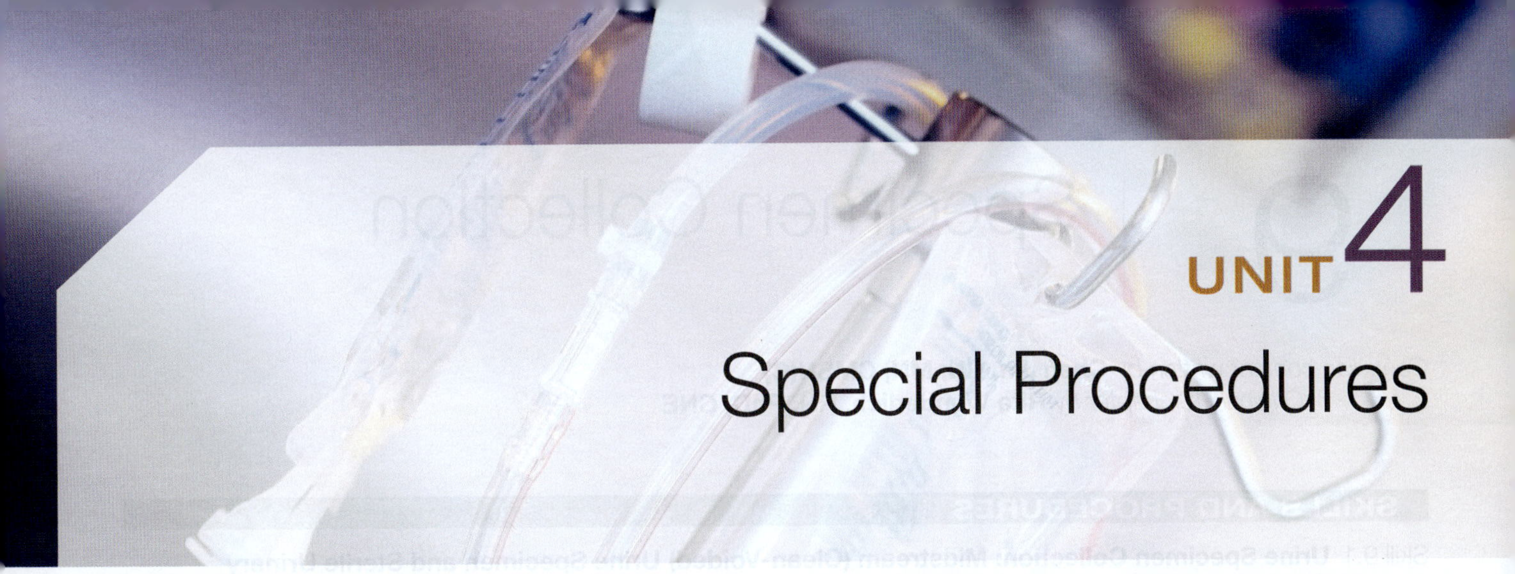

UNIT 4 Special Procedures

Making clinical judgements and decisions about any patient is a complex process, and in many cases the nurse needs to collect additional data from laboratory studies and diagnostic procedures. This information must be included in a patient's health and physical assessment database. It is important to analyze cues from laboratory and diagnostic findings to determine whether problems exist that are affecting the patient's health. It does not matter whether the patient is undergoing a routine physical examination and needs a blood specimen, has a urinary tract infection and needs a clean-voided urinary specimen, or requires a cardiac catheterization–data from these studies provide additional assessment data and cues, which are important in correctly identifying a patient's health problem and nursing diagnoses.

Collecting specimens from patients and preparing patients for diagnostic tests requires more than having knowledge about the procedure and the necessary skills to obtain a specimen. For many of the skills in this unit, you will need to use clinical judgement to assess a patient's ability to assist in specimen collection, identify any cultural considerations when obtaining specimens, and provide patient and family caregiver education to ensure successful specimen collection or prediagnostic procedure preparation and postprocedure care.

Many diagnostic procedures are done in an outpatient setting, and in some instances the time you spend with your patient before the procedure is limited. Before preparing a patient for a procedure, assess your patient's and caregiver's education needs. Does the patient understand the procedure? Are there any positioning requirements for the procedure? Is any local or moderate sedation involved? What type of postprocedure care will be required? To make a sound clinical judgement, a nurse needs to collect and analyze this information and determine an individualized patient and caregiver education plan for preprocedure and postprocedure care.

The chapters in this unit include relevant assessments, planning, implementation, and evaluation for each specimen collection and diagnostic procedure. The amount of data you collect about a patient for a specific specimen collection or diagnostic test depends on environmental factors such as the complexity and urgency of the test. In some situations, a patient may experience a lot of uncertainty and stress related to specimen collection, and even more so with diagnostic procedures. Your patient might be fearful of the outcome. In these situations, your assessment must go beyond the basic assessment steps for a specific specimen collection or diagnostic procedure. Use therapeutic communication skills to holistically and fully assess, understand, and implement nursing interventions to address the patient's fears and anxieties.

As you prepare for any of the skills in this unit, use your clinical judgement to inform your clinical decision making. Consider a patient's presenting condition and any risks for problems to determine whether more assessment data are needed or whether adjustments are necessary to how you prepare the patient for the test or procedure. Analyze the specimen or diagnostic procedure findings, and, as appropriate, communicate the findings to other members of the health care team. Plan and implement individualized nursing interventions to address postprocedure care or abnormal results. Use objective evaluation criteria to determine the patient response to any postprocedure interventions or follow-up care.

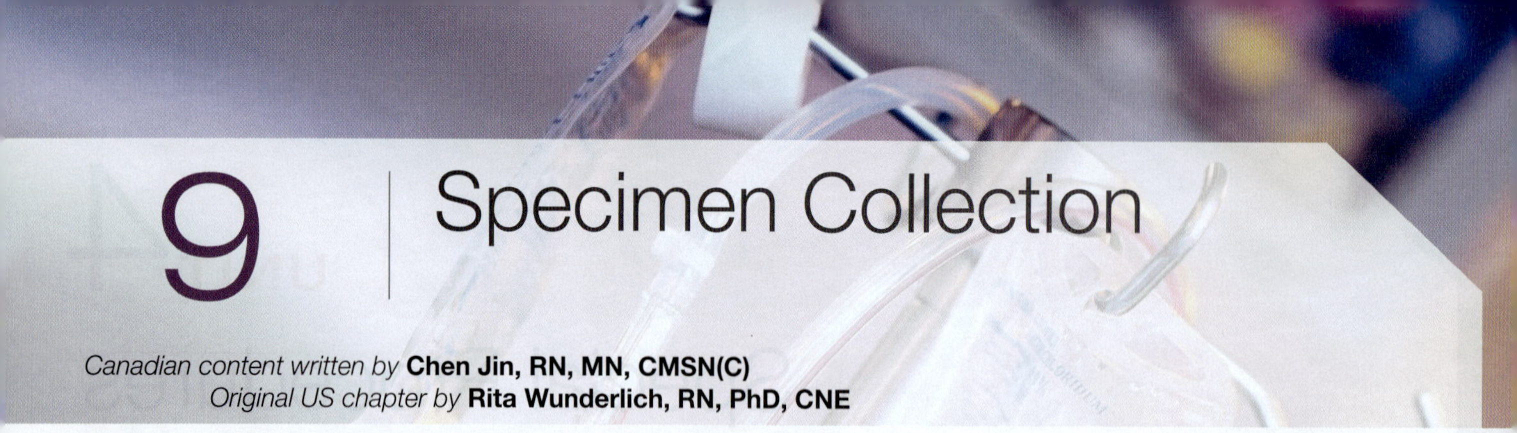

9 Specimen Collection

Canadian content written by **Chen Jin, RN, MN, CMSN(C)**
Original US chapter by **Rita Wunderlich, RN, PhD, CNE**

SKILLS AND PROCEDURES

OBJECTIVES

Mastery of content in this chapter will enable the nurse to:

- Explain the rationale for the collection of each specimen.
- Identify the special conditions necessary for collection of each specimen.
- Provide patient education to promote patient cooperation during specimen collection.
- Identify measures to minimize anxiety and promote safety during specimen collection.
- Describe nursing responsibilities for processing a specimen after collection.
- Document appropriate information in a patient's electronic health record or written record after collection of a specimen.
- Use correct technique for collecting clean-voided, timed, and catheterized urine specimens.
- Use correct technique for collecting specimens and cultures for blood and other body fluids.
- Use correct technique to perform venipuncture.
- Use infection control practices during specimen collection techniques.
- Use correct technique to perform arterial puncture for blood gas measurement.
- Identify nursing responsibility for reporting laboratory results to the health care provider.

MEDIA RESOURCES

- http://evolve.elsevier.com/Canada/Perry/clinicalskills/

PURPOSE

Laboratory test results aid in the diagnosis of health care problems, provide information about the stage and activity of a disease process, and measure a patient's response to therapy. Nurses are accountable for correctly collecting specimens, monitoring patient outcomes, and ensuring that these tests are collected and shared with the interprofessional team in a timely manner.

STANDARDS OF CARE

- Accreditation Canada (2020)—*Required Organizational Practices–2020 Handbook* (https://physicians.nshealth.ca/resources/required-organizational-practices-2020-handbook)
- Public Health Agency of Canada (PHAC, 2021a)—*Canadian Biosafety Guidelines* (https://www.canada.ca/en/public-health/services/canadian-biosafety-standards-guidelines/guidance.html)

- National Collaborating Centre for Infectious Diseases (2020)—*Canadian Public Health Laboratory Network Best Practices for COVID-19 V1.0* (https://nccid.ca/wp-content/uploads/sites/2/2020/05/COVID-Best-Practices-V1.01-v3.pdf)

PRINCIPLES FOR PRACTICE

- Proficiency and judgement in obtaining specimens minimize patient discomfort, promote patient safety, and ensure accuracy and quality of diagnostic procedures.
- Everyone who handles body fluids is at risk for exposure. The use of hand hygiene and personal protective equipment (PPE) is necessary to protect health care workers and patients. Always complete a point-of-care risk assessment for use of PPE (see Chapter 5, Box 5.1). Proper labelling of a container marked as biohazard protects and informs laboratory personnel and others who may come in contact with the specimen (PHAC, 2021a).
- Each employer may establish its own values for each test, which are printed on the employer laboratory forms. When questions arise, consult the employer procedure manual or call the laboratory.

PERSON-CENTRED CARE

- Patients often experience embarrassment or discomfort when giving a sample of body excretions or secretions, especially urine, urogenital, or stool samples. It is important to handle excretions or secretions discretely and provide a patient with as much privacy as possible while practising the principles of trauma-informed care. Given clear instructions, patients can obtain their own specimens of urine, stool, and sputum without unnecessary exposure (MacDonald et al., 2024).
- It is important to practise trauma-informed care with patients who are trauma survivors, as they may have experienced inappropriate or unpleasant touch in the past. Touch, even when appropriate and necessary for providing care, can easily activate a fight, flight, or freeze response. Nurses are often required to touch patients, sometimes in sensitive areas, to collect specimens. Nurses may need to help patients sit up in bed, apply the hospital identification band, listen to their lungs, or examine a wound. Any touch may be activating for a patient and bring up difficult feelings or memories. The triggering of these feelings or memories may lead to increased anxiety and activation of the stress response, which can result in disruptive behaviours and even lead the patient to disconnect from care. Health care providers should always ask permission and obtain verbal consent to touch someone (Fleishman et al., 2019).
- Patients who are 2SLGBTQI+ (Two-Spirit, lesbian, gay, bisexual, transgender, queer, intersex, and additional sexual orientations and gender identities) may encounter uncomfortable situations when asked to collect a specimen. For instance, some health care facilities fail to offer gender-neutral spaces in which to perform specimen collection. It is crucial that health care providers have knowledge of sexual and gender minority–centred care (Institute for Quality Management in Healthcare, 2019). Use gender-inclusive language when referring to different genitalia for specimen collection (e.g., when explaining to the patient how to cleanse for a midstream urine specimen).
- Consider both cultural and language barriers when delegating specimen collection to patients and caregivers. Language barriers make it difficult to explain the purpose of tests and collection techniques. They can lead to inaccurate patient assessment, misdiagnosis and/or delayed treatment, incomplete understanding of the patient's condition and prescribed treatment, or misunderstanding of an investigation (de Moissac & Bowen, 2019). Be sure to use strategies such as diagrams, illustrations, repeated return demonstrations, and interpreters when appropriate.
- Whenever possible, use gender-congruent caregivers when collecting vaginal, rectal, and urinary specimens from patients whose cultural values demand modesty and distinct separation of gender roles.

EVIDENCE-INFORMED PRACTICE

- Hemolysis of blood specimens causes delayed treatment of patients and increases health care costs (Simundic et al., 2020).
- Venipuncture is recommended over the collection of a blood sample from an intravenous (IV) site to prevent hemolysis when possible (Simundic et al., 2020).
- Hemolysis may result from vigorously shaking a blood sample, which invalidates the test (MacDonald et al., 2024). Promptly deliver blood specimens to the laboratory for processing to prevent hemolysis.
- Urine specimens for culture should be processed as soon as possible. If urine specimens cannot be processed within 30 minutes of collection, they should be refrigerated, placed on ice, inoculated into primary isolation medium before transport, or transported in an appropriate urine preservative. Refrigerated specimens should be cultured within 24 hours. Otherwise, growth of bacteria can occur, resulting in higher organism counts, which can falsely be interpreted as positive (BC Guidelines and Protocols Advisory Committee, 2020).
- To effectively promote wound healing, an appropriately performed wound swab can direct the proper treatment for the wound. The Levine technique is the preferred method of wound culture (Orsted et al., 2017).

SAFETY GUIDELINES

- Verify the type of procedure scheduled and the procedure site with the patient.
- Follow routine practices (see Chapter 5) when collecting specimens of blood or body fluids.
- Properly label all specimens and confirm requisitions with patient's identification, date and time the specimen is obtained, name of the test, and source of the specimen/culture for each container.
- Deliver specimens to the laboratory within the recommended time, or ensure that they are stored properly for later transport.
- Follow procedures for special conditions (e.g., iced specimens, special containers with preservatives) required for transport of specimens. Specific prerequisite conditions include fasting and nothing by mouth (NPO), which may be needed before collection of a specimen (MacDonald et al., 2024).
- Know employer policy regarding infection control practices for transportation of all specimen containers containing body substances.
- Follow procedures for medications or dietary intake that may result in some deviations from normal values.
- Follow precautions for collecting specimens from patients who require transmission-based precautions (e.g., protective isolation).

SKILL 9.1 Urine Specimen Collection: Midstream (Clean-Voided) and Sterile Urinary Catheter

Video Clip NSO *Nursing Skills Online Specimen Collection Module 3 / Lessons 1 and 2*

A urinalysis provides information about kidney or metabolic function, nutrition, and systemic diseases. Urine collection uses a variety of methods, depending on the purpose of the urinalysis and the presence or absence of a urinary catheter. Guidelines for assessment, planning, and evaluation are similar, regardless of the method of collection. Routine urinalysis includes measurement of nine or more elements, including urine pH, protein and glucose levels, ketones, specific gravity, white blood cell (WBC) count, and presence of bacteria, blood, or both (MacDonald et al., 2024).

Types of Urine Tests and Specimens

- *A random urine specimen for routine urinalysis* is collected using a specimen "hat" (Fig. 9.1), which is placed under a toilet seat to collect voided urine. The nurse then places approximately 120 mL of urine in a properly labelled specimen container and sends it to the laboratory.
- *A timed urine specimen for quantitative analysis* requires urine to be collected over 2 to 72 hours. The 24-hour timed collection (see Procedural Guideline 9.1) is most common and allows for measurement and quantitative analysis of elements such as amino acids, creatinine, hormones, glucose, and adrenocorticosteroid excretion.
- *A urine specimen for culture and sensitivity (C&S)* is performed to identify whether bacteria are present (culture) and to determine the most effective antibiotic for treatment (sensitivity). Specimens for C&S are collected either as a clean-voided midstream specimen or under sterile technique from a urinary catheter. Urine collected using these methods may also be analyzed for the same components as those measured by routine urinalysis.
- *Chemical properties of urine* are tested by immersing a specially prepared test strip of paper (Chemstrip) into a clean urine specimen. The test detects the presence of glucose, ketones, protein, or blood, which are not normally present in urine (see Procedural Guideline 9.2). When the screening test for the presence of substances in the urine is positive, additional laboratory tests are used to determine a patient's diagnosis or to measure the effectiveness of treatment.

Delegation and Collaboration

The skill of collecting urine specimens may be delegated to an unregulated care provider (UCP), or collaboration may occur with parts of the skill such as monitoring, skill implementation, teaching, and documentation. The nurse may collaborate with the UCP on the following:

- Obtaining the specimens at a specified time when appropriate

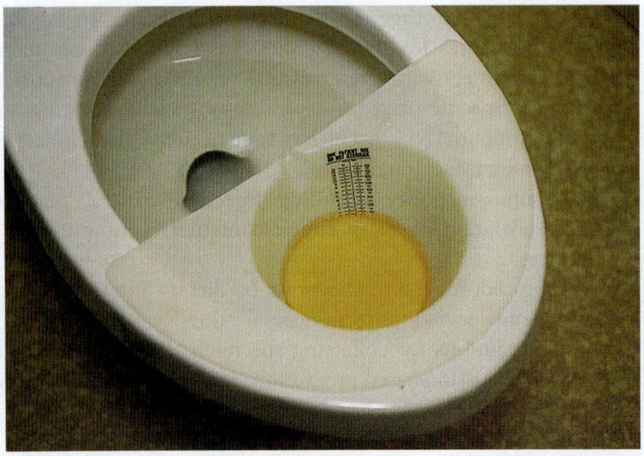

FIG 9.1 Specimen hat.

- Positioning patient as necessary when mobility restrictions are present
- Communicating when the urine is not clear (e.g., contains blood, cloudiness, or excess sediment)
- Communicating when a patient is unable to initiate a stream or has pain or burning on urination

Interprofessional collaboration often occurs with urine specimen collections. Doing so ensures that all health care team members are aware of the need to save all urine when a patient is undergoing a timed urine specimen collection.

Equipment

- Completed identification labels with appropriate patient identifiers
- Completed laboratory requisition
- Small plastic biohazard bag (or container)

Midstream (Clean-Voided) Urine Specimen

- Specimen hat (see Fig. 9.1) or bedpan (for nonambulatory patient)
- Sterile specimen container (Fig. 9.2)
- Urine C&S preservative tube (Fig. 9.3)
- Antiseptic towelettes

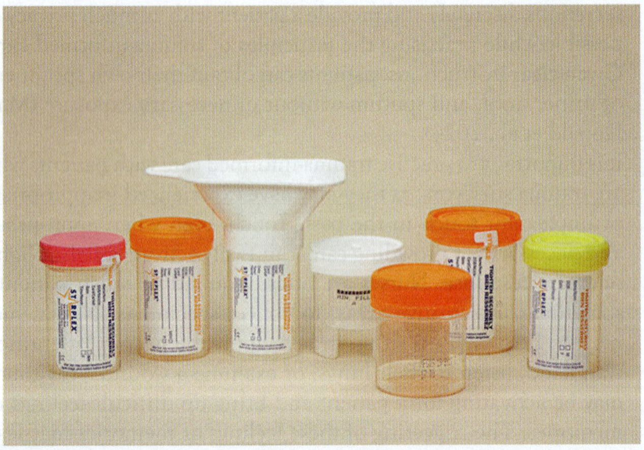

FIG 9.2 Various specimen collection containers. *(Image courtesy Starplex Scientific Inc.)*

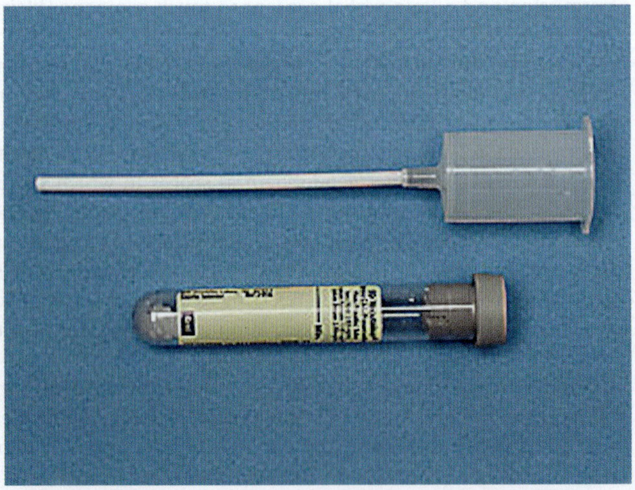

FIG 9.3 Urine C&S preservative tube. *(Courtesy and copyright © Becton Dickinson.)*

- Clean gloves
- Soap, water, washcloth, and towel

Sterile Urine Specimen From Urinary Catheter

- Specimen container (nonsterile for routine urinalysis, sterile for culture)
- 20-mL Luer-Lok syringe for routine urinalysis or 3-mL Luer-Lok syringe for culture
- Antiseptic swab
- Clean gloves
- Clamp

STEP	RATIONALE
ASSESSMENT	
1. Identify patient using at least two person-specific identifiers (e.g., name and date of birth, or name and medical record number) according to employer policy. Compare identifiers with information on patient's medical record and laboratory requisition.	Ensures correct patient. Complies with Accreditation Canada standards and improves patient safety (Accreditation Canada, 2020).
2. Throughout the procedure, the 4 moments for hand hygiene are to be implemented; hand hygiene should occur before initial patient (or patient environment) contact, before an aseptic procedure, after body fluid exposure risk, and after patient (or patient environment) contact. Additional hand hygiene should be performed when hands are visibly soiled.	Proper hand hygiene helps prevent the spread of infectious agents to health care providers.
3. Assess patient's or caregiver's understanding of purpose of test and method of collection.	Allows you to clarify misunderstanding; promotes patient cooperation.
4. Assess patient's ability to help with urine specimen collection (e.g., ability to position self and hold container).	Determines degree of help patient requires.
5. Assess for signs and symptoms of a urinary tract infection (UTI) (frequency, urgency, dysuria, hematuria, flank pain, fever; cloudy, malodorous urine).	These are indicators of a UTI.
6. Refer to employer procedures for specimen collection methods.	Employer policies may vary regarding collection and/or handling of specimens.

NURSING DIAGNOSES

- Potential for infection
- Insufficient knowledge regarding specimen collection

Related factors and risk factors are individualized on the basis of patient's condition or needs.

STEP	RATIONALE
PLANNING	
1. Expected outcomes following completion of procedure:	
• Specimen free of contaminants is collected.	Proper collection technique prevents substances from changing normal characteristics of urine.
• Patient discusses procedure for specimen collection.	Procedure is performed safely.
• Patient discusses purpose and benefits of specimen collection.	Evaluates patient's learning.
IMPLEMENTATION	
1.	Proper hand hygiene helps prevent the spread of infectious agents to health care providers.
2. Check labels and complete laboratory requisition for specimen container.	Organizes procedure.
3. Provide privacy for patient; close curtains around bed or close room door. Allow mobile patients to collect specimen in bathroom.	Privacy allows patient to relax and produce specimen more easily.
4. Collect midstream (clean-voided) urine specimen.	
a. Apply clean gloves. Give patient cleaning towelette or towel, washcloth, and soap to clean perineum, or assist patient with cleaning perineum. Help bedridden patient onto bedpan to facilitate access to perineum. Remove and dispose of gloves.	Reduces transmission of microorganisms. Patients prefer to wash their own perineal areas when possible. Cleaning prevents contamination of specimen after urine passes from urethra.

STEP	RATIONALE
b. Using aseptic technique, open outer package of commercial specimen kit.	Maintains sterility of equipment.
c. Apply clean gloves.	Reduces transmission of microorganisms.
d. Pour antiseptic solution over cotton balls (unless kit contains prepared antiseptic towelettes).	Cotton ball or towelette is used to clean perineum.
e. Open specimen container, maintaining sterility of the inside of the container, and set cap aside with sterile side up. Do not touch inside of cap or container.	Maintains sterility of equipment. Contaminated specimen is most frequent reason for inaccurate reporting of urine C&S.
f. Use aseptic technique to help patient or allow patient to independently clean perineum and collect specimen. Amount of help needed varies with each patient. Inform patient that antiseptic solution will feel cold.	Maintains patient's dignity and comfort.
(1) *Male genitalia:*	
(a) Hold penis with one hand; using circular motion and antiseptic towelette, clean meatus, moving from centre to outside three times with different towelettes (see Step 4f[1][a] illustration). Have uncircumcised patient retract foreskin for effective cleaning of urinary meatus and keep retracted during voiding. Return foreskin when done.	Reduces number of microorganisms at urethral meatus and moves from areas of least to most contamination. Return of foreskin prevents stricture of penis.
(b) If employer procedure indicates, rinse area with sterile water and dry with gauze.	Prevents contamination of specimen with antiseptic solution.
(c) After patient initiates urine stream into toilet or bedpan, have patient pass urine specimen container into stream and collect 90–120 mL of urine (MacDonald et al., 2024) (see Step 4f[1][c] illustration).	Initial urine flushes out microorganisms that normally accumulate at urinary meatus and prevents transfer into specimen.

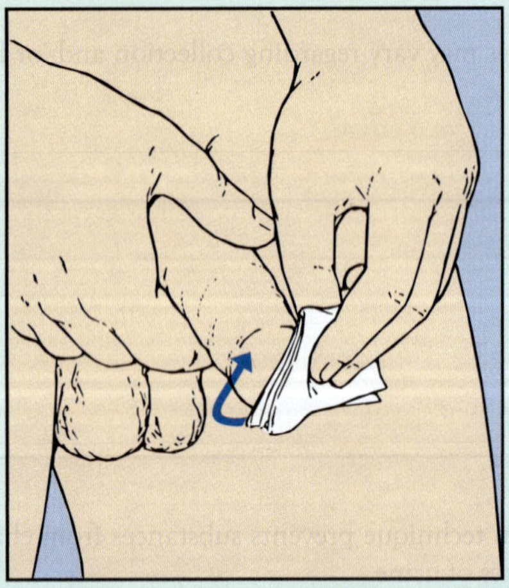

STEP 4F(1)(A) Cleaning technique (male genitalia).

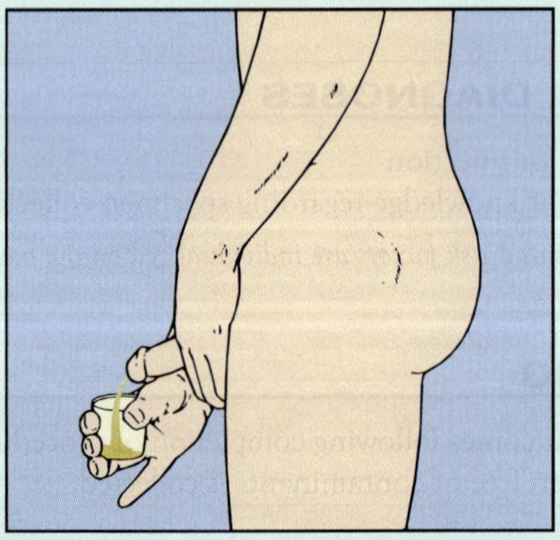

STEP 4F(1)(C) Collecting midstream urine specimen (male genitalia).

STEP	RATIONALE
(2) *Female genitalia:*	
(a) Either nurse or patient spreads labia minora with fingers of nondominant hand.	Provides access to urethral meatus.
(b) With dominant hand, clean urethral area with antiseptic swab (cotton ball or gauze). Move from front (above urethral orifice) to back (toward anus). Use fresh swab each time; clean three times; begin with labial fold farthest from you, then labial fold closest, and then down centre (see Step 4f[2][b] illustration).	Prevents contamination of urinary meatus with fecal material. Cleaning down centre last decreases contamination from labia.
(c) If employer procedure indicates, rinse area with sterile water and dry with cotton ball.	Prevents contamination of specimen with antiseptic solution.
(d) While continuing to hold labia apart, patient initiates urine stream into toilet or bedpan; after stream is achieved, pass specimen container into stream and collect 90–120 mL of urine (MacDonald et al., 2024) (see Step 4f[2][d] illustration).	Initial stream flushes out resident microorganisms that accumulate at urethral meatus and prevents transfer into specimen.

STEP	RATIONALE

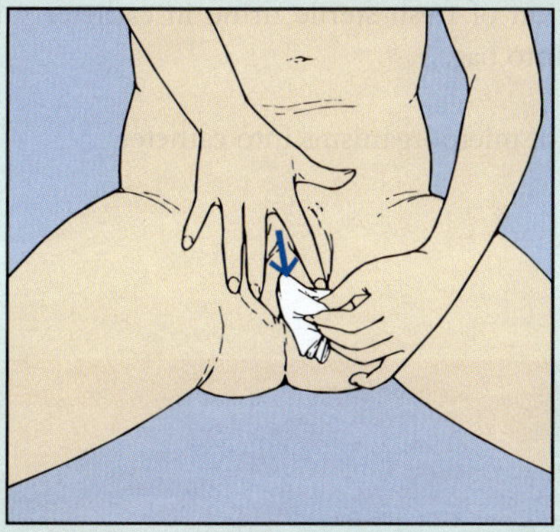

STEP 4F(2)(B) Clean from front to back, holding labia apart (female genitalia).

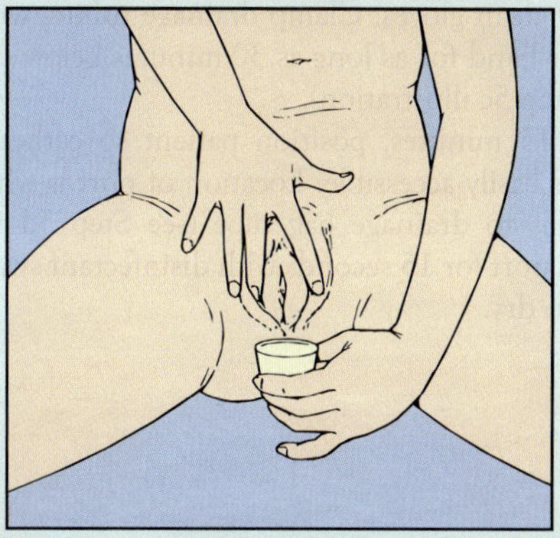

STEP 4F(2)(D) Collecting midstream urine specimen (female genitalia).

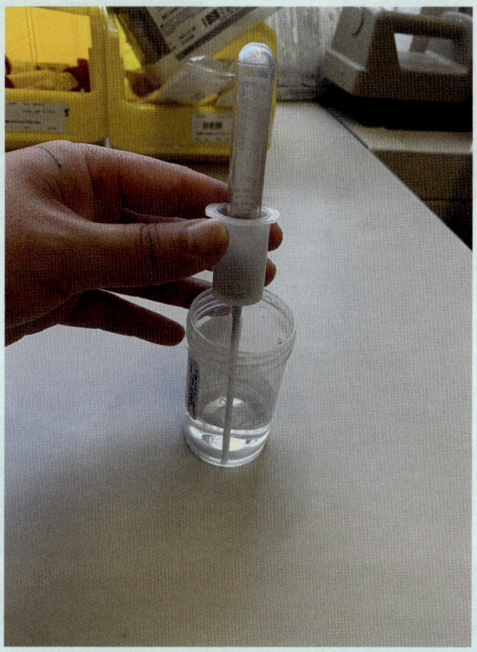

STEP 4J Collecting urine culture and sensitivity (C&S) via preservative tube. *(Image courtesy Mausam Gurung).*

STEP	RATIONALE
g. Remove specimen container before flow of urine stops and before releasing labia or penis. Patient finishes voiding into bedpan or toilet. Offer to help with personal hygiene as appropriate.	Prevents contamination of specimen with skin flora. Prevents sediment from bladder from getting into specimen.
h. Replace cap securely on specimen container, touching only outside.	Retains sterility of inside of container and prevents spillage of urine.
i. Clean urine from exterior surface of container.	Prevents transfer of microorganisms to others.
j. Use the straw to transfer urine into the transport tube (see Step 4j illustration).	
5. Collect urine from in-dwelling urinary catheter.	
a. Explain that you will use a needleless syringe to remove urine through the catheter port and that patient will not experience any discomfort.	Minimizes anxiety when you manipulate catheter and aspirate urine with syringe from catheter port.
b. Explain that you will need to clamp the catheter for 15–30 minutes (MacDonald et al., 2024) before obtaining a urine specimen and that urine cannot be obtained from the drainage bag.	Allows urine to accumulate in catheter. Urine in drainage bag is not considered sterile.

STEP	RATIONALE
c. Apply clean gloves. Clamp drainage tubing with clamp or rubber band for as long as 30 minutes below catheter port (see Step 5c illustration).	Permits collection of fresh sterile urine in catheter tubing rather than draining into bag.
d. After 15 minutes, position patient so catheter sampling port is easily accessible. Location of port is where catheter attaches to drainage bag tube (see Step 5d illustration). Clean port for 15 seconds with disinfectant swab and allow port to dry.	Prevents entry of microorganisms into catheter.

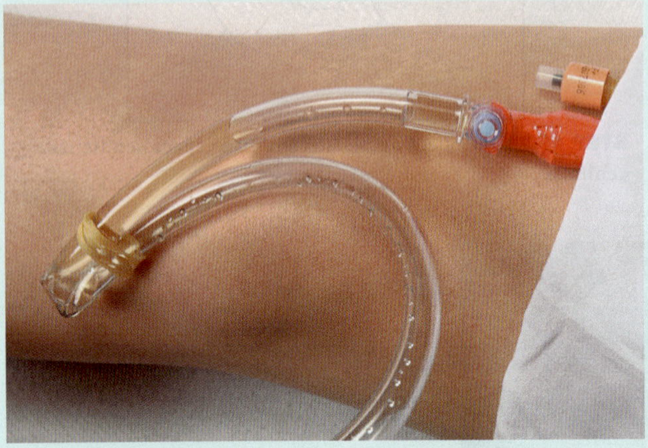

STEP 5C **Rubber band used to clamp drainage tube.**

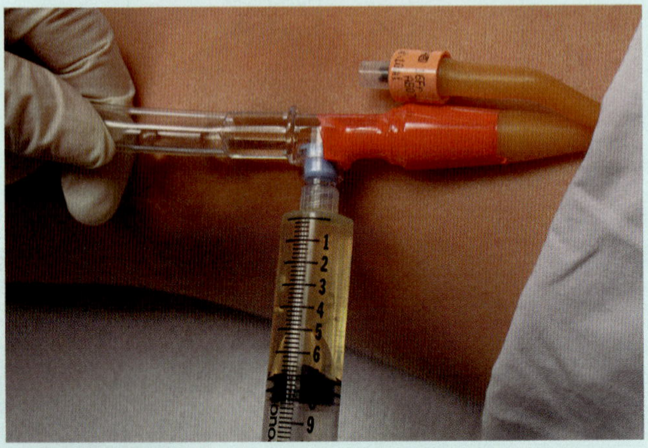

STEP 5D **Access urinary catheter port with Luer-Lok syringe or syringe with blunt plastic valve.**

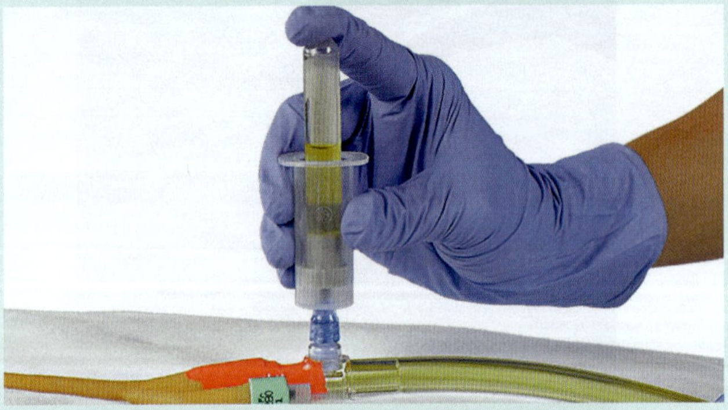

STEP 5E **Access urinary catheter port with Luer-Lok access device.** *(Courtesy and copyright © Becton Dickinson.)*

STEP	RATIONALE
e. Attach needleless Luer-Lok syringe to built-in catheter sampling port. Some needleless ports use a blunt plastic valve or slip-tip syringe inserted into the port diaphragm. For urine culture, collect urine directly using urine C&S preservative tube via Luer-Lok access device (see Step 5e illustration).	Guideline recommends use of Luer-Lok needleless system. Needleless system prevents injury by needle-stick.
f. Withdraw 5–10 mL for culture or 20 mL for routine urinalysis.	Allows collection of urine without contamination. Proper volume is needed to perform test. Increased volume of sample may be required for specific tests.
g. Transfer urine from syringe into clean urine container for routine urinalysis or into sterile urine container for culture.	Prevents contamination of urine during transfer procedure.
h. Place lid tightly on container.	Prevents contamination of specimen by air and loss by spillage.
i. Unclamp catheter and allow urine to flow into drainage bag. Ensure that urine flows freely.	Allows urine to drain by gravity and prevents stasis of urine in bladder.
6. Securely attach label to container (not lid). In patient's presence, confirm label information (two person-specific identifiers, specimen source, and collection date and time). If appropriate, indicate if patient is menstruating.	Ensures that specimen is identified correctly for proper diagnosis (Accreditation Canada, 2020).
7. Dispose of soiled supplies. Remove and dispose of gloves.	Prevents transmission of microorganisms.

STEP	RATIONALE
8. Send specimen and completed requisition to laboratory within 20 minutes. Refrigerate specimen if delay cannot be avoided.	Delay of analysis may significantly alter test results (MacDonald et al., 2024).

EVALUATION

1. Inspect midstream (clean-voided) specimen for contamination with toilet paper or stool.	Contaminants prevent specimen from being used.
2. Evaluate patient's urine C&S report for bacterial growth.	Routine cultures identify organism(s), and sensitivity study identifies antimicrobial medications that may be effective against pathogen.
3. Observe urinary drainage system in catheterized patient to ensure that it is intact and patent.	System must remain closed to remain sterile.
4. **Use teach-back:** "I want to be sure I clearly explained the way to obtain a urine sample. Can you tell me how you would take the sample?" Develop a revised teaching plan if patient or caregiver is unable to teach back correctly.	Determines level of understanding of instructional topic.

Unexpected Outcomes	Related Interventions
1. Urine specimen is contaminated with stool or toilet paper.	• Repeat patient instruction and specimen collection. If unable to obtain specimen through clean voiding, patient may need catheterization (see Chapter 34, Skill 34.1).
2. Patient is unable to void, or urine does not collect in drainage tube.	• Ensure patency of tube, then offer fluids if permitted to enhance urine production.
3. Urine culture reveals bacterial growth (determined by colony count >10 000 organisms/mL).	• Report findings to health care provider. • Administer medications as prescribed. • Monitor patient for fever and dysuria.
4. Lumen leading to balloon that holds catheter in place is punctured.	• Notify health care provider. • Prepare for removal of existing catheter and insertion of new catheter.

Communication and Documentation

- Document collection of specimen in progress notes in electronic health record (EHR) or chart or per employer policy; note method used to obtain specimen, date and time collected, type of test prescribed, appearance, odour and colour of urine, and time sent to laboratory.
- Document your evaluation of patient and caregiver learning.
- Report any abnormal findings to health care provider.

DOCUMENTATION EXAMPLE

25-year-old patient (he/him) arrived in the clinic with dysuria, lower abdominal pain. Urine C&S prescribed. Provided teaching on how to accurately collect sample per employer protocol. 90 mL concentrated, strong odour, midstream urine was collected in the specimen bottle at 1400 hours. The sample was sent to lab at 1415 hours. Patient waiting to see health care provider.

Special Considerations

Teaching

- Explain significance of cleaning genital area before collecting specimen.
- Discuss signs and symptoms of a UTI (e.g., burning or pain with urination, urgency, increased frequency, cloudy urine) with patient and caregiver, if appropriate.
- Self-catheterization may be an alternative for urine collection and taught to patients, if appropriate.

Pediatric

- Urine collection bags may be used with infants and young children who are not toilet trained, for some forms of analysis (such as glucose, ketones, or proteins) (Giannoumis, 2021; May, 2018). Ensure that you cut a small slit in the diaper and pull the urine collection bag through the slit so that collected urine is visible outside the diaper (Fig. 9.4). Remove the bag as soon as the urine specimen is visible (Keenan-Lindsay et al., 2022).
- For some forms of analysis, urine may also be aspirated with a syringe directly from the diaper (Keenan-Lindsay et al., 2022).
- To collect a urine specimen for culture, use the midstream (clean-voided) collection method (May, 2018). Collection using sterile urine-collecting bags or directly from diapers is not recommended because results are often contaminated and therefore inaccurate when analyzing for pathogenic microorganisms (May, 2018). However, it is challenging to collect a urine specimen via the midstream method with infants and younger children; thus,

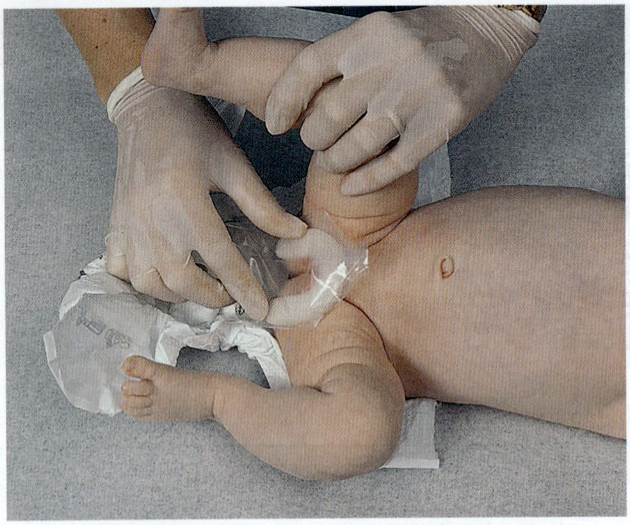

FIG 9.4 **Application of urine collection bag.** *(From Warekois, R. S., Robinson, R., & Primrose, P. B. [2020]. Phlebotomy worktext and procedures manual [5th ed.]. Elsevier.)*

when infection is suspected and an accurate specimen is critical, suprapubic urine aspiration or insertion of a sterile catheter is recommended (Giannoumis, 2021).

Gerontological

- Older persons may need help positioning themselves to obtain a specimen. In confused patients, use interprofessional collaboration to obtain information about how best to help the patient collect a specimen (Boscart et al., 2023).

Care in the Community: Home Management

- Instruct a patient collecting a sample at home to keep it refrigerated or on ice until it reaches the laboratory to minimize bacterial growth before applying it to a culture medium in the laboratory setting.

Procedural Guideline 9.1 *Collecting a Timed Urine Specimen*

Some tests of renal function and urine composition require urine to be collected over 2–72 hours. The 24-hour timed collection method is used most often. It measures elements such as amino acids, creatinine, hormones, glucose, and adrenocorticosteroids. A timed urine collection provides a means to measure the concentration or dilution of urine.

To ensure the accuracy of a 24-hour timed urine specimen, the patient and staff must work together to collect all voided urine in a 24-hour period. Obtain an appropriate container with or without preservative. The type of analysis for the 24-hour timed specimen determines the need for any preservative. The specimen container can be placed in the patient's bathroom or the "soiled" utility room. Post a sign to remind the patient and staff that a test is in progress. Label the specimen container with all appropriate identification information and the number of containers sequentially if more than one container is needed. Documentation and collection of all urine is necessary for an accurate test result.

Delegation and Collaboration

The skill of collecting a timed urine specimen can be delegated to a UCP. The nurse informs the UCP about the following:

- When timed collection begins, proper method to store the collected urine, where to place signs that a timed urine collection is in progress, and saving all urine
- Reporting when blood, mucus, or foul odours are present in the urine specimen or if there is a break in the collection procedure

Equipment

- Large collection bottle with cap that usually contains a chemical preservative
- Bedpan, urinal, specimen hat, bedside commode, or pediatric potty chair
- Graduated measuring container for intake and output (I&O) measurement
- Large basin to hold collection bottle surrounded by ice if immediate refrigeration is required
- Specimen identification label and completed laboratory requisition
- Instructional signs that remind patient and staff of timed urine collection
- Clean gloves
- Plastic biohazard plastic bag or container

Procedural Steps

1. Identify patient using at least two person-specific identifiers (e.g., name and date of birth, or name and medical record number) according to employer policy. Compare identifiers with information on patient's medical record and laboratory requisition (Accreditation Canada, 2020).
2. Throughout the procedure, the 4 moments for hand hygiene are to be implemented; hand hygiene should occur before initial patient (or patient environment) contact, before an aseptic procedure, after body fluid exposure risk, and after patient (or patient environment) contact. Additional hand hygiene should be performed when hands are visibly soiled.
3. Explain the reason for specimen collection, how the patient can help, and that urine must be free of feces and toilet tissue.
4. Place specimen collection container in the bathroom and, if indicated, in a pan of ice. Post signs to remind staff, family and visitors, and patient of timed urine collection on patient's door and toileting area. If patient leaves unit, be sure that personnel in receiving area collect and save all urine.
5. If possible, have patient drink 2–4 glasses of water about 30 minutes before times of collection to facilitate ability to void at the appropriate time for test to begin.
6. Apply clean gloves. Discard the first voided specimen as the test begins. Indicate time test began on laboratory requisition. For accurate results, the patient must begin the test with an empty bladder. Begin collecting all urine for designated time.
7. Measure volume of each voiding if I&O are to be recorded. Place all voided urine in labelled specimen bottle with appropriate additives.

Continued

Procedural Guideline 9.1 *Collecting a Timed Urine Specimen—cont'd*

8. Unless instructed otherwise, keep specimen bottle in specimen refrigerator or container of ice in bathroom to prevent decomposition of urine.
9. Encourage patient to drink 2 glasses of water 1 hour before timed urine collection ends. Encourage patient to empty bladder during last 15 minutes of urine collection period.
10. Apply clean gloves. Collect final specimen at end of collection period. Label specimen (two person-specific identifiers, specimen source, collection date and time, number of bottle) in patient's presence, attach appropriate requisition, and send to laboratory. Remove gloves and discard.
11. Remove signs. Tell patient that specimen collection period is done.

Procedural Guideline 9.2 *Urine Screening for Glucose, Ketones, Protein, Blood, and pH*

Video Clip NSO Nursing Skills Online

Tests for chemical properties of urine are part of the routine urinalysis completed in the laboratory or as a point-of-care test performed at the bedside or in the home. A Multistix reagent test strip may simultaneously be used to assess for up to nine chemical properties: specific gravity, pH, protein, glucose, ketones, blood bilirubin, urobilinogen, leukocytes, and nitrates. The test is easy to perform and causes no pain. This type of screening is used when more detailed laboratory testing is not available (e.g., in a health care provider's office, clinic, or long-term care setting). The use of urine testing for managing blood glucose is no longer recommended but continues to be useful in detecting the presence of ketones in patients with diabetes (Diabetes Canada Clinical Practice Guidelines Expert Committee, 2018). Capillary blood monitoring is an accurate assessment of serum glucose levels (MacDonald et al., 2024).

Delegation and Collaboration

The skill of urine screening for chemical properties can be delegated to a UCP. The nurse informs the UCP to do the following:

- Obtain the specimen correctly (e.g., before meals, following a "double-voided" specimen)
- Report the results of the test or any odour, blood, or mucus in the urine specimen

Equipment

- Bedpan, urinal, specimen hat, bedside commode, or pediatric potty chair
- Container for urine from catheter
- Watch with second hand or digital counter
- Reagent test strip (check expiration date on container)
- Test strip colour chart
- Paper towel
- Clean gloves
- Small biohazard plastic bag for delivery of specimen to a laboratory (or container specified by employer)

Procedural Steps

1. Identify patient using at least two person-specific identifiers (e.g., name and date of birth, or name and medical record number) according to employer policy. Compare identifiers with information on medical record and laboratory requisition (Accreditation Canada, 2020).
2. Determine whether a double-voided specimen is needed for glucose testing. If required, ask the patient to void and discard specimen, then drink a glass of water.
3. Apply clean gloves. Throughout the procedure, the 4 moments for hand hygiene are to be implemented; hand hygiene should occur before initial patient (or patient environment) contact, before an aseptic procedure, after body fluid exposure risk, and after patient (or patient environment) contact. Additional hand hygiene should be performed when hands are visibly soiled.
4. Ask the patient to collect a fresh, random urine specimen. If patient is catheterized, remove a 5- to 10-mL specimen from the catheter port (see Skill 9.1).
5. Immerse end of reagent strip into urine container. Remove the strip immediately and tap it gently against the side of the container to remove excess urine.
6. Hold strip in a horizontal position to prevent mixing of chemical reagents (see Step 6 illustration).

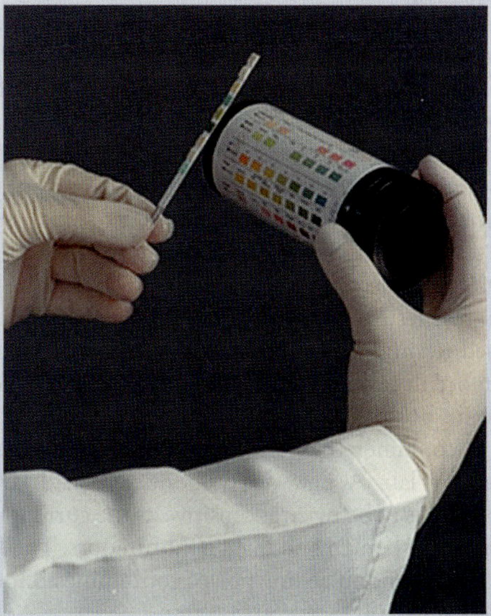

STEP 6 Testing urine using reagent strip.

7. Precisely time the number of seconds specified on container, and compare colour of strip with colour chart on container (Table 9.1).
8. When appropriate, discuss test results with patient. Discard urine. Remove and discard gloves.
9. Record results immediately on appropriate flow sheet. Report reading to health care provider.

Continued

Procedural Guideline 9.2 *Urine Screening for Glucose, Ketones, Protein, Blood, and pH—cont'd*

TABLE 9.1

Example of a Chart for a Reagent Strip*

Test	When to Read	Range of Results
pH	60 seconds	5.0–9.0
Protein	60 seconds	(–) or 3+ (5 g/L)
Glucose	10 seconds (qualitative)	(–) to 4+ (55 mmol/L)
	30 seconds (quantitative)	(–) to 4+ (55 mmol/L)
Ketones	40 seconds	(–) to 3+ (large)
Blood	60 seconds	(–) to 4+ (large)

*Based on Roche Canada's Chemstrip 7 product line.

SKILL 9.2 Measuring Occult Blood in Stool

Video Clip **NSO** *Nursing Skills Online Specimen Collection Module 3 / Lesson 4*

Hemoccult testing is useful for screening for the presence of occult (not visible) blood in the stool for conditions such as colon cancer, bleeding gastrointestinal (GI) ulcers, and localized gastric or intestinal irritation. Use caution; a false-positive result may occur if a patient has ingested red meat within 3 days of testing or is taking certain medications (e.g., iron). A false-negative result may occur if that patient is taking vitamin C (MacDonald et al., 2024). The test measures microscopic amounts of blood in the stool. Normally, a person loses small amounts of blood daily in the feces as a result of minor abrasions of the nasopharyngeal or oral mucosa. If greater than 50 mL of blood enters the feces from the upper GI tract, the blood causes melena (darkening of feces). When blood is present, further testing is indicated to determine the source of the bleeding.

Patients are often instructed on how to collect stool specimens for the test at the home. Only a small amount of stool is needed to perform the test successfully. The common types of stool tests used are the gFOBT (guaiac fecal occult blood test) and the FIT (fecal immunochemical test) (Canadian Cancer Society, 2022). Methods of guaiac-based testing include Hemoccult slides and Hematest tablets. The Hemoccult testing kit is commonly used in the community setting. In some hospitals, a stool sample is collected with a fecal transportation container (Fig. 9.5), and Hemoccult testing is then performed in the lab. A new deoxyribonucleic acid (DNA) stool sample test promises to be twice as sensitive as the current guaiac testing for precancerous benign and malignant tumours. The DNA stool sample test identifies nonbleeding polyps containing abnormal DNA (MacDonald et al., 2024).

Delegation and Collaboration

The skill of testing stool for occult blood can be delegated to a UCP. The nurse informs the UCP to do the following:

- Report immediately if any blood is detected and not to discard stool from a positive test so the nurse may repeat testing

Equipment

- Soap, water, washcloth, and towel
- Paper towel
- Clean gloves
- Wooden applicators

Hemoccult Test

- Fecal container with white spoon cap (see Fig. 9.5) or cardboard Hemoccult slide (Fig. 9.6)
- Hemoccult developing solution

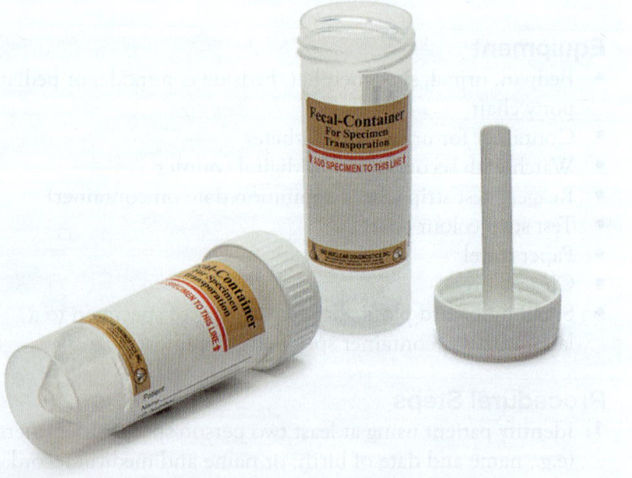

FIG 9.5 Fecal transportation container with white spoon cap. *(Courtesy and copyright © Bio Nuclear Diagnostics Inc.)*

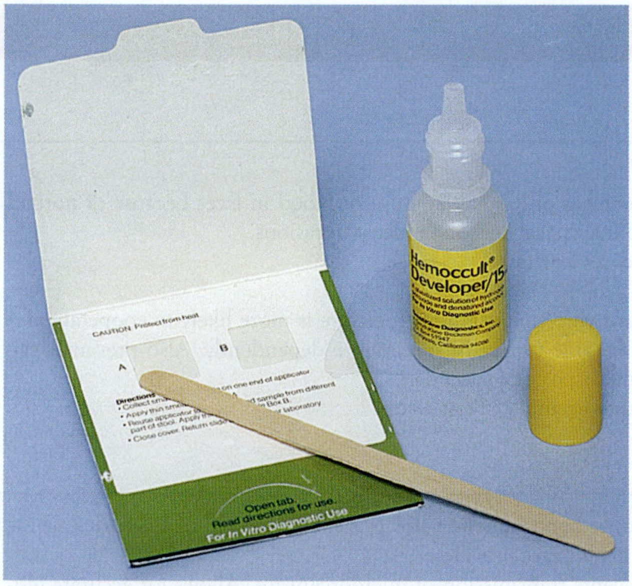

FIG 9.6 Hemoccult testing kit for measuring occult blood.

Hematest

- Hematest tablets (must be protected from moisture, heat, and light)
- Guaiac paper
- Clean container of tap water

STEP	RATIONALE
ASSESSMENT	
1. Identify patient using at least two person-specific identifiers (e.g., name and date of birth, or name and medical record number) according to employer policy. Compare identifiers with information on patient's medical record and laboratory requisition.	Ensures correct patient. Complies with Accreditation Canada standards and improves patient safety (Accreditation Canada, 2020).
2. Throughout the procedure, the 4 moments for hand hygiene are to be implemented; hand hygiene should occur before initial patient (or patient environment) contact, before an aseptic procedure, after body fluid exposure risk, and after patient (or patient environment) contact. Additional hand hygiene should be performed when hands are visibly soiled.	Proper hand hygiene helps prevent the spread of infectious agents to health care providers.
3. Assess patient's or caregiver's understanding of need for stool test.	Provides information on which to base necessary health teaching.
4. Assess patient's ability to cooperate with procedure and collect specimen.	To avoid embarrassment, patients often prefer to collect own stool specimen. Some patients require help.
5. Assess patient's medical history for GI disorders (e.g., history of bleeding, colitis, or hemorrhoids).	Routine screening may be initiated. Hemorrhoids can cause bleeding that may be misinterpreted as upper GI bleeding.
6. Review patient's medications for medications that contribute to GI bleeding.	Anticoagulants increase risk of bleeding in GI tract, even from minor trauma to mucosa. Long-term use of steroids, nonsteroidal anti-inflammatory medications (NSAIDs), and acetylsalicylic acid (Aspirin) can irritate mucosa and result in bleeding (MacDonald et al., 2024).
7. Refer to health care provider's prescriptions for medication or dietary modifications or restrictions before test.	Specimens will be positive if contaminated by menstrual blood, hemorrhoid blood, or povidone–iodine. Diets rich in meats, green leafy vegetables, poultry, and fish may produce false-positive results.

NURSING DIAGNOSES

- Anxiety
- Bowel incontinence
- Constipation
- Insufficient knowledge regarding collection and testing of stool specimen
- Diarrhea

Related factors are individualized on the basis of patient's condition or needs.

STEP	RATIONALE
PLANNING	
1. Expected outcomes following completion of procedure:	
• Test for occult blood is negative.	Patient has only small amount of blood in feces because of normal nasopharyngeal and oral mucosa abrasions.
• Patient discusses purpose and benefits of testing stool for blood.	Validates learning.
2. Explain procedure to patient and caregiver. Discuss reason for specimen collection and how patient can help. Explain that feces must be free of urine and toilet tissue.	Patient who understands procedure is more likely to cooperate and may be able to obtain specimen independently. Also prevents accidental disposal of specimen.
3. Arrange for any needed dietary or medication restrictions.	Ensures accuracy of test results.
IMPLEMENTATION	
1.	Proper hand hygiene helps prevent the spread of infectious agents to health care providers.
2. Apply clean gloves. Obtain uncontaminated stool specimen and place in clean, dry container not contaminated with urine, water, or toilet tissue.	Prevents transmission of microorganisms. Allows for accurate testing when specimen is not contaminated with other products.
3. Use tip of wooden or plastic applicator to obtain small part of feces for Hemoccult slide or fecal transportation container (to send to laboratory).	Small specimen is sufficient for measuring blood content.
4. Measure for occult blood.	
a. Perform Hemoccult slide test:	
(1) Open flap of Hemoccult slide. Apply thin smear of stool on paper in first box.	Guaiac paper inside box is sensitive to fecal blood content.
(2) Using same applicator, obtain second fecal specimen from different part of stool and apply thinly to second box of slide (see Step 4a[2] illustration).	Occult blood from upper GI tract is not always dispersed equally throughout stool. Findings of occult blood are more conclusive for GI bleeding when entire specimen is found to contain blood.
(3) Close slide cover and turn slide over to reverse side. Open cardboard flap and apply 2 drops of Hemoccult developing solution on each box of guaiac paper (see Step 4a[3] illustration).	Developing solution penetrates underlying fecal specimen. Change in colour of guaiac paper indicates presence of blood.

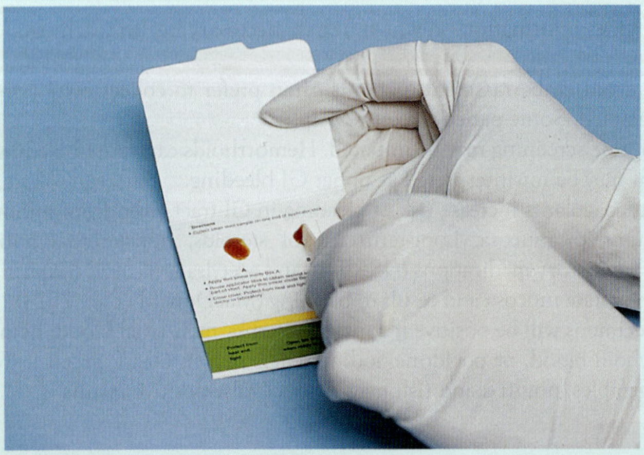

STEP 4A(2) Applying stool specimen to both spots on Hemoccult slide.

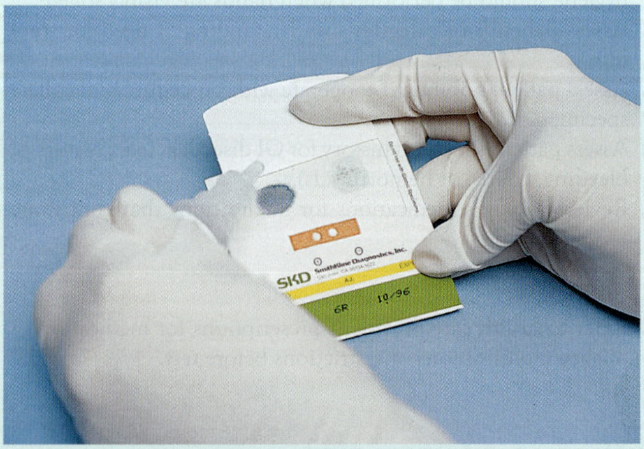

STEP 4A(3) Applying developing solution.

STEP	RATIONALE
(4) Read results of test after 30–60 seconds. Note colour changes.	Ensures correct results. Bluish discoloration indicates occult blood (guaiac positive). No change in colour of guaiac paper indicates negative results.
(5) Dispose of test slide in proper receptacle.	Reduces transfer of microorganisms.
b. Perform test using Hematest tablets:	Tablet contains solid form of developing solution.
(1) Place stool on guaiac paper. Then place Hematest tablet on top of stool specimen. Apply 2–3 drops of tap water to tablet, allowing water to flow onto guaiac paper.	Tap water dissolves Hematest tablet and thus dispenses developing solution over specimen and guaiac paper.

STEP	RATIONALE
(2) Observe colour of guaiac paper within 2 minutes.	Bluish discoloration is guaiac positive. Do not read colour after 2 minutes. False findings may occur.
(3) Dispose of tablet and paper in proper receptacle.	Reduces transfer of microorganisms.
5. Wrap wooden applicator in paper towel, grasp in nondominant hand, and remove gloves over wrapped applicator. Dispose of all equipment in appropriate receptacles.	Reduces transfer of microorganisms.

EVALUATION

1. Note colour changes in guaiac paper.	Reveals blood in feces.
2. **Use teach-back:** "You will need to check your stool two more times for blood when you go home. I want to be sure I explained the procedure correctly. Tell me the steps you will use to collect this specimen." Develop a revised teaching plan if patient or caregiver is unable to teach back correctly.	Determines level of understanding of instructional topic.

Critical Decision Point *A single positive test result does not confirm bleeding or indicate colorectal cancer. It could be caused by various medical conditions. To confirm positive results, the test must be repeated while the patient is on a meat-free, high-residue diet and with more in-depth diagnostic screening, such as colonoscopy* (Canadian Cancer Society, 2022).

3. Note character of stool specimen.	Certain abnormal constituents of stool may be visible.

Unexpected Outcomes	Related Interventions
1. Test for occult blood is positive.	• Continue to monitor patient. • Notify health care provider.

Communication and Documentation

- Document results of test and include stool characteristics in progress notes in EHR or chart.
- Document your evaluation of patient and caregiver learning.
- Report positive test results to health care provider.

DOCUMENTATION EXAMPLE

80-year-old patient (he/him) came to emergency department with history of black stool, dizziness, fatigue. Occult blood test was prescribed to rule out gastrointestinal bleed. Black loose stool was collected and sent to lab at 2100 hours. Advised the patient to report any dark stool, and taught patient importance of slowly getting up from toilet to avoid dizziness.

Special Considerations

Pediatric

- Children who are school age and older are concrete thinkers, are often very curious, and may ask many questions about the test. Answer questions honestly and at the child's level of understanding.
- Allow child to watch, if desired, while performing test (Hockenberry et al., 2024).
- Testing reagent is often poisonous; thus, keep out of reach of small children.

Gerontological

- Older persons may require assistance with positioning themselves to obtain specimen.
- In confused patients, it may be necessary for the caregiver to help the patient collect and test the specimen for blood (Boscart et al., 2023).

Persons With Cognitive or Physical Challenges

- Collecting a stool specimen may elicit different reactions for a person with a cognitive challenge. The caregiver may be a valuable resource in obtaining this specimen.

Care in the Community: Home Management

- Many patients or caregivers are instructed to collect specimens at home and return them to the health care provider's office immediately after collection. Be sure they know infection control principles. Be sure they are aware of diet and medication restrictions before and after the stool collection period.

SKILL 9.3 Measuring Occult Blood in Gastric Secretions (Gastroccult)

Video Clip NSO Nursing Skills Online Specimen Collection Module 3 / Lesson 3

Analysis of gastric secretions or emesis can detect blood that is not always visible. Gastroccult testing helps to reveal bleeding in the esophagus or stomach. The test can verify the presence of blood when gastric contents are red or black or when gastric contents (or vomitus) have the appearance of coffee grounds. The test measures microscopic amounts of blood in the gastric secretions. Gastric aspirate obtained by either nasogastric (NG) tube, nasoenteral (NE) tube, or emesis is an appropriate sample for use with this test. It is a useful diagnostic tool for conditions such as upper GI ulcers or bleeding. Because the test is easy to perform, patients are often taught how to test emesis in the home.

Delegation and Collaboration

The skill of Gastroccult testing can be delegated to a UCP for testing vomitus specimen. You cannot delegate the skill of Gastroccult testing to a UCP if the specimen is collected from an NG or NE tube. The nurse informs the UCP to do the following:

- Report immediately if blood or coffee-ground vomitus is visible in NG or NE tube secretions
- Save specimen for repeat testing

Equipment

- Facial tissues
- Emesis basin
- Wooden applicator or 3-mL syringe
- Catheter tip syringe
- Cardboard Gastroccult test slide
- Gastroccult developing solution
- Clean gloves

STEP	RATIONALE
ASSESSMENT	
1. Identify patient using at least two person-specific identifiers (e.g., name and date of birth, or name and medical record number) according to employer policy. Compare identifiers with information on patient's medical record and laboratory requisition.	Ensures correct patient. Complies with Accreditation Canada standards and improves patient safety (Accreditation Canada, 2020).
2. Throughout the procedure, the 4 moments for hand hygiene are to be implemented; hand hygiene should occur before initial patient (or patient environment) contact, before an aseptic procedure, after body fluid exposure risk, and after patient (or patient environment) contact. Additional hand hygiene should be performed when hands are visibly soiled.	Proper hand hygiene helps prevent the spread of infectious agents to health care providers.
3. Assess patient's or caregiver's understanding of need for test.	Provides information on which to base necessary health teaching.
4. Assess patient's medical history for bleeding or GI disorders.	Routine screening may be initiated.
5. Assess patient's medical history for GI disorders (e.g., history of bleeding, colitis).	Anticoagulants increase risk of bleeding in GI tract, even from minor trauma to mucosa. Long-term use of steroids, NSAIDs, and acetylsalicylic acid (Aspirin) can irritate mucosa.

NURSING DIAGNOSES

- Anxiety
- Insufficient knowledge regarding occult blood testing
- Fear

Related factors are individualized on the basis of patient's condition or needs.

STEP	RATIONALE
PLANNING	
1. Expected outcomes following completion of procedure:	
• Test for occult blood is negative.	Patient has no blood or only small amount of blood in gastric secretions.
• Patient discusses purpose and benefits of testing gastric contents for blood.	Validates learning.
2. Explain procedure to patient and caregiver. Discuss why specimen collection is necessary.	Patient who understands procedure is more likely to be less anxious and more cooperative.
IMPLEMENTATION	
1.	Proper hand hygiene helps prevent the spread of infectious agents to health care providers.
2. Apply clean gloves. Verify NG tube placement (see Chapter 32).	Ensures aspiration of gastric contents.

STEP	RATIONALE

IMPLEMENTATION

STEP	RATIONALE
3. Obtain specimen by disconnecting suction or gravity drainage tube from NG or NE tube. Using a syringe, aspirate 0.5–5 mL of fluid from NG or NE tube.	Only a small amount of specimen is needed. In pediatric settings, even smaller amounts would be required.

Critical Decision Point *Observe specimen. If you find red blood or coffee-ground material, report these findings immediately to health care provider.*

STEP	RATIONALE
4. To obtain sample of vomitus, use 3-mL syringe or wooden applicator to obtain sample from emesis basin.	A small specimen is sufficient for measuring blood content.
5. Perform Gastroccult test:	
a. Using wooden applicator or syringe, apply 1 drop of gastric sample to Gastroccult blood test slide.	Sample must cover test paper for test reaction to occur.
b. Apply 2 drops of commercial developer solution over sample and 1 drop between positive and negative performance monitors (see Step 5b illustration).	

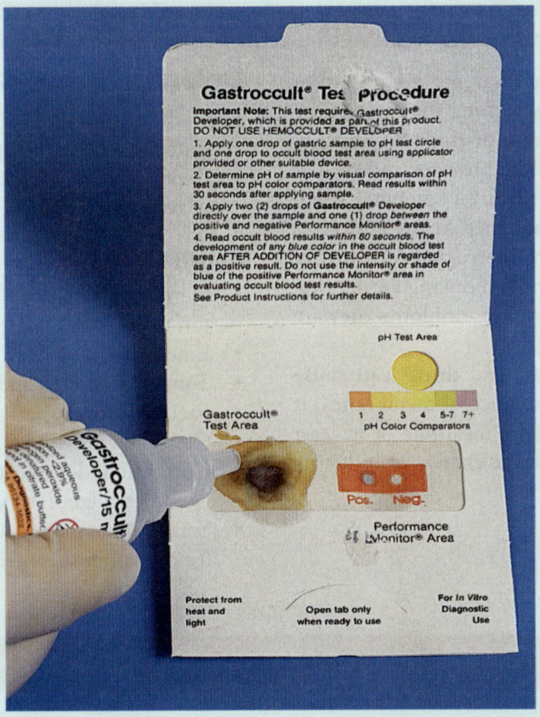

STEP 5B Applying developing solution to Gastroccult test area.

STEP	RATIONALE
c. Verify that performance monitor turns blue in 30 seconds.	Indicates proper function of testing paper.
d. After 60 seconds, compare colour of gastric sample with that of performance monitor.	If sample turns blue, test is positive for occult blood. If sample turns green, sample is negative for occult blood.
e. Dispose of test slide, wooden applicator, and syringe in proper receptacle. If needed, reconnect NG or NE tube to drainage system or suction. Remove gloves.	Reduces transmission of microorganisms.

EVALUATION

STEP	RATIONALE
1. Note character of gastric secretions.	Blood may be visible, or coffee-ground material denoting blood may be observed.
2. Note colour changes on Gastroccult blood test slide.	Reveals blood in gastric secretions.
3. **Use teach-back:** "I want to make sure you know the purpose of the procedure and understand it. Can you tell me what we will need to do to obtain a gastric specimen from your vomitus (or NG/NE tube)?" Develop a revised teaching plan if patient or caregiver is unable to teach back correctly.	Determines level of understanding of instructional topic. Generally, patients only self-test vomitus in the home environment, and not via NG or NE tube.

Unexpected Outcomes	Related Interventions
1. Test for occult blood is positive.	• Continue to monitor patient. • Notify health care provider.

Communication and Documentation

- Document results of test and presence of any unusual characteristics of gastric contents in progress notes in EHR or chart.
- Document your evaluation of patient and caregiver learning.
- Report positive test results to health care provider.

DOCUMENTATION EXAMPLE

Coffee-ground secretion noted in the patient's NG tube; collected sample per employer policy. Performed Gastroccult blood test, test result showed blue. Reported result to health care provider. Informed patient and family to report if patient presents with any lightheadedness, dizziness, stomach pain, or decreased level of consciousness.

Special Considerations

Pediatric

- Children who are school age and older are concrete thinkers, are often very curious, and may ask many questions about the test. Answer questions honestly and at the child's level of understanding. Allow the child to watch, if desired, while test is performed (Hockenberry et al., 2024).

Care in the Community: Home Management

- Many patients or caregivers can perform the Gastroccult test on vomitus. Be sure they know infection control principles.

✦ SKILL 9.4 Collecting Nose and Throat Specimens for Culture

When patients have signs and symptoms of an upper respiratory or sinus infection, and for the purposes of screening for methicillin-resistant *Staphylococcus aureus* (MRSA), a nose or throat culture, or both, is a simple diagnostic tool to identify the presence and type of microorganisms. Other sites may be prescribed for sampling when screening for MRSA. Cultures should be obtained before antibiotic therapy is initiated because antibiotics may interrupt the growth of the organisms in the laboratory. If a patient is receiving antibiotics, notify the laboratory and identify which specific antibiotics they are receiving (MacDonald et al., 2024).

Collection of a specimen from the nose and throat can cause discomfort and gagging because of sensitive mucosal membranes. It is important to collect a throat culture before mealtime or at least 1 hour after eating or drinking to decrease the chance of inducing vomiting.

Delegation and Collaboration

The skill of obtaining specimens from the nose and throat cannot be delegated to a UCP. The nurse informs the UCP to do the following:

- Report shortness of breath, difficulty breathing, and other signs of respiratory distress

Equipment

- Sterile swab(s) in culture transport tube(s) (flexible swab with cotton tip may be used for nasopharyngeal cultures)
- Emesis basin or clean container *(optional)*
- Tongue depressor and penlight
- Facial tissues
- Clean gloves
- Completed identification labels with proper patient identifiers
- Completed laboratory requisition
- Small biohazard plastic bag for delivery of specimen to laboratory (or container specified by employer)

STEP	RATIONALE
ASSESSMENT	
1. Identify patient using at least two person-specific identifiers (e.g., name and date of birth, or name and medical record number) according to employer policy. Compare identifiers with information on patient's medical record and laboratory requisition.	Ensures correct patient. Complies with Accreditation Canada standards and improves patient safety (Accreditation Canada, 2020).
2. Throughout the procedure, the 4 moments for hand hygiene are to be implemented; hand hygiene should occur before initial patient (or patient environment) contact, before an aseptic procedure, after body fluid exposure risk, and after patient (or patient environment) contact. Additional hand hygiene should be performed when hands are visibly soiled.	Proper hand hygiene helps prevent the spread of infectious agents to health care providers.
3. Assess patient's understanding of purpose of procedure and ability to cooperate. You may need help obtaining throat cultures from confused, combative, or unconscious patients.	Provides information on which to base health teaching and assistance. Assistance may be required to ensure nurse safety when obtaining throat cultures from confused or combative patients and patient safety when obtaining a culture from an unconscious patient.
4. Inspect condition of nares and drainage from nasal mucosa and sinuses.	Reveals signs that indicate infection or allergic irritation. Clear drainage usually indicates allergy. Yellow, green, or brown drainage usually indicates infection.

STEP	RATIONALE

ASSESSMENT

STEP	RATIONALE
5. Ask if patient is experiencing postnasal drip, sinus headache or tenderness, nasal congestion, sore throat, or exposure to others with similar symptoms.	Symptoms help reveal nature of problem.
6. Apply clean gloves. Assess condition of posterior pharynx.	Reveals local inflammation or lesions of pharynx.
7. Assess patient for signs of infection, including fever, chills, and/or fatigue.	Infection originating within nasopharynx can become systemic, requiring antibiotic therapy.
8. Review health care provider's prescriptions to determine whether nose, throat, or both cultures are needed.	Prevents exposing patient to unnecessary discomfort of repeated cultures.

NURSING DIAGNOSES

- Acute pain
- Persistent pain
- Insufficient knowledge regarding specimen collection
- Potential for infection

Related factors and risk factors are individualized on the basis of patient's condition or needs.

PLANNING

STEP	RATIONALE
1. Expected outcomes following completion of procedure:	
• There is no bacterial growth in specimens.	Absence of bacterial infection.
• Patient does not experience bleeding of nasal mucosa.	Procedure is atraumatic.
• Specimen is not contaminated.	Evidenced by results of laboratory analysis.
• Patient discusses purpose of nose and throat cultures.	Validates learning.
2. Plan to do culture before mealtime or at least 1 hour after eating.	Procedure often induces gagging; timing decreases patient's chances of vomiting.
3. Explain procedure to patient and caregiver. Discuss reason for specimen collection and how patient can help.	Understanding procedure usually decreases anxiety and promotes cooperation.
4. Explain that patient may have tickling sensation or gagging during swabbing of throat. Nasal swab may create urge to sneeze. Each procedure only takes a few seconds to complete.	Helps patient relax.

IMPLEMENTATION

STEP	RATIONALE
1. Ask patient to sit erect in bed or chair facing you. An acutely ill patient or young child may lie back against bed with head of bed raised to 45-degree angle in semi-Fowler's position. Loosen cap and have swab in tube ready for use.	Provides easy access to nasal or oral structures. Allows nurse to grasp swab easily without danger of contamination. Most commercial tubes have tops that fit securely over end of swab. Allows touching of outer tops without contaminating swab stick.
2.	Proper hand hygiene helps prevent the spread of infectious agents to health care providers.
3. Collect throat culture:	
a. Apply required PPE (see Chapter 5, Box 5.1) (e.g., gloves, a medical mask, a gown, and/or eye protection) (PHAC, 2021b).	For possible, suspected, or confirmed exposure to COVID-19, PPE should be consistent with a minimum of droplet and contact precautions. Reduces transmission of microorganisms.
b. Instruct patient to tilt head backward. For patients in bed, place pillow behind shoulders.	Facilitates visualization of pharynx.
c. Ask patient to open mouth and say "ah." If necessary to visualize pharynx, use penlight and depress tongue with tongue depressor and note inflamed areas of pharynx or tonsils. Depress anterior third of tongue only.	Permits exposure of pharynx, relaxes throat muscles, and minimizes gag reflex. Area to be swabbed should be visualized clearly.

Critical Decision Point *Do not attempt throat culture in a pediatric patient if you suspect acute epiglottitis because trauma from swab might cause increase in edema, resulting in occlusion of airway* (Hockenberry et al., 2024).

STEP	RATIONALE
d. Insert swab without touching lips, teeth, tongue, cheeks, or uvula toward posterior pharynx.	Prevents contamination with organisms from oral cavity (MacDonald et al., 2024).

STEP	RATIONALE
e. Gently but quickly swab posterior pharynx, tonsils, and inflamed areas (see Step 3e illustration).	These areas contain the most microorganisms.
f. Carefully withdraw swab without touching oral structures.	Collects microorganisms from throat tissues without contamination from mouth and tongue.

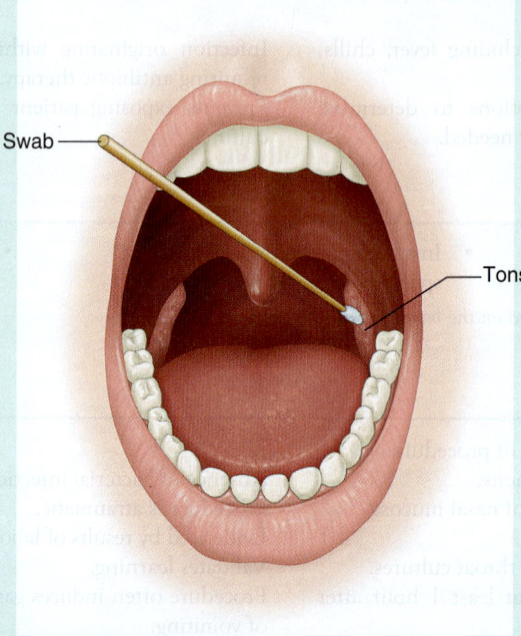

STEP 3E Collecting specimen from posterior pharynx.

STEP	RATIONALE
4. Collect nasal culture:	
a. Apply required PPE as required (see Chapter 5, Box 5.1).	For possible, suspected, or confirmed exposure to COVID-19, PPE should be consistent with a minimum of droplet and contact precautions. Reduces transmission of microorganisms.
b. Encourage patient to blow nose, then check patient's nostrils for patency with penlight. Select nostril with greatest patency. For MRSA, ensure both nostrils are clear.	Clears nasal passages of mucus containing resident bacteria.
c. With patient in sitting position, have patient tilt head backward. Patients in bed should have a small pillow behind shoulders.	Provides access to nasal passages and facilitates visualization of nasal septum and sinuses.
d. Carefully pass swab approximately 2–2.5 cm (0.8–1 inch) into nostril. Rotate swab against the nasal mucosa gently and keep it there for 20–30 seconds (Cadham Provincial Laboratory, 2020). **Note:** If you need to obtain *nasopharyngeal culture*, use special swab that can be flexed downward to reach nasopharynx.	Swab should remain sterile until it reaches area to be cultured. Rotating swab covers all surfaces where exudate is present.
e. Remove swab without touching sides of nasal canal. If screening for MRSA, both left and right nostrils should be sampled with the same swab.	Prevents contamination of swab by resident bacteria.
f. Offer patient facial tissue and/or wash cloth.	Minimizes period of time that patient experiences discomfort.
5. Carefully insert swab into culture transport tube and recap tube securely. If using specific type of culture kit, crush the culture transport tube with fingers at the appropriate area and make sure the specimen is in contact with the medium (see Step 5 illustrations).	Placing swab within culture transport tube maintains life of bacteria for testing. Crushing tube releases culture medium.

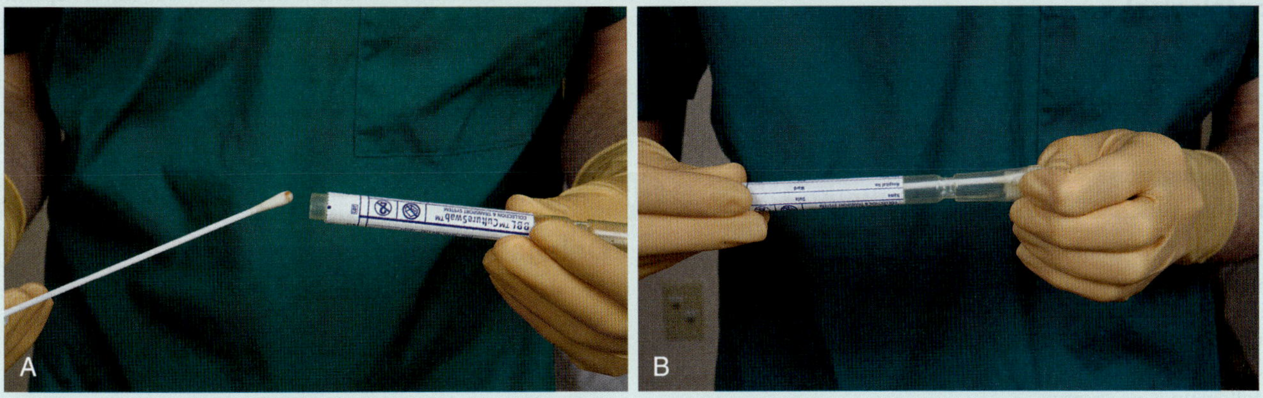

STEP 5 Activating culture tube. A, Place swab into tube. B, Crush tube to release liquid medium.

STEP	RATIONALE
6. Attach completed identification label to culture transport tube and confirm identifiers, specimen source, and collection date and time in front of patient (see employer policy). Note on laboratory requisition if patient is taking antibiotic or if specific organism is suspected (e.g., *Bordetella pertussis*).	Incorrect identification of specimen could result in diagnostic or therapeutic errors.
7. Enclose specimen in biohazard bag and send immediately to laboratory. Remove and dispose of gloves.	Specimen not sent to laboratory immediately or refrigerated allows growth of organisms and inaccurate results.
8. Ensure patient is comfortable.	Provides for patient's comfort.

EVALUATION

1. Check laboratory record for results.	Results reveal type of organisms in nose or pharynx and antibiotics most likely to be effective.
2. **Use teach-back:** "I want to be sure I explained the purpose and procedure for obtaining a throat culture. Please tell me why we are obtaining this culture." Develop a revised teaching plan if patient or caregiver is unable to teach back correctly.	Determines level of understanding of instructional topic.

Unexpected Outcomes	Related Interventions
1. Nose and throat cultures reveal bacterial growth.	• Notify health care provider of findings. • Administer medications as prescribed.
2. Patient experiences minor nasal bleeding.	• Apply mild pressure and ice pack over bridge of nose. • Notify health care provider of patient's condition.
3. Specimen is contaminated.	• Repeat specimen collection.

Communication and Documentation

- Document appearance of nasal and oral mucosal structure and specimen collection, date, time, and disposition in progress notes in EHR or chart.
- Document your evaluation of patient and caregiver learning.
- Report unusual test results to health care provider.

DOCUMENTATION EXAMPLE

67-year-old patient (she/her) admitted to medical unit with congestive heart failure. As part of routine screening, MRSA screening test performed. Explained the purpose and procedure of the test to patient. Observed nasal mucosa is pink, moist, no discharge noted, no septal deviation. Obtained a swab from both nostrils at 1500 hours, and sent to lab at 1530 hours. Patient tolerated procedure well.

Special Considerations

Teaching

- Teach patient that procedure may cause slight discomfort and that gagging is common.
- Discuss reason for time delay in receiving culture results.

Pediatric

- Allow young children to visualize and examine the speculum to help decrease their fear.
- Immobilization of child's head and arms are important when obtaining specimen. You should do this in a firm, gentle, kind manner. Ask another nurse to help if necessary.
- Ask parents to act as coach and suggest that they hold their child on their lap. Do not ask parents to restrain child (Hockenberry et al., 2024).
- Showing tongue depressor and penlight to child and demonstrating how to say "ah" helps to decrease anxiety.

- School-age children will be more cooperative if given opportunity to ask questions about procedure and results.

Gerontological

- Some older persons need help in keeping their mouths open to obtain specimens.
- Some older persons have poor dentition. Take care not to break a tooth, and consider removal of dentures.

Patients With Physical or Cognitive Challenges

- A patient who has intellectual or cognitive challenges may perceive the act of obtaining a nose or throat culture specimen as a threat. Explain the procedure in short and simple sentences. Observe patient for warning signs of increased agitation or combativeness. If these occur, stop the procedure and give the patient time to calm down (Mendes, 2018).

✦ SKILL 9.5 Obtaining Vaginal or Urethral Discharge Specimens

Normally, drainage from the vagina or urethra is thin, nonpurulent, whitish or clear, and small in amount. Factors such as poor hygiene practices can cause an accumulation of discharge. If a patient develops an increased amount of discharge or if there is a change in the character of discharge from the vagina or urethra, health care provider follow-up is necessary.

Patients most commonly requiring cultures of vaginal or urethral discharge have signs and symptoms of a sexually transmitted infection (STI) or urinary tract infection (UTI). Patients suspected of having an STI may be embarrassed by their condition. Show respect and understanding toward the patient. When collecting vaginal or urethral specimens, work quickly and calmly, practising person-centred care to maintain the patient's privacy at all times.

Delegation and Collaboration

The skill of obtaining vaginal or urethral discharge specimens cannot be delegated to a UCP.

Equipment

- Sterile swab in sterile culture tube (commercially available culture tubes have swab and tube with ampule containing special transport medium)
- Sheet, blanket, or paper drape
- Clean gloves
- Penlight or gooseneck lamp
- Completed identification labels with proper patient identifiers
- Completed laboratory requisition
- Small biohazard plastic bag for delivery of specimen to laboratory (or container specified by employer)

STEP	RATIONALE
ASSESSMENT	
1. Identify patient using at least two person-specific identifiers (e.g., name and date of birth, or name and medical record number) according to employer policy. Compare identifiers with information on patient's medical record and laboratory requisition.	Ensures correct patient. Complies with Accreditation Canada standards and improves patient safety (Accreditation Canada, 2020).
2. Throughout the procedure, the 4 moments for hand hygiene are to be implemented; hand hygiene should occur before initial patient (or patient environment) contact, before an aseptic procedure, after body fluid exposure risk, and after patient (or patient environment) contact. Additional hand hygiene should be performed when hands are visibly soiled.	Proper hand hygiene helps prevent the spread of infectious agents to health care providers.
3. Assess patient's understanding of need for specimen collection and ability to cooperate with procedure.	Provides information on which to base necessary health teaching.
4. Apply clean gloves. Assess condition of external genitalia and urethra, meatus, and vaginal orifice. Observe for redness; swelling; verbalization of tenderness; and discharge that is whitish, mucoid, or purulent or a whitish discharge such as cottage cheese. Remove and discard gloves. NOTE: This step may be done during collection.	Reduces transmission of microorganisms. Assessment findings and specimen test results reveal nature of problem.
5. Ask patient about dysuria, localized pruritus of genitalia, or lower abdominal pain.	Symptoms of urinary tract or vaginal infection.
6. If symptoms suggest STI, gather and record patient's sexual history.	Determines sexual activity and whether there has been sexual contact with a person known to have an STI. If culture results are positive, inform patient of need to receive treatment, have sexual partners evaluated if applicable, and refrain from sexual activity during treatment (MacDonald et al., 2024).
7. Refer to health care provider's prescription to determine whether culture is to be vaginal or urethral.	Patient may require one or both types of cultures.

STEP	RATIONALE

NURSING DIAGNOSES

- Acute pain
- Anxiety
- Insufficient knowledge regarding specimen collection
- Potential for infection

Related factors and risk factors are individualized on the basis of patient's condition or needs.

PLANNING

STEP	RATIONALE
1. Expected outcomes following completion of procedure:	
• Specimen is not contaminated.	Results will reveal whether skin cells or mucosal cells have contaminated specimen.
• Vaginal or urethral cultures do not reveal growth of microorganisms.	Evidence of absence of infection.
2. Explain procedure to patient, caregiver, or both. Discuss reason for specimen collection and how patient can help.	Patients who understand procedure are less anxious and more likely to cooperate.
• Instruct patient with female genitalia not to douche 24 hours before culture is obtained.	Douching of vaginal canal would remove discharge-containing pathogens.
• Instruct patient with male genitalia not to urinate 1 hour before urethral culture is obtained.	Urinating by patient with male genitalia washes secretions out of urethra (MacDonald et al., 2024).

IMPLEMENTATION

STEP	RATIONALE
1.	Proper hand hygiene helps prevent the spread of infectious agents to health care providers.
2. Apply clean gloves.	
3. Draw bedside curtains or close room door. Place "Do Not Enter" sign on door (if available).	Provides privacy and demonstrates respect as part of person-centred nursing care.
4. Help patient to proper position, raise gown, and drape body parts to be exposed:	Provides easy access to perineal area. Draping minimizes exposure of body parts, reducing anxiety.
a. *Patient with female genitalia:* Dorsal recumbent position with sheet draped over each leg and genitalia.	
b. *Patient with male genitalia:* Sitting on chair or bed or lying supine with sheet draped across lower trunk and genitalia.	
5. Direct light source onto perineum (may not be needed for patient with male genitalia).	Allows better visualization of external urethral or vaginal structures.
6. Open culture tube and hold swab in dominant hand.	Provides for easier manipulation of swab during culture collection.
7. Instruct patient to breathe slowly and deeply.	Helps patient relax. Tensing of muscles around pelvic floor may cause discomfort during swabbing.
8. Obtain specimens.	
a. *Patient with female genitalia:*	
(1) With nondominant hand, fully separate labia to expose vaginal orifice.	Exposes perineum and ensures that specimen is of vaginal discharge.
(2) Touch tip of swab into discharge pool, being careful not to touch skin or mucosa along perineum or vaginal canal. If no discharge is visible, gently insert swab 1–2.5 cm (0.33–1 inch) into vaginal orifice and rotate before removal.	Discharge contains greatest concentration of microorganisms.
(3) To expose urethral meatus, use nondominant hand to pull gently on labia minora upward and back to separate.	Allows better visualization of urethral orifice.
(4) Use swab; gently apply to tip of meatus where discharge is visible. Avoid touching labia.	Discharge contains greatest concentration of microorganisms.

Critical Decision Point *If discharge near vagina appears different from discharge along perineum, collect separate specimens from each area because, if two organisms are present, they could be cross-contaminated on a single swab. Label specimen with area of patient's body that you swabbed.*

STEP	RATIONALE
b. *Patient with male genitalia:*	
(1) Grasp patient's penis proximal to glans with nondominant hand; if patient is uncircumcised, gently retract foreskin.	Provides clear exposure of urethral meatus.

STEP	RATIONALE
(2) Use dominant hand to hold swab. Apply gently to area of discharge at urinary meatus.	Discharge contains greatest number of microorganisms.
(3) If no discharge is apparent, health care provider may prescribe swab to be introduced into urinary meatus. Hold male genitalia firmly but gently.	Excess manipulation can cause erection.
(4) Return foreskin to natural position.	Tightening of foreskin around shaft of penis can cause localized discomfort, edema, and potential necrosis.
9. Return each swab to culture tube and secure top.	Retains microorganisms within tube.
10. If using commercial culture tube, wrap ampule with gauze to prevent injury to your fingers while crushing. Immediately squeeze end of tube to crush ampule (see Skill 9.4). Push tip of swab into fluid medium.	Medium supports life of microorganisms until culture is analyzed.
11. Remove and discard gloves.	Reduces transmission of microorganisms.
12. Label each culture tube with identification label, affix completed requisition, and confirm identifiers in front of patient (Accreditation Canada, 2020).	Incorrect specimen identification could lead to diagnostic or therapeutic error.
13. Send specimen to laboratory immediately or refrigerate.	Bacteria multiply quickly. Prompt analysis ensures accurate results.
14. Help patient to comfortable position, help with personal hygiene, and remove and discard drape.	Reinforces patient's sense of self-esteem. Reduces transmission of microorganisms.

EVALUATION

1. Review laboratory results for evidence of pathogens.	Results will reveal type of organisms present. Certain organisms are common to vaginal tract. Urethra should be free of microorganisms.
2. Continue to monitor whether discharge is present; if so, observe colour and amount.	Characteristics of discharge indicate specific type of infection.
3. **Use teach-back:** "I want to be sure I explained the purpose and procedure for obtaining this culture. Please tell me the steps of this procedure." Develop a plan for revised patient or caregiver teaching if they are unable to repeat back correctly.	Determines level of understanding of instructional topic.

Unexpected Outcomes	Related Interventions
1. Vaginal or urethral cultures reveal growth of pathogenic microorganisms.	• Notify health care provider of findings and follow new prescriptions. • Continue to monitor patient.
2. Specimen is contaminated with feces or epidermal cells.	• Repeat specimen collection.

Communication and Documentation

- Document types of cultures obtained and date and time sent to laboratory in progress notes in EHR or chart.
- Document your evaluation of patient and caregiver learning.
- Report laboratory results to health care provider.

DOCUMENTATION EXAMPLE

32-year-old patient (she/her) came to the emergency department with symptoms of lower abdominal pain, dysuria, white vaginal discharge, and T 38.9°C orally. Vaginal swab for C&S sample was collected and sent to lab at 1600 hours.

Special Considerations

Teaching

- Discuss sexuality and safer sex practices with patient if appropriate.
- Patients with urethral or vaginal discharge often require instruction about perineal hygiene measures.
- Teach patient proper administration route of prescribed medication (e.g., suppositories, topical) (see Chapter 21).

Pediatric

- A second nurse can help with specimen collection from an infant or young child by gently holding child's legs apart in froglike position. Have parent present to encourage cooperation.
- Ensure parents understand that obtaining a vaginal specimen will not affect virginity of the child.

Patients With Physical or Cognitive Challenges

- Collecting vaginal or urethral culture may elicit different reactions for a person with a cognitive challenge. It may be helpful to have the caregiver assist. Explain procedure in short, clear sentences; carefully consider the needs of the individual; and provide care in a sensitive and respectful manner (Sullivan et al., 2018).
- When a patient has physical challenges, an assistant may be needed to position patient to obtain a culture.

Procedural Guideline 9.3 *Collecting a Sputum Specimen by Expectoration*

Sputum is mucus produced by cells of the lungs, bronchi, and trachea. A specimen is collected either by having a patient cough and expectorate into a sterile specimen container or by suctioning into a sterile sputum trap (see Skill 9.6). In a healthy patient, sputum production is minimal; a disease state can increase the amount and character of sputum. Sputum specimens are collected to identify cancer cells, for C&S, and for acid-fast bacillus (AFB) to diagnose pulmonary tuberculosis. Based on patient's presenting signs and symptoms (e.g., communicable disease) and indications, appropriate PPE may be required for performing the procedure (Shared Health, 2022).

Delegation and Collaboration

The skill of collecting a sputum specimen by expectoration can be delegated to a UCP. The nurse instructs the UCP to do the following:

- Immediately report the presence of blood in the sputum or changes in patient's vital signs

Equipment

- Appropriate PPE based on the patient's condition; transmission-based precautions will be required when caring for patient who has a transmissible disease
- Completed identification labels with appropriate patient identifiers
- Completed laboratory requisition
- Small biohazard plastic bag for delivery of specimen to laboratory (or container as specified by employer)
- Sterile specimen container (screw-capped)
- Clean gloves
- Facial tissues
- Emesis basin *(optional)*
- Toothbrush *(optional)*
- Disinfectant swab *(optional)*

Procedural Steps

1. Identify patient using at least two person-specific identifiers (e.g., name and date of birth, or name and medical record number) according to employer policy. Compare identifiers with information on medical record and laboratory requisition (Accreditation Canada, 2020).
2. Throughout the procedure, the 4 moments for hand hygiene are to be implemented; hand hygiene should occur before initial patient (or patient environment) contact, before an aseptic procedure, after body fluid exposure risk, and after patient (or patient environment) contact. Additional hand hygiene should be performed when hands are visibly soiled.
3. Provide opportunity to rinse mouth with water. Patient should not use mouthwash or toothpaste because the products may alter culture results.
4. Apply clean gloves. Provide sputum cup and instruct patient not to touch the inside of the container.
5. Have the patient take 3 or 4 deep, slow breaths with full exhalation. Then have patient take full inhalation followed immediately by a forceful cough, expectorating sputum directly into specimen container.
6. Repeat until 5–10 mL of sputum (not saliva) has been collected. A minimum of 3 mL must be collected.
7. Secure lid on container tightly. If any sputum is present on outside of container, wipe it off with disinfectant.
8. Offer patient tissues after patient expectorates. Then dispose of tissues and offer mouth care.
9. Remove and dispose of gloves.
10. Securely attach properly completed identification label and laboratory requisition to side of specimen container (not lid). Confirm identifiers in patient's presence.
11. Enclose specimen in a biohazard bag.
12. Send specimen to laboratory immediately.

✦ SKILL 9.6 Collecting a Sputum Specimen by Suction

Video Clip NSO Nursing Skills Online

Sputum is produced by cells lining the respiratory tract. Although production is minimal in the healthy state, disease states can increase the amount or change the character of sputum. Examination of sputum aids in the diagnosis and treatment of several conditions, ranging from simple bronchitis to lung cancer.

Suctioning is often indicated to collect sputum from patients unable to spontaneously expectorate a sample for laboratory analysis. Sometimes suctioning provokes violent coughing, which can induce vomiting and constriction of pharyngeal, laryngeal, and bronchial muscles. In addition, it may cause hypoxemia or vagal overload, causing cardiopulmonary compromise and increased intracranial pressure.

Delegation and Collaboration

The skill of collecting sputum specimens by suction cannot be delegated to a UCP. The nurse instructs the UCP to do the following:

- Notify the nurse if the patient expectorates bloody sputum

Equipment

- Completed identification labels with proper patient identifiers
- Completed laboratory requisition
- Suction device (wall or portable)
- Sterile suction catheter (size 14, 16, or 18 French [Fr] or suction catheter with sleeve [see Chapter 23])
- Sterile gloves and clean gloves
- Sterile water
- In-line specimen container or sputum trap
- Small plastic bag (or a container)
- Oxygen therapy equipment (if indicated)
- Protective eyewear
- Disinfectant wipe

STEP	RATIONALE
ASSESSMENT	
1. Identify patient using at least two person-specific identifiers (e.g., name and date of birth, or name and medical record number) according to employer policy. Compare identifiers with information on patient's medical record and laboratory requisition.	Ensures correct patient. Complies with Accreditation Canada standards and improves patient safety (Accreditation Canada, 2020).
2. Throughout the procedure, the 4 moments for hand hygiene are to be implemented; hand hygiene should occur before initial patient (or patient environment) contact, before an aseptic procedure, after body fluid exposure risk, and after patient (or patient environment) contact. Additional hand hygiene should be performed when hands are visibly soiled.	Proper hand hygiene helps prevent the spread of infectious agents to health care providers.
3. Check health care provider's prescriptions for type of sputum analysis and specifications (e.g., amount of sputum, number of specimens, time of collection, method to obtain). Specimens for AFB require three consecutive morning samples.	Specific test dictates when or how frequently specimens are collected. The ideal time to collect sputum is early morning, before the patient eats, drinks, smokes, brushes teeth, or uses mouthwash, because bronchial secretions tend to accumulate during the night. Bacteria also accumulate as secretions pool.
4. Assess patient's level of understanding of procedure and its purpose.	Provides baseline to establish teaching plan.
5. Assess when patient last ate a meal (or had tube feeding).	It is best to obtain specimen 1–2 hours after or 1 hour before meal to minimize gagging, which can cause vomiting and aspiration.
6. Determine whether patient needs help to obtain specimen.	Positioning, postural drainage, and deep breathing and coughing exercises may improve ability to cough productively. Suctioning is often indicated when patient is unable to cough and expectorate.
7. Assess patient's respiratory status, vital signs, blood pressure, and pulse oximetry.	These data serve as a preprocedural baseline. Active coughing may alter respiratory status. Respiratory status can depend on amount of sputum in tracheobronchial tree.

NURSING DIAGNOSES

- Inadequate airway clearance
- Inadequate breathing pattern
- Insufficient knowledge regarding specimen collection procedures
- Potential for aspiration
- Potential for infection

Related factors and risk factors are individualized on the basis of patient's condition or needs.

STEP	RATIONALE
PLANNING	
1. Expected outcomes following completion of procedure:	
• Patient's respirations are same rate and character before and after procedure.	Specimen collection did not alter respiratory status.
• Patient maintains comfort level and experiences minimal anxiety.	Suctioning tends to cause anxiety.
• Sputum is not contaminated by saliva or oropharyngeal flora.	Sputum must originate from tracheobronchial tree for accurate results.
• Patient discusses purpose and benefit of sputum collection.	Validates learning.
2. Explain procedure and purpose. Instruct patient to breathe normally during suctioning to prevent hyperventilation.	Promotes understanding and cooperation.
IMPLEMENTATION	
1.	Proper hand hygiene helps prevent the spread of infectious agents to health care providers.
2. Apply clean glove to nondominant hand. Prepare suction machine or device and determine whether it functions properly. When performing open deep suctioning via endotracheal tube or tracheostomy tube, apply appropriate PPE (e.g., N95 respirator, eye protection, gloves, and gown) according to employer policy (Shared Health, 2022).	Adequate amount of suction is necessary to aspirate sputum. Deep suction via endotracheal tube or tracheostomy tube is considered to be an aerosol-generating medical procedure.
3. Close curtains or room door.	Provides privacy as part of person-centred care.

STEP	RATIONALE
IMPLEMENTATION	
4. Position in high or semi-Fowler's position for suctioning.	Promotes full lung expansion and facilitates ability to cough.

Critical Decision Point *If patient has surgical incision or localized area of discomfort, have them place pillow or hands firmly over affected area. Splinting of painful area minimizes muscular stretching and discomfort during coughing and thus makes cough more productive.*

STEP	RATIONALE
5. Connect suction tube to adapter on sputum trap. Open sterile water (see Chapter 23).	Establishes suction that passes through sputum trap to aspirate specimen.
6. Using sterile technique, apply sterile glove to dominant hand or use clean glove if suction catheter has plastic sleeve.	Tracheobronchial tree is sterile body cavity. Allows you to manipulate suction catheter without contamination.
7. With gloved hand, connect sterile suction catheter to rubber tubing on sputum trap.	Aspirated sputum will go directly to trap instead of to suction tubing.
8. Lubricate suction catheter tip with sterile water (*with suction off*).	Lubrication allows for easier insertion of catheter.
9. Gently insert tip of suction catheter through nasopharynx, endotracheal tube, or tracheostomy tube without applying suction (see Chapter 23).	Minimizes trauma to airway as catheter is inserted.
10. Gently and quickly advance catheter into trachea. Warn patient to expect to cough.	Entrance of catheter into larynx and trachea triggers cough reflex.
11. As patient coughs, apply suction for 5–10 seconds, collecting 2–10 mL of sputum.	Ensures collection of sputum from deep within tracheobronchial tree. Suctioning longer than 10 seconds can cause hypoxia and mucosal damage.
12. Release suction and remove catheter; turn off suction.	Suction can damage mucosa if applied during withdrawal.
13. Detach catheter from specimen trap and dispose of catheter in appropriate receptacle.	Decreases risk of spreading microorganisms.
14. Secure top on specimen container tightly. For sputum trap, detach suction tubing and connect rubber tubing on sputum trap to plastic adapter (see Step 14 illustration).	Contains microorganisms within container, preventing exposure to personnel handling specimen.

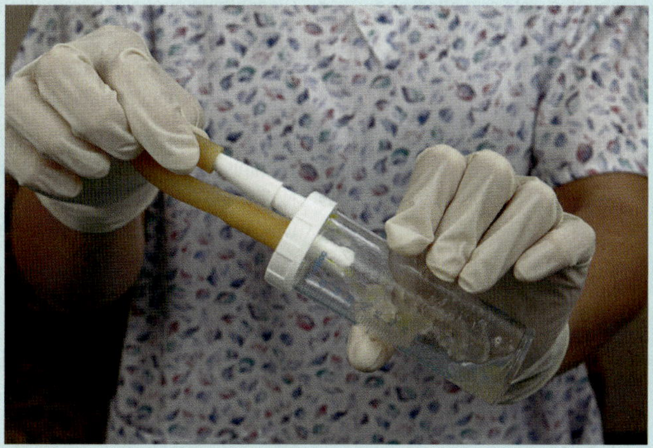

STEP 14 Closing sputum specimen trap.

STEP	RATIONALE
15. If any sputum is present on outside of container, wipe it off with disinfectant.	Prevents spread of infection to people handling specimen.
16. Offer patient tissues after suctioning. Dispose of tissues in emesis basin or appropriate container.	Maintains cleanliness and comfort.
17. Remove and dispose of gloves.	Reduces transmission of microorganisms.
18. Label specimen with identification label on side of specimen container (not lid). Confirm person-specific identifiers in front of patient (Accreditation Canada, 2020). Place specimen in small plastic bag (or container specified by employer) and attach requisition.	Incorrect identification could lead to diagnostic or therapeutic error. Plastic bag or container reduces risk of health care worker's exposure to sputum.
19. Send specimen immediately to laboratory or refrigerate.	Bacteria multiply quickly. Prompt analysis ensures accurate results.

STEP	RATIONALE
20. Apply a new pair of gloves if providing patient with mouth care.	Proper hand hygiene helps prevent the spread of infectious agents to health care providers.
21. Remove gloves and discard.	Promotes comfort.

EVALUATION

1. Observe patient's respiratory status throughout procedure, especially during suctioning. If patient is in distress, measure oxygen saturation with pulse oximeter.	Excessive coughing or prolonged suctioning can alter respiratory pattern and cause hypoxia. Determines oxygenation status.
2. Note anxiety or discomfort in patient.	Procedure can be uncomfortable. If patient becomes short of breath, anxiety will develop.
3. Observe character of sputum: colour, consistency, odour, volume, viscosity, and/or presence of blood.	Characteristics may indicate disease entities.
4. Refer to laboratory reports for test results.	Indicates whether abnormal cells or microorganisms are present in sputum.
5. **Use teach-back:** "I want to make sure you understand this procedure. Can you repeat back to me the steps we need to do to get this sputum sample?" Develop a plan for revised patient or caregiver teaching if they are unable to repeat back correctly.	Determines level of understanding of instructional topic.

Unexpected Outcomes	Related Interventions
1. Patient becomes hypoxic with increased respiratory rate and effort and shortness of breath.	• Discontinue suctioning immediately. • Administer oxygen (if prescribed). • Notify health care provider of patient's condition. • Continue to monitor patient's vital signs and pulse oximetry.
2. Patient remains anxious or reports discomfort from suction catheter.	• Discontinue procedure until stable. • Administer oxygen (if prescribed). • Notify health care provider of patient's change in condition. • Continue to monitor patient's vital signs and pulse oximetry.
3. Patient reports pain when coughing to produce sputum.	• Encourage patient who is recovering from surgical procedure to splint incision before coughing. • Obtain prescription for pain medication as needed (prn). • Inform health care provider of changes in patient's condition.

Communication and Documentation

- Document the method used to obtain specimen, date and time collected, type of test prescribed, and transport to laboratory in progress notes in EHR or chart. Describe characteristics of sputum specimen. Describe patient's tolerance of procedure.
- Report unusual sputum characteristics to nurse in charge or health care provider.
- Document your evaluation of patient and caregiver learning.
- When laboratory reports are available, report abnormal findings to health care provider. If AFB sputum culture is positive, initiate appropriate isolation techniques.
- Most employer policies require nurses to note on specimen requisition if patient is receiving antibiotics.

DOCUMENTATION EXAMPLE

78-year-old patient (he/him) admitted with dyspnea and inability to clear lung secretions. Explained the purpose and procedure of sputum specimen collection to the patient. Using 14 French suction catheter, performed the sputum collection at 1330 hours. Patient tolerated procedure well. Sputum sample was delivered to lab at 1400 hours.

Special Considerations

Teaching

- Demonstrate proper splinting technique for postoperative patients.
- If aerosol treatment is indicated, teach patient purpose of procedure, explaining that it will stimulate coughing and sputum expectoration.

Pediatric

- Children need very clear instructions or demonstration for deep breathing. Infants and young children will be unable to cooperate; aerosol treatment may be indicated.
- Use smaller catheter size for young children. It may be possible to elicit a cough by tickling the back of the throat with the suction catheter.

✦ SKILL 9.7 Obtaining Wound Specimens for Culture

Video Clip **NSO** *Nursing Skills Online Specimen Collection Module 3 / Lesson 5*

When caring for a patient with a wound, assess the condition of the wound and observe for signs of infection. Localized inflammation, tenderness, warmth, and purulent drainage are signs and symptoms of wound infection. Identification of the causative organism confirms an infection and provides guidelines for accurate treatment. A wound specimen is analyzed to determine the type and number of pathogenic microorganisms. Additionally, a specimen may be collected from a wound site or other sites such as the rectum, groin, or nares for the purpose of screening to identify patients colonized by methicillin-resistant *Staphylococcus aureus* (MRSA), vancomycin-resistant enterococci (VRE), or both. Identification of these patients ensures infection prevention measures are put in place.

Collect a wound specimen from fresh exudate in the centre of the wound, from an area of viable tissue (Orsted et al., 2017). Cleansing the wound with sterile normal saline prior to obtaining a sample is necessary to rid the wound of old exudate, and recover specimen at and below the level of the wound bed surface (Orsted et al., 2017). This minimizes the risk of contaminating the sample with skin flora, necrotic tissue, or slough (Orsted et al., 2017). Resident colonies of bacteria on the skin grow in wound exudate and may not be the true causative organisms of infection. Deeper wound tissue specimens provide a collection of bacteria that is a more accurate indication of the causative organisms (Haalboom et al., 2018). Use separate techniques to collect specimens for measuring aerobic versus anaerobic microorganisms. Aerobic organisms grow in superficial wounds exposed to the air. Anaerobic organisms grow deep within body cavities, where oxygen is not normally present.

Delegation and Collaboration

The skill of obtaining wound tissue specimens cannot be delegated to a UCP. The nurse instructs the UCP to do the following:

- Report foul odour, increase in drainage, and increase in temperature or if patient reports discomfort

Equipment

- Sterile swab in culture tube for aerobic culture (with transport medium)
- Sterile swab in culture tube for anaerobic culture (contains carbon dioxide or nitrogen gas)
- 30–60 mL irrigation syringe and 19- to 20-gauge Cathlon
- 5–10 mL safety syringe and 19-gauge needle (for anaerobic culture) (NOTE: Syringe sampling may not be done in some facilities; check employer policy.)
- Two pairs of clean gloves
- Protective eyewear *(optional)*
- Sterile dressing tray and materials to redress wound (determined by type of dressing)
- Paper or plastic disposable bag
- Completed specimen identification label with proper patient identifiers
- Completed laboratory requisition
- Small plastic biohazard bag (or container)

STEP	RATIONALE
ASSESSMENT	
1. Identify patient using at least two person-specific identifiers (e.g., name and date of birth, or name and medical record number) according to employer policy. Compare identifiers with information on patient's medical record and laboratory requisition.	Ensures correct patient. Complies with Accreditation Canada standards and improves patient safety (Accreditation Canada, 2020).
2. Throughout the procedure, the 4 moments for hand hygiene are to be implemented; hand hygiene should occur before initial patient (or patient environment) contact, before an aseptic procedure, after body fluid exposure risk, and after patient (or patient environment) contact. Additional hand hygiene should be performed when hands are visibly soiled.	Proper hand hygiene helps prevent the spread of infectious agents to health care providers.
3. Assess patient's understanding of need for wound culture and ability to cooperate with procedure.	Use data to develop teaching plan. A wound is a painful site. Collection of specimen may cause anxiety or fear.
4. Assess patient for signs of fever, chills, or excessive thirst. Note in medical record laboratory results if WBC count is elevated.	Signs and symptoms indicate systemic infection.
5. Assess patient's pain at wound site using an appropriate pain assessment tool. If patient requires analgesic before dressing changes, give medication 30 minutes before beginning procedure to allow it to reach peak effect.	Pain at wound site often increases with infection.
6. Determine when dressing change is scheduled (see Chapters 39 and 40). Perform wound assessment as part of actual procedure.	
7. Review health care provider's prescriptions for aerobic or anaerobic culture.	Specimens are taken from different sites and placed in different containers, depending on type of culture.

STEP	RATIONALE

NURSING DIAGNOSES

- Acute pain
- Persistent pain
- Reduced tissue integrity
- Insufficient knowledge regarding wound drainage culture procedure
- Anxiety
- Potential for infection
- Potential for injury

Related factors or risk factors are individualized on the basis of patient's condition or needs.

PLANNING

STEP	RATIONALE
1. Expected outcomes following completion of procedure:	
• Wound culture does not reveal bacterial growth.	Wound remains free of pathogenic microorganisms.
• Culture swab is free of contamination from skin bacteria.	Test results indicate type of cells present.
• Patient discusses purpose of and procedure for specimen collection.	Validates learning.
2. Determine whether analgesia is necessary. Administer analgesic 30 minutes before dressing change and/or specimen collection.	Minimizes discomfort during procedure. Provides person-centred care.
3. Explain reason for wound culture and how it will be collected.	Promotes understanding and cooperation and eases anxiety.
4. Explain that patient may feel tickling sensation when wound is swabbed.	Anticipation of expected sensations minimizes anxiety.

IMPLEMENTATION

STEP	RATIONALE
1.	Proper hand hygiene helps prevent the spread of infectious agents to health care providers.
2. Close bedside curtains or door to room.	Provides privacy.
3. Prepare patient environment: sanitize working surface, position patient, adjust height of bed, and turn on lights.	Environmental factors can increase risk for infection and delay wound healing.
4. Prepare sterile field, then add necessary sterile supplies and cleaning solution.	
5. Apply clean gloves.	Gloves minimize exposure to microorganisms.
6. Remove old dressings covering wound. Fold soiled sides of dressing together and dispose. Remove soiled gloves and discard.	Signs indicate wound infection.
7. Apply clean gloves. Observe wound for swelling, separation of wound edges, inflammation, and drainage.	Provides baseline for condition of wound.
8. Thoroughly cleanse/irrigate wound with sterile normal saline or sterile water per employer policy. After cleansing the wound, ensure periwound skin is cleansed from edges outward.	Removes old exudate containing skin flora, preventing possible contamination of specimen. Larger amounts of solution may be required for larger wounds. Cleanse wound, then periwound (clean to dirty) to avoid contamination of the wound.
9. Use sterile gauze to remove excess normal saline or water from the wound surface and use a clean gauze pad for each wipe. Ensure a 1 cm × 1 cm (0.4 inch × 0.4 inch) area of viable wound bed tissue is visible.	Avoids contamination. Ensures that the swab is collected from viable tissue, not necrotic slough, pooled exudates, or eschars (because surface pathogens are often contaminants).
10. Obtain cultures:	
a. Aerobic culture:	
(1) Carefully open sterile swab in culture tube. Rotate tip of swab over 1 cm × 1 cm (0.4 inch × 0.4 inch) area of viable tissue in centre of wound for 5 seconds (Levine technique). Use sufficient pressure to extract exudate from wound. Avoid touching wound edge or periwound skin with swab. Immediately place swab into culture tube and ensure tip of swab is in contact with medium.	For dry wounds, the swab can be premoistened in the transport medium or with sterile normal saline before swabbing wound. The swab should be coated with fresh exudate from wound. If there are multiple wounds in the same location, use separate swabs for each. Medium preserves bacteria until laboratory analysis is complete.
b. Anaerobic culture:	
(1) Take swab from special anaerobic culture tube, swab deeply into draining body cavity, and rotate gently. Remove swab and return to culture tube.	Specimen is taken from deep cavity where oxygen is not present. Carbon dioxide or nitrogen gas keeps organisms alive until analysis is complete. Air injected into tube would cause organisms to die.
Or	
(2) Insert tip of syringe (without needle) into wound and aspirate 5–10 mL of exudate. Attach 19-gauge needle, expel all air, and inject drainage into special culture tube.	Sterile large-bore needle (19-gauge) allows exudate to be transferred from sterile syringe into special culture tube without contamination.

STEP	RATIONALE
IMPLEMENTATION	
11. Remove and dispose of gloves.	Reduces transfer of microorganisms.
12. Perform wound dressing change per health care provider's prescription and/or employer policy, following dressing change skill. Apply new sterile dressing (see Chapters 39 and 40) using aseptic technique.	Protects wound from further contamination; aids in absorbing drainage and debridement of wound.
13. Place correct specimen label on each culture tube. Verify person-specific identifiers in front of patient (Accreditation Canada, 2020). NOTE: Indicate on specimen whether patient is receiving antibiotics.	Ensures correct results for correct patient.
14. Send specimens to laboratory immediately (within 1 hour).	Bacteria multiple rapidly. Prompt analysis ensures accurate results.
15. Remove and dispose of gloves and soiled supplies in appropriate receptacles according to employer policy.	Reduces transmission of microorganisms.
16. Help patient to comfortable position.	Promotes patient's ability to relax.
EVALUATION	
1. Obtain laboratory report for results of cultures.	Report indicates whether pathogenic organisms have been identified.
2. Observe character of wound drainage.	Characteristics can reveal abnormal status and infection.
3. Observe edges of wound for redness and bleeding.	Indicates trauma to healing tissue.
4. **Use teach-back:** "I want to make sure you understand what needs to be done to get this sample. Can you tell me the steps of the procedure?" Develop a revised teaching plan if patient or caregiver is unable to teach back correctly.	Determines level of understanding of instructional topic.

Unexpected Outcomes	Related Interventions
1. Wound cultures reveal bacterial growth.	• Monitor patient for fever, chills, or excessive thirst, which indicate systemic infection. • Inform health care provider of findings.
2. Wound culture is contaminated from superficial skin cells.	• Monitor patient for fever and pain. • Inform health care provider of findings. • Repeat collection of specimen as prescribed.
3. Patient reports increased pain.	• Provide analgesia. • Notify health care provider.

Communication and Documentation

- Document types of specimens obtained, source, and time and date sent to laboratory and describe appearance of wound and characteristics of drainage in progress notes in EHR or chart.
- Report any evidence of infection to the health care provider.
- Document your evaluation of patient and caregiver learning.
- Document patient's reaction to procedure and response to analgesics.

DOCUMENTATION EXAMPLE

Patient admitted with end-stage renal disease, nurse noted a pressure injury at the bottom of right heel with moderate amount of purulent drainage, reported to the health care provider. Wound swab C&S was completed; cleansed the pressure injury with normal saline, 1-cm diameter ulcer, 0.5 cm in depth, purulent discharge, obtained swab at the middle of the ulcer at 1100 hours. Sent the sample to lab at 1120 hours.

Special Considerations

Teaching

- Instruct patient to inform you if procedure causes pain or if you need to stop because patient is unable to tolerate pain.
- Teach patient to assess status of wound for changes and signs and symptoms of infection.

Pediatric

- If procedure is to be performed on a child and is anticipated to be painful, some employers prefer performing it in an area other than the child's room to maintain feeling that child's room is a safe place (Hockenberry et al., 2024).
- It is often helpful to have an additional nurse or other adult available to help with specimen collection in a young child or infant.

Gerontological

- Older persons may need help with positioning to change the dressing and obtain a wound culture. For confused patients, it may be necessary for the caregiver to help with the collection of the specimen (Boscart et al., 2023).

Patients With Physical or Cognitive Challenges

- Changing a dressing and collecting wound culture may elicit different reactions in a person with physical or cognitive challenges, particularly if it causes pain. If possible, give the patient time to process the procedure (Mendes, 2018).

Care in the Community: Home Management

- Teach patient antiseptic practices (e.g., handwashing, disposal of dressings, and clean technique for applying dressing).

✦ SKILL 9.8 Collecting Blood Specimens and Culture by Venipuncture (Syringe and Vacutainer Method)

Video Clip NSO Nursing Skills Online Caring for Central Vascular Access Devices (CVAD) Module 12 / Lesson 2

Blood tests are one of the most common diagnostic aids in the care and evaluation of patients. Tests allow health care providers to screen patients for early signs of physical illness, monitor changes in acute or chronic diseases, and evaluate responses to therapies.

With some employers, the nurse is responsible for collecting blood specimens; however, many employers have specially trained phlebotomists who are responsible for drawing venous blood. Be familiar with your employer's policies and procedures for drawing blood samples.

The three methods of obtaining blood specimens are (1) venipuncture, (2) skin puncture, and (3) arterial puncture. All procedures require sterile technique. Venipuncture is the most common method of obtaining blood specimens. This method involves inserting a hollow-bore needle into the lumen of a large vein to obtain a specimen using either a needle and syringe or a Vacutainer device that allows the drawing of multiple samples. Because veins are major sources of blood for laboratory testing and routes for IV fluid or blood replacement, maintaining their integrity is essential. The nurse needs to be skilled in venipuncture to avoid unnecessary injury to veins.

Skin puncture, also called *capillary puncture*, is the least traumatic method of obtaining a blood specimen. A sterile lancet or needle is used to puncture a vascular area on a finger or earlobe in an adult or child. The nurse places a drop of blood on a test slide, wicks a drop of blood to a test slide, or collects it within a thin glass capillary tube for laboratory analysis. Changes in health care economics and delivery have resulted in the increased use of skin puncture. Point-of-care clinical laboratory tests at the bedside most frequently involve skin puncture (MacDonald et al., 2024).

Blood cultures aid in the detection of bacteria in the blood. It is important that at least two culture specimens be drawn from two different sites. Because bacteremia may be accompanied by fever and chills, blood cultures should be drawn when these symptoms are present (MacDonald et al., 2024). Bacteremia exists when both cultures grow the infectious agent. Only one culture growing bacteria is considered contamination. All cultures should be drawn before antibiotic therapy begins because the antibiotic may interrupt the growth of an organism in the laboratory. If the patient is receiving antibiotics, notify the laboratory and indicate which specific antibiotics the patient is receiving (MacDonald et al., 2024).

Delegation and Collaboration

The skill of collecting blood specimens by venipuncture can be delegated to a specially trained UCP. In some facilities, phlebotomists obtain the venipuncture samples. Employer and government regulations and policies differ regarding personnel who may draw blood specimens. The nurse informs the UCP to do the following:

- Report any patient discomfort or signs of excessive bleeding from the puncture site to the nurse

Equipment

All Procedures

- Clean gloves
- Small pillow or folded towel
- Tourniquet
- Chlorhexidine 2% in 70% alcohol swabs or other antiseptic (check employer policy)
- Sterile 5 cm × 5 cm (2 inch × 2 inch) gauze
- Adhesive bandage or adhesive tape
- Completed identification labels with proper patient identifiers
- Completed laboratory requisition
- Small plastic biohazard bag (or container)
- Sharps container

Venipuncture With Syringe

- Sterile safety needles (20- to 21-gauge for adults; 23- to 25-gauge for children)
- Sterile 10- to 20-mL Luer-Lok syringes
- Blood transfer device (needleless)
- Appropriate blood specimen tubes

Venipuncture With Vacutainer

- Vacutainer with Luer-Lok adapter
- Sterile double needles or butterfly needles (20- to 21-gauge for adults; 23- to 25-gauge for children)
- Appropriate blood specimen tubes

Blood Cultures

- Sterile double needles or butterfly needles (20- to 21-gauge for adults; 23- to 25-gauge for children)
- Two or three 20- to 30-mL sterile syringes
- Culture bottle adapters
- Anaerobic and aerobic culture bottles (check employer policy)

Central Venous Catheter Collection

- Two empty 10-mL sterile syringes
- Sterile 10-mL normal saline flushes
- Vacutainer with Luer-Lok adapter
- Culture bottle adapters
- Appropriate blood specimen tubes

STEP	RATIONALE
ASSESSMENT	
1. Identify patient using at least two person-specific identifiers (e.g., name and date of birth, or name and medical record number) according to employer policy. Compare identifiers with information on patient's medical record and laboratory requisition.	Ensures correct patient. Complies with Accreditation Canada standards and improves patient safety (Accreditation Canada, 2020).
2. Throughout the procedure, the 4 moments for hand hygiene are to be implemented; hand hygiene should occur before initial patient (or patient environment) contact, before an aseptic procedure, after body fluid exposure risk, and after patient (or patient environment) contact. Additional hand hygiene should be performed when hands are visibly soiled.	Proper hand hygiene helps prevent the spread of infectious agents to health care providers.

STEP	RATIONALE
3. Assess patient's understanding of purpose of procedure and ability to cooperate.	Provides data for you to establish teaching plan and provides emotional support. Some patients' past experiences may increase their anxiety.
4. Determine whether special conditions need to be met before specimen collection (e.g., patient allowed nothing by mouth [NPO], specific time for collection in relation to medication given, need to ice specimen).	Some tests require meeting specific conditions to obtain accurate measurement of blood elements (e.g., fasting blood sugar, drug peak and trough level, timed endocrine hormone levels).
5. Assess patient for possible risks associated with venipuncture: anticoagulant therapy, low platelet count, bleeding disorders (history of hemophilia). Review medication history.	Patient history may include abnormal clotting abilities caused by low platelet count, hemophilia, or medications that increase risk of bleeding and hematoma formation.
6. Assess patient for contraindicated sites for venipuncture: presence of IV infusion, hematoma at potential site, arm on side of mastectomy, or hemodialysis shunt.	Drawing specimens from such sites can result in false test results or may injure patient. Samples taken from vein near IV infusion may be diluted or contain concentrations of IV fluids. Postmastectomy patients may have reduced lymphatic drainage in arm on operative side, increasing risk for infection from needle-sticks. Never use arteriovenous shunt to obtain specimens because of risks of clotting and bleeding. Hematoma indicates existing injury to vessel wall.
7. Identify presence of tape sensitivities or latex allergies.	Requires avoiding exposure to these items.
8. Before drawing blood cultures, assess for systemic signs and symptoms of bacteremia, including fever and chills.	Three blood culture samples should be drawn at least 1 hour apart, beginning at the earliest signs of sepsis (MacDonald et al., 2024).
9. Review health care provider's prescriptions for type of tests.	Multiple samples are often needed. A health care provider's prescription is required.

Critical Decision Point *Some specimens have special collection requirements before or after specimen collection; examples follow:*
- *Cryoglobulin levels: Place tube in warm water for transport.*
- *Ammonia and ionized calcium levels: Place tube in ice for transport.*
- *Lactic acid levels: Do not use tourniquet.*
- *Vitamin levels: Avoid exposure of test tube to light.*

NURSING DIAGNOSES

- Anxiety
- Fear
- Insufficient knowledge regarding blood specimen collection process
- Potential for injury
- Potential for infection

Related factors and risk factors are individualized on the basis of patient's condition or needs.

PLANNING

STEP	RATIONALE
1. Expected outcomes following completion of procedure:	
• Venipuncture site shows no evidence of continued bleeding or hematoma after specimen collection.	Indicates that hemostasis is achieved.
• Patient denies anxiety or discomfort.	Explanation relieves anxiety; procedure is performed quickly. Removal of painful stimulus lessens anxiety.
• An adequate sample is collected for testing (see employer policy or laboratory manual).	Appropriate laboratory analysis can be conducted.
• Patient discusses purpose, procedure, and benefits of venipuncture.	Validates learning.
2. Explain procedure to patient: describe purpose of tests; explain how sensation of tourniquet, alcohol swab, and needle-stick will feel.	Anticipatory guidance helps to reduce anxiety.

IMPLEMENTATION

STEP	RATIONALE
1.	Proper hand hygiene helps prevent the spread of infectious agents to health care providers.

STEP	RATIONALE
2. Bring equipment to bedside and organize.	Facilitates procedure.
3. Close bedside curtain or room door.	Provides for privacy. Reduces transmission of infection.
4. Raise or lower bed to comfortable working height.	Reduces strain on your back muscles and improves access to venipuncture site.
5. Help patient to supine or semi-Fowler's position, with patient's arms extended to form straight line from shoulders to wrists. Place small pillow or towel under upper arm. (*Option*: Lower arm briefly so it fills veins in hand and lower arm with blood.)	Helps to stabilize extremity because arms are most common sites of venipuncture. Supported position in bed reduces chance of injury to patient if fainting occurs.
6. Apply tourniquet so it can be removed by pulling an end with single motion.	Tourniquet blocks venous return to heart from extremity, causing veins to dilate for easier visibility.
a. Position tourniquet 5–10 cm (2–4 inches) above venipuncture site selected (antecubital fossa site is most often used).	
b. Cross tourniquet over patient's arm (see Step 6b illustration). You may place it over gown sleeve to protect skin.	Placing tourniquet over gown sleeve protects older person's skin, which is very fragile.
c. Hold tourniquet between your fingers close to arm. Tuck loop between patient's arm and tourniquet so you can grasp free end easily (see Step 6c illustration).	Pull free end to release tourniquet after venipuncture.

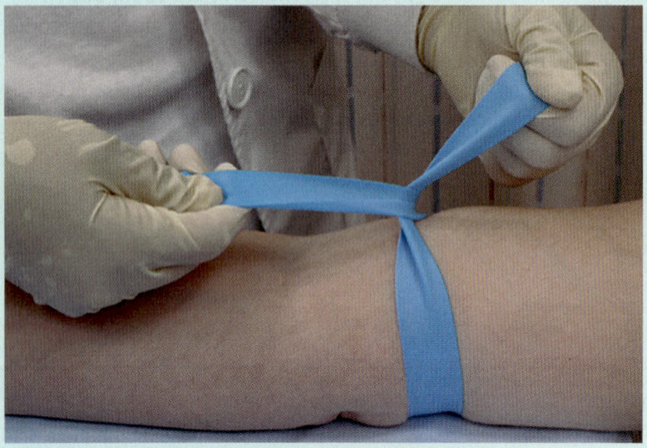

STEP 6B Cross tourniquet over arm.

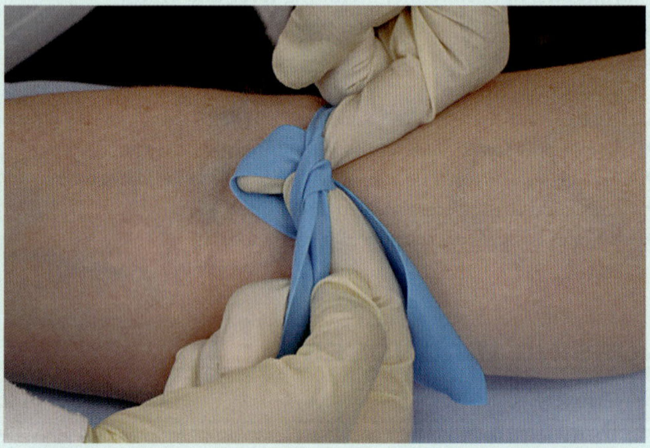

STEP 6C Tuck loop between patient's arm and tourniquet.

Critical Decision Point *Palpate distal pulse (e.g., radial) below tourniquet. If pulse is not palpable, remove tourniquet, wait 60 seconds, and reapply it more loosely. If tourniquet is too tight, pressure will impede arterial blood flow.*

STEP	RATIONALE
7. Do not keep tourniquet on patient longer than 1 minute.	Prolonged tourniquet application causes stasis, localized acidemia, and hemoconcentration (MacDonald et al., 2024).
8. Quickly inspect extremity for best venipuncture site, looking for straight, prominent vein without swelling or hematoma. Of three veins located in antecubital area, median cubital vein is preferred (see Step 8 illustration).	Straight and intact veins are easiest to puncture.
9. Apply clean gloves. Palpate selected vein with finger (see Step 9 illustration). Note whether vein feels firm and rebounds when palpated or if it feels rigid or cordlike and rolls when palpated. Avoid vigorously slapping vein, which can cause vasospasm.	Patent, healthy vein is elastic and rebounds on palpation. Thrombosed vein is rigid, rolls easily, and is difficult to puncture.

STEP	RATIONALE

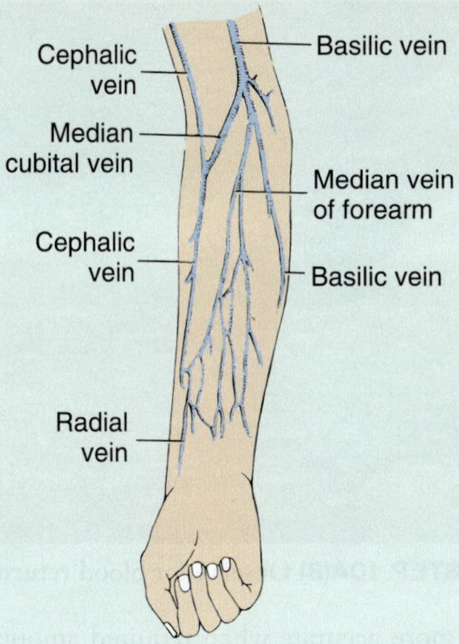

STEP 8 Location of antecubital veins.

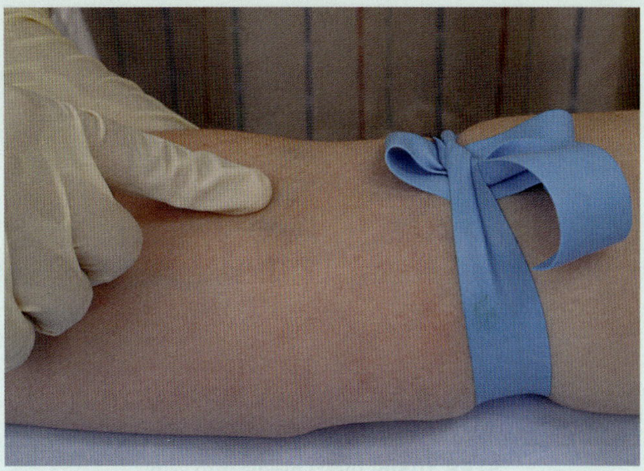

STEP 9 Palpate vein.

10. Obtain blood specimen.

a. Syringe method:

STEP	RATIONALE
(1) Have syringe with appropriate needle securely attached.	Needle must not dislodge from syringe during venipuncture.
(2) Clean site with antiseptic, with first swab moving back and forth on horizontal plane, another swab on vertical plane, and last in circular motion from site outward to form a 5 cm × 5 cm (2 inch × 2 inch) area for 30 seconds. Allow site to dry for approximately 30 seconds.	Antimicrobial agent removes resident bacteria from skin surface so that organisms do not enter puncture site. Drying enables antiseptic to achieve its antimicrobial task and reduces "sting" of venipuncture. Alcohol left on skin can cause hemolysis of sample and retraction of tissue away from puncture site.
(a) If drawing sample for blood alcohol level or blood cultures, use only antiseptic swab rather than alcohol swab.	Ensures accurate test results.
(3) Remove needle cover and inform patient that "stick" lasts only a few seconds.	Patient has better control over anxiety when prepared for what to expect.
(4) Place thumb or forefinger of nondominant hand 2.5 cm (1 inch) below site and gently pull skin taut. Stretch skin steadily until vein is stabilized.	Stabilizes vein and prevents rolling during needle insertion.
(5) Hold syringe and needle at 10- to 30-degree angle from patient's arm with bevel up.	Reduces chance of penetrating both sides of vein during insertion. Bevel up decreases chance of contamination by not dragging bevel opening over skin and allows point of needle to first puncture skin, reducing trauma.
(6) Slowly insert needle into vein, stopping when "pop" is felt as needle enters vein (see Step 10a[6] illustration).	Prevents puncture through vein to opposite side.
(7) Hold syringe securely and pull back gently on plunger.	Holding syringe prevents needle from advancing. Pulling on plunger creates vacuum needed to draw blood into syringe. If plunger is pulled back too quickly, pressure may collapse vein.
(8) Observe for blood return (see Step 10a[8] illustration).	If blood flow fails to appear, needle may not be in vein.

STEP	RATIONALE

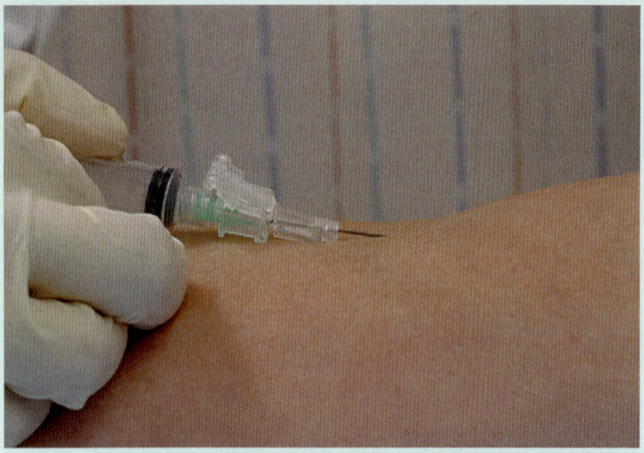

STEP 10A(6) Insert needle into vein.

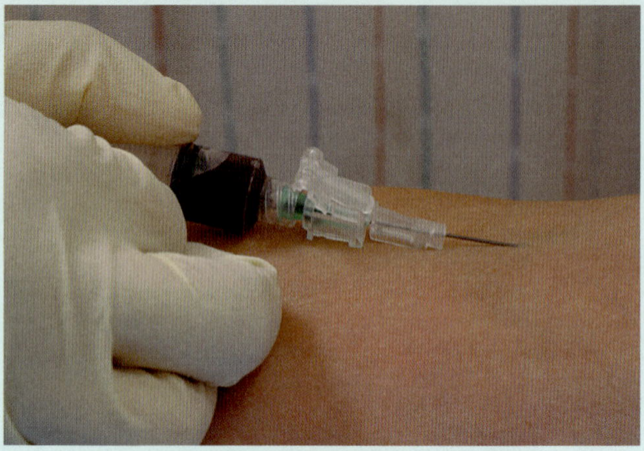

STEP 10A(8) Observe for blood return.

STEP	RATIONALE
(9) Obtain desired amount of blood, keeping needle stabilized.	Test results are more accurate when required amount of blood is obtained. Some tests cannot be performed without minimal blood requirement. Movement of needle increases discomfort.
(10) After obtaining specimen, release tourniquet.	Reduces bleeding at site when needle is withdrawn.
(11) Apply 5 cm × 5 cm (2 inch × 2 inch) gauze over site without applying pressure. Quickly but carefully withdraw needle from vein and apply pressure following removal of needle (see Step 10a[11] illustration) for 2–3 minutes or until bleeding stops. Check for hematoma.	Pressure over needle can cause discomfort. Careful removal of needle minimizes discomfort and vein trauma. Hematoma may cause compression injury (McCall, 2021).
(12) Activate safety cover and immediately discard needle in sharps container.	Prevents needle-stick injury.
(13) Attach blood-filled syringe to needle-free blood transfer device. Attach tube and allow vacuum to fill tube to specified level. Remove and fill other tubes as appropriate (see Step 10a[13] illustration). Gently rotate each tube back and forth per specified tube or test requirements.	Additives prevent clotting. Proper mixing of tubes ensures that culture medium is blended with blood (Alberta Precision Laboratories, 2023). Shaking can cause hemolysis of red blood cells (RBCs). Over-mixing of coagulation tubes may trigger the blood-clotting cascade pathway (Alberta Precision Laboratories, 2023).

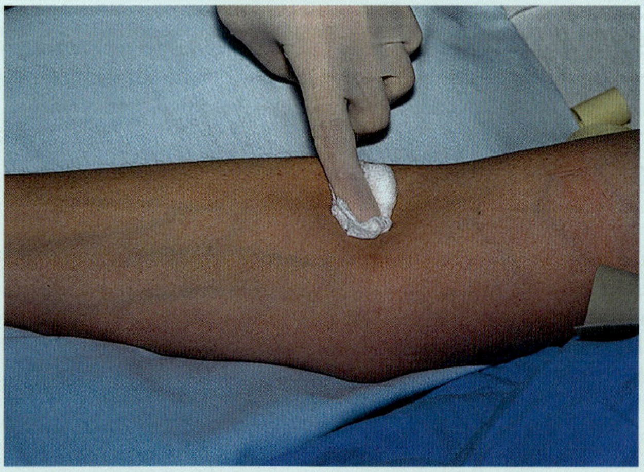

STEP 10A(11) Apply gauze to puncture site.

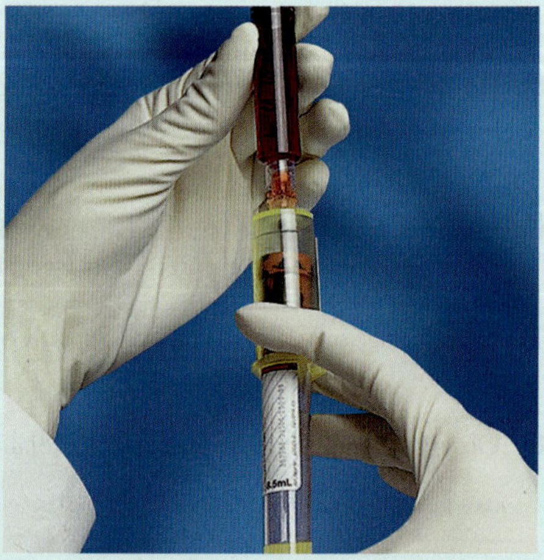

STEP 10A(13) Attach blood-filled syringe to needle-free blood transfer device.

STEP	RATIONALE
b. **Vacutainer system method:**	
(1) Attach double-ended needle or butterfly needle to Vacutainer tube (see Step 10b[1] illustration for double-ended needle).	Long end of needle is used to puncture vein. Short end covered with rubber is inserted into Vacutainer and is used to puncture blood tubes.
(2) Have proper blood tube resting inside Vacutainer device, but do not puncture rubber stopper on tube.	Puncturing causes loss of tube vacuum.
(3) Clean venipuncture site by following Steps10a(2) and 10a(2)(a) for antiseptic swab. Allow to dry.	Cleans skin surface of resident bacteria so organisms do not enter puncture site. Drying maximizes effect of antiseptic.
(4) Remove needle cover and inform patient that "stick" will occur, lasting only a few seconds.	Patient has better control over anxiety when prepared about what to expect.
(5) Place thumb or forefinger of nondominant hand 2.5 cm (1 inch) *below* site and gently pull skin taut. Stretch skin down until vein stabilizes.	Helps to stabilize vein and prevent rolling during needle insertion.
(6) Hold needle at 10- to 30-degree angle from patient's skin with bevel up.	Smallest and sharpest point of needle will puncture skin first. Reduces chance of penetrating sides of vein during insertion. Keeping bevel up causes less trauma to vein.
(7) Slowly insert needle into vein (see Step 10b[7] illustration).	Prevents puncture on opposite side.

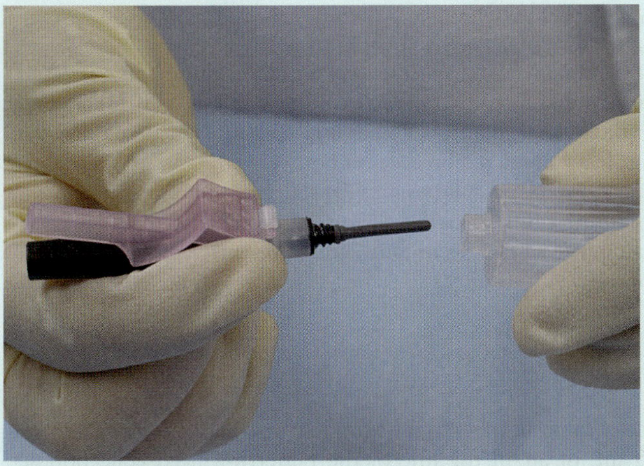

STEP 10B(1) Attach double-ended needle to Vacutainer tube.

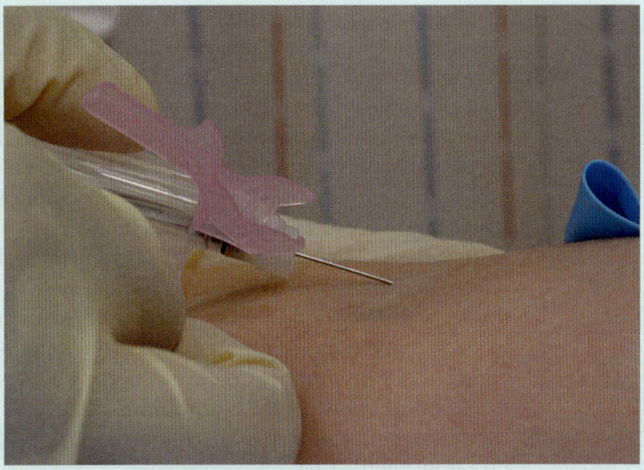

STEP 10B(7) Insert needle into vein.

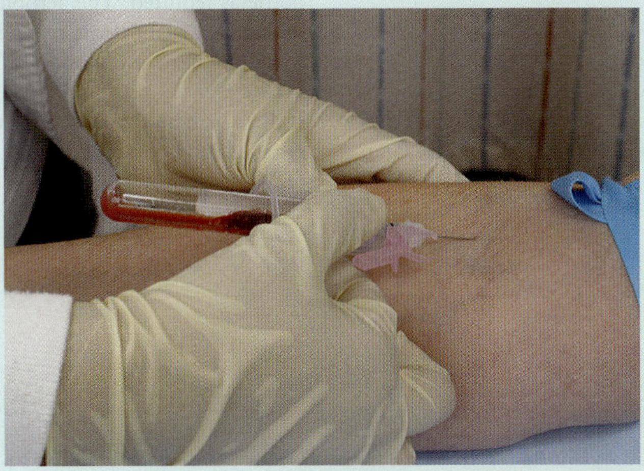

STEP 10B(9) Blood flowing into tube.

STEP	RATIONALE
(8) Grasp Vacutainer securely and advance tube into needle with rubber (do not advance other needle end into vein).	Pushing tube through stopper breaks vacuum and causes flow of blood into tube. If needle in vein advances, vein may become punctured on other side.
(9) Note flow of blood into tube, which should be fairly rapid (see Step 10b[9] illustration).	Failure of blood to appear indicates that vacuum in tube is lost or needle is not in vein.

STEP	RATIONALE
(10) After filling specimen tube, firmly grasp Vacutainer and remove tube. Insert additional tubes as needed (and in the correct order). Gently rotate each tube back and forth per specified tube or test requirements.	Vacuum in tube stops flow at amount to be collected. Grasping prevents needle from advancing or dislodging. Tube should fill completely because additives in certain tubes are measured in proportion to filled tube. Ensures proper mixing with additive to prevent clotting.
(11) After last tube is filled and removed from Vacutainer, release tourniquet.	Reduces bleeding at site when needle is withdrawn.
(12) Apply 5 cm × 5 cm (2 inch × 2 inch) gauze over puncture site without applying pressure, and quickly but carefully withdraw needle with Vacutainer from vein.	Pressure over needle can cause discomfort. Careful removal of needle minimizes discomfort and vein trauma.
(13) Immediately apply pressure over venipuncture site with gauze for 2–3 minutes or until bleeding stops. Observe for hematoma. Tape gauze dressing securely.	Direct pressure minimizes bleeding and prevents hematoma formation. Hematoma may cause compression and nerve injury. Pressure dressing controls bleeding.
(14) Dispose of syringe, needle, gauze, and other supplies in appropriate containers.	Safe disposal of supplies exposed to body fluids prevents transfer of microorganisms.
c. Blood culture:	
(1) Clean venipuncture site as in Step 10a(2) with antiseptic swab or follow employer policy. Allow to dry.	Antimicrobial agent cleans skin surface so that organisms do not enter puncture site or contaminate culture. Drying ensures complete antimicrobial action and decreases stinging.
(2) Remove caps off culture bottles and cleanse tops for 30 seconds with antiseptic. Allow to dry for 1 minute.	Ensures that bottle top is sterile.
(3) Collect required volumes of blood (per employer policy) using syringe method (see Step 10a) with two 20- or 30-mL syringes *or* using a double-ended needle or butterfly needle attached directly to culture bottle via bottle adapter. Ensure collection of specimen from two separate venipuncture sites.	The optimum blood volume level for each culture bottle is 20 mL; the required amount for each culture bottle is 5–10 mL (Steiner et al., 2020). Pediatric volumes and collection methods may vary (e.g., less volume required, fewer bottles, etc.). At least two blood cultures must be collected from two different sites to confirm culture growth (Alberta Precision Laboratories, 2022).
(4) With each specimen, activate needle safety guard and remove and discard needles. If using **syringe method**, replace with new sterile needles and then inject each blood specimen into culture bottles.If using **double-ended needle or butterfly needle**, use bottle adapters to allow direct flow of blood into culture bottles.	Maintains sterile technique and prevents contamination of specimen.
(5) If both aerobic and anaerobic cultures are needed, fill aerobic bottle first.	The aerobic bottle should be filled first because there is about 0.5 mL of air in the line of the butterfly-winged collection set. Sometimes it is difficult to obtain 8–10 mL of blood per culture bottle as required. The aerobic bottle is the more critical bottle to inoculate for laboratory test results (Warekois et al., 2020).
(6) Gently mix blood in each culture bottle.	Mixes medium and blood.
d. Central venous catheter (CVC) collection:	
(1) Select appropriate port on catheter (see Step 10d[1] illustration). Turn off all infusions and clamp lumens.	If there is more than one lumen, select distal lumen, if possible. Prevents dilution of sample with medication or total parenteral nutrition (TPN).

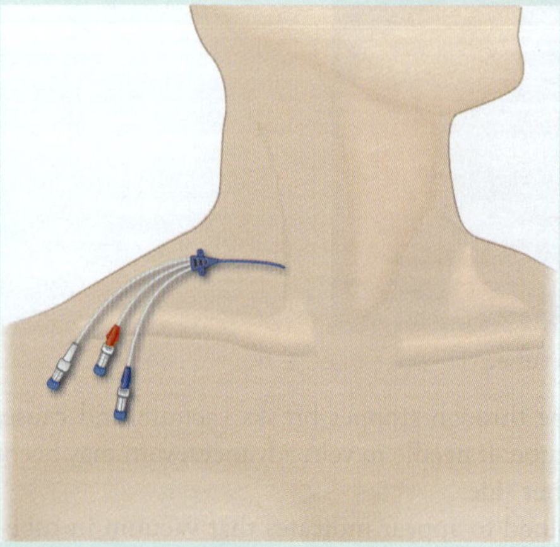

STEP 10D(1) Triple-lumen central venous catheter (CVC); select appropriate distal lumen port.

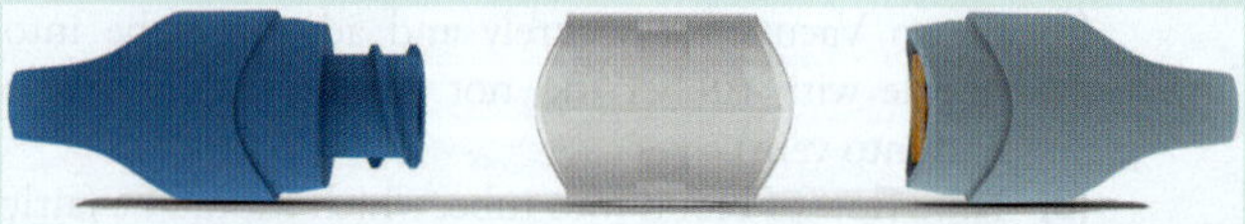

STEP 10D(2) Disinfecting cap system. Disinfects and protects both intravenous (IV) catheter needleless Luer access and end of IV tubing.

STEP	RATIONALE
(2) Cleanse selected port's Luer-Lok access cap with antiseptic and/or remove Luer-Lok disinfecting cap (e.g., DualCap, SwabCap) (see Step 10d[2] illustration). Attach 10-mL prefilled normal saline syringe to selected port. Open clamp. Aspirate for blood return. Flush 10–20 mL normal saline (NS) using turbulent (push–pause) flow (or per employer policy). Do not use syringe smaller than 10 mL.	Antiseptic-impregnated caps are recommended for use in conjunction with frictional antiseptic wiping between applications and access (Fraser Health Authority, 2018). The disinfecting cap eliminates the issue of disinfecting CVC ports adequately. Aspirating and flushing ensures patency of selected lumen and catheter in vein. Check employer policy for specified flushing volume. Pressure from small syringe may damage catheter.
(3) For **syringe method**, use same syringe and immediately aspirate 5–7 mL of blood for discard, reclamp catheter, then remove and discard syringe. Attach 10- to 20-mL Luer-Lok syringe, unclamp catheter, and aspirate desired amount of blood for sample. Reclamp catheter and remove specimen syringe. To transfer blood from syringe to specimen tube, use blood transfer device with Luer-Lok adapter. Attach specimen syringe to blood transfer device via Luer-Lok, then insert tube into blood transfer device.	Discard ensures that blood sample is not contaminated with IV fluids, medication, or other products. Check employer policy for specific discard amounts. Tubes have vacuum and automatically fill to necessary amount.
(4) For **Vacutainer method**, clamp catheter and remove syringe used for flushing. Attach Vacutainer with Luer-Lok adapter, unclamp catheter, and advance tube into Vacutainer to activate blood flow. Allow blood to fill tube, clamp catheter, and discard first tube. Attach specimen tube to Vacutainer, unclamp catheter, and obtain blood specimen (see Step 10d[4] illustration). Remove Vacutainer after all specimens collected.	Tubes have vacuum and automatically fill to necessary amount.
(5) After all specimens have been collected, clamp catheter.	

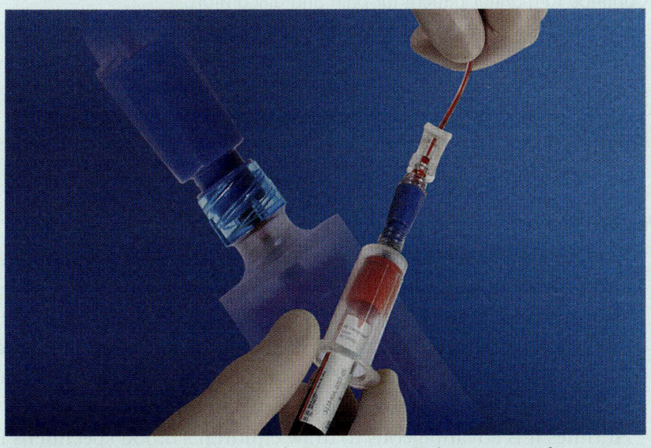

STEP 10D(4) Male Luer-Lok Vacutainer adapter attaches to port; blood draws directly into specimen tubes. *(Courtesy and copyright © Becton Dickinson.)*

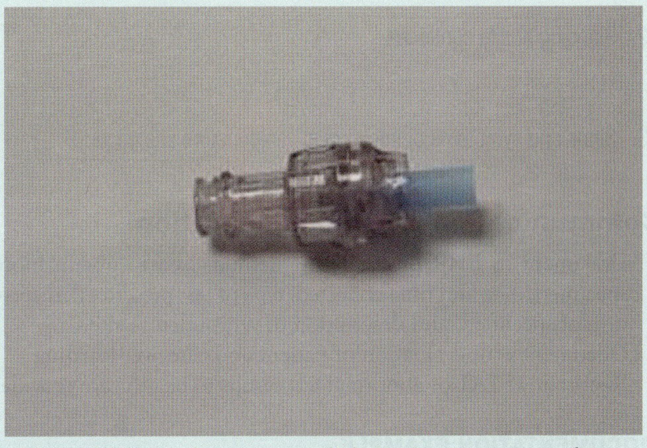

STEP 10D(6) Neutral-pressure cap helps maintain patency of vascular access device. *(Image courtesy of April Ambalina.)*

STEP	RATIONALE
(6) Attach prefilled NS syringe(s) and flush with 10–20 mL NS using push–pause method (volume per employer policy). To lock lumen, ensure correct solution (heparin or saline) and pressure for cap is instilled. Neutral and positive pressure caps are designed for syringe to be removed, and the lumen will be automatically locked. For caps without automatic neutral or positive pressure, hold syringe plunger steady at completion of flush, lock off lumen with clamp, and remove syringe (see Step 10d[6] illustration).	Push–pause creates turbulence that helps to clear lumen. Neutral fluid displacement cap designs (e.g., One-Link [Baxter]) prevent blood from flowing into tip of catheter and forming clot and lowers the risk for bloodstream infections.
(7) Blood tubes contain additives; gently rotate back and forth 8–10 times (or per specific test requirements).	Additives mix with blood to prevent clotting. Shaking can cause hemolysis of RBCs, producing inaccurate test results.

STEP	RATIONALE
11. Check tubes for any sign of external contamination with blood. Decontaminate with antiseptic if necessary.	Prevents cross-contamination. Reduces risk for exposure to pathogens present in blood.
12. Remove gloves after specimen is obtained and any spillage is cleaned.	Reduces risk for exposure to bloodborne pathogens.
13. Help patient to comfortable position, and ensure any infusions are re-established and/or required lumens are locked as prescribed or per employer policy.	
14. Attach completed identification label to each tube and affix proper requisition. Verify identifiers in front of patient (Accreditation Canada, 2020).	Incorrect identification of specimen could result in diagnostic or therapeutic errors.
15. Place specimens in biohazard bag and send to laboratory. Cultures must be sent to laboratory within 30 minutes (MacDonald et al., 2024).	Minimizes spread of microorganisms.

EVALUATION

1. Inspect venipuncture site for homeostasis.	Determines whether bleeding has stopped or hematoma has formed.
2. Determine whether patient is still anxious or fearful.	Some patients require more blood tests in future. Address concerns and let patient express anxiety.
3. Check laboratory report for test results.	Reveals constituents of blood specimen.
4. **Use teach-back:** "I want to be sure you understand the purpose and procedure for obtaining a blood specimen. Tell me why we are collecting this blood specimen." Develop a revised teaching plan if patient or caregiver is unable to teach back correctly.	Determines level of understanding of instructional topic.

Unexpected Outcomes	Related Interventions
1. Hematoma forms at venipuncture site.	• Apply pressure using 5 cm × 5 cm (2 inch × 2 inch) gauze dressing. • Continue to monitor patient for pain and discomfort.
2. Bleeding at site continues.	• Apply pressure to site; patient may also apply pressure. • Monitor patient. • Notify health care provider.
3. Signs and symptoms of infection at venipuncture site occur.	• Notify health care provider.

Communication and Documentation

- Document in EHR or chart the method used to obtain blood specimen, date and time collected, type of test prescribed, disposition of specimen, and description of venipuncture site.
- Document your evaluation of patient and caregiver learning.
- Report any STAT or abnormal test results to health care provider.

DOCUMENTATION EXAMPLE

Patient (she/her) arrived at clinic with fever, chills. Blood cultures were prescribed. Explained the purpose and the procedure to the patient. Using butterfly needle, obtained aerobic and anaerobic samples at right antecubital fossa at 1245 hours; no sign of bleeding at the site. Patient tolerated procedure well. Resting with a warm blanket and call bell within reach. Sample was delivered to lab at 1330 hours.

Special Considerations

Teaching

- Instruct patient to briefly apply pressure to venipuncture site. Patients with bleeding disorders or those undergoing anticoagulant therapy should apply pressure for at least 5 minutes.
- Instruct patient to notify nurse or health care provider if persistent or recurrent bleeding or expanding hematoma develops at venipuncture site.

Pediatric

- Explain procedure to child at developmentally appropriate age and provide atraumatic care (Hockenberry et al., 2024).
- Because children often fear that loss of their blood is a threat to their lives, explain to them that their blood is continually being produced. An adhesive bandage gives them assurance that their blood will not leak out through the puncture site (Hockenberry et al., 2024).
- At times it is advantageous to draw children's blood specimens in a treatment room instead of in their bed or room to maintain the feeling that their room is a safe place (Hockenberry et al., 2024).
- When performing venipuncture on children, explore sources for vein access: scalp, antecubital fossa, saphenous, and hand veins.
- Application of eutectic mixture of local anaesthetics (EMLA) cream to the venipuncture site may be prescribed before the needle-stick to reduce pain in infants and young children (Hockenberry et al., 2024).
- Vacutainers are not recommended for use in children under 2 years of age because of the possible risk of vein collapse.

Gerontological

- Older persons have fragile veins that are easily traumatized during venipuncture. Sometimes application of warm compresses may help in obtaining samples. Use of a small-bore catheter may be beneficial.

✦ SKILL 9.9 Blood Glucose Monitoring

Blood glucose monitoring (BGM) is an essential component of any diabetes mellitus self-management program (Diabetes Canada Clinical Practice Guidelines Expert Committee, 2018). There are different glucose monitoring modalities (Table 9.2) (Cheng et al., 2021). The procedure is less painful than venipuncture, and the ease of the skin puncture method makes it possible for patients to perform this procedure at home. The development of reagent strips, home glucose monitors, and the skin puncture method has revolutionized home care management of patients with diabetes mellitus.

Blood glucose reflectance meters that are lightweight and run on batteries (e.g., Accu-Chek III, OneTouch) (Fig. 9.7) are commonly used in the community. The glucose monitors used in hospitals (e.g., StatStrip; Fig. 9.8) are similar. For individual product operation, please refer to the product user manual and employer policy. After a drop of blood from the skin puncture is dropped or wicked onto a reagent strip, the meter provides an accurate measurement of blood glucose level in 5–50 seconds. Point-of-care blood glucose testing meters must be cleaned and disinfected after each patient use (Choi et al., 2021).

The glucose meters differ in several ways, including amount of blood needed for each test, testing speed, overall size, ability to store test results in memory, cost of the meter, and cost of the test strips. Some larger meters are voice activated, which provides support for older persons or patients with visual impairments. Most meters now allow for the use of an alternative site or forearm capillary testing. Through advancements in technology, an improved method for glucose measurement is now available on the market. A minimally invasive glucose meter, which uses a very small, fine plastic sensor inserted through the abdomen, provides continuous readings of blood glucose levels (Fig. 9.9). One disadvantage is that the patient must wear the meter at all times for continuous glucose monitoring (CGM) (Fig. 9.10). Some newer monitors allow for the use of alternative sites and can be worn externally. People can monitor their blood glucose through monitoring devices or by using their smartphones.

With increasing CGM use among inpatients, the bedside nurse needs to become familiar with this technology and its advantages and limitations. Nurses should be aware that glucose levels measured via CGM (interstitial fluid glucose) lag behind glucose levels measured using capillary glucose. This difference is important when recognizing hypoglycemia and administering insulin (Perez-Guzman et al., 2021). Follow employer policy to facilitate patient use of CGM in the hospital, and follow nursing practice guidelines on care of patients using CGM.

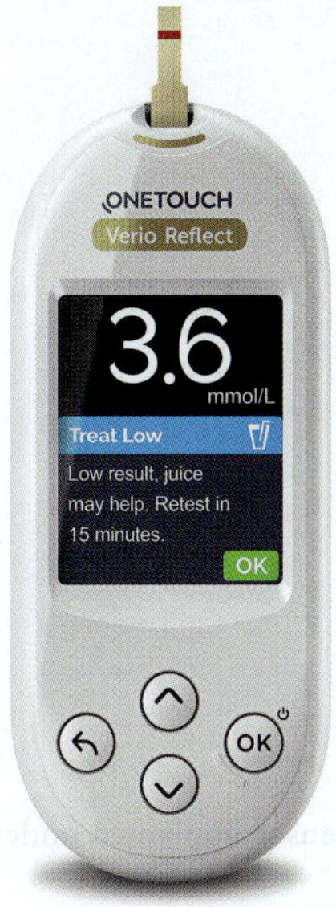

FIG 9.7 **Blood glucose monitor.** (*Courtesy LifeScan IP Holdings, LLC.*)

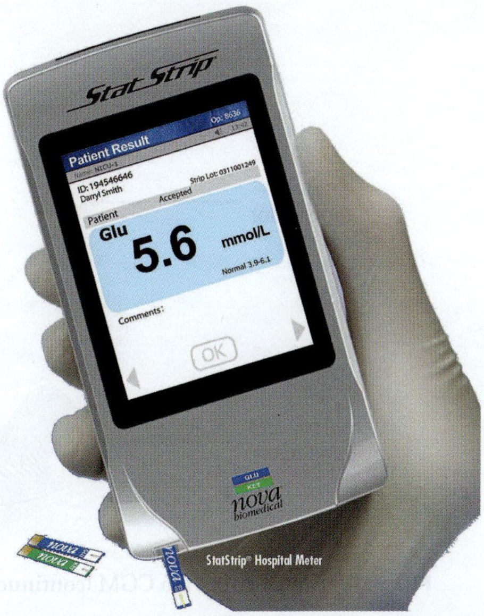

FIG 9.8 **StatStrip blood glucose monitor.** (*Courtesy Nova Biomedical.*)

TABLE 9.2

Current Terminology for Different Glucose Monitoring Modalities

New term	Previous term	Definition
Capillary blood glucose (CBG)	Self-monitored blood glucose (SMBG)	Determination of glucose in the capillary blood using fingersticks
Intermittently scanned continuous glucose monitoring (isCGM)	Flash glucose monitoring (FGM)	Measurement of interstitial fluid glucose via intermittent scanning of sensing device
Real-time continuous glucose monitoring (rtCGM)	Continuous glucose monitoring	Measurement of interstitial fluid glucose via a sensing device that is continuously transmitting the data to a device with real-time display for viewing at any time
Masked continuous glucose monitoring (mCGM)*	Professional continuous glucose monitoring	Measurement of interstitial fluid glucose via a sensing device that stores the data to be retrieved at a later time

*mCGM is a diagnostic tool for use by diabetes care providers, not for diabetes self-management.

From Cheng, A. Y. Y., Feig, D. S., Ho, J., et al. (2021). Blood glucose monitoring in adults and children with diabetes: Update 2021. *Canadian Journal of Diabetes*, *45*(7), 580–587. https://doi.org/10.1016/j.jcjd.2021.07.003

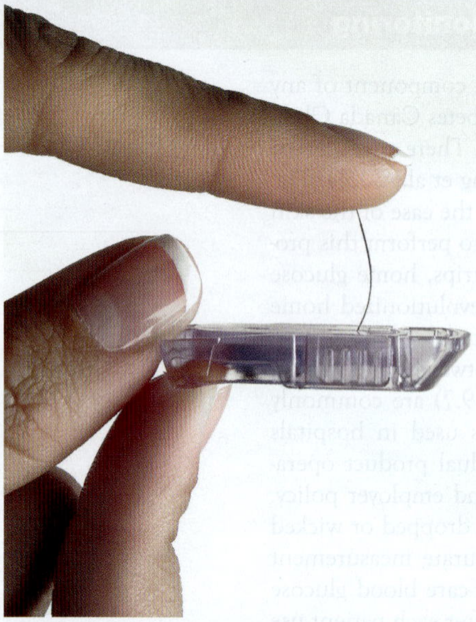

FIG 9.9 Tiny sensor implanted under skin transmits continuous reading to receiver. (*Courtesy DexCom; reprinted with permission.*)

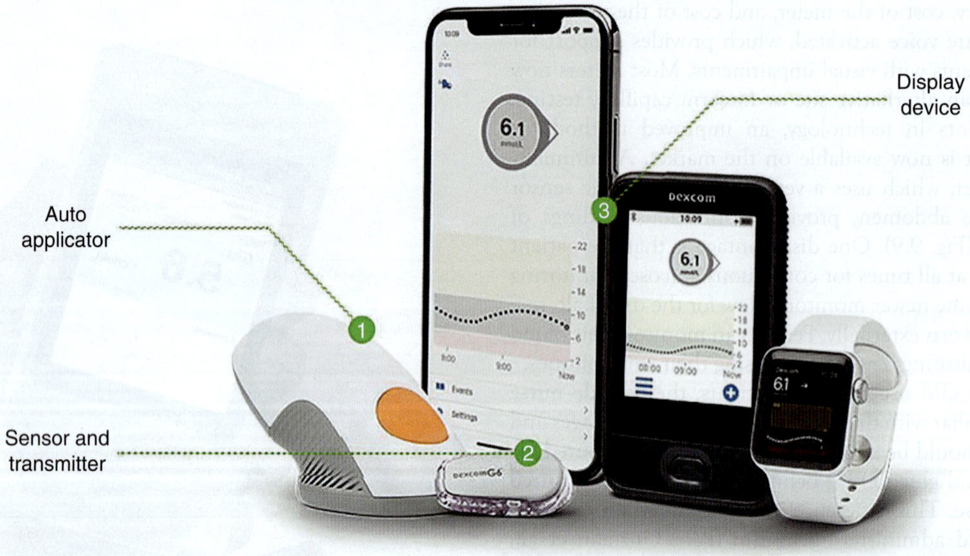

FIG 9.10 The DexCom G6 CGM (continuous glucose monitoring) system. (*Courtesy DexCom; reprinted with permission.*)

Since multiple methods are available to obtain blood samples for glucose testing, it is crucial to clean and disinfect shared equipment after every use to prevent bloodborne pathogen transmission (Centers for Disease Control and Prevention, 2011).

Testing of glycosylated hemoglobin (HbA1c) evaluates the amount of glucose available in the bloodstream over the 120-day lifespan of a red blood cell. HbA1c provides an accurate long-term index of a patient's average blood glucose level drawn by venous puncture (MacDonald et al., 2024).

Delegation and Collaboration

Assessment of a patient's condition cannot be delegated to a UCP. When the patient's condition is stable, the skill of obtaining and testing a sample of blood for blood glucose level may be delegated to a UCP, depending on employer policy. The nurse informs the UCP by doing the following:

- Explaining appropriate sites to use for puncture and when to obtain glucose levels
- Reviewing expected blood glucose levels and when to report unexpected glucose levels to the nurse

Equipment

- Antiseptic swab
- Cotton ball
- Lancet device (either self-activating or button activated)
- Blood glucose meter (e.g., Accu-Chek III, OneTouch)
- Blood glucose test strips appropriate for meter brand used
- Clean gloves
- Sterile 5 cm × 5 cm (2 inch × 2 inch) gauze

STEP	RATIONALE

ASSESSMENT

STEP	RATIONALE
1. Identify patient using at least two person-specific identifiers (e.g., name and date of birth, or name and medical record number) according to employer policy. Compare identifiers with information on patient's medical record.	Ensures correct patient. Complies with Accreditation Canada standards and improves patient safety (Accreditation Canada, 2020).
2. Throughout the procedure, the 4 moments for hand hygiene are to be implemented; hand hygiene should occur before initial patient (or patient environment) contact, before an aseptic procedure, after body fluid exposure risk, and after patient (or patient environment) contact. Additional hand hygiene should be performed when hands are visibly soiled.	Proper hand hygiene helps prevent the spread of infectious agents to health care providers.
3. Assess patient's understanding of procedure and purpose of BGM. Determine whether patient understands how to perform test and its importance in glucose control.	Provides baseline for developing teaching plan.
4. Determine whether specific conditions need to be met before or after collection (e.g., fasting, postprandial, after certain medications, before insulin doses).	Dietary intake of carbohydrates and ingestion of concentrated glucose preparations alter blood glucose levels.
5. Determine whether risks exist (e.g., low platelet count, anticoagulant therapy, bleeding disorders).	Abnormal clotting mechanisms increase risk for local ecchymosis and bleeding.
6. Assess potential puncture site. Inspect site for edema, inflammation, cuts, or sores. Avoid areas of bruising and open lesions. Avoid using hand on side of mastectomy.	Sides of fingers are commonly selected because they have fewer nerve endings. Measurements from alternative sites are meter specific and may be different from those at traditional sites. Puncture site should not be edematous, inflamed, or recently punctured because these factors cause increased interstitial fluid and blood to mix and also increase risk for infection.
7. Review health care provider's prescription for time or frequency of measurement.	Health care provider determines test schedule on the basis of patient's physiological status and risk for glucose imbalance.
8. For patient with diabetes mellitus who performs test at home, assess ability to handle devices. Patient may choose to continue self-testing while in hospital.	Patient's physical health may change (e.g., vision disturbance, fatigue, pain, disease process), preventing them from performing test.

NURSING DIAGNOSES

- Inadequate health maintenance
- Anxiety
- Insufficient knowledge regarding BGM

Related factors are individualized on the basis of patient's condition or needs.

PLANNING

STEP	RATIONALE
1. Expected outcomes following completion of procedure:	
• Puncture site shows no evidence of bleeding or tissue damage.	Hemostasis is achieved. Lancet or needle did not puncture skin too deeply.
• Blood glucose measurements are accurate.	Normal fasting glucose is 4.0–7.0 mmol/L, indicating good metabolic control (Diabetes Canada Clinical Practice Guidelines Expert Committee, 2018). Values may vary slightly; check employer policy.
• Patient can verbalize procedure for self-monitoring blood glucose.	Demonstrates psychomotor learning.
• Patient explains test results.	Validates knowledge.
2. Explain procedure and purpose. Offer patient and caregiver opportunity to practise testing procedures. Provide resources and teaching aids.	Promotes understanding and cooperation.

IMPLEMENTATION

STEP	RATIONALE
1. Instruct patient to perform hand hygiene, including forearm (if applicable), with soap and water. Rinse and dry.	Promotes skin cleansing and vasodilation at selected puncture site. Reduces transmission of microorganisms.
2.	Proper hand hygiene helps prevent the spread of infectious agents to health care providers.

STEP	RATIONALE
3. Position patient comfortably in chair or in semi-Fowler's position in bed.	Ensures easy access to puncture site. Patient assumes position when self-testing.
4. Remove reagent strip from container and tightly reseal cap. Check code or scan barcode on container. Use only test strips recommended for meter. Some newer meters do not require code and/or have disc or drum with 10 or more test strips.	Protects strips from accidental discoloration caused by exposure to air or light.
5. Insert strip into meter (refer to manufacturer directions [see Step 5 illustration]). Do not bend strip. Meter turns on automatically.	Some machines must be calibrated; others require zeroing of timer. Each meter is adjusted differently.

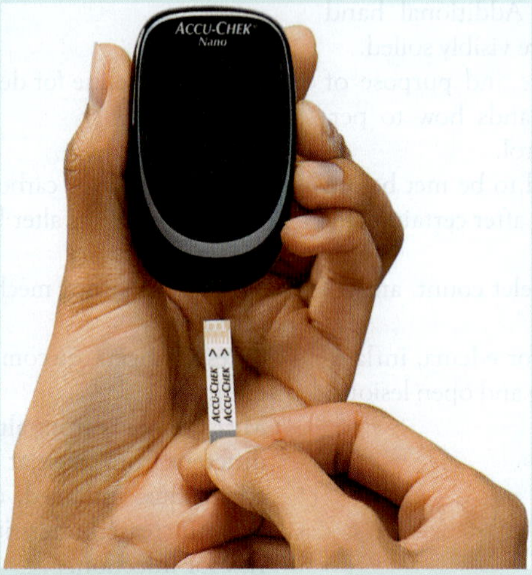

STEP 5 Load test strip into meter. *(Courtesy Accu-Chek Glucometer.)*

STEP	RATIONALE
6. Meter displays code on screen that must match code from test strip vial. In the hospital, follow prompts to input patient identification (ID) after scanning the code on the container. Press proper button on meter to confirm matching codes. Meter is ready for use.	Codes must match for meter to operate. Meters have different messages that confirm that meter is ready for testing and blood can be applied.
7. Apply clean gloves. Prepare single-use lancet or multiple-use lancet device. **Note:** Some meters recommend that this step be completed before preparing test strip. Remove cap from lancet device; insert new lancet. Some lancet devices have disc or cylinder that rotates to new lancet.	Reduces transmission of microorganisms. Never reuse a lancet because of risk for infection.
a. Twist off protective cover on tip of lancet. Replace cap of lancet device.	
b. Cock lancet device, adjusting for proper puncture depth.	Each patient varies as to depth of insertion needed.
8. Obtain blood sample.	
a. Cleanse patient's finger lightly with antiseptic and allow to dry. Choose vascular area for puncture site. In stable adults, select lateral side of finger. Avoid central tip of finger, which has denser nerve supply (MacDonald et al., 2024).	Removes microorganisms. Side of finger is less sensitive to pain.
b. Hold area to be punctured in dependent position. Do not milk or massage finger site.	Increases blood flow to area before puncture. Milking may hemolyze specimen and introduce excess tissue fluid (MacDonald et al., 2024).
c. Hold tip of lancet device against area of skin chosen for test site (see Step 8c illustration). Press release button on device. Some devices allow you to see blood sample forming. Remove device.	Placement ensures that lancet enters skin properly.
d. With some devices, a blood sample begins to appear. Otherwise, gently squeeze or massage fingertip until round drop of blood forms (see Step 8d illustration).	Adequate-size blood sample is needed to test glucose.

STEP	RATIONALE

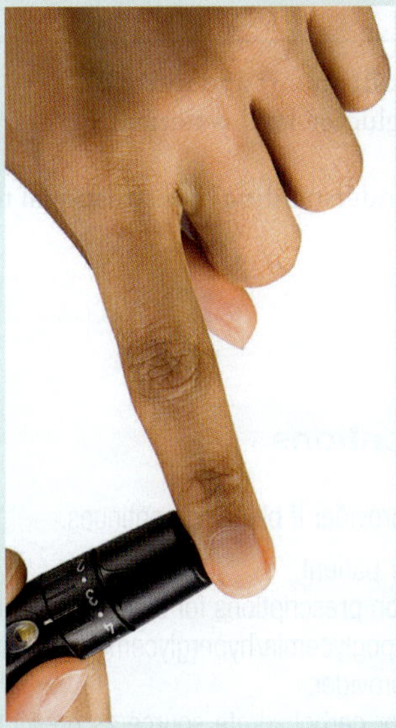

STEP 8C Prick side of finger with lancet. *(Courtesy Accu-Chek Glucometer.)*

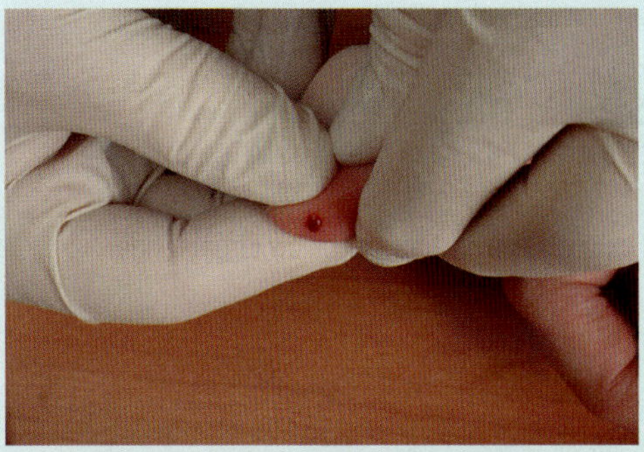

STEP 8D Gently squeeze puncture site until drop of blood forms.

STEP	RATIONALE
9. Obtain test results.	Exposure of blood to test strip for prescribed time ensures proper results.
a. Be sure that meter is still on. Wipe away the first droplet of blood with a cotton ball or gauze. Bring test strip in meter to drop of blood. Blood will be wicked onto test strip (see Step 9a illustration). Follow specific meter instructions to be sure that you obtain adequate sample.	The first drop of blood may be contaminated with the alcohol used for disinfection, which may provide an inaccurate result. Newer meters may no longer require the first drop to be discarded (Perry et al., 2021).

Critical Decision Point *Do not scrape blood onto the test strips or apply it to wrong side of test strip. This prevents accurate glucose measurement.*

b. Blood glucose test result will appear on screen of meter (see Fig. 9.7). Some devices "beep" when completed.

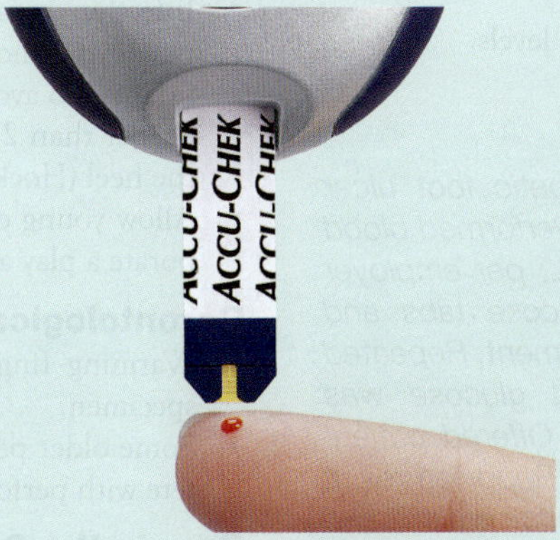

STEP 9A Touch test strip to blood drop. Blood wicks into test strip. *(Courtesy Accu-Chek Glucometer.)*

STEP	RATIONALE
10. Turn meter off. Some meters turn off automatically. Offer patient cotton ball and hold over puncture site until bleeding stops. Dispose of test strip, lancet, cotton ball, and gloves in proper receptacles.	Meter is battery powered. Proper disposal reduces risk for needlestick injury and spread of infection.
11. Discuss test results with patient and encourage questions and eventual participation in care if this is a new diabetes diagnosis.	Promotes participation in and adherence to therapy.

STEP	RATIONALE

EVALUATION

1. Inspect puncture site for bleeding or tissue injury.	Site can be source of discomfort and infection.
2. Compare glucose meter reading with normal blood glucose levels and previous test results.	Determines whether glucose level is normal.
3. **Use teach-back:** "I want to be sure I explained clearly the way to obtain a blood glucose reading. Show me the steps you will use to obtain your blood glucose measurement." Develop a revised teaching plan if patient or caregiver is unable to teach back correctly.	Determines level of understanding of instructional topic.

Unexpected Outcomes	Related Interventions
1. Puncture site is bruised or continues to bleed.	• Apply pressure. • Notify health care provider if bleeding continues.
2. Blood glucose level is above or below target range.	• Continue to monitor patient. • Check for medication prescriptions for deviations in glucose level. • Follow employer hypoglycemia/hyperglycemia protocol. • Notify health care provider. • Administer insulin or carbohydrate source as prescribed, depending on glucose level.
3. Glucose meter malfunctions.	• Review instructions for troubleshooting glucose meter. • Repeat test.

Communication and Documentation

- Document procedure and glucose level in progress notes in EHR or chart or on special flow sheet. Document action taken for abnormal range.
- Document patient response, including appearance of puncture site, in progress notes in EHR or chart.
- Document explanations or teaching provided in progress notes in EHR or chart and evaluation of patient and caregiver learning.
- Document and report abnormal blood glucose levels.

DOCUMENTATION EXAMPLE

Patient (they/them) was admitted with diabetic foot ulcer with symptoms of weakness at 0300 hours. Performed blood glucose test; blood glucose was 3.0 mmol/L; per employer hypoglycemia protocol, administered 3 glucose tabs and monitored for signs and symptoms of improvement. Repeated glucose test after 10 min. Result: Blood glucose was 4.5 mmol/L. Patient stated they felt better. Offered patient two slices of peanut butter on toast and tea. Reported result to health care provider. Will continue to monitor patient and will recheck blood glucose after 15–30 minutes.

Special Considerations

Teaching

- Provide information on where patient with diabetes mellitus can obtain testing supplies. When possible, teach with the same meter that patient will use at home.
- Provide patient with information on where to obtain help if glucose meter has malfunctioned.
- Stress the importance of regularly monitoring blood glucose levels, particularly in patients with diabetes mellitus.

Pediatric

- Allow young children to choose puncture site; outer aspect of heel and great toe are common puncture sites in infants.
- Heel warming helps to obtain specimen from a neonate.
- Infection or abscess of the heel and necrotizing osteochondritis are the most serious complications of heelstick puncture in infants. To avoid osteochondritis, make sure that puncture is not deeper than 2 mm (0.1 inch) and is made at the outer aspect of the heel (Hockenberry et al., 2024).
- Allow young child with parent to demonstrate technique; incorporate a play activity for further understanding.

Gerontological

- Warming fingertips with warm water may facilitate obtaining specimen.
- Some older persons have vision or dexterity problems that interfere with performing self-fingersticks.

Care in the Community: Home Management

- Provide information on correct disposal of sharps in nonpermeable and puncture-resistant container.
- Suggest that patient attend support group if needed.
- Be sure that patient's caregiver can perform test when patient is ill or unable to manipulate devices.
- Teach patient and caregiver how to record findings or retrieve results from the memory of the glucose meters.

✦ SKILL 9.10 Obtaining an Arterial Specimen for Blood Gas Measurement

Effectiveness of oxygenation and ventilation is assessed by measuring arterial blood gases (ABGs). Measurement of ABGs provides valuable information for assessing and managing disturbance in patient's respiration and metabolism (MacDonald et al., 2024). The parameters measured in an ABG include arterial blood pH, partial pressure of oxygen (PaO_2), partial pressure of carbon dioxide ($PaCO_2$), and arterial oxygen saturation (SaO_2).

Each employer has a policy regarding which health care providers can obtain ABG samples. Many employers allow nurses in specialty areas (e.g., critical care) to obtain them; others specify a certified respiratory therapist or a physician, and some require institutional certification of this skill. Always check employer policy.

Delegation and Collaboration

The skill of obtaining an ABG sample cannot be delegated to a UCP. The nurse informs the UCP to do the following:

- Report any bleeding from an arterial puncture site
- Report any changes in patient vital signs, level of consciousness, or restlessness

Equipment

Commercial blood gas kit or individual supplies, including:

- 3-mL heparinized syringe
- 23- or 25-gauge needle with safety guard
- Filter cap (allows expelling of air and retains blood)
- Alcohol swabs (2)
- 5 cm × 5 cm (2 inch × 2 inch) gauze pad
- Tape
- Sodium heparin (1:1 000 solution)
- Cup or plastic bag with crushed ice
- Clean gloves
- Protective eyewear
- Completed identification labels with proper patient identifiers
- Completed laboratory requisition
- Small plastic biohazard bag (or container)

STEP	RATIONALE
ASSESSMENT	
1. Identify patient using at least two person-specific identifiers (e.g., name and date of birth, or name and medical record number) according to employer policy. Compare identifiers with information on patient's medical record.	Ensures correct patient. Complies with Accreditation Canada standards and improves patient safety (Accreditation Canada, 2020).
2. Throughout the procedure, the 4 moments for hand hygiene are to be implemented; hand hygiene should occur before initial patient (or patient environment) contact, before an aseptic procedure, after body fluid exposure risk, and after patient (or patient environment) contact. Additional hand hygiene should be performed when hands are visibly soiled.	Proper hand hygiene helps prevent the spread of infectious agents to health care providers.
3. Assess for factors that influence ABG measurements:	Allows you to eliminate factors that interfere with accurate measurement.
a. Hypoventilation or hyperventilation	Hypoventilation can cause retention of CO_2, and hyperventilation can cause decreased CO_2 levels (Hockenberry et al., 2024).
b. Body temperature	Change in body temperature by as little as 0.6°C (1°F) can alter ABG values (Hockenberry et al., 2024).
4. Identify medications or herbal products that may influence ABG measurement (e.g., anticoagulants, diuretics, St. John's wort).	Certain medications increase risk for bleeding at puncture site or may cause hemoconcentration.
5. Assess respiratory status, including rate, depth, rhythm, adventitious sounds, and use of accessory muscles.	Physical signs and symptoms may indicate need for ABG sample.
6. Review criteria for choosing site for ABG sample.	Prevents causing compromised circulation from puncture.

Critical Decision Point *Factors that contraindicate the use of arterial site include amputation, contractures, localized infection, dressing or cast, mastectomy, or arteriovenous shunts.*

STEP	RATIONALE
a. Assess collateral blood flow. *Perform Allen test.*	Allen test is used to assess collateral circulation before performing arterial puncture on radial artery. A positive Allen test ensures that there is collateral circulation to the hand in case thrombosis of radial artery occurs following puncture (MacDonald et al., 2024).
(1) Have patient make tight fist and raise hand above heart.	Removes as much blood from hand as possible.
(2) Apply direct pressure to both radial and ulnar arteries (see Step 6a[2] illustration).	Obstructs arterial blood flow to hand.
(3) Have patient lower and open hand (see Step 6a[3] illustration).	Fingers and hand should be pale and blanched, indicating lack of arterial blood flow.
(4) Release pressure over ulnar artery; observe colour of fingers, thumbs, and hand (see Step 6a[4] illustration).	Flushing identifies that circulation through the ulnar artery is good and that the ulnar artery alone is capable of providing blood supply to the entire hand. Therefore, you can use the radial artery for puncture.

STEP	RATIONALE

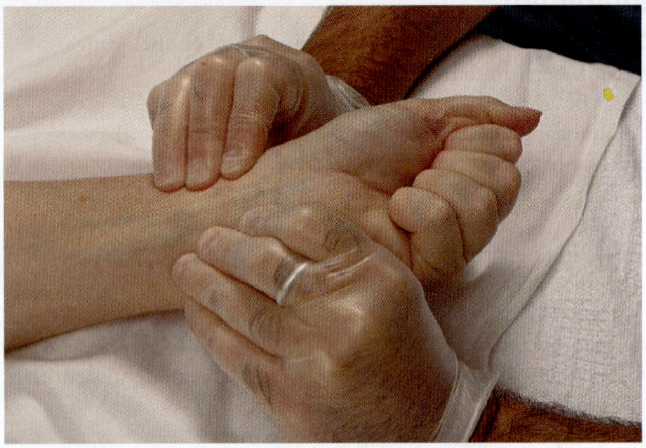

STEP 6A(2) Apply pressure to radial and ulnar arteries.

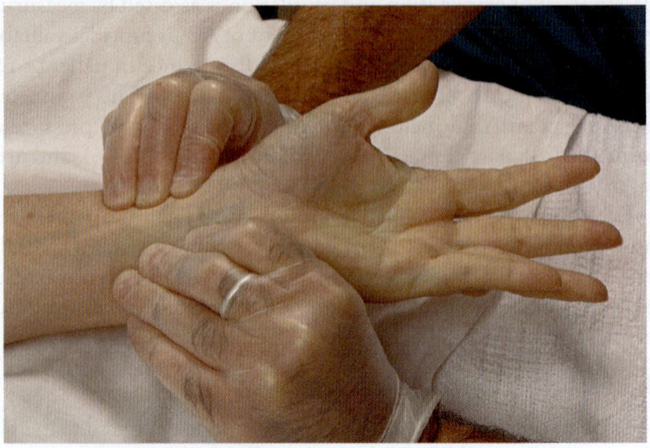

STEP 6A(3) Patient opening hand; note colour.

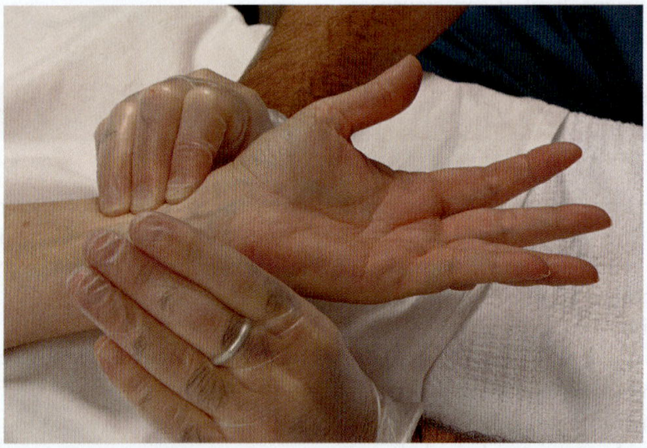

STEP 6A(4) Release pressure over ulnar artery and note colour of hand.

Critical Decision Point *If there is no flushing in 15 seconds, Allen test is negative. You should repeat it on the other arm or choose another artery for puncture* (MacDonald et al., 2024).

STEP	RATIONALE
b. Assess accessibility of vessel.	Palpating, stabilizing, and performing venipuncture of superficial artery is easier. Superficial arteries are located at distal ends of extremities.
c. Assess tissue surrounding artery.	Muscle, tendon, and fat have decreased sensation to pain. Bony periosteum and nerves are highly sensitive to pain.
d. Assess that arteries are not directly adjacent to veins.	Helps reduce chance of venous puncture and possibility of inaccurate samples.
7. Assess arterial sites for use in obtaining specimen.	Arterial blood may be obtained from areas where strong pulses are palpable (i.e., radial, brachial, or femoral artery) (MacDonald et al., 2024).

Critical Decision Point *Previous puncture sites or pre-existing conditions may eliminate potential sites (see employer policy). Artery should be easily accessible.*

STEP	RATIONALE
a. Radial artery	Safest, most accessible site for puncture. It is superficial, is not adjacent to large veins, usually has adequate collateral circulation by ulnar artery, and is relatively painless if periosteum is avoided. Used when Allen test is positive.

STEP	RATIONALE
ASSESSMENT	
b. Brachial artery	Has reasonable collateral blood flow, is less superficial, is more difficult to palpate and stabilize, carries increased risk for venous puncture, and results in increased discomfort for patient if brachial nerve is punctured. It is used when radial artery is inaccessible or Allen test is negative.
c. Femoral artery	Nurses without specialized training should not use this artery. It has no adequate collateral flow if obstructed below inguinal ligament, is difficult to stabilize, is deep, and is directly adjacent to the femoral vein. It is the best artery to use in emergency (e.g., cardiac arrest or hypovolemic shock when pulses are difficult to palpate).
8. Review baseline ABG values for patient.	Provides baseline for comparison and evaluation of therapies.
9. Determine patient's knowledge about ABG procedure.	Obtaining blood specimen is painful. Patient who is knowledgeable will be more cooperative.

NURSING DIAGNOSES

- Reduced gas exchange
- Reduced airway clearance
- Inadequate breathing pattern
- Inadequate peripheral tissue perfusion
- Anxiety
- Insufficient knowledge regarding ABGs
- Potential for injury

Related factors and risk factors are individualized on the basis of patient's condition or needs.

STEP	RATIONALE
PLANNING	
1. Expected outcomes following completion of procedure:	
• Patient's ABG values are within normal range.	Indicates adequate oxygenation.
• Patient's extremity distal to puncture remains warm and pink, has adequate capillary refill, and is free of pain.	Indicates adequate arterial circulation to extremity.
• Patient denies anxiety, and respiratory rate remains within baseline.	Anxiety increases respiratory rate, which can alter ABG results.
• Patient correctly discusses ABG procedure.	Indicates learning.
2. Prepare heparinized syringe (if not in commercial kit).	Heparin mixes with specimen to prevent clotting.
a. Aspirate 0.5 mL sodium heparin (1 000 units/mL) into syringe from vial or ampule.	Prevents blood sample from clotting before reaching laboratory. Excessive heparin can affect pH of arterial sample.
b. Withdraw plunger entire length of syringe. Maintain asepsis.	Coats inside of barrel of syringe with heparin.
c. Eject all heparin in barrel out of syringe.	In hub of syringe 0.15–0.25 mL of sodium heparin remains; 0.05 mL of sodium heparin adequately anticoagulates 1 mL of blood; 0.15 mL adequately anticoagulates 3 mL without affecting pH level.
3. Explain steps and purpose of procedure to patient.	Reduces anxiety and promotes understanding and cooperation.
IMPLEMENTATION	
1.	Proper hand hygiene helps prevent the spread of infectious agents to health care providers.
2. Palpate selected radial, femoral, or brachial site with fingertips.	Determines area of maximal impulse for puncture site.
3. Using radial artery, elevate patient's wrist with small pillow and ask them to extend fingers downward. Stabilize artery through slight hyperextension of wrist.	Flexes wrist and positions radial artery closer to surface. Reduces mobility of artery and makes insertion of needle easier.
4. Apply clean gloves. Clean area of maximal impulse with alcohol swab or antiseptic swab (check employer or manufacturer recommendation). Wipe in circular motion away from site or use back-and-forth strokes. Allow to dry.	Reduces number of resident bacteria on surface of skin. Drying maximizes antibacterial effects.

STEP	RATIONALE
5. Hold 5 cm × 5 cm (2 inch × 2 inch) gauze with same fingers used to palpate artery.	Keeps gauze pad accessible for covering puncture site when necessary.
6. Use corner of sterile gauze pad or alcohol wipe to point to chosen site.	Maintaining location of artery improves likelihood of successful puncture.
7. Hold needle bevel up and insert at 30- to 45-degree angle into artery. Prepare patient for needle-stick because radial sticks are painful.	Angle allows for better arterial flow into needle. Prepared patient will be less likely to withdraw arm.
8. Stop advancing needle when blood is noted returning into hub of needle or syringe.	Quick return of blood indicates that arterial flow is obtained. Prevents puncturing through both sides of artery.
9. Allow arterial pulsations to pump 2–3 mL of blood into heparinized syringe slowly (see Step 9 illustration).	Allowing pulsations to help fill syringe reduces presence of air bubbles in sample. Bubbles alter ABG results.
10. When sampling is complete, hold 5 cm × 5 cm (2 inch × 2 inch) gauze over puncture site, withdraw syringe and needle, and activate safety guard over needle.	Pad minimizes pulling of skin as needle is withdrawn. Decreases contamination from blood and accidental needle-stick.
11. Apply pressure over and just proximal to puncture site with pad (see Step 11 illustration).	Insertion of needle into artery is just proximal to insertion site through skin. Gauze absorbs any blood that might ooze from site.
12. Maintain continuous pressure on and proximal to site for 3–5 minutes (approximately 15 minutes if patient is undergoing anticoagulant therapy or has bleeding disorder) (MacDonald et al., 2024). Have another nurse remove safety needle and attach filter cap to syringe (see Step 15 below) if prolonged pressure is needed.	To avoid hematoma formation, apply and hold pressure or apply a pressure dressing to arterial puncture site for 3–5 minutes (MacDonald et al., 2024). Prevents delay in preparing syringe in ice.

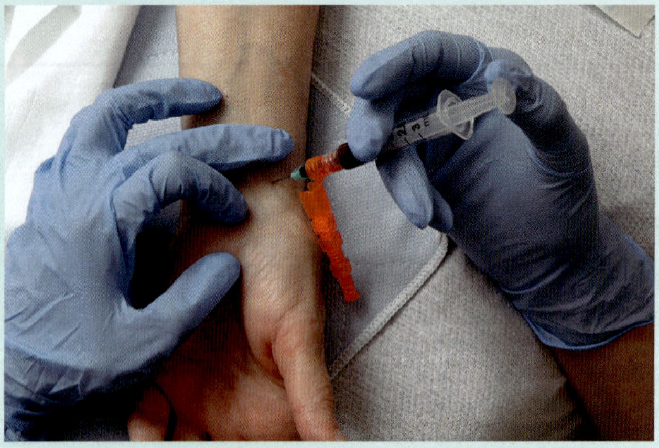

STEP 9 Blood flowing into syringe.

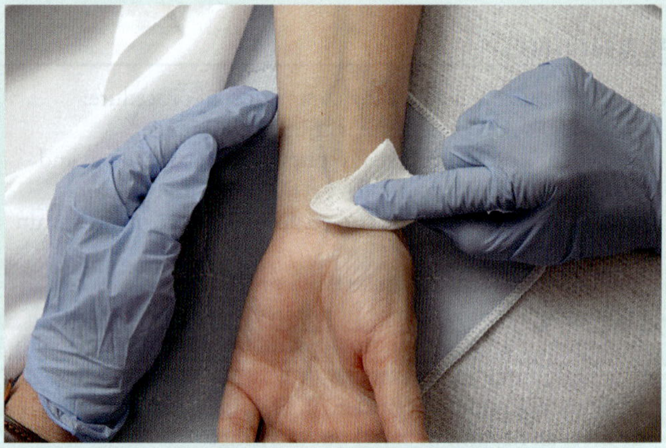

STEP 11 Apply firm pressure to arterial puncture site.

STEP	RATIONALE
13. Visually inspect site for signs of bleeding or hematoma formation.	Determines whether continued need exists to exert pressure. Because artery rather than vein has been accessed, monitor puncture site for bleeding.
14. Palpate artery below or distal to puncture site.	Determines whether pulse quality has changed, indicating alteration in arterial flow.
15. Take syringe, remove safety needle, and discard needle in appropriate biohazard container. Attach filter cap to syringe (available in kit) to expel air or cover tip of syringe with 5 cm × 5 cm (2 inch × 2 inch) sterile gauze to expel air (see employer procedure). Some kits may have all supplies, including syringe with heparin, needle with safety needle cap, and filter cap that allows air (but not blood) to vent (see Step 15 illustration).	Decreases chance of contamination from room air. Air bubbles in specimen can falsely elevate or decrease results, depending on patient's blood gas concentration (Van Leeuwen & Bladh, 2021).

STEP	RATIONALE

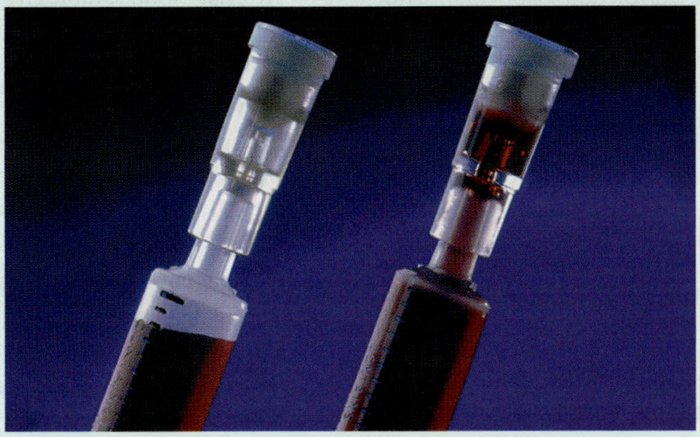

STEP 15 **Filter-Pro Air Bubble Removal Device expels air safely from syringe without accidentally expelling blood and aerosolizing sample.** *(With permission from Smiths Medical, Carlsbad, CA.)*

STEP	RATIONALE
16. Prepare syringe for laboratory analysis (according to employer policy).	
a. Place patient identification label on syringe in front of patient; confirm person-specific identifiers (Accreditation Canada, 2020).	Ensures proper identification of sample.
b. Place syringe in cup of crushed ice (check employer policy).	Failure to place ABG sample on ice can affect results of pH, PaO_2, and $PaCO_2$ (MacDonald et al., 2024).
c. Attach properly labelled laboratory requisition to blood gas sample. Add appropriate patient data (e.g., hemoglobin, mode and flow of supplemental oxygen, and patient's body temperature) (check employer policy).	Prevents mislabelled specimens. Hemoglobin level, supplemental oxygen, and hypothermia or hyperthermia affect PaO_2 and $PaCO_2$ values.
17. Place sample in biohazard bag. Send sample to laboratory immediately.	Prevents alteration in gas tensions resulting from metabolic processes that continue after blood is drawn.
18. Remove gloves and discard.	Reduces transmission of microorganisms.

EVALUATION

1. Inspect puncture site and area distal to puncture site for complications.	An artery can be obstructed, or important structures anatomically juxtaposed to an artery can be penetrated (MacDonald et al., 2024).
2. Review results of sample as soon as possible.	Identifies any abnormality and expedites initiation of treatment.
3. **Use teach-back:** "I want to be sure I explained the way I will obtain your blood sample. Tell me the steps I will use to obtain this specimen." Develop a revised teaching plan if patient or caregiver is unable to teach back correctly.	Determines level of understanding of instructional topic.

Unexpected Outcomes	Related Interventions
1. Patient has abnormal ABG values.	• Continue to monitor patient. • Notify health care provider of findings and obtain further prescriptions.
2. Patient has hematoma formation at puncture site.	• Continue to monitor patient. • Notify health care provider.
3. Puncture site is bruised or continues to bleed.	• Apply pressure. • Notify health care provider if bleeding continues.

Communication and Documentation

- Document results of Allen test, location and condition of puncture site, patient's tolerance of procedure, and disposition of specimen to laboratory in progress notes in EHR or chart.
- Communicate ABG results to health care provider as soon as available.
- Document patient's fraction of inspired oxygen concentration (FiO_2) and any ventilator settings (e.g., tidal volume [Vt], respiratory frequency [RF], mode of ventilation).
- Document your evaluation of patient and caregiver learning.
- Document results of test in progress notes in EHR or chart.

DOCUMENTATION EXAMPLE

Patient (she/her) required ABG result for qualifying home oxygen program; health care provider performed Allen test. The patient's palm colour returned to normal in less than 5 seconds. Successfully obtained left radial artery blood sample, patient tolerated procedure well. Sample was immediately delivered to the lab.

Special Considerations

Teaching

- Teach patient to report numbness, burning, and/or tingling during and after in hand that had radial artery puncture.

Pediatric

- In neonatal and pediatric patients, you can use capillary blood gas. Procedures are similar to those for obtaining heelsticks.
- Neonatal patients, especially premature infants, will often have normal ABG values that differ from those in adults.
- Arterial blood samples from punctures are painful and cause crying and breath holding, which affect the accuracy of ABG values (decreases PaO_2) (Hockenberry et al., 2024).

Gerontological

- Pay special attention during interpretation of ABGs for patients with chronic pulmonary conditions. In these patients, compensatory mechanisms may allow normal pH in face of markedly elevated $PaCO_2$.

Patients With Physical or Cognitive Challenges

- This is a painful procedure, and patients with physical or cognitive challenges may not be able to understand the procedure. Some patients may require medication to reduce any procedure-related anxiety (Mendes, 2018).

✦ REVIEW QUESTIONS

1. *An 88-year-old patient (she/her) is admitted from home to the health care facility. The patient has an in-dwelling Foley catheter. Her urine is dark and cloudy. She is pulling at her Foley catheter, and is restless and confused. Vitals are as follows: temperature: 38.4°C; blood pressure: 88/50 mm Hg; pulse: 128 beats/min.* On the basis of these findings, which laboratory specimens would you expect to obtain?
2. *A patient was diagnosed with type 1 diabetes mellitus 2 years ago. The patient was admitted with diabetic ketoacidosis (DKA) related to an upper respiratory infection associated with a past history of chronic obstructive pulmonary disease (COPD). The patient states that they quit taking insulin because they were nauseated and vomiting. You observe that the patient has multiple puncture sites that are reddened on the central tip of the fingers. The patient states that their fingertips are sore. They are expected to be discharged home the next day.* Which instructions will you provide to the patient to help with self-management of type 1 diabetes mellitus?
3. *This same patient was to be discharged today, but during the night the patient developed shortness of breath. The patient has received multiple respiratory treatments over the past 3 hours, yet you observe that their work of breathing has increased dramatically.* Using SBAR (situation–background–assessment–recommendation), show how you would communicate with the health care team.
4. A urine specimen for culture and sensitivity is being collected from a patient with male genitalia. Which steps should be used to obtain an accurate specimen? (*Select all that apply.*)
   1. Check two person-specific identifiers.
   2. Help patient to perform pericare before the sterile part of the procedure.
   3. Wipe head of the penis back and forth three times with each swab.
   4. Collect 10–20 mL for the sample.
   5. Have patient initially void into a bedpan or clean container.
   6. Have patient hold penis above the sterile specimen cup without touching the container.
5. The nurse is preparing to obtain a throat culture on a 22-year-old patient. Which step(s) would facilitate obtaining an accurate specimen? (*Select all that apply.*)
   1. Placing patient in a sitting position or with head elevated at a 45-degree angle
   2. Having patient lean head forward
   3. Inserting swab without touching lips, teeth, tongue, or cheeks
   4. Swabbing the tonsillar area
   5. Swabbing the uvula
   6. Having patient blow her nose
6. Place the following steps for collecting a sterile urine specimen for culture and sensitivity (C&S) from a Luer-Lok catheter port in the correct order:
   1. Attach Luer-Lok syringe to Luer-Lok port.
   2. Clamp drainage tube with clamp or rubber band for 15 minutes.
   3. Clean catheter entry port and wait for disinfectant to dry.
   4. Unclamp catheter and allow urine to flow into drainage bag.
   5. Aspirate 3 mL of urine into syringe attached to Luer-Lok.

Visit the Evolve site for a complete list of answers to the Review Questions.

✦ NEXT GENERATION NCLEX® (NGN)

For practice with answering exam questions related to unfolding NGN case studies, please consult the Next Generation NCLEX® (NGN)-Style Case Studies for Skills and Techniques on the Evolve website: http://evolve.elsevier.com/Canada/Perry/clinicalskills/

REFERENCES

Accreditation Canada. (2020). *Required organizational practices handbook.* https://physicians.nshealth.ca/resources/required-organizational-practices-2020-handbook

Alberta Precision Laboratories. (2022). *Blood culture collection guideline.* https://www.albertahealthservices.ca/assets/wf/lab/if-lab-tc-blood-culture-collection-guideline-mi6805.pdf

Alberta Precision Laboratories. (2023). *Factors affecting blood test results.* https://www.albertahealthservices.ca/assets/wf/lab/if-lab-tc-cal-factors-affecting-blood-test-results-px-sc250.pdf

BC Guidelines and Protocols Advisory Committee. (2020). *Urinary tract infections in the primary care setting–Investigation.* https://www2.gov.bc.ca/gov/content/health/practitioner-professional-resources/bc-guidelines/urinary-tract-infections

Boscart, V., McCleary, L., Sheiban Taucar, L., et al. (2023). *Ebersole and Hess' gerontological nursing and healthy aging in Canada* (3rd ed.). Elsevier.

Cadham Provincial Laboratory. (2020). *Guide to services 2020.* https://www.gov.mb.ca/health/publichealth/cpl/docs/guide_to_services.pdf

Canadian Cancer Society. (2022). *Screening for colorectal cancer.* https://cancer.ca/en/cancer-information/cancer-types/colorectal/screening

Centers for Disease Control and Prevention. (2011). *Infection prevention during blood glucose monitoring and insulin administration.* https://www.cdc.gov/injectionsafety/blood-glucose-monitoring.html

Cheng, A. Y. Y., Feig, D. S., Ho, J., et al. (2021). Blood glucose monitoring in adults and children with diabetes: Update 2021. *Canadian Journal of Diabetes*, *45*(7), 580–587. https://doi.org/10.1016/j.jcjd.2021.07.003

Choi, S., Choi, S. J., Jeon, B. R., et al. (2021). What we should consider in point of care blood glucose test. Current quality management status of a single institution. *Medicina (Kaunas, Lithuania)*, *57*(3), Article 238. https://doi.org/10.3390/medicina57030238. https://doi.org/10.3390/medicina57030238

de Moissac, D., & Bowen, S. (2019). Impact of language barriers on quality of care and patient safety for official language minority Francophones in Canada. *Journal of Patient Experience*, *3*, 24–32. https://doi.org/10.1177/2374373518769008

Diabetes Canada Clinical Practice Guidelines Expert Committee. (2018). Diabetes Canada 2018 clinical practice guidelines for the prevention and management of diabetes in Canada. *Canadian Journal of Diabetes*, *42*(Suppl. 1), S1–S325. https://guidelines.diabetes.ca/cpg

Fleishman, J., Kamsky, H., & Sundborg, S. (2019). Trauma-informed nursing practice. *Online Journal of Issues in Nursing*, *24*(2), Article 3. https://doi.org/10.3912/OJIN.Vol24No02Man03

Fraser Health Authority. (2018). *Central venous catheters in adult patients–Self-learning module*. https://www.fraserhealth.ca/-/media/Project/FraserHealth/FraserHealth/Health-Professionals/Professionals-Resources/Acute-Care-Orientation/CVC-Self-Learning-Package-v9-June-2018-FINAL.pdf

Giannoumis, M. (2021). Approach to: Pediatric urinary tract infection (UTI). McGill *Journal of Medicine*, *19*(2). https://doi.org/10.26443/mjm.v19i1.312

Haalboom, M., Blokhuis-Arkes, M. H. E., Beuk, R. J., et al. (2018). Wound swab and wound biopsy yield similar culture results: Culture results of swab versus biopsy. *Wound Repair and Regeneration*, *26*(5), 192–199. https://doi.org/10.1111/wrr.12629

Hockenberry, M. J., Duffy, E. A., & Gibbs, K. (2024). *Wong's nursing care of infants and children* (12th ed.). Elsevier.

Institute for Quality Management in Healthcare. (2019). *Care considerations for inclusion of gender diversity within medical laboratory services (version 2.0)*. https://diagnostics.accreditation.ca/Portals/1/Docs/Resources/Education/White%20Paper%20-%20Care%20Considerations%20for%20Inclusion%20of%20Gender%20Diversity%20Within%20Medical%20Laboratory%20Services.pdf

Keenan-Lindsay, L., Sams, C., & O'Connor, C. L. (2022). *Perry's maternal child nursing care in Canada* (3rd ed.). Elsevier Inc.

Macdonald, S., Pagana, K. D., Pagana, T. J., et al. (2024). *Pagana's Canadian manual of diagnostic and laboratory tests* (3rd ed.). Elsevier Inc.

May, O. W. (2018). Urine collection methods in children: Which is the best? *Nursing Clinics of North America*, *53*(2), 137–143. https://doi.org/10.1016/j.cnur.2018.01.001

McCall, R. (2021). *Phlebotomy essentials* (Enhanced 7th ed.). Jones & Bartlett.

Mendes, A. (2018). Meeting the care needs of a person with dementia who is distressed. *British Journal of Nursing*, *27*(4), Article 219. https://doi.org/10.12968/bjon.2018.27.4.219

National Collaborating Centre for Infectious Diseases. (2020). *Canadian Public Health Laboratory Network best practices for COVID-19 V1.0* https://nccid.ca/wp-content/uploads/sites/2/2020/05/COVID-Best-Practices-V1.01-v3.pdf

Orsted, H. L., Keast, D. H., Forest-Lalande, L., et al. (2017/2021). Best practice recommendations for the prevention and management of wounds. *In Foundations of best practice for skin and wound management–A supplement of Wound Care Canada Wounds Canada*. https://www.woundscanada.ca/docman/public/health-care-professional/bpr-workshop/165-wc-bpr-prevention-and-management-of-wounds/file

Perez-Guzman, M. C., Shang, T., Zhang, J. Y., et al. (2021). Continuous glucose monitoring in the hospital. *Endocrinology and Metabolism*, *36*(2), 240–255. https://doi.org/10.3803/EnM.2021.201

Perry, A. G., Potter, P. A., Ostendorf, W., et al. (2021). *Clinical nursing skills and techniques* (10th ed.). Elsevier Canada.

Public Health Agency of Canada (PHAC). (2021a). *Canadian biosafety guidelines*. https://www.canada.ca/en/public-health/services/canadian-biosafety-standards-guidelines/guidance.html

Public Health Agency of Canada (PHAC). (2021b). *Infection prevention and control for COVID-19: Interim guidance for acute healthcare settings*. https://www.canada.ca/en/public-health/services/diseases/2019-novel-coronavirus-infection/health-professionals/infection-prevention-control-covid-19-second-interim-guidance.html

Shared Health. (2022). *Provincial requirements for personal protective equipment (PPE)*. https://sharedhealthmb.ca/files/covid-19-provincial-ppe-requirements.pdf

Simundic, A., Baird, G., Cadamurro, J., et al. (2020). Managing hemolyzed samples in clinical laboratories. *Critical Reviews in Clinical Laboratory Sciences*, *57*(1), 1–21. https://doi.org/10.1080/10408363.2019.1664391

Steiner, K., Baron-Stefaniak, J., Hirschl, A. M., et al. (2020). Education of medical personnel optimizes filling volume of blood culture bottles without negatively affecting microbiology testing. *BMC Health Service Research*, *20*, Article 1105. https://doi.org/10.1186/s12913-020-05959-z

Sullivan, W., Diepstra, H., Heng, J., et al. (2018). Primary care of adults with intellectual and developmental disabilities: 2018 Canadian consensus guidelines. *Canadian Family Physician*, *64*(4), 254–279. https://www.cfp.ca/content/64/4/254

Van Leeuwen, A. M., & Bladh, M. L. (2021). *Davis's comprehensive handbook of laboratory and diagnostic tests with nursing implications* (9th ed.). F. A. Davis.

Warekois, R. S., Robinson, R., & Primrose, P. B. (2020). Special collections and procedures. In *Phlebotomy: Worktext and procedures manual* (5th ed., pp. 218–233). Elsevier.

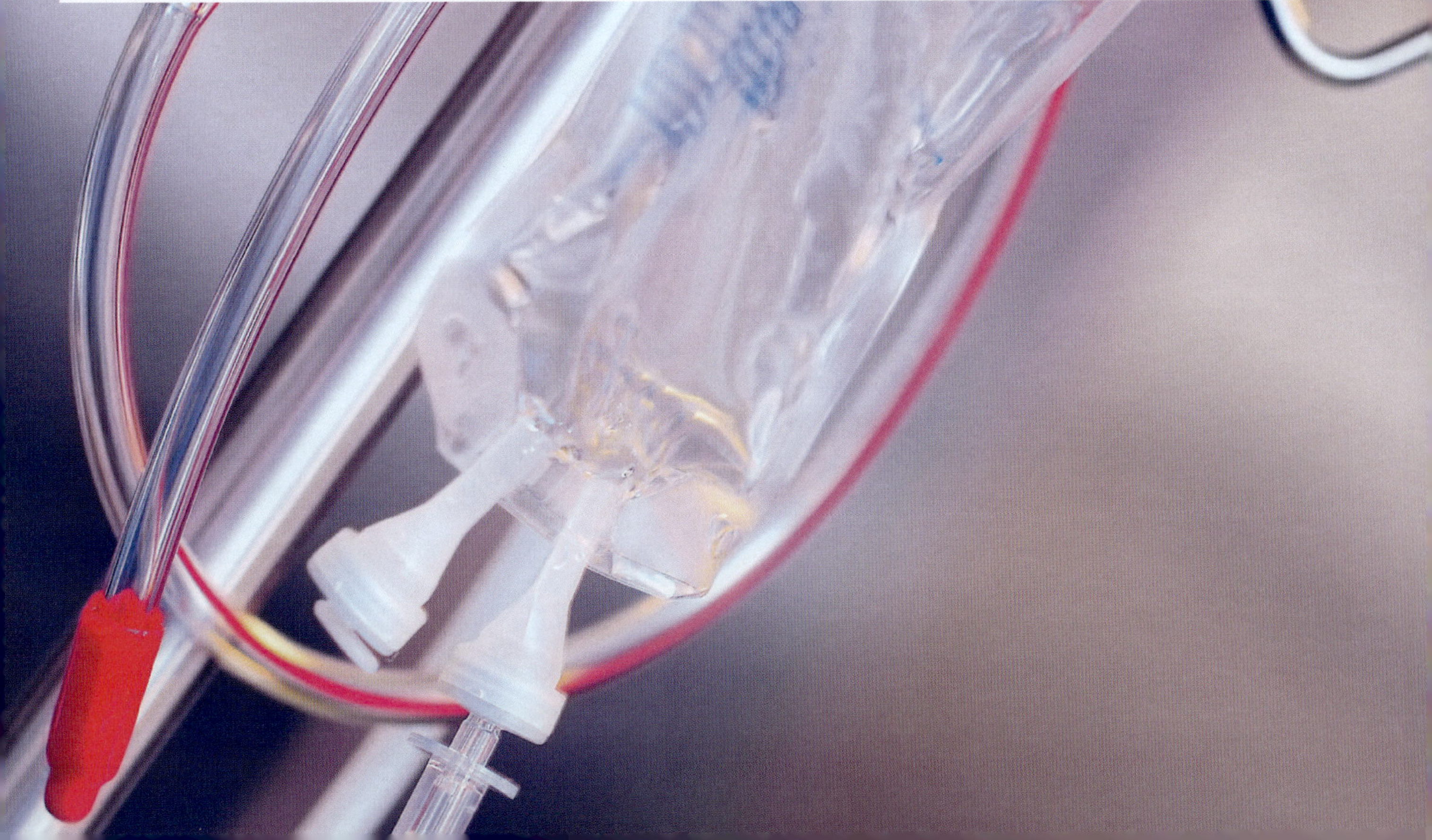

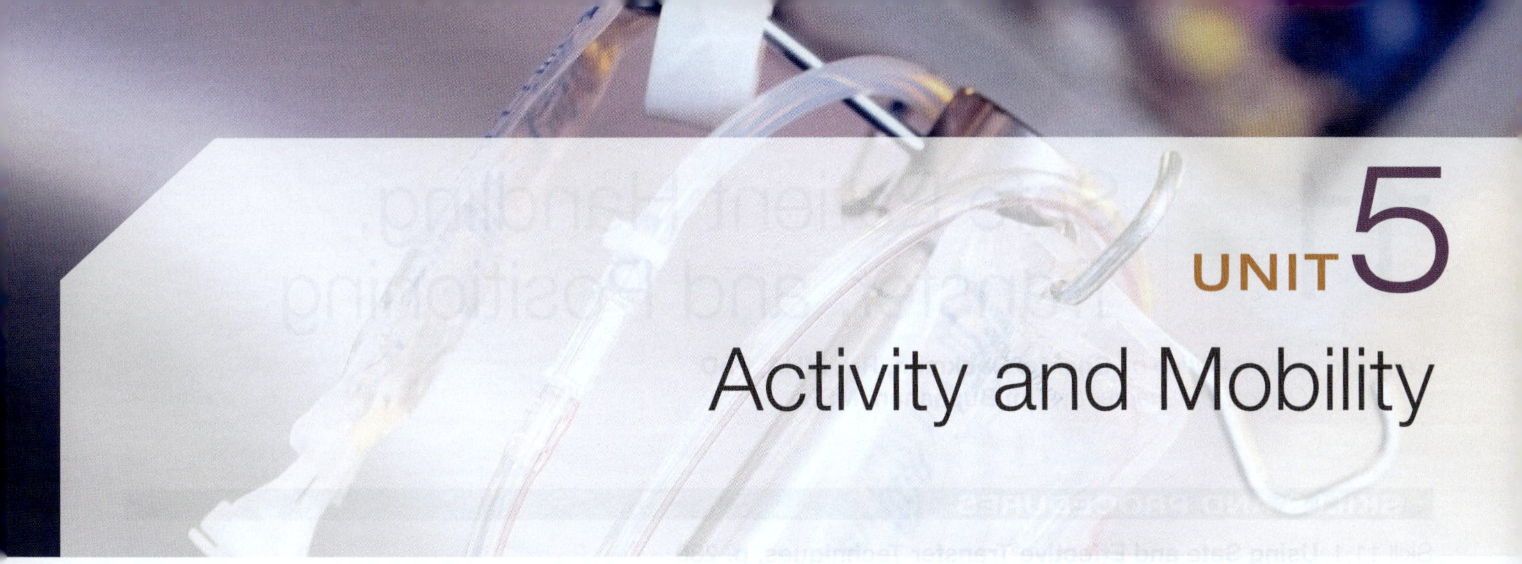

UNIT 5
Activity and Mobility

Safe activity and mobility practices are important for both the health care provider and the patient. Health care agencies are responsible for providing nurses with safety information, training, and resources to use when transferring, positioning, and lifting patients, but it is a nurse's responsibility to use these correctly. A nurse's knowledge about and skills in safe, efficient transfer and positioning techniques and use of assistive equipment ensures safe patient transfer and mobility without injury to the patient or nurse.

To maintain your safety when positioning or transferring patients, you must fully understand and apply the principles for safe patient handling. Prior to moving a patient, use your clinical judgement to assess your knowledge and skill level for safe patient handling, transfer, and positioning. Assess the patient and determine whether they will be able to assist with movement. Consider patient factors such as balance, weight, weight-bearing ability, and cognitive status, as these can either facilitate or impede safe patient positioning. Assess whether the patient can understand directions about positioning. Determine what resources, such as a lift team or hydraulic lift devices, are available. Assess for obstacles in the environment that make positioning difficult. Critically think about your prior experience in safely transferring and positioning patients. What worked? What did not work? What resources did you use? What resources were missing? Determine the number of people needed to safely transfer the patient, and plan and discuss the steps of the procedure before initiating the transfer. Using clinical judgement in the assessment and analysis of data assists in planning and implementing safe patient transfer and positioning.

Safe mobility practices include early progressive activity and exercise. This activity decreases length of hospital stays and improves posthospital rehabilitation. Use your clinical judgement to correctly assess and analyze data to support a mobility plan. For example, data collected in an outpatient setting for stable or recovering patients may include routine activity and frequency of the activity. However, patients recovering from a myocardial infarction will require assessment of activity tolerance because they will need a prescribed, graduated activity plan. Your knowledge about a patient and their disease processes will assist you in assessing and planning appropriate activity. The skills in this unit outline specific mobility exercises and the use of assistive devices. Your clinical judgement guides your clinical decision making in individualizing activity interventions for a patient's level of health and evaluating a patient's response to activity.

However, there are situations in which immobile patients require support surfaces and special beds to prevent complications of immobility. In these situations, patients have conditions such as paralysis, bilateral leg amputations, and obesity that place them at risk for pressure injuries. To provide safe patient care, use your clinical judgement to continually assess and analyze the patient to determine whether a support surface is necessary to prevent pressure injuries. Use your employer's skin care/wound care resource nurse to determine the best surface for each patient. Once the patient is on the support surface, you will need to recognize and analyze cues to determine the patient's response to and tolerance of the support surface.

11 Safe Patient Handling, Transfer, and Positioning

Canadian content written by **Chantal Backman, RN, MHA, PhD**
Original US chapter by **Tim Buchanan, MSN**

SKILLS AND PROCEDURES

OBJECTIVES

Mastery of content in this chapter will enable the nurse to:

- Describe principles of safe patient handling, transfer, and positioning.
- Explain the correct use of body mechanics/techniques to prevent self-injury and promote health care workers' and patients' safety.
- Explain the importance of using mechanical lifts and other assist devices when moving, positioning, and transferring patients.
- Perform an assessment for determining the type of approach to use and amount of help needed to transfer and position patients safely.
- Describe transfer and positioning procedures to follow to ensure patient and nurse safety.
- Describe positioning techniques for the supported Fowler's, supine, prone, 30-degree lateral side-lying, and semiprone positions.
- Describe the procedures for helping a patient move up in bed, helping a patient to a sitting position, logrolling a patient, and transferring a patient from a bed to a chair.

MEDIA RESOURCES

- http://evolve.elsevier.com/Canada/Perry/clinicalskills/

PURPOSE

Health care facilities are required to provide employees with safety information and education to properly transfer, position, and lift patients. The greatest risk factor for overexertion injuries in health care workers is the manual lifting, moving, and repositioning of patients. Such patient tasks occur repeatedly during a nurse's routine shift of care, resulting in high rates of nursing injuries (Baptiste-McKinney & Halvorson, 2018). The use of correct body mechanics, including general principles of good body mechanics (e.g., not bending or twisting at the waist; lifting with the legs while moving stretchers/beds and getting supplies), are important to avoid injuries while placing less strain on the musculoskeletal system. However, relying on proper body mechanics and manual lifting techniques alone is not effective for reducing health care workers' musculoskeletal injuries. A comprehensive safe patient-handling program that combines management commitment with employee involvement, policies, and proper mechanical equipment availability and education is needed (Canadian Centre for Occupational Health and Safety [CCOHS], 2018).

Nurses might need to move, roll, steady, and position patients while using lifting equipment. However, because most musculoskeletal injuries in care facilities are cumulative, any steps taken to minimize the potential for musculoskeletal injuries during patient-handling tasks benefit health care workers. Nurses should always refer to their employer's policies. Many patients have conditions that result in immobility or require limitations in activity imposed by their treatment plan. It is an important nursing role to safely and correctly position and move patients to reduce the risks associated with immobilization such as skin breakdown, pneumonia, and thromboembolism. When performing the skills in this chapter, it is essential to use safe patient-handling techniques.

STANDARDS OF CARE

- Accreditation Canada (2020)—*Required Organizational Practices–2020 Handbook* (https://physicians.nshealth.ca/resources/required-organizational-practices-2020-handbook)
- Canadian Centre for Occupational Health and Safety (CCOHS, 2012)—*Patient Lifts and Worker Risks* (http://www.ccohs.ca/newsletters/hsreport/issues/2012/08/ezine.html)
- Canadian Centre for Occupational Health and Safety (CCOHS, 2018)—*Ergonomic Safe Patient Handling Program* (https://www.ccohs.ca/oshanswers/hsprograms/patient_handling.html)

PRINCIPLES FOR PRACTICE

- Body mechanics are the coordinated effort of the musculoskeletal and nervous systems to maintain balance, posture, and body alignment during lifting, bending, moving, and performing activities of daily living (ADLs).

- The use of safe patient transfer and positioning techniques helps patients achieve an optimal level of independence without resultant injury to health care providers.
- Teaching the use of safe patient-handling equipment in combination with proper body mechanics is more effective than either one in isolation (CCOHS, 2018).
- Patient repositioning is a procedure where a patient is moved to a new position on the same surface (e.g., repositioning in bed or while seated).
- Patient transfers are used to assist a patient who can totally bear weight or at least bear weight with one leg or both arms to move from one surface to another (e.g., from sitting to standing). A transfer assessment is always completed to assess weight-bearing ability, weight, and patient medical conditions.
- Patient lifts are designed to carry the entire weight of the patient and transfer patients from one place to another (e.g., from bed to bath, chair to stretcher). Patient lifts are usually done using mechanical devices (e.g., ceiling lift, sling lift, sit-to-stand lift) (Fig. 11.1).
- Use of lifting/transfer equipment and devices, ergonomic assessments and controls, no-lift policies, and training and education are recommended (Matz, 2019).
- Key principles in determining the proper handling techniques to use for patients include identifying whether a patient is weight bearing and knowing the patient's weight and height, strength, and ability to cooperate and provide help (CCOHS, 2018).
- Patients who are at high risk for complications from improper positioning and injury during transfer include those with poor nutrition, poor circulation, loss of sensation, alterations in bone formation or joint mobility, and impaired muscle development.

PERSON-CENTRED CARE

- Ultimately, it is a patient's choice to increase their mobility and activity level. Practise person-centred nursing care by considering a patient's knowledge, cultural beliefs, and attitudes about the loss of independent activity and the person's willingness to participate in activity when developing a plan of care.

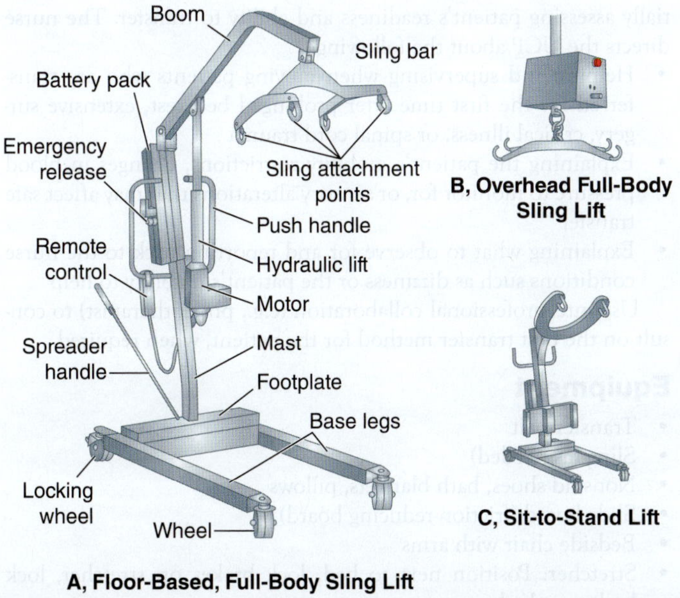

FIG 11.1 Examples of mechanical lifts. A, Floor-based, full-body sling lift. B, Overhead full-body sling lift. C, Sit-to-stand lift. (*From US Food and Drug Administration [FDA]. [n.d.]. Patient lifts: Safety guide [p. 2].* https://www.fda.gov/media/88149/download)

- Use simple language when providing patients information about the complications of immobility and their unique risks.
- Consider the circumstances surrounding a patient's loss of independent activity and mobility to ensure that a plan of care is realistic and attainable.
- Understand to what extent the patient chooses to have a caregiver involved to learn transfer and positioning techniques for care at home.

EVIDENCE-INFORMED PRACTICE

There is more evidence available about the techniques necessary to reduce workplace injuries within health care facilities.

- Inpatient health care facilities have some of the highest rates of injury and illness among all industries. In 2021, the health and social services industry had 67 685 lost time claims out of the 277 217 total claims made in Canada (Association of Workers' Compensation Boards of Canada, 2021).
- CCOHS (2018) has provided guidelines for how to complete an ergonomics hazard assessment based on patient population, patient-handling tasks, and physical environment. It is critical to educate health care staff about devices, equipment, and patient-handling policies.
- Most organizations have developed "no-lift" policies that discourage manual lifting and require the use of safe handling of equipment and devices as needed (CCOHS, 2018; Occupational Health Clinic for Ontario Workers Inc., 2022).
- Many provinces have implemented safe patient-handling and mobility programs to improve safety for patients and health care workers in order to mitigate the risk associated with patient handling or mobility activities (e.g., Nova Scotia Health, 2022).
- Knowledge about safe, efficient transfer and positioning techniques (Box 11.1) and proper use of assistive equipment and devices promotes safe patient transfer without injury to a patient or health care worker (CCOHS, 2018).

SAFETY GUIDELINES

- Know how physiological influences on body alignment and mobility affect patients throughout the lifespan. Inactive older persons are at risk for muscle atrophy, loss of bone mass, contractures of joints, and pressure injury (Boscart et al., 2023).
- Always promote the patient's independence when possible (e.g., decision making for time to perform activities) while safely adhering to any prescribed rehabilitation plan.

BOX 11.1

Principles of Safe Body Mechanics When Transferring and Positioning Patients

Mechanical lifts and lift teams are essential when a patient is unable to help. When a patient is able to help, remember these principles:

- The lower the centre of gravity, the greater the stability of the nurse.
- The equilibrium of an object is maintained as long as the line of gravity passes through its base of support.
- Facing the direction of movement prevents abnormal twisting of the spine.
- Dividing balanced activity between arms and legs reduces the risk for back injury.
- Leverage, rolling, turning, and pivoting require less work than lifting.
- When friction is reduced between the object to be moved and the surface on which it is moved, less force is required to move it.

- Control the factors that can indirectly affect body mechanics by making the environment safe. Cluttered hallways and bedside areas increase a patient's risk of falling (see Chapter 42). To avoid patient injury, clear the immediate environment of any obstacles where a patient will stand/walk.
- Arrange equipment (e.g., intravenous [IV] lines, feeding tubes, Foley catheter) so that it will not interfere with the transfer process.
- Mentally review the steps of a transfer before beginning to ensure the safety of both the patient and the nurse. This mental review assists the nurse in determining the amount and type of assistance required for transfer, including type of transfer equipment and the number of personnel it will take to safely transfer and prevent harm or injury.
- Assess a patient's range of motion. Contractures or spasticity limit joint and muscle mobility; take care not to position a patient's limb in an unnatural position. This could result in injury or dysfunction of the affected limb (see Chapter 12).
- Determine a patient's level of sensory perception (vision and hearing) because this affects the person's ability to cooperate during transfer and lifting procedures (see Chapter 8).
- Loss of sensation increases vulnerability to the hazards of immobility because of the inability to sense pain or the need for repositioning.
- Use assistive equipment and devices to transfer and position patients safely.

BOX 11.2

Bedrail Safety Tips

A patient can get trapped in the bedrails of a hospital bed.

Before Using Bedrails

- Assess whether a patient would benefit from the use of bedrails.
- Know the potential areas of entrapment (within the rail, under the rail, between the rail and the mattress, between split bedrails, between the end of the rail and the side edge of the headboard or footboard, and between the headboard or footboard and the end of the mattress).
- Make sure the mattress is the right size.
- Use a mattress with raised foam edges.
- Contact the manufacturer for the product safety information and ensure regular maintenance of the bedrail latching system.

When Using Bedrails

- Lower sections of the bedrail (if possible).
- Make sure all latches are securely fastened.
- Monitor patient regularly and report any bed-related incidents.

- Evaluate patient for correct body alignment and pressure injury risks after a transfer.
- Know the risk factors for bed entrapment in the hospital or long-term care facility and in home health care, and how to prevent it (Box 11.2) (Government of Canada, 2015).
- Educate patients and caregivers about how equipment functions in order to reduce their anxiety and enlist their cooperation.

✦ SKILL 11.1 Using Safe and Effective Transfer Techniques

NSO *Nursing Skills Online Safety Module 1 / Lesson 3*

Safe and effective transfer is a nursing skill for assisting dependent patients or patients with restricted mobility to attain positions to regain or maintain optimal independence. For example, transferring from a bed to a chair promotes physical activity to maintain and improve joint motion, increase strength, promote circulation, relieve pressure on the skin, and improve urinary and respiratory functions (see Chapter 12). It also benefits a patient psychologically by increasing social activity and mental stimulation and providing a change in environment (Power-Kean et al., 2023).

Safe transfer involves the use of friction-reducing devices, which fall into three categories: air-assisted transfer devices, friction-reducing slide sheets and tubes, and transfer and roller type boards (Baptiste-McKinney & Halvorson, 2018). Such devices provide patient comfort during the transfer and repositioning process. The use of friction-reducing devices also promotes in-bed mobility, potentially reduces risk for pressure injuries, provides ease of movement for patients and caregivers, and reduces the spinal load during a transfer (Baptiste-McKinney & Halvorson, 2018). However, it is critical that the correct techniques be used.

When preparing to transfer patients, consider the type of problems that may develop. For example, a patient who has been immobile for several days or longer may be weak or dizzy or may develop orthostatic hypotension (decreased blood pressure) when transferred to a chair. To ensure safe patient transfers, always use a gait or transfer belt or an appropriate lift and obtain assistance when transferring patients. Many people place a transfer belt on a person incorrectly (by putting it around the person's waist). Not only can this cause the person discomfort, but it can also decrease the transfer's efficiency and effectiveness. A transfer belt, when used properly, should fasten snugly around the patient's lower abdomen-hip area, as close as possible to their centre of gravity. Follow the principles of proper body mechanics (Box 11.1) when you are required (within safe patient-handling guidelines) to lift a patient or any patient care equipment. The guidelines will reduce lumbar injury. Remember that injuries are not only related to lifting. Activities that involve bending and twisting (e.g., carrying supplies and equipment and pushing and pulling equipment) can also cause injury.

Delegation and Collaboration

The skill of effective transfer techniques can be delegated to an unregulated care provider (UCP). The nurse is responsible for initially assessing patient's readiness and ability to transfer. The nurse directs the UCP about the following:

- Helping and supervising when moving patients who are transferred for the first time after prolonged bed rest, extensive surgery, critical illness, or spinal cord trauma
- Explaining the patient's mobility restrictions, changes in blood pressure to monitor for, or sensory alterations that may affect safe transfer
- Explaining what to observe for and reporting back to the nurse conditions such as dizziness or the patient's inability to help

Use interprofessional collaboration (e.g., physiotherapist) to consult on the best transfer method for the patient, when required.

Equipment

- Transfer belt
- Sling (as needed)
- Nonskid shoes, bath blankets, pillows
- Slide board (friction-reducing board)
- Bedside chair with arms
- Stretcher: Position next to bed, lock brakes on stretcher, lock brakes on bed
- Mechanical/hydraulic lift: Use frame, canvas strips or chains, and hammock or canvas strips; stand-assist lift device
- Sphygmomanometer and stethoscope
- Clean gloves (if there is risk of soiling)

STEP	RATIONALE
ASSESSMENT	
1. Identify patient using at least two person-specific identifiers (e.g., name and date of birth, or name and medical record number) according to employer policy.	Ensures correct patient. Complies with Accreditation Canada's standards and improves patient safety (Accreditation Canada, 2020).
2. Throughout the procedure, the 4 moments for hand hygiene are to be implemented; hand hygiene should occur before initial patient (or patient environment) contact, before an aseptic procedure, after body fluid exposure risk, and after patient (or patient environment) contact. Additional hand hygiene should be performed when hands are visibly soiled.	Proper hand hygiene helps prevent the spread of infectious agents to health care providers.
3. Review medical record or directly assess physical capacity of a patient to transfer and help with transfer (see Chapter 8). Assess the following:	Determines patient's ability to tolerate and help with transfer and whether special adaptive techniques or safe-handling devices are necessary.
a. Muscle strength (legs and upper arms) through active range of motion	Immobile patients have decreased muscle strength, tone, and mass. Affects ability to bear weight, raise body, and thus help with transfer.
b. Joint mobility and contracture formation	Immobility or inflammatory processes (e.g., arthritis) may lead to contracture formation and impaired joint mobility.
c. Paralysis or paresis (spastic or flaccid)	Patient with central nervous system (CNS) damage may have bilateral paralysis (requiring transfer by swivel bar, sliding bar, mechanical lift) or unilateral paralysis, which requires belt transfer to strong side. Weakness (paresis) requires stabilization of knee while transferring. Flaccid arm must be supported with sling during transfer.
d. Bone continuity (trauma, amputation) or calcium loss from long bones	Patients with trauma to one leg or hip may be unable to bear weight when transferred. Amputees may use sliding board to transfer. Osteoporosis increases risk for injury.
4. Refer to medical record for most recent recorded weight and height for patient.	These factors are used to determine whether mechanical transfer device or friction-reducing device is needed for transfer.
5. Assess for the following: history of previous fall; whether the patient has a fear of falling; and the presence of weakness, dizziness, or orthostatic hypotension (e.g., previously on bed rest, first time arising from supine position after surgical procedure, history of dizziness when arising).	Determines risk for fainting or falling during transfer. Previous fall history is a fall risk factor, and having a fear of falling can alter one's gait and security in walking. The move from supine to vertical position with a decrease of 20 mm Hg or more in systolic blood pressure (BP) results in orthostatic hypotension (Tyerman & Cobbett, 2023). Neurogenic orthostatic hypotension is a sustained reduction BP upon standing that is caused by autonomic dysfunction, and it is common among patients with neurodegenerative disorders (e.g., Parkinson's disease). In this situation, a systolic BP drop ≥20 mm Hg (or ≥10 mm Hg diastolic) upon standing, with little or no compensatory increase in heart rate, is consistent with neurogenic orthostatic hypotension (Biswas et al., 2019).
6. Assess medical record for patient's level of fatigue and activity tolerance during previous transfers. Assess endurance by noting patient's participation in ADLs.	Estimates ability of patient to participate in transfer. Planned rest periods before transfer may enhance function.
7. Assess patient's proprioceptive function (awareness of posture and changes in equilibrium):	Determines stability of patient's balance for transfer.
a. Ability to maintain balance while sitting in bed or on side of bed	Determines risk of fainting or falling during transfer.
b. Tendency to sway or position self to one side	Patients with brain dysfunction may have proprioceptive losses. This may cause them to lean to one side or lose balance during transfer.
8. Assess patient's sensory status, including adequacy of vision and hearing and presence of peripheral sensation loss (see Chapter 8).	Determines influence of sensory loss on ability to make transfer. Visual field loss decreases patient's ability to see in direction of transfer. Peripheral sensation loss decreases proprioception. Patients with visual and hearing losses need transfer techniques adapted to deficits.

Critical Decision Point *Patients with hemiplegia may "neglect" one side of the body (inattention to or unawareness of one side of body or environment), which distorts perceptions of the visual field.*

STEP	RATIONALE
9. Assess patient for pain (e.g., joint discomfort, muscle spasm), and measure level of pain using appropriate pain rating scale. Offer prescribed analgesic 30 minutes before transfer.	Pain reduces patient's motivation and ability to be mobile. Pain relief before transfer enhances patient participation (Booker et al., 2021).

STEP	RATIONALE
10. Assess patient's cognitive status:	Determines patient's ability to follow directions and help during transfer.
a. Ability to follow verbal instructions	May indicate that patient is at risk for injury.
b. Short-term memory	Patient with short-term memory deficit may have difficulty with transfer, initial learning, or consistent performance.
c. Recognition of physical deficits and limitations to movement	Patient's knowledge of deficits can help you plan a safe transfer.

Critical Decision Point *Patients with certain conditions that affect cognition, such as dementia, head trauma, or degenerative neurological challenges, may have perceptual cognitive defects that create safety risks. If the patient has difficulty comprehending, simplify instructions by describing one step at a time and maintain consistency.*

STEP	RATIONALE
11. Assess patient's level of motivation, such as their eagerness versus unwillingness to be mobile.	Altered psychological states often reduce patient's desire to engage in activity.
12. Assess previous mode of transfer (if applicable).	Determines mode of transfer and help required to provide continuity.
13. Just before transfer, assess patient's vital signs.	Vital sign changes such as increased pulse and respiration may indicate activity intolerance (see Chapter 7). A patient with low BP may not tolerate a sudden position change and is at risk for orthostatic hypotension. Provides baseline to determine tolerance to transfer.
14. Refer to safe-handling algorithm (available in most facilities) to determine whether a lift device or mechanical transfer device is needed and the number of people needed to help with transfer. *Do not start procedure until all required caregivers are available.*	Ensures safe patient handling, reducing risk of injury to patient and caregivers.

NURSING DIAGNOSES

- Acute or persistent pain
- Acute confusion
- Reduced physical mobility
- Reduced stamina
- Reduced skin integrity
- Potential for falls
- Potential for injury

Related factors and risk factors are individualized on the basis of patient's condition or needs.

PLANNING

STEP	RATIONALE
1. Expected outcomes following completion of procedure:	
• Patient sits on side of bed without dizziness, weakness, or orthostatic hypotension.	Precautions during transfer prevent vascular compromise.
• Patient tolerates increased activity.	Gradual increase in number of transfers and period of time out of bed increases tolerance and endurance.
• Patient can bear more weight.	Repeated transfers usually result in improved endurance and greater independence of patient.
• Patient transfers without injury.	Use of proper techniques prevents injury.
• Patient transfers with minimal discomfort.	Transfer procedures are performed correctly.
2. Assess environment for tripping hazards (e.g., equipment, cords, IV lines, etc.) before proceeding with transfer.	Promotes patient and nurse safety.
3. Explain to patient (in simple language) how you are going to prepare for transfer technique and safety precautions to be used. Explain benefits and reasons for getting up in a chair. Do so in a way that matches patient's beliefs and values regarding recovery or maintaining health.	Provides for clearer understanding by patient. Motivates patient to be involved in transfer.
4. Close room curtains or door.	Provides for patient privacy.
5. Get additional caregivers, necessary lift or transfer device, or both, to perform transfer.	Safe-handling algorithms (see employer policy) determine number of caregivers and type of devices needed to transfer a patient if lifting is required.

STEP	RATIONALE

IMPLEMENTATION

STEP	RATIONALE
1. Help patient from supine to sitting position on edge of bed with bed positioned so that top of mattress is even with your elbows. (See Chapter 12, Procedural Guideline 12.3, Step 13 with illustrations.)	Reduces strain on your back.
2. Allow patient to sit on side of bed for a few minutes. Have patient alternately flex and extend feet, move lower legs up and down. Ask if patient feels dizzy; if so, check BP. Have patient relax and take a few deep breaths until dizziness subsides and balance is gained. If dizziness lasts more than 60 seconds, or if systolic BP has dropped ≥20 mm Hg within 3 minutes of sitting upright, return patient to bed. Recheck BP.	Allows patient's circulation to equilibrate to reduce chance of orthostatic hypotension.

Critical Decision Point *Remain in front of patient until the person regains balance, and continue to provide physical support to weak or cognitively impaired patient.*

STEP	RATIONALE
3. Transfer patient from bed to chair. *Option:* Apply clean gloves if bed linen is soiled.	
a. Have chair in position at 45-degree angle with one side against bed, facing foot of bed.	Positions chair with easy access for transfer.
b. Place bed in low position or to point where patient's feet are comfortably on the floor and hips and knees at a 90-degree angle. Help patient apply stable, nonskid shoes/socks.	Provides patient stability when transferring. Shoes/socks prevent slipping on floor.
c. If patient has partial weight-bearing capacity with upper body strength or caregiver must lift more than 15.9 kg (35 lb), use mechanical lift or transfer aid with minimum of two or three caregivers (Matz, 2019) (see Step 3c illustration). Follow manufacturer lift guidelines to apply.	The use of mechanical lift devices is strongly recommended to transfer a patient to reduce risk for musculoskeletal injury (CCOHS, 2018).

Critical Decision Point *If patient demonstrates weakness or paralysis on one side of the body, place chair on their strong side.*

STEP	RATIONALE
d. If patient has partial weight-bearing capacity, is cooperative and able to stand, and has upper body strength, use stand-and-pivot technique with one caregiver.	
(1) Apply transfer belt (see Step 3d[1] illustration). Be sure that it completely circles waist. Place belt low and be sure that it is snug. Avoid placing belt over any IV lines, incisions, or drainage tubes. You may need to adjust belt once patient stands.	Transfer belt allows you to maintain stability of patient during transfer and reduces risk of falling (Matz, 2019; WorkSafeNB, 2015).
(2) Place patient's weight-bearing (or strong) leg under the patient and the weak (or non-weight-bearing) foot forward.	Patient will stand on stronger (or weight-bearing) leg initially, raising torso.

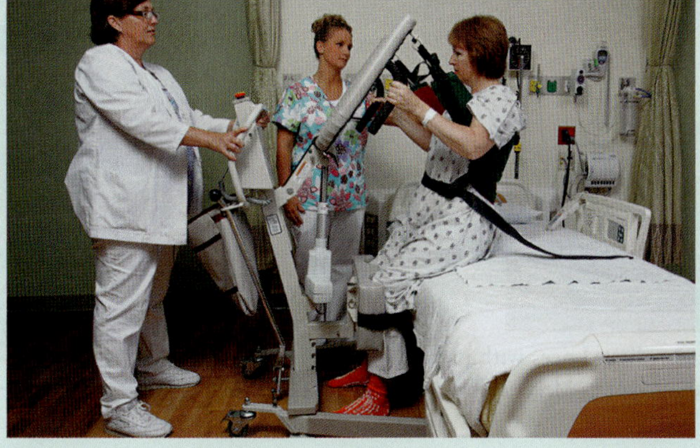

STEP 3C Patient grasps handles as nurse turns on motorized lift.

STEP	RATIONALE
(3) Spread your feet apart. Flex hips and knees, aligning knees with patient's knees.	Ensures balance with wide base of support. Flexing knees and hips lowers your centre of gravity to object to be raised; aligning knees with those of patient allows for stabilization of knees when patient stands.
(4) Grasp transfer belt with both hands, keeping your palms up, along patient's sides (see Step 3d[4] illustration).	Transfer belt allows you to move patient at centre of gravity. Patients should never be lifted by or under their arms.
(5) Rock patient up to standing position on count of three while straightening hips and legs and keeping knees slightly flexed (see Step 3d[5] illustration). While rocking patient in back-and-forth motion, make sure that your body weight is moving in the same direction as patient's, to ensure that you and patient are moving in same direction simultaneously. Unless contraindicated, patient may be instructed to use hands to push up, if applicable.	Rocking motion gives patient's body momentum and requires less muscular effort to lift the person.

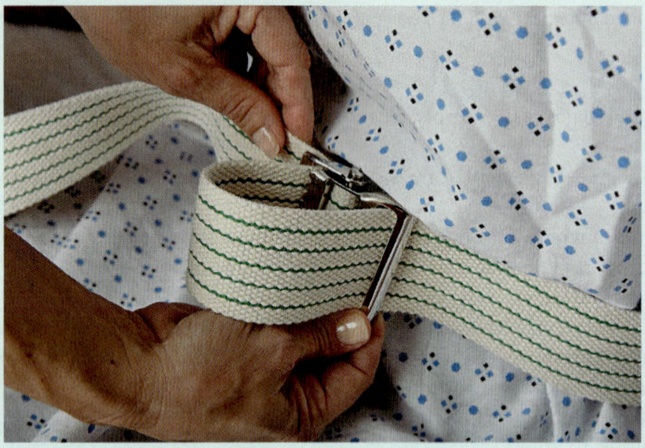

STEP 3D(1) **Application of transfer belt.**

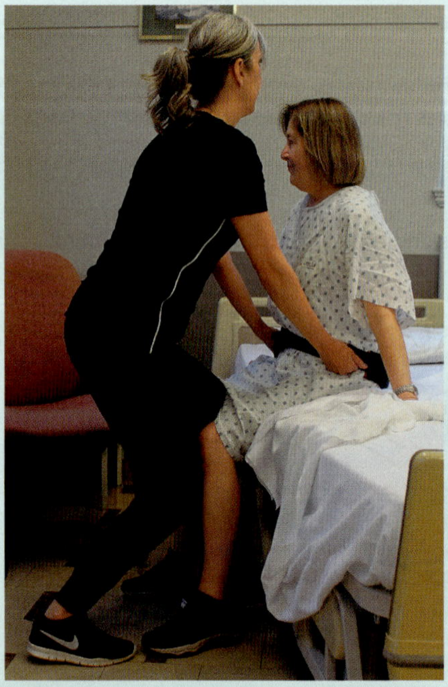

STEP 3D(4) **Nurse flexes hips and knees, aligns knees with patient's knee, and grasps transfer belt palms up.** (*Courtesy Melanie Deveau and Jackie Hartigan-Rogers.*)

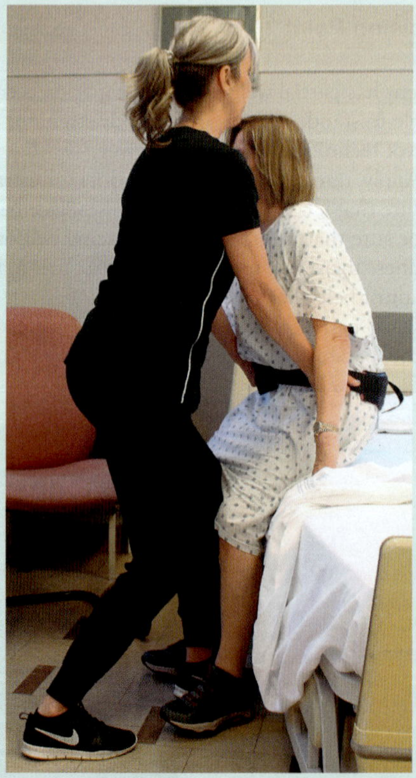

STEP 3D(5) **Nurse rocks patient (who is able to help) to standing position.** (*Courtesy Melanie Deveau and Jackie Hartigan-Rogers.*)

STEP	RATIONALE
(6) Maintain stability of patient's weakened leg with your knee.	Ability to stand can often be maintained in weak limb with support of knee to stabilize.
(7) Pivot on foot farthest from chair.	Maintains support of patient while allowing adequate space for patient to move.
(8) Instruct patient to use armrests on chair for support and ease into chair (see Step 3d[8] illustration).	Increases patient stability.
(9) Flex hips and knees while lowering patient into chair.	Prevents injury from poor body mechanics.
(10) Assess patient for proper alignment in sitting position. Provide support for weakened extremity. Sling or lap board can be used to support an injured or flaccid arm. Stabilize leg with bath blanket or pillow.	Prevents injury to patient from poor body alignment.
(11) Proper alignment for sitting position: Head is erect, and vertebrae are in straight alignment. Body weight is evenly distributed on buttocks and thighs. Thighs are parallel and in horizontal plane. Both feet are supported on floor, and ankles are comfortably flexed. A 2.5- to 5-cm (1- to 2-inch) space is maintained between edge of seat and popliteal space on posterior surface of knee.	Prevents stress on intravertebral joints. Prevents increased pressure over bony prominences and reduces damage to underlying musculoskeletal system.
e. If patient is unable to cooperate (regardless of ability to bear weight) or has no upper body strength, use ceiling or floor hydraulic lift to transfer patient from bed to chair.	Research supports use of mechanical lifts to prevent musculoskeletal injuries (CCOHS, 2018). Use of ceiling-mounted lifts is a popular choice because of availability of lift in each patient's room (see Step 3e illustration).

Critical Decision Point *Patients with new hip replacements who have hip precautions should not be using a Hoyer lift because it may promote hip flexion of 90 degrees, which is contraindicated for patients with posterior hip precautions.*

STEP	RATIONALE
(1) Bring mechanical floor lift to bedside or lower ceiling lift and position properly.	Ensures safe elevation of patient off bed.

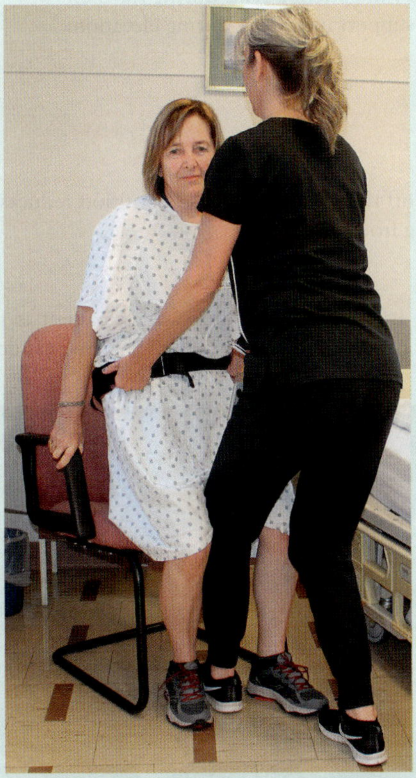

STEP 3D(8) Patient uses armrests and is guided to sit in chair. (*Courtesy Melanie Deveau and Jackie Hartigan-Rogers.*)

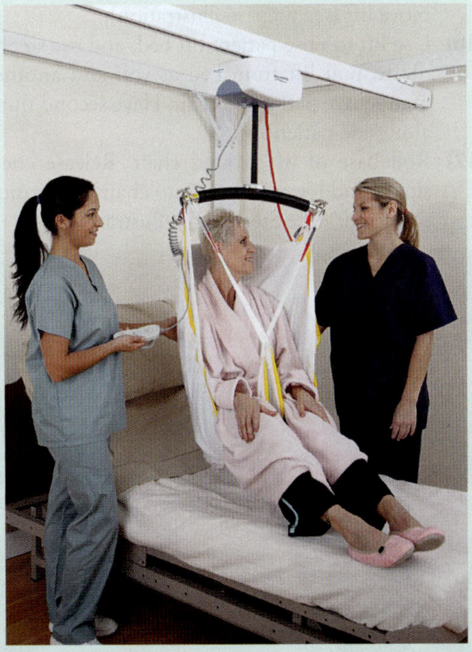

STEP 3E Ceiling lift. (*Courtesy Waverly Glen Systems, a Prism Medical Co.*)

STEP	RATIONALE
(2) Position chair near bed and allow adequate space to manoeuvre the lift.	Prepares environment for safe use of lift and subsequent transfer.

Critical Decision Point *If patient demonstrates weakness or paralysis on one side of the body, place chair on patient's strong side.*

STEP	RATIONALE
(3) Raise bed to high position with mattress flat. Lower side rail on side near chair.	Ensures proper body mechanics.
(4) Have second nurse positioned at opposite side of bed.	Maintains patient safety, preventing fall from bed.
(5) Roll patient on side away from you.	Positions patient for placement of lift sling.
(6) Place hammock or canvas strips under patient to form sling. With two canvas pieces, lower edge fits under patient's knees (wide piece), and upper edge fits under patient's shoulders (narrow piece).	Two types of seats are supplied with a mechanical/hydraulic lift: hammock style is better for patients who are flaccid, weak, and need support; canvas strips can be used for patients with normal muscle tone. Hooks should face away from patient's skin. Place sling under patient's centre of gravity and greatest part of body weight.
(7) Roll patient back toward you as second nurse pulls hammock (straps) through.	Ensures that sling is in proper position before lift.
(8) Return patient to supine position. Be sure that hammock or straps are smooth over bed surface. Sling should extend from shoulders to knees (hammock) to support patient's body weight equally.	Completes positioning of patient on mechanical/hydraulic sling.
(9) Remove patient's eyeglasses, if worn.	Swivel bar is close to patient's head and could break eyeglasses.
(10) Place horseshoe base of floor lift under patient's bed (on side with chair).	Positions lift efficiently and promotes smooth transfer.
(11) Lower horizontal bar to sling level by following manufacturer directions. Lock valve if required.	Positions hydraulic lift close to patient. Locking valve prevents injury to patient.
(12) Attach hooks on strap (chain) to holes in sling. Short chains or straps hook to top holes of sling; longer chains hook to bottom of sling (see manufacturer directions).	Secures hydraulic lift to sling.
(13) Elevate head of bed to Fowler's position.	Positions patient in sitting position.
(14) Have patient fold arms over chest.	Prevents injury to patient's arms during transfer.
(15) If the lift is electric, push the button to raise the patient off the bed. If the lift is a nonelectric lift, pump the hydraulic handle using long, slow, even strokes until patient is raised off bed (see Step 3e[15] illustration). For ceiling lift, turn on control device to move lift (see Step 3e illustration).	Ensures safe support of patient during elevation.
(16) Use lift to raise patient off bed, and use steering handle to pull lift from bed as you and another nurse manoeuvre patient to chair. Have second nurse stand alongside patient.	Lifts patient off the bed safely; nurse's position reduces any risk of patient falling from sling.
(17) Roll base of lift around chair. Release check valve slowly and lower patient into chair (see manufacturer directions) (see Step 3e[17] illustration).	Positions lift in front of chair into which patient is to be transferred. Safely guides patient into back of chair as seat descends.

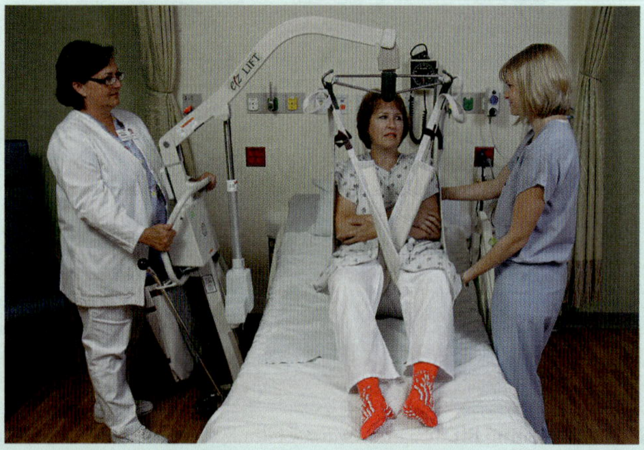
STEP 3E(15) Patient lifted in hydraulic lift above bed.

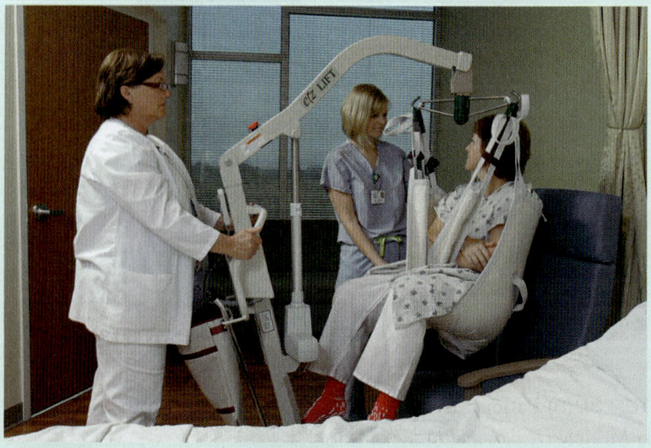
STEP 3E(17) Use of hydraulic lift to lower patient into chair.

STEP	RATIONALE
(18) Close check valve as soon as patient is down in chair and straps can be released.	If valve is left open, boom may continue to lower and injure patient.
(19) Remove straps and roll mechanical/hydraulic lift out of patient's path.	Prevents damage to skin and underlying tissues.
(20) Check patient's sitting alignment and correct if necessary.	Prevents injury from poor posture.
4. Perform lateral transfer from bed to stretcher:	The three-person lift for horizontal transfer from bed to stretcher is no longer recommended and is, in fact, discouraged (Matz, 2019). Physical stress can be decreased significantly by using a slide board or friction-reducing board positioned under drawsheet beneath patient. In addition, patient is more comfortable with this method.
a. Determine whether patient can assist.	Patient's strength and weight determine how much help is required for safe transfer. During any patient-transferring task, if any caregiver is required to lift more than 15.9 kg (35 lb) of patient's weight, patient is considered fully dependent and an assist device is used (Matz, 2019; Occupational Safety and Health Association, 2014).
(1) If patient can assist, caregiver is only needed to stand by for safety, with stretcher and bed locked as patient moves to stretcher. Surface of stretcher should be 1.3 cm (0.5 inches) lower for lateral move.	
(2) If patient is partially or not at all able to help and is <90.7 kg (<200 lb), use friction-reducing device, lateral transfer board, or roller board.	
(3) If patient is partially or not at all able to help and is >90.7 kg (>200 lb), use a ceiling lift with supine sling or a mechanical lateral-transfer device, or air-assisted device with three caregivers.	

Critical Decision Point *Air-assisted devices float patients from an air-layered surface directly across to another surface (bed, stretcher). They can also be used for repositioning. Indicated for patients with compromised skin integrity, pressure injuries, multiple traumas, burns, oncology patients experiencing severe pain, and bariatric patients* (Baptiste-McKinney & Halvorson, 2018).

STEP	RATIONALE
b. Lateral transfer with friction-reducing device—slide board (see Step 4b illustration), roller board, or air-assisted device:	Maintains alignment of spinal column. Ensures that bed does not move inadvertently.

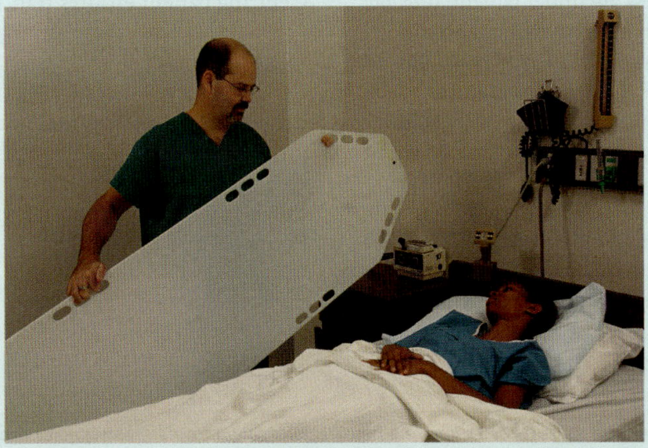

STEP 4B Slide board.

STEP	RATIONALE
(1) Apply clean gloves if there is risk of soiling. Lower head of bed as much as patient can tolerate. Be sure to lock bed brakes.	Reduces transmission of microorganisms.
(2) Cross patient's arms on chest.	Prevents injury to arms during transfer.
(3) Lower side rails. To place transfer device (slide or roller board) or deflated air-assisted mattress under patient, position two nurses on side of bed toward which patient will be turned. Position third nurse on other side of bed.	Distributes weight equally between nurses.
(4) Fanfold drawsheet on both sides.	Provides strong handles to grip drawsheet without slipping.

STEP	RATIONALE
(5) On count of three, logroll patient onto side toward the two nurses. Turn patient as one unit with smooth, continuous motion.	Maintains body in alignment, preventing stress on any part.
(6) Place transfer device (slide or roller board) or deflated mattress of air-assisted device under drawsheet (see Step 4b[6] illustration). Spread out deflated mattress on bed under patient as you would a new sheet.	Prevents friction from contact of skin with board.

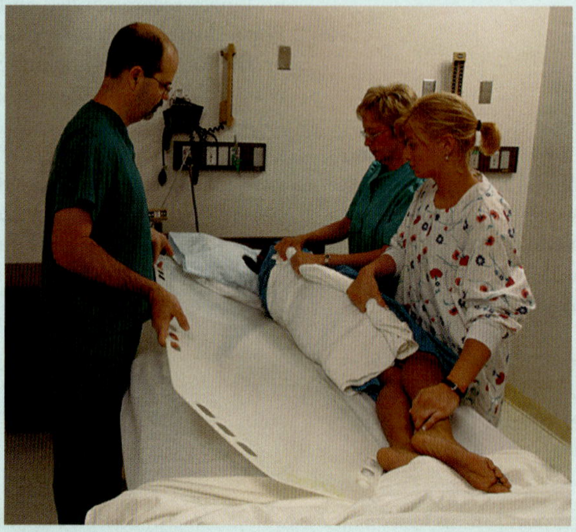

STEP 4B(6) Caregivers placing slide board under drawsheet.

STEP	RATIONALE
(7) Advise patient that they will be rolling over hard or irregular surface. Ask patient to stay aligned as they roll toward the one nurse on other side of bed. Gently roll patient back onto transfer device (slide or roller board).	
(8) Be sure board and mattress are under patient. (*Option:* Roll out the deflated air mattress so that it is positioned over bed mattress.) Then position patient supine so that they are centred over the board or mattress.	Centring patient ensures transfer of torso and lower extremities.
(9) Ensure stretcher surface is 1.3 cm (0.5 inches) lower than bed. Lock brakes on stretcher. Instruct patient not to move.	Ensures that stretcher does not move inadvertently during transfer.
(10) *Option*: At this time, inflate the mattress.	Provides for smooth transfer with no shear force.
(11) Two nurses position themselves on side of stretcher while third nurse positions self on side of bed without stretcher. All three nurses place feet wide apart, with one foot slightly in front of the other, and grasp the friction-reducing device.	Promotes easy transfer.

Critical Decision Point *For patients with stage III or IV pressure injuries, take care to avoid shearing force against skin. A nurse may also be positioned at the head of patient's bed to protect and support the person's head and neck if patient is weak or unable to help.*

STEP	RATIONALE
(12) Holding the edges of board or air-inflated mattress and one nurse counting to three, the two nurses slide the board or mattress, positioning patient onto stretcher (see Step 4b[12], illustration A). The third nurse guides the board or mattress in place. *Option:* Inflate air-assisted device and slide patient across bed onto stretcher (see Step 4b[12], illustrations *B* and *C*).	Slide board remains stationary, provides slippery surface to reduce friction, and allows patient to transfer easily to stretcher.

STEP	RATIONALE

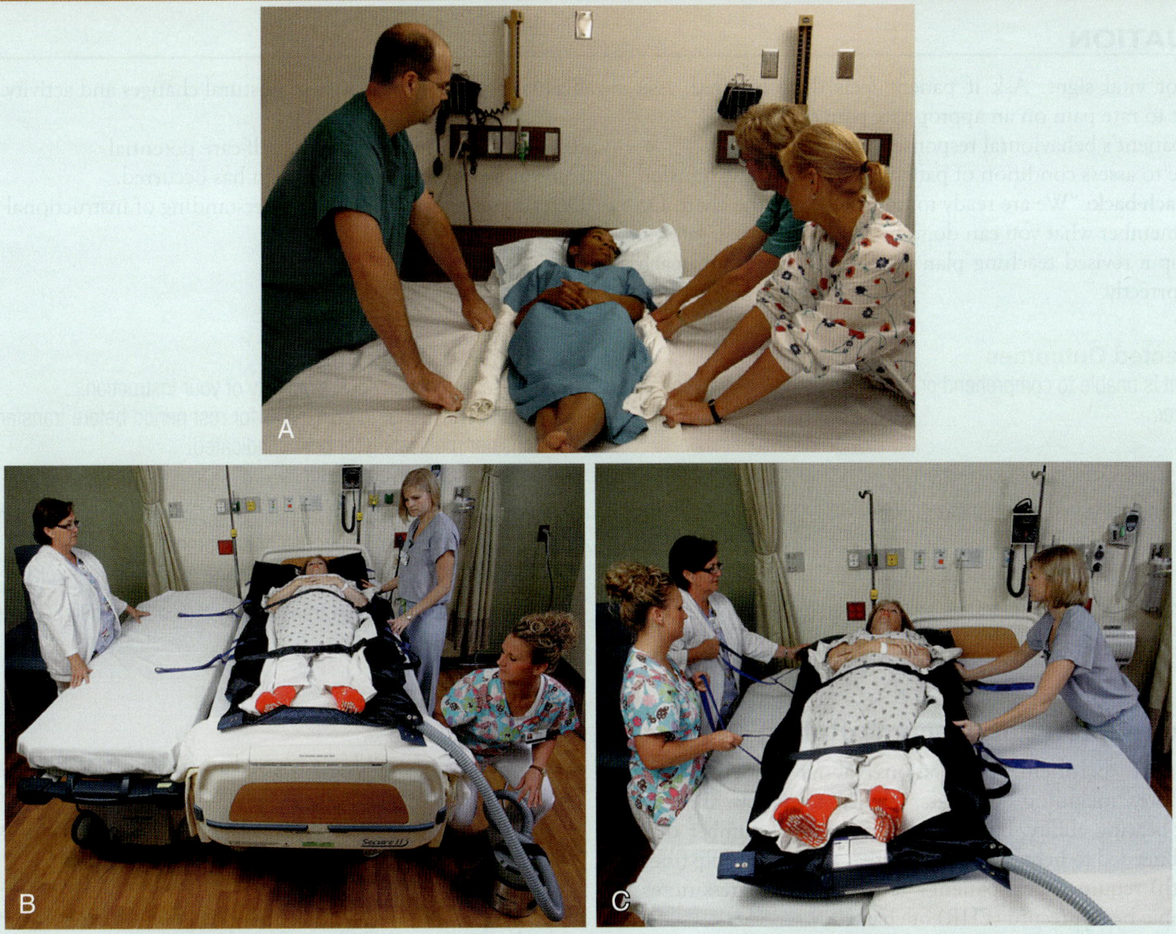

STEP 4B(12) A, Transfer of patient to stretcher using slide board. B, Inflating air-assisted transfer device. C, Transfer of patient using air-assisted transfer device.

Critical Decision Point *Air-assisted devices have a limitation. Once a transfer begins, the friction-reduction capability contributes to an increase in momentum, making it more difficult to stop the transfer. Use caution to be sure the patient does not slide beyond or even off the stretcher or bed to which the patient is being transferred* (Baptiste-McKinney & Halvorson, 2018).

STEP	RATIONALE
(13) Position patient in centre of stretcher. Raise head of stretcher if not contraindicated. Raise stretcher side rails. Cover patient with blanket.	Provides for patient comfort.
c. **Bariatric lateral transfer to and from bed or stretcher:**	
(1) If patient can fully assist, use minimum of two caregivers.	If a bariatric patient is about to fall, little can be done by a caregiver to prevent the fall. Caregiver should be prepared to move any items out of the way that could cause injury. Try to protect patient's head. Transfer toward stronger side. Use of mechanical devices ensures patient and caregiver safety.
(2) If patient can only partially or not at all assist, use a sliding board with slide sheet, mechanical floor-based lift, bariatric ceiling lift with supine sling, or air-assisted friction-reducing device with a minimum of three caregivers (Baptiste-McKinney & Halvorson, 2018).	

Critical Decision Point *When used in combination with slide boards, a slide sheet may be of value, as use of a sliding board alone often does not function well owing to the high level of friction created by a patient's body mass.*

STEP	RATIONALE
5. After transferring patient to bed, chair, or stretcher, be sure patient is positioned comfortably with nurse call bell within patient's reach.	Restores comfort and sense of well-being. Ensures patient can call for assistance if needed, promotes safety, and prevents falls.
6. Remove and dispose of gloves (if used).	Reduces transmission of microorganisms.

STEP	RATIONALE
EVALUATION	
1. Monitor vital signs. Ask if patient feels dizzy or tired. Ask patient to rate pain on an appropriate pain scale.	Evaluates patient's response to postural changes and activity.
2. Note patient's behavioural response to transfer.	Reveals level of motivation and self-care potential.
3. Be sure to assess condition of patient's skin after next transfer.	Determines whether injury to skin has occurred.
4. Use teach-back: "We are ready to transfer you to the chair. Do you remember what you can do to help us transfer you safely?" Develop a revised teaching plan if patient is unable to teach back correctly.	Determines patient's level of understanding of instructional topic.

Unexpected Outcomes	Related Interventions
1. Patient is unable to comprehend or is unwilling to follow directions for transfer.	• Reassess continuity and simplicity of your instruction. • If patient is tired or in pain, allow for rest period before transferring. • Consider medicating for pain if indicated. • Consider using hydraulic lift.
2. Patient sustains injury on transfer.	• Evaluate incident that led to injury (e.g., inadequate assessment, change in patient status, improper use of equipment). • Complete adverse event/incident report according to employer policy.
3. Patient is unable to stand for the time required to transfer to chair.	• Consider use of a lateral transfer board (see Procedural Guideline 11.1) or hydraulic lift.

Communication and Documentation

- Document pertinent observations about patient transfer procedure, including weakness, ability to follow directions, weight-bearing ability, balance, ability to pivot, number of personnel needed to help, assist device used, amount of help (muscle strength) required, and patient's response, in progress notes in electronic health record (EHR) or chart.
- Document your evaluation of patient and caregiver learning.
- Communicate transfer ability and help needed during hand-off report or to other caregivers.
- Use interprofessional collaboration to discuss patient progress or remission and revise the plan of care as required (e.g., collaborate with physiotherapist, occupational therapist).

DOCUMENTATION EXAMPLE

Patient is ambulating safely with a two-wheel walker and weight bearing as tolerated. Patient is a one-person assist to bed from chair if not using walker. Patient teaching completed re: safety precautions with walker. Physiotherapist patient teaching completed re: how to get up from the bed and walk with walker. Patient states they have no pain; sitting in chair in room reading a book.

Special Considerations

Teaching

- Teach patient and caregiver the importance of increasing activity out of bed.
- Instruct caregiver on how to assess a patient's tolerance to increased activity.
- Inform patient that use of mechanical transfer devices is for comfort and safety.

Pediatric

- Whenever possible, it is good to transport a child by stretcher, stroller, or wheelchair outside confines of room to increase environmental stimuli and provide social contact with others (Hockenberry et al., 2024).
- Children confined to bed for any length of time, such as those in traction, need to have dependent skin surfaces assessed at least three times in a 24-hour period.

Gerontological

- A health concern that threatens the function of an older person is the risk for falls (Boscart et al., 2023). Concern increases when an older person enters a health care facility. Assess the patient for the risk for falls on admission and implement a protocol to prevent falls (Tyerman & Cobbett, 2023) (see Chapter 14).

Care in the Community: Home Management

- Have caregiver practise and demonstrate transfer skills to achieve success before taking patient home. Alternatively, have patient (if living alone) practise transfer skills in bed that will be used at home. Teach patient to transfer to a chair with arms for ease of rising and sitting. Home should be free of hazards (e.g., throw rugs, electric cords in walkways, slippery floors). If wheelchair is used as chair, access must be possible through all doorways, and space for transfer must be available in bedroom and bathroom (see Chapter 42).
- Aids that enhance transfer ability are shower stools, elevated commodes, handrails on tub, and nonskid shower surface. Medical supply stores provide excellent information and catalogues of such supplies.

Procedural Guideline 11.1 *Wheelchair Transfer Techniques*

Video Clip

Transferring a patient from a bed to a wheelchair encompasses most of the same principles discussed in Skill 11.1. The following procedural guideline focuses on the safety precautions that need to be considered when a weight-bearing patient is using a wheelchair. This technique is common when hospitalized patients are taken by wheelchair to procedures. Several additional steps must be taken to maintain the safety of a patient and for the nurse to avoid injury when transferring a patient from or to a wheelchair (Fairchild et al., 2022). Check wheelchair locks, wheels, and footplates for proper functioning before use.

Delegation and Collaboration

The skill of transferring a patient to or from a wheelchair can be delegated to a UCP. The nurse directs the UCP about the following:

- Assessing and supervising when moving patients who are transferring for the first time after prolonged bed rest, extensive surgery, critical illness, or spinal cord trauma
- Explaining the patient's mobility restrictions, changes in BP, or sensory alterations that may affect safe transfer

Collaborate with interprofessional health care team (e.g., physiotherapist, occupational therapist) about proper type of wheelchair for a patient and best transfer technique.

Equipment

- Transfer belt
- Nonskid shoes
- Wheelchair
- Transfer board

Procedural Steps

1. Identify patient using at least two person-specific identifiers (e.g., name and date of birth, or name and medical record number) according to employer policy.
2. Throughout the procedure, the 4 moments for hand hygiene are to be implemented; hand hygiene should occur before initial patient (or patient environment) contact, before an aseptic procedure, after body fluid exposure risk, and after patient (or patient environment) contact. Additional hand hygiene should be performed when hands are visibly soiled.
3. Review medical record to assess patient's weight, height, and strength; cognition; level of pain; and balance during previous transfer. Or complete a full assessment (see Skill 11.1) to determine patient's ability to help with transfer.
4. Explain to patient the steps you will be taking to help in transfer.
5. Check wheelchair locks, wheels, and footplates for proper functioning before use.
6. Transferring patient from a wheelchair to a bed (patient is cooperative and weight bearing) using pivot technique:
   a. Adjust the height of the bed to the level of the seat of the wheelchair.
   b. Position wheelchair at a 45-degree angle next to the bed midway between the head and foot of the bed, with the wheelchair facing toward the foot of the bed. Remove the armrest nearest the side of the bed.
   c. Lock both wheels of the wheelchair. Locks are located above the rims of the wheels. Push handle forward to lock.
   d. Raise the footplates.
   e. Place a transfer belt on patient. Be sure that it completely encircles patient's waist. Place the belt low and be sure that it is snug. Avoid placing the belt over any IV lines, incisions, or drainage tubes.
   f. Have patient place their hands on armrests and stand by as you have them move to the front of the wheelchair.
   g. Stand slightly in front of patient to guard and protect the person throughout the transfer.
   h. Instruct patient to stand on a count of three as you place both hands (palms up) under transfer belt while bending your knees.
   i. Allow patient to stand a few seconds to ensure that they are not dizzy and have good balance. Pivot with patient as the person turns to face away from the side of the bed. Then have patient sit on the edge of the mattress. Be sure patient is firmly sitting and not slipping off edge of the bed.
   j. With patient sitting on edge of the bed, place your arm nearest the head of the bed under their shoulder while supporting the head and neck. Place your other arm under patient's knees. Bend your knees and keep your back straight.
   k. Tell patient to help lift the legs when you begin to move. On a count of three, standing with a wide base of support, raise patient's legs as you pivot their body and lower the shoulders onto the bed. Remember to keep your back straight.
   l. Help patient return to a comfortable position in bed.
7. Transferring patient from a wheelchair to a bed (patient is non-weight-bearing and unable to stand but is cooperative and has upper body strength) using transfer board:
   a. Follow Steps 6a through 6e.
   b. If possible, have the seat of the wheelchair level with the top of the bed mattress. Position a transfer board by placing it across the bed to the chair so the patient can slide across it. Be sure the board overlaps the chair and mattress so that it will not slip out of place. Then have patient use their hands on wheelchair arms to raise their hips up, and place the other part of the board under the patient's buttock that is closest to the bed (see Step 7b illustration).

Continued

Procedural Guideline 11.1 *Wheelchair Transfer Techniques—cont'd*

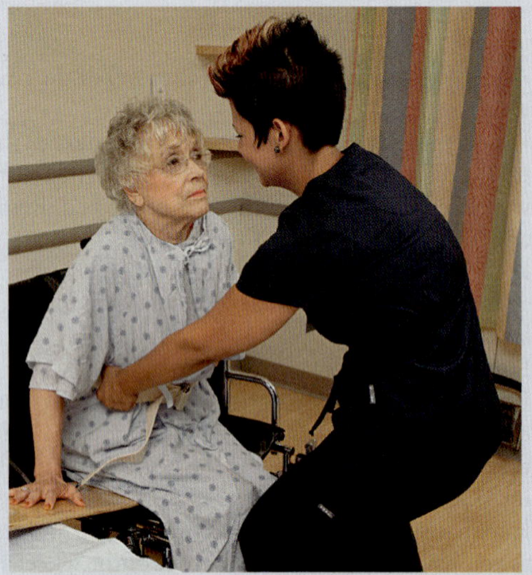

STEP 7B Patient transfer from wheelchair to bed using a lateral transfer board.

c. Stand in front of patient and have the person move to the front of the wheelchair.
d. Place your legs on the outside of the patient's legs. Be sure that patient's feet are on the floor. Grasp the transfer belt (palms up) along both of patient's sides. Have patient place one hand on the slide board and the other on the mattress surface.
e. Bend your knees and, on a count of three, have patient use the arms to slide across the board from the chair to the bed. If patient is struggling to move across the board, try to have them lean their head and shoulders in the direction opposite to the way they want their hips to move.
f. Have patient sit on edge of bed slightly above where the bed bends when elevated. This prevents having to move patient up in bed.
g. Assist patient by raising their legs as you pivot their body, moving their legs back onto the mattress, and position in comfortable position.
h. Raise side rails (as appropriate), lower bed to lowest position, and place nurse call system within easy reach.

8. Monitor vital signs after patient has been transferred. Ask if patient feels dizzy or fatigued.
9. Note patient's behavioural response to transfer.
10. **Use teach-back:** "I want to be sure I explained what to do as I move you from the chair to the bed. Tell me how you can help move to the bed." Develop a revised teaching plan if patient is unable to teach back correctly.
11. Document patient's ability to tolerate transfer (fatigue, level of pain) and level of assistance required.

✦ SKILL 11.2 Moving and Positioning Patients in Bed

Video Clip NSO *Nursing Skills Online Safety Module 1 / Lesson 3*

Correctly positioning patients in bed is crucial for maintaining their body alignment and comfort; preventing injury to their musculoskeletal and integumentary systems; and providing sensory, motor, and cognitive stimulation. A patient with impaired mobility, decreased sensation, impaired circulation, or lack of voluntary muscle control can suffer damage to the musculoskeletal and integumentary systems while lying down. Immobilized patients require vigilant nursing care with frequent repositioning to reduce the risk of physical complications, including pressure injuries, reduced ventilation, muscle contractures, and deep vein thrombosis. Proper positioning with correct body alignment minimizes these risks. The term *body alignment* refers to the condition of the joints, tendons, ligaments, and muscles in various body positions. When the body is aligned, whether standing, sitting, or lying, no excessive strain is placed on these structures. Patients contribute to repositioning through their own frequent movement. Often patients adopt positions that increase their pressure injury risk. Patients routinely slip down in bed, so routine monitoring of patient positions is important. Caregivers are at risk for injury during positioning of patients in bed. It is important to follow your employer's safe-handling algorithms and use appropriate repositioning devices.

Delegation and Collaboration

The skills of moving and positioning patients in bed and maintaining correct body alignment can be delegated to a UCP. The nurse directs the UCP about the following:

- Explaining about any moving and positioning restrictions (e.g., avoid prone position, patient has one-sided weakness) and type of safe patient-handling devices needed
- Designating specific times throughout the shift that the UCP must reposition the patient
- Providing information regarding patient's individual needs for body alignment (e.g., patient with spinal cord injury), ability to help, and number of other caregivers needed to help

Equipment

- Pillows, drawsheet
- Appropriate safe patient-handling assistive device (e.g., friction-reducing device, ceiling lift, or mechanical floor lift)
- Therapeutic boots/splints (*optional*)
- Trochanter roll
- Sandbag
- Hand rolls
- Clean gloves

STEP	RATIONALE
ASSESSMENT	
1. Identify patient using at least two person-specific identifiers (e.g., name and date of birth, or name and medical record number) according to employer policy.	Ensures correct patient. Complies with Accreditation Canada's standards and improves patient safety (Accreditation Canada, 2020).
2. Throughout the procedure, the 4 moments for hand hygiene are to be implemented; hand hygiene should occur before initial patient (or patient environment) contact, before an aseptic procedure, after body fluid exposure risk, and after patient (or patient environment) contact. Additional hand hygiene should be performed when hands are visibly soiled.	Proper hand hygiene helps prevent the spread of infectious agents to health care providers.
3. Assess patient's range of motion (ROM) (see Chapters 8 and 12) and current body alignment while patient is lying down.	Provides baseline data for later comparisons. Determines ways to improve position and alignment.
4. Assess for risk factors that contribute to complications of immobility:	Increased risk factors require patient to be repositioned more frequently.
a. *Reduced sensation:* Cerebrovascular accident (CVA), spinal cord injury, or neuropathy	With reduced sensation, patient has difficulty moving and poor awareness of involved body part. Patient is unable to position body part and protect it from pressure.
b. *Impaired mobility:* Traction, arthritis, CVA, spinal cord injury, hip fracture, joint surgery, or other contributing disease processes	Traction, bone fractures, surgery, or arthritic changes of affected extremity result in decreased ROM. Loss of function caused by CVA or spinal cord injury can lead to contractures.
c. *Impaired circulation:* Arterial insufficiency	Decreased circulation predisposes patient to pressure injury.
d. *Age:* Very young child, older person	Premature and young infants require frequent turning because their skin is fragile. Normal physiological changes associated with aging predispose older persons to developing complications of immobility.
5. Assess patient's level of consciousness.	Determines need for special aids or devices. Patients with altered levels of consciousness may not understand instructions and may be unable to help with positioning.
6. Assess patient for presence of pain; rate using appropriate pain rating scale.	Pain reduces patient's motivation and ability to be mobile. Pain relief before transfer enhances patient participation (Booker et al., 2021).
7. Assess condition of patient's skin, especially over bony prominences. Know patient's Braden score and risk of developing a pressure injury.	Provides baseline to determine effects of positioning.
8. Refer to patient's EHR or chart for most recent recorded weight and height.	Factors needed to determine whether mechanical lift, mechanical transfer device, or friction-reducing device is needed for moving patient up in bed.
9. Assess patient's physical ability to help with moving and positioning, which may be affected by age, level of consciousness, disease process, strength, ROM, and coordination.	Enables you to use patient's mobility, strength, and coordination during positioning. Determines need for additional help. Ensures patient and nurse safety.
10. Assess for sensory loss (vision and hearing) (see Chapter 8).	Deficits affect patient's ability to cooperate during repositioning procedures.
11. Apply clean gloves (as needed) to assess for presence of incisions, drainage tubes, and equipment (e.g., traction). Empty drainage bags before positioning. Remove and dispose of gloves.	Reduces transmission of microorganisms. Alters positioning procedure and type of position in which to place patient. Eliminates barriers to moving patient.
12. Assess motivation of patient and ability of caregivers to participate in moving and positioning if patient is to be discharged home.	Indicates whether instruction is necessary before discharge.
13. Check health care provider's prescriptions before positioning patient.	Some positions may be contraindicated in certain situations (e.g., spinal cord injury; hip fracture; respiratory difficulties; certain neurological conditions; presence of incisions, drains, or tubing).

STEP	RATIONALE

NURSING DIAGNOSES

- Acute confusion
- Reduced physical mobility
- Reduced stamina
- Reduced skin integrity
- Potential for impaired skin integrity

Related factors and risk factors are individualized on the basis of patient's condition or needs.

PLANNING

STEP	RATIONALE
1. Expected outcomes following completion of procedure:	
• Patient retains ROM.	Correct positioning allows patient to achieve optimal joint mobility and alignment.
• Patient's skin shows no evidence of breakdown.	Frequent position changes decrease occurrence of skin breakdown.
• Patient's comfort level increases.	Proper positioning reduces stress on joints.
• Patient's level of independence in completing ADLs increases.	Maintaining good body alignment and joint mobility increases patient's overall mobility. Patient with inadequate joint mobility may need help to carry out ADLs.
2. If patient perceives their pain to be enough to avoid movement, offer an analgesic 30 minutes (if prescribed) before repositioning.	Will lessen discomfort when positioning extremities. NOTE: An analgesic may not be available as frequently as a patient requires turning.
3. Remove all pillows and devices used in previous position.	Reduces interference from bedding during positioning procedure.
4. Get additional caregivers and/or necessary lift or transfer device to perform positioning.	Safe-handling algorithms (see employer policy) determine number of caregivers and type of devices needed to position a patient if lifting is required.
5. Explain positioning procedure to patient using plain language.	Helps decrease anxiety and increase cooperation.
6. Close door to room or bedside curtains.	Provides for patient privacy.

IMPLEMENTATION

STEP	RATIONALE
1. Raise level of bed to comfortable working height, level with your elbows.	Raises level of work toward nurse's centre of gravity and reduces risk for back injuries.
2. Assist patient to move up in bed:	This is not a one-person task unless patient can help completely. Pulling patients who have migrated in bed carries an extremely high risk of caregiver injury (Matz, 2019).
a. Determine whether the patient can assist.	Determines degree of risk in repositioning patient and technique required to safely help patient.
(1) Patient is fully able to assist:	Promotes patient independence.
(a) Stand at bedside to help with positioning of tubing and equipment as patient moves.	
(b) Have patient place feet flat on mattress, grasp either side rails or overhead trapeze and, on a count of three, lift hips up and push legs so body moves up in bed.	
(2) Patient is partially able to assist:	
(a) Encourage patient to help using friction-reducing device (e.g., slide board).	Repositioning device reduces friction as patient is moved up in bed.
(b) Patient weighs <90.7 kg (<200 lb): Use friction-reducing sheet or slide board and two or three caregivers.	
(c) Patient weighs >90.7 kg (>200 lb): Use friction-reducing device and at least three caregivers.	
i. *Using a friction-reducing device (three nurses):* Position patient supine with head of bed flat. A nurse stands on each side of bed.	Prevents friction from contact of skin with board.
ii. Remove pillow from under head and shoulders and place it at head of bed.	
iii. Turn patient side to side to place friction-reducing device under drawsheet on bed, with device extending from shoulders to thighs/ankles.	

STEP	RATIONALE
iv. Return patient to supine position.	
v. Have two caregivers grasp drawsheet (one on each side of bed) firmly and have third nurse hold onto end of friction-reducing device.	Slide board remains stationary, provides slippery surface to reduce friction, and allows patient to move up in bed easily.
vi. Place feet apart with forward-backward stance. Flex knees and hips. On count of three, shift weight from front to back leg and move patient and drawsheet to desired position up in bed (see Step 2a[2][c][vi] illustration).	Positions patient smoothly without exerting shear force against skin and without risk of injury to nurses.
(3) Patient unable to assist:	
(a) Use appropriate number of caregivers and appropriate safe-handling devices (e.g., supine sling with ceiling lift or floor-based lift and two or more caregivers).	Repositioning patients manually is associated with high risk of musculoskeletal injury (Matz, 2019).

Critical Decision Point *Protect patient's heels from shearing force by having another caregiver lift heels while moving patient up in bed.*

STEP	RATIONALE
3. Position patient in bed in one of the following positions, ensuring correct body alignment and protecting pressure areas.	Prevents injury to patient's musculoskeletal system and integument. Even positioning patient side to side requires use of safe-handling techniques.
a. Determine whether patient can assist.	Determines degree of risk in repositioning patient and the technique required to safely help patient.
b. With patient lying supine, move them up in bed following Steps 2a(1)–(3).	
c. Position patient in supported semi-Fowler's (see Step 3c illustration) or Fowler's position:	
(1) With patient lying supine, elevate head of bed 45–60 degrees if not contraindicated.	Increases comfort, improves ventilation, and increases patient's opportunity to socialize or relax.
(2) Rest head against mattress or on small pillow.	Prevents flexion contractures of cervical vertebrae.
(3) Use pillows to support arms and hands if patient does not have voluntary control or use of hands and arms.	Prevents shoulder dislocation from effect of downward pull of unsupported arms, promotes circulation by preventing venous pooling, and prevents flexion contractures of arms and wrists.
(4) Position small pillow at lower back.	Supports lumbar vertebrae and decreases flexion of vertebrae.
(5) Place small pillow or roll under thighs.	Prevents hyperextension of knee and occlusion of popliteal artery from pressure from body weight.
(6) Support calves with pillows.	Heels should not be in contact with bed to prevent prolonged pressure of mattress on heels. This is sometimes referred to as *floating* heels.
d. Position hemiplegic patient in supported semi-Fowler's or Fowler's position:	

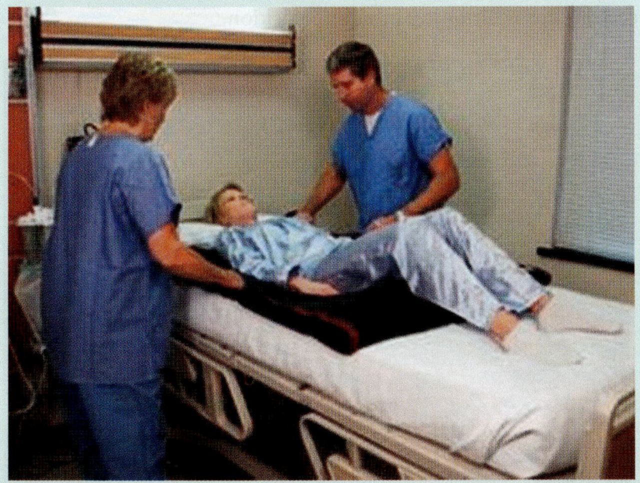

STEP 2A(2)(C)(vi) Moving patient and drawsheet to desired position up in bed. (*From EZ Way, Inc., Clarinda, IA.*)

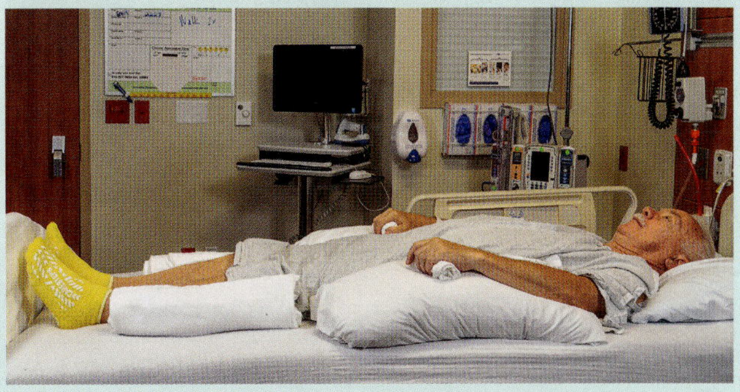

STEP 3C Supported semi-Fowler's position.

STEP	RATIONALE
Critical Decision Point *A patient who has had a cerebrovascular accident (CVA) may have problems with muscle tone that could affect your ability to position them appropriately. Consider consulting with physiotherapist or occupational therapist for special limb braces.*	
(1) Elevate head of bed 45–60 degrees.	Increases comfort, improves ventilation, and increases patient's opportunity to relax. Adjust head of bed according to patient's condition. For example, those with increased risk for pressure injury remain at 30-degree angle (see Chapter 39).
(2) Position patient in Fowler's position as anatomically straight as possible.	Counteracts tendency to slump toward affected side. Improves ventilation and cardiac output; decreases intracranial pressure. Improves patient's ability to swallow, and helps prevent aspiration of food, liquids, and gastric secretions.
(3) Position head on small pillow with chin slightly forward. If patient is totally unable to control head movement, avoid hyperextension of neck.	Prevents hyperextension of neck. Too many pillows under head may cause or worsen neck flexion contracture.
(4) Provide support for involved arm and hand by placing arm away from patient's side and supporting elbow with pillow.	Paralyzed muscles do not automatically resist pull of gravity as they normally do. As a result, shoulder subluxation, pain, and edema may occur.
(5) Place rolled blanket (trochanter roll) firmly alongside patient's legs.	Ensures proper alignment. Prevents external rotation of hips, which contributes to contractures.
(6) Support feet in dorsiflexion with therapeutic boots, splints, or sandbag.	Prevents plantar flexion contractures or footdrop by positioning patient's ankle in neutral dorsiflexion. Positions foot so heel is aligned in opening of splint to prevent pressure. Other therapeutic boots or splints are manufactured with thick padding to cushion heel and prevent pressure injury.
e. Position patient in supported supine position:	
(1) Place patient supine with head of bed flat.	Necessary for properly aligning patient.
(2) Place small, rolled towel under lumbar area of back.	Provides support for lumbar spine.
(3) Place pillow under upper shoulders, neck, and head.	Maintains correct alignment and prevents flexion contractures of cervical vertebrae.
(4) Place trochanter rolls or sandbags parallel to lateral surface of patient's thighs.	Reduces external rotation of hip.
(5) Place patient's feet in dorsiflexion with therapeutic boots, splints, or sandbag (see Step 3e[5] illustration).	Maintains feet in dorsiflexion. Prevents plantar flexion contractures or footdrop.
(6) Place pillows under pronated forearms, keeping upper arms parallel to patient's body (see Step 3e[6] illustration).	Reduces internal rotation of shoulder and prevents extension of elbows. Maintains correct body alignment.
(7) Place hand rolls in patient's hands. Consider physiotherapy collaboration for use of hand splints.	Reduces extension of fingers and abduction of thumb. Maintains thumb slightly adducted and in opposition to fingers.
f. Position hemiplegic patient in supine position:	
(1) Place head of bed flat.	Necessary for positioning in supine position.

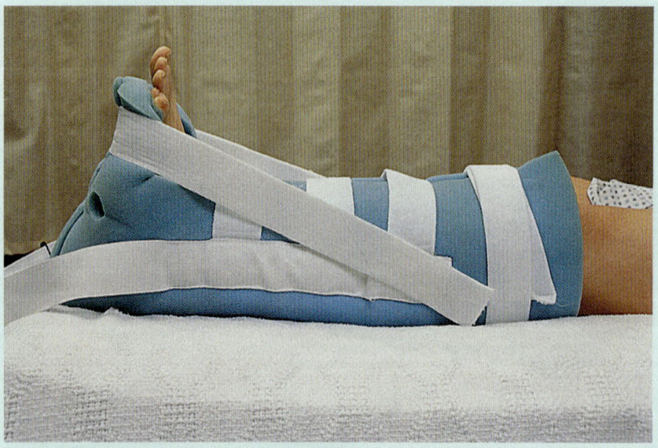

STEP 3E(5) Foot boot with lower leg extension.

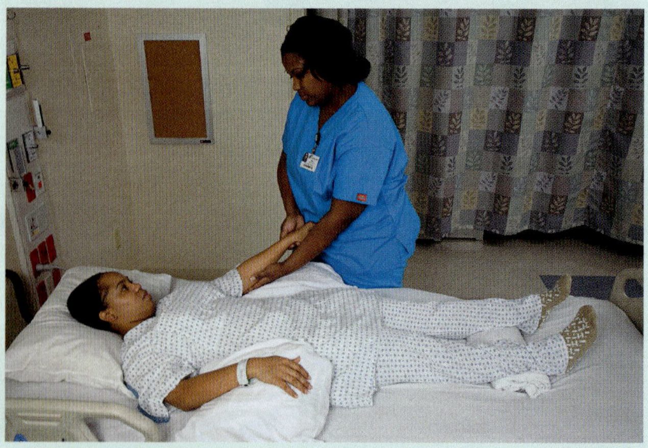

STEP 3E(6) Supported supine position with pillows in place.

STEP	RATIONALE
(2) Place folded towel or small pillow under shoulder of affected side.	Decreases possibility of pain, joint contracture, and subluxation. Maintains mobility in muscles around shoulder to permit normal movement patterns.
(3) Keep affected arm away from body with elbow extended and palm up. Position affected hand in one of recommended positions for flaccid or spastic hand. (Alternative is to place arm out to side, with elbow bent and hand toward head of bed.)	Maintains mobility in arm, joints, and shoulder to permit normal movement patterns. (Alternative position counteracts limitation of ability of arm to rotate outward at shoulder [external rotation]. External rotation must be present to raise arm overhead without pain.)
(4) Place folded towel under hip of involved side.	Diminishes effect of spasticity in entire leg by controlling hip position.
(5) Flex affected knee 30 degrees by supporting it on pillow or folded blanket.	Slight flexion breaks up abnormal extension pattern of leg. Extensor spasticity is most severe when patient is supine.
(6) Support feet with soft pillows at right angle to leg.	Maintains foot in dorsiflexion and prevents footdrop. Pillows prevent stimulation to ball of foot by hard surface, which has tendency to increase muscle tone in patient with extensor spasticity of lower extremity.
g. Position patient in 30-degree lateral (side-lying) position (two nurses):	This position is recommended to prevent development of pressure injury by reducing direct contact of trochanter with support surface (see Chapter 39).
(1) Lower head of bed completely or as low as patient can tolerate. One nurse on each side of bed.	Provides position of comfort for patient and removes pressure from bony prominences on back.
(2) Lower side rail, then position patient on side of bed opposite to the direction in which patient is to be turned. Move upper trunk, supporting shoulders first; then move lower trunk, supporting hips.	Provides room for patient to turn to side.
(3) Flex patient's knee that will not be next to mattress, after being turned. Keep foot on mattress. Place one hand on patient's upper bent leg near hip and other hand on patient's shoulder.	Use of leverage makes turning to side easy.
(4) Using knee and hip for leverage, roll patient onto side toward you.	Rolling decreases trauma to tissues. In addition, patient is positioned so leverage on hip makes turning easy.
(5) Place pillow under patient's head and neck.	Maintains alignment. Reduces lateral neck flexion. Decreases strain on sternocleidomastoid muscle.
(6) Nurse facing patient's back places hands under patient's dependent shoulder and brings shoulder blade forward.	Prevents patient's weight from resting directly on shoulder joint.
(7) Position both arms in slightly flexed position. Support upper arm with pillow level with shoulder; other arm, by mattress.	Decreases internal rotation and adduction of shoulder. Supporting both arms in slightly flexed position protects joint. Ventilation improves because chest is able to expand more easily.
(8) Place hands under dependent hip and bring hip slightly forward so angle from hip to mattress is approximately 30 degrees.	The 30-degree lateral position reduces pressure on trochanter; designed to prevent pressure injury.
(9) Place small tuck-back pillow behind patient's back. (Make by folding pillow lengthwise. Smooth area is slightly tucked under patient's back.)	Provides support to maintain patient on side.
(10) Place pillow under semiflexed upper leg, supporting leg so it is level with hip from groin to foot (see Step 3g[10] illustration).	Flexion prevents hyperextension of leg. Maintains leg in correct alignment. Prevents pressure on bony prominences.
(11) Place sandbags parallel to plantar surface of dependent foot. May use ankle-foot orthotic on feet if available.	Maintains dorsiflexion of foot.
h. Position patient in semiprone position:	
(1) Lower head of bed completely.	Provides for proper body alignment while patient is lying down.
(2) Place patient supine on side of bed opposite to the direction in which they are to be turned. Move upper trunk, supporting shoulders first, followed by moving lower trunk, supporting hips.	Prepares patient for position.
(3) Move to other side of bed and turn patient on side. Place in lateral position, with patient lying partially on abdomen, dependent shoulder lifted out, and arm placed at patient's side.	

STEP	RATIONALE

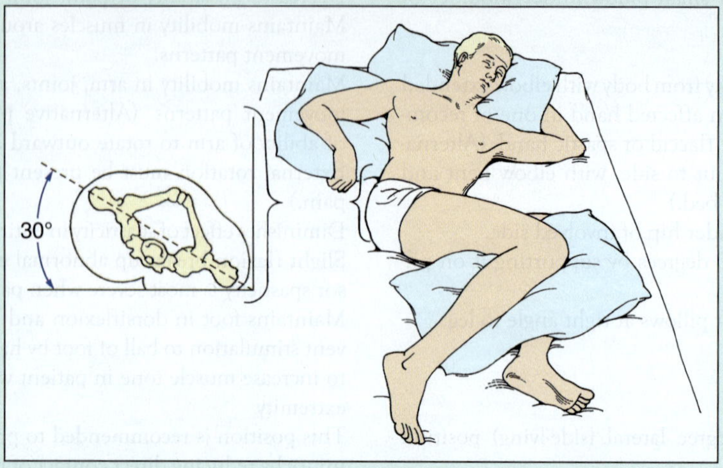

STEP 3G(10) Thirty-degree lateral position with pillows in place.

STEP	RATIONALE
(4) Place small pillow under patient's head.	Maintains proper alignment and prevents lateral neck flexion.
(5) Place pillow under flexed upper arm, supporting arm level with shoulder.	Prevents internal rotation of shoulder. Maintains alignment.
(6) Place pillow under flexed upper legs, supporting leg level with hip.	Prevents internal rotation of hip and adduction of leg. Flexion prevents hyperextension of leg. Reduces mattress pressure on knees and ankles.
(7) Place sandbags parallel to plantar surface of foot (see Step 3h[7] illustration).	Maintains foot in dorsiflexion. Prevents plantar flexion contractures or footdrop.
i. Logroll patient (three nurses):	

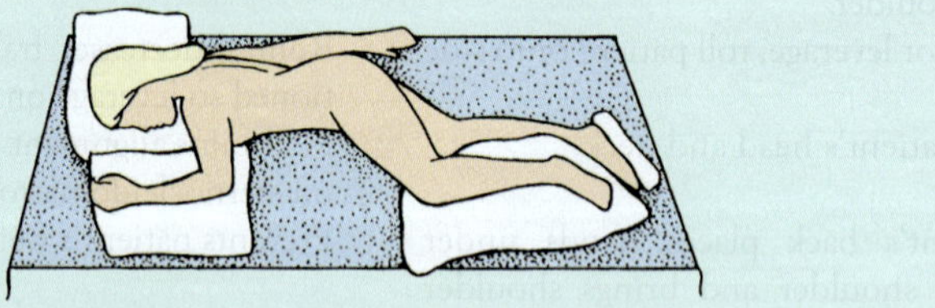

STEP 3H(7) Sandbag supporting right foot in dorsiflexion.

Critical Decision Point *A nurse can have the UCP assist when there is a health care provider's prescription to logroll a patient. Patients with a spinal cord injury or those recovering from neck, back, or spinal surgery often need to keep the spinal column in straight alignment to prevent further injury.*

STEP	RATIONALE
(1) Place small pillow between patient's knees.	Prevents tension on spinal column and adduction of hip.
(2) Cross patient's arms on chest.	Prevents injury to arms.
(3) Position two nurses on side toward which patient is to be turned and one nurse on side where pillows are to be placed (see Step 3i[3] illustration).	Distributes weight equally between nurses during turning.
(4) Fanfold drawsheet along backside of patient.	Provides strong handles to grip drawsheet without slipping.
(5) With one nurse grasping drawsheet at lower hips and thighs and the other nurse grasping drawsheet at patient's shoulders and lower back, roll patient as one unit in a smooth, continuous motion on count of three (see Step 3i[5] illustration).	Maintains proper alignment by moving all body parts at the same time, preventing tension or twisting of spinal column.
(6) Nurse on opposite side of bed places pillows along length of patient for support (see Step 3i[6] illustration).	Maintains patient in side-lying position.

STEP	RATIONALE
(7) Gently lean patient as a unit back toward pillows for support. Place patient's feet in therapeutic boots or splints if appropriate.	Ensures continued straight alignment of spinal column, preventing injury. Prevents foot drop.
4. Raise side rails (as appropriate) and lower bed to lowest position. Ensure nurse call system is within easy reach.	Promotes safety and prevents falls. Ensures patient can call for assistance if needed.

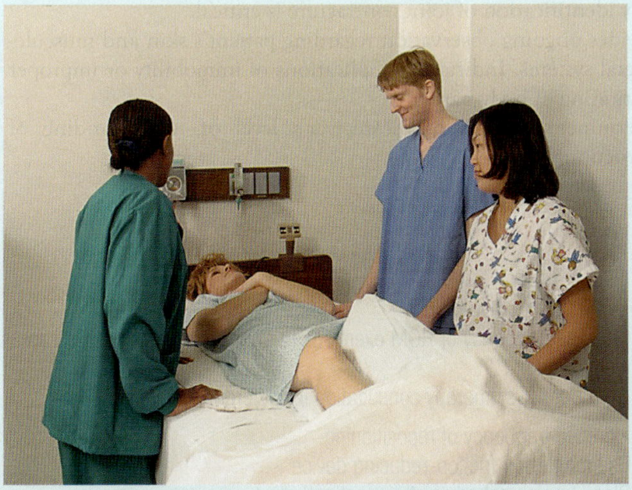

STEP 3I(3) Preparing patient for logrolling.

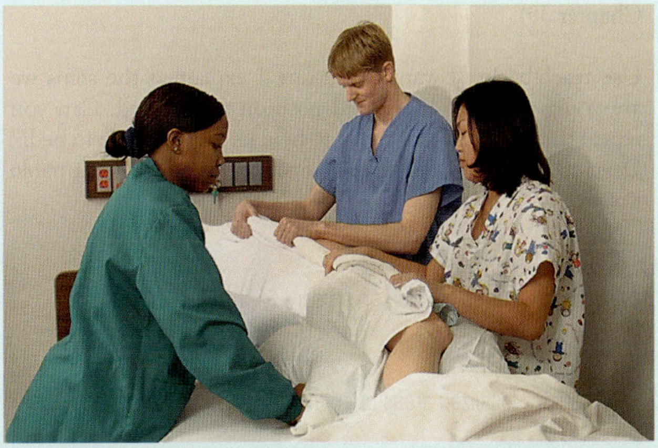

STEP 3I(6) Placing pillows along patient's back for support.

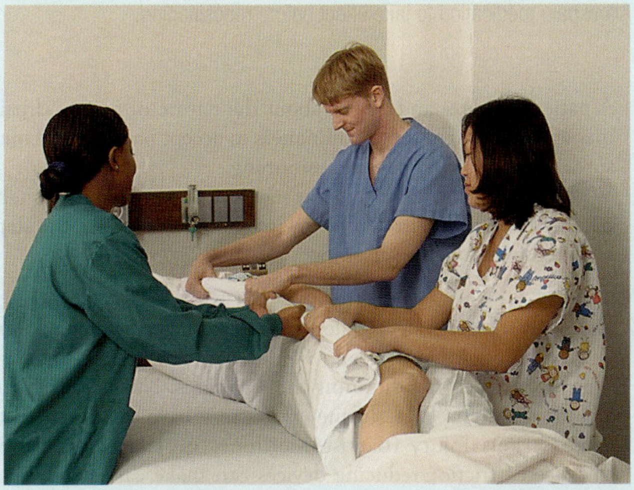

STEP 3I(5) Logrolling patient onto side.

STEP	RATIONALE

EVALUATION

STEP	RATIONALE
1. Assess patient's body alignment, position, and level of comfort. Patient's body should be supported by adequate mattress, and vertebral column should be without observable curves.	Determines effectiveness of positioning. Additional supports (e.g., pillows, bath blankets) may be added or removed to promote comfort and correct body alignment.
2. Observe for changes in joint ROM.	Early identification of joint contracture is critical.
3. Observe for areas of erythema or breakdown involving skin (see Chapter 39).	Provides ongoing observation regarding patient's skin and musculoskeletal systems. Indicates complications of immobility or improper positioning of body part.
4. Use teach-back: "I want to be sure I explained the steps we are going to use to move and position you in bed. Can you repeat the steps you can follow to help us move you up in bed?" Develop a revised teaching plan if patient or caregiver is unable to teach back correctly.	Determines patient's and caregiver's level of understanding of instructional topic.

Unexpected Outcomes	Related Interventions
1. Joint contractures develop or worsen.	• Increase frequency of ROM exercises to affected and immobilized areas (see Chapter 12). • Consider physiotherapy consultation for different positioning.
2. Skin shows localized areas of erythema and breakdown.	• Increase frequency of repositioning. • Use a different friction-reducing device. • Place turning schedule above patient's bed.
3. Patient avoids moving.	• Medicate with analgesia as prescribed by health care provider to ensure patient's comfort before moving. • Allow pain medication to take effect before repositioning.

Communication and Documentation

- Document in progress notes in EHR or chart: time and position change of patient throughout shift, observations (e.g., condition of skin, joint movement, patient's ability to help with positioning), and whether positioning devices are needed.
- Document your evaluation of patient and caregiver learning.
- Communicate observations during hand-off report and document in progress notes in EHR or chart.
- Communicate skin or joint complications to health care provider.

Special Considerations

Teaching

- Teach caregiver how to position patient, especially when caring for infant, young child, or confused or unconscious patient.
- Teach patient ways to help with positioning and provide opportunity for return demonstration.
- Teach patient and caregiver signs and symptoms of pressure injury and contractures.
- A patient's values and beliefs about the nature of pain and pain management might affect willingness to accept pain control measures needed for frequent repositioning.
- With patients who are in any way sensitive to personal contact, be patient and explain in depth why it is necessary to take the steps required for proper positioning.

Pediatric

- Owing to the generally smaller size and frame of young children, it is common for nurses and family members to use the basic draw sheet when repositioning these patients. Nurses will manually lift children. These lifting efforts may have the potential to cause serious injury (Baptiste-McKinney & Halvorson, 2018). The use of friction-reducing devices can make care tasks much more comfortable and prevent injury.

Gerontological

- Reposition older persons at least every 1 to 2 hours and maintain a regular program of ROM exercises (Tyerman & Cobbett, 2022).

✦ REVIEW QUESTIONS

A 37-year-old patient (he/him) who may have suffered a spinal cord injury in a motor vehicle accident is admitted to the health care institution. He has sustained multiple deep lacerations on his face and trunk and facial fractures of the maxillary and zygomatic bones. He has a cervical collar in place. He rates his pain at 9 on a scale of 0 to 10 (with 0 = no pain and 10 = worst pain ever). He weighs approximately 88 kg (193.6 lb). You are preparing to transfer him to a stretcher. The emergency department nurse was extremely busy and was unable to provide a complete report. Review Questions 1 to 3 relate to the case study presented here.

1. Which other information would you obtain about this patient before safely transferring him to a stretcher?
2. The unregulated care provider (UCP) states that the patient wants to be turned and that he will be glad to reposition him without help. The health care provider's prescription is for logrolling until the computed tomography (CT) scan is completed and injury to the neck and spine is ruled out. What is the appropriate, safe action in response to turning the patient? Explain your answer.
3. The patient continues to feel pain at a level of 7 after receiving pain medication, and his heart rate is 118 beats/min compared with a baseline of 82. The patient states, "I can't take this pain anymore." He refuses to go to radiology for this procedure. Write an SBAR (situation–background–assessment–recommendation) for communicating this situation.
4. A patient is to sit up in a chair for breakfast 1 day after abdominal surgery per the health care provider's prescriptions. Which of the following would you select to ensure a safe transfer while facilitating cooperation from the patient? (*Select all that apply.*)
   1. Offer pain medication 30 minutes before transferring patient.
   2. Assess presence of weakness, dizziness, and muscle strength.
   3. Determine need for safe patient-handling device.
   4. Ask the UCP to transfer patient to the chair.
   5. Follow prescription to transfer patient even though patient is refusing.
5. Place the following steps in the correct sequence to facilitate safe transfer from wheelchair to bed.
   1. Position wheelchair at a 45-degree angle next to bed.
   2. Stand by as you have patient move to front of wheelchair.
   3. Raise footplates and apply transfer belt.
   4. Lock wheelchair.
   5. Position self slightly in front of patient.
   6. Have patient stand as you place both hands under transfer belt and pivot to side of bed.
   7. Adjust height of bed to level of wheelchair seat.
6. Place the following steps in the correct sequence for safe use of a mechanical/hydraulic lift to transfer patients from bed to chair.
   1. Release check valve slowly and lower patient into chair.
   2. Roll patient back toward you as second nurse pulls hammock (straps) through holes.
   3. Position chair near bed and allow adequate space to manoeuvre lift.
   4. Attach hooks on strap to holes in sling.
   5. Roll patient onto side toward second nurse and position sling under patient.
   6. Use lift to raise patient off bed and steering handle to pull lift from bed and manoeuvre to chair.
   7. Place horseshoe base of floor lift under patient's bed and lower horizontal bar to sling level.
   8. Roll patient supine onto canvas seat.

Visit the Evolve site for a complete list of answers to the Review Questions.

✦ NEXT GENERATION NCLEX® (NGN)

For practice with answering exam questions related to unfolding NGN case studies, please consult the Next Generation NCLEX® (NGN)-Style Case Studies for Skills and Techniques on the Evolve website: http://evolve.elsevier.com/Canada/Perry/clinicalskills/

REFERENCES

Accreditation Canada. (2020). *Required organizational practices handbook.* https://physicians.nshealth.ca/resources/required-organizational-practices-2020-handbook

Association of Workers' Compensation Boards of Canada. (2021). *National Work Injury/Disease Statistics Program (NWISP): Lost time claims–injury/disease.* https://awcbc.org/en/statistics/

Baptiste-McKinney, A., & Halvorson, B. (2018). The use of friction-reducing devices in a safe patient handling and mobility program. *International Journal of Safe Patient Handling & Mobility, 8*(3), 132–141. https://sphmjournal.com/product/use-friction-reducing-devices-safe-patient-handling-mobility-program/

Biswas, D., Karabin, B., & Turner, D. (2019). Role of nurses and nurse practitioners in the recognition, diagnosis, and management of neurogenic orthostatic hypotension: A narrative review. *International Journal of General Medicine, 12,* 173–184. https://doi.org/10.2147/IJGM.S170655

Booker, S. Q., Herr, K. A., & Horgas, A. L. (2021). A paradigm shift for movement-based pain assessment in older adults: Practice, policy and regulatory drivers. *Pain Management Nursing, 22*(1), 21–27. https://doi.org/10.1016/j.pmn.2020.08.003

Boscart, V., McCleary, L., Sheiban Taucar, L., et al. (2023). *Ebersole and Hess' gerontological nursing and healthy aging in Canada* (3rd ed.). Elsevier.

Canadian Centre for Occupational Health and Safety (CCOHS). (2012). *Patient lifts and worker risks.* https://www.ccohs.ca/newsletters/hsreport/issues/2012/08/ezine.html [Seminal Reference]

Canadian Centre for Occupational Health and Safety (CCOHS). (2018). *Ergonomic safe patient handling program.* https://www.ccohs.ca/oshanswers/hsprograms/patient_handling.html

Fairchild, S. L., & O'Shea, R. K. (2022). *Pierson and Fairchild's principles and techniques of patient care* (7th ed.). Elsevier.

Government of Canada. (2015). *Hospital bed safety.* https://www.canada.ca/en/health-canada/services/drugs-medical-devices/hospital-bed-safety.html [Seminal Reference]

Hockenberry, M. J., Duffy, E. A., & Gibbs, K. (2024). *Wong's nursing care of infants and children* (12th ed.). Elsevier.

Matz, M. (2019). *Patient handling and mobility assessments: A white paper* (2nd ed.). The Facility Guidelines Institute. https://www.fgiguidelines.org/wp-content/uploads/2019/10/FGI-Patient-Handling-and-Mobility-Assessments_191008.pdf

Nova Scotia Health. (2022). *Safe patient handling and mobility program.* https://library.nshealth.ca/InjuryPrevention#s-lg-box-12487534

Occupational Health Clinic for Ontario Workers Inc. (2022). *Patient handling for healthcare workers.* https://www.ohcow.on.ca/edit/files/general_handouts/Healthcare%20Workers%20Patient%20Handling.pdf

Occupational Safety and Health Association. (2014). *Safe patient handling–preventing musculoskeletal disorders in nursing homes.* OSHA Publication 3108. https://www.osha.gov/Publications/OSHA3708.pdf [Seminal Reference]

Power-Kean, K., Zettel, S., El-Hussein, M. T., et al. (2023). *Huether and McCance's understanding pathophysiology* (2nd ed.). Elsevier Inc.

Tyerman, J., & Cobbett, S. (Eds.) (2023). *Lewis's medical-surgical nursing in Canada: Assessment and management of clinical problems* (5th ed.). Elsevier Canada.

WorkSafeNB. (2015). *Transfer belts.* https://www.worksafenb.ca/media/1783/transferdist-1.pdf [Seminal Reference]

12 Exercise, Mobility, and Immobilization Devices

Canadian content written by **Shawna Ryan, RN, COHN, MN**
Original US chapter by **Patricia A. Potter, RN, MSN, PhD, FAAN**

SKILLS AND PROCEDURES

OBJECTIVES

Mastery of content in this chapter will enable the nurse to:

- Describe the implications of preventing deconditioning and deep vein thrombosis in patient care.
- Describe the evidence that supports early activity and exercise in patient care.
- Explain how to plan a safe exercise program for a patient.
- Describe indications for performing range-of-motion exercises.
- Describe risk factors related to the development of deep vein thrombosis.
- Identify complications that may develop in a patient wearing either elastic stockings or a sequential compression device.
- Identify significant assessment data to be noted before assisting with exercise and ambulation.
- Demonstrate assisting with ambulation, assisting with ambulation with the use of an assistive device, assisting with range-of-motion exercises, and applying elastic stockings and a sequential compression device.
- Develop teaching plans for safety in the home while using an ambulation aid, applying and monitoring effects of elastic stockings and sequential compression devices, and performing range-of-motion exercises.

MEDIA RESOURCES

- http://evolve.elsevier.com/Canada/Perry/clinicalskills/

PURPOSE

Regular physical activity and exercise contribute to patients' physical and emotional well-being while at the same time positively impacting their psychosocial health (MacDonald & Jakubec, 2021; San Román-Mata et al., 2020). Regular physical activity and exercise should apply in the care of patients in all settings. Functional decline (e.g., the loss of the ability to perform self-care or activities of daily living [ADLs]) may result not only from illness or adverse treatment effects but also from deconditioning. Deconditioning is associated with inactivity and can lead to generalized weakness, impaired aerobic capacity, and cognitive impairment within a short period of time (Chen et al., 2022). Deconditioning results in numerous physical changes and is a particular risk for hospitalized patients who spend most of their time in bed, even when they are able to walk. Nurses can play an important role in increasing the overall activity of patients across the continuum of care to minimize the effects of deconditioning (Coles et al., 2020). In addition to deconditioning, patients with limited mobility are at risk of developing thromboembolic disease and deep vein thrombosis (DVT) (Box 12.1). The promotion of early exercise and mobility in health care settings and as a daily therapy for patients is basic to competent nursing practice.

STANDARDS OF CARE

- Accreditation Canada (2020)—*Required Organizational Practices—2020 Handbook* (https://physicians.nshealth.ca/resources/required-organizational-practices-2020-handbook)
- Canadian Association of Critical Care Nurses (CACCN, 2018)—*Position Statement: Patient- and Family-Centred Care* (https://caccn.ca/wp-content/uploads/2019/10/PS062018PSPFCCare.pdf)
- Centers for Disease Control and Prevention (2022)—*What Is Venous Thromboembolism?* (https://www.cdc.gov/ncbddd/dvt/facts.html)
- Registered Nurses' Association of Ontario (RNAO, 2017)—*Preventing Falls and Reducing Injury From Falls* (https://rnao.ca/bpg/guidelines/prevention-falls-and-fall-injuries)

BOX 12.1

Risk Factors for Deep Vein Thrombosis

Injury to a Vein, Often Caused By:
- Fractures
- Severe muscle injury
- Major surgery (e.g., involving the abdomen, pelvis, hip, or legs)

Decreased Blood Flow, Often Caused By:
- Confinement to bed (e.g., caused by a medical condition or after surgery)
- Limited movement (e.g., a cast on a leg to help heal an injured bone)
- Sitting for a long time, especially with crossed legs
- Paralysis

Increased Estrogen, Often Caused By:
- Birth control pills
- Hormone replacement therapy, sometimes used after menopause
- Pregnancy, for up to 6 weeks after giving birth

Certain Chronic Medical Illnesses, Such As:
- Heart disease, lung disease, cancer and its treatment, inflammatory bowel disease (Crohn's disease or ulcerative colitis)

Other Factors, Including:
- Previous DVT or PE
- Family history of DVT or PE
- Age (risk increases as age increases)
- Obesity
- A catheter located in a central vein
- Inherited clotting factors

DVT, Deep vein thrombosis; *PE,* pulmonary embolism.

From Centers for Disease Control and Prevention. (2022). *What is venous thromboembolism?* https://www.cdc.gov/ncbddd/dvt/facts.html

- Registered Nurses' Association of Ontario (RNAO, 2010)—*Strategies to Support Self-Management in Chronic Conditions: Collaboration With Clients* (https://rnao.ca/bpg/guidelines/strategies-support-selfmanagement-chronic-conditions-collaboration-clients)

PRINCIPLES FOR PRACTICE

- Older persons are at greater risk of losing muscle mass, strength, and power; developing orthostatic hypotension, decubitus ulcers, syncope, and confusion; and experiencing fractures and functional incontinence because of decreased mobility from bed rest (Liu et al., 2018; Parola et al., 2021; Smith et al., 2020).
- Early mobility and activity reduce impairment in cardiovascular and metabolic functioning, and lower the risk for pulmonary complications, development of pressure injury, and elimination alterations (Alaparthi et al., 2020; Coles et al., 2020; Liu et al., 2018).
- Changes in a patient's mobility and activity can result from a variety of health problems (e.g., musculoskeletal, cardiovascular, and neurological) and therapeutic reasons (e.g., prescribed bed rest or reduced activity from sedation). Direct nursing measures help to maintain or restore optimal mobility and decrease the hazards associated with immobility.
- It is important to act aggressively and to implement early activity and mobility once patients are physiologically stable and able to respond to verbal stimulation (Coles et al., 2020).
- When caring for patients with reduced mobility, consider that there may be profound psychosocial and developmental effects (Wheatley et al., 2020). Across the lifespan, immobilization often leads to emotional, intellectual, sensory, and sociocultural alterations. For younger and older persons alike, immobility may alter employment, family role functions, and social interactions. Such changes can lead to altered self-concept, lowered self-esteem, and depression.

PERSON-CENTRED CARE

Person-centred care in nursing practice involves integrating the whole person as a partner in care (CACCN, 2018). In exercise and mobility, person-centred care is realized when the nurse:

- Empowers and promotes the patient's proactive and preferred level of engagement in their health (CACCN, 2018). It is important to assess each patient's expectations concerning activity and exercise and determine their perception of what is normal or acceptable.
- Assesses a patient's level of physical and emotional comfort as well as their basic safety needs before implementing activity or exercise therapies (CACCN, 2018; RNAO, 2017). Patients with pain, nausea, or fatigue have little motivation to engage in physical activity. Patients who are anxious or afraid of injury often resist participation.
- Is sensitive to the nonmedical aspects of care (culture, beliefs, values, and spirituality) (CACCN, 2018). When assisting with exercises or ambulation, the nurse must recognize that these activities may place patients in compromising positions. Provide privacy (e.g., clothing, blanket, privacy curtains around bed) to preserve the patient's dignity and enhance participation.

EVIDENCE-INFORMED PRACTICE

- It is estimated that more than half of all patients hospitalized are at increased risk for the development of venous thromboembolism (VTE). Current evidence supports the following early nonpharmacological interventions in addition to pharmacological prophylaxis to prevent VTE (Bircher & Chowdhury, 2020):
  - Early ambulation
  - Mechanical methods of VTE prevention (e.g., intermittent pneumatic compression, graduated compression stockings, venous foot pump)
  - Continuation of prophylaxis until the patient is ambulatory or discharged
  - Pharmacological prophylaxis for patients at low risk of bleeding who have at least one risk factor for the development of VTE (e.g., prolonged immobility ≥3 days, age ≥60 years of age, previous VTE)
  - A formal program in health care agencies for VTE prevention
- Immobility and the resultant deconditioning of hospitalized patients have led to greater efforts within hospitals to adopt evidence-informed early progressive mobility protocols:
  - Schallom and colleagues (2020) examined the impact of an interdisciplinary mobility protocol in seven specialty intensive care units. The results indicate that early patient mobilization benefits include increased mobility levels, a significant decrease in intensive care unit length of stay, and decreased delirium. Complications resulting from early mobilization were minimal.
  - In a systematic review of the literature, it was found that safe and effective interventions that support early mobilization and physiotherapy can have a significant impact on functional outcomes in the critical care setting (Alaparthi et al., 2020; Negro et al., 2018). In critical care units and immediate post-acute environments, the mobilization of critically ill but stable

patients who have required a period of mechanical ventilation can be done safely with minimal risk to patients.

- Even though the evidence strongly supports the benefits of early mobilization in a variety of health care settings, adhering to the protocol is not always consistent owing to institutional, nurse, patient, and treatment barriers such as nurse-to-patient ratio, knowledge deficit, illness severity, and presence of tubes and drains (Coles et al., 2020). In a study designed to address the challenges with implementing early mobilization protocols, researchers found that using evidence-informed practice to address these barriers was effective for enhancing postoperative recovery of patients who had abdominal surgery (Coles et al., 2020). More research is needed in this area, but early mobilization is becoming a more common practice.
- Across the continuum of care, physical activity and exercise are integral aspects for older populations and those with chronic and neuromuscular diseases (i.e., multiple sclerosis [MS], Parkinson's disease, diabetes mellitus) who are negatively affected by immobility. Whether patients are hospitalized or situated in the community, the integration of physical activity and exercise can promote health and prevent risks such as falls.
- Hendrich (2021) has advocated that mobility is a predictor of health-related quality of life among older persons and that preserving mobility requires equal focus on other aspects of a care plan.
- Exercise leads to enhanced quality of life, improved cognition, and independence as well as reduced fatigue, anger, and depression among people with MS (Multiple Sclerosis Society of Canada, 2022).

SAFETY GUIDELINES

- Obtain and become familiar with any type of assistive device to be used. Know how to properly prepare and use a device so you can teach patients or caregivers how to use it safely and correctly.
- Prior to any mobilization, prepare yourself, the patient, the environment, and the equipment. Ensure that the patient's vital signs are stable, that pain is controlled, and that their energy level supports activity. Obtain assistance from other personnel as needed, ensure the environment is clear from clutter, use safe patient-handling devices, and have the patient wear flat, nonskid shoes or socks.
- Assess the patient's cognitive status for their ability to follow mobility instructions as well as their fear of falling. Ask patients about their fear of falling and whether they have fallen recently, and identify ways to reduce falling risks.
- Use appropriate clinical guidelines (see employer protocols) for assessing level of mobility (Chapter 11) and advancing a patient's activity level. Interprofessional collaboration is required to ensure a coordinated, holistic approach to mobility decision making for the patient, with shared, complementary responsibilities among members of the health care team (MOVE Canada, 2022).
- Know a patient's care plan for discharge planning. A patient may need to continue the exercise regimen or use an assistive device for their care in the community setting.

✦ SKILL 12.1 Promoting Early Activity and Exercise

Regular physical activity is strongly linked to improved physical and mental health and healthy development of Canadians of all ages, regardless of whether a chronic disease or disability is present (Government of Canada, 2018). As a nurse, you may work in a variety of settings with the opportunity to engage patients in mobility and plan health promotion activities. It is crucial to educate patients and caregivers about the importance of regular physical activity and exercise and how these activities can be incorporated into daily routines.

In health care settings, interprofessional health care members have made a concerted effort to increase patients' activity and mobility levels as soon as possible, to prevent deconditioning and other complications of immobilization. Early progressive mobility protocols are the standard of care for critical care patients as well as for those on general nursing units and across the continuum of care (see employer policy for protocols) (Coles et al., 2020). However, the success and progression of these protocols require tailoring of early mobility to the individual's condition (Coles et al., 2020; Liu et al., 2018). While the positive impact of early mobilization is recognized, nurses often have difficulty routinely helping patients ambulate because of overall patient care demands and heavy workload, lack of access to equipment, or lack of familiarity with transfer skills and training (see Chapter 11) (Alaparthi et al., 2020). Some hospitals have designated special mobility teams or mobility assistants to engage patients in early ambulation and activity. Successful implementation of early progressive mobility protocols and improved patient outcomes are linked to interprofessional collaboration in which all members of the interprofessional team are involved in mobility decisions (Brock et al., 2018; Hodgson et al., 2018). The interprofessional team includes, but is not limited to, the nurse, respiratory therapist, physiotherapist, physician, pharmacist, and patient.

Delegation and Collaboration

The skill of promoting early activity and exercise for patients can be delegated to an unregulated care provider (UCP) trained in transfer and assisted ambulation skills. Across health care settings (e.g., hospitals, long-term care facilities, home, and community settings), the nurse directs the UCP by doing the following:

- Explaining the level of progressive mobility that a patient has achieved
- Explaining any restrictions in prescribed range-of-motion (ROM) exercises (see Procedural Guideline 12.1)
- Explaining whether there are any weight-bearing precautions or whether the patient needs to use assistive devices
- Explaining criteria to use to stop assisted ambulation or sitting if the patient cannot tolerate activity

Equipment

- Inpatient: Pulse oximeter, gait belt, patient-specific mobility tools, and assistive devices (see Skill 12.2)
- Outpatient: Patient-specific mobility tools and assistive devices, dependent on type of exercise recommended (e.g., 2.2-kg [5-lb] weights, resistance bands)

STEP	RATIONALE
ASSESSMENT	
1. Identify patient using at least two person-specific identifiers (e.g., name and date of birth, or name and medical record number) according to employer policy.	Ensures correct patient. Complies with Accreditation Canada's standards and improves patient safety (Accreditation Canada, 2020).
2. Throughout the procedure, the 4 moments for hand hygiene are to be implemented; hand hygiene should occur before initial patient (or patient environment) contact, before an aseptic procedure, after body fluid exposure risk, and after patient (or patient environment) contact. Additional hand hygiene should be performed when hands are visibly soiled.	Proper hand hygiene helps prevent the spread of infectious agents to health care providers.
3. Review patient's health record for: • Baseline mobility and functional history • Mobility restrictions and weight-bearing status • Medical history conditions that influence or contraindicate mobility/exercise (e.g., dysrhythmias, recent myocardial infarction, stroke, paralyzed extremity, neuromuscular disease, peripheral neuropathy, current pregnancy) • Health care provider's prescription for early mobility or exercise program	Examples of conditions that may contraindicate or require adjustments to activity. Patients should have medical clearance to begin an activity/exercise program.
4. Assess patient's beliefs, values, and perceptions regarding current health status and confidence in being capable of performing exercise.	Perceived self-efficacy is a judgement of capability. The outcomes that people anticipate depend largely on their judgements of how well they will be able to perform in given situations (Hodgson et al., 2018; RNAO, 2010; Simpson et al., 2021).
5. Gather baseline assessment of vital signs and oxygen saturation (if available).	Allows you to assess patient's ability to participate in activity/exercise and evaluate patient's response to activity/exercise.
6. Assess patient's pain level using an appropriate pain rating scale (see Chapter 16 for pain assessment resources).	Determines whether there is need for an analgesic before mobilizing or ambulating patient. Allows you to counsel patient as to best time to attempt more strenuous exercise.
7. Complete a patient mobility assessment (see Chapter 11) within 24 hours of admission (MOVE Canada, 2022).	Allows you to minimize injury to self and patient, determine whether it is safe to mobilize a patient independently, and determine whether assistive devices are required.
8. Implement early progressive mobility protocol specific to the acuity of your patient (e.g., critical care).	Mobility protocols are established for acute care patients with specific protocols for critical care. Different mobility protocols and policies exist for various levels of care.

Critical Decision Point *Terminate physical activity when:*

- *Heart rate is greater than a 20% increase in resting value or less than 40 beats/min or greater than 130 beats/min.*
- *Oxygen saturation shows greater than 4% drop from baseline or less than 88–90%.*
- *Blood pressure: Systolic pressure is greater than 180 mm Hg or greater than 20% decrease in systolic/diastolic or orthostatic hypotension.*
- *Respirations are less than 5 breaths/min or greater than 40 breaths/min.*

Terminate exercise if dizziness lasts 60 seconds or fainting or diaphoresis occurs; change in breathing pattern occurs with increase in accessory muscle use, extreme fatigue, or severe dyspnea with respiratory rate greater than baseline by more than 20 breaths/min (Bassett et al., 2021; Wahba et al., 2022; Yang et al., 2021).

STEP	RATIONALE
9. Perform a multisystem assessment (e.g., cardiac, respiratory, musculoskeletal, and neurological) and safety screening (Alaparthi et al., 2020; Coles et al., 2020; Yu et al., 2021).	If high-risk clinical features are present, then consultation should take place with the health care provider and team prior to mobilization. Allows you to assess patient's ability to participate in activity/exercise.
Cardiac status: Assess patient's myocardial stability. • No evidence of active myocardial ischemia has occurred over last 24 hours. • No dysrhythmia requiring new antidysrhythmic drug has occurred over last 24 hours. • Heart rate is >40 beats/min and <130 beats/min. • Stable blood pressure (systolic >90 mm Hg or no change of more than 30 mm Hg) (Bassett et al., 2021; Yang et al., 2021).	Ensures cardiac stability. Exercise can initiate ischemic attack or worsen dysrhythmias (Bassett et al., 2021; Yang et al., 2021).
• No increase of any inotrope/vasopressor agents has occurred for last 2 hours (Yang et al., 2021).	Change in inotrope/vasopressor dose could lead to adverse effects, including tachycardia, dysrhythmias, and blood pressure changes such as orthostatic hypotension (Bassett at al., 2021; Burchum & Rosenthal, 2021).

STEP	RATIONALE
Respiratory status: Assess oxygenation status; must be adequate on: • Fraction of inspired oxygen (FiO_2) ≤60% • Positive end-expiratory pressure (PEEP) (on ventilator) <10 cm H_2O • Respiratory rate <30 breaths/min (Wittmer et al., 2021) • Oxygen saturation ≥90% (Bassett et al., 2021)	Activity assessment criteria allow for early ambulation (Yang et al., 2021).
Musculoskeletal: No unstable major fractures or large open wounds (Bassett et al., 2021)	Healing of unstable fractures and wounds can be compromised if mobilized too early or incorrectly (Tyerman & Cobbett, 2023).
Neurological status: • Patient engages to voice of caregiver. • Patient responds appropriately to verbal stimulation and commands. • No evidence of spinal precautions, open lumbar drains, or uncontrolled seizures.	Patient must be alert, responsive, and able to follow directions (Yang et al., 2021).
10. Assessment to facilitate transition and support of mobility/exercise in community.	
a. Identify patient's activity/exercise history: • "Which type of regular daily exercise do you perform at home?" • "Do you exercise or play a sport at least three times a week? How often in a week do you exercise, and how would you describe the intensity of this exercise (i.e., breathless, sweating, increased heart rate)?" • "How long have you been exercising regularly?"	Provides information on patient's motivation or willingness to exercise regularly. Allows you to plan exercise that complements and advances patient's activity level.
b. Ask patient to what extent they enjoy exercising and what their beliefs are about their ability to exercise.	Factors positively associated with adult physical activity (Astle & Duggleby, 2024).
c. Determine whether patient has social support from peers, family, friends, or spouse.	Factors positively associated with adult physical activity (Astle & Duggleby, 2024).
d. Determine whether patient has access to facility or area to exercise. Is their neighbourhood considered safe?	Absence of facility or sense of safety discourages activity/exercise.
e. Consider these factors in your assessment: patient's age, income level, time available to exercise, rural resident, overweight, being disabled.	Factors negatively associated with adult participation in activity (Astle & Duggleby, 2024).
f. Have patient rate quality of life based on current activity level.	Serves as baseline to measure long-term benefits of exercise.

NURSING DIAGNOSES

- Acute pain
- Persistent pain
- Readiness for enhanced health management
- Reduced physical mobility
- Reduced stamina

Related factors are individualized on the basis of patient's condition or needs.

PLANNING

STEP	RATIONALE
1. Expected outcomes following completion of procedure: • Inpatient: Patient will progress from sitting on edge of bed to sitting in chair 20 minutes three times a day (TID). • Inpatient: Patient will gradually increase ambulation distance during hospital stay. • Outpatient: Patient will identify and develop an exercise and activity program to perform. • Outpatient: Patient will demonstrate adherence to exercise/activity plan at home. • Patient will report a perceived improvement in overall mobility and quality of life (NOTE: Some employers may use a scale for measurement).	Early mobility protocol is designed with progressive levels of exercise to promote improved patient function and cognition; reduce length of hospital stay, complications of illness, and bed rest; and improve patient's perceived quality of life. Relevant and appropriate exercise plan increases adherence.
2. Inpatient: Consult with physiotherapy regarding role in protocol to provide planned active resistance exercise for patients. Consult physiotherapist on types of exercises suited for patient's mobility restrictions.	Progressive resistance exercise (PRE) is a method of increasing ability of muscles to generate force.
3. All patients: Explain benefits and reasons for activity/exercise. Do so in a way that matches patient's beliefs and values regarding recovery or maintaining health.	Exercise self-efficacy is an important predictor of the adoption and maintenance of exercise behaviours. Self-efficacy is the belief and conviction that one can perform a given activity successfully (Hodgson et al., 2018; RNAO, 2010; Simpson et al., 2021).

STEP	RATIONALE
4. Inpatient: Explain precautions that will be taken to prevent falls during ambulation (gait belt, assisted walking, monitoring for dizziness).	Patient may have a fear of falling. Explanation may relieve anxiety.
5. Inpatient: As patient progresses to ambulating, try to schedule ambulation around patient's other activities.	Avoids overexertion of patient. Organizes nursing care activities.

IMPLEMENTATION

STEP	RATIONALE
1.	Proper hand hygiene helps prevent the spread of infectious agents to health care providers.
2. Early progressive mobility protocol: Each patient starts at a different level, depending on their medical status and ability to participate in mobility. *Stage 1: Patient unstable* • Initiate passive ROM exercises TID (see Procedural Guideline 12.1). Turn patient every 2 hours. • Help patient to sitting position in bed (e.g., stretcher chair or elevating head of bed to 30 degrees) and maintain for 20 minutes TID, or as tolerated. • Obtain a physiotherapy consultation if patient is alert to determine whether strengthening exercises are indicated.	This level is designed for patients who are medically unstable to tolerate activity or have bed rest prescriptions because of a medical condition.
Stage 2: Patient stable • Continue passive/active ROM exercises TID. • Turn patient every 2 hours. • Help patient to sitting position in bed and maintain for 20–30 minutes TID. • Initiate sitting patient on edge of bed or lift patient to chair. • Dependent with ADLs. • Obtain physiotherapy consultation for mobility/strengthening program (e.g., active resistance exercise).	Patient begins to progress, patient is starting to be able to sit independently on edge of bed or tolerate sitting up in a chair. Principles of active resistance exercise: (1) perform small number of repetitions until fatigue, (2) allow sufficient rest between exercises for recovery, and (3) increase resistance as ability to generate force increases. Evidence indicates that PRE improves function and strength and reduces pain, which can improve quality of life and ability to do everyday tasks (Lightfoot et al., 2022).
Stage 3: Patient stable • Patient is able to do active ROM exercises TID. • Patient is able to turn self every 2 hours and assist with ADLs. • Help patient to sitting position in bed and maintain for 20 minutes TID; sitting on edge of bed unsupported (but supervised). • Active transfer to chair with the patient sitting up in chair 20–30 minutes TID (use mechanical lift, as needed). • Physiotherapy to continue with strengthening program as prescribed.	Patient progresses to transfer training, prewalking activities. Patient can still be in critical care unit (CCU) during this phase or on nursing unit.
Stage 4: Patient stable • Patient is able to do active ROM exercises TID. • Patient is able to turn self every 2 hours and assist with ADLs. • Active transfer to chair with patient sitting up in chair 1–2 hours TID sitting on edge of bed unsupported (but supervised). • Physiotherapy to continue with strengthening program. • Initiate ambulation. Apply gait belt (if needed). Have patient ambulate (marching in place, walking in halls) (see Procedural Guideline 12.3 and Skill 12.2). **Note:** Ambulation time and distance should increase daily during hospitalization.	Patients can still be in CCU during this phase or out on general nursing unit. Progression of mobility (amount of help required and distance walked) should occur until hospital discharge.

STEP	RATIONALE
Stage 5: Patient stable • Patient is able to turn self. • Patient is able to do active leg and arm exercises. • Patient is active in ADLs. • Sitting in chair at bedside minimum of 2 hours, or as tolerated TID. • Continue to increase ambulation time and distance (5–10 metres) with aides or staff assistance and wheelchair follow as required. *Stage 6: Patient stable* • Same as stage 5; patient able to progress in distance and frequency of walking with assistance as required.	
3. Exercise and activity promotion	
a. Initiate an exercise program that contains any of the following components: • Warm-up (5–10 minutes) • Strengthening exercises • Endurance physiotherapy • Balance exercises • Flexibility exercises • Cool-downs Consider consulting physiotherapy to help develop a complete exercise program that would fit the needs of your patient. A good overview of physical activity guidelines across the lifespan can be found at http://csepguidelines.ca/.	Warm-up directs needed blood flow to muscles and prepares body for exercise. Warming up is important for preventing injury. Flexibility exercises help prevent tightness of muscles and improve joint ROM. Loss of ROM or muscle tightness can impede a person's function. Cool-downs help body recover from exercises.
b. Recommend strength training for adults.	Strength training improves muscle strength and bone density and can be beneficial for older persons.
c. The Heart and Stroke Foundation of Canada (2022) recommends moderate to vigorous aerobic exercise totalling at least 150 minutes per week in bouts of 10 minutes or more. Include activities of light, moderate, and vigorous effort (e.g., light walking; easy gardening; climbing stairs; playing sports; jogging, swimming, or biking).	Designed to improve overall cardiovascular health.
d. Recommend balance exercises for older persons to decrease risk for falls. Ensure patient has something sturdy nearby to hold onto (wall or chair) if they become unsteady. • Perform exercises: standing on one foot, walking heel to toe, balance walking, back leg raises, side leg raises. Have patient do strength exercises (back leg raises, side leg raises) 2 or more days per week, but not on any 2 days in a row (National Institute on Aging, 2020; RNAO, 2017).	Helps improve person's balance while standing or sitting and may decrease risk for falls.
e. Recommend that patient perform cool-down (5–10 minutes) after exercising: • Quadriceps stretch • Hamstring/calf stretch • Chest and arm stretch • Neck, upper back, and shoulder stretch	Stretching help muscles relax and become more flexible.

EVALUATION

1. Measure vital signs and oxygen saturation during activity/exercise and compare findings with baseline.	Determines patient's exercise tolerance.

Critical Decision Point *Each employer (or even each CCU) may have different screening criteria based on the population that it commonly sees.*

STEP	RATIONALE
2. Evaluate patient's pain severity using appropriate pain rating scale (e.g., on a scale of 0–10, 0 being no pain and 10 being worst pain ever) (see Chapter 16 for pain assessment resources).	Exercises can increase muscle discomfort.
3. Monitor number of steps or estimated distance during walking.	Provides objective measure of ambulation progression.
4. After patient has reached each stage of mobility protocol or after patient in the community has been exercising for at least 2–3 months, evaluate level of confidence in performing exercises.	Determines self-efficacy and likelihood of continued participation in exercise.
5. Use teach-back: "We've talked about doing a warm-up and cool-down as part of your exercise plan. Tell me why each one is important." Develop a revised teaching plan if patient or caregiver is unable to teach back correctly.	Determines patient's and caregiver's level of understanding of instructional topic.

Unexpected Outcomes	Related Interventions
1. Patient has abnormal vital sign response or decrease in oxygen saturation, requiring termination of exercise. (In community settings, be sure that patient or caregiver knows patient's normal pulse range and when to terminate exercise.)	• Return patient to chair or bed immediately using safe patient-handling principles. • Notify health care provider. • Continue to monitor vital signs until patient's condition stabilizes.
2. Patient develops chest pain or discomfort during exercise.	• Return patient to chair or bed immediately using safe patient-handling principles. • Notify health care provider. • Use interprofessional collaboration and prepare for possible electrocardiogram. • Continue to monitor vital signs until patient's condition stabilizes. • In community setting, have caregiver call 9-1-1.

Communication and Documentation

- Document in the patient medical record or clinic record the results of patient screening, type of exercise implemented, pre-exercise and postexercise assessments, and patient's tolerance in progress notes in electronic health record (EHR) or chart.
- Document your evaluation of patient and caregiver learning.
- Report to health care provider any signs or symptoms indicative of exercise intolerance.

DOCUMENTATION EXAMPLE

Patient postop day 1 following inguinal hernia repair. Completed premobility assessment on patient at 1000 hours. Baseline vitals: B/P 124/86, T 36.5 C (oral), P 74, R 20. Oxygen saturation 98% on room air. Pain 3/10. Gait belt applied to patient's waist. Patient tolerated sitting on edge of bed with no dizziness reported. Assisted patient to ambulate approximately 10 metres. Patient tolerated activity well with no increase in pain and no dizziness. Gait and balance stable. Post ambulation vitals stable: B/P 128/86, T 36.5 C (oral), P 76, R 23. Oxygen saturation 98% on room air. Patient states pain remains the same, 3/10.

Special Considerations

Teaching

- Teach patients that physically active occupations can count toward meeting the key guidelines for physical activity, as can active transportation choices (walking or bicycling). All types of aerobic activities can count, as long as they are of sufficient intensity (e.g., mowing the lawn, vacuuming).
- In the inpatient setting, teach caregivers how to be a coach for encouraging and safely assisting patients with ambulation (see employer policy).
- Inform patients of the benefits of early mobilization and how it specifically relates to their recovery (e.g., reduced length of stay in CCU, fewer days in hospital).

Gerontological

- As part of their weekly physical activity, older persons should do multicomponent physical activity that includes balance training as well as aerobic and muscle-strengthening activities.
- Older persons should determine their level of effort for physical activity relative to their level of fitness.
- Older persons with chronic conditions should understand whether and how their conditions affect their ability to do regular physical activity safely.
- When older persons cannot do 150 minutes of moderate-intensity aerobic activity a week because of chronic conditions, they should be as physically active as their abilities and conditions allow.

Care in the Community: Home Management

- Teach patient or caregiver how to measure carotid or radial pulse (see Chapter 7, Skill 7.7), what a normal range is for patient, how to monitor exercise tolerance, and when to notify health care provider about problems.
- Have patient or caregiver keep diary to record exercise activities, progression, and patient response.

Procedural Guideline 12.1 *Performing Range-of-Motion Exercises*

Range-of-motion (ROM) refers to the distance or amount of freedom a joint can be moved in a certain direction (e.g., rotating, bending, or twisting). ROM exercises may be active, passive, or active assisted. They are active if a patient can move the limb against gravity, active assisted when a caregiver is needed to help the patient move the limb against gravity, and passive when the exercises are performed by a caregiver. Always encourage patients to be as active and independent as possible in every aspect of ADLs. Incorporate active ROM exercises into a patient's ADLs (Table 12.1), and incorporate passive ROM into bathing and feeding activities. Collaborate with patients to develop schedules for ROM activities.

Delegation and Collaboration

The skill of performing ROM exercises can be delegated to a trained UCP. Patients with spinal cord injuries, burns, or orthopedic trauma usually require assistance from professional nurses or physiotherapists to perform ROM exercises. The nurse directs the UCP to do the following:

- Perform exercises slowly and provide adequate support to each joint being exercised
- Not exercise joints beyond the point of resistance or to the point of fatigue or pain
- Be aware of a patient's individual limitations or pre-existing conditions such as arthritis that affect ROM

Equipment

- No mechanical or physical equipment needed
- Clean gloves *(optional)*

Procedural Steps

1. Identify patient using at least two person-specific identifiers (e.g., name and date of birth, or name and medical record number) according to employer policy (Accreditation Canada, 2020).
2. Throughout the procedure, the 4 moments for hand hygiene are to be implemented; hand hygiene should occur before initial patient (or patient environment) contact, before an aseptic procedure, after body fluid exposure risk, and after patient (or patient environment) contact. Additional hand hygiene should be performed when hands are visibly soiled.
3. Review patient's chart for physical assessment findings that could affect the performance of ROM exercises (e.g., pain in joint, skin integrity or presence of wound near joint, presence of deformity; level of consciousness and ability to attend); health care provider prescriptions (e.g., any ROM restrictions for medical reasons); medical diagnosis, medical history, and progress.
4. Obtain data on patient's baseline joint function. Observe for obvious limitations in joint mobility, redness, or warmth over joints; joint tenderness; deformities, or edema.
5. Determine patient's or caregiver's readiness to learn (e.g., desire to learn, perceived ability to perform exercise, perceived benefit of exercise). Explain in plain language reason for the ROM exercises, and describe and demonstrate exercises to be performed.
6. Assess patient's level of comfort using an appropriate pain rating scale (see Chapter 16) before exercises. Determine whether patient would benefit from pain medication before beginning ROM exercises; then administer analgesic 30 minutes before exercise.
7. Apply clean gloves if wound drainage or skin lesions are present.
8. Help patient to a comfortable position, preferably sitting or lying down.
9. When performing passive ROM exercises (Table 12.2), support joint by holding distal part of extremity or using cupped hand to support joint (see Step 9 illustrations).

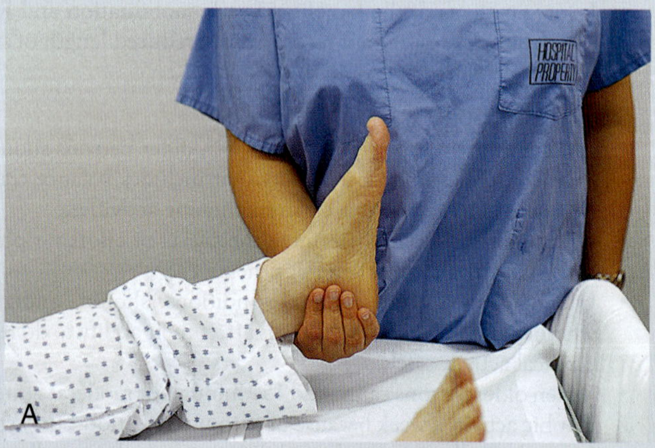

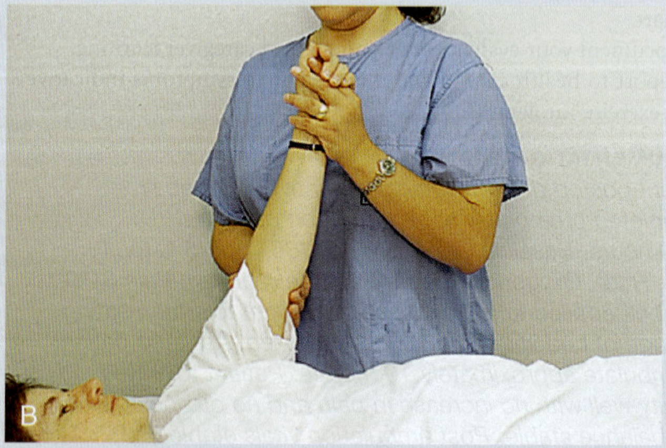

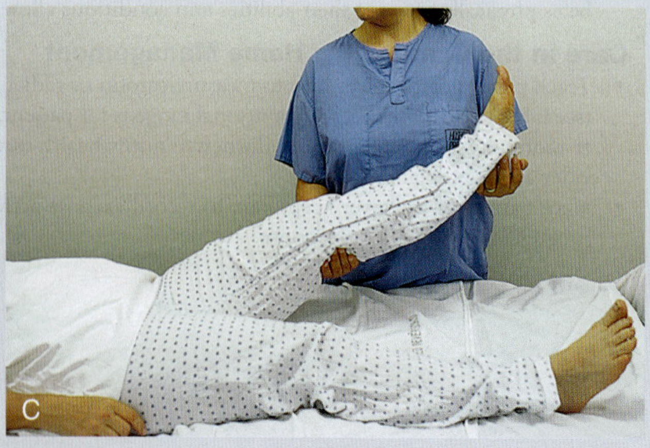

STEP 9 A, Support joint by holding distal and proximal areas adjacent to joint. B, Support joint by cradling distal part of extremity. C, Use cupped hand to support joint.

Procedural Guideline 12.1 *Performing Range-of-Motion Exercises—cont'd*

10. Complete exercises in head-to-toe sequence. Repeat each movement five times during exercise period. Inform patient how these exercises can be incorporated into ADLs (see Table 12.1).

Critical Decision Point *When resistance is noted within a joint, do not force joint motion. Consult with health care provider or physiotherapist.*

11. Observe patient performing ROM activities.
12. Remove gloves, if worn.
13. Measure joint motion as needed to determine level of improvement.
14. Evaluate patient during exercise by having them rate the severity of pain on a pain scale.
15. **Use teach-back:** "Let's review what I discussed about ways to practise ROM at home. Tell me some exercises you can do at home." Develop a revised teaching plan if patient or caregiver is unable to teach back correctly.
16. Document exercises performed and patient's tolerance in progress notes in EHR or chart.

TABLE 12.1

Incorporating Active Range-of-Motion Exercises Into Activities of Daily Living

Joint Exercised	Activity of Daily Living	Movement
Neck	Nodding head "yes"	Flexion
	Shaking head "no"	Rotation
	Moving right ear to right shoulder	Lateral flexion
	Moving left ear to left shoulder	Lateral flexion
Shoulder	Reaching to turn on overhead light	Flexion, extension
	Reaching to bedside stand for book	Hyperextension
	Rotating shoulders toward chest	Internal rotation
	Rotating shoulders toward back	External rotation
Elbow	Eating, bathing, shaving, grooming	Flexion, extension
Wrist	Eating, bathing, shaving, grooming	Flexion, extension, ulnar/radial deviation
Fingers and thumb	All activities requiring fine-motor coordination (e.g., writing, eating, painting)	Flexion, extension, abduction, adduction, opposition
Hip	Walking	Flexion, extension, hyperextension
	Moving to side-lying position	Flexion, extension, abduction
	Moving from side-lying position	Extension, adduction
	Rolling feet inward	Internal rotation
	Rolling feet outward	External rotation
Knee	Walking	Flexion, extension
	Moving to and from side-lying position	Flexion, extension
Ankle	Walking	Dorsiflexion, plantar flexion
	Moving toe toward head of bed	Dorsiflexion
	Moving toe toward foot of bed	Plantar flexion
Toes	Walking	Extension, hyperextension
	Wiggling toes	Abduction, adduction

Continued

Procedural Guideline 12.1 *Performing Range-of-Motion Exercises—cont'd*

TABLE 12.2
Range-of-Motion Exercises

Body Part	Type of Joint	Type of Movement	Range (Degrees)	Primary Muscles
Neck, cervical spine	Pivotal	Flexion: Bring chin to rest on chest.	45	Sternocleidomastoid
	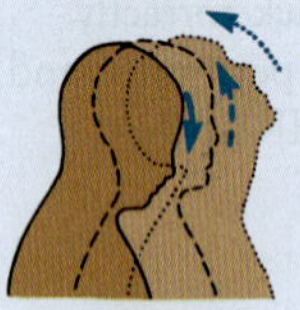	Extension: Return head to erect position.	45	Trapezius
		Hyperextension: Bend head back as far as possible.	10	Trapezius
	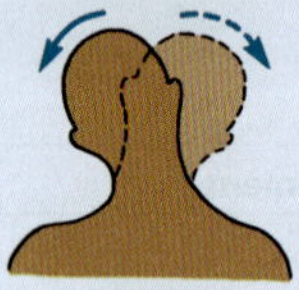	Lateral flexion: Tilt head as far as possible toward each shoulder.	40–45	Scalenus
	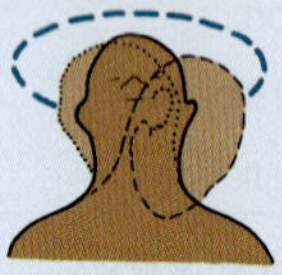	Rotation: Turn head as far as possible in circular movement.	180	Sternocleidomastoid, upper trapezius
Shoulder	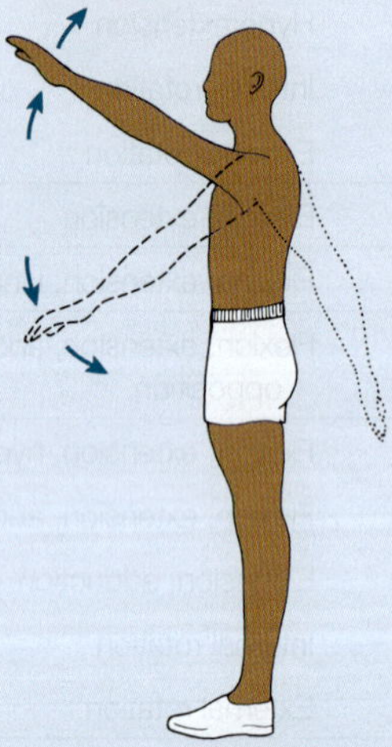	Horizontal flexion: Swing arm horizontally forward.	130	Coracobrachialis, deltoid, pectoralis major
		Horizontal extension: Swing arm horizontally backward.	45	Latissimus dorsi, teres major, triceps brachii
		Abduction: Bring arm up sideways.	180	Supraspinatus, deltoid, trapezius, and serratus anterior
		Adduction: Bring arm toward midline of the body.	45	Pectoralis major, triceps, teres major
		Shoulder extension: Move arm behind body, keeping elbow straight.	0–60	Latissimus dorsi, teres major, deltoid
	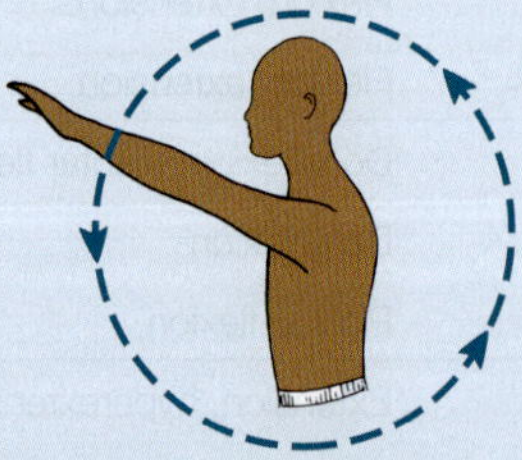	Circumduction: Move arm in full circle (circumduction is combination of all movements of ball-and-socket joint).	360	Deltoid, coracobrachialis, latissimus dorsi, teres major
Elbow	Hinge	Flexion: Bend elbow so lower arm moves toward its shoulder joint and hand is level with shoulder.	150	Biceps brachii, brachialis, brachioradialis
	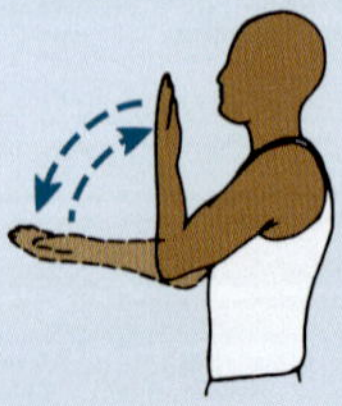	Extension: Straighten elbow by lowering hand.	150	Triceps brachii

Procedural Guideline 12.1 *Performing Range-of-Motion Exercises—cont'd*

TABLE 12.2

Range-of-Motion Exercises—cont'd

Body Part	Type of Joint	Type of Movement	Range (Degrees)	Primary Muscles
Forearm	Pivotal 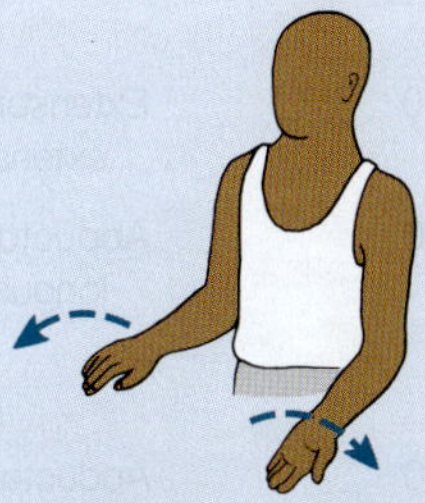	Supination: Turn lower arm and hand so palm is up.	70–90	Supinator, biceps brachii
		Pronation: Turn lower arm so palm is down.	70–90	Pronator teres, pronator quadratus
Wrist	Condyloid 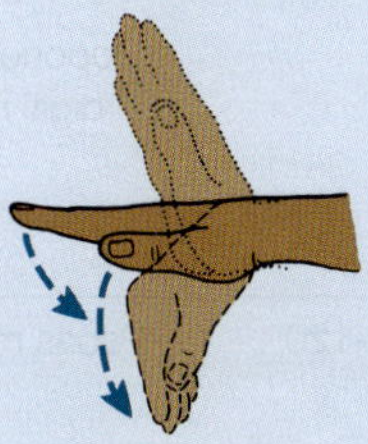	Flexion: Move palm toward inner aspect of forearm.	80–90	Flexor carpi ulnaris, flexor carpi radialis
		Extension: Move fingers and hand posterior to midline.	70–80	Extensor carpi radialis brevis, extensor carpi radialis longus, extensor carpi ulnaris
		Hyperextension: Bring dorsal surface of hand back as far as possible.		Extensor carpi radialis brevis, extensor carpi radialis longus, extensor carpi ulnaris
	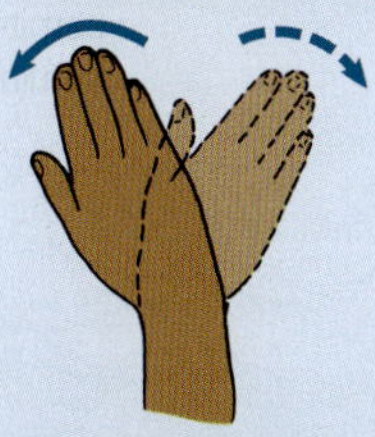	Radial deviation: Bend wrist medially toward thumb.	Up to 30	Flexor carpi radialis brevis, extensor carpi radialis brevis, extensor carpi radialis longus
		Ulnar deviation: Bend wrist laterally toward fifth finger.	30	Flexor carpi ulnaris, extensor carpi ulnaris
Fingers	Condyloid hinge 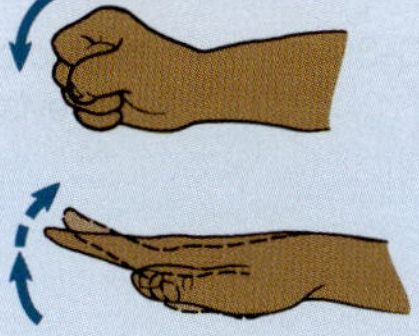	Flexion: Make fist.	90	Lumbricales, interosseus volaris, interosseus dorsalis
		Extension: Straighten fingers.	90	Extensor digiti quinti proprius, extensor digitorum communis, extensor indicis proprius
		Hyperextension: Bend fingers back as far as possible.	30–60	Extensor digitorum
	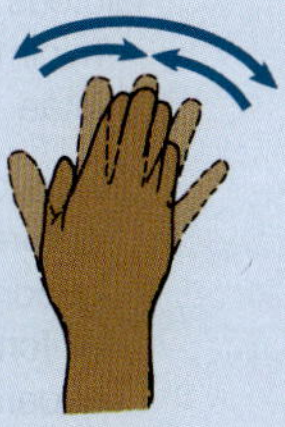	Abduction: Spread fingers apart.	30	Interosseus dorsalis
		Adduction: Bring fingers together.	30	Interosseus volaris

Continued

Procedural Guideline 12.1 *Performing Range-of-Motion Exercises—cont'd*

TABLE 12.2

Range-of-Motion Exercises—cont'd

Body Part	**Type of Joint**	**Type of Movement**	**Range (Degrees)**	**Primary Muscles**
Thumb	Saddle 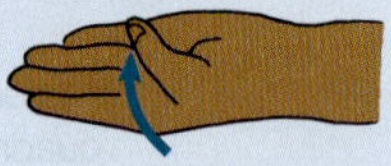	Flexion: Move thumb across palmar surface of hand.	90	Flexor pollicis brevis
		Extension: Move thumb straight away from hand.	90	Extensor pollicis longus, extensor pollicis brevis
		Abduction: Extend thumb laterally (usually done when placing fingers in abduction and adduction).	30	Abductor pollicis brevis and longus
		Adduction: Move thumb back toward hand.	30	Adductor pollicis obliquus, adductor pollicis transversus
	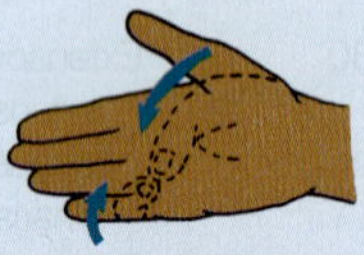	Opposition: Touch thumb to each finger of same hand.		Opponens pollicis, opponens digiti minimi
Hip	Ball and socket 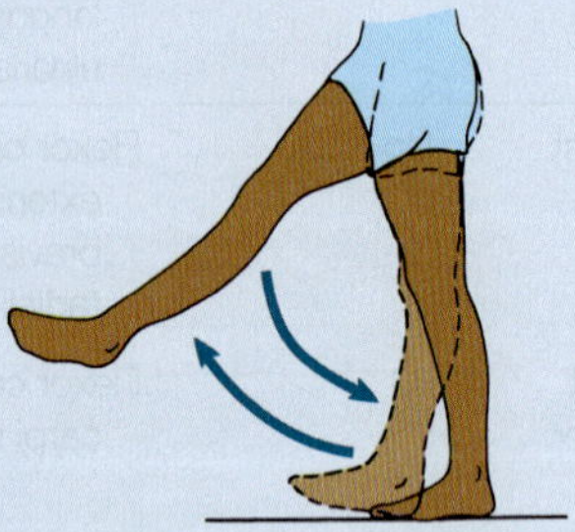	Flexion: Move leg forward and up.	110–120	Psoas major, iliacus, sartorius
		Extension: Move leg back beside other leg.	90–120	Gluteus maximus, semitendinosus, semimembranosus
	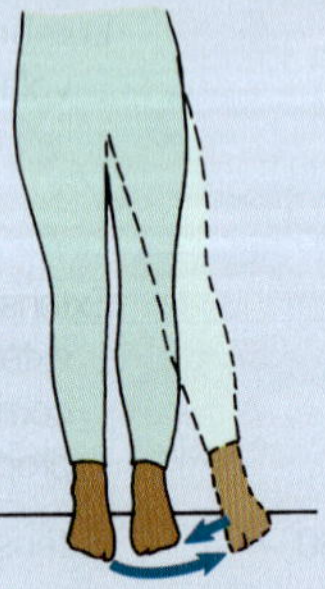	Abduction: Move leg laterally away from body.	30–50	Gluteus medius, gluteus minimus
		Adduction: Move leg back toward midline position and beyond if possible.	20–30	Adductor longus, adductor brevis, adductor magnus
	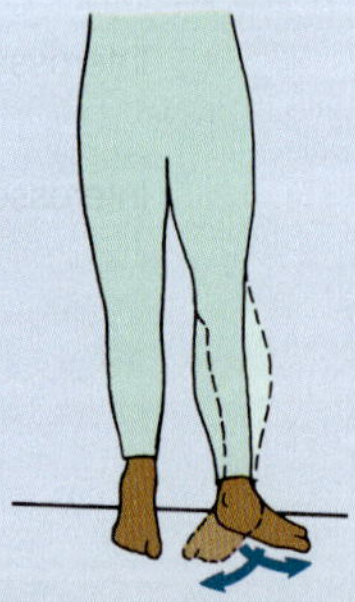	Internal rotation: Turn foot and leg toward other leg.	45	Gluteus medius, gluteus minimus, tensor fasciae latae
		External rotation: Turn foot and leg away from other leg.	45	Obturatorius internus, obturatorius externus, quadratus femoris, piriformis, gemellus superior and inferior, gluteus maximus

Procedural Guideline 12.1 *Performing Range-of-Motion Exercises—cont'd*

TABLE 12.2

Range-of-Motion Exercises—cont'd

Body Part	Type of Joint	Type of Movement	Range (Degrees)	Primary Muscles
	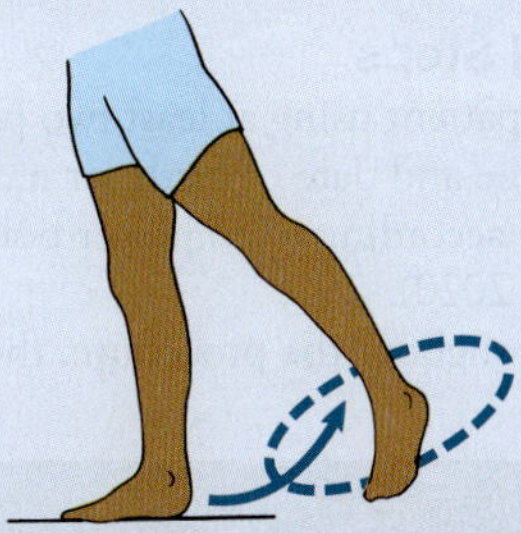	Circumduction: Move leg in circle.	120–130	Psoas major, gluteus maximum, gluteus medius, adductor magnus
Knee	Hinge 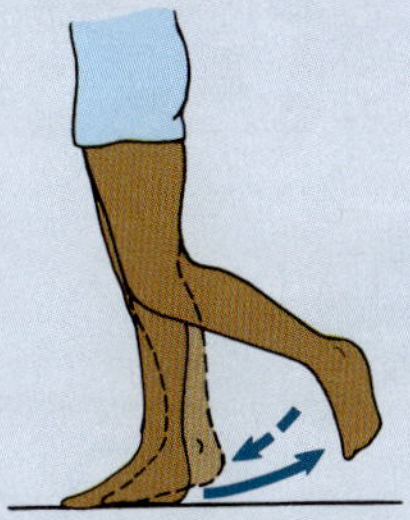	Flexion: Bring heel back toward back of thigh.	120–130	Biceps femoris, semitendinosus, semimembranosus, sartorius
		Extension: Return leg to floor.	120–130	Rectus femoris, vastus lateralis, vastus medialis, vastus intermedius
Ankle	Hinge 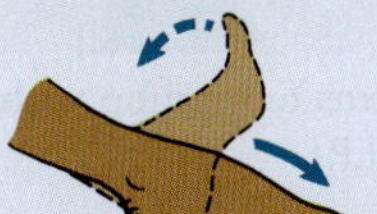	Dorsal flexion: Move foot so toes are pointed upward.	20–30	Tibialis anterior
		Plantar flexion: Move foot so toes are pointed downward.	45–50	Gastrocnemius, soleus
Foot	Gliding 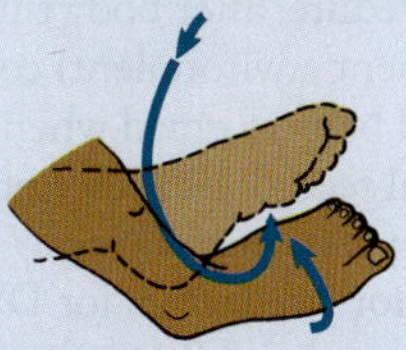	Inversion: Turn sole of foot medially.	35 or less	Tibialis anterior, tibialis posterior
		Eversion: Turn sole of foot laterally.	10 or less	Peroneus longus, peroneus brevis
Toes	Condyloid 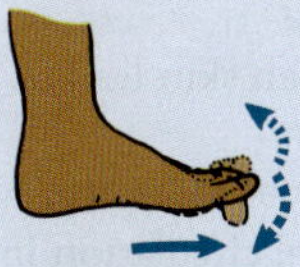	Flexion: Curl toes downward.	30–60	Flexor digitorum, lumbricalis pedis, flexor hallucis brevis
		Extension: Straighten toes.	30–60	Extensor digitorum longus, extensor digitorum brevis, extensor hallucis longus
	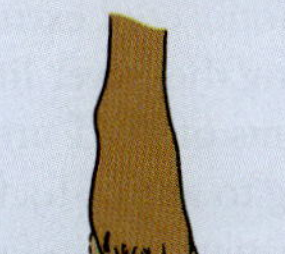	Abduction: Spread toes apart.	15 or less	Abductor hallucis, interosseus dorsalis
		Adduction: Bring toes together.	15 or less	Adductor hallucis, interosseus plantaris

Continued

Procedural Guideline 12.2 *Applying Graduated Compression (Elastic) Stockings and Sequential Compression Device*

Video Clip

The development of deep vein thrombosis (DVT) is a hazard of immobility. Common risk factors include conditions that influence Virchow's triad: hypercoagulability (e.g., clotting disorders, fever, dehydration); venous wall abnormalities (e.g., orthopedic surgery, varicose veins); and blood flow stasis (e.g., immobility, obesity, pregnancy) (Lurie et al., 2019; Tyerman & Cobbett, 2023). Signs of DVT include swelling in the affected leg (rarely swelling in both legs); warm, cyanotic skin; and pain in the leg that often starts in the calf and can feel like cramping or soreness. If DVT is suspected, keep patient calm and quiet in bed and notify the health care provider.

If patients are at high risk for DVT, mechanical thromboprophylaxis (use of elastic stockings or intermittent sequential compression devices [SCDs]) is a recommended form of therapy (Bircher & Chowdhury, 2020; Nicholson et al., 2020; Tamowicz et al., 2019), especially in patients after surgery.

Anticoagulant medication is the best approach for preventing DVTs; however, early ambulation, adequate hydration, wearing compression stockings or intermittent SCDs, and using foot pumps are equally important (Badireddy & Mudipalli, 2021; Bircher & Chowdhury, 2020). All intermittent compression systems have a simple objective (i.e., to squeeze blood from the underlying deep veins, which, if the valves are competent, will be displaced proximally). On deflation of the cuff, the veins will refill and, because of the intermittent nature of the system, will ensure periodic flow of blood through the deep veins if there is a supply (Berszakiewicz et al., 2020). Compression stockings appear to function mainly by preventing distension of veins. Reduction of edema and leg pain during the day is accomplished while wearing elastic stockings (Lee et al., 2020). SCDs pump blood into deep veins, thus removing pooled blood and preventing venous stasis. A venous plexus foot pump promotes venous return by pumping blood through compression, mimicking the natural action of walking (Fig. 12.1). The combination of stockings and foot compression has been shown to be more effective than stockings alone in reducing the incidence of both DVT and pulmonary embolism (Petersen et al., 2022).

Delegation and Collaboration

The skill of applying and maintaining graduated compression stockings and intermittent SCDs or mobile compression devices (MCDs) may be delegated to a UCP. The nurse initially determines the size of elastic stockings and assesses the patient's lower extremities for any signs and symptoms of DVT or impaired circulation. The nurse directs the UCP to do the following:

- Remove the SCD sleeves (exception: MCDs may remain on) before allowing a patient to get out of bed
- Report to the nurse if one calf appears larger than the other or is red or hot, if the patient has calf pain, or if there are signs of skin breakdown or allergic reactions to elastic (redness, itching, or irritation)

Equipment

- Tape measure
- Graduated compression stockings
- SCD/MCD insufflator with air hoses attached, adjustable Velcro compression stockings/SCD sleeve (*Option:* Cotton stockinette with MCD)
- Compression device pump
- Hygiene supplies

Procedural Steps

1. Identify patient using at least two person-specific identifiers (e.g., name and date of birth, or name and medical record number) according to employer policy (Accreditation Canada, 2020).
2. Throughout the procedure, the 4 moments for hand hygiene are to be implemented; hand hygiene should occur before initial patient (or patient environment) contact, before an aseptic procedure, after body fluid exposure risk, and after patient (or patient environment) contact. Additional hand hygiene should be performed when hands are visibly soiled.

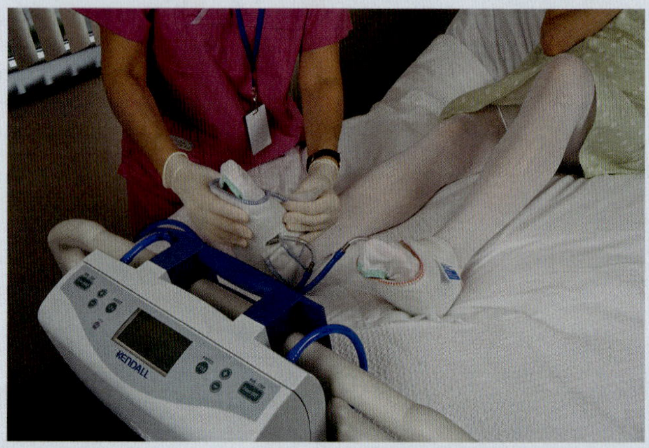

FIG 12.1 Venous plexus foot pump with bedside controls. *(Courtesy Tyco Healthcare Group LP.)*

3. Review medical record for prescription for SCDs/MCDs or graduated compression stocking.
4. Assess patient for risk factors for DVT (see Box 12.1) (Centers for Disease Control and Prevention, 2020).
5. Assess for contraindications for use of elastic stockings or compression devices:
   a. Dermatitis or open skin lesions on area to be covered by stockings/sleeves.
   b. Recent skin graft to lower leg.
   c. Decreased arterial circulation in lower extremities as evidenced by cyanotic, cool extremities or gangrenous conditions affecting the lower limb(s).
   d. If signs or symptoms of DVT are present, do not manipulate the leg to apply stockings.
6. Assess condition of patient's skin (area to be covered by stockings) and circulation to the legs. Palpate pedal pulses, note any palpable veins, and inspect skin over lower extremities for edema, skin discoloration, warmth, and presence of lesions.
7. Obtain health care provider's prescription.
8. Assess patient's or caregiver's knowledge of previous use of elastic or sequential compression stockings.
9. Explain procedure and reason for applying elastic stockings or SCDs/MCDs.

Procedural Guideline 12.2 *Applying Graduated Compression (Elastic) Stockings and Sequential Compression Device—cont'd*

10. Position patient in supine position.
11. Bathe patient's legs as needed. Dry thoroughly.
12. Apply graduated compression stocking:
    a. Use tape measure to measure patient's leg to determine proper elastic stocking size (follow package directions).
    b. *Optional:* Apply a small amount of powder or cornstarch to legs, provided patient does not have sensitivity.
    c. Turn elastic stocking inside out: Place one hand into stocking, holding heel of stocking. Take other hand and pull stocking inside out until the heel is reached (see Step 12c illustration).
    d. Place patient's toes into foot of elastic stocking up to the heel, making sure that stocking is smooth (see Step 12d illustration).
    e. Slide remaining part of stocking over patient's foot, making sure that toes are covered. Make sure that foot fits into toe-and-heel position of stocking. Stocking will now be right side out (see Step 12e illustration).
    f. Slide stocking up over patient's calf until sock is completely extended. Be sure that stocking is smooth and that no ridges or wrinkles are present (see Step 12f illustration).
    g. Instruct patient not to roll stockings partially down, to avoid wrinkles and crossing legs, and to elevate legs while sitting.

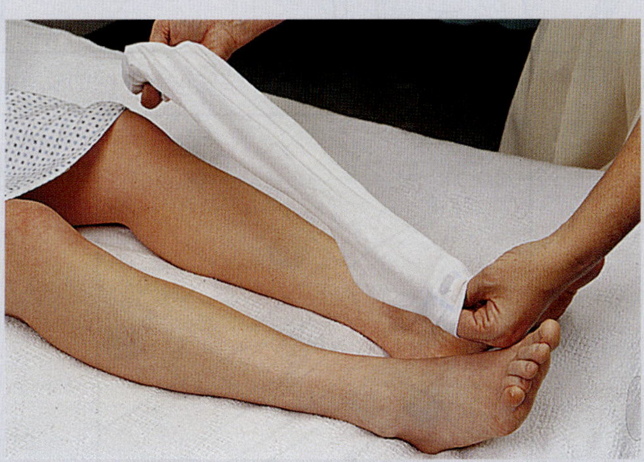

STEP 12C Turn stocking inside out; hold heel and pull through.

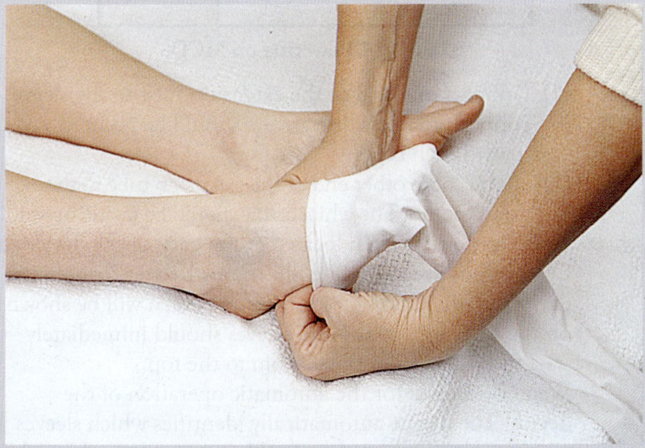

STEP 12D Place toes into foot of stocking.

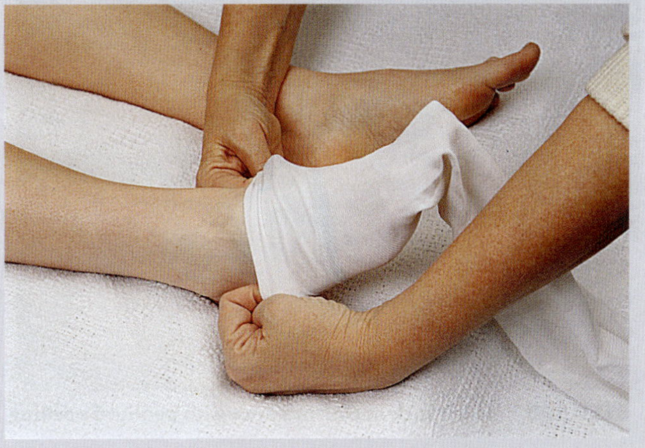

STEP 12E Slide remaining part of stocking over foot.

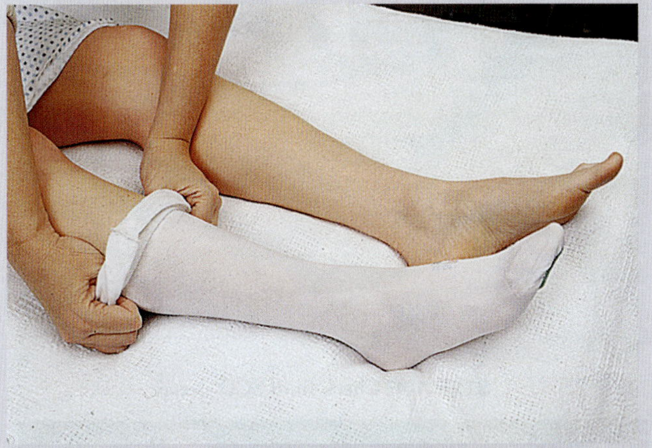

STEP 12F Slide sock up leg until completely extended.

13. Apply SCD sleeve(s):
    a. Remove SCD sleeve from plastic cover; unfold and flatten on bed.
    b. Arrange SCD sleeve under patient's leg according to leg position indicated on inner lining of sleeve.
    c. Place patient's leg on SCD sleeve. Back of ankle should line up with ankle marking on inner lining of sleeve.
    d. Position back of knee with popliteal opening on inner sleeve (see Step 13d illustration).
    e. Wrap SCD sleeve securely around patient's leg. Check fit of SCD sleeve by placing two fingers between patient's leg and sleeve (see Step 13e illustration).
    f. Attach SCD sleeve connector to plug on mechanical unit. Arrows on connector line up with arrows on plug from mechanical unit (see Step 13f illustration).
    g. Turn on mechanical unit. Green light indicates that unit is functioning. Monitor functioning SCD through one full cycle of inflation and deflation.

Continued

Procedural Guideline 12.2 *Applying Graduated Compression (Elastic) Stockings and Sequential Compression Device—cont'd*

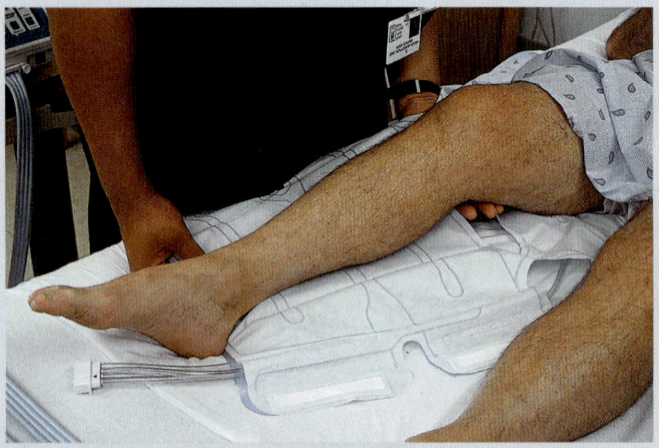

STEP 13D Position back of patient's knee with popliteal opening.

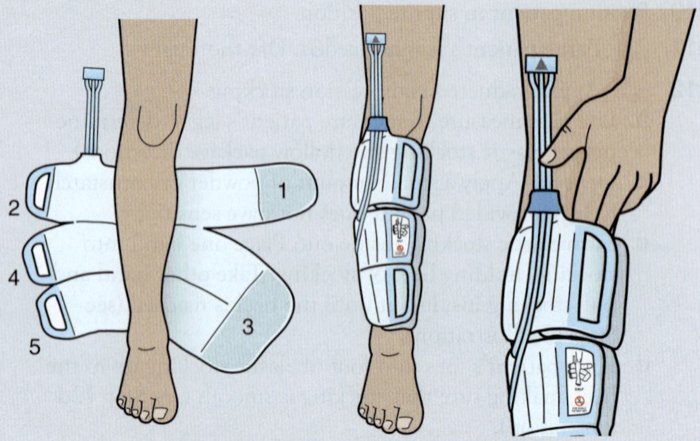

STEP 14C Application of sleeve to calves.

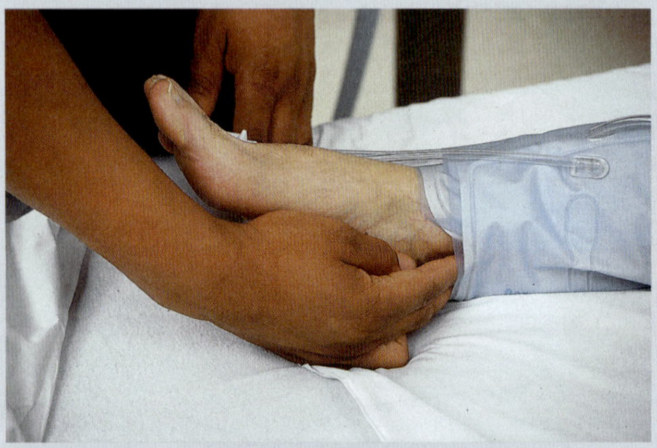

STEP 13E Check fit of SCD sleeve.

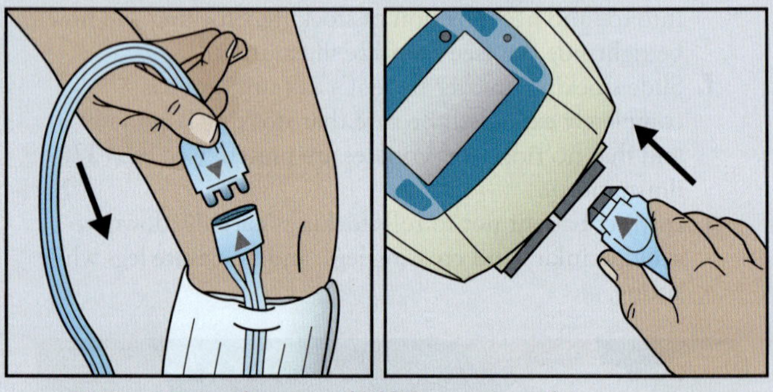

STEP 14D Application of MCD connector hose to pump.

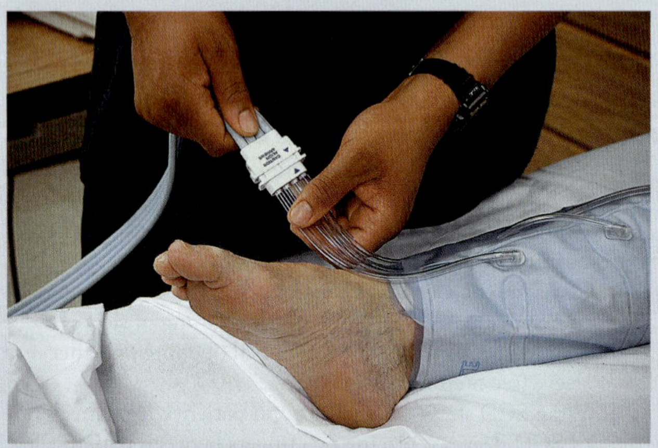

STEP 13F Align arrows when connecting plug to mechanical unit.

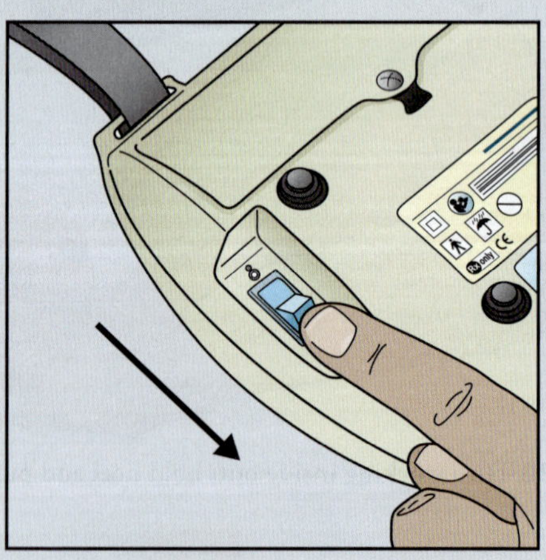

STEP 14E Powering on MCD.

14. Apply MCD sleeve:
    a. A cotton stockinette is provided along with the calf sleeves. Apply over patient's calves.
    b. Wrap the sleeve smoothly around the patient's calf and fasten it beginning at the top, moving toward the bottom.
    c. Place two fingers between patient's calf and sleeve to be sure it is snug but not too tight (see Step 14c illustration).
    d. The device has two identical extension tubes (see Step 14d illustration). Use either end of the extension tube to connect to the sleeve or device pump.
        (1) Connect one end of the extension tube to the sleeve connector. The white arrows should be pointed toward each other.
        (2) Connect the other end of the extension tube to the device pump. The white arrow should be facing upward.
    e. Press the power switch located at the back of the device to ON position (see Step 14e illustration). After turning the device on, the Configuration Setup Screen will be shown on the LCD screen and the sleeves should immediately start to inflate, from the bottom to the top.
    f. Wait 60 seconds for the automatic operation of the device. The device automatically identifies which sleeves are connected, selects the suitable treatment mode, and will display information on the main LCD screen.

Procedural Guideline 12.2 *Applying Graduated Compression (Elastic) Stockings and Sequential Compression Device—cont'd*

15. Position patient comfortably. When wearing MCD sleeves, a patient may walk with device in place (see Step 15 illustration).

Critical Decision Point *Caution patient not to exit bed and walk with SCDs in place. Have patient call for assistance. However, patient may walk with MCD in place.*

16. Remove compression stockings or SCD/MCD sleeves at least once per shift (e.g., long enough to inspect skin for irritation or breakdown and determine patient's comfort level).

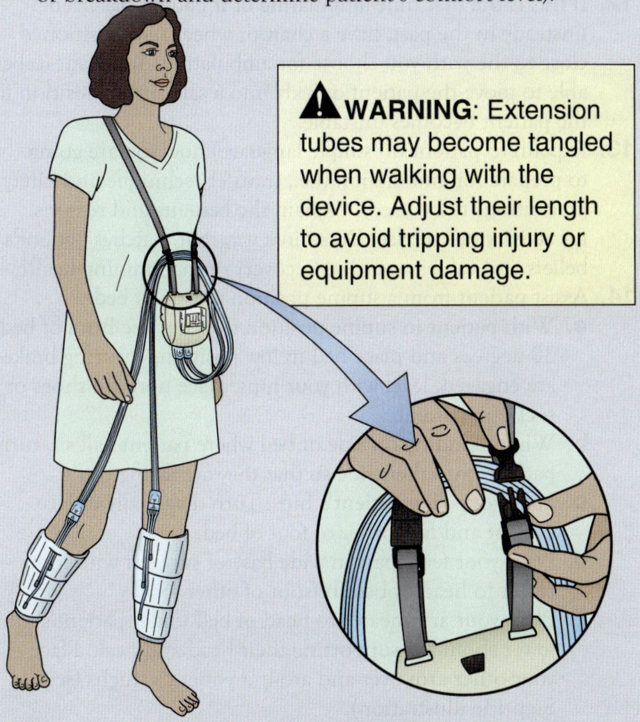

STEP 15 Walking with MCD.

17. Evaluate skin integrity and circulation to patient's lower extremities as prescribed (see employer policy).

18. Educate patient and caregiver about how to care for elastic stockings (keep two pairs and wash one daily) and precautions to take to prevent DVT at home (Government of Alberta, 2022):

- Stay active and move around as much as possible.
- When sitting for long periods of time, such as when travelling for more than 4 hours:
  - Get up and walk around every 2–3 hours.
  - Drink plenty of water.
  - Exercise legs while sitting by raising and lowering heels while keeping toes on the floor, raising and lowering toes while keeping heels on the floor, tightening and releasing leg muscles.
  - Wear loose-fitting clothes.

19. **Use teach-back:** "I want to be sure you understand why you have elastic stockings. Tell me in your own words the reasons why you are wearing these stockings." Develop a revised teaching plan if patient or caregiver is unable to teach back correctly.

20. Document condition of lower extremities, application of stockings or SCD/MCD, patient education, and patient response in progress notes in EHR or chart.

Procedural Guideline 12.3 *Assisting With Ambulation (Without Assistive Devices)*

Video Clip

Patients who are immobile for even a short time often require help with ambulation. Having patients ambulate early after immobilization is important in preventing deconditioning. The benefits of ambulation include maintenance of muscle tone, strength, and joint flexibility and function of the respiratory, circulatory, and gastrointestinal systems. Although these benefits are well established, patient ambulation requires interprofessional collaboration around decision making related to when and how to ambulate and should always be preceded by assessing the patient's fall risk (see Chapter 13). Using a gait belt to assist a patient in ambulation increases patient safety and decreases a patient's fall risk.

When helping a patient up and out of bed or a chair, there is a risk for orthostatic hypotension. Orthostatic hypotension or postural hypotension is a decrease in blood pressure that occurs when a patient changes from a horizontal to a vertical position. A decrease in blood pressure greater than 20 mm Hg in systolic pressure or 10 mm Hg in diastolic pressure with symptoms of dizziness, light-headedness, nausea, tachycardia, pallor, and fainting indicates orthostatic hypotension (Tyerman & Cobbett, 2023). Orthostatic hypotension is common among older persons. Although it can be related to the aging process, orthostatic hypotension may also result from a variety of factors, such as anemia, adverse effects of medications, deconditioning, infection, and systemic disease (Palma & Kaufmann, 2020). When a patient moves from a lying to a sitting position, instruct them to dangle their legs on the side of the bed (sitting on the edge of the bed while moving their legs back and forth) and make sure their feet can touch the floor to allow the circulatory system to equilibrate and thus minimize the onset of orthostatic hypotension. After leg dangling, have the patient stand; if they tolerate standing without dizziness, proceed with ambulation.

Continued

Procedural Guideline 12.3 *Assisting With Ambulation (Without Assistive Devices)—cont'd*

Use safety precautions before and during ambulation to control for orthostatic hypotension and subsequent falling.

Delegation and Collaboration

The skill of assisting patients with ambulation can be delegated to a UCP. The nurse directs the UCP to do the following:

- Have a patient dangle legs following lying in bed and check patient's blood pressure before ambulation
- Immediately return a patient to the bed or chair if nauseated, dizzy, pale, or diaphoretic, and report these signs and symptoms to the nurse immediately
- Apply safe, nonskid shoes or socks on the patient, and ensure that the environment is free of clutter and that there is no moisture on the floor before ambulating patient

Equipment

- Gait belt
- Nonskid shoes or socks

Procedural Steps

1. Identify patient using at least two person-specific identifiers (e.g., name and date of birth, or name and medical record number) according to employer policy (Accreditation Canada, 2020).
2. Throughout the procedure, the 4 moments for hand hygiene are to be implemented; hand hygiene should occur before initial patient (or patient environment) contact, before an aseptic procedure, after body fluid exposure risk, and after patient (or patient environment) contact. Additional hand hygiene should be performed when hands are visibly soiled.
3. Review medical record for patient's most recent activity experience, including distance ambulated, use of any assistive device, tolerance to activity, balance, and gait. Note any medications, chronic illnesses, presence of foot or leg deformity, or history of falling, all of which may influence patient's ability to ambulate independently.
4. Review most recently recorded weight for patient; this may indicate need for help from another care provider.
5. Review medical record for any history of or risks for orthostatic hypotension; identify medications or conditions that may place patient at risk.
6. Review health care provider's prescription for activity; note any mobility or weight-bearing restrictions.
7. Determine the best time to ambulate, considering other scheduled activities such as bathing or other medical procedures.
8. Check patient's environment for any barriers or safety risks. When walking, it is helpful within a hospital or rehabilitation centre to walk in an area where handrails are on the walls and chairs are nearby.
9. Assess patient's physical readiness to ambulate (see employer's protocol for mobility assessment and fall risk assessment [see Chapter 13]):
   a. Assess baseline resting heart rate, blood pressure, oxygen saturation (when available), and respirations.
   b. If patient's strength and endurance have been affected by illness or deconditioning, assess ROM and muscle strength (see Chapter 8) of lower extremities while in bed.
   c. Ask if patient feels excessively tired or is currently experiencing any pain. Determine source and severity of pain using an appropriate pain rating scale (see Chapter 16). This may delay ambulation. Offer an analgesic 30 minutes before ambulation to improve patient's tolerance to exercise.

Critical Decision Point *Do not administer an analgesic that could make the patient feel dizzy.*

10. Assess patient's level of response to commands. Is the patient able to understand instructions and cooperate during ambulation? Also assess patient's views and perceptions regarding current state of health and willingness to participate in activity.
11. Assess patient for any visual, hearing, or perceptual deficits that may affect their ability to follow instructions.
12. If this is the first time ambulating or if patient has been unsteady in the past, have a chair or wheelchair positioned close to the path you choose for ambulation. You want to be able to move the patient quickly into a safe sitting position if the patient becomes unstable.
13. Explain to patient (in simple language) how you are going to prepare for ambulation (i.e., transfer technique and safety precautions to be used). Explain the benefits and reasons for activity or exercise. Do so in a way that matches patient's beliefs and values regarding recovery or maintaining health.
14. Assist patient from a supine position to side of bed:
    a. With patient in supine position in bed, raise head of bed 30 degrees and place bed in low position, ensuring brakes are engaged, level with your hips. Place nonskid shoes or socks on patient.
    b. While standing on side of bed where patient will sit, turn patient onto their side so that they are facing you.
    c. Stand opposite patient's hips. Turn diagonally to face patient and far corner of foot of bed.
    d. Place your feet apart in wide base of support with foot closer to head of bed in front of other foot.
    e. Place your arm nearer to head of bed under patient's lower shoulder, supporting their head and neck. Place your other arm over and around patient's thighs (see Step 13e illustration).

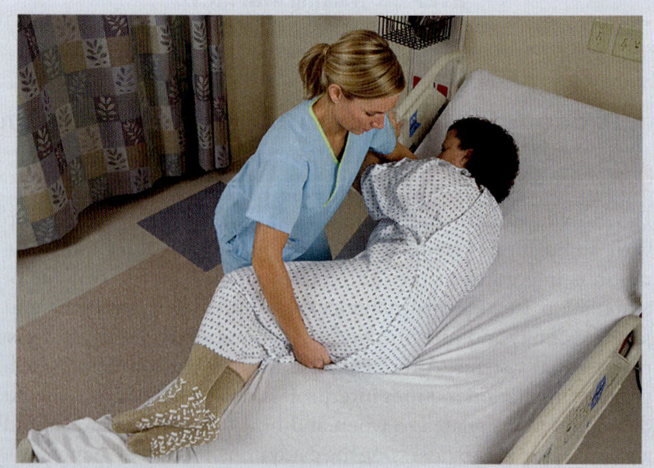

STEP 13E **Nurse places arm over patient's thigh and other arm under patient's shoulder.**

    f. Move patient's lower legs and feet over side of bed. Pivot weight onto your rear leg as you allow patient's upper legs to swing downward (see Step 13f illustration). At same time, continue to shift weight to your rear leg and elevate patient's trunk to the upright position.

Procedural Guideline 12.3 *Assisting With Ambulation (Without Assistive Devices)—cont'd*

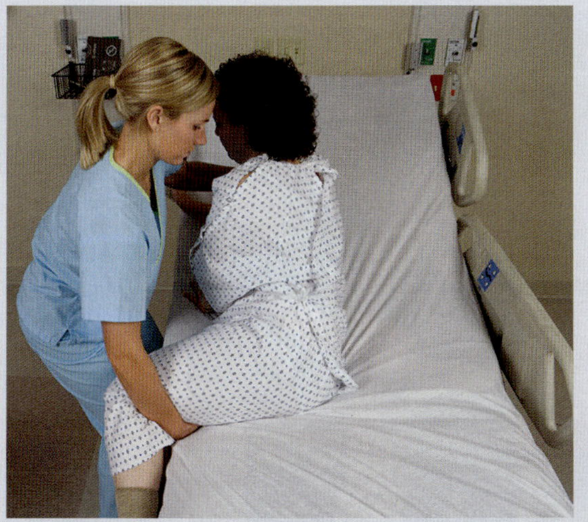

STEP 13F Nurse shifts weight to rear leg and elevates patient to sitting position.

15. Allow patient to sit on side of bed for a few minutes. Have patient alternately flex and extend feet and move lower legs up and down (see Step 14 illustration). Ask if patient feels dizzy; if so, check the blood pressure. Have patient relax and take a few deep breaths until dizziness subsides and balance is gained. If dizziness lasts more than 60 seconds, return patient to lying position in bed (Jones & Kuritzky, 2018). Recheck blood pressure.

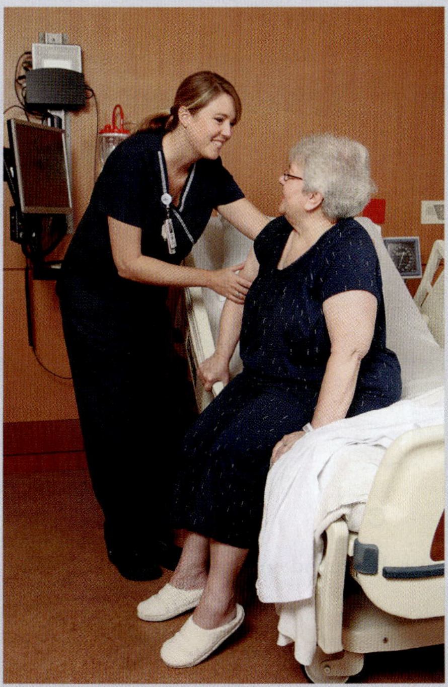

STEP 14 Patient sits on side of bed.

16. Apply gait belt around patient's waist. Be sure that it completely encircles the waist. Place belt low and be sure that it is snug. Avoid placing it over any intravenous (IV) lines, incisions, or drainage tubes. You may need to adjust it once patient stands. Hold onto belt along patient's back with your palm facing up. The gait belt controls patient's centre of mass during mobility, controls descent if a fall occurs, and reduces the chance of grabbing patient's upper extremities.
17. Help patient into standing position at bedside. Have patient stand fully erect with shoulders back and looking ahead (not at floor). Next, assess patient's ability to bear weight and balance.
18. If patient is unsteady, place in chair or return to bed immediately and obtain additional help.
19. If patient has an IV line, place IV pole on same side as patient's arm where the infusion is located. Instruct patient where to hold and push the pole while walking.
20. If a Foley catheter is present, empty drainage bag before ambulating patient. You or patient will carry bag below the level of patient's bladder. Sometimes you can pin the bag in the proper position on patient's gown. Be sure that there is no tension on the tubing.
21. Set a mutual goal with patient about how far or how long to ambulate. Walk a distance that patient can tolerate (see employer policy). Plan to increase ambulation time and distance during successive walks, as patient can tolerate.
22. Stand on patient's unaffected side and slightly behind. If assistive device (e.g., cane, walker) is used (see Skill 12.2), stand on patient's affected side and slightly behind.
23. Grasp gait belt firmly with palm facing up (see Step 22, illustration A). Take a few steps, supporting patient with one hand on the gait belt and the other under the elbow of patient's flexed arm (see Step 22, illustration B). *Optional:* Use ambulation lift or ceiling lift with a gait harness for a more dependent patient who is now walking for first time after being in bed.
24. Have patient take a few steps forward. Then assess their strength and balance before continuing.
25. When ambulating down a hallway, position patient between yourself and the wall. Encourage use of handrail (if present).
26. Observe how patient walks (posture, gait, balance, coordination) and evaluate activity tolerance to ambulation (i.e., measure pulse and respirations and compare with baseline).
27. If patient starts to fall (see Step 27 illustrations):
    a. Grasp patient's gait belt with both hands around their waist with palms up. Stand with feet apart for a broad base of support (see Step 27, illustration A).
    b. Extend one leg, pull patient against you, and guide the patient to slide down your leg as you ease them to the floor (see Step 27, illustration B). *Caution:* If patient is obese, do not risk personal injury.
    c. Bend your knees and lower your body as patient slides to floor (see Step 27, illustration C).
    d. Stay with patient until help arrives.
28. Once patient has completed the walk, return them to a bed or chair and help them assume a comfortable position.
29. Record time or distance ambulated, any changes in vital signs, and patient's tolerance (symptoms such as pain and fatigue) in progress notes in EHR or chart.

Continued

Procedural Guideline 12.3 *Assisting With Ambulation (Without Assistive Devices)—cont'd*

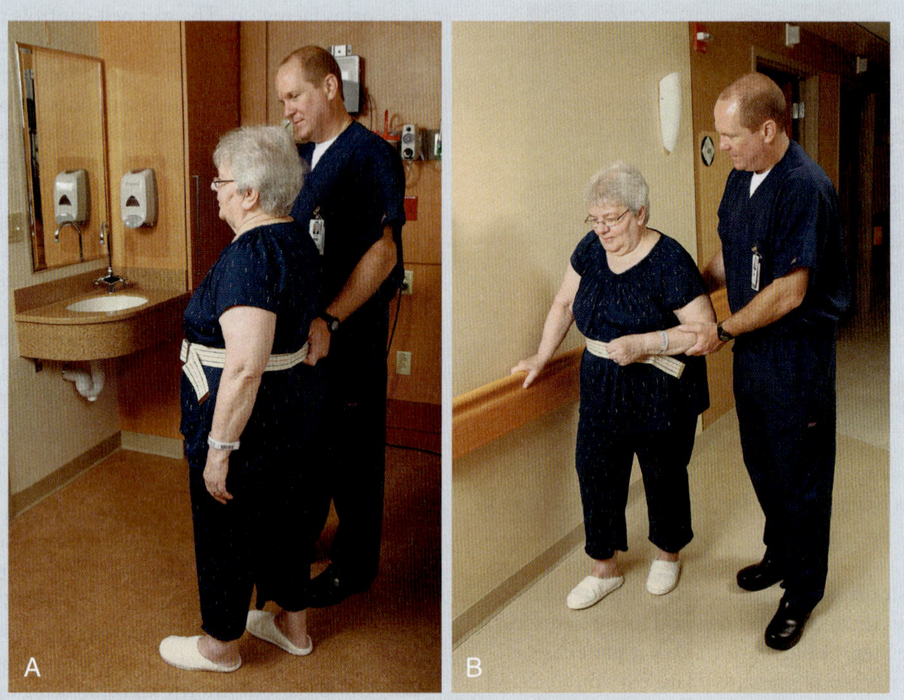

STEP 22 A, Nurse grasps gait belt firmly. B, Nurse helps patient by providing support under patient's flexed arm.

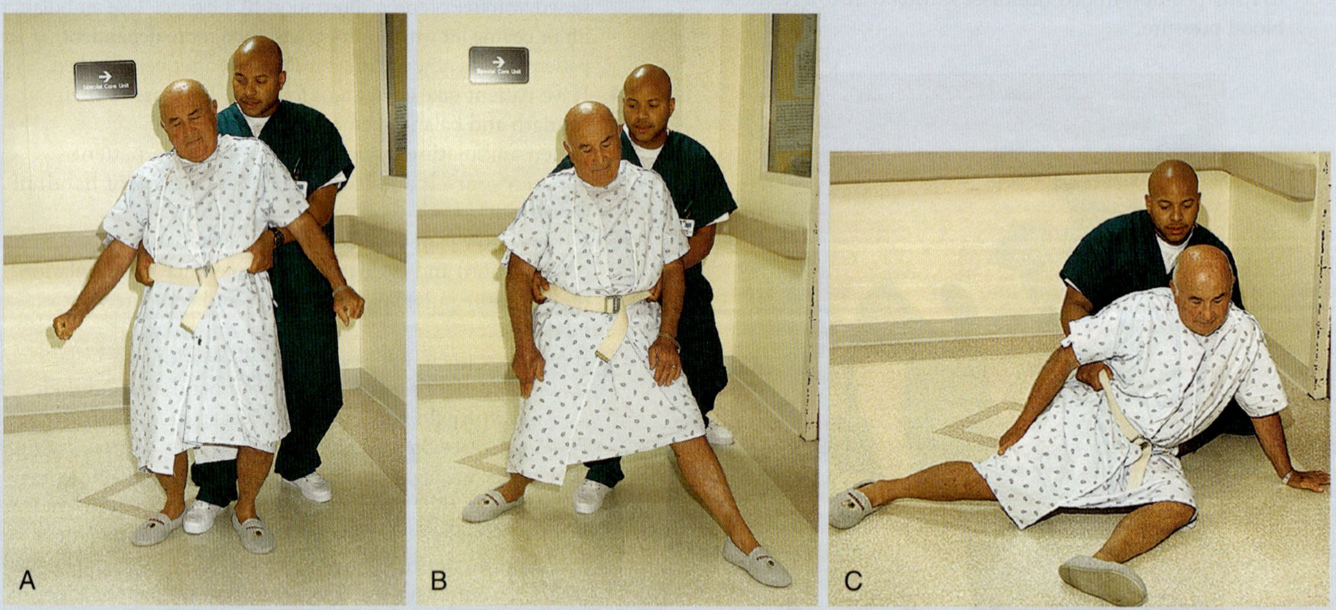

STEP 27 A, Grasp gait belt and stand with feet apart to provide broad base of support. B, Extend one leg and let patient slide against it to floor. C, Bend knees to lower body as patient slides to floor.

✦ SKILL 12.2 Assisting With Use of Canes, Walkers, and Crutches

An assistive device is any device that is designed, made, or adapted to help a person perform a particular task or function. For example, canes, crutches, and walkers are assistive devices for walking. An assistive device increases stability during ambulation; supports weak extremities; or reduces the load on weight-bearing structures such as hips, knees, or ankles. These devices range from standard canes, which provide balance and minimal physical support, to crutches and walkers, which are used by patients with weight-bearing limitations on one or more of their legs.

A physiotherapist should be consulted to help choose the proper assistive device, fit the device, and instruct the patient on the correct technique. Selection of an appropriate device depends on a patient's age, diagnosis, muscular coordination, weight-bearing status, and ease of manoeuverability. Use of assistive devices may be temporary (e.g., during recovery from a fractured extremity or orthopedic surgery) or permanent (e.g., a patient with paralysis or permanent weakness of the lower extremities). As a nurse, you help patients use their devices correctly during ambulation. When helping a patient with an assistive device ambulate, always have a gait belt on the patient and stand slightly behind and off to the side of the patient (on the patient's affected side).

Canes are lightweight, easily movable devices that extend about waist high and are made of wood or metal. They help to maintain balance by widening the base of support. There are three types of canes. The standard crook cane has a half circle handle and provides the least support for patients requiring only minimal assistance to walk. The tripod cane (pyramid cane) has three legs, and the quad cane has four legs; the additional legs provide a wider base of support. These types of canes are useful for patients with unilateral or partial leg paralysis. They also have the advantage of standing alone, freeing the arms to help a patient rise from a chair.

A crutch is a wooden or metal staff that reaches from the ground almost to the axilla. Crutches remove weight from one leg. They are used by patients who must transfer more weight to their arms than is possible with canes. There are two types of crutches: axillary and Lofstrand. Patients of all ages often use axillary crutches short term for various weight-bearing limitations on the lower extremities. A Lofstrand crutch has a handgrip and a metal band that fits around a patient's forearm. Both the metal band and the handgrip are adjusted to fit a patient's height. This type of crutch is useful for patients with a permanent disability such as paraplegia (Astle & Duggleby, 2024; Tyerman & Cobbett, 2023). The metal armband stabilizes and helps to guide the crutch. It also allows patients to use their hands for other activities such as opening doors without dropping the crutches. The anterior opening of the band allows patients to free themselves of the crutches if a fall occurs.

A walker is a lightweight, movable device that stands about waist high and consists of a metal frame with handgrips, four widely placed sturdy legs, and one open side. It provides a wide base of support and the greatest stability and security during walking. A walker can be used by a patient who is weak, has a weight-bearing limitation on a lower extremity, or has problems with balance. Most of the walkers that are used today are wheeled walkers. These walkers have two wheels on the front posts or four wheels on all posts of the walker, making them easier to use and requiring less energy to move them. This design is safer to use for patients with balance disorders because a patient keeps all four posts on the floor at all times. In contrast, a standard walker (no wheels, only the four posts) requires a patient to have the balance to lift up the walker to advance it. Patient education and safety for walkers should include proper adjustment for the patient's height and ability, knowledge of how to use the braking system, and the intended use.

Delegation and Collaboration

The skill of assisting patients with ambulation can be delegated to a UCP. The nurse should conduct the initial assessment when the patient is ambulating for the first time. The nurse directs the UCP to do the following:

- Have a patient dangle their legs after lying in bed before ambulation
- Immediately return a patient to the bed or chair if the patient is nauseated, dizzy, pale, or diaphoretic, and report these signs and symptoms to the nurse immediately.
- Apply safe, nonskid shoes on the patient, and ensure that the environment is free of clutter and that there is no moisture on the floor before the patient ambulates.
- Interprofessional collaboration (e.g., physiotherapist) can help determine the appropriate assistive device and type of gait to be used by patient.

Equipment

- Ambulation device (crutch, walker, cane)
- Safety device (gait belt)
- Well-fitting, flat, nonskid shoes for patient
- Goniometer *(optional)*

STEP	RATIONALE
ASSESSMENT	
1. Identify patient using at least two person-specific identifiers (e.g., name and date of birth, or name and medical record number) according to employer policy.	Ensures correct patient. Complies with Accreditation Canada's standards and improves patient safety (Accreditation Canada, 2020).
2. Throughout the procedure, the 4 moments for hand hygiene are to be implemented; hand hygiene should occur before initial patient (or patient environment) contact, before an aseptic procedure, after body fluid exposure risk, and after patient (or patient environment) contact. Additional hand hygiene should be performed when hands are visibly soiled.	Proper hand hygiene helps prevent the spread of infectious agents to health care providers.
3. Complete assessment steps in Procedural Guideline 12.3, Steps 1–12.	Determines patient's ability to ambulate with a device and readiness for learning necessary gaits and precautions.
4. Determine patient's or caregiver's understanding of type of device to be used in ambulating.	Allows patient to verbalize concerns. Patient who has been immobile may be hesitant to ambulate. Caregiver may be hesitant to learn how to help with ambulation.
5. Assess degree of assistance that patient needs. Consult with physiotherapy to make this recommendation.	For safety, another person may be needed initially to help with patient ambulation. Allow patient as much independence as possible.

STEP	RATIONALE

NURSING DIAGNOSES

- Reduced physical mobility
- Altered health management
- Fatigue
- Potential for falls
- Potential for injury
- Reduced knowledge regarding use of assistive device
- Reduced stamina
- Willingness for enhanced health management

Related factors and risk factors are individualized on the basis of patient's condition or needs.

PLANNING

STEP	RATIONALE
1. Expected outcomes following completion of procedure:	
• Patient ambulates using assistive device without injury.	Appropriate level of assistance with device ensures patient's safety.
• Patient is able to ambulate without excessive fatigue or dizziness and with return of vital signs to baseline 3–5 minutes after rest.	Assistive device chosen requires minimal exertion. Patient tolerates exercise.
• Patient demonstrates correct use of assistive device, gait pattern, and weight-bearing status.	Demonstrates learning and physical ability to use device.
2. Explain to patient how you are going to prepare for ambulation (e.g., transfer technique out of bed and safety precautions to be used while walking). Explain benefits and reasons for activity/exercise. Do so in a way that matches patient's educational level and beliefs and values regarding recovery or maintaining health.	Exercise self-efficacy is an important predictor of the adoption and maintenance of exercise behaviours. Self-efficacy is a belief and conviction that one can successfully perform a given activity (Hodgson et al., 2018; RNAO, 2010; Simpson et al., 2021).
3. Explain and demonstrate specific gait technique to patient or caregiver.	Teaching and demonstration enhance learning, reduce anxiety, and encourage cooperation.
4. Check for appropriate height and fit of assistive device. If physiotherapist has seen patient, the device should be at appropriate height. **Note:** This step is usually done when patient is standing at side of bed and is stable.	Ensures that patient is able to ambulate successfully without injury using device.
a. *Cane measurement:* Cane should extend from greater trochanter of the hip to floor while cane is held 15 cm (6 inches) from foot. Allow 15- to 30-degree elbow flexion. Cane handle should fit comfortably in palm of hand.	If cane is too short, patient has difficulty supporting weight and is bent over and uncomfortable. As weight is taken on by hands and affected leg is lifted off floor, complete extension of elbow is needed.
b. *Crutch measurement:* Includes three areas: patient's height, distance between crutch pad and axilla, and angle of elbow flexion. Use one of two methods:	Promotes optimal support and stability.
(1) Standing: Position crutches with crutch tips at 15 cm (6 inches) to side and 15 cm in front of patient's feet (tripod position). Crutch pads should be 5–6.25 cm (2–2.5 inches) or 3–4 finger widths under axilla (Astle & Duggleby, 2024) (see Step 4b[1] illustration).	Radial nerve passes under axillary area superficially. If crutch is too long, it places pressure on axilla and radial nerve. Injury to radial nerve causes paralysis of elbow and wrist extensors, commonly called *crutch palsy*. In addition, if crutch is too long, shoulders are forced upward, and patient cannot push body off the ground. If ambulation device is too short, patient is bent over and uncomfortable.

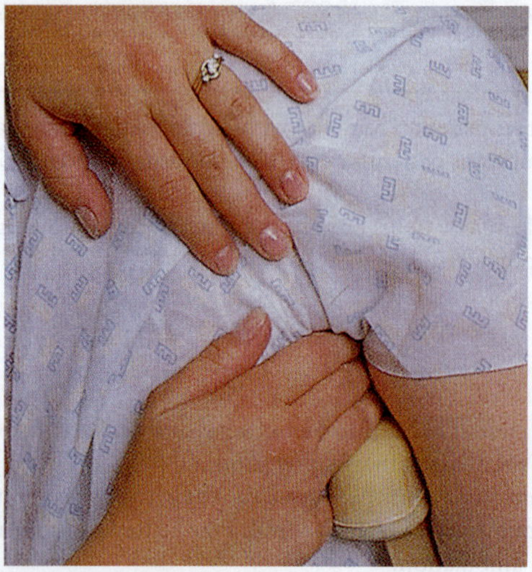

STEP 4B(1) Crutch pad is 3 to 4 finger widths under axilla.

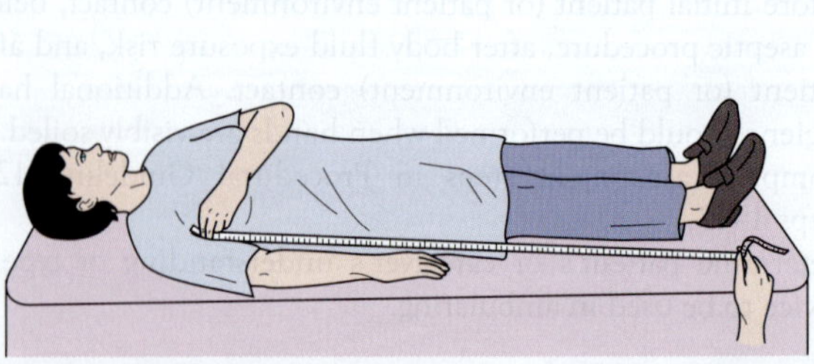

STEP 4B(2) Measuring length of crutch with patient in bed.

STEP	RATIONALE
(2) Supine: Crutch pad is approximately 5–6.25 cm (2–2.5 inches) or 3–4 finger widths under axilla, with crutch tips positioned 15 cm (6 inches) lateral to patient's heel (see Step 4b[2] illustration).	
(3) Height of handgrip must be adjusted so patient's elbow is flexed 15–30 degrees or it sits at approximately height of wrist crease. Both height of crutch and handgrip dimensions are adjustable on a well-made crutch.	Low handgrips cause radial nerve damage. High handgrips cause elbow to be sharply flexed, decreasing strength and stability of arms. This allows patient to fully extend the elbow when taking a step.
c. *Walker measurement:* When patient relaxes arms at side of body and stands up straight, top of walker should line up with crease on inside of wrist (Astle & Duggleby, 2024). Elbows should flex about 15–30 degrees when standing inside walker, with hands on handgrips.	Walker should be at proper height so that patient does not bend forward. Patient must have sufficient strength to be able to move walker.
5. Make sure that ambulation device has rubber tips.	Prevents device from slipping.

Critical Decision Point *Remove obstacles from pathways, including throw rugs (in the home), fall pads, and electrical cords, and wipe up any spills immediately. Avoid crowds. Crowds increase the risk that patient will lose balance (e.g., increased risk that crutch, cane, or walker will be kicked or jarred).*

IMPLEMENTATION

STEP	RATIONALE
1.	Proper hand hygiene helps prevent the spread of infectious agents to health care providers.
2. If using crutches, have patient report any tingling or numbness in upper torso.	Helps indicate whether crutches are being used incorrectly or are wrong size.
3. Help patient from lying position to side of bed (see Procedural Guideline 12.3, Step 14) or up from chair.	Ensures that patient is stable and ready to ambulate.
4. Allow patient to sit on edge of bed for a few minutes. Have patient alternately flex and extend feet and move lower legs. Ask if patient feels dizzy. Have patient relax and take a few deep breaths until dizziness subsides and balance is gained.	Determines ability to tolerate standing. If dizziness lasts more than 60 seconds, this may indicate orthostatic hypotension; return patient to bed (Jones & Kuritzky, 2018; Wahba et al., 2022). Recheck blood pressure.
5. Apply gait belt around patient's waist. Be sure that it completely encircles patient's waist. Place belt low and be sure that it is snug. You may need to adjust belt once patient stands. Hold belt along patient's back with your palms facing up as patient walks.	Belt controls patient's centre of mass during mobility, controls descent if a fall occurs, and reduces chance of grabbing patient's upper extremities.
6. Help patient stand at bedside. Reassess height of device to make sure that it is correct size. Have patient stand fully erect with shoulders back and looking ahead (not at floor). At this time, assess patient's ability to bear weight and balance (e.g., Does patient have discomfort or unsteady stance?).	Ensures that patient begins ambulation with correct posture and position.
7. If patient is unsteady, seat patient in chair or return to bed immediately.	Patient may require strengthening exercises or evaluation of balance by a physiotherapist.
8. Decide with patient how far to ambulate.	Determines mutual goal.
9. Implement ambulation around patient's other activities.	Taking scheduled rest periods between activities reduces patient fatigue.
10. Helping patient walk with cane (steps are the same with standard, tripod, or quad cane):	
a. Have patient hold cane on unaffected side. Direct patient to place cane forward 10–15 cm (4–6 inches) and slightly to the side of the foot, keeping body weight on both legs. Allow approximately 15- to 30-degree elbow flexion.	Offers most support when on stronger side of body. Cane and weaker leg work together with each step.
b. To begin, have patient move cane forward about 15–25 cm (6–10 inches), keeping body weight on both legs.	Distributes body weight equally.
c. Instruct patient to advance involved leg forward, even with the cane. The cane and affected leg swing and strike the ground at the same time.	Body weight is supported by cane and strong leg.
d. Have patient advance strong leg 15–25 cm (6–10 inches) past cane.	Aligns patient's centre of gravity. Returns patient body weight to equal distribution.

STEP	RATIONALE
e. Have patient move involved leg forward, even with strong leg, which can go as far forward as bad leg or slightly past it.	
f. Repeat sequences as patient tolerates. Once comfortable, have patient advance cane and weak leg together.	
11. Helping patient crutch walk by using appropriate crutch gait:	To use crutches, patient supports self with hands and arms; therefore, ability to balance body in upright position and stamina are necessary. Type of crutch gait depends on patient's weight-bearing status.
a. Four-point gait:	This is the most stable crutch gait. It provides at least three points of support at all times. Patient must be able to bear weight on both legs. Patient moves each leg alternately with each opposing crutch so three points of support are always on floor. Often used when patient has some form of paralysis (e.g., children with spastic cerebral palsy) (Hockenberry et al., 2024). May also be used for arthritic patients.
(1) Begin in tripod position (see Step 11a[1] illustration). Have patient place the crutch tips about 4–6 inches (10–15 cm) to the side and in front of each foot (Astle & Duggleby, 2024). Have patient place weight on handgrips, not under arms.	Improves balance by providing wide base of support. Patient should have posture of erect head and neck, straight vertebrae, and extended hips and knees.
(2) Move right crutch forward 10–15 cm (4–6 inches) (see Step 11a[2], illustration A).	Crutch and foot position similar to arm and foot position during normal walking.

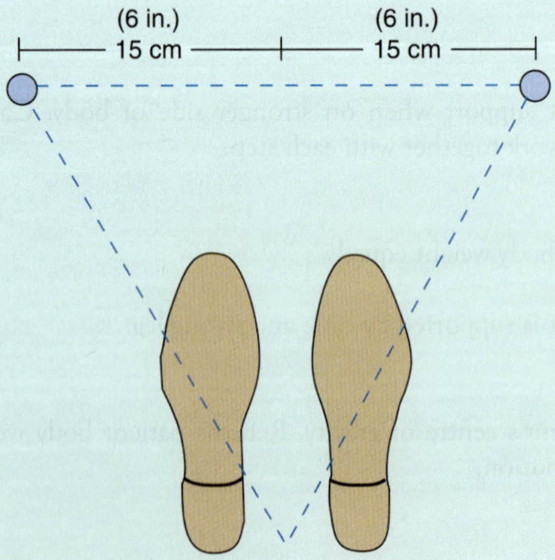

STEP 11A(1) Tripod position.

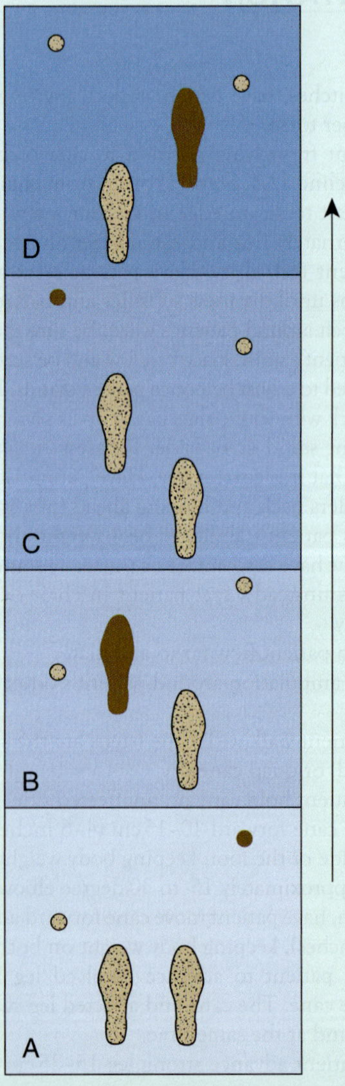

STEP 11A(2) Four-point gait. Solid feet and crutch tips show foot and crutch tip movement in each of four phases. (Read from bottom to top.) A, Right tip moves forward. B, Left foot moves toward left crutch. C, Left crutch tip moves forward. D, Right foot moves toward right crutch.

STEP	RATIONALE
(3) Move left foot forward to level of left crutch (see Step 11a[2], illustration *B*).	
(4) Move left crutch forward 10–15 cm (4–6 inches) (see Step 11a[2], illustration *C*).	
(5) Move right foot forward to level of right crutch (see Step 11a[2], illustration *D*).	
(6) Repeat sequence.	
b. Three-point gait (see Step 11b illustrations):	Requires patient to bear all weight on one foot. Weight is borne on strong leg and then on both crutches. Affected leg does not touch ground during early phase of three-point gait. May be useful for patient with broken leg or sprained ankle.
(1) Begin in tripod position (see Step 11b, illustration A), with patient standing on weight-bearing foot.	Improves patient's balance by providing wide base of support.
(2) Advance both crutches and involved leg, keeping foot of involved leg off floor (see Step 11b, illustration *B*).	
(3) Move weight-bearing leg forward, stepping on floor (see Step 11b, illustration C).	
(4) Repeat sequence.	
c. Two-point gait (see Step 11c illustrations):	Requires at least partial weight bearing on each foot. Is faster than four-point gait. Requires more balance because only two points support body at one time.
(1) Begin in tripod position (see Step 11c, illustration A).	Improves patient's balance by providing wide base of support.
(2) Move left crutch and right foot forward (see Step 11c, illustration B).	Crutch movements are similar to arm movement during normal walking; patient moves crutch at same time as opposing leg.
(3) Move right crutch and left foot forward (see Step 11c, illustration C).	
(4) Repeat sequence.	
d. Swing-to gait:	Used by patients whose lower extremities are paralyzed or who wear weight-supporting braces on their legs.
(1) Begin in tripod position.	This is the easier of two swinging gaits. It requires ability to partially bear body weight on both legs.

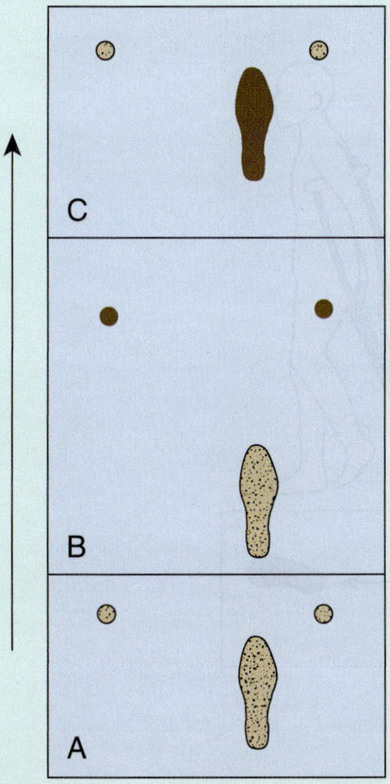

STEP 11B Three-point gait with weight borne on unaffected right leg. Solid foot and crutch tips show weight bearing in each phase from A to C. (Read from bottom to top.)

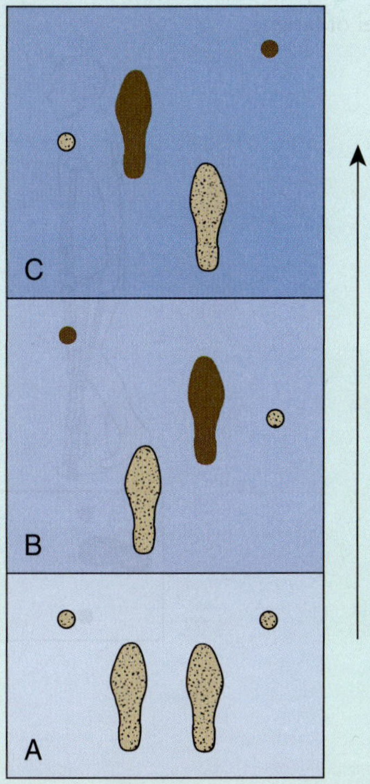

STEP 11C Two-point gait. Solid areas indicate weight-bearing leg and crutch tips from A to C. (Read from bottom to top.)

STEP	RATIONALE
(2) Move both crutches forward. (3) Lift and swing legs to crutches, letting crutches support body weight. (4) Repeat two previous steps.	
e. Swing-through gait (see Step 11e illustration): (1) Begin in tripod position. (2) Move both crutches forward. (3) Lift and swing legs through and beyond crutches. (4) Repeat sequence.	Requires that patient have ability to bear partial weight on both feet. Improves patient's balance by providing wide base of support. Initial placement of crutches increases patient's base of support so, when body swings forward, patient is moving centre of gravity toward additional support provided by crutches.
12. Helping patient climb stairs with a railing using crutches (partial weight bearing, one leg):	Climbing stairs with use of a railing is safest way for patient with crutches to ascend stairs.

Critical Decision Point *There is a risk of falling using this technique. Monitor patient's balance carefully. See option below.*

STEP	RATIONALE
a. Have patient begin in tripod position, standing on weight-bearing leg.	Improves patient's balance by providing wide base of support.
b. Patient transfers body weight to crutch.	Prepares patient to transfer weight to strong leg when ascending first stair.
c. Have patient hold handrail with one hand (strong leg next to railing). As the nurse, you carry crutch positioned next to handrail. Patient holds other crutch.	Ensures patient safety.
d. Have patient support weight evenly between the handrail and crutch (see Step 12d illustration).	Achieves balance.
e. Patient next places some weight on crutches and then steps up to first step with weight-bearing foot (see Step 12e illustration). Have patient get balance.	
f. Patient then straightens uninvolved knee and lifts body weight, bringing crutches and affected leg up the stair.	
g. Repeat sequence of steps until patient reaches top of stairs (see Step 12f illustration). Observe patient's balance and level of fatigue.	

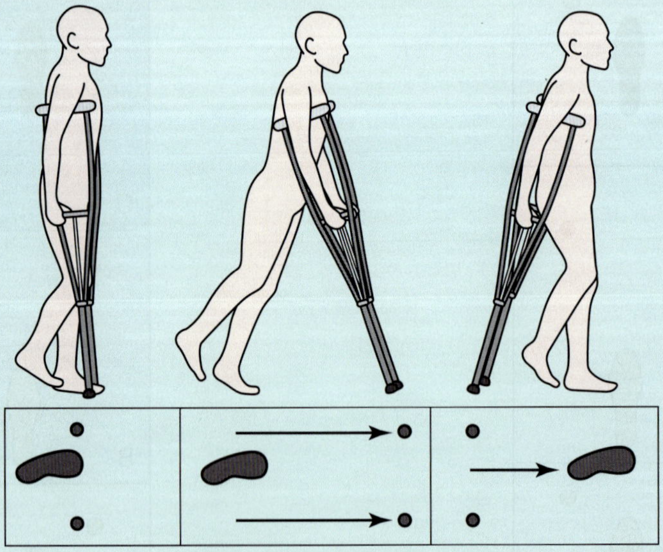

STEP 11E Swing-through gait.

STEP	RATIONALE

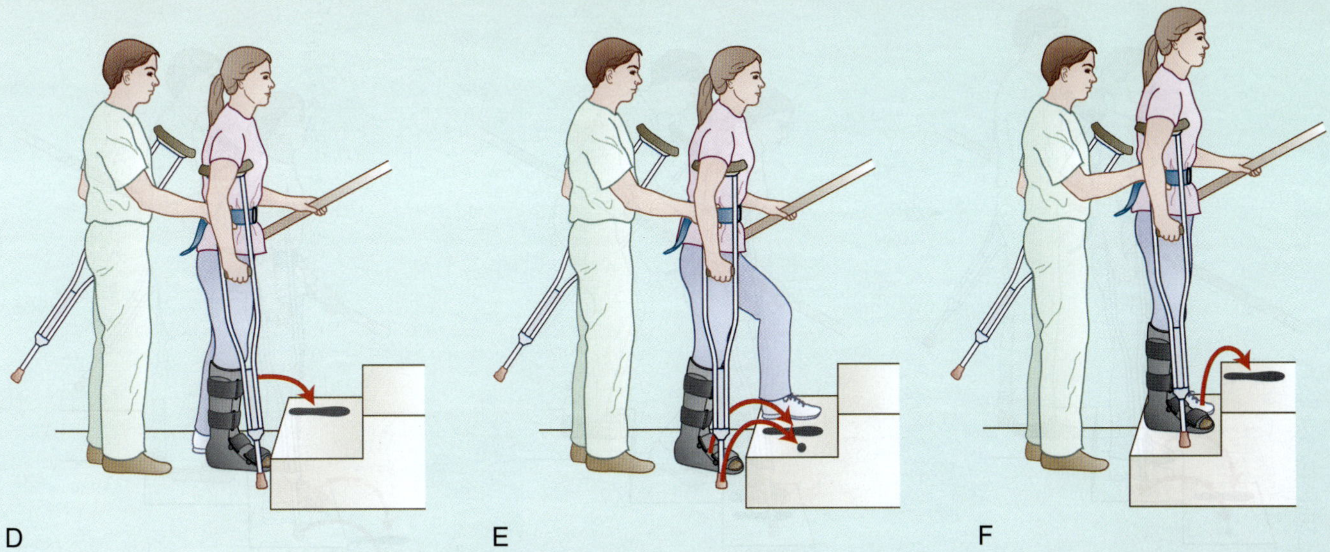

STEP 12 (D–F) Ascending stairs with crutches.

h. *Option:* Have patient sit on the lower stair. If distance and reach allows, place crutches at the top of the staircase. If this isn't possible, have patient place crutches as far up the stairs as they can. Then patient will move them to the top as they progress up the stairs (Astle & Duggleby, 2024).

Rationale: Reaching for inaccessible crutches could lead to a fall. Moving up by seat avoids risks of losing balance and tripping on stairs.

(1) In the seated position, have patient reach behind with both arms.

(2) Then have patient use arms and weight-bearing foot or leg to lift up one step.

(3) Repeat this process one step at a time.

13. Helping patient descend stairs with a railing with crutch (partial weight bearing, one leg):

Critical Decision Point *There is a risk of falling using this technique. Monitor patient's balance carefully. See option below.*

a. Begin in tripod position.

Rationale: Improves patient's balance by providing wide base of support.

b. Patient transfers body weight to strong leg and aligns with crutches.

Rationale: Prepares patient to release support of body weight maintained by crutches.

c. Have patient hold handrail with one hand (involved leg next to railing). As the nurse, you carry crutch positioned next to handrail (see Step 13c illustration). Patient holds other crutch.

d. Have patient bend their strong knee while moving crutch and involved leg down a step (see Step 13d illustration).

e. Patient then supports their weight evenly between handrail and crutch (see Step 13e illustration). Be sure that patient has good balance.

f. Have patient slowly bring involved leg down one step. Caution patient not to hop.

Rationale: Hopping could injure leg and create risk for fall.

g. *Option:* Have patient sit on the top step. Place crutches down the stairs by sliding them to the lowest possible point on the stairway. Then continue to move them down as patient progresses down the stairs (Astle & Duggleby, 2024).

Rationale: Reaching for inaccessible crutches could lead to a fall. Moving down by seat avoids risk of losing balance and falling down stairs.

(1) In the seated position, have patient reach behind with both arms.

(2) Have patient use arms and weight-bearing foot or leg to lift themselves down one step.

(3) Repeat this process one step at a time.

STEP	RATIONALE

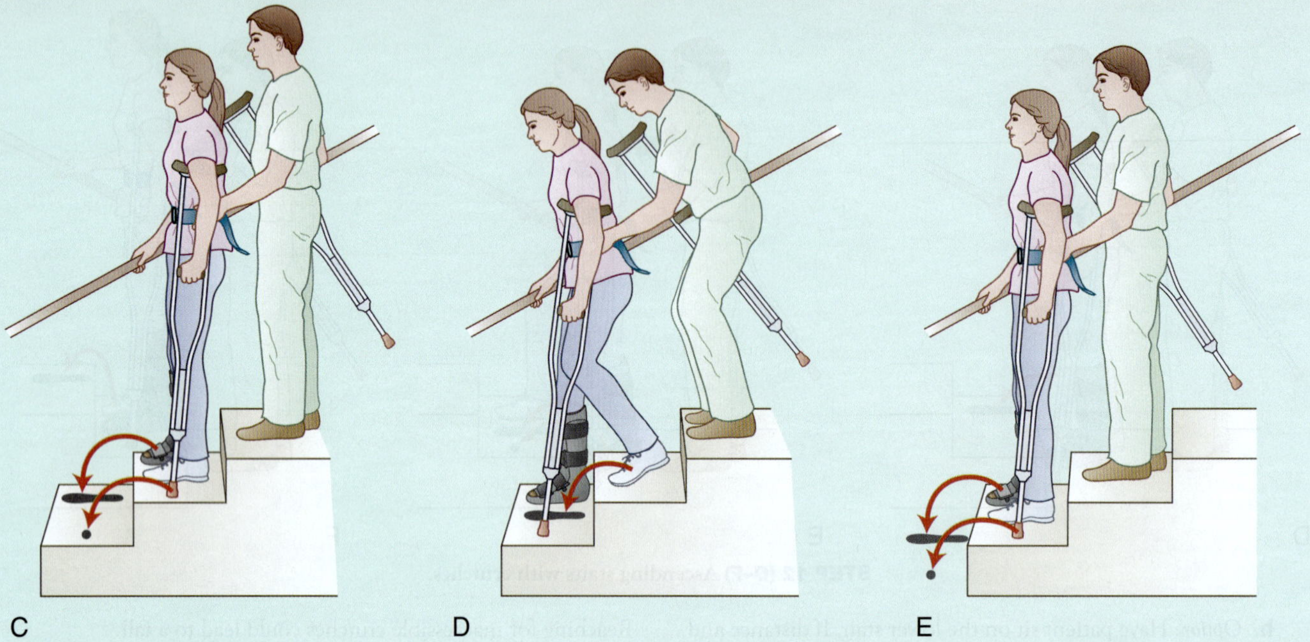

STEP 13 (C–E) Descending stairs with crutches.

STEP	RATIONALE
14. Helping patient ambulate with walker:	Patients who are able to bear partial weight use walkers.
a. Have patient stand straight in centre of walker and grasp handgrips on upper bars.	Patient balances self before attempting to walk.
b. Have patient move walker a comfortable distance forward, about 15–20 cm (6–8 inches). Patient then takes step forward with involved leg first and follows through with good leg. Instruct patient not to advance leg past the front bar of walker. If patient has equal strength in both legs, it makes no difference which leg advances first.	Provides broad base of support between walker and patient. Patient then moves centre of gravity toward walker. Keeping all four feet of walker on floor is necessary to prevent tipping walker.
c. If patient is unable to bear weight on involved leg, have them slowly hop to centre of walker using strong leg, supporting weight on hands.	
d. Instruct patient not to try to climb stairs with walker unless they have a specific walker for steps.	Patient should use handrails as alternative. Using walker could cause a fall.
15. After patient ambulates, help them back to bed or chair and help assume comfortable position.	Prevents transmission of infection.

EVALUATION

1. After ambulation, obtain patient's vital signs, observe skin colour, and ask about comfort and energy levels.	Evaluates how patient tolerated procedure and whether there was progress in ambulation. Assesses stage of patient's illness and degree of convalescence when evaluating process.
2. Evaluate patient's subjective statements regarding experience.	Evaluates activity tolerance.
3. Evaluate patient's gait pattern: Observe body alignment in standing position and balance during gait.	Determines whether patient is using supportive aids for ambulation correctly. Keep in mind patient's previous manner of ambulating when assessing gait.
4. **Use teach-back:** "You have done well walking with your walker. We reviewed with your partner how to place a gait belt. I talked about why it is important for your partner to use a gait belt to help you at first. Can both of you tell me why a gait belt is important?" Develop a revised teaching plan if patient or caregiver is unable to teach back correctly.	Determines patient's and caregiver's level of understanding of instructional topic.

Unexpected Outcomes	Related Interventions
1. Patient is unable to ambulate because of fear of falling, physical discomfort, upper body muscles that are too weak to use ambulation device, or lower extremities that are too weak to support body.	• Consult with physiotherapist about possible exercise program to strengthen muscles or other alternative methods that patient can use for ambulation. • Provide analgesic for discomfort. • Discuss with patient fears or concerns about walking using assistive device.
2. Patient sustains an injury.	• Notify health care provider. • Return patient to bed if injury is such that it is safe to do so. • Document per employer policy.
3. When using cane or walker, patient bends over and does not stand up straight.	• Reinforce correct posture.

Communication and Documentation

- Document in the patient medical record the assessment findings, type of assistive device and gait patient used, amount of help required, distance walked, and activity tolerance in progress notes in EHR or chart.
- Document your evaluation of patient and caregiver learning.
- Immediately report any injury sustained during attempts to ambulate, alteration in vital signs, or inability to ambulate to nurse in charge or health care provider.

DOCUMENTATION EXAMPLE

Patient ambulated independently with use of 4-wheeled walker for approximately 12 metres at 1100 hours. Vital signs pre-ambulation: B/P 120/76, P 68, R 22, oxygen saturation on room air 97%. Patient stood erect at walker with gait steady and balance stable. Patient indicated no pain pre or post ambulation. Post vital signs: B/P 126/80, P 70, R 23, oxygen saturation on room air 97%. Activity tolerated well.

Special Considerations

Teaching

- Instruct patient to do exercises such as squeezing a rubber ball, raising and lowering both arms in a slow and rhythmic manner while holding weights, chair push-ups, and pull-ups, all of which help strengthen upper extremities.
- Teach patients who use a walker to examine the frame daily. When inspecting a walker, the patient should observe for signs of bending or deformation of the frame, protruding screws that can scratch, and loose or missing screws that weaken the joints of the frame. Assess handgrips for any cracks or signs of being loose, and ensure proper function of brakes on wheeled walkers.
- Teach patients to use the arms of a chair rather than the assistive device to give them leverage when getting up from a chair; the device is likely to tip if used for this purpose.
- Blistering or soreness of the hands can result from continual pressure between the hand and the handle of a crutch. Advise patient to release pressure intermittently and wear gloves or pad the handle to reduce friction.
- Instruct patient that, if wearing shoes with varying heel sizes, the crutches, canes, and walkers may need to be adjusted to maintain the proper height.
- Caution patients when using an assistive device: *Don't look down.* Look straight ahead as you normally do when you walk. *Don't walk on slippery surfaces.* Avoid snowy, icy, or rainy conditions. *Don't put any weight on the affected foot* if your doctor has so advised (Astle & Duggleby, 2024).
- For assistive devices such as motorized scooters, patients and caregivers should know how to properly operate the equipment, apply brakes, and adhere to safety standards. Safety information can be accessed through the Canada Safety Council (https://canadasafetycouncil.org/motorized-scooters-and-other-devices/) and Transport Canada (https://www.tc.gc.ca/eng/motorvehiclesafety/tp-tp2436-rs200803-menu-374.htm). Health Canada offers guidance on purchasing assistive devices (https://www.canada.ca/en/health-canada/services/healthy-living/your-health/lifestyles/seniors-aging-assistive-devices.html).

Pediatric

- For rehabilitation of a small child who has not yet learned to walk or who is unsteady, special crutches with three or four legs provide the needed stability to allow the child to maintain an upright posture and learn to walk (Hockenberry et al., 2024).
- Another option for children who are just learning to walk would be front- or rear-rolling walkers.

Gerontological

- The Public Health Agency of Canada and the Canadian Society for Exercise Physiology (CSEP) have many resources and guidelines about physical activity for older persons. Both agencies offer tips that care providers can use to motivate patients (see https://www.canada.ca/en/public-health/services/health-promotion/healthy-living/physical-activity/physical-activity-tips-older-adults-65-years-older.html; https://csepguidelines.ca/guidelines/adults-65/).

Care in the Community: Home Management

- Teach patient how to use the ambulation aid on various terrains (e.g., carpet, stairs, rough ground, inclines). Teach how to manoeuvre around obstacles such as doors and how to use the aid when transferring to and from a chair, toilet, and tub.
- Teach caregivers how to help and what to observe to ensure that an assistive device is used correctly.
- Teach patient to conduct safety and maintenance checks of ambulation devices on a routine basis.

✦ SKILL 12.3 Care of a Patient With an Immobilization Device

Immobilization devices increase stability of bones and joints, support an extremity, or reduce the load on weight-bearing structures such as hips, knees, or ankles (Table 12.3). A splint immobilizes and protects a body part. Slings provide support, immobilization, and elevation of the arm or shoulder following injury or surgery. An abduction splint or pillow is used after hip replacement surgery to maintain a patient's legs in an abducted position so that the new joint remains stable. Cloth and foam splints, known as immobilizers, provide long-term immobilization (Fig. 12.2). Orthotic devices or orthoses maintain joint(s) in a position that enables a patient to maximize the movement they can produce (facilitation); prevent, correct, or compensate for deformity or contracture; and reduce weight or forces being taken through a limb.

Medical device–related pressure injuries can result from the use of devices designed and applied for diagnostic or therapeutic purposes. In the case of immobilization devices or orthotics, the resultant pressure injury generally conforms to the pattern or shape of the device (Berlowitz, 2020). It is a nursing responsibility to carefully assess the skin prior to device placement, ensure that the device supports an extremity as intended, and evaluate the condition of the skin on an

TABLE 12.3
Immobilization Devices

Device	Uses and Benefits	Features
Soft splints	• Temporary splints reduce pain and prevent tissue damage from further motion immediately after an injury (e.g., fracture or sprain). • Air splints, Thomas splints, and improvised splints from material on hand are examples of temporary splints applied in emergency situations.	• Available commercially or can be made for almost any body part. • Velcro or buckle closures permit these devices to be adjusted to fit a body part of almost any size and shape.
Moulded splints	• Provide support to patients with chronic injuries or diseases such as arthritis. • Maintain the body part in a functional position to prevent contractures and muscle atrophy during the period of disuse.	• Made of plastic, which can be cleaned with a washcloth and warm soap and water. • Can be removed quickly for assessment of the skin or a wound.
Abduction pillow	• Permits a patient to be turned without changing the position of the healing limb. • Prevents dislocation of the hip prosthesis.	• Easily removed for nursing care (e.g., skin care, dressing changes, and neurovascular assessments).
Immobilizers	• Immobilizers treat sprains and dislocations that do not require complete and continuous immobilization in a cast or traction.	• Common types of immobilizers include cervical collars (soft or hard), belt-type shoulder immobilizers, and knee immobilizers.
Braces	• Support weakened structures during weight bearing. • Chest and abdominal braces (Boston brace) immobilize the thoracic and lumbar vertebral column to treat scoliosis (curvature of the spine). • Lumbar braces support lumbar and sacral tissues after spinal surgery. • Leg and foot braces hold the thigh, leg, and foot in functional positions for weight bearing and ambulation.	• Made of sturdy materials such as leather, metal, and moulded plastic.

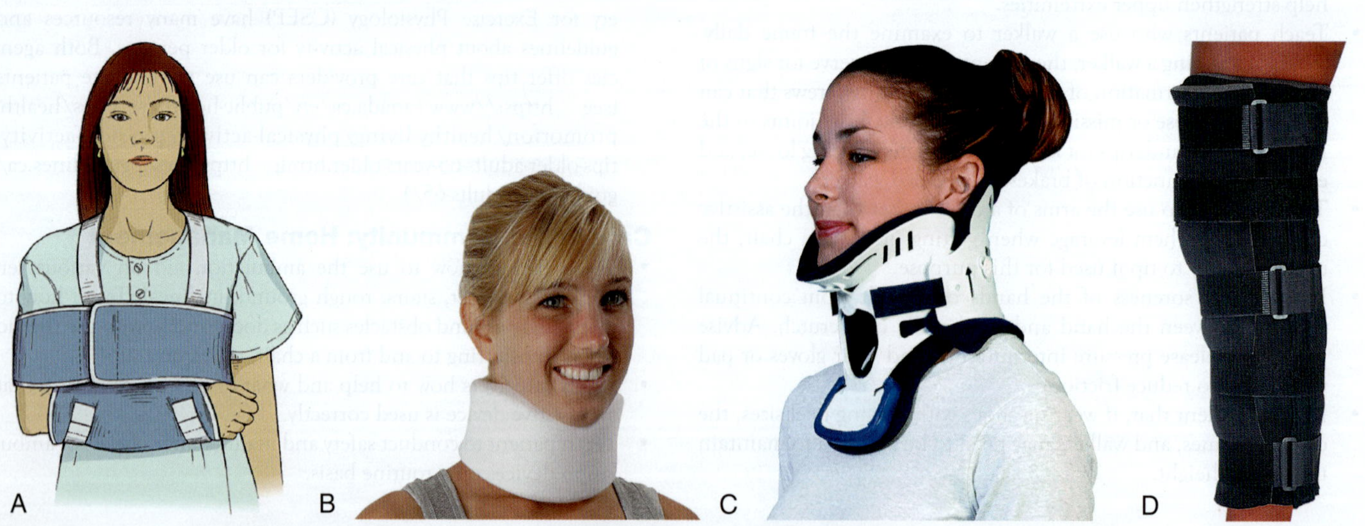

FIG 12.2 **Examples of immobilizers. A, Shoulder/arm immobilizer. B, Soft cervical collar. C, Hard cervical collar. D, Knee immobilizer.** (*A from Chudnofsky, C. R., & Chudnofsky, A. S. [2020]. Roberts and Hedges' Clinical procedures in emergency medicine and acute care. Elsevier;* **B–D** *used with permission from Össur Americas. All rights reserved.*)

ongoing basis. In addition, if a device is applied too tightly or incorrectly, there can be compression, causing reduction in circulation to the extremity.

Delegation and Collaboration

The skill of caring for a patient wearing a brace, splint, or sling can be delegated to a UCP. The nurse directs the UCP about the following:

- Reviewing prescribed schedule of wear and activities permitted while patient is in the brace, splint, or sling
- Reviewing any special observations that might be required based on device
- Informing the nurse if patient experiences pain, rubbing, or pressure from the brace, splint, or sling or if a change occurs in the condition of patient's skin under device

Equipment

Brace, splint, or commercially prepared sling; cotton shirt or gown; clean gloves; cotton webbing or bandage *(optional)*; towel, washcloth, soap, and basin with water

STEP	RATIONALE
ASSESSMENT	
1. Identify patient using at least two person-specific identifiers (e.g., name and date of birth, or name and medical record number) according to employer policy.	Ensures correct patient. Complies with Accreditation Canada's standards and improves patient safety (Accreditation Canada, 2020).
2. Throughout the procedure, the 4 moments for hand hygiene are to be implemented; hand hygiene should occur before initial patient (or patient environment) contact, before an aseptic procedure, after body fluid exposure risk, and after patient (or patient environment) contact. Additional hand hygiene should be performed when hands are visibly soiled.	Proper hand hygiene helps prevent the spread of infectious agents to health care providers.
3. Review patient's medical history, previous and current activity level, description of the condition requiring immobilization, and medical order for device.	Reveals patient's current and previous health status and purpose of immobilization. Medical order required for use of devices.
4. Inspect area of skin in contact with immobilization device or area that will be covered by newly applied device (apply clean gloves if there is risk of contact with body fluids).	Reduces transmission of microorganisms. Provides baseline to monitor for skin breakdown. Immobile and older persons are particularly vulnerable.

Critical Decision Point *When assessing medical device–related pressure injuries, remove only those devices that can be safely removed. "Nonremovable" devices includes those that are not normally removed during patient care (e.g., casts) and in situations in which the patient has a health care provider prescription to "not remove." Skin under the edges of nonremovable devices can be assessed if it can be done without displacing the device.*

STEP	RATIONALE
5. Palpate temperature, pulse, and sensation of extremity distal to where device is to be applied.	Provides baseline to measure circulation and sensorineural status. Reduces transmission of microorganisms.
6. Assess patient's and/or caregiver's knowledge and experience with immobilization devices.	Determines whether there is a need for patient education.
7. Assess patient's level of pain using an appropriate pain assessment tool.	Provides a baseline to determine whether immobilization device affects comfort.
8. Refer to occupational therapy or physiotherapy to determine type of device to be used, desired position, and amount of activity and movement permitted.	Provides direction in proper fit and use of device.
PLANNING	
1. Expected outcomes following completion of procedure:	
• Patient's skin remains intact, warm, without signs of pressure and with normal sensation.	Device applied correctly without skin irritation.
• Patient and caregiver verbalize purpose, correct application, and care of the device.	Demonstrates learning.
• Patient reports a temporary increase in pain (using appropriate pain scale) during device application.	Normal response to device application.
• Patient uses the device correctly, including schedule of wear, activity limitations, and positioning.	Able to perform self-care while wearing device.
2. Provide privacy by closing room curtains or doors and prepare environment.	Ensures comfortable, organized environment.
3. Explain to patient and caregiver purpose of device and how it will be applied.	Promotes understanding needed for self-care of device.
IMPLEMENTATION	
1.	Proper hand hygiene helps prevent the spread of infectious agents to health care providers.

STEP	RATIONALE
2. Assist patient to a comfortable position: apply upper extremity brace/splint/sling with patient sitting upright; apply lower extremity brace with patient lying down.	Facilitates correct, aligned placement of brace/splint/sling.
3. Apply clean gloves if there is risk of contact with body fluids. Prepare skin that will be enclosed in brace/splint/sling by cleaning skin with soap and water; rinse, pat dry, and change any dressings (if present). If applying a back brace, put a thin cotton shirt or gown on patient. Ensure that there are no wrinkles to cause pressure.	This protects skin and keeps brace clean. Smooth cotton clothing between the brace and skin protects skin from irritation and absorbs moisture.
4. Inspect device for wear, damage, or rough edges.	Decreases potential for skin breakdown and maintains correct alignment.
5. Apply brace/splint/sling as directed by health care provider, orthotist, physiotherapist, or occupational therapist. Be sure application provides for the alignment and support indicated in the order:	Proper application of the brace/splint/sling is important to avoid skin breakdown, pressure injuries, neurovascular compromise, calluses, or worsening of deformity.
a. Apply even tension on any bandage or gauze padding that is ordered to be applied against skin; wrap distal to proximal.	Prevents trapping of blood and fluid distal to immobilization device.
b. Prevent padding from gathering or bunching.	Prevents irritation to underlying tissues.
c. Support joints when you position and apply the device.	Reduces risk of musculoskeletal injury during movement.
6. Apply commercial sling:	Commercially available slings secure arm to chest for added support and have padding on strap for comfort.
a. Be sure correct size is chosen. Place elbow into close side of sling, aligning arm into sling and slipping wrist and hand through open side of sling or through separate Velcro enclosure (see Fig. 12.2, A).	
b. Enclose Velcro strap around arm, place strap around patient's neck, and tighten buckle until it fits snugly.	
c. Position arm so that the hand and forearm are higher than elbow.	
7. Remove and dispose of gloves.	Reduces transmission of microorganisms.
8. Teach patient and caregiver prescribed schedule of wear and activities while in device as directed by health care provider, physiotherapist, or occupational therapist.	Proper use of brace/splint/sling facilitates healing and mobility and reduces pain and stress.
9. Reinforce instruction regarding signs to report to health care provider: skin breakdown, pressure, or rubbing.	Device may need to be adjusted. Changes may also be required because of growth or atrophy, when muscles regain or lose strength, or after reconstructive surgery.
10. Teach patient/caregiver how to care for brace/splint/sling:	Maintains integrity of device.
a. When not in use, store metal braces upright in a safe but easily accessible location.	Prevents deformity or bending of brace.
b. Store splints of moulded materials away from heat.	Prevents melting and deformation of splint.
c. Treat any leather material with leather preservative.	Prevents drying or cracking.
d. Keep brace clean, dry, and in good working order. Clean plastic parts with a damp cloth and thoroughly dry. Clean metal brace joints with a pipe cleaner, and oil weekly. Remove rust with steel wool, and clean metal parts with a solvent.	Maintains function and integrity of devices.
11. Assist patient in ambulating with brace/splint/sling in place.	Determines whether patient is able to ambulate safely.
12. Observe while patient or caregiver applies and removes brace/splint/sling.	Promotes patient independence; demonstration confirms level of learning skill.
13. Help patient to comfortable position.	Gives patient sense of well-being.
14. Place nurse call system in an accessible location within patient's reach.	Ensures patient can call for assistance if needed and promotes safety and prevents falls.
15. Raise side rails (as appropriate) and lower bed to lowest position.	Ensures patient safety.
16. Dispose of supplies or dirty linen.	Reduces transmission of microorganisms.

STEP	RATIONALE

EVALUATION

STEP	RATIONALE
1. Inspect care of skin underneath device for redness or skin breakdown. If allowed, removed device briefly to assess skin thoroughly.	Monitors for development of pressure injury.
2. Palpate temperature, pulse, sensation of extremity distal to device. Check capillary refill by pressing on toe or finger (see Step 2 illustration).	Screens for changes in circulation due to compression of device against skin.

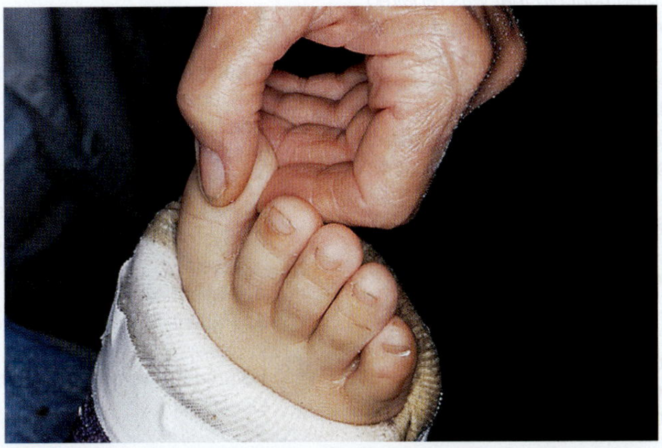

STEP 2 Inspecting toe to assess capillary refill.

STEP	RATIONALE
3. Inspect alignment of the limb after application of device.	Device is designed to support limb in a stable position.
4. Ask patient to rate level of pain after device application, using an appropriate pain assessment tool.	Application of device may cause temporary discomfort, but eventually the support it offers reduces pain.
5. Use teach-back: "I want to be sure I explained clearly the need for the brace/splint/sling, how to maintain the device, and the limitations of this device. Can you tell me how you will use this brace/splint/sling safely?" Develop a revised teaching plan if patient is unable to teach back correctly.	Teach-back is an evidence-based health literacy intervention that promotes patient engagement, patient safety, adherence, and quality. The goal of teach-back is to ensure that you have explained medical information clearly so that patients and their families understand what you communicated to them (Agency for Healthcare Research and Quality, 2020).

Unexpected Outcomes	Related Interventions
1. Patient reports increased severity in pain after application of the device.	• Reposition extremity. • Administer analgesics as ordered to maintain patient's comfort level. • Increase frequency of neurovascular checks. • Inform health care provider.
2. Patient develops area of pressure, redness, or skin breakdown.	• Inspect device for proper fit and positioning and for areas of damage, wear, and rough edges. • Notify health care provider. • Notify orthoptist, physiotherapist, or occupational therapist so that adjustments to device can be made.

Communication and Documentation

- Document in the patient medical record or clinic record assessments of skin integrity, neurovascular status, application of and type of device, schedule of wear, activity level, movement permitted, patient's tolerance of procedure, and instructions given to patient and caregiver in progress notes in EHR or chart.
- Document your evaluation of patient's or caregiver ability to apply device, ambulate, and remove device.
- Report to health care provider any unexpected outcomes.

Special Considerations

Teaching

- When a patient has an immobilization device, instruct the patient to inspect skin daily for pressure or areas of breakdown. Involve family or caregiver as appropriate.
- Give patients a list of medical suppliers in the community to obtain new sling or elastic wrap for splints.

Pediatric

- If a child's extremity has been immobilized for a long time, perform upper body strengthening exercises to condition and strengthen arms and shoulders (Hockenberry et al., 2024).
- Monitor children closely to ensure that they do not remove an immobilization device.
- Recognize that bracing in adolescents affects body image and self-esteem.

Gerontological

- Lightweight immobilization devices are less restrictive for older persons.
- Older persons may have decreased sensation, so carefully assess fit of immobilization device (Boscart et al., 2023).

Care in the Community: Home Management

- Remind patient to inspect and clean immobilization device weekly.

✦ REVIEW QUESTIONS

A 72-year-old patient (she/her) was transferred out of the critical care unit (CCU) following a motor vehicle accident and has progressed through stages 1 and 2 of an early mobility protocol to stage 3, where she will sit in a chair for 20 minutes. She had a fractured right hip that was repaired in surgery and has multiple bruises causing discomfort in her right shoulder and chest area. During surgery, she had significant blood loss. She has been in the CCU for 3 days. Her heart rate per minute since being hospitalized has ranged from 72 to 94, BP 118–146/72–84 mm Hg, and respirations 18 to 26 breaths/minute. The nurse is helping the patient with active range-of-motion (ROM) exercises before getting her to sit on the side of the bed.

Review Questions 1 to 3 relate to the case study presented here.

1. What should be included in the nurse's assessment before getting the patient up to sit in a chair? (*Select all that apply.*)
   1. Assess the patient's beliefs, values, and perceptions regarding exercise.
   2. Assess the patient's ROM and strength.
   3. Complete a set of vitals before ambulation.
   4. Ask the patient's spouse how much the patient exercises at home.
   5. Assess the patient's most recent laboratory results.

2. The patient develops a fever in the afternoon and refuses to get out of bed. She reports pain at a level of 7 on a scale of 0–10. You are concerned that the patient may be at risk for deep vein thrombosis (DVT). Which risk factors does the patient have for developing DVT? (*Select all that apply.*)
   1. Immobility
   2. Fever
   3. Pain
   4. Hip surgery
   5. History of hypertension

3. The nurse assesses the patient's legs for signs of a developing DVT. Which of the following assessment measures would be used to monitor for DVT? (*Select all that apply.*)
   1. Palpation of skin temperature
   2. Auscultation for a bruit
   3. Measurement of calf circumference
   4. Range of motion of right leg

4. Place the following steps for a four-point crutch gait in the correct order.

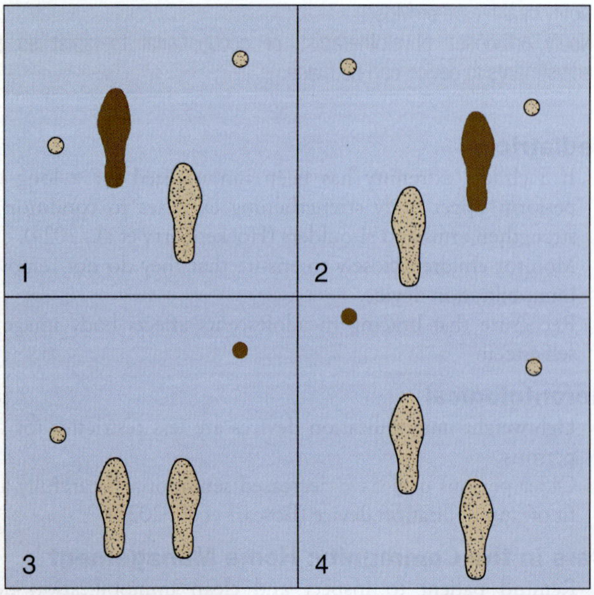

5. Which tips should you recommend to patients for preventing DVT in the home environment? (*Select all that apply.*)
   1. Avoid sitting for any period of time longer than 2–3 hours.
   2. Limit fluid intake while travelling.
   3. Wear loose-fitting clothes if travelling for more than 4 hours.
   4. When sitting, always keep your legs crossed.
   5. Perform foot exercises when flying in a plane for more than 4 hours.

6. A patient is placed on an early progressive mobility protocol. After the nurse helps the patient sit in a chair for 15 minutes, which data indicate to the nurse that the patient needs to return to bed immediately? (*Select all that apply.*)
   1. Patient is dizzy for 15 seconds.
   2. Respiratory rate increases over baseline by 4 breaths/min.
   3. Systolic blood pressure falls 30 mm Hg below baseline systolic level.
   4. Patient expresses severe fatigue.
   5. Patient becomes diaphoretic.

Visit the Evolve site for a complete list of answers to the Review Questions.

✦ NEXT GENERATION NCLEX® (NGN)

For practice with answering exam questions related to unfolding NGN case studies, please consult the Next Generation NCLEX® (NGN)-Style Case Studies for Skills and Techniques on the Evolve website: http://evolve.elsevier.com/Canada/Perry/clinicalskills/

REFERENCES

Accreditation Canada. (2020). *Required organizational practices handbook.* https://physicians.nshealth.ca/resources/required-organizational-practices-2020-handbook

Agency for Healthcare Research and Quality. (2020). *Teach-back: Intervention.* https://www.ahrq.gov/patient-safety/reports/engage/interventions/teachback html

Alaparthi, G. K., Gatty, A., Samuel, S. R., et al. (2020). Effectiveness, safety, and barriers to early mobilization in the intensive care unit. *Critical Care Research & Practice, 2020*, Article 7840743. https://doi.org/10.1155/2020/7840743

Astle, B. J., & Duggleby, W. (2024). *Potter and Perry's Canadian fundamentals of nursing* (7th ed.). Elsevier.

Badireddy, M., & Mudipalli, V. R. (2021). Deep venous thrombosis prophylaxis. *StatPearls.* https://www.ncbi.nlm.nih.gov/books/NBK534865/

Bassett, S. M., Jordan, J. L., & Weeks, D. L. (2021). Safety and efficacy of early ambulation on an alternative oxygen delivery device for patients receiving bedside heated humidified high-flow nasal cannula therapy. *Cardiopulmonary Physical Therapy Journal, 32*(3), 97–105. https://doi.org/10.1097/CPT.0000000000000147

Berlowitz, D. (2020). Prevention of pressure-induced skin and soft tissue injury. *UpToDate.* https://www.uptodate.com/contents/prevention-of-pressure-induced-skin-and-soft-tissue-injury

Berszakiewicz, A., Sieroń, A., Krasiński, Z., et al. (2020). Compression therapy in venous diseases: Current forms of compression materials and techniques. *Postepy Dermatologii i Alergologii, 37*(6), 836–841. https://doi.org/10.5114/ada.2019.86991

Bircher, A., & Chowdhury, A. (2020). Current DVT prophylaxis: A review. *Orthopaedics and Trauma, 34*(3), 161–167. https://doi.org/10.1016/j.mporth.2020.03.010

Boscart, V., McCleary, L., Sheiban Taucar, L., et al. (2023). *Ebersole and Hess's gerontological nursing and healthy aging in Canada* (3rd ed.). Elsevier.

Brock, C., Marzano, V., Green, M., et al. (2018). Defining new barriers to mobilisation in a highly active intensive care unit—Have we found the ceiling? An observational study. *Heart & Lung, 47*(4), 380–385. https://doi.org/10.1016/j.hrtlng.2018.04.004

Burchum, J. R., & Rosenthal, L. D. (2021). *Lehne's pharmacology for nursing care* (11th ed.). Elsevier.

Canadian Association of Critical Care Nurses (CACCN). (2018). *Position statement: Patient- and family-centred care.* https://caccn.ca/wp-content/uploads/2019/10/PS062018PSPFCCare.pdf

Centers for Disease Control and Prevention. (2022). *What is venous thromboembolism?* https://www.cdc.gov/ncbddd/dvt/facts.html

Chen, Y., Almirall-Sánchez, A., Mockler, D., et al. (2022). Hospital–associated deconditioning: Not only physical, but also cognitive. *International Journal of Geriatric Psychiatry*, *37*(3). https://doi.org/10.1002/gps.5687

Coles, S., Erdogan, M., Higgins, S. D., et al. (2020). Impact of an early mobilization protocol on outcomes in trauma patients admitted to the intensive care unit: A retrospective pre-post study. *Journal of Trauma and Acute Care Surgery*, *88*(4), 515–521. https://doi.org/10.1097/TA.0000000000002588

Government of Alberta. (2022). *Compression stockings: How to use them*. https://myhealth.alberta.ca/health/medications/pages/conditions.aspx

Government of Canada. (2018). *A common vision for increasing physical activity and reducing sedentary living in Canada: Let's get moving*. https://www.canada.ca/content/dam/phac-aspc/documents/services/publications/healthy-living/lets-get-moving/pub-eng.pdf

Heart and Stroke Foundation of Canada. (2022). *How much physical activity do you need?* https://www.heartandstroke.ca/healthy-living/stay-active/how-much-physical-activity-do-you-need

Hendrich, A. L. (2021). CE: Reimagining injurious falls and safe mobility. *American Journal of Nursing*, *121*(9), 34–44. https://doi.org/10.1097/01.NAJ.0000790188.10474.10

Hockenberry, M. J., Duffy, E. A., & Gibbs, K. (2024). *Wong's nursing care of infants and children* (12th ed.). Elsevier.

Hodgson, C. L., Capell, E., & Tipping, C. J. (2018). Early mobilization of patients in intensive care: Organization, communication and safety factors that influence translation into clinical practice. *Critical Care*, *22*(1), 77–77. https://doi.org/10.1186/s13054-018-1998-9

Jones, J., & Kuritzky, L. (2018). Recognition and management of orthostatic hypotension in primary care. *Journal of Family Practice*, 67(Suppl. 8), S25–S30.

Lee, Y., Kim, K., Kang, S., et al. (2020). Compression stocking length effects on oedema, pain, and satisfaction in nursing students: A pilot randomized trial. *Healthcare*, *8*(2), Article 149. https://doi.org/10.3390/healthcare8020149

Lightfoot, C. J., Vadaszy, N., Watson, E. L., et al. (2022). Perceptions and experiences of a progressive resistance exercise program in people with chronic kidney disease. *Nephrology Nursing Journal*, *49*(1), 19–27.

Liu, B., Moore, J. E., Almaawiy, U., et al. (2018). Outcomes of mobilisation of vulnerable elders in Ontario (MOVE ON): A multisite interrupted time series evaluation of an implementation intervention to increase patient mobilization. *Age and Ageing*, *47*(1), 112–119. https://doi.org/10.1093/ageing/afx128

Lurie, J. M., Maximilian, C. Y., Subramaniam, S., et al. (2019). Virchow's triad in "silent" deep vein thrombosis. *Journal of Vascular Surgery: Venous and Lymphatic Disorders*, *7*(5), 640–645. https://doi.org/10.1016/j.jvsv.2019.02.011

MacDonald, S. A., & Jakubec, S. L. (2021). *Stanhope and Lancaster's community health nursing in Canada* (4th ed.). Elsevier.

MOVE Canada. (2022). *Mobilization*. https://www.movescanada.ca/mobilization/

Multiple Sclerosis Society of Canada. (2022). *Exercise and physical activity*. https://mssociety.ca/hot-topics/exercise-and-physical-activity

National Institute on Aging. (2020). *How older adults can get started with exercise*. https://www.nia.nih.gov/health/how-older-adults-can-get-started-exercise

Negro, A., Cabrini, L., Lembo, R., et al. (2018). Early progressive mobilization in the intensive care unit without dedicated personnel. *Canadian Journal of Critical Care Nursing*, *29*(3), 26–31. https://www.caccn.ca/files/CJCCN/29-3-2018%20CJCCN.pdf

Nicholson, M., Chan, N., Bhagirath, V., & Ginsberg, J. (2020). Prevention of venous thromboembolism in 2020 and beyond. *Journal of Clinical Medicine*, *9*(8), 2467. https://doi.org/10.3390/jcm9082467

Palma, J.-A., & Kaufmann, H. (2020). Management of orthostatic hypotension. *Continuum*, *26*(1), 154–177. https://doi.org/10.1212/CON.0000000000000816

Parola, V., Neves, H., Duque, F. M., et al. (2021). Rehabilitation programs for bedridden patients with prolonged immobility: A scoping review protocol. *International Journal of Environmental Research and Public Health*, *18*(22), Article 12033. https://doi.org/10.3390/ijerph182212033

Petersen, M. L., Vázquez, F. J., & Mayer, H. F. (2022). Mechanical thromboprophylaxis alone in body contouring surgery for post massive weight loss patients: Is this good enough? *Aesthetic Plastic Surgery*, *46*(1), 248–254. https://doi.org/10.1007/s00266-021-02449-3

Registered Nurses' Association of Ontario (RNAO). (2010). *Strategies to support self-management in chronic conditions: Collaboration with clients*. https://rnao.ca/sites/rnao-ca/files/Strategies_to_Support_Self-Management_in_Chronic_Conditions_-_Collaboration_with_Clients.pdf

Registered Nurses' Association of Ontario (RNAO). (2017). *Preventing falls and reducing injury from falls* (4th ed.). https://rnao.ca/sites/rnao-ca/files/bpg/FALL_PREVENTION_WEB_1207-17.pdf

San Román-Mata, S., Puertas-Molero, P., Ubago-Jiménez, J. L., & González-Valero, G. (2020). Benefits of physical activity and its associations with resilience, emotional intelligence, and psychological distress in university students from southern Spain. *International Journal of Environmental Research and Public Health*, *17*(12), Article 4474. https://doi.org/10.3390/ijerph17124474

Schallom, M., Tymkew, H., Vyers, K., et al. (2020). Implementation of an interdisciplinary AACN early mobility protocol. *Critical Care Nurse*, *40*(4), e7–e17. https://doi.org/10.4037/ccn2020632

Simpson, D. B., Jose, K., English, C., et al. (2021). Factors influencing sedentary time and physical activity early after stroke: A qualitative study. *Disability and Rehabilitation*, *44*(14), 3501–3509. https://doi.org/10.1080/09638288.2020.1867656

Smith, T. O., Sreekanta, A., Walkeden, S., et al. (2020). Interventions for reducing hospital-associated deconditioning: A systematic review and meta-analysis. *Archives of Gerontology and Geriatrics*, *90*, Article 104176. https://doi.org/10.1016/j.archger.2020.104176

Tamowicz, B., Mikstacki, A., Urbanek, T., et al. (2019). Mechanical methods of venous thromboembolism prevention: From guidelines to clinical practice. *Polish Archives of Internal Medicine*, *129*(5), 335–341. https://dx.doi.org/10.20452/pamw.4482

Tyerman, J., & Cobbett, S. (Eds.). (2023). *Lewis's medical–surgical nursing in Canada: Assessment and management of clinical problems* (5th ed.). Elsevier Canada.

Wahba, A., Shibao, C. A., Muldowney, J. A. S., et al. (2022). Management of orthostatic hypotension in the hospitalized patient: A narrative review. *The American Journal of Medicine*, *135*(1), 24–31. https://doi.org/10.1016/j.amjmed.2021.07.030

Wheatley, C., Wassenaar, T., Salvan, P., et al. (2020). Associations between fitness, physical activity and mental health in a community sample of young British adolescents: Baseline data from the fit to study trial. *BMJ Open Sport & Exercise Medicine*, *6*(1), e000819–e000819. https://doi.org/10.1136/bmjsem-2020-000819

Wittmer, V. L., Paro, F. M., Duarte, H., et al. (2021). Early mobilization and physical exercise in patients with COVID-19: A narrative literature review. *Complementary Therapies in Clinical Practice*, *43*, Article 101364. https://doi.org/10.1016/j.ctcp.2021.101364

Yang, R., Zuo, D., Zhang, C., et al. (2021). Safety assessment criteria for early active mobilization in mechanically ventilated ICU subjects. *Respiratory Care*, *66*(2), 307–315. https://doi.org/10.4187/respcare.07888

Yu, X., Wu, Y., & Ning, R. (2021). The deep vein thrombosis of lower limb after total hip arthroplasty: What should we care. *BMC Musculoskeletal Disorders*, *22*(1), 547–547. https://doi.org/10.1186/s12891-021-04417-z

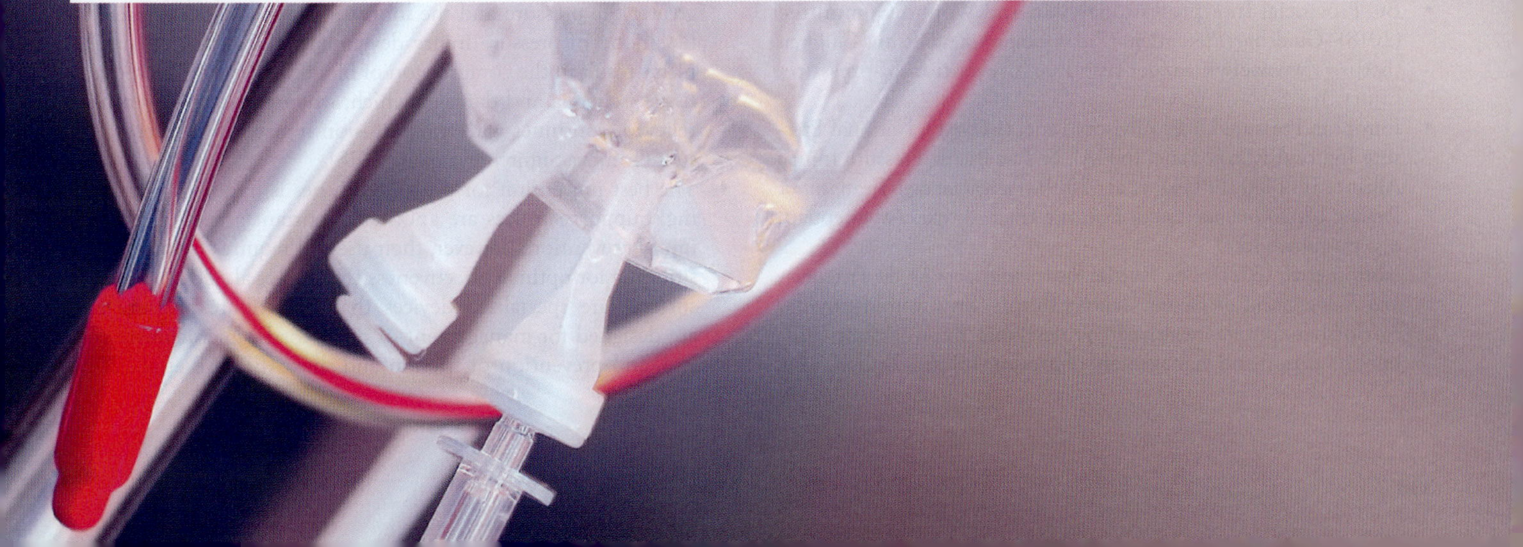

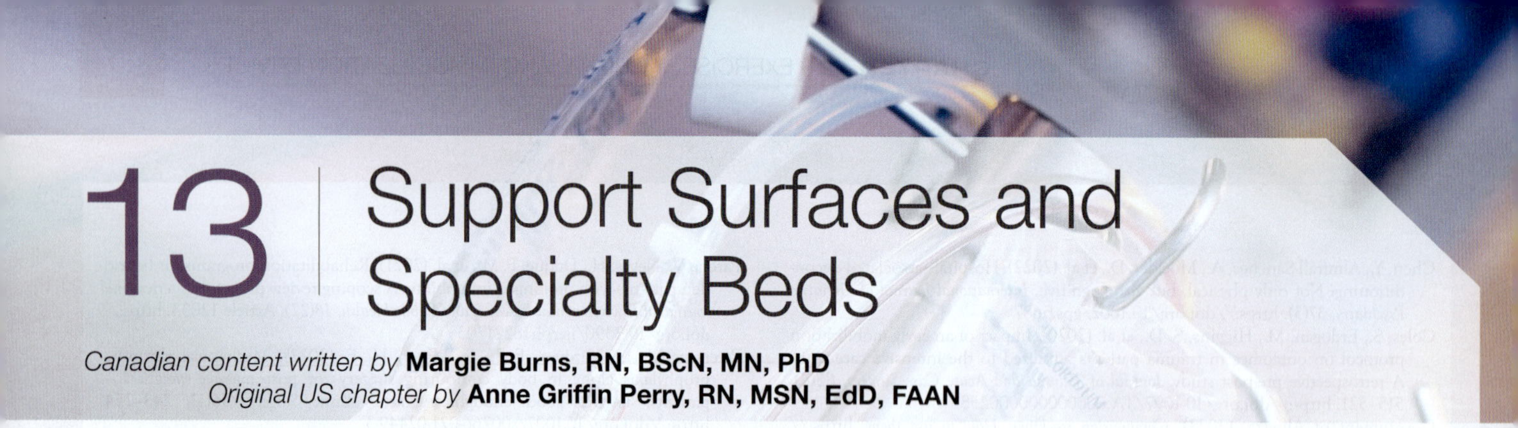

13 Support Surfaces and Specialty Beds

Canadian content written by **Margie Burns, RN, BScN, MN, PhD**
Original US chapter by **Anne Griffin Perry, RN, MSN, EdD, FAAN**

SKILLS AND PROCEDURES

OBJECTIVES

Mastery of content in this chapter will enable the nurse to:

- Identify the different types of support surfaces and specialty beds used for pressure redistribution.
- Explain why preventive nursing care is still essential when using support surfaces and specialty beds.
- Describe guidelines for placing patients on support surfaces and specialty beds.
- Compare the differences between mattress overlays and mattress replacements.
- Describe mechanisms by which skin breakdown can occur on a specialty bed, a support surface mattress, or a wheelchair seat cushion.
- Describe the steps for correct placement of a patient on a specialty bed or a support surface mattress.

MEDIA RESOURCES

- http://evolve.elsevier.com/Canada/Perry/clinicalskills/

PURPOSE

Despite increasing technological advances in health care, pressure injuries remain a major problem that affects patient comfort, length of stay in a health care facility, and health care costs. Interprofessional collaboration is key to reducing pressure injuries, with nurses at the forefront of their prevention and treatment in health care settings (Norton et al., 2021; Yilmazer & Bulut, 2019). Indeed, the clinical judgement of nurses and subsequent interventions directly impact patient outcomes, and the prevention of pressure injuries is an indicator of quality care (Lovegrove et al., 2022; Serraes et al., 2018; Yilmazer & Bulut, 2019).

STANDARDS OF CARE

- BC Provincial Interprofessional Skin and Wound Committee (2018)—*Guideline: Prevention of Pressure Injury in Adults and Children* (https://www.clwk.ca/get-resource/prevention-of-pressure-injury/)
- European Pressure Ulcer Advisory Panel (EPUAP), National Pressure Injury Advisory Panel (NPIA), & Pan Pacific Pressure Injury Alliance (PPPIA) (EPUAP et al., 2019)—*Prevention and Treatment of Pressure Ulcers/Injuries: Quick Reference Guide* (https://www.epuap.org/pu-guidelines/)
- Norton et al. (2021)—*Best Practice Recommendations for the Prevention and Management of Pressure Injuries* (http://www.woundscanada.ca/docman/public/health-care-professional/bpr-workshop/172-bpr-prevention-and-management-of-pressure-injuries-2/file)

PRINCIPLES FOR PRACTICE

- The factors that contribute to pressure injury formation are both extrinsic (e.g., pressure, moisture, friction, shear, and medical devices) and intrinsic (e.g., malnutrition, loss of sensation, impaired mobility, aging skin, impaired neurological status, infection, acute illness, incontinence, vascular disease, and pain) (Registered Nurses' Association of Ontario [RNAO], 2011, as cited in Norton et al., 2021). Pressure injuries are localized injuries to the skin, underlying tissue, or both, usually over a bony prominence, because of pressure or pressure in combination with friction or *shear* (which is the damage to tissue caused by opposing parallel forces) (Norton et al., 2021). In supine adults, the lateral heel and sacrum are the sites most at risk for pressure injury (Tomova-Simitchieva et al., 2018).
- The major cause of pressure injuries is unrelieved pressure. The greater the pressure and the longer it is applied, the greater the likelihood of pressure injury development. Pathological mechanisms result in the compression of blood vessels with subsequent tissue ischemia and damage, which, when pressure is eventually relieved, continues with a reperfusion injury to the affected tissues (Tomova-Simitchieva et al., 2018).
- The best prevention for pressure injuries is frequent repositioning. Support surfaces are another important aspect of pressure injury prevention; however, their use still requires frequent repositioning for optimal effectiveness (Norton et al., 2021). Support surfaces are specialized devices that redistribute pressure and are designed for management of tissue loads, microclimate control, and prevention of friction and shear (EPUAP et al., 2019;

Tomova-Simitchieva et al., 2018). Microclimate is the mean skin temperature, skin moisture, and air flow between the patient's skin and the support surface (Tomova-Simitchieva et al., 2018). Support surfaces are used in acute, rehabilitative, long-term, and home care settings. Support surfaces reduce pressure by redistributing it over a larger surface area. There are two ways in which a support surface reduces pressure. The first is preventive, in which pressure is not consistently reduced below 32 mm Hg (e.g., foam, air, or gel overlay). The second is therapeutic, in which pressure is consistently reduced below 32 mm Hg (e.g., powered overlay air mattress or low-air-loss mattress).

- Preventive surfaces are for patients at risk for skin breakdown and partial-thickness injury.
- Therapeutic surfaces are for patients at high risk for pressure injury development or for those with existing pressure injuries (BC Provincial Interprofessional Skin and Wound Committee, 2018; Norton et al., 2021). Support surfaces are one intervention for redistributing pressure; they are used in conjunction with other pressure injury risk-reduction strategies (see Chapter 39), including frequent repositioning.
- To prevent pressure injuries, essential linkages of care include the completion of a risk assessment (e.g., Braden Scale [see Chapter 39] for adults and Braden Q scale for pediatrics [BC Provincial Interprofessional Skin and Wound Committee, 2018]) followed by critical thinking and clinical decision making to implement appropriate interventions (Lovegrove et al., 2018).
- While it has not been determined which type of support surface is most effective in preventing pressure injuries (Choi et al., 2021; Serraes et al., 2018), it is agreed that—in addition to repositioning—individuals at high risk for pressure injury should be placed on a pressure-redistribution support surface (BC Provincial Interprofessional Skin and Wound Committee, 2018; EPUAP et al., 2019).
- Specialty support surfaces are an important part of pressure injury prevention (Tomova-Simitchieva et al., 2018). Pressure-redistribution surfaces can be made from a variety of materials including foam, air cells, or water bags; can be powered or nonpowered; and are classified as either reactive or active surfaces (Shi et al., 2021; Tomova-Simitchieva et al., 2018). Reactive surfaces passively redistribute the patient's body weight yet maintain a constant pressure on the skin (Shi et al., 2021). Active surfaces mechanically, and regularly, adjust pressures applied to the patient's skin to actively redistribute pressure (Shi et al., 2021).
- Several support surfaces also reduce friction, shear, and moisture. Support surfaces with a slick surface help decrease friction and shear. Surfaces with porous covers allow airflow, which reduces moisture, resulting in decreased risk for skin maceration. Table 13.1 provides a comparison of support surfaces.
- Frequent repositioning, which temporarily relieves pressure, is the backbone of prevention protocols. No bed or mattress eliminates

TABLE 13.1

Support Surfaces

Category and Mechanism of Action	Indications for Use	Advantages	Disadvantages
Support Surfaces and Overlays			
Foam Overlay (Available as an Overlay or in a Full Mattress)			
Reduces pressure; the cover (top) can reduce friction and shear. Base height of 7.5–10 cm (3–4 inches); see manufacturer guidelines regarding amount of body weight supported	Use for moderate- to high-risk patients	One-time charge No setup fee Cannot be punctured Available in various sizes (e.g., bed, chair, operating room table) Little maintenance Does not need electricity	Elevated body temperature Hot and may trap moisture Limited lifespan Plastic protective sheet needed for incontinent patients or patients with draining wounds Not indicated for those with existing stage 3 or 4 pressure injuries
Water Overlay (Available as an Overlay or in a Full Mattress)			
Reduces pressure and pressure points because surface provides flotation with pressure reduction by redistributing patient's weight evenly over entire support surface	Use for high-risk patients	Readily available Some control over motion sensations Easy to clean	Easily punctured Heavy Fluid motion may make procedures (e.g., dressing changes, CPR) difficult Maintenance needed to prevent microorganism growth Patient transfers out of bed are difficult Difficult to raise and lower head of bed
Gel Overlay			
Reduces pressure and pressure points because surface provides flotation by redistributing patient's weight evenly over entire support surface	Use for moderate- to high-risk patients Use for patients who are wheelchair dependent	Low maintenance Easy to clean Multiple-patient use Impermeable to needle punctures	Heavy Expensive Lacks airflow for moisture control Variable friction control
Nonpowered Air-Filled Overlay			
Reduces pressure by lowering mean interface pressure between patient's tissue and mattress	Use for moderate- to high-risk patients Use for patients who can reposition themselves	Easy to clean Multiple-patient use Low maintenance Potential repair of some air-filled products Durable	Damaged by punctures from needles and sharps Requires routine monitoring to determine adequate inflation pressure Patient transfers out of bed are difficult

Continued

TABLE 13.1

Support Surfaces—cont'd

Category and Mechanism of Action	Indications for Use	Advantages	Disadvantages
Low-Air-Loss Overlay (Available as an Overlay or in a Full Mattress)			
Maintains constant and slight air movement against patient's skin; also assists in managing the heat and humidity (microclimate) of the skin	Use for moderate- to high-risk patients	Easy to clean Maintains constant inflation Deflates to facilitate transfer and CPR Moisture control Fabric covering overlay is air permeable, bacteria impermeable, and waterproof Reduces shear and friction Setup provided by manufacturer	Damaged by needles and sharps Noisy Requires electricity, but some are available with short backup battery In home may need to purchase backup generator in case of loss of electrical power
Specialty Beds			
Air-Fluidized Bed			
Bedframe contains silicone-coated beads and provides pressure redistribution by the fluid-like medium that is created by forcing air through beads, resulting in immersion and envelopment of the patient	Use for high-risk patients Use for patients with stage 3 or 4 pressure injuries or burns	Less frequent turning or repositioning Improved patient comfort Quickly becomes firm for CPR or other treatments when device is turned "off" Reduces shear, friction, and edema to site May facilitate management of copious wound drainage or incontinence Setup provided by manufacturer	Continuous circulation of warm, dry air may increase patient risk for dehydration Possible increase in room temperature Patient may experience disorientation Patient transfer difficult Heavy Expensive May not be wide enough for use with obese patients or patients with contractures Patient cannot lie prone because of risk of suffocation
Low-Air-Loss Bed			
Bedframe with series of connected air-filled pillows; flow of air controls amount of pressure in each pillow and assists in managing the heat and humidity (microclimate) of the patient's skin	Use for patients who need pressure relief, those who cannot be repositioned frequently, or those who have skin breakdown on more than one surface Contraindicated in patients with unstable spinal column	Can raise and lower head and foot of bed Easy transfer in and out of bed Less frequent turning schedule Pillows can be transferred to stretcher with patient Setup provided by manufacturer	Portable motor is noisy Bed surface material is slippery; patients can easily slide down mattress or out of bed when being transferred
Kinetic Therapy			
Provides continuous passive motion to promote mobilization of pulmonary secretions and low air loss, which provides pressure relief	Use primarily for patients needing spinal stabilization Should not be used when patient is hemodynamically unstable	Reduces pulmonary complications associated with restricted mobility Reduces risk for urinary stasis and urinary tract infections Reduces venous stasis	Does not reduce shear or moisture. Cannot be used with cervical or skeletal traction Possible motion sickness initially Possible sensations of claustrophobia

CPR, Cardiopulmonary resuscitation.

Data from McNichol, L. L., Ratliff, C., & Yates, S. (2022). *Wound, Ostomy, and Continence Nurses Society core curriculum: Wound management* (2nd ed.). Wolters Kluwer. Wound, Ostomy, and Continence Nurses Society (WOCN). (2016). *Guideline for prevention and management of pressure ulcers (injuries)* (2nd ed.).

the need for competent, person-centred nursing care and a regular, consistent repositioning regime. Repositioning frequency is guided by the patient's individual care needs, such as their level of activity and mobility, skin and tissue tolerance, medical condition, and degree of pain or comfort (EPUAP et al., 2019). Use lift teams and lifting devices to transfer patients from a regular bed to a special support surface (see Chapter 11). Although useful, turning devices still injure soft tissues, requiring a nurse to be especially observant for signs of pressure formation.

PERSON-CENTRED CARE

- When making decisions about the best support surface for a patient, you must first complete a thorough patient assessment, including individual needs, health care provider preferences, and location of the patient.
- Person-centred nursing care is required to ensure that the features of the support surface match a patient's unique pressure-reduction needs and circumstances.
- Always describe to a patient and caregiver which interventions will be instituted and allow time for questions as needed.
- Some cultural groups may hesitate to ask questions or ask for help, especially when they have limited proficiency in the province/territory's official language. When this is the situation, provide for an interpreter early.
- Educate the patient and caregiver on all of the features of the support surface, provide a demonstration, and observe return demonstration of these features.

EVIDENCE-INFORMED PRACTICE

- Evidence suggests that pressure-redistribution surfaces are effective in preventing pressure injuries (Tomova-Simitchieva et al., 2018).
- Nurses play a central role in implementing interventions to prevent pressure injuries beginning with identification of at-risk patients and implementation of interventions, such as frequent repositioning of the patient and use of an appropriate pressure-redistribution support surface (de Labachelerie et al., 2022; Serraes et al., 2018; Yilmazer & Bulut, 2019).
- Pressure-redistribution surfaces serve as adjuncts to prevent pressure injuries but do not replace the need for regular patient repositioning (Norton et al., 2021).
- There is insufficient evidence to support one specific pressure-redistribution surface or design over another for the prevention of pressure injuries (Choi et al., 2021).
- Consider using a silicone dressing over bony prominences to prevent pressure injuries in at-risk patients (EPUAP et al., 2019; Norton et al., 2021).
- For patients at risk of pressure injuries, low-friction materials such as lifting or slider sheets should be used to reduce friction and shear (EPUAP et al., 2019; Norton et al., 2021).
- High-specification gel or air mattresses are likely more effective in preventing pressure injuries than standard hospital foam mattresses (Tomova-Simitchieva et al., 2018).
- Encourage patients to be up as soon as medically possible in a specialty chair or wheelchair equipped with a tailored support surface for pressure relief.
- Measure seat cushions so they are properly fitted to the person's body type and chair size to prevent friction and pressure.
- Pressure-redistribution surfaces should be used in the operating room for individuals who have, or are at risk of developing, a pressure injury (BC Provincial Interprofessional Skin and Wound Committee, 2018; EPUAP et al., 2019).

SAFETY GUIDELINES

- Using a valid and reliable tool (e.g., Braden Scale [Lovegrove et al., 2018]), perform a complete patient assessment on admission to determine the patient's risk for pressure injuries (BC Provincial Interprofessional Skin and Wound Committee, 2018; Norton et al., 2021) (see Chapter 39).
  - For adults with a Braden score of 18 or less, and children with a Braden Q score of 15 or less, repeat the patient assessment every shift (or daily if in a rehabilitation unit, at each visit if receiving clinic or home care, and weekly if in residential care) (BC Provincial Interprofessional Skin and Wound Committee, 2018; Norton et al., 2021).
  - For adults with a Braden score of 19 or greater, and children with a Braden Q score of 16 or greater, repeat patient assessment every shift if in the emergency department or critical care unit, daily in acute inpatient units, with bathing in rehabilitation units or residential care facilities, and during clinical or home care visits if the patient's condition has deteriorated (BC Provincial Interprofessional Skin and Wound Committee, 2018; Norton et al., 2021).
  - In any care setting, with any previous risk assessment score, repeat the patient assessment whenever the patient's condition has deteriorated or they have been transferred or admitted to hospital (BC Provincial Interprofessional Skin and Wound Committee, 2018; Norton et al., 2021).
- Select a support surface based on the patient's risk of developing pressure injuries, such as impaired mobility, need for microclimate control, reduction of shear, and size and weight of patient.
- Know the reason for and extent of a patient's reduced mobility. A patient who is not easy to reposition or who has pressure injuries involving multiple surfaces benefits from pressure-redistribution support devices.
- To prevent medical device–associated pressure injuries, devices should be carefully chosen and fitted appropriately (EPUAP et al., 2019). Following application of medical devices, skin around and under the device should be regularly monitored for pressure injury (EPUAP et al., 2019; Norton et al., 2021).
- Continue to provide basic prevention care measures against the hazards of immobility (e.g., regular skin assessment, turning, correct positioning, or range-of-motion exercises).
- Use safe patient-handling techniques and proper body mechanics when positioning or working with patients (see Chapter 11).
- Follow all safety measures to prevent injury to patients from accidental falls or improper positioning when placing them on specialty beds or mattresses.
- Educate caregivers about the advantages and disadvantages and methods of operation of all support devices to ensure their proper use in all settings.
- Use interprofessional collaboration (e.g., wound care nurse, physiotherapist) to maximize preventive strategies and patient safety.

Procedural Guideline 13.1 *Selection of a Pressure-Redistribution Support Surface*

Delegation and Collaboration

The selection of a pressure-redistribution support device cannot be delegated to an unregulated care provider (UCP).

Collaborate with the interprofessional health care team to determine the optimal support surface. Collaborate with discharge planning and social work services to ensure patient is provided with the correct support services required upon discharge.

Equipment

- Pressure injury risk assessment tool (see employer policy) (see Chapter 39)
- Body chart, tape measure, and/or camera to document existing areas of impaired skin integrity
- Documentation form or electronic health record (EHR)
- Skin care products

Procedural Steps

1. Identify patient using at least two person-specific identifiers (e.g., name and date of birth, or name and medical record number) according to employer policy.
2. Throughout the procedure, the 4 moments for hand hygiene are to be implemented; hand hygiene should occur before initial patient (or patient environment) contact, before an aseptic procedure, after body fluid exposure risk, and after patient (or patient environment) contact. Additional hand hygiene should be performed when hands are visibly soiled.
3. Assess patient's risk for skin breakdown using an appropriate risk assessment tool (e.g., for adult patient, Braden Scale score ≤18 indicates "at risk"; for pediatric patient, Braden Q score ≤16 indicates "at risk" and ≤9 indicates "very high risk" (see Chapter 39, Tables 39.1 and 39.2).

Continued

Procedural Guideline 13.1 *Selection of a Pressure-Redistribution Support Surface—cont'd*

4. Assess patient's existing pressure injuries, including location, stage, areas of blistering, abnormal reactive hyperemia, and abrasion.
5. Consider the following risk factors and comorbidities: advanced age, altered perception, diabetes, fever, poor dietary intake, hemodynamic instability, hypoperfusion, hypoxemia, obesity, edema, and abnormal laboratory blood results (EPUAP et al., 2019; RNAO, 2011, as cited in Norton et al., 2021).
6. Assess patient's level of comfort using an appropriate pain rating scale (e.g., scale of 0 [no pain] to 10 [worst pain ever]).
7. Determine the need for a pressure-reduction surface from assessment data. Place "at-risk" patients on a pressure-redistribution surface rather than on a standard mattress (BC Provincial Interprofessional Skin and Wound Committee, 2018; Tomova-Simitchieva et al., 2018).
8. Identify patient factors when selecting an appropriate surface:
   a. Braden Scale score ≤18 (adult) and Braden Q scale ≤16 (pediatric).
   b. Does the patient need pressure redistribution (e.g., the patient cannot be repositioned or there is an existing pressure injury)?
   c. Is the surface needed for short- or long-term care? A short-term surface is usually needed for an acute illness and hospitalization, while a long-term surface is usually needed for extended or home care.
   d. What is the potential comfort level achieved by the surface? If the patient is sensitive to noise, a device with a loud motor will increase discomfort.
   e. Are the patient and caregiver cooperative and adherent to repositioning? In addition, are they aware that a support surface should never replace repositioning? Is adequate help available for repositioning? In a home setting, a support surface is often necessary when the caregiver or patient is unable to reposition independently or help with repositioning.
   f. Does the support surface have the potential to interfere with the patient's independent functioning? The height of the overlay and its soft edge may affect the patient's ability to transfer, and a high-air-loss bed is not appropriate for a patient who needs to get in and out of bed frequently.
   g. What are the patient's financial resources?
   h. If the patient is using the device in the home, what are the environmental limitations? Will the home and existing electrical service accommodate the surface selected? Can the caregiver in the home manage the surface?
   i. How durable is the product? Is the surface easy to puncture? Can the surface be easily cleaned?
   j. Does the patient need pressure-relief surfaces in a chair or wheelchair? Has the family or caregiver been instructed on appropriate inflation of the device? An evidence- and consensus-based algorithm to guide selection of an appropriate support surface based on individual patient needs has been developed by the Wound, Ostomy, and Continence Nurses Society (WOCN, n.d.) and is available at https://algorithm.wocn.org/#home.
9. Choose the appropriate surface (see Table 13.1).
   a. Specialized support surfaces redistribute pressure over a larger area, thereby reducing pressure injury (Tomova-Simichieva et al., 2018). Specialized support surfaces are indicated for patients who are at risk of developing a pressure injury (BC Interprofessional Skin and Wound Committee, 2018; EPUAP et al., 2019; Tomova-Simichieva et al., 2018) or have an existing pressure injury/injuries (BC Interprofessional Skin and Wound Committee, 2018; EPUAP et al., 2019). Additionally, because patients are unconscious and unable to reposition themselves during surgery (Basli & Van Giersbergen, 2021), pressure-redistribution surfaces must be used on the operating table for patients who have a pressure injury or are at risk of developing a pressure injury (BC Interprofessional Skin and Wound Committee, 2018; EPUAP et al., 2019).
   b. While it has not been established which specialized support surface is most effective in preventing pressure injuries (Choi et al., 2021; Serraes et al., 2018), air support surfaces may be more effective than standard mattresses or pressure-reducing foam mattresses (Serraes et al., 2018). However, this benefit may be limited to the short term and not impact the longer-term risk of developing pressure injuries (Nixon et al., 2019). Therefore, it is suggested that high-specification foam mattresses be used for patients at risk of developing pressure injuries and that higher technology support surfaces be considered when these foam mattresses fail to prevent a pressure injury (Nixon et al., 2019).
   c. Assess the effectiveness of the specialized support surface twice daily (BC Interprofessional Skin and Wound Committee, 2018). For static overlay mattresses only, assess for bottoming out—that is, the support surface is ineffective and the patient is sitting or lying directly on the underlying structure or frame of the chair/bed—by placing a hand between the patient's bony prominence and the support surface and assessing for adequate cushion (BC Interprofessional Skin and Wound Committee, 2018).

Critical Decision Point *Hand checks are a satisfactory but subjective method of assessing for "bottoming out" of static air overlay mattresses* ***only****. The hand check method is inappropriate for replacement mattresses and integrated bed systems (bedframe and support surfaces)* (Call et al., 2015; WOCN, 2016).

   d. When excess moisture is a potential risk, a gel or air support surface is more effective at improving skin microclimate by reducing heat and moisture than standard mattresses are Tomova-Simitchieva et al., 2018).
10. Check employer policy regarding implementation of a support surface:
    a. Obtain a health care provider's prescription. This is usually required for a patient to obtain third-party reimbursement.
    b. Use interprofessional collaboration (e.g., case manager, social worker) to help patient and caregiver obtain the required surface product.
    c. Use interprofessional collaboration (e.g., home care nurse, discharge planner) if the device is anticipated for long-term use. Specific procedures and evaluations are needed for continuity of surface when patient is transitioning care to an extended care facility or discharged home.
11. Apply clean gloves. Inspect condition of skin regularly according to employer policy to evaluate changes in skin and effectiveness of therapy.
12. Inspect existing pressure injuries for evidence of healing.
13. Observe for side effects associated with the specific pressure-reducing surface (e.g., nausea, dizziness).
14. Remove and discard gloves.
15. Document pressure injury risk assessment and skin assessment in patient's EHR or chart.
16. Document the support surface selected and patient response to the surface in patient's EHR or chart.

✦ SKILL 13.1 Placing a Patient on a Support Surface

There are numerous support surfaces available to reduce pressure on tissues overlying bony prominences. These devices are recommended for preventive measures for patients with reduced mobility and risk of developing pressure injuries. Most of these devices are easy to apply and keep clean. The extent to which these devices actually reduce pressure and prevent skin breakdown is highly variable.

Support surfaces are categorized as mattress (or wheelchair) overlays (Fig. 13.1), mattress replacements, or specialty beds. An overlay rests on top of a hospital mattress and uses foam, air, water, gel, or combinations of these products to provide pressure relief. Mattress overlays and mattress replacements are either nonpowered (e.g., foam, gels) or powered (e.g., alternating-pressure surfaces).

A flotation pad is made of a silicone or polyvinyl-chloride gel enclosed in a vinyl-covered square. The pad serves as an artificial layer of fat to protect bony surfaces such as the sacrum and greater trochanters. These flotation pads are available for the bed or wheelchair (Fig. 13.2).

There are two types of foam mattresses. One is the foam mattress overlay, which has a flat smooth surface, foam rubber peaks (egg-crate, Fig. 13.3), or a cut surface. Place one on top of a bed mattress, and place a sheet over the foam mattress pad overlay to prevent soiling and provide ease of cleaning. The second type is the high-specification foam specialty mattress, which completely replaces the hospital mattress and is covered by a loose-fitting cover intended to protect the mattress and minimize friction and shear. Some of the newer foam mattresses are made of memory foam and have an increased lifespan. The memory foam moulds to the shape of the body and reduces pressure to the area in contact with the foam.

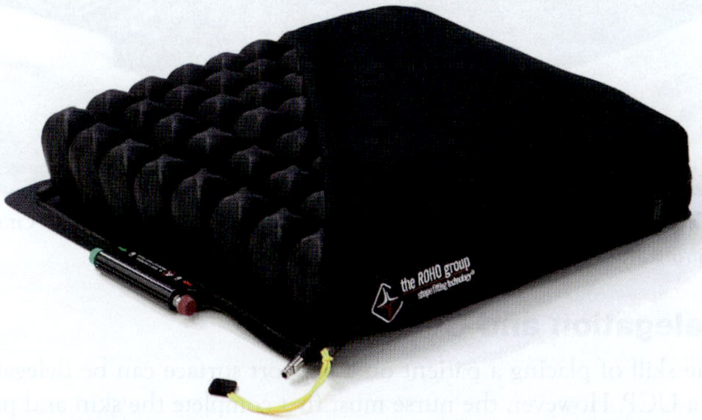

FIG 13.1 ROHO cushion for wheelchair. (*© ROHO Group. Reprinted with permission. All rights reserved.*)

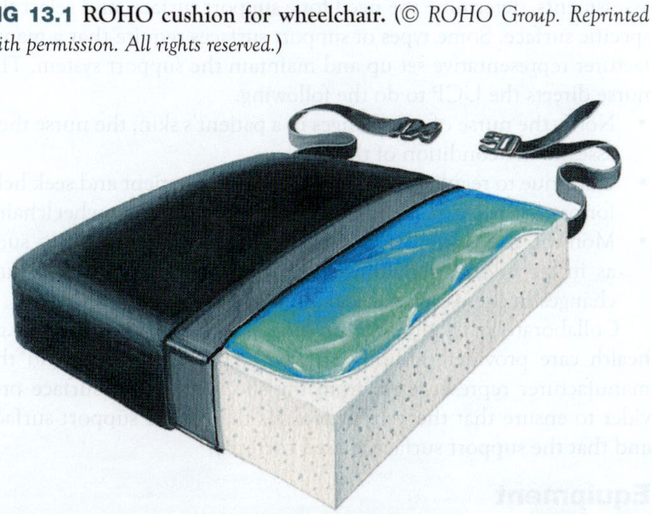

FIG 13.2 Gel cushion for wheelchair. (*© Skil-Care Corp. Reprinted with permission. All rights reserved.*)

One type of air mattress is fully integrated into the hospital bed or designed to be placed in a wheelchair (Fig. 13.4). The nurse can adjust this bed surface to a patient's comfort level by adding or removing air through buttons within the patient's reach; alternatively, pressures can be automatically adjusted to a patient's position and movement when in the automatic mode. Always use a bedsheet to cover an air mattress to prevent skin from touching the plastic surface. Always be cautious of patient safety: overinflation may cause the patient to fall or "flip" out of the bed; underinflation could result in patient entrapment (i.e., the patient is "trapped" between the mattress and the bed rail).

Air mattress overlays are either nonpowered or powered and consist of interconnected air cells or cushions inflated using a motorized blower (Fig. 13.5). More complex air mattresses contain several layers of tubes or support cells. These mattresses use a pressure-cycling device to intermittently inflate and deflate or to maintain a constant inflation and slight air movement in the mattress.

A nonpowered support surface is inflated with a simple air blower after placing the mattress on a bed. An integrated air mattress connects with a pressure-cycling device that intermittently inflates and deflates sections of the mattress, creating a cycling effect that minimizes pressure on bony prominences (Fig. 13.6).

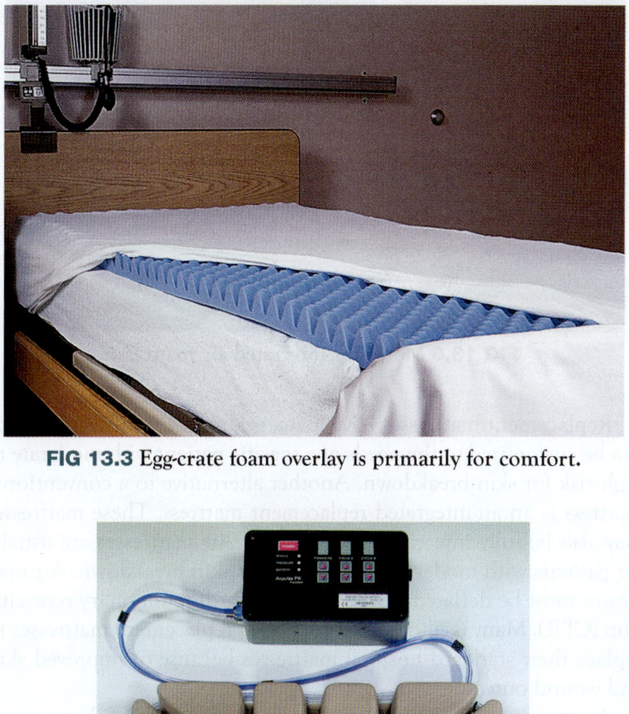

FIG 13.3 Egg-crate foam overlay is primarily for comfort.

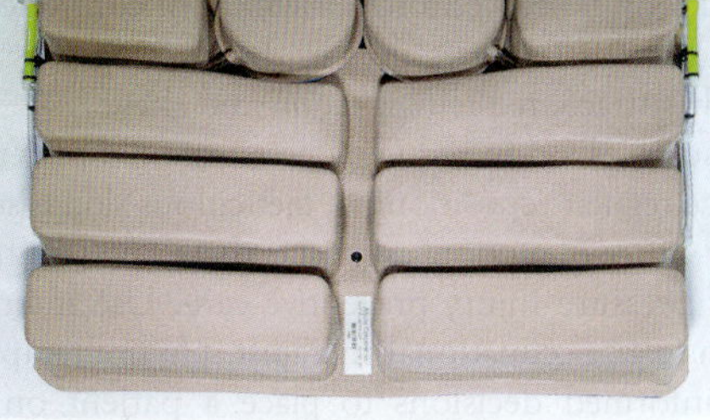

FIG 13.4 Air-filled cushion for wheelchair. (*© Aquila Corporation. Reprinted with permission. All rights reserved.*)

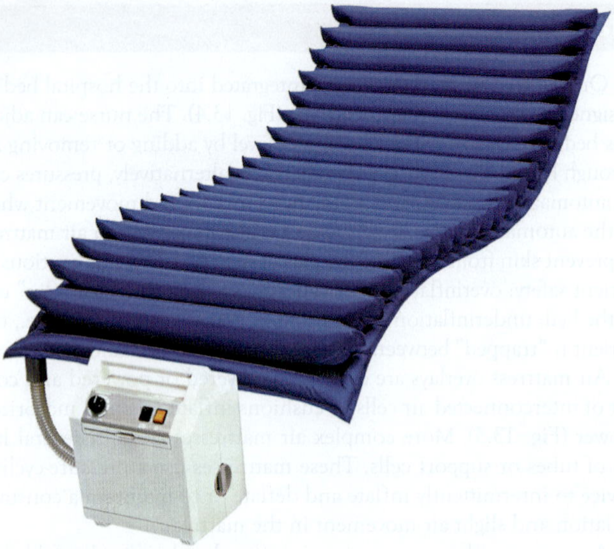

FIG 13.5 **Dynamic air mattress overlay.** (© 2002 *Hill-Rom Services. Reprinted with permission. All rights reserved.*)

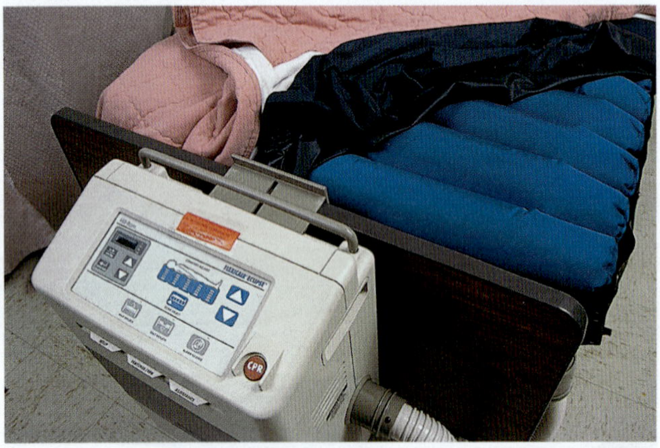

FIG 13.6 **Motor for integrated air mattress.**

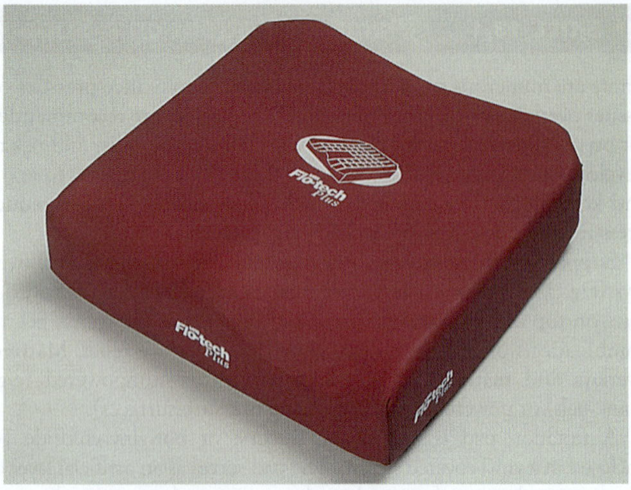

FIG 13.7 **Low-pressure seat cushion.** (*Reproduced with permission from Medical Support Systems Ltd.*)

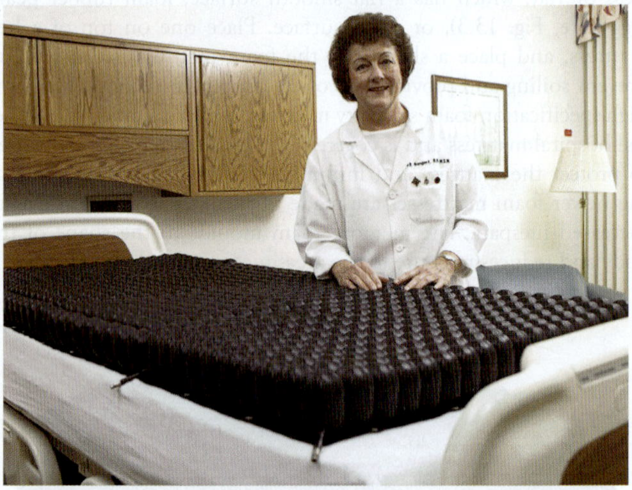

FIG 13.8 **ROHO dry flotation mattress for bed.** (© *The ROHO Group. Reprinted with permission. All rights reserved.*)

Replacement mattresses have foam, gel, air, or fluid sections that can be customized to the needs of a specific patient with moderate to high risk for skin breakdown. Another alternative to a conventional mattress is an air-integrated replacement mattress. These mattresses may also be fully integrated into the bed. Air mattresses are usually for patients with moderate to high risk for skin breakdown. Air mattresses must be deflated before initiating cardiopulmonary resuscitation (CPR). Many facilities have purchased replacement mattresses to replace their standard hospital mattresses because of improved skin and wound outcomes.

Another preventive intervention is a pressure-redistribution seat cushion (Fig. 13.7) overlaid on a wheelchair or chair (EPUAP et al., 2019), or a dry, nonpowered flotation mattress system (Fig. 13.8) that can be overlaid on a bed. Through a system of controlled dynamics, a cushion maintains low pressures by distributing pressure across a patient's body surface, reducing friction and shear.

Support surfaces aid in reducing pressure on a patient's skin but do not replace regular repositioning, meticulous skin assessment and skin care, or range-of-motion exercises; these interventions are the hallmarks of pressure injury preventive care. Use interprofessional collaboration (e.g., occupational therapist, physiotherapist) to arrive at evidence-informed decisions to place a patient on a pressure-redistribution surface and to determine which support surface is best for the patient (see Procedural Guideline 13.1).

Delegation and Collaboration

The skill of placing a patient on a support surface can be delegated to a UCP. However, the nurse must first complete the skin and pain assessments, determine the need for a support surface, and select the specific surface. Some types of support surfaces require that a manufacturer representative set up and maintain the support system. The nurse directs the UCP to do the following:

- Notify the nurse of any changes in a patient's skin; the nurse then assesses the condition of the skin
- Continue to regularly turn and reposition a patient and seek help for patient position changes as necessary in bed or a wheelchair
- Monitor the normal functioning of the support device, such as inflation and deflation cycles, and report to the nurse any changes in these cycles or leakage of air, water, or gel

Collaborate with the interprofessional health care team (e.g., health care provider, wound care nurse, physiotherapist) and the manufacturer representative from the specific support surface provider to ensure that the patient receives the correct support surface and that the support surface is used correctly.

Equipment

- Pressure injury risk-assessment tool (see employer policy) (see Chapter 39)

- Mattress and/or chair overlay support surface of choice: foam overlays, air mattress overlay, bed with integrated surface, air-integrated replacement mattress
- Sheet(s)
- Clean gloves (if soiled linen is being handled)
- Standard bedframe (with mattress) if overlay is to be used *(optional)*

STEP	RATIONALE
ASSESSMENT	
1. Identify patient using at least two person-specific identifiers (e.g., name and date of birth, or name and medical record number) according to employer policy.	Complies with Accreditation Canada's standards and assures that patients receive the care that is meant for them (Accreditation Canada, 2020).
2. Throughout the procedure, the 4 moments for hand hygiene are to be implemented; hand hygiene should occur before initial patient (or patient environment) contact, before an aseptic procedure, after body fluid exposure risk, and after patient (or patient environment) contact. Additional hand hygiene should be performed when hands are visibly soiled.	Proper hand hygiene helps prevent the spread of infectious agents to health care providers.
3. Determine patient's risk for pressure injury formation using a valid assessment tool (e.g., Braden Scale) and assess for risk factors for pressure injuries (e.g., nutritional deficits, shear stress, friction, alterations in mobility and sensory perception, moisture, and abnormal serum albumin and hemoglobin levels) (see Chapter 39).	The prevention of pressure injuries begins with an accurate assessment that guides subsequent interventions (Lovegrove et al., 2018).

Critical Decision Point *Patients with unstable conditions do not always tolerate the turning or positioning required for thorough assessment or the application of a support surface mattress. For critically ill patients who may become unstable during repositioning, turn the patient slowly to allow physiological adaptation to the movement* (BC Provincial Interprofessional Skin and Wound Committee, 2018; EPUAP et al., 2019).

STEP	RATIONALE
4. Perform skin assessment (see Chapters 8 and 39). Inspect condition of skin, especially over dependent sites and bony prominences.	Provides baseline to determine change in skin integrity or in existing pressure injury.
5. Assess patient's level of comfort using an appropriate pain rating scale.	Provides baseline to determine patient's response to therapy and comfort needs.

Critical Decision Point *For patients experiencing pain, administer prescribed analgesics a sufficient amount of time prior to performing care activities involving movement* (BC Provincial Interprofessional Skin and Wound Committee, 2018; Norton et al., 2021).

STEP	RATIONALE
6. Assess patient's understanding of purpose of support surface.	Misconceptions affect patient's cooperation in use of mattress.
7. Verify health care provider's prescription for type of support surface.	Health care provider's prescription is usually required to ensure third-party payment of support surface.

NURSING DIAGNOSES

- Insufficient peripheral tissue perfusion
- Reduced physical mobility
- Reduced skin integrity
- Pain (acute, chronic)
- Insufficient knowledge regarding use of support surface mattress
- Potential for impaired skin integrity
- Potential for infection

Related factors and risk factors are individualized on the basis of patient's condition or needs.

STEP	RATIONALE
PLANNING	
1. Expected outcomes following completion of procedure:	
• Patient's skin is without erythema or mottling.	Mottling represents hypoxia, which is an abnormal physiological response in tissues under pressure.
• Existing pressure injury shows signs of healing.	Skin remains free of new pressure injuries. Support surface does not interfere with circulation to dependent areas.
• Patient expresses improved level of comfort.	Equalized pressures have eliminated localized areas of discomfort.
• Patient is removed from therapeutic surface when risk for pressure injuries decreases.	Provides for efficient, cost-effective care while maintaining high-quality outcomes.
2. Explain purpose of mattress and method of application to patient and caregiver.	Reduces anxiety and promotes cooperation.
3. Close room door or bedside curtain.	Provides patient privacy and demonstrates person-centred care during application of mattress to bed or transfer to alternative bed.

STEP	RATIONALE
IMPLEMENTATION	
1. Apply clean gloves (if linens are soiled or wet). Get help to position patient or mattress as needed.	Reduces transmission of microorganisms. Assistance from other caregivers reduces risk for friction and shear in transfer to new surface.
2. Apply support surface to bed or prepare alternative bed (bed may be occupied or unoccupied). Keep sharp objects away from air mattress or air-surface bed.	
a. Replacing mattress:	
(1) Apply mattress to bedframe after removing standard hospital mattress.	Hospital mattress needs to be stored. In some instances, mattress replacements are standard procedure.
(2) Apply sheet over mattress. Keep linens between surfaces to a minimum.	Sheet reduces soiling.
b. Preparing an air mattress/overlay:	
(1) Apply deflated mattress flat over surface of bed mattress. (There may be directions on pad indicating which side to place up.)	Provides smooth, even surface.
(2) Bring any plastic strips or flaps around corners of bed mattress.	Secures air mattress in place.
(3) Attach connector on air mattress to inflation device. Inflate mattress to proper air pressure as determined by air pump or blower.	Mattresses vary as to requiring one-time or continuous inflation cycle. Check inflation daily. Manufacturer directions indicate desired air pressure designed to distribute patient's body weight evenly. Directions are included with each mattress.
(4) Place sheet over air mattress, being sure to eliminate all wrinkles.	Prevents soiling of mattress; reduces direct contact of skin with plastic surface. Wrinkles can cause pressure.

Critical Decision Point *Layers of linen or padding should be in correct order to support a healthy skin microclimate. Only use bedding or seat coverings that are recommended for use with specialty support surfaces* (BC Provincial Interprofessional Skin and Wound Committee, 2018; Norton et al., 2021).

STEP	RATIONALE
(5) Check air pumps to be sure that pressure cycle alternates.	Alternating airflow mattress produces intermittent cycling, inflating only parts of mattress at any one time. Intermittent cycle continually alternates pressure against skin and soft tissue.
(6) Help patient transfer in and out of bed.	Mattress surface is less firm and slippery. This makes it difficult for some patients to transfer from bed to chair or stretcher.
c. Using an air-surface bed:	
(1) Obtain and place linen on bed.	In some instances, an air-surface bed is available in patient rooms. If not, an ordering system exists to obtain one as needed (see employer policy).
(2) Place switch in "prevention" mode.	In "prevention" mode, surface pressures change automatically with patient position to equalize pressure and eliminate points of pressure.

Critical Decision Point *Most pressure-relieving beds are equipped with a CPR switch to instantly lower head section from an elevated position and deflate the mattress to provide a firm surface for chest compressions (Fig. 13.9). Note this information on the patient's record.*

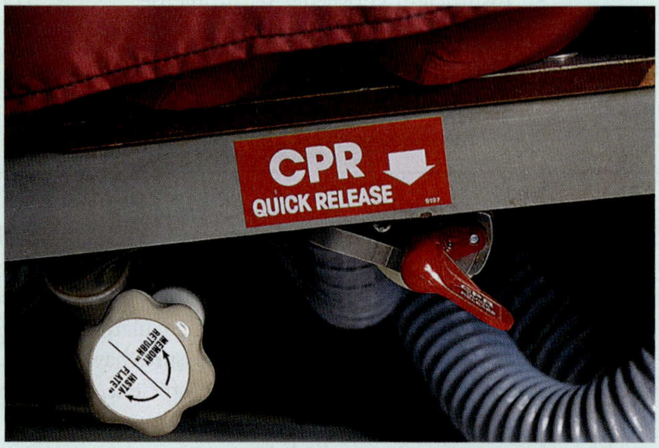

FIG 13.9 Cardiopulmonary resuscitation (CPR) switch deflates low-air-loss bed to provide hard surface.

STEP	RATIONALE
3. Position patient comfortably as desired over support surface. Reposition frequently, according to employer policy.	Location of existing pressure injury/injuries might limit choice of positioning (EPUAP et al., 2019). Reposition the patient to a position that relieves pain, and avoid positioning patient onto reddened areas or sites of existing pressure injuries (BC Provincial Interprofessional Skin and Wound Committee, 2018).
4. Remove and dispose of gloves in appropriate receptacle.	Reduces transmission of microorganisms.

EVALUATION

STEP	RATIONALE
1. Reassess patient's risk for pressure injury formation at routine intervals.	Documents change in status, which is critical for evaluating continued need for therapeutic surface.
2. Inspect and compare condition of patient's skin every 8 hours (or according to employer policy) to determine changes in skin integrity, pressure injury status, and effectiveness of support surface.	Determines whether pressure sores develop or whether condition of existing sores changes.
3. Ask patient to rate comfort on an appropriate pain rating scale.	If pressure-relief mattress is effective, patient generally experiences less discomfort.
4. Evaluate functioning of support surface periodically.	If signs of wear or reduced functioning are noted, remove the specialized support surface from use and request that maintenance assess its functioning and suitability for continued use (McNichol et al., 2020).
5. Use teach-back: "I want to be sure I explained why we put your mother on this specialty bed. Tell me why we placed her on this type of bed." Develop a revised teaching plan if caregiver is unable to teach back correctly.	Determines caregiver's level of understanding of instructional topic.

Unexpected Outcomes	Related Interventions
1. Patient develops localized areas of abnormal reactive hyperemia for longer than 30 minutes, mottling, swelling, and tenderness with evidence of skin breakdown.	• Modify skin care regimen. • Increase frequency of skin assessment. • Increase types of pressure-relief interventions. • Check for proper inflation of support surface. • Revise turning schedule. • Consult with skin care expert. • Notify health care provider.
2. Existing pressure areas fail to heal or increase in size or depth.	• Modify skin care regimen. • Revise turning schedule. • Consult with skin care expert. • Notify health care provider.
3. Patient expresses discomfort while on support surface.	• Evaluate need for analgesia or mild sedation. • Evaluate need to modify support surface. • Reposition patient more frequently. • Unless contraindicated, provide back massage. Avoid rubbing areas at risk for pressure injury such as bony prominences (BC Provincial Interprofessional Skin and Wound Committee, 2018; EPUAP et al., 2019).

Communication and Documentation

- Document type of support surface applied, extent to which patient tolerated procedure, and condition of patient's skin in progress notes in EHR or chart and/or skin assessment flow sheet.
- Document your evaluation of patient and caregiver learning.
- Report evidence of pressure injury formation to nurse in charge or health care provider.

DOCUMENTATION EXAMPLE

Patient premedicated with morphine 10 mg SUBCUT via butterfly to left upper arm 30 minutes prior to transfer to air mattress overlay using ceiling lift and sling by 2 staff members and writer. Patient tolerated procedure well and denies discomfort at present. Skin appears intact with slight redness noted to coccyx. Discussed importance of maintaining skin integrity and options for prevention of skin breakdown with patient and caregiver.

Special Considerations

- Fall prevention strategies include use of a bed alarm and keeping the bed in a low position with the brakes locked and bottom rails down (if the bed has a split rail) (RNAO, 2017). These interventions do not have strong evidence to support their use, and therefore clinical decision making should guide which interventions are used when providing individualized patient care (RNAO, 2017).
- Fall prevention mats are associated with an increased risk for falls among hospitalized adult patients (Bittencourt et al., 2017, as cited in Canada's Drug and Health Technology Agency [CADTH], 2018).

Teaching

- Explain risks of immobility and pressure injury formation to patient and caregivers (see Chapter 39).
- Instruct in proper use of body mechanics, positioning, and pressure-relief methods.
- Explain purpose and function of the pressure-redistribution surface. Include reminder that the surface augments care and does not replace the need for turning and pressure-relief manoeuvres.
- Explain precautions regarding sharp objects and fire hazards.

Pediatric

- Use a pressure injury risk assessment tool that has been developed specifically for use in children (see Chapter 16).
- Encourage family members to provide pressure-redistribution care such as holding and repositioning the child (BC Provincial Interprofessional Skin and Wound Committee, 2018).
- The child's ability to communicate their perception of pressure is influenced by their developmental level and ability to communicate (Norton et al., 2021).
- Parent or guardian can support children in being able to express their pain and treatment preferences related to pressure injuries and reinforce why a specialty bed is needed (Hockenberry et al., 2024).

Gerontological

- Implement preventive measures because an older person's skin is drier, thinner, and less pressure sensitive, increasing the risk for skin breakdown.
- Adding mattress overlays changes the bed height. Use care when transferring and teaching caregiver to transfer a patient from bed to chair.

Patients With Physical or Cognitive Challenges

- Support surfaces should be chosen with special attention to an enhanced impact on skin microclimate; shear reduction; pressure-redistribution capabilities; and a surface area wide enough to turn the patient without rolling into the bedrails (EPUAP et al., 2019).
- Patients living with obesity may require a bariatric bed, which is a specialized bed designed to support increased weight and provide additional comfort. For these patients, friction and shear injuries are more likely because of the drag of heels and sacrum during transfer (Norton et al., 2021).
- Practise person-centred care and engage in respectful dialogue when caring for patients living with physical or cognitive challenges, recognize any societal stigma and biases, and maintain a patient's dignity at all times.

Care in the Community: Home Management

- Most of the devices may be adapted for home use on a standard twin bed or hospital bed.
- Base selection on patient needs and environmental audit as part of person-centred care in the community. For example, a patient on total bed rest who smokes is not an ideal candidate for a foam mattress because of the potential for fire; a patient with pets that sleep in the bed is not suited for an air-filled mattress because of the risk for puncture.
- Address concerns in the home setting related to the need for a backup generator or other plan to maintain the support surface during power outages.

✦ SKILL 13.2 Placing a Patient on a Specialty Bed

Air-suspension beds are designed for patients who are immobile or confined to bed. The air-suspension bed supports a patient's weight on air-filled cushions. There are two types of systems: low air loss and high air loss. A low-air-loss system minimizes pressure and reduces shear. Low-air-loss support surfaces are effective in heat and moisture control and thus impact the skin microclimate (Tomova-Simitchieva et al., 2018). Specialized foam mattresses should be used for patients at risk for a pressure injury; however, if this support surface is not effective, higher technology air support surfaces are indicated (Nixon et al., 2019). If a patient has stage 3 or 4 pressure injuries, a low-air-loss bed or air-fluidized bed should be considered (EPUAP et al., 2019).

High-air-loss beds provide for selective drying and do not increase insensible fluid losses. For patients requiring high air loss under a body part (e.g., under the buttocks), high-air-loss cushions can be substituted. It is also possible to adapt the air-suspension beds to individual patient needs with specialty cushions for positioning, foot support, and lateral arm supports.

Another adaptation of the air-suspension bed is the kinetic low-air-loss bed (Fig. 13.10). This bed is used in critical care areas and can provide a pressure-relief surface while rotating approximately 30 to 35 degrees continuously. Do not use this surface with a patient who has an unstable spine or who is in traction.

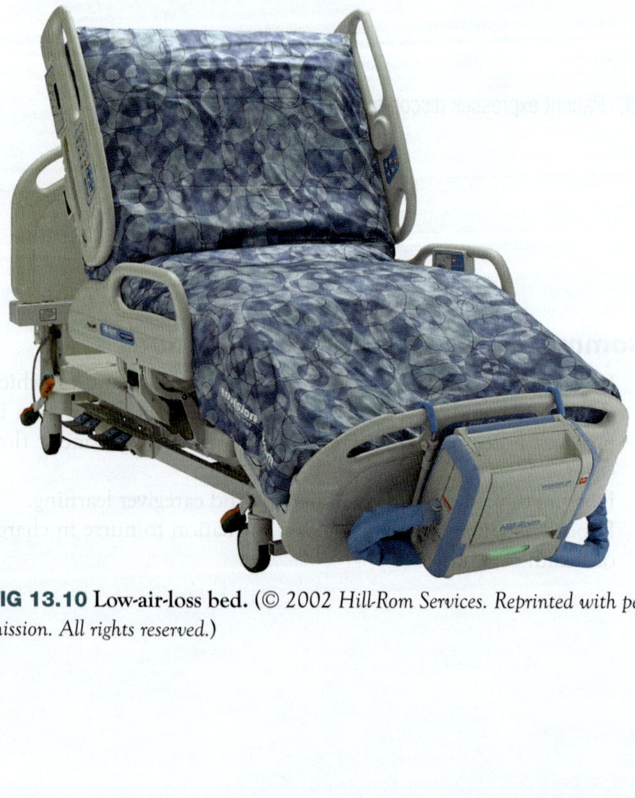

FIG 13.10 Low-air-loss bed. (*© 2002 Hill-Rom Services. Reprinted with permission. All rights reserved.*)

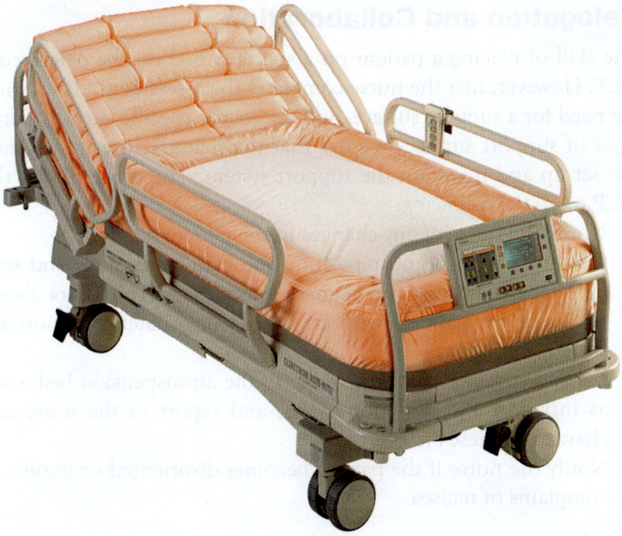

FIG 13.11 **Combination air-fluidized, low-air-loss bed.** (© *2008 Hill-Rom Services. Reprinted with permission. All rights reserved.*)

An air-fluidized or combination bed is a powered device designed to distribute a patient's weight evenly over its support surface (Fig. 13.11). In this type of system, pressure redistribution occurs by a fluid-like medium that is created by forcing air through beads (microspheres). The bed minimizes pressure and reduces shearing force and friction through the principle of fluidization. Fluidization occurs when air is forced upward through these microspheres toward the surface of the mattress and the patient's body, resulting in the patient essentially floating on the top of the mattress (Arnold et al., 2020). Air-fluidized beds are effective in promoting positive outcomes (e.g., faster and complete healing, reduced rate of pressure injury–related admissions) for patients with stage 2 or greater pressure injuries compared with other active support surfaces and standard hospital mattresses (Haesler, 2018).

Air-fluidized beds are useful in the care of patients who require minimal movement to prevent skin damage by shearing force and for patients who experience significant pain when being turned or positioned (e.g., burn patients, those who have undergone extensive skin grafts or have existing pressure injuries, and victims of multiple trauma). Patients tend to perspire and lose body fluids while on the bed because the surface of the filter sheet warms. As patients perspire, moisture is quickly absorbed into the circulating microspheres. Diaphoresis often goes undetected; thus, insensible fluid loss is not always evident until a patient develops fluid and electrolyte imbalances. Therefore, the nurse needs to monitor the patient's fluid balance status carefully.

Head-of-bed position changes are not possible with some conventional fluidized beds. Use foam wedges to elevate the head. Combinations of fluidized-low-air-loss beds that allow head-of-bed elevation are also available. These beds use air to lift the upper body while the lower body stays on a fluidized bed surface. The weight of the bed structure makes transport extremely difficult. A pediatric version of this bed is available.

A valuable resource in the care of a patient who is living with morbid obesity (a person who weighs more than 45.4 kg [100 lb] above ideal weight) is the bariatric bed (Fig. 13.12). The bariatric bed can allow upright or sitting positions, patient transport, and in-bed scale use. It is equipped with hand controls that allow self-positioning and facilitate independence for an obese patient. The full-function hand controls also allow the nurse to change the bed position and thus facilitate care while reducing risk for injury when staff move a patient. The in-bed scale provides the nurse with a means to obtain accurate weights and thus improves health care and patient dignity. The bed is slightly wider than a standard hospital bed, yet is within the guidelines for standard door width, which allows movement into and out of a room without difficulty. Because the bariatric bed is capable of supporting weights up to 453.6 kg (1 000 lb) (Hill-Rom Services, 2022), it provides a stable, balanced surface that limits hospital liability should the standard bedframe collapse or the electric motor burn out.

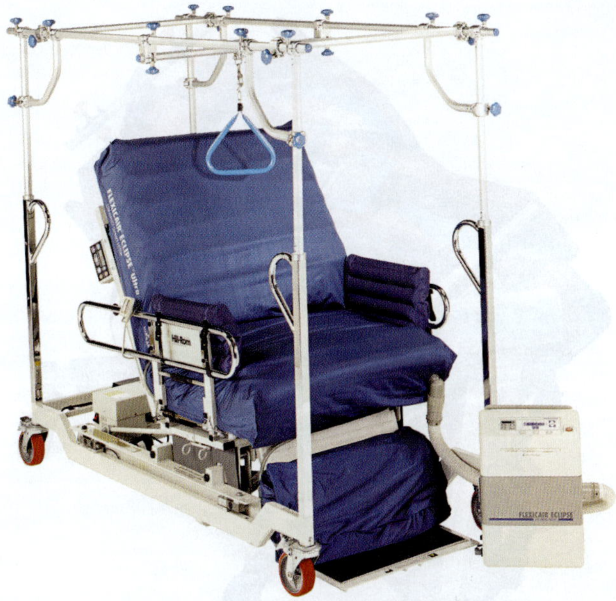

FIG 13.12 **Bariatric bed with low-air-loss mattress replacement.** (© *2008 Hill-Rom Services. Reprinted with permission. All rights reserved.*)

A limitation of this bed is the lack of pressure reduction or relief in the mattress. An at-risk patient who is obese needs to have some type of pressure-redistribution mattress placed on the bariatric bed. Choices for pressure redistribution include air or gel type mattresses and low-air-loss replacement systems. These beds also have CPR switches, which permit an immediate hard surface for chest compressions.

The Rotokinetic bed helps maintain skeletal alignment while providing constant rotation (Fig. 13.13). It is used in the care of patients with spinal cord injuries or multiple traumas. The support structure of the bed outlines the body parts and maintains proper alignment when secured properly. This bed improves skeletal alignment with constant side-to-side rotation up to 90 degrees. It rotates from side to side at a 60- to 90-degree angle every 7 minutes. The nurse may adjust turning angles to meet a patient's needs. Constant rotation reduces pressure injury development and stimulates body systems. It is recommended that the bed stay in the rotation mode for at least 20 hours a day. There is an emergency lever that can quickly interrupt rotation when needed. To initiate CPR, return the bed to the horizontal position and lock in place.

The constant motion often leads to sensory distress for patients, especially older persons. This sensory effect is associated with the constant kinetic stimulation, the limited visual field, and inner ear disequilibrium. Be aware of these complications and provide necessary emotional support.

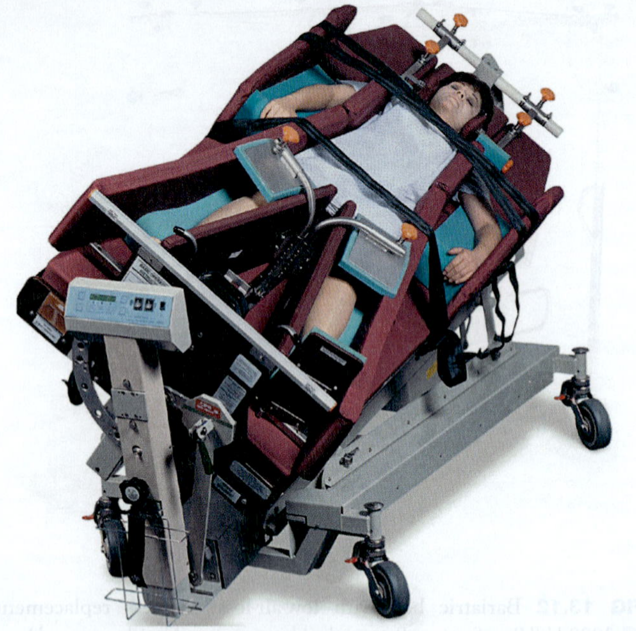

FIG 13.13 Rotokinetic bed. (*RotoRest. Courtesy Kinetic Concepts, San Antonio, TX.*)

Delegation and Collaboration

The skill of placing a patient on a specialty bed can be delegated a UCP. However, first the nurse completes the assessment, determines the need for a support surface, and selects the specific surface. Some types of support surfaces require that the manufacturer representative set up and maintain the support system. The nurse directs the UCP to do the following:

- Notify the nurse of any changes in the patient's skin
- Continue to turn and reposition the patient regularly and seek help for patient position changes as necessary. This is not always necessary for patients who are placed on a lateral-rotation air-suspension bed.
- Monitor the normal functioning of the air-suspension bed, such as inflation and deflation cycles, and report to the nurse any changes in these cycles
- Notify the nurse if the patient becomes disoriented or restless or complains of nausea

Equipment

- Disposable bed pads, if indicated
- Clean gloves (*optional*)
- Foam positioning wedges, if indicated
- Special sheet (if appropriate; supplied by manufacturer)
- Mechanical lift (if indicated)

STEP	RATIONALE
ASSESSMENT	
1. Identify patient using at least two person-specific identifiers (e.g., name and date of birth, or name and medical record number) according to employer policy.	Complies with Accreditation Canada's standards and assures that patients receive the care that is meant for them (Accreditation Canada, 2020).
2. Throughout the procedure, the 4 moments for hand hygiene are to be implemented; hand hygiene should occur before initial patient (or patient environment) contact, before an aseptic procedure, after body fluid exposure risk, and after patient (or patient environment) contact. Additional hand hygiene should be performed when hands are visibly soiled.	Proper hand hygiene helps prevent the spread of infectious agents to health care providers.
3. Determine patient's risk for pressure injury formation using a valid assessment tool (e.g., Braden Scale) and assess for risk factors for pressure injuries (e.g., nutritional deficits, shear stress, friction, alterations in mobility and sensory perception, moisture, and abnormal serum albumin and hemoglobin levels) (see Chapter 39).	The prevention of pressure injuries begins with an accurate assessment that guides subsequent interventions (Lovegrove et al., 2018).
4. Identify patients who will benefit from air-suspension therapy or air-fluidized therapy (e.g., immobilized or burn patients).	Determines that patient receives correct type of bed for their needs.
5. Assess risk for complications from air-fluidized beds:	
a. Dehydration	Patients may become dehydrated with use of this bed because of insensible fluid loss.
b. Aspiration	Inability to elevate head of bed is limited to placing foam wedges under patient's head and shoulders.
c. Difficulty with patient positioning	Repositioning is limited to use of foam wedges.
d. Level of orientation	Patients may be at risk of developing delirium from dehydration and floating sensation with air-fluidized bed.

Critical Decision Point *Patients with unstable conditions do not always tolerate turning or positioning required for thorough assessment or the application of a support surface mattress.*

STEP	RATIONALE
6. Inspect condition of skin, especially over dependent sites and bony prominences. Note appearance of existing pressure injury and determine stage of injury (see Chapter 39).	Provides baseline to determine patient's response to therapy and comfort needs.
7. Assess patient's level of comfort using an appropriate pain rating scale.	Provides baseline to determine patient's response to therapy and comfort needs.

Critical Decision Point *For patients experiencing pain, administer prescribed analgesics a sufficient amount of time prior to performing care activities involving movement* (BC Provincial Interprofessional Skin and Wound Committee, 2018; Norton et al., 2021).

STEP	RATIONALE
8. Verify health care provider's prescription for type of support surface.	Health care provider's prescription is usually required to ensure third-party payment of support surface.
9. Review patient's serum electrolyte levels if available.	Movement of air through mattress increases patient's risk for dehydration (McNichol et al., 2021).
10. Determine whether patient needs to be weighed frequently.	Scales are available in some air-suspension beds and as under-bed units for patients who need to be weighed frequently or those who cannot be moved for weighing.

NURSING DIAGNOSES

- Insufficient peripheral tissue perfusion
- Insufficient knowledge regarding use of support surface mattress
- Insufficient fluid volume
- Reduced physical mobility
- Reduced skin integrity
- Pain (acute, chronic)
- Potential for impaired skin integrity

Related factors and risk factors are individualized on the basis of patient's condition or needs.

PLANNING

STEP	RATIONALE
1. Expected outcomes following completion of procedure:	
• Patient's skin is without erythema or mottling.	Mottling represents hypoxia, which is an abnormal physiological response in tissues under pressure.
• Existing pressure injury shows signs of healing.	Skin remains free of new pressure injuries. Support surface does not interfere with circulation to dependent areas.
• Patient expresses improved level of comfort.	Equalized pressures have eliminated localized areas of discomfort.
• Patient is removed from therapeutic surface when risk for pressure injuries decreases.	Provides for efficient, cost-effective care while maintaining high-quality outcomes.
2. Explain purpose of mattress and method of application to patient and caregiver.	Reduces anxiety and promotes cooperation.
3. Review instructions provided by manufacturer.	Promotes safe and correct use of bed.
4. Obtain additional personnel needed to transfer patient to bed.	Ensures safety by having sufficient personnel for transfer.
5. For patients with moderate to severe pain, premedicate approximately 30 minutes before transfer to bed.	Promotes patient's comfort during transfer to bed (BC Provincial Interprofessional Skin and Wound Committee, 2018; Norton et al., 2021).
6. Close room door or bedside curtain.	Provides patient privacy and demonstrates person-centred care during application of mattress to bed or transfer to alternative bed.

IMPLEMENTATION

STEP	RATIONALE
1. Apply clean gloves (if linens are soiled or wet). Get help to position patient or mattress as needed.	Reduces transmission of microorganisms. Assistance from other caregivers reduces risk for friction and shear in transfer to new surface.
2. Transfer patient to bed using appropriate transfer techniques (see Chapter 11). Bed surface is sometimes slippery; thus, do not attempt transfers without help.	Appropriate safe patient-handling techniques maintain alignment and reduce risk for injury during procedure. Manufacturer representative adjusts bed to patient's height and weight.
3. Once patient has been transferred, turn bed on by depressing switch; regulate temperature.	Releasing Instaflate or turning on bed allows pressure cushions to adjust automatically to preset levels to minimize pressure, friction, and shear.
4. Position patient and perform range-of-motion exercises as appropriate.	Promotes comfort and reduces contracture formation.

STEP	RATIONALE
5. To turn patient, position bedpans, or perform other therapies, turn on Instaflate or other setting. Once you have completed the procedure, release Instaflate. With air-fluidized bed, use foam wedges to position patient as needed.	Instaflate firms bed surface to facilitate turning and handling of patient. Patient does not receive pressure relief while bed is in this mode.
6. Use special features of bed as needed.	
a. Scales	Facilitates ability to obtain routine weights.
b. Portable transport units to maintain inflation when primary power is interrupted	Provides for continuous pressure reduction.
c. Specialty cushions for positioning, providing pressure relief, reducing moisture, preventing patient from sliding down in bed, or relieving weight from orthopedic devices	Reduces pressure, friction, and shearing forces.
d. Lateral rotation (Fig. 13.14), which allows approximately 30 degrees of turning	Underinflation or improper functioning of certain overlays may result in tissue damage. Likewise, overinflation can result in too firm a surface and create pressure damage.

Critical Decision Point *A patient should never be placed in prone position on an air-fluidized bed because of the chance of suffocation.*

STEP	RATIONALE
7. Assess effectiveness of pressure-relief mattress or seat cushion by placing hand beneath support surface under a bony prominence.	"Bottoming out" occurs when the support surface is inadequate, or fails, and the patient is in direct contact with the frame of the bed or chair (BC Provincial Interprofessional Skin and Wound Committee, 2018).
8. Remove and dispose of gloves in appropriate receptacle.	Reduces transmission of microorganisms.

EVALUATION

1. Reassess patient's risk for pressure injury formation at routine intervals.	Documents change in status, which is critical for evaluating continued need for therapeutic surface.
2. Inspect and compare condition of patient's skin every 8 hours (or according to employer policy) to determine changes in skin integrity, pressure injury status, and effectiveness of support surface.	Determines whether pressure sores develop or whether condition of existing sores changes.
3. Ask patient to rate comfort or pain using an appropriate pain rating scale.	If pressure-relief mattress is effective, patient generally experiences less discomfort.
4. Evaluate functioning of support surface periodically, according to employer policy.	Regular inspection of mechanical components of mattress ensures proper functioning.
5. Use **teach-back:** "I want to be sure I explained why your bed is in this position. Tell me why we placed your bed sideways and how you might feel." Develop a revised teaching plan if patient or caregiver is unable to teach back correctly.	Determines patient's and caregiver's level of understanding of instructional topic.

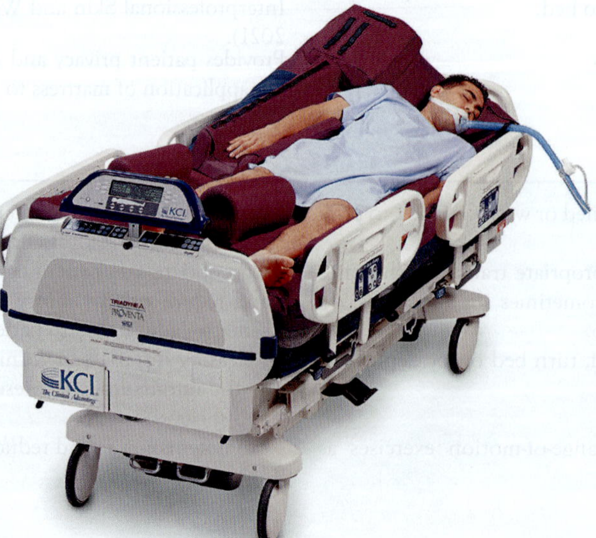

FIG 13.14 Lateral rotation bed. (*Tria Dyne™ Therapy System. Courtesy KCI Licensing, Inc., 2013.*)

Unexpected Outcomes	Related Interventions
1. Existing areas of skin breakdown or pressure areas fail to heal or increase in size and depth.	• Modify skin care regimen. • Increase frequency of skin assessment. • Change types of pressure-relief interventions. • Check for proper inflation of support surface. • Revise turning schedule. • Consult with skin care expert. • Notify health care provider.
2. Patient becomes nauseated.	• Provide short-term antiemetic such as prochlorperazine. If using lateral rotation, obtain antiemetic prescription around the clock. • If using lateral rotation, decrease cycle frequency. • Notify health care provider.

Communication and Documentation

- Document transfer of patient to bed, amount of help needed for transfer, tolerance of procedure, and condition of skin in progress notes in EHR or chart and/or skin assessment flow sheet.
- Document your evaluation of patient and caregiver learning.
- Report changes in condition of skin, level of orientation, and electrolyte levels to health care provider.

DOCUMENTATION EXAMPLE

Patient noted to be incontinent of a large amount of urine. Lasix 80 mg PO administered at 0800 hours. Skin care completed and sheets changed with assist of 3 including writer. Pressure areas assessed and a stage 3 pressure injury on coccyx was noted. During repositioning, patient noted to be disorientated to place and time and able to only minimally assist with turning. Morning blood results checked and K+ noted to be 3.4 mmol/L. Charge nurse and health care provider notified re: stage 3 pressure injury, patient disorientation, and hypokalemia.

Special Considerations

- Fall prevention strategies include use of a bed alarm and keeping the bed in a low position with the brakes locked and bottom rails down (if the bed has a split rail) (RNAO, 2017). These interventions do not have strong evidence to support their use, and therefore clinical decision making should guide which interventions are used when providing individualized patient care (RNAO, 2017).
- Fall prevention mats are associated with an increased risk for falls among hospitalized adult patients (Bittencourt et al., 2017, as cited in CADTH, 2018).

Teaching

- Explain function and purpose of specialty support surface or bed.
- Explain the need to continue to change position at intervals to diminish the effects of immobility.
- Explain the need for adequate fluid intake because bed surfaces sometimes contribute to dehydration.

Pediatric

- The air-suspension bed is used commonly with older children and for children with significant burns. Make sure that instructions are age appropriate and include any restrictions, such as raising the head of the bed.
- Parent or guardian needs to know that the child will have some dizziness or nausea when first placed on the air-fluidized or other specialty bed. This effect is due to the flotation sensation and will disappear as the child becomes adjusted to the bed.

Gerontological

- Some hospitalized older persons experience misperceptions of their environment that are intensified by the constant flotation of these types of beds. Proprioception abnormalities affecting older persons are the result of nervous system and muscle changes (McNichol et al., 2021).

Patients With Physical or Cognitive Challenges

- Patients with physical or cognitive challenges, or those who are confused, may have difficulty adjusting to specialty beds, especially beds that give the patient a sensation of movement and/or increase noise in the environment (Sullivan et al., 2018). Observe these patients for increased confusion, which may result in the need to consider other specialty bed options.

Care in the Community: Home Management

- The air-fluidized bed is extremely heavy (up to 954 kg [2 100 lb]); therefore, the company leasing the bed needs to inspect the home for accessibility and structural support to ensure safe use.
- Use interprofessional collaboration (e.g., social worker, home care case manager) to determine third-party reimbursement. Thorough documentation of skin condition is essential in obtaining reimbursement.
- A version of the air-fluidized bed is available for rent or purchase for home use; the bed rental company is responsible for proper cleaning.
- Instruct caregiver in importance of maintaining patient hydration and skin care.
- Instruct caregiver regarding steps to take in the event of a power failure. This may include purchasing a backup generator for the home.

✦ REVIEW QUESTIONS

The nurse is assigned to admit a 48-year-old patient who was involved in a motor vehicle accident that resulted in quadriplegia, causing loss of sensation and movement below the neck. The patient is unable to change positions or transfer without help. The patient has a language barrier, and communicating instructions about the patient's care is difficult. The nurse has arranged for the services of a qualified interpreter to help breach the language barrier. Following interprofessional collaboration (e.g., physiotherapy, social services), the health care provider prescribes an air-suspension bed with lateral rotation because the patient has some blistering over bony prominences and the patient's impaired mobility and sensation increase the risk of developing pressure injuries. The patient begins experiencing a small amount of nausea and restlessness when they are initially placed on the air-suspension bed.

Review Questions 1 to 4 relate to the case study presented here.

1. When this patient indicates sudden dizziness, the nurse checks their vital signs and notes that they are hypotensive and tachycardic. What should the nurse's initial actions be?
2. While conducting a skin assessment, the nurse notices skin breakdown over the coccyx and left hip, even though this patient has received meticulous skin care and routine repositioning. What is the appropriate nursing action to take first?
3. The patient continues to experience nausea and dizziness on the air-suspension bed. Using SBAR (situation–background–assessment–recommendation), show how you would communicate with the health care team about this patient.
4. The patient is discharged to home with home health care. The patient has been prescribed an air-celled cushion that will move with the patient (i.e., a ROHO cushion) and is taught to self-adjust the inflation during the day when they are in a wheelchair. The caregiver notes that the patient has small areas of continuing redness on their ischia. The caregiver should do which of the following? (*Select all that apply.*)
   1. Report the situation to the nurse or case manager immediately.
   2. Instruct the patient not to change the chair cushion inflation.
   3. Check for proper inflation of the cushion.
   4. Re-inflate the cushion appropriately while the patient is sitting on it and wait to re-evaluate the skin condition later.
   5. Increase frequency of checking the patient's skin.
5. Place the following steps for applying an air mattress overlay in the correct order.
   1. Check air pumps to be sure that pressure cycle alternates.
   2. Bring any plastic strips or flaps around corners of bed mattress.
   3. Apply deflated mattress flat over surface of bed mattress.
   4. Place sheet over air mattress, being sure to eliminate all wrinkles.
   5. Attach connector on air mattress to inflation device and inflate to proper pressure.
6. The nurse is caring for a patient on an air-fluidized bed. Which complications should the nurses assess for in this patient? (*Select all that apply.*)
   1. Back pain from lack of firm support
   2. Dehydration from the amount of warm circulating air
   3. Problems moving the patient out of bed because of body submersion
   4. Lack of healing of the pressure injury because of high skin and bed pressures
   5. Difficulty moving the bed to another location because of its weight

Visit the Evolve site for a complete list of answers to the Review Questions.

✦ NEXT GENERATION NCLEX® (NGN)

For practice with answering exam questions related to unfolding NGN case studies, please consult the Next Generation NCLEX® (NGN)-Style Case Studies for Skills and Techniques on the Evolve website: http://evolve.elsevier.com/Canada/Perry/clinicalskills/

REFERENCES

Accreditation Canada. (2020). *Required organizational practices handbook*. https://physicians.nshealth.ca/resources/required-organizational-practices-2020-handbook

Arnold, M., Yanez, C., & Yanez, B. (2020). Wound healing in the long-term acute care setting using an air-fluidized therapy/continuous low-pressure therapeutic bed. *The Journal of Wound, Ostomy and Continence Nursing, 47*(3), 284–290. https://doi.org/10.1097/WON.0000000000000646

Basli, A. A., & Van Giersbergen, M. Y. (2021). Comparison of interface pressures on three operating table support surfaces during surgery. *Journal of Tissue Viability, 30*(3), 410–417. https://doi.org/10.1016/j.jtv.2021.04.006

BC Provincial Interprofessional Skin and Wound Committee. (2018). *Guideline: Prevention of pressure injury in adults and children*. BC Patient Safety and Quality Council. https://www.clwk.ca/buddydrive/file/guideline-prevention-of-pressure-injuries-2017-november-final/

Call, E., Deppisch, M., Jordan, R., et al. (2015). *Hand check method: Is it an effective method to monitor support surfaces for bottoming out? A National Pressure Ulcer Advisory position statement*. National Pressure Ulcer Advisory Panel. https://cdn.ymaws.com/npuap.site-ym.com/resource/resmgr/position_statements/hand-check-position-statemen.pdf [Seminal Reference]

Canada's Drug and Health Technology Agency. (2018, March 19). *Falls prevention mats for patients in health care settings: Clinical effectiveness and guidelines*. https://www.cadth.ca/sites/default/files/pdf/htis/2018/RB1202%20Falls%20Prevention%20Mats%20Final.pdf

Choi, J. S., Hyun, S. Y., & Chang, S. J. (2021). Comparing pressure injury incidence based on repositioning intervals and support surfaces in acute care settings: A quasi-experimental pragmatic study. *Advances in Skin & Wound Care, 34*(8), 1–6. https://doi.org/10.1097/01.ASW.0000755912.27170.9a

de Labachelerie, C., Viollet, E., Alonso, S., et al. (2022). Comparison of interface pressures in two dynamic pressure ulcer prevention supports (NIMBUS 3 and SUMMIT): A randomized controlled trial. *Journal of Tissue Viability, 31*(1), 11–15. https://doi.org/10.1016/j.jtv.2021.09.002

European Pressure Ulcer Advisory Panel (EPUAP), National Pressure Injury Advisory Panel (NPIAP), & Pan Pacific Pressure Injury Alliance (PPPIA). (2019). *Prevention and treatment of pressure ulcers/injuries: Quick reference guide*. https://www.epuap.org/pu-guidelines/

Haesler, E. (2018). Evidence summary: Pressure injuries: Active support surfaces for preventing and treating pressure injuries. *Wound Practice & Research, 26*(1), 50–51. https://journals.cambridgemedia.com.au/application/files/3015/8518/8556/summary.pdf

Hill-Rom Services. (2022). *Compella™ bariatric bed*. https://www.hillrom.ca/en/products/compella-bariatric-bed/

Hockenberry, M. J., Duffy, E. A., & Gibbs, K. (2024). *Wong's nursing care of infants and children* (12th ed.). Elsevier.

Lovegrove, J., Fulbrook, P., Miles, S., et al. (2022). Effectiveness of interventions to prevent pressure injury in adults admitted to intensive care settings: A systematic review and meta-analysis of randomized controlled trials. *Australia Critical Care, 35*, 186–203. https://doi.org/10.1016/j.aucc.2021.04.007

Lovegrove, J., Miles, S., & Fulbrook, P. (2018). The relationship between pressure ulcer risk assessment and preventative interventions: A systematic review. *Journal of Wound Care, 27*(12), 862–875. https://doi.org/10.12968/jowc.2018.27.12.862

McNichol, L. L., Mackey, D., Watts, C., et al. (2020). Choosing a support surface for pressure injury prevention and treatment. *Nursing, 50*(2), 41–44. https://doi.org/10.1097/01.NURSE.0000651620.87023.d5

McNichol, L. L., Ratliff, C., & Yates, S. (2021). *Wound, Ostomy, and Continence Nurses Society core curriculum: Wound management* (2nd ed.). Wolters Kluwer.

Nixon, J. Smith, I. L., Brown, S., et al. (2019). Pressure relieving support surfaces for pressure ulcer prevention (PRESSURE 2): Clinical and health economic results of a randomized controlled trial. *EClinical Medicine, 14*, 42–52. https://doi.org/10.1016/j.eclinm.2019.07.018

Norton, L., Smith, I. L., Brown, S., et al. (2021). Best practice recommendations for the prevention and management of pressure injuries. *Wounds Canada*. https://www.woundscanada.ca/docman/public/health-care-professional/bpr-workshop/172-bpr-prevention-and-management-of-pressure-injuries-2/file

Registered Nurses' Association of Ontario (RNAO). (2017). *Preventing falls and reducing injury from falls* (4th ed.). https://rnao.ca/bpg/guidelines/prevention-falls-and-fall-injuries

Serraes, B., van Leen, M., Schols, J., et al. (2018). Prevention of pressure ulcers with a static air support surface: A systematic review. *International Wound Journal, 15*(3), 333–343. https://doi.org/10.1111/iwj.12870

Shi, C., Dumville, J. C., Cullum, N., et al. (2021). Foam surfaces for preventing pressure ulcers. *Cochrane Database of Systematic Reviews, 2021*(5), CD013621. https://doi.org/10.1002/14651858.CD013621.pub2

Sullivan, W. F., Diepstra, H., Heng, J., et al. (2018). Primary care of adults with intellectual and developmental disabilities: 2018 Canadian consensus guidelines. *Canadian Family Physician, 64*(4), 254–279. https://www.cfp.ca/content/64/4/254

Tomova-Simitchieva, T., Lichterfeld-Kottner, A., Blume-Peytavi, U., et al. (2018). Comparing the effects of 3 different pressure ulcer prevention support surfaces on the structure and function of heel and sacral skin: An exploratory cross-over trial. *International Wound Journal, 15*, 429–437. https://doi.org/10.1111/iwj.12883

Wound, Ostomy, and Continence Nurses Society (WOCN). (n.d.). *An evidence- and consensus-based support surface algorithm*. https://algorithm.wocn.org/#home

Wound, Ostomy, and Continence Nurses Society (WOCN). (2016). *Guideline for prevention and management of pressure ulcers (injuries)* (2nd ed.). [Seminal Reference]

Yilmazer, T., & Bulut, H. (2019). Evaluating the effects of a pressure injury prevention algorithm. *Advances in Skin & Wound Care*, 32(6), 278–284. https://doi.org/10.1097/01.ASW.0000553597.18658.6b

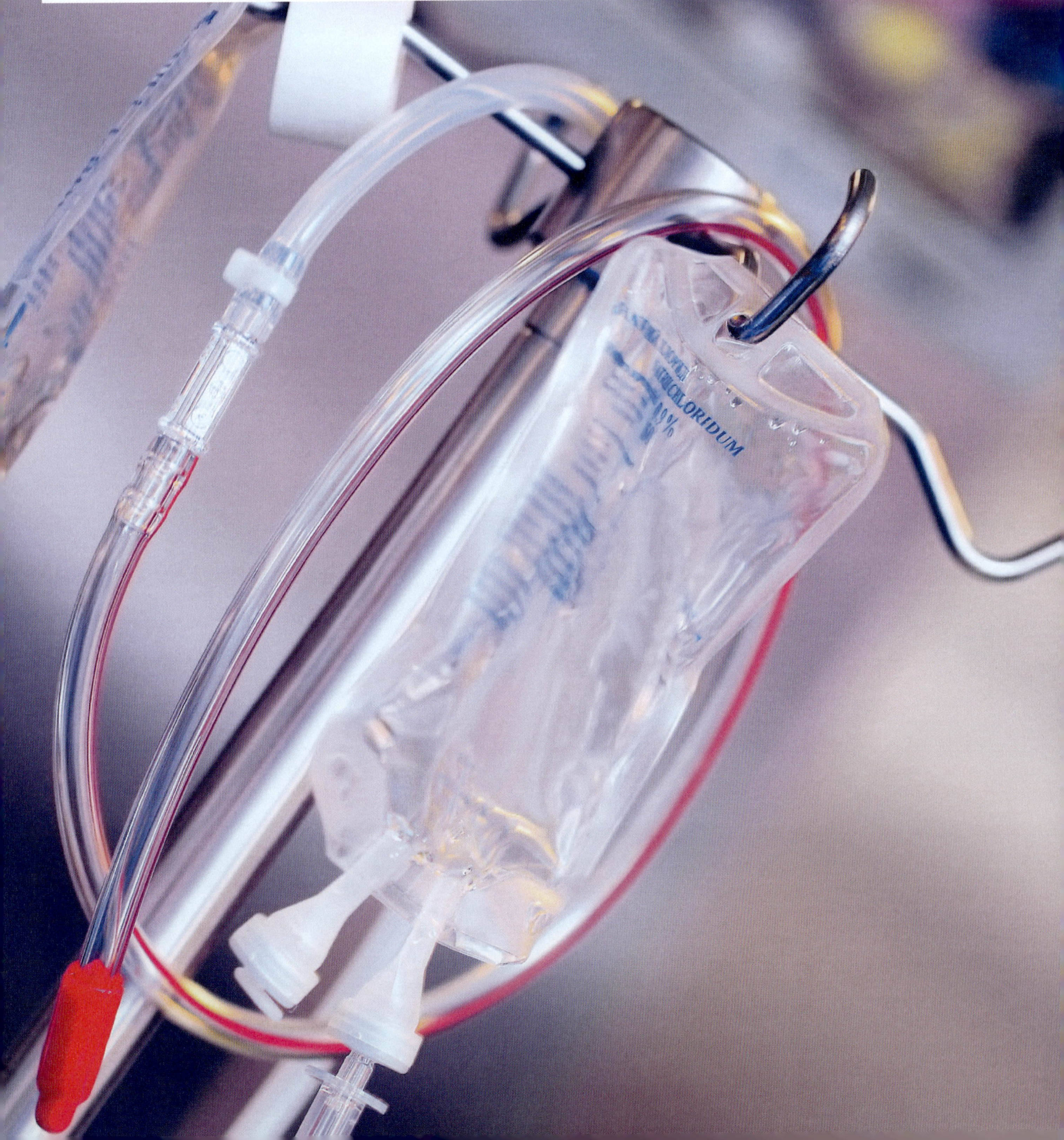

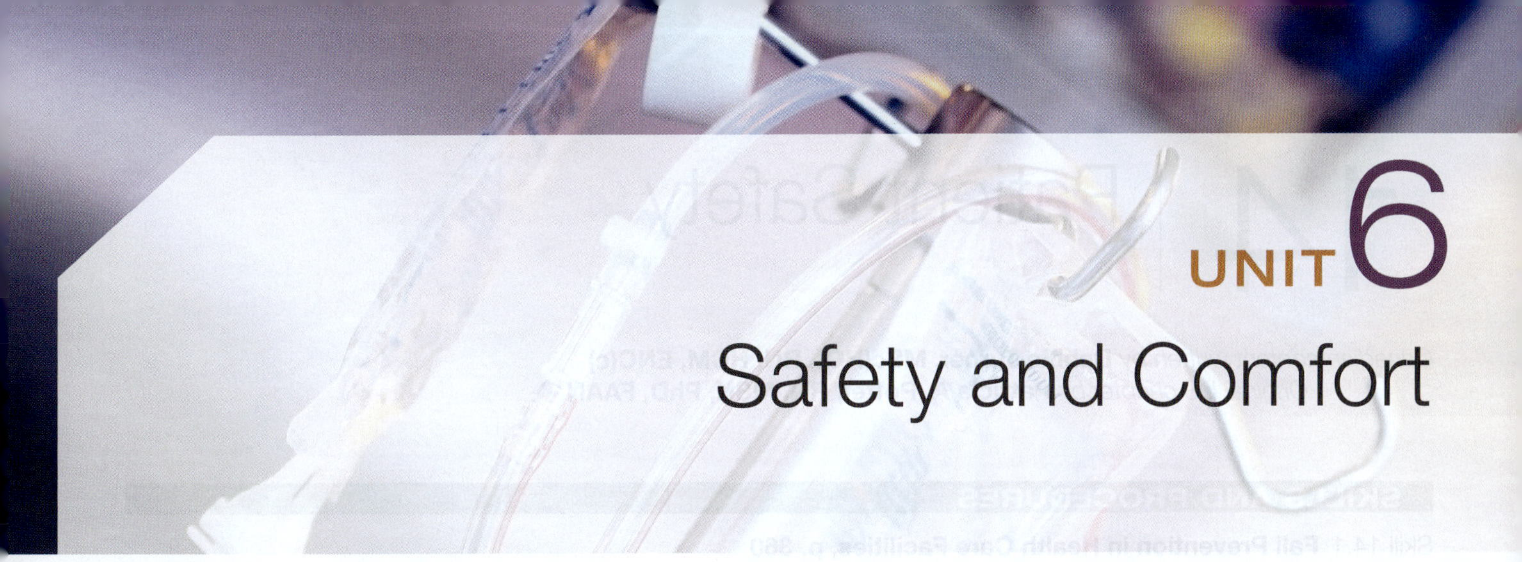

UNIT 6

Safety and Comfort

Patient safety and comfort are two important basic human needs. Managing a patient's health care environment, reducing risks for patient injury, and knowing how to respond in hazardous emergency situations require good clinical judgement and decision making. Critical thinking applied during patient assessment identifies patient safety risks so that you can identify problems accurately and take appropriate precautions based on your scientific knowledge and evidence-informed safety standards. For example, assessment of a patient's risk factors compared with the common risk factors associated with falls offers direction for specific steps to take to prevent patient falls. If a nurse assesses that a patient has visual problems and an unsteady gait, the nurse applies knowledge of the types of interventions that best match the risks. Having night lights in bathrooms and marking the edges of stairs in bright yellow are appropriate for patients with visual alterations. Use of handrails on stairs and elimination of throw rugs are interventions suited to patients with gait problems. Safety procedures must be patient centred to be effective.

Comfort is one of the most common patient needs that nurses manage. When you care for a patient experiencing pain or other uncomfortable symptoms, direct the patient's assessment based on knowledge of the physiology of pain and the patient's condition, the mechanisms in which pain therapies relieve pain, and the patient's unique presentation of their pain experience. Your own experience in assisting patients with pain management is also valuable in making clinical judgements for subsequent patients. A patient-centred approach to assessment allows patients to make decisions about methods for pain relief and thus assists you in selecting appropriate nonpharmacological versus pharmacological comfort measures. Critical thinking applied to pain management requires anticipation of the symptoms and physical changes patients may experience based on their clinical conditions. When a patient has pain related to an arthritic knee, pharmacological measures for pain relief in addition to safe support for ambulation are required. If the patient's pain is from a surgical incision, then pharmacological measures and physical support of the incision to minimize stress are necessary.

Procedures such as patient-controlled analgesia (PCA), epidural analgesia, and local anaesthesia pumps require the use of critical thinking to ensure patient safety. Because PCA is self-managed by a patient, a priority is providing the patient with the information necessary to ensure safe medication administration. Critical thinking involves applying assessment data about a patient's ability and readiness to manipulate the PCA device to judge the appropriateness of the therapy for the patient. Epidural analgesia is an invasive procedure. Part of skill competency in this case is implementing strict safety precautions to reduce the patient's risk for infection.

Therapeutic nurse–patient relationships are key to the effective implementation of nursing skills. Such relationships are crucial when supporting patients who are in need of end-of-life or palliative care. Good clinical judgements are based on understanding the patient and family as a unit. A thorough assessment of the emotional, social, and physical impact of a terminal or long-term chronic condition on the patient and family unit and the application of knowledge about the grief response allow you to choose appropriate palliative and end-of-life support measures.

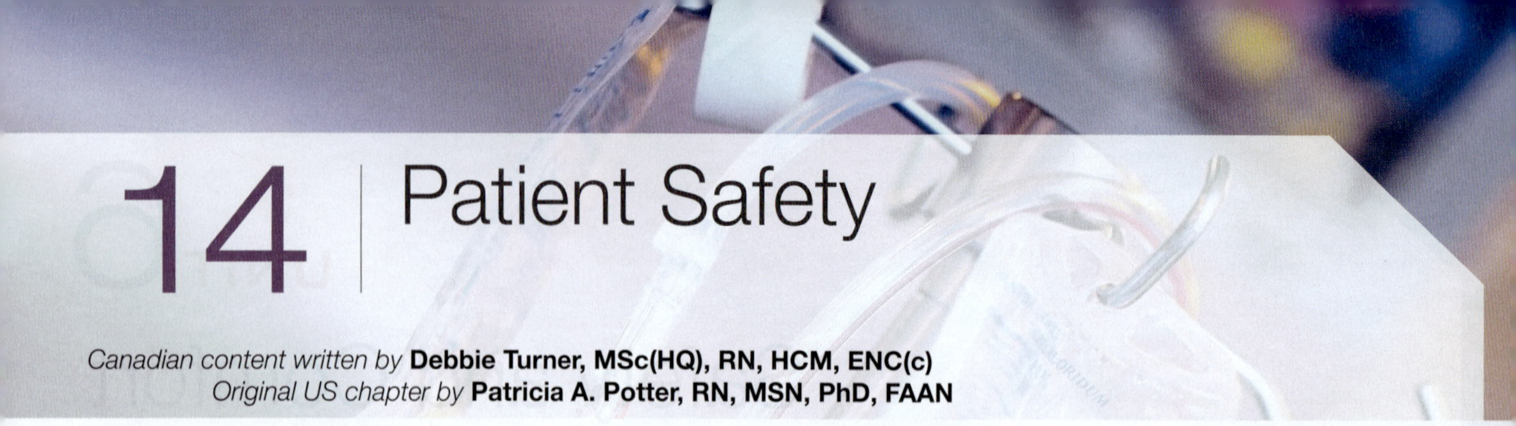

14 Patient Safety

Canadian content written by **Debbie Turner, MSc(HQ), RN, HCM, ENC(c)**
Original US chapter by **Patricia A. Potter, RN, MSN, PhD, FAAN**

SKILLS AND PROCEDURES

Skill 14.1 **Fall Prevention in Health Care Facilities, p. 360**
Skill 14.2 **Designing a Restraint-Free Environment, p. 369**
Skill 14.3 **Applying Physical Restraints, p. 372**
Skill 14.4 **Seizure Precautions, p. 379**
Procedural Guideline 14.1 **Fire, Electrical, and Chemical Safety, p. 384**

OBJECTIVES

Mastery of content in this chapter will enable the nurse to:

- Identify the features of a culture of safety.
- Explain the importance of national standards for patient safety.
- Describe current evidence in fall prevention.
- Explain the importance of a fall risk assessment in providing for patient safety.
- Describe nursing interventions specific for reducing patients' risks for falls.
- Describe steps in the design of a restraint-free environment.
- Describe nursing interventions taken in the event of a fire, electrical shock, or chemical spill.
- Explain precautions used to prevent injury in patients who are restrained.
- Describe nursing interventions for a patient who experiences generalized seizures.
- Describe methods to evaluate safety interventions.

MEDIA RESOURCES

- http://evolve.elsevier.com/Canada/Perry/clinicalskills/

PURPOSE

Improving patient safety and the quality of health care delivery is a national priority (Healthcare Excellence Canada, 2019). Health care that is provided in a safe environment, in which nurses practise safety-related skills, reduces the risk for illness and injury and contains the costs of health care by preventing extended lengths of treatment and hospitalization, improving or maintaining a patient's functional status, and increasing the patient's sense of well-being. As part of the interprofessional health care team, nurses are accountable to implement all activities that support a patient-centred culture of safety. Key features of a *culture of safety* are the determination to achieve consistently safe operations in health care, transparency in reporting adverse events and near misses without fear of punishment, interprofessional and caregiver collaboration for quality improvement, and adequate resources to address identified safety concerns (Healthcare Excellence Canada, 2019).

STANDARDS OF CARE

- Accreditation Canada (2020)–*Required Organizational Practices–2020 Handbook* (https://physicians.nshealth.ca/resources/required-organizational-practices-2020-handbook)
- Canadian Institute for Health Information (CIHI, 1996–2022)–*Patient Safety* (https://www.cihi.ca/en/patient-safety)
- Healthcare Excellence Canada (2019)–*Strengthening Commitment for Improvement Together: A Policy Framework for Patient Safety* (https://www.patientsafetyinstitute.ca/en/toolsResources/PolicyFrameworkforPatientSafetyCanada/Documents/PolicyFramework%20Document%20ENG%20FINAL.pdf)
- Healthcare Excellence Canada (2022)–*Our Strategy: Shaping the Future of Quality and Safety. Together.* (https://www.healthcareexcellence.ca/en/about/about-us/our-strategy/)
- Registered Nurses' Association of Ontario (RNAO, 2017)–*Preventing Falls and Reducing Injuries From Falls*, 4th edition (https://rnao.ca/bpg/guidelines/prevention-falls-and-fall-injuries)

PRINCIPLES FOR PRACTICE

- The integration and implementation of evidence-informed nursing skills and procedures promote a safer health care environment and improve patient outcomes.
- The nurse is responsible for incorporating critical thinking skills when using the nursing process, assessing each patient and the environment for hazards that threaten safety, and planning and intervening appropriately to maintain a safe environment, thus contributing to a culture of safety.

- Safe patient care is a priority, with a focus on managing safety risks, reducing the incidence of adverse health care–associated conditions, and reducing harm from inappropriate care (Healthcare Excellence Canada, 2019).
- The Healthcare Excellence Canada (n.d.) SHIFT to Safety program is designed to assist patients and families in advocating for their health care safety, enable health care providers to prioritize safety when caring for patients, and create a positive patient safety culture. (In 2022, the Canadian Patient Safety Institute [CPSI] and the Canadian Foundation for Healthcare Improvement [CFHI] amalgamated to become a new organization called *Healthcare Excellence Canada*.)
- A culture of safety is established when the employer's actions, through the adoption of evidence-informed policies, shift from a "blaming" to a "thank you" attitude following the identification and reporting of adverse events (Healthcare Excellence Canada, 2019).
- As a health care provider, it is essential to share information about any patient injury, learn from errors, and participate in the trending and evaluation of those errors for quality improvement (Health Canada, 2022a).
- When an adverse event (including a near miss) is identified, the nurse takes immediate steps to protect the safety and dignity of patients. Nurses must be aware of provincial and territorial legislation and Standards of Nursing Practice that may include direction about disclosure and reporting (Canadian Nurses Association, 2017).
- Being involved in an adverse event can be devastating for the nurse, patient, and family. It is estimated that up to 50% of interprofessional health care team members experience second victim syndrome at some point in their careers. The psychological impact of an error may be similar to that which characterizes post-traumatic stress disorder (PTSD), causing the person to feel self-doubt in their ability to perform at work and worry about their potentially negative impact on future patients (Institute for Safe Medication Practices Canada, 2017).

PERSON-CENTRED CARE

- Person-centred care is an approach to health care that focuses on the patient rather than on their illness or disease. It involves partnering with patients to enable them to be active participants and have a voice in the design and delivery of the care they receive, and providing timely evidence-informed care in a respectful context in order to improve their health care experience (Montague et al., 2019).
- Being hospitalized or living in a care facility may place patients at risk for injury because of the unfamiliar and confusing environment. Normal life cues such as a bed without side rails and the direction one usually takes to the bathroom are absent. Thought processes and coping mechanisms are affected by physical and psychological illness and the accompanying emotions. Thus, patients are more vulnerable to injury.
- For patients of diverse cultural backgrounds, vulnerability to injury may be intensified. It is a nurse's responsibility to diligently protect all patients, regardless of their cultural background. Most adverse events are related to failures of communication. Health care providers must be particularly attentive to communication during assessment. For example, the nurse must use approaches that recognize a patient's cultural background (e.g., using an interpreter or simple language) so that appropriate questions can be raised to clearly reveal health behaviours and risks.
- Nurses enhance a patient's safety by considering the whole person and seeing each care situation through "the patient's eyes," not just from a nurse's perspective. The following are some specific person-centred safety guidelines:
    - Nurses should empower patients to express their goals for health care and to share information that enables the patient to make informed decisions (Montague et al., 2019).
    - When restraints are needed, the nurse needs to clarify their meaning to the patient and family. Always use a "least restraints" approach and behaviour management techniques, including a comprehensive risk assessment protocol (Canadian Nurses Protective Society, 2021).
    - The nurse collaborates with family members in accommodating a patient's cultural perspectives regarding restraints. Removing restraints when family members are present shows respect and caring for a patient.
    - Nurses should be familiar with employer restraint policies. It is important to identify potential areas for negotiation with a patient's and family's preferences, such as using a mitten instead of arm restraints.
    - Nurses need to inform patients and family members of the reasons a patient is at risk of falling. It is important for patients to know their risks, the options that exist to promote safety, and the consequences of not following precautions.

EVIDENCE-INFORMED PRACTICE

Significant research continues in the area of fall prevention, both in community and health care settings.

- Young patients with neurological changes who have impaired gait and balance or medium-to-severe motor disability are at increased risk of falling. Patients who are relatively independent and still involved in challenging activities have an increased exposure to fall risk. Improperly fitted canes and walkers, wheelchair characteristics, and environmental hazards are significant environmental risk factors (RNAO, 2017).
- In health care settings, multifactorial fall prevention programs (using multiple fall prevention strategies) that incorporate a patient education component reduce both the number of falls and the number of recurrent fallers (Heng et al., 2020).
- Older persons should be screened routinely for relevant risk factors for falling. These individuals will most likely benefit from a fall prevention program targeted to their risk factors (e.g., frailty, polypharmacy, multimorbidity, vitamin D status, and home hazards). Not all fall prevention strategies are useful for all patients (Berry & Kiel, 2022).
- Exercise can significantly reduce the number of falls among older persons with and without cognitive impairment in community and facility-based settings (Berry & Kiel, 2022).
- Vitamin D and calcium supplementation, home visits, and adjustments within the living environment can reduce the risk for falls among older persons in noninstitutional settings (Berry & Kiel, 2022). Including an occupational therapist or physiotherapist in a home-hazard assessment may have added benefit.
- Patient- and nurse-specific risk factors, such as nurse–patient ratios and level of nursing experience, contribute to a higher incidence of falls (Bowden et al., 2019).
- A safety priority for Accreditation Canada (2020) is falls prevention. Fall prevention programs may include team education, risk assessments, balance and strength training, vision care, medication evaluation, physical environment assessments, behavioural assessments, and bed exit alarms. Fall prevention programs

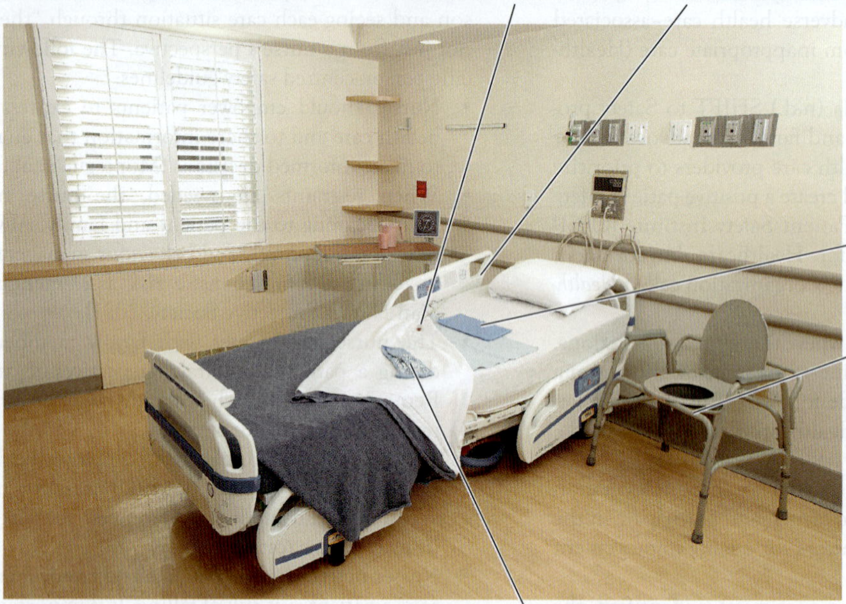

FIG 14.1 Safe patient room environment with bed in low position, bed alarm activated, nonskid footwear available, call light in place, and bedside commode positioned along bedside.

need to be interprofessional, collaborative, and person centred to minimize fall injury. Accreditation Canada (2020) identifies three tests for falls prevention adherence:

- Universal fall precautions are identified and implemented to ensure a safe environment.
- Team members and volunteers are educated, and patients and caregivers are provided with information to prevent falls and reduce injuries from falling.
- The effectiveness of fall prevention and injury reduction precautions and education are evaluated to inform improvements when indicated.

SAFETY GUIDELINES

- Accurate patient identification is crucial for ensuring patient safety before any procedures are carried out. Use at least two person-specific identifiers (Accreditation Canada, 2020).
- Safety begins with a patient's immediate environment (Fig. 14.1). Always keep a bed in the low position and a bed alarm activated, and use necessary fall prevention strategies. The call-light or bed-control system allows patients to adjust bed positions and to signal caregivers for help. Explain to patients and visitors how to operate the call system correctly, and then use teach-back to confirm their understanding by having them demonstrate use of the device. Also ensure the patient environment has adequate lighting, appropriate room temperature, good ventilation, and minimal noise to contribute to a safe patient environment.
- Always be alert to conditions within a patient's environment that pose risks for patient injury (e.g., personal care items out of reach, hazards along walking paths, liquid spilled on the floor, poorly functioning equipment).
- Do not use workarounds when performing skills or procedures. A workaround occurs when a person improvises or works around intended work practices.
- Communicate clearly to other health care providers the plan of care, including test results, procedures to be performed, procedures completed, and patient response.

✦ SKILL 14.1 Fall Prevention in Health Care Facilities

NSO *Nursing Skills Online Safety Module 1 / Lesson 1*

Falls are a recurrent problem in health care facilities that affect patients, families, visitors, care providers, and the health care system. A fall may result in fractures, bruises, lacerations, or internal bleeding, leading to increased diagnostic tests and treatments, extended hospital stays, and discharge to rehabilitation or long-term care instead of home. Approximately 4% of all adverse events in Canadian hospitals are related to injuries from falls (CIHI, 2022). Fall prevention involves completing a fall risk assessment of the person and the environment to inform safe patient care.

Risk factors for falls are numerous, complex, and interactive. Each person may have a combination of risk factors according to life circumstance, health status, health behaviours, economic status, social supports, and environment. Older persons are at increased risk for falls owing to chronic and acute health conditions, physical or cognitive challenges, inadequate nutrition, and social isolation (Boscart et al., 2023). As a nurse, your role is to assess these factors in each patient and determine the most suitable preventive interventions that match the patient's risks and behaviour.

Healthcare Excellence Canada (2015) defines *never events* as "patient safety incidents that result in serious harm or death, and that can be prevented by using organizational checks and balances" (p. 4). It has identified 15 pan-Canadian "never events," which are incidents that should never occur in a health care setting. One of these "never events" is patient death or serious harm as a result of transport of a frail patient or a patient with dementia, where protocols were not followed to ensure that the patient was left in a safe environment. Organizations are encouraged to report "never events" and to share best practices and quality improvement successes in order to enhance patient safety.

Fall prevention is not simple. The Fall Prevention/Injury Reduction Intervention Model (Fig. 14.2) focuses on providing a safe environment, assistance with mobility, fall risk reduction, and engagement with the patient and family (Healthcare Excellence Canada & RNAO, 2018). The RNAO (2017) has issued a detailed list of the components involved in preventing falls (Box 14.1).

Another area of risk includes wheelchair-related falls involving older persons and those living with disabilities. Patients fall from wheelchairs because of unlocked brakes, overreaching, sliding, tipping the chair, and unassisted transfers. Wheelchair-related injuries from falls include fractures, concussions, dislocations, amputations, and serious head and spinal injuries. An example of a wheelchair characteristic that increases the risk for falls is having smaller and

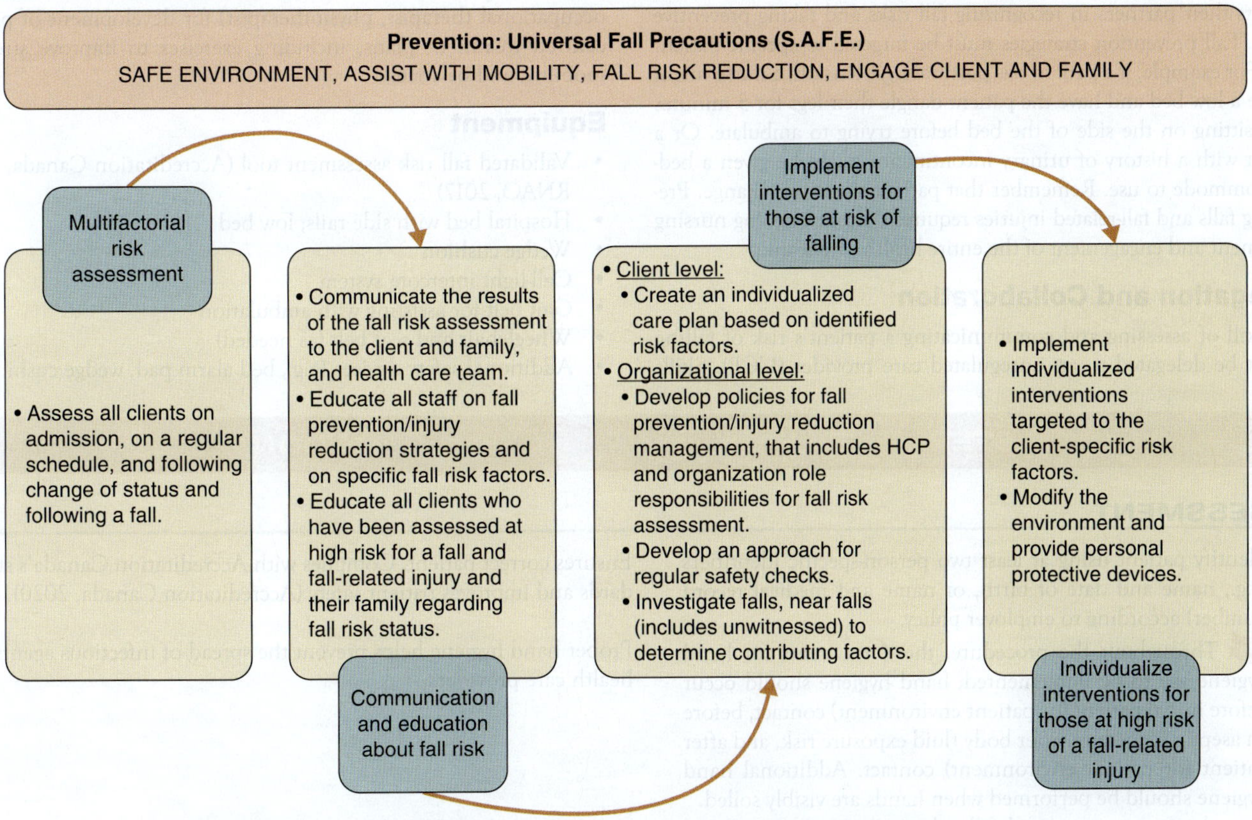

FIG 14.2 Healthcare Excellence Canada/RNAO Fall Prevention/Injury Reduction Intervention Model. HCP, Health care provider. (*From Healthcare Excellence Canada & Registered Nurses' Association of Ontario. [2018]. Reducing falls and injuries from falls: Getting started kit–Evidence update [p. 5].* https://www.patientsafetyinstitute.ca/en/toolsResources/Pages/Falls-resources-Getting-Started-Kit.aspx)

BOX 14.1

Components of Evidence-Informed Universal Falls Precautions

- Environmental modifications:
  - Implement universal falls precautions; modify equipment and other factors in the physical and structural environment
  - Bedrails in low position; nurse call light placed within reach
- Exercise interventions and physical training:
  - Core strength training, Pilates exercise training, muscle strengthening, stepping training, perturbation-based balance training (lower-limb strengthening exercises)
  - Exergaming (interactive gaming)
  - Fall prevention exercise programs
  - Foot and ankle exercises that strengthen and stretch the foot and ankle
  - Individualized exercise or physiotherapy
  - Interactive cognitive–motor interventions
- Footwear:
  - Nonslip shoes; thin, hard-soled footwear with high collars
- Multifaceted podiatry care:
  - Footwear assessment
  - Customized insoles
  - Foot and ankle exercises
- Pacemakers
- Whole-body vibration for postmenopausal women
- Cognitive–motor interference (training for the performance of two simultaneous tasks to prevent falls)
- Continence management (e.g., prompted elimination management schedule)
- Medication management (be aware of medications associated with falling)
- Rounding (e.g., hourly) as a strategy to proactively meet the person's needs and prevent falls
- Vitamin D supplementation

Adapted from Registered Nurses' Association of Ontario. (2017). *Preventing falls and reducing injuries from falls* (4th ed.). https://rnao.ca/sites/rnao-ca/files/bpg/FALL_PREVENTION_WEB_1207-17.pdf

harder front wheels, as these cause a chair to tip when they strike uneven terrain. Caregivers also put themselves at risk for injury by not handling patients correctly or not asking for help. Injuries can occur while caregivers transfer patients who are agitated, fearful, unsteady, or too weak to transfer. Tripping over the front foot or leg rest and leaning over the back of the wheelchair to engage or disengage the wheel lock are common sources of injury.

It is important for nurses to identify patients' fall risks and communicate these risks to patients, their visitors, and members of the health care team. Person-centred care is important, with nurses making patients their partners in recognizing fall risks and taking preventive action. Fall prevention strategies must be targeted to specific patient risks. For example, if a patient has postural hypotension, a nurse might choose a low bed and have the patient dangle their legs for 5 minutes while sitting on the side of the bed before trying to ambulate. Or a patient with a history of urinary incontinence might be given a bedside commode to use. Remember that patient situations change. Preventing falls and fall-related injuries requires diligent ongoing nursing assessment and engagement of the entire health care team.

Delegation and Collaboration

The skill of assessing and communicating a patient's risk of falling cannot be delegated to an unregulated care provider (UCP). Skills used to prevent falls can be delegated. The nurse directs the UCP by doing the following:

- Explaining a patient's mobility limitations and specific fall prevention measures needed to minimize risks
- Teaching specific environmental safety precautions to use (e.g., bed locked in low position, call light within reach)
- Explaining patient behaviours (e.g., disorientation, wandering, anxiety) that are precursors to falls and that should be reported immediately

Collaborate with the interprofessional health care team (e.g., occupational therapist, physiotherapist) for development of person-centred treatment plans, including exercises to improve strength, mobility, and balance.

Equipment

- Validated fall risk assessment tool (Accreditation Canada, 2020; RNAO, 2017)
- Hospital bed with side rails; low bed
- Wedge cushion
- Call-light intercom system
- Gait belt for assisting with ambulation
- Wheelchair and seat belt (as needed)
- Additional safety devices (e.g., bed alarm pad, wedge cushion)

STEP	RATIONALE
ASSESSMENT	
1. Identify patient using at least two person-specific identifiers (e.g., name and date of birth, or name and medical record number) according to employer policy.	Ensures correct patient. Complies with Accreditation Canada's standards and improves patient safety (Accreditation Canada, 2020).
2. Throughout the procedure, the 4 moments for hand hygiene are to be implemented; hand hygiene should occur before initial patient (or patient environment) contact, before an aseptic procedure, after body fluid exposure risk, and after patient (or patient environment) contact. Additional hand hygiene should be performed when hands are visibly soiled.	Proper hand hygiene helps prevent the spread of infectious agents to health care providers.
3. Complete a person-centred fall risk assessment using critical thinking and clinical judgement. Be sensitive to the population being screened: patient's age (over 65), presence of comorbidities, altered memory and cognition, incontinence or urinary frequency and urgency, reduced hearing and vision, orthostatic hypotension, arthritis, impaired gait, weak lower extremities, poor balance, fatigue, need for transfer assistance, and decreased peripheral sensation (Healthcare Excellence Canada & RNAO, 2018). Also assess for risk for injury during fall (e.g., vitamin D level, osteoporosis, bleeding tendency).	A variety of physiological factors predispose patients to falling and injury from falling. There are a variety of fall risk assessment tools. Those with a greater number of risk factors are less likely to be sensitive because all patients will be found to be at risk. Tools based on the risk factors of a population (e.g., older persons, oncology, or neurological patient) are more likely to be sensitive to predicting falls.

Critical Decision Point *Do not ask patient to provide a self-report of balance, gait, or ability to ambulate. Ask patient to walk a short distance and observe each factor.*

STEP	RATIONALE
4. Assess level of patient's pain using an appropriate rating scale (e.g., on a scale from 0 to 10, with 0 being no pain, and 10 being worst pain ever).	Pain has been shown to be a risk factor for falls (Boscart et al., 2023).
5. Determine whether patient has a history of recent falls or other injuries within the home. Use an appropriate risk assessment tool to identify high-risk patients (e.g., St. Thomas Risk Assessment Tool in Falling Elderly Inpatients [STRATIFY], Morse Fall Scale, Hendrich II Fall Risk) (Heng et al., 2020).	Symptoms are helpful in identifying the cause of falls. Onset, location, and activity associated with a fall provide further details about causative factors and how to prevent future falls.

STEP	RATIONALE
6. Review patient's medications (including over-the-counter [OTC] medications and herbal products) for use of antidepressants, sedatives and hypnotics (especially benzodiazepines), anxiolytics, beta blockers, diuretics, antihypertensives, neuroleptics, anti-Parkinson's medications, hypoglycemics, nonsteroidal anti-inflammatories, opioids, antipsychotics, and laxatives. Assess for polypharmacy (e.g., over four medications, duplicate medications, medications inappropriate for condition) (Healthcare Excellence Canada & RNAO, 2018).	Effects of certain medications and use of multiple medications increase risk for falls and injury (Healthcare Excellence Canada & RNAO, 2018).

Critical Decision Point *If patient is on multiple medications, collaborate with health care provider and pharmacist about possibility of reducing or adjusting doses.*

STEP	RATIONALE
7. Assess patient for fear of falling: Consider those over 70 years of age, female, lower income, or single and have poor perceived general health (Kiel, 2022).	Fear of falling is interrelated with incidence of falls, change in way patient walks, curtailment of activities, immobility, functional dependence, and falls with serious injury (Healthcare Excellence Canada & RNAO, 2018).
8. Perform the "timed up-and-go" (TUG) test if patient is able to ambulate. At a minimum, observe patient walk in room (with or without help). Steps for TUG dual assessment: • Give patient verbal instructions to stand up from a chair, walk 3 metres (10 feet) as quickly and safely as possible (cross a line marked on the floor), turn around, walk back, and sit down. • Have patient rise from straight-back chair without using arms for support. • Begin counting. • Observe patient's postural stability, gait, stride length, and sway. • Have patient return to chair and sit down without using arms for support. Check time elapsed. • For accuracy, a patient should have one practice trial that is not included in the score. The patient must use the same assistive device each time they are tested to be able to compare scores.	The TUG test is a simple and quick clinical, performance-based measure of lower-extremity function, mobility, and fall risk, useful even with healthy adults (Jeong et al., 2019). It quantifies a patient's functional mobility. Observing a patient's walk allows you to determine whether gait and posture are normal. The TUG test is a measure of physical and cognitive performance. Ability to follow simple instructions measures cognitive function. A TUG time >10 seconds indicates an increased risk of falling for hospitalized patients (Jeong et al., 2019), while ≥13.5 seconds indicates the risk for individuals in community settings (Heng et al., 2020). Recent evidence suggests that there should be three trials of the TUG test, and the scores averaged to determine the most accurate result (Heng et al., 2020).
9. Assess condition of equipment (e.g., legs on bedside commode, tips of walker).	Equipment in poor repair increases risk for fall.
10. Assess patient's medical history for osteoporosis, use of anticoagulants, history of previous fracture, cancer, and recent chest or abdominal surgery.	Factors increase likelihood of injury from fall.
11. Use person-centred approach to determine what patient knows about risks of falling and steps that they can take to prevent falls.	Knowledge of fall risks influences one's ability to take necessary precautions in reducing falling. Matching interventions with factors that patient perceives as relevant may increase success in preventing falls.
12. If patient is assessed to be a fall risk, apply colour-coded wristband (see Step 12 illustration). Some facilities institute fall risk signs on doors.	Colour-coded bands (e.g., yellow, blue–check employer policy) are easily recognizable.

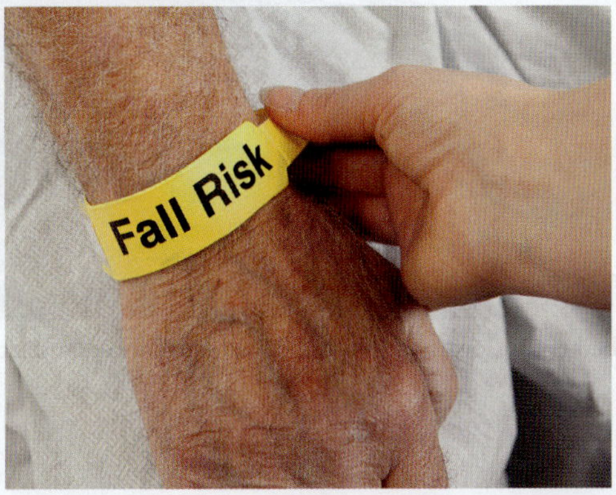

STEP 12 Fall risk armband alerts health care staff to patient's risk of falling.

STEP	RATIONALE
13. If patient is in a wheelchair, assess their level of comfort, fatigue, boredom, mental status, or level of engagement with others.	These factors can cause patient to make an attempt to exit wheelchair without help.

NURSING DIAGNOSES

- Acute or persistent pain
- Reduced physical mobility
- Inadequate transfer ability
- Reduced urinary elimination
- Reduced stamina
- Reduced memory
- Potential for falls
- Potential for injury
- Potential for trauma

Related factors and risk factors are individualized on the basis of patient's condition or needs.

PLANNING

STEP	RATIONALE
1. Expected outcomes following completion of procedure:	
• Patient's environment is free of hazards	Hazards predispose patients to tripping and falls.
• Patient and/or caregiver is able to identify fall risks.	Patient awareness of risks promotes cooperation and understanding of fall prevention plan.
• Patient and/or caregiver verbalizes understanding of fall prevention interventions.	Demonstrates person-centred care by involving patient and caregiver in decisions about preventive strategies.
• Patient does not experience a fall or injury.	Fall precautions show success in preventing falls.
2. Gather equipment.	Organizes care. Reduces transmission of microorganisms.
3. Explain what you plan to do. Specifically discuss reasons that patient is at risk of falling. Include caregivers (as appropriate) in discussion. Provide privacy. Be sure that patient is comfortable.	Reduces patient anxiety and promotes cooperation. Results in fall prevention measures that are person centred and not just routine. Younger patients are very independent and often believe that they are not likely to fall.

IMPLEMENTATION

STEP	RATIONALE
1. Conduct hourly purposive rounding on all patients to determine status of pain, need to toilet, and need to relocate personal items for easy reach; provide pain relief intervention.	Provides nurses with surveillance mechanism to purposefully keep patients safe and comfortable by proactively meeting their needs. Research that associates rounding with fall reduction needs to be more rigorous (RNAO, 2017).
2. Adjust bed to low position with wheels locked (see Step 2 illustration).	Height of bed allows ambulatory patient to get in and out of bed easily and safely. Pads provide nonslip surface on which to stand.

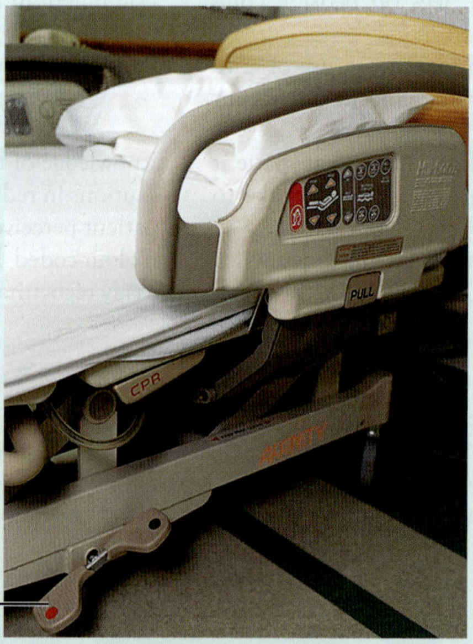

STEP 2 Hospital bed should be kept in lowest position with wheels locked and side rails up (as appropriate).

STEP	RATIONALE
3. Encourage use of properly fitted skidproof footwear. *Optional:* Place nonslip padded floor mat on exit side of bed.	Prevents falls due to slipping on floor.
4. Orient patient to surroundings, call light, and routines to expect in plan of care.	Orientation to room and plan of care provides familiarity with environment and activities to anticipate.
a. Provide patient's hearing aid and glasses. Be sure that each is functioning and clean. If patient indicates visual or hearing problems, refer to appropriate health care provider.	Enables patient to remain alert to conditions in environment.
b. Place call-light and bed-control system in an accessible location within patient's reach. Explain and demonstrate how to turn system on and off at bedside and in bathroom (see Step 4b illustration). Have patient perform return demonstration.	Knowledge of location and use of call light is essential for patient to be able to call for help quickly. Reaching for an object when in bed can lead to an accidental fall.
c. Explain to patient and caregiver when and why to use call system (e.g., report pain, get out of bed, go to bathroom). Provide clear instructions to patient and caregiver regarding mobility restrictions.	Increases likelihood that patient will call for help and that nurse will be able to respond to patient's needs in a timely way.
5. Safe use of side rails:	
a. Explain to patient and caregiver reason for using side rails (i.e., moving and turning self in bed safely).	Promotes cooperation.
b. Check employer policy regarding side rail use.	
(1) *Dependent, less mobile patients:* In bed with two side rails, keep both rails up. (NOTE: Rails on newer hospital beds allow for room at foot of bed for patient to safely exit bed, or may only have two upper side rails.) In bed with four side rails, leave two upper rails up.	Side rails are restraint devices if they immobilize or reduce ability of a patient to move their arms, legs, body, or head freely.
(2) *Patient able to get out of bed independently:* In bed with two side rails, keep only one rail up. In bed with four side rails, leave two upper side rails up. Place nonslip padded floor mats at exit side of bed.	Allows for safe exit from bed.
6. Make patient's environment safe:	
a. Remove excess equipment, supplies, and furniture from rooms and halls.	Reduces likelihood of falling or tripping over objects.
b. Keep floors free of clutter and obstacles (e.g., intravenous [IV] pole, electrical cords), particularly path to bathroom.	Reduces likelihood of falling or tripping over objects.
c. Coil and secure excess electrical, telephone, and any other cords or tubing.	Reduces risk of entanglement.
d. Clean all spills promptly. Post sign indicating wet floor. Remove sign when floor is dry (usually done by housekeeping).	Reduces risk of falling on slippery, wet surfaces.
e. Ensure adequate glare-free lighting; use a night light at night.	Glare may be a problem for older persons because of vision changes.

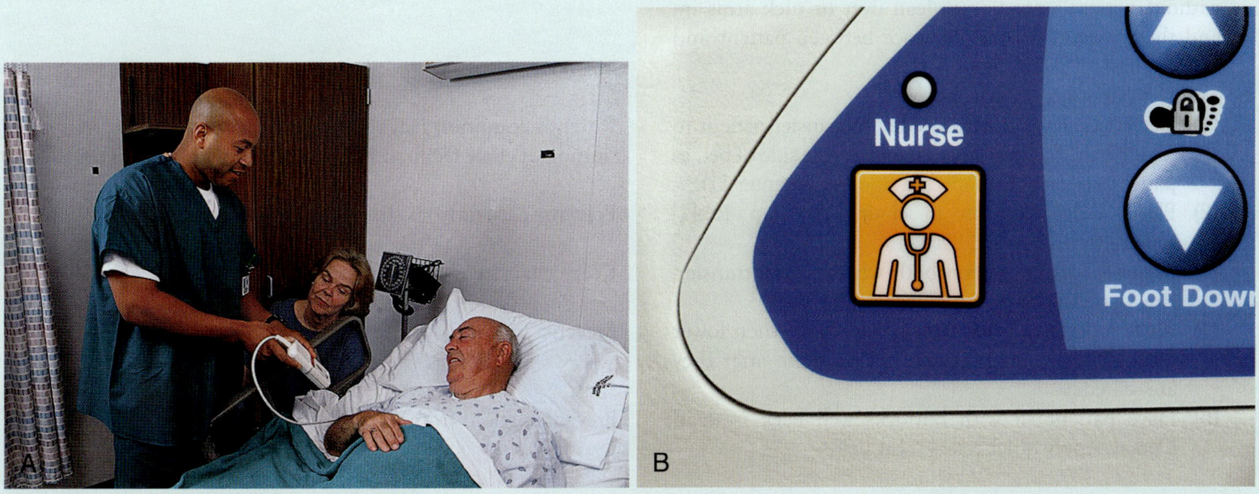

STEP 4B A, Nurse demonstrates use of call light to patient. B, Nurse call system within bed.

STEP	RATIONALE
f. Have assistive devices (e.g., cane, walker, bedside commode) on exit side of bed. Have chair back of commode placed against wall of room if possible.	Provides added support when transferring out of bed. Stabilizes commode.
g. Arrange personal items (e.g., water pitcher, telephone, reading materials, dentures) within patient's easy reach and in logical way.	Facilitates independence and self-care; prevents falls related to reaching for hard-to-reach items.
h. Secure locks on beds, stretchers, and wheelchairs.	Prevents accidental movement of devices during patient transfer.
7. Provide comfort measures; offer ordered analgesics for patients experiencing pain.	Pain can be a factor causing patients to exit bed; thus, pain relief is essential. However, be cautious, as opioids increase fall risk.
8. Interventions for patients at moderate-to-high risk of falling (based on fall risk assessment):	
a. Prioritize call-light responses to patients at high risk using team approach, with all staff having responsibility to respond.	Ensures rapid response by health care provider when patient calls for help.
b. Establish elimination schedule, using bedside commode when appropriate.	Proactive elimination scheduling keeps patients from being unattended with sudden urge to use toilet.

Critical Decision Point *The need for elimination is a common event leading to a patient's fall* (Berry & Kiel, 2022).

STEP	RATIONALE
c. Stay with patient (standing outside bathroom unless patient status indicates you must remain in the bathroom).	Patients often try to get up to stand and walk back to their beds from the bathroom without help.
d. Place patient in Geri chair or wheelchair with wedge cushion. Use wheelchair only for transport, not for sitting for extended period.	Maintains alignment and comfort and makes it difficult to exit chair.
e. Use low bed that has low height above floor and apply floor mats.	Reduces fall-related injuries.
f. Activate bed alarm for patient.	Alarm activates when patient rises off sensor. Alarm sounds alert to staff.
g. Confer with physiotherapy on feasibility of gait training, strength and balance training, and regular weight-bearing activities.	Exercise can reduce falls, fall-related fractures, and several risk factors for falls in individuals with low bone density and in older persons. Strength and balance training has been shown to reduce the rate of injurious falls in older persons (Berry & Kiel, 2022).
h. Use sitters or restraints only when alternatives are exhausted.	A sitter is a nonprofessional staff member or volunteer who stays in a patient room to closely observe patients who are at risk of falling. Restraints should be used only as final option (see Skill 14.2).
9. When ambulating patient, have patient wear a gait belt or walking sling and walk along their side (see Chapter 12).	Safe patient-handling techniques (e.g., use of walking sling or gait belt) allows for safe patient ambulation and prevention of injury to you and patient.
10. Safe use of wheelchair:	
a. Be sure that wheelchair is correct fit for patient: Patient's thighs are level while sitting, feet flat on floor; back of chair comes up to mid-shoulder; elbows rest on armrests without patient's needing to lean over or tuck arms in; and there are two fingers of space between patient and side of chair.	Correctly fitted chair promotes comfort, making it less likely that patient will to try to exit it.
b. Transfer patient to wheelchair.	
(1) Determine level of help needed to transfer patient to wheelchair. Position wheelchair on same side of bed as patient's strong or unaffected side (see Chapter 11).	Patient's condition may require more than a one-person assist. Positioning of chair facilitates patient's ability to help in transfer.
(2) Place wedge cushion in chair (see Step 10b[2] illustration).	Prevents patient from slipping out of chair.
(3) Securely lock brakes on both wheels when transferring patient into or out of wheelchair.	Keeps chair steady and secure.
(4) Raise footplates before transfer to chair; then lower footplates, placing patient's feet on them after they are seated.	Prevents tripping over footplate.
(5) Have patient sit with buttocks well back in seat. *Option:* Apply quick-release seat belt.	Prevents patient from sliding out of chair.

STEP	RATIONALE
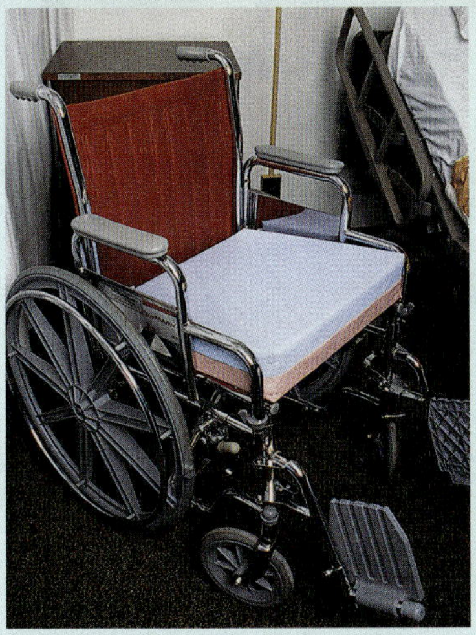 **STEP 10B(2)** Wheelchair with footplates raised and wedge cushion in place.	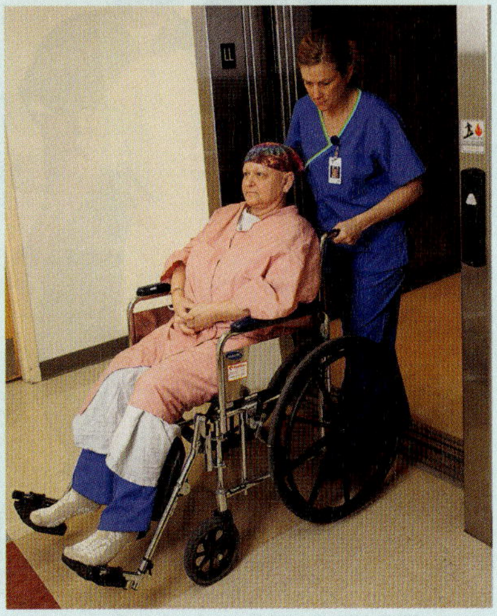 **STEP 10B(6)** Nurse backing wheelchair into elevator.
(6) Back wheelchair into and out of elevator or door, leading with large rear wheels first (see Step 10b[6] illustration).	Prevents smaller front wheels from catching in crack between elevator and floor, causing chair to tip.
c. Manage patient's pain, and do not allow patient to sit in wheelchair for an extended period; provide alternative sitting option.	Reduces the restlessness and discomfort that can lead to wheelchair exit.
11. Remove unnecessary supplies.	

EVALUATION

STEP	RATIONALE
1. Ask patient and caregiver to identify patient's fall risks.	Demonstrates learning.
2. Ask patient and caregiver to describe fall prevention interventions that are implemented.	Demonstrates learning.
3. Evaluate patient's ability to use assistive devices such as walker or bedside commode.	Adjustments in devices may become necessary.
4. Evaluate for changes in motor, sensory, and cognitive status and review if any falls or injuries have occurred.	May require different interventions to be added. Fall outcomes determine success of plan.
5. Use teach-back: "I want to be sure I explained clearly to you why you are more likely to fall than other patients. Tell me some of those reasons." Develop a revised teaching plan if patient or caregiver is unable to teach back correctly.	Determines patient's and caregiver's level of understanding of instructional topic.

Unexpected Outcomes	Related Interventions
1. Patient and caregiver are unable to identify fall risks or fall prevention strategies.	• Reinforce identified risks with patient and review safety measures with caregiver.
2. Patient starts to fall while ambulating with nurse or caregiver.	• Put both arms around patient's waist or grasp gait belt. • Stand with feet apart to provide broad base of support (see Chapter 12). • Extend one leg and let patient slide against it to floor (Fig. 14.3, *A*). • Bend knees and lower body as patient slides to floor (see Fig. 14.3, *B*).
3. Patient found after falling.	• Call for assistance. • Assess patient for injury and stay until help arrives. • Notify primary health care provider and caregiver. • Complete report as indicated by employer. • Evaluate patient's environment and risk factors; revise fall prevention plan as needed.

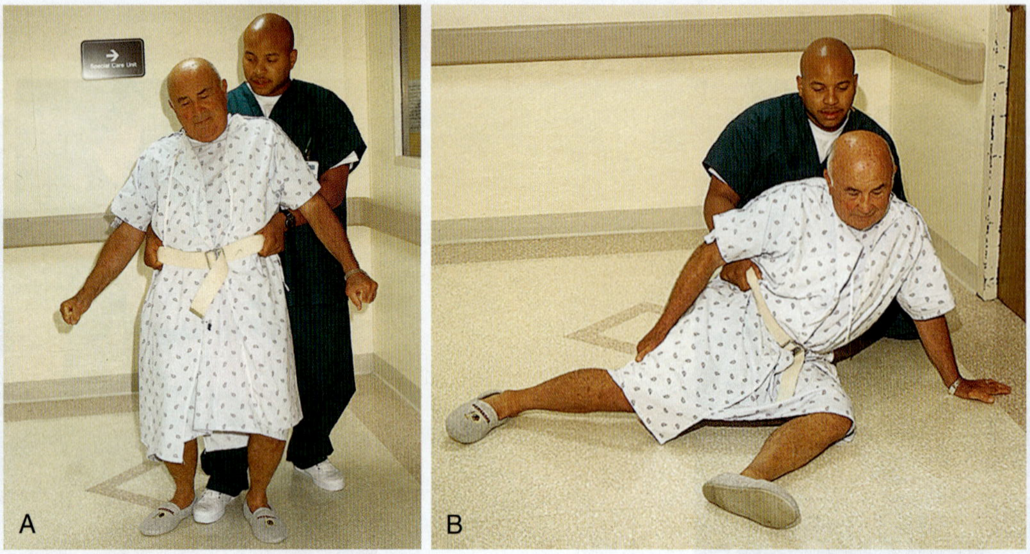

FIG 14.3 A, Stand with feet apart to provide broad base of support; extend one leg against which patient can slide to floor. B, Bend knees and lower body as patient slides to floor.

Communication and Documentation

- Document fall risk assessment findings, specific interventions used to prevent falls, and patient's response to teach-back in care plan on flow sheet or in progress notes in electronic health record (EHR) or chart.
- Report to health care personnel specific risks to patient's safety and measures taken to minimize risks.
- Document your evaluation of patient and caregiver learning.
- If a fall occurs, document a description of the fall as given by patient or you as witness. Be sure to include baseline assessment, any injuries noted, tests or treatments given, follow-up care, and additional safety precautions taken after fall. Complete report per employer policy.

DOCUMENTATION EXAMPLE

Patient found on floor at bedside. States to writer that they were getting up to use the commode when their legs "gave out." Patient screened as low fall risk on admission. Patient alert and oriented, denies head injury or neck pain. Assisted back to bed with 2 staff. Vital signs and head-to-toe assessment completed. Patient indicates left hip pain. Redness noted over left greater trochanter. No obvious deformity, rotation, or shortening noted, and patient able to lightly weight-bear when assisted back to bed. Fall risk assessment repeated with additional fall precautions implemented. Health care provider notified. Postfall investigation completed. Patient education provided on the importance of calling staff for assistance. Patient verbalized understanding to call staff.

Special Considerations

Teaching

- The National Council on Aging website has educational resources on fall prevention for older persons and caregivers (https://www.ncoa.org/caregivers/health/prevention/falls-prevention).
- Encourage patients to have annual vision and hearing examinations. Adaptive devices such as a hearing aid or glasses are sometimes necessary or need modification.
- Emphasize to patients the need to always look ahead when ambulating and use good posture.
- Teach patients how to use assistive devices and keep them in good repair.

Pediatric

- Encourage parents to follow best practices for fall prevention among children (Alberta Health Services, n.d.):
  - *Play safely.* Be sure playground equipment that a child uses is designed and maintained properly and that there is a safe, soft landing surface below; optimal equipment height to reduce risk of head injury is 1.5 metres (5 feet).
  - *Make the home safer.* Use home safety devices such as guards on windows that are above ground level, stair gates, and guard rails. Canadian legislation prohibits the use of baby walkers.
  - *Keep sports safe.* Be sure that a child wears protective gear such as wrist guards, knee and elbow pads, and a helmet for biking or skating when playing active sports.
  - *Supervision is key.* Supervise young children at all times around fall hazards, whether at home or out to play.
- Keep side rails of hospital beds down to allow toddlers and preschoolers easy exit and decrease the need to crawl over the rails (Hockenberry et al., 2024).
- When caring for infants, keep a hand on the child when you turn away from the bedside.

Gerontological

- Interventions to improve balance confidence, including multicomponent behavioural group interventions and exercise (including tai chi), have shown benefits for older persons (Berry & Kiel, 2022).

Patients With Physical or Cognitive Challenges

- An area of fall risk includes wheelchair-related falls resulting from unlocked brakes, overreaching, sliding, tipping the chair, and unassisted transfers. Wheelchair-related injuries from falls include fractures, concussions, dislocations, amputations, and serious head and spinal injuries.
- Caregivers are also at risk for injury from not handling patients correctly or not asking for help. Injuries can occur while caregivers transfer patients who are agitated, fearful, unsteady, or too weak to transfer.

Care in the Community: Home Management

- See Chapter 42, "Safety in the Community."

✦ SKILL 14.2 Designing a Restraint-Free Environment

Video Clip NSO *Nursing Skills Online Safety Module 1 / Lesson 2*

A physical restraint is any physical, environmental, or chemical (e.g., anxiolytic, sedative) measure that restricts the movement or controls the behaviour of a patient (College of Nurses of Ontario [CNO], 2022). Evidence suggests that the use of restraints increases the severity of falls. Best practice is a least-restraint policy that requires all possible alternative interventions to be exhausted before deciding to use a restraint (CNO, 2022).

Because physical and chemical restraints restrict a patient's physical activity or normal access to the body, serious and often fatal complications can develop, especially when patients try to get out of restraints. As a nurse, always be aware of employer policy related to the use of restraints. Creating a restraint-free environment allows you to implement interventions to reduce wandering and risk for patient falls. *A restraint-free environment is the first goal of care for all patients.*

Patients at risk for falls or wandering present special safety challenges. Wandering is a common problem in patients who are confused or disoriented (e.g., patients with dementia). Interrupting a wandering patient can increase their distress. Wandering is a persistent problem in long-term care settings. Common strategies to manage wandering include environmental adaptations, use of signalling tags, distraction, social interaction, regular exercise, and circular design of a patient care unit. More frequent observation of patients, involvement of family during visitation, and frequent reorientation are also helpful measures.

Delegation and Collaboration

The skills of assessing patient behaviours and orientation to the environment and determining the type of restraint-free interventions to use cannot be delegated to a UCP. Actions for promoting a safe environment can be delegated to UCPs. The nurse directs the UCP about the following:

- Using specific diversional or activity measures for making the environment safe
- Applying appropriate alarm or monitoring devices
- Reporting patient behaviours and actions (e.g., confusion, getting out of bed unassisted, combativeness) to the nurse

Collaborate with the interprofessional health care team (e.g., speech therapist, occupational therapist, physiotherapist) for exercise options and activities that provide meaningful stimulation.

Equipment

- Visual or auditory stimuli (e.g., calendar, clock, radio, photos, CD or MP3 player, television, smartphone)
- Diversional activities (e.g., puzzle, game, audiobooks, DVD)
- Wedge cushion
- Wraparound belt
- *Options:* Electronic bracelet or pressure pad alarm sensor; bed enclosure system

STEP	RATIONALE
ASSESSMENT	
1. Identify patient using at least two person-specific identifiers (e.g., name and date of birth, or name and medical record number) according to employer policy.	Ensures correct patient. Complies with Accreditation Canada's standards and improves patient safety (Accreditation Canada, 2020).
2. Throughout the procedure, the 4 moments for hand hygiene are to be implemented; hand hygiene should occur before initial patient (or patient environment) contact, before an aseptic procedure, after body fluid exposure risk, and after patient (or patient environment) contact. Additional hand hygiene should be performed when hands are visibly soiled.	Proper hand hygiene helps prevent the spread of infectious agents to health care providers.
3. Assess patient's medical history for dementia, depression, or delirium. Use an appropriate assessment tool (e.g., Confusion Assessment Method [CAM], Nursing Delirium Screening Scale [Nu-DESC]). Signs and symptoms include acute onset and fluctuating course of symptoms, inattention, impaired level of alertness, and a disturbance of cognition (e.g., disorientation, memory impairment, or alteration in language) (American Psychiatric Association, 2016; Heinrich et al., 2019).	Delirium is associated with adverse outcomes, including increased patient morbidity and mortality and increased costs (Heinrich et al., 2019).
4. Assess patient's behaviour (e.g., orientation, level of consciousness, ability to understand and follow directions, resistant behaviours, restlessness, agitation), balance, gait, vision, hearing, bowel and bladder routine, level of pain, electrolyte and blood count values, and presence of orthostatic hypotension.	Accurate assessment identifies patients with safety risks and the physiological causes for patient behaviours that prompt caregivers to use restraints. Ensures proper selection of nonrestraint interventions.
5. Review OTC and prescribed medications (see Skill 14.1) that pose risk for falls. Assess for interactions and untoward effects.	Medication interactions or adverse effects often contribute to falling or altered mental status.
6. Assess patient's or caregiver's knowledge of condition and prescribed treatments.	Knowledge of treatment protocols and rationales increases patient's cooperation.

STEP	RATIONALE
7. For patients who wander or have known dementia, assess for cognitive decline using Mini-Mental State Examination (MMSE) (see Chapter 42).	Determines cause and nature of wandering, which leads to effective intervention selection.
8. Assess degree of wandering behaviour using Revised Algase Wandering Scale (RAWS) (Chiu et al., 2011).	The RAWS is a valid and reliable measure overall and is used to evaluate patient behaviours relative to persistent walking, spatial disorientation, and eloping behaviour subscales (Varshawsky & Traynor, 2021).
9. For patients with dementia, ask family or friends about their usual communication style and cues to indicate pain, fatigue, hunger, and need to urinate or defecate.	Enables person-centred care to identify individual patient cues for which patient behaviours often prompt wandering when need is unmet.
10. Inspect condition of any therapeutic medical devices.	Patients who become restless, agitated, or confused will attempt to remove medical devices and then become candidates for physical restraint.

NURSING DIAGNOSES

- Wandering
- Insufficient knowledge regarding need for least-restraint environment
- Potential for falls
- Potential for injury
- Potential for trauma

Related factors and risk factors are individualized on the basis of patient's condition or needs.

PLANNING

STEP	RATIONALE
1. Expected outcomes following completion of procedure:	
• Patient is injury-free and does not inflict injury on others while in restraint-free environment.	Alternative interventions are successful in reducing agitation and preventing injury or least-restraint use.
• Patient does not remove a therapeutic medical device.	

IMPLEMENTATION

STEP	RATIONALE
1. Orient patient and caregiver to surroundings, introduce to staff, and explain all treatments and procedures. Be sure that patient is able to read your name badge.	Promotes patient understanding and cooperation.
2. Assign same staff to care for patient as often as possible. Encourage family and friends to stay with patient. In some facilities, volunteers are effective companions.	Increases familiarity with individuals in patient's environment, decreasing anxiety and restlessness. Companions are helpful and prevent patient from being alone.
3. Place patient in room that is easily accessible to caregivers, close to nurses' station.	Allows for frequent observation to reduce falls among high-risk patients.
4. Be sure that patient is wearing glasses, hearing aid, or other sensory-aid devices and that all are functioning.	Improves patient's level of orientation to environment.
5. Provide visual and auditory stimuli meaningful to patient (e.g., clock, calendar, radio, CD, or MP3 player [with patient's choice of music], television, and family pictures).	Orients patient to day, time, and physical surroundings. Stimuli must be individualized for this strategy to be effective.
6. Anticipate patient's basic needs (e.g., elimination needs, relief of pain, relief of hunger) as quickly as possible; conduct hourly rounding (RNAO, 2017).	Providing basic needs in timely fashion decreases patient discomfort, anxiety, restlessness, and incidence of falls.
7. Provide scheduled ambulation, chair activity, and elimination (e.g., during rounding, ask patient about elimination needs). Organize treatments so patient has uninterrupted periods throughout the day.	Regular opportunity to void avoids risk of patient trying to reach bathroom alone. Provides for sleep and rest periods. Constant activity overstimulates patients.
8. Position IV catheters, urinary catheters, and tubes and drains out of patient view. Use camouflage by wrapping IV site with bandage or stockinette. Place undergarments on patient with urinary catheter or cover abdominal feeding tubes and drains with loose abdominal binder.	Maintains medical treatment and reduces patient access to tubes and lines.
9. Decrease wandering: Eliminate stressors from environment such as cold at night, changes in daily routines, and extra visitors.	Reduced stress allows patient's energy to be channelled more appropriately.

STEP	RATIONALE
10. Use stress reduction techniques such as back rub, massage, and guided imagery (see Chapter 16).	Reduces anxiety and restlessness.
11. Use diversional activities: puzzles, games, music therapy, pet therapy, activity apron, performing purposeful activity (e.g., folding towels, drawing, and colouring). Be sure that it is an activity in which patient has interest. Involve caregiver (if appropriate).	Meaningful diversional activities provide distraction, help reduce boredom, and provide tactile stimulation. Minimize occurrences of wandering.
12. Position patient on wedge cushion and apply wraparound belt (see Step 12 illustration).	Cushion prevents slipping in chair and makes it difficult for patient to get out of chair without help. Wraparound belt allows patient to lift flap for self-release.
13. Use pressure-sensitive bed or chair pad with alarms:	Alarms alert staff to patient who is standing or rising from bed or chair without help.
a. Explain use of device to patient and caregiver.	
b. When patient is in bed, position device so it is correctly positioned under patient's mid-to-low back or buttocks.	Alarm activates sooner if placed under patient's back. By the time buttocks are off sensor, patient may be almost out of bed.
c. Test alarm by applying and releasing pressure.	Ensures that alarm is audible through call-light system.
14. Place electronic monitoring bracelet on wrist of patient with dementia.	Tag in bracelet contains radio-frequency circuit that communicates with detection sensor usually installed at an exit door or elevator. Distance between tag and monitor is constantly measured with an alarm, which sounds when predetermined distance is exceeded.
15. Place wandering patient in bed enclosure system (see Step 15 illustration).	Restraint alternative allows patient freedom of movement within protected environment.
16. Ensure patient is comfortable.	
17. Collaborate with physiotherapy, speech, and occupational therapy for activities that provide stimulation and exercise.	Involvement in meaningful and purposeful activities reduces tendency to wander. Exercise improves balance and coordination.
18. Minimize invasive treatments (e.g., tube feedings, blood sampling) as much as possible.	Stimuli increase patient's restlessness.

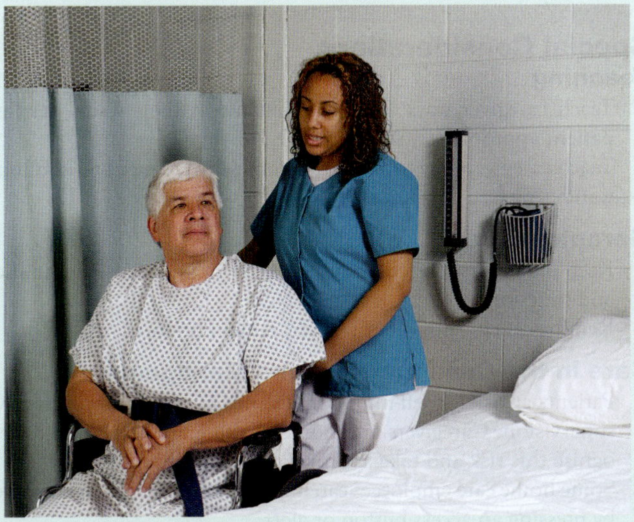

STEP 12 Wraparound belt. *(iStockphoto/nano)*

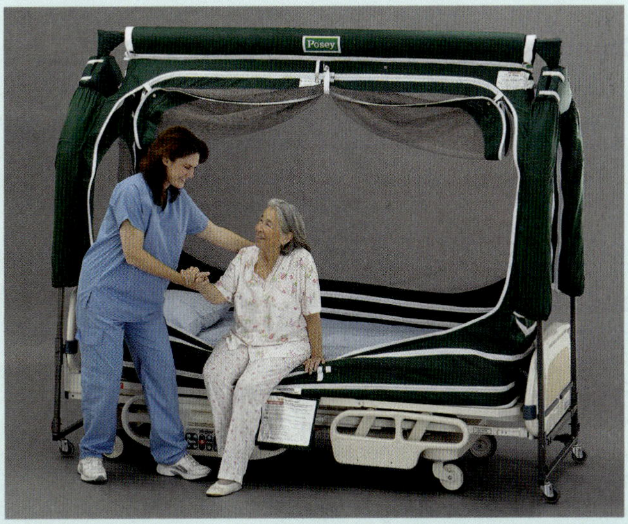

STEP 15 Bed enclosure system. *(Courtesy Posey Company, Arcadia, CA.)*

STEP	RATIONALE
EVALUATION	
1. Monitor patient's behaviour routinely.	Will determine whether agitation, wandering, or attempt to remove medical devices has been prevented.
2. Observe patient for any injuries.	Patient should be injury-free.
3. Observe patient's behaviour toward staff, visitors, and other patients.	Ensures that patient's behaviour does not cause injury to others.
4. **Use teach-back:** "We've talked about what we are doing to reduce your husband's wandering. Tell me ways you can help. I want to be sure you understand." Develop a revised teaching plan if caregiver is unable to teach back correctly.	Determines caregiver's level of understanding of instructional topic.

Unexpected Outcomes	Related Interventions
1. Patient displays behaviours that increase risk for injury to self or others.	• Review episodes for pattern (e.g., activity, time of day) that indicates alternatives that would eliminate behaviour. • Discuss with all caregivers and family alternative interventions.
2. Patient sustains injury or is agitated and places others at risk for injury.	• Notify health care provider. • Complete report according to employer policy. • Identify alternative measures for safety or behavioural control. • Apply physical restraint (see Skill 14.3) only after all possible alternatives have been exhausted.
3. Patient wanders away from facility.	• Be prepared to follow employer policy, which should include whom to notify; who will search for patient; which areas will be searched and their priority; who will notify authorities, if necessary; who will notify family members; and who will coordinate search efforts.

Communication and Documentation

- Document restraint alternatives used, patient behaviours that relate to cognitive status, and interventions to mediate these behaviours in progress notes in EHR or chart.
- Document your evaluation of caregiver learning.

DOCUMENTATION EXAMPLE

Patient agitated, yelling out, and banging on furniture. Patient refused to allow writer to obtain vital signs. Patient is alert but not able to accurately tell writer where they are. Patient reoriented to person, place, and time. Cognitive assessments completed. Patient denies needing to use the washroom. Water and blanket offered to patient. Patient sitting in recliner chair and moved to a room closer to nursing station to allow close monitoring. Substitute decision maker (SDM) at bedside with patient. Patient teaching provided to SDM with instructions to call staff for help if patient becomes agitated again. SDM appropriately demonstrated to staff how to call for help. Will continue to frequently monitor patient's cognitive behaviour.

Special Considerations

Teaching

- Teach caregiver ways to involve patient in their visits, keeping patient appropriately stimulated.
- Teach caregiver how to adapt the home environment to minimize wandering (see Chapter 42).

Gerontological

- Keep older persons active and ambulatory to increase endurance and function.
- Reminiscence helps older persons remain oriented.

Care in the Community: Home Management

- Patients at risk for self-injury or violence to others need intensive supervision. Caregivers and home health employees need to recognize this risk and take appropriate preventive measures.
- Some home care employees can immediately access their employer by pressing an access button or alert.
- Nurses should also assess for signs of violence or the presence of weapons.
- Defuse anger by displaying a calm and caring demeanour.
- Avoid behaviours that may be interpreted by patient as aggressive (e.g., getting close, speaking loudly, moving quickly).
- Have caregiver set up an area in the home where it is safe for an older person to wander.

✦ SKILL 14.3 Applying Physical Restraints

Video Clip **NSO** *Nursing Skills Online Safety Module 1 / Lesson 2*

In health care settings, restraints are most commonly used to prevent the disruption of therapy. Restraints are used in critical care settings, where patients who are seriously ill often unknowingly attempt to remove endotracheal tubes, IV catheters, urinary catheters, and feeding tubes (Freeman et al., 2018). Unplanned removal of endotracheal tubes has been found to be associated with agitation, inadequate sedation, and reduced patient surveillance by health care staff; however, the effectiveness of the use of physical restraints in adult critical care areas has not been established (Freeman et al., 2018). Nurses often pursue prescriptions for restraints when they are concerned that disruption of therapy can significantly injure patients; however, a least-restraint approach is best practice. Nurses need to implement approaches to appropriately secure medical devices and prevent accidental removal without using restraints (e.g., ensure endotracheal tube is anchored correctly; IV line is secured; long-sleeved robe covers IV insertion site). The use of physical and chemical restraints in long-term care has been associated with concerns about patient behaviours (e.g., wandering and aggression) and fall risks and a shortage of nurse staffing (fewer staff to monitor patient safety).

The least-restraint directive is best practice in facilities across Canada. Healthcare Excellence Canada (2015) had considered adding "patient death or serious harm caused by the use of restraints …" (p. 11) as a "never event," but did not do so because restraints are sometimes needed for both patient and health care provider safety, and they were concerned about balancing benefits with risk of harm (e.g., preventing patient falls). Accreditation Canada (2020) requires health care facilities to have restraint policies and procedures.

For example, in Ontario, the *Patient Restraints Minimization Act* (2001) directs hospitals and other facilities to ensure that any patient who is under restraint, confined, or on whom a monitoring device is used is properly monitored and subject to regular assessment within a defined period of time (c. 16, s. 8).

Restraints are used for a variety of reasons, such as protecting patients from harming themselves or others. Restraints should only be used when all other prevention, de-escalation, and crisis management strategies have failed to keep the patient safe (CNO, 2022).

Restraints are a temporary way to keep patients safe. However, there is no evidence that they prevent falls, reduce wandering, or prevent medical devices from being pulled out. Research has shown that patients suffer fewer injuries if left unrestrained (Berry & Kiel, 2022). The use of mechanical or physical restraints requires a health care provider's prescription and must be based on a face-to-face patient assessment. The nurse must ensure that the patient or caregiver is aware of restraint use and its rationale because there is a potential liability from restraint use in the absence of informed consent (Healthcare Excellence Canada, 2017).

Extreme caution is required in their application when there is no other option to manage the undesired behaviour. Chemical restraint, or *acute control medication* (ACM), refers to "the administration of psychotropic medication in situations where a person may have already lost behavioural control or where there is imminent risk of loss of control in behaviour that will lead to harm to self or others" (Healthcare Excellence Canada, 2017, p. 4).

Delegation and Collaboration

The skills of assessing a patient's behaviour and level of orientation, the need for restraints, and the appropriate restraint type, as well as continually assessing the patient's behaviour while a restraint is in place, cannot be delegated to a UCP. Applying and routinely checking a restraint can be delegated to a UCP. The nurse directs the UCP by doing the following:

- Reviewing correct placement of the restraint and how to routinely check the patient's circulation, skin condition, and breathing
- Reviewing when and how to change a patient's position and provide range-of-motion (ROM) exercises, elimination assistance, and skin care
- Instructing the UCP to notify the nurse immediately if there is a change in the patient's level of agitation, skin integrity, circulation of extremities, or breathing

The nurse collaborates with the interprofessional health care team (e.g., physiotherapist, IV nurse) regarding the patient behaviour leading to the use of restraints and how the patient reacts when a restraint is removed for therapy.

Equipment

- Proper restraint (e.g., belt, wrist, mitten)
- Padding (if needed)

STEP	RATIONALE
ASSESSMENT	
1. Identify patient using at least two person-specific identifiers (e.g., name and date of birth, or name and medical record number) according to employer policy.	Ensures correct patient. Complies with Accreditation Canada's standards and improves patient safety (Accreditation Canada, 2020).
2. Throughout the procedure, the 4 moments for hand hygiene are to be implemented; hand hygiene should occur before initial patient (or patient environment) contact, before an aseptic procedure, after body fluid exposure risk, and after patient (or patient environment) contact. Additional hand hygiene should be performed when hands are visibly soiled.	Proper hand hygiene helps prevent the spread of infectious agents to health care providers.
3. Assess for underlying cause(s) of agitation and cognitive impairment leading to patient-initiated medical device removal (Freeman et al., 2018):	
a. Assess for life-threatening physiological impairments.	Physiological alterations might lead to accidental patient-initiated medical device removal (Freeman et al., 2018). Identification of conditions might lead to more appropriate medical or pharmacological treatment, eliminating need for restraints (see Skill 14.2).
b. Assess for respiratory and neurological conditions, fever and sepsis, hypoglycemia and hyperglycemia, alcohol or substance withdrawal, and fluid and electrolyte imbalance.	

STEP	RATIONALE
c. Notify health care provider of change in mental status and compromised physiological status.	
d. Obtain baseline or premorbid cognitive function from caregivers.	Caregivers provide an excellent source of information for patient's behaviour patterns and past history.
e. Establish whether patient has history of dementia or depression.	
f. Review medications (including OTC and herbal therapy) that cause risk of falling to identify interactions or adverse effects.	
g. Review current laboratory values.	
4. Assess patient's current behaviour (e.g., confusion, disorientation, agitation, restlessness, combativeness, inability to follow directions, or repeated removal of tubing, dressing, or other therapeutic devices). Does patient create a risk to other patients?	If patient's behaviour continues despite treatment or restraint alternatives, use of least restrictive restraint is indicated.
5. If restraint alternatives failed earlier, confer with a health care provider. Review employer policies and provincial/territorial laws regarding restraints. Obtain the current health care provider's prescription, which must include purpose, type, location, and time or duration of restraint. Determine whether signed consent for use of restraint is necessary (see employer policy). Some policies require that the prescription be renewed according to time limits for a maximum of 24 consecutive hours (Healthcare Excellence Canada, 2017).	A health care provider's prescription for least restrictive type of restraint is required (Accreditation Canada, 2020).

Critical Decision Point *A licensed independent health care provider responsible for the care of the patient evaluates the patient in person within 1 hour of the initiation of restraint used for the management of violent or self-destructive behaviour that jeopardizes the physical safety of the patient, staff, or others. A registered nurse or a physician assistant may conduct the in-person evaluation if they are trained in accordance with the requirements and consult with the aforementioned health care provider after the evaluation as determined by facility policy. Always use the least restrictive restraint possible (e.g., mitts, elbow extenders)* (Healthcare Excellence Canada & RNAO, 2018).

STEP	RATIONALE
6. Review manufacturer instructions for restraint application before entering patient's room. Determine most appropriate size of restraint.	You need to be familiar with all devices used for patient care and protection. Incorrect application of a restraint device can result in patient injury or death.

NURSING DIAGNOSES

- Potential for injury
- Potential for trauma

Risk factors are individualized on the basis of patient's condition or needs.

PLANNING

STEP	RATIONALE
1. Expected outcomes following completion of procedure:	
• Patient maintains intact skin integrity, pulses, temperature, colour, and sensation of restrained body part.	Restraints are applied and monitored correctly.
• Patient is free from injury.	Restraints are removed in a timely manner.
• Patient's therapy (e.g., IV tube, catheters) is uninterrupted.	Disruption of therapy causes patient injury, pain, or discomfort and increases risk for infection.
• Patient maintains self-esteem and sense of dignity.	Physical restraints have a detrimental effect on psychosocial well-being of patient.
• Restraint is discontinued as soon as possible.	Limits period of time patient is at risk for injury.
2. Gather equipment and perform hand hygiene.	Promotes organization and reduces transmission of microorganisms.
3. Explain what you plan to do and why. Provide privacy.	Reduces patient anxiety and promotes cooperation.

STEP	RATIONALE
IMPLEMENTATION	
1. Adjust bed to proper height and lower side rail on side of patient contact. Be sure that patient is comfortable and in proper body alignment.	Allows you to use proper body mechanics and prevents injury during restraint application. Positioning prevents contractures and neurovascular injury while restraint is in place.
2. Inspect area where restraint is to be placed. Note whether there is any nearby tubing or device. Assess condition of skin, sensation, adequacy of circulation, and range of joint motion.	Restraints sometimes compress and interfere with functioning of devices or tubes. Assessment provides baseline to monitor patient's response to restraint.
3. Pad skin and bony prominences (as necessary) that will be under restraint.	Reduces friction and pressure from restraint to skin and underlying tissue.
4. Apply proper-sized restraint. **Note:** Refer to manufacturer directions.	
a. *Mitten restraint:* Thumbless mitten device restrains patient's hands. Place hand in mitten, being sure that Velcro strap is around wrist and not forearm (see Step 4a illustration).	Prevents patient from dislodging or removing medical device, removing dressings, or scratching but allows greater movement than wrist restraint. It is considered a restraint alternative if untethered and patient is physically and cognitively able to remove it.
b. *Elbow restraint (freedom splint):* Restraint consists of rigidly padded fabric that wraps around arm and is closed with Velcro. The upper end has a clamp that hooks to sleeve of patient's gown or shirt (see Step 4b illustration). Insert arm so elbow joint rests against padded area, keeping joint extended.	Commonly used with infants and children to prevent elbow flexion (e.g., with IV line placed in antecubital fossa). Restraint keeps elbow extended, making it difficult to remove or disrupt a medical device.
c. *Belt or body restraint:* Have patient in sitting position in bed. Apply belt over clothes, gown, or pyjamas. Be sure to place restraint at waist, not chest or abdomen. Slot in belt may be positioned in front for limited movement or rear for increased movement. Remove wrinkles or creases in clothing. Bring ties through slots in belt. Help patient lie down in bed. Have patient roll to side, and avoid applying belt too tightly. Ensure that straps secured to bedframe are snug so that belt does not slide to sides of bed (see Step 4c[a] illustrations). *Option:* Apply restraint net if intent is to limit patient turning (see Step 4c, illustration *B*).	Restrains centre of gravity and prevents patient from rolling off stretcher, sitting up while on stretcher, or falling out of bed. Tight application interferes with ventilation if belt moves up over abdomen or chest.
d. *Extremity (ankle or wrist) restraint:* Restraint made of soft quilted material or sheepskin with foam padding. Wrap limb restraint around wrist or ankle with soft part toward skin and secure snugly (not tightly) in place by Velcro strap (see Step 4d, illustration A). Insert two fingers under secured restraint (see Step 4d, illustration *B*).	Restraint is designed to immobilize one or all extremities. Maintains immobilization of extremity to protect patient from fall or accidental removal of therapeutic device (e.g., IV tube, Foley catheter). Tight application interferes with circulation and potentially causes neurovascular injury.

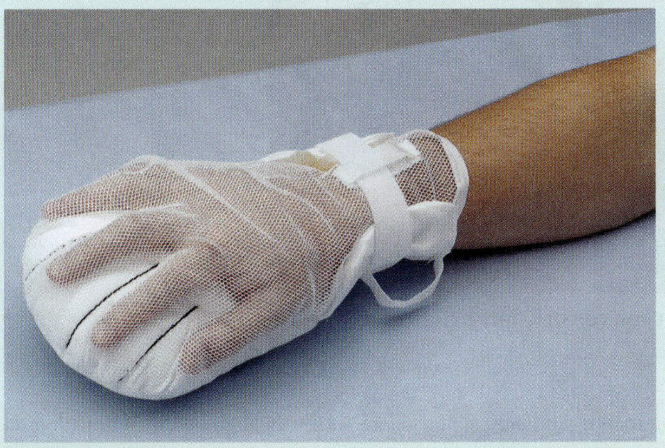

STEP 4A Mitten restraint. *(From Sorrentino, S. A., & Remmert, L. N. [2021]. Mosby's textbook for nursing assistants [10th ed.]. Elsevier.)*

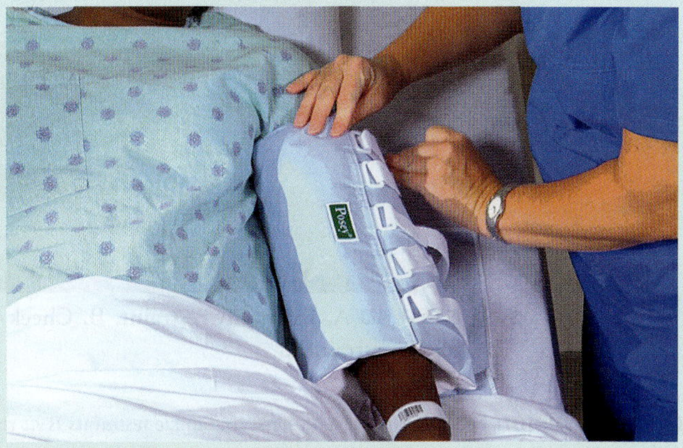

STEP 4B Freedom elbow restraint. *(Courtesy Posey Company, Arcadia, CA.)*

STEP	RATIONALE

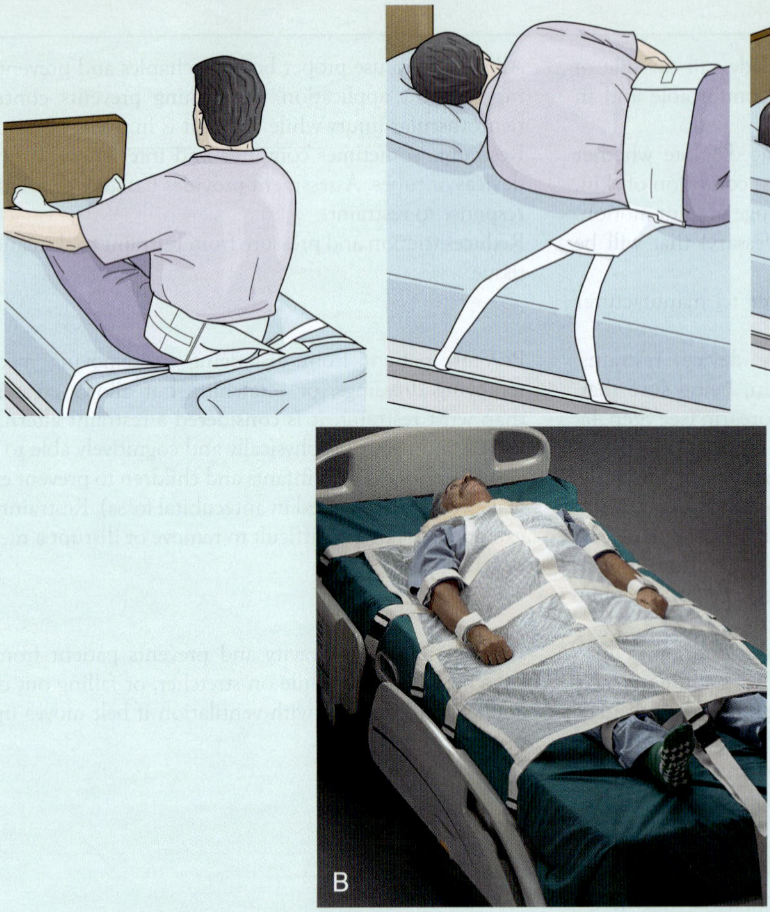

STEP 4C A, Properly applied belt restraint allows patient to turn in bed. B, Option: Restraint with net limits patient's ability to turn. *(A, From Sorrentino, S. A., & Remmert, L. N. [2021]. Mosby's textbook for nursing assistants [10th ed.]. Elsevier; B, Courtesy Posey Company, Arcadia, CA.)*

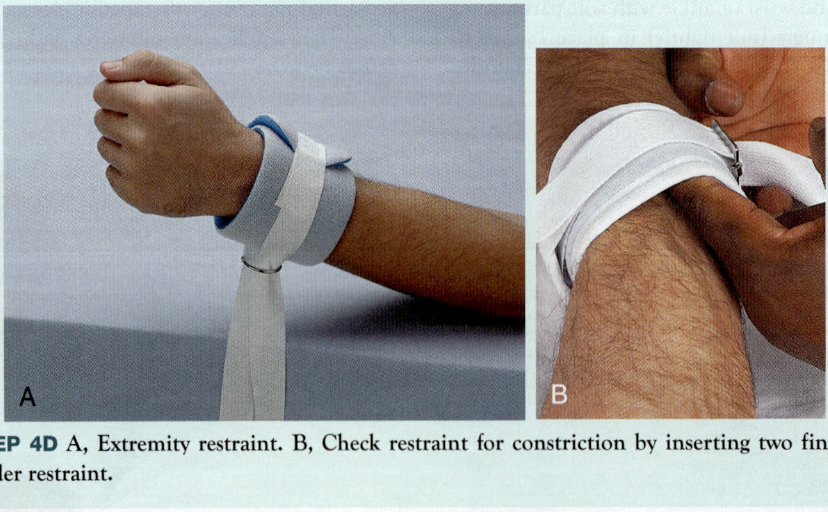

STEP 4D A, Extremity restraint. B, Check restraint for constriction by inserting two fingers under restraint.

Critical Decision Point *Patient with wrist and ankle restraints is at risk for aspiration if positioned supine. Place patient in lateral position or with head of bed elevated rather than supine.*

STEP	RATIONALE
5. Attach restraint straps to part of bed frame that moves when raising or lowering head of bed. Be sure that straps are secure. *Do not attach to side rails.* Attach restraint to chair frame for patient in chair or wheelchair, being sure that buckle is out of patient's reach.	Properly positioned strap does not tighten and restrict circulation when bed is raised or lowered.

STEP	RATIONALE
6. Secure restraints on bed frame with quick-release buckle (see Step 6 illustration). *Do not tie strap into a knot.* Be sure that buckle is out of patient reach.	Allows for quick release in emergency.

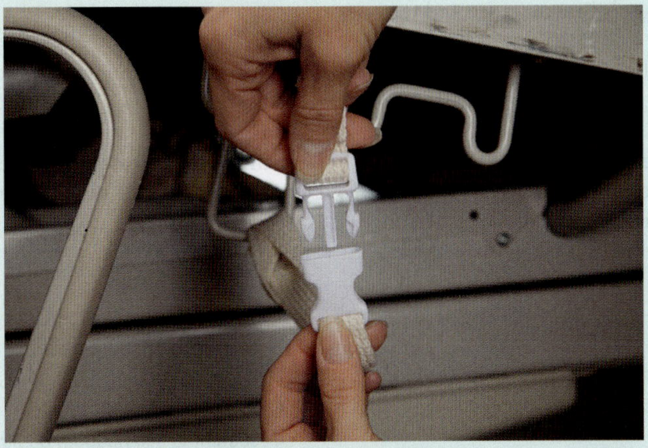

STEP 6 Quick-release buckle makes it easier to disconnect and evacuate patients in an emergency.

STEP	RATIONALE
7. Double-check and insert two fingers under secured restraint one more time. Assess proper placement of restraint, including skin integrity, pulses, skin temperature and colour, and sensation of restrained body part.	Provides baseline to later evaluate if injury develops from restraint.
8. Assess patient and remove restraint during hourly rounding or more frequently, as determined by employer policy. Reposition patient, provide comfort, assess patient need for elimination, and evaluate patient condition each time. If patient is violent or noncompliant, remove one restraint at a time or have staff assistance while removing restraints.	Provides opportunity to attend to patient's basic needs and determine need for continuation.

Critical Decision Point *Do not leave a patient who is violent or aggressive unattended while restraints are off.*

STEP	RATIONALE
9. Secure call-light or intercom system within patient's reach.	Allows patient, family, or caregiver to get help quickly.
10. Leave bed or chair with wheels locked. Keep bed in lowest position.	Prevents bed or chair from moving if patient tries to get out. If patient falls with bed in lowest position, this reduces chance of injury.

EVALUATION

1. After application, evaluate patient for signs of injury every 15–30 minutes (check employer policy) (e.g., circulation, vital signs, ROM, physical and psychological status, and readiness for discontinuation).	Frequent evaluation prevents injury to patient and ensures removal of restraint at earliest possible time. Frequency of monitoring guides staff in determining appropriate intervals for evaluation based on patient's needs and condition, type of restraint used, risk associated with use of chosen intervention, and other relevant factors.
2. Evaluate patient's need for elimination, nutrition and fluids, and hygiene, and release restraint at hourly rounding.	Prevents injury to patient and attends to basic needs.
3. Evaluate patient for any complications of immobility.	Early detection of skin irritation, restricted breathing, or reduction in mobility prevents serious adverse events.

STEP	RATIONALE
4. Evaluate patient within 1–4 hours after initiation of restraints (depending on employer policy).	Determines patient's immediate situation, reaction to restraints, medical and behavioural condition, and need to continue or terminate restraints.
5. After 24 hours, before writing a new prescription, health care provider who is responsible for patient's care must see and reassess patient.	Ensures that restraint application continues to be medically appropriate.
6. Observe IV catheters, urinary catheters, and drainage tubes to ensure that they are positioned correctly and that therapy remains uninterrupted.	Reinsertion is uncomfortable and increases risk for infection or interrupts therapy.
7. Observe patient's behaviour and reaction to presence of restraint.	Restraints can increase restlessness and agitation, resulting in harm.
8. Use teach-back: "We've talked about the reason we're using restraints on your father. Tell me that reason. I want to be sure you understand." Develop a revised plan if caregiver is unable to teach back correctly.	Determines caregiver's level of understanding of instructional topic.

Unexpected Outcomes	Related Interventions
1. Patient experiences impaired skin integrity.	• Evaluate need for continued use of restraint and if alternatives can be used. • If restraint is still needed, be sure that it is applied correctly and provide adequate padding. • Check skin under restraint for abrasions and remove restraints more often. Provide appropriate skin care and change wet or soiled restraints.
2. Patient becomes more confused or agitated.	• Determine cause of behaviour and eliminate if possible; consult with health care provider. • Determine need for more or less sensory stimulation and make any stimulation meaningful. • Reorient as needed and try restraint-free options.
3. Patient has neurovascular injury (e.g., cyanosis, pallor, and coldness of skin or subjective symptoms of tingling, pain, or numbness).	• Remove restraint immediately, stay with patient, and have health care provider notified. • Protect extremity from further injury.

Communication and Documentation

- Document nursing interventions and restraint alternatives tried on restraint flow sheet or in progress notes in EHR or chart.
- Document your evaluation of caregiver learning.
- Document purpose for restraint, type and location, time applied, time restraint ended, and routine observations made every 15 minutes (e.g., skin colour, pulses, sensation, vital signs, behaviour) in flow sheets or progress notes.
- Document patient's level of orientation and behaviour after restraint application. Document times patient was evaluated, attempts to use alternatives, and patient's response when restraint was removed.

DOCUMENTATION EXAMPLE

Patient remains in 5-point restraints as prescribed because of risk of physical violence to self and others. Continues to be agitated, thrashing about on stretcher and yelling/threatening staff. Security present for 1:1 safety watch. Restraint use assessed. Patient able to move all 4 limbs spontaneously and on command. Circulation, sensation, movement (CSM) intact for all 4 limbs. Restraints secure. Vital signs attempted. Patient refusing vital signs; alert and orientated, breathing spontaneously at a rate of 20 breaths/min, speech clear. Skin warm, pink, and dry. Pupils appear equal. Will trial a release of a restraint once agitation decreases. Behavioural reassessment completed.

Special Considerations

Teaching

- Explain thoroughly to patient and caregiver the use of restraints. Caution caregiver against removing, repositioning, or retying restraint.

Pediatric

- Limit the use of restraints to clinically appropriate and adequately justified situations (e.g., examination or treatment that involves the head and neck) after exhausting all appropriate alternatives. Remain with infant while restrained and remove restraint immediately after treatment is completed.
- When a child needs to be restrained for a procedure, it is best if the person applying the restraint is not the child's parent or guardian.
- When an infant or small child requires a restraint, a mummy wrap using a blanket or sheet effectively controls their movements (Hockenberry et al., 2024).

Gerontological

- Restrained older persons often respond with anger, fear, depression, humiliation, demoralization, discomfort, and resignation.
- Consider the risks associated with restraints (e.g., pressure injuries, impaired strength and balance) for older persons (Boscart et al., 2023). All of the complications of immobility are amplified, leading to greater risk for functional decline.

Patients With Physical or Cognitive Challenges

- In general, patients who have physical and cognitive challenges can be restrained only to control behaviours that create an emergency or crisis situation.

Care in the Community: Home Management

- Much of the evidence available relating to the use of restraints has been derived from acute and chronic care facilities, not from the home setting. The caregiver has a different role in the home setting and more influence related to care decisions (Scheepmans et al., 2018).
- Caregivers should be educated about the importance of frequently checking on the patient when restraints are used in order to ensure safety. In home settings, restraints often involve use of equipment that is already in the person's home instead of professional equipment (e.g., placing a chair close to the table) (Scheepmans et al., 2018).

✦ SKILL 14.4 Seizure Precautions

The incidence of Canadians living with epilepsy has risen, likely owing to increased rates of diagnosis and decreased mortality. Epilepsy is a brain disorder where abnormal bursts of electrical activity result in seizures (Public Health Agency of Canada, 2019). *Seizures* are the sudden, abnormal, uncontrolled electrical discharge of neurons in the brain that interfere with normal function (Tyerman & Cobbett, 2023). Seizures are classified as focal, generalized, or unknown onset (Pack, 2019). The International League Against Epilepsy revised the operational classification of seizure types to adopt more transparent names when classifying seizures (Pack, 2019):

- **Focal onset**—Patient may be aware or have impaired awareness; motor versus nonmotor onset; focal aware seizure (prior term *simple partial seizure*); focal impaired awareness seizure (prior term *complex partial seizure*); focal to bilateral tonic-clonic (prior term *partial onset with secondary generalization*); hyperkinetic seizure (agitated thrashing or leg pedalling movements); focal seizures can have emotional manifestations (e.g., fear, joy).
- **Generalized onset**—Can be motor (e.g., tonic-clonic) or nonmotor (absence); myoclonic-tonic-clonic seizure is common in juvenile epilepsy.
- **Unknown onset**—Can be motor (e.g., tonic-clonic) or nonmotor; referred to as an unclassified seizure and can include additional features (e.g., tonic-clonic, epileptic spasms, behaviour arrest). An unknown onset seizure may later become classified as a focal or generalized seizure.

Prolonged seizures last between 5 and 30 minutes, whereas status epilepticus is defined as 30 minutes or more of continuous clinical or electrographic (shown on an electroencephalogram [EEG]) seizure activity or multiple episodes with no recovery between seizures (Madhiyazhagan, 2021). Once a seizure lasts more than 5 minutes, it is recommended that treatment protocols be initiated to minimize the risk of permanent damage (Madhiyazhagan, 2021). It is a critical care emergency. Status epilepticus can be convulsive (rhythmic jerking of the extremities), nonconvulsive (activity on EEG), or repetitive focal motor signs not associated with altered awareness.

Traditionally, patients who have a seizure are immediately placed in the side-lying semi-prone position to prevent aspiration of oral secretions (Crawshaw & Cock, 2020). This approach is still a standard of practice. Refer to employer policy for positioning guidelines.

The current practice guidelines for patients with status epilepticus include the following (Madhiyazhagan, 2021; Tyerman & Cobbett, 2023):

- Ensure patent airway when patient loses consciousness.
- Provide noninvasive airway protection and gas exchange with head positioning, keeping the airway patent and administering oxygen (see Chapters 23 and 25).
- Monitor vital signs, level of consciousness, oxygen saturation, Glasgow Coma Scale, and pupil size and reactivity, according to employer policy.
- Establish an IV route for emergency medications.
- When seizure begins to subside, intubation (insertion of an artificial airway) should be attempted only if gas exchange is compromised or if patient is believed to have increased intracranial pressure; never force an airway between a patient's clenched teeth.
- Administer IV dextrose if patient is hypoglycemic.

Delegation and Collaboration

The skill of assessing a patient's risk for seizures cannot be delegated to a UCP. However, the skills for making a patient's environment safe and the ongoing care of patients on seizure precautions can be delegated. The nurse directs the UCP about the following:

- The patient's prior seizure history and factors that may trigger a seizure
- Taking immediate action in the event of a seizure by protecting the patient from falling or injury, not trying to restrain the patient, and not placing anything into the mouth
- Informing the nurse immediately when seizure activity develops
- Observing the patient's seizure pattern

Equipment

- Seizure pads for side rails and headboard
- Suction machine and oral Yankauer suction catheter
- Oral airway
- Oxygen via nasal cannula or face mask
- Equipment for vital signs, pulse oximetry, and blood glucose testing (see Chapter 7)
- Equipment for IV insertion (see Chapter 29)
- Emergency antiepileptic medications:
  - For emergent conditions, benzodiazepines such as IV lorazepam, midazolam for intramuscular (IM) administration (also nasal or buccal), rectal diazepam; for urgent treatment, oral valproate sodium or phenytoin, IV midazolam terminate seizures with fewer adverse effects (Madhiyazhagan, 2021)
  - Clean gloves
  - Equipment for vital signs, pulse oximetry, and blood glucose monitoring

STEP	RATIONALE

ASSESSMENT

STEP	RATIONALE
1. Identify patient using at least two person-specific identifiers (e.g., name and date of birth, or name and medical record number) according to employer policy.	Ensures correct patient. Complies with Accreditation Canada's standards and improves patient safety (Accreditation Canada, 2020).
2. Throughout the procedure, the 4 moments for hand hygiene are to be implemented; hand hygiene should occur before initial patient (or patient environment) contact, before an aseptic procedure, after body fluid exposure risk, and after patient (or patient environment) contact. Additional hand hygiene should be performed when hands are visibly soiled.	Proper hand hygiene helps prevent the spread of infectious agents to health care providers.
3. Assess patient's seizure history (e.g., new diagnosis, seizure within last year), knowledge of precipitating factors (e.g., emotional stress, sleep deprivation), frequency of seizures, presence of aura (e.g., metallic taste, perception of breeze blowing on face, or noxious odour), body parts affected, and sequence of events if known. Use family as resource if necessary.	Knowledge about seizure history and nature of seizures allows you to eliminate triggers that cause seizure, anticipate onset of seizure activity, and take appropriate safety measures.
4. Assess for medical and surgical conditions, including history of head trauma, electrolyte disturbances (e.g., hypoglycemia, hyperkalemia), heart disease, excess fatigue, and alcohol or caffeine consumption. Also assess for any bleeding tendencies.	Common conditions that lead to seizures or worsen existing seizure condition. Bleeding conditions could predispose patient to injury during seizure.
5. Assess medication history (e.g., antidepressants and antipsychotics). Assess for patient's adherence to anticonvulsants and therapeutic medication levels if test results are available.	Certain medications lower seizure threshold. Seizure medications must be taken as prescribed and not stopped suddenly. Stopping or changing dose may precipitate seizure activity.
6. Inspect patient's environment for potential safety hazards (e.g., extra furniture or equipment). Keep bed in low position, side rails up at head of bed.	Protects patient from injury sustained by striking head or body on furniture or equipment.
7. Assess patient's individual and cultural perspective about the meaning of seizures and their treatment.	Demonstrates person-centred care. Some cultures may follow different caring practices for a person with seizures.

NURSING DIAGNOSES

- Nonadherence
- Insufficient knowledge regarding seizure precautions
- Potential for aspiration
- Potential for injury
- Potential for inadequate airway clearance
- Reduced self-concept

Related factors and risk factors are individualized on the basis of patient's condition or needs.

PLANNING

STEP	RATIONALE
1. Expected outcomes following completion of procedure:	
• Patient remains free of traumatic injury while experiencing seizure.	Seizure precautions prevent patients from incurring injury from a fall or seizure.
• Patient's airway remains patent during seizure activity.	Airway occlusion and aspiration are potential complications of seizure activity.
• Patient does not experience lowered sense of self-concept following seizure episode.	Loss of bowel or bladder control is common in generalized seizures, causing patient to feel embarrassment or shame.
2. Inform patient and appropriate caregiver that patient is on seizure precautions.	May help to relieve patient and caregiver anxiety.

STEP	RATIONALE

IMPLEMENTATION

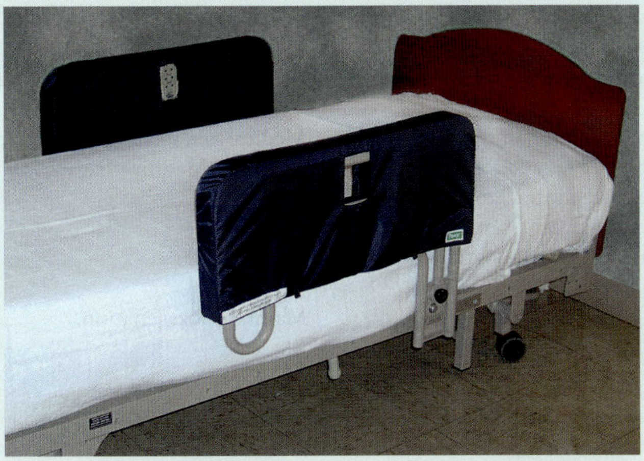

STEP 1 Padded side rails for patients at risk for head injury.

STEP	RATIONALE
1. For patients with history of seizures, keep bed in lowest position with side rails up (see employer policy). Pad rails if patient is at risk for head injury. Have oral suction and oxygen equipment ready for use.	Modifications to environment minimize risk of injury from seizure activity or related fall. Use padded side rails only when patient is at risk for head injury (see Step 1 illustration).
2. Place patient with history of seizures in room close to nurse's station or room with video monitor.	Improves likelihood of quick response with emergency equipment.
3. Focal or generalized seizure response.	
a. Position patient safely.	
(1) If patient is standing or sitting, guide them to floor and protect head by cradling it in your lap or place pillow under head. Position patient to keep head tilted to maximize breathing (if able). Try to position patient on side *but do not force*. Do not lift patient from floor to bed during seizure.	Position protects patient from aspiration and traumatic injury, especially head injury.
(2) If patient is in bed, turn them onto side (*do not force*) and raise side rails.	
b. Note time seizure began and call for help immediately to have staff member bring emergency cart to bedside and clear surrounding area of furniture. Provide airway protection and gas exchange by positioning head. Have health care provider notified immediately.	Timing and description of seizure may help in ultimate identification of type of seizure. Establishing and protecting airway when patient loses consciousness must occur immediately (Pack, 2019).
c. Keep patient in side-lying position (if possible), supporting head and keeping it flexed slightly forward.	Position prevents tongue from blocking airway and promotes drainage of secretions, reducing risk of aspiration.
d. Do not restrain patient; if patient is flailing limbs, hold them loosely. Loosen restrictive clothing or gown to aid breathing.	Prevents musculoskeletal injury. Promotes free ventilatory movement of chest and abdomen.
e. *Never force any object into patient's mouth*, such as fingers, medicine, tongue depressor, or airway, when teeth are clenched.	Prevents injury to mouth and possible aspiration.

Critical Decision Point *Injury can result from forcible insertion of a hard object into patient's mouth. Soft objects break and become aspirated. Insert a bite block or oral airway in advance if you recognize the possibility of a generalized seizure.*

STEP	RATIONALE
f. If possible, provide privacy. Have staff control flow of visitors in area.	Embarrassment is common after a seizure, especially if others witnessed it.
g. Observe sequence and timing of seizure activity. Note type of seizure activity (tonic, clonic, staring, blinking); whether more than one type of seizure occurs; level of consciousness; character of breathing; presence of incontinence; presence of autonomic signs of lip smacking, mastication, or grimacing; rolling of eyes.	Continued observation helps to document, diagnose, and treat seizure disorder.

STEP	RATIONALE
h. As patient regains consciousness, assess vital signs and reorient and reassure them. Explain what happened and answer patient's questions. Stay with patient until fully awake.	Informing patients of type of seizure activity experienced helps them to participate knowledgeably in their care. Some patients remain confused for a period of time after seizure or become violent.
4. Status epilepticus is a critical care emergency.	
a. Follow Steps 3a–3c to stabilize airway and call emergency team.	Ensures rapid response and management of airway and breathing.
b. Assist health care provider with intubation (introduction of endotracheal tube or oral airway) (see Chapter 23) if oxygen saturation is compromised or elevated intracranial pressure is suspected. (NOTE: Apply clean gloves if timing allows.) Health care provider on team will intubate patient when jaw is relaxed (between seizure activity).	Medical emergency requires rapid response. Airway establishes oxygenation (Madhiyazhagan, 2021; Pack, 2019).
c. Access and administer oxygen; turn on suction equipment; keep airway patent with oral suctioning (if possible).	Maintains oxygenation.

Critical Decision Point *Never place hands in patient's mouth during a seizure. The patient may accidently bite your fingers. Do not force any type of airway into mouth.*

STEP	RATIONALE
d. Have another nurse on team monitor vital signs and oxygen saturation according to employer policy, and have team member perform fingerstick to check blood glucose (Madhiyazhagan, 2021).	Necessary to monitor and support baseline vital signs and determine whether patient is hypoglycemic (common cause of seizure).
e. Member of team will prepare for and insert IV catheter (if one is not in place) with 0.9% sodium chloride infusing and administer IV antiseizure medications (see Chapter 29).	Provides route for IV medication to stop seizure and for fluid resuscitation (Madhiyazhagan, 2021).
f. As seizure begins to subside, suction patient's airway if secretions have accumulated. If oral airway was inserted, be sure that it remains in correct position. Continue oxygen administration.	Maintains open airway and oxygenation.
g. Keep patient in side-lying position of comfort in bed with side rails up and bed in lowest position.	Provides for continued safety to reduce risk for aspiration of secretions as patient regains consciousness and lessens risk for fall with injury if patient tries to exit bed.
5. As patient regains consciousness, reorient and reassure them. Explain what happened and provide quiet, nonstimulating environment (e.g., lights low, minimal care interruptions). Place call-light or intercom system within reach. Instruct patient not to get out of bed without help.	Provides for continued safety. Patients are often confused and lethargic following seizure. They are at risk for falls if they attempt to get out of bed.
6. Clean up patient care area; dispose of used supplies.	Reduces transmission of microorganisms.

EVALUATION

1. Check vital signs and oxygen saturation every 15 minutes post-seizure and maintain patent airway.	Determines patient's cardiopulmonary status and response to seizure episode.
2. Recheck blood glucose per health care provider prescription.	Determines whether normal blood glucose level has been reached.
3. Examine patient for injury, including oral cavity (broken teeth, laceration of tongue or mucosa) and extremities.	Determines presence of any traumatic injuries resulting from seizure activity.

Critical Decision Point *If onset of seizure was not witnessed and you suspect that patient fell and struck head, treat as a closed head injury or spinal injury. Place a cervical collar on patient before attempting to turn or reposition.*

4. Evaluate patient's mental status after seizure (level of consciousness, confusion, hallucinations). Encourage them to verbalize feelings.	Temporary mental status changes are common following seizure. Therapeutic interaction enables patient to recognize feelings associated with having a seizure disorder.
5. Help health care provider as needed conduct neurological examination of patient and collect any ordered blood tests (see Chapter 9).	Evaluates for potentially life-threatening metabolic alterations (Tyerman & Cobbett, 2023).

Unexpected Outcomes	Related Interventions
1. Patient suffers traumatic injury.	• Continue to protect patient from further injury. • Notify health care provider immediately. • Administer prescribed treatments. • Reassess patient's environment to ensure that environment is free of safety hazards. • Complete required employer documentation.
2. Patient aspirates oral secretions.	• Turn onto side, insert oral airway (if possible; see Chapter 23), and apply suction to remove material in oral pharynx and maintain patent airway. • Administer oxygen as needed per order.

Communication and Documentation

- Document in progress notes in EHR or chart what you observed before, during, and after seizure. Provide detailed description of the type of seizure activity and sequence of events (e.g., motor activity, level of consciousness, vital signs and oxygen saturation, colour, movement of extremities, incontinence, patient's status immediately following seizure, and time frame of events).
- Document treatments administered: establishment of IV line, fluid infusing, stabilization of airway.
- Alert health care provider immediately as seizure begins. Status epilepticus is a critical care emergency that requires immediate interprofessional collaboration.

DOCUMENTATION EXAMPLE

Patient heard to be making inaudible sounds, altered level of consciousness with shaking involving all extremities witnessed by writer. Pillows placed alongside rails to minimize potential for patient injury. Oxygen applied per health care prescription to maintain O_2 sat levels. Patient incontinent of urine. Bed linens changed and personal care provided to patient. Vital signs obtained following seizure were within normal limits; continuously monitoring airway. Head to toe assessment completed. PERRLA, patient alert and oriented, moving all limbs spontaneously, and verbalizing they feel tired.

Special Considerations

Teaching

- Inform an adult with an unprovoked first seizure that their seizure recurrence risk is greatest early within the first 2 years (21–45%). The patient's health care provider is likely to prescribe immediate antiepileptic drug (AED) therapy to reduce recurrence risk within the first 2 years (Perucca et al., 2018).
- Patients need to know that antiseizure medications help control epilepsy. Warn them to take prescribed medications regularly. They should never stop medications suddenly because this precipitates seizures.
- Advise patient to avoid alcohol, which is often incompatible with anticonvulsive medications and intensifies central nervous system depression.
- Proper oral hygiene and frequent dental care are necessary when patient takes phenytoin long term because gingival hyperplasia is an adverse effect.
- Encourage patient to wear a medical alert bracelet or carry identification card noting presence of seizure disorder and listing medications taken.
- Fatigue, stress, and illness can potentiate seizures. Teach patients to eat a balanced diet regularly, get adequate sleep, and consult their health care provider promptly when ill.
- A seizure disorder usually imposes driving limitations. It is recommended that a waiting period of 6–12 seizure-free months elapse before patient attempts to drive or operate dangerous equipment (refer to specific provincial/territorial law).

Pediatric

- Teach parents what to observe for in their child's seizure.
- Child should wear a medical alert bracelet noting presence of a seizure disorder.
- Encourage children with severe atonic seizures (abrupt loss of muscle tone, often dropping to floor) to wear helmets to protect them when they fall.

Gerontological

- Older persons often have symptoms that make it difficult to recognize a seizure disorder. Confusion lasting several days, receptive and expressive speech problems, and unusual behaviours are often the result of a seizure.
- Older persons metabolize some antiseizure medications more slowly, allowing medications to accumulate and possibly result in toxicity. Consult a pharmacist for specific information.
- If patient has dentures, do not try to remove them during a seizure. If they loosen, tilt head slightly forward and remove after seizure.

Care in the Community: Home Management

- Instruct caregiver about steps to take when patient experiences a seizure.
- Complete a fall risk assessment in the patient's home to decrease the potential for injury in the event of a fall.
- Until a seizure condition is well controlled (usually for at least 1 year), make sure that patient does not take a tub bath or engage in activities such as swimming unless another person is present.
- Refer patient to Epilepsy Canada or a community resource for support groups.

Procedural Guideline 14.1 *Fire, Electrical, and Chemical Safety*

Surgical safety checklists mitigate preventable patient harm relative to intraoperative procedures, including surgical fires. Sentinel events involving fire are typically electrical or anaesthetic related and are not limited to the operating room setting (Cramer et al., 2020). Smoking-related fires pose a significant risk because of unauthorized smoking in beds or bathrooms. Healthcare Excellence Canada's (2015) "never event" list includes "patient death or serious harm due to an accidental burn" (p. 7) from oxygen fires; unintended burns occurring during surgery; and heat or cold burns from assisted bathing, the use of hot or cold packs, and wound care. In the home setting, oxygen-related fires are a risk for patients requiring oxygen therapy (see Chapter 23). Health care facilities routinely check and maintain all electrical devices. Every biomedical device (e.g., suction machine, infusion pump) must have a safety inspection sticker with an expiration date applied to it. Electrical equipment in good working order requires a three-prong electrical plug for proper grounding. If a patient brings an electrical device to a hospital, an engineer must inspect the device for safe wiring and function before use. Always discourage patients from bringing nonessential electrical devices (e.g., hair dryers or electric toothbrushes) into a health care facility. Many patients living with physical challenges use battery chargers for mobility equipment function. These devices need to be inspected by hospital engineers as well. Prevention is the key to fire safety. Always comply with employer smoking policies, use equipment correctly, and keep combustible materials away from heat sources.

Chemicals in many medications (e.g., chemotherapy medications), anaesthetic gases, cleaning solutions, and disinfectants are potentially toxic. They injure the body after skin or mucous membrane (e.g., eyes) contact, ingestion, or vapour inhalation. The Workplace Hazardous Materials Information System (WHMIS) (Health Canada, 2022b) regulates hazard classification and requirements for labels and safety data sheets (SDS) (previously called *material safety data sheets*) for each hazardous chemical in the workplace. An SDS form contains information about the properties of the particular chemical and handling the substance in a safe manner (Table 14.1).

Delegation and Collaboration

The skill of fire, electrical, and chemical safety can be delegated to a UCP. Interprofessional collaboration is a priority in an emergency situation. In the event of fire, collaborate with the fire department; in an electrical or chemical event, collaborate with the safety officer of the facility. The nurse directs the UCP to do the following:

- Identify patients requiring the most help to evacuate or protect
- Be aware of any risks for chemical exposure

Equipment

Fire

- Appropriate fire extinguisher for fire: type A, B, C, or ABC

Chemical

- Appropriate personal protective equipment (PPE): Clean gloves, mask, gown
- SDS form

Procedural Steps

1. Review employer policies for rapid response to fire, electrical, and chemical emergency. Know your responsibilities, such as initiating fire alarm and patient evacuation.
2. Know the location of fire alarms, emergency equipment (e.g., fire extinguishers), SDS forms, emergency eyewash stations, and emergency exit routes.
3. Assess patient's mental status and ability to ambulate, transfer, or move to anticipate the procedures that will be needed to evacuate the patient.
4. Be alert to situations that increase the risk of fire (e.g., a patient on oxygen charging a cell phone while in bed). Regularly check a patient room for electrical or fire hazards.
5. Know which patients are on oxygen. Oxygen delivery may be shut off in the event of a severe fire.
6. Inspect equipment for current maintenance sticker. Check electrical equipment for basic safety features (i.e., intact cords and plugs, intact casing). Know employer process for tagging and reporting broken or unsafe equipment.
7. **Fire safety:**
   a. Follow the acronym *RACE:*
      (1) **R**escue patient from immediate injury by removing from area or shielding from fire to avoid burns.
      (2) **A**ctivate fire alarm immediately. Follow employer policy for alerting staff to respond. (In many situations perform steps 1 and 2 simultaneously by using call system to alert staff while you help patients at risk.)
      (3) **C**ontain the fire by:
         (a) Closing all doors and windows
         (b) Turning off oxygen and electrical equipment
         (c) Placing wet towels along base of doors
      (4) **E**vacuate patients:
         (a) Direct ambulatory patients to walk by themselves to a safe area. Know the fire exits and emergency evacuation route.
         (b) If patient is on life support, maintain respiratory status manually (bag-valve mask) until patient is removed from fire area.
         (c) Move bed-bound patients by stretcher, bed, or wheelchair.
         (d) For patients who cannot walk or ambulate, use these options:
            (i) Place on blanket and drag patient out of area of danger.
            (ii) Use two-person swing: Place patient in sitting position and have two staff members form a seat by clasping forearms together. Lift patient into "seat" and carry out of area of danger (see Step 7a[4][d][ii], illustrations A and *B*).

Procedural Guideline 14.1 *Fire, Electrical, and Chemical Safety—cont'd*

Critical Decision Point *Consider the patient's weight and size when choosing an evacuation carry. Use safe patient-handling techniques. Have a staff member help to avoid injury.*

(e) If fire department personnel are on the scene, they will help with evacuation of patients.

b. Extinguish fire using appropriate fire extinguisher: type A for ordinary combustibles (e.g., wood, cloth, paper, most plastics); type B for flammable liquids (e.g., gasoline, grease, paint, anaesthetic gas); type C for electrical equipment; type ABC for any type of fire (most common extinguisher in use). To use an extinguisher, follow the acronym *PASS*:

(1) **P**ull the pin (see Step 7b[1], illustration *A*).
(2) **A**im nozzle at base of fire (see Step 7b[1], illustration *B*).
(3) **S**queeze extinguisher handles (see Step 7b[1], illustration *C*).
(4) **S**weep from side to side to coat area evenly.

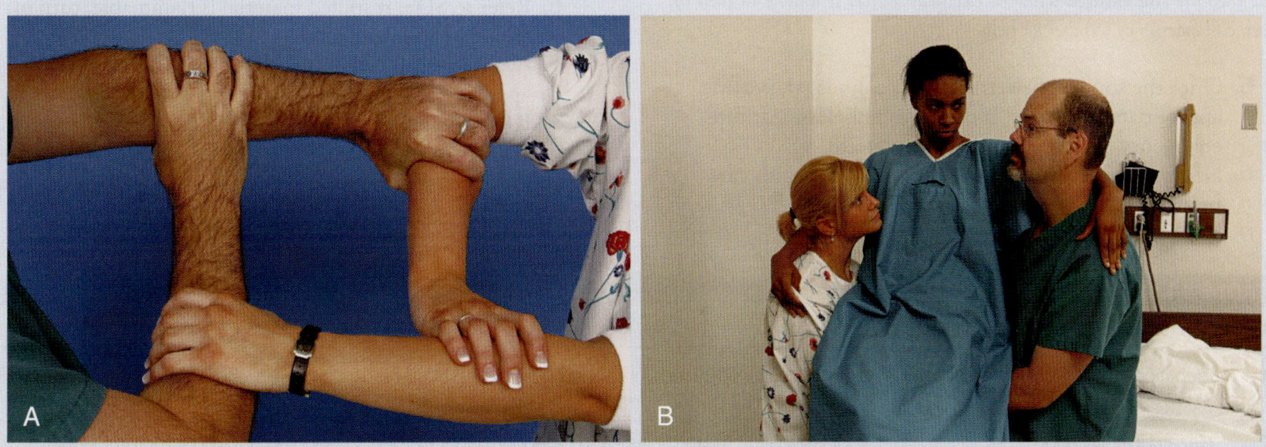

STEP 7A(4)(D)(II) A, Hands positioned to form two-person evacuation swing. B, Patient seated firmly on swing and holding shoulders of nurses for evacuation.

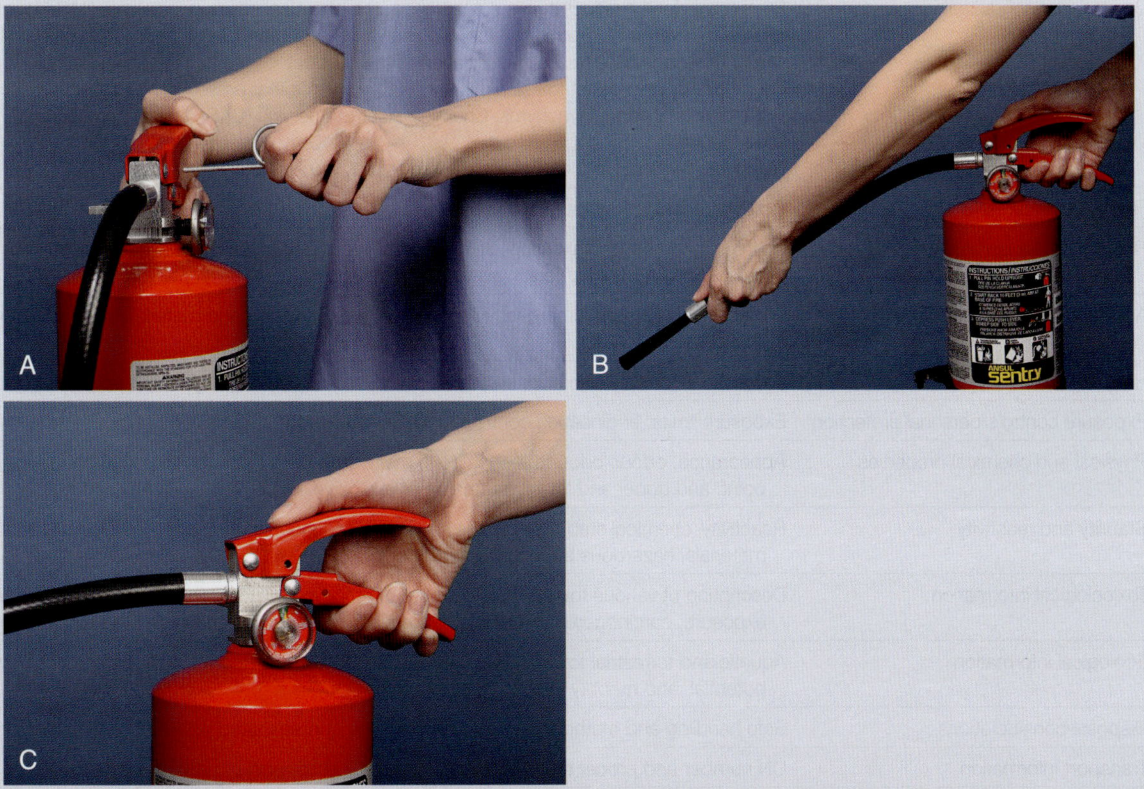

STEP 7B(1) A, Pull safety pin from fire extinguisher. B, Aim nozzle of hose at base of fire. C, Squeeze handle while sweeping side to side with nozzle.

Continued

Procedural Guideline 14.1 *Fire, Electrical, and Chemical Safety—cont'd*

c. Most facilities have fire doors that are held open by magnets and close automatically when a fire alarm sounds. Fire doors should never be blocked.

8. **Electrical safety:**
   a. If patient receives an electrical shock, immediately turn off power to electrical source and assess for presence of a pulse. *Caution:* When disengaging electrical source, check for presence of water on floor.

Critical Decision Point *Do not touch a person who is being shocked while they are still engaged with the electrical source. If unable to turn off power, call emergency number for help.*

   b. Once the source of electricity is disconnected, provide appropriate assistance. If patient is pulseless, institute emergency resuscitation (see Chapter 28).
   c. Notify emergency personnel and patient's health care provider.
   d. If patient has a pulse and remains alert and oriented, obtain vital signs and assess the skin for signs of thermal injury.
9. **Chemical safety:**
   a. Attend to any person exposed to a chemical. Treat chemical splashes to the eyes immediately; flush eyes using clean, lukewarm tap water for 15–20 minutes; stand under a shower or place head under running faucet. Remove contact lenses if flushing does not remove them (see Chapter 19).
   b. Notify people in the immediate area of the spill and evacuate all nonessential personnel from area.
   c. Refer to SDS; if spilled material is flammable, turn off electrical and heat sources.
   d. Avoid breathing vapours of spilled material; apply appropriate respirator.
   e. Use appropriate PPE (refer to SDS) to clean up a spill.
   f. Dispose of any materials used in cleanup as hazardous waste.
10. Follow employer policy for reporting any fire and document accordingly.

TABLE 14.1

Safety Data Sheets Requirement Summary

1	Identification	Product identifier, recommended use and restrictions on use, supplier contact information, emergency phone number
2	Hazard identification	Classification (hazard class and category), label elements (including hazard pictogram, signal word, hazard statement, and precautionary statements) and other hazards (e.g., thermal hazards)
3	Composition/ingredients information	For a hazardous product that is a substance: the chemical name, synonyms, CAS No. and the chemical name of impurities, stabilizing solvents, and stabilizing additives where classified and that contribute to the classification of the product For a hazardous product that is a mixture: for ingredients that present a health hazard, the chemical name, synonyms, Chemical Abstract Service (CAS) registry number, and concentration **Note:** Confidential business information rules may apply.
4	First aid measures	First aid measures by route of exposure as well as most important symptoms or effects
5	Firefighting measures	Suitable (and unsuitable) extinguishing media, specific hazards, special equipment, and precautions for fire fighters
6	Accidental release measures	Protective equipment, emergency procedures, and methods and materials for containment and cleanup
7	Handling and storage	Precautions for safe handling, conditions for storage, including any incompatibilities
8	Exposure controls/personal protection	Exposure limits, engineering controls, and personal protective equipment
9	Physical and chemical properties	Appearance, odour, odour threshold, pH, melting/freezing point, boiling point and range, flash point, and upper and lower flammable or explosive limits
10	Stability and reactivity	Reactivity, chemical stability, possible hazardous reactions, conditions to avoid, incompatible materials, hazardous decomposition products
11	Toxicological information	Description of various toxic effects by route of entry, including effects of acute or chronic exposure, carcinogenicity, reproductive effects, and respiratory sensitization
12	Ecological information	Aquatic and terrestrial toxicity (if available), persistence and degradability, bioaccumulative potential, and mobility in soil
13	Disposal considerations	Safe handling and methods of disposal, including contaminated packaging
14	Transport information	UN number and proper shipping name, hazard classes, packing group
15	Regulatory information	Safety, health, and environmental regulations specific to the product
16	Other information	Other information, including date of the latest revision of the SDS

From Eversafe Media Inc. (2017). *WHMIS 2015 safety data sheets*. https://eversafetraining.com/whmis-2015-safety-data-sheets/

REVIEW QUESTIONS

A 72-year-old patient (he/him) was admitted to an acute medicine division. The patient has diabetes mellitus, heart disease, and arthritis and has been admitted for acute pneumonia. His home medications include an oral hypoglycemic (glyburide), a nonsteroidal anti-inflammatory drug (NSAID), and a laxative. He has symptoms of fever (39.4°C), productive cough with dark yellow mucus, and chest pain when breathing and coughing. His appetite has been poor. He has an intravenous (IV) line running with D_5NS at 80 mL/hr. He reports feeling very tired. The nurse observes that he is having difficulty standing up from the bed and needs help to walk to the nearby bedside commode. The health care provider schedules a colonoscopy to investigate the new development of blood in his stool and abdominal cramping. The patient is placed on nothing by mouth (NPO) status until after the colonoscopy. It has been 7 hours since the test was ordered, and the patient has not eaten.

Review Questions 1 to 3 relate to the case study presented here.

1. Identify the factors that place the patient at risk of falling and recommend three fall prevention strategies appropriate for this patient.
2. The nurse enters the room to find the patient lying in bed, unresponsive to verbal command, and exhibiting tonic and clonic movement of his extremities. What is the first step the nurse should take and why? What likely caused the seizure?
3. The patient begins to awaken from the seizure. He knows his name but is confused about the date and time. He asks, "What happened?" Blood glucose is 3.2 mmol/L. How would the nurse report the patient's clinical situation using SBAR (situation–background–assessment–recommendation)?
4. A 42-year-old patient is on an orthopedic floor following a compound fracture of the lower leg. The patient's leg is in a splint enclosed with an Ace bandage. The nurse enters the room and discovers fire in the bedside garbage can. Place in the correct order the following actions that should be taken by the nurse:
   1. The nurse turns off the oxygen source at the head of the bed.
   2. The nurse gets help from a staff member, transfers the patient into a wheelchair, and moves the patient to a different room.
   3. The nurse moves the patient's bed away from the garbage can.
   4. The nurse hits the emergency button in the room and instructs the unit clerk to report a fire emergency.
5. The nurse is caring for an older person with progressive dementia. The nurse is concerned about the patient's risk of wandering. Which of the following interventions would be appropriate for this patient? (*Select all that apply.*)
   1. Determine from family the patient's usual communication style and cues to indicate hunger or need to go to bathroom.
   2. Provide a diversional activity that family reports patient enjoys.
   3. Place patient in a bed enclosure.
   4. Use soft wrist restraints for the patient when restlessness increases.
   5. Control room temperature and reduce number of care routines.
6. A nurse is assessing an older patient who reports falling a month ago at home, with no injury sustained. Which of the following would the nurse assess about the previous fall? (*Select all that apply.*)
   1. The medications the patient is currently taking
   2. The location of the fall in the home
   3. The patient's medical conditions
   4. The activity the patient was engaged in just before the fall
   5. Whether the patient had dizziness or weakness just before falling

Visit the Evolve site for a complete list of answers to the Review Questions.

NEXT GENERATION NCLEX® (NGN)

For practice with answering exam questions related to unfolding NGN case studies, please consult the Next Generation NCLEX® (NGN)-Style Case Studies for Skills and Techniques on the Evolve website: http://evolve.elsevier.com/Canada/Perry/clinicalskills/

REFERENCES

Accreditation Canada. (2020). *Required organizational practices handbook.* https://physicians.nshealth.ca/resources/required-organizational-practices-2020-handbook

Alberta Health Services. (n.d.). *Preventing falls: Injury prevention and safety, information for health professionals.* https://www.albertahealthservices.ca/injprev/Page15787.aspx

American Psychiatric Association. (2016). Neurodevelopmental disorders. In *Diagnostic and statistical manual of mental disorders* (5th ed., text rev.). https://doi.org/10.1176/appi.books.9780890425787.x01_Neurodevelopmental_Disorders

Berry, S., & Kiel, D. (2022). Falls: Prevention in nursing care facilities and the hospital setting. *UpToDate.* https://www.uptodate.com/contents/falls-prevention-in-nursing-care-facilities-and-the-hospital-setting

Boscart, V., McCleary, L., Sheiban Taucar, L., et al. (2023). *Ebersole and Hess' gerontological nursing and healthy aging in Canada* (3rd ed.). Elsevier.

Bowden, V., Bradas, C., & McNett, M. (2019). Impact of level of nurse experience on falls in medical surgical units. *Journal of Nursing Management, 27*(4), 833–839. https://doi.org/10.1111/jonm.12742

Canadian Institute for Health Information (CIHI). (1996–2022). *Patient safety.* https://www.cihi.ca/en/patient-safety [Seminal Reference]

Canadian Institute for Health Information (CIHI). (2022). *Patient harm in Canadian hospitals? It does happen* [Infographic]. https://www.cihi.ca/en/patient-harm-in-canadian-hospitals-it-does-happen

Canadian Nurses Association. (2017). *Code of ethics for registered nurses.* https://hl-prod-ca-oc-download.s3-ca-central-1.amazonaws.com/CNA/2f975e7e-4a40-45ca-863c-5ebf0a138d5e/UploadedImages/documents/Code_of_Ethics_2017_Edition_Secure_Interactive.pdf

Canadian Nurses Protective Society. (2021). *InfoLAW: Patient restraints.* https://cnps.ca/article/patient-restraints/

Chiu, Y., Hsu, W.-C., & Algase, D. L. (2011). Validation of the Chinese revised algase wandering scale-community version for persons with dementia in northern Taiwan. *Aging & Mental Health, 15*(2), 243–251. https://doi.org/10.1080/13607860903046511 [Seminal Reference]

College of Nurses of Ontario (CNO). (2022). *Understanding restraints.* https://www.cno.org/en/learn-about-standards-guidelines/educational-tools/restraints/

Cramer, J. D., Balakrishnan, K., Roy, S., et al. (2020). Intraoperative sentinel events in the era of surgical safety checklists: Results of a national survey. *Otolaryngology-Head and Neck Surgery, 4*(4), 1–13. https://doi.org/10.1177/2473974X20975731

Crawshaw, A., & Cock, H. (2020). Medical management of status epilepticus: Emergency room to intensive care unit. *Seizure: European Journal of Epilepsy, 75,* 145–152. https://doi.org/10.1016/J.seizure.2019.10.006

Eversafe Media Inc. (2017). *WHMIS 2015 safety data sheets.* https://eversafetraining.com/whmis-2015-safety-data-sheets/

Freeman, S., Yorke, J., & Dark, P. (2018). Patient agitation and its management in adult critical care: A systematic review and narrative synthesis. *Journal of Clinical Nursing, 27*(7–8), e1284–e1308. https://doi.org/10.1111/jocn.14258

Health Canada. (2022a). *Canada's Vigilance Program.* https://www.canada.ca/en/health-canada/services/drugs-health-products/medeffect-canada/canada-vigilance-program.html

Health Canada. (2022b). Workplace *Hazardous Materials Information System (WHMIS).* https://www.canada.ca/en/health-canada/services/environmental-workplace-health/occupational-health-safety/workplace-hazardous-materials-information-system.html

Healthcare Excellence Canada. (n.d.). *SHIFT to safety.* http://www.patientsafetyinstitute.ca/en/About/Programs/shift-to-safety/Pages/default.aspx

Healthcare Excellence Canada. (2015). *Never events for hospital care in Canada.* https://www.patientsafetyinstitute.ca/en/toolsResources/NeverEvents/Pages/default.aspx [Seminal Reference]

Healthcare Excellence Canada. (2017). *Mental health care: Seclusion and restraint.* Patient Safety Education Program. https://www.patientsafetyinstitute.ca/en/education/PatientSafetyEducationProgram/PatientSafetyEducationCurriculum/MentalHealthModules/Pages/Mental-Health-Care-Seclusion-and-Restraint.aspx [Seminal Reference]

Healthcare Excellence Canada. (2019). *Strengthening commitment for improvement together: A policy framework for patient safety*. https://www.patientsafetyinstitute.ca/en/toolsResources/PolicyFrameworkforPatientSafetyCanada/Documents/PolicyFramework%20Document%20ENG%20FINAL.pdf

Healthcare Excellence Canada & Registered Nurses' Association of Ontario. (2018). *Reducing falls and injuries from falls: Getting started kit–Evidence update*. https://www.patientsafetyinstitute.ca/en/toolsResources/Pages/Falls-resources-Getting-Started-Kit.aspx

Heinrich, T., Kato, H., Emanuel, C., et al. (2019). Improving the validity of nurse-based delirium screening: A head-to-head comparison of nursing delirium-screening scale and short confusion assessment method. *Psychosomatics*, *60*(2), 172–178. https://doi.org/10.1016/j.psym.2018.09.002

Healthcare Excellence Canada. (2022). *Our strategy: Shaping the future of quality and safety. Together.* https://www.healthcareexcellence.ca/en/about/about-us/our-strategy/

Heng, H., Jazayeri, D., Shaw, L., et al. (2020). Hospital falls prevention with patient education: A scoping review. *BMC Geriatrics*, 20, Article 140. https://doi.org/10.1186/s12877-020-01515-w

Hockenberry, M., Duffy, E. A., & Gibbs, K. (2024). *Wong's nursing care of infants and children* (12th ed.). Elsevier.

Institute for Safe Medication Practices Canada. (2017). The second victim: Sharing the journey toward healing. *ISMP Canada Safety Bulletin*, *17*(9), 1–6. https://www.ismp-canada.org/download/safetyBulletins/2017/ISMPCSB2017-10-SecondVictim.pdf

Jeong, S., Shin, D. W., Han, K., et al. (2019). Timed up-and-go test is a useful predictor of fracture incidence. *Bone*, *127*, 474–481. https://doi.org/10.1016/j.bone.2019.07.018

Kiel, D. (2022). Falls in older persons: Risk factors and patient evaluation. *UpToDate*. http://www.uptodate.com/contents/falls-in-older-persons-risk-factors-and-patient-evaluation

Madhiyazhagan, M. (2021). Time is brain: Review of emergency management of status epilepticus in adults. *Current Medical Issues*, *19*(4), 269–273. https://doi.org/10.4103/cmi.cmi_53_21

Montague, T., Nemis-White, J., Aylen, J., et al. (2019). Canada's evolving Medicare: Patient-centred care. *Healthcare Quarterly*, *22*(2), 27–31. https://www.longwoods.com/content/25908/healthcare-quarterly/canada-s-evolving-medicare-patient-centred-care

Pack, A. M. (2019). Epilepsy overview and revised classification of seizures and epilepsies. *Epilepsy*, *25*(2), 306–321. https://doi.org/10.1212/CON.0000000000000707

Patient Restraints Minimization Act, S.O. 2001, c. 16. https://www.ontario.ca/laws/statute/01p16 [Seminal Reference]

Perucca, P., Scheffer, I. E., & Kiley, M. (2018). The management of epilepsy in children and adults. *The Medical Journal of Australia*, *208*(5), 226–233. https://doi.org/10.5694/mja17.00951

Public Health Agency of Canada. (2019). *Epilepsy in Canada*. https://www.canada.ca/en/public-health/services/publications/diseases-conditions/epilepsy.html

Registered Nurses' Association of Ontario (RNAO). (2017). *Preventing falls and reducing injuries from falls* (4th ed.). https://rnao.ca/sites/rnao-ca/files/bpg/FALL_PREVENTION_WEB_1207-17.pdf [Seminal Reference]

Scheepmans, K., de Casterlé, B. D., Paquay, L., et al. (2018). Restraint use in older adults in home care: A systematic review. *International Journal of Nursing Studies*, *79*, 122–136. https://doi.org/10.1016/j.ijnurstu.2017.11.008

Tyerman, J., & Cobbett, S. (Eds.). (2023). *Lewis's medical-surgical nursing in Canada: Assessment and management of clinical problems* (5th ed.). Elsevier Canada.

Varshawsky, A., & Traynor, V. (2021). Graphic designed bedroom doors to support dementia wandering in residential care homes: Innovative practice. *Dementia*, *20*(1), 348–354. https://doi.org/10.1177/1471301219868619

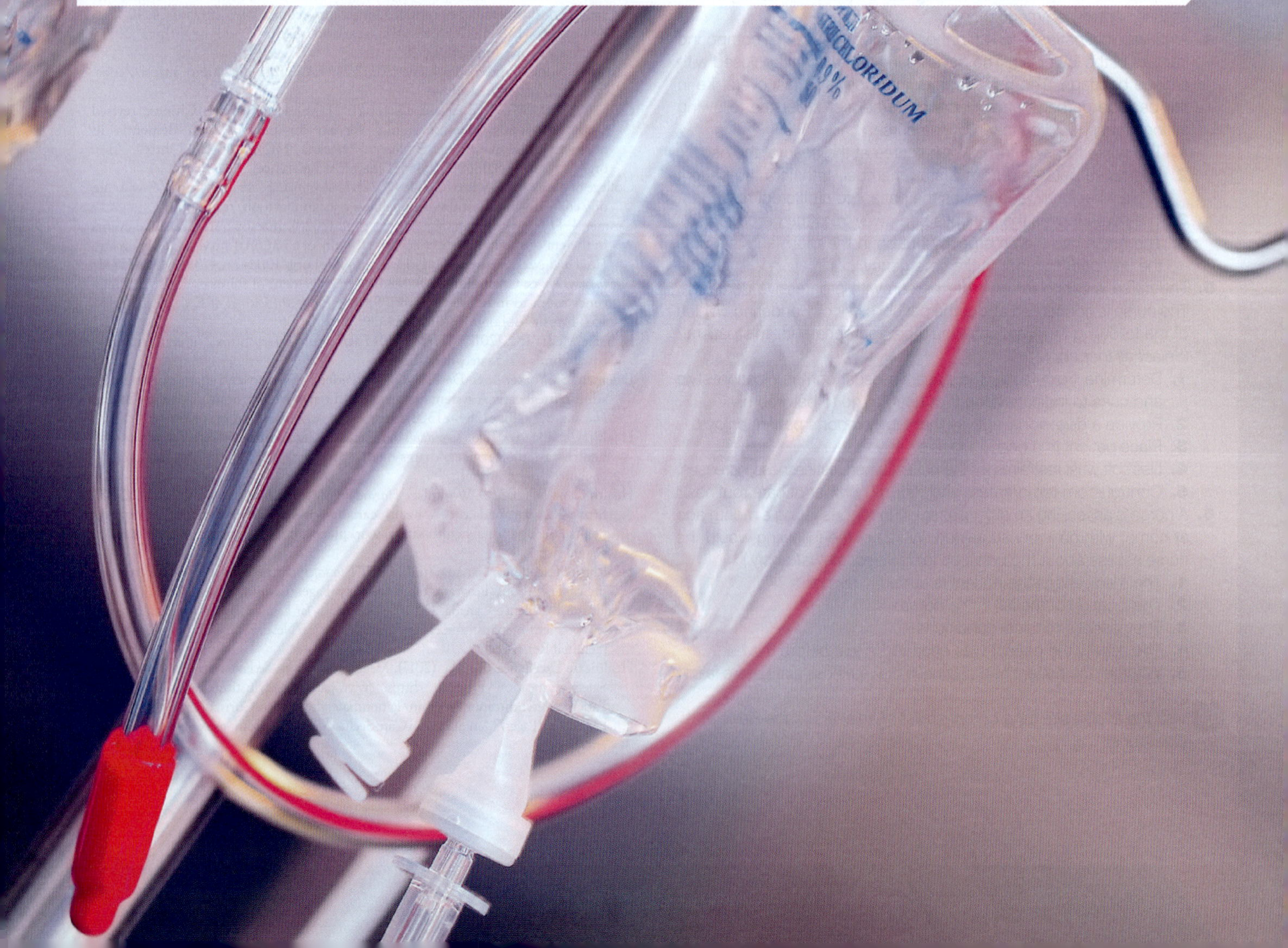

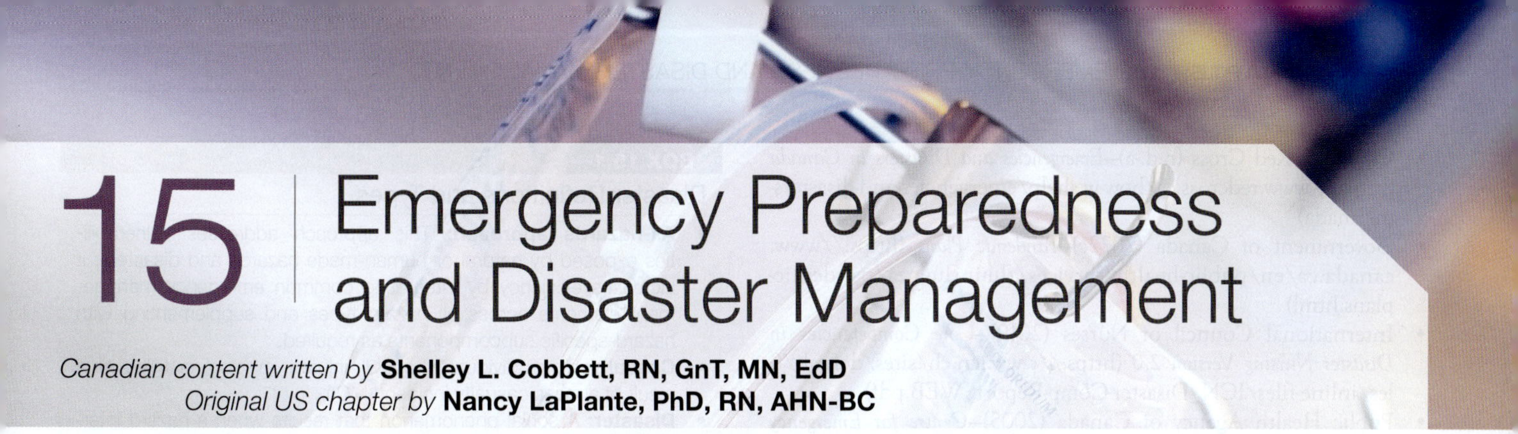

15 Emergency Preparedness and Disaster Management

Canadian content written by **Shelley L. Cobbett, RN, GnT, MN, EdD**
Original US chapter by **Nancy LaPlante, PhD, RN, AHN-BC**

SKILLS AND PROCEDURES

OBJECTIVES

Mastery of content in this chapter will enable the nurse to:

- Describe elements of emergency preparedness and disaster management, including prevention and mitigation, preparedness, response, and recovery.
- Describe the characteristics of different types of disasters.
- Identify actions to take in the event of biological, chemical, or radiation exposure.
- Explain guidelines for patient care in the event of a mass casualty incident.
- Identify components of the START and JumpSTART triage systems.
- Describe factors related to the mental health and well-being of patients, nurses, and health care providers postdisaster.

MEDIA RESOURCES

- http://evolve.elsevier.com/Canada/Perry/clinicalskills/

PURPOSE

The incidence of natural and human-made disasters and infectious diseases continues to rise throughout the world, increasing the likelihood and frequency of these events happening in Canada. Recent massive wildfires in Lytton, British Columbia (Canadian Red Cross, 2022), and Fort McMurray, Alberta, were unlike any fires seen before within our borders (Canadian Red Cross, 2017). Although natural disasters—the ice storms in New Brunswick, severe flooding in Quebec and Ontario, and the threat of earthquakes in British Columbia—continue to be cause for concern, the global COVID-19 pandemic declared by the World Health Organization (WHO) in March 2020 has emphasized the need for emergency preparedness at the municipal, provincial/territorial, and federal levels. This *pandemic* (worldwide spread of a new disease) has changed the reality for people around the world. Coronavirus disease (COVID-19) is an infectious disease caused by SARS-CoV-2, a newly discovered strain of coronavirus (World Health Organization [WHO], n.d.-a). Most recently, the monkeypox virus (MPV), a virus that belongs to the *Orthopoxvirus* genus (which includes the variola virus [smallpox virus]), is currently endemic in 10 countries in West and Central Africa, with its presence having been identified on every continent other than Antarctica (Cohen, 2022). Although it is early in the evolution of MPV, some epidemiologists indicate it may be a new global threat (Cohen, 2022). The recent COVID-19 pandemic and the evolving MPV endemic have demonstrated how important it is that both the general public and health care providers understand the implications of any form of disaster and how to respond. Chapter 5 describes the type of precautions health care providers take to protect from exposure to pathogens such as COVID-19.

Canadian emergency management adopts an all-hazards approach to address natural and human-made disasters. Pandemics and epidemics can also be disasters, as was realized with the global COVID-19 pandemic. Regardless of the cause of the disaster, it is of paramount importance that we have well-educated health care providers who are skilled in disaster preparedness and emergency management and are able to effectively educate the public and deliver care to diverse populations at times of crisis. Nurses, as members of the interprofessional health care team, play a key role in the coordination and implementation of emergency preparedness and disaster management. Postdisaster mental health and well-being are important to assess in patients, nurses, and members of the interprofessional health care team. Many factors may adversely affect mental health status postdisaster—for example, social and economic losses, emotional suffering, the extent of property damage, loss of loved ones, lack of preparedness, and impact of the disaster on one's personal and professional life (Makwana, 2019). The psychological effects of disasters are often more pronounced among children, women, and older persons. Mao and Agyapong (2021) identified the vulnerability and protective social determinant factors that impact mental health and resiliency in disaster survivors. These factors included gender, age, ethnicity, social support, and socioeconomic status. Information gathered from the many postdisaster evaluations that have occurred in recent years has provided a considerable body of knowledge and experience to improve the response of an entire health care team and the many agencies and individuals involved in a disaster response.

STANDARDS OF CARE

- Canadian Nurses Association (2012)—*Position Statement: Emergency Preparedness and Response* (https://www.cna-aiic.ca/en/nursing/nursing-tools-and-resources/emergency-preparedness)

- Canadian Red Cross (n.d.-a)—*Emergencies and Disasters in Canada* (https://www.redcross.ca/how-we-help/emergencies-and-disasters-in-canada)
- Government of Canada (2022c)—*Pandemic Plans* (https://www.canada.ca/en/public-health/services/flu-influenza/pandemic-plans.html)
- International Council of Nurses (2019)—*Core Competencies in Disaster Nursing Version 2.0* (https://www.icn.ch/sites/default/files/inline-files/ICN_Disaster-Comp-Report_WEB.pdf)
- Public Health Agency of Canada (2005)—*Centre for Emergency Preparedness and Response* (https://www.canada.ca/en/public-health/services/emergency-preparedness-response/centre-emergency-preparedness-response.html)
- Public Safety Canada (2017)—*An Emergency Management Framework for Canada*, Third edition (https://www.publicsafety.gc.ca/cnt/rsrcs/pblctns/2017-mrgnc-mngmnt-frmwrk/index-en.aspx)

PRINCIPLES FOR PRACTICE

- A disaster is any unexpected event, the effect of which leads to significant destruction, adverse consequences, or both (Box 15.1).
- Surveillance of the public by the WHO focuses on current health threats, such as outbreaks of measles and COVID-19 (Box 15.2).
- There are two main types of disasters: natural and human-made. If the public is not adequately protected, the spread of vector-borne disease can create a natural disaster.
- The main purpose of the *Emergency Management Framework for Canada* (the Framework) (Public Safety Canada, 2017) is to save lives, preserve the environment, and protect property and the economy. The Framework includes information used to assist with collaborative management to enhance the four interdependent emergency management components: prevention and mitigation, preparedness, response, and recovery from potential threats and disaster events.
- *Prevention and mitigation* are focused on eliminating, reducing, or adapting to the risk of disasters; *preparedness* is the state of readiness to respond to a disaster situation and manage its consequences prior to the disaster occurring; *response* is the ability to act during, immediately before, and after a disaster to minimize suffering and losses; and *recovery* is restoration of conditions to an acceptable level postdisaster (Public Safety Canada, 2017).
- Effective implementation of the four emergency management components is based on an evidence-informed risk assessment, strong public awareness, and community engagement, all of which are key attributes of societal resilience (Public Safety Canada, 2017).
- An all-hazards approach is used to identify, analyze, and prioritize potential natural and human-made threats, considering vulnerabilities, potential consequences, and means to mitigate the risks (Public Safety Canada, 2022a).
- The Canadian Red Cross is an invaluable resource in the event of a disaster. The organization provides assistance in disaster situations for people's basic needs, including family reunification, emergency lodging, reception and information, emergency food, emergency clothing, and personal services (Canadian Red Cross, n.d.-c).
- Most disasters in Canada have been local (community, municipal, provincial) in nature but can be declared to be national under the *Emergencies Act (1985)*, allowing the implementation of special measures to ensure safety and security and to amend other Acts as required.
- Canada's *Emergencies Act* can be used in response to an urgent, temporary, and critical emergency that seriously endangers the health and safety of Canadians and that cannot be dealt with effectively by any other federal, provincial, or territorial law (Fig. 15.1). For example, the *Emergencies Act* was declared on February 14, 2022, and then revoked on February 23, 2022, in response to the ongoing blockades and protests taking place in Ottawa and at some border crossings (Feldman, 2022).
- Promoting effective emergency preparedness and response requires collaboration between all levels of government and interprofessional collaboration among nongovernmental agencies such as the health, social services, safety, transportation, meteorology, and voluntary sectors (e.g., Canadian Red Cross, St. John Ambulance) (Canadian Nurses Association, 2012). Nurses play a vital role on the interprofessional team related to emergency preparedness and response.
- Some provincial nursing regulatory agencies have regulations that allow a person who is authorized to practise nursing as a registered nurse in another jurisdiction in Canada or the United

BOX 15.1

Disaster Definitions and Types

- **All-hazards approach:** This approach addresses vulnerabilities exposed by natural or human-made hazards and disasters; it increases efficiency by integrating common emergency management elements across all hazard types and supplementing with hazard-specific subcomponents as required.
- **Casualty:** Any individual who is ill, injured, missing, or killed as a result of a mass casualty incident (MCI).
- **Disaster:** A social phenomenon that results when a hazard intersects with a vulnerable community, overwhelming or exceeding the community's ability to cope, and may cause serious harm to safety, health, welfare, property, or environment.
- **Emergency:** A present or imminent event that requires immediate coordination of actions concerning persons or property to protect the health, safety, or welfare of people, or to limit damage to property or the environment.
- **Emergency management:** The management of emergencies involving all hazards, including activities and risk management measures related to prevention and mitigation, preparedness, response, and recovery.
- **Emergency preparedness:** Efforts taken prior to an emergency to help support event response, help reduce the impacts of events, and help identify opportunities for future prevention and mitigation efforts.
- **Hazard:** A potentially damaging physical event, phenomenon, or human activity that may cause injury or death, property damage, social and economic disruption, or environmental degradation.
- **Hazardscape:** The cumulative emergency management environment, consisting of all hazards, risks, vulnerabilities, and capacities.
- **Mass casualty incident (MCI):** Any event or situation (e.g., bombing of a public area) that results in multiple casualties and deaths; exists when health care needs exceed health care resources.
- **Threat:** The presence of a hazard and an exposure pathway to threats that may be natural or human induced, accidental or intentional.
- **Triage:** The process of selecting and prioritizing patients based on the urgency of their need for care; can occur in agency settings (Canadian Triage and Acuity Scale [CTAS]) or community settings (START and JumpSTART triage).
- **Vulnerability:** Conditions determined by physical, social, economic, and/or environmental factors or processes that increase the susceptibility of a community to the impact of hazards.

Adapted from Public Safety Canada. (2017). *An Emergency Management Framework for Canada* (3rd ed., pp. 20–23); Public Safety Canada. (2022). *Emergency management.* https://www.publicsafety.gc.ca/cnt/mrgnc-mngmnt/index-en.aspx

BOX 15.2

Coronavirus Disease (COVID-19)

- Coronavirus disease (COVID-19) is an infectious disease caused by a new strain of coronavirus, SARS-CoV-2, which was first detected in December 2019.
- Most people infected with SARS-CoV-2 will experience mild to moderate gastrointestinal or respiratory illness and recover without requiring special treatment. Older persons and those with underlying medical concerns (e.g., cardiovascular disease, diabetes, chronic respiratory disease, cancer) are more likely to develop serious illness.
- COVID-19 symptoms include cough, fever or chills, shortness of breath or difficulty breathing, muscle or body aches, sore throat, new loss of taste or smell, diarrhea, headache, fatigue, nausea or vomiting, and congestion or runny nose.
- COVID-19 can be severe, and in some cases has caused death.
- The best way to prevent and slow transmission is to be well informed about the COVID-19 virus, the disease it causes, and how it spreads.
- It is possible to become infected through contact with an asymptomatic person.
- Protect yourself and others from infection by wearing a mask, maintaining physical distance of 2 metres when possible, washing hands frequently, and avoiding touching your face.
- The COVID-19 virus spreads primarily through aerosolized droplets of saliva or discharge from the nose when an infected person coughs or sneezes, so it is important that you also practice respiratory etiquette (e.g., by coughing into a flexed elbow).
- There are two types of tests for COVID-19:
  - Viral or diagnostic test: A viral test determines whether a person is currently infected with the coronavirus. This is the test a person will receive if a doctor refers them for a COVID-19 test based on symptoms and other factors (e.g., comorbidities).
  - Antibody test: An antibody test can show whether a person was previously exposed to or infected with the virus and whether the body has created antibodies in an attempt to defend itself. It takes at least 12 days after exposure for the body to make enough antibodies to show up on a test.

Data from World Health Organization. (2023). *Coronavirus disease (COVID-19) pandemic.* https://www.who.int/emergencies/diseases/novel-coronavirus-2019

States to practise nursing in the province during an emergency (e.g., College of Registered Nurses of Manitoba). A nurse who is eligible for Canadian Nurses Protective Society (CNPS) services and moves to another Canadian jurisdiction to do emergency work remains eligible for CNPS services (CNPS, 2020).

- The National Public Alerting System (NPAS) is a collaborative initiative among the federal–provincial–territorial governments and industry partners that provides the capability to rapidly warn the public of imminent or actual hazards using various communication modalities (Public Safety Canada, 2020b) (Fig. 15.2). A public awareness campaign, Alert Ready, provides information on the types of alerts that can be issued, wireless device compatibility, and what to do if an alert occurs.
- As of April 6, 2018, the NPAS has wireless and smartphone capabilities (for more information, see https://www.alertready.ca/).
- Incident Command System Canada (ICS Canada, 2012) has outlined an incident communications plan that addresses preparedness planning related to equipment, systems, and protocols necessary to achieve integrated voice and data communications in the event of a disaster. On an individual level, the 9-1-1 system can be activated.
- The Incident Command System (ICS) is designed to enable effective, efficient incident management through integration of facilities, equipment, personnel, procedures, and communications within a common organizational structure (ICS Canada, 2012). Refer to Fig. 15.3 for an example of a hospital ICS.
- A mass casualty incident (MCI) occurs when the number of casualties, or the rate of their arrival, overwhelms the local health care system, where the needs of people exceed the local resources and capabilities (DeNolf & Kahwaji, 2021).
- The Canadian Disaster Database (CDD) describes disasters that have affected Canada since the 1900s (excluding war) (Public Safety Canada, 2022b).
- The Public Health Agency of Canada funds the National Emergency Strategic Stockpile (NESS), which provides health and social service supplies quickly to provinces and territories when their own resources are depleted during an emergency. There is a central depot in Ottawa, and several supply centres are located across Canada (Public Health Agency of Canada, 2022).
- Support resources required during a disaster include human resources, agencies, facilities, supplies, and vehicles. Support is for the victims of disaster and all health care providers involved. Support is holistic, encompassing the body, mind, and spirit. Health care providers (including nurses, first responders, and physicians) are at risk for post-traumatic stress disorder (PTSD).
- Health care providers care for the worried well (those frightened by the events) and sick and injured individuals (including the walking wounded) already admitted to the hospital or emergency department (ED).
- Acute care facility EDs must have an emergency disaster plan and protocols to address high patient volume and surges in the ED (Accreditation Canada, 2020) as well as internal disasters.
- Health care facilities need to be competent in disaster preparedness and management at all levels of the health care system. For example, facilities must have clear plans related to incident command, triage, MCIs or mass gatherings, and hazardous materials (Canadian Association of Emergency Physicians [CAEP], 2020).
- Even with a well-developed acute care facility disaster preparedness and management plan, coping with the consequences of a disaster is a complex challenge. Trained health care providers who work in tandem with frontline emergency personnel and community resources are best positioned to lead institutions to better disaster preparedness (CAEP, 2020).
- The WHO (2011) has provided a hospital emergency response checklist for an all-hazards approach.
- Canada has aligned the Workplace Hazardous Materials Information System (WHMIS) with the Globally Harmonized System of Classification and Labelling of Chemicals (GHS) (Canadian Centre for Occupational Health and Safety, 2022) and developed pictograms for easy identification of potential health hazards (Fig. 15.4).
- Climate change is affecting health and increasing the transmission of vector-borne diseases by ticks and mosquitos, which spread disease from human to human (e.g., malaria or dengue fever) or from animals to humans (e.g., West Nile virus, Lyme disease) (Government of Canada, 2022a, 2022b). Guidelines for nursing education on climate-driven vector-borne diseases include relevant, evidence-informed principles to provide care and support to those affected by these diseases (Canadian Association of Schools of Nursing, 2020).
- Public Safety Canada (2020b) has developed the Regional Resilience Assessment Program, a comprehensive risk assessment program for owners and operators of critical infrastructure (CI) facilities within the 10 CI sectors in Canada, one of which is the health care sector.
- The Canadian Red Cross (n.d.-a), in partnership with Indigenous peoples across Canada, has developed a culturally appropriate

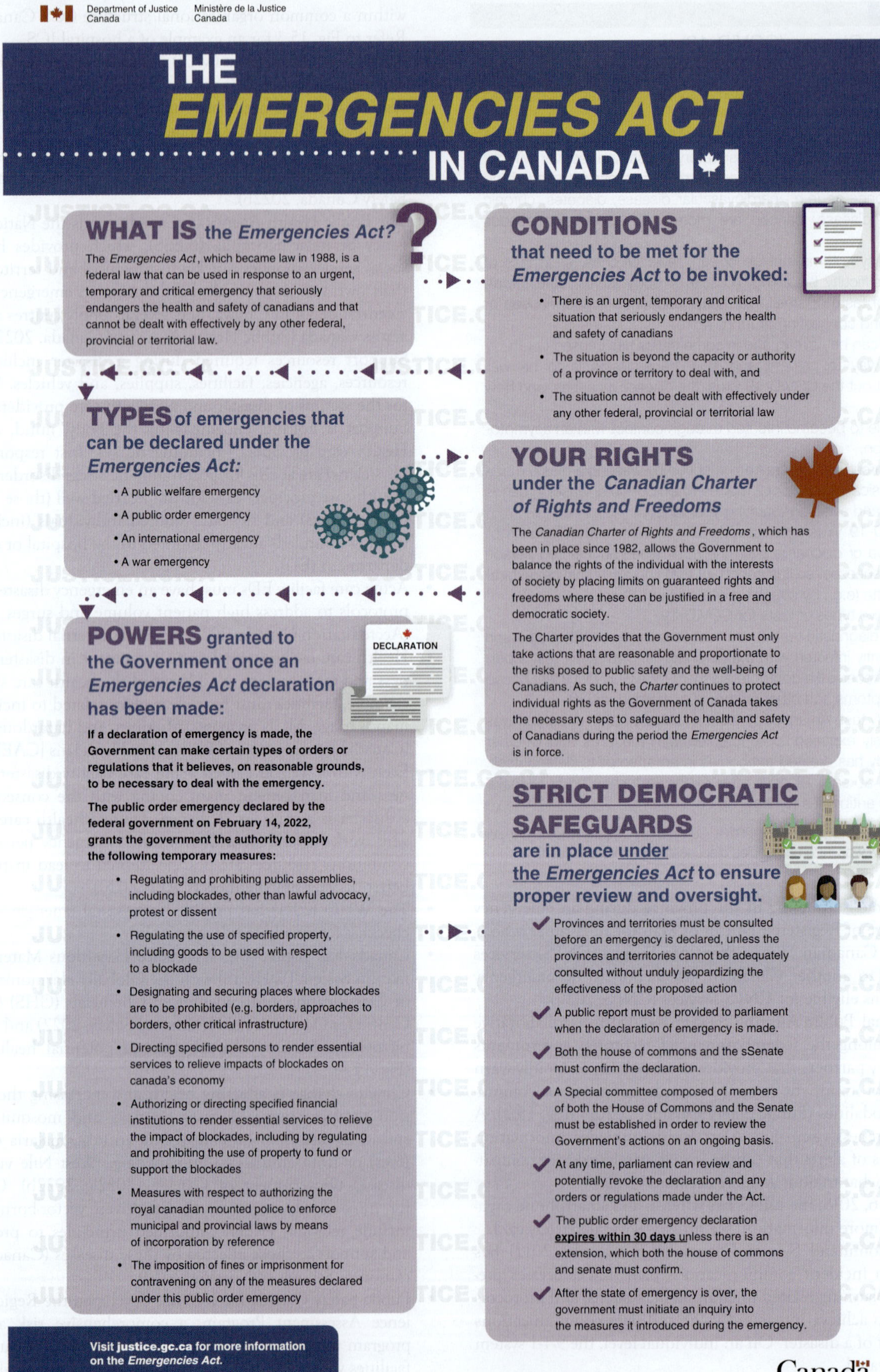

FIG 15.1 Canada's *Emergencies Act* infographic. (From Government of Canada. [2022]. *The Emergencies Act in Canada*. https://www.justice.gc.ca/eng/csj-sjc/ea_infog-lu_infog.html)

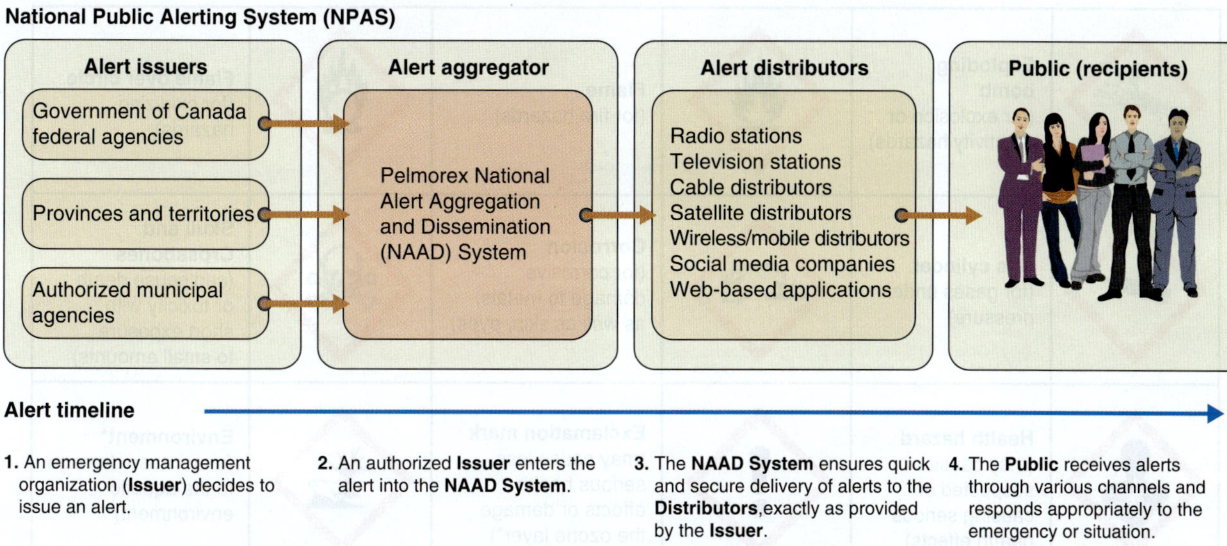

FIG 15.2 National Public Alerting System. (*From Public Safety Canada. [2020]. National Public Alerting System. https://www.publicsafety.gc.ca/cnt/mrgnc-mngmnt/mrgnc-prprdnss/ntnl-pblc-lrtng-sstm-en.aspx*)

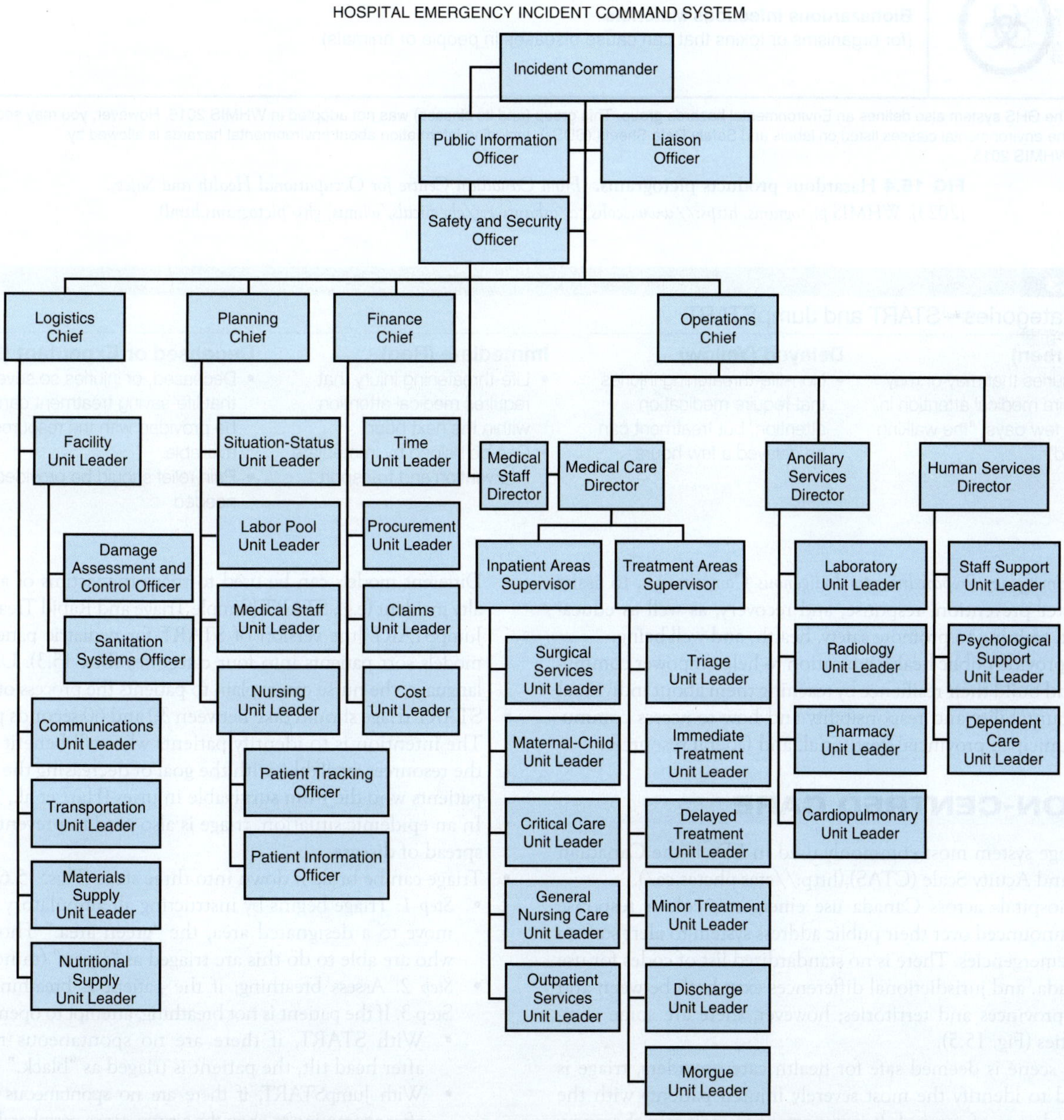

FIG 15.3 A hospital emergency incident command system prepares all response teams to work smoothly in a disaster situation.

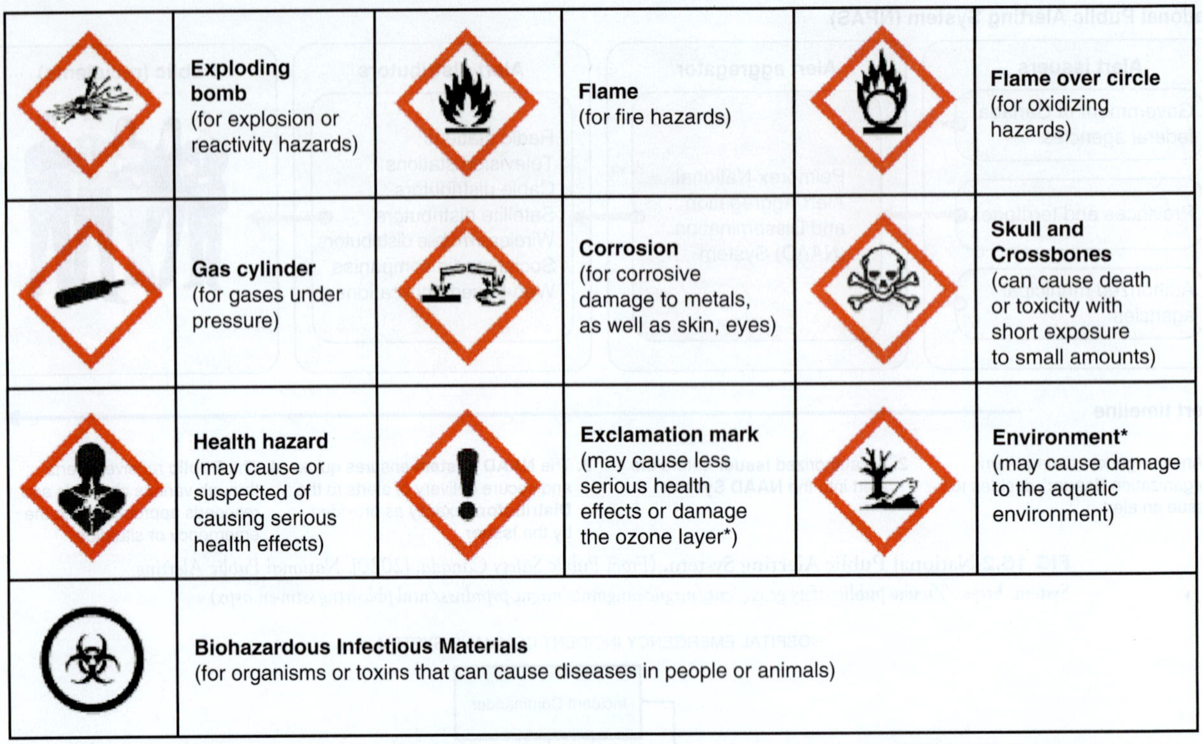

* The GHS system also defines an Environmental hazards group. This group (and its classes) was not adopted in WHMIS 2015. However, you may see the environmental classes listed on labels and Safety Data Sheets (SDSs). Including information about environmental hazards is allowed by WHMIS 2015.

FIG 15.4 **Hazardous products pictograms.** (*From Canadian Centre for Occupational Health and Safety. [2023]. WHMIS pictograms. https://www.ccohs.ca/oshanswers/chemicals/whmis_ghs/pictograms.html*)

BOX 15.3

Triage Categories—START and JumpSTART

Minor (Green)	Delayed (Yellow)	Immediate (Red)	Deceased or Expectant (Black)
• Minor injuries that may or may not require medical attention in the next few days; "the walking wounded"	• Non–life-threatening injuries that require medication attention, but treatment can be delayed a few hours	• Life-threatening injury that requires medical attention within the next hour • Can be helped by immediate intervention and transport	• Deceased, or injuries so severe that life-saving treatment cannot be provided with the resources available • Pain relief should be provided as needed

guide, *Emergency Preparedness for Indigenous Communities*, to assist in disaster prevention, response, and recovery, as well as education and training to promote safety, health, and well-being.

- Nurses provide public health education to help empower communities and build their resilience by teaching them about individual self-accountability and responsibility and how to access community, municipal, provincial/territorial, and federal resources.

PERSON-CENTRED CARE

- The triage system most commonly used in EDs is the Canadian Triage and Acuity Scale (CTAS) (http://ctas-phctas.ca/).
- Many hospitals across Canada use emergency colour response codes announced over their public address system to alert staff to on-site emergencies. There is no standardized list of codes for use in Canada, and jurisdictional differences exist both between and within provinces and territories; however, there are some commonalities (Fig. 15.5).
- Once a scene is deemed safe for health care providers, triage is initiated to identify the most severely injured patients with the greatest chance of survival. It is important to maintain therapeutic communication while conveying caring and compassion.
- Different models can be used to triage the victims of a mass casualty incident (e.g., START [Simple Triage and Rapid Treatment] and JumpSTART [the version of START for pediatric patients]). Both models sort patients into four categories (Box 15.3). Using simple language, the nurse can explain to patients the process of triage.
- START triage should take between 30 and 60 seconds per patient. The intention is to identify patients who will benefit most from the resources available, with the goal of decreasing the number of patients who die from survivable injuries (Hart et al., 2018).
- In an epidemic situation, triage is also used to prevent secondary spread of disease.
- Triage can be broken down into three steps (Figs. 15.6 and 15.7):
  - *Step 1:* Triage begins by instructing all ambulatory patients to move to a designated area, the "green area." Those patients who are able to do this are triaged as "green" (minor).
  - *Step 2:* Assess breathing; if the patient is breathing, move to Step 3. If the patient is not breathing, attempt to open the airway.
    - With START, if there are no spontaneous respirations after head tilt, the patient is triaged as "black."
    - With JumpSTART, if there are no spontaneous respirations after attempting to open the airway, assess peripheral pulse. If no pulse, the patient is triaged as black. If the patient has a palpable

COLOUR	EMERGENCY	COLOUR	EMERGENCY
Red	Fire	Pink	Pediatric emergency
Blue	Cardiac arrest	White	Violent person/hostage
Green	Evacuation	Black	Bomb threat
Yellow	Missing adult	Brown	Hazardous substance
Orange	External disaster; mass casualty	Grey	External air exclusion
Silver	Person with a weapon	Amber	Missing child

FIG 15.5 Hospital emergency colour response codes. (*Adapted from Quinte Health Care. [2022]. Emergency codes. https://www.qhc.on.ca/emergency-codes-p2134.php*)

pulse, five assisted ventilations (15 seconds) are given; if spontaneous respirations return, the patient is triaged as "red." If there is no return of respirations, the patient is triaged as black.

  - *Step 3*: Assess respiratory rate, perfusion, and mental status.
- A common mnemonic that can assist with differentiating between the triage categories of "yellow" and "red" for START is RPM-30-2-Can Do. To be triaged as yellow, the patient must have a respiratory rate under 30 breaths/min, capillary refill must be under 2 seconds, and mental status must be adequate; that is, the patient "can do" what they are asked. If any one of these three criteria are not met, the patient is triaged as red.
- The mnemonic for JumpSTART is RPM-30-2-Can Do-15-45 to reflect the differences in the normal respiratory rates between children and adults. Pediatric patients who are breathing under 15 breaths/min or over 45 breaths/min are triaged as red.
- During triage, the nurse provides psychological support to survivors as well as physical care. The nurse must remain calm and assess a patient's immediate psychological response. Some patients present with dissociative symptoms such as disorientation, depression, anxiety, psychosis, and an inability to care for self.
- Community engagement is key to successfully controlling people's responses during disasters; establishing trust is essential. The inclusivity and compassion conveyed by those working in communities experiencing a disaster allows for a more successful disaster recovery. Regardless of cultural differences and potential language difficulties, it is important for health care professionals to use culturally sensitive care when working in disaster situations. Professional interpreters become an important resource.
- Some disaster events result in a changed culture for individuals, families, communities, and populations. Once a disaster has struck, there can be a sense of vulnerability that causes increased fear and a sense of insecurity.

EVIDENCE-INFORMED PRACTICE

- With the increased frequency of all types of disasters globally, all nurses must be prepared to deal with a variety of disaster situations and the resulting physical and mental effects that these have on the victims and communities. Although attention to emergency preparedness has increased, research, including a recent systematic review by Labrague et al. (2018), has showed that globally nurses are often underprepared, which has implications for policy, education, and practice:
  - Nurses in Bangladesh and Laos felt unprepared to treat disaster victims without a physician, while nurses in Cambodia and Solomon Islands felt unprepared to perform assessments related to biological and chemical agents (Labrague et al., 2018).
  - Nurses in the Philippines felt they were not sufficiently prepared and were not confident in responding effectively to any disasters. Although nurses in Sweden felt prepared to deal with emergencies, they scored low on disaster readiness, disaster response, and disaster evaluation (Labrague et al., 2018; Langan et al., 2019).

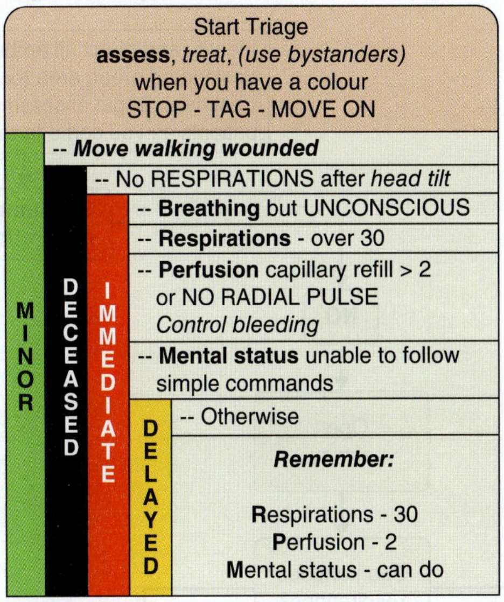

FIG 15.6 START triage. (*From https://disastermedicine.wordpress.com/03-mass-triage/*)

  - Policy implications concern the need to increase the confidence and preparation of the workforce. Practice implications focus on the knowledge of nurses with experience who can mentor others and the provision of time to practise in mock drills (Langan et al., 2019). Nursing education needs to ensure that disaster content is in the curriculum at all levels of education to raise awareness and encourage further learning (Labrague et al., 2018).
  - In a Canadian study by Nowell et al. (2021), researchers found that collaboration and teamwork helped increase nurses' confidence in their ability to provide effective patient care during a disaster. When nurses lacked confidence, they experienced a state of chaos and anxiety, whereas those nurses who expressed confidence in their abilities to cope and provide care during a pandemic were reported to be in a calmer state of acceptance.
- Older persons and children are most vulnerable to the physiological stresses and psychological responses caused by natural disasters and can benefit from targeted postdisaster care plans. The question remains as to how prepared the older-person population is for natural disasters.
- Age-related changes in older persons (e.g., decline in sensory, cognitive, and functional abilities), social isolation, the lack of support systems to assist during a disaster, and potentially limited financial resources place older persons at increased risk during disasters. For example, inability to access routine medical care or chronic disease management during a disaster, medication shortages, or lack of access to nutrition and fresh water can intensify chronic conditions, leading to an increase in morbidity and mortality among older persons (Gilmartin et al., 2019).
- Children who are exposed to disasters experience a range of physical and psychological effects that are often linked to family

and social contexts and to developmental age and stage. Children do not necessarily experience long-term effects postdisaster, especially if provided with adequate treatment and support (Grolnick et al., 2018). Postdisaster mental health care for children is of utmost importance–detection, treatment, and prevention of adverse mental health effects in both the immediate and long-term postdisaster periods are critical.

SAFETY GUIDELINES

When considering all forms of disaster, there are basic safety guidelines for a nurse or other health care provider to follow:

- Be prepared to shelter in place if required (Box 15.4).
- The first priority at any disaster scene is to protect oneself and other team members. The second priority is to protect the public, patients, and the environment (Box 15.5).

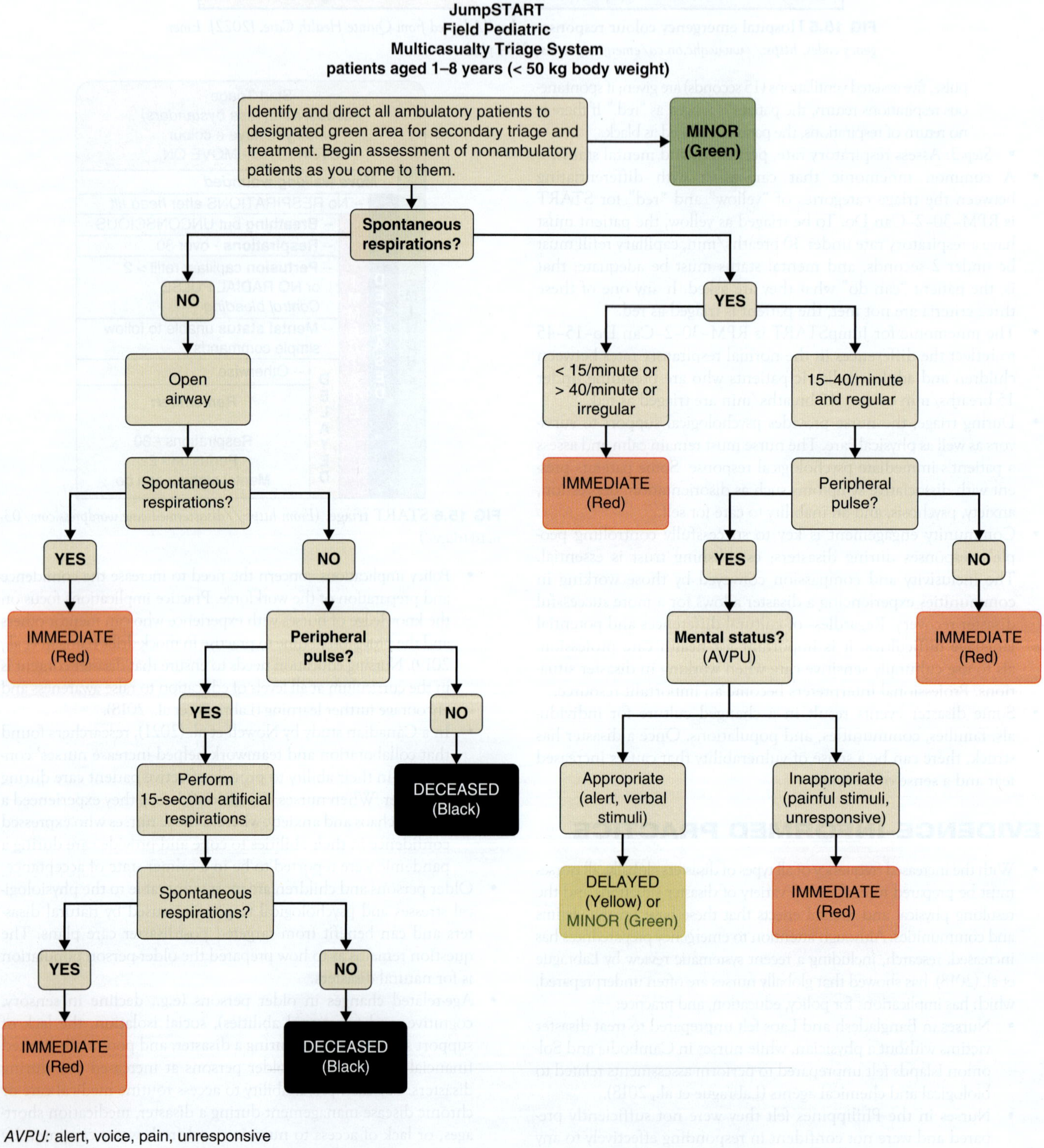

FIG 15.7 **JumpSTART triage.** *(From Fire Fighting in Canada. [2007]. EMS focus: Handling the mass casualty incident, creating order out of chaos [Figure 2]. https://www.firefightingincanada.com/emergency-disaster-management/ems-focus-oct.-06-cff-1448)*

BOX 15.4

Guidelines for Sheltering in Place

Be prepared to shelter in place:

- Remain in your home or office.
- Close and lock all windows and exterior doors.
- Turn off all fans and heating and air-conditioning systems.
- Close fireplace damper if applicable.
- Get your emergency preparedness kit.
- Go to an interior room that is above ground level, if possible one with no windows. With chemical environmental contamination, an above-ground location is best because some chemicals are heavier than air and may seep into basements even when windows are closed.
- Use duct tape to seal all cracks around the door and any vents into the room.
- Monitor emergency reports and stay put until it is announced that all is safe or an evacuation order has been issued.
- Additional supplies may be required, depending on the reason for sheltering in place—for example, in a pandemic, a thermometer, non-Aspirin pain reliever, acetaminophen, bleach.

Adapted from Public Safety Canada. (2022). *During an emergency*. https://www.getprepared.gc.ca/cnt/hzd/drng-en.aspx

BOX 15.5

Safety and Security

- Trained emergency personnel (e.g., firefighters and police) are responsible for the safety and security of a disaster scene.
- Call 9-1-1 if emergency personnel have not already been notified.
- Do not disturb the scene; key evidence could be lost or contaminated.
- A health care facility becomes a secondary disaster site when contaminated by the agent from the original disaster scene. For example, a patient exposed to radiation who then enters a health care facility prior to decontamination may inadvertently contaminate health care providers and others.

- It is essential that rescue and health care workers avoid becoming victims. This may go against one's initial instinct to help others, but first responders must wait until a disaster scene is secured and all safety precautions are taken.
- Assessing hazards is more important than knowing the exact cause of a disaster; an MCI can result in secondary hazards that come in many forms (Box 15.6).
- The potential for public alarm and major disruption of everyday life is enormous. Nurses must be prepared to implement crisis intervention and stress management techniques.
- In an MCI, most people, whether contaminated, exposed, or not, will self-triage and go directly to a local hospital, bypassing triage and treatment. Plans are needed to transfer patients to other medical facilities.
- Use of personal protective equipment (PPE) minimizes the risk for contact with contaminated materials or individuals. Proper use of advanced forms of PPE requires training, fitting, and an understanding that not all PPE protects against all potential hazards. Most employers require annual fit testing for PPE masks.
- When used inappropriately, PPE becomes a hazard (e.g., dehydration; decreased vision, mobility, and ability to communicate). Some of these hazards occur because the user is unable to eat, drink, or go to the bathroom while using advanced forms of PPE.
- PPEs are categorized by levels A to D, for the level of safety provided:
  - Level A—Selected when the greatest level of skin, respiratory, and eye protection is required. At this level, maximum protection is provided: a self-contained breathing apparatus, total encapsulating chemical-protective suit, coveralls, undergarments, chemical-resistant boots and gloves, hard hat, and disposable protective suit worn over the encapsulating suit. Practical limitations include limited air supply (20–50 minutes) and heat stress. Highly trained personnel use level A protection in heavily contaminated areas. If you are not wearing this type of protection and you are near an area where level A PPE is being used, get out or do not enter it.
  - Level B—Provides the highest level of respiratory protection but lower level of skin protection. Used by trained responders, this PPE includes a self-contained breathing apparatus; hooded chemical-resistant suit; and face, boot, and glove protection. Level B protection also requires training and fitting.
  - Level C—First responders and hospital personnel are trained and fitted to use level C protection, which involves knowing the concentration and type of airborne substance(s) and the criteria for using air-purifying respirators. Level C constitutes the use of full-face or half-mask air-purifying respirators (e.g., N95 mask), hooded chemical-resistant clothing, and protective gloves and boots. Because of the garment protection worn with levels A, B and C, the user is at risk for dehydration and hyperthermia.
  - Level D—Standard work uniforms or work clothes are appropriate and used for nuisance contamination only. The users must wear coveralls and chemical-resistant shoes, and, depending on the contaminant, gloves, goggles, mask, face shield, and hard hats may also be worn. There is no respiratory protection. It is important to implement routine practices when using level D protection. Depending on the circumstances, gown, cap, eye protection, mask, gloves, and shoe covers may be required.
- The most recently labelled level of protection is BioPPE. BioPPE requires the use of standard work clothes along with contact and respiratory protection. Double gloving and an N95 mask (or better) are recommended (see Chapter 5). BioPPE protection is not adequate when caring for patients exposed to toxic chemicals; however, it provides adequate protection against radiological and biological agents.
- Hand hygiene that includes washing with soap and water followed by use of an alcohol gel is important at all levels.

BOX 15.6

Potential Hazards at the Scene of a Disaster

- Downed power lines
- Smoke and toxic gases
- Debris that can result in trauma
- Fractured or leaking gas lines
- Fire resulting in burns
- Structural collapse
- Blood and other body fluids
- Inclement weather
- Hazardous materials
- Chemical, biological, radiological, or nuclear exposure
- Flooding and the threat of drowning
- Explosion, particularly secondary explosions
- Snipers
- Darkness
- Infection
- High-velocity projectiles and the pressure wave after an explosion
- Becoming incapacitated and being unable to protect yourself or patients

✦ SKILL 15.1 Care of a Patient After Biological or Chemical Exposure

Bioterrorism involves the intentional use of biological agents to cause illness and death in a population. Common routes of bioterrorism include adding the agent to food or water and using aerosolized agents. The use of biological agents is a considerable terrorist threat because they are easy to disperse and can affect large numbers of people at a relatively low cost (Box 15.7). Incubation periods and common initial clinical symptoms make detection of a biological attack difficult. Some biological attacks are unannounced or covert, and the onset of symptoms is delayed by an incubation period (i.e., the time between exposure and onset of symptoms). Biological agents have variable incubation periods from 1 or 2 days to several weeks, during which some of these agents may be transmitted as an infected patient exposes others. The mode of transmission of the biological agent determines the severity of the disaster. Recognition of bioterrorism is a challenge because early signs and symptoms mimic the flu or produce a rash that can be mistaken for a viral illness (Fig. 15.8, *A–B*). Sometimes several biological agents are disseminated at the same time, further confusing the issue. To understand how to protect yourself from becoming a victim, you need to understand the mode of transmission and precautions to take for biosafety (Table 15.1).

A chemical disaster is the dispersal of a toxic chemical agent into the environment. The mechanism of dispersal is not always known. In fact, the dispersal mechanism, such as an explosion or fire, can be a secondary terrorist attack designed to create greater fatalities. Explosions spread a toxic chemical in uncontrolled directions, creating more victims. Symptoms from chemical exposure are usually apparent within minutes, but some are delayed up to 24 hours. Early recognition of a chemical event is a priority because nurses will need to administer many chemical antidotes quickly. Toxic chemical incidents, like biological events, are often unannounced or covert. Terrorists often intend for chemical agents to cause mass casualties and induce fear and mass hysteria.

Chemical events are generally confined to small areas, although larger dispersal of these agents may occur (e.g., via a crop duster). The nature and scale of contamination depends on the state of the agent used (e.g., gas versus liquid), characteristics of the chemical used (e.g., heavier or lighter than air), and where the event occurs (e.g., indoors, where ventilation systems affect dispersal, or outdoors, where wind and velocity affect speed and direction of dispersal). For safety reasons, rescue workers should be upwind and uphill from a toxic chemical disaster scene to avoid exposure. The exception is when cyanide gas has been released. Cyanide is lighter than air and thus will travel uphill. Although cyanide has the unique smell of bitter almonds, the presence of this odour is rare among published cases of cyanide poisoning (Parker-Cote et al., 2018).

Because symptoms are almost immediate, victims need to be evacuated as quickly as possible from a contaminated zone to a decontamination zone. Appropriate PPE protects rescue workers. Before decontamination, victims are a potential source of contamination for rescue workers. Nurses need to protect themselves against toxic chemical contamination when in contact with a contaminated patient. Secondary contamination is high with toxic chemical incidents. Table 15.2 summarizes chemical warfare agents, presenting symptoms, and untreated course of exposure.

The rapid chemical decontamination of the victims of a toxic chemical incident is more important than determining the exact toxic chemical. When rapid decontamination is needed, trained personnel are required. Decontamination is either gross or technical, and generally occurs at the scene. A hospital provides decontamination when a contaminated individual presents for treatment. Interprofessional collaboration is required so that staff can take appropriate precautions to avoid becoming victims themselves.

BOX 15.7

Potential Bioterrorism Agents and Diseases

- Anthrax (*Bacillus anthracis*)
- Botulism (*Clostridium botulinum* toxin)
- Brucellosis (*Brucella* species)
- *Chlamydia psittaci* (psittacosis)
- Ebola virus hemorrhagic fever
- Epsilon toxin of *Clostridium perfringens*
- *Escherichia coli* O157:H7 (*E. coli*)
- Food safety threats (e.g., *Salmonella* species, *E. coli* O157:H7, *Shigella*)
- Plague (*Yersinia pestis*)
- Q fever (*Coxiella burnetii*)
- *Salmonella* species (salmonellosis)
- *Shigella* (shigellosis)
- Tularemia (*Francisella tularensis*)
- Typhoid fever (*Salmonella Typhimurium*)
- Variola major virus (smallpox)
- *Vibrio cholerae* (cholera)
- Viral hemorrhagic fevers (filoviruses [Ebola, Marburg] and arenaviruses [Lassa, Machupo])
- Water safety threats (e.g., *Vibrio cholerae*, *Cryptosporidium parvum*)

Data from Centers for Disease Control and Prevention. (2018). *Bioterrorism agents/diseases*. https://emergency.cdc.gov/agent/agentlist-category.asp

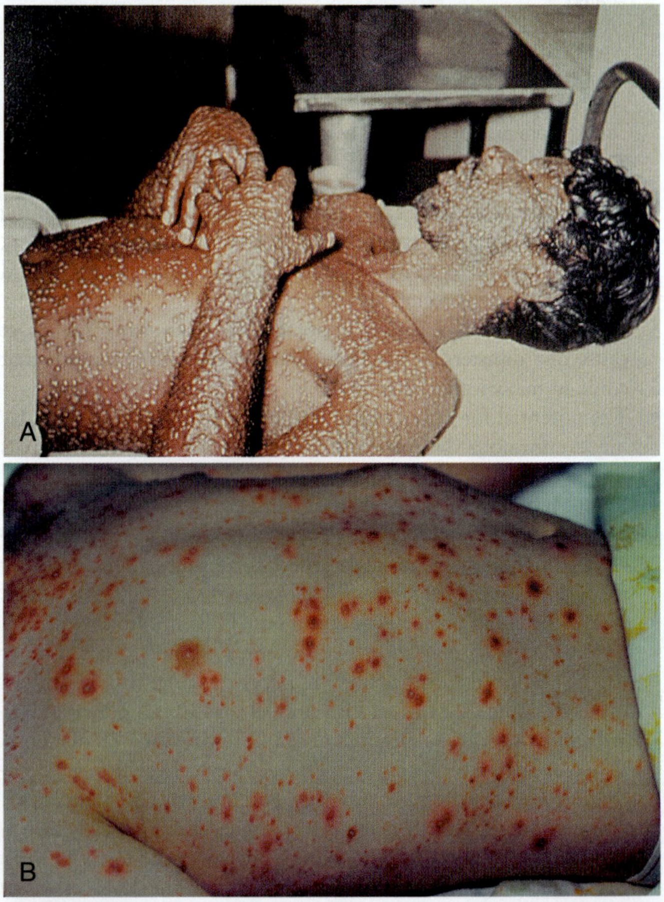

FIG 15.8 Differences in distribution of smallpox versus chickenpox. A, Man with smallpox. B, Chickenpox covering patient torso. (*A, Courtesy CDC/NIP/Barbara Rice. B, Courtesy David Effron, MD.*)

TABLE 15.1

Summary of Selected Class A Biological Warfare Agents

Disease/ Infectious Agent	Form and Incubation/Onset of Symptoms	Untreated Course of Disease: Early-Onset Symptoms	Untreated Course of Disease: Late-Onset Symptoms	Probable Route of Contamination for Use as a Biological Warfare Agent	Treatment of Mass Casualties	Prophylaxis/ Vaccine
Bacterial Biological Agents						
Anthrax *Bacillus anthracis*, a Gram-positive bacillus that can remain stable in spore form	Inhalation or pulmonary (usually within 48 hours, but may incubate for up to 60 days)	Febrile flulike symptoms (malaise, low-grade fever, dry cough, and headache)	Severe respiratory distress, hemodynamic failure, and death	Aerosol; no person-to-person transmission	Ciprofloxacin or doxycycline	Ciprofloxacin or, if susceptible, doxycycline; vaccine available but in short supply
	Cutaneous (1–12 days)	Local urticaria; painless papular lesions usually located on head, forearms, or hands	Papular lesions become vesicular, later developing black eschar and edema	Person-to-person transmission through direct contact with skin lesions		
	Gastrointestinal (1–7 days)	Abdominal pain, nausea, vomiting, and diarrhea	Gastrointestinal bleeding, fever; usually followed by toxic sepsis and death	Contaminated food and/or water		
Plague Acute, severe bacterial infection secondary to a Gram-negative bacillus, *Yersinia pestis*	Bubonic Onset of symptoms dependent on route of transmission (1–6 days)	Swollen, tender lymph nodes (most notable femoral and inguinal), high fever, rapid pulse	Hypotension, extreme exhaustion, death	Aerosol and then human-to-human by droplet inhalation	Ciprofloxacin or doxycy-cline	Ciprofloxacin or doxycycline; no vaccine available at present time
	Pneumonic (1–6 days)	High fever, chills, tachycardia, headache	Fulminate pneumonia (foamy hemoptysis, tachypnea, and dyspnea), sepsis, and death			
Botulism Anaerobic Gram-positive bacillus that produces a potent muscle-paralyzing neurotoxin	Foodborne (12–36 hours)	Nausea, vomiting, diarrhea	Symmetrical cranial nerve paralysis, descending flaccid paralysis (progressive paralysis of arms, respiratory muscles, and legs), and death	Contaminated food	Passive immunization (antitoxin); supportive care	Passive immunization (antitoxin); antitoxin available in short supply
	Inhalational (2 hours–8 days)	No fever, no changes in mental status	Symmetrical cranial nerve paralysis, descending flaccid paralysis (progressive paralysis of arms, respiratory muscles, and legs), and death	Inhalation of aerosolized toxin		
Typhoidal tularemia *Francisella tularensis*, an extremely infectious bacterium	Contaminated water or food or via aerosol distribution (1–14 days)	Flulike symptoms (headache, cough, fever and chills, malaise)	Pharyngeal ulcers, pleuritic chest pain, pneumonia, pericarditis, respiratory failure, sepsis, and death	Inhalation of aerosolized bacteria	Ciprofloxacin or doxycycline	Ciprofloxacin or doxycycline; vaccine available, only limited supply; vaccine offers incomplete protection

Continued

TABLE 15.1
Summary of Selected Class A Biological Warfare Agents—cont'd

Disease/ Infectious Agent	Form and Incubation/Onset of Symptoms	Untreated Course of Disease: Early-Onset Symptoms	Untreated Course of Disease: Late-Onset Symptoms	Probable Route of Contamination for Use as a Biological Warfare Agent	Treatment of Mass Casualties	Prophylaxis/ Vaccine
Major Viral Biological Agent of Concern—Smallpox						
Smallpox variola virus	Distribution via airborne droplets, aerosols, and fomites (7–17 days; weaponized smallpox when delivered aerosolized has an incubation period of only 3–5 days)	Acute viral symptoms (high fever, myalgia, headache, and backache)	Continued viral symptoms, high fever, prostration, synchronous onset of rash progressing from macules to papules to vesicles, and eschar formation. Vesicles more abundant on extremities and face, and all develop at the same time; pustules appear on palms of hands and soles of feet (unlike chickenpox)	Transmitted person to person by large droplets; therefore, spread may be by inhalation of aerosolized virus, oral secretions, infected human vector exposure, or exposure to contaminated objects	Supportive therapy only (ventilator)	None; vaccine available in short supply

TABLE 15.2
Summary of Selected Chemical Warfare Agents

Chemical Agent	Onset of Symptoms	Untreated Course of Chemical Exposure
"Lethal" agents—nerve agents (tabun, sarin, soman, and VX)	Symptoms are generally immediate.	Pinpoint pupils; shortly thereafter, salivation, runny nose, dyspnea, chest tightness, nausea, muscle twitching, coma, seizures, and death
"Blood" agents—hydrogen cyanide	Rapid onset of symptoms, though cyanide poisoning is sometimes associated with the smell of bitter almonds.	Death caused by asphyxiation
"Blister" agents—mustard and lewisite	Symptoms may be immediate or delayed.	Skin irritation and blistering
"Choking" agents—phosgene and chlorine	Symptoms can be immediate or delayed up to 24 hours.	Coughing, choking, and disruption in pulmonary function that can lead to death

Delegation and Collaboration

The skill of assessing a patient exposed to a biological or chemical agent cannot be delegated to an unregulated care provider (UCP). The nurse directs the UCP to do the following:

- Use appropriate PPE to prevent exposure during care activities
- Use proper techniques for handling a body after death to prevent contamination

Equipment

Choice of equipment depends on the specific biological or chemical agent. The following is a general list of supplies that might be used:

- Biohazard bags with label
- Soap and water
- 0.5% diluted bleach or an approved germicidal agent
- Negative-pressure room (high-efficiency particulate air [HEPA] filtration may be required) with anteroom
- Appropriate PPE
- Scissors or other tool to cut off clothing
- Equipment for physical examination
- Oxygen therapy
- Airway maintenance supplies
- Intravenous (IV) therapy supplies
- Isolation equipment/room, depending upon the nature of the exposure and its route of transmission

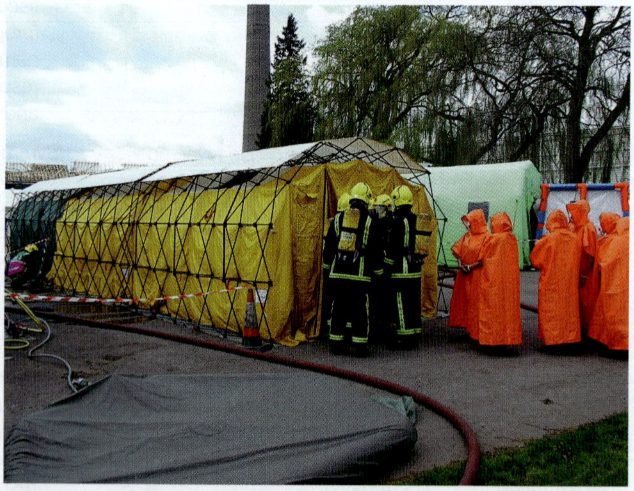

FIG 15.9 **Inflatable decontamination shower for ambulatory victims.** (*Courtesy Professional Protection Systems, Ltd.*)

- Decontamination room or area; large volumes of water, decontamination shower (Fig. 15.9); adult decontamination rooms may not meet the needs of children requiring decontamination; decontamination areas for ambulatory victims will not meet the needs of those who are not ambulatory.

STEP	RATIONALE
ASSESSMENT	
1. Identify patient using at least two person-specific identifiers (e.g., name and date of birth, or name and medical record number) according to employer policy.	Ensures correct patient. Complies with Accreditation Canada's standards and improves patient safety (Accreditation Canada, 2020).
2. Throughout the procedure, the 4 moments for hand hygiene are to be implemented; hand hygiene should occur before initial patient (or patient environment) contact, before an aseptic procedure, after body fluid exposure risk, and after patient (or patient environment) contact. Additional hand hygiene should be performed when hands are visibly soiled. Don proper PPE.	Proper hand hygiene helps prevent the spread of infectious agents to health care providers.
3. Conduct focused health history and physical examination (e.g., skin assessment; pulmonary assessment: oxygen saturation, lung sounds, sputum character; cardiac: heart sounds; gastrointestinal [GI]: nausea, vomiting, diarrhea; neurological: movement of extremities, Glasgow Coma Scale, reflexes). Review history of patient's presenting symptoms and determine whether a pattern exists (see Chapter 8). Observe for presence of liquid on patient's skin, mucous membranes, or clothing, and for odour (e.g., chlorine), assessing the condition of skin to determine severity of exposure.	Symptom identification and clustering data help to accurately determine exposure to type of biological or chemical agent and patient's response.
4. Measure patient's vital signs and include assessment of pain using an appropriate pain rating scale.	Provides baseline to later evaluate patient's response to therapy.
5. Review results of diagnostic tests and consult with health care provider.	Initial signs and symptoms of exposure to biological agent suggest common disorders (e.g., flu). Further review of diagnostic findings helps to rule out other common disorders.
6. Assess patient for pre-existing health risks (e.g., history of heart disease, pulmonary disease, cancer) that complicate effects of exposure to biological agent.	Patients with pre-existing medical conditions often require additional treatment or are at greater risk for death.
7. Remain calm. Listen to patient and assess their immediate psychological response after exposure. Some patients present with dissociative symptoms (e.g., feeling as though they are "not there" or sensing that everything is outside of the person): disorientation, depression, anxiety, psychosis, and inability to care for self. Even without direct exposure to a biological or chemical agent, many individuals, spurred by feelings of fear and doom, present for emergency services.	Aids in providing appropriate crisis intervention and stress management. Remaining calm and projecting confidence while assessing individuals for clinical symptoms reduce anxiety of the ill and worried well as they experience the general sense of panic associated with a biological or chemical exposure.
8. Identify and gather all patient contact information (names, addresses, and phone numbers) before the patient leaves the ED.	All patient contacts need to be identified for proper follow-up by the public health department. Often patients will self-triage and transport to the ED.
9. Identify employer resources available (e.g., critical-incident stress-debriefing teams, counsellors, psychiatric and mental health nurse practitioners).	Expert resources help to assess extent of the psychological impact of disaster.

Critical Decision Point *Consider that a biological or toxic chemical event has occurred when large numbers of ill persons present who have unexplained yet similar symptoms; when there are unexplained deaths, particularly among young and healthy populations; when there is an unusual pattern associated with the symptoms (e.g., geographical, seasonal, patient population); when a patient fails to respond to traditional therapy; or when a single patient presents with symptoms suggestive of an uncommon agent (e.g., anthrax or smallpox). Once you suspect a biological or chemical event, notify incident command immediately. The primary objective for initial care of a chemical event may be decontamination. This is achieved by removing clothing, scrubbing the skin, and hydrolysis (a process of chemical dilution using large volumes of water).*

STEP	RATIONALE

NURSING DIAGNOSES

- Reduced airway clearance
- Inadequate swallowing
- Reduced gas exchange
- Decreased cardiac output
- Acute pain
- Reduced skin integrity
- Acute confusion
- Nausea
- Anxiety/fear
- Post-trauma syndrome
- Potential for imbalanced body temperature
- Potential for imbalanced fluid volume
- Potential for peripheral neurovascular dysfunction

Related factors and risk factors are individualized on the basis of patient's condition or needs.

PLANNING

STEP	RATIONALE
1. Expected outcomes following completion of procedure:	
• Patient is comforted.	In some cases, care is only palliative, with comfort as the focus. Do not underestimate the value of *comfort as care*.
• Patient's vital signs return to baseline.	When there are no underlying medical conditions and *if* the patient's disease process is responsive to treatment (when available), vital signs will normalize. However, this may take days or weeks.
• Patient's work of breathing decreases.	Indicates improved gas exchange and cardiac output.
• Patient's skin integrity returns to baseline or no new injury develops.	Antibiotic and antitoxin therapy will aid in resolution or healing of lesions over time; minimizes exposure of skin to chemical agent and reduces severity and extent of lesions.
• Patient's level of consciousness (LOC) returns to baseline.	Treatment measures restore neurological function and oxygenation status.
• Patient's mental health status returns to pretrauma level of functioning.	Crisis intervention successfully reduces patient's anxiety, fear, and dissociative symptoms.
2. Dispense timely and accurate information, including decontamination (if appropriate): accurate description of agent to which patient has been exposed and implications for patient and family.	Information relieves anxiety and fear.

IMPLEMENTATION

STEP	RATIONALE
1. Continue wearing PPE applied before assessment. Follow required transmission-based precautions. (See Table 15.1 for route of contamination.) Prepare for decontamination and isolation if required.	Reduces transmission of microorganisms and the likelihood of additional secondary sites of contamination.

Critical Decision Point *Only trained personnel using required PPE may decontaminate patients with toxic chemical contamination. Hold victims outside decontamination area until preparations have been completed for decontamination. If patient is grossly contaminated, consider decontamination before entry into building.*

STEP	RATIONALE
2. Decontaminate patient (see emergency policies).	
a. Act quickly; avoid touching contaminated parts of clothing as much as possible.	Prevent your own contamination.
b. Remove all clothing from patient. CAUTION: Do not pull clothing over patient's head; instead, cut garments off.	Cutting off clothing prevents contamination of head and hair.
c. Use large amounts of soap and/or water to wash patient thoroughly.	Leads to biological or chemical dilution and, in some cases, prevents patient death.
d. If patient's eyes are burning or vision is blurred, rinse eyes with plain water for 10–15 minutes. If patient wears contacts, remove and place with contaminated clothing; do not reinsert into eyes. Wash eyeglasses with soap and water; reapply when completed.	Flushes toxins from eyes.
3. Establish airway and administer oxygen if needed (see Chapter 23).	Various agents (e.g., pulmonary anthrax) commonly cause respiratory problems that may result in altered gas exchange.
4. Control bleeding.	Various agents can cause extensive bleeding.

STEP	RATIONALE
5. Administer appropriate antibiotics, antitoxins, or appropriate chemical agent treatment protocol.	Various biological agents are commonly treated with ciprofloxacin and/or doxycycline. Appropriate chemical agent protocol varies with patient exposure.
6. Administer immunizations (e.g., in the event of smallpox).	Administration of the smallpox vaccine is the only known method to prevent the development of smallpox in an exposed person. If administered within 4 days of exposure, the vaccine usually prevents smallpox symptoms. If administered 4–7 days after exposure, the vaccine may decrease the severity of the disease (Hussain, 2018).
7. Administer fluid and nutrition therapy (see Chapters 29 and 33).	Biological agents commonly cause GI disturbances that sometimes result in dehydration.
8. Dispose of patient's contaminated clothing in appropriate biohazard bag and seal (see employer policy).	Reduces likelihood of secondary biological or chemical contamination.
9. Provide supportive care (e.g., comfort measures, including pain management) (see Chapters 16 and 17).	Some victims that have been exposed to a biological or chemical agent will not survive; palliative care is essential (see Chapter 17).
10. After leaving patient area, remove most heavily contaminated items first. Peel off gown and gloves, roll inside out, and dispose of them.	Avoids contamination of self, others, and environment. Reduces transmission of microorganisms.
11. Remove face shield from behind and dispose of safely. Remove goggles and mask from behind. Place goggles in container for reprocessing; dispose of mask safely.	
12. Counsel patient and family about acute and potential long-term psychological effects of exposure. Offer access to trained counsellors. Support survivors of a disaster by identifying resources available.	Reaction of patients will include shock, fear, and immobilization. Long-term psychological effects can arise without proper counselling. Social support networks foster coping in the days following a disaster.

Critical Decision Point *Interprofessional collaboration between health care providers and other rescue workers is required to create an ongoing plan to manage patients exposed to a biological or chemical agent while continuing to care for other patients at the health care facility seeking care for illness unrelated to the current* MCI.

EVALUATION

1. Observe for improved airway maintenance, breathing, circulation, LOC, and neurological functioning.	Evaluates patient's response to available treatment and supportive care.
2. Evaluate vital signs and level of pain.	Evaluates patient's response to treatment and determines whether comfort measures are effective.
3. Inspect condition of patient's skin; note character of lesions or extent of blistering.	Evaluates patient's response to antibiotic therapy and determines extent of healing.
4. Ask patient, "Tell me how you feel right now." Check level of orientation and ability to conduct conversation.	Evaluates patient for changes that suggest either improvement in or deterioration of psychological status.

Unexpected Outcomes	Related Interventions
1. Patient's physical or psychological symptoms progress.	• Notify health care provider. • Notify mental health treatment team. • Remain calm, offer reassurance, and protect self and others from physical harm. • Continue to provide comfort care.
2. Patient death occurs.	• When handling bodies, consider continued risk for contamination; make sure that everyone is fully informed regarding proper procedure.
3. Secondary contamination of rescue workers.	• Rescue workers must immediately remove their clothing, scrub their bodies, and use copious amounts of soap and water, according to employer policy. Provide clean clothes. Report symptoms to a health care provider or nursing supervisor.

Communication and Documentation

- Report suspected cases of a biological or chemical incident to health care provider following employer protocol. In the event of an ED exposure to a communicable disease, the department will be locked down immediately. Public health officials (e.g., the public health officer) will determine whether the hospital should be locked down.
- Document patient's status, decontamination and treatment procedures, and response to treatment and comfort measures.
- Use disaster checklists to quickly document specific data regarding patient status, treatment administered, and response to treatment and comfort measures.
- Report any unexpected outcome to health care provider in charge.

DOCUMENTATION EXAMPLE

Patient presented ambulatory to ED with symptoms of burning feeling in their eyes. Sclera of eyes noted to be slightly reddened. Patient states that they got household bleach splashed in their eyes when cleaning at home and immediately flushed the eyes with cool water for 5 minutes. Vital signs normal. Pain 3 on a scale of 1 to 10. No redness or rash noted around eye area. Denies any breathing issues or vision problems. Sought care to ensure that home treatment was appropriate. Eyes flushed with lukewarm water × 15 minutes. Patient stated that the burning and pain was gone and asked about further treatment. HCP indicated that no further treatment is required unless visual changes are experienced. Patient explained visual changes that they were to monitor for to this writer. Patient advised to wear sunglasses when outside for the next 24–48 hours. Patient left ambulatory with family member.

Special Considerations

Teaching

- Preparation for an MCI goes a long way toward preventing casualties and chaos. Public education of the likelihood of a mass casualty biological or chemical event is necessary and includes information about types of biological and chemical agents, mode of transmission/dissemination, symptoms, treatment, and locations of shelters, disaster treatment sites, and how to shelter in place (see Box 15.4).
- Preparedness includes teaching individuals, families, and communities about resilience and the ability to care for themselves when support services are not available or are inaccessible.
- Health care providers need an opportunity to debrief after a disaster to help avoid psychological complications such as PTSD.
- Encourage families to prepare for the unexpected (see Care in the Community: Home Management).

Pediatric

- Children are an especially vulnerable population, and many facets influence the impact of a disaster on children. These facets often include age, sex, family dynamics, and level of exposure to the disaster (Hockenberry et al., 2024).
- Children have both physical and emotional needs during disasters. They often show stress-related symptoms and may have temporary changes in behaviour after a disaster (Hockenberry et al., 2024).
- To avoid becoming a secondary victim, emergency responders need to consider potential contamination of children before picking them up and holding them. Often, decontamination consists of providing fresh air and a large volume of low-pressure warm water. Observe children for potential hypothermia because they are more susceptible.
- Adult decontamination facilities do not always meet the needs of children. The special PPE worn by rescue workers may frighten young children. The cleaning process and possible separation from uncontaminated parents will likely cause considerable stress and anxiety. Additional health care workers are often necessary to ensure that adequate decontamination has taken place. Verbal encouragement and praise are effective in facilitating the process.
- Many disasters result in the need to relocate, which creates stress and unique challenges in children. Stress may be increased by changes in children's cultural, psychological, and social environment. Reactions of their parents and other family members contribute to how well the child will cope with relocation and whether or not they will be able to stay connected with friends and familiar activities (Hockenberry et al., 2024).
- Children are very vulnerable to the adverse effects of environmental chemicals and toxins because (1) kilogram for kilogram, children take in larger doses of toxins through food, water, and air; (2) children's organ systems are less mature and thus unable to remove some of the toxins; and (3) their life expectancy is longer, and long-term effects of exposure to toxins are unknown (Hockenberry et al., 2024).
- Disasters disrupt critical infrastructure (CI) and may cause large-scale displacement, leading to unsafe water, lack of access to health care, and decreases in vector control and infectious agents (WHO, n.d.-b). Outbreaks of communicable diseases have been reported after natural disasters, and children are more likely to develop infections secondary to immature immune systems (Hockenberry et al., 2024).
- Families should be kept together after a disaster. Family togetherness offers reassurance to a child and lessens fears of being abandoned and unprotected (Hockenberry et al., 2024).
- The media has an enormous influence over children and may affect development and behaviour. Encourage parents to limit their children's exposure to media reports of the disaster and to watch television with them whenever possible to clarify information and answer questions (Hockenberry et al., 2024).
- The death of a child is always traumatic; parents may have a compelling need to be present during pediatric resuscitation and at the time of death; ideally, you should allow it. It is important for nurses to be present to explain what is happening and facilitate the grieving process (Hockenberry et al., 2024).

Gerontological

- Under disaster conditions, triage older persons according to injuries, not age.
- Because older persons often have several concurrent illnesses, exposure to a biological or chemical agent often worsens these conditions and results in the need for more immediate care than an initial triage may suggest.
- Older persons are vulnerable during a disaster; they have higher rates of severe illness and mortality, have difficulty accessing essential services, are exposed to ageism, and experience stress and anxiety during times of confinement (United Nations Economic Commission for Europe, 2020).

Patients With Physical or Cognitive Challenges

- Collaboration with government organizations is critical for developing strategies to make emergency communications and related announcements accessible to people with physical or cognitive challenges (Kim & Zakour, 2018).

Care in the Community: Home Management

- Assemble a disaster kit before disaster strikes. The Canadian Red Cross and Public Safety Canada (2022c) offer information on how to assemble a disaster preparedness kit (Box 15.8).
- Individuals with special needs (e.g., hearing impairment, impaired mobility, special diets) and individuals without vehicles require additional planning to be prepared for a disaster.
- Post emergency telephone numbers by the telephone, enter them in smartphone contacts, and teach children how and when to call 9-1-1.
- Family members need to establish a meeting place away from the home in case they cannot stay in their home or cannot reach their home during a disaster.
- Remain isolated and advise friends and relatives not to visit if family members are symptomatic.
- Instruct family members to use the appropriate PPE needed to protect the family; this can include sheltering in place.
- Maintain strict hand hygiene for both well and symptomatic family members after using the bathroom, before eating and drinking, and after contact with pets.
- When a sick individual's symptoms worsen, transport them to the nearest designated hospital.
- Change a sick person's clothing and bed linens frequently; wash them separately from those of other family members using any commercial detergent.
- Disinfect surfaces that the symptomatic person comes in contact with. Use an appropriate disinfectant (e.g., Lysol), especially when surfaces are soiled by blood or other body fluids.

BOX 15.8

Basic Emergency Kit

- Water (at least 2 litres of water per person per day; minimum 72-hour supply)
- Food that won't spoil (e.g., canned food, energy bars, dried food, peanut butter, rice); replace food in your kit every year
- Manual can opener
- Extra keys to your car and house
- Some cash in small denominations
- A copy of your emergency plan and contact information
- Battery-operated or crank flashlight and radio
- Fresh batteries
- Matches in waterproof container
- Candles
- First aid kit
- Emergency blanket
- Sanitation and hygiene items (e.g., hand sanitizer, toiletries, toilet paper)
- Cell phone and chargers
- Copies of personal documents (e.g., birth certificates, deed to home, passport)
- Duct tape
- Household chlorine bleach or water-purifying tablets
- Basic tools
- A whistle
- If applicable, medications, infant formula, equipment for persons with disabilities, pet supplies

Adapted from Public Safety Canada. (2022c). *Emergency kits*. https://www.getprepared.gc.ca/cnt/kts/index-en.aspx

- Family caregivers need to get plenty of rest, drink fluids frequently, and eat a healthy diet. If the caregiver develops symptoms, obtain appropriate medical care immediately.
- Keep upwind and uphill from the release of any chemical agents unless it is cyanide.

✦ SKILL 15.2 Care of a Patient After Radiation Exposure

Radiological events differ from nuclear events. A radiological event is the dispersal of radioactive material via a "dirty bomb," by deliberate contamination of food or water supplies, or over the terrain. A nuclear event involves a device that releases nuclear energy in an explosive manner as a result of a nuclear chain reaction. Radiation affects the body in many ways, depending on the level of exposure. High levels of radiation exposure cause a person to develop acute radiation syndrome (ARS) with symptoms of vomiting, diarrhea, erythema, and changes in blood cell counts (Barabanova et al., 2019).

Radiation comes in a variety of forms. Alpha particles are the least dangerous, travelling only a few centimetres in the air. They do not penetrate materials easily and are harmful only if ingested. An individual's clothing blocks alpha particles from reaching the skin. Beta particles penetrate a short distance into the skin. Protective clothing is necessary for protection. Gamma rays pose the greatest health risk because the waves penetrate deeply, causing severe burns and internal injury. Lead shielding protects against gamma rays. Blasts caused by a nuclear explosion cause not only injury from radiation exposure but also traumatic injuries and burns. Some victims will present with many combined forms of injury requiring treatment. The sooner symptoms begin to appear, the greater a patient's exposure to the radiation. Early symptoms (i.e., within a few hours) suggest that an individual has received a lethal dose of radiation.

Nuclear incidents usually result in widespread destruction requiring specialized equipment and resources at the scene to assess structural damage and levels of radioactivity. Radiological events usually cover much smaller areas, but they are often difficult to define. Specialized equipment and training are required to assess the source of radioactivity, determine the scope of contamination, and perform decontamination. During a nuclear emergency, individuals may be instructed to shelter in place. Individuals who were outside during the nuclear emergency are to remove clothes, seal them in a plastic bag, rinse hair and body in a shower, and then don clean clothes from a closed drawer or closet (Public Safety Canada, 2020a).

Delegation and Collaboration

The skill of assessing and caring for a patient exposed to a radiological agent cannot be delegated to a UCP. The nurse directs the UCP to do the following:

- Use appropriate PPE to prevent exposure
- Use techniques for handling a body after death to prevent contamination

Equipment

- Decontamination room or area
- Scissors or other tool to cut off clothing
- Clothing containers; type depends on the kind of radiological exposure
- Appropriate PPE for use by personnel in area of radiation release
- Appropriate PPE for health care workers in health care facilities (i.e., surgical masks, N95 masks recommended if available)
- Radiation meter available to survey hands and clothing at frequent intervals
- Equipment for select specimen collection
- Equipment for physical examination

STEP	RATIONALE

ASSESSMENT

STEP	RATIONALE
1. Identify patient using at least two person-specific identifiers (e.g., name and date of birth, or name and medical record number) according to employer policy.	Ensures correct patient. Complies with Accreditation Canada's standards and improves patient safety (Accreditation Canada, 2020).
2. Throughout the procedure, the 4 moments for hand hygiene are to be implemented; hand hygiene should occur before initial patient (or patient environment) contact, before an aseptic procedure, after body fluid exposure risk, and after patient (or patient environment) contact. Additional hand hygiene should be performed when hands are visibly soiled. Don proper PPE.	Proper hand hygiene helps prevent the spread of infectious agents/radiiological particles to health care providers.

Critical Decision Point *Before assessment, a specially trained technician conducts a radiation survey of the patient, initially scanning the face, hands, and feet with a radiation survey instrument. If meter results are positive, a thorough survey (5–8 minutes per person) is conducted.*

STEP	RATIONALE
3. Assess patient's symptoms by performing a focused health history and physical examination (see Skill 15.1).	Symptom identification and clustering of data are first steps to determine patient's condition and response to radiation.
4. Measure patient's vital signs and include assessment of pain on an appropriate pain scale (e.g., on a scale of 0 to 10, where 0 is no pain and 10 is worst pain ever).	Provides baseline to later evaluate patient's response to therapy.

Critical Decision Point *Do not touch a wound if you suspect the presence of radioactive fragments.*

STEP	RATIONALE
5. Assess patient for pre-existing medical conditions that will complicate effects of the radiological exposure. Symptoms of ARS include vomiting, headache, diarrhea, erythema, and changes in blood cell counts (Barabanova et al., 2019).	Patients with pre-existing medical conditions can require additional treatment or are at greater risk for death.
6. Determine patient's allergies, specifically allergy for iodine sensitivity.	Patients with iodine sensitivity need to avoid taking potassium iodide, the treatment of choice for radioactive iodine exposure.
7. Assess individual psychological response to radiological event. Some patients present with dissociative symptoms (e.g., feeling as though they are "not there," sensing that experiences are outside the person): disorientation, depression, anxiety, psychosis, and an inability to care for self. Ask patient, "How do you feel now?" Determine level of orientation, ability to follow conversation.	Enables appropriate crisis intervention and stress management. Remaining calm and projecting confidence while assessing individuals for clinical symptoms versus feeling of panic go a long way toward reducing anxiety of the ill and worried well, as they experience the general sense of panic associated with a radiological event.
8. Identify employer resources available (e.g., critical-incident stress-debriefing teams, counsellors, psychiatric and mental health nurse practitioners).	Expert resources assess extent of psychological impact of disaster.

Critical Decision Point *A radiological event is the event most feared by most individuals. Many are uneducated regarding the dangers of and differences among radiation materials. Health care facilities will likely have many anxious, frightened individuals who can potentially create a danger to the environment. Assess individuals for signs of psychological distress. Early identification of symptoms and stress management interventions can help prevent an individual or mass panic response.*

NURSING DIAGNOSES

- Acute pain
- Inadequate fluid volume
- Diarrhea
- Anxiety/fear
- Nausea
- Potential for post-trauma syndrome
- Potential for infection
- Reduced tissue integrity

Related factors and risk factors are individualized on the basis of patient's condition or needs.

STEP	RATIONALE

PLANNING

STEP	RATIONALE
1. Expected outcomes following completion of procedure:	
• Patient is comforted.	In some cases, the only care that is available is palliative.
• Patient is successfully decontaminated.	Decontamination procedures remove radioactive materials from patient's skin.
• Patient's vital signs return to baseline.	When there are no underlying medical conditions and *if* the patient's disease process is responsive to treatment (when available), vital signs will return to normal within days or weeks.
• Patient is free of nausea and diarrhea.	GI alterations following radiation exposure typically respond to antidiarrheal and antiemetic medications.
• Patient's skin integrity returns to baseline.	Radiological burns are minimized through successful decontamination procedures.
• Patient's immune system (e.g., complete blood count [CBC]) returns to baseline.	Exposure to radiation is minimized successfully.
• Patient's work of breathing decreases.	Indicates improved gas exchange and cardiac output.
2. Explain care to patient and family. Explain your role, orient to location and activities to perform, explain what patient has experienced, and ask, "How are you feeling right now?" Assure them that the health care provider will see them shortly.	Crisis intervention re-establishes patient's orientation and sense of reality.

IMPLEMENTATION

STEP	RATIONALE
1. Continue wearing PPE applied during assessment. Prepare for decontamination. **Note:** Only trained personnel should use required PPE to decontaminate patients with radiological contamination.	Reduces likelihood of secondary radiological contamination to untrained personnel attempting decontamination.
2. Provide for patient privacy by closing room curtains or door.	Prevents anxiety or embarrassment when clothes are removed.
3. Decontaminate patient:	
a. Remove patient's clothing.	Normally eliminates up to 90% of contamination.
b. Wash patient's skin thoroughly with water and soap, taking care not to abrade or irritate the skin.	Use of large amounts of water is critical in decontamination.
Use tepid decontamination water. Cover wounds with waterproof dressings to avoid spread of radioactivity (Radiation Emergency Medical Management [REMM], 2023b).	Water that is too cold will close pores, and water that is too hot enhances absorption of radioactive materials or can cause a thermal burn (REMM, 2023b).
c. Have radiation technician resurvey patient after washing. Rewash as necessary.	Determines whether residual radiation is present.
d. Isolate and cover any area of skin that is still positive for radiation by using plastic bag or wrap.	Area is washed until no further reduction in contamination is achieved (verified by survey instrumentation) and then covered to reduce exposure of health care workers.
4. Bag and tag patient's contaminated clothing for further evaluation and place in an appropriate biohazard container.	Reduces likelihood of secondary contamination when you use containers designed to contain radiological particles.

Critical Decision Point *Interprofessional collaboration is required to create an ongoing plan to manage patients exposed to radiological materials while continuing to care for patients at the health care facility seeking care for illness unrelated to the current nuclear or radiological event.*

STEP	RATIONALE
5. Prepare for possibly obtaining CBC, urinalysis, fecal specimen, and swabs of body orifices (see Chapter 9).	CBC establishes baseline to assess changes in patient's immunological status over time. A health care provider who suspects internal contamination will order collection of urine, feces, and body orifice swabs to analyze for radionuclides.
6. Treat symptoms according to ordinary treatment practices: provide IV fluid support, antidiarrheal therapies, antiemetic medications, and potassium iodide tablets.	Patient exposed to radiation is at risk for GI alterations and fluid imbalance. Treatment is directed at minimizing or removing internal contamination (inhalation, ingestion, or absorption through open wounds) (REMM, 2023a).
7. Remove most heavily contaminated items first. Peel off gown and gloves, roll inside out, and dispose of them.	Avoids contamination of self, others, and environment. Reduces transmission of microorganisms/radiological particles.
8. Remove face shield from behind and dispose of safely. Remove goggles and mask from behind. Place goggles in container for reprocessing; dispose of mask safely.	
9. Counsel patient and family on both acute and potential long-term psychological effects of exposure. Offer access to professional counsellors.	Reaction of patients to exposure includes shock, immobilization, and fear. Long-term psychological effects can arise without proper counselling.

STEP	RATIONALE
EVALUATION	
1. Observe skin integrity, fluid balance, respiratory and GI status, LOC, and neurological functioning. Look for improvement of other radiological agent–specific symptoms. Evaluate vital signs.	Evaluates patient's physical response to available treatment and supportive care.
2. Monitor CBC and other laboratory tests.	Determines patient's immune response.
3. Evaluate patient's LOC, orientation, and ability to relate events. Ask if patient remembers what has occurred; observe affect.	Determines whether psychological status has improved.

Unexpected Outcomes	Related Interventions
1. Secondary contamination of rescue workers occurs.	• Institute appropriate decontamination of worker.
2. Patient's symptoms progress despite appropriate treatment.	• Notify health care provider in charge. • Continue to provide comfort care.
3. Patient's psychological state deteriorates, with development of disorientation, suicidal ideation, or violence toward others.	• Notify mental health treatment team. • Remain calm, offer reassurance, and protect self and others from physical harm. • Continue to provide comfort care (see Chapter 17).
4. Patient death occurs.	• When handling bodies, consider continued risk for contamination; make sure that everyone is fully informed about proper procedure. • If the deceased is known or suspected to be contaminated, all people handling the body will wear PPE and a personal dosimeter. • When delegating preparation of the deceased, consider the level of training of those managing the body.

Communication and Documentation

- Document patient's status, treatment provided, response to treatment, and comfort measures in the patient's chart.
- Record patient and family response to instruction.
- Report immediately the presence of open wound and any suspected radioactive fragment to health care provider in charge.
- Communicate any unexpected outcomes to health care provider.

Special Considerations

Teaching

- See Skill 15.1 Teaching considerations.

Pediatric

- Children are vulnerable to radiation because (1) their organ systems are more sensitive than those of adults and (2) they have a longer expected lifespan over which to develop complications from the radiological exposure.
- See Skill 15.1 for further pediatric considerations.

Gerontological

- Some older persons have many concurrent illnesses, which can be worsened by radiological agents. The older person may therefore need more immediate care than initial triage had indicated.
- See Skill 15.1 for further gerontological considerations.

Care in the Community: Home Management

- When a radiological or nuclear event becomes reality, information could be broadcast on the radio, television, or social media sites; listen for special instructions, including appropriate means for sheltering in place.
- Keep upwind and uphill from the release of radioactive materials.
- See Skill 15.1 for further home management considerations.

✦ REVIEW QUESTIONS

Victims of an explosion at a chemical plant are arriving in the emergency department (ED). Authorities state that the identity of the substance is currently unknown, but there were reports of a "funny smell" earlier in the day. Review Questions 1 to 3 relate to the case study presented here.

1. Which safety measures should the nurses take to protect themselves and the other patients in the ED from exposure to the chemical agent?

2. The nurse on the scene has been asked to triage the remainder of the victims using the START triage system. Place the following patients in order of highest priority to lowest priority:

1. A 22-year-old with cyanosis, a respiratory rate of 35, and confusion
2. A 14-year-old with a diffuse red rash on the extremities
3. A 56-year-old with controlled bleeding of deep lacerations received from falling debris
4. A 41-year-old with full-thickness burns on 50% of the body

3. One of the final victims to arrive in the ED is an 85-year-old patient with a history of angina and prostate cancer. The patient, who lives alone in an apartment in a retirement community, has audible wheezes on assessment and is able to answer all questions clearly. Vital signs are as follows: pulse: 96 beats/min, irregular; respiratory rate: 28 breaths/min; O_2 saturation: 88%. The patient's electrocardiogram (ECG) on admission to the ED reveals a possible anterior wall myocardial infarction (MI). Using SBAR (situation–background–assessment–recommendation), show how you would communicate with the health care team about this patient's condition.
4. The nurse is caring for a patient who had a biological exposure. Which actions can the nurse direct the unregulated care provider (UCP) to complete? (*Select all that apply.*)
   1. Conduct a focused health history.
   2. Handle the body after death.
   3. Review diagnostic test results.
   4. Gather and wear personal protective equipment (PPE).
   5. Administer a decontamination shower.
5. The nurse caring for a patient after radiation exposure suspects that the patient is suffering a psychological response. Which of the following findings would lead the nurse to make this determination? (*Select all that apply.*)
   1. Disorientation to place and time
   2. Heightened self-care practices
   3. Depression related to the exposure
   4. Inability to follow a conversation
   5. Planning for a family vacation
6. The nurse is caring for a patient who was exposed to a chemical agent and needs to be decontaminated. Place the following steps in the correct order:
   1. Wash patient with soap and water.
   2. Dispose of contaminated clothing.
   3. Remove contaminated clothing.
   4. Administer intravenous (IV) fluids.
   5. Rinse eyes with plain water.
   6. Initiate treatment for chemical agent.

Visit the Evolve site for a complete list of answers to the Review Questions.

NEXT GENERATION NCLEX® (NGN)

For practice with answering exam questions related to unfolding NGN case studies, please consult the Next Generation NCLEX® (NGN)-Style Case Studies for Skills and Techniques on the Evolve website: http://evolve.elsevier.com/Canada/Perry/clinicalskills/

REFERENCES

Accreditation Canada. (2020). *Required organizational practices handbook.* https://physicians.nshealth.ca/resources/required-organizational-practices-2020-handbook

Barabanova, A. V., Bushmanov, A. J., & Kotenko, K. V. (2019). Acute radiation sickness from Chernobyl. In *Earth systems and environmental sciences.* Elsevier. https://doi.org/10.1016/B978-0-12-409548-9.12128-1

Canadian Association of Emergency Physicians. (2020). *CAEP position paper on hospital disaster preparedness–Executive summary.* https://caep.ca/wp-content/uploads/2020/03/CAEP-Position-Statement-on-Disaster-Preparedness-Full-Statement-FINAL.pdf

Canadian Association of Schools of Nursing. (2020). *Guidelines for undergraduate nursing education on climate-driven vector-borne diseases.* https://www.casn.ca/wp-content/uploads/2020/04/VB-Disease-Doc-web.pdf

Canadian Centre for Occupational Health and Safety. (2022). *WHMIS/GHS/(M)SDS.* https://www.ccohs.ca/topics/legislation/WHMIS/

Canadian Nurses Association. (2012). *Position statement: Emergency preparedness and response.* https://www.cna-aiic.ca/en/nursing/nursing-tools-and-resources/emergency-preparedness [Seminal Reference]

Canadian Nurses Protective Society (CNPS). (2020). *Legal considerations when nursing in a pandemic.* https://cnps.ca/article/Legal-Considerations-Nursing-Pandemic/

Canadian Red Cross. (n.d.-a). *Emergencies and disasters in Canada.* https://www.redcross.ca/how-we-help/emergencies-and-disasters-in-canada

Canadian Red Cross. (n.d.-b). *Emergency preparedness for Indigenous communities.* https://www.redcross.ca/how-we-help/emergencies-and-disasters-in-canada/be-ready-emergency-preparedness-and-recovery/emergency-preparedness-for-indigenous-communities

Canadian Red Cross. (n.d.-c). *How we help.* https://www.redcross.ca/how-we-help

Canadian Red Cross. (2017, May 23). *Recovery continues in Fort McMurray as Red Cross releases Alberta fires one year report.* https://www.redcross.ca/about-us/red-cross-stories/2017/recovery-continues-in-fort-mcmurray-as-red-cross-releases-alberta-fires-one-year-report

Canadian Red Cross. (2022). *2021 British Columbia fires.* https://www.redcross.ca/how-we-help/current-emergency-responses/2021-british-columbia-fires

Centers for Disease Control and Prevention. (2018). *Bioterrorism agents/diseases.* https://emergency.cdc.gov/agent/agentlist-category.asp

Cohen, J. (2022). Monkeypox is a new global threat. African scientists know what the world is up against. *Science.* https://doi.org/10.1126/science.add2880

DeNolf, R., & Kahwaji, C. (2021). EMS mass casualty management. *StatPearls.* https://www.ncbi.nlm.nih.gov/books/NBK482373/

Emergencies Act, RSC 1985, c. 22 (4th Supp.). https://laws-lois.justice.gc.ca/eng/acts/e-4.5/page-1.html

Feldman, S. (2022, February 22). *The Emergencies Act: Parliament's role during a national emergency.* HillNotes, Library of Parliament. https://hillnotes.ca/2022/02/22/the-emergencies-act-parliaments-role-during-a-national-emergency/

Gilmartin, M., Spurlock, W. R., Foster, N., et al. (2019). Improving disaster preparedness, response and recovery for older adults. *Geriatric Nursing, 40*(4), 445–447. https://doi.org/10.1016/j.gerinurse.2019.07.006

Government of Canada. (2022a). *Climate change and health.* https://www.canada.ca/en/health-canada/services/climate-change-health.html

Government of Canada. (2022b). *Infectious diseases and climate change.* https://www.canada.ca/en/health-canada/services/climate-change-health/infectious-diseases.html

Government of Canada. (2022c). *Pandemic plans.* https://www.canada.ca/en/public-health/services/flu-influenza/pandemic-plans.html

Grolnick, W., Schonfeld, D. J., Schreiber, M., et al. (2018). Improving adjustment and resilience in children following a disaster: Addressing research challenges. *American Psychologist, 73*(3), 215–229. https://doi.apa.org/doi/10.1037/amp0000181

Hart, A., Nammour, E., Mangolds, V., et al. (2018). Intuitive versus algorithmic triage. *Prehospital and Disaster Medicine, 33*(4), 355–361. https://doi.org/10.1017/S1049023X18000626

Hockenberry, M., Duffy, E. A., & Gibbs, K. (2024). *Wong's nursing care of infants and children* (12th ed.). Elsevier.

Hussain, A. (2018). Smallpox treatment and management. *Medscape.* https://emedicine.medscape.com/article/237229-treatment

Incident Command System Canada. (2012). *Incident Command System operational description.* https://www.icscanada.ca/images/upload//ICS%20OPS%20Description2012.pdf

International Council of Nurses. (2019). *Core competencies in disaster nursing version 2.0.* https://www.icn.ch/sites/default/files/inline-files/ICN_Disaster-Comp-Report_WEB.pdf

Kim, H., & Zakour, M. (2018). Exploring the factors associated with the disaster preparedness of human service organizations serving persons with disabilities. *Human Service Organizations: Management, Leadership & Governance, 42*(1), 19–32. https://doi.org/10.1080/23303131.2017.1380737

Labrague, L. J., Hammad, K., Gloe, D. S., et al. (2018). Disaster preparedness among nurses: A systematic review of literature. *International Nursing Review, 65*(1), 41–53. https://doi.org/10.1111/inr.12369

Langan, J. C., Lavin, R. P., Griffin, A. R., et al. (2019). From brainstorming to strategic plan: The framework for the society for the advancement of disaster nursing: A work in progress. *Nursing Administration Quarterly, 43*(1), 84–93. https://doi.org/10.1097/NAQ.0000000000000335

Makwana, N. (2019). Disaster and its impact on mental health: A narrative review. *Journal of Family Medicine and Primary Care, 8*(10), 3090–3095. https://doi.org/10.4103/jfmpc.jfmpc_893_19

Mao, W., & Agyapong, V. I. O. (2021). The role of social determinants in mental health and resilience after disasters: Implications for public health policy and practice. *Frontiers in Public Health, 9*, Article 658528. https://doi.org/10.3389/fpubh.2021.658528

Nowell, L., Dhingra, S., Andrews, K., et al. (2021). A grounded theory of clinical nurses' process of coping during COVID-19. *Journal of Clinical Nursing, 2021*, 1–12. https://doi.org/10.1111/jocn.15809

Parker-Cote, J., Rizer, J., Vakkalanka, J. P., et al. (2018). Challenges in the diagnosis of acute cyanide poisoning. *Clinical Toxicology, 56*(7), 609–617. https://doi.org/10.1080/15563650.2018.1435886

Public Health Agency of Canada. (2005). *Centre for Emergency Preparedness and Response.* https://www.canada.ca/en/public-health/services/emergency-preparedness-response/centre-emergency-preparedness-response.html [Seminal Reference]

Public Health Agency of Canada. (2022). *National Emergency Strategic Stockpile (NESS).* https://www.canada.ca/en/public-health/services/emergency-preparedness-response/national-emergency-strategic-stockpile.html

Public Safety Canada. (2017). *An Emergency Management Framework for Canada* (3rd ed.). https://www.publicsafety.gc.ca/cnt/rsrcs/pblctns/2017-mrgnc-mngmnt-frmwrk/index-en.aspx [Seminal Reference]

Public Safety Canada. (2020a). *National Public Alerting System.* https://www.publicsafety.gc.ca/cnt/mrgnc-mngmnt/mrgnc-prprdnss/ntnl-pblc-lrtng-sstm-en.aspx

Public Safety Canada. (2020b). *Regional Resilience Assessment Program.* https://www.publicsafety.gc.ca/cnt/ntnl-scrt/crtcl-nfrstrctr/rrap-faq-en.aspx

Public Safety Canada. (2022a). *All-Hazards Risk Assessment.* https://www.publicsafety.gc.ca/cnt/mrgnc-mngmnt/mrgnc-prprdnss/ll-hzrds-rsk-ssssmnt-en.aspx

Public Safety Canada. (2022b). *The Canadian Disaster Database.* https://www.publicsafety.gc.ca/cnt/rsrcs/cndn-dsstr-dtbs/index-en.aspx

Public Safety Canada. (2022c). *Emergency kits.* https://www.getprepared.gc.ca/cnt/kts/index-en.aspx

Radiation Emergency Medical Management (REMM). (2023a). *Internal contamination: Via digestive tract–animation.* US Department of Health and Human Services. https://remm.hhs.gov/contamimage_5.htm

Radiation Emergency Medical Management (REMM). (2023b). *Procedures for radiation decontamination.* US Department of Health and Human Services. https://remm.hhs.gov/ext_contamination.htm

United Nations Economic Commission for Europe. (2020). Older persons in emergency situations. *UNECE Policy Brief on Ageing, 25,* 1–21. https://reliefweb.int/sites/reliefweb.int/files/resources/ECE_WG1_36_PB25.pdf

World Health Organization (WHO). (n.d.-a). *Coronavirus disease (COVID-19).* https://www.who.int/health-topics/coronavirus#tab=tab_1

World Health Organization (WHO). (n.d.-b). *Water sanitation and health.* https://www.who.int/teams/environment-climate-change-and-health/water-sanitation-and-health/environmental-health-in-emergencies/humanitarian-emergencies

World Health Organization (WHO). (2011). *Hospital emergency response checklist: An all-hazards tool for hospital administrators and emergency managers.* https://www.euro.who.int/__data/assets/pdf_file/0008/268766/Hospital-emergency-response-checklist-Eng.pdf [Seminal Reference]

World Health Organization (WHO). (2023). *Coronavirus disease (COVID-19) pandemic.* https://www.who.int/emergencies/diseases/novel-coronavirus-2019

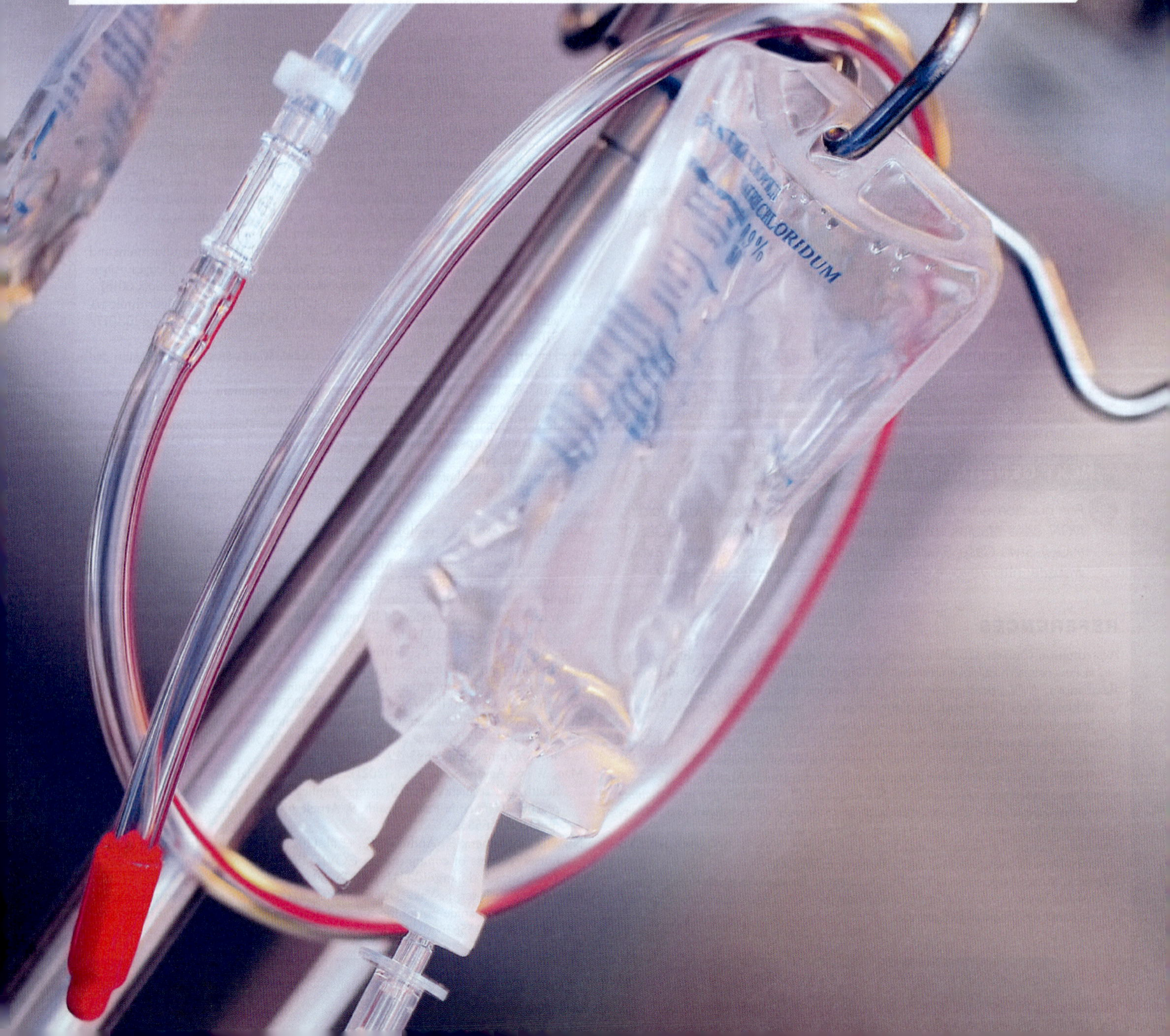

16 Pain Assessment and Management

Canadian content written by **Monakshi Sawhney, RN(EC), NP(Adult), MN, PhD**
Original US chapter by **Patricia A. Potter, RN, MSN, PhD, FAAN**

SKILLS AND PROCEDURES

OBJECTIVES

Mastery of content in this chapter will enable the nurse to:

- Understand the components of a pain assessment.
- Assess adverse effects of analgesics.
- Describe how an initial pain assessment allows the nurse to provide a patient with basic comfort measures.
- Identify and discuss various nonpharmacological pain relief measures.
- Assess and implement nonpharmacological measures to relieve pain.
- Describe the process for delivering medication through a patient-controlled analgesia device.
- Assess a patient receiving epidural analgesia.
- Assess a patient receiving a peripheral nerve block.
- Evaluate the effectiveness of pain management techniques.

MEDIA RESOURCES

- http://evolve.elsevier.com/Canada/Perry/clinicalskills/

PURPOSE

Pain is the most common reason that people seek health care; yet, it is often under-recognized, misunderstood, and inadequately treated. The International Association for the Study of Pain (IASP) defines *pain* as "an unpleasant sensory and emotional experience associated with, or resembling that associated with, actual or potential tissue damage" (Raja et al., 2020). This definition of pain is supported by six additional key concepts that expand upon the definition. The additional concepts are as follows (Raja et al., 2020):

1. Pain is a personal experience influenced by biological, psychological, and social factors.
2. Pain is more than a neurological response (i.e., it is more than the activity of sensory neurons).
3. An individual's understanding of pain changes over the lifespan and through life experience.
4. Clinicians need to respect an individual's experience of pain.
5. Pain can be a catalyst for change and adaptation; however, it can also have a negative impact on function and social and psychological well-being.
6. Pain can be expressed either verbally or through behaviours; there are many ways to express pain.

Acute pain is defined as a response to and experience of unpleasant stimuli. It motivates behaviours to avoid potential or actual tissue damage. It is recent in onset and self-limiting. Acute pain generally lasts from hours to days or a month after the precipitating event. It resolves as tissue healing occurs (Health Quality Ontario, 2018a; Kent et al., 2017). *Chronic pain* is defined as pain that lasts longer than 3 months or past the time of normal tissue healing (Health Quality Ontario, 2020). It can impact the person's physical, psychological, and social well-being. Many people in Canada experience chronic pain. Based on data from the Canadian Community Health Survey, the prevalence of chronic pain in individuals aged 12 years and older is estimated to be 21% (Shupler et al., 2019). Approximately 7.6 million Canadians are living with chronic pain, including 1 out of every 5 children or youth, and 1 out of every 3 people over the age of 65 years (Canadian Pain Task Force, 2021). As Canada's population continues to age, the prevalence of chronic pain is expected to increase.

The patient is the only one who knows whether pain is present and what the experience is like. Your role as a nurse is to recognize the unique nature of pain for each patient and to help select appropriate therapies. The skills in this chapter emphasize the importance of using critical thinking along with an integrated approach that considers both nonpharmacological (including physical and psychological interventions) and pharmacological therapies in managing a patient's pain.

STANDARDS OF CARE

- Canadian Anesthesiologists' Society (Dobson et al., 2023)–*Guidelines to the Practice of Anesthesia* (https://www.cas.ca/en/practice-resources/guidelines-to-anesthesia)

- Health Canada (Canadian Pain Task Force, 2021)—*An Action Plan for Pain in Canada* (https://www.canada.ca/content/dam/hc-sc/documents/corporate/about-health-canada/public-engagement/external-advisory-bodies/canadian-pain-task-force/report-2021-rapport/report-rapport-2021-eng.pdf)
- Health Quality Ontario (2018a, 2018b, 2018c)—*Opioid Prescribing for Acute Pain; Opioid Prescribing for Chronic Pain; Opioid Use Disorder* (https://www.hqontario.ca/Evidence-to-Improve-Care/Quality-Standards/View-All-Quality-Standards)
- Health Services Organization and Solutions for Kids in Pain (2023)—*Pediatric Pain Management Standard* (https://healthstandards.org/uncategorized/hso-and-skip-release-the-first-pediatric-pain-management-standard/)
- Michael G. DeGroote National Pain Centre (2017)—*Canadian Guideline for Opioids for Chronic Noncancer Pain* (https://healthsci.mcmaster.ca/npc/guidelines)
- Registered Nurses' Association of Ontario (2013)—*Best Practice Guideline: Assessment and Management of Pain* (https://rnao.ca/bpg/guidelines/assessment-and-management-pain)
- Royal College of Anaesthetists (2020)—*Best Practice in the Management of Epidural Analgesia in the Hospital Setting* (https://fpm.ac.uk/sites/fpm/files/documents/2020-09/Epidural-AUG-2020-FINAL.pdf)

PRINCIPLES FOR PRACTICE

- Addressing chronic pain requires multiple and diverse approaches. The Canadian Pain Task Force (2021) has outlined six goals as part of their recommended action plan (Box 16.1). Their recommendations build upon system improvement efforts at the federal, provincial/territorial, and regional levels.
- Patients' cognitive impairments represent special challenges to pain assessment. Carefully observe a patient's behaviour and nonverbal responses to pain when they are unable to self-report (Box 16.2).
- Pain that patients experience can be acute (transient), chronic (persistent), or both, including cancer and noncancer pain.
- Pain can be classified as nociceptive or neuropathic. *Nociceptive pain* is defined as pain that occurs as a result of damage to tissues (not nerves) and is due to activation of pain-sensing nerves (International Association for the Study of Pain [IASP], 2020). Some words that patients use to describe nociceptive pain include dull, aching, sore, and sharp. *Neuropathic pain* is defined as pain that occurs as a result of damage from nerves either in the peripheral or central nervous system. Neuropathic pain is a clinical description (and not a diagnosis), and it requires a demonstrable lesion or a disease (IASP, 2020). Some words that patients use to describe neuropathic pain include burning, electric shocks, numb, and tingling.

BOX 16.1

The Canadian Pain Task Force: An Action Plan for Pain

In 2019, the Canadian Pain Task Force (CPTF) was established by Health Canada to provide advice to guide the federal government in assessing and recommending an improved approach for the prevention and management of chronic pain. Multiple and diverse approaches are needed to address chronic pain, including changes in policies and regulation, programs, practices, and attitudes. The *Action Plan for Pain in Canada* outlines actions that are needed to improve outcomes for people living with chronic pain and to reduce the impact on families, communities, and society. Recommendations are focused around six primary goals:

1. Pain is recognized as a public health priority and coordination of action across jurisdictions spurs collaboration, leadership, and support to ensure a consistent approach to pain throughout Canada.
2. People have equitable and consistent access to a continuum of timely, evidence-informed, and person-centred pain care and supports across jurisdictions.
3. People living with pain and health professionals have the knowledge, skills, and educational supports to appropriately assess and manage pain based on population needs. The broader community understands pain as a legitimate, biopsychosocial condition and stigma is reduced.
4. Pain research and related infrastructure enables discovery, catalyzes innovation, and results in the translation of knowledge into real world impact.
5. Data enables effective monitoring of pain and facilitates improvement of health system quality.
6. There is improved and equitable access to services for populations disproportionately impacted by pain.

BOX 16.2

Pain Assessment in Nonverbal Patients

Recommended Assessment Approaches

- Attempt a self-report of pain using simple yes/no responses or vocalizations or a numerical rating scale.
- Search for the potential cause of pain by using physical examination techniques (e.g., palpation).
- Assume that pain is present after ruling out other causes (e.g., infection or constipation).
- Identify pathological conditions or procedures that may cause pain.
- Observe patient behaviours (e.g., confusion, pacing, facial expressions, vocalizations, body movements such as guarding) that indicate pain. These vary based on patient's developmental level.
- Ask caregivers whether the patient's current behaviour (e.g., crying out, restlessness) is different from their customary behaviour. This change in behaviour may signal pain.
- Attempt an analgesic trial if pathological conditions or procedures that may induce pain are present.

Using a Behavioural Pain Assessment Tool

- Use reliable and valid tools (e.g., Critical Care Pain Observation Tool [CPOT], Pain Assessment Checklist for Seniors With Limited Ability to Communicate [PACSLAC-II], Pain Assessment in Advanced Dementia [PAINAD] scale) to recognize the presence or absence of pain, and provide a rating of pain severity in nonverbal critically ill patients and older persons with impaired cognition (Gélinas, 2016; Horgas, 2017; Tsai et al., 2018).
- Select an appropriate pain assessment scale for each patient (e.g., visual analogue scale, FACES Pain Scale or FACES Pain Scale–Revised); no one scale is required for all specific groups of patients.
- Vital signs are not sensitive indicators for the presence of pain.
- An electronic Pain Assessment Tool (ePAT) app was recently developed to provide point-of-care facial recognition technology for detecting facial microexpressions that are indicative of pain, as well as the presence of pain-related behaviours (voice, movement, behaviour, activity, and body). An analysis revealed a sensitivity of 96.1% and accuracy of 95%, supporting the clinical usefulness of the ePAT for identifying pain in patients with moderate to severe dementia (Hoti et al., 2018).

Adapted from Gélinas, C. (2016). Pain assessment in the critically ill adult: Recent evidence and new trends. *Intensive and Critical Care Nursing, 34*, 1–11; Herr, K., Coyne, P. J., Key, T., et al. (2011). Pain in the nonverbal patient: Position statement with clinical practice recommendations. *Pain Management Nursing, 7*(2), 44–52; Hoti, K., Atee, M., & Hughes, J. D. (2018). Clinimetric properties of the electronic Pain Assessment Tool (ePAT) for aged-care residents with moderate to severe dementia. *Journal of Pain Research, 11*, 1037–1044; Tsai, I. P., Jeong, S. Y.-S., & Hunter, S. (2018). Pain assessment and management for older patients with dementia in hospitals: An integrative literature review. *Pain Management Nursing, 19*(1), 54–71.

- The most effective pain management combines nonpharmacological and pharmacological strategies. The classes of analgesics include (1) nonopioids and nonsteroidal anti-inflammatory drugs (NSAIDs), (2) opioids (traditionally called *narcotics*), and (3) adjuvants or coanalgesics (e.g., antidepressants and muscle relaxants) that enhance analgesics or have analgesic properties.
- Implementation of pain management strategies, including administering nonpharmacological and pharmacological measures in a timely manner, is imperative for optimal relief. Pain is easier to manage before it becomes severe.
- The current approach to acute and chronic pain management is to provide *multimodal analgesia*, which combines medications with at least two different mechanisms of action and nonpharmacological strategies so that pain control can be optimized (Health Quality Ontario, 2018a, 2018b; Paladini & Varrassi, 2021).
- Practise person-centred care and explore with the patient nonpharmacological (complementary/integrative) strategies to manage pain; nonpharmacological approaches generally do not require a health care provider prescription (check employer policy) and encourage the patient to actively participate in achieving a higher level of comfort and, in some instances, freedom from pain.

PERSON-CENTRED CARE

- Pain management should be person centred, with nurses practising patient advocacy, patient empowerment, compassion, and respect. Caring for patients in pain requires recognition that pain can and should be relieved.
- Teaching the patient and their family about pain treatment and having an attitude of dignity and caring will enable the nurse to individualize a patient's pain control plan.
- Pain is unique to each individual. It is important to recognize all factors influencing a patient's pain and to integrate them into an individualized plan for pain management. A timely, factual, and accurate pain assessment requires that the nurse work closely with patients and their families. Be objective, listen carefully, and assess any symptoms that a patient expresses.
- Effective communication and caring are key to gathering all the information needed to accurately determine the character of a patient's pain and its impact. Knowing these factors will help you as a nurse to intervene effectively to manage your patient's pain.
- A patient's cultural background can influence their recognition of pain, expression of pain, when to seek treatment, and which treatments are desirable (Orhan et al., 2018). Practising person-centred care enables the nurse to choose proper pain assessment tools for completing a culturally sensitive pain assessment. It is important to ask each patient about specific cultural considerations regarding pain expression and management; avoid cultural stereotypes.
- In some cultures, there may not be a specific word for pain; there are only descriptors for pain. Therefore, a pain scale may not work for all cultures, and it is important to be able to assess how the person describes pain.
- Explore a patient's beliefs about pain and discomfort. For example, cultures with a holistic world view of health and illness mix religious or spiritual aspects, what they consider natural, and the supernatural in their belief systems. Use interpreters to explain pain assessment tools and help patients report their pain as needed.
- Every patient with pain, including those with opioid use disorder, has the right to be treated with dignity, respect, and high-quality pain assessment and management (Health Quality Ontario, 2018c).
- When patients with acute pain have pre-existing chronic pain conditions, assessment and management should focus on effective analgesia. This includes the use of pharmacological and nonpharmacological strategies and the prevention of withdrawal (Health Quality Ontario, 2018a).

EVIDENCE-INFORMED PRACTICE

In a systematic review by Skelly and colleagues (2018), 202 studies of noninvasive nonpharmacological treatments for five common chronic pain conditions (chronic low back pain; chronic neck pain; osteoarthritis of the knee, hip, or hand; fibromyalgia; and tension headache) were examined. The results demonstrated that exercise, multidisciplinary rehabilitation, acupuncture, cognitive behavioural therapy, and mind–body practices were most consistently associated with slight to moderate improvements in function and pain control for specific chronic pain conditions. Nursing implications to consider from these evidence-informed studies include the following:

- Apply evidence that is relevant to everyday practice for the specific patients for whom you care.
- Complete comprehensive pain assessments (Skill 16.1) to understand each patient's unique pain experience in order to tailor interventions.
- Collaborate with patients to use nonpharmacological interventions (Skill 16.2) in addition to pharmacological and medical treatment measures. Use nonpharmacological interventions that patients perceive as being potentially helpful.

SAFETY GUIDELINES

- Patients who receive opioids (by any route, such as oral, intramuscular [IM], subcutaneous, intravenous [IV], epidural) need to be monitored for signs and symptoms of oversedation and respiratory depression. Excess sedation (difficult to arouse) precedes respiratory depression, especially in "opioid-naive" patients (i.e., patients who have never taken opioids for any reason or who have not taken opioids in the past 5 weeks) (Rosenquist, 2022). Use of a standard sedation scale can help prevent respiratory depression as it aids in observing and intervening for oversedation.
- Monitor activities such as standing, ambulation, and transfer to a chair if the patient has received an opioid. Assess patient's blood pressure, pulse, and respirations before initiating activity.
- If a patient has undergone an outpatient procedure, educate the patient and caregiver about precautions: the patient cannot drive for 24 hours; the caregiver may need to provide help with ambulation or take precautions to make the home environment safe.
- Monitor for potential adverse effects of opioid analgesics and recommend or institute supportive measures (e.g., addition of stool softener or high-fibre diet for adverse effect of constipation).
- If a patient is receiving epidural analgesia, infusion lines should not have any medication ports and should be labelled clearly and identified to prevent accidental connection with tubing of a different type (e.g., IV line, tube feeding, blood infusion line) (Galligan, 2020; Institute for Safe Medication Practices Canada [ISMP Canada], 2015). Follow these guidelines:
  - Limit access to epidural lines to health care providers with proper education and competence. There can be serious ramifications of misconnections, infections, occlusions, or misadministration of medications.
  - Trace an epidural catheter line from the access site into the patient's body all the way to the end source of an infusion or capped access port before connecting or reconnecting tubing or administering a medication.

BOX 16.3

Opioid Use Disorder and Pain Treatment

Opioid use disorder is defined as "a problematic pattern of opioid use leading to clinically significant impairment or distress, with at least two of the following criteria occurring within a 12-month period" (American Psychiatric Association, 2022). It includes the following 11 criteria:

1. Opioids are taken in larger amounts or over a longer period than was intended.
2. There is a persistent desire or unsuccessful effort to cut down or control opioid use.
3. A great deal of time is spent in activities necessary to obtain or use the opioid or to recover from its effects.
4. There are symptoms of craving, which includes a strong desire or urge to use opioids.
5. Recurrent opioid use results in a failure to fulfill role obligations.
6. Opioid use continues even when the person experiences persistent or recurrent social or interpersonal problems caused or made worse by the effects of opioids.
7. Important social, occupational, or recreational activities are given up or reduced because of opioid use.
8. Recurrent opioid use occurs even in situations in which physical hazards exist.
9. Opioid use continues despite knowing that a persistent or recurring physical or psychological problem, likely to have been caused or made worse by the substance, exists.
10. Tolerance, as defined by either of the following:
    a. A need for increased amounts of opioids to achieve the desired effect.
    b. A diminished effect with continued use of the same amount of an opioid.
11. Withdrawal, as manifested by either of the following:
    a. The characteristic opioid withdrawal syndrome.
    b. Opioids (or a closely related substance) are taken to relieve or avoid withdrawal symptoms.

Individuals with an opioid use disorder should receive care that is respectful of their rights and dignity and that promotes shared decision making (Health Quality Ontario, 2018c). They should also be treated with the same degree of respect and privacy as any other person. Adequate pain management should not be withheld from a patient for fear of worsening addiction or relapse of addiction (Canadian Pain Task Force, 2021). However, these patients should be monitored carefully.

- Communicate any practice changes, including dressing location and type of tubing and connectors, with all members of the health care team who are providing care to the patient.
- Patients currently receiving opioids for chronic pain require reassessment of any new pain or increased pain (Box 16.3). Use interprofessional collaboration to address pharmacological and nonpharmacological therapies to ensure that all team members are aware of at-home (individualized) dosages and therapies.
- Drug–drug interactions, including enhanced or reduced effects or adverse effects, often occur with the multiple medication use required by people with chronic pain. This practice is termed *rational polypharmacy* or *multimodal analgesia* (Paladini & Varrassi, 2021).
- Be knowledgeable about your employer's policy regarding the frequency of pain assessment and timing for follow-up assessments. A patient who is receiving opioids within an acute care facility requires frequent assessment during the first 24 hours.

✦ SKILL 16.1 Pain Assessment and Basic Comfort Measures

Video Clip

An accurate and comprehensive pain assessment is necessary to identify the nature of pain, the patient's perception of pain, and the effects of pain on their lifestyle, as well as to offer clues regarding the cause of the pain. A thorough assessment enables nurses to arrive at proper nursing diagnoses and select appropriate pain relief therapies. Effectively managing a patient's pain does not mean eliminating it; however, it does mean getting it to an acceptable level for the patient. Pain management requires that the nurse work with the patient to prevent pain whenever possible and identify an acceptable intensity of pain and other factors that pain can influence, especially sleep, that allow maximum patient function.

Nurses use the nursing process to recognize distinct and unique differences in patient perceptions and responses to pain. The nursing process offers a guide in providing person-centred care—getting to know a patient and developing an individualized plan of care.

Delegation and Collaboration

Assessment of a patient's pain cannot be delegated to an unregulated care provider (UCP). UCPs may identify to the nurse when a patient is in pain. The nurse is responsible for completing a pain assessment. UCPs may provide selected nonpharmacological strategies (e.g., back rubs, heat or cold application) as instructed by the nurse and according to employer policy. The nurse directs the UCP to do the following:

- Eliminate environmental conditions that worsen pain (e.g., an excessively warm, noisy room).
- Provide maximum rest periods for patient; a written schedule for caregivers to follow is ideal.
- Turn and place patients in a position of comfort at least every 2 hours or remind patients to turn themselves. Encourage patient to use a pillow for splinting if needed.
- Observe for and report to the nurse behavioural signs of pain for patients who are unable to self-report (see Box 16.2).
- Screen for pain during patient transfer or other activity that might provoke pain.

Collaborate with the interprofessional health care team (e.g., a clinical nurse specialist, pain management nurse) for further assessment of patients who present with chronic, intractable pain; pain that is not responding to treatment; and cases of multiple pain sources.

Equipment

- Pain rating scale (check employer policy)

STEP	RATIONALE
ASSESSMENT	
1. Identify patient using at least two person-specific identifiers (e.g., name and date of birth, or name and medical record number) according to employer policy.	Ensures correct patient. Complies with Accreditation Canada's standards and improves patient safety (Accreditation Canada, 2020).
2. Throughout the procedure, the 4 moments for hand hygiene are to be implemented; hand hygiene should occur before initial patient (or patient environment) contact, before an aseptic procedure, after body fluid exposure risk, and after patient (or patient environment) contact. Additional hand hygiene should be performed if hands are visibly soiled.	Proper hand hygiene helps prevent the spread of infectious agents to health care providers.
3. Assess patient's risk for pain (e.g., those undergoing invasive procedures, anxious patients, history of chronic illness, those unable to communicate).	Allows you to anticipate patient's needs and intervene in a timely manner, possibly preventing pain.
4. Ask patient if they are in pain. Observe for nonverbal indicators of pain; ask significant others if they believe patient is in pain. Older persons and patients from various cultures may not admit to having pain. Try using other words, such as *hurt* or *discomfort*, or use a professional interpreter if a language difference exists.	There is no objective test to measure pain. The patient's self-report of pain is the best way to assess pain. Recognizes that cultural differences exist in how pain is expressed.
5. Examine site of patient's pain or discomfort when possible. Inspect (discoloration, swelling, drainage), palpate (change in temperature, area of altered sensation, painful area, areas that trigger pain), and assess range of motion of involved joints. Percussion and auscultation can help to identify abnormalities (e.g., underlying mass or lung crackles) and determine cause of pain (see Chapter 8). *When assessing abdomen, always auscultate first and then inspect and palpate.*	Reveals nature of pain and directs you toward appropriate interventions.
6. Assess physical, behavioural, and emotional signs and symptoms of pain:	Signs and symptoms may reveal source and nature of pain. Nonverbal responses to pain are useful in assessing pain in patients who are cognitively impaired or nonverbal Pain in an older person requires careful, comprehensive assessment, diagnosis, and management (Schofield, 2018).
a. Moaning, crying, whimpering, groaning, vocalizations **b.** Decreased activity **c.** Facial expressions (e.g., grimace, clenched teeth) **d.** Change in usual behaviour (e.g., less active, irritable) **e.** Abnormal gait (e.g., shuffling) and posture (e.g., bent, leaning) **f.** Guarding a body part **g.** Diaphoresis **h.** Changes in sleep patterns	
i. Decreased gastrointestinal (GI) motility, constipation, nausea, and vomiting	Unrelieved acute pain can cause stimulation of the parasympathetic nervous system, which decreases GI tract activity (Swift, 2018).
j. Insomnia, anorexia, and fatigue	
k. Depression, hopelessness, anger, fear, social withdrawal	Patients with chronic pain often have depression. This combination can increase perception and intensity of pain (Canadian Pain Task Force, 2021).

Critical Decision Point *Physiological responses (e.g., tachycardia, hypertension) to acute pain are of short duration and return to normal within minutes. Be aware that a patient with chronic pain does not usually exhibit physical signs and symptoms. Avoid use of physiological responses alone to determine pain therapy selected, even with acute pain* (Erden et al., 2018).

STEP	RATIONALE
7. Assess characteristics of pain. Follow employer policy regarding frequency of assessment. Use the OPQRSTUV pain assessment:	This acronym guides clinicians in collecting complete information about patient's pain experience (Eloge et al., 2018).
a. Onset (e.g., "When did the pain start?")	Identifies when the pain first began.
b. Provocative/Palliative factors (e.g., "What makes your pain better or worse?"): Consider patient's experience with over-the-counter (OTC) medications (including herbal and topical) that help to reduce pain.	Identifies nature and source of pain and what patient uses to reduce discomfort. Combination of interventions is often most effective approach to pain relief.
c. Quality: Use open-ended questions (e.g., "Tell me what your pain feels like.")	Helps to determine underlying pain mechanism (e.g., somatic versus neuropathic pain).

STEP	RATIONALE
ASSESSMENT	
d. Region/Radiation (e.g., "Show me everywhere your pain is."). Have patient use finger (if possible) to point out areas of pain.	Identify location of pain and possible causative factors for acute or transient pain.
e. Severity: Use valid pain rating scale appropriate to patient's age, language skills, developmental level, culture, and comprehension (see Step 7e illustration). Ask patient to rate pain at rest, before any intervention, and when they are moving or engaged in care activity. Pain intensity may be determined with a numerical scale, categorical scale, or pictorial scale. For patients with dementia or those who cannot express themselves verbally, use observational pain assessment scales such as the Pain Assessment Checklist for Seniors With Limited Ability to Communicate (PACSLAC-II) (Table 16.1) and the Pain Assessment in Advanced Dementia (PAINAD) scale (Natavio et al., 2020).	An appropriate pain rating scale is reliable, is easily understood, and reflects changes in pain intensity.
f. Timing: Ask patient if pain is constant, intermittent, continuous, or a combination. Does pain increase during specific times of day, with particular activities, or in specific locations?	Environmental stimuli such as loud noises, bright lights, strong odours, or temperature extremes sometimes alter patient's response to pain.
g. Understanding and Use: What is patient's understanding of the pain and how is it affecting them and their family (e.g., the impact on activities of daily living [ADLs], work, relationships, and enjoyment of life)? What strategies (including medications) have they used to manage pain recently and in the past?	Provides important baseline information to gauge effectiveness of pain management interventions. Allows for a comprehensive assessment of medications, including prescription medications, OTCs, herbal/dietary supplements, recreational drugs, and alcohol (Eloge et al., 2018). This includes the use of cannabis or cannabinoids. A clinical practice guideline for medical cannabis or cannabinoids for chronic pain makes a weak (cautious) recommendation to offer a trial of noninhaled medical cannabis in addition to standard care for people living with chronic cancer or noncancer pain (Busse et al., 2021).
h. Value: Are there any values or beliefs that the patient or family has regarding pain? What are the patient's goals?	This informs person-centred care and helps identify any cultural or personal beliefs that impact pain and pain management.
8. Assess patient's health and illness history and type of therapies successfully used to relieve pain (e.g., medications, OTC products, heat and cold therapies).	History provides information for type of therapies to use for patient's specific situation. Many patients do not mention using OTC products for fear of being criticized or because they do not want them taken away.
9. Assess patient's response to previous pharmacological interventions, especially ability to function (e.g., sleeping, eating, and other ADLs). Determine whether any analgesic adverse effects are likely based on medication and patient's previous responses (e.g., itching or nausea).	Determines extent to which therapies have or have not been successful in the past. Some adverse effects, especially pruritus (itching), which can occur with morphine, are often poorly tolerated by patient and indicate need to identify another analgesic.
10. Assess for allergies to medications, with focus on analgesics.	Some patients with asthma or an allergy to Aspirin are also allergic to other NSAIDs (Simon, 2022).

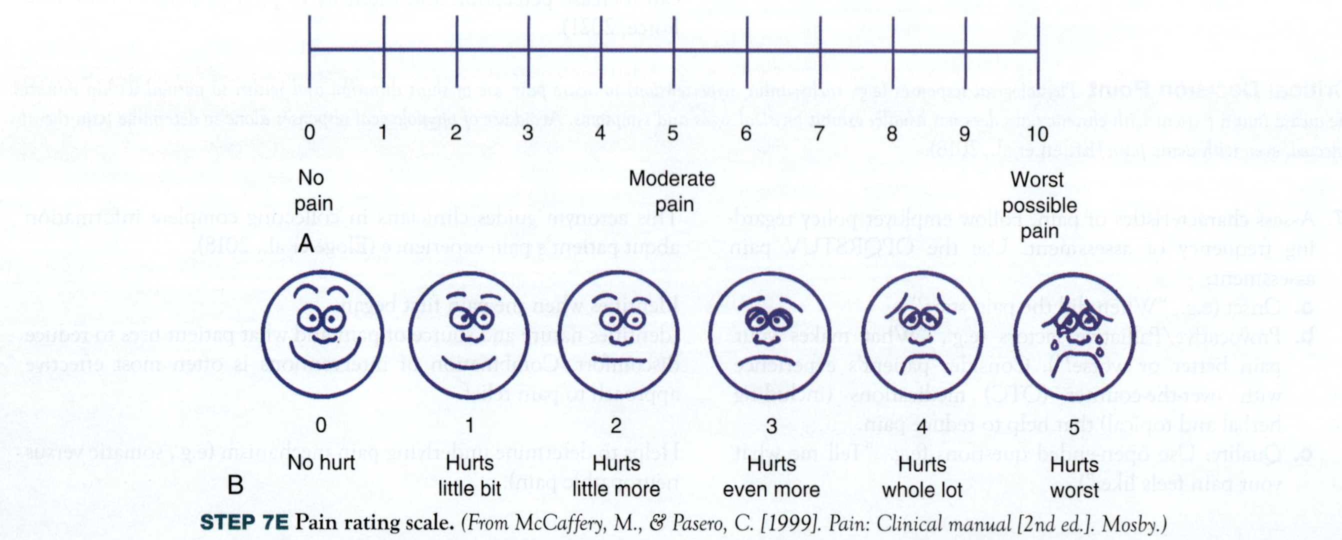

STEP 7E **Pain rating scale.** *(From McCaffery, M., & Pasero, C. [1999]. Pain: Clinical manual [2nd ed.]. Mosby.)*

TABLE 16.1

Pain Assessment Checklist for Seniors With Limited Ability to Communicate (PACSLAC-II)

Date of Assessment: Time:	Check if present
Facial Expressions	
1. Grimacing	
2. Tighter face	
3. Pain expression	
4. Increased eye movement	
5. Wincing	
6. Opening mouth	
7. Creasing forehead	
8. Lowered eyebrows or frowning	
9. Raised cheeks, narrowing of the eyes, or squinting	
10. Wrinkled nose and raised upper lip	
11. Eyes closing	
Verbalizations and Vocalizations	
12. Crying	
13. A specific sound for pain (e.g., "ow," "ouch")	
14. Moaning and groaning	
15. Grunting	
16. Gasping or breathing loudly	
Body Movements	
17. Flinching or pulling away	

Date of Assessment: Time:	Check if present
18. Thrashing	
19. Refusing to move	
20. Moving slowly	
21. Guarding sore area	
22. Rubbing or holding sore area	
23. Limping	
24. Clenched fist	
25. Going into fetal position	
26. Stiff or rigid posture	
27. Shaking or trembling	
Changes in Interpersonal Interactions	
28. Not wanting to be touched	
29. Not allowing people near	
Changes in Activity Patterns or Routines	
30. Decreased activity	
Mental Status Changes	
31. Are there mental status changes that are due to pain and are not explained by another condition (e.g., delirium due to medication, etc.)?	
Total Score (add up checkmarks)	

From Chan, S., Hadjistavropoulos, T., Williams, J., & Lints-Martindales, A. (2014). Evidence-based development and initial validation of the Pain Assessment Checklist for Seniors With Limited Ability to Communicate-II (PACSLAC-II). *Clinical Journal of Pain, 30*(9), 816–824. https://geriatricpain.org/sites/geriatricpain.org/files/2020-06/PACSLAC%20II%20Checklist.pdf. Reproduced with permission. The PACSLAC-II is copyrighted by Sarah Chan, Shannon Fuchs-Lacelle, and Thomas Hadjistavropoulos and may not be reproduced without permission. For permission to reproduce the PACSLAC-II contact Thomas.Hadjistavropoulos@uregina.ca, who is authorized to grant permission on behalf of all of the copyright holders. The developers of the PACSLAC-II specifically disclaim any liability arising directly or indirectly from use or application of the PACSLAC-II. Use of the PACSLAC-II may not be appropriate for some patients and the PACSLAC-II is not a substitute for a thorough assessment by a qualified health professional. The PACSLAC-II (like other observational pain assessment tools) is a screening tool and not a definitive indicator of pain. As such, sometimes it may fail to identify pain and other times it may incorrectly signal the presence of pain. The PACSLAC-II should be used by qualified health care staff within the context of their broader knowledge and examination of the patient.

STEP	RATIONALE

NURSING DIAGNOSES

- Acute pain
- Reduced stamina
- Anxiety
- Chronic pain
- Insufficient knowledge regarding alternative pain therapies
- Altered sleep pattern
- Fatigue
- Fear
- Reduced physical mobility
- Inadequate coping
- Potential for constipation

Related factors and risk factors are individualized on the basis of patient's condition or needs.

PLANNING

STEP	RATIONALE
1. Expected outcomes following implementation of a pain management intervention:	
• Patient verbalizes full or partial relief from pain.	Patient's self-report of pain is single most reliable indicator of pain (Raja et al., 2020).
• Patient displays nonverbal behaviours such as relaxed face and absence of squinting.	Nonverbal behaviours can be valid and reliable indicators of pain and pain relief in patients who are cognitively impaired (Natavio et al., 2020).
• Patient reports improvement in sleep, nutritional intake, physical activity, and personal relationships.	Adequate pain relief usually permits patient to participate in usual ADLs.
2. Set pain-intensity goal with patient (when able).	Pain is unique to each individual. Patient sets individual goal for tolerable pain severity (Health Quality Ontario, 2020).

STEP	RATIONALE
IMPLEMENTATION	
1. Apply clean gloves (if indicated).	Reduces transmission of microorganisms.
2. Prepare patient's environment.	
• Temperature suited to patient	Temperature and sound extremes can enhance patient's perception of pain.
• Sound	
• Lighting	Bright or very dim lighting can aggravate pain sensation.
• Eliminate unnecessary interruptions and coordinate care activities; allow for rest.	Fatigue increases pain perception.
3. Teach patient how to use pain rating scale. Explain range of intensity scores and how they relate to measure pain.	Accurate reporting by patient or family improves ongoing pain assessment, treatment, and evaluation.
4. Prepare and administer appropriate pain-relieving medications (nonopioids, opioids, coanalgesics, or multimodal combination) per health care provider's prescription (see Chapter 20). Choice of medication depends on patient's condition. For example, postoperative pain is often treated initially with opioids or acetaminophen and an NSAID (which provide effective nonopioid analgesia for postoperative patients).	Nonopioids are effective for mild to moderate pain. Patients with chronic pain are typically prescribed multimodal therapy (more than one type of analgesic) for pain relief.
5. Remove or reduce painful stimuli.	Reduction of pain stimuli and pressure receptors maximizes responses to pain-relieving interventions.
a. Help patient turn and reposition to comfortable position with good body alignment.	Reduces stress on musculoskeletal system.
b. Smooth wrinkles in bed linens.	Reduces pressure and irritation to skin.
c. Loosen constrictive bandages (if appropriate to purpose of bandage) or loosen or remove devices (e.g., blood pressure cuff, elastic hose, or sequential stockings).	Bandage or device encircling extremity can restrict circulation and cause pain (see Chapter 40).
d. Reposition underlying tubes or equipment.	Removes pressure on skin.
e. Use pillows as needed for alignment and positioning support (see Step 5e illustration).	Helps maintain position that reduces strain on muscles and pressure areas.
6. Teach patient how to splint over painful site using either a pillow or hand.	Splinting reduces pain by minimizing muscle movement at time of stress.
a. Explain purpose of splinting.	Promotes patient's cooperation.
b. Place pillow or blanket over site of discomfort and help patient place hands firmly over area of discomfort (see Step 6b illustration).	Splinting immobilizes painful area.

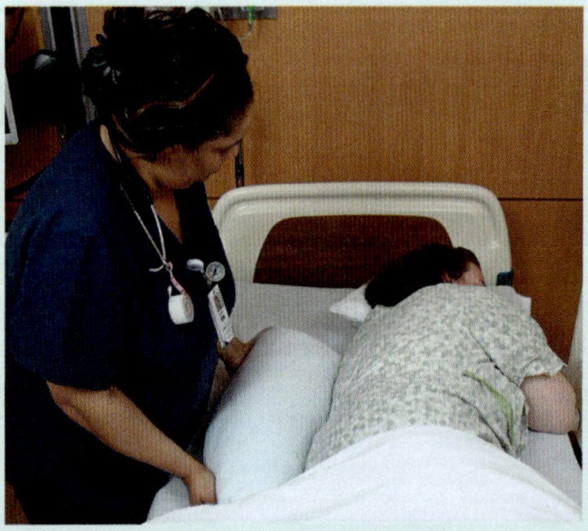

STEP 5E Positioning patient in side-lying lateral position for comfort.

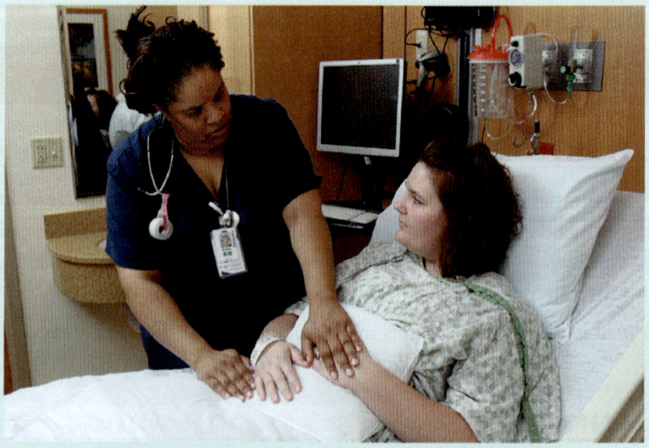

STEP 6B Patient shown how to splint painful area.

STEP	RATIONALE
IMPLEMENTATION	
c. Have patient hold area firmly while coughing, deep breathing, and turning.	Splinting decreases movement and subsequent pain during activity.
7. Reduce or eliminate emotional factors that increase pain experiences (see Skill 16.2). Use biopsychosocial treatments: cognitive behavioural and/or behavioural therapies.	Helps patients relax. Thoughts influence feelings, which change perception and behaviours, including a perception of pain relief (Tang, 2018). Psychological approaches to the management of chronic pain emphasize neuromodulation as a long-term therapy (Turk & Gatchel, 2018).
a. Offer information that reduces anxiety (e.g., explaining cause of pain, if known).	
b. Offer patient the opportunity to use distraction techniques (e.g., prayer, music, television, singing to self, counting) (if appropriate, see Box 16.4).	Serves as form of distraction.
c. Spend time to allow patient to talk about pain and answer questions. Listen attentively.	Conveys caring as part of person-centred care.
8. If used, remove and dispose of gloves in appropriate receptacle.	Reduces transmission of microorganisms.
EVALUATION	
1. Within 1 hour of an intervention (e.g., after repositioning or after a medication reaches its peak effect), ask patient to describe level of relief using a pain rating scale (e.g., Numeric Rating Scale from 0 to 10, with 0 = no pain and 10 = worst pain ever).	Evaluates and documents effectiveness of pain-relieving interventions in timely manner.
2. Compare patient's current pain with personally set pain-intensity goal.	Helps to determine appropriate changes to pain management plan. Makes patient active participant in care.
3. Compare patient's ability to function and perform ADLs before and after pain interventions.	Contributes to determining effectiveness of pain-relieving interventions, especially in nonverbal patients.
4. Observe patient's nonverbal behaviours.	Determines effectiveness of pain-relieving interventions.
5. Evaluate for analgesic adverse effects.	Adverse effects of analgesics may be controlled by reducing dose, increasing time intervals, or administering other medications.
6. Use **teach-back:** "We discussed different ways to manage pain. How could you use nondrug ways to manage your pain at home?" Develop a revised teaching plan if the patient is unable to teach back correctly.	Determines patient's level of understanding of instructional topic.

Unexpected Outcomes	Related Interventions
1. Patient verbalizes continued pain that exceeds pain-intensity goal or displays nonverbal behaviour reflecting worsening pain.	• Repeat complete pain assessment. • Implement different nonpharmacological pain relief measures. • Ask patient and caregivers which alternatives might be helpful. • Notify health care provider.
2. Patient experiences unexpected or adverse reaction to medication.	• Assess unexpected effects on patient. • Notify health care provider immediately. • Be prepared to administer antidote if indicated (e.g., antiemetic, antihistamine, opioid-reversing agent such as naloxone). • Monitor for effectiveness of antidote; antidote may have shorter half-life than opioid; repeat dose of antidote may be needed. • Complete adverse reaction documentation according to employer policy.

BOX 16.4

Nonpharmacological Strategies for Pain Management*

Relaxation and Power of the Mind
- Self-comfort
- Progressive muscle relaxation
- Biofeedback
- Breathing exercises
- Music relaxation
- Visual imagery

Put Your Body to Work
- Exercise
- Yoga
- Tai chi
- Pacing activities
- Energy conservation
- Body mechanics

Spirituality and Reflection
- Engaging in religious practices (praying)
- Humour
- Setting aside time to focus on what *is*
- Sharing your stress with others
- Journalling
- Smudging, use of tobacco
- Sweat lodge

What to Do When Pain Flares
- Cold and hot therapies
- Ball therapy
- Contrast baths
- Massage
- Acupressure, acupuncture
- Distraction

*Can be used in conjunction with analgesia medications.

DOCUMENTATION EXAMPLE

44-year-old patient is postoperative day 2 following a right open nephrectomy. The patient was assessed while lying in bed. The incision to the right side of lateral aspect of the abdomen is covered with a dry dressing, which is dry and intact. The patient is not presenting any nonverbal indicators of pain. Bowel sounds are present in all 4 quadrants of the abdomen, with a minimum of 3 gurgling sounds heard. Patient states they have no nausea or vomiting, and they have been sleeping well. Pain assessment findings include: onset of pain occurred on the day of surgery, the pain is provoked when moving, especially when getting out of bed, the pain is palliated or relieved with analgesics and rest, the quality of the pain is dull at rest and sharp with movement, the region of the pain is right side of the abdomen around the incision, the severity of the pain is 2/10 at rest and 5/10 with moving out of bed, the pain subsides to 3/10 once the patient gets out of bed and is walking, timing of the pain is with movement. The patient's understanding of the pain is that it is related to the surgery and will subside as healing takes place. They state they do value nonpharmacological pain management options, but understand that oral analgesics may also be required for a short period of time to help manage the pain. The patient has an allergy to penicillin and has an allergy bracelet on right wrist. The patient takes acetaminophen occasionally for infrequent mild headaches. Acetaminophen 1 000 mg and hydromorphone 1 mg PO were administered 30 minutes ago in anticipation of getting out of bed, walking, and sitting in the chair. Patient was assisted out of bed, walked in the hallway with supervision, and is currently sitting in the chair with the call bell in reach. Patient was instructed to sit in the chair for 30 min, and to use the call bell if they need assistance.

Communication and Documentation

- Document the quality and intensity of the pain before an intervention, the pain relief therapies used, any patient or family education provided, and patient response to interventions in progress notes in electronic health record (EHR) or chart.
- Document your evaluation of the patient's understanding and knowledge.
- Document inadequate pain relief (not reaching goal), a reduction in patient function, and adverse effects from pain interventions (pharmacological and nonpharmacological) in the EHR or chart. Communicate these findings to the health care provider.

Special Considerations

Teaching

- Review patient's and caregiver's understanding of the pain assessment tool and how to use it when providing pain therapies.
- Explain to patient and caregiver the behavioural changes that may result from pain (e.g., change in activity level, splinting a body part, decreased social interaction).
- Ask patient and caregiver about fear of addiction, a common primary concern, or other misconceptions that could undermine patient's pain relief (Table 16.2).

Pediatric

- Some children are reluctant to report pain because they have misconceptions about the cause of their pain or they fear the consequences (e.g., another painful procedure or an injection).
- Infants and children experience pain but respond to it differently than adults. Infants and children who do not have the ability to self-report their pain are at risk of having their pain go unrecognized. A valid observational pain assessment tool such as the Face Legs Activity Cry Consolability-revised (FLACC-r) scale, the Children's Hospital of Eastern Ontario Pain Scale (CHEOPS), or the COMFORT/COMFORT scale (Andersen et al., 2017) should be used.
- Parents are helpful when assessing their child's pain and planning pain relief therapies. Most parents know how their child exhibits pain and which pain relief interventions have been successful.
- Children with verbal skills can rate their level of pain on the FACES Pain Scale, FACES Pain Scale–Revised (see https://www.iasp-pain.org/resources/faces-pain-scale-revised/), pain rating scale, or Numeric Rating Scale (0–10). The Numeric Rating Scale (0–10) can be used in children over the age of 7 years (Birnie et al., 2019). The absolute value of a pain-intensity score is not as important as the changes in scores in each individual child. In clinical use with children, a change in pain of 2 out of 10 (i.e., a change of one face) represents the least change that can be considered clinically significant when using FACES Pain Scale–Revised (Birnie et al., 2019).
- Pharmacological pain management is safe and effective in pediatric patients when the dose is calibrated according to the child's weight; however, evidence cautions that this practice may be inappropriate for children who are obese (Ameer & Weintraub, 2018).

Gerontological

- Older persons who are able to express themselves can use self-report pain scales. In addition, assessment should include how the pain is affecting function, sleep, appetite, activity, mood, and relationships with others (Boscart et al., 2023).

TABLE 16.2

Misconceptions: Barriers to the Assessment and Treatment of Pain

Misconception	Correction
The best judge of the existence and severity of a patient's pain is the health care provider or nurse caring for the patient.	The patient's self-report is the most reliable indicator of the existence and intensity of pain.
Clinicians should use their personal opinions and beliefs about the truthfulness of a patient to determine their true pain status.	Allowing each clinician to act on personal beliefs presents the potential for different pain assessments by different clinicians, leading to different interventions from each clinician. This results in inconsistent and often inadequate pain management. A patient's self-report of pain is the standard for pain assessment.
Visible signs, either physiological or behavioural, always accompany pain and can be used to verify its existence and severity.	Even with severe pain, periods of physiological and behavioural adaptation occur, leading to periods of minimal or no observable signs of pain. Lack of pain expression does not necessarily mean lack of pain.
The pain rating scale commonly used in daily clinical practice is the Numeric Rating Scale (NRS) (a scale from 1 to 10, where 1 = no pain and 10 = worst pain ever).	The preferred pain rating scale depends on a patient's cognitive and physical ability, culture, developmental level, and availability, as well as employer policy.
Older persons with cognitive impairment are unable to use pain rating scales.	When an appropriate pain rating scale is used and a patient is given sufficient time to process information and respond, many older persons with cognitive impairment can use a pain rating scale.
If patients hurt enough, they will tell you.	Patients are often hesitant to report pain for fear of being labelled as complainers, hypochondriacs, or addicts.
Psychosocial interventions alone reduce or alleviate pain.	Nonpharmacological interventions are synergistic with medications but are not a substitute for pharmacological management of pain if needed.

Adapted from Pasero, C., & McCaffery, M. (2011). *Pain assessment and pharmacological management*. Mosby.

- Practise person-centred care and take the time required when explaining a pain assessment scale.
- Pain is not a natural occurrence of aging, although older persons are at risk of experiencing more pain-producing conditions.
- Nonverbal older persons experiencing pain are at high risk for inadequate pain relief (Natavio et al., 2020). Ensure that your assessment is thorough, and evaluate a patient's response critically.

Care in the Community: Home Management

- Consider home conditions that improve sleep, such as type of bed and environmental stimuli. A supportive bed and quiet environment enhance sleep and promote pain management.
- Families are the main support for older persons. Educate them about causes of painful conditions, common misconceptions about use of analgesics, type of pain medications appropriate for the patient, and how to support medication adherence.

✦ SKILL 16.2 Nonpharmacological Pain Management

Effective pain management does not always mean the elimination of pain. A variety of nonpharmacological therapies are available to directly lessen a patient's pain and provide additive relief when analgesics are administered. Nonpharmacological interventions can be used in any health care setting, and there is evidence of their efficacy in providing pain relief (Health Quality Ontario, 2018a, 2018b). These interventions are used in combination with, not in place of, pharmacological interventions. Nonpharmacological techniques diminish the physical effects of pain, alter a patient's perception of pain, and provide a patient with a greater sense of control.

Nonpharmacological interventions are appropriate for patients who experience anxiety or fear, would like to avoid or reduce pharmacological pain management interventions, or have inadequate or incomplete pain relief with pharmacological interventions alone. Nurses can help patients manage their pain by teaching them to add a variety of nonpharmacological techniques for self-care (Box 16.4). Patients and families today are more aware of complementary techniques and should be encouraged to continue whatever has helped them. Nurses practising person-centred care are mindful that every person responds differently and encourage patients to try different techniques.

Relaxation and Guided Imagery

Relaxation and guided imagery help to relieve acute and chronic pain, anxiety, and depression. The deep, slow breathing associated with relaxation, performed alone or in combination with the focused concentration of guided imagery, influences autonomic and pain processing, essential features in the modulation of sympathetic arousal and pain perception (Turk & Gatchel, 2018). Relaxation has been shown to be effective in reducing many types of pain (e.g., acute, chronic, surgical, cancer) (Tick et al., 2018). Relaxation and guided imagery provide patients with self-control when pain occurs. In guided imagery, a person draws on personal memories, dreams, and visions to create an image in the mind; concentrates on that image; and gradually becomes less aware of pain. Focus of the imagination helps patients change their perceptions about their disease, treatment, and healing ability, which helps relieve pain, tension, or stress. Choosing images that patients find pleasant requires a careful assessment. For example, a scene of rolling waves at the seashore is restful to one patient but may be frightening to another.

Cutaneous Stimulation

Massage

A gentle massage or back rub, a form of cutaneous stimulation, is the application of touch and movement to muscles, tendons, and ligaments without manipulation of the joints. A proper massage not only blocks perception of pain impulses but also helps relax muscle tension and spasm that otherwise might increase pain. Massage therapy can produce a relaxation response that creates a calm state and enhances the ability to rest (Tick et al., 2018). Massage hastens the elimination of wastes stored in muscles, improves oxygenation of tissues, and stimulates the relaxation response in the nervous system. A superficial massage of the back, shoulders, and lower part of the neck is sometimes referred to as a back rub. Offering a back rub after a bath or before a patient prepares for sleep promotes relaxation and comfort. An effective back rub takes 3 to 6 minutes and is an important intervention for decreasing pain and improving sense of well-being. Patients outside of the hospital setting may benefit from massage therapy from a registered massage therapist.

Heat and Cold

Heat and cold applications are placed on the skin to relieve pain and promote healing by improving circulation and reducing edema. The selection of heat versus cold varies with a patient's preference and condition. The application of heat or cold in a facility or home health environment requires a health care provider's prescription. Although the physiological responses to heat and cold differ, superficial heat or cold applications provide comfort in conditions such as muscle spasms, strains, and localized joint pain (see Chapter 41 for a review of heat and cold therapy).

Distraction

Distraction is a technique that diverts an individual's attention away from mild or moderate pain sensation. It can be used alone to manage mild pain or with analgesics to manage brief bouts of severe pain, such as pain related to procedures (Scheffler et al., 2017; Tyerman & Cobbett, 2023). By introducing meaningful stimuli, the nurse helps a patient consciously attend to only one stimulus, thus diverting the attention away from pain. There are internal and external distraction techniques. Internal techniques include having patients count, sing to themselves, pray, or repeat statements in their head, such as "I can cope." External techniques include changing a patient's activity, virtual reality, listening to music, reading, walking, playing a musical instrument, or watching a comedy program (Scheffler et al., 2017). Therapeutic communication with a nurse is another example of distraction. When the distraction is removed, a patient may have a heightened awareness of pain.

Delegation and Collaboration

Assessment of a patient's pain cannot be delegated to a UCP. The skill of nonpharmacological pain management strategies can be delegated. The nurse directs the UCP by doing the following:

- Identifying and explaining which nonpharmacological measures work best for a patient
- Explaining how to adapt strategies to patient restrictions (e.g., massage in side-lying versus prone position)
- Instructing the UCP to report worsening of a patient's pain

Equipment

- Pain rating scale
- *Massage:* Lotion or oil (consider aromatherapy lotion), folded sheet, bath towel
- *Relaxation:* Patient's music preference and device to play music (e.g., radio, MP3 or CD player, smartphone, etc.)
- *Distraction:* Based on patient preference (e.g., reading material, puzzles, video or computer games)

STEP	RATIONALE
ASSESSMENT	
1. Identify patient using at least two person-specific identifiers (e.g., name and date of birth, or name and medical record number), according to employer policy.	Ensures correct patient. Complies with Accreditation Canada's standards and improves patient safety (Accreditation Canada, 2020).
2. Throughout the procedure, the 4 moments for hand hygiene are to be implemented; hand hygiene should occur before initial patient (or patient environment) contact, before an aseptic procedure, after body fluid exposure risk, and after patient (or patient environment) contact. Additional hand hygiene should be performed if hands are visibly soiled.	Proper hand hygiene helps prevent the spread of infectious agents to health care providers.
3. Assess patient's language level and values they have regarding alternative pain relief approaches. Identify descriptive terms that you will use when guiding patient through relaxation or guided imagery.	Ensures that care is person centred and culturally appropriate. Establishes connection with patient to enhance your ability to guide relaxation.
4. Assess character of patient's pain (see Skill 16.1) and review findings to consider cause for pain.	Establishes baseline to determine effects of intervention. Helps determine whether nonpharmacological approaches are appropriate.
5. Assess facial expressions, nonverbal indications of discomfort (e.g., grimacing, frowning, voice tone), body position and movement (e.g., restlessness, muscle tension), and patient's self-report (see Skill 16.1).	Serves as baseline to evaluate effectiveness of pain relief measures. Overt signs and symptoms are usually not present with chronic pain. Physical signs and symptoms indicate change in comfort level.
6. Apply gloves when drainage is present. Examine site of patient's pain or discomfort. Include inspection (discoloration, swelling, drainage), palpation (change in temperature, area of altered sensation, painful area, areas that trigger pain), and range of motion of involved joints (if applicable).	Clinical observations may clarify information from patient. Site of discomfort may direct you to specific types of pain relief measures.
7. Assess character of patient's respirations.	Establishes baseline. Relaxation techniques focus on breathing.
8. Review health care provider prescription for pain relief (if required by employer).	In some facilities, a prescription is necessary to perform nonpharmacological therapies.
9. Assess patient's understanding of pain and willingness to receive nonpharmacological pain relief measures.	Participation increases effectiveness of pain relief measure. If patient is reluctant to try activity, provide information about suggested therapy.

STEP	RATIONALE
ASSESSMENT	
10. Assess preferred patient activities (e.g., puzzles, crocheting or knitting, game on electronic device, board games, music, or relaxation tape).	Demonstrates person-centred care and improves likelihood that distraction will be effective.
11. Assess type of image patient would prefer to use in guided imagery.	Prevents use of image that could frighten patient.
12. Review any restrictions in patient's mobility or positioning.	Determines whether massage is appropriate and position to have patient assume.

NURSING DIAGNOSES

- Acute pain
- Anxiety
- Chronic pain
- Reduced stamina
- Insufficient knowledge regarding nonpharmacological methods of pain control
- Inadequate coping
- Powerlessness

Related factors are individualized on the basis of patient's condition or needs.

PLANNING

STEP	RATIONALE
1. Expected outcomes following completion of procedures:	
• Patient demonstrates and describes pain relief measures.	Demonstrates patient understanding and learning.
• Patient is relaxed and comfortable after technique as evidenced by slow, deep respirations; calm facial expressions; calm tone of voice; relaxed muscles; relaxed posture.	Nonpharmacological strategies help patient relax and experience less discomfort. Physiological response to relaxation procedures and massage is deep relaxation.
• Patient reports pain relief as assessed by a valid and reliable pain rating scale or tool.	Patient's subjective report is most reliable indicator of presence of pain.
2. Explain purpose of technique and what you expect of patient during activity. Explain how to use pain rating scale (Skill 16.1).	Proper explanation of activity enhances patient participation. Accurate reporting of pain by patient improves your evaluation and treatment.
3. Set mutual pain-intensity goal with patient (when able) for rest and during routine care activities.	Patient sets individual goal for tolerable pain severity.
4. Plan time to perform technique when patient is able to concentrate (e.g., after voiding or awakening from nap).	Increases opportunity for success.
5. Administer an analgesic 30 minutes before implementing a nonpharmacological therapy.	Patient is able to gain level of comfort needed to perform nonpharmacological therapies.

IMPLEMENTATION

STEP	RATIONALE
1. Prepare patient's environment:	Contributes to safe patient environment.
• Temperature suited to patient • Sound	Temperature and sound extremes can enhance patient's perception of pain.
• Lighting	Bright or very dim lighting can aggravate pain sensation.
• Minimize interruptions and coordinate care activities; allow for rest.	Fatigue increases pain perception.
2. Massage:	

Critical Decision Point *Massage is contraindicated in cases of muscle, bone, or joint injury, or in bruised, swollen, or inflamed areas.*

STEP	RATIONALE
a. Place patient in comfortable position such as prone or side-lying. Have patients with difficulty breathing lie on side of bed with head of bed elevated.	Enhances relaxation and exposes areas to be massaged.
b. Adjust bed to comfortable position for you; lower upper side rail on side where you are standing. Drape patient to expose only area that you will massage.	Ensures proper body mechanics and prevents strain on back.
c. Turn on music to patient's preference.	Promotes relaxation.

STEP	RATIONALE
IMPLEMENTATION	
d. Ensure that patient is not allergic to lotion; warm lotion in hands or in basin of warm water. NOTE: If you massage head and scalp, delay use of lotion until completed.	Warm lotion is soothing, and warmth helps to produce local muscle relaxation.
e. Choose stroke technique based on desired effect or body part.	Ensures fuller relaxation of body part.

Critical Decision Point *Use very gentle massage with patients who are unable to communicate because they cannot tell you if massage becomes uncomfortable.*

STEP	RATIONALE
(1) Effleurage: Massaging upward and outward from vertebral column and back again (see Step 2e[1] illustration).	Light, gliding stroke used without manipulating deep muscles smooths and extends muscles, increases nutrient absorption, and improves lymphatic and venous circulation.
(2) Pétrissage: Fascicles of muscles are kneaded, lifted, grasped, squeezed, rolled, and released (see Step 2e[2] illustration).	Kneading tense muscle groups promotes relaxation and stimulates local circulation.
(3) Friction	Strong circular strokes bring blood to surface of skin, increasing local circulation and loosening tight muscle groups.
f. Encourage patient to breathe deeply and relax during massage.	Potentiates effects of massage.
g. Standing behind patient, stimulate scalp and temples.	
h. Supporting patient's head, use friction to rub muscles at base of head.	Strong circular strokes (friction) stimulate local circulation and relaxation.
i. Reposition if needed. With patient in supine position, massage hands and arms as appropriate.	Releases tension in hands and arms. Hand massage decreases cortisol and increases relaxation (Maratos et al., 2017).
(1) Support hand and apply friction to palm using both thumbs.	
(2) Support base of finger and work each finger in corkscrew-like motion.	
(3) Complete hand massage using effleurage strokes from fingertips to wrist.	
(4) Knead muscles of forearm and upper arm between thumb and forefinger.	Encourages relaxation; enhances circulation and venous return.
j. After determining that patient has no neck injury or condition that contraindicates neck manipulation, massage neck as appropriate:	
(1) Place patient in prone position unless contraindicated.	Provides access to neck muscles.
(2) Knead each neck muscle between thumb and forefinger.	Reduces tension that often localizes in neck muscles.
(3) Gently stretch neck by placing one hand on top of shoulders and other at base of head. Gently move hands away from one another.	Helps relax muscle body.
k. Massage back as appropriate:	Patient with back injury, surgery, or epidural infusion should not receive back massage.
(1) Assist patient to prone position unless contraindicated; side-lying position is an option.	Provides access to muscle groups in back.
(2) Do not allow hands to leave patient's skin.	Continuous contact with surface of skin is soothing and stimulates circulation to tissues. Breaking contact with skin can startle patient.

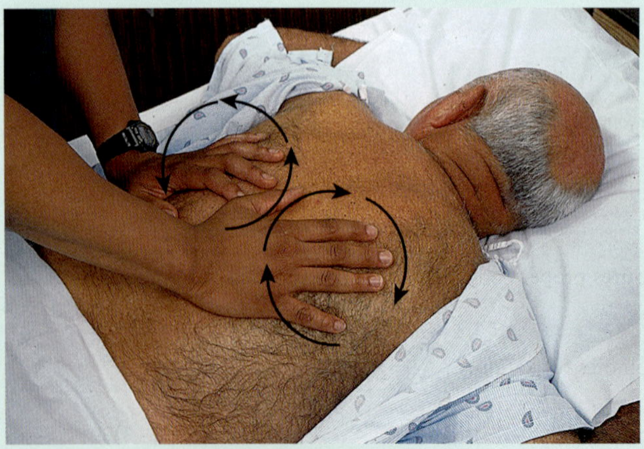

STEP 2E(1) Effleurage.

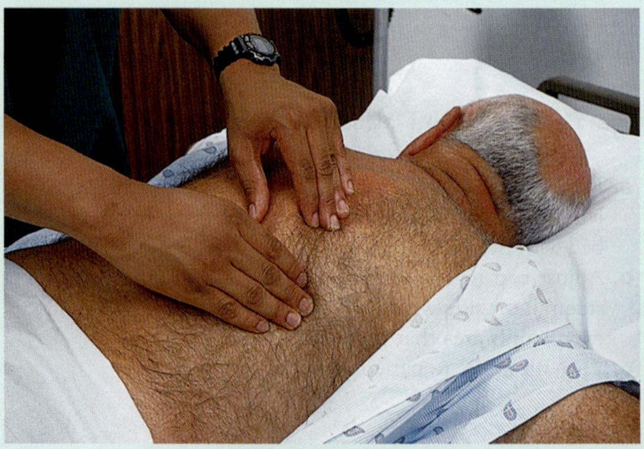

STEP 2E(2) Pétrissage.

STEP	RATIONALE
IMPLEMENTATION	
(3) Apply hands first to sacral area; massage in circular motion. Stroke upward from buttocks to shoulders. Massage over scapulas with smooth, firm stroke. Continue in one smooth stroke to upper arms and laterally along sides of back down to iliac crest (see Step 2k[3] illustration). Continue massage pattern for 3 minutes.	General, firm pressure applied to all muscle groups promotes relaxation.
(4) Use effleurage along muscles of spine in upward and outward motion.	Massage follows distribution of major muscle groups.
(5) Use pétrissage on muscles of each shoulder toward front of patient.	Area often tightens because of tension.
(6) Use palms in upward and outward circular motion from lower buttocks to neck.	Brings blood to surface of skin.
(7) Knead muscles of upper back and shoulder between thumb and forefinger.	These muscles are thick and can be massaged vigorously.
(8) Use both hands to knead muscles up one side of back and then the other.	
(9) End massage with long, stroking effleurage movements.	Most soothing of massage movements.
l. Massage feet as appropriate:	
(1) Place patient in supine position.	Returns patient to comfortable anatomical position.
(2) Hold foot firmly. Support ankle with one hand or support sides of foot with each hand while performing massage.	Maintains joint stability and prevents injury during massage.
(3) Make circular motions with thumb and fingers around bones of ankle and top of foot.	All massage strokes help to relax muscles.
(4) Trace space between tendons with firm finger pressure, moving from toe to ankle.	
(5) Massage sides and top of each toe.	
(6) Use top of fist to make circular motions on bottom of foot.	
(7) Knead sides of foot between index finger and thumb.	
(8) Conclude with firm, sweeping motions over top and bottom of foot.	Strokes that are too light may tickle.
m. Tell patient that you are ending massage.	Informs and prepares patient to inhale and exhale deeply.
n. When procedure is complete, instruct patient to inhale deeply and exhale. Caution them to move slowly after resting for a few minutes.	Returns patient to more awake and alert state. When deeply relaxed, patient may experience dizziness on arising too rapidly and may need time for vessels to redistribute blood supply.
o. Wipe excess lotion or oil from patient's body with bath towel.	Excess lotion or oil can irritate skin and lead to breakdown.
p. Return bed to low position and raise side rails as appropriate when massage is finished.	Side rails cannot be used as a restraint.

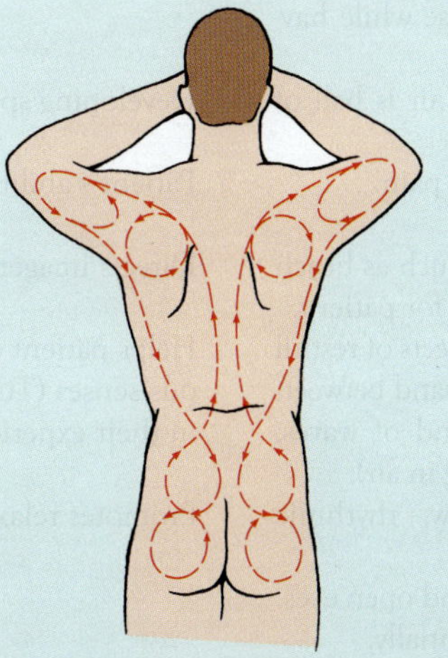

STEP 2K(3) Circular massage of the back.

STEP	RATIONALE
IMPLEMENTATION	
3. Progressive relaxation with deep breathing:	
a. Have patient assume comfortable sitting position (sitting with feet uncrossed) or lie in supine position with small pillow under head.	Maximizes ability to relax.
b. Instruct patient to take several slow, deep, diaphragmatic breaths. It may help to have patient close their eyes.	Increased oxygen lessens anxiety and prevents shortness of breath with relaxation breathing technique. Prevents hyperventilation. Eye closure maintains patient focus on exercise.
c. Explain as follows: "The air coming in through your nose should move downward into your lower belly. Let your belly expand fully. Now breathe out through your mouth (or your nose, if that feels more natural). Alternate normal and deep breaths several times. Pay attention to how you feel when you breathe in and breathe out normally and when you breathe deeply. Shallow breathing feels tense and constricted, while deep breathing helps you relax."	Patient able to focus on exercise with your coaching. Becoming mindful of how body feels can enhance relaxation.
d. Continue the exercise: "To practise, put one hand on your abdomen, just below your belly button. Feel your hand rise about an inch each time you breathe in and fall about an inch each time you breathe out. Your chest will rise slightly, too, along with your belly. Remember to relax your belly so that each time you breathe in, it expands fully. As you breathe out slowly, let yourself sigh out loud."	Allows patient to master slow, deep breathing.
e. Observe patient and caution against hyperventilation.	Causes patient to eliminate more carbon dioxide than is produced, and consequently results in respiratory alkalosis and elevated blood pH. Patient becomes dizzy and light-headed.
f. Coach patient to locate any area of muscle tension and alternate tightening and relaxing all muscle groups for 6–7 seconds, beginning at feet and working upward toward head.	Relaxation is an integrated response associated with diminished sympathetic nervous system arousal; decreased muscle tension is desired outcome.
(1) Instruct patient to tighten muscles during inhalation and relax muscles during exhalation.	Relaxation decreases pulse and respiration rates and blood pressure and helps reduce anxiety (Turk & Gatchel, 2018).
(2) As each muscle group relaxes, ask patient to enjoy relaxed feeling and allow mind to drift and think how nice it is to be relaxed. Have patient breathe deeply.	Allows opportunity to enjoy feelings of relaxation.
(3) Calmly explain during exercise that patient may feel sensations of tingling, heaviness, floating, or warmth as relaxation occurs.	Prevents anxiety if sensation occurs without warning.
(4) Have patient continue slow, deep breaths throughout exercise.	
(5) When finished, have patient inhale deeply, exhale, and move about slowly after resting for a few minutes.	Returns patient to more awake and alert state. Rising too rapidly can cause dizziness.
4. Guided imagery:	
a. Direct patient through guided imagery exercise while having them focus on an image. Example follows:	
(1) Instruct patient to imagine that inhaled air is ball of healing energy.	Developing specific images helps to remove pain perception.
(2) Imagine that inhaled air travels to area of pain.	Patient's ability to concentrate decreases pain perception.
b. Alternatively, you may direct imagery.	
(1) Ask patient to imagine a pleasant place, such as beach or mountains. Choose an image peaceful for patient.	Directs imagery after selection of restful place.
(2) Direct patient to experience all sensory aspects of restful place (e.g., for beach: warm breeze, warm sand between toes, warmth of sunshine, rhythmic sound of waves, smell of salt air, gulls gliding and swooping in air).	Helps patient concentrate and relax through stimulation of numerous senses (Turk & Gatchel, 2018). Make sure that it is something in their experience, not just yours.
(3) Direct patient to continue deep, slow, rhythmic breathing.	Promotes relaxation through muscle relaxation.
(4) Direct patient to count to three, inhale, and open eyes. Suggest that patient move about slowly initially.	

STEP	RATIONALE
IMPLEMENTATION	
c. Provide patient time to practise the exercise without interruption. Recordings of relaxation exercises are available almost everywhere; libraries are an excellent source.	Guided imagery requires an intense level of concentration that takes time to achieve.
5. Distraction:	
a. Direct patient's attention away from pain by involving them in a distraction technique.	Redirection of attention can alter emotional or cognitive aspects of pain (Turk & Gatchel, 2018).
(1) Music: Play selection for approximately 30 minutes in location where patient is comfortable. Set volume or loudness at comfortable level. Use music of patient's choosing. Emphasize listening to rhythm, and adjust volume as pain increases or decreases.	Music creates positive psychological outcomes, including decreased anxiety and depression (Turk & Gatchel, 2018).
(2) Direct patient to give detailed account of an event or story; describe pleasant memories.	Focus on details of event enhances distraction from painful stimulus.
(3) Provide activity (e.g., puzzle, computer game, reading material) at time when patient is relaxed.	Engagement in activity requires level of comfort for participation.
(4) Engage patient in meaningful conversation; encourage participation of family members and visitors.	Visitors can help direct attention away from mild to moderate pain. Rarely is someone in severe pain able to use distraction.
6. Remove and dispose of any supplies.	Reduces transmission of microorganisms.
EVALUATION	
1. Observe character of respirations, body position, facial expression, tone of voice, mood, mannerisms, and verbalization of discomfort.	Determines effectiveness of procedure, level of relaxation, degree of pain relief achieved, and which procedures were most effective.
2. Ask patient to use pain rating scale to rate comfort level.	Measures change in pain intensity.
3. Observe patient perform pain management techniques.	Confirms learning.
4. Use teach-back: "I want to be sure I explained some techniques for reducing pain without using medication. Tell me what technique you might want to try." Develop a revised teaching plan if patient or caregiver is unable to teach back correctly.	Determines patient's and caregiver's level of understanding of instructional topic.

Unexpected Outcomes	Related Interventions
1. Patient is unable to concentrate on technique because pain intensity is unchanged or escalating or demonstrates nonverbal behaviours indicative of pain.	• Evaluate character of pain and determine whether further analgesia is necessary. • Ensure that environment is conducive to learning and using technique. • Consult with health care provider on increase in dose or alternate medication. • Consider different technique or combination of complementary strategies.

Communication and Documentation

- Document assessment findings, procedure and technique(s) used, preparation given to patient, patient's response to procedure or technique, change in overall condition, and further comfort needs related to event in progress notes in EHR or chart. Incorporate pain relief technique into nursing care plan.
- Communicate patient's response to nonpharmacological interventions to the staff at change of shift or in care plan meeting.
- Document your evaluation of patient and caregiver learning.
- Communicate any unusual responses to techniques (e.g., uncontrolled or aggravated pain or muscle spasms) to health care provider.

Special Considerations

Teaching

- Provide patient information about each nonpharmacological therapy, including purpose, rationale for how pain is relieved, and how patient can maximize benefits. If UCP performs massage, you still need to provide patient education.
- Some techniques require more practice before patients achieve results. Pharmacological intervention is sometimes required to lessen pain so patient can relax.
- Teach patient to rest between periods of activity at home and hospital because fatigue increases pain perception.
- Teach caregiver how to perform massage (if not contraindicated) as part of home care.

Pediatric

- Nonpharmacological pain management therapies can be used successfully with children. Adapt distraction and relaxation strategies to the developmental level of the child (e.g., use a pacifier for an infant, offer reading or playing a recording of a favourite story for a preschooler, encourage a teenager to listen to music with headphones) (Hockenberry et al., 2024). Play therapists are good resources for appropriate distraction techniques.
- Because children usually have an active imagination, relaxation is often a powerful adjuvant in pain control.

- Parents are very helpful in providing pain relief. For example, they provide comfort to their child by their presence, engaging in conversation, and holding and cuddling their child.

Gerontological

- Visual, hearing, cognitive, and motor impairments make it difficult for older persons to be able to effectively use procedures such as distraction, relaxation, or guided imagery. Make certain that glasses, hearing aids, and other assistive devices are in place.
- Pain management in older persons may be challenging and requires an interprofessional team approach that involves nonpharmacological and pharmacological strategies (Buowari, 2021).
- Older persons are often reluctant to report pain, and they generally under-report pain (Buowari, 2021).
- Untreated pain in older persons interferes with all aspects of the older person's life (physical, psychological, social), and this can lead to poor quality of life (Buowari, 2021).

Care in the Community: Home Management

- Family members need to collaborate in planning time to reduce noise and other stimuli in the home. Doing so promotes patient relaxation and the effectiveness of other nonpharmacological techniques.

✦ SKILL 16.3 Monitoring Patients Receiving Patient-Controlled Analgesia

▶ *Video Clip*

Patient-controlled analgesia (PCA) is a method of pain management that permits patients to self-administer analgesic medications (usually opioids, such as morphine, hydromorphone, or fentanyl). It is important to understand the analgesic equivalence (equianalgesia) associated with opioids to ensure their safe delivery. For example, hydromorphone is more potent than morphine, and fentanyl is more potent than both morphine and hydromorphone; therefore, the dose delivered to a patient will be adjusted on the basis of the opioid. PCA is a method of analgesic administration for acute and chronic pain, including conditions such as postoperative pain, cancer, and end-of-life pain. The goal is to maintain a constant plasma level of analgesic. The most common route of using PCA involves IV or subcutaneous medication administration.

PCA devices can be programmed to deliver a patient demand (bolus) dose, a continuous infusion (basal rate), or both. The effectiveness and safety of PCA are dependent on providing a bolus dose that provides analgesia while minimizing adverse effects. Other safety measures include having control limits for the total dosage that can be administered each hour and having a timing control (lockout period) that regulates the minimum interval (e.g., 10 minutes between doses) (Pastino & Lakra, 2022).

Patients who will be using PCA need to understand how, why, and when to self-administer a medication. To receive the preprogrammed bolus dose of analgesic medication, the patient must push the applicable button attached to the PCA pump. Monitoring levels of sedation is essential with the use of PCA. This is especially true for most patients who are "opioid naive" (i.e., those who have never taken opioids for any reason or who have not taken opioids in the past 5 weeks). In addition, oversedation is a risk in patients with obstructive sleep apnea (OSA) (brief cessation of respirations during sleep) or in patients with undiagnosed sleep apnea who are obese (Pastino & Lakra, 2022). Assessment of patient sedation levels is critical.

The advantages of PCA can include achieving more constant serum levels of an opioid and avoiding peaks and troughs of a large bolus. Patients may report improved satisfaction with pain management related to the ability to control when they receive their opioid analgesic and the fast onset of the pain medicine. Concerns involving PCA use are patient-related errors, pump failure, or health care provider errors. Patients may misunderstand how PCA therapy works, mistake the PCA button for a nurse call button, or have caregivers operate the demand button. A pump may fail to deliver a medication on demand or have a faulty alarm or low battery. Health care providers may incorrectly program a dose, concentration, or rate. Other errors include failing to clamp or unclamp tubing, improperly loading a syringe or cartridge, failing to monitor for adverse effects or overdose, and not responding to alarms. PCA requires careful monitoring; nurses should never try to operate it without fully understanding the model in use. Many employers require an independent double-check by two nurses when initiating a PCA, changing the dose, or discontinuing the pump medications.

Delegation and Collaboration

The skill of administering PCA cannot be delegated to a UCP. The nurse directs the UCP to do the following:

- Notify the nurse if the patient has a change in health status or increased pain or identifies that someone other than the patient is administering the PCA dose on behalf of the patient

Equipment

- PCA pump and tubing
- Identification label and time tape (may come attached and completed by pharmacy)
- Needleless connector
- Alcohol swab
- Adhesive tape
- Clean gloves (when applicable)
- Equipment for vital signs and pulse oximeter, or capnography (CO_2) (if available) monitoring equipment

STEP	RATIONALE
ASSESSMENT	
1. Identify patient using at least two person-specific identifiers (e.g., name and date of birth, or name and medical record number) according to employer policy.	Ensures correct patient. Complies with Accreditation Canada's standards and improves patient safety (Accreditation Canada, 2020).
2. Throughout the procedure, the 4 moments for hand hygiene are to be implemented; hand hygiene should occur before initial patient (or patient environment) contact, before an aseptic procedure, after body fluid exposure risk, and after patient (or patient environment) contact. Additional hand hygiene should be performed if hands are visibly soiled.	Proper hand hygiene helps prevent the spread of infectious agents to health care providers.

STEP	RATIONALE

ASSESSMENT

STEP	RATIONALE
3. Check accuracy and completeness of medication administration record (MAR) or computer printout with health care provider's prescription for patient's name, name of medication, dose, frequency of medication (continuous or demand or both), and lockout period. Check medical record for patient's history of medication allergies and typical reactions. Review medication in a drug reference manual.	Health care provider prescription required for administration of opioid medication. Ensures that patient receives right medications. Avoids placing patient at risk for allergic reaction. Understanding medications before administering them helps prevent medication errors (Hanson & Haddad, 2021).
4. Assess patient's pain (see Skill 16.1). Also assess patient's ability to use the PCA control and their cognitive status for ability to understand purpose of PCA and how to use device.	Reduces transmission of microorganisms. Reveals source and nature of pain and factors that may increase pain. Determines patient's ability to use PCA safely and correctly.
5. Assess for conditions that predispose patients to adverse effects from opioids. Known, untreated, or unknown OSA poses a significant risk for respiratory depression (Chang et al., 2022; Kawada, 2019)	Assessment should be completed before surgery by anaesthesia using the STOP-Bang questionnaire (Chang et al., 2022; Kawada, 2019). Identification of such conditions enables the interprofessional team to take appropriate actions to minimize adverse effects.
6. Apply clean gloves. Assess patency of IV access and surrounding tissue for inflammation or swelling (see Chapter 29).	Reduces transmission of microorganisms. IV line needs to be patent for safe administration of pain medication. Confirmation of placement of IV catheter and integrity of surrounding tissues ensures that medication is safely administered.

Critical Decision Point *Be aware that nausea is not an allergic reaction, and it can be managed. Pruritus alone is not an allergic reaction; it is common to opioid use and can be managed. Hives, shortness of breath, difficulty breathing, and pruritus occurring together may indicate an allergic reaction that requires immediate intervention.*

STEP	RATIONALE
7. Assess patient's knowledge and perceived effectiveness of previous pain management strategies, especially previous PCA use.	Response to pain control strategies helps identify learning needs and affects patient's willingness to try therapy.

NURSING DIAGNOSES

- Acute pain
- Anxiety
- Chronic pain
- Insufficient knowledge regarding use of PCA
- Fear
- Inadequate coping
- Reduced physical mobility

Related factors are individualized on the basis of patient's condition or needs.

PLANNING

STEP	RATIONALE
1. Expected outcomes following completion of procedure:	
• Patient verbalizes pain relief.	Subjective measure of pain relief.
• Patient rates pain lower on pain scale.	Subjective measure of pain relief as stated by patient.
• Patient exhibits relaxed facial expression and body position.	Nonverbal cues of pain relief.
• Patient remains alert and oriented.	Indicates freedom from overly sedating effects of opioids. Sleepiness is usually from fatigue and not necessarily a sign of oversedation. Difficulty waking or rousing a patient could be the first sign of opioid-induced respiratory depression.
• Patient increasingly participates in self-care activities.	Suggests successful pain relief.
• Patient correctly operates PCA device.	Demonstrates safe and appropriate use of PCA.
2. Collect appropriate equipment. Draw curtains around patient's bed or close door to room.	Aids in organization. Maintains patient privacy.

IMPLEMENTATION

STEP	RATIONALE
1. Obtain PCA analgesic (prepared by pharmacy). Check label of medication two times; when removed from storage and when preparing for assembly.	Follows 10 rights of medication administration to be sure of correct medication. *This is the first and second check for accuracy.*
2. At the patient's side, compare MAR or computer printout with name of medication on drug cartridge. Do an independent double-check with another nurse and confirm the prescription and correct setup of PCA. The independent double-check should include verifying the prescription and the device independently and not just examining the existing setup.	Ensures that correct patient receives right medication. *This is the third check for accuracy.*

STEP	RATIONALE
IMPLEMENTATION	
3. Explain the purpose and demonstrate function of PCA to patient and caregiver as follows:	Reinforces person-centred care and enables patient participation in care and independence in pain control. Preoperative education about PCA therapy improves postoperative pain relief.
a. Explain type of medication in device.	
b. Explain that self-dosing aids in managing pain prior to repositioning, walking or coughing, and deep breathing.	
c. Explain safety features of PCA: pump is programmed to deliver a prescribed type and dose of pain medication, lockout interval, and 1- to 4-hour dosage limits. Explain how lockout time prevents overdose.	Maintains patient's safe use of PCA.
d. Demonstrate to patient how to push medication demand button (see Step 3d illustration). Instruct caregiver to refrain from pushing PCA button to give medication.	It is important that the patient has the knowledge to safely operate the PCA and that they be the only person pushing the medication demand button (i.e., not the caregiver).
e. Instruct patient to notify nurse of possible adverse effects, problems in obtaining pain relief, changes in severity or location of pain, alarm sounding, or questions.	
4. Apply clean gloves. Check the medication vial or medication bag for accurate labelling and precipitate.	Reduces transmission of microorganisms. Avoids medication error and injury to patient.
5. Position patient comfortably to be sure that IV or central line site is accessible.	Ensures unimpeded flow of infusion.
6. Insert drug cartridge into infusion device (see Step 6 illustration) and prime tubing.	Locks system and prevents air from infusing into IV tubing.

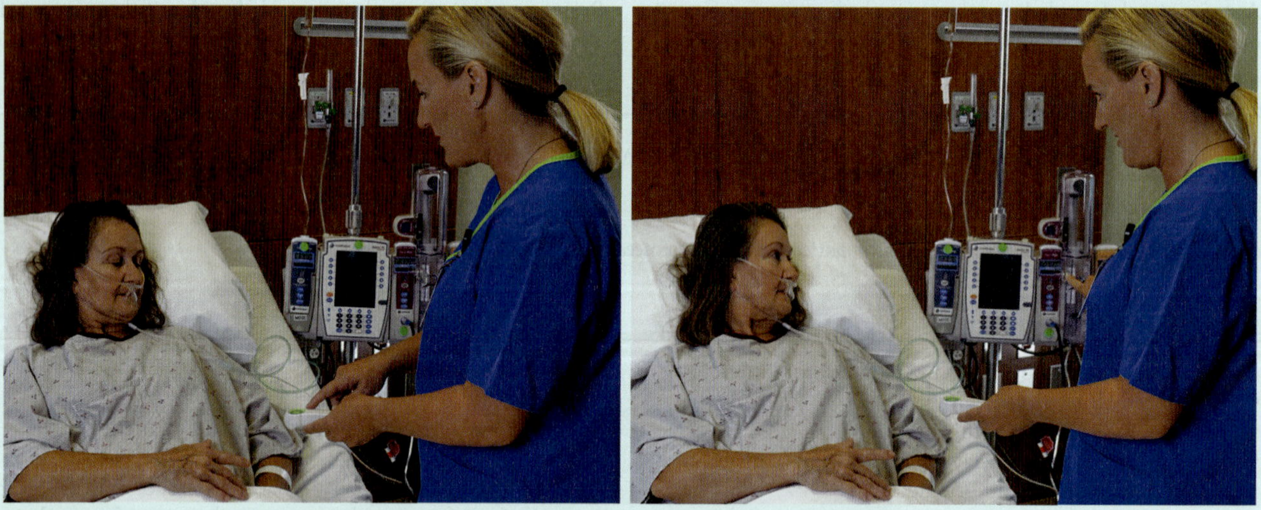

STEP 3D Patient learns how to press PCA device button.

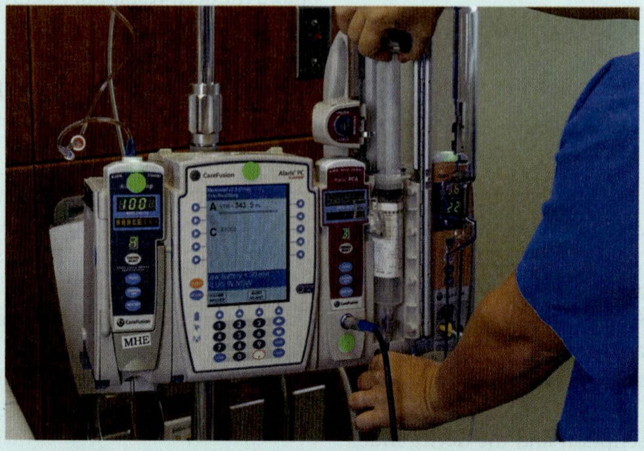

STEP 6 Nurse inserting drug cartridge into PCA device.

IMPLEMENTATION

STEP	RATIONALE
7. Attach needleless adapter to tubing adapter of patient-controlled module.	Needed to connect with IV line.
8. Wipe injection port of maintenance IV line vigorously with alcohol or antiseptic for 15 seconds and allow to dry.	Minimizes entry of surface microorganisms during needle insertion, reducing risk of catheter-related bloodstream infection.
9. Insert needleless adapter into injection port nearest patient (at Y-site of peripheral IV or central line, or connect to its own IV site). Avoid any possibility that PCA tubing could be used to administer direct IV. for another medication.	Establishes route for medication to enter main IV line. Needleless systems prevent needle-stick injuries. Prevents medication interaction and incompatibility.
10. Secure connection and anchor PCA tubing with tape. Label PCA tubing.	Prevents dislodging of needleless adapter from port. Facilitates patient's ability to ambulate. Label prevents error from connecting tubing from different device to PCA.
11. Program computerized PCA pump as prescribed to deliver prescribed medication dose and lockout interval. Have second nurse check setting. (NOTE: Recheck with oncoming nurse during shift hand-off to ensure line reconciliation.)	Ensures safe, therapeutic medication administration. With appropriate dose intervals (e.g., 10 minutes), usually an appreciable analgesic effect and/or mild sedation is achieved before patient can access the next dose; thus, there is less risk for oversedation and respiratory depression.
12. Discard gloves and supplies in appropriate containers.	Reduces transmission of microorganisms. The federal *Controlled Drugs and Substances Act* regulates the control and dispensation of opioids for all institutions.
13. If patient is experiencing pain, have patient demonstrate use of PCA system; if not, have patient repeat instructions given earlier.	Repeating instructions reinforces learning. Checking patient's understanding through return demonstration helps you determine patient's level of understanding and ability to manipulate device.
14. To discontinue PCA:	
a. Check prescription for discontinuation. Obtain necessary information from pump for documentation; note date, time, amount infused, and amount of medication wasted and reason for wastage.	Two nurses must witness and document the wastage of opioids (formerly called narcotics) to meet the requirements of the *Controlled Drugs and Substances Act.*
b. Apply clean gloves. Turn off pump. Disconnect PCA tubing from primary IV line, but maintain IV access.	Reduces transmission of microorganisms. Ensures continuation of IV infusion.
c. Dispose of empty cartridge, tubing, and gloves according to employer policy.	

EVALUATION

STEP	RATIONALE
1. Use appropriate pain rating scale to evaluate patient's pain intensity following treatments and procedures according to employer policy.	Determines response to PCA dosing. Documenting "PCA effective" is not an adequate documentation of a patient's pain level.
2. Observe patient for nausea or pruritus.	Common adverse effects of opioid.
3. Monitor patient's level of sedation, vital signs, and pulse oximetry or capnography per employer policy.	Patient is at highest risk during the first 24 hours of use. Excess sedation (difficult to arouse) precedes respiratory depression.
4. Have patient demonstrate dose delivery.	Evaluates skill in use of PCA.
5. Evaluate number of attempts (number of times patient pushed button), delivery of demand doses (number of times medication actually given and total amount of medication delivered in particular time frame), and basal dose if prescribed, following employer policy.	Helps to evaluate effectiveness of PCA dose and frequency in relieving pain. Maintains compliance with *Controlled Drugs and Substances Act.*
6. **Use teach-back:** "I want to be sure I explained how PCA will help with your pain and how you should use the device. Tell me the steps you will use to activate the PCA." Develop a revised teaching plan if patient is unable to teach back correctly.	Determines patient's level of understanding of instructional topic.

Unexpected Outcomes	Related Interventions
1. Patient verbalizes continued or worsening discomfort or displays nonverbal behaviours indicative of pain.	• Perform complete pain reassessment. • Assess for possible other causes of discomfort or additional complications, other than pain. • Inspect IV site for possible catheter occlusion or infiltration. • Evaluate number of attempts and deliveries initiated by patient. • Check that maintenance of IV fluid is running continuously. • Evaluate pump for operational problems. • Consult with health care provider.
2. Patient is sedated and not easily aroused.	• Stop PCA. • Notify health care provider. • Elevate head of bed 30 degrees unless contraindicated. • Instruct patient to take deep breaths. • Apply oxygen at 2 L/min per nasal cannula (if prescribed). • Assess vital signs, oxygen saturation, and/or capnography. • Evaluate amount of opioid delivered. • Ask caregivers if they pressed button without patient's knowledge. • Review MAR for other possible sedating medications. • Prepare to administer an opioid-reversing agent. • Observe patient frequently.
3. Patient unable to manipulate PCA device to maintain pain control.	• Consult with health care provider regarding alternative medication route or possibly a basal (continuous) dose.

Communication and Documentation

- Document the medication, concentration, dose (basal and/or demand), time started, lockout time, amount of IV solution infused, and remaining solution in progress notes in EHR or chart. Use special PCA documentation forms, if available.
- Document findings of the assessment of patient response to analgesia on PCA medication form, in progress notes in EHR or chart, according to employer policy. This includes vital signs, oximetry or capnography, sedation status, pain rating, and status of vascular access site.
- Communicate signs of oversedation to health care provider immediately.
- Document evaluation of patient learning.

Teaching

- Provide instructions on how to use PCA prior to starting the PCA pump. If the patient is having surgery, provide education before surgery.
- Encourage patients to push button on the PCA pump before the pain is severe. Teach the patient to use PCA bolus prior to activities or procedures that will increase pain.
- Explain regimen to caregivers so they can support and coach patient (but ensure that they refrain from pushing the bolus button for patient).
- Inform patient of nonpharmacological pain management strategies (see Box 16.4) that supplement or enhance pharmacological intervention (see Skill 16.2).

Pediatric

- PCA is an effective means of pain control in children who can understand the concept. When selecting children for PCA use, consider a patient's developmental level, cognitive level, and motor skills. PCA use is safe and effective for patients as young as 5 years old; however, it is most often used with adolescents (Soffin & Liu, 2018). From a developmental perspective, use of PCA is particularly effective with adolescents because it leads to feelings of control.
- Although controversial, some employers have provided specific guidelines and training to allow parents and nurses to push the button for children too young or unable to use the device on their own. When this is allowed, the concept of patient control is negated, and the inherent safety of PCA needs to be monitored (Hockenberry et al., 2024).

Gerontological

- Older persons sometimes appear more sensitive to analgesics and experience more opioid adverse effects (Boscart et al., 2023). Older persons' reduced renal and liver function slows opioid metabolism and excretion. This causes a faster peak effect and a longer duration of action of the opioid. Dosages should be started low and titrated upward slowly until pain relief is achieved (Galicia-Castillo & Weiner, 2022).
- If patient confusion occurs while using PCA, notify health care provider (may need a prescription to lower the dose or lengthen the lockout time). Refusing to provide analgesia is not the answer; confusion may be caused by pain (Pasero & McCaffery, 2011).

Patients With Physical or Cognitive Challenges

- Patients with a cognitive challenge may benefit from using IV PCA; however, they may require more careful assessment prior to initiation and require ongoing monitoring, including:
  - Assessing whether the patient can effectively use PCA, including completing a formal cognitive assessment along with determining level of consciousness and orientation.
  - Determining and documenting whether the patient can understand, demonstrate, and recall how to use the PCA device correctly.
  - Assessing whether the PCA is being used appropriately to manage pain. Some patients with a cognitive impairment may push the PCA button when they do not have pain. Alternatively, patients may only use PCA when reminded by nurses or other health care providers, therefore not optimizing their pain management (Licht et al., 2009).
- For patients with physical challenges (such as arthritis/weakness in the hands), the traditional handset for the PCA devices (PCA button) can be changed to a handset that is easier to use.

✦ SKILL 16.4 Monitoring Patients Receiving Epidural Analgesia

Epidural analgesia is highly effective for controlling acute pain during labour; after surgery; or after trauma to the chest, abdomen, pelvis, or lower limbs. It has the potential to provide excellent pain relief, minimal adverse effects, and high patient satisfaction when compared with other methods of analgesia (Bos et al., 2017). Patient-controlled epidural analgesia (PCEA) has been shown to provide excellent control of labour and postoperative pain (Motamed, 2022). Use of PCEA is safe and efficient, and complications from this technique are rare. Epidural opioids reduce the total amount of opioid medication required to control pain and thus produce fewer opioid-related adverse effects. However, if epidural analgesia is not managed correctly, it can cause serious complications; safe and effective management requires a coordinated interprofessional approach (Bos et al., 2017).

The epidural space contains a network of vessels, nerves, and fat between the vertebral column and the dura mater, the outermost meninges covering the spinal cord (Fig. 16.1). Analgesics delivered into this space are distributed by (1) diffusion through the dura mater into the cerebrospinal fluid (CSF), where they act directly on the receptors in the dorsal horn of the spinal cord; (2) blood vessels in the epidural space, where they are delivered systemically; and (3) absorption into the fat in the epidural space, creating a depot where the analgesia is slowly released systemically. An analgesic acts by binding to opiate receptors in the dorsal horn of the spinal column, thus blocking pain impulse transmission to the cerebral cortex (Hernandez et al., 2018).

Opioids and local anaesthetics, separately or in combination, are used in epidural analgesia. Opioids are delivered close to their site of action (central nervous system) and thus require much smaller doses to achieve the same pain relief (Galligan, 2020). Common opioids administered via epidural include morphine, hydromorphone, fentanyl, and sufentanil. These opioids differ in their lipophilic "fat-soluble" and hydrophilic "water-soluble" properties, which affect absorption rate and duration of action. Fentanyl and sufentanil are lipophilic, causing them to have a quicker onset and shorter duration of action (2 hours). Morphine and hydromorphone are hydrophilic, resulting in longer onset and duration of action (24 hours) (Hernandez et al., 2018).

The patient is placed in the lateral side-lying or sitting position with the shoulders and hips in alignment and the hips and head flexed during insertion of an epidural catheter. An anaesthesia provider, using sterile technique, typically places a catheter into the epidural space below the second lumbar vertebra, where the spinal cord ends (Fig. 16.2). However, epidurals may also be placed at the thoracic level of the spinal cord. Temporary or short-term catheters are not sutured in place and exit from the insertion site on the back. A catheter intended for permanent or long-term use is "tunnelled" subcutaneously and exits on the side of the body (Fig. 16.3) or on the abdomen. Tunnelling reduces infection and catheter dislodgement. A sterile occlusive dressing covers the catheter exit site and is secured to the patient. An X-ray film confirms epidural catheter placement.

A health care provider administers epidural medication intermittently via a bolus, or the patient can inject the medication intermittently on demand (PCEA) through a pump. An epidural infusion can also be given continuously via a controlled delivery system such as an implanted infusion pump (Bos et al., 2017). The use of epidural opioids requires astute nursing observation and care; thus, most institutions require specialized training for nurses who will manage epidural analgesia. Nursing students involved in helping with the care of patients receiving epidural analgesia must understand all safety principles.

The catheter poses a threat to patient safety because of its anatomical location, its potential for migration through the dura, and its proximity to spinal nerves and vessels. Catheter migration into the subarachnoid space can produce dangerously high medication levels. Frequent complications include hypotension, respiratory depression, motor block, urinary retention, pruritus, and superficial infection around a catheter. *Do not administer other supplemental opioids or sedatives when patients are on an epidural.* The combined effect adds to the risk for respiratory depression. In many facilities, anaesthesia providers are the only health care providers who may initiate epidural opioid infusions or administer a medication bolus.

Delegation and Collaboration

The skill of epidural analgesia administration cannot be delegated to a UCP.

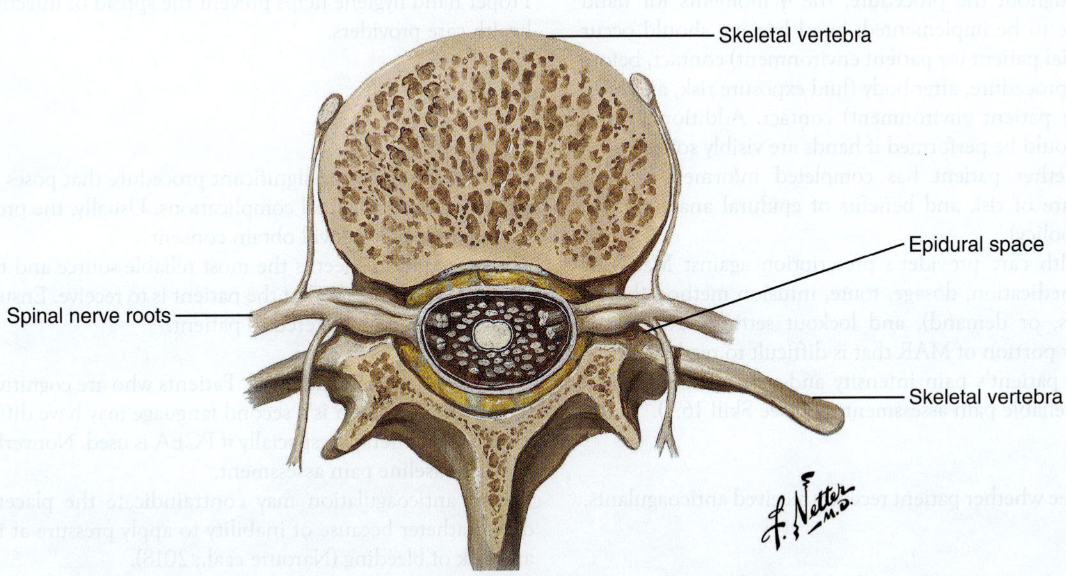

FIG 16.1 Anatomical drawing of epidural space. *(Reprinted from www.netterimages.com © Elsevier Inc. All rights reserved.)*

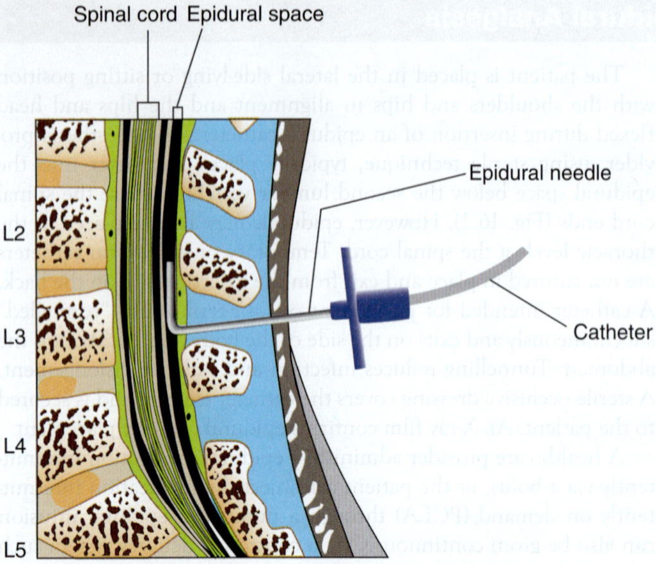

FIG 16.2 Placement of epidural catheter.

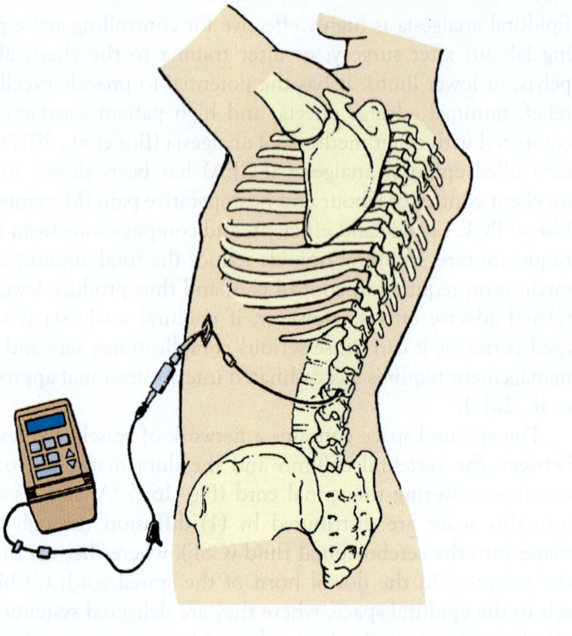
FIG 16.3 Epidural catheter attached to ambulatory infusion pump. *(Image courtesy Astra Zeneca Pharmaceuticals, Wilmington, DE. All rights reserved.)*

Equipment

- Clean or sterile gloves.
- Premixed preservative-free epidural analgesic medications as prescribed by health care provider for use in IV infusion pump (usually prepared by pharmacy).
- Clean or sterile gloves.
- Infusion pump and compatible tubing (do not use Y-ports for infusion; some infusion pumps have colour-coded tubing for intraspinal use).
- Antibacterial filter
- Tape
- Label (for tubing and injection port)
- Equipment for vital signs and pulse oximetry or capnography (see employer policy)

STEP	RATIONALE
ASSESSMENT	
1. Identify patient using at least two person-specific identifiers (e.g., name and date of birth, or name and medical record number) according to employer policy).	Ensures correct patient. Complies with Accreditation Canada's standards and improves patient safety (Accreditation Canada, 2020).
2. Throughout the procedure, the 4 moments for hand hygiene are to be implemented; hand hygiene should occur before initial patient (or patient environment) contact, before an aseptic procedure, after body fluid exposure risk, and after patient (or patient environment) contact. Additional hand hygiene should be performed if hands are visibly soiled.	Proper hand hygiene helps prevent the spread of infectious agents to health care providers.
3. Assess whether patient has completed informed consent and is aware of risk and benefits of epidural analgesia (see employer policy).	Epidural analgesia is a significant procedure that poses risks for serious and potentially fatal complications. Usually, the provider who is placing the epidural will obtain consent.
4. Verify health care provider's prescription against MAR for name of medication, dosage, route, infusion method (bolus, continuous, or demand), and lockout settings. Recopy or reprint any portion of MAR that is difficult to read.	The prescription sheet is the most reliable source and the only legal record of medications that the patient is to receive. Ensures that right medication is administered to patient.
5. Assess the patient's pain intensity and pain quality using a valid and reliable pain assessment tool (see Skill 16.1).	Establishes baseline pain level. Patients who are cognitively impaired or for whom English is a second language may have difficulty understanding the therapy, especially if PCEA is used. Nonverbal responses provide baseline pain assessment.
6. Check to see whether patient recently received anticoagulants.	Recent anticoagulation may contraindicate the placement of epidural catheter because of inability to apply pressure at insertion site and risk of bleeding (Narouze et al., 2018).
7. Assess whether patient routinely takes herbal medications; document complete list.	Some herbal medications interfere with the clotting mechanism (e.g., garlic, Dong Quai, ginkgo biloba) (Narouze et al., 2018).

STEP	RATIONALE

ASSESSMENT

Critical Decision Point *Contraindications to epidural analgesia include coagulopathies, abnormal clotting test results, compromised immunity, history of multiple abscesses, increased intracranial pressure, and sepsis. Additional contraindications include skeletal or spinal abnormalities* (Chawla, 2021).

STEP	RATIONALE
8. Assess for history of medication allergies.	Avoids placing patient at risk for allergic reaction.
9. Assess patient's sedation level by assessing level of wakefulness or alertness, ability to follow commands, and drowsiness.	Establishes baseline before first dose. Assessment of sedation level is more reliable for detecting early opioid-induced respiratory depression than assessment of decreased respiratory rate. Sedation always precedes respiratory depression from opioids.
10. Assess rate, pattern, and depth of respirations; pulse oximetry or capnography; blood pressure and temperature (see Chapter 7).	Establishes baseline of circulatory and oxygenation status. Opioids can cause hypotension. Infection is complication of epidurals, reflected by fever.
11. Assess initial motor and sensory function of lower extremities (see Chapter 8). Test sensation to cold in the dermatomes associated with the expected area of sensory block. Assess motor function by having the patient flex both feet and knees and raise each leg off bed. Pay special attention to patients with pre-existing sensory or motor abnormalities.	Establishes baseline. Ongoing monitoring of motor and sensory status ensures that neural blockage is not affecting function (Galligan, 2020).

Critical Decision Point *For all patients on PCEA, assess for sensory and motor function before ambulation or transfer.*

STEP	RATIONALE
12. Inspect catheter insertion site for redness, warmth, tenderness, swelling, and drainage. Apply sterile gloves when removing occlusive dressing.	Catheter sites are at risk for local infections. Purulent drainage is sign of infection. Clear drainage may indicate CSF leaking from punctured dura. Bloody drainage may indicate that catheter entered blood vessel. Report and document as per employer policy.
13. Follow catheter tubing and check connection site with epidural tubing. Verify that catheter is secured to patient's skin from back, side, or front. Be sure that catheter is connected securely to IV tubing. Remove gloves.	Prevents catheter dislodgement or migration. Ensures tubing is connected to the correct place. Tubing misconnections cause severe patient injury and death if the wrong medication infuses into the epidural space.

Critical Decision Point *Note that in most health care settings, the pharmacy prepares and provides the medication and infusion bag.*

STEP	RATIONALE
14. Check patency of epidural tubing. Check infusion pump for proper calibration and operation.	Kinked or clamped tubing interrupts analgesic infusion.

Critical Decision Point *Note that epidural infusions should be labelled "For Epidural Use Only"* (ISMP Canada, 2015). *Infusion pumps should be configured specifically for epidural analgesia with preset limits for maximum infusion rate and bolus size; lockout time should be standardized if used for PCEA.*

NURSING DIAGNOSES

- Acute pain
- Anxiety
- Chronic pain
- Reduced stamina
- Insufficient knowledge regarding epidural analgesia
- Reduced physical mobility
- Potential for infection
- Potential for injury

Related factors and risk factors are individualized on the basis of patient's condition or needs.

PLANNING

STEP	RATIONALE
1. Expected outcomes following completion of procedure:	
• Patient verbalizes pain relief within 30–60 minutes of initiating epidural infusion.	Indicates that medication and dose are effective in relieving pain, catheter is intact, and equipment is functioning properly in compliance with health care provider's prescription.
• Patient has no headache during epidural infusion or after discontinuation.	Indicates that catheter is in epidural space. No CSF leakage.
• Patient's blood pressure remains within normal range (normotensive), and heart rate remains at or above baseline.	Indicates absence of some of the circulatory adverse effects of epidural opioids.

STEP	RATIONALE
PLANNING	
• Patient is alert, oriented, and easily aroused.	Indicates absence of excessive sedation or oversedation.
• Patient's respirations are regular, of adequate depth, and ≥10 breaths/min. Pulse oximetry SpO_2 ≥95%.	Indicates adequate ventilation and reduced risk for respiratory depression from opioids.
• Patient voids without difficulty; averages a minimum of 30 mL/hr.	Indicates absence of urinary retention (potential opioid adverse effect).
• Patient has no or minimal pruritus and no paresthesia of lower extremities.	Indicates absence of potential adverse effect of epidural medications.
• Epidural system remains intact and functioning.	Infusion system is patent; no interruption in medication delivery to epidural space.
2. Explain purpose and function of epidural analgesia and expectations of patient during procedure (e.g., ask patient to call for help before getting out of bed). Demonstrate to patient how to use pump on demand (when appropriate).	Proper explanation enhances patient cooperation and helps with effective results.
3. Place patients receiving epidural analgesia close to the nurses' station.	Ensures close supervision during infusion.
IMPLEMENTATION	
1. Check label of medication carefully against MAR or computer printout two times. NOTE: Pharmacy prepares medication for pump.	Reduces transmission of microorganisms. Ensures safe and appropriate medication administration. *This is the first and second check for accuracy.*
2. When receiving patient during hand-off or when helping during insertion by anaesthesia provider, apply an "epidural line" label to the epidural infusion tubing. Be sure that there are no Y-ports on tubing. Epidural infusions should be labelled "For Epidural Use Only."	Labelling helps to ensure that analgesic is administered into correct line and the epidural space (ISMP Canada, 2015). Epidural infusion system between pump and patient should be considered closed, with no injection or Y-ports.
3. At the bedside, recheck patient identity and compare MAR or computer printout with name of medication on drug container.	Ensures that right patient receives right medication. *This is the third check for accuracy.*
4. Before initiating analgesia, clarify purpose of epidural and demonstrate how it functions to patient and caregiver.	Proper explanation enhances patient cooperation with administering a demand dose and improves likelihood of effective results.
5. Apply clean gloves. Administer infusion; anaesthesia provider typically starts or administers first dose. Thereafter, nurse maintains infusion.	Reduces transmission of microorganisms.
a. Continuous infusion:	Tubing filled with solution and free of air bubbles avoids air embolus.
(1) Attach container of diluted preservative-free medication to infusion pump tubing and prime tubing (see Chapter 22).	
(2) Insert tubing into infusion pump (see Chapter 22) and attach distal end of tubing to antibacterial filter; then connect to epidural catheter using aseptic technique.	Pump propels fluid through tubing. Filter reduces entrance of microorganisms into infusion line.
(3) Check infusion pump for proper calibration, setting, and operation. Many facilities require two nurses to check settings as an independent double-check.	Ensures that patient is receiving proper dosing.
(4) Tape all connections. Start infusion (see Chapter 22).	Taping maintains secure closed system to prevent infection.
b. Administer bolus dose of analgesic via infusion pump.	Done if the patient is experiencing pain (usually by anaesthesia provider).
(1) While helping anaesthesia provider, perform Steps 5a(1)–5a(4). Adjust infusion pump setting for required bolus amount. Initiate pump to deliver prescribed bolus.	Prevents accidental infusion of an overdose.
c. Administer dose on demand (bolus button) when using PCEA.	Gives patient control over administration of analgesic.
(1) While helping anaesthesia provider, perform Steps 5a(1)–5a(4). Set pump for lockout time (as prescribed).	
(2) Have patient initiate demand dose as needed.	

STEP	RATIONALE
IMPLEMENTATION	
6. Explain that nurses will monitor patient's response to epidural analgesic routinely. Also instruct patient on signs or problems to report to nurse (e.g., pruritus, inability to pass urine, change in sensation).	Builds trust to encourage patient to be partner in care.
7. Keep an IV line patent for 24 hours after epidural analgesia has ended.	Provides route for any emergency medications such as naloxone or lipids.
8. Remove and dispose of gloves in appropriate receptacle.	Reduces transmission of microorganisms.
9. Before removal of epidural catheter, check for presence of therapeutic anticoagulation. Check employer policy for removal while patient is receiving anticoagulation therapy.	Removal of epidural catheter while patient is anticoagulated increases risk for spinal hematoma because of anticoagulation and inability to compress vessels.
EVALUATION	
1. Evaluate patient's pain severity using a valid pain rating scale, and evaluate the location and quality of the pain.	Evaluates effectiveness of epidural infusion.
2. Evaluate blood pressure and heart rate; respiratory rate, rhythm, depth, and pattern; pulse oximetry or capnography; and sedation level based on patient's clinical condition. Generally measured more frequently in first 12 hours of infusions (e.g., hourly) (see employer policy), after bolus infusions or changes of infusion rate, and in periods of cardiovascular or respiratory instability.	Oversedation occurs before respiratory depression and should be monitored closely to prevent respiratory depression (Motamed, 2022). Postural hypotension, vasodilation, and heart rate changes may occur from pain or medication adverse effects (Chawla, 2021).
3. Help patient when changing positions.	Protects patient in case of postural hypotension.
4. Evaluate catheter insertion site every 2–4 hours for redness, warmth, tenderness, swelling, or drainage. Note character of drainage (e.g., bloody, clear, or purulent). Do not remove dressing unless you are discontinuing the epidural catheter.	Bloody drainage may occur if catheter has migrated into a vessel. Report immediately and treat as emergency (Galligan, 2020).
5. Inspect epidural site for disruption or displacement of catheter.	Could lead to infusion of medication into higher level of spinal cord.
6. Observe for pruritus, especially of face, head, neck, and torso. Inform patient that this is a side effect but is often not an allergic response.	Pruritus is assessed with opioid use (Motamed, 2022).
7. Observe for nausea and vomiting and presence of headache. Note any nonverbal signs of headache (grimacing, massaging head, positional changes in pain).	Nausea from epidural analgesia worsens by movement. Headache and CSF leakage may occur from a dural puncture. The headache is often worse when patient is sitting upright than when they are lying down.
8. Monitor intake and output. Evaluate for bladder distension and urinary frequency or urgency. Consult with health care provider for possible need for intermittent catheterization.	Prevents urinary retention.
9. Evaluate for motor weakness or numbness and tingling of lower extremities (paresthesias).	Reducing epidural dose (per prescription) may help eliminate unwanted motor and sensory deficits.
10. **Use teach-back:** "We discussed the adverse effects or problems that you might have from the epidural medicine that is running. Which effects should you tell me about?" Develop a revised teaching plan if patient or caregiver is unable to teach back correctly.	Determines patient's and caregiver's level of understanding of instructional topic.

Unexpected Outcomes	Related Interventions
1. Patient states that pain is still present or has increased. Primary causes are insufficient medication dose or catheter blockage, breakage, or improper position.	• Check all tubing, connections, medication doses, and pump settings. • Inform the health care provider if the pain is not well controlled. • Confer with health care provider on adequacy of medication dose and offer breakthrough analgesia as prescribed.
2. Patient is sedated or not easily aroused.	• Stop epidural infusion and elevate patient's head of bed 30 degrees (unless contraindicated). *Stay with patient and call for help.* • Notify health care provider and prepare to administer opioid-reversing agent naloxone per health care provider's prescription. • Monitor all vital signs, pulse oximetry, capnography, and sedation level continuously until patient is easily aroused.

Unexpected Outcomes	Related Interventions
3. Patient experiences periods of apnea; or respirations are less than 10 breaths/min, shallow, or irregular (check employer policy).	• Instruct patient to take deep breaths. • Stop epidural infusion, stay with patient, and call for help. Notify health care provider. • Prepare to administer opioid-reversing agent (naloxone) per health care provider's prescription (see employer policy). • Monitor at least every 30 minutes until respirations are at least 8 or more per minute and of adequate depth for 2 hours.
4. Patient reports sudden headache. Clear drainage is present on epidural dressing, or more than 1 mL of fluid is aspirated from catheter.	• Stop infusion or bolus dosing. Stay with patient and call for help. • Notify health care provider.
5. Patient experiences minimal urinary output, urinary frequency or urgency, bladder distension, pruritus, or nausea and vomiting.	• Consult with health care provider about reducing dose of opioid and discuss treatment for adverse effects.

Communication and Documentation

- Document medication, dose, method of administration (bolus, demand, or continuous), and time given (if injection) or time begun and ended (if demand or continuous) on appropriate medication record in the EHR or chart. Specify concentration and diluent.
- With continuous or demand infusion, obtain and document pump readout (frequency according to employer policy).
- Document assessments of patient's status in progress notes in EHR or chart and/or on appropriate flow sheet, including vital signs, pulse oximetry/capnography, intake and output, sedation level, pain severity score, neurological status, appearance of epidural site, presence or absence of adverse reactions to medication, and presence or absence of complications resulting from placement and maintenance of epidural catheter.
- Report any adverse reactions or complications to health care provider immediately.
- Document your evaluation of patient and caregiver learning.

Special Considerations

Teaching

- Describe catheter placement and purpose to patient as appropriate. Drawing or showing pictures often helps.
- Teach patient and caregivers the purpose, action, and signs and symptoms of adverse reactions to opioid or local anaesthetic. Teach when and which signs and symptoms to report to a nurse.
- Teach patient to report pain level with acceptable (to patient) pain scale.
- Inform patient of other pain management strategies that supplement or enhance pharmacological intervention (e.g., imagery, distraction, relaxation).
- Some patients may attempt to ambulate without help or overdo other activities. Caution them to call for a nurse to help with any activity until it is determined they are safe to ambulate independently. Explain that the first attempt to ambulate may feel awkward related to decreased sensation, but motor (leg) function should be unaffected.

Pediatric

- Apply EMLA (eutectic mixture of local anaesthetics) cream to the epidural site a minimum of 60 minutes before catheter insertion.
- Dosing regimens for children must be adapted for age and weight, with maximum dosage clearly defined to minimize cumulative local anaesthetic toxicity (Ocay et al., 2018).
- Hourly assessments are recommended, especially in the first 12 hours. There should be regular review of need for infusion, especially after 48 hours.

Gerontological

- Older persons are at the same risk for complications and medication adverse effects as other adult patients.

Care in the Community: Home Management

- Patients needing long-term therapy are discharged with a tunnelled catheter. Before considering catheter placement and care in the home, assess patient's fine-motor skills, cognitive ability, and stage of disease and prognosis and the degree of involvement of caregiver.
- Teach patient and caregiver proper dosage and administration of medication. Evaluating patient's technique for catheter care, administering medication, and reinforcing instructions are priorities.
- Teach patient and caregiver aseptic technique for medication administration as needed and for all catheter care procedures, including dressing changes. Instruct patient to change dressing every week (refer to employer policy). Teach signs and symptoms of infection and instruct patient to report to nurse or health care provider immediately should signs and symptoms appear.
- Teach patient and caregiver about signs and symptoms of adverse reactions to medication being used and interventions to alleviate mild adverse effects in the home.
- Provide patient and caregiver with phone numbers of health care providers to contact in an emergency and resources in the community.

✦ SKILL 16.5 Monitoring Patients Receiving Peripheral Nerve Blocks

During surgery for procedures such as hip or knee arthroplasty, shoulder repair or arthroscopy, breast reconstruction, and abdominal surgery, some anaesthesiologists and surgeons may administer a single shot or continuous peripheral nerve block (Biswas et al., 2018; Ilfeld, 2017). Surgeons may infiltrate local anaesthetics into the wound bed.

When a continuous peripheral nerve block is used, a catheter is put in place close to a nerve. Local anaesthetic is infused into the catheter through a pump (e.g., bupivacaine or ropivacaine). The local anaesthetic is infused continuously to "bathe" the specific nerve or nerve plexus responsible for pain at the surgical site, thus maintaining analgesia during and after surgery. Patients may still require oral analgesics, but the total dosage is often reduced. Pumps that are used for peripheral nerve blocks may be programmed to deliver a continuous infusion or may include a patient demand or PCA feature.

Assessment of patients who receive peripheral nerve blocks includes assessing pain intensity, location, and quality. The site of the nerve block should be assessed for any bruising or hematoma. If a patient is receiving a continuous peripheral nerve block, the site should also be assessed to ensure the infusion catheter is intact (Ilfeld & Mariano, 2018). In patients who undergo upper or lower extremity surgery, assessment also includes checking for sensory and motor block. Patients who have received a lower extremity block are at risk of falling because of the potential motor block they may experience.

Assessment and care of a patient who has received a peripheral nerve block require a coordinated interprofessional approach. With patients undergoing surgery, peripheral nerve blocks are usually initiated preoperatively. Using interprofessional collaboration, the patient is provided with education and prepared for the procedure. After surgery, interprofessional collaboration maximizes patient safety and is used to assess the patient's pain, mobility, and activities of daily living and to provide patient education.

Patients may be discharged home with an ambulatory pump or a disposable pump to deliver local anaesthetics for peripheral nerve blocks. A disposable pump is one-time use only, used for a few days, allowing patients to control their postoperative pain with a local anaesthetic infusion at home. Patients and their caregivers learn how to remove the catheter at home. Nursing care focuses on assessment of catheter site and connections, evaluation of local anaesthetic adverse effects, and patient teaching.

Delegation and Collaboration

The skill of managing local anaesthetic infusion pump analgesia in facilities cannot be delegated to a UCP. If the patient is going home with a peripheral nerve block, it is important to provide patient and caregiver teaching on how to manage the nerve block.

Equipment

- Pump in place from surgery

Teaching Home Removal of Peripheral Nerve Block Catheter

- Clean gloves
- Sterile 10 cm × 10 cm (4 inch × 4 inch) gauze pads
- Adhesive bandage
- Tape
- Plastic bag

STEP	RATIONALE
ASSESSMENT	
1. Identify patient using at least two person-specific identifiers (e.g., name and date of birth, or name and medical record number) according to employer policy.	Ensures correct patient. Complies with Accreditation Canada's standards and improves patient safety (Accreditation Canada, 2020).
2. Throughout the procedure, the 4 moments for hand hygiene are to be implemented; hand hygiene should occur before initial patient (or patient environment) contact, before an aseptic procedure, after body fluid exposure risk, and after patient (or patient environment) contact. Additional hand hygiene should be performed if hands are visibly soiled.	Proper hand hygiene helps prevent the spread of infectious agents to health care providers.
3. Apply clean gloves and assess surgical dressing and site of catheter insertion. Dressing should be dry and intact.	Reduces transmission of microorganisms. Determines whether catheter is placed properly.
4. Be sure that catheter tubing is correctly labelled; then assess catheter connection. Be sure that it is secure. Teach patient and caregiver that if the catheter becomes detached, do *not* reattach or reinsert; instead, notify surgeon immediately.	Reattachment could lead to infection. Tubing misconnections could lead to infusion of inappropriate medications into surgical wound site.
5. Perform a complete pain assessment (see Skill 16.1).	Provides baseline to determine efficacy of analgesia.
6. Review the operative report or anaesthetic record for position of catheter.	Confirms catheter location with your own observation.
7. Read medication label on device and compare to MAR and the health care provider's prescription.	Provides information regarding type of anaesthetic, concentration, volume, flow rate, date and time prepared.
8. Assess for presence of blood backing up in tubing. If blood is present, stop infusion and notify health care provider. Remove gloves and dispose of them in appropriate receptacle.	Indicates possible displacement of catheter into blood vessel.
9. Determine level of extremity activity that patient can perform per health care provider's prescriptions.	Excessive activity can cause catheter displacement.
10. Confirm patient allergies (should be completed preoperatively and intraoperatively). Assess for signs of local anaesthetic toxicity: hypotension, dizziness, tremor, severe itching, swelling of skin or throat, irregular heartbeat, palpitations, confusion, ringing in ears, muscle twitching, numbness around mouth, metallic taste, seizure.	Early identification of toxicity prevents or lessens possibility of complications. Local anaesthetics can have serious systemic effects (El-Boghdadly et al., 2018).
11. Assess patient's and caregiver's knowledge of infusion pump.	Assesses level of teaching and support required.

STEP	RATIONALE

NURSING DIAGNOSES

- Acute pain
- Anxiety
- Insufficient knowledge regarding purpose of infusion pump
- Reduced physical mobility
- Potential for infection

Related factors and risk factors are individualized on the basis of patient's condition or needs.

PLANNING

STEP	RATIONALE
1. Expected outcomes following completion of procedure:	
• Patient verbalizes full or partial relief from pain.	Patient's self-report of pain is single most reliable indicator of pain.
• Patient achieves reduction of nonverbal behaviours indicative of pain, such as grimacing, clenching teeth, rocking.	Nonverbal behaviours are valid and reliable indicators of pain in absence of self-report (Tyerman & Cobbett, 2023).
• Patient moves about in bed, sleeps and eats better, is more active, and communicates easily with family and friends.	Adequate pain relief allows patient to participate in ADLs.
• Patient or caregiver verbalizes correct procedure for catheter removal.	

IMPLEMENTATION

STEP	RATIONALE
1. When repositioning or ambulating patient, use caution. Do not pull on the catheter.	Avoids catheter dislodgement.
2. When preparing patient for discharge, it may be necessary for you to connect the catheter to a smaller pump for use at home (depending on type of pump). One example is a pump about the size of a baby bottle. When pump is connected, the balloon inside pump is full of medication, and plunger is all the way to the top. As medication infuses, balloon inside pump shrinks, and plunger goes down.	
3. Teach patient or caregiver what to observe and how to prepare for removal of catheter at home (may also be done by community health nurse).	
a. Explain how to perform hand hygiene and apply clean gloves.	Reduces transmission of microorganisms.
b. Have patient assume relaxed position in bed or chair with lower extremity in normal alignment.	Relaxes joint muscles, reducing traction from muscle tension, and provides distraction.
c. Apply clean gloves, and provide clean gloves to patient or caregiver. Have patient or caregiver gently lift adhesive dressing covering catheter insertion site and remove any remaining tape.	Reduces transmission of microorganisms. Exposes catheter insertion site.
4. Teach patient or caregiver how to remove catheter.	
a. Explain to patient or caregiver to place 10 cm × 10 cm (4 inch × 4 inch) gauze over site, grasp catheter as close as possible to where it enters skin, and gently pull it out with steady motion. This should cause little discomfort or resistance. A small amount of blood or fluid drainage is normal.	Prevents breakage of catheter.
b. Instruct patient or caregiver to look for mark (e.g., black dot) on end of catheter tip and hold new sterile gauze using pressure over the site for 2–5 minutes.	Indicates complete removal of catheter. Achieves hemostasis.

Critical Decision Point *Patients receiving anticoagulants may require pressure to be applied longer than 5 minutes.*

STEP	RATIONALE
c. Instruct patient or caregiver to wash skin to remove any surgical soap or adhesive near the site and then apply bandage.	Cleanses insertion site.
d. Inform patient or caregiver to place catheter in plastic bag, remove and dispose of gloves, and tie bag before discarding in garbage. Lastly, instruct patient or caregiver to perform hand hygiene.	Reduces transmission of microorganisms.

STEP	RATIONALE
IMPLEMENTATION	
5. Explain to patient that any remaining numbness should go away within 24 hours after catheter is removed.	Allows patient and caregiver to anticipate progress and recognize problems.
6. Remind patient or caregiver of follow-up appointment with surgeon.	Increases patient adherence.
EVALUATION	
1. Ask patient to rate pain intensity using appropriate pain assessment scale at both rest and with activity.	Determines patient response to local infusion of medication.
2. Observe for signs of adverse medication reaction and report any signs immediately.	Local analgesics can cause systemic adverse effects if absorbed into the bloodstream (El-Boghdadly et al., 2018).
3. Observe patient's position, mobility, relaxation, participation in ADLs, and any nonverbal behaviours.	Indicates successful pain management.
4. Inspect condition of surgical dressing.	Wet dressing indicates possible catheter migration out of wound, especially if drainage is clear.
5. **Use teach-back:** "It is important for you to remove the catheter at home correctly. Explain to me the steps to take to remove the catheter." Develop a revised teaching plan if patient or caregiver is unable to teach back correctly.	Determines patient's and caregiver's level of understanding of instructional topic.

Unexpected Outcomes	Related Interventions
1. Patient verbalizes pain intensity greater than previously determined goal or demonstrates nonverbal behaviours indicative of pain. Catheter may be displaced or clogged, or surgical site may be developing complications.	• Check reservoir for presence of medication. • Check patency of tubing. • Notify health care provider.
2. Patient reports symptoms of local anaesthetic adverse reaction (bleeding, arrhythmias, weakness or numbness of affected area, seizure, confusion, infection, drowsiness, ringing in ears), possible hypersensitivity to local anaesthetic, displacement of catheter into vein, or pump failure (releasing too much medication into site).	• Stop infusion (El-Boghdadly et al., 2018). • Notify health care provider.

Communication and Documentation

- Document medication and concentration, date catheter inserted, and type of demand feature (continuous or demand) in MAR in EHR or chart.
- Document location of catheter, patient's pain rating, response to anaesthetic, and additional comfort measures given in progress notes in EHR or chart.
- Document additional analgesics necessary to control pain on MAR in EHR or chart.
- Document any adverse reactions to local anaesthetic (El-Boghdadly et al., 2018) in progress notes in EHR or chart and report to health care provider.
- Communicate any damp dressing or displaced catheter to surgeon.
- Document your evaluation of patient and caregiver learning.

Special Considerations

Teaching

- Provide preoperative teaching about purpose before patient goes to operating room.
- If pump being used includes a PCA component through the peripheral nerve block catheter, instruct patient to depress button as needed to manage pain.
- Instruct patient to inform nurse if pain exceeds pain-intensity goal because additional oral and/or intravenous analgesics may be administered to manage pain.

Pediatric

- Local continuous infusion pumps have been used for children undergoing orthopedic surgery. Instruct parents and the child as described in "Care in the Community: Home Management." Explain special precautions to avoid dislodging the catheter.

Gerontological

- Continuous dosing is sometimes administered, but demand doses require a mentally competent adult. In addition, take special precautions to protect the catheter.

Care in the Community: Home Management

- Instruct patient and caregiver to notify the health care provider immediately if the peripheral nerve block catheter has excessive fluid or bleeding on the dressing occurs; if patient has signs of anaesthetic reaction, including arrhythmias, weakness, or numbness of affected area, seizure, confusion, drowsiness, or ringing in the ears; or if signs of infection develop (redness and tenderness at catheter site, drainage, or fever). Provide written copy of instructions.
- Provide verbal and written instructions regarding how and when to discontinue device when at home.
- Provide instructions regarding any restrictions to extremity movement after surgery.
- Provide patient information about each nonpharmacological therapy (see Skill 16.2), including purpose, rationale for how pain is relieved, and how patient can maximize benefits.
- Teach patient to rest between periods of activity at home and in hospital because fatigue increases pain perception.

✦ REVIEW QUESTIONS

A 56-year-old account executive (they/them) underwent a colectomy (removal of a portion of colon) this morning. The patient returns from the operating room with an epidural catheter connected to an epidural pump set to deliver 5 mL/hr of ropivacaine 0.2% with hydromorphone 0.1 mg/mL, with a patient-controlled bolus of 2 mL every 20 minutes prn (as needed). The patient has been able to follow instructions and self-administer analgesic doses correctly. The nurse caring for the patient knows to assess for adverse effects of the epidural analgesic.

Review Questions 1 to 4 relate to the case study presented here.

1. It is approximately 10 hours after surgery, and the patient has not been able to pass urine. The nurse assesses them by scanning the patient's bladder, determining there is approximately 500 mL of urine in the bladder. Considering the patient's clinical situation, what could explain their symptoms?

2. The patient's vital signs are BP 132/86 mm Hg; pulse 84 beats/min, regular; R 20 breaths/min, temperature 37.6°C. The epidural and surgical dressings are intact. Abdomen is assessed with mild discomfort over bladder owing to inability to pass urine during the last 10 hours. The patient describes their pain as aching and sometimes sharp and rates their pain along their abdominal incision as 5/10 on a scale of 0–10. The patient's partner is visiting and asks if there is a way they can be helpful. Describe ways that the partner can help promote pain relief. Using SBAR (situation–background–assessment–recommendation), show how you would communicate with the health care team about this patient.

3. The patient is scheduled to stand up at the bedside within 6 hours of returning from surgery. Describe measures the nurse can institute to enhance the patient's ability to safely mobilize and then return to bed more comfortably.

4. On the second day after surgery, the patient's epidural infusion is discontinued, and they are placed on oral analgesics to manage the pain. Prescriptions: acetaminophen PO 1 000 mg q6h, pregabalin PO 25 mg q12h, and hydromorphone 1–3 mg PO q6h prn. The patient's vital signs are stable: BP 125/76 mm Hg; pulse 74 beats/min, regular; R 16 breaths/min; temperature 37.2°C. Abdomen is assessed and the surgical dressing is intact; the nurse auscultates bowel sounds in all four quadrants. The patient describes their pain as aching and sometimes sharp, and rates the pain they feel along the abdominal incision as 5/10 on a scale of 0–10. What could the nurse do to help the patient manage their pain?

5. The nurse is caring for an older person who has peripheral neuropathy causing ongoing nerve pain. In addition, the patient has discomfort in their back from osteoarthritis. The nurse's assessment reveals that the patient has reduced hearing and is cognitively alert. Which of the following statements accurately describe guidelines for how to select pain relief therapies for this patient? (*Select all that apply.*)

1. A cognitive behavioural strategy would likely not be effective for this patient.
2. Work with patient to determine the combination of analgesics and/or adjuvants prescribed that is most effective in relieving pain.
3. Explain to the patient that initial opioid dosages will be high and then tapered down to achieve pain relief.
4. Be certain that patient's hearing aid is in place before practising guided imagery.
5. Plan a quiet time to provide the patient with a body massage.

6. The nurse is caring for a patient who is receiving morphine by way of patient-controlled analgesia. The nurse has just completed measuring the patient's respirations and pulse oximetry. The nurse reviews the patient's medical record to identify their risk for oversedation. Which of the following factors increase a patient's risk for oversedation? (*Select all that apply.*)

1. A patient who has received an opioid for pain within the last 2 months
2. A patient who is cognitively impaired
3. A patient who has a history of obstructive sleep apnea
4. A patient who has an allergy to opioids
5. A patient who is opioid naive

7. In the space below, fill in the rationale for each step that explains how to instruct a patient or caregiver in the proper way to remove a peripheral nerve block catheter at home.

STEP	RATIONALE
Explain how to perform hand hygiene.	
Have patient or caregiver gently lift the adhesive dressing covering the catheter insertion site and remove any remaining tape.	
Explain to patient or caregiver to grasp the catheter as close as possible to where it enters the skin and gently pull it out. Inspect catheter to ensure it is intact.	
Instruct patient or caregiver to hold pressure over the site for 5 minutes, then apply an adhesive bandage.	
Explain to patient that any remaining numbness should go away within 24 hours after the catheter is removed.	

Visit the Evolve site for a complete list of answers to the Review Questions.

✦ NEXT GENERATION NCLEX® (NGN)

For practice with answering exam questions related to unfolding NGN case studies, please consult the Next Generation NCLEX® (NGN)-Style Case Studies for Skills and Techniques on the Evolve website: http://evolve.elsevier.com/Canada/Perry/clinicalskills/

REFERENCES

Accreditation Canada. (2020). *Required organizational practices handbook.* https://physicians.nshealth.ca/resources/required-organizational-practices-2020-handbook

Ameer, B., & Weintraub, M. (2018). Pediatric obesity: Influence on drug dosing and therapeutics. *The Journal of Clinical Pharmacology, 58*(S10), S94–S107. https://doi.org/10.1002/jcph.1092

American Psychiatric Association. (2022). *Diagnostic and statistical manual of mental disorders* (5th ed., text rev.). https://dsm.psychiatryonline.org/doi/book/10.1176/appi.books.9780890425787

Andersen, R. D., Langius-Eklöf, A., Nakstad, B., et al. (2017). The measurement properties of pediatric observational pain scales: A systematic review of reviews. *International Journal of Nursing Studies, 73*, 93–101. https://doi.org/10.1016/j.ijnurstu.2017.05.010 [Seminal Reference]

Birnie, K., Hundert, A. S., Lalloo, C., et al. (2019). Recommendations for selection of self-report pain intensity measures in children and adolescents: A systematic review and quality assessment of measurement properties. *Pain, 160*(1), 5–18. https://doi.org/10.1097/j.pain.0000000000001377

Biswas, A., Perlas, A., Ghosh, M., et al. (2018). Relative contribution of adductor canal block and intrathecal morphine to analgesia and functional recovery after total knee arthroplasty. *Regional Anesthesia and Pain Medicine*, *43*(2), 154–160. https://doi.org/10.1097/aap.0000000000000724

Bos, E. M. E., Hollmann, M. W., & Lirk, P. (2017). Safety and efficacy of epidural analgesia. *Current Opinion in Anesthesiology*, 30(6), 736–742. https://doi.org/10.1097/ACO.0000000000000516

Boscart, V., McCleary, L., Sheiban Taucar, L., et al. (2023). *Ebersole and Hess' gerontological nursing and healthy aging in Canada* (3rd ed.). Elsevier.

Buowari, D. Y. (2021). Pain management in older persons. In S. Amornyotin (Ed.), *Update in geriatrics*. IntechOpen. https://doi.org/10.5772/INTECHOPEN.93940

Busse, J. W., Vankrunkelsven, P., Zeng, L., et al. (2021). Medical cannabis or cannabinoids for chronic pain: A clinical practice guideline. *British Medical Journal*, *374*, n2040. https://doi.org/10.1136/bmj.n2040

Canadian Pain Task Force. (2021). *An action plan for pain in Canada*. Health Canada. https://www.canada.ca/content/dam/hc-sc/documents/corporate/about-health-canada/public-engagement/external-advisory-bodies/canadian-pain-task-force/report-2021-rapport/report-rapport-2021-eng.pdf

Chan, S., Hadjistavropoulos, T., Williams, J., & Lints-Martindales, A. (2014). Evidence-based development and initial validation of the pain assessment checklist for seniors with limited ability to communicate-II (PACSLAC-II). *The Clinical Journal of Pain*, 30(9), 816–824. https://geriatricpain.org/sites/geriatricpain.org/files/2020-06/PACSLAC%20II%20Checklist.pdf [Seminal Reference]

Chang, J. L., Goldberg, A. N., Alt, J. A., et al. (2022). International consensus statement on obstructive sleep apnea. *International Forum of Allergy & Rhinology* [Advance online publication]. https://doi.org/10.1002/alr.23079

Chawla, J. (2021). Epidural nerve block. *Medscape*. https://emedicine.medscape.com/article/149646-overview#a1

Dobson, G., Chau, A., Denomme, J., et al. (2023). Guidelines to the practice of anesthesia: Revised edition 2023. *Canadian Journal of Anesthesia*, *70*(1), 16–55. https://link.springer.com/article/10.1007/s12630-022-02368-0

El-Boghdadly, K., Pawa, A., & Chin, K. J. (2018). Local anesthetic systemic toxicity: Current perspectives. *Local and Regional Anesthesia*, *11*, 35–44. https://doi.org/10.2147/LRA.S154512

Eloge, J., Napier, T. C., & Dantz, B. (2018). OPQRST(U): Integrating substance use disorders or "Use" into the medical history. *Substance Abuse*, *39*(4), 505–508. https://doi.org/10.1080/08897077.2018.1469104

Erden, S., Demir, N., Ugras, G. A., et al. (2018). Vital signs: Valid indicators to assess pain in intensive care unit patients? An observational, descriptive study. *Nursing and Health Sciences*, *20*(4), 502–508. https://doi.org/10.1111/nhs.12543

Galicia-Castillo, M., & Weiner, D. (2022). Dosing and selected characteristics of analgesic drugs for treatment of persistent pain in older adults. *UpToDate*. https://www.uptodate.com/contents/image?imageKey=ANEST%2F95621

Galligan, M. (2020). Care and management of patients receiving epidural analgesia. *Nursing Standard*, *35*(12), 77–82. https://doi.org/10.7748/ns.2020.e11573

Gélinas, C. (2016). Pain assessment in the critically ill adult: Recent evidence and new trends. *Intensive and Critical Care Nursing*, *34*, 1–11. https://doi.org/10.1016/j.iccn.2016.03.001 [Seminal Reference]

Hanson, A., & Haddad, L. M. (2021). Nursing rights of medication administration. *StatPearls*. https://www.ncbi.nlm.nih.gov/books/NBK560654/

Health Quality Ontario. (2018a). *Opioid prescribing for acute pain: Care for people 15 years of age and older*. Queen's Printer for Ontario. http://www.hqontario.ca/portals/0/documents/evidence/quality-standards/qs-opioid-acute-pain-clinician-guide-en.pdf

Health Quality Ontario. (2018b). *Opioid prescribing for chronic pain: Care for people 15 years of age and older*. Queen's Printer for Ontario. http://www.hqontario.ca/portals/0/documents/evidence/quality-standards/qs-opioid-chronic-pain-clinician-guide-en.pdf

Health Quality Ontario. (2018c). *Opioid use disorder: Care for people 16 years of age and older*. Queen's Printer for Ontario. http://www.hqontario.ca/portals/0/documents/evidence/quality-standards/qs-opioid-use-disorder-clinician-guide-en.pdf

Health Quality Ontario. (2020). *Chronic pain: Care for Adolescents, adults, and children*. Queen's Printer for Ontario. https://www.hqontario.ca/Portals/0/documents/evidence/quality-standards/qs-chronic-pain-quality-standard-en.pdf

Health Services Organization and Solutions for Kids in Pain. (2023). *Pediatric pain management standard*. https://healthstandards.org/uncategorized/hso-and-skip-release-the-first-pediatric-pain-management-standard/

Hernandez, G. A., Grant, M. C., & Wu, C. L. (2018). Epidural opioids for postoperative pain. In H. T. Benzon, S. N. Raja, S. M. Fishman, et al. (Eds.), *Essentials of pain medicine* (4th ed., pp. 129–133). Elsevier. https://doi.org/10.1016/C2014-0-03837-3

Hockenberry, M. J., Duffy, E. A., & Gibbs, K. (2024). *Wong's nursing care of infants and children* (12th ed.). Elsevier.

Horgas, A. L. (2017). Pain assessment in older adults. *Nursing Clinics of North America*, *52*(3), 375–385. https://doi.org/10.1016/j.cnur.2017.04.006 [Seminal Reference]

Hoti, K., Atee, M., & Hughes, J. D. (2018). Clinimetric properties of the electronic Pain Assessment Tool (ePAT) for aged-care residents with moderate to severe dementia. *Journal of Pain Research*, *11*, 1037–1044. https://doi.org/10.2147/jpr.s158793

Ilfeld, B. (2017). Continuous peripheral nerve blocks: An update of the published evidence and comparison with novel, alternative analgesic modalities. *Anesthesia & Analgesia*, *124*(1), 306–334. https://doi.org/10.1213/ANE.0000000000001581

Ilfeld, B. M., & Mariano, E. R. (2018). Continuous peripheral nerve blocks. In H. T. Benzon, S. N. Raja, S. M. Fishman, et al. (Eds.), *Essentials of pain medicine* (4th ed., pp. 135–146). Elsevier. https://doi.org/10.1016/C2014-0-03837-3

Institute for Safe Medication Practices Canada (ISMP Canada). (2015). *Ontario critical incident learning: Resources to sustain incident learning*. https://www.ismp-canada.org/download/ocil/ISMPCONCIL2015-13_IncidentLearning.pdf [Seminal Reference]

International Association for the Study of Pain (IASP). (2020). *Terminology*. https://www.iasp-pain.org/resources/terminology/

Kawada, T. (2019). Lung function, sleep-disordered breathing and stroke. *European Journal of Neurology*, *26*(4), Article e47. https://doi.org/10.1111/ene.13834

Kent, M. L., Tighe, P. J., Belfer, I., et al. (2017). The ACTTION-APS-AAPM Pain Taxonomy (AAAPT) multidimensional approach to classifying acute pain conditions. *The Journal of Pain*, *18*(5), 479–489. https://doi.org/10.1016/j.jpain.2017.02.421

Licht, E., Siegler, E. L., & Reid, M. C. (2009). Can the cognitively impaired safely use patient-controlled analgesia? *Journal of Opioid Management*, *5*(5), 307–312. https://doi.org/10.5055/jom.2009.0031 [Seminal Reference]

Maratos, F., Duarte, J., Barnes, C., et al. (2017). The physiological and emotional effects of touch: Assessing a hand-massage intervention with high self-critics. *Psychiatry Research*, *25*, 221–227. https://doi.org/10.1016/j.psychres.2017.01.066

Michael G. DeGroote National Pain Centre. (2017). *Canadian guideline for opioids for chronic noncancer pain*. https://healthsci.mcmaster.ca/npc/guidelines

Motamed, C. (2022). Clinical update on patient-controlled analgesia for acute postoperative pain. *Pharmacy*, *10*(1), Article 22. https://doi.org/10.3390/pharmacy10010022

Narouze, S., Benzon, H. T., Provenzano, D., et al. (2018). Interventional spine and pain procedures in patients on antiplatelet and anticoagulant medications (2nd ed.): Guidelines from the American Society of Regional Anesthesia and Pain Medicine, the European Society of Regional Anaesthesia and Pain Therapy, the American Academy of Pain Medicine, the International Neuromodulation Society, the North American Neuromodulation Society, and the World Institute of Pain. *Regional Anesthesia and Pain Medicine*, *43*(3), 225–262. https://doi.org/10.1097/AAP.0000000000000700

Natavio, T., McQuillen, E., Dietrich, M. S., et al. (2020). A comparison of the Pain Assessment Checklist for Seniors With Limited Ability to Communicate (PACSLAC) and Pain Assessment Advanced Dementia Scale (PAINAD). *Pain Management Nursing*, *21*, 502–509. https://doi.org/10.1016/j.pmn.2020.04.001

Ocay, D. D., Otis, A., Teles, A. R., et al. (2018). Safety of patient-controlled analgesia after surgery in children and adolescents: Concerns and potential solutions. *Frontiers in Pediatrics*, *6*, Article 336. https://doi.org/10.3389/fped.2018.00336

Orhan, C., Van Looveren, E., Cagnie, B., et al. (2018). Are pain beliefs, cognitions, and behaviors influenced by race, ethnicity, and culture in patients with chronic musculoskeletal pain: A systematic review. *Pain Physician*, *21*, 541–558. https://www.painphysicianjournal.com/current/pdf?article=NTUwMw%3D%3D&journal=114

Paladini, A., & Varrassi, G. (2021). Multimodal pharmacological analgesia in pain management. In V. Waisundara, I. Banjari, & J. Balkić (Eds.), *Pain management: Practices, novel therapies, and bioactives*. IntechOpen. https://doi.org/10.5772/intechopen.93620

Pasero, C., & McCaffery, M. (2011). *Pain assessment and pharmacological management*. Mosby. [Seminal Reference]

Pastino, A., & Lakra, A. (2022). Patient-controlled analgesia. *StatPearls*. https://www.ncbi.nlm.nih.gov/books/NBK551610/

Raja, S. N., Carr, D. B., Cohen, M., et al. (2020). The revised International Association for the Study of Pain definition of pain: Concepts, challenges, and compromises. *Pain*, *161*(9), 1976–1982. https://doi.org/10.1097/j.pain.0000000000001939

Rosenquist, R. (2022). Use of opioids in the management of chronic non-cancer pain. *UpToDate*. https://www.uptodate.com/contents/use-of-opioids-in-the-management-of-chronic-non-cancer-pain

Royal College of Anaesthetists. (2020). *Best practice in the management of epidural analgesia in the hospital setting*. https://fpm.ac.uk/sites/fpm/files/documents/2020-09/Epidural-AUG-2020-FINAL.pdf [Seminal Reference]

Scheffler, M., Koranyi, S., Meissner, W., et al. (2017). Efficacy of non-pharmacological interventions for procedural pain relief in adults undergoing burn wound care: A systematic review and meta-analysis of randomized controlled trials. *Burns*,

44(7), 1709–1720. https://doi.org/10.1016/j.burns.2017.11.019 [Seminal Reference]

Schofield, P. (2018). The assessment of pain in older people: UK national guidelines. *Age and Ageing*, *47*(Suppl. 1), i1–i22. https://doi.org/10.1093/ageing/afx192

Shupler, M. S., Kramer, J. K., Cragg, J. J., et al. (2019). Pan-Canadian estimates of chronic pain prevalence from 2000 to 2014: A repeated cross-sectional survey analysis. *The Journal of Pain*, *20*(5), 557–565. https://doi.org/10.1016/j.jpain.2018.10.010

Simon, R. (2022). NSAIDs (including Aspirin): Allergic and pseudoallergic reactions. *UpToDate*. https://www.uptodate.com/contents/nsaids-including-aspirin-allergic-and-pseudoallergic-reactions

Skelly, A. C., Chou, R., Dettori, J. R., et al. (2018). *Noninvasive nonpharmacological treatment for chronic pain: A systematic review.* Comparative effectiveness review No. 209. AHRQ Publication No. 18-EHC013-EF. US Department of Health and Human Services. https://effectivehealthcare.ahrq.gov/sites/default/files/pdf/nonpharma-chronic-pain-cer-209.pdf

Soffin, E. M., & Liu, S. S. (2018). Patient-controlled analgesia. In H. T. Benzon, S. N. Raja, S. M. Fishman, et al. (Eds.), *Essentials of pain medicine* (4th ed., pp. 117–122). Elsevier. https://doi.org/10.1016/B978-0-323-40196-8.00013-9

Swift, A. (2018). Understanding pain and the human body's response to it. *Nursing Times*, *114*(3), 22–26.

Tang, N. Y. K. (2018). Cognitive behavioural therapy in pain and psychological disorders: Towards a hybrid future. *Progress in Neuro-Psychopharmacology and Biological Psychiatry*, *87*(Part B), 281–289. https://doi.org/10.1016/j.pnpbp.2017.02.023

Tick, H., Nielsen, A., Pelletier, K. R., et al. (2018). Evidence-based nonpharmacological strategies for comprehensive pain care: The consortium pain task force white paper. *Explore*, *14*(3), 177–211. https://doi.org/10.1016/j.explore.2018.02.001

Tsai, I. P., Jeong, S. Y.-S., & Hunter, S. (2018). Pain assessment and management for older patients with dementia in hospitals: An integrative literature review. *Pain Management Nursing*, *19*(1), 54–71. https://doi.org/10.1016/j.pmn.2017.10.001

Turk, D., & Gatchel, R. (2018). *Psychological approaches to pain management* (3rd ed.). Guilford Press.

Tyerman, J., & Cobbett, S. (Eds.). (2023). *Lewis's medical-surgical nursing in Canada: Assessment and management of clinical problems* (5th ed.). Elsevier Inc.

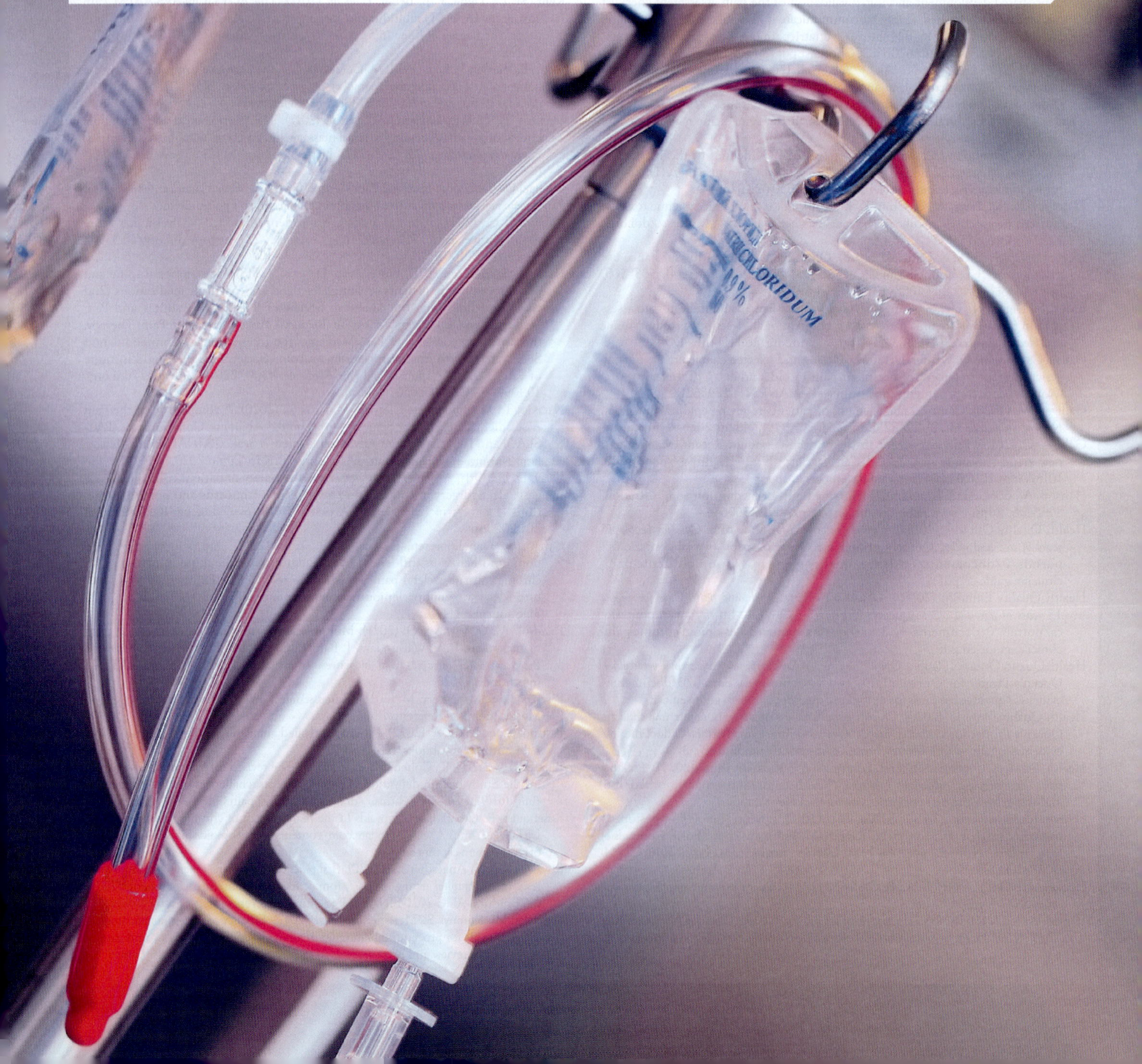

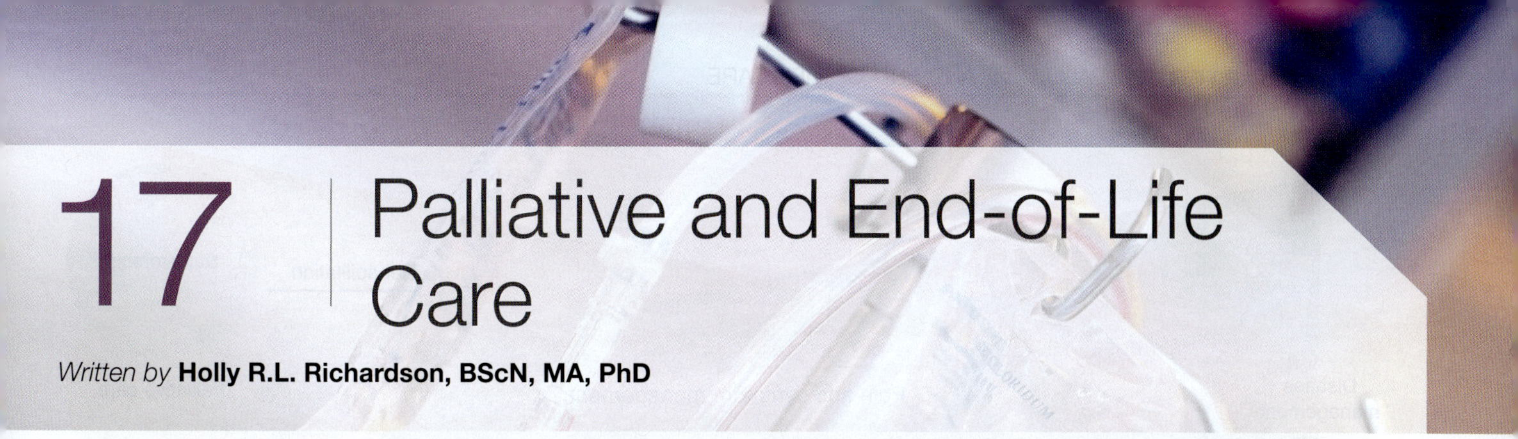

17 | Palliative and End-of-Life Care

Written by **Holly R.L. Richardson, BScN, MA, PhD**

SKILLS AND PROCEDURES

OBJECTIVES

Mastery of content in this chapter will enable the nurse to:

- Explain the philosophy and principles of an integrated palliative approach to care.
- Differentiate between hospice palliative care and end-of-life care.
- Describe approaches to goals of care conversations.
- Describe approaches to optimizing comfort and quality of life.
- Describe approaches to psychosocial and spiritual care at the end of life.
- Explain physiological changes typical of impending death.
- Explain the nurse's role in response to requests for medical assistance in dying.
- Describe the nurse's role in assisting patients and families in grief associated with serious illness and death.
- Describe the process of postmortem care.
- Explain a nurse's role in facilitating autopsy and organ and tissue donation requests.

MEDIA RESOURCES

- http://evolve.elsevier.com/Canada/Perry/clinicalskills/

PALLIATIVE CARE IN CANADA

The World Health Organization (WHO) defines *palliative care* as follows:

> *An approach that improves the quality of life of patients (adults and children) and their families who are facing problems associated with life-threatening illness. It prevents and relieves suffering through the early identification, correct assessment and treatment of pain and other problems, whether physical, psychosocial, or spiritual.*
>
> (WHO, 2020, para. 1)

Palliative care is culturally safe and sensitive, equitable, person-centred collaborative care—provided in any setting to patients of any age with serious, life-limiting illnesses—that addresses the physical, emotional, spiritual, social, and practical concerns of both patients and their caregivers to enhance quality of living, dignity in death, and healthy grieving.

In Canada, the terms *hospice* and *palliative care* are used interchangeably. Unfortunately, both terms are often associated with end-of-life care, leading to an erroneous belief that hospice palliative care (HPC) is relevant only to those in the end stages of a life-limiting illness. This has led to debate about the need to use alternate terms to describe this approach to care. The Canadian Hospice Palliative Care Association (CHPCA), which provides leadership, advocacy, and a national voice for HPC in Canada, endorses the synonymous use of the terms, both of which include end-of-life and bereavement care. Further, the CHPCA states that some may view hospice as community-based rather than hospital-based care. For example, hospice care is often delivered in a limited number of residential hospices (homelike care facilities) that are partially funded through charitable donations (CHPCA, 2022). People who receive care in residential hospices are often in an advanced stage of illness or nearing the end of life, which may also conflate the term hospice with end-of-life care. By contrast, the Canadian Virtual Hospice (https://www.virtualhospice.ca/) uses the term *hospice* to describe their multitude of online resources to support people of all ages and their families at any stage of a life-limiting illness. Despite synonymous use of these terms in Canada, the term *palliative care* has been adopted by the federal government in describing the need for an *integrated palliative approach* to care, as described in this section.

HPC is evolving in Canada. Since June 17, 2016, eligible Canadians have had the right to choose medical assistance in dying (MAiD) (Bill C-14, *An Act to Amend the Criminal Code and to Make Related Amendments to Other Acts [Medical Assistance in Dying]*, 2016). When this law was enacted, there was not universal access to quality palliative care. This raised concerns that MAiD might be viewed as the only option for some Canadians to relieve their suffering. In response to this gap in essential care, the *Framework on Palliative Care in Canada* Act was enacted on December 12, 2017 (Bill C-277, *An Act Providing for the Development of a Framework on Palliative Care in Canada*, 2017). Since this time, the WHO has declared palliative care a human right (WHO, 2020).

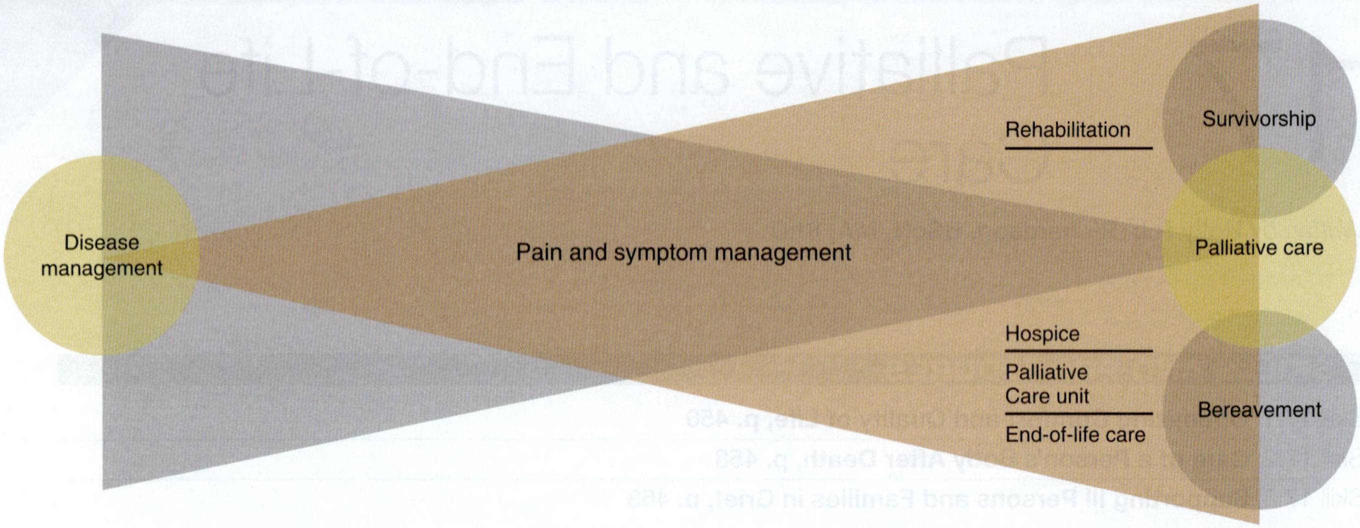

FIG 17.1 The Bow Tie Model—An integrated palliative approach. *(From Hawley, P. H. [2014]. The Bow Tie Model of 21st century palliative care. Journal of Pain and Symptom Management, 47[1], 2–5. Reprinted with permission.)*

The aims of the *Framework on Palliative Care in Canada Act* are to ensure universal and equitable access to quality palliative care by defining palliative care; identify health care provider and informal caregiver education needs; support palliative care providers; draw on existing frameworks, strategies, and best practices across the country to inform framework development; do research and collect data to evaluate progress in meeting the palliative care needs of Canadians; and evaluate the need for re-establishment of funding for initiatives to oversee this work (Bill C-277, 2017). These aims have resulted in an evolving Framework on Palliative Care in Canada (Health Canada, 2018) and an action plan (Health Canada, 2019) that builds on this framework. Another key document for understanding the direction of HPC in Canada is *The Way Forward National Framework: A Roadmap for an Integrated Palliative Approach to Care* (CHPCA, 2015), developed by the CHPCA in conjunction with the Quality End-of-Life Care Coalition of Canada (QELCCC) and the Canadian government.

An important aim of an integrated palliative approach is to initiate palliative care early in the course of a life-limiting illness and in all settings, not merely in those that specialize in HPC. A cultural shift is required whereby nurses and other health care providers—regardless of setting—would possess and apply basic requisite palliative care competencies. Nurses can advocate for this cultural shift by educating the public and other health care providers on how to "ADOPT principles EARLY in a person's life-limiting condition, ADAPT strategies to meet patient and family needs, and EMBED practices into usual care in settings not specialized in palliative care" (iPANEL, 2018, para. 1). A series of infographics and videos developed by the group iPANEL (Initiative for a Palliative Approach in Nursing: Evidence and Leadership) are tools that were designed for nurses to facilitate change in their various care areas (iPANEL, 2018). Fig. 17.1 illustrates a model of the continuum of care in which palliative care, along with curative treatments, is initiated early for a person with a life-limiting illness. In this model, palliative care is integrated throughout the trajectory of the illness, which includes recovery, end of life, and bereavement.

An integrated palliative approach to care requires a team comprising a variety of professional and essential caregivers (e.g., volunteers, pharmacists, social workers, paramedics, designated informal caregivers, physicians, spiritual care providers, and unregulated care providers [UCPs]). To ensure seamless transitions in care, it is imperative to coordinate ongoing collaboration and communication among team members and between teams located in various settings (e.g., chronic/acute, primary, specialty, long-term, and home care, as well as jails/prisons, shelters, and the streets) and sectors (e.g., non-profit, volunteer, justice). A cultural shift to an integrated palliative approach also requires that nurses and other health care providers—regardless of setting—possess and apply basic palliative care competencies. Coordinated collaboration involves understanding the scope and skills of each team member and assigning roles according to the needs of the ill person and family and the availability of team members in the care setting.

Over the past decade, palliative care competency frameworks have provided educators and practitioners with guidance in the development of requisite shared and discipline-specific competencies at general and specialty levels of care. Based on interprofessional competency documents developed by experts in Quebec, Nova Scotia, British Columbia, Ontario, and Alberta, the Canadian Partnership Against Cancer and Health Canada (2021) published the Canadian Interdisciplinary Palliative Care Competency Framework, outlining competencies for nurses, generalist physicians, social workers, personal support workers, and volunteers. Box 17.1 contains a list of the 12 competency domains of this Canadian palliative care competency framework. To better understand the competencies for health care providers not listed there, see the Nova Scotia Palliative Care Competency Framework (Nova Scotia Health Authority, 2017).

Interprofessional collaboration includes, but is not limited to, team rounds, where expressed needs of the family are discussed and where team members decide on the best approaches and the appropriate team member(s) to follow up with the family. For example, although nurses may be the first to identify psychosocial and spiritual issues and may provide immediate support, team discussions or consultations give nurses the opportunity draw on the expertise of the social worker, psychologist, or spiritual care provider for follow-up on complex or unresolved issues. Shared documentation records can facilitate interprofessional collaboration and communication, and digital records would allow for communication across settings. Historically, nurses have played a vital role in the care of patients and families experiencing serious, life-limiting illness, death, and grief. Nurses are also ideally positioned to identify illness transitions and approaching death and be proactive in assessing for unmet needs. The Gold Standards Framework Proactive Identification Guidance (PIG) (Thomas et al., 2022), the Supportive and Palliative Care

Indicators Tool (SPICT) (Piers et al., 2021), and the Palliative Performance Scale (PPS) (Canadian Partnership Against Cancer & Health Canada, 2021; Victoria Hospice, 2022a) are useful for determining transitions in care and predicting the need for an increased palliative focus or a specialty palliative care consult. Consultation with a specialty palliative care team is another example of collaboration, in which a primary or secondary health care team consults a tertiary palliative care team for expert advice or involvement to address complex or unmet needs. Fig. 17.2 illustrates palliative pathways with varying needs for consultation with specialty palliative care teams.

STANDARDS OF CARE

The following are links to seminal documents within the evolution of HPC in Canada. The CHPCA's *Standards and Norms of Practice* web page provides links to national principles and norms of practice, including those for use in pediatric care. Accompanying these documents is a model to guide the development of HPC services in Canada, pan-Canadian gold standards for palliative home care, and nursing standards of practice. More recently, national palliative care competencies were developed based on provincial competency documents that provide national guidance for educators of palliative care volunteers and health practitioners in selected disciplines. The final link is an example of a provincial palliative care competency document that outlines shared and discipline-specific competencies for numerous other disciplines. It is imperative to know the shared and discipline-specific competencies of team members to enhance shared care, ensure appropriateness of the provider to meet patient and family needs, and use health care resources appropriately.

- Canadian Hospice Palliative Care Association (CHPCA, n.d.)—*Standards and Norms of Practice* (https://www.chpca.ca/resource/norms/)
- Canadian Partnership Against Cancer & Health Canada (2021)—*The Canadian Interdisciplinary Palliative Care Competency Framework* (https://s22457.pcdn.co/wp-content/uploads/2021/07/palliative-care-competency-framework-EN.pdf)
- Nova Scotia Health Authority (2017)—*The Nova Scotia Palliative Care Competency Framework: A Reference Guide for Health Professionals and Volunteers* (https://library.nshealth.ca/ld.php?content_id=34202519)

BOX 17.1

The Canadian Interdisciplinary Palliative Care Competency Domains

The following domains are those under which specific nursing competencies are listed. See the link to the full document at the end of this box. Note that the competency document was developed in collaboration with Indigenous organizations and communities and is broad in its inclusiveness. Ongoing collaboration is needed to identify specific requisite competencies as well as gaps and opportunities related to meeting the palliative care needs of Indigenous communities.

1. Principles of a palliative approach to care
2. Cultural safety and humility
3. Communication
4. Optimizing comfort and quality of life
5. Care planning and collaborative practice
6. Last days and hours
7. Loss, grief, and bereavement
8. Self-care
9. Professional and ethical practice
10. Education, evaluation, quality improvement, and research
11. Advocacy
12. Virtual care

From Canadian Partnership Against Cancer & Health Canada. (2021). *The Canadian Interdisciplinary Palliative Care Competency Framework.* https://s22457.pcdn.co/wp-content/uploads/2021/07/palliative-care-competency-framework-EN.pdf

PRINCIPLES FOR PRACTICE

The guiding principles of our national palliative care framework can be found in Box 17.2. Palliative care should be introduced early in the course of a life-limiting illness or frailty and may be provided in conjunction with other life-sustaining treatments, such as surgery and chemotherapy. A palliative approach to care involves helping ill people of any age, and in any setting, achieve an optimal quality of life and to live as actively as possible until death. This approach includes attending to suffering, recognizing and proactively managing pain and symptoms early on, and identifying when burdens of treatment outweigh benefits or when treatment is misaligned with the ill person's and family's goals and preferences.

The ill person identifies who their family is, which may include those who are not related biologically or through marriage. The family is affected by the illness and death and may also be involved

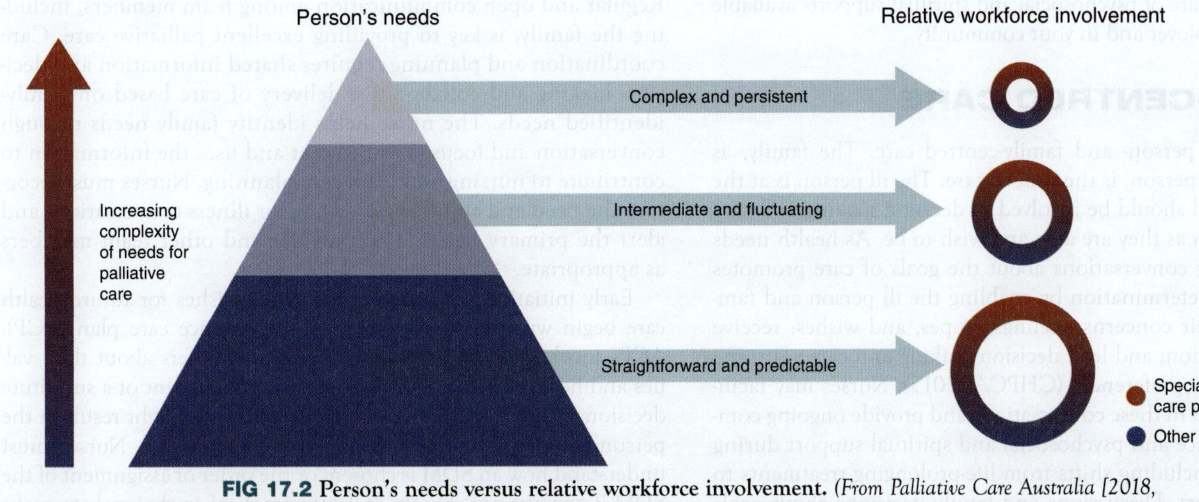

FIG 17.2 **Person's needs versus relative workforce involvement.** *(From Palliative Care Australia [2018, January]. Palliative care service development guidelines [Fig. 3.2]. https://palliativecare.org.au/wp-content/uploads/dlm_uploads/2018/02/PalliativeCare-Background-to-Service-Delivery-2018_v3.pdf. Reprinted with permission.)*

BOX 17.2

Guiding Principles of Palliative Care in Canada

- Palliative care is person- and family-centred care.
- Death, dying, grief, and bereavement are a part of life.
- Caregivers are both providers and recipients of care.
- Palliative care is integrated and holistic.
- Access to palliative care is equitable.
- Palliative care recognizes and values the diversity of Canada and its peoples.
- Palliative care services are valued, understood, and adequately resourced.
- Palliative care is high-quality and evidence-based.
- Palliative care improves quality of life.
- Palliative care is a shared responsibility.

in decision making according to the ill person's wishes or when the ill person lacks capacity to direct care themselves. Family members often become informal caregivers in addition to their other roles and responsibilities, resulting in increased risk for caregiver burnout. Nurses need to develop relationships with the ill person's family and/or designated caregivers to develop care plans that include support of the family and caregivers throughout illness, dying, and bereavement. Developmental needs of children also require special consideration. Therefore, ongoing, holistic assessment of the family along with psychosocial, spiritual, informational, and practical support are needed to maintain family wellness. As the end of life approaches, palliative care continues in the facilitation of a peaceful death and in bereavement support for the family that aligns with their spiritual and cultural preferences.

To nurture your capacity as a nurse to remain compassionately engaged with patients and family members, you must also care for yourself physically, spiritually, and emotionally. Explore your own attitudes and beliefs about death and dying, and recognize how past experiences with suffering, death, and dying might affect your ability to be emotionally present and provide quality palliative care. Recognize signs of compassion fatigue in self and colleagues, and develop strategies to prevent it and cope with personal emotional responses to caring for dying persons and their families. One such strategy includes being aware of psychosocial and spiritual supports available through your employer and in your community.

PERSON-CENTRED CARE

Palliative care is person- and family-centred care. The family, as defined by the ill person, is the unit of care. The ill person is at the centre of care and should be involved in decision making and care planning as much as they are able and wish to be. As health needs change, revisiting conversations about the goals of care promotes dignity and self-determination by enabling the ill person and family to express their concerns, feelings, hopes, and wishes; receive relevant information; and lead decision making and care planning according to their preferences (CHPCA, 2015). Nurses may facilitate or be involved in these conversations and provide ongoing compassionate presence and psychosocial and spiritual support during life transitions, including shifts from life-prolonging treatments to a focus on comfort. Discussions and family decisions about goals of care should be accurately documented and communicated to the teams involved.

CULTURAL SAFETY

Culture influences the meaning of illness, pain, and suffering; how one expresses grief; and ideas about an afterlife. Given the wide range of cultural beliefs that exist, it is important to first engage in self-reflection on your own cultural and personal beliefs about loss and death and explore common end-of-life cultural or religious practices of others. Do not assume an ill person or family adheres to the practices of their identified culture or religion. Instead, practise cultural humility. Be comfortable with not knowing, and engage in respectful curiosity, asking what cultural, spiritual, or religious practices are important to the person and family and how to best incorporate these into their plan of care. For further guidance on spiritual assessment, see the list of useful assessment tools compiled by the VHA Office of Patient-Centered Care and Cultural Transformation (Rindfleisch, n.d.).

When death is near, provide families with the opportunity to engage in cultural, spiritual, or religious rites, rituals, or practices that bring peace and meaning to the experience. Interprofessional collaboration may include a consult with an appropriate spiritual care provider, with the family's permission, to ensure that end-of-life rights and rituals are carried out according to cultural and religious needs. *Living My Culture* (Canadian Virtual Hospice, n.d.) is also a useful resource for exploring the palliative and end-of-life experiences of a variety of cultural groups in Canada.

Practise openness and sensitivity to exploring the unique end-of-life needs and preferences of all families, considering age, gender, sexual orientation, cognitive and physical ability, ethnicity, language, culture, spiritual or religious practices, and preferred lifeways. Family culture also affects communication patterns and roles. Nurses need to understand how families prefer to receive information and the roles they will play in caregiving and decision making. For example, members of some cultures may prefer that information about treatment and prognosis be filtered through a family member, and in some families a designated head of the family may make health care decisions on behalf of ill family members. For these reasons, it is important to practise person-centred care and ask how the ill person prefers to receive and process health information and make important health decisions.

COMMUNICATION AND COLLABORATIVE CARE PLANNING

Regular and open communication among team members, including the family, is key to providing excellent palliative care. Care coordination and planning requires shared information and decision making and collaborative delivery of care based on family-identified needs. The nurse helps identify family needs through conversation and focused assessment and uses the information to contribute to nursing and team care planning. Nurses must recognize the need and appropriate timing for illness conversations and alert the primary health care provider and other team members as appropriate.

Early initiation of conversations about wishes for future health care begin with the development of an advance care plan (ACP). ACPs involve conversations with significant others about their values and health care preferences and the appointment of a substitute decision maker (SDM) in advance of events that might result in the person's inability to make decisions for themselves. Nurses must understand how an SDM is chosen, or the order of assignment of the SDM if one was not chosen, and support them in their role to make decisions based, as much as possible, on the wishes and preferences of the incapacitated ill or injured person. Nurses should be aware of the associated legal considerations in the province or territory in which they practise.

ACPs can provide a sense of control, prevent unwanted health care interventions, and reduce stress and uncertainty for others when making life-and-death decisions on behalf of an ill or injured person. Note that ACPs may need revisions as health care and life situations change and that the capacity of a patient to make health care decisions may decline as the end of life approaches. Nurses can assist any adult, ill or healthy, to develop an ACP by utilizing the tools developed by Advance Care Planning Canada (2022a), which can be found at https://www.advancecareplanning.ca. A copy of the ACP should be placed on the medical record (see employer policy), and the person should be encouraged to provide a copy to the primary health care provider and family.

ACPs often include decisions about whether to initiate cardiopulmonary resuscitation (CPR) (see Chapter 28) or allow natural death (AND). Verbal "do not resuscitate" (DNR) or AND requests should be documented in the medical record according to employer policy and will likely include wishes about the level of care–that is, comfort only or information about when and how to intervene in specific health situations. In instances where a person is in an advanced stage of illness, is frail, or has multiple comorbidities, the outcomes of CPR are often unsuccessful or result in increased suffering (Advance Care Planning Canada, 2022b). Helping families understand possible outcomes can alleviate the pressure to initiate CPR in these cases and assist the family in making a decision that is in the best interest of the ill person. Resources for helping families making decisions about CPR are available online (Advance Care Planning Canada, 2022b). Another useful tool for documenting and communicating end-of-life care wishes is a Medical Orders for Scope of Treatment (MOST) and related documents, developed by the Interior Health regional health authority in British Columbia (Interior Health, 2020). It is important to note, however, that an ACP is a legal document and that it overrides any documentation on clinical tools. Therefore, it is important to ensure that any ACPs in existence are updated appropriately to match current wishes and clinical documentation. It is also important to refer to provincial laws and regulations when engaging in advance care planning. Provincial advance care planning tools are available at http://advancecareplanning.ca.

Goals of care conversations take place in the context of illness. They should be initiated early and be revisited whenever health needs change in response to progressing disease or lack of response to treatments. Goals of care conversations begin with an understanding of what the ill person and family know about the illness and prognosis, how they prefer to receive information (and in how much detail), and how they wish to be involved in decision making (Ariadne Labs, 2021). Informed decision making requires an understanding of the illness and prognosis while weighing the benefits and burdens of treatment options based on what could happen as the illness progresses. Ariadne Labs (2021) has created a serious-illness conversation guide and other resources to help facilitate goals of care conversations; the guide has been adopted or adapted by many provincial health programs. Note that ethnicity, religion, and culture influence attitudes toward life-sustaining treatments.

Ongoing conversations about goals of care can prevent the need for decision making in times of crisis and uncertainty. However, despite planning for future possibilities, there are times when decisions need to be made in the moment. These in-the-moment conversations about treatment decisions are guided by the same principles used in goals of care planning.

Ethical and Legal Considerations

Nurses can help avoid ethical dilemmas by maintaining ongoing, open communication with the health care team and family about needs and goals of care. An integrative review found end-of-life care to be the most common ethical dilemma faced by nurses, with communication about prognosis, inadequate palliation, questions of potential healing, and futility identified as the main sources of concern (Rainer et al., 2018). The nurse may also suggest an ethical consult in intractable ethical dilemmas. First and foremost, the nurse has an ethical duty to act in the best interest of patients and must adhere to provincial/territorial laws and regulations (i.e., MAiD, child and family services acts, adult protection acts, and personal directives acts). However, what is best for the patient is not always easily determined. The following is an outline of some of the more contentious ethical issues in end-of-life care.

Decisions About Initiating and Discontinuing Treatment

Goals of care conversations often involve decisions to forego the initiation of medical interventions or to stop treatments that have already begun. Ethically, there is no difference between not initiating and stopping treatments, although it may be more difficult to discontinue interventions that have been started and are essential to life (e.g., mechanical ventilation). In futile situations, it may help families to weigh the benefits and burdens in relation to the ill person's values and quality of life and to consider the implications of starting or continuing treatments that prolong life (and perhaps suffering) versus facilitating a peaceful death. Respecting family decisions, despite personal and professional reservations, promotes dignity and prevents distress that can persist into bereavement and possibly complicate the grieving process. In situations where families are not ready to forego the initiation of treatment that is unlikely to be of benefit, time-limited treatment trials with specific guidelines for evaluation can be offered. This gives the family the sense of doing everything possible while having time to prepare for the eventual death.

Palliative Sedation and the Principle of Double Effect

Palliative sedation is a legally acceptable means of relieving intractable suffering in the terminally ill person by intermittent or continuous administration of sedating medications such as midazolam by a palliative or pain specialist to reduce consciousness. This may be coupled with adjuncts such as continuous opioids to control pain or breathlessness or neuroleptics for delirium (Bhyan et al., 2022). Although difficult to verify empirically, some argue that palliative sedation hastens death (Bhyan et al., 2022; Rodrigues et al., 2018). However, the principle of double effect has been used as ethical justification for palliative sedation for intractable suffering, whether physical, psychological, or existential. The *principle of double effect* maintains that the nature and intent of the action must be good (i.e., to relieve suffering), that the bad effect must not be the cause of the desired outcome (i.e., hastening death to relieve suffering), that the good effect outweighs the bad effect (i.e., relief of suffering outweighs the risk of hastened death), and that there are no other viable means of achieving the desired effect (Bhyan et al., 2022; Rodrigues et al., 2018). For example, in providing palliative sedation to alleviate intractable pain or other symptoms, the intent is to relieve suffering. Intractable symptoms are those that have been unresponsive to conventional treatments, necessitating sedation as a last resort to relieve them. The bad effect, which may be death in some cases, is not the route to achieve the desired outcome of relieving suffering, and the benefit of relief from suffering outweighs the possibility of a hastened death. The principle of double effect, therefore, has long provided ethical reasoning for palliative sedation to be an acceptable means of relieving intractable suffering at the end of life.

Medical Assistance in Dying

Since June 2016, it has been legally permissible for eligible Canadians to request and receive MAiD in order to relieve intractable suffering by intentionally hastening death. Requests for MAiD are prompted by suffering and compromised quality of life. Requests for or questions about MAiD may arise during routine care by the nurse. Responding to requests for MAiD requires an ability to be with suffering and explore its sources while adhering to federal/provincial/territorial laws, regulatory body guidelines, employer policies, and ethical practices.

The nurse's role in MAiD is to acknowledge patients' requests with compassion and without judgement. Sitting with them and asking what led them to ask about MAiD at this time is one way to open the conversation. Assessing suffering with empathy and exploring the patient's end-of-life needs, hopes, and concerns enables the nurse to learn what is important to the person and to identify gaps in care. The nurse can then ask permission to share this information with the patient's most responsible care provider (i.e., physician, nurse practitioner) so that further discussion about wishes, needs, and eligibility can guide informed decision making. Maintaining confidentiality and gaining permission to share the context of the MAiD request with necessary care providers is of utmost importance.

Nurses and other health care providers are legally able to assist with MAiD, but they also have the right to conscientiously object to being involved based on deeply held personal beliefs and values. If the nurse objects to being involved in the care of a person who is requesting MAiD, they must not share their personal rationale with the patient; instead, they must ensure continued quality care until another care provider assumes responsibility. This relates to the nurse's duty to care and the ethical edict to not abandon patients. Useful practice resources on MAiD include the *Code of Ethics for Registered Nurses* (Canadian Nurses Association, 2017), Health Canada's website on MAiD (Health Canada, 2023a), accountability and liability information concerning the provision of MAiD (Canadian Nurses Protective Society, 2021), and provincial and territorial contact information for end-of-life care services (Health Canada, 2023b).

Self-Care and Fitness to Practice

Ethical and moral dilemmas can impact nurses and other health care providers in profound ways. Moral distress arises when a person may know the right thing to do but is unable to act, or is prevented from acting, in concert with their moral and ethical beliefs (Dorman & Raffin Bouchal, 2020). More specifically, moral distress relates to a person's inability to take the action they feel is right, accompanied by feelings of helplessness and perceived suffering (Dorman & Raffin Bouchal, 2020). Moral residue results when each experience of moral distress stays with the person, suggesting that perhaps this lingering moral residue exacerbates moral distress when navigating subsequent moral dilemmas. If left unacknowledged, moral distress and moral residue can impact the nurse's ability to give compassionate, quality care and lead to deterioration in the nurse's physical, psychosocial, and spiritual health (Dorman & Raffin Bouchal, 2020).

Moral distress is also associated with "nurse burnout and patient care avoidance" (Wolcott Altaker et al., 2018, p. 295). Therefore, it is imperative for the nurse to be mindful of personal feelings and responses to moral and ethical dilemmas and to attend to personal well-being. Moral distress may be addressed by debriefing with the team when moral and ethical dilemmas arise, finding support through specialized ethics teams or employee assistance programs and counselling, or using personal wellness supports that assist with making meaning of morally complex situations.

Not only is self-care necessary to meet nursing standards related to fitness to practice, but it is also listed as a nursing palliative care competency (see Box 17.1). Specifically, nurses must reflect on their own attitudes, beliefs, and experiences related to suffering, death, and dying and understand how these may impact their care of patients who are suffering or at the end of life. Knowing where to find resources to support oneself and the team and being able to recognize signs of distress while caring for oneself and colleagues is a core palliative care competency for nurses in Canada (Canadian Partnership Against Cancer & Health Canada, 2021). Another self-care competency specific to palliative care nurses is being able to recognize and respond to compassion fatigue in oneself and others. Compassion fatigue is emotional exhaustion and desensitization that results when nurses are exposed to ongoing trauma and suffering (Henson, 2020; Jarrad & Hammad, 2020). Like moral distress and moral residue, compassion fatigue can lead to physical, psychosocial, and spiritual health problems (Henson, 2020). Seeking help and caring for oneself and others in ways that reduce stress and assist in finding meaning and purpose in one's work are ways that can prevent compassion fatigue and enable nurses to provide safe, compassionate, and quality palliative care.

✦ SKILL 17.1 Optimizing Comfort and Quality of Life

Proactive and timely management of patients' symptoms and related distress are key to optimizing comfort and quality of life. Patients living with life-limiting illness experience multiple, complex physical symptoms and often have various emotional, relational, practical, and spiritual concerns. Total pain, a concept introduced by palliative care pioneer Dame Cicely Saunders, describes how physical pain and symptoms are indivisible from the psychosocial, emotional, and spiritual experiences of the person, and how each domain affects the other (Wood, 2021). Supporting patients begins by understanding the impact of these symptoms and concerns on patients' and their families' lives from their shared and individual points of view. Through careful assessment, nurses can identify needs and provide information and education to enable self-management while drawing on health care team expertise to assist families in taking full advantage of the benefits of palliative care to enhance quality of life.

Delegation and Collaboration

The nurse draws on the expertise of all team members, including the patient and designated caregivers, in supporting and managing symptoms and related distress. Some supportive care can be delegated to an unregulated care provider (UCP). However, the nurse must conduct the initial assessments and develop the nursing plans of care. The nurse directs the UCP to do the following:

- Notify the nurse if the ill person reports new symptoms or if existing symptoms worsen or change
- Notify the nurse if the ill person or family reports or exhibits signs of distress or if they have questions about the care plan
- Provide or assist with basic comfort care, such as positioning, room temperature control, hygiene, and mouth care
- Report possible adverse effects of medications, as instructed by the nurse
- Speak to unconscious or dying persons because hearing is the last sense to diminish

Equipment

- Personal care items most preferred by patient
- Comfort and hygiene products
- Clean gloves

STEP	RATIONALE
ASSESSMENT	
1. Identify patient using at least two person-specific identifiers (e.g., name and date of birth, or name and medical record number) according to employer policy.	Ensures correct patient. Complies with Accreditation Canada's standards and improves patient safety (Accreditation Canada, 2020).
2. Throughout the procedure, the 4 moments for hand hygiene are to be implemented; hand hygiene should occur before initial patient (or patient environment) contact, before an aseptic procedure, after body fluid exposure risk, and after patient (or patient environment) contact. Additional hand hygiene should be performed when hands are visibly soiled.	Proper hand hygiene helps prevent the spread of infectious agents to health care providers.
3. Ask patients to describe symptoms in their own words. Use open-ended prompts such as the following: • "Describe your leg pain to me." • "Tell me how you are sleeping since you started taking this medicine."	Symptoms are personal perceptions experienced only by the patient. Open-ended questions lead to more detailed, patient-specific concerns and priorities.
Allow sufficient time for patients to describe their symptoms and encourage them to say more: • "You've told me about your leg pain. Do you have pain anywhere else?" • "Is there anything else concerning to you?"	Ensures a more complete assessment. Prevents you from making assumptions about patient's symptoms, prematurely stopping the assessment process.
4. Use employer-approved pain and symptom assessment tools. The Edmonton Symptom Assessment System (ESAS) (Cancer Care Ontario, 2010) uses a 0–10 scale to measure the patient's current perception of a myriad of symptoms and includes anterior and posterior body outlines for locating areas of pain (Canadian Partnership Against Cancer & Health Canada, 2021). It can be completed by a caregiver, a health care provider, or the ill person, independently or with help. The Palliative Performance Scale (PPS) (Victoria Hospice, 2022a) is useful for assessing functional ability and as a prognostic tool (Canadian Partnership Against Cancer & Health Canada, 2021). It measures the ill person's ability to ambulate, participate in activity or work, perform self-care, and eat or drink, as well as their level of consciousness. It measures each domain in increments of 10, with 0 meaning death and 100 meaning full function. The domain scores are added up and the total is converted to a score out of 100. The final score is reported as a percentage and can be useful in determining when care needs are increasing or when death is approaching.	Consistent use of a standard assessment scale helps determine changes in symptoms and evaluate effectiveness of interventions. Tools that can be filled out by the ill person or caregivers enable self-monitoring and care.
5. Assess patient's emotional and spiritual health. Does the patient feel anxious, sad, depressed, bored, lonely, or understimulated? Ask questions such as "How has your declining health been affecting your…(e.g., life, relationships, emotions, sense of self, spiritual health, well-being, etc.)?"	Pain and other physical symptoms can cause and be exacerbated by emotional, relational, and spiritual issues. See Cicely Saunders's concept of "total pain" described earlier in the introduction to Skill 17.1.
6. Assess patient's pain severity using an employer-approved assessment scale and evaluate pain characteristics. Assess behaviour in patients who are nonverbal or cognitively impaired using an approved assessment tool (see Chapter 16).	Consistent use of a standard pain scale helps assess changes in patient pain levels and evaluate effectiveness of pain interventions.
7. If patient cannot self-report pain, observe for these symptoms (American Cancer Society, 2019): • Noisy breathing—Laboured, harsh, or rapid breaths • Making pained sounds—Including groaning, moaning, or expressing hurt • Facial expressions—Looking sad, tense, or frightened; frowning or crying • Body language—Tension, clenched fists, knees pulled up, inflexibility, restlessness, or looking like they are trying to get away from the hurt area • Body movement—Changing positions to get comfortable but can't	Patients unable to report or verbalize pain show nonverbal signs of pain. Patients who are nonverbal or cognitively impaired are unable to report pain and are at risk of having their pain go untreated or undertreated. Sometimes behavioural cues such as increased distress, agitation, or changes in activity patterns or interactions with others may indicate underlying pain or other symptoms. Be sure to compare behaviours with typical behaviours for that person.

STEP	RATIONALE
ASSESSMENT	
8. Assess for feeling of breathlessness (does patient feel that they are getting enough air?), respiratory rate, breathing patterns, and lung sounds. Assess for presence of airway secretions.	Dyspnea, air hunger, or shortness of breath results from metabolic or respiratory changes. Near the end of life, Cheyne-Stokes respirations are common; this abnormal breathing pattern is characterized by alternating periods of apnea and hyperpnea.
9. Observe condition of skin, especially back, heels, and buttocks (see Chapter 8).	Decreased nutrition, hydration, peripheral circulation, and activity level can contribute to skin breakdown.
10. Inspect patient's oral cavity, including mucosa, tongue, and teeth (see Chapter 8).	Dehydration, difficulty swallowing, and inflammation of mouth are common at the end of life.
11. Assess bowel function (see Chapter 35).	
a. Determine usual bowel elimination pattern (frequency, character, usual time of day) and effectiveness of usual bowel management routines.	Patients experience constipation because of decreased fluid and fibre intake, immobility, age, disease processes, or medications such as opioids (Mooney et al., 2019). Patients who have diarrhea are at risk for dehydration.
b. If patient is passing liquid stool, assess for presence of fecal impaction (see employer policy).	Watery stool leaking around blockage indicates fecal impaction.
c. Review medication regimens, prescriptions, and over-the-counter medications known to cause constipation (e.g., opioids, antacids).	Medications can alter bowel elimination patterns. Diarrhea results from infections, diseases, or medications (e.g., antibiotics or chemotherapy). Change in therapy might be necessary.
d. Identify typical food and fluid intake over 1 week and patient's activity levels.	Oral intake and activity levels influence bowel elimination patterns.
12. Assess urinary elimination (see Chapter 34) and ability to control urination. If incontinent, assess for skin breakdown or patient discomfort.	Urinary incontinence may result from delirium, urinary tract infection, medications, immobility, or severe constipation (Farrington & Murphy, 2019).
13. Assess patient's appetite, ability to swallow, and for presence of nausea or vomiting. Use standardized tool for assessment if available (Collett & Chow, 2019).	Medications, pain, depression, disease progression, or decreased blood flow to digestive organs near death often contribute to nausea, vomiting, and decreased appetite.
a. Consider presence of nausea in patients receiving enteral feedings.	Patients who have decreased consciousness are unable to report nausea.
14. Assess daily food and fluid intake in relation to patient's condition and preferences.	Nutrition screening helps identify deficits and allows for interventions to be carried out to improve nutritional status.
15. Use descriptive scale to assess fatigue (e.g., scale with descriptors—none, moderate, severe). Ask if fatigue limits patient's ability to perform desired activities.	Fatigue is the most common symptom of progressive illness and has a profound impact on quality of life (O'Neil-Page et al., 2019).
16. Assess for terminal delirium in patients near death (e.g., confusion, restlessness, and/or agitation, with or without day-night reversal).	Allows you to identify this condition and implement interventions to keep patient safe and decrease patient and family distress (Goldberg et al., 2019).
a. Consider whether patient has pain, nausea, dyspnea, full bladder or bowel, poor sleep patterns, anxiety, or joint pain from immobility.	Risk factors for presence of delirium are common physical problems that need to be treated or ruled out as causative factors.
b. Review medical record for hypercalcemia, hypoglycemia, hyponatremia, or dehydration.	Metabolic imbalances can cause restlessness or delirium.
c. Review patient's medications.	Unintended responses to medications result in changed activity states.
d. Determine whether patient has unresolved emotional or spiritual issues. Refer to spiritual care provider, psychologist, social worker, or other team member, as needed.	Spiritual and emotional distress may contribute to restlessness or increased pain.

NURSING DIAGNOSES

The priority of diagnoses is dependent on the ill person's (or family's) perception of symptoms and whether death is near. For example, irregular and noisy breathing and reduced peripheral tissue perfusion (as evidenced by mottled extremities) are normal in the last days and hours of life.

- Inadequate breathing pattern—less of a priority if expected and not distressing
- Reduced peripheral tissue perfusion—less of a priority if expected
- Persistent pain
- Acute pain
- Anxiety
- Constipation
- Diarrhea
- Nausea
- Fatigue—the person may rate this as very distressing, and therefore it may be a greater priority.
- Reduced stamina
- Total urinary incontinence
- Bowel incontinence
- Inadequate hydration of oral mucous membranes
- Inadequate swallowing
- Potential for constipation
- Spiritual distress
- Inadequate coping
- Compromised family coping

Related factors and risk factors are individualized on the basis of patient's condition or needs.

STEP	RATIONALE
PLANNING	
1. Expected outcomes following completion of procedure:	
• Patient reports acceptable level of pain.	Indicates pain control.
• Patient reports feeling warm and comfortable.	Warming interventions help reverse effects of reduced peripheral circulation.
• Patient reports comfortable eating and drinking patterns.	Optimal food and fluid intake are based on patient preferences and comfort.
• Patient has soft, formed bowel movements.	Indicates adequate bowel function and peristaltic activity.
• Skin remains free of irritation or breakdown.	Interventions to protect skin from immobility and bowel or urinary incontinence are effective.
• Patient is not restless.	Therapies have calming effect.
• Patient reports less distress from fatigue.	Energy conservation methods are effective; patient adjusts to changes in activity level.
• Patient experiences less respiratory distress.	Patient is less apprehensive and breathes easily.
• The patient reports they are at peace.	Indicates absence of emotional and spiritual distress.
IMPLEMENTATION	
1. Provide pain relief. Use a multimodal approach. Invite the use of cultural and spiritual practices and traditional medicines, according to patient's wishes.	Nonpharmacological measures supplement pain medication and can increase patient comfort. Cultural and spiritual practices and traditional healing aim to bring comfort. Pain and other physical symptoms can cause and be exacerbated by emotional, relational, and spiritual issues. See Cicely Saunders's concept of "total pain" described earlier in the introduction to Skill 17.1.
a. Administer prescribed analgesics and adjuvants. Confer with the prescriber and recommend an around-the-clock (ATC) dosing schedule, especially if pain is anticipated for most of the day. A variety of extended- or controlled-release oral opioid formulations (dosing intervals of 8, 10, 12, or 24 hours) and transdermal patches (72 hours) are effective.	Opioids should be given on a fixed dosage schedule ATC rather than prn, with doses given before pain returns (Burchum & Rosenthal, 2019). An ATC medication lessens the severity of end-of-dose pain, allowing patient to sleep through the night, and reduces "clock watching" for the next dose. Extended-release medications maintain constant serum opioid concentration, minimizing toxic and subtherapeutic concentrations (Burchum & Rosenthal, 2019).
b. Draw on team expertise and utilize pharmacological as well as nonpharmacological and complementary and integrative medicine approaches where appropriate (e.g., massage, acupuncture, music therapy, mind–body approaches, cultural and spiritual practices) (see Chapter 16).	Use of complementary therapies can help alleviate symptoms and related suffering and give patients and families a sense of self-efficacy (Meyer & Ring, 2019).
c. Provide patient and family education on causes and patterns of pain and safety of opioid use and explain interventions.	Encourages patient autonomy and reduces emotional distress, clarifying misinformation about opioid therapies.
d. Reassess patient's pain 1 hour after administration of pain medication or complementary therapy.	Determines whether desired effect of medication or complementary treatment has been achieved and whether patient has reduced pain level.
2. Provide general comfort measures.	
a. Provide bath and skin care based on patient's preferences and hygiene needs (see Chapter 18). NOTE: Daily baths are not always desired or necessary at end of life if they cause discomfort, fatigue, or increased pain.	Clean skin promotes comfort and reduces risk of skin breakdown.
b. Provide eye care and use artificial tears in patients with decreased consciousness (see Chapter 19).	Eye irritation causes pain. Blink reflex diminishes near death, causing drying of cornea.
c. Reposition bed-bound patients regularly, or according to the person's goals of care and wishes and be sure to premedicate if movement causes pain (Samuriwo, 2019). Do not position on tubes or other objects. Keep skin clean and dry. Also ensure adequate hydration and nutrition according to goals of care and wishes.	Prolonged, even slight pressure from weight of patient's body or objects causes skin injury. There is significant risk for pressure injuries in older persons and in those experiencing inadequate hydration and nutrition, immobility, and incontinence. Risk increases in the last couple of weeks before death owing to physiological shutdown (Samuriwo, 2019). In advanced states of illness or frailty, some wounds cannot be healed (Samuriwo, 2019), although control of pain, odour, and exudate can prevent reduced quality of life (see Chapter 39).

STEP	RATIONALE
IMPLEMENTATION	
3. Provide oral hygiene after meals and at bedtime while patient is awake and more frequently in mouth-breathing or unconscious patients (see Chapter 18).	Oral mucosa integrity is needed for normal swallowing and to minimize anorexia and malnutrition. Mouth rinses remove oral debris and clean the mouth. Dehydration develops as patient experiences metabolic changes and fluid intake declines.
a. Use antifungal oral rinses as prescribed or sodium bicarbonate or normal saline rinses.	Patients near death breathe through the mouth, which dries oral mucosa.
b. Moisten lips with nonpetroleum balm.	Prevents skin breakdown.
4. Initiate bowel management regimen to reduce risk for constipation or diarrhea.	Interventions improve peristalsis in constipation, soften fecal mass, and decrease abdominal discomfort.
a. Give patients whatever fluids they enjoy if medically tolerated. Near end of life, patient may refuse fluids. Do not force fluid intake.	Decreased blood flow to intestines at end of life causes lack of appetite and anorexia.
b. Encourage regular physical activity (e.g., walking) if tolerated.	Research has shown that physical activity seems to improve quality of life for people throughout chronic illness, including at the end of life (Meyer & Ring, 2019).
c. Administer daily stool softener or laxative, especially in patients using opioids for pain management.	Constipation is a side effect of regular opioid administration.
d. In case of diarrhea, provide low-residue diet; treat infections or discontinue medications if possible. Administer antidiarrheal medications. Patients with persistent diarrhea require rigorous skin care to promote comfort and prevent skin breakdown.	Treatments reduce incidence and severity of diarrhea, reducing the risk of dehydration.
5. Manage urinary incontinence with intervention appropriate for patient's conditions (e.g., condom catheter, adult incontinence pads [see Chapter 34]).	Urinary output declines near death, making it possible to manage incontinence without an in-dwelling catheter.
Critical Decision Point *For bed-bound patients consider an in-dwelling catheter only if skin integrity, patient preference, or fatigue from bed changes becomes an issue.*	
6. Toward the end of life, offer patient favourite foods in amount and at times they desire. Do not overly encourage patient to eat.	Patients may experience gastrointestinal (GI) distress, dry mouth, or other symptoms related to their disease process, which may contribute to decreased oral intake. In addition, patients nearing final hours of life decrease their oral intake because of slowing of bodily functions or altered level of consciousness.
a. Treat nausea by administering antiemetics intravenously or rectally as prescribed. As nausea subsides, offer clear liquids and ice chips. Avoid caffeinated liquids, milk, and fruit juices.	GI mucosa tolerates clear liquids more readily. Certain liquids increase stomach acidity.
7. Manage fatigue.	Taking rest breaks during activity will help conserve energy. Tired patients need help and monitoring to ensure patient safety.
a. Help patient identify valued or desired tasks and preferred times of day to perform tasks and determine how to conserve energy for only those tasks. Help with activities of daily living. Eliminate extra steps in activities.	
b. Explain care activities before performing them and include patient in setting daily schedule.	Minimizes anxiety and maintains patient's autonomy and involvement.
c. Discuss with patient easy ways to incorporate exercise (e.g., yoga, walking, biking, and swimming) into daily activities.	Research has shown that physical activity seems to improve quality of life for people throughout chronic illness, including at the end of life (Meyer & Ring, 2019).
8. Support patient's breathing efforts.	
a. Position for comfort in semi-Fowler's or Fowler's position.	Promotes maximal ventilation, lung expansion, and drainage of secretions.
b. Elevate head to facilitate postural drainage. Turn from side to side to mobilize and drain secretions. Suction only if necessary.	Deep airway suctioning causes discomfort and is not effective in reducing airway noise or secretion clearance (Harman et al., 2022).
c. Provide prescribed antimuscarinic medications.	Anticholinergic (i.e., antimuscarinic) medications reduce saliva and excessive secretions, thus decreasing noisy respirations (Donesky, 2019), but they should be initiated before excessive secretions begin to be effective.

STEP	RATIONALE
IMPLEMENTATION	
d. Stay with patients experiencing dyspnea or air hunger. Use interventions that patients perceive as relieving their shortness of breath (choice of oxygen-delivery modes, fan near face, body position). Administer opioids or anxiolytics as prescribed. Benzodiazepines may also be administered for anxiety related to dyspnea. Keep room cool with low humidity.	Sharing control with patients reduces anxiety that contributes to feelings of air hunger. Morphine is the medication of choice for dyspnea, decreasing respiratory rate, and decreasing anxiety (Donesky, 2019).
9. Manage restlessness.	
a. Keep patient's room quiet with soft lighting and at comfortable temperature. Offer caregivers the opportunities to maintain close contact. Encourage use of soft music, prayer, or reading from patient's favourite book.	Reduces unnecessary external stimulation and provides comforting space. Privacy allows caregivers the chance to provide verbal assurances and touch; physical touch may provide comfort and reassurance.
b. Use least-sedating pharmacological options to control restlessness. Consult with health care team about titrating a medication (e.g., lorazepam). Discontinue all nonessential medications. Use subcutaneous, transdermal, sublingual, or rectal medication delivery routes.	Reduces delirium without making patient unconscious. Control of restlessness relieves family's concern that patient is in pain, distress, or danger. Determine cause of delirium, if possible, to decrease use of medication (Harman et al., 2022).
10. Manage anxiety.	
a. Provide counselling and supportive therapy. Consult with prescribing health care provider for benzodiazepines, the medications of choice. Offer available counselling services (e.g., spiritual care, psychologist, social worker).	Counselling improves patient and family understanding of the disease and its expected course and is used to identify strengths and coping strategies.

Critical Decision Point **CAUTION:** *The use of benzodiazepines in very old persons can result in paradoxical agitation, confusion, disinhibition, and increased risk for falls and may not result in the desired effect (i.e., relief of insomnia or anxiety)* (Gerlach, 2018).

STEP	RATIONALE
EVALUATION	
1. Ask patient to rate pain using an employer-approved assessment scale and evaluate pain characteristics. Assess behaviour in patients who are nonverbal or cognitively impaired using an approved assessment tool (see Chapter 16).	Determines extent of pain relief.
2. Ask patient to describe mouth comfort and inspect oral cavity.	Evaluates condition of oral cavity and ability to chew, swallow, and speak.
3. Evaluate frequency of defecation; after patient defecates, inspect feces.	Determines status of bowel function and character of stool.
4. Observe skin condition.	Determines whether skin tears or areas of pressure or maceration are present.
5. Ask patient to rate fatigue (scale ranging from none to moderate to severe, or ESAS) and compare with baseline. Observe for fatigue or shortness of breath when patient performs activities.	Determines whether patient is less distressed with activity.
6. Observe patient's respiratory patterns and ask if breathing is easy and comfortable.	Determines whether respiratory distress is relieved.
7. Observe patient's behaviour or ask caregiver to report on it. Note level of restlessness.	Determines level of comfort and extent of restlessness.
8. Use **teach-back:** "I want to be sure I explained that we want to control your pain, and this requires you to describe it. Tell me what the numbers on the pain scale mean. Tell me when is a good time to let me know about your pain before it gets too severe." Develop a revised teaching plan if patient or caregiver is unable to teach back correctly.	Determines patient's and caregiver's level of understanding of instructional topic.

Unexpected Outcomes	Related Interventions
1. One or several symptoms remain unresolved, with patient reporting little or no relief.	• Increase frequency of or change an intervention. • Try combination therapies.
2. Patient becomes anxious, fearful, or exhausted because of continued symptoms.	• Give patient therapy choices and try different interventions. • Elicit support from other team members (e.g., spiritual care, psychology, social work). • Explain goals of therapies and possible reasons for symptoms. • Answer call lights quickly and explain plan of care throughout the day.

Communication and Documentation

- Document detailed descriptions of patient symptoms in progress notes in electronic health record (EHR) or chart and/or appropriate flow sheets. Use consistent descriptors for comparison over time.
- Report unexpected new symptoms or uncontrolled existing symptoms to health care provider and document appropriately. Document psychosocial, emotional, spiritual, and practical concerns and interventions and consult appropriate team members when necessary.
- Document conversations about treatment decisions.
- Document cultural and spiritual preferences for care, including those specific to dying, death, and aftercare, and develop and document a plan to realize patient and family wishes.
- Document your evaluation of patient and caregiver learning.
- Document type of interventions used and patient's response in progress notes in EHR or chart. Note successful interventions in the care plan.

DOCUMENTATION EXAMPLE

Patient awake at 0200 hours. Stated they were unable to sleep. Wondered aloud why this is happening and what they did to deserve this suffering and began to weep. Writer responded empathetically and explored the meaning of the comment. Patient expressed guilt and regret for past actions and a wish to reconcile with their estranged adult child, Kerry. Writer explored what being a parent means to them and their relationship with Kerry. Acknowledged the love they feel for Kerry and explored possible approaches to reconciliation. Asked if they would like to talk to someone on the team to help them work through this issue. Patient stated they felt better after talking and that they are going to reach out to Kerry. Will check back with patient tomorrow evening to assess progress with issue and provide emotional support.

Special Considerations

Teaching

- Involve the patient and designated caregivers in planning and caregiving. With proper instruction and support, they can perform most symptom management interventions, perform personal care (e.g., bathing, oral hygiene), and administer medications and treatments in the home setting. Assessment of readiness to learn and the impact of taking on self-care or additional caregiver roles is important to prevent undue caregiver stress.

Pediatric

- Teach parents how to recognize and assess pain in a nonverbal child.
- Be honest and use developmentally appropriate language to answer children's questions about their own or a loved one's illness.
- Encourage questions and keep children informed of changes in their own or their loved one's illness according to their cues.
- Maintain routines and usual childhood activities as much as possible.
- Encourage involvement of children in their own caregiving and decision making based on their ability, needs, and readiness (Hockenberry et al., 2024).
- Suggestions to assist therapeutic conversations with pediatric patients and family members can be found in *Talking With Children and Youth About Serious Illness* (McClement & Stenekes, 2019).

Gerontological

- Include older persons in conversations and accommodate communication limits (e.g., hearing deficits).
- Older persons need companionship and maintenance of self-esteem. Detached caregiver behaviours such as being slow to respond to physical discomforts, failing to keep room odour-free, and speaking in hushed tones of voice are often perceived by the person as abandonment. Encourage a family member, friend, sitter, or volunteer to stay with the patient during the night. Some older persons who have developed a lifestyle around aloneness prefer solitude. Demonstrate person-centred care by being sensitive to a patient's preferences (Boscart et al., 2023).
- Assessing and addressing pain in an older person who is cognitively impaired or nonverbal is sometimes difficult and involves proactive symptom management.
- Patients at the end of life or with dementia lose their capacity to report adverse effects, call for help, evaluate treatments, or make decisions. Among the risks is poor symptom management and patient falls. Use effective communication with those with cognitive impairment and be aware of likely causes of anxiety, fear, and resistance to care when carrying out interventions. Ensure safety measures are in place.

Care in the Community: Home Management

People with chronic and life-limiting illnesses and end-of-life care needs are living everywhere in our communities, and as the ill person's needs increase, informal caregivers such as family members take on added roles and responsibilities. Although caregiving can be fulfilling, mounting and unrelenting responsibilities, stress, role strain, and isolation can lead to overwhelm and ill health among designated caregivers. Alarmingly, the COVID-19 pandemic has exacerbated this risk. Therefore, it is crucial for nurses to assess caregivers, explore health and practical needs, and facilitate access to resources and support. Although there are many assessment tools that can be used, the Zarit Burden Interview is the most-studied validated tool that has been reliable across different ethnicities and in various illness situations (Duchesne, 2018). Nurses can access this tool online (https://dementiapathways.ie/_filecache/edd/c3c/89-zarit_burden_interview.pdf). A great caregiving guide for Canadian families can also be accessed online (Order of St. Lazarus Canada & CHPCA, 2019). The Canadian government offers benefits for caregivers, for which patients and caregivers may be eligible (Health Canada, 2022).

Despite available resources and supports for caregivers, large gaps remain. Furthermore, the pandemic has exacerbated and exposed pre-pandemic systemic gaps and inequities in palliative care across the country, particularly among people who are marginalized and underserved and those receiving care in the home and in community settings. Key findings of stakeholder engagement activities involving palliative care patients, caregivers, and experts from a variety of disciplines and sectors (Health Canada, 2021) identify these groups as being the most affected by the pandemic and as facing the greatest barriers to accessing quality palliative care. These stakeholders have also highlighted other systemic gaps and provided suggested solutions and tools that evolved from learning from the pandemic (Health Canada, 2021).

In summary, the areas needing attention include *stuff*: access to medication, personal protective equipment, and supplies; *staff*: mobilizing, educating, and supporting staff; *space*: optimizing inpatient bed usage, supporting care at home, and avoiding unnecessary transfers; *system*: triaging and coordinated collaboration of interprofessional (and unregulated) care providers (and volunteers) from inside and outside the traditional health care system and sector; *sedation*: use of palliative sedation for intractable symptoms, *separation*:

reducing isolation and increasing connection to family, care providers, and grief and bereavement supports and resources; *equity:* improving access to quality, culturally appropriate palliative care for marginalized and underserved groups; and *communication:* enhanced communication regarding advance care planning and goals of care, as well as between and among care providers and the patient and family (Health Canada, 2021).

END-OF-LIFE CARE

Nurses need to recognize a patient's transition to the end-of-life and active dying phases and communicate to the patient and family the expectation of imminent death. This is a good time to revisit conversations about preferences for end-of-life care. The Palliative Performance Scale (PPS) (Victoria Hospice, 2022a) is useful in determining when death is nearing.

Allow young children to visit a dying parent, sibling, or grandparent if desired. Encourage parents to express their concerns about how to talk about death and loss with their children. Do not use euphemisms to describe death to children. Instead, use the words *die, dying,* or *died.* Offer resources such as storybooks to help parents explain death to children. Helpful resources can be found on the Canadian Virtual Hospice's website (https://www.virtualhospice.ca/).

Care in the Community: Home Management

If a home death is planned, help families to prepare for this. Ensure presence of all necessary equipment as well as a medication kit containing common medications needed for symptom management at the end of life. Ensure that there is a plan in place for the pronouncement of death and removal of the deceased from the home.

For an expected home death, a letter can be written by the physician, or nurse practitioner in some provinces, informing the coroner/medical examiner's office and the funeral home of the expected death. There is no legal requirement that a physician pronounce the death. If an expected death occurs in a hospital, long-term care facility, or other facility, the nurse should adhere to employer policy on pronouncement of death (Canadian Medical Protective Association [CMPA], 2019). For home deaths, advise the family not to call emergency responders at the time of death to avoid invoking procedures necessary to investigate unexpected or suspicious deaths.

Educate the patient and family members about the signs of imminent death, what to expect, and how to recognize and attend to discomfort (Table 17.1). Ensure that the family has access to around-the-clock support if the patient plans to die at home. Educating a person and family about what to expect during the final days or hours can alleviate anxiety and promote a more positive death experience for all involved. Consider the type of support that family members will need at the time of death and make arrangements. Useful resources for families include *Remaining at Home: Things to Consider,* a brief guide to dying at home (Stenekes & Streeter, 2023), and Victoria Hospice's (2022b) psychosocial assessment tool.

TABLE 17.1

Physical Signs and Symptoms in the Final Stages of Dying

Physical Signs and Symptoms	Rationale	Intervention
Coolness, colour, and temperature change in hands, arms, feet, and legs; mottling of legs; perspiration	Peripheral circulation diminished as blood shunts to vital organs Patient may feel cool to touch, but core temperature normal	Place socks on feet. Cover with light blanket. Do not use electric blanket because person is unable to report excess heat.
Increased sleeping	Decreased energy, psychological withdrawal, medications	Spend time with person; hold their hand. Speak to person, even if there is no response. Maintain compassionate presence with the person and family. This, in itself, can be very therapeutic.
Disorientation, confusion of time, place, person	Metabolic changes, medications, changing sleep–wake cycles, decreased oxygenation	Identify self by name; reorient person to time and place. Decrease environmental stimuli.
Incontinence of bladder and/or bowel	Decreased muscle tone and consciousness	Change bedding as appropriate. Use bed pads; try not to use in-dwelling catheters.
Upper airway secretions; noisy respirations	Decreased cough reflex, inability to expectorate secretions or clear throat, relaxation of glottis, decreased muscle tone	Elevate head with pillow or raise head of bed; turn head to side to drain secretions. Suction minimally. Administer anticholinergics as prescribed.
Restlessness	Metabolic changes and decrease in oxygen to brain	Calm patient by speech and action; reduce light, rub back, stroke arms, or read aloud. Do not use restraints.
Decreased intake of food and fluids, nausea	Blood shunted away from gastrointestinal (GI) tract, causing decreased GI motility and anorexia; ketosis	Do not force patient to eat or drink; give ice chips or popsicles if desired. Provide mouth care.

Adapted from Boscart, V., McCleary, L., Sheiban Taucar, L., et al. (2023). *Ebersole and Hess' gerontological nursing and healthy aging in Canada* (3rd ed.). Elsevier.

✦ SKILL 17.2 Care of a Person's Body After Death

At the time of death, nurses provide compassionate care to patients and family members through their presence, by offering information, guidance, and support and by facilitating communication. In addition, nurses provide postmortem care (i.e., care of the person's body after death) in a dignified, respectful manner, consistent with a patient's religious and cultural practices and the local law (National Consensus Project for Quality Palliative Care, 2018).

Organ donation is another important nursing consideration near the time of death that is influenced by cultural or religious beliefs and legislation. While the Canadian government is responsible for ensuring the safety of donated organs, provinces and territories have specific guidelines and procedures as well as laws regarding consent. With the exception of some provinces (e.g., Nova Scotia), explicit rather than presumed consent is required in Canada, and donors can give prior consent by indicating this on their health card or driver's licence or through a registry. In the absence of prior consent, the next of kin can give consent. Even with prior consent of the donor, agreement of the family is sought before organ procurement (Norris, 2021).

In the case of vital organ donation (e.g., heart, lungs, liver, pancreas, small bowel, or kidneys), a patient must remain on life support until the organs are surgically removed. A nurse's role in organ procurement includes helping to identify potential organ donors, providing care for the donor's body, and caring for the family throughout the donation process (Findlater & Thomson, 2018). Family members often need help understanding the terms *neurologically determined death (NDD)*, which is the irreversible loss of consciousness and the ability to breathe, and *death by circulatory determination (DCD)*, in which critically ill ventilator-dependent patients have a very poor prognosis for recovery or quality of life and are hence removed from mechanical ventilation (Trillium Gift of Life Network, n.d.). Because life support keeps the deceased's organs functioning until they can be retrieved, families may incorrectly believe that the patient is still alive. For that reason, it is crucial for families to understand the meaning of NDD and DCD so they can make informed decisions with minimal distress. Tissues such as eyes, bone, and skin are retrieved from deceased patients not on life support, and there may be special care of the deceased person in preparation for donation. Although nurses must follow provincial and territorial laws and protocols regarding organ and tissue donation, useful information, resources, and tools relevant to the Canadian context can be found at Ontario's Trillium Gift of Life Network (https://www.giftoflife.on.ca/en/professionals.htm).

Because of the sensitive nature of making requests for organ donation, professionals educated in organ procurement often assume that responsibility. They inform family members of their options for donation and that making a donation does not delay funeral arrangements. Nurses may facilitate the organ donation request by providing a private place to have the conversation and by helping to identify the SDM to be involved in the request. Sometimes nurses notify the local donor registry to determine whether a patient qualifies for organ donation because certain medical conditions prohibit donation. Nurses also reinforce explanations of the donation procedure and inform the family about how the deceased's body will be cared for. Above all, nurses must honour the family's cultural and religious practices and support their final decision. Donor families often report that donating organs helped them in their grief and that they felt positive about the experience.

The second procedure of legal and medical significance often performed after a death is an autopsy, or postmortem examination. An autopsy, the surgical dissection of a person's body after death, helps determine the exact cause and circumstances of a death, discovers the pathway of a disease, or provides research data. It is not performed in every death. Provincial laws determine when autopsies are required, but they are usually performed in circumstances of unexpected, unexplained deaths (e.g., when death occurs within 24 hours of hospital admission; unexpected death in the home) and deaths resulting from accidents or drugs (CMPA, 2022).

Certification of death and completion of the death certificate are also guided by provincial/territorial legislation and should be completed as soon as possible after the death. In cases that do not require reporting, physicians and, in some regions, certified nurse practitioners who have knowledge of the person's illness leading up to the death can complete the death certificate. Each province/territory uses either the coroner or medical examiner's system to determine the process for investigation and which deaths are considered reportable (CMPA, 2019, 2022).

Delegation and Collaboration

The skill of caring for a person's body after death can be delegated to a UCP. However, it is often easier for the nurse and UCP to work together in providing postmortem care. The nurse directs the UCP to do the following:

- Follow employer policy and the law in cases of autopsy or organ and tissue donation
- Honour family cultural or religious rituals when performing postmortem care
- Handle the person's body with dignity and respect for privacy

Equipment

- Clean gloves and isolation gown
- Plastic bag for hazardous waste disposal
- Washbasin, washcloth, warm water, and bath towel
- Clean gown or disposable gown for the deceased's body as indicated by employer policy
- Shroud kit with name tags
- Syringes for removing urinary catheter
- Scissors
- Small pillow or towel
- Paper tape, gauze dressings
- Paper bag, plastic bag, or other suitable receptacle for patient's belongings to be returned to family members
- Valuables envelope

STEP	RATIONALE
ASSESSMENT	
1. Identify patient, ensuring arm-band information matches patient medical record.	Ensures correct patient.
2. Ask the responsible health care provider to establish the time of death and determine the need for an autopsy. If an autopsy is planned or the death was unexpected or unusual, use special precautions to preserve evidence (see local law and employer policy). In these instances, and in those in which death occurs within 24 hours of admission to hospital, all tubes and medical equipment should be left in place.	Validates the patient's death. Autopsy can determine cause of death and reveal more about a disease. When an autopsy is not required by law, a patient's legal representative and the health care provider or designated requester must complete and sign an autopsy consent form (Alberta Precision Laboratories, 2015).
3. Throughout the procedure, the 4 moments for hand hygiene are to be implemented; hand hygiene should occur before initial patient (or patient environment) contact, before an aseptic procedure, after body fluid exposure risk, and after patient (or patient environment) contact. Additional hand hygiene should be performed when hands are visibly soiled.	Proper hand hygiene helps prevent the spread of infectious agents to health care providers.
4. Determine whether family members or significant others are present and whether they have been informed of the death. Identify patient's SDM (next of kin or durable power of attorney [DPOA]).	Verifies that family has been notified of patient's death, and avoids inappropriate communication of this sensitive information.
5. Determine whether patient's SDM has been asked about organ and tissue donation, and validate that a donation request form has been signed. Notify organ request team per policy.	It is important to check provincial regulations, as varying policies pertaining to consent for organ donation exist. For example, federal guidelines require documentation that explicit consent has been given, whereas in Nova Scotia, consent is implied, and one must opt out of the choice for organ donation (Norris, 2021).
6. Provide family members and friends with a private place to gather. Give them time to ask questions (including those about medical care) or discuss grief.	Creates safe environment for grieving family. Questions provide information about how they are coping with loss and their needs.
7. Ask family members whether they have requests for preparation or viewing of the deceased (e.g., washing and positioning of the deceased, special clothing, shaving). Determine whether they wish to be present or help with care of the deceased.	Respects individuality of patient and family and supports their right to having cultural or religious values and beliefs upheld. Provides closure for those who wish to help with care of the deceased.
8. Contact support person (e.g., spiritual care, social work) to stay with family members not helping to prepare the deceased. Implement in timely manner a bereavement care plan after patient's death when family remains the focus of care (National Consensus Project for Quality Palliative Care, 2018).	Provides family support during an emotional time.
9. Consult health care provider's prescription for special care directives or specimens that are to be collected.	Specimens may be used in determining cause of death.
10. Apply clean gloves, gown, or protective barriers.	Reduces transmission of microorganisms.
11. Assess general condition of the person's body and note presence of dressings, tubes, and medical equipment. (If leaving room at this time, remove personal protective equipment and discard in appropriate receptacles.)	Validates whether tissue damage was present before postmortem care. Reduces transmission of microorganisms.
12. Ensure patient comfort before leaving patient room.	

NURSING DIAGNOSES

For patients:

- Potential for impaired skin integrity

For family members and significant others:

- Inadequate coping
- Compromised family coping
- Potential for complicated grief
- Powerlessness
- Insufficient knowledge regarding organ donation
- Grieving

Related factors and risk factors are individualized on the basis of the patient's, the family's, and significant others' needs.

STEP	RATIONALE

PLANNING

STEP	RATIONALE
1. Expected outcomes following completion of procedure:	
• Deceased's body is free of new skin damage.	Careful handling of the deceased prevents lacerations, bruises, or abrasions during postmortem care.
• Family and significant others are able to express grief.	Family and significant others feel supported through their loss.

Critical Decision Point *Immediately after death and before proceeding with other activities, place the deceased's body in a supine position and straighten the limbs* (Horst, 2019). *This will prevent livor mortis from occurring in the face and other areas visible to the family during viewing. Livor mortis is purplish discoloration of skin due to pooling of blood in dependent areas that occurs within 30 minutes after death and can last up to 12 hours* (Claridge, n.d.). *Proper positioning also prevents unnatural alignment of the body prior to rigor mortis, which is the stiffening of the body that occurs within about 2 hours of the death and lasts for about 36–48 hours* (Claridge, n.d.). *A pillow may be used in preparation for family viewing if needed.*

STEP	RATIONALE
2. Position patient supine in bed, arms at sides, in a private room if possible. If patient has a roommate, explain and move roommate to another location temporarily.	Provides staff with larger area for postmortem care and for family members to gather in a private setting.

Critical Decision Point *"Washing and positioning the deceased is best done where death occurs before stiffening of the body (rigor mortis) sets in. Rigor mortis happens within two to seven hours after death"* (Horst, 2019, para. 5).

STEP	RATIONALE
3. A patient's death must be certified as soon as possible by someone in authority (e.g., physician or, in some jurisdictions, a certified nurse practitioner). This person completes forms certifying the cause, time, and place of death. The legal form is necessary for life insurance and financial and property issues.	These steps make it possible for an official death certificate to be prepared.
4. Direct UCP to gather needed equipment and arrange at bedside.	Because this is often an emotional time for family members, organized, efficient care is important.

IMPLEMENTATION

STEP	RATIONALE
1. Identify patient using at least two person-specific identifiers (e.g., name and date of birth, or name and medical record number) according to employer policy. Tag the deceased person's body and leave tag in place as directed by employer policy.	Ensures correct patient. Complies with Accreditation Canada's standards and improves patient safety (Accreditation Canada, 2020).
2. Help family members notify others of the death. Promptly notify the mortuary, as chosen by the family, and discuss plans for postmortem care.	Following a death, grieving persons have difficulty focusing on details and often need guidance. Being informed increases the family's sense of control.
3. If patient is donating tissue, consult employer policy for guidelines related to care of the deceased person's body.	Retrieval of tissues (e.g., eyes, bone, skin) may require special procedures.
4. Apply clean gloves, gown, or protective barriers.	Reduces transmission of microorganisms.

Critical Decision Point *If caregivers are assisting with postmortem care, make sure they wear gowns and gloves to protect themselves from exposure to body fluids.*

STEP	RATIONALE
5. Remove in-dwelling devices (e.g., urinary catheter, endotracheal tube). Disconnect and cap off (no need to remove) intravenous lines. *Do not remove in-dwelling devices in cases of autopsy* (follow employer policy).	Creates normal appearance for family viewing of the deceased. Removing intravenous catheters allows fluids to leak. Removal of tubes and lines is contraindicated if an autopsy is planned.
6. Clean the mouth and clean and replace dentures as soon as possible. If dentures cannot be replaced, send them with the deceased in clearly labelled denture cup and transport together to mortuary. If culturally appropriate, close mouth with rolled-up towel under chin (Horst, 2019).	Gives face more natural appearance. If dentures are not replaced, it can be very difficult later for workers at funeral home to place dentures.
7. Place small pillow under head or position according to cultural preferences. Do not tie hands together on top of the person's body. Check employer policy regarding need to secure hands and feet. Use only circular gauze bandaging to secure appendages.	Patient appears natural. Weight of limp arms causes skin damage and discoloration if hands are tied. Some employers require securing limbs to prevent tissue damage when the deceased person is being moved.

IMPLEMENTATION

STEP	RATIONALE
8. Close eyes by applying light pressure for up to a few minutes (Horst, 2019). Some cultures prefer that eyes remain open. Use saline-moistened gauze if corneal or eye donation is to take place.	Closed eyes convey to some people a more peaceful and natural appearance. Damp gauze prevents corneal drying.
9. Groom and arrange hair into preferred style, if known. Remove any clips, hairpins, or rubber bands. Do not shave patient. Some faith groups may prohibit shaving.	Hard objects damage or discolour face and scalp.
10. Wash soiled body parts. In some cultures, it is common practice for family members to wash the body of the deceased.	Prepares the deceased person for viewing and reduces odours. Mortuary personnel provide complete bath. Inviting participation in postmortem care according to family wishes respects cultural practices.
11. Remove soiled dressings and replace with clean dressings, using paper tape or circular gauze bandaging.	Changing dressings controls odours and creates more acceptable appearance. Paper tape minimizes skin damage when tape is removed.

Critical Decision Point *Turning a recently deceased person to the side sometimes causes the flow of exhaled air. This is a normal event and not a sign of life.*

STEP	RATIONALE
12. Place absorbent pad under buttocks.	Relaxation of sphincter muscles at time of death causes release of urine or feces.
13. Place clean gown on the deceased. Some employers require gown removal before placing deceased in shroud.	Provides privacy and prepares the deceased for viewing.
14. Identify personal belongings that stay with deceased and those to be given to family.	Prevents loss of valuable or meaningful property.
15. If family requests viewing, respect individual cultural practices. Otherwise, place clean sheet over the deceased person up to chin with arms outside covers. Remove medical equipment from room. Provide soft lighting and chairs.	Maintains respect for patient and those viewing deceased. Prevents exposure of body parts. Removing medical equipment provides more peaceful, natural setting.
16. Allow mourners time alone with the deceased person to say goodbye. Help facilitate spiritual and cultural end-of-life practices (i.e., preplan with facilities management to pause smoke alarms and sprinkler systems to enable burning of sacred medicines). Some families may want time to sit quietly with the deceased person, console each other, and share memories. Some cultural practices include maintaining silence at the time of death, whereas others express grief with intense emotional displays, loud wailing, or "falling out." Do not rush any grieving process. Provide space for large families and support the inclusion of important community members.	Compassionate and culturally sensitive and safe care provides family members with opportunity for healing. Ensure privacy and a safe environment, (e.g., provide a chair at bedside for family member who might collapse).
17. After mourners leave, remove linens and gown per employer policy. Place the deceased in shroud provided by the employer (Fig. 17.3).	Shroud protects injury to skin, avoids exposure of the deceased, and provides barrier to protect against potentially contaminated body fluids.
18. Place identification label on outside of shroud if required by employer policy. Follow employer policy for marking a deceased's body that poses an infectious risk to others. Remove and dispose of personal protective equipment.	Ensures proper identification of the deceased. Reduces exposure of morgue and mortuary staff to contamination.
19. Arrange prompt transportation of the deceased to the mortuary. If you anticipate a delay, transport deceased to the morgue. If the death occurred at home, inform the family of proper positioning and that a cool room temperature will help maintain the condition of the deceased's body.	Mortuary personnel obtain best results if embalming occurs before full rigor mortis (i.e., stiffening of body after death).

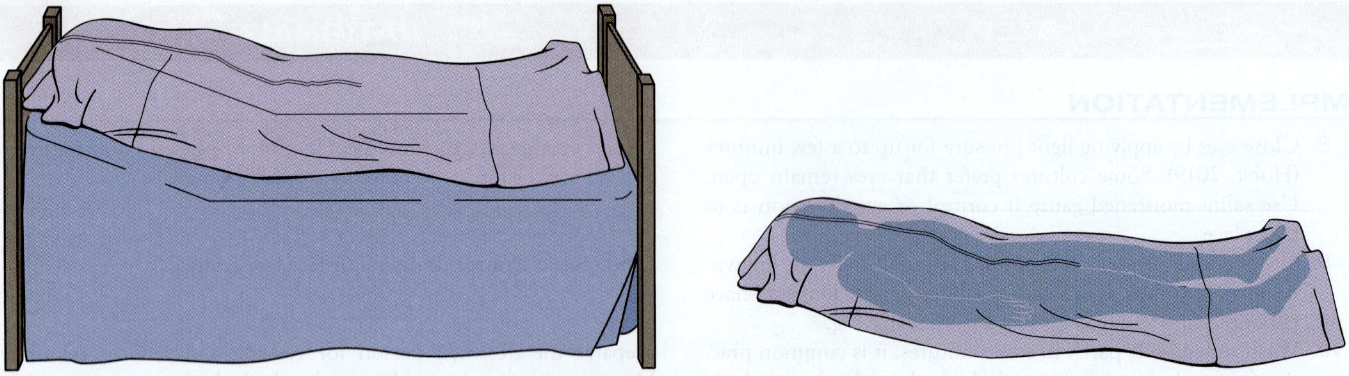

FIG 17.3 Deceased person in shroud.

STEP	RATIONALE

EVALUATION

1. Observe family members', friends', and significant others' responses to the loss.	The need for referral or help is based on evaluation of person's unique response to loss.
2. Note appearance and condition of deceased's skin during caregiving.	Provides information for postmortem care documentation.

Unexpected Outcomes	Related Interventions
1. A family member becomes immobilized with grief and has difficulty functioning.	• Enlist the help of a family member or trusted friend to provide direction and support.
2. A grieving person becomes agitated and threatens or strikes out against others.	• Call for assistance from a psychiatric nurse practitioner, spiritual care provider, or social worker who has a relationship with the family. • Enlist help from security staff or crisis intervention professional if safety is a concern.

Communication and Documentation

- Document time of death in the progress notes in EHR or chart, describe any resuscitative measures taken (if applicable), and note the name of the professional certifying the death.
- Document any special preparation of the deceased for autopsy or organ/tissue donation. Note whom you called and who made the request for organ/tissue donation.
- Document names of mortuary and names of family members consulted at the time of death and their relationship to the deceased.
- Document on appropriate form personal articles left on the deceased (e.g., teeth or glasses), jewellery taped to skin, or tubes and lines left in place. Note how valuables and personal belongings were handled and who received them. Secure signatures as required by employer policy.
- Document time the deceased was transported and the destination. Note the location of identification tags.

DOCUMENTATION EXAMPLE

Patient died peacefully in bed with adult child (Kerry) at the bedside. Death pronounced at 0735 hours by Dr. E. Heron. Other children (Jeremy and Jeff) were called and are on their way. Social worker called to be available to support the family. No religious or spiritual care desired. Provided comfort to Kerry and asked if and how they would like to be involved in caring for their mother. Kerry stated they would like to wash their mother's hair and face and then wait in the lounge for siblings. Assisted Kerry with care and talked about their mother, then Kerry left with the social worker to wait for siblings. Cleansed and positioned the deceased's body per protocol. Skin intact and free of scratches and bruises except for a 3 mm × 4 mm open area on coccyx. Applied gauze with micropore paper tape. Prepared the deceased for viewing by the family. Support provided to family in their grieving.

Special Considerations

Pediatric

- Offer family members, especially parents, opportunities to be with the child throughout the dying process and help with death aftercare.
- Parents frequently want to hold their child after death. Parents of deceased newborns often want a memento of their baby (e.g., picture, article of clothing, footprint, or lock of hair). Make every effort to honour parent requests.

Gerontological

- Some older persons have very small families and surviving circles of friends. Nurses and other care providers are sometimes the only human presence during death. Arrange for someone to be with the person when death is imminent.

End-of-Life Care in the Community: Home Management

- After death of patient at home, follow employer guidelines for postmortem care and transfer and for disposal of durable medical equipment (e.g., tubing, needles, syringes), soiled dressings or linens, and medications. Instruct family members in safe and proper handling and disposal of medical waste.

✦ SKILL 17.3 Supporting Ill Persons and Families in Grief

Grief experiences during serious illness and at the end of life can have profound physical, psychological, social, and spiritual impacts on dying people, family members, friends, and caregivers. Grief associated with serious illness or death may arise at any time. Hospitalization, chronic illness, and disability involve multiple losses. Hospitalized people lose privacy and control over normal routines and lifeways. With chronic illness, a person's body no longer functions as it once did, leading to possible loss of independence, self-esteem, and social roles. Declining ability and threat of end of life may create isolation from usual social supports, and death separates people from the physical presence of a person in their lives. Family and friends may also grieve these cumulative losses along with the patient. Grief may be caused by losing the person they once knew and the role they played in their life, witnessing a person's decline and suffering, or facing the ultimate loss of the person through death itself. The family is the unit of care throughout the illness and becomes the sole focus of care following the death.

Grief

Grief is the emotional response to a loss that varies according to one's personal experiences, psychological makeup, cultural expectations, and spiritual beliefs. Coping with the grief associated with death involves a period of mourning, which is the outward social expression of grief and the behaviours associated with loss (Corless & Meisenhelder, 2019). Mourning practices and rituals help grieving individuals adapt to loss, receive social support, adjust, and go forward in life without the deceased. Most mourning rituals are culturally influenced, learned practices. Bereavement—the state of grief and sadness that a person experiences after a loved one dies—is often considered the socially recognized period in which those legally or biologically closest to the deceased attend to personal and practical matters related to the death (Corless & Meisenhelder, 2019).

As a nurse, supporting the bereft after a death begins with being attentively and compassionately present. Take time to acknowledge the death and honour the person who died. This may include offering condolences and sharing memories of the deceased or simple warmth, empathy, and respect for the patient's and family's wishes as you care for them and the deceased. Assessment of the family for bereavement risk is important in order to identify where grief and bereavement supports may be needed. In recent years, the risk for grief complications has been exacerbated by the COVID-19 pandemic owing to people's isolation from practical and social supports and the impact of restrictions placed on gathering to commemorate the deceased and other after-death rituals and practices (Diolaiuti et al., 2021; Morris et al., 2020). This experience has underscored the importance of assessing a family's social supports and ongoing professional bereavement supports where needed.

Although there are no standardized tools to assess risk for complicated grief, the Bereavement Risk Assessment Tool (BRAT) (Victoria Hospice, 2008) is commonly used in Canada for predicting the possible need for additional follow-up or resources to support a grieving family. It is also important to understand the various types of grief. Normal or uncomplicated grief is evidenced by a variety of physical, cognitive, emotional, and behavioural responses that are as varied as the individuals experiencing them. Some people do not report feeling distressed or depressed, while others feel distressed for a lifetime without negative consequences. Grieving people may also need reassurance that their responses are common reactions to loss. For example, it is not uncommon for family members to feel the presence of the deceased person and to yearn for their return (Corless & Meisenhelder, 2019). An uncomplicated grief experience often helps a person mature and develop life perspective, although some people may prefer not to process the emotional experience of grief and focus instead on resilience, growth, or positive outcomes after a loss.

Anticipatory grief is an unconscious process that occurs before an actual loss or death and involves gradual disengagement from what is being lost. For example, if a dying process is lengthy, the person and family prepare for death before it occurs and sometimes, but not always, display fewer common grief responses at the time of death (Corless & Meisenhelder, 2019).

Complicated grief is characterized by prolonged and intense grieving and is associated with poor mental health outcomes and reduced function and quality of life (Diolaiuti et al., 2021). While some clinicians and scholars resist pathologizing grief, others see the need to intervene early to prevent poor health outcomes. For example, the 5th edition of the *Diagnostic and Statistical Manual of Mental Disorders* introduced "Persistent Complex Bereavement Disorder" (PCBD) as a pathological state characterized by severe and persistent grief and mourning reactions. PCBD is included within the category of "Other Specified Trauma- and Stressor-Related Disorders" (Diolaiuti et al., 2021, p. 2). Despite the urge to identify PCBD, there are no agreed-upon criteria with which to do so.

Delegation and Collaboration

The skills of assessing patients' or family members' grief reactions and designing appropriate interventions cannot be delegated to a UCP. The nurse directs the UCP to do the following:

- Inform the nurse when a patient or family member exhibits behaviour commonly associated with grief (e.g., crying, anger, withdrawal)
- Form supportive relationships with patients and families and inform the nurse when patients or family members have questions or concerns
- Alert the nurse to the arrival of designated caregivers so the nurse can discuss the plan of care and offer support

STEP	RATIONALE
ASSESSMENT	
1. Sit near patient/family in a quiet, private location. Centre yourself and establish quiet, compassionate presence. Establish eye contact. Be aware that use of sustained eye contact in some cultures conveys disrespect or may cause discomfort. Recognize the needs of people who have been marginalized, discriminated against, and historically traumatized, and provide a space of openness, respect, and safety.	A willingness to be present with another in their suffering expresses compassion and offers opportunities for healing (Borneman & Brown-Saltzman, 2019). Privacy protects confidentiality and promotes a sense of safety for people when they are expressing their thoughts and emotions. Recognizing needs and providing a safe space contributes to culturally safe practice and prevents compounded traumas.

STEP	RATIONALE
2. Consider the influence of a person's cultural background on communication and honour wishes about communication. Apply principles of plain language and health literacy during assessment (National Consensus Project for Quality Palliative Care, 2018).	Individual differences influence grief responses and communication styles (Corless & Meisenhelder, 2019). Stress impacts the ability to absorb health information.
3. Determine whether the loss was sudden or unexpected and how much time has elapsed since the loss.	Unexpected loss is a risk factor for complicated grief (Diolaiuti et al., 2021). Intense grief or grief that interferes with daily functioning many months after a loss may be an indicator of complicated grief (Diolaiuti et al., 2021).
4. Listen carefully to the person's story and observe their responses to understand the significance of the loss to the patient or family member, identify concerns, and assess their ability to sustain hope and move forward in life. Provide empathy and use open-ended questions such as the following: • "How are you handling this unexpected loss?" • "Tell me how your loss affects you as a person." • "What provides you with hope to move forward?" • "What gives your life meaning?"	Develops trust in a caring relationship. Actively listening to patient's/family's concerns and being attentive to feelings and needs convey empathy and compassion. Complicated grief is highly associated with feelings of role confusion, loss of meaning, loneliness (Malgaroli et al., 2018), and unexpected losses (Diolaiuti et al., 2021). Hope and meaning are expressions of the spiritual that intertwine with experiences of grief. Knowing the source of priority concerns will assist the nurse in identifying appropriate team members to provide follow-up (i.e., psychologist, social worker, spiritual care provider).
5. Combine knowledge of natural human responses to grief with observation of behaviours. Normalize and support a wide range of emotions. Clarify observations by sharing them, as in the following examples: • "You've mentioned several times that you feel hopeless." • "It seems that this is hard for you to talk about." • "I can see this loss has turned your world upside down."	Normalizing contributes to acceptance of feelings and the freedom to express them. Sharing observations confirms accuracy of observations, validates the griever's feelings, and prompts them to continue sharing.
6. Encourage the person to describe the loss and its impact on quality of life (e.g., "You said your diagnosis changed your life forever. Tell me more.").	Listening to person's description helps to minimize assumptions.
7. Ask the person to describe the coping strategies they use most often in difficult times. Examples: • "How have you handled loss in the past?" • "Who usually supports you in times like these?"	Familiar, effective coping strategies are often helpful in the current crisis, loss, or grief experience. This draws on the person's inherent strengths and supports.
8. Assess spiritual needs, beliefs, and resources. Focus on aspects likely to be involved (e.g., trust, feelings of connectedness, life meaning and purpose, faith/belief, and hope). Refer to specific spiritual assessment tools mentioned at the beginning of this chapter under "Cultural Safety."	Identifies person's spiritual beliefs and values. Enables patient autonomy by identifying beliefs and preferences for care or rituals related to faith or spirituality that enhance healing. Offers a greater understanding of person's culture and values to ensure culturally safe care.

NURSING DIAGNOSES

- Inappropriate denial
- Hopelessness
- Compromised family coping
- Death anxiety
- Anxiety
- Fear
- Potential for complicated grieving
- Potential for spiritual distress
- Potential for caregiver role strain
- Readiness for enhanced hope
- Readiness for enhanced coping
- Readiness for enhanced family coping
- Grieving

Related factors and risk factors are individualized on the basis of patient's condition or needs.

PLANNING

STEP	RATIONALE
1. Expected outcomes following interventions	
• Person maintains relationships with supportive and significant people.	Supportive social networks contribute to healing and prevent loneliness. Supports feelings of connectedness.
• Person expresses grief in keeping with their cultural and spiritual practices.	Person retains cherished values and ways of being.
• Person uses healthy and effective coping strategies.	Effective and healthy coping strategies enable healing and sense of self-efficacy.
• Person maintains normal life routines.	Maintaining life routines keeps the person engaged with living.
• Person identifies sense of acceptance and peace.	Indicates coping with loss.

STEP	RATIONALE
IMPLEMENTATION	
1. Show an empathic understanding of the person's feelings, acknowledge needs, and recognize strengths. Provide compassionate presence.	Promotes trust, caring, compassion, and empathy. Recognizing strengths gives person sense of self-efficacy.
2. Offer information about patient's illness and treatment or death. Clarify misunderstandings or misinformation. Use culturally appropriate language and simple terms.	Misunderstanding adds to person's uncertainty, anxiety, and suffering.
3. Encourage person to sustain relationships with others to help maintain independence and receive necessary help. Include patient-identified support people in discussions.	Affiliation with others offers support and helps person stay engaged in life.
4. Help patient achieve short-term goals (e.g., symptom relief, task completion, resolution of relational problems, adaptation to loss of function).	Helping people identify and meet their personal goals contributes to their quality of life.
a. Help grievers prepare for the days and weeks following a death by providing grief and bereavement support and practical information and resources.	Assists grievers to move forward and provides information and support to facilitate healthy grieving.
5. Provide frequent opportunities to express fears and concerns. Be attentive to expressions of intense emotions.	Emotions change quickly and frequently during stress and complicate communication for nurses and patients.
6. Provide education and support. Discuss procedures, plan of care, and anticipated changes. Use interprofessional collaboration as appropriate to support patient's needs and preferences.	Reduces anxiety, provides comfort, and promotes person-centred care. Utilizes specialized skills of team members and facilitates holistic and comprehensive care.
7. Provide instruction on relaxation strategies: mindfulness-based stress reduction, guided imagery, meditation, hand massage, healing touch (see Chapter 16).	Complementary therapies have been shown in select cases to relieve anxiety and effectively reduce stress, thus providing useful coping strategies (Stomski et al., 2018).
8. For the person who is dying, encourage visits with loved ones, life review with stories or photographs, or projects such as organizing photo albums or journal writing. (For bereft families, see Skill 17.2)	Reviewing positive and negative events in one's life allows a person to find meaning in their experiences, resolve conflicts, and come to a place of acceptance (Borneman & Brown-Saltzman, 2019).
9. Facilitate patient's religious/spiritual practices and connections with faith community. Use prayer or music and provide a listening presence. Make a referral to a spiritual care provider if appropriate and desired by the family.	Spiritual interventions help patients maintain hope and connect with the core of their identity. Spiritual interventions can decrease anxiety, promote a sense of peace, and help patients find meaning in their life (Rosa, 2019).
EVALUATION	
1. Note descriptions of relationships and activities with others.	Provides information on extent to which relational ties are maintained.
2. Observe behaviours during ongoing interactions.	Evaluates ability to express grief and coping.
3. Elicit perceptions of benefit gained from use of coping interventions.	Evaluates efficacy of interventions.
4. Discuss progress toward performing routine activities at home and adaptation to loss.	Evaluates achievement of desired goals or need for goal revision.

Unexpected Outcomes	Related Interventions
1. Person does not acknowledge loss and shows signs of extreme sorrow, anger, withdrawal, or denial.	• Consider referral to a team member with specialized skills in grief counselling (e.g., nurse practitioner, psychologist, spiritual care provider, social worker).
2. Person does not receive needed support from their social network.	• Share and validate observations of relational strain or person's concern over relational interactions. • Consider referral to a team member who has specialized skills in grief counselling.

Communication and Documentation

- Document interventions used to support patient and family coping and note verbal and nonverbal responses in progress notes in EHR or chart.
- Communicate grief reactions to members of the interprofessional/interdisciplinary team and determine who will provide follow-up, if necessary.

DOCUMENTATION EXAMPLE

All children of the deceased were present in the lounge with the social worker at 0830 hours. Introduced myself and provided condolences to Kerry's siblings. Invited family to spend time with their mother and remained for 25 minutes recounting memories of their mother and providing comfort. Kerry was especially distraught and was being comforted by siblings. Kerry stated that they "wished they hadn't stayed away so long," admonishing themselves for their choices. Provided comfort and relayed to Kerry how their mother spoke so lovingly of them, and the peace and joy their mother found when Kerry responded positively to a request for reconciliation. Kerry continued to sob, stating, "I just wish we had done this sooner." Siblings hugged and consoled Kerry. Gave family some private time and gathered grief and bereavement resources. Informed the social worker of the need for follow-up with Kerry. Will continue to collaborate with family to develop bereavement plan.

Special Considerations

Teaching

- Give caregivers and family members basic information about common grief responses and how to offer or find support. Coach them on ways to provide physical, emotional, and spiritual support to the patient and to one another (e.g., providing basic hygiene to ill persons, listening attentively, avoiding false reassurances, allowing for the expression of difficult emotions, talking about normal family activities).

Pediatric

- Children's understanding of death differs from that of adults and is influenced by age and developmental level. Respect parents' wishes about when and what to tell children about illness or death. When discussing sensitive topics with children, encourage parents to offer caring explanations at a level a child can understand. Avoid using euphemisms for death. Instead, use the words *die* or *died* to prevent confusion, especially among young children.
- Play therapy or drawing helps children express thoughts, emotions, or fears about illness or death.
- Be alert to all family members' grief reactions because they may feel guilt, resentment, or helplessness with the illness or death of a sibling, child, or grandchild. Facilitate communication with family members who must be separated from an ill child.
- SDMs, usually the parents, need to make health care decisions for infants and young children. Some decisions are difficult because outcomes for children are often unpredictable.

Gerontological

- Losing a spouse after a long and satisfying relationship is very difficult and is essentially a loss of self. The mourning is as much for oneself as for the individual (Boscart et al., 2023).
- Intense grief may cause a temporary decrease in cognitive function that can manifest as confusion (Boscart et al., 2023).
- Many older persons have coexisting medical conditions that add to their symptom burden. They also have lived long enough to have experienced cumulative losses, including members of their family and community, which may complicate their grief experience.

✦ REVIEW QUESTIONS

You are caring for an older person who has been hospitalized for abdominal pain, anorexia, weight loss, and weakness. The patient was treated 10 years earlier for prostate cancer. Test results now confirm that the patient has a large tumour in their abdomen and the cancer has spread to the lymph nodes. No medical interventions are available to cure the disease. When you enter the room, the patient tells you in an angry voice that they want to transfer to a different hospital where people will help them fight their cancer. Review Questions 1 to 3 relate to the case study presented here.

1. Which of the following nursing responses is most appropriate?
   1. "I'll let your doctor know how you're feeling. Right now, let me take your blood pressure."
   2. "The news of your illness progression has upended your world. Tell me what you understand about your prognosis and how this is affecting you?"
   3. "You have every right to seek a second opinion, although I'm not sure where you would get one."
   4. "It sounds like you're upset. I'll call your family to come and be with you."
   5. "We have the best doctors here, and I don't think you'll get a different opinion elsewhere."
2. The next day the patient reports mild abdominal pain and mentions that they have not had a bowel movement for 3 days. The patient's partner reports to you that the patient has not had anything to eat or drink for 24 hours.
   1. What might be the cause of the patient's inability to have a bowel movement?
   2. List three interventions to provide.
3. Four weeks later you take care of this patient again. Their symptoms include weight loss, anorexia, worsening abdominal pain, depression, and anxiety. The patient's partner tells you that the nurse practitioner asked them whether they would be open to a consult with the specialist palliative care team. The partner says to you, "I'm still not sure whether palliative care would be best for us." Which key points would you include in a discussion with the patient and partner about palliative care? Using SBAR (situation–background–assessment–recommendation), show how you would communicate your assessment to the other health care providers.
4. The nurse is caring for a patient with cancer who has been admitted to the palliative care unit. What are the goals of palliative care? (*Select all that apply.*)
   1. Physical symptom management
   2. Facilitating maintenance of cultural and spiritual preferences
   3. Curative care
   4. Extending life as long as possible
   5. Providing a dignified death
   6. Improving quality of life
5. A nurse suggests that the patient receive a consult with a specialist palliative care team for symptom management related to anxiety and increasing pain. A family member asks the nurse whether this means that the patient is dying. What should the nurse tell the patient and family about the care the patient is receiving? (*Select all that apply.*)
   1. Palliative care and end-of-life care are the same thing.
   2. Palliative care is for any patient, any time, with any chronic disease, in any setting.
   3. A specialty palliative care team helps regular caregivers manage complex symptoms.
   4. Palliative care interventions relieve suffering and the symptoms of illness and treatment.
6. A nurse has the responsibility of managing a deceased patient's postmortem care. Arrange the steps for postmortem care in the proper order.
   1. Bathe the deceased's body.
   2. Collect any needed specimens.
   3. Remove all drains and in-dwelling tubes.
   4. Position the deceased person for viewing.
   5. Speak to the family members about their possible participation.
   6. Confirm that a request for organ/tissue donation and/or autopsy has been made.
   7. Notify a support person (e.g., spiritual care provider, bereavement specialist) for the family.
   8. Accurately tag the deceased, indicating their identity and any safety issues regarding infection control.

Visit the Evolve site for a complete list of answers to the Review Questions.

✦ NEXT GENERATION NCLEX® (NGN)

For practice with answering exam questions related to unfolding NGN case studies, please consult the Next Generation NCLEX® (NGN)-Style Case Studies for Skills and Techniques on the Evolve website: http://evolve.elsevier.com/Canada/Perry/clinicalskills/

REFERENCES

Accreditation Canada. (2020). *Required organizational practices handbook.* https://physicians.nshealth.ca/resources/required-organizational-practices-2020-handbook

Advance Care Planning Canada. (2022a). *Advance care planning in Canada.* https://www.advancecareplanning.ca

Advance Care Planning Canada. (2022b). *CPR decision aids.* https://www.advancecareplanning.ca/resource/cpr-decision-aids/

Alberta Precision Laboratories. (2015). *Autopsy information for next of kin.* https://www.albertaprecisionlabs.ca/hp/Page13871.aspx [Seminal Reference]

American Cancer Society. (2019). *Physical changes as you near the end of life.* https://www.cancer.org/treatment/end-of-life-care/nearing-the-end-of-life/physical-symptoms.html

Ariadne Labs. (2021). *Serious illness conversation guide.* https://www.ariadnelabs.org/serious-illness-care/for-clinicians/

Bhyan, P., Pesce, M. B., Shrestha, U., et al. (2022). Palliative sedation in patients with terminal illness. *StatPearls.* https://www.ncbi.nlm.nih.gov/books/NBK470545/

Bill C-14, *An Act to Amend the Criminal Code and to Make Related Amendments to Other Acts (Medical Assistance in Dying)*, 42nd Parliament, 1st session, 2016. https://www.parl.ca/LegisInfo/en/bill/42-1/C-14 [Seminal Reference]

Bill C-277, *An Act Providing for the Development of a Framework on Palliative Care in Canada*, 42nd Parliament, 1st session, 2017. https://www.parl.ca/DocumentViewer/en/42-1/bill/C-277/royal-assent [Seminal Reference]

Borneman, T., & Brown-Saltzman, K. (2019). Meaning in illness. In B. R. Ferrell, & J. A. Paice (Eds.), *Oxford textbook of palliative nursing* (5th ed., pp. 456–466). Oxford University Press. https://doi.org/10.1093/med/9780190862374.003.0036

Boscart, V., McCleary, L., Sheiban Taucar, L., et al. (2023). *Ebersole and Hess' gerontological nursing and healthy aging in Canada* (3rd ed.). Elsevier.

Burchum, J. R., & Rosenthal, L. D. (2019). *Lehne's pharmacology for nursing care* (9th ed.). Elsevier.

Canadian Hospice Palliative Care Association (CHPCA). (n.d.). *Standards and norms of practice.* https://www.chpca.ca/resource/norms

Canadian Hospice Palliative Care Association (CHPCA). (2015). *The way forward national framework: A roadmap for an integrated palliative approach to care.* http://www.hpcintegration.ca/media/60044/TWF-framework-doc-Eng-2015-final-April1.pdf [Seminal Reference]

Canadian Hospice Palliative Care Association (CHPCA). (2022). *Hospice palliative care: FAQs.* https://www.chpca.ca/about-hpc/

Canadian Medical Protective Association (CMPA). (2019). *Completing medical certificates of death: Who's responsible?* https://www.cmpa-acpm.ca/en/advice-publications/browse-articles/2016/completing-medical-certificates-of-death-who-s-responsible

Canadian Medical Protective Association (CMPA). (2022). *Understanding the role of coroners and medical examiners.* https://www.cmpa-acpm.ca/en/advice-publications/browse-articles/2013/understanding-the-role-of-coroners-and-medical-examiners

Canadian Nurses Association. (2017). *Code of ethics for registered nurses.* https://www.cna-aiic.ca/en/nursing/regulated-nursing-in-canada/nursing-ethics [Seminal Reference]

Canadian Nurses Protective Society. (2021). *Medical assistance in dying: What every nurse should know*. https://cnps.ca/article/medical-assistance-in-dying-what-every-nurse-should-know/

Canadian Partnership Against Cancer & Health Canada. (2021). *The Canadian interdisciplinary palliative care competency framework*. https://www.partnershipagainstcancer.ca/topics/palliative-care-competency-framework/

Canadian Virtual Hospice. (n.d.). *Living my culture*. https://livingmyculture.ca/culture/

Cancer Care Ontario. (2010). *Edmonton Symptom Assessment System*. http://cancercaresoutheast.ca/edmonton-symptom-assessment-system-esas [Seminal Reference]

Claridge, J. (n.d.). *Rigor mortis and lividity*. https://www.exploreforensics.co.uk/rigor-mortis-and-lividity.html

Collett, D., & Chow, K. (2019). Nausea and vomiting. In B. R. Ferrell, & J. A. Paice (Eds.), *Oxford textbook of palliative nursing* (5th ed., pp. 149–162). Oxford University Press. https://doi.org/10.1093/med/9780190862374.003.0012

Corless, I. B., & Meisenhelder, J. B. (2019). Bereavement. In B. R. Ferrell, & J. A. Paice (Eds.), *Oxford textbook of palliative nursing* (5th ed., pp. 390–404). Oxford University Press. https://doi.org/10.1093/med/9780190862374.003.0031

Diolaiuti, F., Marazziti, D., Beatino, M. F., et al. (2021). Impact and consequences of COVID-19 pandemic on complicated grief and persistent complex bereavement disorder. *Psychiatry Research*, 300, Article 113916. https://doi.org/10.1016/j.psychres.2021.113916

Donesky, D. A. (2019). Dyspnea, cough, and terminal secretions. In B. R. Ferrell, & J. A. Paice (Eds.), *Oxford textbook of palliative nursing* (5th ed., pp. 217–229). Oxford University Press. https://doi.org/10.1093/med/9780190862374.003.0016

Dorman, J. D., & Raffin Bouchal, S. (2020). Moral distress and moral uncertainty in medical assistance in dying: A simultaneous evolutionary concept analysis. *Nursing Forum*, *55*(3), 320–330. https://doi.org/10.1111/nuf.12431

Duchesne, V. (2018). *Caregiver stress: Supporting caregivers in primary care*. eMentalHealth.ca. https://primarycare.ementalhealth.ca/index.php?m=fpArticle&ID=56036

Farrington, N., & Murphy, C. (2019). Bladder management in palliative care. In B. R. Ferrell, & J. A. Paice (Eds.), *Oxford textbook of palliative nursing* (5th ed., pp. 230–237). Oxford University Press. https://doi.org/10.1093/med/9780190862374.003.0017

Findlater, C., & Thomson, E. M. (2018). Organ donation and management of the potential organ donor. *Anesthesia and Intensive Care Medicine*, *16*(7), 315–320. https://doi.org/10.1016/j.mpaic.2015.04.013

Gerlach, L. B., Wiechers, I. R., & Maust, D. T. (2018). Prescription benzodiazepine use among older adults: A critical review. *Harvard Review of Psychiatry*, *26*(5), 264–273. https://doi.org/10.1097/HRP.0000000000000190

Goldberg, W., Mahr, G., Williams, A. M., et al. (2019). Delirium, confusion, and agitation. In B. R. Ferrell, & J. A. Paice (Eds.), *Oxford textbook of palliative nursing* (5th ed., pp. 319–329). Oxford University Press. https://doi.org/10.1093/med/9780190862374.003.0023

Harman, S. M., Bailey, F. A., & Walling, A. M. (2022). Palliative care: The last hours and days of life. *UpToDate*. http://www.uptodate.com/contents/palliative-care-the-last-hours-and-days-of-life

Health Canada. (2018). *Framework on palliative care in Canada*. https://www.canada.ca/en/health-canada/services/health-care-system/reports-publications/palliative-care/framework-palliative-care-canada.html

Health Canada. (2019). *Action plan on palliative care: Building on the framework on palliative care in Canada*. https://www.canada.ca/en/health-canada/services/health-care-system/reports-publications/palliative-care/action-plan-palliative-care.html

Health Canada. (2021). *Home and community-based palliative care: Shaping the future from lessons learned during the COVID-19 pandemic*. https://cdnhomecare.ca/wp-content/uploads/2021/06/Home-and-Community-based-Palliative-Care-Shaping-the-Future-from-Lessons-Learned-during-the-COVID-19-Pandemic_JUN25.pdf

Health Canada. (2022). *Benefits for caregivers*. https://www.canada.ca/en/financial-consumer-agency/services/caring-someone-ill/benefits-tax-credits-caregivers.html

Health Canada. (2023a). *Medical assistance in dying*. https://www.canada.ca/en/health-canada/services/medical-assistance-dying.html

Health Canada. (2023b). *Provincial and territorial contact information for end-of-life care services*. https://www.canada.ca/en/health-canada/services/provincial-territorial-contact-information-links-end-life-care.html

Henson, J. S. (2020). Burnout or compassion fatigue: A comparison of concepts. *Medsurg Nursing*, 29(2), 77–81, 95.

Hockenberry, M., Duffy, E. A., & Gibbs, K. (2024). *Wong's nursing care of infants and children* (12th ed.). Elsevier.

Horst, G. R. (2019). *Care of the body after death*. https://www.virtualhospice.ca/en_US/Main+Site+Navigation/Home/Topics/Topics/Final+Days/Care+of+the+Body+After+Death.aspx

Interior Health. (2020). *Medical Orders for Scope of Treatment (MOST): Frequently asked questions: Public resource*. https://www.interiorhealth.ca/sites/default/files/PDFS/most-faq-public-resource.pdf

iPANEL. (2018). *Initiative for a Palliative Approach in Nursing: Evidence and Leadership*. https://www.uvic.ca/research/groups/palliative/projects/current/ipanel.php

Jarrad, R. A., & Hammad, S. (2020). Oncology nurses' compassion fatigue, burnout, and compassion satisfaction. *Annals of General Psychiatry*, *19*(22). https://doi.org/10.1186/s12991-020-00272-9

Malgaroli, M., Maccallum, F., & Bonanno, G. A. (2018). Symptoms of persistent complex bereavement disorder, depression, and PTSD in a conjugally bereaved sample: A network analysis. *Psychological Medicine*, *48*(14), 2439–2448. https://doi.org/10.1017/S0033291718001769

McClement, S., & Stenekes, S. (2019). *Talking with children and youth about serious illness*. https://www.virtualhospice.ca/en_US/Main+Site+Navigation/Home/Topics/Topics/Communication/Talking+with+Children+and+Youth.aspx

Meyer, M., & Ring, M. (2019). Complementary and integrative therapies in palliative care. In B. R. Ferrell, & J. A. Paice (Eds.), *Oxford textbook of palliative nursing* (5th ed., pp. 361–370). Oxford University Press. https://doi.org/10.1093/med/9780190862374.003.0028

Mooney, S. N., Patel, P., & Buga, S. (2019). Bowel management: Constipation, diarrhea, obstruction, and ascites. In B. R. Ferrell, & J. A. Paice (Eds.), *Oxford textbook of palliative nursing* (5th ed., pp. 186–205). Oxford University Press. https://doi.org/10.1093/med/9780190862374.003.0014

Morris, S. E., Moment, A., & deLima Thomas, J. (2020). Caring for bereaved family members during the COVID-19 pandemic: Before and after the death of a patient. *Journal of Pain and Symptom Management*, 60(2), e70–e74. https://doi.org/10.1016/j.jpainsymman.2020.05.002

National Consensus Project for Quality Palliative Care. (2018). *Clinical practice guidelines for quality palliative care* (4th ed.). https://www.nationalcoalitionhpc.org/wp-content/uploads/2018/10/NCHPC-NCPGuidelines_4thED_web_FINAL.pdf

Norris, S. (2021, October 25). *Consent for organ donation in Canada*. HillNotes, Library of Parliament. https://hillnotes.ca/2021/10/25/consent-for-organ-donation-in-canada/

Nova Scotia Health Authority. (2017). *The Nova Scotia palliative care competency framework: A reference guide for health professionals and volunteers*. https://library.nshealth.ca/ld.php?content_id=34202519 [Seminal Reference]

O'Neil-Page, E., Dean, G. E., & Anderson, P. R. (2019). Fatigue. In B. R. Ferrell, & J. A. Paice (Eds.), *Oxford textbook of palliative nursing* (5th ed., pp. 132–139). Oxford University Press. https://doi.org/10.1093/med/9780190862374.003.0010

Order of St. Lazarus Canada & Canadian Hospice Palliative Care Association. (2019). *A caregiver's guide: A handbook about end-of-life care*. https://www.stlazarus.ca/docs/publications/caregivers_guide_2019_en.pdf

Piers, R., De Brauwer, I., Baeyens, H., et al. (2021). Supportive and Palliative Care Indicators Tool prognostic value in older hospitalised patients: A prospective multicentre study. *BMJ Supportive & Palliative Care*. https://doi.org/10.1136/bmjspcare-2021-003042 [Online ahead of print]

Rainer, J., Schneider, J. K., & Lorenz, R. A. (2018). Ethical dilemmas in nursing: An integrative review. *Journal of Clinical Nursing*, 27(19–20), 3446–3461. https://doi.org/10.1111/jocn.14542

Rindfleisch, J. A. (n.d.). *Whole health: Change the conversation. Clinical tool: Spiritual assessment tools*. VHA Office of Patient-Centered Care and Cultural Transformation. https://www.va.gov/WHOLEHEALTHLIBRARY/docs/M11_Spiritual_Assessment_Tools.pdf

Rodrigues, P., Crokaert, J., & Gastmans, C. (2018). Palliative sedation for existential suffering: A systematic review of argument-based ethics literature. *Journal of Pain and Symptom Management*, *55*(6), 1577–1590. https://doi.org/10.1016/j.jpainsymman.2018.01.013

Rosa, W. (2019). Spiritual care intervention. In B. R. Ferrell, & J. A. Paice (Eds.), *Oxford textbook of palliative nursing* (5th ed., pp. 447–455). Oxford University Press. https://doi.org/10.1093/med/9780190862374.003.0035

Samuriwo, R. (2019). Enhancing end-of-life skin care to prevent pressure ulcers in primary care: Key considerations for nurses. *Journal of Community Nursing*, 33(3), 56–60. https://www.jcn.co.uk/journals/issue/06-2019/article/enhancing-end-of-life-skin-care-to-prevent-pressure-ulcers-in-primary-care

Stenekes, S., & Streeter, L. (2023). *Remaining at home: Things to consider*. https://www.virtualhospice.ca/en_US/Main+Site+Navigation/Home/Topics/Topics/Decisions/Remaining+at+home_+Things+to+consider.aspx

Stomski, N., Petterson, A., Kristjanson, L., et al. (2018). The effect of self-selected complementary therapies on cancer patients' quality of life and symptom distress: A prospective cohort study in an integrative oncology setting. *Complementary Therapies in Medicine*, 37, 1–5. https://doi.org/10.1016/j.ctim.2018.01.006

Thomas, K., Watson, M., Wilson, J. A., et al. (2022). *The gold standards framework proactive identification guidance (PIG)* (7th ed.). National Gold Standards Framework Centre for End of Life Care. https://goldstandardsframework.org.

uk/cd-content/uploads/files/PIG/Proactive%20Identification%20Guidance%20v7%20(2022).pdf
Trillium Gift of Life Network. (n.d.). *Determination of death.* Ontario Health. https://www.giftoflife.on.ca/en/professionals.htm#hp-neuro1
Victoria Hospice. (2008). *Bereavement Risk Assessment Tool (BRAT).* BCGuidelines.ca. https://www2.gov.bc.ca/assets/gov/health/practitioner-pro/bc-guidelines/palliative3_appendix_e.pdf [Seminal Reference]
Victoria Hospice. (2022a). *Clinical tools for professionals: Palliative Performance Scale.* https://victoriahospice.org/how-we-can-help/clinical-tools/
Victoria Hospice. (2022b). *Clinical tools for professionals: Psychosocial assessment.* https://victoriahospice.org/how-we-can-help/clinical-tools/
Wolcott Altaker, K., Howie-Esquivel, J., & Cataldo, J. K. (2018). Relationships among palliative care, ethical climate, empowerment, and moral distress in intensive care unit nurses. *American Journal of Critical Care, 27*(4), 295–302. https://doi.org/10.4037/ajcc2018252
Wood, J. (2021). Cicely Saunders, "total pain" and emotional evidence at the end of life. *Medical Humanities, 48*, 411–420. https://doi.org/10.1136/medhum-2020-012107
World Health Organization (WHO). (2020, August 5). *Palliative care.* https://www.who.int/news-room/fact-sheets/detail/palliative-care

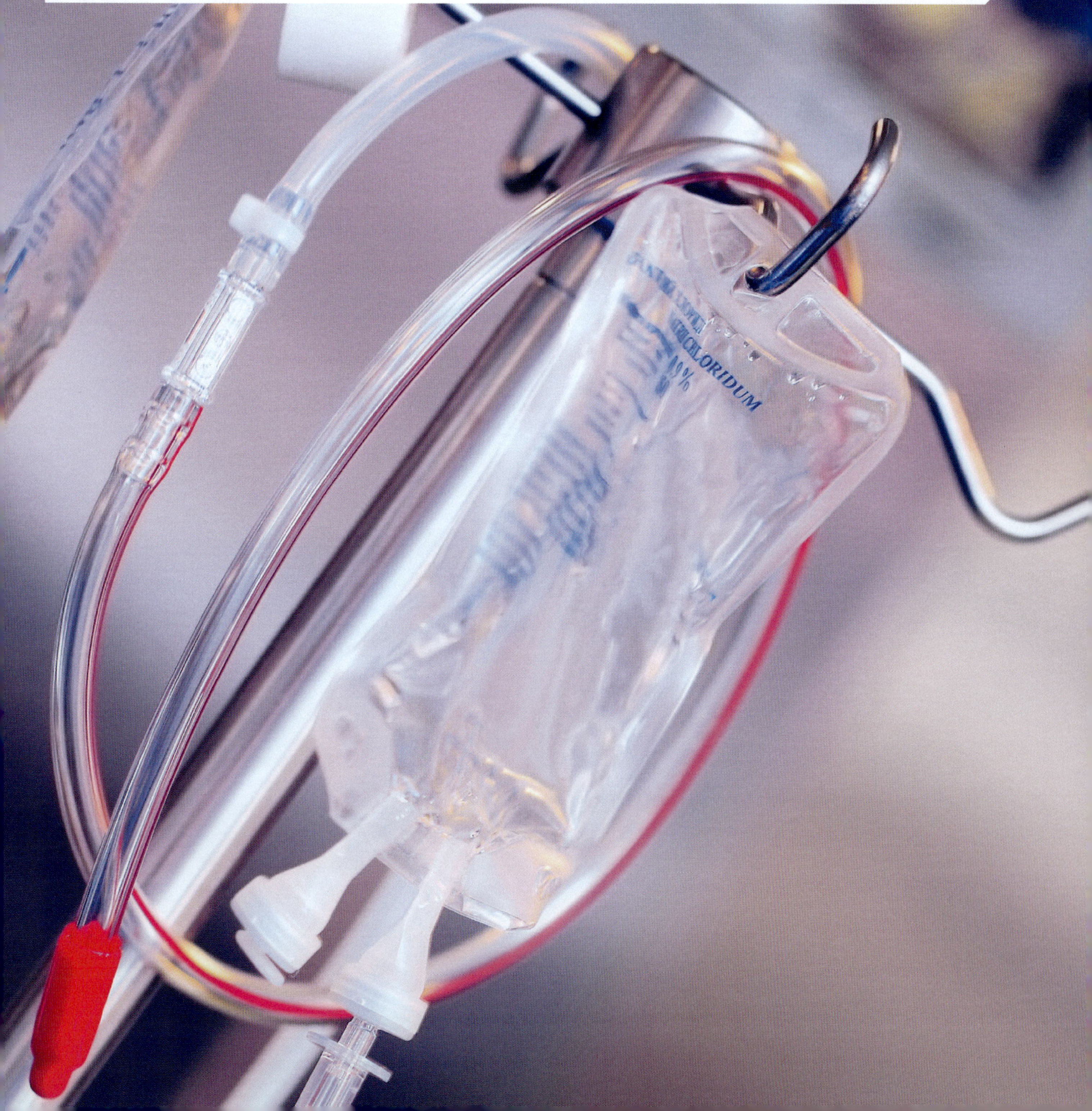

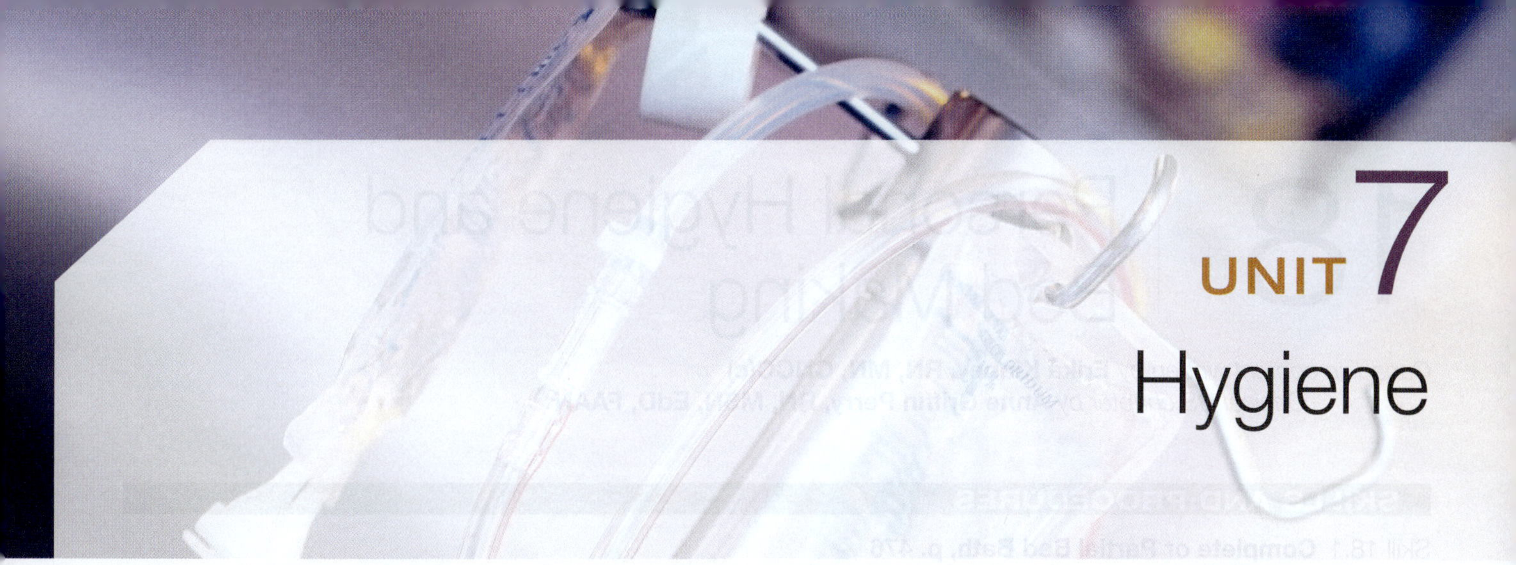

UNIT 7
Hygiene

Adequate and complete hygiene is important for a patient's health and level of comfort. Hygiene is a basic human need that requires a patient's participation whenever possible. Prior to providing any hygiene, gather complete assessment data about your patient's hygiene practices and preferences (e.g., specific products, time preferences). Recognize cultural considerations regarding personal hygiene practices or the need for gender-congruent caregivers. Asking your patients or their caregiver about hygiene practices not only promotes hygiene but also provides patient-centred care.

All of the skills associated with bathing are intimate and at times can be embarrassing for a patient. Before initiating any personal hygiene procedure, assess your patient and identify cues that indicate any embarrassment or discomfort in having someone provide this care. Take the time to explain how you will maintain patient privacy and confidentiality and why it is important that a health care provider perform this care. When you assist a patient with personal hygiene, you have the opportunity to fully assess your patient's skin, mobility, and independent functioning.

During bathing, use your clinical judgement to conduct focused skin assessments to determine any risk for or actual pressure injuries. Analyze any assessment cues to determine what skin care protocols are needed or if you need to use an employer's skin care or wound care nurse as a resource. Also focus your assessment on the patient's comfort and mobility. If the patient is in pain, administer an analgesic 20 to 30 minutes before bathing. Determine whether the patient can physically assist with bathing or whether it is difficult for them to change positions. This information will help you plan for the type of bath to provide and future position changes or transfer.

Bathing provides an opportunity to perform nail and foot care. Know what type of nail care requires a health care provider's prescription—for example, patients with diabetes mellitus and other peripheral vascular diseases. Prior to implementing any nail or foot care, use clinical judgement to assess and analyze data about any existing or at-risk nail or foot problems. Assess the skin on the feet for any pressure or tissue injuries. Identify cues, such as the inability to perceive sensation or decreased pulses, that could indicate impaired circulation, which also increases your patient's risk for skin or tissue injuries. Do not overlook cues that indicate poorly fitting shoes, such as blisters or calluses.

Oral hygiene is necessary to promote good oral health and prevent complications associated with health conditions. When you care for unconscious or debilitated patients, recognize their risk for infection and/or aspiration to guide your assessment. These patients need regular and specific oral hygiene practices. Clinical judgement will allow you to adapt a skill to meet the patient's needs. For example, if a patient cannot fully expectorate mucus from the mouth, do you offer an oral suction device that the patient can use or do you have a caregiver learn how to provide suctioning? Analyze any assessment cues to determine frequency and type of oral hygiene.

Hair care supports a patient's comfort, appearance, and sense of well-being. Prior to implementing any hair care, it is important to assess for any cultural considerations, as cutting or shaving hair may be forbidden. Assess your patient's hair and scalp or any cues that indicate a problem—for example, dandruff, head lice, or hair loss. When problems are identified, plan and implement measures to reduce or treat the problem. For example, persons with facial hair need this hair to be kept free of food and secretions. Brushing and combing a patient's hair reduces matting and tangling. Blood, dressings, and diaphoresis leave a sticky residue and oil on the hair that must be removed. Hair care interventions may seem basic, but they are very important in promoting your patient's sense of well-being.

18 Personal Hygiene and Bed Making

Canadian content written by **Erika Kinney, RN, MN, CNCC(c)**
Original US chapter by **Anne Griffin Perry, RN, MSN, EdD, FAAN**

SKILLS AND PROCEDURES

OBJECTIVES

Mastery of content in this chapter will enable the nurse to:

- Describe clinical guidelines to use for providing personal hygiene to patients.
- Identify principles of aseptic technique applied while administering a bed bath.
- Administer a complete bed bath.
- Explain precautions to take when assisting patients with a tub bath or shower.
- Explain precautions for minimizing transmission of infection during hygienic care.
- Identify clinical guidelines to follow when administering oral hygiene.
- Explain differences in providing oral hygiene for dependent patients versus unconscious patients.
- Identify clinical guidelines for administering hair, nail, and foot care.
- Comb, brush, and shampoo the hair of a bed-bound patient.
- Shave a patient safely.
- Identify risk factors for foot and nail problems.
- Safely administer nail care.
- Change the linen on an unoccupied bed and on an occupied bed.

MEDIA RESOURCES

- http://evolve.elsevier.com/Canada/Perry/clinicalskills/

PURPOSE

Hygiene is important for promoting and preserving physical and mental health. When the nurse delivers hygiene to a patient, it is an excellent time to discuss health-related concerns, perform a physical assessment, and provide patient education. Providing personal hygiene is also necessary for a person's comfort, safety, and sense of well-being.

STANDARDS OF CARE

- Accreditation Canada (2020)—*Required Organizational Practices–2020 Handbook* (https://physicians.nshealth.ca/resources/required-organizational-practices-2020-handbook)
- Alzheimer Society of Canada (ASC, 2022)—*Bathing* (https://alzheimer.ca/en/help-support/im-caring-person-living-dementia/providing-day-day-care/personal-care/bathing)
- Canadian Dental Association (CDA, n.d.-e)—*Your Oral Health* (https://www.cda-adc.ca/en/oral_health/index.asp)
- Wounds Canada (Orsted et al., 2017/2021)—*Best Practice Recommendations for the Prevention and Management of Wounds* (https://www.woundscanada.ca/docman/public/health-care-professional/165-wc-bpr-prevention-and-management-of-wounds/file)

PRINCIPLES FOR PRACTICE

- Regular bathing of all patients is essential to maintaining skin integrity by promoting circulation and hydration.

- When bathing people with dementia, it is important to balance the need for patient independence and privacy with the requirement to ensure that the patient is safe (ASC, 2022; Mendes, 2018).
- When providing patient hygiene, maintain a patient's privacy and comfort and encourage patients to participate in their hygiene care.
- Bathing the patient is an excellent opportunity to perform a complete skin assessment.

PERSON-CENTRED CARE

- As a nurse, always convey sensitivity and respect for a patient's cultural beliefs and habits in the way you provide hygiene. For example, some cultures value female modesty, and the patient or family may therefore request caregivers of the same gender (Giger & Haddad, 2021).
- Skin problems cause changes that affect a patient's appearance and body image. Be sensitive to a patient's feelings while caring for skin problems.
- Determine whether a patient's ethnicity requires that certain customs be followed when providing personal hygiene.
- Be sure to take each patient's preferences into consideration when providing hygiene. Simply asking patients about their preferences (e.g., products to use, best time to perform aspects of hygiene) can create a more trusting and nurturing environment.
- Be aware of cultural considerations and assess the patient's self-care ability in order to provide culturally sensitive, person-centred care.
- By recognizing and understanding distressed behaviours, the nurse can preserve patient dignity and maintain safety while bathing patients with dementia (Mendes, 2018). Shifting the focus of care from the tasks of bathing to the needs and abilities of the patient helps promote person-centred care, can minimize apprehension, and makes the bathing experience as pleasant as possible for the patient (ASC, 2022).

EVIDENCE-INFORMED PRACTICE

- Recent evidence supports the use of daily bathing with chlorhexidine gluconate (CHG) to reduce the rate of health care–associated infections (HAIs), including central line–associated bloodstream infections (CLABSIs) (Gall et al., 2020; Musuuza et al., 2019).
- Results from multiple studies conducted in various settings (long-term care, critical care units, and noncritical care units) support daily bathing with 2 to 4% CHG bathing solutions (as prepackaged cloths or liquid CHG soap in water) because it substantially reduces colonization and bloodstream HAIs, including methicillin-resistant *Staphylococcus aureus* (MRSA) and vancomycin-resistant *enterococci* (VRE) infections (Frost et al., 2018; Gall et al., 2020; Huang et al., 2019).
- CHG bathing products are also used as preoperative or preprocedure skin preparations in many facilities to reduce the incidence of surgical site infections (SSIs) (Tingley & Lê, 2021).
- If using liquid CHG soap in bath water, it is important to reserve a bath basin for bathing only and not for storage. The use of CHG solutions should be avoided in patients with a CHG allergy and for bathing above the jawline or on skin that is broken (Agency for Healthcare Research and Quality [AHRQ], 2022).

SAFETY GUIDELINES

- Patients who are totally dependent on someone else require help with personal hygiene or must learn or adapt to new hygiene techniques. When providing personal hygiene, important safety principles to follow are prevention of infection and of patient injury.
- Keep all items for personal care and hygiene within a patient's reach. When the head of the bed is raised, the bedside stand is usually not within easy reach and must be moved forward. If a patient must leave the bed to go to the bathroom, be sure that there is a clear pathway to prevent falls.
- Use clean gloves when you anticipate contact with nonintact skin or mucous membranes or when there is or may likely be contact with drainage, secretions, excretions, or blood. Additional precautions requiring other personal protective equipment (PPE) may be necessary, depending on the patient's condition (see Chapter 5).
- To reduce the risk of infection, always perform hygiene measures moving from most clean to least clean or dirty areas. This often requires a change of gloves and performing hand hygiene during care activities.
- When using water or solutions for hygiene care, be sure to test the solution temperature to prevent burn injury. This is especially important for patients with reduced sensation, such as those with diabetes mellitus, peripheral neuropathy, or spinal cord injury. It is also important for patients who are unable to communicate.
- To avoid injury when performing hygiene care, use principles of body mechanics and safe patient handling (see Chapter 11), and assess the patient's ability to participate in care by using an appropriate assessment tool (e.g., Mini-Mental State Examination [MMSE], Barthel ADL Index, Functional Independence Measure).
- The nurse is responsible and accountable for assessing and evaluating a patient before and after care to detect unexpected outcomes and to give proper direction to unregulated care providers (UCPs) when delegating hygiene care.
- Monitor laboratory findings such as coagulation studies before administering oral care to prevent bleeding.

THE SKIN

The skin is the largest organ in the human body; it protects the body from heat, light, injury, and infection. It serves to (1) help regulate body temperature; (2) store water, vitamin D, and fat; (3) help sense pain and other stimuli; and (4) prevent the entry of bacteria. Three primary layers make up the skin: the epidermis, dermis, and subcutaneous tissue. The skin covers the entire surface of the body and is continuous with the mucous membranes of the mouth, eyes, ears, nose, vagina, and rectum. Thorough hygiene is essential to maintain the integrity and function of each skin layer.

The epidermis, or outer skin layer, is the first line of defence against external injury and infection. Sebum, an oily substance secreted from sebaceous glands in the hair follicles, provides an acidic coating. This acidic coating protects the epidermis against penetration by chemicals and microorganisms. It also minimizes loss of water and plasma proteins.

Two types of sweat glands, the eccrine and apocrine glands, are distributed over the surface of the skin. Eccrine glands secrete a watery fluid (sweat) that helps control temperature through evaporation. The apocrine glands secrete sweat in the axillary and genital areas. Bacterial decomposition of sweat from the apocrine glands is what produces body odour.

The subcutaneous tissue layer contains blood vessels, nerves, lymph tissue, and loose connective tissue filled with fat cells. Fatty tissue insulates the body. Subcutaneous tissue also provides support for upper skin layers.

Bacteria reside on the outer surface of the skin. Rather than causing disease, these resident bacteria are normal flora that prevent disease-causing microorganisms from reproducing. Because certain areas of the skin are regularly exposed to environmental irritants and the skin is an active immune organ sensitive to physiological changes in the body, some skin problems commonly occur (Table 18.1).

THE MOUTH

The oral cavity, which is lined with a normally moist and intact light pink mucous membrane, contains the teeth and gums. The membranous lining protects underlying organs; secretes mucus to keep the oral cavity lubricated; and absorbs water, salts, and other solutes.

TABLE 18.1
Common Skin Problems

Problem	Characteristics	Implications	Interventions
Dry skin 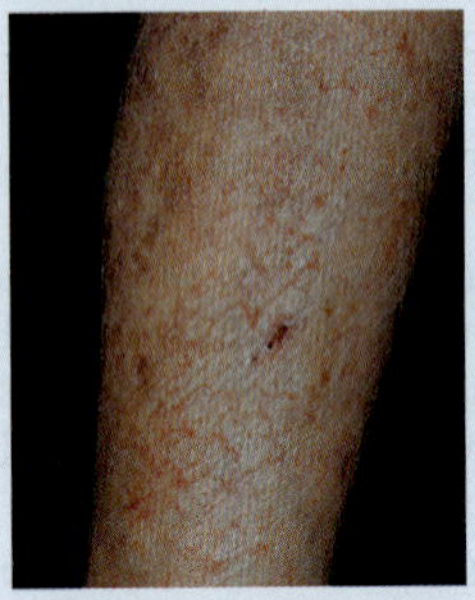	Flaky, rough texture caused by lack of moisture in outer stratum corneum, resulting in less pliable epidermis; most common on anterior surfaces of lower legs, knees, elbows, and backs of hands	Skin may crack, bleed, and become inflamed. As a result, redness, pruritus, and discomfort may develop.	Effective treatment of dry skin involves bathing with warm, not hot, water and use of moisturizers (nonpetroleum), rather than limiting frequency of bathing. Use super-fatted soap (e.g., Dove) for cleaning. Rinse body thoroughly of all soap because residue left can cause irritation and breakdown. Add moisture to air using humidifier. Increase fluid intake when skin is dry.
Acne 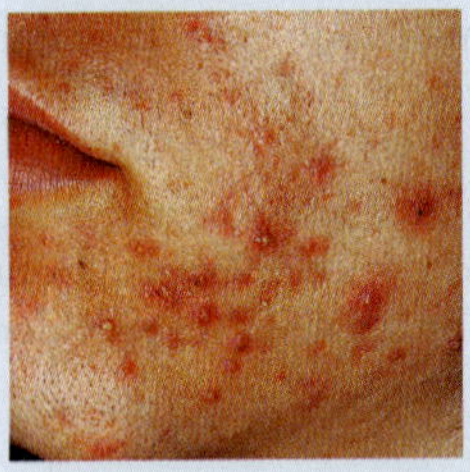 *(From James, W. D., et al. [2007]. Andrew's diseases of the skin: Clinical dermatology [10th ed.]. Saunders.)*	Inflammatory, papulopustular skin eruption, usually involving bacterial breakdown of sebum; appears on face, neck, shoulders, and back	Infected material within pustule can spread if area is squeezed or picked. Permanent scarring can result.	Wash hair and skin each day with warm water and soap to remove oil. Use cosmetics sparingly because oily cosmetics or creams accumulate in pores and tend to make condition worse. Implement necessary dietary restrictions by eliminating foods found to aggravate condition. Use prescribed topical antibiotics for severe acne.
Hirsutism 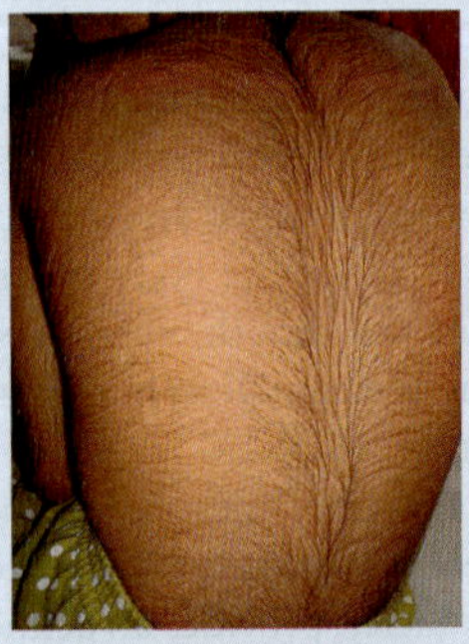 *(From Goyal, D., et al. [2010]. Coffin–Siris syndrome with Mayer–Rokitansky–Küster–Hauser syndrome: A case report. Journal of Medical Case Reports, 4, 354.)*	Excessive growth of body and facial hair	May cause negative body image.	Shaving is safest method to remove hair. Electrolysis and laser permanently remove hair. Tweezing and bleaching are temporary.
Skin rashes 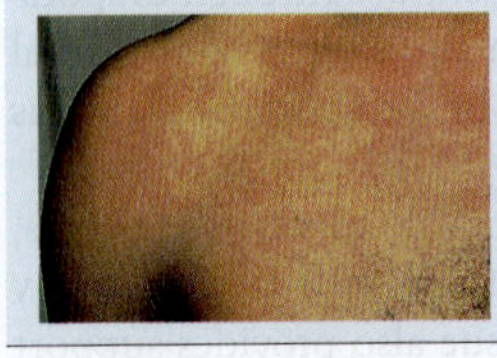	Skin eruption that results from overexposure to sun or moisture or from allergic reaction; may be flat or raised, localized or systemic, pruritic or nonpruritic	If skin is continually scratched, inflammation and infection may occur. Rashes also cause discomfort.	Wash area thoroughly and apply antiseptic spray or lotion to prevent further itching and aid healing process. Warm or cold soaks may relieve inflammation.

TABLE 18.1

Common Skin Problems—cont'd

Problem	Characteristics	Implications	Interventions
Contact dermatitis 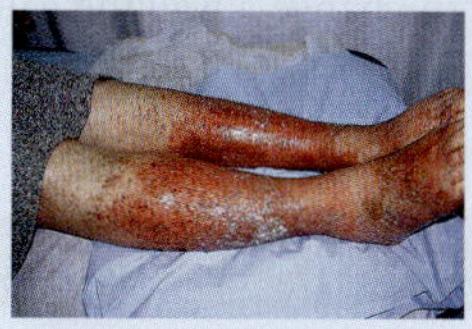 *(From Lewis, S. L., et al. [2011]. Medical-surgical nursing: Assessment and management of clinical problems [8th ed.]. Mosby.)*	Acute or chronic eczematous rash characterized by abrupt onset with well-defined geometric margins of erythema, pruritus, pain, and appearance of scaly, oozing lesions; appears on head, neck, scalp, hands, legs, dorsum of feet, and trunk	Dermatitis is often difficult to eliminate because the person is usually in continual contact with substance causing skin reaction. Substance may be hard to identify.	Identify and avoid contributing agents (e.g., cleaners, poison ivy or poison oak, cosmetics, latex, shoes/rubber). Treatment consists of removing contributing agent, if identified, and applying over-the-counter topical steroids or calamine lotion. In some cases, steroids may be prescribed. Tepid baths may also provide relief.
Abrasion 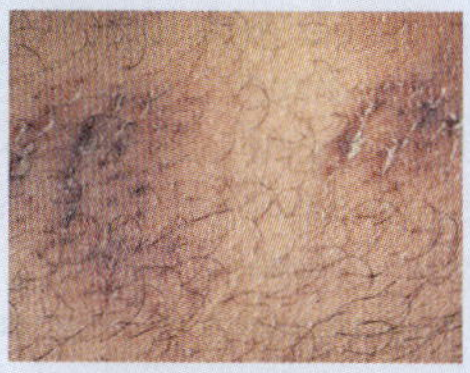 *(From Cottran, S. R., et al. From the teaching collection of the Department of Dermatology, University of Texas, Southwestern Medical School, Dallas, TX.)*	Scraping or rubbing away of epidermis may result in localized bleeding and later weeping of serous fluid	Infection occurs easily as result of loss of protective skin layer.	Nurses should keep nails short and not wear jewellery when providing care to avoid patient injury. Wash abrasions with mild soap and water. Dressing or bandage could increase risk for infection because of retained moisture.

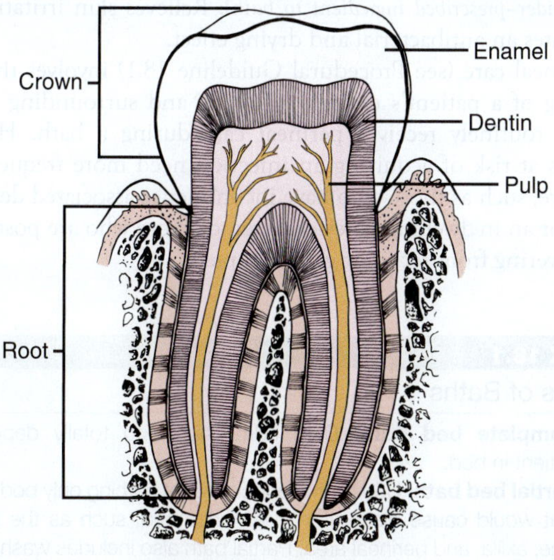

FIG 18.1 Normal tooth.

Saliva, a clear viscous fluid secreted by the mucous and salivary glands of the mouth, helps to prevent dental caries and plaque formation and lubricates the oral cavity. Lubrication of the oral cavity aids in chewing and swallowing. Saliva provides a means for removing cellular and bacterial debris that can cause infection, particularly fungal infection (Marques et al., 2021). Hyposalivation results in dry mouth, or xerostomia, and affects taste, swallowing, digestion, nutrition, and denture fit (Marques et al., 2021).

The teeth are organs of chewing (i.e., mastication). Dentin, a hard, ivory-like substance that surrounds the pulp cavity, forms the major part of a tooth (Fig. 18.1). A layer of enamel, visible in the oral cavity, covers the upper part of the tooth, or crown. The periodontal membrane, just below the gum margins, surrounds the tooth root and holds it firmly in place. A tooth receives its blood, lymph, and nerve supply from the base of the tooth socket within the jaw. Healthy teeth are smooth, shiny, and properly aligned.

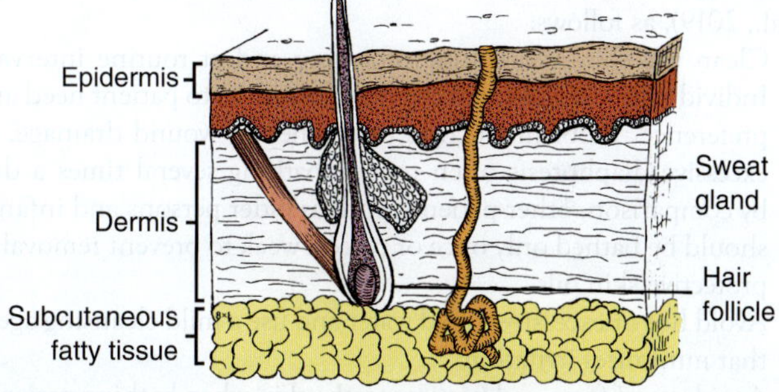

FIG 18.2 Cross-section of hair follicle and supporting structures.

The gums, or gingivae, are mucous membranes with underlying supportive fibrous tissue. They encircle the necks of erupted teeth to hold them firmly in place. The gums normally are pink, moist, firm, and relatively inelastic.

EYES, EARS, AND HAIR

Hair grows from follicles located within the dermis of the skin (Fig. 18.2). Tiny blood vessels supply nourishment for each follicle for normal hair growth. Each hair has a shaft extending from the follicle. A sebaceous gland inside each follicle secretes sebum, an oily substance that lubricates the hair and scalp. The hair shaft is normally shiny and pliant and is not excessively oily, dry, or brittle. The primary function of hair is to act as the first line of protection. For example, hair protects the scalp from injury. Eyebrows and eyelashes protect the eyes from foreign particles. Personal hygiene related to the eyes and ears is covered in Chapter 19.

Special hair-care practices focus on caring for the scalp, axilla, and pubic areas. Hair growth, distribution, and pattern are indicators of a person's health status. Hormonal changes, emotional and physical stress, aging, intake of toxins (e.g., arsenic, cocaine), gender, ethnicity, nutrition, infection, and certain diseases affect hair characteristics. A person's appearance and sense of well-being often depend on the way the hair looks and feels. Illness or disability sometimes prevents patients from maintaining daily hair care.

THE NAILS

The nails are epithelial tissues that grow from the root of the nail bed, located in the skin at the nail groove. A normal, healthy nail is transparent, smooth, and convex, with a pink nail bed and translucent white tip. A normal colour indicates adequate oxygenation to peripheral tissues. Pigment deposits or bands are common in the nail beds of patients with dark skin. The feet and nails require special care to prevent infection, odour, and injury. Problems typically result from abuse or poor care. Foot pain can often change a walking gait, causing strain on different muscle groups.

✦ SKILL 18.1 Complete or Partial Bed Bath

Video Clip

Bathing removes sweat, oil, dirt, and microorganisms from the skin. It also stimulates circulation and provides a refreshed and relaxed feeling. For some patients, a bath is a time for socialization and pleasure, especially for those who are bedridden or seriously disabled. It is important to encourage patients to actively participate in bathing, while being mindful of any limitations they may have and ensuring a safe environment (see Chapter 14).

Wound Care Canada highlights the importance of skin care in the prevention and management of pressure injuries and the essential role of interprofessional collaboration in maintaining skin integrity (Orsted et al., 2017/2021). The National Pressure Injury Advisory Panel (NPIAP), the European Pressure Ulcer Advisory Panel (EPUAP), and the Pan Pacific Pressure Injury Alliance (PPPIA) provide clinical practice guidelines with evidence-informed recommendations for the prevention and treatment of pressure injuries, including sound principles for good bathing techniques (EPUAP et al., 2019), as follows:

- Clean the skin at the time of soiling and at routine intervals. Individualize frequency of cleaning according to patient need and preference. Problems such as incontinence, wound drainage, or excessive diaphoresis often require bathing several times a day; by comparison, other patients, such as older persons and infants, should be bathed only once or twice a week to prevent removal of protective skin oils.
- Avoid hot or excessively cold water and use a mild cleansing agent that minimizes irritation.
- Avoid use of force and friction on the skin when bathing patients. Do not massage reddened areas, especially over bony prominences, because this can promote pressure injury formation.
- Minimize environmental factors that lead to skin drying, such as low humidity (<40%) and exposure to cold. Depending on a patient's age and physical condition, maintain room temperature between 20 and 23°C. Infants, older persons, and acutely ill patients may need a warmer temperature. However, certain critically ill patients require cooler room temperatures to lower the metabolic demands of the body. Controlling drafts and eliminating lingering odours from draining wounds, vomitus, bedpans, or urinals also improve a patient's comfort.
- Use bathing as a time to interact with and assess a patient. When giving a complete bath, perform a physical assessment of all body systems and discuss issues of concern for a patient.
- During bathing, help patients through normal joint range-of-motion (ROM) exercises to promote circulation and joint integrity.
- For patients who tire easily, consider giving a partial instead of complete bed bath.
- There are two categories of baths: cleansing and therapeutic. Cleansing baths include the bed bath, tub bath, sponge bath at the sink, shower, and prepackaged disposable bed bath (Box 18.1). The type of cleansing bath to use depends on the assessment of a patient's physical capabilities and the degree of hygiene required. When a person is unable to perform personal care because of illness or disability, the nurse is responsible for helping with bathing. The nurse can also clean and groom the patient's hair, shave a patient, and clean the nails during or immediately after a bath.

Health care providers generally prescribe therapeutic baths for a specific effect, such as soothing the skin or promoting the healing process. Types of therapeutic baths include the following:

- *Sitz bath:* Cleans and reduces pain and inflammation of perineal and anal areas. Used for patients who have undergone rectal or perineal surgery or childbirth or who have local irritation from hemorrhoids or fissures. Patient sits in a special tub or basin (see Chapter 41).
- *Medicated bath (addition of over-the-counter, herbal, or health care provider–prescribed ingredient to bath):* Relieves skin irritation and creates an antibacterial and drying effect.

Perineal care (see Procedural Guideline 18.1) involves thorough cleaning of a patient's external genitalia and surrounding skin. A patient routinely receives perineal care during a bath. However, patients at risk of acquiring an infection need more frequent perineal care, such as those who have incontinence-associated dermatitis (IAD) or an in-dwelling Foley catheter, or those who are postpartum or recovering from rectal or genital surgery.

BOX 18.1

Types of Baths

- **Complete bed bath:** Bath administered to totally dependent patient in bed.
- **Partial bed bath:** Bed bath that consists of bathing only body parts that would cause discomfort if left unbathed, such as the hands, face, axilla, and perineal area. Partial bath also includes washing the back and providing a back rub. Partial bed bath is administered to dependent patients in need of partial hygiene or self-sufficient bedridden patients who are unable to reach all body parts.
- **Sponge bath at the sink:** Involves bathing from a bath basin or sink, with patient sitting in a chair. The patient is able to perform part of the bath independently. The nurse helps with hard-to-reach areas.
- **Tub bath:** Involves immersion in a tub of water, which allows more thorough washing and rinsing than a bed bath. Patients may require nurse's help. Some facilities have tubs equipped with lifting devices that facilitate positioning dependent patients in the tub.
- **Shower:** Patient sits or stands under a continuous stream of water. The shower provides more thorough cleaning than a bed bath but can be tiring.
- **Disposable bed bath/travel bath:** The bag bath contains several soft, nonwoven cotton cloths that are premoistened in no-rinse solution and heated before use. The bag bath offers an alternative because of the ease of use, reduced time bathing, and patient comfort (Matsumoto et al., 2019).

Delegation and Collaboration

The skill of assessing a patient's skin, pain level, and ROM cannot be delegated to an unregulated care provider (UCP). Bathing is a fundamental nursing skill and the responsibility of a registered nurse (RN) or licensed/registered practical nurse (LPN/RPN) and provides many opportunities for patient assessment. This skill may be delegated to a UCP. The nurse instructs the UCP about the following:

- Not massaging reddened skin areas during bathing
- Contraindications to soaking a patient's feet
- Reporting any signs of impaired skin integrity to the nurse
- Proper ways to position patients with musculoskeletal limitations or an in-dwelling Foley catheter or other equipment (e.g., intravenous [IV] tubing)

Collaborate with interprofessional health care team members (e.g., wound care nurse) to identify specific bathing and skin care interventions when patients have a pressure injury or are at increased risk for a pressure injury from reduced mobility and sensation, poor nutrition, or medical devices (see Chapters 39 and 40).

Equipment

- Washcloths and bath towels
- Bath blanket
- Bar or liquid soap, or 120 mL bottle of 4% CHG (dispensed in a single bath-sized bottle)
- Toiletry items (deodorant, lotion)
- Disposable wipes
- Warm water
- Clean hospital gown or patient's own pyjamas or gown
- Laundry bag
- Clean gloves
- Wash basin
- Eye patch/shield and nonallergenic tape (for unconscious patient)

STEP	RATIONALE
ASSESSMENT	
1. Identify patient using at least two person-specific identifiers (e.g., name and date of birth, or name and medical record number) according to employer policy.	Ensures correct patient. Complies with Accreditation Canada's standards and improves patient safety (Accreditation Canada, 2020).
2. Throughout the procedure, the 4 moments for hand hygiene are to be implemented; hand hygiene should occur before initial patient (or patient environment) contact, before an aseptic procedure, after body fluid exposure risk, and after patient (or patient environment) contact. Additional hand hygiene should be performed when hands are visibly soiled.	Proper hand hygiene helps prevent the spread of infectious agents to health care providers.
3. Assess room environment for safety (e.g., check room for spills; make sure that equipment is working properly; and ensure that bed is in locked, low position).	Identifies safety hazards in patient environment that could cause or potentially lead to harm (LeLaurin & Shorr, 2019).
4. Assess patient's fall risk status (if partial bathing out of bed or self-bath is to be performed) (see Chapter 14).	Allows for anticipation of needed precautions, such as having patient sit on chair in front of basin.
5. Assess patient's tolerance for bathing: activity tolerance, comfort level, musculoskeletal function, and presence of shortness of breath.	Determines patient's ability to perform or tolerate bathing and type of bath to administer (e.g., tub bath, bed bath).
6. Assess patient's cognitive and functional status using appropriate tools to assess self-care ability. For patients with suspected dementia, observe behaviour and any signs of distress, especially after telling patient it is bath time.	Functional status assesses a patient's capacity for self-bathing and how much supervision or help is needed to accomplish activities of daily living (ADLs). Every attempt should be made to avoid bathing people against their will (ASC, 2022).

Critical Decision Point *Patients with dementia may become agitated. Observe for behaviours such as restlessness, yelling, and fighting with caregivers.*

STEP	RATIONALE
7. Assess patient's visual status, ability to sit without support, hand grasp, and ROM of extremities (see Chapter 8).	Further determines degree of help needed for bathing.
8. Assess for presence and position of external medical device or equipment (e.g., IV line or oxygen tubing).	Affects how the patient will be positioned and aids in planning bathing activities.
9. Assess patient's usual bathing routine. How often does the person bathe? Do they usually shower or bath? What time of day? Does the person use any special products, robes, towels, or equipment during bathing (e.g., scented soaps, music, back brush, or sponge) to make the experience more enjoyable? Is the person concerned about loss of privacy?	Demonstrates person-centred care and encourages patient to participate in self-care. Promotes patient's comfort and willingness to cooperate. Using a patient's established routine may reduce agitation in a patient with dementia.
10. Ask if patient has noticed any problems related to condition of skin and genitalia.	Provides information to direct physical assessment of skin and genitalia during bathing. Also influences selection of skin care products.
11. Before or during bath, assess condition of patient's skin. Note presence of dryness (indicated by flaking, redness, scaling, and cracking), excessive moisture, inflammation, or pressure injuries (see Chapter 39).	Provides baseline for comparison of skin integrity over time.

STEP	RATIONALE
ASSESSMENT	
12. Identify risks for skin impairment: older age, immobilization, reduced sensation, nutrition and hydration, excessive skin moisture or drainage, shear or friction on skin, vascular insufficiencies, presence of external devices. *Option:* Use a pressure injury assessment tool (e.g., Braden Scale; see Chapter 39).	Risk factors increase the likelihood of injury to the skin because of pressure, impaired tissue synthesis, softening of or friction on tissues, and impaired circulation.
13. Assess patient's comfort using an appropriate pain assessment scale (e.g., 0–10 pain scale).	Bath can soothe and comfort patient. Provides baseline measure.
14. Assess patient's knowledge and perceptions of the importance of skin hygiene, preventive measures to take, and common skin problems encountered (see Table 18.1).	Determines patient's willingness to learn and type of instruction required.
15. Review medical record for prescriptions for specific precautions concerning patient's movement or positioning and whether there is a prescription for a therapeutic bath. Note and confirm with patient any allergies or sensitivities to bath products.	Prevents accidental injury to patient during bathing activities. Determines level of help that patient needs. Prevents allergic reactions to hygiene products during bathing.

NURSING DIAGNOSES

- Bathing/self-care deficit
- Reduced stamina
- Reduced physical mobility
- Reduced skin integrity
- Inadequate knowledge regarding skin care
- Potential for impaired skin integrity
- Potential for infection

Related factors are individualized on the basis of patient's condition or needs.

STEP	RATIONALE
PLANNING	
1. Expected outcomes following completion of procedure:	
• Skin is free of excretions, drainage, or odour.	Skin is clean.
• Skin shows decreased redness, cracking, flaking, and scaling.	Indicates reduction in skin dryness.
• Joint ROM remains same or improves from previous measurement.	Repeated ROM exercise during bathing helps prevent contractures and promotes joint movement.
• Patient expresses sense of comfort and relaxation.	Bath relaxes patient and removes sources of discomfort.
• Patient tolerates bath without fatigue or chilling.	Fatigue during bathing indicates worsening of chronic cardiopulmonary conditions.
• Patient describes benefits and techniques of proper hygiene and skin care.	Demonstrates learning with ability to repeat back to demonstrate understanding.
2. Explain procedure and ask patient for suggestions on how to prepare supplies. If partial bath, ask how much of bath patient wishes to complete.	Promotes patient's cooperation, participation, and promotion of self-care as appropriate.
3. Adjust room temperature and ventilation, close room doors and windows, and draw room divider curtain.	Warm room that is free of drafts prevents rapid loss of body heat during bathing. Privacy provides for patient's mental and physical comfort.
4. Prepare equipment and place supplies on bedside table. If it is necessary to leave room, be sure that call light is within patient's reach, bed is in low position, and wheels are locked.	Avoids interrupting procedure or leaving patient unattended to retrieve missing equipment. Provides for patient safety.

Critical Decision Point *Never leave the bedside without ensuring that the appropriate number of side rails have been raised (see employer policy). The number of side rails depends on the patient's fall risk assessment; however, having all side rails raised may be considered a restraint if the patient is unable to lower the rail.*

STEP	RATIONALE
IMPLEMENTATION	
1. Offer patient bedpan or urinal. Apply clean gloves to help patient as needed. Provide toilet tissue and dispose of any excrement properly. Dispose of gloves. Provide patient towel and moist washcloth.	Patient feels more comfortable after voiding. Reduces transmission of microorganisms. Prevents interruption of bath.
2. If patient has nonintact skin or skin is soiled with drainage, excretions, or body secretions, apply new pair of clean gloves before beginning bath.	Reduces transmission of microorganisms.

STEP	RATIONALE
IMPLEMENTATION	
3. Raise bed to comfortable working height. Lower side rail closest to you and help patient assume comfortable supine position, maintaining body alignment. Bring patient toward side closest to you (with patient staying supine).	Aids access to patient. Maintains patient's comfort throughout procedure. Uses proper body mechanics, thus minimizing strain on back muscles. If patient is overweight, get help from another caregiver or use lift device for positioning (see Chapter 11).
4. Place bath blanket over patient. Have patient hold top of bath blanket, and remove top sheet from under bath blanket without exposing patient. Place soiled linen in laundry bag.	Blanket provides warmth and privacy. Take care to avoid linen contacting uniform.
5. Remove patient's gown or pyjamas.	Provides full exposure of body parts during bathing.
a. If gown has snaps on sleeves, simply unsnap and remove gown without pulling IV tubing (if present).	Avoids disruption of IV therapy or IV infusion flow rate.
b. If gown has no snaps and if an extremity is *injured* or has reduced mobility, begin removal from *unaffected* side first.	Undressing unaffected side first allows easier manipulation of gown over body part with reduced ROM.
c. If patient has an IV line and gown with no snaps, remove gown from arm *without* IV line first. Then remove gown from arm with IV line (see Step 5c, illustration *A*). Pause IV fluid infusion by pressing appropriate sensor on IV pump. Remove IV tubing from pump; use regulator to slow IV infusion. Remove IV bag from pole (see Step 5c, illustration *B*) and slide IV bag and tubing through arm of patient's gown (see Step 5c, illustration *C*). Rehang IV bag (see Step 5c, illustration *D*), reconnect tubing to pump, open regulator clamp, and restart IV fluid infusion by pressing appropriate sensor on IV pump. If IV fluids are infusing by gravity, check IV flow rate and regulate if necessary. *Do not disconnect IV tubing to remove gown.*	Manipulation of IV tubing and bag can disrupt IV infusion flow rate.

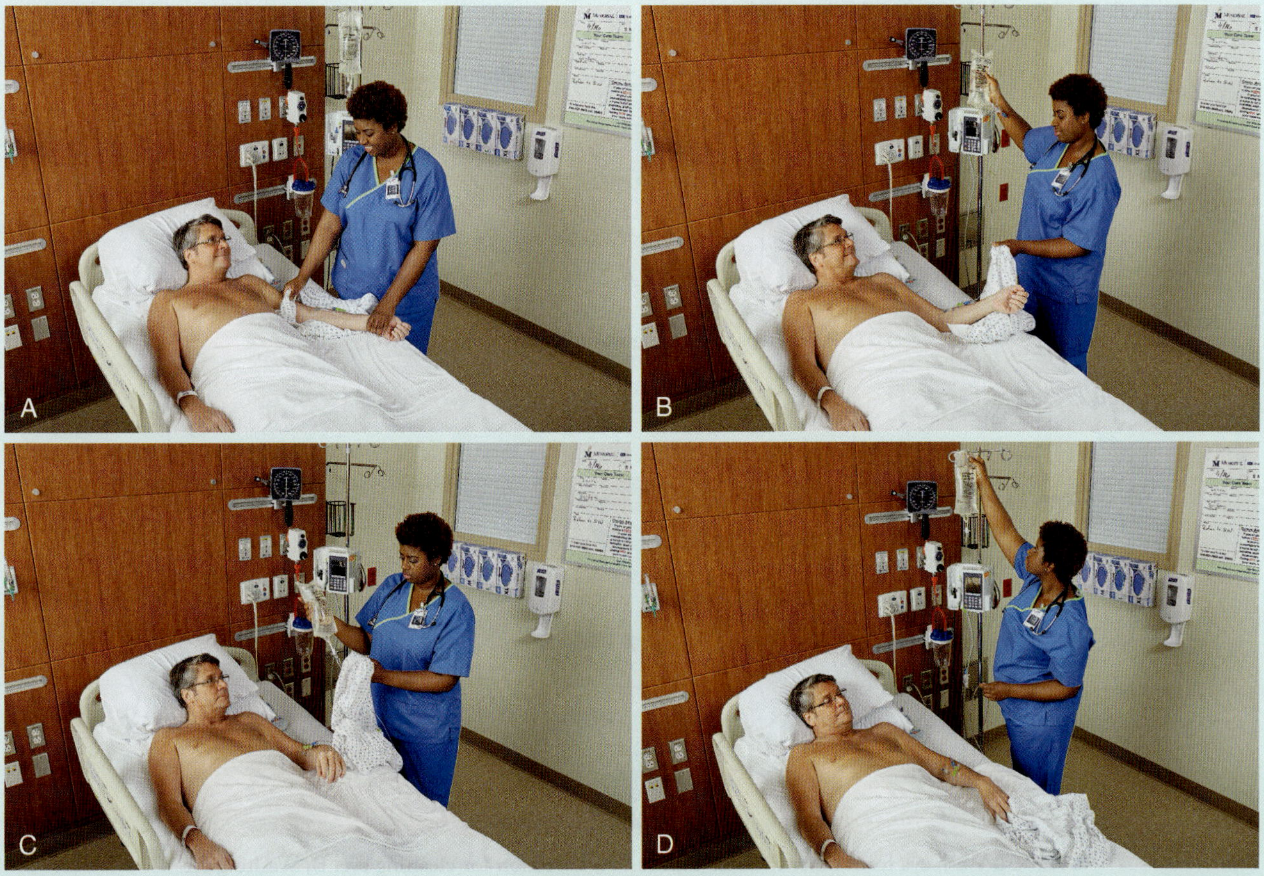

STEP 5C A, Remove patient's gown. B, Remove IV bag from pole. C, Slide IV tubing and bag through arm of patient's gown. D, Rehang IV bag.

STEP	RATIONALE
IMPLEMENTATION	
6. Raise side rail. Lower bed temporarily to lowest position and raise on return after you fill wash basin two-thirds full with warm water. Place basin along with supplies on over-bed table and position over patient's bed. Check water temperature by placing your forearm in the water, by using a handheld thermometer, or by having patient place fingers in water to ensure it is not too hot or too cool.	Raising side rail and lowering bed maintains patient's safety. Warm water promotes comfort, relaxes muscles, and prevents unnecessary chilling. Use of over-bed table allows you to move to opposite side of bed without having to move equipment. Testing water temperature prevent burns to skin.
7. Lower side rail. Remove pillow (if tolerated). Raise head of bed (HOB) 30–45 degrees if allowed. Place bath towel under patient's head. Place second bath towel over patient's chest.	Removal of pillow makes it easier to wash patient's ears and neck. Placement of towels prevents soiling of bed linen and bath blanket.
8. Wash face.	

Critical Decision Point *Do not use bath water with 4% liquid CHG added or 2% CHG bathing cloths* (see Procedural Guideline 18.2) *on the eyes or face* (AHRQ, 2022).

STEP	RATIONALE
a. Ask if patient is wearing contact lenses. You may choose to remove them at this time.	Prevents accidental injury to eyes.
b. Form a mitt with washcloth (see Step 8b illustration); immerse in water and wring thoroughly.	Mitt retains water and heat better than loosely held washcloth; keeps cold edges from brushing against patient and prevents splashing.
c. Wash patient's eyes with plain warm water, using a clean area of cloth for each eye and bathing from inner to outer canthus (see Step 8c illustrations). Soak any crusts on eyelid for 2 to 3 minutes with warm, damp cloth before attempting removal. Dry around eyes thoroughly but gently.	Soap irritates eyes. Use of separate sections of mitt reduces infection transmission. Bathing eye gently from inner to outer canthus prevents secretions from entering nasolacrimal duct. Pressure causes internal injury.

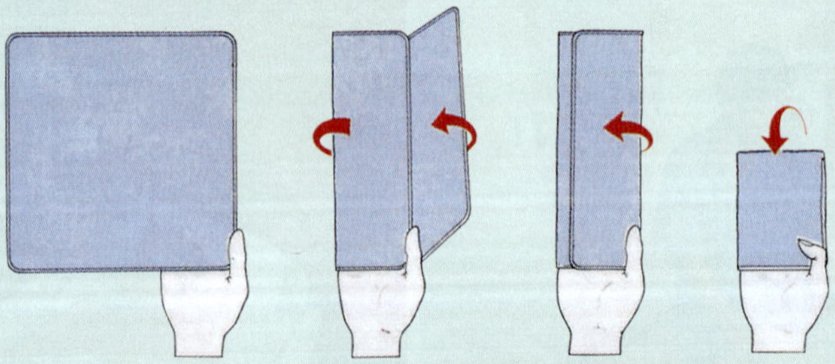

STEP 8B Steps for folding washcloth to form a mitt.

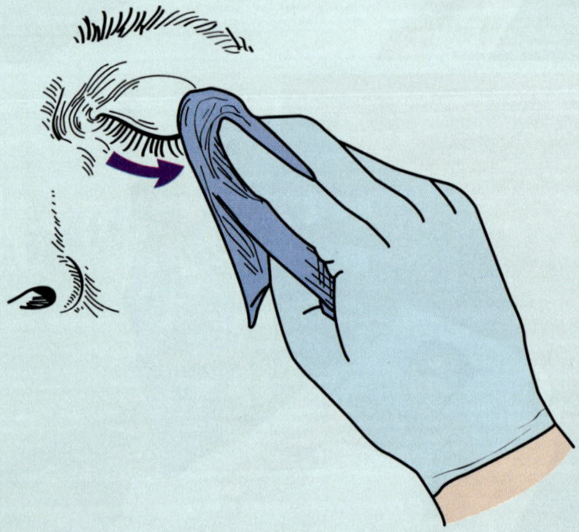

A

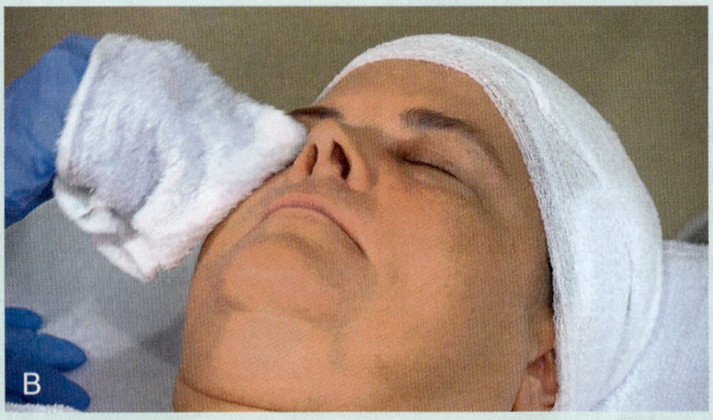

B

STEP 8C Wash eye from inner to outer canthus. A, Direction for cleaning eye. B, Washing eye from inner to outer canthus.

STEP	RATIONALE

IMPLEMENTATION

STEP	RATIONALE
d. Ask if patient prefers to use soap on face. Otherwise wash, rinse, and dry forehead, cheeks, nose, neck, and ears without using soap. Ask patients with facial hair whether they want to be shaved (see Procedural Guideline 18.4).	Soap tends to dry face, which is exposed to air more than other body parts.
e. Provide eye care for unconscious patient.	Patients who are unconscious have lost the normal protective corneal reflex of blinking, increasing the risk for corneal drying, abrasions, and eye infection.
(1) Instill eye drops or ointment per health care provider's prescription (see Chapter 19).	
(2) In the absence of blink reflex, keep eyelids closed. Close eye gently, using back of your fingertip, before placing eye patch or shield. Place tape over patch or shield. Do not tape eyelid.	When blink reflex is absent, patient loses a protective mechanism. Keeping eyelids closed maintains eye moisture and prevents injury.
9. Wash upper extremities and trunk. *Option:* Change bath water at this time. Prepare CHG bathing solution per employer policy, or use no-rinse CHG cloths.	Evidence shows that CHG use in daily bathing can reduce incidence of HAIs (Huang et al., 2019; Musuuza et al., 2019).

Critical Decision Point *When using CHG, use one washcloth or wipe for washing each major body part. Then dispose of cloth and use a new cloth for the next body part* (AHRQ, 2022). *Dipping cloth back into basin contaminates solution and makes CHG less effective. Do not rinse after bathing with CHG solution. Allow CHG to dry on the skin to achieve antimicrobial effects.*

STEP	RATIONALE
a. Remove bath blanket from patient's arm that is closest to you. Place bath towel lengthwise under arm and wash using long, firm strokes from distal to proximal (fingers to axilla).	Long, firm strokes promote venous return.
b. Raise and support arm above head (if possible) to wash axilla, rinse, and dry thoroughly (see Step 9b illustration). Apply deodorant to underarms as needed or desired.	Movement of arm exposes axilla and exercises normal ROM of joint. Deodorant controls body odour.
c. Move to other side of bed and repeat steps with other arm.	

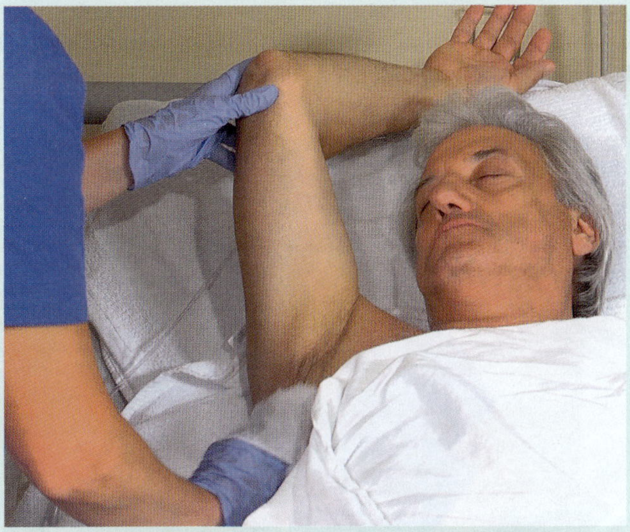

STEP 9B Position of patient's arm for washing axilla.

STEP	RATIONALE
IMPLEMENTATION	
d. Cover patient's chest with bath towel and fold bath blanket down to umbilicus. Bathe chest with long, firm strokes. If patient has breasts, take special care when bathing skin under patient's breasts, lifting upward if necessary while bathing underneath breast. Rinse if using soap and water and dry well.	Draping prevents unnecessary exposure of body parts. Towel maintains warmth and privacy. Secretions and dirt collect easily in areas of tight skinfolds. Skin under breasts is vulnerable to excoriation if not kept clean and dry.
10. Wash hands and nails.	
a. Fold bath towel in half and lay it on bed beside patient. Place basin on towel. Immerse patient's hand in water. Allow hand to soak for 3–5 minutes before cleaning fingernails (see Skill 18.4). Remove basin and dry hand well. Repeat for other hand. **Note:** Do not soak fingers of patients who have diabetes mellitus.	Soaking softens cuticles and calluses of hand, loosens debris beneath nails, and enhances feeling of cleanliness. Thorough drying removes moisture from between fingers. Soaking hands of patient with diabetes mellitus can lead to maceration and increase risk for infection.
11. Check temperature of bath water and change water if necessary; otherwise continue.	Warm water maintains patient's comfort.

Critical Decision Point *If using CHG solution in bath water, do not discard water. One bottle of CHG soap is sufficient for a complete bath.*

STEP	RATIONALE
12. Wash abdomen.	
a. Place bath towel lengthwise over chest and abdomen. (You may need two towels.) Fold bath blanket down to just above pubic region. Bathe, rinse, and dry abdomen with special attention to umbilicus and skinfolds of abdomen and groin. Keep abdomen covered between washing and rinsing. Dry well.	Keeping skinfolds clean and dry helps prevent odour and skin irritation. Moisture and sediment that collects in skinfolds predispose skin to maceration.
b. Apply clean gown or pyjama top by dressing affected side first. *Option:* You may omit this step until completion of bath.	Maintains patient's warmth and comfort. Allows easier manipulation of gown over body part with reduced ROM.

Critical Decision Point *If one extremity is injured or immobilized, always dress affected side first.*

STEP	RATIONALE
13. Wash lower extremities.	
a. Cover chest and abdomen with top of bath blanket. Expose near leg by folding blanket toward midline. Be sure that other leg and perineum remain draped. Place bath towel under leg as you support patient's knee and ankle.	Prevents overexposure. Method of placement supports patient's joint.
b. Wash leg using long, firm strokes from ankle to knee and knee to thigh (see Step 13b illustration). Assess condition of extremities.	Promotes circulation and venous return. Assessment is key to identifying signs and symptoms of venous thrombosis.

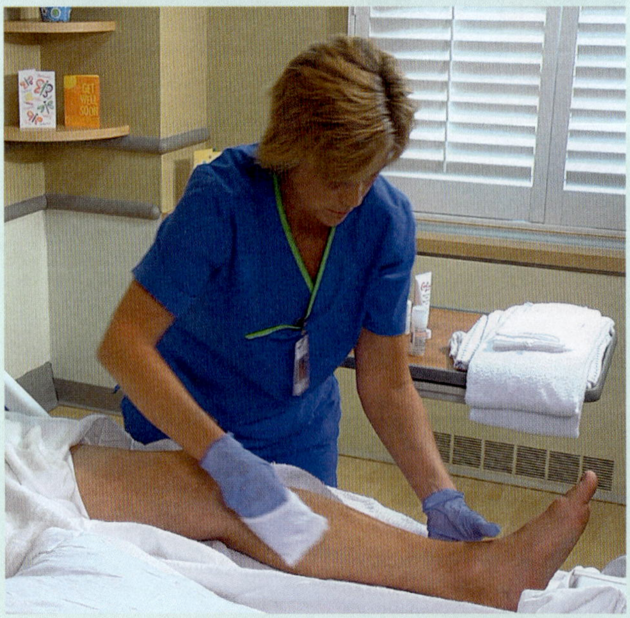

STEP 13B Washing patient's leg.

STEP	RATIONALE

IMPLEMENTATION

Critical Decision Point *During the bath, assess for signs of warmth, redness, swelling, tenderness, and pain in the lower extremities because these might be early signs of a venous thromboembolism (VTE).*

STEP	RATIONALE
c. Clean foot, making sure to bathe between toes. Dry toes and feet completely.	Secretions and moisture are often present between toes, predisposing patient to maceration and skin breakdown.
d. Raise side rail; remove towel; move to opposite side of bed, lower side rail, place dry towel under second leg, and repeat Steps 13b and 13c for other leg and foot. Apply a light layer of moisturizing lotion to both feet; avoid leaving excess lotion between toes. When finished, remove used towel.	Moisturizers are effective in reducing dry skin; however, in excess they can cause maceration.
e. Cover patient with bath blanket, raise side rail, and change bath water (if using plain soap and water).	Decreased bath water temperature causes chilling. Clean water reduces transmission of microorganisms.
14. Wash back.	
a. Apply clean gloves (if not already applied). Lower side rail. Help patient assume prone or side-lying position, using safe patient-handling techniques (see Chapter 11) (as applicable). Place towel lengthwise along patient's side.	Reduces transmission of microorganisms. Exposes back and buttocks for bathing.
b. If fecal material is present, enclose in fold of underpad or toilet tissue and remove with disposable wipes.	Skinfolds near buttocks and anus may contain fecal secretions and microorganisms.
c. Keep patient draped by sliding bath blanket over shoulders and thighs during bathing. Wash, rinse, and dry back from neck to buttocks with long, firm strokes. Pay special attention to folds of buttocks and anus.	Maintains warmth and prevents unnecessary exposure.
d. Clean buttocks and anus, washing front to back (see Step 14d illustration). Clean, rinse, and dry area thoroughly. If needed, place clean, absorbent pad under patient's buttocks.	Cleaning buttocks after back prevents contamination of water.
15. While patient is supine, provide perineal care (see Procedural Guideline 18.1).	

Critical Decision Point *At end of bath, skin may feel sticky for a few minutes. Do NOT wipe off. Allow skin to air dry* (AHRQ, 2022).

STEP	RATIONALE
16. Massage back if patient desires.	Promotes patient relaxation.
17. Clean and file nails as needed (check employer policy) (see Skill 18.4).	
18. Apply body lotion to skin and topical moisturizing agents to dry, flaky, reddened, or scaling areas. NOTE: If using CHG solution for bathing, only use a product compatible with CHG (AHRQ, 2022).	Dry skin results in reduced pliability and cracking. Moisturizers help prevent skin breakdown.

Critical Decision Point *Massage is contraindicated in the presence of acute inflammation, over bony prominences, and where there is the possibility of damaged blood vessels or fragile skin* (EPUAP et al., 2019). *Massage of the legs is also contraindicated because of the possible presence of a blood clot, which could become dislodged.*

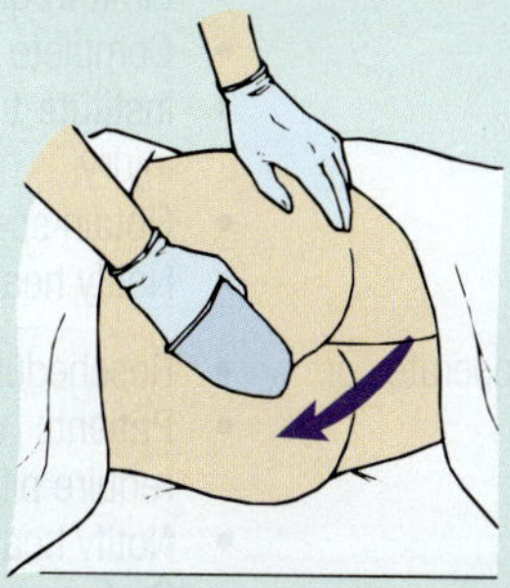

STEP 14D Clean buttocks and anus, washing front to back.

STEP	RATIONALE
IMPLEMENTATION	
19. Remove and dispose of gloves in appropriate receptacle. Help patient complete grooming if requested (e.g., combing hair, shaving).	Reduces transmission of microorganisms. Promotes patient's body image.
20. Check function and position of external devices (e.g., indwelling catheters, nasogastric tubes, IV lines, braces).	Ensures that bathing activities did not disrupt systems.
21. Replace top bed linen by pulling sheet and bedspread from foot of bed to cover patient before removing bath blanket. Apply gloves if linen is soiled. *Option*: Make occupied bed at this time (see Procedural Guideline 18.6).	Maintains patient warmth and privacy.
22. Place bed in low, locked position and raise appropriate number of side rails so they do not restrain patient from exiting bed safely. Make sure that patient is in comfortable position with call light and personal possessions in reach.	Maintains patient safety. Reaching for call light or personal items can lead to a fall.
23. Disinfect/rinse and dry bed basin according to employer policy. This is especially important if using CHG solution. CAUTION: Do not use basin for CHG as storage container for supplies.	Reduces transmission of microorganisms. Evidence has shown that basins are frequently contaminated with microbes and are a possible source for the spread of HAIs (Haque et al., 2020).

EVALUATION

1. Observe skin; pay particular attention to areas that were previously soiled, reddened, flaking, scaling, or cracking or that showed early signs of breakdown. Inspect areas normally exposed to pressure.	Bathing should leave skin clean and clear. If there are signs of skin irritation (e.g., redness, blistering), take steps to reduce pressure.
2. Observe ROM during bathing.	Measures joint mobility.
3. Ask patient to rate level of comfort (using an appropriate pain rating scale).	Determines changes in level of comfort during bathing.
4. Ask if patient feels tired (on a scale of 0–10, with 0 = not tired at all and 10 = the most tired ever).	Measures tolerance to bathing activity.
5. **Use teach-back:** "I want to be sure I explained the importance of keeping your skin clean, especially while in the hospital. Tell me why we want to bathe you daily." Develop a revised teaching plan if patient or caregiver is unable to teach back correctly.	Determines patient's and caregiver's level of understanding of instructional topic.

Unexpected Outcomes	Related Interventions
1. Areas of excessive dryness, rashes, irritation, or pressure injury appear on skin.	• Review employer skin care policy regarding special cleansing and moisturizing products. • If using CHG soap, it may become necessary to reduce frequency of bathing. Sensitivity to CHG is rare. • Limit frequency of complete baths. • Complete pressure injury assessment (see Chapter 39). • Institute turning and positioning measures to keep patient off pressure injury. • Obtain special bed surface if patient is at risk for skin breakdown. • Notify health care provider and/or obtain wound consultation.
2. Patient becomes excessively tired and unable to cooperate or participate in bathing.	• Reschedule bathing for a time when patient is more rested. • Patients with cardiopulmonary conditions and breathing difficulties require pillow or elevated HOB during bathing. • Notify health care provider about changes in patient's fatigue level. • Perform hygiene measures in stages between scheduled rest periods.

Unexpected Outcomes	Related Interventions
3. Patient seems unusually restless or expresses discomfort.	• Use less stressful method of bathing, such as a disposable bath (see Procedural Guideline 18.2). • Consider analgesia before bathing. • Schedule rest periods before bathing.

Communication and Documentation

- Document procedure, observations (e.g., breaks in skin, inflammation, or areas of pressure injury), level of patient participation, and how the patient tolerated procedure in progress notes in electronic health record (EHR) or chart.
- Report evidence of alterations in skin integrity because patient may require special skin care.
- Document evaluation of patient and caregiver learning.

DOCUMENTATION EXAMPLE

Complete bed bath performed with minimal assistance from patient. No abnormal skin findings noted. Will continue to monitor skin integrity and perform preventative turning and positioning every 2 hours, and skin care PRN.

Special Considerations

Teaching

- Teach patients how to inspect surfaces between skinfolds and explain the signs of irritation or breakdown. Use simple language.
- Consider the need to include a caregiver in learning the bathing process. Plan for a return demonstration.

Pediatric

- Some adolescents require or prefer more frequent bathing as a result of their more active sebaceous glands.
- Young adolescents with female genitalia should learn basic perineal hygiene measures and understand why they are predisposed to urinary tract infections.
- To maintain safety when bathing children, they must be supervised at all times, and water temperature should be checked with your elbow or wrist to ensure that it is not too hot (Health Canada, 2018).

Gerontological

- Older persons with incontinence need meticulous skin care to reduce IAD and the risk of infection. The use of barrier creams is sometimes recommended to keep the skin intact and free from infections.
- If patients have signs of dementia, they may consider caregiver behaviour to be an assault. Awareness of situations that can trigger agitation—such as overstimulation, a change in routine, or feelings that their dignity has been offended—are important in preventing and managing potential aggressive behaviour (Mendes, 2018).
- When bathing a patient with dementia, follow these guidelines (ASC, 2022):
  - Practise person-centred nursing care by maintaining the patient's normal routine as much as possible.
  - Provide adequate lighting and prepare the bath ahead of time.
  - Encourage toileting prior to bathing to reduce the chances of incontinence in the bath.
  - Do not rush, and speak in a low, pleasant voice, giving information before and throughout the bathing process.
  - If agitation occurs, use distraction; bring up a pleasant topic or use other distraction such as music, singing, holding an object, or eating.
  - Concentrate on the person's feelings and reactions. Pay attention and do not converse with others.

Care in the Community: Home Management

- Type of bath chosen depends on assessment of the home, availability of running water, and condition of bathing facilities.
- In the home, set up equipment according to patient's established routines.
- Patients at risk for falls may benefit from the following safety measures:
  - Installation of grab bars in shower
  - Adhesive strips applied to shower or tub floor
  - Addition of a shower chair or placement of a chair or stool in the tub or shower

Long-Term Care

- Tubs in long-term care settings frequently come equipped with electronic thermometers to measure water temperature. The tubs also have hydraulic lifts to help residents into the tub.

Procedural Guideline 18.1 *Perineal Care*

Perineal care involves thorough cleaning of the patient's external genitalia and surrounding skin. A patient routinely receives perineal care during a complete bed bath (see Skill 18.1). However, patients who have fecal or urinary incontinence, an in-dwelling Foley catheter, or rectal or genital surgery may need more frequent perineal care. This is especially important for reducing catheter-associated urinary tract infection (CAUTI) in patients with in-dwelling Foley catheters. Wear clean gloves during perineal care because of the risk of contact with infectious organisms present in fecal, urinary, or vaginal secretions. To avoid embarrassing the patient, act in a professional and sensitive manner and always provide patient privacy.

Delegation and Collaboration

The skill of performing perineal care can be delegated to a UCP. The nurse instructs the UCP to do the following:

- Avoid any physical restriction that affects proper positioning of patient
- Properly position a patient with an in-dwelling Foley catheter
- Inform the nurse of any perineal drainage, excoriation, or rash

Equipment

- Washcloths, bath towels, and bath blanket
- Cleaning product for bath (CHG cloths are safe to be used for perineal and catheter care) (AHRQ, 2022)

Continued

Procedural Guideline 18.1 *Perineal Care—cont'd*

- Disposable wipes and wash basin
- Warm water
- Laundry bag
- Waterproof pad or bedpan
- Clean gloves
- Additional supplies when perineal care is provided other than during a bath: cotton balls or swabs, solution bottle or container filled with warm water or prescribed rinsing solution, and waterproof bag

Procedural Steps

1. Identify patient using at least two person-specific identifiers (e.g., name and date of birth, or name and medical record number) according to employer policy (Accreditation Canada, 2020).
2. Throughout the procedure, the 4 moments of hand hygiene are to be implemented; hand hygiene should occur before initial patient (or patient environment) contact, before an aseptic procedure, after body fluid exposure risk, and after patient (or patient environment) contact. Additional hand hygiene should be performed when hands are visibly soiled.
3. Assess environment for safety (e.g., check room for spills; make sure that equipment is working properly; and ensure that bed is in locked, low position).
4. Assemble supplies. Provide privacy, and explain procedure and its importance for preventing infection.
5. Apply clean gloves. Place basin with warm water and cleansing solution on over-bed table.
6. Providing perineal care for an individual with female genitalia:
   a. If patient can manoeuvre and handle washcloth, allow them to clean perineum on their own.
   b. Help patient assume dorsal recumbent position. Note restrictions or a limitation in patient's positioning. Position waterproof pad under patient's buttocks.
   c. Drape patient with bath blanket placed in shape of a diamond.
   d. Fold both outer corners of bath blanket up around patient's legs onto abdomen and under hip (see Step 6d illustration). Lift lower tip of bath blanket when you are ready to expose the perineum.

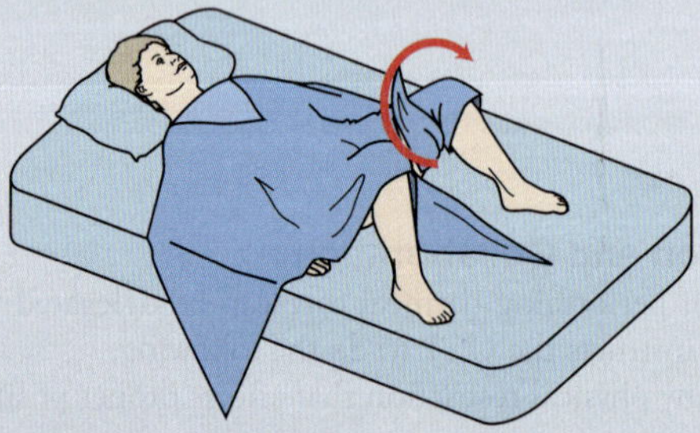

STEP 6D Drape patient for perineal care.

   e. Wash and dry patient's upper thighs. (Note: If employer uses CHG solution for perineal care, do not rinse; allow to dry.)
   f. Wash labia majora. Use nondominant hand to gently retract labia from thigh. Use dominant hand to wash carefully in skinfolds. Wipe in direction from perineum to rectum (front to back). Repeat on opposite side using separate section of washcloth or new washcloth. Rinse and dry area thoroughly.
   g. Gently separate labia with nondominant hand to expose urethral meatus and vaginal orifice. With dominant hand, wash downward from pubic area toward rectum in one smooth stroke (see Step 6g illustration). Use separate section of cloth for each stroke. Clean thoroughly over labia minora, clitoris, and vaginal orifice. Avoid tension on in-dwelling catheter if present and clean area around it thoroughly.

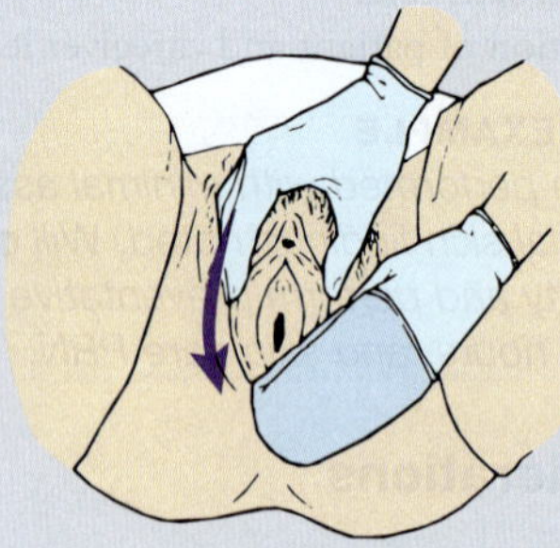

STEP 6G Clean from perineum to rectum (front to back).

   h. Rinse and dry area thoroughly, using front-to-back method.
   i. If patient uses bedpan, pour warm water over perineal area and dry thoroughly. (Exception: Do not rinse if using CHG.)
   j. Fold lower corner of bath blanket back between patient's legs and over perineum. Ask patient to lower legs and assume comfortable position.
7. Providing perineal care for an individual with male genitalia:
   a. If patient is able to manoeuvre and handle washcloth, allow them to clean perineum on their own.
   b. Help patient to supine position. Note restriction in mobility.
   c. Fold lower half of bath blanket up to expose upper thighs. Wash and dry thighs.
   d. Cover thighs with bath towels. Raise bath blanket to expose genitalia. Gently raise penis and place bath towel underneath. Gently grasp shaft of penis. If patient is uncircumcised, retract foreskin. If patient has an erection, defer procedure until later.
   e. Wash tip of penis at urethral meatus first. Using circular motion, clean from meatus outward (see Step 7e illustration). Discard washcloth and repeat with clean cloth until penis is clean. Rinse and dry gently and thoroughly. (Exception: Do not rinse if using CHG.)

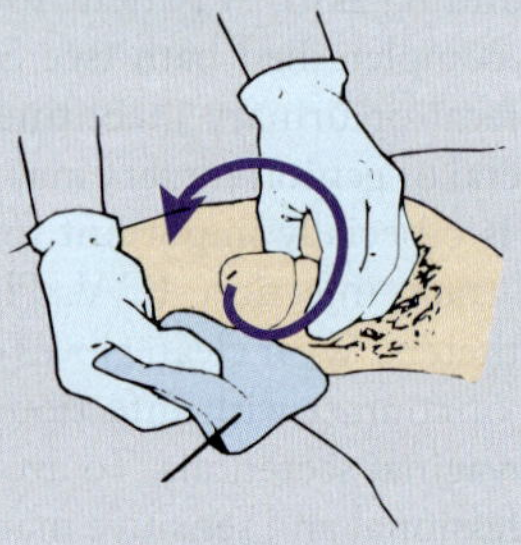

STEP 7E Use circular motion to clean tip of penis.

Procedural Guideline 18.1 *Perineal Care—cont'd*

f. Return foreskin to its natural position.

Critical Decision Point *After administering perineal care for patients with an uncircumcised penis, make sure that foreskin is in its natural position. This position is extremely important in patients with decreased sensation in their lower extremities. Tightening of foreskin around shaft of penis causes local edema and discomfort and, if not corrected, may cause permanent urethral damage.*

g. Take a new washcloth and gently clean shaft of penis and scrotum by having patient abduct legs. Pay special attention to underlying surface of penis. Lift scrotum carefully and wash underlying skinfolds. Rinse and dry thoroughly. (EXCEPTION: Do not rinse if using CHG.)

h. Fold bath blanket back over patient's perineum and help them get into a comfortable position.

8. Avoid placing tension on an in-dwelling catheter, if present, and clean around it thoroughly during procedure.
9. Observe perineal area for any irritation, redness, or drainage that persists after perineal hygiene.
10. Dispose of gloves and used supplies in proper receptacles.
11.
12. **Use teach-back:** "We talked about how to wash your genital area to reduce the chance of infection. Describe for me how to wash your genital area." Develop a revised teaching plan if patient or caregiver is unable to teach back correctly.

Procedural Guideline 18.2 *Use of Disposable Bed Bath, Tub, or Shower*

The use of disposable washcloths impregnated with an antiseptic solution such as CHG is common in acute care hospitals, especially in critical care settings. However, the cloths can be used in any setting. CHG cloths should be used for all bathing purposes, including once-a-day full-body bathing, incontinence care, or any other reasons for additional cleaning (AHRQ, 2022). CHG can replace soap and water baths because it is effective at cleaning and removing bacteria, and the antiseptic binds to the skin for persistent antibacterial activity lasting 24 hours (AHRQ, 2022).

Although showers are available to patients in acute care, tub and shower bathing are more common in long-term care settings. When patients use a tub or shower, follow guidelines to maintain patient safety to prevent falls.

Delegation and Collaboration

The skill of bathing a patient in a tub or shower or using disposable cloths for bathing can be delegated to a UCP. The nurse instructs the UCP to do the following:

- Avoid massaging reddened skin areas during bathing
- Use proper positioning for patients with musculoskeletal limitations or an in-dwelling Foley catheter or other equipment (e.g., IV tubing)
- Report changes in skin or perineal area or signs of impaired skin integrity to the nurse

Equipment

- Washcloths and bath towels (for tub or shower), bath blanket, cleaning product, toiletry items (deodorant, lotion), disposable wipes, clean hospital gown or patient's own pyjamas or gown, and laundry bag
- Prepackaged, disposable bathing cloths
- Clean gloves

Procedural Steps

1. Identify patient using at least two person-specific identifiers (e.g., name and date of birth, or name and medical record number) according to employer policy (Accreditation Canada, 2020).
2. Throughout the procedure, the 4 moments for hand hygiene are to be implemented; hand hygiene should occur before initial patient (or patient environment) contact, before an aseptic procedure, after body fluid exposure risk, and after patient (or patient environment) contact. Additional hand hygiene should be performed when hands are visibly soiled.
3. Assess environment for safety (e.g., check room for spills; make sure that equipment is working properly; and ensure that bed is in locked, low position) and provide privacy.
4. Assess degree of help patient will need for bathing, risk of falling (e.g., ability to stand, get into a tub), patient's risk for skin breakdown, and presence of allergy or sensitivity to bathing solution (e.g., CHG) (see Skill 18.1).
5. Apply clean gloves. Arrange supplies and toiletry items at bedside if using bathing cloths; otherwise, prepare supplies and equipment in patient's bathroom or in shower room.
6. Bathing cloths: (All of Step 6 follows the AHRQ [2022] universal bathing protocol for skin decolonization to prevent HAIs. This approach is used commonly in critical care and acute care hospitals.)
   a. Adjust room temperature and ventilation, close room doors and windows, and draw room divider curtain.
   b. Position patient supine or in a position of comfort. Use a bath blanket to drape areas of body not being cleaned as bath proceeds (see Skill 18.1).
   c. Help patient remove old gown (see Skill 18.1).
   d. *Option:* Warm package of bathing cloths in a microwave, following package directions. Do not use a microwave that is used for food preparation. The cleaning pack contains six premoistened cloths.

Critical Decision Point *Check temperature of cloth after warming and have patient check as well to prevent burns to the skin.*

   e. Use all six bathing cloths in the following order (see Step 6e illustration), positioning and using drapes as described in Skill 18.1:

Continued

Procedural Guideline 18.2 *Use of Disposable Bed Bath, Tub, or Shower—cont'd*

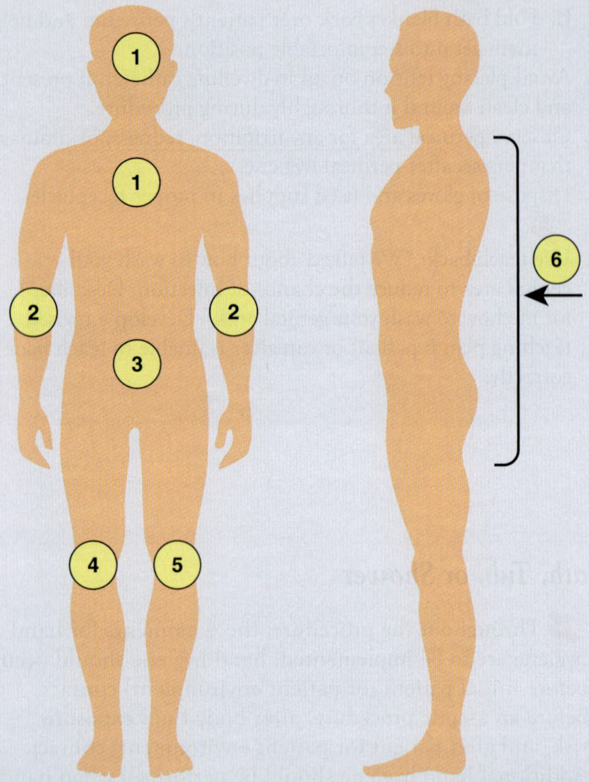

STEP 6E **Order for use of six bathing cloths.** *From Agency for Healthcare Research and Quality. (2022). Section 10-7: Patients with devices: Prevent infections during your hospital stay: BATHE daily with chlorhexidine (CHG) cloths. AHRQ Pub. No. 20[22]-0036. https://www.ahrq.gov/sites/default/files/wysiwyg/hai/abate/handouts/patient-chg-bathing.pdf*

- **(1)** Cloth 1: Face, neck, and chest. Avoid eyes and ear canals.
- **(2)** Cloth 2: Both shoulders, arms, and hands.
- **(3)** Cloth 3: Abdomen and then groin/perineum.
- **(4)** Cloth 4: Right leg and foot.
- **(5)** Cloth 5: Left leg and foot.
- **(6)** Cloth 6: Back of neck, back, and then buttocks.

f. Firmly massage skin with CHG cloth. Tell patient that the skin may feel sticky for a few minutes.

g. Ensure thorough cleaning of soiled areas such as the neck, skinfolds, and perineal areas. CHG is safe to use on perineal areas, including external mucosa. It is also safe for superficial wounds, including stage 1 and stage 2 decubitus pressure injuries.

h. Do NOT rinse, wipe off, or dry with another cloth. Allow skin to air dry.

i. CHG cloths have built-in moisturizers. Skin may feel sticky for a few minutes.

j. If additional moisturizer is needed, use only CHG-compatible products.

k. Dispose of leftover cloths, help patient to comfortable position, and assist in applying clean gown.

7. Tub bath or shower:

a. Assess patient's fall risk; consider patient's physical ability to stand and get into tub, and review prescriptions for precautions concerning their movement or positioning. A health care provider's prescription usually is needed for tub bath or shower.

b. Check tub or shower for availability and cleanliness. Use cleaning techniques outlined in employer policy if necessary. Place nonslip mat on tub or shower bottom. Place skid-proof disposable bath mat or towel on floor in front of tub or shower.

c. Place hygiene and toiletry items within easy reach of tub or shower.

d. Help patient to bathroom if necessary. Have them wear a robe and skid-proof slippers to bathroom.

e. Demonstrate how to use call signal for help. Place "occupied" sign on bathroom door. Close door.

f. Fill bathtub halfway with warm water. Check temperature of bath water, have patient test it, and adjust it if it is too warm or too cold. Explain which faucet controls hot water.

Critical Decision Point *Do not use bath oil in tub water because it makes tub slippery and can cause a fall.*

g. If patient is taking shower, turn shower on and adjust water temperature before they enter the shower stall. Use shower seat or tub chair if available (see Step 7g illustration).

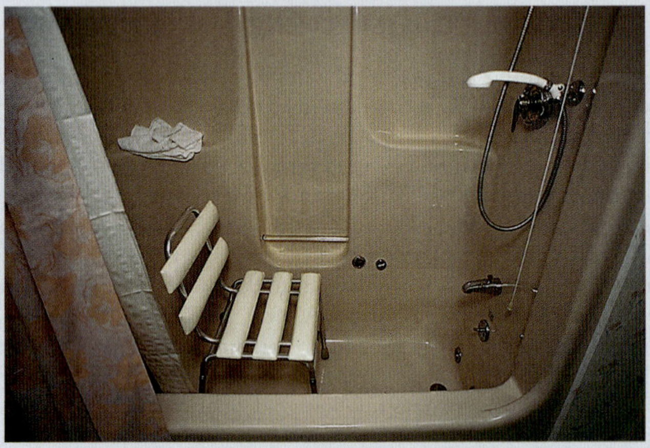

STEP 7G **Shower seat for patient safety.**

h. Tell patient that you will not allow them to remain in tub longer than 20 minutes. Provide privacy for patient and check on patient every 5 minutes, if patient health status indicates that it is safe to leave them alone. Remove and dispose of gloves.

i. Apply clean gloves. Return to bathroom when patient signals, and knock before entering.

j. For patient who is unsteady, drain tub of water before they attempt to get out. Place bath towel over patient's shoulders. Help them get out of tub as needed, and assist with drying. If possible, have a shower chair available for patient to sit on.

k. Help patient as needed to don clean gown or pyjamas, slippers, and robe. (In home, extended care, or rehabilitation setting, encourage patient to wear regular clothing.)

l. Help patient to room and to comfortable position in bed or chair. Leave call light in reach.

m. Clean tub or shower, remove soiled linen, and discard of disposable supplies according to employer policy.

n. Remove and dispose of gloves.

8. Evaluate condition of patient's skin. Pay attention to areas that were previously soiled, reddened, flaking, or scaling or showing signs of breakdown.

9. Ask patient to rate level of fatigue and comfort.

✦ SKILL 18.2 Oral Hygiene

Maintenance of daily oral hygiene, including brushing, flossing, and rinsing, is essential for the prevention and control of plaque-associated oral diseases. In addition to preventing inflammation and infection, oral hygiene promotes comfort, ease of swallowing for better food intake, and verbal communication. Brushing removes food particles, plaque (the cause of dental caries), and bacteria from the teeth; massages the gums; and relieves discomfort from unpleasant odours and tastes. Flossing removes tartar that collects at the gum line. Rinsing removes dislodged food particles and excess toothpaste.

When a patient becomes ill, many factors influence the need for oral hygiene. Offer oral hygiene assistance as required. Plan the frequency of care based on a patient's clinical condition and the condition of their oral cavity. For example, a stroke patient who has difficulty swallowing may require care as often as every 4 hours; a patient on a ventilator will require special care to reduce the chances of developing ventilator-associated pneumonia (VAP) (see Skill 18.3).

In addition to recommendations for the general population, there are oral-care regimens designed to relieve discomfort and facilitate healing of chemotherapy- and radiation therapy–related mucositis, stomatitis, and xerostomia. These types of oral lesions are very painful and interfere with a patient's nutrition. Specific regimens are discussed later in this chapter.

Delegation and Collaboration

The skill of providing oral hygiene (including tooth brushing, flossing, and rinsing) can be delegated to a UCP. However, the nurse is responsible for assessing the patient's gag reflex to determine whether the patient is at risk for aspiration. The gag reflex is triggered when an object touches the back of the mouth, causing contraction of muscles in the throat. The nurse instructs the UCP about the following:

- Types of changes in oral mucosa (e.g., presence of lesions or open areas) to observe for and report to the nurse
- Reporting patient's complaints of pain or occurrence of bleeding during oral care
- Being aware of special precautions such as aspiration precautions, including:
  - Keeping HOB raised 30 to 45 degrees
  - Explaining need to report excessive coughing or choking during procedure
- Not flossing when a patient has a bleeding tendency

Equipment

- Soft-bristled toothbrush (hard-bristled toothbrush damages enamel and gums)
- Nonabrasive fluoride toothpaste or dentifrice
- Dental floss
- 0.12% CHG (*optional*; see employer policy)
- Tongue depressor
- Penlight
- Water glass with cool water, straw
- Normal saline or an essential oil–antiseptic mouth rinse (*optional*)
- Emesis basin
- Bath towels to place over patient's chest; paper towels
- Clean gloves
- *Option:* Moisturizing lubricant for lips

STEP	RATIONALE
ASSESSMENT	
1. Identify patient using at least two person-specific identifiers (e.g., name and date of birth, or name and medical record number) according to employer policy.	Ensures correct patient. Complies with Accreditation Canada's standards and improves patient safety (Accreditation Canada, 2020).
2. Throughout the procedure, the 4 moments for hand hygiene are to be implemented; hand hygiene should occur before initial patient (or patient environment) contact, before an aseptic procedure, after body fluid exposure risk, and after patient (or patient environment) contact. Additional hand hygiene should be performed when hands are visibly soiled.	Proper hand hygiene helps prevent the spread of infectious agents to health care providers.
3. Assess environment for safety (e.g., check room for spills; make sure that equipment is working properly; and ensure that bed is in locked, low position).	Identifies safety hazards in patient environment that could cause or potentially lead to harm (LeLaurin & Shorr, 2019).
4. Apply clean gloves. Instruct patient not to bite down during assessment of oral cavity. Using a penlight and tongue depressor, inspect integrity of lips, teeth, buccal mucosa, gums, palate, and tongue (see Chapter 8).	Reduces transmission of microorganisms. Determines status of patient's oral cavity and extent of need for oral hygiene. Provides baseline to determine change after hygiene.
5. Identify presence of common oral problems.	Helps determine type of hygiene and information that patient requires for self-care.
a. *Dental caries:* Chalky-white discoloration of tooth or presence of brown or black discoloration	
b. *Gingivitis:* Inflammation of gums	May indicate periodontal disease.
c. *Periodontitis:* Receding gum lines, inflammation, gaps between teeth	May indicate periodontal disease.
d. *Halitosis:* Bad breath	May indicate periodontal disease.
e. *Cheilosis:* Cracking lips	
f. *Stomatitis:* Inflammation of mouth tissues or structures	
g. *Mucositis:* Inflammation of oral mucous membrane	
h. Dry, cracked, coated tongue	
6. Remove and dispose of gloves.	Prevents transmission of microorganisms.

STEP	RATIONALE

ASSESSMENT

STEP	RATIONALE
7. Review medical record and assess patient's risk for oral hygiene problems:	Certain conditions increase likelihood of impaired oral cavity integrity and need for preventive care.
a. Dehydration: Inability to take fluids or food by mouth; health care provider's prescription prohibiting food or fluids by mouth (NPO) for a procedure or because of patient's condition. It is extremely important to perform regular oral care when a patient is NPO.	Causes excess drying and fragility of mucous membranes and lips; increases accumulation of thick secretions on tongue and gums.
b. Presence of nasogastric or oxygen tubes; mouth breathers	Causes drying of mucosa.
c. Chemotherapeutic medications	Medications kill rapidly multiplying cells, including sloughing of normal cells lining oral cavity. Mucositis with ulcers and inflammation can develop.
d. Radiation therapy to head and neck	Reduces salivary flow and lowers pH of saliva; leads to stomatitis and tooth decay (National Cancer Institute [NCI], 2021).
e. Presence of artificial airway (e.g., endotracheal tube)	Tube irritates gums and mucosa. Excess secretions accumulate on teeth and tongue.
f. Blood-clotting disorders (e.g., leukemia, aplastic anemia)	Predisposes patient to inflammation and bleeding of gums.
g. Oral surgery, trauma to mouth	Break in mucosa increases risk for infection. Vigorous brushing can disrupt suture lines.
h. Aging	With advancing age, mucosa becomes thin and less elastic.
i. Chemical injury	Results from irritants such as alcohol, tobacco, acidic foods, or adverse effects of medications (e.g., antibiotics, steroids, antidepressants).
j. Diabetes mellitus	Predisposes patient to dry mouth, gingivitis, periodontal disease, and loss of teeth.
8. Determine patient's oral hygiene practices.	Identifies errors in patient's technique, deficiencies in preventive oral hygiene, patient's level of knowledge regarding dental care.
a. Frequency of tooth brushing and flossing	The CDA (n.d.-b, n.d.-c) recommends brushing teeth at least twice a day with CDA-approved fluoridated toothpaste and once-a-day flossing.
b. Type of toothpaste, dentifrice, and mouth rinse used (assess if CHG is indicated for use)	Mouthwashes and oral-care products with CDA seal of recognition demonstrate oral health benefits (CDA, n.d.-c).
c. Last dental visit and frequency of visits	The CDA recommends regular dental visits; however, frequency of visits can vary for each patient and should be determined by their dentist (CDA, n.d.-c).
9. Assess patient's ability to grasp and manipulate toothbrush.	Determines level of help required from nurse. Some older patients or people with musculoskeletal or nervous system alterations are unable to hold toothbrush with a firm grip or manipulate brush. Large-handled toothbrushes or a toothbrush handle pushed through a small rubber ball may be of help.

NURSING DIAGNOSES

- Bathing/self-care deficit
- Impaired oral mucous membrane
- Deficient knowledge regarding oral hygiene care
- Risk for infection

Related factors are individualized on the basis of patient's condition or needs.

PLANNING

STEP	RATIONALE
1. Expected outcomes following completion of procedure:	
• Patient expresses feeling of mouth cleanliness.	Hygiene measures remove secretions and thickened mucosa.
• Oral cavity structures have normal characteristics: • Oral mucosa is moist, intact, and of normal colour. • Gums are pink, firm, and adherent to neck of teeth. • Teeth are clean, smooth, and shiny. • Tongue is pink, without secretions or coating.	Hygiene measures maintain integrity of teeth and healthy oral mucosa.
• Patient describes correct oral hygiene techniques.	Demonstrates understanding of instruction.
• Patient makes choices regarding hygiene procedure and helps by flossing and brushing.	Demonstrates ability to manage self-care.
2. Gather equipment and supplies at bedside.	Avoids interrupting procedure or leaving patient unattended to retrieve missing equipment.
3. Explain procedure to patient and discuss preferences regarding use of hygiene aids.	Some patients feel uncomfortable about having nurse care for their basic needs. Patient involvement with procedure minimizes anxiety.

STEP	RATIONALE

IMPLEMENTATION

1. Close room doors and draw room divider curtain.	Reduces transmission of microorganisms. Privacy ensures patient's mental and physical comfort.
2. Arrange supplies on bedside table so they are within easy reach.	Creates organized workspace.
3. Raise bed to comfortable working height. Raise HOB to at least semi-Fowler's position (unless contraindicated) and lower side rail. Move patient or help patient move close to side from which you choose to work. A side-lying position can be used.	Raising bed and positioning patient promote good body mechanics and prevent nurse from having muscle strain. Semi-Fowler's position helps prevent patient from choking or aspirating. **Note:** If patient is overweight, use safe handling techniques (see Chapter 11).
4. Place towel over patient's chest.	Prevents soiling of patient's gown.
5. Apply clean gloves.	Reduces transmission of microorganisms.
6. Apply toothpaste to brush bristles. Hold brush over emesis basin. Pour small amount of water over toothpaste.	Moisture aids in distribution of toothpaste over tooth surfaces.
7. Patient may help by brushing. Hold toothbrush bristles at 45-degree angle to gum line (see Step 7 illustration). Be sure that tips of bristles rest against and penetrate (gently) under gum line. Brush inner and outer surfaces of upper and lower teeth by brushing from gum to crown of each tooth. Clean biting surfaces of teeth by holding top of bristles parallel with teeth and brushing gently back and forth (see Step 7 illustration). Brush sides of teeth by moving bristles back and forth (see Step 7 illustration).	Angle allows brush to reach all tooth surfaces and clean under gum line where plaque and tartar accumulate. Back-and-forth motion loosens food particles caught between teeth and along chewing surfaces.
8. Have patient hold brush at 45-degree angle and lightly brush over surface and sides of tongue (see Step 8 illustration). Avoid initiating gag reflex.	Microorganisms collect and grow on surface of tongue and contribute to bad breath. Gagging may cause aspiration of toothpaste.
9. Allow patient to rinse mouth thoroughly with water by instructing them to take several sips of water (may use straw), swish water across all tooth surfaces, and spit into emesis basin. Use this time to observe patient's brushing technique and teach importance of brushing teeth twice a day.	Rinsing removes food particles.
10. Have patient rinse teeth with antiseptic mouthwash for 30 seconds. Then have them spit rinse into emesis basin.	Oral rinsing with an alcohol-free mouthwash, as a complement to brushing and flossing, helps reduce plaque, gingivitis, and/or tartar formation on the teeth (American Dental Association, 2019).
11. Help to wipe patient's mouth.	Promotes sense of comfort.

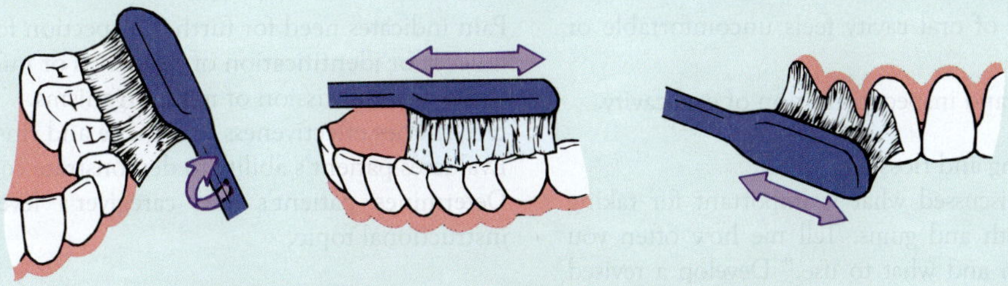

STEP 7 Directions of brush for tooth brushing.

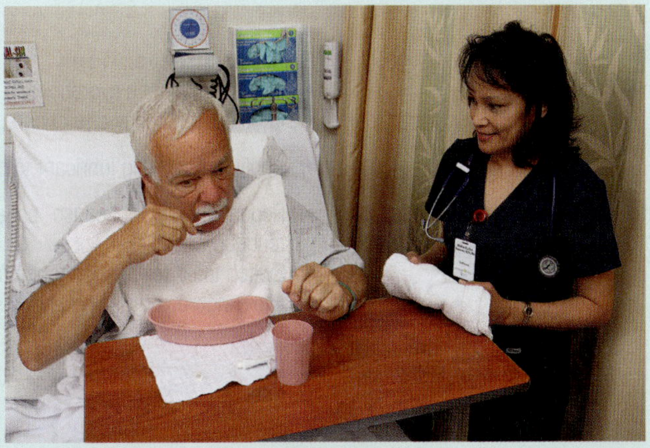

STEP 8 Nurse observes patient's tooth-brushing technique, including brushing of tongue.

STEP	RATIONALE

IMPLEMENTATION

12. Allow patient to floss. Floss between all teeth. Hold floss against tooth while moving it up and down sides of teeth. Instruct patient on importance of daily flossing (see Step 12 illustrations).	Flossing once daily removes plaque and decay-causing bacteria between teeth and under gum line, preventing gum disease. Immunocompromised patients are sometimes on precautions that prohibit use of floss or Waterpik because of potential to dislodge bacteria and cause bleeding of gums.

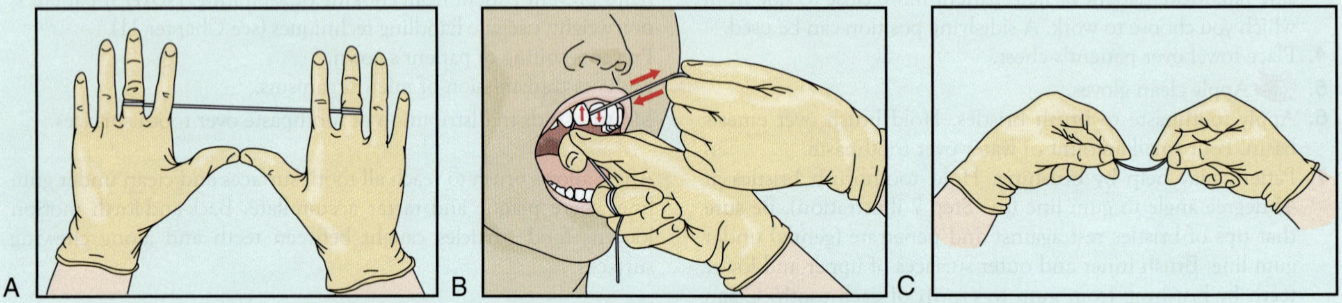

STEP 12 **Flossing. A, Dental floss is held between middle fingers to floss upper teeth. B, Floss is moved in up-and-down motions between teeth. Floss is moved up and down from crown to gum line. C, Floss is held with index fingers to floss lower teeth.**

13. Allow patient to rinse mouth thoroughly with cool water and spit into emesis basin. Help to wipe the mouth. Apply moisturizing lubricant to lips (if patient desires).	Rinsing removes plaque and tartar from oral cavity.
14. Help patient to comfortable position with call light in reach, remove emesis basin and over-bed table, raise side rail if appropriate, and lower bed to original position.	Provides for patient comfort and safety.
15. Wipe off bedside table, discard soiled linen in dirty laundry bag, remove soiled gloves, and return equipment to proper place.	Proper disposal of soiled equipment prevents spread of infection.

EVALUATION

1. Ask patient if any area of oral cavity feels uncomfortable or irritated.	Pain indicates need for further inspection for possible breaks in oral mucosa or identification of stomatitis or infection.
2. Apply clean gloves and inspect condition of oral cavity.	Reduces transmission of microorganisms. Determines effectiveness of hygiene and rinsing.
3. Observe patient brushing and flossing.	Evaluates patient's ability to demonstrate correct technique.
4. **Use teach-back:** "We discussed what is important for taking proper care of your teeth and gums. Tell me how often you should brush your teeth and what to use." Develop a revised teaching plan if patient or caregiver is unable to teach back correctly.	Determines patient's and caregiver's level of understanding of instructional topic.

Unexpected Outcomes	Related Interventions
1. Mucosa is dry and inflamed. Tongue has thick coating.	• Increase patient's hydration. • Increase frequency of oral care, focusing on tongue brushing.
2. Cheilosis—lips are dry and cracked.	• Apply moisturizing lubricant to patient's lips.
3. Gum margins are retracted from teeth, with localized areas of inflammation. Bleeding occurs around gum margins.	• Report findings because patient may have an underlying bleeding tendency. • Switch to softer-bristled toothbrush or sponge toothette. • Avoid vigorous brushing and flossing.

Unexpected Outcomes	Related Interventions
4. Mucosa becomes inflamed from repeated chemotherapy administration, and a lesion from sloughing of tissue develops. These conditions can also be caused by radiation therapy used to treat head and neck cancers.	• Determine best-practice oral regimen for mucositis and stomatitis. Common regimens used to promote healing and comfort include: • Use fluoride toothpaste. • Use one of the following rinses made with salt and/or baking soda (NCI, 2021): • 5 mL (1 tsp) salt in 1 L (4 cups) of water • 5 mL (1 tsp) baking soda in 250 mL (1 cup) of water • 2.5 mL (0.5 tsp) salt and 30 mL (2 tbsp) baking soda in 1 L (4 cups) of water • An antibacterial rinse two to four times a day for gum disease; rinse for 1–2 minutes • If dry mouth (xerostomia) and hyposalivation occur, additional rinses to increase moisture may be used. Brushing and gentle flossing should be continued as well.

Communication and Documentation

- Document procedure on basic care checklist in progress notes in EHR or chart.
- Record condition of oral cavity in progress notes in EHR or chart.
- Document your evaluation of patient and caregiver learning.
- Report bleeding, pain, or presence of lesions to nurse in charge or health care provider.

DOCUMENTATION EXAMPLE

Oral hygiene provided for patient with minimal assistance. Alcohol-free antiseptic mouth rinse used. No bleeding, pain, or lesions noted in oral cavity, and patient reports mouth feels fresh and clean. Patient verbalized understanding of importance of regular oral hygiene.

Special Considerations

Teaching

- Educate patients about methods to prevent tooth decay (e.g., reduce intake of carbohydrates, especially sweet, sticky snacks between meals; brush within 30 minutes of eating sweets; rinse mouth thoroughly with water or alcohol-free antiseptic mouth rinse; use fluoride toothpaste). Use simple language and available teaching materials at proper literacy level.
- Educate patients to visit a dentist regularly (based on dentist's recommendations) for professional cleaning and oral examination; frequency of visits varies for each patient and should be determined by their dentist (CDA, n.d.-c).
- When teaching special oral-care regimens, include caregiver.
- Avoid mints if conditions of the mouth are associated with ulcerations of the oral mucosa.

Pediatric

- Every infant should receive an oral health risk assessment from their primary health care provider or qualified health care provider within 6 months of the eruption of the first tooth or by 12 months of age (CDA, n.d.-d).
- Oral hygiene measures should be started before a child has a tooth. The goal is to wipe gums and teeth. Tooth brushing should be performed for children by a parent twice daily, using a soft toothbrush of age-appropriate size and the correct amount of fluoridated toothpaste (CDA, n.d.-a).
- Children under 3 years should have their teeth brushed by an adult. Using fluoridated toothpaste is determined by level of risk of developing tooth decay. If a child is low risk, their teeth can be brushed with a toothbrush moistened with water. Otherwise, a minimal amount (size of grain of rice) of fluoridated toothpaste can be used. For children aged 3 to 6 years, a small amount (size of a green pea) of fluoridated toothpaste is recommended (CDA, n.d.-a).
- Teach parents that infants should not be put to bed with a bottle; this causes tooth decay and ear infections. Limit snacks to three or four per day. Avoid giving sugary snacks and drinks and sticky candy.

Gerontological

- Several normal age-related changes occur in the oral cavity. Thinning of the oral mucosa and decreased vascularity of the gingivae predispose older persons to injury and periodontal disease. Loss of tissue elasticity and decreased mass and strength of the muscles make chewing more difficult. Loss of the alveolar bone can loosen natural teeth.
- The number of taste buds declines with advancing age. To enhance the taste of food, some older persons choose salty and sugary foods, which erode tooth enamel and expose dentin.
- It is recommended that an adult not smoke, chew tobacco, or use snuff. Smoking may impair blood flow to the gums, reducing the amount of oxygen and nutrients to the tissues and making them more vulnerable to infection. Chemicals in tobacco smoke cause inflammation and cell damage and can weaken the immune system. Nicotine is toxic to cells that make new connective tissue and also increases the production of an enzyme that breaks down tissue (National Institute of Dental and Craniofacial Research, 2018).
- Some older persons may find it difficult to maintain good oral hygiene with flossing and brushing because of decreased dexterity and decreasing eyesight.

Care in the Community: Home Management

- During the initial home visit, document the condition of a patient's mouth, teeth, and gums as part of a comprehensive health assessment, thus providing a baseline for assessing the patient's ability to comply with special diets and fluid intake and carry out oral hygiene practices.

Procedural Guideline 18.3 *Care of Dentures*

Oral bacteria from multiple strains and *Candida* species are found on acrylic dentures (Fujinami et al., 2021). Encourage patients who wear dentures to continue to care for them and to provide this care as frequently as they would for natural teeth. Loose dentures can cause discomfort and make it difficult for patients to chew food and speak clearly. Routine denture care reduces the risk for gingival infection. Offer dental care after every meal and before a patient goes to bed. Some patients are unable to care for their dentures, and nurses become responsible for providing denture and oral care. Dentures are a patient's personal property; be sure to handle them with care because they are easy to break. Reinsert them as soon as possible. Note that it is common for patients to choose to not wear their dentures during an acute illness.

Delegation and Collaboration

The skill of performing denture care can be delegated to a UCP. The nurse instructs the UCP to do the following:

- Avoid the use of hot or excessively cold water when caring for dentures
- Inform the nurse if there are cracks in dentures
- Inform the nurse if the patient has any oral discomfort

Equipment

- Soft-bristled toothbrush or denture toothbrush
- Denture dentifrice or denture paste (regular toothpaste may be abrasive to dentures), denture adhesive (optional)
- Glass of water
- Emesis basin or sink
- 10 cm × 10 cm (4 inch × 4 inch) gauze
- Washcloth
- Denture cup (for storage)
- Clean gloves

Procedural Steps

1. Identify patient using at least two person-specific identifiers (e.g., name and date of birth, or name and medical record number) according to employer policy (Accreditation Canada, 2020).
2. Throughout the procedure, the 4 moments for hand hygiene are to be implemented; hand hygiene should occur before initial patient (or patient environment) contact, before an aseptic procedure, after body fluid exposure risk, and after patient (or patient environment) contact. Additional hand hygiene should be performed when hands are visibly soiled.
3. Assess environment for safety (e.g., check room for spills; make sure that equipment is working properly; and ensure that bed is in locked, low position).
4. Assess patient to ensure dentures fit and for any gum or mucous membrane tenderness or irritation. Ask patient about denture care and product preferences.
5. Determine if patient has necessary dexterity to clean dentures independently or requires help.
6. Position patient comfortably sitting up in bed or help them walk from bed to chair placed in front of sink.
7. Fill emesis basin with tepid water. (If using sink, place washcloth in bottom of sink and fill sink with approximately 2.5 cm [1 inch] of water.)
8. Apply clean gloves.
9. Ask patient to remove dentures. If patient is unable to do this independently, grasp upper plate at front with thumb and index finger wrapped in gauze and pull downward. Gently lift lower denture from jaw and rotate one side downward to remove from patient's mouth. Place dentures in emesis basin or sink lined with washcloth and 2.5 cm (1 inch) of water.
10. Apply cleaning agent to brush and brush surfaces of dentures (see Step 10 illustration). Hold dentures close to water. Hold brush horizontally and use back-and-forth motion to clean biting surfaces. Use short strokes from top of denture to biting surfaces to clean outer teeth surfaces. Hold brush vertically and use short strokes to clean inner teeth surfaces. Hold brush horizontally and use back-and-forth motion to clean undersurface of dentures (see Skill 18.2).

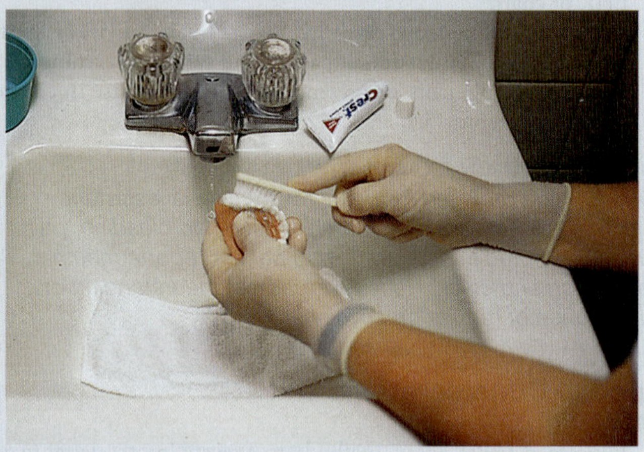

STEP 10 **Brushing surface of dentures.**

11. Rinse thoroughly in tepid water. If water is too cold, dentures can crack. If it is too hot, dentures can become warped and no longer fit.
12. Some patients use an adhesive to seal dentures in place. Apply a thin layer to undersurface before inserting, if requested by patient.
13. If patient needs help with inserting dentures, moisten upper denture and press firmly to seal it in place. Insert moistened lower denture (if applicable). Ask if dentures feel comfortable.
14. Some patients prefer to store their dentures to give gums a rest and reduce risk for infection. Store in tepid water in enclosed, labelled denture cup. Keep denture cup in a secure place labelled with patient's name to prevent loss when not worn (e.g., at night, during surgery).
15. Dispose of supplies. Remove and discard gloves.
16. Return patient to a comfortable position. Leave call light in reach.

✦ SKILL 18.3 Performing Mouth Care for an Unconscious or Debilitated Patient

Unconscious or debilitated patients pose challenges because of their risk for alterations of the oral cavity from drying of the mucous membrane, thickened secretions, and the inability to eat or drink. They are susceptible to infection because of the change in the normal flora of the oral cavity and are at risk for infection because of increased plaque formation from the dryness of the mouth and decreased salivation. Dryness of the oral mucosa is also caused by mouth breathing and oxygen therapy. Respiratory secretions often are thick and place patients at risk for ineffective airway clearance, requiring oral suction (see Chapter 23). Debilitated patients are also at risk for aspiration. Although saliva production is decreased, saliva is present and can pool in the back of the oral cavity, which is a contributing factor for aspiration in patients with reduced gag reflexes. The secretions in the oral cavity change very rapidly to Gram-negative pneumonia-producing bacteria if aspiration occurs.

The critically ill patient with an endotracheal tube who is on mechanical ventilation is at risk for VAP as a result of continuous aspiration of microorganisms that are able to colonize in the respiratory tract or equipment (Tran & Butcher, 2019). Some patients require mouth care as often as every 1 to 2 hours until the mucosa returns to normal. Proper hygiene requires keeping the mucosa moist and removing secretions as they accumulate in the back of the throat. Many hospitals use an oral-care bundle to reduce incidence of VAP, which may include using a CHG mouth rinse (check employer policy), and keeping the HOB elevated 30 to 45 degrees or more unless contraindicated to prevent aspiration of oral secretions.

Because many debilitated patients have either a reduced or an absent gag reflex as a result of change in consciousness or a neurological injury, providing oral care requires protecting patients from choking and aspiration. The safest technique is to have two nurses provide care. One nurse provides oral care while another nurse suctions oral secretions, as necessary, with a Yankauer suction tip (see Chapter 23). A UCP may assist the nurse with oral care and suctioning. It is important to evaluate the level and frequency of oral care daily during assessment of the oral cavity. Routine suctioning of the mouth and pharynx is required to manage oral secretions to reduce the risk for aspiration.

Delegation and Collaboration

The skill of providing oral hygiene to an unconscious or debilitated patient can be delegated to a UCP. The nurse is responsible for assessing a patient's gag reflex. The nurse instructs the UCP to do the following:

- Have another caregiver help the UCP and properly position patient for mouth care
- Be aware of special precautions, such as aspiration precautions
- Use an oral suction catheter for clearing oral secretions (see Skill 25.1)
- Report signs of impaired integrity of oral mucosa to the nurse
- Report any bleeding of mucosa or gum or excessive coughing or choking to the nurse

Equipment

- Small pediatric soft-bristled toothbrush, toothette sponges, or suction toothbrushes for patients for whom brushing is contraindicated
- Antibacterial solution per employer policy
- Fluoride toothpaste
- Water-based mouth moisturizer
- Tongue blade
- Penlight
- Oral suction equipment
- Oral airway (uncooperative patient or patient who shows bite reflex)
- Water-soluble lip lubricant
- Water glass with cool water
- Face and bath towel
- Emesis basin
- Clean gloves

STEP	RATIONALE
ASSESSMENT	
1. Identify patient using at least two person-specific identifiers (e.g., name and date of birth, or name and medical record number) according to employer policy.	Ensures correct patient. Complies with Accreditation Canada's standards and improves patient safety (Accreditation Canada, 2020).
2. Throughout the procedure, the 4 moments for hand hygiene are to be implemented; hand hygiene should occur before initial patient (or patient environment) contact, before an aseptic procedure, after body fluid exposure risk, and after patient (or patient environment) contact. Additional hand hygiene should be performed when hands are visibly soiled.	Proper hand hygiene helps prevent the spread of infectious agents to health care providers.
3. Assess environment for safety (e.g., check room for spills; make sure that equipment is working properly; and ensure that bed is in locked, low position).	Identifies safety hazards in patient environment that could cause or potentially lead to harm (LeLaurin & Shorr, 2019).
4. Apply clean gloves and assess for presence of gag reflex by placing tongue blade on back half of tongue.	Reduces transmission of microorganisms. Helps in determining aspiration risk.

Critical Decision Point *Patients with impaired gag reflex still require oral care; however, they have a higher risk for aspiration. Keep suction equipment available when caring for patients who are at risk for aspiration.*

STEP	RATIONALE

ASSESSMENT

STEP	RATIONALE
5. Inspect condition of oral cavity (see Chapter 8).	Determines condition of oral cavity and need for hygiene. Establishes baseline to show improvement following oral care.
6. Remove and dispose of gloves in proper receptacle.	Reduces transmission of microorganisms.
7. Assess patient's risk for oral hygiene problems (see Skill 18.2).	Certain conditions increase likelihood of alterations in integrity of oral cavity mucosa and structures, necessitating more frequent care.
8. Assess patient's respirations or oxygen saturation.	Helps in early recognition of aspiration.

NURSING DIAGNOSES

- Impaired oral mucous membrane
- Risk for aspiration
- Risk for infection

Related factors are individualized on the basis of patient's condition or needs.

PLANNING

STEP	RATIONALE
1. Expected outcomes following completion of procedure:	
• Oral cavity structures have normal characteristics: buccal mucosa and tongue are pink, moist, and intact; gums are moist and intact; teeth are clean, smooth, and shiny; tongue is pink and without coating; lips are moist, smooth, and without cracks.	Degree of improvement in condition of oral cavity following oral hygiene depends on extent of secretions or changes that existed before care.
• Debilitated patient expresses feeling of mouth cleanliness.	Comfort achieved.
• Oropharynx remains clear of secretions.	Secretions removed, thus avoiding aspiration.
2. Gather equipment and supplies at bedside.	Avoids interrupting procedure or leaving patient unattended to retrieve missing equipment.
3. Explain procedure to patient or caregiver if present.	Even debilitated or intubated patients are usually able to hear. Explanation can reduce anxiety.

IMPLEMENTATION

STEP	RATIONALE
1. Pull curtain around bed or close room door.	Provides privacy.
2. Apply clean gloves.	Reduces transmission of microorganisms.
3. Place towel on over-bed table and arrange equipment. If needed, turn on suction machine and connect tubing to suction catheter.	Prevents soiling of tabletop. Equipment prepared in advance ensures smooth, safe procedure. Supplies being within reach creates organized workspace.
4. Raise bed to appropriate working height; lower side rail.	Use of good body mechanics with bed in high position prevents injury.
Unless contraindicated (e.g., head injury, neck trauma), position patient in side-lying position. Turn patient's head toward mattress in dependent position with HOB elevated at least 30 degrees.	Allows secretions to drain from mouth instead of collecting in back of pharynx. Prevents aspiration. If patient is overweight, follow safe handling techniques for positioning (see Chapter 11).
5. Place towel under patient's head and emesis basin under chin.	Prevents soiling of bed linen.
6. Remove dentures or partial plates if present.	Allows for thorough cleaning of prosthetics later. Provides clearer access to oral cavity.
7. If patient is uncooperative or having difficulty keeping mouth open, insert an oral airway (see Chapter 28). Insert upside down and turn airway sideways and over tongue to keep teeth apart. Insert when patient is relaxed, if possible. Do not use force.	Prevents patient from biting down on nurse's fingers and provides access to oral cavity.

Critical Decision Point *Never place fingers into the mouth of an unconscious or debilitated patient because this may occlude the airway and could cause caregiver injury as a result of the patient's bite response.*

STEP	RATIONALE

IMPLEMENTATION

STEP	RATIONALE
8. Clean mouth using brush moistened in water. Apply toothpaste or use antibacterial solution first to loosen crusts. Hold toothbrush bristles at 45-degree angle to gum line. Be sure that tips of bristles rest against and penetrate gently under gum line. Brush inner and outer surfaces of upper and lower teeth by brushing from gum to crown of each tooth; clean biting surfaces of teeth by holding top of bristles parallel with teeth and brushing gently back and forth (see Skill 18.2). Brush sides of teeth by moving bristles back and forth. Use toothette sponge if patient has bleeding tendency or use of toothbrush is contraindicated. Suction any accumulated secretions. Moisten brush with clean water or antibacterial solution to rinse. Clean lips and mucosa with toothette (see Step 8 illustration). Use brush or toothette to clean roof of mouth, gums, and inside cheeks. Gently brush tongue but avoid stimulating gag reflex (if present). Repeat rinsing several times and use suction to remove secretions. Use towel to dry off lips.	Brushing action removes food particles between teeth and along chewing surfaces and crusts for mucosa. Do not use commercial swabs because they do not clean teeth. Repeated rinsing removes all debris and helps to moisten mucosa. Suction removes secretions and fluids that collect in posterior pharynx, thus reducing aspiration risk.
9. Apply thin layer of water-soluble moisturizer to lips (see Step 9 illustration).	Lubricates lips to prevent drying and cracking.

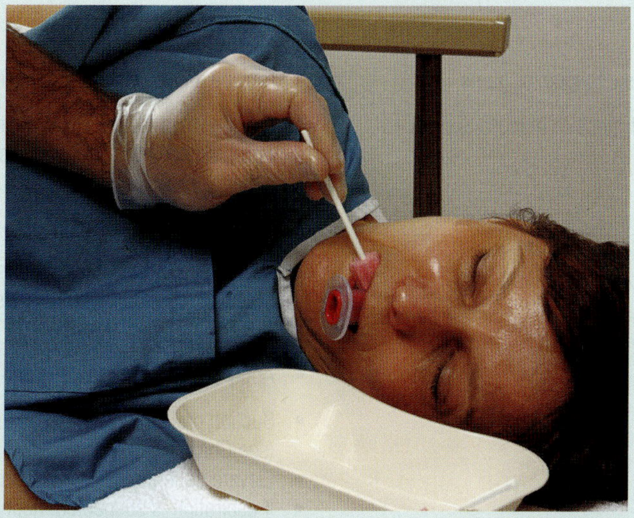

STEP 8 Cleaning lips and mucosa around oral airway with toothette.

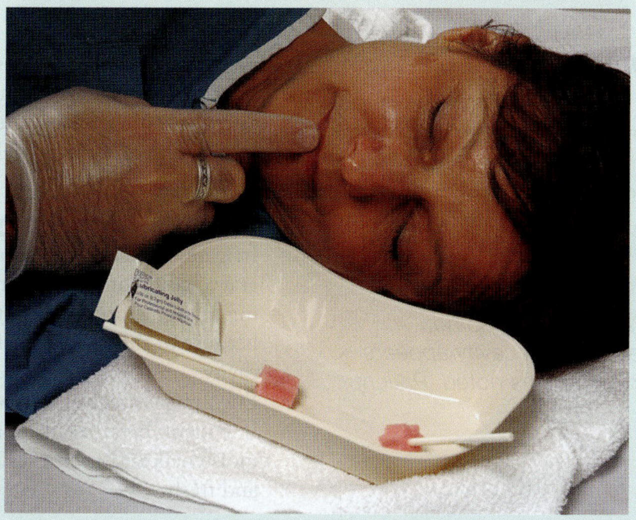

STEP 9 Application of water-soluble moisturizer to lips.

STEP	RATIONALE
IMPLEMENTATION	
10. Inform patient that procedure is completed. Return patient to comfortable and safe position.	Provides meaningful stimulation to unconscious or less responsive patient.
11. Raise side rails as appropriate and return bed to locked, low position. Leave call light in reach.	Reduces patient's risk of falling from bed.
12. Clean equipment and return it to its proper place. Place soiled linen in dirty laundry bag.	Proper disposal of soiled equipment prevents spread of infection.
13. Remove and dispose of gloves in proper receptacle.	Reduces transmission of microorganisms.
EVALUATION	
1. Apply clean gloves and use tongue blade and penlight to inspect oral cavity.	Reduces transmission of microorganisms. Determines efficacy of cleaning. Once thick secretions are removed, underlying inflammation or lesions may be revealed.
2. Ask patient (if able to respond) if mouth feels clean.	Evaluates level of comfort.
3. **Use teach-back:** "I explained what is needed to reduce your partner's risk of choking on secretions in his throat. Tell me the ways you will prevent choking when you give mouth care at home." Develop a revised teaching plan if patient or caregiver is unable to teach back correctly.	Determines patient's and caregiver's level of understanding of instructional topic.

Unexpected Outcomes	Related Interventions
1. Secretions or crusts remain on mucosa, tongue, or gums.	• Provide more frequent oral hygiene.
2. Localized inflammation or bleeding of gums or mucosa is present.	• Provide more frequent oral hygiene with toothette sponges. • Apply water-based mouth moisturizer to provide moisture and maintain integrity of oral mucosa. • Chemotherapy and radiation can cause mucositis (inflammation of mucous membranes in mouth) because of sloughing of epithelial tissue. Room-temperature saline rinses, bicarbonate and sterile water rinses, and oral care with a soft-bristled toothbrush decrease severity and duration of mucositis.
3. Lips are cracked or inflamed.	• Apply moisturizing gel or water-soluble lubricant to lips more often.
4. Patient aspirates secretions.	• Suction oral airway as secretions accumulate to maintain airway patency (see Chapter 23). • Elevate patient's HOB to facilitate breathing. • If aspiration is suspected, notify health care provider. Prepare patient for chest X-ray film examination.

Communication and Documentation

- Document procedure, appearance of oral cavity, presence of gag reflex, and patient's response to procedure in medical record in progress notes in EHR or chart.
- Document your evaluation of patient and caregiver learning.
- Report any unusual findings (e.g., bleeding, ulceration, choking response) to nurse in charge or health care provider.

DOCUMENTATION EXAMPLE

Oral hygiene provided to patient. No gag reflex noted; suction available throughout procedure. Oral cavity appears intact with no bleeding, lesions, or ulcerations noted. Patient tolerated procedure well.

Special Considerations

Teaching

- It is important that caregivers understand how to provide good oral care when required for a patient in the home. Instruction in how to perform mouth care enables the caregiver to understand how to protect the patient from aspirating while thoroughly cleaning the oral cavity. Use the teach-back technique by observing the caregiver perform mouth care procedure effectively or asking them to describe the procedure.

Care in the Community: Home Management

- Irrigate oral cavity with bulb syringe; if unavailable, substitute gravy baster or large syringe. Caution caregiver against instilling a large amount of water or rinsing agent in the oral cavity because of the risk for aspiration. Observe caregiver irrigate oral cavity.
- Encourage caregiver to clean patient's mouth at least twice a day. If patient breathes through mouth, a soft-bristled toothbrush moistened and used every 1 to 2 hours will keep mouth moist and fresh.

Procedural Guideline 18.4 *Hair Care—Combing and Shaving*

A person's comfort, appearance, and sense of well-being can be influenced by how their hair looks and feels. Brushing, combing, and shaving are basic hygiene measures for all patients unable to provide their own self-care. Most long-term care facilities have beauty shops where patients can go for professional hair care. An immobilized patient's hair soon becomes tangled if not brushed or combed regularly. Dressings may leave sticky adhesive, blood, or antiseptic solutions on the hair. Diaphoresis leaves hair oily and unmanageable. Proper hair care is important to a person's body image.

Certain chemotherapy medications and radiation therapy cause loss of hair (alopecia). Many patients choose to wear a wig; however, some choose to wear hair scarves or turbans. Table 18.2 describes common hair and scalp conditions and nursing interventions.

Dependent patients with beards or moustaches need help keeping facial hair clean, especially after eating. Shaving facial hair is a task most individuals prefer to do for themselves daily. Because some religions and cultures forbid cutting or shaving any body hair, it is important to obtain consent from these patients. Make sure to be aware if patients are at risk of bleeding before shaving.

Delegation and Collaboration

The skills of combing and shaving can be delegated to a UCP. The nurse instructs the UCP to do the following:

- Properly position a patient with head or neck mobility restrictions
- Report how the patient tolerated the procedure and any concerns (e.g., neck pain)
- Use an electric razor for any patient at risk of bleeding tendencies

TABLE 18.2

Hair and Scalp Problems

Characteristics	Implications	Interventions
Dandruff—Scaling of scalp accompanied by itching; in severe cases, dandruff occurs on eyebrows	Dandruff causes embarrassment; if it enters eyes, conjunctivitis may develop.	Shampoo regularly with medicated shampoo; in severe cases, obtain health care provider's advice.
Ticks—Small grey-brown parasites that burrow into skin and suck blood	Ticks transmit several diseases, including Rocky Mountain spotted fever, Lyme disease, and tularemia.	Do not pull ticks from skin because sucking apparatus remains behind and may cause skin to become infected; placing drop of oil on tick or covering it with petrolatum eases removal; oil suffocates tick.
Pediculosis capitis (head lice)—Tiny grey-brown–white parasitic insects that attach to hair strands; about size of a sesame seed; nits or eggs look like oval particles attached at an angle to hair shaft; bites or pustules may be observed behind ears and at hairline	Head lice are difficult to remove and, if not treated, may spread to furniture and other people.	Check entire scalp. Use medicated shampoo for eliminating lice or permethrin (Nix), available as a crème rinse. *Caution against use of products containing lindane because the ingredient is toxic and known to cause adverse reactions* (National Pediculosis Association, 2023). Remove patient's clothing before treatment and apply new clothing following treatment. Repeat treatment according to product directions. Check hair for nits and comb with nit comb for 2–3 days until sure all lice and nits have been removed. Manual removal of lice is the best option when treatment has failed. Vacuum infested areas of home. Wash linens in hot water and dry for at least 30 minutes.
Pediculosis corporis (body lice)—Tend to cling to clothing; thus, may not be easily seen; suck blood and lay eggs on clothing and furniture	Patient itches constantly; scratches on skin may become infected; hemorrhagic spots may appear on skin where lice are sucking blood. Lice may spread to other people.	Patient should bathe or shower thoroughly; after skin is dried, apply lotion for eliminating lice; after 12–24 hours another bath or shower should be taken; bag infested clothing or linen until laundered. Vacuum items that cannot be washed.
Pediculosis pubis (crab lice)—Found in pubic hair; grey-white with red legs	Lice may spread through bed linen, clothing, furniture, or sexual contact.	Shave hair from affected area; clean the same way as for body lice; if lice were sexually transmitted, partner must be notified.
Hair loss (alopecia)—Balding patches in periphery of hairline; hair becomes brittle and broken; caused by diseases, medication adverse effects, and improper use of hair care products and hair styling devices	Patches of uneven hair growth and loss alter patient's appearance.	Offer patients access to scarves, hairpieces, or wigs. Stop hair care practices that damage hair.

Continued

Procedural Guideline 18.4 *Hair Care—Combing and Shaving—cont'd*

Equipment

Hair Care

- Wide-tooth comb and hairbrush

Shaving With Razor

- New disposable or electric razor
- Clean gloves
- Bath towel(s), mirror, washcloth, wash basin
- Shaving cream or soap, aftershave lotion (if patient desires and it is not contraindicated)

Moustache Care

- Scissors; brush or comb
- Bath towel
- Gooseneck lamp or overhead light

Procedural Steps

1. Identify patient using at least two person-specific identifiers (e.g., name and date of birth, or name and medical record number) according to employer policy (Accreditation Canada, 2020).
2. Throughout the procedure, the 4 moments for hand hygiene are to be implemented; hand hygiene should occur before initial patient (or patient environment) contact, before an aseptic procedure, after body fluid exposure risk, and after patient (or patient environment) contact. Additional hand hygiene should be performed when hands are visibly soiled.
3. Inspect condition of hair and scalp. Inspect for presence of any infestation (e.g., pediculosis). **Note:** Apply clean gloves and gown if infestation is suspected.
4. Discard gloves and perform hand hygiene after inspection.
5. Assess patient's hair care and shaving product preferences (e.g., shampoo, aftershave lotion, skin conditioner).
6. Assess if patient has bleeding tendency. Review medical history, medications, and laboratory values (e.g., platelet count, anticoagulation studies).

Critical Decision Point *A patient with bleeding risk should use an electric razor.*

7. Assess patient's ability to manipulate comb, brush, or razor.
8. Gather equipment and supplies at patient's bedside. Explain your intent to provide hair or beard care. Ask patient to explain during procedure what they will use to comb hair or shave. Ask patient to indicate if they are uncomfortable during the procedure.
9. Position patient sitting in chair or up in bed with head elevated 45–90 degrees (as tolerated).
10. Provide privacy; close door or pull curtain. Arrange supplies at bedside table and adjust lighting.
11. Apply clean gloves if necessary.
12. Combing and brushing hair:
    a. Part hair into two sections and then separate it into two more sections (see Step 12a illustrations).

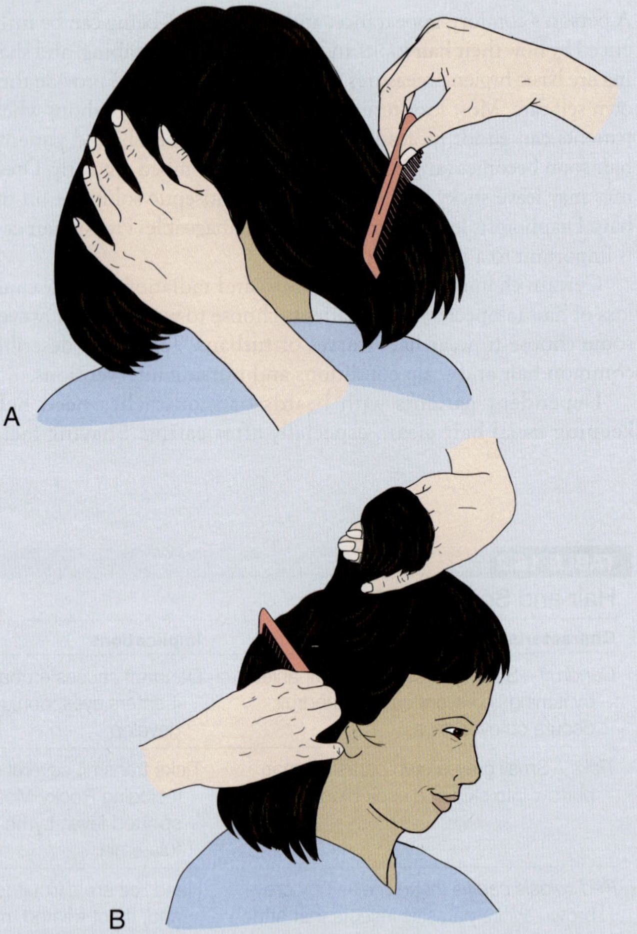

STEP 12A Parting hair. A, Part hair down the middle and divide it into two main sections. B, Part main section into two smaller sections.

    b. Brush or comb from scalp toward hair ends.
    c. Moisten hair lightly with water, conditioner, or alcohol-free detangle product before combing.
    d. Move fingers through hair to loosen any larger tangles.
    e. Using a wide-tooth comb, start on either side of head and insert comb with teeth upward to hair near scalp. Comb through hair in circular motion by turning wrist while lifting up and out. Continue until all hair is combed through and comb into place to shape and style.
13. Shaving with disposable razor:
    a. Place bath towel over patient's chest and shoulders.
    b. Run warm water in wash basin. Check water temperature.
    c. Place washcloth in basin and wring out thoroughly. Apply cloth over patient's entire face for several seconds.
    d. Apply approximately 0.6 cm (0.25 inches) shaving cream or soap to patient's face. Smooth cream evenly over sides of face, on chin, and under nose.
    e. Hold razor in dominant hand at 45-degree angle to patient's skin. Begin by shaving across one side of patient's face using short, firm strokes in direction that

Procedural Guideline 18.4 *Hair Care—Combing and Shaving—cont'd*

hair grows (see Step 13e illustration). Use nondominant hand to gently pull skin taut while shaving. Ask patient if they feel comfortable.

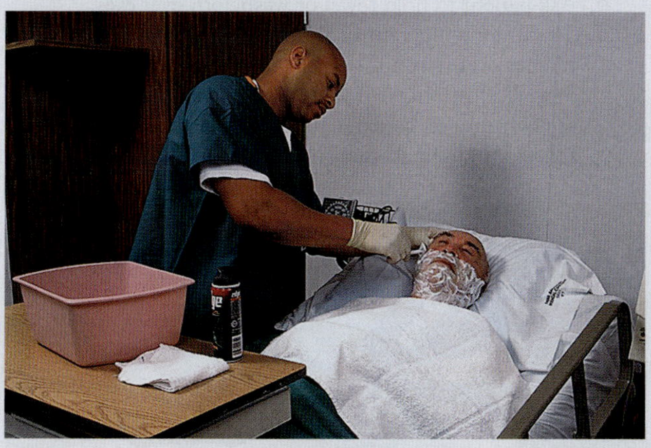

STEP 13E Shaving patient using short, firm strokes.

f. Dip razor blade in water because shaving cream accumulates on edge of blade.
g. After all facial hair is shaved, rinse face thoroughly with warm, moistened washcloth.
h. Dry face thoroughly and apply aftershave lotion if desired. Remove towel.

14. Shaving with electric razor:
    a. Place bath towel over patient's chest and shoulders.
    b. Apply skin conditioner or pre-shave preparation.
    c. Turn razor on and begin by shaving across side of face. Gently hold skin taut while shaving over surface of skin. Use gentle downward stroke of razor in direction of hair growth.
    d. After completing shave, remove towel and apply aftershave lotion as desired unless contraindicated.
15. Moustache and beard care:
    a. Place bath towel over patient's chest and shoulders.
    b. If necessary, gently comb moustache or beard.
    c. Allow patient to use mirror and direct areas to trim with scissors.
    d. After completing, remove towel.
16. Help patient assume desired comfortable position. Leave call light in reach.
17. Return reusable equipment to proper place. Discard soiled linen in dirty laundry bag. Remove gloves and discard in appropriate receptacle.
18. Ask patient how the hair and scalp feel.
19. Inspect condition of shaved area and skin underneath beard or moustache. Look for areas of localized bleeding from cuts and areas of dryness.
20. Ask patient if face feels clean and comfortable.
21. **Use teach-back:** "I want to be sure I explained to you the risks of using a regular razor at home. Tell me what type of razor you should use and why this is important. Tell me the things to watch for with a bleeding tendency." Develop a revised teaching plan if patient or caregiver is unable to teach back correctly.

Procedural Guideline 18.5 *Hair Care—Shampooing*

The frequency of shampooing depends on the condition of the hair and a person's daily routines and cultural preferences. Dry hair, which commonly results from aging and protein deficiency, requires less frequent shampooing than oily hair. In some health care facilities, the nurse needs a health care provider's prescription to shampoo a patient who is dependent or has limited mobility because it is challenging to find ways to shampoo the hair without causing injury to a patient's neck.

Remind hospitalized patients that more frequent shampooing is necessary when they remain in bed for extended periods of time, have excessive perspiration, or undergo treatments that leave blood or solutions in the hair. Two types of shampooing are available for patients: (1) traditional shampoo and water and (2) a disposable dry shampoo cap. Patients who are able to sit in a chair in front of a sink can be shampooed. Make sure that a patient's condition does not contraindicate neck hyperextension. Exercise caution with patients who have suffered neck injuries because flexion and hyperextension of the neck could cause further injury. In addition, patients with positional vertigo are not able to tolerate neck hyperextension if it increases their dizziness. A folded towel placed under the neck on the edge of the sink provides added comfort.

If a patient cannot sit in a chair or be transferred to a stretcher, shampoo the hair with the patient in bed, using traditional shampoo and water or a disposable shampoo product.

Delegation and Collaboration

The skill of shampooing the hair of bed-bound patients and the use of a disposable shampoo product can be delegated to a UCP. The nurse instructs the UCP about the following:

- Proper way to position a patient with a head or neck mobility restriction
- Knowledge of care for lice, stressing steps to take to prevent transmission to other patients

Equipment

- Bath towels
- Clean gloves, clean gown (*optional*) (if patient has known head lice)
- Clean comb and brush

Regular Shampoo

- Washcloth
- Shampoo, hair conditioner (*optional*); hydrogen peroxide and saline (*optional*)
- Water pitcher with warm water
- Plastic shampoo board, wash basin
- Bath blanket, waterproof pad

Continued

Procedural Guideline 18.5 *Hair Care—Shampooing—cont'd*

Disposable Shampoo

- Disposable shampoo cap product

Procedural Steps

1. Identify patient using at least two person-specific identifiers (e.g., name and date of birth, or name and medical record number) according to employer policy (Accreditation Canada, 2020).
2. Throughout the procedure, the 4 moments for hand hygiene are to be implemented; hand hygiene should occur before initial patient (or patient environment) contact, before an aseptic procedure, after body fluid exposure risk, and after patient (or patient environment) contact. Additional hand hygiene should be performed when hands are visibly soiled.
3. Inspect condition of hair and scalp before beginning shampoo. This determines whether special shampoos or treatments are necessary (e.g., dandruff, lice, removal of blood). If draining head wounds are suspected, apply clean gloves. If lice are present, the patient may be placed on contact precautions. Check employer policy.
4. Review medical record to confirm that there are no contraindications to the procedure. Check employer policy for health care provider prescriptions as needed. Certain medical conditions, such as head and neck injuries, spinal cord injuries, and arthritis, place a patient at risk for injury during shampooing because of positioning and manipulation of the patient's head and neck.
5. Assess environment for safety (e.g., check room for spills; make sure that equipment is working properly; and ensure that bed is in locked, low position) (LeLaurin & Shorr, 2019).
6. Explain procedure to patient using simple language.
7. Assemble equipment at bedside, including pitcher with warm water.
8. Provide privacy by closing room door or curtain dividers. Raise bed to comfortable working height, and lower side rail on side where you will stand.
9. Shampooing bed-bound patient with shampoo board:
   a. Apply clean gloves. Place waterproof pad under patient's shoulders, neck, and head.
   b. Position patient supine with head and shoulders at top edge of bed. Place shampoo board under patient's head and wash basin under end of trough spout (see Step 9b illustration). Be sure that trough spout extends beyond edge of mattress.

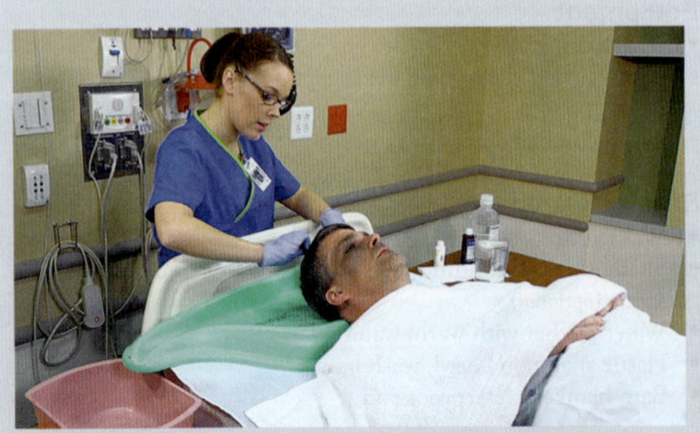

STEP 9B Patient positioned over shampoo board.

   c. Place rolled towel under patient's neck and bath towel over patient's shoulders.
   d. Brush and comb patient's hair.
   e. Ask patient to hold towel or washcloth over eyes.
   f. Test water temperature. Slowly pour water from pitcher over hair until it is completely wet (see Step 9f illustration). If hair contains matted blood, apply hydrogen peroxide to dissolve clots and rinse with saline. Apply small amount of shampoo.

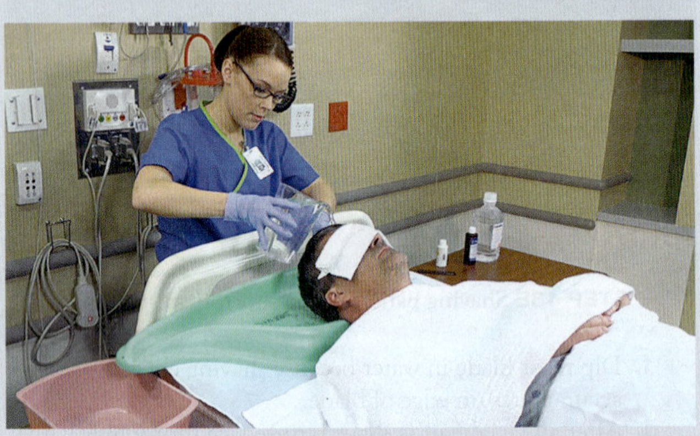

STEP 9F Nurse pouring water over patient's hair.

   g. Work up lather with both hands. Start at hairline and work toward back of neck. Lift head slightly with one hand to wash back of head. Shampoo sides of head. Massage scalp by applying pressure with fingertips.
   h. Rinse hair with water. Make sure that water drains into basin. Repeat rinsing until hair is free of soap. (If you need to refill pitcher, raise side rail when leaving bedside.)
   i. Apply conditioner if requested and rinse hair thoroughly.
   j. Wrap patient's head in bath towel. Dry face with cloth used to protect eyes. Dry off any moisture along neck or shoulders.
   k. Dry patient's hair and scalp. Use second towel if first one becomes saturated.
   l. Comb hair to remove tangles and dry with dryer if desired.
   m. Apply oil preparation or conditioning product to hair if desired by patient.
   n. Variation for patients with coarse, curly hair: Condition hair after washing. To untangle hair, use wide teeth of comb. Beginning at nape of neck, comb small subsections of hair, starting at hair ends. Continue to work through small sections until hair is free of tangles.
   o. Help patient to comfortable position and complete styling of hair. Leave call light in reach.
   p. Dispose of and store supplies as appropriate. Remove gloves and discard in appropriate receptacle.
10. Shampooing with disposable shampoo product:
   a. Patient can be sitting on chair or in bed. Apply clean gloves.
   b. Comb hair to remove any tangles or debris.
   c. Open package, apply cap, and secure all hair beneath cap (see Step 10c illustration).

Procedural Guideline 18.5 *Hair Care—Shampooing—cont'd*

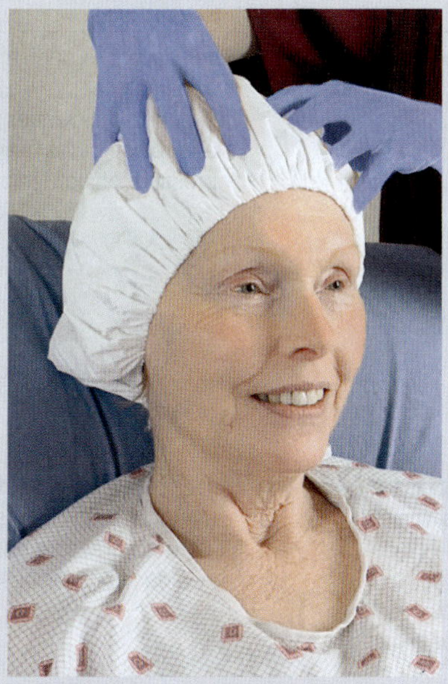

STEP 10C Patient wearing disposable shampoo cap.

d. Massage head through cap. Check fitting around head to maintain correct fit.
e. Massage for 2–4 minutes according to directions on package; additional time may be required for longer hair or hair matted with blood.
f. Discard cap in garbage; do not dispose of cap in toilet because it may clog plumbing.
g. If patient desires, towel-dry hair. Brush or comb patient's hair.
h. Remove gloves.
i. Help patient to comfortable position with call light in reach.

11. Inspect condition of hair and scalp.
12. **Use teach-back:** "During the shampoo we discussed ways to reduce the risk of getting exposed to lice in your home. Tell me three ways to reduce the chance of exposing yourself and others to lice." Develop a revised teaching plan if patient or caregiver is unable to teach back correctly.

✦ SKILL 18.4 Performing Nail and Foot Care

The best time to provide nail and foot care is during a patient's daily bath. Many facilities require a health care provider's prescription before the nurse can trim nails, and some require special certification to provide nail care (check employer policy). Feet and nails often require special care to prevent infection, odours, pain, and injury to soft tissues. Often, people are unaware of foot or nail problems until discomfort or pain occurs. Common foot and nail problems are presented in Table 18.3. For proper foot and nail care, instruct patients to protect the feet from injury, keep them clean and dry, and wear appropriate footwear. Instruct patients how to properly inspect the feet for lesions, dryness, or signs of infection. To maintain and promote foot and nail health, patients should visit a podiatrist when necessary. This is especially important for patients with foot disorders, peripheral vascular diseases (PVDs), or diabetes mellitus; older persons; and patients who are immunocompromised.

Patients most at risk of developing serious foot problems are those with peripheral neuropathy and PVD. These two disorders, commonly found in patients with diabetes mellitus, cause a reduction in blood flow to the extremities and a loss of sensory, motor, and autonomic nerve function. As a result, a patient is unable to feel heat and cold, pain, pressure, and positioning of the foot or feet. The reduction in blood flow impairs healing and increases risk of infection. The development of diabetic foot ulcers has three contributing factors: (1) peripheral neuropathy (changes in the function and efficiency of the nerves); (2) ischemia (decrease in the blood flow related to plaque formation in arteries); and (3) a pivotal event (trauma caused by banging the toe or stepping on a foreign object). If foot ulcers do not heal, they can become infected quickly and lead to gangrene and subsequent amputation.

Delegation and Collaboration

The skill of providing nail and foot care to patients *without diabetes mellitus* or *circulatory compromise* can be delegated to a UCP. The nurse instructs the UCP about the following:

- Not trimming patient's nails (unless permitted by employer policy or health care provider prescription)
- Special considerations for patient positioning
- Reporting any breaks in skin, redness, numbness, swelling, or pain to the nurse

The nurse collaborates with the interprofessional health care team (e.g., a podiatrist or foot care specialist) to identify specific procedure for foot care for patients with PVD, diabetes mellitus, and foot ulcers or injuries.

Equipment

- Wash basin
- Emesis basin
- Washcloth and towel
- Nail clippers (check employer policy)
- Soft nail or cuticle brush
- Plastic applicator stick
- Emery board or nail file
- Body lotion
- Disposable bath mat
- Clean gloves

TABLE 18.3

Common Foot and Nail Problems

Condition	Characteristics	Implications	Interventions
Callus 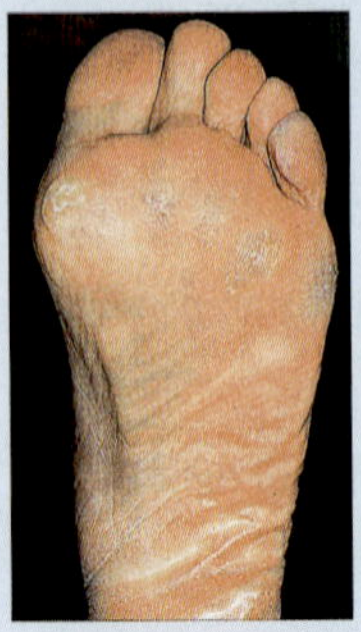	Thickened part of epidermis, consisting of mass of horny, keratotic cells; usually flat, painless, and found on undersurface of foot or palm of hand; caused by local friction or pressure	Foot calluses may cause discomfort when wearing tight-fitting shoes.	Refer patient to podiatrist; do not self-treat. Use of orthotic devices cushions and redistributes weight and pressure off calluses.
Corns 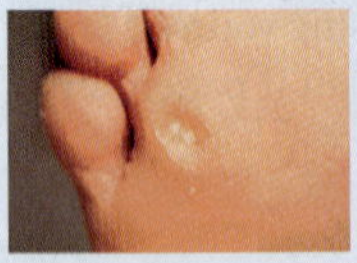	Keratosis caused by friction and pressure from shoes; mainly on toes, over bony prominence; usually cone-shaped, round, and raised; calluses with painful core	Conical shape compresses underlying dermis, making it thin and tender. Pain is aggravated by tight-fitting shoes. Patients may suffer alteration in gait because of pain.	Refer patient to podiatrist. Avoid use of oval corn pads, which increase pressure on toes. Use wider, softer shoes.
Plantar warts 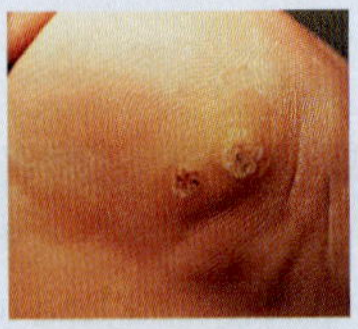	Fungating lesions on sole of foot caused by papillomavirus	Warts may be contagious, are painful, and make walking difficult.	Refer patient to podiatrist.
Athlete's foot (tinea pedis) 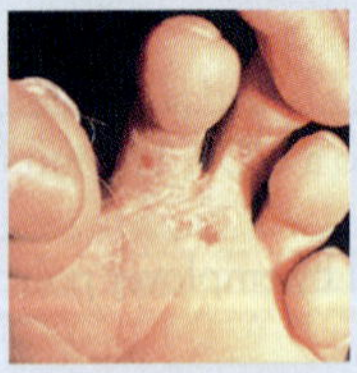	Fungal infection of foot; scaliness and cracking of skin between toes and on soles of feet; small blisters containing fluid may appear, apparently induced by constricting footwear	Athlete's foot can spread to other body parts, especially hands. It is contagious and frequently recurs.	Feet should be well ventilated. Drying feet well after bathing and applying powder help prevent infection. Wearing clean socks or stockings reduces incidence. Health care provider may prescribe application of topical antifungal agents.
Ingrown nails 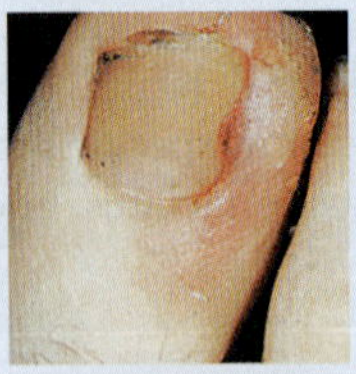	Toenail or fingernail growing inward into soft tissue around nail; results from improper nail trimming, poor shoe fit, or heredity	Ingrown nails can cause localized pain when pressure is applied.	Treatment is frequent warm soaks (**Exception:** patients with diabetes mellitus) in antiseptic solution and removal of part of nail that has grown into skin. Teach patient proper nail-trimming techniques. Refer to podiatrist.
Paronychia 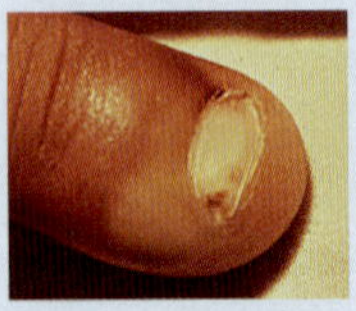	Inflammation of tissue surrounding nail after hangnail or other injury; occurs in people who frequently have their hands in water; common in patients with diabetes mellitus	Area can become infected.	Treatment is warm compresses or soaks (**Exception:** patients with diabetes mellitus) and local application of antibiotic ointments. Paronychia can be prevented by careful manicuring.
Foot odours	Result of excess perspiration promoting microorganism growth and possibly faulty foot hygiene or improper footwear	Excess perspiration causes discomfort.	Frequent washing, use of foot deodorants and powders, and clean footwear prevent or reduce this problem.

STEP	RATIONALE
ASSESSMENT	
1. Identify patient using at least two person-specific identifiers (e.g., name and date of birth, or name and medical record number) according to employer policy.	Ensures correct patient. Complies with Accreditation Canada's standards and improves patient safety (Accreditation Canada, 2020).
2. Throughout the procedure, the 4 moments for hand hygiene are to be implemented; hand hygiene should occur before initial patient (or patient environment) contact, before an aseptic procedure, after body fluid exposure risk, and after patient (or patient environment) contact. Additional hand hygiene should be performed when hands are visibly soiled.	Proper hand hygiene helps prevent the spread of infectious agents to health care providers.
3. Assess environment for safety (e.g., check room for spills; make sure that equipment is working properly; and ensure that bed is in locked, low position).	Identifies safety hazards in patient environment that could cause or potentially lead to harm (LeLaurin & Shorr, 2019).
4. Apply clean gloves. Inspect all surfaces of fingers, toes, feet, and nails. (NOTE: This can be done during the bath.) Pay close attention to areas of dryness, inflammation, or cracking. Also inspect areas between toes, and heels and soles of feet. Inspect socks for stains.	Reduces transmission of microorganisms. Integrity of feet and nails determines frequency and level of hygiene required. Heels, soles, and sides of feet are prone to irritation from ill-fitting shoes. Socks may become stained from bleeding or draining ulcer.
5. Assess circulation to extremities bilaterally: inspect colour of skin; palpate temperature of toes, feet, and fingers and capillary refill of nails; palpate radial and ulnar pulse of each hand and dorsalis pedis pulse of foot; note character and symmetry of pulses (see Chapters 7 and 8). Remove and dispose of gloves in appropriate receptacle.	Extremities should always be assessed bilaterally to check for symmetry. Circulatory alterations often change integrity of nails and increase patient's chance of localized infection when break in skin integrity occurs.
6. Observe patient's walking gait (when appropriate). Have patient walk down the hall or walk in a straight line while wearing comfortable shoes or slippers (if able). Ask if patient has pain when walking (using an appropriate pain scale).	Alterations in bony structures of feet may cause pain, imbalance, and unsteady gait.
7. Ask if patient has history of leg pain on walking that is relieved with rest.	Claudicating pain is related to ischemia with diabetic and neuropathic disorders.
8. Ask if patient uses nail polish and polish remover frequently.	Chemicals in these products cause excessive dryness of nails.
9. Assess type of footwear patient wears: Does patient wear socks? Compression hose? Are shoes tight or ill fitting? Are garters or knee-high nylons worn? Is footwear clean?	Some types of shoes and footwear predispose patient to foot and nail problems (e.g., infection, areas of friction, ulcerations).
10. Identify patient's risk for foot or nail problems.	Certain conditions increase likelihood of foot or nail problems (e.g., diabetes mellitus, being immunocompromised).
a. Older person	Poor vision, lack of coordination, or inability to bend over contributes to difficulty in performing foot and nail care. Normal physiological changes of aging can result in brittle nails. Discoloured, thickened, and deformed nails can indicate infection, fungus, or disease (Centers for Disease Control and Prevention, 2022).
b. Diabetes mellitus	Vascular changes reduce blood flow to peripheral tissues. Break in skin integrity places patient with diabetes mellitus at high risk for skin infection.
c. Heart failure, renal disease	Both conditions increase tissue edema, particularly in dependent areas (e.g., feet). Edema reduces blood flow to neighbouring tissues.
d. Cerebrovascular accident (stroke)	Presence of residual foot or leg weakness or paralysis results in altered walking patterns. Altered gait pattern causes increased friction and pressure on feet.
11. Assess for use of home remedies.	It is always a good idea to evaluate a patient's self-care routine. Patient's personal care practices may overlap or clash with prescribed medical treatment. Collaborate with patient, when possible, to ensure best outcome possible.
a. Over-the-counter (OTC) liquid preparations to remove corns or warts	Patients with diabetes mellitus or circulatory insufficiency should seek professional treatment and avoid self-treating.
b. Cutting corns or calluses with razor blade or scissors	Carries risk of cutting skin, which can lead to infection.
c. Use of oval corn pads	May exert pressure on toes, thereby decreasing circulation to surrounding tissues. Seek professional treatment.

STEP	RATIONALE
ASSESSMENT	
d. Application of adhesive tape	Skin of older person is thin and delicate and prone to tearing when adhesive tape is removed.
12. Assess patient's ability to care for nails or feet: visual alterations, fatigue, and musculoskeletal weakness.	Extent of patient's ability to perform self-care determines degree of help required from nurse and need to educate caregiver.

NURSING DIAGNOSES

- Bathing/self-care deficit
- Reduced physical mobility
- Reduced skin integrity
- Reduced tissue perfusion
- Inadequate knowledge regarding foot and nail care
- Potential for infection

Related factors are individualized on the basis of patient's condition or needs.

STEP	RATIONALE
PLANNING	
1. Expected outcomes following completion of procedure:	
• Nails are smooth. Cuticles and tissues surrounding nails are clear and of normal colour. Surfaces of feet are smooth.	Excess skin layers are removed. Nail integrity and cleanliness are maintained.
• Patient walks freely, without pain or unusual gait.	Foot care removes excess skin layers or shortens nails so that patient can walk more comfortably.
• Patient explains or demonstrates nail care correctly.	Patient learns self-care skill.
2. Gather equipment and supplies at bedside on over-bed table.	Avoids interrupting procedure or leaving patient unattended to retrieve missing equipment. Easy access to equipment prevents delays.
3. Explain procedure to patient, including fact that proper soaking of nails on hands requires several minutes in warm water. EXCEPTION: Patients with diabetes mellitus should not soak hands or feet.	Patient must be willing to place fingers in basin for up to 10 minutes. Patient may become anxious or tired.
4. Obtain health care provider's prescription for cutting nails (check employer policy). Obtaining prescription for podiatry consultation should be initiated if patient has diabetes mellitus, peripheral neuropathy, or PVD.	Patient's skin may be cut accidently. Certain patients are more at risk for infection, depending on their medical condition. A podiatrist should assess and develop a regular schedule for nail care for patients with vascular insufficiency or peripheral neuropathy.
IMPLEMENTATION	
1. Apply clean gloves.	Reduces transmission of microorganisms.
2. Pull curtain around bed or close room door to provide privacy.	Maintaining patient's privacy reduces anxiety.
3. Help ambulatory patient sit in chair and place disposable bath mat on floor under patient's feet. Help bed-bound patient to supine position with HOB elevated 45 degrees, then place waterproof pad on mattress (keep side rail up until ready to begin).	Sitting in chair facilitates immersing feet in basin. Bath mat protects feet from exposure to soil or debris.
4. Fill wash basin with warm water. Test water temperature. Place basin on floor or lower side rail and then place basin on pad on mattress. Have patient immerse feet. If patient has diabetes mellitus, peripheral neuropathy, or PVD, go to Step 13 to begin foot care.	Prevents accidental burns to patient's skin.

Critical Decision Point *Patients who have diabetes mellitus, peripheral neuropathy, or PVD should not soak their hands and feet because of the increased risk for maceration, which makes skin susceptible to infection.*

STEP	RATIONALE
5. Adjust over-bed table to low position and place it over patient's lap.	Easy access prevents accidental spills.
6. Fill emesis basin with warm water and place basin on towel on over-bed table. Test water temperature.	Warm water softens fingernails and thickened epidermal cells. Prevents accidental burns to patient's skin.
7. Instruct patient to place fingers in emesis basin and arms in comfortable position.	Prolonged positioning causes discomfort unless normal anatomical alignment is maintained.

STEP	RATIONALE
IMPLEMENTATION	
8. Allow feet and fingernails to soak 5–10 minutes. If patient has diabetes mellitus, peripheral neuropathy, or PVD, skip this step and go straight to Step 9.	Goal is to soften debris beneath nails so it can be removed easily.
9. Clean gently under fingernails with end of plastic applicator stick while fingers are immersed (see Step 9 illustration).	Removes debris under nails that harbours microorganisms.
10. Use soft cuticle brush or nailbrush to clean around cuticles to decrease overgrowth.	Nailbrush helps prevent inflammation and injury to cuticles. The cuticle slowly grows over the nail and must be pushed back with a soft nail brush regularly.
11. Remove emesis basin and dry fingers thoroughly.	Thorough drying impedes fungal growth and prevents maceration of tissues.

Critical Decision Point *Check employer policy for appropriate process for cleaning beneath nails. Do not use an orange stick or end of cotton swab; these may splinter and can cause injury.*

STEP	RATIONALE
12. Check employer policy on nail care regarding filing and trimming. Trim nails straight across at level of finger or follow curve of finger, ensuring that you do not cut down into nail grooves (see Step 12 illustration). Use disposable emery board and file nails to ensure that there are no sharp corners.	Trimming straight across avoids skin overgrowth at nail edges, which can lead to ingrown nails or infection. Filing nails straight across eliminates sharp nail edges, minimizing risk that nail can injure an adjacent finger.
13. Move over-bed table away from patient. Begin foot care by scrubbing callused areas of feet with washcloth.	Provides easier access to feet. Friction removes dead skin layers.
14. Clean between toes with washcloth.	
15. Dry feet thoroughly and trim or cut toenails (see Step 12).	Moisture can cause skin maceration.
16. Apply lotion to feet and hands. Rub in thoroughly. Do not leave excess lotion between toes.	Lotion lubricates dry skin by helping to retain moisture.
17. Help patient back to bed and into comfortable, safe position, leaving call light within reach.	
18. Sanitize or dispose of equipment according to employer policy. Emery boards should be disposable. Dispose of soiled linen in dirty laundry bag. Remove gloves and discard in appropriate receptacle.	Reduces transmission of infection.

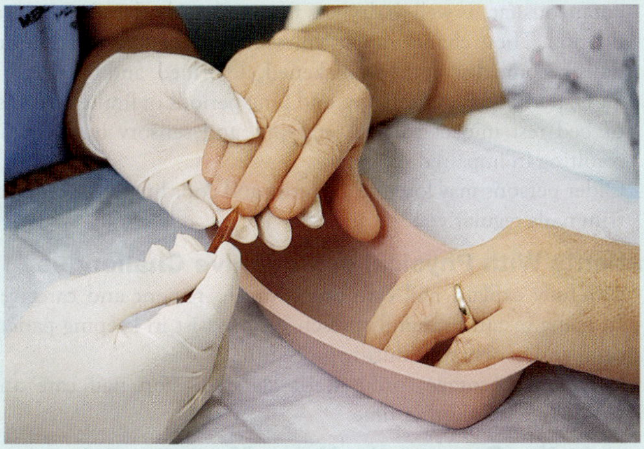

STEP 9 Clean under fingernails.

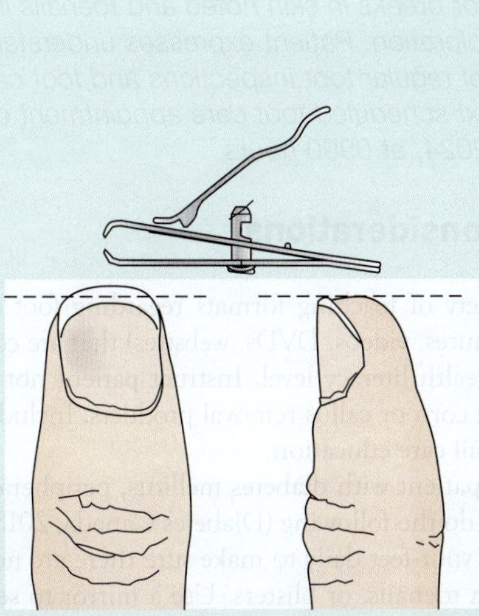

STEP 12 Trim nails straight across when using nail clipper.

STEP	RATIONALE
EVALUATION	
1. Inspect nails, areas between fingers and toes, and surrounding skin surfaces.	Inspection enables evaluation of condition of skin and nails and any remaining rough nail edges.
2. If possible, have patient stand and walk and rate any pain.	Evaluates whether nail care removed excess skin or uneven nail surfaces that can cause discomfort.
3. Observe patient's walk after foot and nail care.	Evaluate level of comfort and mobility achieved.
4. **Use teach-back:** "We discussed how to prevent infection in the skin around your nails. This is important because you have diabetes. Tell me the tips you should follow to protect your feet from infection." Develop a revised teaching plan if patient or caregiver is unable to teach back correctly.	Determines patient's and caregiver's level of understanding of instructional topic.

Unexpected Outcomes	Related Interventions
1. Cuticles and surrounding tissues are inflamed and tender to touch.	• Repeat nail care. • Evaluate need for antifungal cream.
2. Localized areas of tenderness occur on feet with calluses or corns at point of friction.	• Change in footwear or corrective foot surgery may be needed for permanent improvement in calluses or corns. • Refer patient to podiatrist.
3. Ulcerations involving toes or feet may remain.	• Institute wound care policies (see Chapter 39). • Consult with wound care specialist and/or podiatrist. • Increase frequency of assessment and hygiene.

Communication and Documentation

- Document procedure and observations of condition of nails and skin around nails in medical record in progress notes in EHR or chart.
- Report any expressed discomforts, breaks in skin, or ulcerations to nurse in charge or health care provider.
- Document your evaluation of patient and caregiver learning.

DOCUMENTATION EXAMPLE

Foot and nail care provided. No foot ulcerations, tenderness, or breaks in skin noted and toenails intact with no discoloration. Patient expresses understanding of importance of regular foot inspections and foot care. Will return for next scheduled foot care appointment on August 22, 2024, at 0900 hours.

Special Considerations

Teaching

- Use a variety of teaching formats regarding foot and nail care (e.g., brochures, videos, DVDs, websites) that are consistent with patient's health literacy level. Instruct patient not to walk barefoot or use corn or callus removal products. Include caregiver in foot and nail care education.
- Instruct a patient with diabetes mellitus, peripheral neuropathy, or PVD to do the following (Diabetes Canada, 2018):
  - Inspect your feet daily to make sure there are no cuts, cracks, ingrown toenails, or blisters. Use a mirror to see the bottom of your feet or ask someone to check them for you. Wash your feet in warm water. Dry them carefully, especially between the toes. Apply lotion to heels and soles.
  - Clean cuts or scratches with mild soap and water. Cover with dry dressing for sensitive skin. Trim toenails straight across and file sharp edges.
  - Wear fresh, clean socks. When possible, wear white socks, as you will be able to see any drainage.
  - Wear well-fitting shoes. They should be supportive and have low heels, and should not pinch or rub.
  - Elevate feet when sitting, and wiggle your toes and ankles for a few minutes several times a day to improve blood flow in your feet and legs.
  - Exercise regularly to improve circulation.

Pediatric

- Teach a parent/guardian how to assess a child's nails and trim them to prevent the child from scratching their skin.
- Use appropriate-sized clippers for infants and small children (check employer policy). *Do not use scissors.*

Gerontological

- Changes in aging skin include thinning of the epidermis and subcutaneous fat, as well as dryness from reduced oil and sweat production. These changes are often evident in the feet. In addition, nails become discoloured, thickened, deformed, and brittle.
- PVD, peripheral neuropathy, and long periods of limited exercise or bed rest impact balance, stability, and sensory impairment, resulting in impaired mobility.
- Older persons may lose the dexterity and coordination needed to trim nails regularly.

Patients With Physical or Cognitive Challenges

- Carefully explain nail care procedure to patient and caregiver. In many instances, family presence can assist in keeping patient calm and cooperative during procedure.
- If patient becomes confused or agitated, stop nail care and reschedule for another time.

Care in the Community: Home Management

- Assess the home for any areas where a person could accidently injure the feet, such as rugs, objects that block pathways, or uneven walks or flooring.
- Encourage patients to not go barefoot or wear open-toed shoes.
- *Alternative therapy:* Apply moleskin to friction areas of the foot or feet or wrap small pieces of lambswool around toes to reduce irritation from corns or bunions.
- Place contact information for podiatrist, health care provider, and home care nurse close by for easy access.

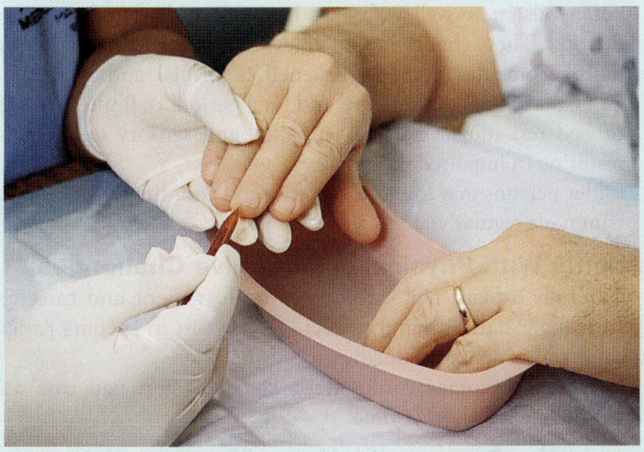

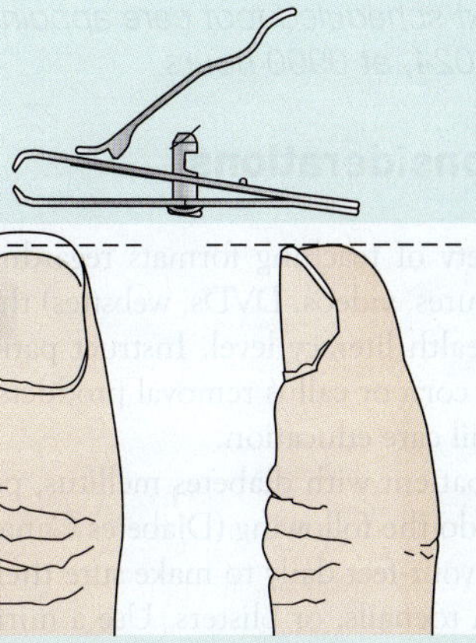

Procedural Guideline 18.6 *Making an Occupied Bed*

The hospital bed is the piece of equipment a patient uses most. It should be comfortable, safe, and adaptable to various positions. The typical hospital bed consists of a firm mattress on a metal frame that can be raised or lowered horizontally. The frame is divided into three sections so that the operator can raise and lower the head and foot of the bed separately and incline the entire bed with the head up or down. Table 18.4 shows common bed positions. Each bed sits on four casters that allow health care workers to move the bed easily. Each caster may have a brake to make sure the bed is stationary. Beds have side rails that can be raised or lowered by pushing or pulling a knob located on both sides of the bed. Research shows that the risk for patient falls is greater when side rails on both sides of a bed are raised, because patients try to climb over the rails to exit the bed. Raising only one rail (when there are only two) or three (when there are four rails) gives patients an exit and therefore the ability to move independently.

At times, it is necessary to make a bed that is occupied by a patient who cannot tolerate being out of bed. If a patient is confined to bed, the bed should be made in a way that conserves time and the patient's energy. A patient's weight, ability to move and turn, pain acuity, and restrictions related to clinical condition or treatment all affect the number of individuals who need to be involved in making an occupied bed. It is essential to use safe patient-handling techniques when turning and positioning a patient over bed linen (see Chapter 11). For a patient in severe pain, an analgesic administered 30–60 minutes before the bed is made can control pain and maintain comfort.

A patient who is unable to get out of bed should still be encouraged to participate in bed-making activities as much as possible. For example, if the patient can turn, help in moving up in bed, or hold top sheets during application, have them do so. These activities help maintain a patient's strength and mobility and allow participation in hygiene care.

Delegation and Collaboration

The skill of making an occupied bed can be delegated to a UCP. The nurse instructs the UCP about the following:

- Any position or activity restrictions that apply
- Looking for wound drainage or loosened equipment that might be found in the bed linens
- Understanding when to obtain help from other caregivers for positioning a patient during linen change and the importance of using good body mechanics and supporting patient alignment
- Using special precautions (e.g., aspiration precautions [see Chapter 31] or positioning for tube-feeding infusion [see Chapter 32]) when positioning a patient during bed making.

Equipment

- Linen bags
- Mattress pad (change only when soiled)
- Bottom sheet (flat or fitted)
- Drawsheet (optional)
- Top sheet, blanket, bedspread, pillowcases
- Waterproof pads (optional)
- Clean gloves (if linen is soiled or there is risk of exposure to body fluids)
- Antiseptic cleanser
- Washcloth

Procedural Steps

1. Review medical record and assess restrictions in mobility or positioning of patient.
2. Throughout the procedure, the 4 moments for hand hygiene are to be implemented; hand hygiene should occur before initial patient (or patient environment) contact, before an aseptic procedure, after body fluid exposure risk, and after patient (or patient environment) contact. Additional hand hygiene should be performed when hands are visibly soiled.
3. Assess environment for safety (e.g., check room for spills; make sure that equipment is working properly; and ensure that bed is in locked position and that appropriate number of side rails are raised) and close room door or divider curtain to provide privacy.
4. Apply clean gloves if patient has been incontinent or if drainage is present on linen.
5. Explain procedure to patient, noting that they will be asked to turn over layers of linen.
6. Raise bed to a comfortable working height; lower HOB as tolerated, keeping patient comfortable. Remove call light.

Critical Decision Point *If patient is on aspiration precautions or receiving tube feeding, maintain HOB 30 degrees or higher.*

7. Lower side rail on side where you are standing. Loosen all top linen. Remove bedspread and blanket separately, leaving patient covered with top sheet. If blanket or spread is soiled, place in linen bag. If items are to be reused, fold into square and place over back of chair.
8. Cover patient with clean bath blanket by unfolding it over top sheet. Have patient hold top edge of bath blanket or tuck blanket under shoulders. Grasp top sheet under bath blanket at patient's shoulders and bring sheet down to foot of bed. Remove sheet and discard in dirty laundry bag.
9. Position patient on far side of bed, turned onto side and facing away from you. NOTE: This step is when another caregiver can help you by standing at bedside across from you. Encourage patient to use side rail to turn. Adjust pillow under patient's head.
10. Ensure there is no tension on any external medical devices.
11. Loosen bottom linens, moving from head to foot. Fanfold or roll any cloth pads, drawsheet (if present), and bottom sheet (in that order) toward patient. Tuck edges of old linen just under patient's buttocks, back, and shoulders (see Step 11 illustration). Do not fanfold mattress pad (if it is to be reused). Remove any disposable pads and discard in receptacle.

Continued

Procedural Guideline 18.6 *Making an Occupied Bed—cont'd*

TABLE 18.4

Common Bed Positions

Position	**Description**	**Uses**
Fowler's 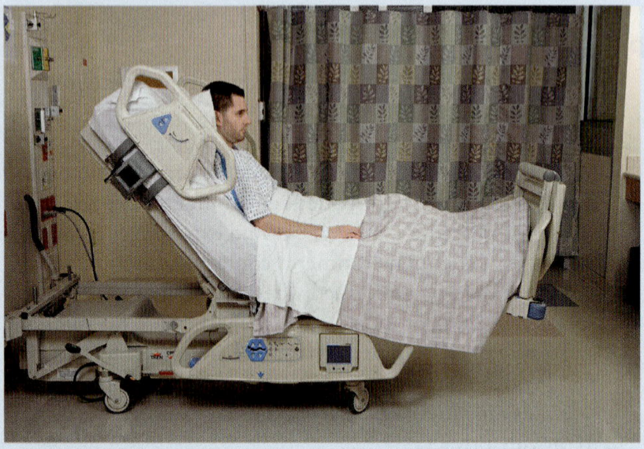	Head of bed raised to angle of 45–90 degrees; semi-sitting position; foot of bed may also be raised at knee	Preferred while patient eats; used during nasogastric tube insertion and nasotracheal suction; promotes lung expansion
Semi-Fowler's 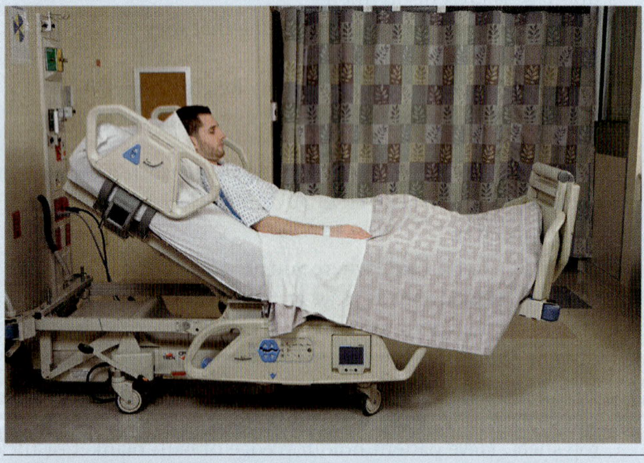	Head of bed raised approximately 30–45 degrees; incline less than Fowler's position; foot of bed may also be raised at knee	Promotes lung expansion; relieves strain on abdominal muscles Used when patients receive gastric feedings to reduce risk for aspiration
Trendelenburg's 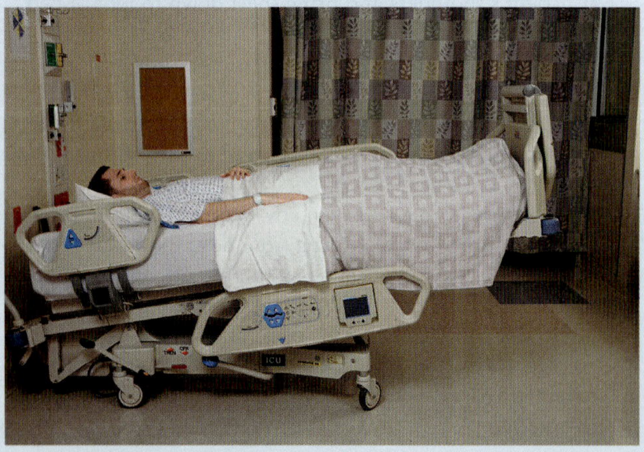	Entire bedframe tilted with head of bed down	For postural drainage; facilitates venous return in patients with poor peripheral perfusion

Procedural Guideline 18.6 *Making an Occupied Bed—cont'd*

TABLE 18.4
Common Bed Positions—cont'd

Position	Description	Uses
Reverse Trendelenburg's 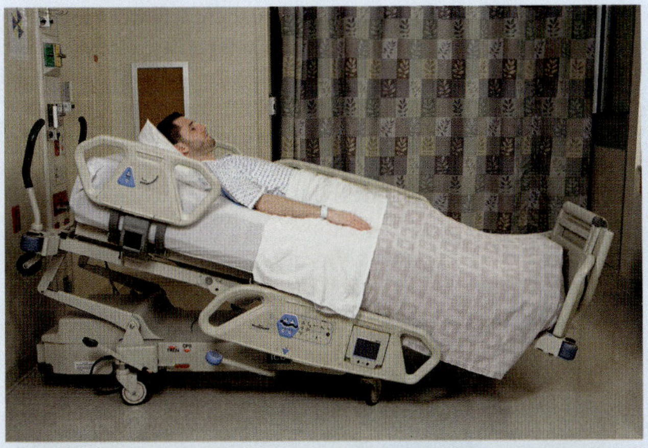	Entire bedframe tilted with foot of bed down	Used infrequently; promotes gastric emptying and prevents esophageal reflux
Supine or flat 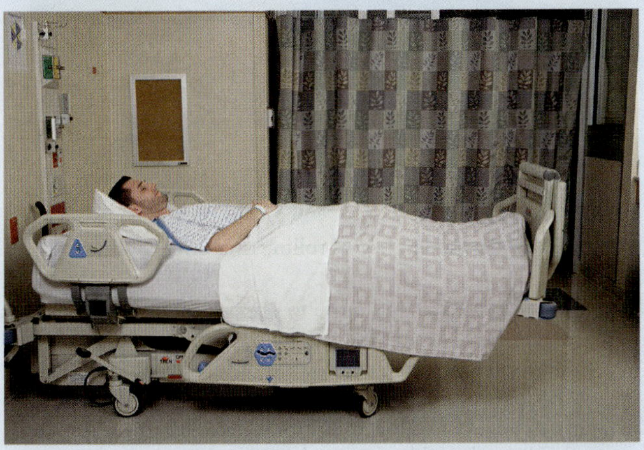	Entire bedframe horizontally parallel with floor	For patients with vertebral injuries and in cervical traction; position used for patients who are hypotensive and generally preferred by patients for sleeping

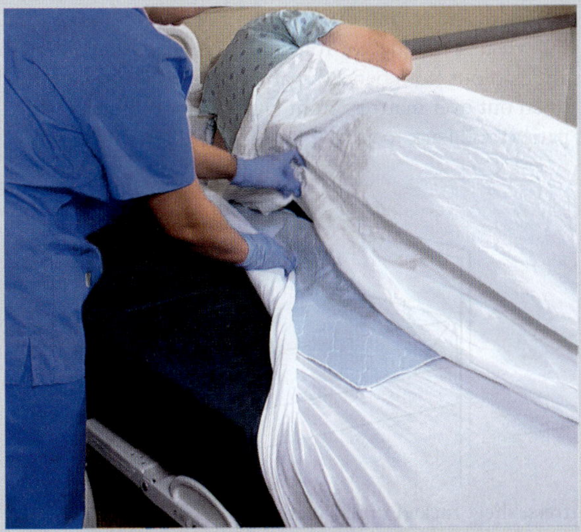

STEP 11 Tuck all soiled linen from one side of bed alongside patient's back.

12. Clean, disinfect, and dry mattress surface if it is soiled or has moisture (see employer policy).
13. Apply clean linens to the exposed half of bed in separate layers. When needed, start with a new mattress pad by placing it lengthwise with centre crease in middle of bed. Fanfold pad to centre of bed alongside patient. Repeat process with bottom sheet.
14. Pull new fitted sheet smoothly over mattress corner at top and bottom of bed. If using a flat sheet, allow edge of sheet to hang about 25 cm (10 inches) over mattress edge at HOB. Be sure that lower hem of bottom flat sheet lies seam down and with bottom edge of mattress.
15. If bottom sheet is flat, mitre top corner at HOB. Face HOB diagonally. Place hand away from HOB under top corner of mattress, lift, and with other hand tuck edge of bottom sheet smoothly under mattress so side edges of sheet above and below mattress meet when brought together.
16. If bottom sheet is flat, mitre top corner at HOB.

Continued

Procedural Guideline 18.6 *Making an Occupied Bed—cont'd*

a. Face HOB diagonally. Place hand away from HOB under top corner of mattress, near mattress edge, and lift.
b. With other hand, tuck top edge of bottom sheet smoothly under mattress so side edges of sheet above and below mattress meet when brought together.
c. To mitre a corner, pick up top edge of sheet at about 45 cm (18 inches) from top end of mattress (see Step 16c illustration).

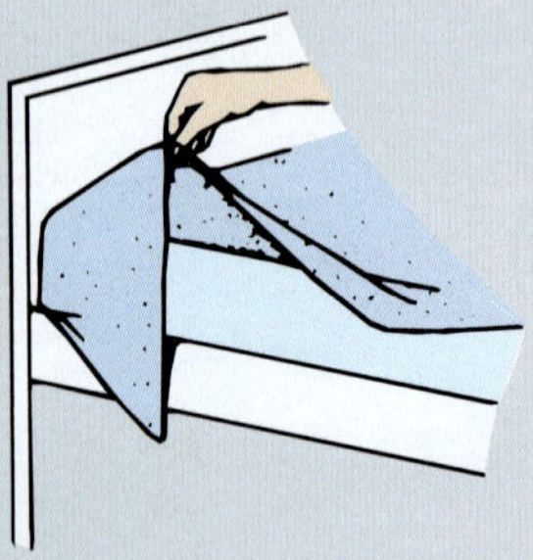

STEP 16C Top edge of sheet picked up.

d. Lift sheet and lay it on top of mattress to form a neat triangular fold, with lower base of triangle even with mattress side edges (see Step 16d illustration).

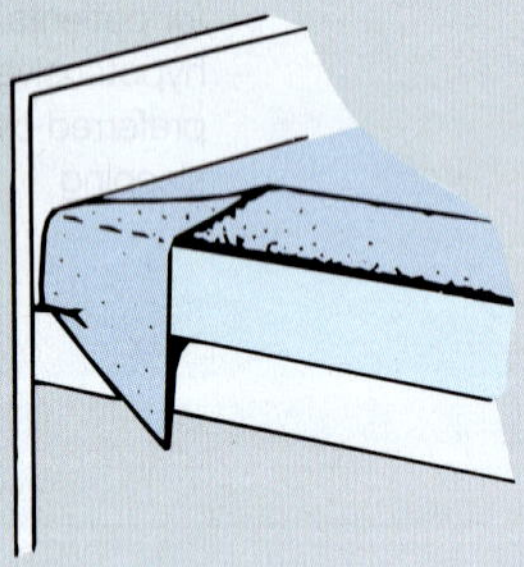

STEP 16D Sheet on top of mattress in a triangular fold.

e. Tuck lower edge of sheet, which is hanging free below the mattress, under the mattress. Tuck with palms down without pulling triangular fold.
f. Hold part of sheet covering side of mattress in place with one hand (see Step 16f illustration). With other hand, pick up top of triangular linen fold and bring it down over side of mattress. Tuck under mattress with palms down without pulling fold (see Step 16f illustration).

17. Tuck remaining part of sheet under mattress, moving toward foot of bed. Keep linen smooth.

18. Place new drawsheet along middle of bed lengthwise. Fanfold or roll drawsheet on top of clean bottom sheet. Tuck under patient's buttocks and torso without touching old linen.

19. Add waterproof pad (absorbent side up) over drawsheet with seam side down. Fanfold toward patient. Continue to keep clean and soiled linen separate. Also keep linen under patient as flat as possible because patient will need to roll over old and new layers of linen when you are ready to make other side of bed.

20. Advise patient that they will be rolling over a thick layer of linens. Keeping patient covered, ask patient to roll toward you slowly over layers of linen and to not raise the hips (see Step 20 illustration). Stress the need to roll while staying aligned.

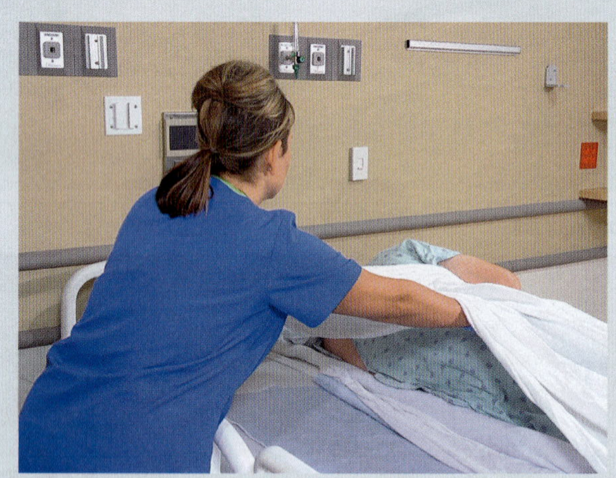

STEP 20 Patient begins rolling over layers of linen.

21. Now raise side rail and move to opposite side of bed. *Option:* The caregiver helping you can help position patient. Have patient roll away from you toward other side of bed, over all of the folds of linen. Again, have patient keep hips still.

22. Loosen edges of soiled linen from under mattress. Remove soiled linen by folding into a bundle or square.

23. Hold linen away from your body and place it in laundry bag.

24. Clean, disinfect, and dry other half of mattress as needed.

25. Pull clean, fanfolded or rolled mattress pad; sheet; drawsheet; and pad out from beneath patient toward you. Smooth all linen out over mattress from HOB to foot of bed. Help patient roll back to supine position and reposition pillow.

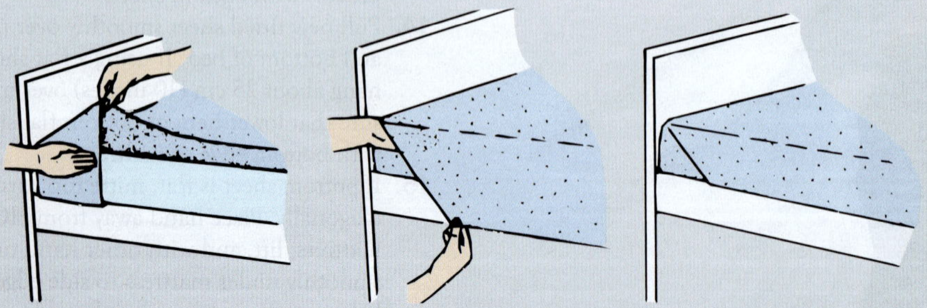

STEP 16F Triangular fold placed over side of mattress; sheet tucked under mattress.

Procedural Guideline 18.6 *Making an Occupied Bed—cont'd*

26. If bottom sheet is fitted, pull corners over mattress edges. If flat sheet is used, mitre top corner of bottom flat sheet (see Steps 16a–16f).
27. Facing side of bed, grasp remaining edge of bottom flat sheet. Lean back slightly, keep back straight, and pull while tucking excess linen under mattress from HOB to foot of bed. Avoid lifting mattress during tucking.
28. Smooth fanfolded drawsheet over bottom sheet (tucking is optional). Smooth waterproof pads, making sure that bed surface is wrinkle free.
29. Place top sheet over patient with vertical centrefold lengthwise down middle of bed and with seam side of hem facing up. Open sheet out from head to foot and unfold over patient. Be sure that top edge of sheet is even with top edge of mattress.
30. Place clean or reused bed blanket on bed over patient. Make sure that top edge is parallel with top edge of sheet and 15–20 cm (6–8 inches) from edge of top sheet. Raise side rail.
31. Go to other side of bed. Lower side rail. Spread sheet and blanket out evenly.
32. Have patient hold onto sheet and blanket while you remove bath blanket; discard in linen bag.
33. Make cuff by turning edge of top sheet down over top edge of blanket.
34. Make horizontal toe pleat; stand at foot of bed and fanfold in sheet and blanket 5–10 cm (2–4 inches) across bed. Pull sheet and blanket up from bottom to make fold approximately 15 cm (6 inches) from bottom edge of mattress.
35. Standing at side of bed, tuck in remaining part of sheet and blanket under foot of mattress. Tuck top sheet and blanket together. Be sure that toe pleats are not pulled out.
36. Make modified mitred corner with top sheet and blanket. Follow Steps 16a–16f. After making triangular fold, do not tuck tip of triangle (see Step 36 illustration).
37. Go to other side of bed. Repeat Steps 35 and 36.
38. Change pillowcase. Have patient raise head. While supporting neck with one hand, remove pillow. Allow patient to lower head. Remove soiled pillowcase and place in linen bag. Grasp clean pillowcase at centre of closed end. Gather case, turning it inside out over the hand holding it. With the same hand, pick up middle of one end of pillow. Pull pillowcase down over pillow with other hand. Do not hold pillow against your uniform. Be sure that pillow corners fit evenly into corners of case. Reposition pillow under patient's head.
39. Place call light within patient's reach on bedrail or pillow; return bed to locked, low position; and raise side rail (as needed).
40. Place all linen in dirty laundry bag. Remove and dispose of gloves in appropriate receptacle. Arrange and organize patient's room.
41. During procedure, inspect skin for areas of irritation. Observe patient for signs of fatigue, dyspnea, pain, or other sources of discomfort.

Procedural Guideline 18.7 *Making an Unoccupied Bed*

A bed may be made with the patient out of the bed (unoccupied) or in the bed (occupied). In some settings, bed linen is not changed every day; however, any wet or soiled linen must always be changed promptly. Moisture on bed linen can easily lead to skin breakdown. An unoccupied bed is one left open with the top sheets fanfolded down. A postoperative surgical bed is prepared for patients returning from the operating room (OR) or procedural area. The bed is left with the top sheets fanfolded lengthwise and not tucked in, to facilitate a patient's transfer from a stretcher. A closed bed, which is made with the top sheets pulled up to the head of the bed, is made by the housekeeping department after a patient is discharged and the bed is cleaned.

Delegation and Collaboration

The skill of making an unoccupied bed can be delegated to a UCP. The nurse instructs the UCP about the following:

- Position or activity restrictions that apply to patient's ability to get out of and back into bed
- The type of special linen to use if patient is on an airflow mattress

Equipment

- Linen/laundry bags
- Mattress pad (change only when soiled)
- Bottom sheet (flat or fitted)
- Drawsheet (optional)
- Waterproof pads (optional)
- Top sheet, blanket, bedspread, pillowcases
- Clean gloves (if linen is soiled or if there is risk of exposure to body fluids)
- Antiseptic cleanser
- Washcloth

Procedural Steps

1. Throughout the procedure, the 4 moments for hand hygiene are to be implemented; hand hygiene should occur before initial patient (or patient environment) contact, before an aseptic procedure, after body fluid exposure risk, and after patient (or patient environment) contact. Additional hand hygiene should be performed when hands are visibly soiled.
2. Assess environment for safety (e.g., check room for spills; make sure that equipment is working properly; and ensure that bed is in locked, low position).
3. If patient is still in the bed, pull room divider curtain or close room door to provide privacy. Follow steps for transferring patient to bedside chair or recliner (see Chapter 11).
4. Lower remaining side rails on bed and raise bed to comfortable working position.

Continued

Procedural Guideline 18.7 *Making an Unoccupied Bed—cont'd*

5. Apply clean gloves if linen is soiled with body fluids. Remove all linen, hold away from uniform, and place in laundry bag. Avoid shaking or fanning linen.
6. Straighten mattress and wipe off any moisture with a washcloth moistened in antiseptic solution (consult employer's housekeeping guidelines). Dry thoroughly.
7. Apply all bottom linen on one side of bed before moving to opposite side.
   a. For fitted sheet: Make sure that fitted sheet is placed smoothly over mattress and top and bottom mattress edge. Fit corners on one end and then the other.
   b. For flat sheet: Place sheet over mattress. Allow about 25 cm (10 inches) to hang over side mattress edge. Lower hem of sheet should lie seam down, even with bottom edge of mattress. Pull remaining top part of sheet over top edge of mattress. While standing at HOB, mitre top corner of bottom sheet (see Procedural Guideline 18.6, Steps 16a–16f). Tuck remaining part of flat bottom sheet under mattress.
   c. *Optional:* Apply drawsheet and/or waterproof pad, laying centrefold along middle of bed lengthwise. Smooth drawsheet/pad over mattress. Tuck excess edge of drawsheet under mattress, keeping palms down.
8. Move to opposite side of bed. Repeat Step 7.
9. Place top sheet over bed with vertical centrefold lengthwise down middle of bed. Open sheet out from head to foot, being sure that top edge of sheet is even with top edge of mattress. *Optional:* Spread a blanket or bedspread evenly over top sheet in same fashion.
10. Standing on one side at foot of bed, lift mattress corner slightly with one hand and with other hand tuck top sheet and blanket or bedspread under mattress.
11. Make modified mitred corner with top sheet, blanket, and bedspread. After making triangular fold, leave tip of triangle untucked (see Procedural Guideline 18.6, Step 36).

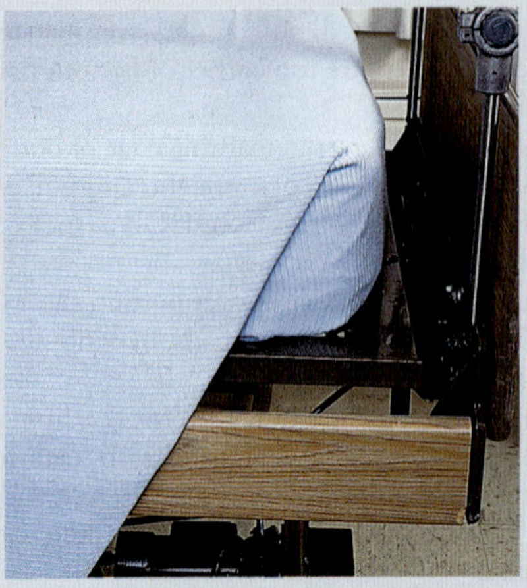

STEP 36 Modified mitred corner.

12. Make cuff by turning edge of top sheet down over top edge of blanket and bedspread.
13. Standing on one side at foot of bed, lift mattress corner slightly with one hand and with other hand tuck top sheet, blanket, and bedspread under mattress. Be sure that toe pleats are not pulled out.
14. Make modified mitred corner with top sheet, blanket, and bedspread. After making triangular fold, do not tuck tip of triangle (see Procedural Guideline 18.6, Step 36).
15. Go to other side of bed. Spread sheet, blanket, and bedspread out evenly. Make cuff with top sheet and blanket (closed bed). Make modified corner at foot of bed. Alternatively, fanfold sheet, blanket, and bedspread at foot of bed, with top layer ready to be pulled up (this leaves an open bed). *Optional:* Make horizontal toe pleat; stand at foot of bed and fanfold in sheet 5–10 cm (2–4 inches) across bed. Pull sheet up from bottom to make fold approximately 15 cm (6 inches) from bottom edge of mattress.
16. Apply clean pillowcase.
17. Place call light within patient's reach on bedrail or pillow and return bed to lowest position, allowing for patient transfer. Help patient to bed.
18. Place linen bag in dirty laundry bag. Remove and dispose of gloves in appropriate receptacle.

✦ REVIEW QUESTIONS

A 78-year-old patient (he/him) has a 3-year history of type 1 diabetes mellitus and hypertension. The patient was just discharged after 5 days of hospitalization with diagnoses of healing right-heel ulcer and controlled hypertension. The discharge summary notes that he requires help with daily dressing changes for the ulcer. He lives alone and can perform all routine activities of daily living (ADLs). During the initial home visit, the patient's vital signs were as follows: temperature: 37°C; pulse, 86 beats/min; blood pressure, 135/85 mm Hg; respiratory rate, 30 breaths/min. The community health nurse noted a right-heel ulcer measuring 2 cm × 2 cm (0.8 inches × 0.8 inches); no drainage was noted. A 10 cm × 10 cm (4 inch × 4 inch) dressing was applied, covered, and wrapped with gauze cling wrap. The nurse assessed that, although the patient understands the need for the daily dressing changes, he is unable to state which precautions are needed to prevent any recurrence.

Review Questions 1 to 3 relate to the case study presented here.

1. List three actions the patient should follow for maintaining good foot care.
2. Which factor places this patient at risk for oral problems?
   1. Break in mucosa and disruption of suture lines with vigorous brushing.
   2. Mucosa becomes thin and less elastic.
   3. Irritation of oral mucosa.
   4. Dryness of mouth with gingivitis.
3. Using SBAR (situation–background–assessment–recommendation), show how the nurse would communicate with the health care team about this patient's status.
4. The nurse is caring for a critically ill patient who has an endotracheal tube and is on mechanical ventilation. Which of the following

factors places the patient at risk for ventilator-associated pneumonia (VAP)? (*Select all that apply.*)

1. The mucous inside the artificial airway grows Gram-negative bacteria.
2. An endotracheal tube bypasses normal airway defences, leading to a change in the normal oral flora.
3. A critically ill patient often has a reduced gag reflex.
4. The presence of an endotracheal tube makes it impossible to suction oral secretions.
5. Critically ill patients have an abnormal amount of mucosa released in the oral cavity.

5. Which of the following actions are steps used when making an unoccupied bed? (*Select all that apply.*)

1. Raise bed to working height.
2. Wear clean gloves at all times.
3. Apply all bottom linen on one side of bed before moving to opposite side.
4. Remove soiled linen and place on the floor.
5. Tuck top sheet and blanket in at bottom of bed using a modified mitred corner.
6. Keep top blanket at head of bed when procedure is completed.
7. Make horizontal toe pleat with all top layers of linen.

6. Place the following steps for providing oral care to a debilitated patient in the correct order.

1. Remove dentures or partial plates if present.
2. Apply thin layer of water-soluble moisturizer to lips.
3. Perform hand hygiene and apply clean gloves.
4. Brush inner and outer surfaces of upper and lower teeth by brushing from gum to crown of each tooth; then clean biting surfaces of teeth.
5. If needed, turn on suction machine and connect tubing to suction catheter.
6. Position patient in side-lying position with head turned toward mattress in dependent position.
7. If patient is uncooperative or having difficulty keeping mouth open, insert an oral airway.

Visit the Evolve site for a complete list of answers to the Review Questions.

✦ NEXT GENERATION NCLEX® (NGN)

For practice with answering exam questions related to unfolding NGN case studies, please consult the Next Generation NCLEX® (NGN)-Style Case Studies for Skills and Techniques on the Evolve website: http://evolve.elsevier.com/Canada/Perry/clinicalskills/

REFERENCES

Accreditation Canada. (2020). *Required organizational practices–2020 handbook.* https://physicians.nshealth.ca/resources/required-organizational-practices-2020-handbook

Agency for Healthcare Research and Quality. (2022). *Standardized nursing protocol: Bed bathing with 2% chlorhexidine (CHG) no-rinse bathing cloths and showering with 4% CHG liquid soap.* https://www.ahrq.gov/sites/default/files/wysiwyg/hai/abate/nursing-protocols/nursing-chg-bed-bathing.pdf

Alzheimer Society of Canada. (2022). *Bathing.* https://alzheimer.ca/en/help-support/im-caring-person-living-dementia/providing-day-day-care/personal-care/bathing

American Dental Association. (2019). *Oral health topics: Mouthrinse (mouthwash).* https://www.ada.org/resources/research/science-and-research-institute/oral-health-topics/mouthrinse-mouthwash

Canadian Dental Association. (n.d.-a). *Dental care for children: Cleaning teeth.* https://www.cda-adc.ca/en/oral_health/cfyt/dental_care_children/cleaning.asp

Canadian Dental Association. (n.d.-b). *Flossing and brushing.* http://www.cda-adc.ca/en/oral_health/cfyt/dental_care_seniors/flossing_brushing.asp

Canadian Dental Association. (n.d.-c). *Oral health–Good for life.* https://www.cda-adc.ca/en/oral_health/cfyt/good_for_life/

Canadian Dental Association. (n.d.-d). *Your child's first visit.* https://www.cda-adc.ca/en/oral_health/cfyt/dental_care_children/first_visit.asp

Canadian Dental Association. (n.d.-e). *Your oral health.* https://www.cda-adc.ca/en/oral_health/index.asp

Centers for Disease Control and Prevention. (2022). *Fungal nail infections.* https://www.cdc.gov/fungal/nail-infections.html

Diabetes Canada. (2018). *A step towards good health.* https://www.diabetes.ca/diabetes-and-you/healthy-living-resources/foot-care/a-step-towards-good-health

European Pressure Ulcer Advisory Panel, National Pressure Injury Advisory Panel, & Pan Pacific Pressure Injury Alliance. (2019). *Prevention and treatment of pressure ulcers/injuries: Quick reference guide.* https://www.internationalguideline.com/static/pdfs/Quick_Reference_Guide-10Mar2019.pdf

Frost, S., Hou, Y. C., Lombardo, L., et al. (2018). Evidence for the effectiveness of chlorhexidine bathing and healthcare-associated infections among adult intensive care patients: A trial sequential meta-analysis. *BMC Infectious Diseases, 18,* 679. https://doi.org/10.1186/s12879-018-3521-y

Fujinami, W., Nishikawa, K., Ozawa, S., et al. (2021). Correlation between the relative abundance of oral bacteria and Candida albicans in denture and dental plaques. *Journal of Oral Biosciences, 63*(2), 175–183. https://doi.org/10.1016/j.job.2021.02.003

Gall, E., Long, A., & Hall, K. (2020). Chlorhexidine bathing strategies for multidrug-resistant organisms: A summary of recent evidence. *Journal of Patient Safety, 16*(3), S16–S22. https://doi.org/10.1097/PTS.0000000000000743

Giger, J., & Haddad, L. (2021). *Transcultural nursing: Assessment and intervention* (8th ed.). Elsevier.

Haque, M., McKimm, J., Sartelli, M., et al. (2020). Strategies to prevent healthcare-associated infections: A narrative overview. *Risk Management and Healthcare Policy, 13,* 1765–1780. https://doi.org/10.2147/RMHP.S269315

Health Canada. (2018). *Bath safety.* https://www.canada.ca/en/health-canada/services/infant-care/bath-safety.html

Huang, S. S., Septimus, E., Kleinman, K., et al. (2019). Chlorhexidine versus routine bathing to prevent multidrug-resistant organisms and all-cause bloodstream infections in general medical and surgical units (ABATE infection trial): A cluster-randomised trial. *The Lancet, 393*(10177), 1205–1215. https://doi.org/10.1016/S0140-6736(18)32593-5

LeLaurin, J. E., & Shorr, R. (2019). Preventing falls in hospitalized patients: State of the science. *Clinical Geriatric Medicine, 35*(2), 273–283. https://doi.org/10.1016/j.cger.2019.01.007

Marques, J. G., Rozan, C., Proença, L., et al. (2021). Assessment of hyposalivation, xerostomia, and oral health-related quality of life in polymedicated patients. *Medical Sciences Forum, 5*(1), 6. https://doi.org/10.3390/msf2021005006

Matsumoto, C., Nanke, K., Furumura, S., et al. (2019). Effects of disposable bath and towel bath on the transition of resident skin bacteria, water content of the stratum corneum, and relaxation. *American Journal of Infection Control, 47*(7), 811–815. https://doi.org/10.1016/j.ajic.2018.12.008

Mendes, A. (2018). Meeting the care needs of a person with dementia who is distressed. *British Journal of Nursing, 27*(4), 219. https://doi.org/10.12968/bjon.2018.27.4.219

Musuuza, J., Guru, P., O'Horo, J. C., et al. (2019). The impact of chlorhexidine bathing on hospital-acquired bloodstream infections: A systematic review and meta-analysis. *BMC Infectious Diseases, 19,* 416. https://doi.org/10.1186/s12879-019-4002-7

National Cancer Institute. (2021). *Oral complications of chemotherapy and head/neck radiation (PDQ)–Health professional version.* https://www.cancer.gov/about-cancer/treatment/side-effects/mouth-throat/oral-complications-hp-pdq

National Institute of Dental and Craniofacial Research. (2018). *Older adults and oral health.* https://www.nidcr.nih.gov/health-info/for-older-adults

National Pediculosis Association. (2023). *Child care providers guide to controlling head lice.* https://www.headlice.org/comb/what-are-head-lice-and-nits/head-lice-removal/child-care-providers-guide-to-controlling-head-lice/

Orsted, H. L., Keast, D. H., Forest-Lalande, L., et al. (2017/2021). Best practice recommendations for the prevention and management of wounds. In *Foundations of best practice for skin and wound management: A supplement of wound care Canada.* https://www.woundscanada.ca/docman/public/health-care-professional/165-wc-bpr-prevention-and-management-of-wounds/file

Tingley, K., & Lê, M. (2021). CADTH health technology review: Chlorhexidine gluconate for skin preparation during catheter insertion and surgical procedures. *Canadian Journal of Health Technologies, 1*(18). https://www.cadth.ca/sites/default/files/pdf/htis/2021/RC1375%20CHG%20Wipes%20Final.pdf

Tran, K., & Butcher, R. (2019). *CADTH rapid response report: Summary with critical appraisal: Chlorhexidine for oral care: A review of clinical effectiveness and guidelines.* https://www.cadth.ca/sites/default/files/pdf/htis/2019/RC1064%20Chlorhexidine%20for%20oral%20care%20Final.pdf

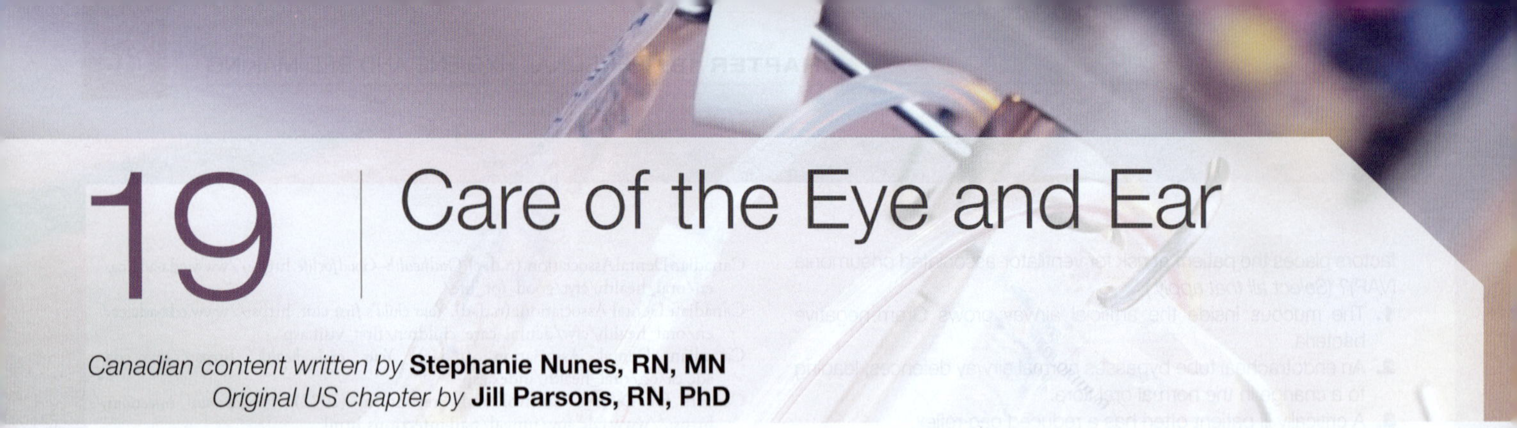

19 Care of the Eye and Ear

Canadian content written by **Stephanie Nunes, RN, MN**
Original US chapter by **Jill Parsons, RN, PhD**

SKILLS AND PROCEDURES

OBJECTIVES

Mastery of content in this chapter will enable the nurse to:

- Explain safety guidelines used in the care of eye and ear prostheses.
- Identify person-centred care guidelines used in caring for eye and ear prostheses.
- Correctly remove, store, clean, and insert a contact lens.
- Correctly perform eye and ear irrigations.
- Describe techniques that determine whether a hearing aid functions properly.
- Correctly remove, clean, and reinsert a hearing aid.

MEDIA RESOURCES

- http://evolve.elsevier.com/Canada/Perry/clinicalskills/

PURPOSE

Vision and hearing are two special senses that help people carry out all daily and recreational activities. Risks to a patients' eye or ear structures or function can alter independence, safety, body image, and self-confidence. The skills in this chapter show how to help patients protect their vision and hearing and use artificial sensory devices correctly to replace or restore sensory function.

STANDARDS OF CARE

- Canadian Academy of Audiology (n.d.-a)—*Reports, Scope, Guidelines, and Position Statements* (https://canadianaudiology.ca/professional-resources/guidelines-and-position-statements/)
- Canadian Association of Optometrists (CAO, n.d.)—*Frequency of Eye Examinations* (https://opto.ca/document/frequency-of-eye-examinations)
- Canadian Hearing Services (2023)—*Services for You* (https://www.chs.ca/service-for-you)

PRINCIPLES FOR PRACTICE

- Meaningful sensory stimuli help people learn about their environment.
- Receiving and understanding environmental stimuli promotes healthy functioning.
- Alteration in a patient's vision and hearing affects health literacy, independence, and adherence to medical and pharmacological therapies.
- Artificial sensory aids can restore some vision and hearing loss. However, these aids must fit and work properly for patients to function optimally in their environments.
- When caring for patients who use aids to help with visual or auditory loss, it is important that the nurse and the health care team, along with the patient and their caregivers, understand how to clean and care for these aids. Breakage or loss of an aid is expensive, with Canadians paying anywhere from $1 200 to $6 000 per hearing aid. Prices of hearing aids vary owing to several factors, including hearing aid manufacturer, province, type of hearing loss, and style of hearing aid. Often, these costs are not covered under public health insurance plans (Group Enroll, 2021).

PERSON-CENTRED CARE

- When a patient is without visual or hearing devices, communication is altered, and the patient is isolated socially and becomes more dependent (Mick et al., 2018).
- The noises within hospitals, rehabilitation centres, and skilled nursing facilities make hearing difficult. Hard flooring surfaces, medical equipment, televisions, and the constant need to speak with other health care providers all produce noise.
- Hearing-impaired patients need time to adjust to their hearing aid. For example, increased background noise makes hearing with an aid even more difficult. The noisy environments of hospitals and other health care facilities further contribute to adjustment to hearing aids (Mick et al., 2018).

- When a patient has auditory impairments, the increased background noise in an unfamiliar environment often makes a patient more anxious and decreases their ability to adjust to new surroundings.
- The widespread use of masks during the COVID-19 pandemic has greatly complicated the daily life of patients with auditory impairments and increases acute stress (Kaya et al., 2021).
- As a nurse, at times you can use touch to get the attention of a patient with severe visual loss or decreased hearing. Practise person-centred care and ask patients if touch is acceptable.
- Understand the cause of a person's sensory loss and then determine the patient's own perception of the reason for the loss.
- Identify a patient's usual practices in using and maintaining sensory assistive devices.

EVIDENCE-INFORMED PRACTICE

- Dual sensory impairment (DSI), the concurrent loss of vision and hearing, has the potential to cause a decline in mobility, self-care, and cognitive function, or contribute to acute confusion or depression and increased mortality risk (Mick et al., 2018).
- DSI in rehabilitation or long-term care settings affects a patient's independence, socialization, and success in using assistive devices and rehabilitation services (Assi et al., 2021).
- Mounting evidence indicates that there are central effects of biological aging and peripheral pathology that affect a person's neural detection of sound, which occurs as early as middle age. Even once hearing loss is suspected, there is an average delay of 7 years before an individual seeks screening and intervention (Ramage-Morin et al., 2019).
- Identify patients at risk of hearing impairments according to the following criteria: male over age 65, male or female over age 75, resident in an assisted living facility, existing visual impairment, chronic ear infection, prolonged exposure to loud noises, and use of ototoxic medication (Ramage-Morin et al., 2019).
- Vision loss includes people who are blind or partially blind, including those without sight from birth and those who are "legally blind" (best corrected visual acuity ≤20/200 and/or a visual field <20 degrees). Vision loss can include other forms of impairment, such as nystagmus, a condition that reduces vision and depth perception (Canadian National Institute for the Blind, n.d.).
- Patients with DSI have unique communication needs that require a thorough assessment (Mick et al., 2018).

SAFETY GUIDELINES

- As a nurse, whenever you care for patients with sensory alterations, safety is a priority. Anticipate how the sensory alteration places a patient at risk for injury (e.g., ability to manoeuvre through the home, climb stairs, and respond to alarms).
- Select interventions based on the type of sensory alteration, patient preference, and patient safety.
- Interprofessional collaboration related to the plan of care for a patient with sensory alterations is beneficial to maximize patient safety and ensure optimal patient care.
- Orient the patient to any new environment or changes within an existing environment to minimize safety hazards (e.g., visual loss affects a patient's ability to see the edge of the stairs). In addition, educate caregivers about the best way to help the patient adapt to sensory alterations.
- When patients have visual impairments, they may have difficulty with tasks requiring visual detail (e.g., reading prescriptions or syringe scales). Visual impairment can increase the risk for improper administration of medications in the home setting. In addition, certain eye conditions such as cataracts and macular degeneration cause a patient difficulty when their eyes adjust to changes in contrast and brightness.
- Provide additional time for patients with hearing loss to ask repeated questions about their care or upcoming procedure.
- If a patient must sign a consent form for a procedure or surgery, be sure to have a method to verify that the patient read, heard, and understood the procedure.

Procedural Guideline 19.1 *Eye Care for Unconscious Patients*

Unconscious patients do not have the natural protective mechanisms of blinking and eye lubrication to protect the cornea. Critically ill patients often develop ocular surface disorders such as exposure keratopathy. Critically ill patients are often on mechanical ventilators and thus heavily sedated, which alters the normal blinking reflex. The hospital environment (e.g., exposure to air conditioning, low air humidity) also increases patient susceptibility to developing dry eyes or other ocular surface disorders (Ahmadinejad et al., 2020; de Araujo et al., 2019).

The blinking reflex flushes debris out of the eye. When patients are heavily sedated or in a coma, tear production is reduced, thus decreasing the normal lubrication of the corneal surface. Tears maintain a moist environment, lubricate the eyes, wash away foreign material and cell debris, prevent organisms from adhering to the ocular surface, and transport oxygen to the outer eye surface. When a patient's normal protective eye mechanisms are not effective, eye care is an important component of nursing care. Left unprotected, damage to the ocular surface can occur. This damage includes corneal scarring, infection, premature cataract formation, and vision changes. Simple eye hygiene measures such as moisture chambers, lubrication, and corneal surface protection are the best interventions to decrease the risk for or prevent damage to the cornea (Ahmadinejad et al., 2020).

Delegation and Collaboration

The skill of providing basic eye care for a comatose patient can be assigned to an unregulated care provider (UCP). However, it is the nurse's responsibility to assess a patient's eyes and administer the sterile lubricant. The nurse instructs the UCP to do the following:

- Adapt the skill for specific patients (e.g., using skin-sensitive tape to affix eye pads)
- Immediately report any eye drainage or irritation to the nurse for further assessment

Equipment

- Clean gloves
- Warm water
- Normal saline solution

Continued

Procedural Guideline 19.1 *Eye Care for Unconscious Patients—cont'd*

- Clean washcloth
- Cotton balls
- Eye pads or patches
- Paper tape
- Eyedropper bulb syringe
- Sterile lubricant or eye preparations as prescribed
- *Option:* A moisture chamber (e.g., polyethylene covers, swimming goggles, shields, pads, or eye patch seals off the eye from the environment [Li & Zhou, 2022]) may also be used; verify with employer policy.

Procedural Steps

1. Identify patient using at least two person-specific identifiers (e.g., name and date of birth, or name and medical record number) according to employer policy (Accreditation Canada, 2020).
2. Throughout the procedure, the 4 moments for hand hygiene are to be implemented; hand hygiene should occur before initial patient (or patient environment) contact, before an aseptic procedure, after body fluid exposure risk, and after patient (or patient environment) contact. Additional hand hygiene should be performed when hands are visibly soiled.
3. Observe patient's eyes for drainage, irritation, redness, and lesions. Apply clean gloves if drainage is present.
4. Always explain each step of the procedure. It is unknown how much an unconscious patient can hear; thus, it is important to continually orient a patient to any procedure.
5. Assess for blink reflex (see Chapter 8).
6. Examine the pupils; determine whether pupils are equal and round and reactive to light and accommodation (PERRLA) (see Chapter 8).
7. Observe patient's eye movements, noting symmetry of movement.
8. Explain procedure to patient and caregiver.
9. Position patient in supine position.
10. Use clean washcloth or cotton balls moistened with warm water or saline and gently wipe each eye from inner to outer canthus. Use a separate, clean cotton ball or corner of the washcloth for each eye to avoid potential cross-contamination of bacteria between eyes.

Critical Decision Point *Be sure water is warm, not hot, to avoid damaging patient's eyes.*

11. Use an eyedropper to instill the prescribed lubricant (e.g., saline, methylcellulose, liquid tears) as prescribed, wiping away any excess lubricant.
12. If the blink reflex is absent, gently close patient's eyes and apply moisture chamber according to employer policy. Secure patch, being careful not to tape patient's eyes.
13. Dispose of excess material, remove gloves, and dispose in appropriate receptacle.
14. Remove eye pads or patches every 4 hours (or as prescribed), and observe condition of patient's eyes for drainage, irritation, redness, and lesions.
15. Document assessment on flow sheet or in progress notes in electronic health record (EHR) or chart.
16. Notify health care provider if signs of irritation or infection are present.

DOCUMENTATION EXAMPLE

Patient remains unresponsive. Scheduled q4h eye care performed. Previous moisture chamber, eye patch removed. Bilateral eyes assessed, no blink reflex. Eyes appear healthy, no discharge noted. Eyes cleansed with clean washcloth and warm water. No lubricant prescribed. New eye patch secured over each eye. Patient tolerated well and will perform next scheduled eye care at 1800 hours.

Procedural Guideline 19.2 *Taking Care of Contact Lenses*

A contact lens is a thin, concave disc that fits directly over the cornea of the eye. It is transparent over at least the pupil and may be colourless or tinted. Contact lenses correct refractive errors of the eye or abnormalities in the shape of the cornea that distort vision. They are relatively easy to apply and remove.

Today, rigid gas permeable (RGP) and soft contact lenses are available. RGP lenses are smaller than soft lenses, and initial awareness of the lens is present; total comfort usually occurs within a couple of weeks. RGP lenses are removed at the end of the day. Daily disposable soft contact lenses are made of malleable plastic polymers and cover the entire cornea and a small rim of the sclera. Contact lenses must accommodate patient needs for comfort, vision correction, and convenience and must be prescribed by an eye care professional (CAO, 2023). Usually, if a patient is not able to provide self-care related to contact lenses while hospitalized, the patient will wear eyeglasses.

It is important to remember that all lenses must be removed periodically to prevent infection and corneal damage and that proper cleaning is necessary before reinserting a lens. As contact lenses are worn, secretions and foreign matter adhere to the lens surface (CAO, 2023). It is extremely important to determine whether patients wear contact lenses, particularly when they are admitted to hospitals or agencies in unresponsive or confused states. If a seriously ill patient is wearing contact lenses and this fact goes undetected, severe corneal injury can result.

Delegation and Collaboration

The skill of taking care of contact lenses can be assigned to a UCP. However, it is the nurse's responsibility to assess a patient's eyes. The nurse directs the UCP to do the following:

- Know a patient's specific type of contact lens, including cleaning solutions and routine, wear schedule, storage, and replacement schedule
- Report immediately to the nurse any eye pain or discomfort, redness, swelling, tearing, or drainage
- Carefully handle the lens to prevent damage and injury

Continued

Procedural Guideline 19.2 *Taking Care of Contact Lenses—cont'd*

Equipment
- Bath towels or waterproof pads
- Sterile saline solution
- Sterile lens care solution(s) for cleaning, disinfecting, and rinsing
- Sterile wetting or conditioning solution (depends on care regimen)
- Sterile enzyme solution (depends on care regimen)
- Flashlight or penlight
- Clean lens storage container
- Suction cup *(optional)*
- Powder-free, clean gloves

Procedural Steps
1. Identify patient using at least two person-specific identifiers (e.g., name and date of birth, or name and medical record number) according to employer policy (Accreditation Canada, 2020).
2. Throughout the procedure, the 4 moments for hand hygiene are to be implemented; hand hygiene should occur before initial patient (or patient environment) contact, before an aseptic procedure, after body fluid exposure risk, and after patient (or patient environment) contact. Additional hand hygiene should be performed when hands are visibly soiled.
3. Inspect patient's eyes or ask patient whether contact lens is in place.

Critical Decision Point *If a patient is unconscious or confused, the nurse must assess for the presence of contact lenses, which are often difficult to detect if they are colourless (not tinted).*

4. Determine whether patient can manipulate and hold contact lenses and whether glasses are available for periods when contacts are not in use. Determine patient's usual routine for wearing, cleaning, and storing lenses.
5. Assess patient for any unusual visual signs or symptoms (e.g., change in visual acuity, blurred vision, halos, photophobia).
6. Review types of medication prescribed for patient: sedatives, hypnotics, muscle relaxants, antihistamines, or another medication that decreases blink reflex and subsequent lubrication of cornea.
7. Explain procedure to patient.
8. Verify expiration date of all solutions and assemble equipment at bedside.
9. Be sure that your fingernails are short and smooth.
10. Position patient in supine or high-Fowler's position in bed.
11. Apply clean gloves. Place towel just below patient's face.
12. Removing lenses:
    a. Removal of soft lens: Follow Steps 1 through 6 for each eye.
        (1) If you are unable to visualize the lens, shine a penlight or flashlight sideways onto the eye to locate the position of the lens.
        (2) Add 2 or 3 drops of sterile saline solution to patient's eye.
        (3) If possible, ask patient to look straight ahead. Retract lower eyelid and expose lower edge of lens.
        (4) Use pad of index finger to slide lens off cornea down onto lower sclera (white of the eye).
        (5) Pull upper eyelid down gently with thumb of other hand and compress lens slightly between thumb and index finger.
        (6) Gently pinch lens and lift out without allowing edges to stick together. Place lens in storage case.

Critical Decision Point *If lens edges stick together, place lens in palm and soak thoroughly with sterile saline solution. Gently roll lens with index finger in back-and-forth motion. If necessary, soak lens in storage solution, which may return lens to normal shape.*

    b. Removal of hard lenses: Follow Steps 1 through 6 for each eye.
        (1) Inspect the eye to be sure that lens is positioned directly over the cornea. If you are unable to visualize the lens, shine a penlight or flashlight sideways onto the eye to locate position of the lens.

Critical Decision Point *If lens is not positioned directly over the cornea, have patient close eyelid, place index and middle fingers of one hand on eyelid just beside the lens and beneath, and gently attempt to massage lens back into place. If lens cannot be repositioned, an immediate referral to an ophthalmologist is needed.*

        (2) Place index finger on outer corner of patient's eye and gently draw skin back toward ear.
        (3) Ask patient to blink. Do not release pressure until blink is completed.

Critical Decision Point *For patients unable to open eye or blink on command, use a lens suction cup to remove lens from eye. Gently apply suction cup to lens surface and lift out.*

        (4) If lens does not dislodge, gently retract eyelid beyond edge of lens. Press lower eyelid gently against lower edge of lens to dislodge lens.
        (5) Allow both eyelids to close slightly and grasp lens as it rises from the eye. Cup lens in hand.
        (6) Inspect lens to be sure that it is intact. Place it in storage container.
    c. After lenses are removed, inspect eye for redness, pain, or swelling of eyelids or conjunctiva; discharge; or excess tearing.
13. Cleaning and storage: Typical cleaning and disinfecting of contact lenses (verify specific method for lenses):
    a. Apply 1 or 2 drops of cleaning solution to lens in palm of hand. Using index finger (soft lenses) or little finger (rigid lenses), rub lens gently but thoroughly on both sides for 20–30 seconds.
    b. Holding lens over emesis basin, rinse thoroughly with recommended rinsing solution.

Critical Decision Point *Only use solutions for cleaning and disinfecting that have been prescribed* (CAO, 2023). *Do not use tap or bottled water. Do not use saline solution. Follow prescriber's instructions and schedules.*

    c. Place lens in proper storage case compartment: "R" for right lens and "L" for left. Rigid lenses are placed inside facing up.
    d. Fill with recommended disinfectant or storage solution.
    e. Secure cover(s) over storage case. Label case with patient's name and medical record number.
14. Inserting lenses:
    a. Inserting a soft lens: Follow Steps 1 through 6 for each eye.

Continued

Procedural Guideline 19.2 *Taking Care of Contact Lenses—cont'd*

(1) Remove right lens from storage case and rinse with recommended rinsing solution; inspect lens for foreign materials, tears, and other damage.
(2) Hold lens on tip of index finger of dominant hand with concave side up.
(3) Inspect lens from side at eye level to ensure that it is not inverted (see Step 14a[3] illustration).

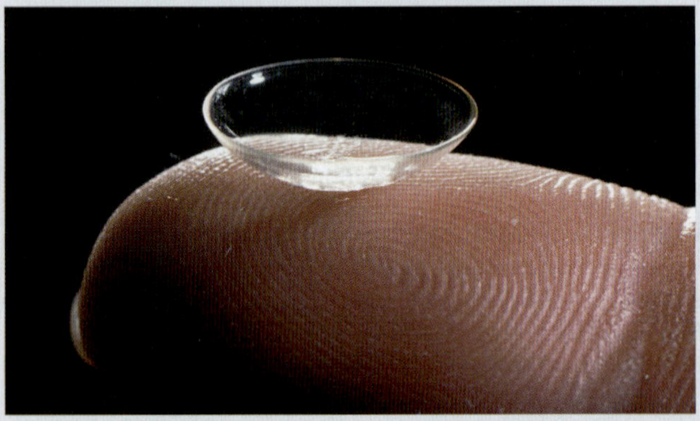

STEP 14A(3) Correct position of soft lens before insertion.

(4) Using middle or index finger of opposite hand, retract upper lid until iris is exposed (see Step 14a[4] illustration). Using middle finger of hand holding the lens, pull down lower lid.

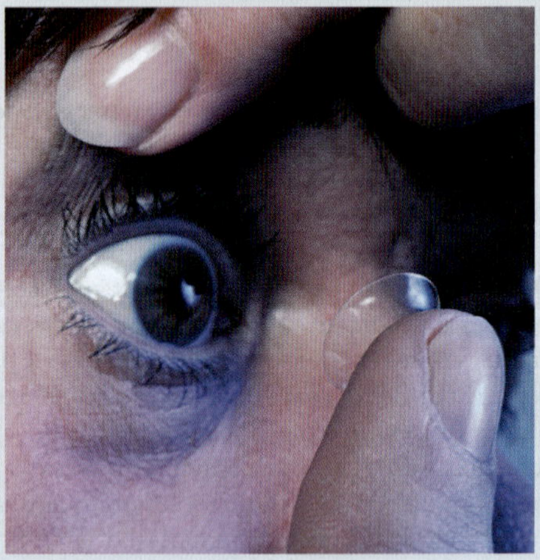

STEP 14A(4) Correct position of hands for soft lens insertion.

(5) Instruct patient to look straight ahead and focus on an object in the distance. Gently place lens directly on cornea and release lids slowly, starting with lower lid.
(6) Ask the patient to close eyes briefly and avoid blinking.

b. Inserting a rigid lens: Follow Steps 1 through 7 for each eye.
(1) Remove right lens from storage case; attempt to lift lens straight up.
(2) Hold lens on tip of index finger of dominant hand with concave side up.
(3) Inspect lens to ensure that it is moist, clean, clear, and free of chips or cracks.
(4) Wet lens surfaces with a few drops of prescribed wetting solution.
(5) Using middle finger of hand holding lens, pull down lower lid (see Step 14b[5] illustration).

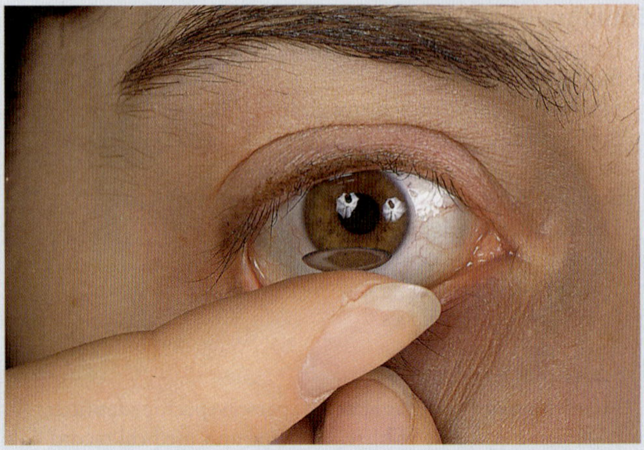

STEP 14B(5) Hand position for rigid lens insertion.

(6) Instruct patient to look straight ahead and focus on an object in the distance (see Step 14b[6] illustration). Gently place lens directly on cornea and release lids slowly, starting with lower lid.

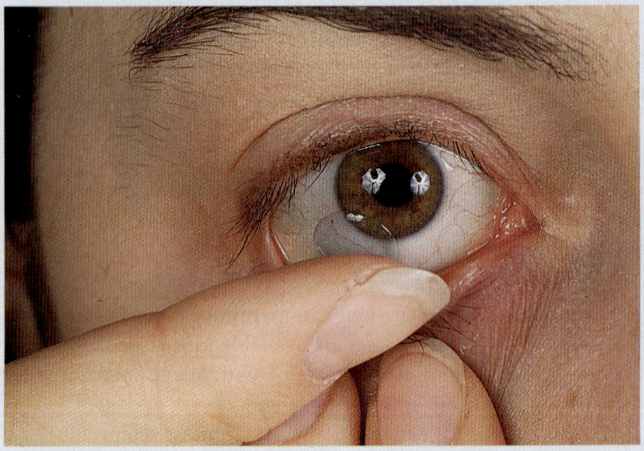

STEP 14B(6) Instruct patient to look straight ahead and focus on an object in the distance.

15. Inspect eye to ensure that lens is on cornea.

Critical Decision Point *If lens is on sclera rather than cornea, ask patient to slowly close eye and look toward the lens. Gentle pressure on the eyelid may help to centre the lens on the cornea. Ask patient to blink a few times.*

16. Ask patient to close eyes briefly and avoid blinking.
17. Ask patient to cover other eye with hand and report whether vision is clear and lens is comfortable.
18. Repeat procedure to insert lens in other eye.
19. Discard solution from storage case and rinse case thoroughly with sterile lens storage solution. Sterilize or replace case as recommended by manufacturer. Allow case to air dry. Dispose of towel, remove gloves, and dispose in appropriate receptacle.
20. Ask patient if lens feels comfortable after removal and reinsertion of lenses.
21. Ask patient if there is blurred vision, pain, or foreign body sensation.
22. Observe eye for drainage or redness.
23. **Use teach-back:** "I want to be sure you understand how to clean your contact lenses. Describe for me the way to clean your lenses." Develop a revised teaching plan if patient or caregiver is unable to teach back correctly.

✦ SKILL 19.1 Eye Irrigation

Chemical injuries to the eye are often work related, caused by common household cleaning solutions or other fumes and aerosols. Chemical burns happen twice as often in children 1–2 years of age than in adults (Bizrah et al., 2019). Acid burns such as bleach, toilet cleaners, and battery fluid cause a haze on the cornea, which often clears, and there is a good chance of recovery. Alkaline burns such as lye, ammonia, and dishwasher detergent often cause permanent injury to the eye. Alkaline burns cause very rapid, irreversible damage (Sharma et al., 2018; Soleimani & Naderan, 2020). A chemical injury to the eye is an emergency and requires flushing the eye with copious amounts of irrigation fluid. Cool tap water is recommended because it is effective, is immediately available for first aid, initially helps to dilute the concentration of the chemical, and can shorten healing time. Tap water irrigation is also used in emergency situations when a foreign object has entered the eye. It is important to flush out the eye with clean water or saline while seeking medical care (Fig. 19.1). Irrigate immediately with copious amounts of cool water, saline, or lactated Ringer's solution for a minimum of 30 minutes to minimize corneal damage (Sharma et al., 2018). If the person wears a contact lens that did not wash out with the irrigation, have them try to remove the lens. The goal in treating ocular chemical injury is to prevent or reduce visual loss caused by the burn (Sharma et al., 2018).

Delegation and Collaboration

The skill of eye irrigation cannot be delegated to a UCP. The nurse directs the UCP to do the following:

- Report any patient complaint of discomfort or excess tearing following irrigation

Equipment

- Emergency: Cool tap water
- Prescribed irrigating solution: Volume usually 30–180 mL at 32–38°C (90–100°F). (For chemical flushing, use normal saline or lactated Ringer's solution in large volume to provide continuous irrigation for 15 minutes.)
- pH test strip
- Sterile basin or bag of solution
- Curved emesis basin
- Waterproof pad or towel
- 10 cm × 10 cm (4 inch × 4 inch) gauze pads
- Soft bulb syringe, eyedropper, or intravenous (IV) tubing
- Clean gloves
- Penlight
- Medication administration record (MAR)

STEP	RATIONALE
ASSESSMENT	
1. In acute emergent situations: Use copious amounts of clear, cool water (normal saline, or lactated Ringer's if quickly available) to flush eyes for at least 30 minutes (Sharma et al., 2018).	Minimizes corneal damage (Sharma et al., 2018).
2. If not an immediate emergency: Identify patient using at least two person-specific identifiers (e.g., name and date of birth, or name and medical record number) according to employer policy.	Ensures correct patient. Complies with Accreditation Canada's standards and improves patient safety (Accreditation Canada, 2020).
3. Throughout the procedure, the 4 moments for hand hygiene are to be implemented; hand hygiene should occur before initial patient (or patient environment) contact, before an aseptic procedure, after body fluid exposure risk, and after patient (or patient environment) contact. Additional hand hygiene should be performed when hands are visibly soiled.	Proper hand hygiene helps prevent the spread of infectious agents to health care providers.

Critical Decision Point *When eye irrigation is an emergency treatment for a chemical burn, follow employer protocol (i.e., usually copious eye irrigation with cool water, normal saline, or lactated Ringer's solution). When possible, determine the chemical. However, do not stop to obtain a history or perform an eye examination. Irrigation is the immediate treatment; delays in irrigation by as little as 20 seconds have been associated with more severe injury in alkaline burns. Once the acute phase is over, an irrigation solution that buffers alkali or acid chemical is then selected, and further examination of the eye is possible* (Sharma et al., 2018).

STEP	RATIONALE
4. Review health care provider's medication prescription, including solution to be instilled and affected eye(s) (right, left, or both) to receive irrigation.	Ensures safe and correct administration of irrigant.
5. Obtain history of injury to assess reason for eye irrigation (e.g., type of injury, when it occurred).	Determines amount and type of solution and immediacy of need for treatment.
6. Determine patient's ability to open affected eye.	Spasm of the eyelid or pain makes opening the eye difficult. Local anaesthetics such as proparacaine or tetracaine cause topical numbness and are used before eye examination procedures.
7. If time permits, do a complete eye examination, including determining whether pupils are equal and round and reactive to light and accommodation (PERRLA) (see Chapter 8). Have patient look in all directions to determine whether there are any visible foreign bodies.	Provides baseline information and determines presence of any foreign bodies.

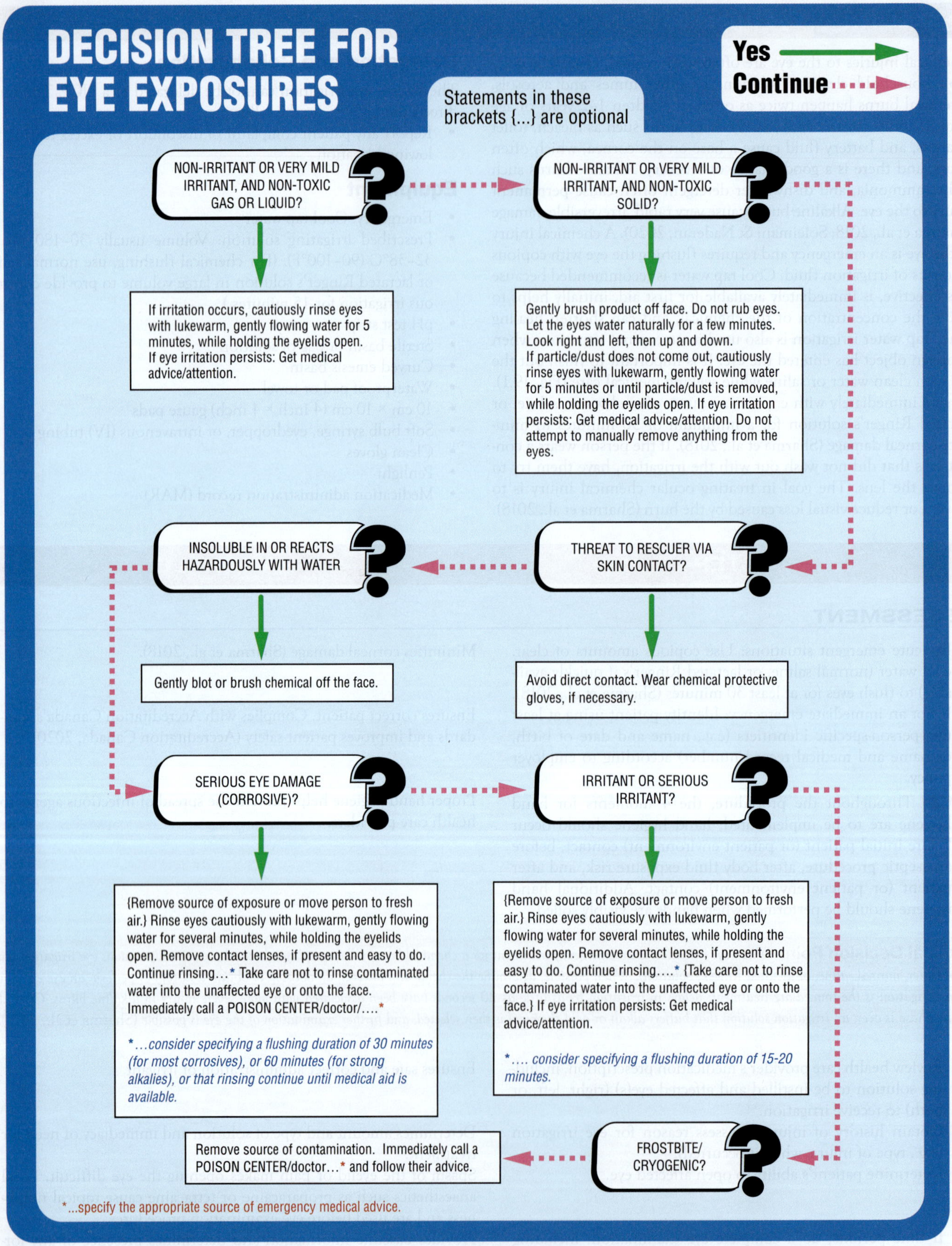

FIG 19.1 **Decision tree for eye exposures.** (*From Canadian Centre for Occupational Health and Safety. [2012]. The Safety Data Sheet–A guide to first-aid recommendations. https://www.ccohs.ca/products/publications/firstaid/*)

STEP	RATIONALE

ASSESSMENT

STEP	RATIONALE
8. Observe eye for redness, excessive tearing, discharge, and swelling. Ask patient about symptoms of itching, burning, pain, blurred vision, or photophobia.	Establishes baseline signs and symptoms.
9. Ask patient to rate level of pain using an appropriate pain rating scale (e.g., on a scale of 0–10, with 0 = no pain, and 10 = the worst pain ever).	Establishes baseline for level of pain.
10. Assess patient's ability to cooperate.	Determines level of assistance needed.

NURSING DIAGNOSES

- Acute pain
- Eyelid edema
- Potential for infection
- Potential for injury

Related factors and risk factors are individualized on the basis of patient's condition or needs.

PLANNING

STEP	RATIONALE
1. Expected outcomes following completion of procedure:	
• Patient demonstrates minimal anxiety during and after irrigation.	Potential for anxiety and pain is high during emergency.
• Patient verbalizes reduced pain, burning, or itching and improved visual acuity after irrigation.	Reflects effectiveness of procedure in removing irritant.
• Patient maintains normal pupillary reaction and eye movement after irrigation.	Reflects effectiveness of procedure in minimizing exposure to irritant and preventing eye damage.
2. Discuss procedure with patient.	Decreases patient anxiety.
3. Check accuracy and completeness of each MAR with health care provider's written prescription. Check patient's name, irrigation solution name and concentration, route of administration, and time for administration. Compare MAR with label of eye irrigation solution.	The prescription sheet is the most reliable source and only legal record of medications or procedures that patient is to receive. Ensures that patient receives correct medication.
4. Assemble supplies at bedside.	Provides easy access to supplies.
5. Help patient to side-lying position on side of affected eye. Turn head toward affected eye. If both eyes are affected, place patient supine for simultaneous irrigation of both eyes.	Position facilitates flow of solution from inner to outer canthus, preventing contamination of unaffected eye and nasolacrimal duct.

IMPLEMENTATION

STEP	RATIONALE
1. Apply clean gloves.	Reduces transmission of microorganisms. Protects hands from chemical irritants.
2. Remove any contact lens, if possible (see Procedural Guideline 19.2). Remove gloves after contact lens is removed. Reapply new gloves.	Prompt removal of lenses is needed to safely and completely irrigate foreign substances from patient's eyes. Removal of gloves following contact lens removal prevents reintroduction of chemical transferred from lens to glove.

Critical Decision Point *In an emergency, such as first aid for a chemical burn, do not delay by removing patient's contact lens before irrigation. Do not remove lens unless rapid swelling is occurring. Flush eye from the inner to outer canthus with cool tap water immediately* (Soleimani & Naderan, 2020).

STEP	RATIONALE
3. Explain to patient that eye can be closed periodically and that no object will touch it.	Informing patients what to expect decreases anxiety and reassures them.
4. Place towel or waterproof pad under patient's face and curved emesis basin just below patient's cheek on side of affected eye.	Catches irrigation fluid.
5. Using gauze moistened with prescribed solution (or normal saline), gently clean visible secretions or foreign material from eyelid margins and eyelashes, wiping from inner to outer canthus.	Minimizes transfer of material into eye during irrigation. Prevents secretions from entering nasolacrimal duct.

STEP	RATIONALE
IMPLEMENTATION	
6. Explain next steps to patient and encourage relaxation: **a.** With gloved finger gently retract upper and lower eyelids to expose conjunctival sacs. **b.** To hold lids open, apply gentle pressure to lower bony orbit and bony prominence beneath eyebrow. Do not apply pressure over eye.	Retraction minimizes blinking and allows irrigation of conjunctiva.
7. Hold irrigating syringe, dropper, or IV tubing approximately 2.5 cm (1 inch) from inner canthus.	Direct contact with irrigation equipment may injure eye.
8. Ask patient to look toward brow. Gently irrigate eye with steady stream toward lower conjunctival sac, moving from inner to outer canthus (see Step 8 illustration).	Minimizes force of stream on patient's cornea. Flushes irritant out and away from the other eye and nasolacrimal duct.

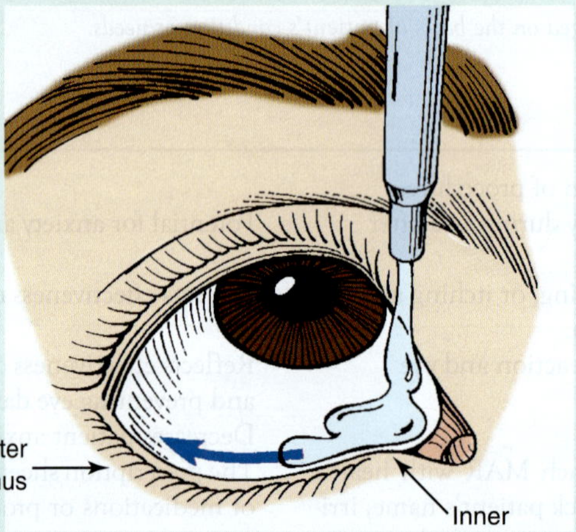

STEP 8 Irrigation of eye from inner to outer canthus.

STEP	RATIONALE
9. Reinforce importance of procedure, and encourage patient by using calm, confident, soft voice.	Reduces anxiety.
10. Allow patient to blink periodically.	Lid closure moves secretions from upper conjunctival sac.
11. Continue irrigation with prescribed solution volume or time or until secretions are cleared. (NOTE: In emergent situation, an irrigation of 30 minutes or more is needed to flush chemicals.)	Assessment of eye secretion pH may be necessary if eye was exposed to an acidic or basic solution during injury (Soleimani & Naderan, 2020).
12. Blot excess moisture from eyelids and face with gauze or towel.	
13. Dispose of soiled supplies, remove gloves, and dispose in appropriate receptacle.	Reduces transmission of microorganisms.
EVALUATION	
1. Observe for verbal and nonverbal signs of anxiety during irrigation.	Verifies that patient is adequately comforted.
2. Assess patient's comfort level after irrigation.	Verifies effective removal of irritant.
3. Inspect eye for movement and to determine if PERRLA.	Impaired reaction to light, accommodation, or movement may indicate injury.
4. Ask patient about improved visual acuity. Have patient read written material.	Corneal damage from irritant can result in altered visual acuity (e.g., blurred vision, cloudiness).
5. Use teach-back: "I want to be sure I explained why it is important that I clean your eyes this way. Tell me the purpose of cleaning your eyes in this manner." Develop a revised teaching plan if patient and caregiver are unable to teach back correctly.	Determines patient's and caregiver's level of understanding of rationale for eye irrigation.

Unexpected Outcomes	Related Interventions
1. Anxiety.	• Reinforce rationale for irrigation. • Allow patient to close eye periodically during irrigation. • Instruct patient to take slow, deep breaths.
2. Patient has pain or foreign body sensation in eye following irrigation, excessive tearing, or photophobia.	• Advise patient to close eye and avoid eye movement. • Immediately notify health care provider or eye care practitioner.

Communication and Documentation

- Document in progress notes in EHR or chart the condition of eye and patient's report of pain and visual symptoms. Record amount and type of irrigation in patient's MAR.
- Document your evaluation of patient and caregiver learning.
- Report continuing symptoms of pain or blurred vision.

DOCUMENTATION EXAMPLE

Patient presented to ED with chemical injury to left eye. Complaining of acute pain, 8/10, burning sensation. No pain to right eye. Left eye cleansed with normal saline moistened gauze. No debris noted. Eyelid retracted and eye irrigated with normal saline for 15 minutes. Patient tolerated procedure well and was able to read education pamphlet afterward with no changes to visual acuity. Patient reported that pain was now 2/10 and improving. Health care provider to see patient for further assessment.

Caring for a Patient With a Prosthetic Eye

- Prosthetic eyes are made from various materials. In the past, glass was the most common material, but it is rarely used today. Poly(methyl methacrylate) (PMMA) is now preferred because of its durability, availability, and minimal cost (Cafiero-Chin et al., 2015).
- A detailed history is required related to the patient's wearing habits, how often the prosthesis is used, and in which manner the prosthesis is to be removed and cleaned.
- Removal of the prosthetic device is similar to removal of a hard contact lens. A small suction device can be used, or it can be removed manually. When removing manually, the prosthesis should be pushed up over the lower eyelid, allowing the device to slip out from the bottom (Cafiero-Chin et al., 2015).
- To replace the prosthesis, the top is inserted first by pushing up under the upper eyelid and sliding the lower portion under the lower eyelid (Cafiero-Chin et al., 2015).

Special Considerations

Teaching

- Help patient identify potential hazards at home and work and the steps to take to prevent accidents. Personal protective eyewear, such as goggles, face shields, safety glasses, or full-face respirators, must be used when an eye hazard exists. The eye protection chosen for specific work situations depends on the nature and extent of the hazard, the circumstances of exposure, other protective equipment used, and personal vision needs (Canadian Centre for Occupational Health and Safety, 2019).
- Review first aid procedures for eye emergencies with patient and caregiver.
- Instruct patient to not press or rub an injured eye.
- Instruct patient to consult with ophthalmologist before reinserting contact lens.

Pediatric

- A child with a foreign body or chemical in the eye may panic. It may be necessary to restrain the child to safely and quickly irrigate the eye.

Care in the Community: Home Management

- If the injury occurred in the workplace, refer to the safety data sheet (SDS) of the Workplace Hazardous Materials Information System (WHMIS), as applicable.

✦ SKILL 19.2 Ear Irrigation

The common indications for irrigation of the external ear are presence of foreign bodies or buildup of cerumen (earwax) in the ear canal. The procedure is not without potential hazards. Usually, irrigations are performed with liquid warmed to body temperature to avoid vertigo or nausea caused by vestibular stimulation. Ear irrigations are effective when the use of commercial drops is unsuccessful in removing cerumen buildup (Oyama, 2019). The greatest danger during ear irrigation is trauma to the tympanic membrane if irrigant is forced into the ear canal under pressure. Damage to the external auditory meatus may occur by scratching of the lining of the canal if a patient suddenly moves or if there is inadequate control of the irrigating syringe. Drying the ear improperly may lead to acute otitis externa (infection of the outer ear).

Ear emergencies can include the presence of foreign bodies, insect bites, or percussion injuries. In addition, a patient can have damage from inside the ear, which includes blood and drainage. Sometimes the cause of bloody drainage may be the result of a head or neck injury. If a head or neck injury is suspected, immobilize the patient. Cover the outside of the ear with a sterile dressing (if available), get medical help immediately, and do not irrigate the ear. In addition, do not irrigate the ear if an organic object (e.g., vegetable), battery, or polystyrene ball is present in the canal; there is a history of ruptured tympanic membrane; or a patient has otitis externa, previous ear surgery (e.g., mastoidectomy), or very hard cerumen (van Wyk, 2022).

Delegation and Collaboration

The skill of administering ear irrigation cannot be delegated to a UCP. The nurse directs the UCP to do the following:

- Immediately report any potential side effects of ear irrigation (e.g., pain, drainage, dizziness)
- Help a patient when ambulating because some vertigo may be present, which increases a patient's risk of falling

Equipment

- Clean gloves
- Otoscope *(optional)*
- Irrigation or bulb syringe
- Basin for irrigating solution (Use sterile basin if sterile irrigating solution is used [when tympanic membrane is ruptured].)
- Emesis basin for drainage or irrigating solution exiting the ear
- Towel
- Cotton balls or 10 cm × 10 cm (4 inch × 4 inch) gauze
- Prescribed irrigating solution warmed to body temperature, mineral oil, or over-the-counter softener
- Medication administration record (MAR) (print or electronic)

STEP	RATIONALE

ASSESSMENT

STEP	RATIONALE
1. Identify patient using at least two person-specific identifiers (e.g., name and date of birth, or name and medical record number) according to employer policy. Compare identifiers with information on patient's MAR or medical record.	Ensures correct patient. Complies with Accreditation Canada's standards and improves patient safety (Accreditation Canada, 2020).
2. Throughout the procedure, the 4 moments for hand hygiene are to be implemented; hand hygiene should occur before initial patient (or patient environment) contact, before an aseptic procedure, after body fluid exposure risk, and after patient (or patient environment) contact. Additional hand hygiene should be performed when hands are visibly soiled.	Proper hand hygiene helps prevent the spread of infectious agents to health care providers.
3. Review health care provider's medication prescription, including solution to be instilled and affected ear(s). Note: The abbreviations AU (for right ear), AS (for left ear), and AD (for both ears) are no longer acceptable (Institute for Safe Medication Practices Canada, 2018); specific ears are to be written out.	Ensures safe and correct administration of medication.
4. Review medical record for history of ruptured tympanic membrane, placement of myringotomy tubes, or surgery of the auditory canal.	These conditions contraindicate irrigation.
5. Inspect pinna and external auditory meatus for redness, swelling, drainage, abrasions, and presence of cerumen or foreign objects.	Findings provide baseline to monitor effects of medication or solution.
a. Always attempt to remove foreign objects in ear by first simply straightening ear canal.	This may cause object to fall out.

Critical Decision Point *If vegetable matter such as a dried bean or pea is occluded in the canal, do not perform irrigation. The material can swell on contact with water and cause further damage to the canal* (Grigg & Grigg, 2018).

STEP	RATIONALE
6. Use otoscope to inspect deeper parts of auditory canal and tympanic membrane. Caution: Do not push an object further into the ear canal.	Verifies whether tympanic membrane is intact.
7. Ask if patient is experiencing pain, using a scale of 0–10 (where 0 = no pain, and 10 = the worst pain ever).	Pain is symptomatic of external ear infection or inflammation.
8. Note patient's ability to hear clearly.	Occlusion of auditory canal by cerumen or foreign object can impair hearing.
9. Review patient's knowledge of purpose for irrigation and normal care of ears.	May indicate need for instruction regarding hygiene.

NURSING DIAGNOSES

- Pain (acute or chronic)
- Insufficient knowledge regarding purpose for irrigation
- Potential for injury

Related factors and risk factors are individualized on the basis of patient's condition or needs.

PLANNING

STEP	RATIONALE
1. Expected outcomes following completion of procedure:	
• Patient denies pain during instillation.	Fluid is properly instilled.
• Patient demonstrates hearing conversation more clearly in affected ear.	Obstruction in ear canal is resolved.
• Patient can discuss purpose of irrigation and describe correct ear care techniques.	Feedback reflects patient's learning.
• Patient's canal is clear of cerumen, foreign material, and discharge.	Inflammation, irritation, and occlusion of canal are relieved.

STEP	RATIONALE

PLANNING

2. Check accuracy and completeness of each MAR with health care provider's written medication or procedure prescription. Check patient's name, medication name and dosage, route of administration, and time for administration. Compare MAR with label of ear irrigation solution.	The prescription sheet is the most reliable source and only legal record of medications or procedures that patient is to receive. Ensures that patient receives correct medication.
3. If patient is found to have impacted cerumen, instill 1 or 2 drops of oil (olive or mineral) or over-the-counter softener into ear twice a day for 2–3 days before irrigation.	Loosens cerumen and ensures easier removal during irrigation.
4. Explain procedure. Prepare patient that irrigation may cause sensation of dizziness, ear fullness, and warmth.	Prepares patient to anticipate effects of irrigation and promotes cooperation.
5. Arrange supplies at bedside. Close curtain or room door.	Helps nurse perform procedure smoothly. Maintains privacy.

IMPLEMENTATION

1. Help patient to sitting or lying position with head turned toward affected ear. Place towel under patient's head and shoulder, and have patient, if able, hold emesis basin under affected ear.	Position minimizes leakage of fluids around neck and facial area. Solution will flow from ear canal to basin.
2. Pour prescribed irrigating solution into basin. Check temperature of solution by pouring small drop on your inner forearm. NOTE: If sterile irrigating solution is used, a sterile basin is required.	
3. Apply clean gloves. Gently clean auricle and outer ear canal with gauze or cotton balls. Do *not* force drainage or cerumen into ear canal.	Reduces transmission of microorganisms and prevents infected material from re-entering ear canal. Forceful instillation of solution into occluded canal can cause injury to eardrum.
4. Fill irrigating syringe with solution (approximately 50 mL).	Enough fluid is needed to provide a steady irrigating stream.
5. For adults and for children over 3 years old, gently pull pinna up and back. In children aged 3 years or younger, pinna should be pulled down and back (Grigg & Grigg, 2018). Adults can lie supine. Place tip of irrigating device just inside external meatus. Leave space around irrigating tip and canal.	Pulling pinna straightens external ear canal. Prevents obstruction of canal with device, which can lead to increased pressure on tympanic membrane.
6. Slowly instill irrigating solution by holding tip of syringe 1 cm (0.5 inches) above opening to ear canal. Direct fluid toward superior aspect of ear canal. Allow it to drain out into basin during instillation. Continue until canal is cleaned or solution is used (see Step 6 illustration).	Slow instillation prevents buildup of pressure in ear canal and ensures contact of solution with all canal surfaces.

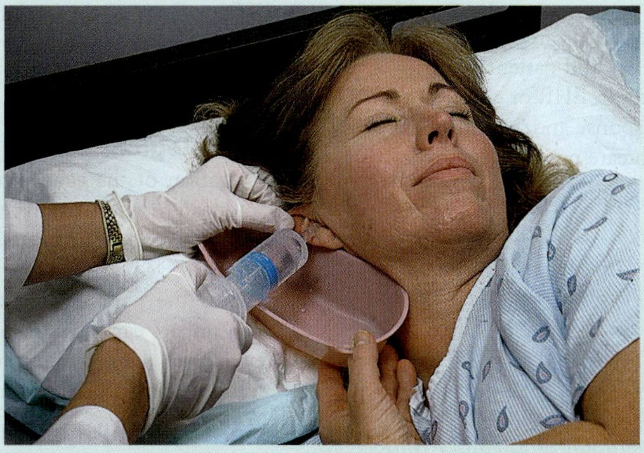

STEP 6 Tip of syringe does not occlude ear canal during irrigation.

STEP	RATIONALE
IMPLEMENTATION	
7. Maintain flow of irrigation in steady stream until pieces of cerumen or exudate flow from canal.	Constant flow of fluid loosens cerumen.
8. Periodically ask if patient is experiencing pain, nausea, or vertigo.	Symptoms indicate that irrigating solution is too hot or too cold or instilled with too much pressure.
9. Drain excessive fluid from ear by having patient tilt head toward affected side.	Excess fluid may promote microorganism growth if not drained.
10. Dry outer ear canal gently with cotton ball. Leave cotton ball in place for 5–10 minutes.	Drying prevents buildup of moisture that can lead to otitis externa.
11. Help patient to sitting position.	Maintains comfort.
12. Remove gloves and dispose of supplies in appropriate receptacle.	Reduces transmission of infection.
EVALUATION	
1. Ask patient if pain is noted during instillation of solution.	Fluid instilled improperly under pressure causes discomfort.
2. Ask patient about sensations of light-headedness or dizziness.	Instillation of fluid into ear can cause some light-headedness or dizziness, which can put patient at risk of falling.
3. Reinspect condition of meatus and canal.	Determines whether solution relieves symptoms and removes foreign materials.
4. Assess patient's hearing acuity.	Determines whether hearing is improved.
5. **Use teach-back:** "I want to be sure you understand how to safely insert the syringe to clean an ear. Show me how you would do this for your mother." Develop a revised teaching plan if caregiver is unable to teach back correctly.	Determines caregiver's level of understanding of instructional topic.

Unexpected Outcomes	Related Interventions
1. Patient indicates increased ear pain during irrigation.	• Rupture of eardrum may have occurred. Stop irrigations and notify health care provider immediately.
2. Ear canal remains occluded with cerumen.	• Repeat irrigation.
3. Foreign body remains in ear canal.	• Refer to auditory specialist if foreign object remains after irrigation.

Communication and Documentation

- Document the procedure, amount of solution instilled, time of administration, and ear receiving irrigation on flow sheet or in progress notes in EHR or chart.
- Document your evaluation of patient and caregiver learning.
- Document appearance of external ear and patient's hearing acuity on flow sheet or in progress notes in EHR or chart.
- Report adverse effects or patient response and/or withheld medications to nurse in charge or health care provider.

DOCUMENTATION EXAMPLE

Patient presented ambulatory to clinic for annual cerumen irrigation. Denies acute concerns. Patient is accurately able to explain purpose of mineral oil instillation for impacted cerumen to this writer. Patient positioned supine and 2 drops of mineral oil instilled into each ear bilaterally. Cotton ball placed in each ear. Patient assisted to seated position and did not complain of any vertigo. Instructed to leave cotton ball in ears for 10–15 minutes. Patient left ambulatory with plan to return next year for follow-up cerumen care.

Special Considerations

Teaching

- Instruct patient that cerumen has an antibacterial effect that maintains an acid pH in the auditory canal.
- Instruct patients to clean ears daily with a washcloth, soap, and warm water.
- Warn patients against placing objects (including cotton swabs) into ear canal.

Pediatric

- When cleaning the ear of a small child, be certain that child's head is immobilized to prevent puncturing eardrum. It may be necessary to have child's parent or staff participate (Grigg & Grigg, 2018).

Gerontological

- Irrigation of the ear can trigger a cough during the procedure and lead to tinnitus and vertigo (Schumann et al., 2022). Perform irrigation according to employer policy and be attentive to patient safety.
- Assess the patient's mental state and physical dexterity. Both can impact ear hygiene and otic medication adherence. Ask the patient to demonstrate the skill and assist the patient with self-administration, as appropriate.

Patients With Physical or Cognitive Challenges

- Patient groups that are vulnerable or unlikely to comment about earwax or loss of hearing—such as people with cognitive challenges—need to have their ears and hearing regularly assessed.

Care in the Community: Home Management

- Instruct patient to use a clean bulb syringe for irrigation. Mineral oil drops or over-the-counter otic preparations can help with removal of cerumen.

✦ SKILL 19.3 Care of Hearing Aids

Hearing is vital for normal communication and orientation to sounds in the environment. Hearing impairment is most common in older persons. Many patients do not seek professional help for this impairment, nor do they consistently wear aids (Ramage-Morin et al., 2019). According to Statistics Canada (2021), 38% of adults aged 20–79 have at least slight hearing loss in one or both ears; persons aged 60–79 were 78% more likely to have hearing loss than younger adults; and males have a higher incidence of hearing loss than females.

Initially, a person with hearing loss may deny the condition or think that there is a stigma attached to the actual hearing loss or the need for a hearing aid (Ruusuvuori et al., 2021). Any hearing loss has social implications, and the person may not engage in social activities. In addition, in social situations, people with a hearing aid often believe that, once their aid is observed, they are viewed as an older person and as having weakened cognitive competence (Ruusuvuori et al., 2021). There are also many safety considerations. Not only do people with hearing loss have difficulty hearing where sounds are coming from, but they also have difficulty hearing or understanding speech (e.g., during patient education); as a result, they may not manage their symptoms or therapies safely (Ramage-Morin et al., 2019).

When a patient has a hearing aid, the nurse's role is to understand how it functions and how to help the patient care for it. It is the role of a hearing professional to determine which type of aid the patient needs and how to establish the best auditory settings for each individual patient . For people with hearing loss, a proper hearing aid improves the ability to hear and understand spoken words. Several styles of hearing aids are currently available to patients (Table 19.1). Hearing aids amplify sound so that can be heard at a more effective level. All hearing aids have four basic components:

1. A microphone, which receives and converts sound into electrical signals
2. An amplifier, which increases the strength of the electrical signal
3. A receiver, which converts the strengthened signal back into sound
4. A power source (batteries)

Hearing aids do not all work the same. The two main types of electronic hearing aids are analogue and digital. Analogue technology converts sound waves into electrical waves, which are amplified. These are custom built to meet the needs of the user and programmed by the manufacturer according to the specifications of the audiologist. Digital technology converts sound waves into numerical codes. The aid is programmed to amplify some frequencies more than others. Digital technology allows the hearing aid to communicate with a number of external devices, including smartphones and Bluetooth technology (Chasin, 2015).

It is a challenge to adjust one's communication style to accommodate a patient with a hearing impairment. Practise person-centred care using the patient as a resource for identifying the communication techniques that they find most helpful. Be sure that a patient can see your face; speak slowly in a normal tone; and rephrase rather than repeat if they cannot understand you. Also remember that a patient may be unable to hear alerts, such as fire alarms or overhead announcements.

Delegation and Collaboration

The skill of caring for a hearing aid can be delegated to a UCP. The nurse directs the UCP to do the following:

- Report ear pain, inflammation, drainage, odour, or changes in hearing
- Identify alternative ways to communicate with a patient while the aid is not in use
- Learn how to carefully handle the aid to prevent damage or injury

Equipment

- Soft towel and washcloth
- Facial tissues
- Brush or wax loop
- Storage case
- Warm water and soap
- Spare battery (size depends on aid) *(optional)*
- Clean gloves (if drainage present)

STEP	RATIONALE
ASSESSMENT	
1. Identify patient using at least two person-specific identifiers (e.g., name and date of birth, or name and medical record number) according to employer policy.	Ensures correct patient. Complies with Accreditation Canada's standards and improves patient safety (Accreditation Canada, 2020).
2. Throughout the procedure, the 4 moments for hand hygiene are to be implemented; hand hygiene should occur before initial patient (or patient environment) contact, before an aseptic procedure, after body fluid exposure risk, and after patient (or patient environment) contact. Additional hand hygiene should be performed when hands are visibly soiled.	Proper hand hygiene helps prevent the spread of infectious agents to health care providers.
3. Determine whether patient can hear clearly with hearing aid by talking slowly and clearly in normal tone of voice.	Inability to hear may indicate a problem with the hearing aid or battery or that the particular model is no longer effective for patient.
4. Ask if patient is able to manipulate and hold hearing aid, or, preferably, observe patient insert aid independently.	Determines level of assistance required in care.
5. Assess if hearing aid is working by removing it from patient's ear. Close battery case and turn volume slowly to high. Cup hand over hearing aid. If you hear a squealing sound (feedback), it is working. If no sound is heard, replace batteries and test again.	May indicate malfunctioning of hearing aid.

TABLE 19.1

Types of Hearing Aids

Type	Advantages	Disadvantages	Cautions
In-the-ear (ITE) hearing aids fit completely in the outer ear and are used for mild to severe hearing loss. 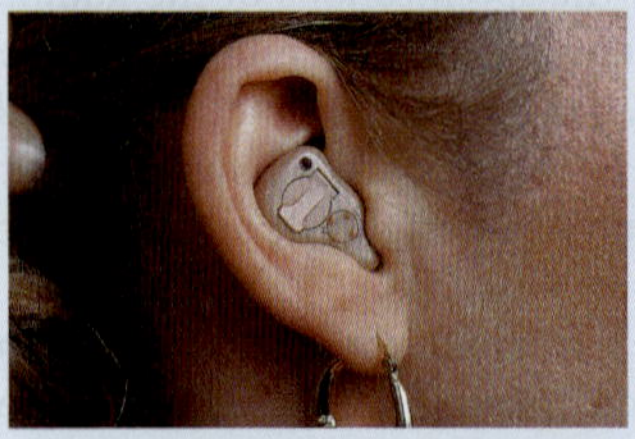	Design of the aid can improve sound transmission through telephone calls. Some ITEs have a *telecoil*, which is a magnetic circuit that allows users to receive sound through the circuitry of the hearing aid instead of the microphone.	ITE aids are damaged by cerumen and ear drainage, and their small size can cause adjustment problems and feedback. They cannot be used with many assistive listening devices.	Not usually worn by children because the casings need to be replaced as the ear grows.
Behind-the-ear (BTE) hearing aids are worn behind the ear and are connected to a plastic ear mould that fits inside the outer ear. Used for mild to profound hearing loss. 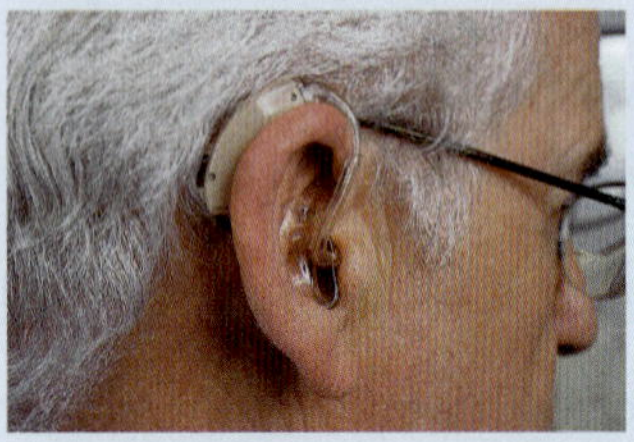	Sound travels through the ear mould into the ear. Useful for persons with chronic ear infections, excess cerumen, or small ear canals. Can be used with a variety of other assistive devices.	Improperly fitted BTE ear moulds can cause feedback, a whistling sound caused by the fit of the hearing aid.	May not be appropriate for children or adults who are active in sports because of potential for damage to the device.
Open-fit hearing aids are customized to fit the size and shape of the ear canal and are best used for persons with mild to moderate high-frequency hearing loss. 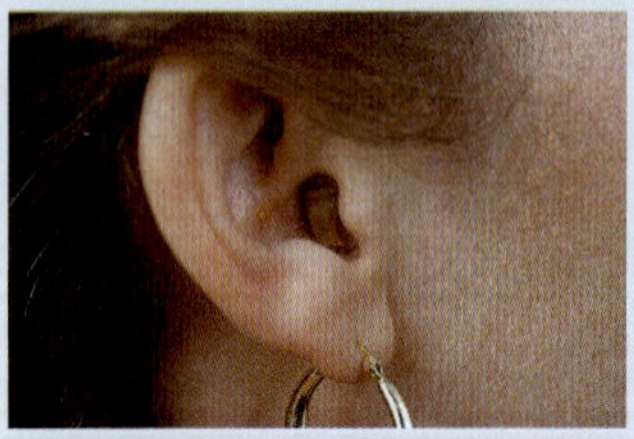	Amplifier and electronics can sit behind the ear, and a slim tube with a small tip is placed in the ear canal.	Because of their small size, canal aids may be difficult for the user to adjust and remove and may not be able to hold additional devices such as a telecoil.	Expensive and not recommended for children. Can also be damaged by cerumen and ear drainage.
Contralateral routing of signal (CROS) is designed for persons with one ear that is unaidable.	Microphone is placed on the unaidable ear and sound is routed to a hearing aid in the other ear.	Does not fully restore ability to localize sounds in space but provides useful sound information to the person.	CROS can be used in children, depending on their age and environment.

Data from Canadian Academy of Audiology. (n.d.-a). *Hearing aids, implants and other devices*. https://canadianaudiology.ca/for-the-public/hearing-aids-and-implants/#what-kinds-of-hearing-aids-are-there; National Institute on Deafness and Other Communication Disorders. (2022, October 11). *Hearing aids*. https://www.nidcd.nih.gov/health/hearing-aids

STEP	RATIONALE
ASSESSMENT	
6. Determine patient's usual routine for caring for their hearing aid.	Provides information as to how patient cares for device, and identifies patient preferences.
7. Assess patient for any unusual physical or auditory signs or symptoms (pain, itching, redness, discharge, odour, tinnitus, decreased acuity). If hearing is reduced, ask the following: When did this start? Is it present all the time? Does the quality of hearing acuity change with male or female voices? Adult or children's voices?	May indicate injury, infection, or cerumen accumulation.
8. Inspect ear mould for cracked or rough edges.	Improperly fitted hearing aids cause irritation or discomfort to external ear canal.

STEP	RATIONALE
ASSESSMENT	
9. Inspect for accumulation of cerumen around aid and plugging of opening in aid.	Cerumen can block sound reception (Schumann et al., 2022).
10. Assess patient's knowledge of and routines for cleaning and caring for hearing aid.	Determines adherence to and knowledge of self-care.

NURSING DIAGNOSES

- Reduced verbal communication
- Insufficient knowledge regarding hearing aid care
- Potential for injury
- Potential for situational low self-esteem

Related factors and risk factors are individualized on the basis of patient's condition or needs.

STEP	RATIONALE
PLANNING	
1. Expected outcomes following completion of procedure:	
• Patient verbalizes comfort after removal and reinsertion of hearing aid.	Hearing aid is removed or inserted properly and positioned correctly.
• Patient responds appropriately to normal conversation and environmental sounds.	Hearing aid and batteries are operational. Aid is secure and unobstructed.
• Patient demonstrates proper care of hearing aid.	Learning is achieved.
2. Discuss procedure with patient. Explain all steps before removing aid.	Patient can help in planning by explaining additional tips for care. Patient may be confused or anxious if verbal instructions are given after removal of hearing aid.
3. Assemble supplies at bedside. Place towel over work area.	Provides easy access to supplies. Towel catches hearing aid if accidently dropped and prevents breakage.
4. Have patient assume supine, side-lying, or sitting position in bed or chair.	Provides easy access for nurse. Promotes patient comfort.

STEP	RATIONALE
IMPLEMENTATION	
1. Apply clean gloves if patient has ear drainage.	Reduces transmission of microorganisms.
2. Removing and cleaning hearing aid(s):	
a. Patient or nurse turns hearing aid(s) volume off, usually by turning volume control to left. Then, grasp aid securely and gently remove device following natural ear contour.	Prevents feedback (whistling) during removal. Prevents dropping of hearing aid. Prevents injury to ear.

Critical Decision Point *Some hearing aids, such as the completely-in-canal (CIC) device, do not have a volume control but are turned off by opening the battery door. Other aids have the volume control located on the remote. Be sure that the patient knows the importance of having the volume turned off when the aid is not in use.*

STEP	RATIONALE
b. Hold hearing aid over towel and wipe exterior with tissue to remove cerumen.	Prevents breakage or damage if hearing aid is dropped. Cerumen may irritate canal and interfere with fit.
c. Inspect all openings in hearing aid for accumulated cerumen. Carefully remove cerumen with wax loop or other device supplied with hearing aid.	Cerumen may block sound from receiver. It may also block pressure equalization channel and create feeling of ear pressure.

Critical Decision Point *The pressure equalization channel is a tiny hole through the entire length of the ear mould; it should be clear for the entire length. The receiver points into the ear through another opening. It is easily damaged. NEVER insert anything into the receiver port!*

STEP	RATIONALE
d. Inspect ear mould for rough edges or any frays in cords.	May irritate ear canal.
e. Open battery door, place hearing aid in labelled storage container, and allow it to air dry.	Allows drying of internal components. Protects against breakage and loss.
f. Assess ear for redness, tenderness, discharge, or odour.	Signs may indicate injury or infection.
g. Repeat procedure for other hearing aid if bilateral.	

STEP	RATIONALE
IMPLEMENTATION	
h. Place towel beneath patient's ear(s). Wash ear canal(s) with washcloth moistened in soap and water. Rinse and dry.	Absorbs excess water. Removes cerumen from ear canal. Removes soap residue and water that may harbour microbes or damage aid.
i. Dispose of towels, remove gloves, and dispose in appropriate receptacle.	Reduces transmission of microorganisms.
j. If storing hearing aid(s), place each in dry storage case with desiccant material. Label case with patient's name and medical record number. If there is more than one hearing aid, note right or left. Indicate in patient's medical record where hearing aid is stored.	Protects hearing aid against damage, moisture, and breakage. Documents how and where hearing aid is stored.
3. Inserting hearing aid(s):	
a. Remove hearing aid(s) from storage case and check battery (see assessment). Check that volume is off.	
b. Identify hearing aid as either right (marked "R," or red colour-coded) or left (marked "L," or blue colour-coded).	Proper orientation prevents damage and injury.
c. When possible, allow patient to insert hearing aid. Otherwise, hold hearing aid with thumb and index finger of dominant hand so canal (long part with holes) is at bottom. Insert pointed end of ear mould into ear canal. Follow natural ear contours to guide hearing aid into place.	Prevents dropping of hearing aid. Proper positioning prevents injury. Pulling on ear may distort canal and make insertion more difficult.
d. Anchor any separate pieces, as in the case of behind-the-ear (BTE) hearing aid or body aid.	Prevents pieces from falling and breaking.
e. Adjust or have patient adjust volume gradually to comfortable level for talking to patient in regular voice 0.9–1.2 metres (3–4 feet) away. Rotate volume control toward nose to increase volume and away from nose to decrease volume.	Gradual adjustment prevents discomfort and injury to ear.
f. Repeat insertion for other hearing aid if bilateral.	
g. Close and store case. Remove and dispose of gloves.	Preserves desiccant. Prevents loss. Reduces transmission of microorganisms.

EVALUATION

1. Ask patient to rate level of comfort after removal or insertion.	Verifies proper technique and positioning.
2. Observe patient during normal conversation and in response to environmental sounds.	Verifies that aid is operational, correctly positioned, unobstructed, and effective.
3. Use teach-back: "I want to be sure you understand what I showed you about how to remove, clean, and reinsert your father's hearing aid. Let's take time now so you can show me how to do it." Develop a revised teaching plan if caregiver is unable to teach back correctly.	Determines caregiver's level of understanding of instructional topic.

Unexpected Outcomes	Related Interventions
1. Patient is unable to hear conversations or environmental sounds. Patient's verbal responses are inappropriate.	• Check function, type, and placement of battery and replace if indicated. • Increase volume if adjustable. • Inspect hearing aid and ear canal for cerumen blockage. • Refer to audiologist for reassessment.
2. Patient experiences discomfort or pain, inflammation, drainage, or odour from affected ear.	• Remove hearing aid and inspect for sharp or rough edges. Refer to provider for repair. • Assess ear for signs of injury or infection. • Confirm correct R or L placement. Reposition hearing aid.

Communication and Documentation

- Document removal of hearing aid, storage location if not reinserted after cleaning, and patient's preferred communication techniques on flow sheet or in progress notes in EHR or chart. If family takes hearing aid home, be sure that this information is documented.
- Document your evaluation of patient and caregiver learning.
- Report any signs or symptoms of infection or injury or sudden decrease in hearing acuity.

DOCUMENTATION EXAMPLE

Removed patient's left hearing aid at HS. Prior to removal, patient stated their preferred method of communication was verbal communication with staff speaking slightly louder. Writer removed left hearing aid; aid assessed and appeared to be intact. Battery door opened and placed inside patient's personal hearing aid container. Container labelled with patient's medical record number and name. Hearing aid container left on patient's nightstand. Left ear assessed, no redness, tenderness, or odour. Patient comfortable, call bell within reach.

Special Considerations

Teaching

- Instruct family that batteries are toxic if swallowed and to keep them away from pets and children.
- Patients should insert the hearing aid after their hair has dried and any hairspray has been applied. Heat from the hair dryer or perfumes and hairspray can damage the hearing aid.
- Dogs in particular and cats are attracted to the smell of used hearing aids. Advise patient to protect the hearing aids and their pets by properly storing the aids out of reach.
- Encourage patients to identify helpful communication tips and teach them to others. Many patients find facial cues informative. Speakers must:
  1. Face patient, stay within 0.9–1.2 metres (3–4 feet) away, and keep hands away from mouth
  2. Get patient's attention before speaking
  3. Rephrase rather than repeat when a patient cannot understand
  4. Reduce background noise or move to a quiet area

Pediatric

- Children are more often fitted with BTE hearing aids because the ear canal is still growing.
- The aid is made less conspicuous with hair styling or becomes a statement of fashion and personality with a brightly coloured or transparent case.
- Children need help to prevent acoustic feedback (whistling), which they are unable to hear. This is usually eliminated by removing and reinserting the device and making sure that no hair is caught between the ear mould and canal or lowering the volume of the device (Hockenberry et al., 2024).

Gerontological

- Advise patient to protect the hearing aid from water, alcohol, hair-spray or cologne, perspiration, rain, and snow and to avoid exposing it to extremes of temperature.
- Encourage patient to store hearing aids and batteries with desiccant or in an electronic dryer to prolong aid's life, minimize repairs, and preserve batteries.
- The small size of some hearing aids may make them difficult to manipulate, particularly for individuals with decreased dexterity or visual acuity. Consult an audiologist to identify a hearing aid that accommodates a patient's particular needs.

Care in the Community: Home Management

- Determine presence and willingness of caregiver to perform necessary care of hearing aid if required.
- Assess patient's home and determine need for special precautions given patient's hearing status.

✦ REVIEW QUESTIONS

A 68-year-old patient (he/him) and his partner have two grown children who are themselves married with children. The patient has worn bilateral in-the-ear (ITE) hearing aids for the last 10 years. He knows how to care for the hearing aids, and is comfortable and satisfied with them. When the aids are working well, he notes that he hears his family and co-workers clearly, has minimal distortion in large gatherings, and is able to distinguish emergency sirens and car horns when driving. Three weeks ago, he had an upper respiratory tract infection, and since that time both he and his partner have noticed changes in his hearing acuity. He is now visiting his primary care clinic to see what can be done with his hearing before going back to the audiologist.

Review Questions 1 to 4 relate to the case study presented here.

1. The patient thinks that he has diminished hearing in the left ear and senses drainage from that ear. Which assessments should the nurse complete?
2. Their preschool- and school-age grandchildren visit frequently and are curious about the hearing aids. Neither the patient nor his partner remembers any patient education regarding hearing aid safety related to young children. What should the nurse include in a teaching session regarding hearing aid safety?
3. During assessment of the left ear, the nurse identifies excessive wax, purulent drainage, and a cloudy tympanic membrane. Using SBAR (situation–background–assessment–recommendation), communicate this information to the health care team.
4. The nurse decides to check the functioning of the hearing aid. Place the following steps in the appropriate order for cleaning the hearing aid:
   1. Wash ear canal.
   2. Place hearing aid in storage case.
   3. Perform hand hygiene and apply clean gloves.
   4. Grasp aid securely and remove from ear following natural ear contour.
   5. Use brush to clean holes in aid.
   6. Have patient turn hearing aid volume off.
5. Which important nursing responsibilities pertain to eye irrigation? (*Select all that apply.*)
   1. Irrigating the eye immediately in emergent situations
   2. Removing dried secretions with moistened gauze
   3. Gently securing the eyelids with paper tape
   4. Checking for the pupillary response
   5. Preventing injury to the patient's corneas
6. When caring for a patient who is hearing impaired, which approaches best facilitate communication? (*Select all that apply.*)
   1. Speaking slightly more loudly than usual
   2. Speaking slightly more slowly using a normal tone
   3. Standing so patient can see the nurse's face
   4. Rephrasing rather than repeating
   5. Using hand gestures to help explain what is being said

Visit the Evolve site for a complete list of answers to the Review Questions.

✦ NEXT GENERATION NCLEX® (NGN)

For practice with answering exam questions related to unfolding NGN case studies, please consult the Next Generation NCLEX® (NGN)-Style Case Studies for Skills and Techniques on the Evolve website: http://evolve.elsevier.com/Canada/Perry/clinicalskills/

REFERENCES

Accreditation Canada. (2020). *Required organizational practices–2020 handbook.* https://physicians.nshealth.ca/resources/required-organizational-practices-2020-handbook

Ahmadinejad, M., Karbasi, E., Jahani, Y., et al. (2020). Efficacy of simple eye ointment, polyethylene cover, and eyelid taping in prevention of ocular surface disorders in critically ill patients: A randomized clinical trial. *Critical Care Research and Practice, 2020,* Article 6267432. https://doi.org/10.1155/2020/6267432

Assi, L., Ehrlich, J. R., Zhou, Y., et al. (2021). Self–reported dual sensory impairment, dementia, and functional limitations in Medicare beneficiaries. *Journal of the American Geriatrics Society, 69*(12), 3557–3567. https://doi.org/10.1111/jgs.17448

Bizrah, M., Yusuf, A., & Ahmad, S. (2019). An update on chemical eye burns. *Eye, 33*(9), 1362–1377. https://doi.org/10.1038/s41433-019-0456-5

Cafiero-Chin, M., Marques, C., & Danz, H. J. (2015). Ocular prosthesis: Indications to management. *Canadian Journal of Optometry, 77*(2), 24–32. https://doi.org/10.15353/cjo.77.507

Canadian Academy of Audiology. (n.d.-a) *Hearing aids, implants and other devices.* https://canadianaudiology.ca/for-the-public/hearing-aids-and-implants/#what-kinds-of-hearing-aids-are-there

Canadian Academy of Audiology. (n.d.-b). *Reports, scope, guidelines, and position statements.* https://canadianaudiology.ca/professional-resources/guidelines-and-position-statements/

Canadian Association of Optometrists. (n.d.). *Frequency of eye examinations.* https://opto.ca/document/frequency-of-eye-examinations

Canadian Association of Optometrists. (2023, March 18). *Wear and care for contact lenses.* https://opto.ca/health-library/wear-care-for-contact-lenses

Canadian Centre for Occupational Health and Safety. (2019). *Personal protective equipment: Eye and face protectors.* https://www.ccohs.ca/oshanswers/prevention/ppe/glasses.html

Canadian Hearing Services. (2023). *Services for you.* https://www.chs.ca/service-for-you

Canadian National Institute for the Blind. (n.d.). *What is blindness?* https://www.cnib.ca/en/sight-loss-info/blindness/what-blindness?region=on

Chasin, M. (2015). Hearing aids—from here to eternity and beyond: An article written for the hard of hearing consumer and their family. *Canadian Audiologist, 2*(2). https://canadianaudiologist.ca/issue/volume-2-issue-2-2015/hearing-aids-from-here-to-eternity-and-beyond-an-article-written-for-the-hard-of-hearing-consumer-and-their-families/

de Araujo, D., Silva, D. V. A., Rodrigues, C. A. O., et al. (2019). Effectiveness of nursing interventions to prevent dry eye in critically ill patients. *American Journal of Critical Care, 28*(4), 299–306. https://doi.org/10.4037/ajcc2019360

Grigg, S., & Grigg, C. (2018). Removal of ear, nose and throat foreign bodies: A review. *Australian Journal of General Practice, 47*(10), 682–685. https://doi.org/10.31128/ajgp-02-18-4503

Group Enroll. (2021, July 6). *Hearing aid prices in Canada: Costs, financing, and saving tips.* https://groupenroll.ca/hearing-aid-prices-in-canada/

Hockenberry, M., Duffy, E. A., & Gibbs, K. (2024). *Wong's nursing care of infants and children* (12th ed.). Elsevier.

Institute for Safe Medication Practices Canada. (2018). *Do not use: Dangerous abbreviations, symbols, and dose designations.* https://www.ismp-canada.org/download/ISMPCanadaListOfDangerousAbbreviations.pdf

Kaya, S., Senli, F. D., Mecit, H., et al. (2021). A study on stress and resilience among hearing-impaired people during the COVID-19 pandemic. *International Journal of Clinical Practice, 75*(11), Article e14861. https://doi.org/10.1111/ijcp.14861

Li, T., & Zhou, H. (2022). Effect of polyethylene cover for preventing corneal injury in critically ill patients: A meta-analysis. *Computational and Mathematical Methods in Medicine, 2022,* Article 6578229. https://doi.org/10.1155/2022/6578229

Mick, P., Parfyonov, M., Wittich, W., et al. (2018). Associations between sensory loss and social networks, participation, support, and loneliness. Analysis of the Canadian longitudinal study on aging. *Canadian Family Physician, 64,* e33–e41. http://www.cfp.ca/content/64/1/e33

National Institute on Deafness and Other Communication Disorders. (2022, October 11). *Hearing aids.* https://www.nidcd.nih.gov/health/hearing-aids

Oyama, L. C. (2019). Foreign bodies of the ear, nose and throat. *Emergency Medicine Clinics of North America, 37*(1), 121–130. https://doi.org/10.1016/j.emc.2018.09.009

Oyama, L. C. (2019). Foreign bodies of the ear, nose and throat. *Emergency Medicine Clinics of North America, 37*(1), 121–130. https://doi.org/10.1016/j.emc.2018.09.009

Ramage-Morin, P., Banks, R., Pineault, D., et al. (2019). Unperceived hearing loss among Canadians aged 40 to 79. *Health Reports, 30*(8), 11–20. Statistics Canada Catalogue No. 82-003-X. https://www150.statcan.gc.ca/n1/en/pub/82-003-x/2019008/article/00002-eng.pdf

Ruusuvuori, J. E., Aaltonen, T., Koskela, T., et al. (2021). Studies on stigma regarding hearing impairment and hearing aid use among adults of working age: A scoping review. *Disability & Rehabilitation, 43*(3), 436–446. https://doi.org/10.1080/09638288.2019.1622798

Schumann, J., Toscano, M. L., & Pfleghaar, N. (2022). *Ear irrigation.* StatPearls. https://www.ncbi.nlm.nih.gov/books/NBK459335/

Sharma, N., Kaur, M., Agarwal, T., et al. (2018). Treatment of acute ocular chemical burns. *Survey of Ophthalmology, 63*(2), 214–235. https://doi.org/10.1016/j.survophthal.2017.09.005

Soleimani, M., & Naderan, M. (2020). Management strategies of ocular chemical burns: Current perspectives. *Clinical Ophthalmology, 14,* 2687–2699. https://doi.org/10.2147/OPTH.S235873

Statistics Canada. (2021, October 20). *Hearing health of Canadian adults* [Infographic]. https://www150.statcan.gc.ca/n1/pub/11-627-m/11-627-m2021077-eng.htm

van Wyk, F. (2022, October 27). Cerumen impaction removal. *Medscape.* https://emedicine.medscape.com/article/1413546-overview

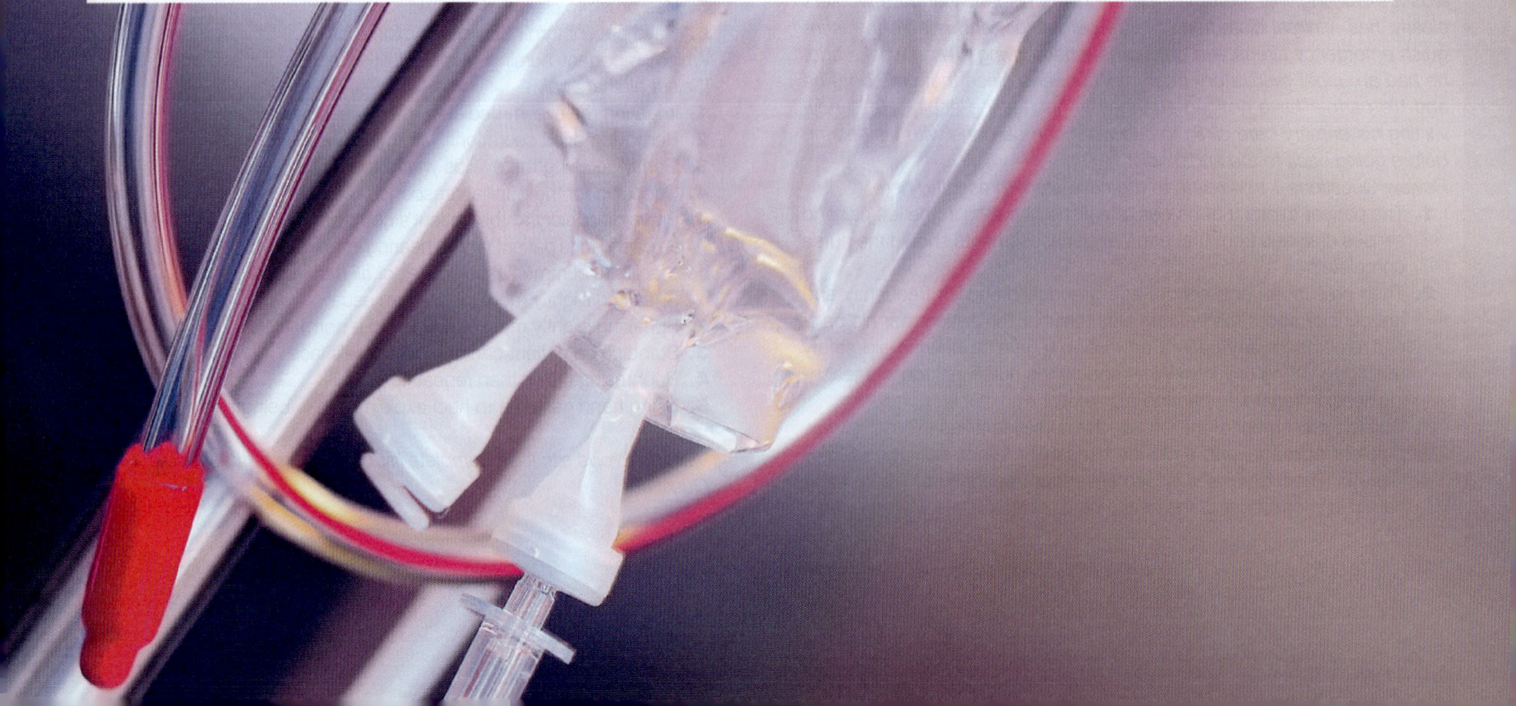

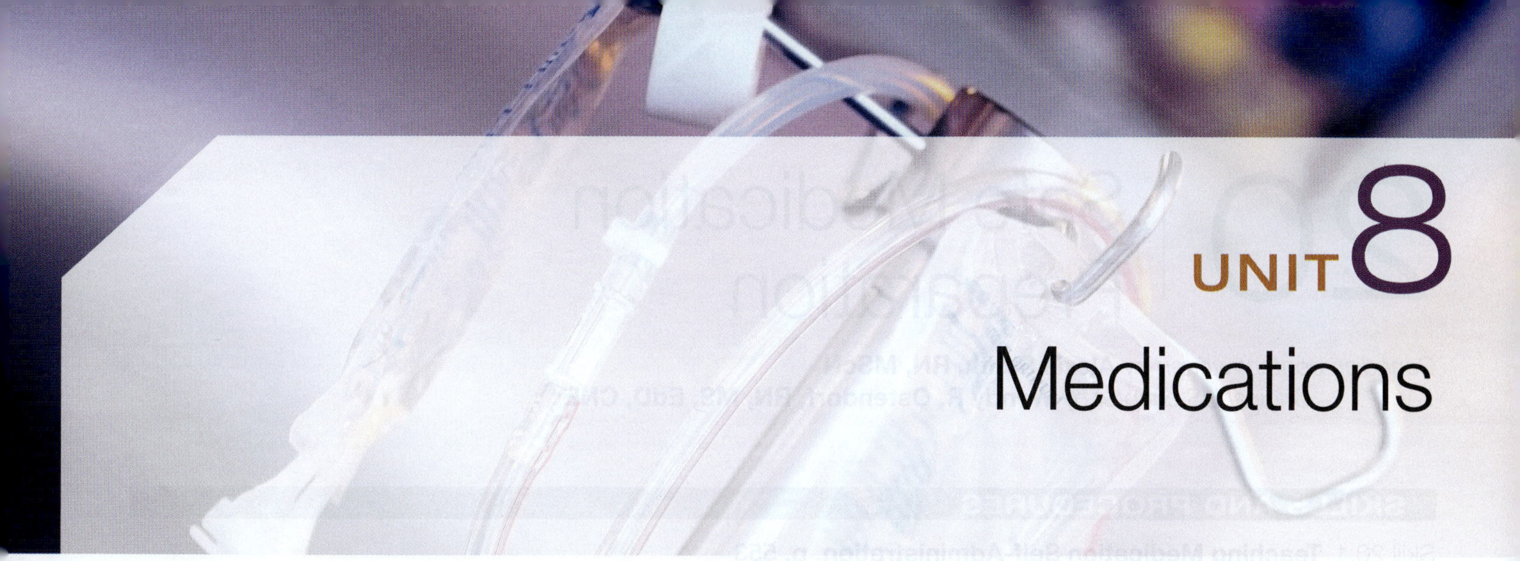

UNIT 8
Medications

Safe medication administration is a complex process that requires critical thinking and sound clinical judgement. You apply knowledge of pharmacological concepts, types of medication actions, expected therapeutic effects, adverse effects, and unexpected reactions in making decisions about preparation and administration of medications. Each patient will present clinical conditions, physical risk factors, and a knowledge level that will require you to adapt your approach in how you educate them about medications. When you perform one of the medication administration skills in this unit, you will apply critical thinking in making clinical judgements about how to safely and accurately prepare and administer medications for patients.

Administration of medications is a time-sensitive and time-pressured nursing action. Safe medication preparation practices include having a quiet, uninterrupted environment to review and prepare all medication orders. In addition to having a thorough pharmacological knowledge base, you must know the nursing implications for each medication, read the label on a medication container, and compare with the health care provider's prescription; accurately calculate and double-check dosages, especially for high-risk medications; and review the need for any preadministration assessments. When you prepare any medication for a patient, you are the individual responsible for administering that medication.

Safe medication preparation practices provide standards to use when assessing a patient so that you can determine whether a medication order is accurate and appropriate for the patient. You apply clinical judgement to ensure that you practise the 10 rights of medication preparation: the right medication is used; the right dose is available; the medication is administered to the right patient by the right route and at the right time; right education; right assessment; right for patient refusal; and following administration, there is the right documentation and evaluation of medication administration.

Prior to administering any medications, assess the patient and use clinical judgement to determine whether any modifications are needed. For example, a patient with facial paralysis may have difficulty swallowing a pill but can safely handle the medication when mixed in a soft food. Use clinical judgement to guide your clinical decision making to determine whether the tablet can be safely crushed, whether the contents of a capsule containing the same medication can be removed, or whether the medication comes in a liquid form. Then, obtain a prescription from the health care provider to administer the medication in the modified format.

In another example, you assess the patient's skin prior to administering a topical analgesic patch. You note that the area underneath the existing patch is excessively dry, blistered, and slightly red. These cues indicate that you need to select a different site for patch placement and provide skin care to the area of tissue injury. This is necessary because topical medications are absorbed through the patient's skin, and impairments to the patient's skin and/or underlying tissue can impede the therapeutic effect.

Inhaled medications are absorbed through a patient's respiratory tract. Inhalation is an effective drug delivery system because it places the medication at the site of action. However, the success of inhaled medications depends on the patient's proper use of the inhaler. For positive patient outcomes, use astute assessment skills and clinical judgement to observe the patient as they use the inhaler, and identify cues to determine whether they are using the inhaler device properly or whether further patient education is necessary.

Administering any parenteral medication is complex because of its invasive nature. In addition to safe medication practices, you need to apply knowledge of basic skin, musculoskeletal, and venous system anatomy in order to safely administer parenteral medications. Use your assessment skills to identify the correct injection site, and observe and analyze patient data cues, such as edema, injury, rash, and so on, that determine whether the site is unacceptable for an injection. Your assessment should also lead to clinical judgements regarding patient positioning. Can the patient assist with positioning or is another health care provider needed to assist?

Safe medication practices are essential to ensuring successful medication therapies, improving patient outcomes, and reducing medication errors. These practices rely on using critical thinking, which involves applying knowledge and experience, coupled with competent medication administration skills. Patients can change quickly, environmental factors add to the complexity of any task, and new medications become available, but the one condition that ensures safe medication practice is the use of clinical judgement to guide your clinical decisions. When administering and preparing medications, apply critical thinking to make appropriate patient assessments, analyze cues derived from the assessment data to identify any problem areas, and then form clinical judgements needed to plan and implement safe medication practices. Once medications have been given, document and evaluate the patient's response to all types of medications.

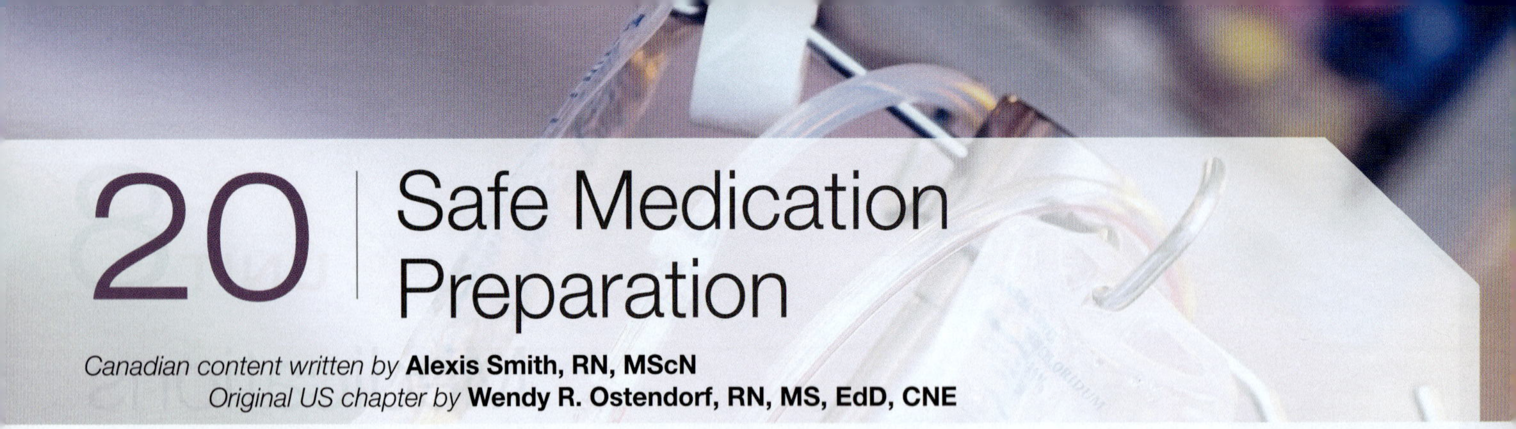

20 Safe Medication Preparation

Canadian content written by **Alexis Smith, RN, MScN**
Original US chapter by **Wendy R. Ostendorf, RN, MS, EdD, CNE**

SKILLS AND PROCEDURES

Skill 20.1 **Teaching Medication Self-Administration, p. 553**

OBJECTIVES

Mastery of content in this chapter will enable the nurse to:

- Describe nursing roles and responsibilities in medication administration.
- Describe the general goals of medication administration.
- Describe factors that contribute to medication errors.
- Differentiate among different types of medication actions.
- List and discuss the 10 rights of medication administration.
- Identify the system of measurement for a given prescribed medication.
- Accurately calculate medication doses.
- Describe the safety features of medication delivery systems.
- Identify guidelines for safe administration of medications.
- Implement nursing actions to prevent medication errors.
- Describe medication error disclosure requirements.
- Explain methods used to educate patients about prescribed medications and self-administration.

MEDIA RESOURCES

- http://evolve.elsevier.com/Canada/Perry/clinicalskills/

PURPOSE

Safe and accurate medication administration is a challenging and important nursing responsibility. All professional nurses need to understand the implications of medication administration. Safe medication administration requires the application of good judgement, critical thinking, and clinical decision-making skills to thorough patient assessment. It also requires an understanding of pharmacotherapeutics, pharmacokinetics, growth and development, nutrition, and mathematics. Nurses are also responsible for teaching a patient and caregiver about medications and their side effects, and for evaluating a patient's and caregiver's ability to administer medications at home.

STANDARDS OF CARE

- Accreditation Canada (2020)—*Required Organizational Practices–2020 Handbook* (https://physicians.nshealth.ca/resources/required-organizational-practices-2020-handbook)
- Healthcare Excellence Canada (n.d.)—*Medication Safety* (https://www.patientsafetyinstitute.ca/en/About/PatientSafetyForwardWith4/pages/medication-safety.aspx)
- Institute for Safe Medication Practices (ISMP) and ISMP Canada:
  - ISMP (2020)—*Oral Dosage Forms That Should Not Be Crushed* (https://www.ismp.org/recommendations/do-not-crush)
  - ISMP (2022b)—*Key Elements of Safe Medication Use* (https://www.ismp.org/ten-key-elements)
  - ISMP Canada (n.d.)—*ISMP Canada Activities for the CMIRPS* (https://www.ismp-canada.org/cmirps/)
  - ISMP Canada (2014)—*Preventable Medication Errors–Look-Alike/Sound-Alike Drug Names* (https://www.ismp-canada.org/download/PharmacyConnection/PC2014-02-Spring_LookalikeSoundalike.pdf)
  - ISMP Canada (2018)—*Do Not Use. Dangerous Abbreviations, Symbols, and Dose Designations* (https://www.ismp-canada.org/download/ISMPCanadaListOfDangerousAbbreviations.pdf)
- Provincial Nursing Association Medication Guidelines (examples):
  - British Columbia College of Nurses and Midwives (2020)—*Medication: Practice Standard for Registered Nurses* (https://www.bccnm.ca/RN/PracticeStandards/Pages/medication.aspx)
  - Nova Scotia College of Nursing (2022)—*Medication Guidelines for Nurses* (https://cdn1.nscn.ca/sites/default/files/documents/resources/MedicationGuidelines.pdf)

PRINCIPLES FOR PRACTICE

Pharmacological Concepts

Medication Names

NSO *Nursing Skills Online Safe Medication Administration Module 5 / Lesson 1*

Some medications have as many as three different names. The chemical name describes the medication composition and molecular structure, such as *N*-acetyl-para-aminophenol, commonly known as Tylenol. The chemical name is rarely used in clinical practice. A manufacturer that first develops a medication provides the generic name (e.g., acetaminophen is the generic name for Tylenol). A medication trade name, or brand name, is used to market the medication. The registered trademark symbol (®) is placed at the end of the trade name to indicate that a manufacturer has claimed the name as a trademark and registered it with the appropriate government agency (e.g., Tempra®, Tylenol®).

Canadian medication databases such as Health Canada's Drug Product Database or the *Compendium of Pharmaceuticals and Specialties* are accessible electronically and can be used to search for medications by generic or trade name.

Many companies choose brand and generic names that are easy to remember. These names can sometimes be very similar, which contributes to medication errors. ISMP Canada (2014) has identified several look-alike/sound-alike medications with similar names and spelling, such as Celebrex for arthritis and Celexa for depression; Lamictal for epilepsy and Lamisil for fungal infections; Losec for ulcers and Lasix for fluid retention. Another measure that has been implemented to help reduce the confusion around medications with similar names includes the use of TALL-man lettering (ISMP Canada, 2016), wherein capital letters are used in specific parts of a word to emphasize dissimilarities in medication names. For example, TEGretol (for seizures) can be confused with TRENtal, which is prescribed for intermittent claudication; the TALL-man letters "TEG" and "TREN" emphasize the difference in the medication names.

Classification

Medications with similar characteristics are grouped together by class. Medication classification indicates the effect of a medication on a body system, the symptoms the medication relieves, or the desired effect of the medication. For example, patients with type 2 diabetes mellitus often take oral hypoglycemic medications to control their blood glucose levels. The sulfonylureas are one class of 11 medications used to treat hyperglycemia. Some medications are part of more than one class. For example, acetaminophen is an analgesic, an antipyretic, and an anti-inflammatory medication.

Medication Forms

Medications are available in a variety of forms or preparations. The form of the medication determines its route of administration. The composition of a medication influences its absorption and metabolism. Many medications are made in several forms, such as tablets, caplets, or suppositories. When administering a medication, be certain to use the proper form (Table 20.1).

Pharmacokinetics

Pharmacokinetics is the study of how medications enter the body, reach their site of action, are metabolized, and exit the body. Understanding pharmacokinetics allows you to properly time medication administration, select an administration route, and judge a patient's response to medications. *Absorption* is the passage of medication molecules into the blood from the site of administration. Factors that influence the rate of absorption include the administration route, ability of a medication to dissolve, blood flow to the administration site, body surface area, and lipid solubility of a medication (Table 20.2). After a medication is absorbed, it is distributed to tissues and organs and finally to the site of medication action. The rate and extent of distribution depend on circulation, cell membrane permeability, and protein binding. Any condition that alters these factors may impact distribution, such as poor perfusion (e.g., heart failure). A medication must pass through biological membranes to reach certain organs. Some membranes are barriers to the passage of medications. For example, the blood–brain barrier allows only fat-soluble medications to pass into the brain and cerebrospinal fluid. The degree to which medications bind to serum proteins, such as albumin, affects distribution. Most medications bind to albumin to some extent. When this happens, the protein-bound medications are unable to exert pharmacological activity. Only the unbound, or "free," medication is active. Older persons and patients with liver disease or malnutrition have reduced albumin, which increases their risk for medication toxicity.

After a medication reaches its site of action, it is metabolized into a less active or inactive form. Biotransformation occurs under the influence of enzymes that detoxify, degrade (break down), and remove biologically active chemicals. Most biotransformation occurs in the liver, although the lungs, kidneys, blood, and intestines also play a role. Some patients (e.g., older persons and those living with chronic disease) are at risk for medication toxicity if their organs cannot metabolize medications effectively.

The final aspect of pharmacokinetics is *excretion*, the process by which medications exit the body through the lungs, exocrine glands, bowel, kidneys, and liver. The chemical makeup of a medication determines the organ of excretion. For example, gaseous and volatile compounds such as alcohol and nitrous oxide exit through the lungs. The site of excretion poses implications for nursing care. For example, when medications exit through sweat glands, the nurse needs to provide skin care to reduce irritation. Nurses must know whether a medication is excreted through the intestines because the administration of laxatives or enemas increases peristalsis, accelerates excretion, and thus lessens the time for medication effects. The kidneys are the main organs for medication excretion; thus, when patients have reduced renal function, they are at risk for medication toxicity.

Pharmacotherapeutics

Pharmacotherapeutics is the study of the therapeutic uses and effects of medications. Medications vary in the way they act and their types of action. Patients do not always respond in the same way to each successive dose of a medication. Sometimes the same medication causes very different responses in different patients. Therefore, it is essential to understand all the effects that medications have on patients.

Therapeutic Effects

Each medication has a therapeutic effect (i.e., the intended or desired physiological response of a medication). For example, morphine sulphate, an analgesic, is administered to relieve a patient's pain. Sometimes a single medication has many therapeutic effects. For example, acetaminophen relieves pain and reduces fever and tissue inflammation. Knowing the desired therapeutic effect for each medication allows the nurse to provide patient education and accurately evaluate its desired effect.

Adverse Effects

Adverse drug events or effects (ADEs) are unintended, undesirable, and often unpredictable. Although at times the effects are apparent immediately, unfortunately, they often take weeks or months to develop. Early clinical recognition is the important first step in identification. ADEs range from mild (e.g., rashes or photosensitivity to light) to potentially fatal (anaphylaxis). Prompt recognition and reporting of ADEs prevent serious injury to patients. Always assess patients who may be at high risk for an ADE, such as pregnant women and patients with chronic disorders (e.g., hypertension, epilepsy, heart disease, psychoses) (Burchum & Rosenthal, 2019). All ADEs must be reported according to employer policy and national reporting structures (see "Reporting Medication Errors" and "Medication Error Disclosure," later in this chapter). The *Protecting Canadians From Unsafe Drugs Act* (Vanessa's Law) was passed in November 2014 and was the basis for a Health Canada (2019b) regulation that mandates reporting of serious adverse medication reactions and medical device incidents by hospitals. Hospitals are accountable for identifying clear internal roles and responsibilities for health care providers to meet mandatory reporting regulations (Health Canada, 2019b). Health care providers may also report ADEs and medical device incidents to the Canada Vigilance Program at Health Canada; the

TABLE 20.1

Forms of Medication

Form	Description
Medication Forms Commonly Prepared for Administration by Oral Route	
Solid Forms	
Caplet	Shaped like a capsule and coated for ease of swallowing
Capsule	Medication encased in a gelatin shell
Tablet	Powdered medication compressed into a hard disc or cylinder
Enteric coated	Coated tablet that does not dissolve in stomach; coating dissolves in intestine, where medication is absorbed
Liquid Forms	
Elixir	Clear fluid containing water and alcohol; often sweetened
Extract	Concentrated medication form made by removing the active part of the medication from its components. Extracts are prepared as a syrup or dried form of pharmacologically active medication, usually made by evaporating solution
Aqueous solution	Substance dissolved in water and syrups
Aqueous suspension	Finely dissolved medication particles in liquid medium must be shaken; when left standing, particles settle to bottom of container
Syrup	Medication dissolved in concentrated sugar solution
Tincture	Alcohol extract from plant or vegetable
Other Oral Forms and Terms Associated With Oral Preparations	
Troche (lozenge)	Flat, round tablet that dissolves in mouth to release medication; not meant for ingestion
Aerosol	Aqueous medication sprayed and absorbed in mouth and upper airway; not meant for ingestion
Sustained release	Tablet or capsule that contains small particles of a medication coated with material that provides medication over an extended period of time
Controlled release	Medication that maintains constant levels in blood or tissue and promotes localization of the medication at a specific site; its release follows a specific, predetermined pattern
Medication Forms Commonly Prepared for Administration by Topical Route	
Ointment (salve or cream)	Semisolid, externally applied preparation, usually containing one or more medications
Liniment	Usually contains alcohol, oil, or soapy emollient applied to skin
Lotion	Semiliquid suspension that usually protects, cools, or cleanses skin
Paste	Medication preparation that is thicker than ointment; absorbed through skin more slowly than ointment; often used for skin protection
Transdermal patch or disc	Medicated disc or patch embedded with medication that is applied to skin Medication absorbed through skin over a designated period of time (e.g., 24 hours)
Medication Forms Commonly Prepared for Administration by Parenteral Route	
Solution	Sterile preparation that contains water or normal saline with one or more dissolved compounds
Powder	Sterile particles of medication that are dissolved in a sterile liquid (e.g., water, normal saline) before administration
Medication Forms Commonly Prepared for Instillation Into Body Cavities	
Suppository	Solid dosage form mixed with gelatin and shaped in form of a pellet for insertion into body cavity (rectum or vagina) Suppository is absorbed when it melts by reaching body temperature
Intraocular disc	Small, flexible oval (similar to a contact lens) consisting of two soft outer layers and a middle layer containing medication; slowly releases medication when moistened by ocular fluid

TABLE 20.2

Medication Absorption

Absorption Factor	Physiological Effects
Route of administration	Topical applications on skin absorb slowly. Medications applied to mucous membranes and respiratory airways absorb quickly. Oral medications pass through the gastrointestinal tract and absorb slowly. The intravenous route produces the most rapid absorption because the medication is available immediately when it enters the systemic circulation.
Ability to dissolve	Solutions and liquid suspensions absorb more readily than tablets or capsules. Acidic medications pass through the gastric mucosa rapidly and absorb rapidly, whereas basic medications (pH >7.0) do not absorb before reaching the small intestine.
Blood flow	When the administration site contains a rich blood supply, medications absorb rapidly.
Body surface area	A medication in contact with a large surface area (e.g., small intestine) absorbs faster than one in contact with smaller surface area (e.g., stomach).
Lipid solubility	Medications that are highly lipid soluble absorb more readily.

Canadian Institute for Health Information's National System for Incident Reporting; ISMP Canada; and the World Health Organization's Global Patient Safety Alerts.

Side Effects

Every medication has the potential to cause harm. No medication is totally safe and absolutely free from nontherapeutic effects. Side effects are predictable and often unavoidable secondary effects produced at a usual therapeutic medication dose. They are either harmless or cause injury. The intensity of side effects is often dose dependent. If the side effects are serious enough to outweigh the benefits of the therapeutic action of a medication, the health care provider will likely discontinue the medication. Patients commonly stop taking medications because of side effects such as anorexia, nausea, vomiting, dizziness, drowsiness, dry mouth, constipation, and diarrhea. Nurses must direct patients to report any side effect to the health care provider following patient teaching on expected side effects. Health care providers report side effects to Health Canada using the online Side Effect Reporting Form, as part of the Canada Vigilance Program. This program is administered by Health Canada to investigate ADEs in order to monitor the safety of medications over time (Health Canada, 2022).

Toxic Effects

Toxic effects develop after prolonged intake of a medication or when a medication accumulates in the blood because of impaired metabolism or excretion. Excess amounts of a medication within the body sometimes have lethal effects, depending on the action of the medication. For example, toxic levels of morphine, an opioid, cause severe respiratory depression and death. Antidotes are available to treat specific types of medication toxicity. For example, naloxone, an opioid antagonist, reverses the effects of opioid toxicity.

Idiosyncratic Reactions

An idiosyncratic reaction is an unpredictable effect in which a patient overreacts or underreacts to a medication or has a reaction different from normal. Predicting which patients will have an idiosyncratic response is impossible. For example, lorazepam is an antianxiety medication that may cause agitation and delirium when given to an older person.

Allergic Reactions

Allergic reactions are also adverse unpredictable responses to a medication. Exposure to an initial dose of a medication causes a patient to become sensitized immunologically. The medication acts as an antigen, which causes antibodies to be produced. With repeated administration, a patient develops an allergic response to the medication, its chemical preservatives, or a metabolite. An allergic reaction ranges from mild to severe, depending on the patient and the medication (Table 20.3). Among the different classes of medications, antibiotics cause a high incidence of allergic reactions (Blumenthal et al., 2019). Severe or anaphylactic reactions, which are life threatening, are characterized by sudden constriction of bronchiolar muscles, edema of the pharynx and larynx, severe wheezing, and shortness of breath. Some patients become severely hypotensive, necessitating emergency resuscitation measures.

It is common practice for hospitalized patients with known medication allergies to have their allergy information recorded in a clearly identifiable place. This allows all caregivers to be aware of each patient's allergies. In many facilities, this information is recorded in a special section of the electronic health record (EHR), on the front of a patient's hard-copy medical record or chart, in the medication administration record (MAR), or on a specially designed label that is applied to the front of a patient's chart. Patients also receive colour-coded allergy identification bands to wear on their wrists.

! SAFETY ALERT Patient allergies should be recorded on *every page* of the MAR (follow employer policy). Nurses are responsible for assessing, verifying, and updating patient allergy information in the health record before administering any medication.

Always record a patient's allergies according to employer policy. Patients who are cared for in other settings (e.g., home or community clinics) and have a known history of an allergy to a medication or substance should wear a medical alert bracelet or necklace, which alerts all health care providers to these allergies in case a patient is found unconscious or is unable to communicate (Fig. 20.1). Many patients who report having an allergy to a medication do not in fact have a true allergy, but rather have experienced a severe side effect or an ADE. It is important for the nurse to be aware of the difference between a true allergy and a side effect. Ask the patient to describe the type of reaction they experienced and offer them examples, such as nausea (side effect) versus hives (allergic reaction).

Medication Tolerance and Dependence

Medication tolerance occurs when the body gets used to a medication over time. It is usually noted clinically when patients receive the same medication for long periods and require higher doses to produce the desired therapeutic effect. Medications such as opium alkaloids (e.g., morphine) and nitrates and substances such as ethyl alcohol and heroin are known to produce tolerance. Patients hospitalized for acute episodes of illness usually do not develop tolerance. It may take a month or longer for tolerance to occur.

Medication tolerance is not the same as medication dependence. Two types of medication dependence exist: psychological (or addiction) and physiological. In psychological dependence, a patient desires the medication for a benefit other than the intended effect. Physiological dependence is a physiological adaptation to a medication that manifests as intense physical disturbance when the medication is withdrawn. When patients receive medications for a short time, such as for postoperative pain, dependence is rare.

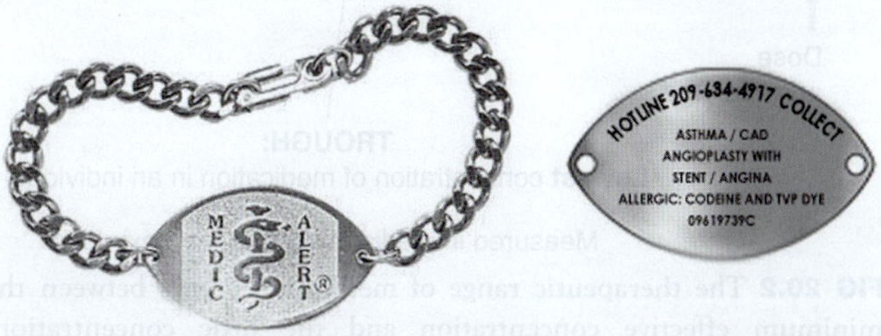

FIG 20.1 MedicAlert bracelet. (*From Astle, B. J., & Duggleby, W. [Eds.]. [2024]. Potter and Perry's Canadian fundamentals of nursing [7th ed.]. Elsevier.*)

TABLE 20.3

Mild to Severe Allergic Reactions

Symptom	Description
Urticaria (hives)	Raised, irregularly shaped skin eruptions with varying sizes and shapes; reddened margins and pale centres
Rash	Small, raised vesicles that are usually reddened; often distributed over the entire body
Pruritus	Itching of the skin; accompanies most rashes
Rhinitis	Inflammation of mucous membranes lining the nose, causing swelling and a clear, watery discharge

Medication Interactions

When one medication modifies the action of another medication, it is referred to as a *medication interaction*. Medication interactions are common in individuals taking many medications. Some medications increase or diminish the action of other medications and alter the way in which another medication is absorbed, metabolized, or eliminated from the body. When two medications have a synergistic effect, their combined effect is greater than the effect of one medication taken separately. For example, alcohol is a central nervous system depressant that has a synergistic effect when combined with antihistamines, antidepressants, and opioids. Sometimes a medication interaction is the desired effect. Health care providers often combine medications to create an interaction that has a therapeutic effect. For example, a patient with hypertension may receive several medications such as diuretics and vasodilators, which act together to control blood pressure when one medication alone is not effective.

Medication Dose Responses

A medication undergoes absorption, distribution, metabolism, and excretion after administration. Medications take time to enter the bloodstream, except when administered intravenously. When a medication is prescribed, the goal is a constant blood level within a safe therapeutic range. The minimum effective concentration (MEC) is the plasma level of the medication below which the effect of the medication does not occur. The toxic concentration is the level at which toxic effects occur. The safe therapeutic range is between the MEC and the toxic concentration (Fig. 20.2). When a medication is administered repeatedly, its serum level fluctuates between doses. The highest level is called the *peak concentration*, and the lowest level is called the *trough concentration*. After peaking, the serum concentration falls progressively. With intravenous (IV) infusions, the peak concentration occurs quickly, but the serum level also begins to fall

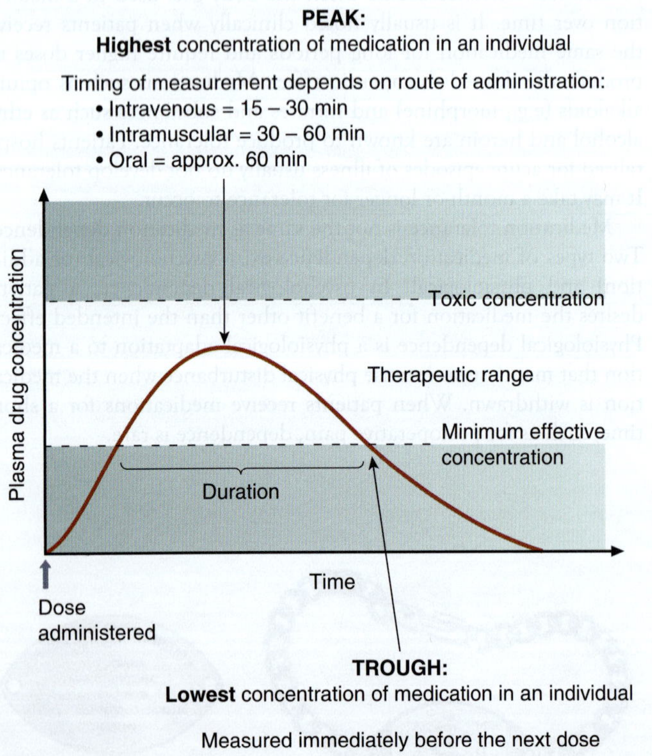

FIG 20.2 **The therapeutic range of medication occurs between the minimum effective concentration and the toxic concentration.** (*Adapted from Burchum, J., & Rosenthal, L. [2016]. Lehne's pharmacology for nursing care [9th ed.]. Saunders.*)

immediately. Some medication doses (e.g., vancomycin or gentamicin) are based on peak and trough serum levels. A patient's trough level is drawn as a blood sample 30 minutes before administering the medication, and the peak level is drawn whenever the medication is expected to reach its peak concentration. The results of the blood test reveal whether the medication is reaching its therapeutic blood level.

All medications have a biological half-life, which is the time it takes for excretion processes to lower the serum medication concentration by half. To maintain a therapeutic plateau, a patient needs to receive regular fixed doses. For example, pain medications are most effective for some cancer patients when they are given around the clock (ATC) rather than when a patient intermittently complains of pain, because the ATC approach allows the body to maintain an almost constant level of pain medication (Burchum & Rosenthal, 2019). After an initial medication dose, the patient receives each successive dose once the previous dose reaches its half-life. The patient and nurse need to follow regular dosage schedules and administer prescribed doses at correct intervals. The following time intervals of medication action allow the nurse to anticipate the effect of a medication:

- *Onset of medication action:* Time it takes after a medication is administered for it to produce a response
- *Peak action:* Time it takes for a medication to reach its highest effective peak concentration
- *Trough:* Minimum blood serum concentration of medication reached just before the next scheduled dose
- *Duration of action:* Length of time during which a medication is present in a concentration great enough to produce a therapeutic effect
- *Plateau:* Blood serum concentration reached and maintained after repeated, fixed doses

Reporting Medication Errors

Medication errors often harm patients because of inappropriate medication use. Errors include inaccurate prescribing; administering the wrong medication via the wrong route or at the wrong time; administering extra doses; and failing to administer a medication. Medication errors are affected by professional practice, health care product design, and procedures and systems such as product labelling and distribution. When an error occurs, the patient's safety and well-being become the top priority. A nurse assesses and examines the patient's condition and notifies the health care provider of the incident as soon as possible. Once the patient is stable, the nurse reports the incident to the appropriate person in the facility (e.g., manager or supervisor).

As a nurse, you are professionally responsible and ethically accountable for reporting all medication errors. This includes errors that resulted in harm to the patient, no harm to the patient, and near misses (a potential error that was identified by the health care provider before it could cause harm to the patient). A written report is completed, usually within 24 hours of an incident (see employer policy). This report (e.g., incident report, adverse event report) is an internal audit tool and not a permanent part of the medical record. To legally protect interprofessional team members and the facility, do not refer to this report in the progress notes in the EHR or chart. Facilities use these reports to track patterns and initiate performance improvement programs as needed. Depending on the circumstances and the severity of the outcome, the nurse or facility may be responsible for reporting the incident to the Canada Vigilance Program and ISMP Canada (Health Canada, 2019a).

As a nurse, you should feel comfortable in reporting an error and not fear repercussions from managerial staff. The consequences of a medication error depend on several factors, including previous work performance, consequences to the patient, and the nurse's response to the error. Outcomes of reporting an error include a patient safety or quality improvement review, employee discipline, professional discipline, and/or a civil lawsuit (Canadian Nurses Protective Society [CNPS], 2021). Even when a patient suffers no harm from a medication error, the facility can still learn why the mistake occurred and what to do in the future to avoid similar errors. Most medication errors can be avoided by applying the principles of the 10 rights of medication administration (CNPS, 2021). There are a number of strategies that you can implement to prevent medication errors (Box 20.1).

Medication Error Disclosure

Patient and family disclosure of medication errors (including harmful incidents, no-harm incidents, and near misses) is based on principles of patient safety, openness, transparency, accountability, and compassion (Healthcare Excellence Canada, 2011). Accreditation Canada (2020) has a Required Organizational Practice (ROP) for disclosure called *patient safety incident disclosure* (formerly called *adverse or sentinel events disclosure*). Facilities must implement a formal and transparent policy and process of disclosure to patients, which include support mechanisms for patients/families and care of interprofessional health team members. Under Canada's Constitution, each province and territory is responsible for its own liability laws. The first Canadian "apology legislation" was passed in 2006 by British Columbia (MacDonald & Attaran, 2009). Since that time, other provinces have followed suit. Be familiar with the apology legislation in the province or territory in which you practise nursing, as well as your employer-specific policies. Current literature; national and international best practices; and ethical, professional, and legal considerations all support open and honest disclosure of patient safety incidents (Healthcare Excellence Canada, 2011). Disclosing a patient safety incident to the patient and family demonstrates respect and person-centred care, contributes to a culture of safety, and facilitates safe and appropriate clinical care.

BOX 20.1

Steps to Prevent Medication Errors

- Always follow the 10 rights of medication administration.
- Only prepare medications for one patient at a time.
- Be sure to read labels at least three times (comparing MAR with label): When removing medication from storage, before taking to patient's room, and before giving medication.
- Use at least two person-specific identifiers every time you administer medications (e.g., patient name, date of birth, hospital number).
- Do not allow any other activity to interrupt administration of medication to a patient (e.g., phone call, pager, discussion with other staff).
- Double-check all calculations and other high-risk medication administration processes (e.g., patient-controlled analgesia) and verify with another nurse.
- Research and question unusual dosages; consider consulting with a pharmacist and clarifying with the health care provider.
- Do not interpret illegible handwriting; clarify with the health care provider.
- Question unusually large or small doses.
- Document all medications as soon as they are given.
- When you have made or discovered an error, reflect on what went wrong and ask how you could have prevented it. Complete a written report per employer policy.
- Evaluate the context or situation in which a medication error occurred. This helps determine whether nurses have the necessary resources for safe medication administration.
- When repeated medication errors occur within a work area, identify and analyze the factors that may have caused the errors and take corrective action.
- Attend in-service programs on the medications you commonly administer.
- Ensure that you are well rested when caring for patients. Nurse fatigue is associated with increased medication errors (Dykstra et al., 2016; Schroers et al., 2021).
- Practise person-centred care when administering medications. Address patients' concerns about medications before administering them (e.g., concerns about their appearance or side effects).
- Follow established employer policies and procedures when using technology to administer medications (e.g., ADS and bar-code scanning). Medication errors occur when nurses "work around" the technology (e.g., override alerts without thinking about them) (Lee & Kang, 2021).

ADS, Automated dispensing system; *MAR*, medication administration record.

Routes of Administration

The route prescribed for administering a medication (Table 20.4) depends on its properties and desired effect and on a patient's physical and mental condition. Because of what a nurse knows about each patient, the nurse needs to collaborate with a health care provider to determine the best route for a patient's medical condition. Table 20.5 summarizes the factors that influence the choice of administration routes.

Medication Distribution

Health care providers (e.g., physicians, pharmacists, nurse practitioners, and registered nurses [in some jurisdictions]) write medication prescriptions, pharmacists dispense medications, and nurses verify and deliver medications to patients. *Verification* is the system of three checks to ensure safe medication administration. The first check, performed by the health care provider, confirms that the right medication is being prescribed for the right purpose. The pharmacist performs the second check, ensuring that the medication is appropriate and prescribed correctly and then provided to the unit correctly. The nurse performs the third check by verifying the medication before administration with the three checks for accuracy to be sure that it is appropriate and prescribed correctly.

A number of technologies for medication distribution have the potential to reduce medication errors and ADEs. These technologies include computerized provider order entry (CPOE), automated dispensing system (ADS), bar coding, and smart infusion devices with dose-error reduction systems (Strudwick et al., 2018).

TABLE 20.4

Routes of Medication Administration

Route	Description
Nonparenteral	
Oral, buccal	By mouth/mucous membrane, or through gastric tube per employer policy
Sublingual	Under the tongue
Topical	On the skin (as a cream or patch) and eyedrops/eardrops
Suppository	Into the rectum or vagina
Parenteral	
Intramuscular (IM)	Into a muscle
Subcutaneous (SUBCUT)	Into the subcutaneous tissue of the skin
Intradermal (ID)	Into the dermis of the skin
Epidural	Into the epidural space
Intravenous (IV)	Into a vein

TABLE 20.5

Factors Influencing Choice of Administration Routes

Advantages	Disadvantages/Contraindications
Oral, Buccal, Sublingual Routes	
Routes are easy and comfortable to administer, convenient, economical; may produce local or systemic effects; and rarely cause anxiety for patient.	Routes are avoided when patient has alterations in GI function (e.g., nausea and vomiting), with reduced GI motility (after general anaesthesia or bowel inflammation), and with surgical resection of part of GI tract. Gastric secretions destroy some medications. Oral administration is contraindicated in patients who are NPO and unable to swallow (e.g., patients with neuromuscular disorders, esophageal strictures, and mouth lesions). Consult health care provider and employer policy on administration of oral medications when patient has gastric suction or before certain diagnostic tests or surgery. An unconscious or confused patient is unable or unwilling to swallow or hold sublingual medication under tongue or buccal medication in cheek. Oral medications sometimes irritate lining of GI tract, discolour teeth, or have an unpleasant taste.
Subcutaneous, Intramuscular, Intravenous, Intradermal, Epidural Routes	
Routes provide means of administration when oral medications are contraindicated. More rapid absorption occurs than with topical or oral routes.	There are risks for introducing infection, and medications are expensive. Some patients experience pain from repeated needle-sticks. Avoid subcutaneous, IM, and ID routes in patients with bleeding tendencies. There is risk for tissue damage with subcutaneous injections.
IV infusion provides medication delivery when patient is critically ill or long-term therapy is necessary. If peripheral perfusion is poor, IV route is preferred over injections.	IV and IM routes have higher absorption rates, thus putting patients at higher risk for reactions.
Epidural provides excellent pain control.	It limits mobility during administration, and there is risk for infection.
Skin	
Topical	
Topical skin applications provide primarily local effect. Route is usually painless. Limited side effects occur.	Extensive applications often require dressings that are bulky for a patient who is attempting to manoeuvre. Do not apply to skin if abrasions are present, unless that is the reason for order. Medications can be absorbed by person applying them if gloves are not worn. Apply new gloves for each topical product application.
Transdermal	
Transdermal applications provide prolonged systemic effects with limited side effects.	Application leaves oily or pasty substance on skin and may soil clothing. Some patients have sensitivity to adhesive. Ensure safe disposal of patch when removed, per employer policy.
Mucous Membranes (Includes Eyes, Ears, Nose, Vaginal, Rectal, Buccal, and Sublingual Routes)	
Therapeutic effects are provided by local application to involved sites. Aqueous solutions are readily absorbed and capable of causing systemic effects.	Mucous membranes are highly sensitive to some medication concentrations. Insertion of rectal and vaginal medications often cause embarrassment.
Mucous membranes provide route of administration when oral medications are contraindicated.	Rectal suppositories are contraindicated if patients have had rectal surgery or if active rectal bleeding is present. If eardrum is ruptured, otic medications are usually contraindicated.
Inhalation	
Inhalation provides rapid relief for local respiratory problems. An inhaled form of insulin is also available. Route provides easy access for introduction of general anaesthetic gases.	Some local agents cause serious systemic effects. If patients are unable to administer inhaler correctly, medication is ineffective. Inhalation is difficult to learn for older persons and children.
Intraocular Disc	
Route is advantageous in that it does not require frequent administration (e.g., as for eyedrops). Patient can also wear disc when sleeping or swimming. Dry eyes do not affect medication delivery.	Local reactions such as tearing, itching, or redness of the eyes occur. Patient needs to know how to insert disc into and remove from eye. Medication is often expensive. Medication is contraindicated in patients with eye infections.

GI, Gastrointestinal; *ID*, intradermal; *IM*, intramuscular; *IV*, intravenous; *NPO*, nothing by mouth.

Computerized Provider Order Entry

CPOE is a system that allows health care providers to enter orders (prescriptions) for medications electronically, eliminating the need for written prescriptions. CPOE increases the accuracy and legibility of medication orders, creates evidence-informed order sets, and strengthens nursing documentation and coordination of care (Elshayib & Pawola, 2020). Decision support software integrated into a CPOE system allows for automatic medication allergy checks, dosage indications, baseline laboratory result checks, and identification of potential medication interactions. When a health care provider enters a prescription through CPOE, the information immediately transmits to the pharmacy and ultimately to the patient's MAR without the need for written transcription.

Distribution Systems

Systems for storing and distributing medications vary. Facilities providing nursing care have special areas for stocking and dispensing medications. Examples of storage areas include special medication rooms, portable locked carts, computerized medication cabinets, and individual storage units next to patients' rooms. Medication storage areas must be locked when unattended.

Unit Dose

A unit-dose system uses an ADS or cart containing a drawer with a 24-hour supply of medications for each patient. Each drawer has a label with the name of the patient and the designated room. The unit dose is the prescribed dose of medication that the patient receives at one time. Each medication form is separately wrapped in a plastic, foil, or paper container. Liquid doses come in prepackaged foil or plastic cups (e.g., for use in long-term care or the home setting). The cart also contains limited amounts of stock medication for special situations. At a designated time each day, the pharmacist or a pharmacy technician refills the drawers in the cart with a fresh supply. Controlled substances are not stored in the individual patient drawer; they are kept in a larger locked drawer or ADS for security. A unit-dose system is designed to reduce the number of medication errors and saves steps in dispensing medications.

Automated Medication Dispensing System

ADSs are variations of unit-dose and floor stock systems (Fig. 20.3). The systems within the health care facility are networked with one another and with other computer systems in the facility (e.g., computerized medical record). ADSs control the dispensing of all medications, including opioid narcotics. Each nurse uses a security code or bioidentification (i.e., their fingerprint) to access the system. Once logged onto the ADS, the nurse selects a patient's name and medication profile. The nurse then selects the medication, dosage, and route from a list displayed on the computer screen. The system opens the medication drawer or dispenses the medication to the nurse and records the event. If the system is connected to the patient's EMR, information about the medication (e.g., name, dose, time) and the name of the nurse who retrieved it from the ADS are recorded.

The bar code medication administration (BCMA) system is often used to identify the patient, the medication, and the identification tag of the nurse administering the medication before recording this information in the patient's EMR. Facilities that implement ADS with BCMA often reduce the incidence of medication errors (Zheng et al., 2020).

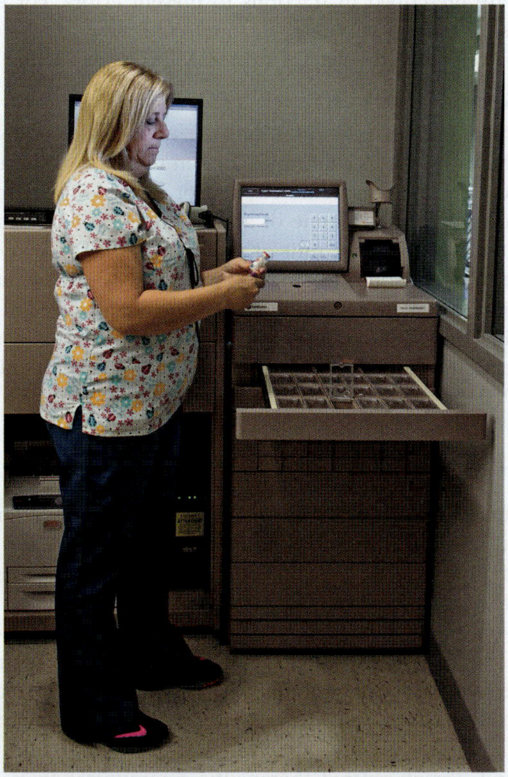

FIG 20.3 Automated medication dispensing system. (*From Davis, K., & Guerra, T. [2019]. Mosby's pharmacy technician: Principles and practice [5th ed.]. Elsevier.*)

Special Handling of Controlled Substances

As a nurse, you are responsible for following the laws and regulations overseeing the administration of controlled substances (e.g., opioids). Violations of the federal *Controlled Drugs and Substances Act* may result in fines, imprisonment, and loss of licence. Facility policies for the proper storage and distribution of controlled substances require the use of computerized systems for these substances (Box 20.2).

Handling Chemotherapy Medications

A common treatment for cancer is chemotherapy, treatment that involves the use of antineoplastic medications. These medications act by killing cells that divide rapidly, one of the main properties of most cancer cells. Chemotherapy is administered via IV and orally. The Canadian Association of Nurses in Oncology (CANO, 2017) standards for chemotherapy nursing practice aim to improve both patient and nurse safety related to administration of these medications. Nurses must undergo certification to administer IV chemotherapy. However, oral chemotherapy is becoming more common and can be administered by a registered nurse.

All forms of chemotherapy pose exposure risks to health care providers, patients, and their caregivers (CANO, 2017). Physically touching a chemotherapy tablet is dangerous. Chemotherapy is highly toxic, not only to cancer cells but also to normal cells. Chemotherapy medications cause DNA damage that leads to cell death or cell growth arrest. The damage to others may not be known for months or years because the injuries could include cancer, birth

BOX 20.2

Guidelines for Safe Opioid Administration and Control

- All controlled medications and substances are stored in a securely locked, substantially constructed cabinet (i.e., ADS) or a locked room.
- Authorized nurses carry a set of keys or an individual computer entry code for the ADS.
- An inventory record is used each time a controlled substance is dispensed. Records are often kept electronically and provide an accurate, ongoing account of the medications used, wasted, and remaining. If you find a discrepancy, correct and report it immediately.
- Use a special inventory record to document a patient's name, date, name of medication, dose, time of medication administration, and signature of nurse dispensing the medication.
- A second nurse witnesses disposal of the unused part if a nurse gives only part of a dose of a controlled substance. Computerized systems record the nurses' names electronically. If paper records are kept, both nurses sign their names on the form. Follow employer policy for appropriate waste of opioids. Do not place wasted part of medications in sharps containers.

ADS, Automated dispensing system.

defects, or immune dysfunction. It is critical that health care providers, patients, and caregivers use proper protective techniques to avoid exposure to oral chemotherapy tablets. A patient excretes chemotherapy chemicals through urine, stool, vomit, sweat, and saliva. When patients self-administer chemotherapy at home, families should be warned of the dangers of exposure. Nurses should follow their employer policies on cytotoxic precautions and protocols. Exposure to oral chemotherapeutic agents during preparation, administration, or disposal can be an occupational risk to health care workers (CANO, 2017). Guidelines for health care providers, patients, and caregivers about how to handle these medications safely and appropriately are essential:

- In health care agencies, cytotoxic agents should be stored in a designated area per the manufacturer's instructions and separately from noncytotoxic agents.
- Use gloves that have been tested for chemotherapy or hazardous medication use and double-glove when indicated, when preparing and handling chemotherapy medications, and after handling the chemotherapy agent or bodily secretions (Canadian Association of Provincial Cancer Agencies, 2015).
- Perform thorough hand hygiene before and after glove application.
- Do NOT crush, cut, or split chemotherapy medications.
- The health care agency must have a spill management and waste disposal policy in place (CANO, 2017).
- Don and dispose of personal protective equipment (PPE) per employer policy (CANO, 2017).

Bar Coding

EHR technology is used to improve patient care quality and coordination by providing health care providers with easier access to patient information in a secure format. The use of electronic bar codes on medication labels and packaging has the potential to improve patient safety in a number of ways. Bar codes are electronically linked to a hospital computer system. A patient's MAR entered into the computer database and encoded in the patient's wristband is accessible to a nurse through a handheld device. The device scans the patient's wristband and then displays the MAR. When administering a medication, the nurse scans the bar code on the medication and the patient's medical record number on the wristband. The computer processes the scanned information, charts it, and updates the patient's MAR record appropriately. The use of bar codes improves the accuracy of patient identification, provides alerts to potential medication error, and improves medical record keeping.

Systems of Medication Measurement

NSO *Nursing Skills Online Safe Medication Administration Module 5 / Lesson 3*

The proper administration of medication depends on the nurse's ability to compute medication doses accurately and measure medications correctly. A careless mistake, such as misplacing a decimal point or adding a zero to a dosage, can lead to fatal errors. The health care provider and patient depend on nurses to check doses before administering medications. The most common medication measurement system is the metric system, although sometimes household systems of measurement (e.g., 1 cup, 1 teaspoon) are used.

Metric System

As a decimal system, the metric system is the most logically organized of the measurement systems. Metric units are easy to convert and compute through simple multiplication and division. Each basic unit of measure is organized into units of 10. Multiplying or dividing by 10 forms secondary units. In multiplication, the decimal point moves to the right; in division, the decimal moves to the left. For example:

$$10\,\text{mg} \times 10 = 100\,\text{mg}$$

$$10\ \text{mg} \div 10 = 1\ \text{mg}$$

The basic units of measurement in the metric system are the metre (length), the litre (volume), and the gram (weight). For medication calculations, you will primarily use volume and weight units. In the metric system, lowercase or capital letters designate the basic units and subdivisions of units:

Gram = g or Gm

Litre = l or L

Milligram = mg

Millilitre = mL

Microgram = mcg (do NOT use "µg" [ISMP Canada, 2018])

When writing medication dosages in metric units, health care providers and nurses use either fractions or multiples of a unit. Convert fractions to decimals:

500 mg or 0.5 g, not 1/2 g

10 mL or 0.01 L, not 1/100 L

Many actual or potential medication errors occur because of the use of fractions or decimal points. Use practice standards when medications are prescribed in fractions to prevent errors. For example, never use a trailing zero (e.g., 1.0 mg), and always include a zero before a decimal point (e.g., 0.1 mL) (ISMP Canada, 2018).

Solutions

Solutions of various concentrations are used for injections, irrigations, and infusions. A solution is a given mass of a solid substance dissolved in a known volume of fluid or a given volume of liquid dissolved in a known volume of another fluid. Solutions are available in units of mass per unit of volume (e.g., g/mL or g/L). The concentration of a solution can also be expressed as a percentage or a proportion (e.g., a 10% solution is 10 g of solid dissolved in 100 mL of solution, and a 1/1 000 solution represents a solution containing 1 g of solid dissolved in 1 000 mL of liquid or 1 mL of liquid mixed with 1 000 mL of another liquid).

PERSON-CENTRED CARE

- A nurse's responsibility when administering medications safely must include interprofessional collaboration and effective communication with health care team members, patients, and caregivers.
- Patients are an important resource for understanding the knowledge they have about their medications, their perceptions about the effects of medications, and their expectations for treatment.
- Consider factors that influence a patient's abilities to communicate effectively, such as anxiety, pain, hearing, or cultural background. Person-centred therapeutic communication is essential to nursing practice and critical in safe medication administration.

- A new scientific field, *pharmacogenetics*, involves the study of the genetic influence on medication response that occurs owing to inherited metabolic defects or deficiencies. The most common mechanism of genetic influence on medications is an alteration in medication metabolism. The outcome is either a reduced benefit or increased toxicity of the medication (Burchum & Rosenthal, 2019).
- A patient's culture, values, level of education, and prior experience with medication therapy and the caregiver's influence on the patient's actions may significantly influence medication response, reporting of side effects, and adherence. For example, in some cultures it is not common to report gastrointestinal problems; thus, some patients may not report nausea, vomiting, and bowel changes related to medication use.
- Use of herbal and homeopathic remedies can alter response to a medication; therefore, all supplements should be reported to the provider.
- As a nurse, you cannot detect a genetic abnormality or be aware of all personal factors that may impact medication therapy. However, you can learn to become aware of cultural differences to better monitor medication therapy.
- Use sound clinical decision making related to medication prescription and administration to reduce overall bias, including flawed social, biological, and genetic assumptions that have a history in race-based diagnosis and treatment (Goodman & Brett, 2021). Best practice is to use a person-centred approach when administering medications.

Safe Medication Administration

Standards are actions that help ensure safe nursing practice. Standards for medication administration are set by health care facilities, the nursing profession, regulatory bodies, and other organizations (Box 20.3). Most facilities have procedure manuals that contain policies about which medications nurses can and cannot deliver. The types and dosages that nurses may administer often vary from unit to unit within a facility. Provincial and territorial professional nursing association standards apply to the practice of safe medication administration. As a nurse, you can prevent medication errors by ensuring effective interprofessional collaboration and by following the rules of medication administration (which in the literature range from 5 to 10 rights [Rohde & Domm, 2017]) consistently every time you administer medications. Many medication errors are linked in some way to an inconsistency in adhering to the following 10 rights:

1. Right patient
2. Right medication
3. Right dose
4. Right route
5. Right time
6. Right education
7. Right to refuse
8. Right assessment
9. Right evaluation
10. Right documentation

Right Patient

Medication errors often occur because one patient gets a medication intended for another patient. Therefore, a key step in administering medications safely is being sure to give the right medication to the right patient. It is difficult to remember every patient's name and face. Before giving a medication to a patient, always use at least two person-specific identifiers (Accreditation Canada, 2020). Acceptable patient identifiers include the patient's name, an identification number assigned by a health care facility such as the medical record number, and the patient's date of birth. Do not use a patient's room number as an identifier. The required identification process mandates collecting patient identifiers reliably when a patient is first admitted to a health care facility. Once identifiers are assigned to a patient (e.g., putting identifiers on an armband and placing the armband on the patient), a nurse uses them to match the patient with the patient name on the MAR.

To identify a patient correctly in an acute care setting, at the patient's bedside compare the patient identifiers on the MAR with those on their identification bracelet (Fig. 20.4). Asking patients to state their full name and identification information provides a third way to verify that you as the nurse are giving medications to the right patient. If an identification bracelet becomes smudged or illegible or is missing, get a new one for the patient. In health care settings where patients do not have an identification bracelet (e.g., long-term care facility), nurses must adhere to best medication practice and use a system to verify the patient's identification with at

BOX 20.3

Safe Medication Practices

- Accurate patient (client) identification using at least two person-specific identifiers (two patient identifiers) (neither can be patient's room number) when providing care, treatment (e.g., medications), or services.
- Improve the effectiveness of communication among caregivers (e.g., use of situation–background–assessment–recommendation (SBAR).
- For verbal or telephone prescriptions, require read-back verification of the complete prescription or test result by the person receiving the prescription/test result.
- Standardize a "Do Not Use" list of abbreviations, acronyms, symbols, and dose designations.
- Improve the safety of using medications.
- Identify and at a minimum annually review a list of look-alike/sound-alike medications used by the organization.
- Before a procedure, label all medications and medication containers (e.g., syringes) that are not labelled. This task should be completed in areas where medicines and supplies are set up, such as on and off the sterile field in perioperative and other procedural settings. Labels include medication name, strength, amount, expiration date when not used within 24 hours, and expiration time when expiration occurs in less than 24 hours.
- Use extra precautions with patients who take anticoagulants. Use only oral unit-dose products and premixed infusions. When heparin is administered intravenously and continuously, use programmable infusion pumps with dose-error reduction systems.
- Maintain and communicate accurate patient medication information.
- Accurately and completely reconcile medications across the continuum of care.
- Ensure there is a process for comparing the patient's current medications with those prescribed for the patient while they are under the care of the health care facility.
- Communicate a complete list of the patient's medications to the next provider of service when a patient is referred or transferred to another setting, service, or level of care. Also provide the complete list to the patient on discharge from the facility.
- Practise person-centred care and encourage patients' active involvement in their own care.
- Use SBAR as a communication strategy to communicate with the interprofessional team.

Adapted from Accreditation Canada. (2021). *Medication management standards*. https://store.accreditation.ca/products/medication-management-standards; Institute for Safe Medication Practices. (2022a). *2020–2021 ISMP Targeted Medication Safety Best Practices for Hospitals*. https://www.ismp.org/guidelines/best-practices-hospitals

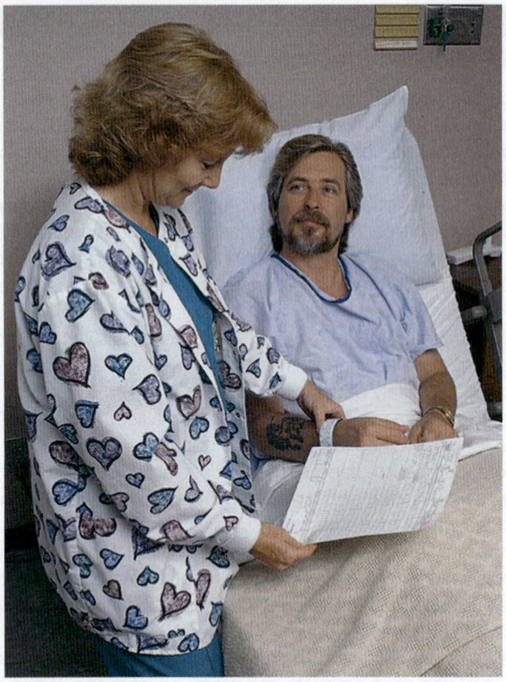

FIG 20.4 Before administering any medications, check patient's identification and allergy bracelets.

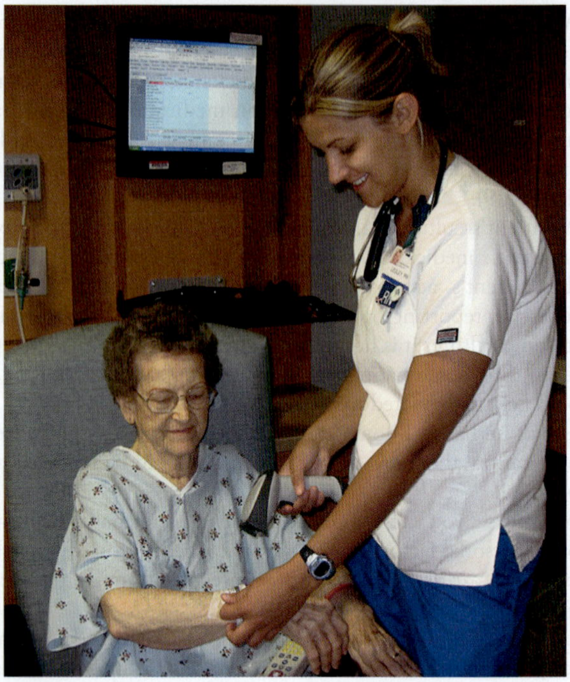

FIG 20.5 Nurse using bar-code scanner to identify patient during medication administration.

least two person-specific identifiers, one of which should include the resident's picture, before administering medications.

In addition to using two person-specific patient identifiers, some facilities use a wireless bar-code scanner to help identify the right patient (Fig. 20.5). This system requires the nurse to scan a personal bar code that is commonly placed on the nurse's name badge first. Then, a bar code is scanned from the single-dose medication package. Finally, the nurse scans the patient's armband. All of this information is stored in the computer for documentation purposes. The system helps prevent medication errors because it adds another step to ensure that the right patient receives the right medication.

Right Medication

The second step of safe medication practice is ensuring you are administering the right medication.

Nurses must have a medication prescription ("order") before administering medications to a patient. Some health care providers write prescriptions by hand in a patient's chart. However, many agencies use CPOE, eliminating the need for handwritten prescriptions and enhancing patient safety (Lin et al., 2017). Regardless of how a prescription is received, the nurse needs to compare the health care provider's orders with the MAR or electronic MAR (eMAR) when the medication is initially prescribed. Nurses verify medication information whenever new MARs are written or distributed or when patients transfer from one nursing unit or health care setting to another (Accreditation Canada, 2021).

ISMP Canada (2018) has published a list of *Dangerous Abbreviations, Symbols, and Dose Designations* to increase patient safety (see Box 4.2). Nurses are responsible for using correct abbreviations and verifying that the prescription was transcribed accurately.

Verbal and telephone prescriptions may be required when written or electronic communication between the health care provider and nurse is not possible. When nurses receive a verbal or telephone prescription, they write or enter the information on the health care provider's prescription sheet. The nurse then repeats back the prescription for verification and documents that the repeat-back occurred. The name of the health care provider and the nurse's

BOX 20.4

Guidelines for Verbal, Telephone, Text, and Email Prescriptions

- Only employer-authorized staff may receive and record prescriptions that are not written.
- Clearly identify patient's name, room number, and diagnosis.
- Although increasing numbers of health care providers are using mobile devices to communicate prescriptions, this type of communication is discouraged, given the risk of violation of confidential health information and incomplete communication of patient status (Walker et al., 2019). Always refer to your employer's policy related to prescriptions received via a mobile device.
- Telephone orders for chemotherapy are not accepted unless they address holding or discontinuing the medication.
- Repeat back all verbal and telephone prescriptions to the health care provider, and follow all employer policies (i.e., two nurses to review and sign).
- Use clarification questions to avoid misunderstandings.
- Document either "verbal order" or "telephone order," including date and time, name of patient, and complete prescription; write the name of the health care provider and sign your name.
- Health care provider co-signs the prescription within the time frame required by the facility (usually 24 hours; verify employer policy).

signature are included. The health care provider will countersign the order at a later time, usually within 24 hours after making it (see employer policy). Box 20.4 provides guidelines for safely taking verbal, telephone, text, and email prescriptions for medications.

Common types of medication prescriptions based on frequency and/or urgency of medication administration include prn (as needed) and single (one-time) prescriptions, which include stat and now prescriptions. Each prescription needs to include the patient's name, date prescribed, medication name, strength and dosage, route, dose frequency, and time(s) of administration. Standing prescriptions and prescriptions to resume previous medications are no longer supported as best practice (Accreditation Canada, 2021) and have been replaced with preprinted or electronic order sets and protocols (College of Registered Nurses of Alberta, 2018). Order sets provide the prescriber with a choice of medications or treatments that apply to a specific patient population. The ISMP has established guidelines for the development of standardized order sets. A protocol guides clinical decision making related to prescriptions or interventions for specific health care issues.

A medication can be prescribed to be given only when a patient requires or requests it (i.e., prn). Administration of this medication depends on nursing assessment based on indication noted in the prn prescription. A prn prescription usually has a minimum interval set for the time of administration.

Single (one-time) prescriptions are common for preoperative medications or medications given before diagnostic procedures. The medication is prescribed to be given only once at a specified time. A stat prescription means that a single dose of medication is given immediately and only once. Stat prescriptions are used for emergencies when a patient's condition changes suddenly. A now prescription is more specific than a one-time prescription and is used when a patient needs a medication quickly but not as soon as a stat prescription. When nurses receive a now prescription, they have up to 90 minutes to give the medication (see employer policy). Range prescriptions are used when a patient's need for medication varies; however, there continue to be concerns about providing enough guidance to nurses, while still allowing them to address the individual needs of a patient (Accreditation Canada, 2021). An example of a poorly written range prescription is "give morphine sulphate 2 to 6 mg IV direct every 2 to 4 hours prn for pain." This prescription is not specific with regard to guidelines needed to give a correct dose. A range prescription must provide objective measures for nurses to use to determine the correct dose. An example of a clearly written range prescription is "give acetaminophen 325 mg–650 mg every 4 hours prn pain. For pain rated as 1–5, 325 mg; for pain rated as 5–10, 650 mg." A range prescription should include specific indications (e.g., pain-rating score, temperature level). Once a dosage is chosen and administered with a range order, follow employer policy regarding use of any portion of the remainder of the range dose within that same time frame.

As a nurse, once you determine that the information on the patient's MAR is accurate, use the MAR to prepare and administer medications. When preparing medications from bottles or containers, *compare the label of the medication container with the MAR three times:* (1) before removing the container from the supply drawer or shelf, (2) as the amount of medication prescribed is removed from the container, and (3) at the patient's bedside before administering the medication to the patient. Always prepare medications from clearly labelled containers (Accreditation Canada, 2021). With unit-dose prepackaged medications, check the label with the MAR when taking medications out of the medication-dispensing system. Finally, verify all medications at the patient's bedside with the patient's MAR and following verification of right patient using two patient identifiers (Accreditation Canada, 2021).

If a patient questions a medication, stop and recheck to be certain that there is no mistake. An alert patient or caregiver will know whether a medication is different from those received before. In most cases, either the prescription has changed or the medication is now being manufactured by a different company. However, attention to a patient's question is how errors are identified and prevented. The similar physical appearances of some medications with respect to colour, size, and shape have led to medication errors. Generic medications are often prescribed as a more cost-efficient substitution for brand-name medications. However, there may be dramatic differences in the appearance of generic medications, depending on the manufacturer (Health Canada, 2018). Patients may be confused as to why their medication has a different colour or shape when the prescription is refilled. However, medications are found under a variety of different names, and nurses must be careful to obtain the exact name and spelling before administering a medication.

At the time of admission, when transferring a patient to a different unit, and when discharging a patient from a hospital, the nurse needs to assess the patient's medication regimen, especially if the person was admitted to the hospital because of a problem with medication self-administration. A key strategy to reduce medication errors at transition points is the process of medication reconciliation. Medication reconciliation is a three-step process: the health care team (1) works with the patient and/or caregiver to generate a best possible medication history (BPMH), (2) identifies and resolves medication discrepancies, and (3) communicates a complete and accurate list of medications (Accreditation Canada, 2021). Patients often leave the hospital with a basic knowledge of their medications but are unable to safely self-administer them once they return home. When patients enter a health care facility, it is critical for health care providers to have an accurate list of the medications that patients are currently prescribed to take and any over-the-counter (OTC) medications being used.

Right Dose

The unit-dose system is designed to minimize errors. When a medication is prepared from a larger volume or strength than needed or when the health care provider prescribes a system of measurement different from that which the pharmacist supplies, the chance of error increases. After calculating the doses of high-risk medications such as insulin or warfarin, the nurse may need to compare the calculation with one done independently by a second nurse (check employer policy). This is especially important if it is an unusual calculation or involves a potentially toxic medication.

After calculating doses, prepare medications accurately. Use syringes and sealed droppers when it is necessary to measure medications accurately. For example, ISMP (2022a) recommends the use of an oral syringe that measures in millilitres (mL). If an oral solution is available only in a bulk size (such as a bottle) or if the patient-specific dose is less than the unit-dose amount (e.g., dose is 3 mL when the unit-dose product is 5 mL), the pharmacy should prepare the patient-specific dose in an oral syringe (or cup) and dispense it to the unit (ISMP, 2022a). Nurses are no longer encouraged to pour medications into graduated cups because of the risk of medication errors. When preparing medication in an oral syringe, draw up the medication slowly to prevent air bubbles from entering the syringe. Air displaces the medication and leads to inaccurate doses.

Medication errors can occur when pills need to be split. Studies show that the accuracy of split tablets is questionable, even if a tablet is scored (ISMP, 2006). In addition, in the home setting, patients may assume that tablets in containers have already been split when they have not or patients may split them again when they have been split already (ISMP, 2006).

To promote patient safety in some inpatient settings, pharmacists split medications, label and package them, and return them to the nurse for administration.

Tablets are sometimes crushed and mixed with food. Be sure to clean the crushing device completely before crushing the tablet. Remnants of previously crushed medications increase concentration of the medication or result in a patient receiving part of an unprescribed medication. Mix crushed medications with very small amounts of food or liquid. Do not use a patient's favourite foods or liquids because medications alter their taste and decrease the patient's desire for them. This is especially a concern for pediatric patients. *Always check to determine whether a medication can be crushed* (see Chapter 21). Some medications have special coatings that prevent them from being absorbed too quickly (e.g., enteric-coated or slow-release medications). These medications should not be crushed. Refer to the "do not crush" list* (ISMP, 2020) to ensure that a medication is safe to crush.

Right Route

The health care provider's prescription must designate a route of administration. If the route of administration is missing or if the specified route is not the recommended route, consult the health care provider immediately. Recent evidence shows that medication errors involving the wrong route are common. For example, enteral and parenteral medications may become confused in the pediatric setting where liquid medications are frequently given orally. When oral medications are prepared in parenteral syringes, there is an increased risk of giving an oral medication through the parenteral route (ISMP, 2022a). The injection of a liquid intended for oral use produces local complications such as sterile abscess or fatal systemic effects. Medication companies label parenteral medications "for injectable use only." Label the syringe after preparing a medication, include the location if appropriate (e.g., right eye), and always use different syringes for enteral and parenteral medication administration (ISMP, 2022a).

Right Time

Safe medication administration involves adherence to prescribed doses and dosage schedules. Some facilities set schedules for medication administration. However, nurses are able to alter this schedule based on knowledge about a medication. For example, at some facilities, medications that are taken once a day are given at 0900 hours. However, if a medication works best when given at bedtime, the nurse administers it before the patient goes to sleep. In addition, acute care agencies use guidelines from the ISMP and Accreditation Canada (2021) to determine safe, effective, and timely administration of scheduled medications. Facilities need clear policies to determine which medications are not eligible for scheduled dosing times and must be given at precise times (e.g., stat doses, first-time or loading doses, one-time doses). Time-sensitive medications require standardized administration schedules (Accreditation Canada, 2021). With time-sensitive medications (e.g., antibiotics, anticoagulants, insulin), early or delayed administration of maintenance doses of more than 30 minutes before or after the scheduled dose will most likely cause harm or result in subtherapeutic responses in a patient. Non–time-sensitive medications include medications in which the timing of administration most likely will not affect the desired effect of the medication if the medication is given 1 to 2 hours before or after its scheduled time. Thus, nurses need to administer time-sensitive–scheduled medications at a precise time or within 30 minutes before or after the scheduled time. Non–time-sensitive medications are administered within 1 to 2 hours of their scheduled time. Nurses must know their employer's policies about the timing of medications to ensure that they administer medications at the right time (ISMP, 2011).

Nurses must also know why a medication is prescribed for a certain time of the day and whether they are able to alter the time schedule. For example, two medications are prescribed, one q8h (every 8 hours) and the other 3 times per day. Both medications are scheduled 3 times a day over 24 hours. The health care provider intends for the nurse to give the q8h medication as time sensitive to maintain its therapeutic blood levels. In contrast, the nurse needs to give the other medication during waking hours. Each facility has a recommended time schedule for medications prescribed at frequent intervals. Nurses need to be aware of timing between prn medication doses and must carefully calculate whether another dose can be administered per the prescription.

Nurses need to give priority to medications that must act at certain times. For example, give insulin at a precise interval before a meal. Give antibiotics on time to maintain therapeutic blood levels. Some medications require the nurse's clinical judgement to determine the proper time for administration. Administer a prn sleeping medication when the patient is ready for bed. Always document whenever there is a call to the patient's health care provider to obtain a change in a medication prescription.

When preparing patients for discharge, help them plan schedules based on preferred medication intervals, the pharmacokinetics of the medication, and the patient's daily schedule. For patients who have difficulty remembering when to take medications, make a chart that lists the times when they should take each medication or prepare a special container to hold each timed dose.

Right Education

The nurse must ensure they have adequate information about the medication being administered and research any medications they are unfamiliar with. Prior to administering a medication, it is important for the nurse to inform the patient of what the medication is, its desired effects, and any side effects.

Right to Refuse

A patient (or legal guardian) has the right to refuse any medication. The nurse should inform the patient or guardian of the consequences of not receiving the prescribed medication. The nurse needs to verify that the information is understood using teach-back techniques and develop a revised teaching plan if the patient (or guardian) is unable to correctly identify the consequences of not taking the medication. The nurse must notify the health care provider that the prescribed medication has been refused and then document the patient's or guardian's refusal of the medication, the teaching that was completed related to the consequences of not taking the medication, and that the health care provider has been notified.

Right Assessment

Prior to administering a medication, the nurse should properly assess the patient to determine that the medication is safe and appropriate. For example, when administering digoxin, the nurse needs to assess the patient's pulse; if the pulse is below 60 beats/min (50 beats/min in some facilities—always check employer policy), the nurse must withhold the dose. The nurse must also ask the patient whether they have any allergies. If a medication is unsafe or inappropriate to administer, the nurse is to notify the health care provider who prescribed the medication. The nurse documents that the medication was not administered, the reason why it was not administered, and that the health care provider was notified.

Right Evaluation

After the medication has been administered, the nurse should assess the patient for any side effects or ADEs, as well as for effectiveness of the medication. For example, when medicating a patient for pain, it is important for the nurse to reassess the patient's pain 30 to 45 minutes after administering the medication. The nurse should compare the patient's premedication status with their postmedication status and document the patient's response to the medication.

Right Documentation

Accurate documentation allows nurses and other health care providers to communicate with one another and improves medication safety. Many medication errors result from inaccurate documentation. Therefore, always document accurately at the time of administration and verify any inaccurate documentation before administering medications. To ensure the right documentation, first make sure that the information on the patient's MAR corresponds exactly with

---

*The ISMP removed the "do not crush" list from its website on November 17, 2022. The organization encourages health care providers and institutions to maintain, update, and periodically review oral dosage forms that may require alteration.

the health care provider's prescription and the label on the medication container. Written prescriptions and medication forms must include the patient's name; the name of the prescribed medication; and the medication dosage, route, and frequency. If there is any question about a medication prescription because it is incomplete, illegible, vague, or not understood, contact the health care provider before administering the medication. Nurses have a duty to question a medication prescription that is unclear or unusual (CNPS, 2021).

Nurses should never document that they have administered a medication until they have actually given it. They need to document the name of the medication, the dose, the time of administration, and the route on the patient's MAR as soon as it is administered.

Also document the site of any injections and the patient's response to medications. The nurse should document whether the medication had the desired therapeutic effect and whether the patient experienced ADEs or side effects. For example, if pain medication is administered, the nurse must reassess and document whether the medication was effective in controlling pain. Efforts to ensure accurate and timely documentation help provide safe care.

Medication Preparation

It is legally advisable to administer only the medications that you as the nurse prepare. Administering a medication prepared by another health care provider increases the opportunity for errors. You must perform several steps before actual administration of medications, including interpreting medication labels, converting measurement units within a system or between systems, and calculating medication doses. The importance of checking similar names and verifying the correct medication cannot be overemphasized.

Interpreting Medication Labels

Medication labels include several basic pieces of information: the trade name of the medication in large letters, the generic name in smaller letters, the form of the medication, the dosage, the expiration date, the lot number, and the name of the manufacturer (Fig. 20.6).

Clinical Calculation

To administer medications safely, nurses use their mathematical skills to safely calculate dosages and mix solutions. This skill is important because medications are not always dispensed in the unit of measure in which they are prescribed. Medication companies package and bottle medications in standard dosages. For example, a patient's health care provider prescribes 20 mg of a medication that is packaged in 40-mg vials. The nurse is responsible for converting available units of volume and weight to the desired doses. Therefore, the nurse needs to be aware of approximate equivalents in all major measurement systems and make use of conversion tables. In addition to medication administration, nurses use volume and weight conversions in a variety of other nursing activities. These include converting fluid ounces to millilitres to measure intake and output (I&O) and converting volume equivalents to calculate IV flow rates.

Conversions Within One System. Converting measurements within one system is relatively easy; simply divide or multiply in the metric system. For example, to change milligrams to grams, divide by 1 000 or move the decimal three points to the left.

$$1\,000 \text{ mg} = 1 \text{ g}$$

$$350 \text{ mg} = 0.35 \text{ g}$$

To convert litres to millilitres, multiply by 1 000 or move the decimal three points to the right.

$$1 \text{ L} = 1\,000 \text{ mL}$$

$$0.25 \text{ L} = 250 \text{ mL}$$

Dosage Calculations. Dosage calculations are necessary when the dose on the medication label differs from the dose prescribed. There are several dose-calculation methods, including using a formula (Box 20.5), dimensional analysis (Box 20.6), and ratio and proportion (Box 20.7). The most common are the ratio–proportion method and use of a formula.

The Formula Method. Dose prescribed: Gentamicin 50 mg IM
Medication available: 100 mg in 1 mL
Step 1.

$$\frac{\text{Dose prescribed}}{\text{Dose on hand}} \times \text{Volume/Vehicle} = \text{Amount to administer}$$

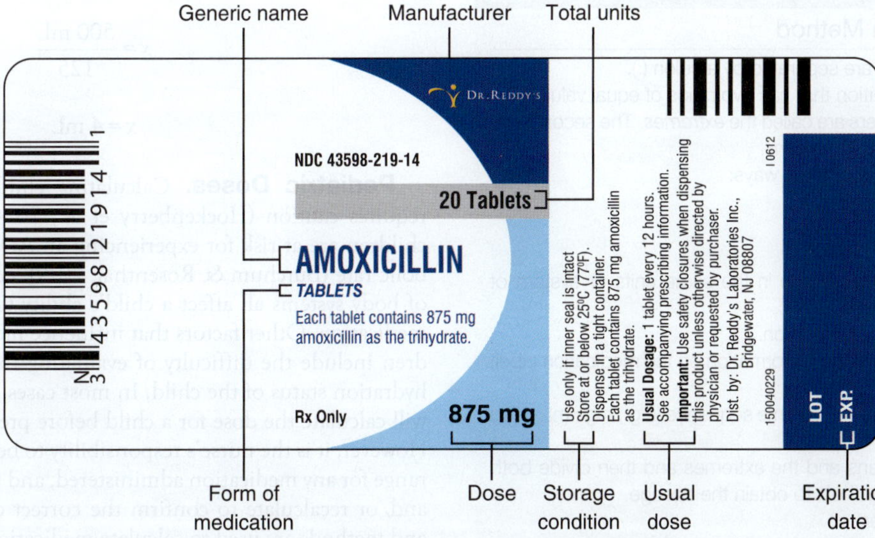

FIG 20.6 Interpreting medication label. (*Courtesy Dr. Reddy's Laboratories, Inc.*)

BOX 20.5

Formula Method

$$\frac{D}{H} \times V = \text{Amount to give}$$

D is the desired dose or the dose prescribed (e.g., 250 mg of penicillin PO 4 times daily).

H is the medication dose on hand or available for use. The dose is on the medication label (e.g., penicillin tablets 250 mg each).

V is the volume (liquid) or vehicle (number of tablets, capsules) that delivers the available dose.

PO, By mouth.
Note: The desired dose (*D*) and the on-hand dose (*H*) must be in the same unit of measurement. If they are in different units, you must convert them before completing the formula.

BOX 20.6

Dimensional Analysis

Use the following steps to solve medication problems using dimensional analysis:

1. Identify the unit of measure that you need to administer. For example, if you are giving a pill, it will usually be a tablet or capsule; for parenteral or oral medications, the unit is millilitres.
2. Estimate the answer in your mind.
3. Place the name or appropriate abbreviation for *x* on the left side of the equation (e.g., *x* tablet, *x* mL).
4. Place available information from the problem in a fraction format on the right side of the equation. Place the abbreviation or units that matches what you are going to administer (determined in Step 1) in the numerator.
5. Look at the medication prescription and add other factors into the problem. Set up the numerator so that it matches the units in the previous denominator.
6. Cancel out like units of measurement on the right side of the equation. You should end up with only one set of units in the equation, and it should match the units on the left side of the equation.
7. Reduce to the lowest terms if possible and solve the problem or solve for *x*. Label your answer.
8. Compare your estimate from Step 2 with your answer in Step 7.

BOX 20.7

The Ratio–Proportion Method

1. The numbers in a ratio are separated by a colon (:).
2. A proportion is an equation that has two ratios of equal value.
3. The first and last numbers are called the *extremes*. The second and third numbers are called the *means*.
4. Write a proportion in one of three ways:
   a. 1:2 = 5:10
   b. 1:2 :: 5:10
   c. 1/2 = 5/10
5. Make sure that all the terms are in the same units or system of measurement.
6. Label all the terms in the proportion.
7. Place the ratio you know (e.g., information on the medication label) first.
8. Put the terms of the ratio in the same sequence (e.g., mg : mL = mg : mL).
9. Cross-multiply the means and the extremes and then divide both sides by the number for the *x* to obtain the dosage.
10. Always label the answer.

Step 2. Calculate your answer:

$$\frac{50\ \text{mg}}{100\ \text{mg}} \times 1\ \text{mL} = 0.5\ \text{mL}$$

Dimensional Analysis Method. This method is used when the dose prescribed has the same label as the dose available.

Dose prescribed: Salazopyrin PO 0.5 g
Tablets available: 0.25 g per tablet
Step 1. The starting factor is 0.5 g.
The answer label is tablets (i.e., How many tablets should be given?).
Step 2. Formulate the conversion equation:
The equivalent needed is 1 tablet = 0.25 g.

$$\frac{0.5\ \text{g}}{1} \times \frac{1\ \text{tablet}}{0.25\ \text{g}} = \#\ \text{of tablets}$$

Cancel labels (g). Note: If properly written, all labels except the answer label will cancel.

Step 3. Solve the equation. Reduce the numerical values and multiply the numerators and denominators. Therefore, 2 tablets should be given for a dose of 0.5 g of Salazopyrin.

Ratio–Proportion Method. A ratio indicates the relationship between two numbers.

Dose prescribed: Phenytoin solution 100 mg PO
Medication available: 125 mg/5 mL
Step 1. Set up the proportion:

$$\frac{125\ \text{mg}}{5\ \text{mL}} = \frac{100\ \text{mg}}{x\ \text{mL}}$$

Step 2. Cross-multiply the equation:

$$125x = 100 \times 5$$

$$125x = 500$$

Step 3. Divide both sides by the number before *x*:

$$\frac{125x}{125} = \frac{500\ \text{mL}}{125}$$

$$x = \frac{500\ \text{mL}}{125}$$

$$x = 4\ \text{mL}$$

Pediatric Doses. Calculating children's medication doses requires caution (Hockenberry et al., 2024). Evidence shows that children are at risk for experiencing an ADE because of their metabolic rate (Burchum & Rosenthal, 2019). Age, weight, and maturity of body systems all affect a child's ability to metabolize and excrete medication. Other factors that influence medication dosages in children include the difficulty of evaluating the desired effect and the hydration status of the child. In most cases, the health care provider will calculate the dose for a child before prescribing the medication. However, it is the nurse's responsibility to be aware of the safe dosage range for any medication administered, and the nurse should recheck and/or recalculate to confirm the correct dose. Different formulas and methods are used to calculate medication doses in children. The

BOX 20.8

Safe Medication Administration in Older Persons

- Consult with the health care provider to keep the medication plan as simple as possible (Burchum & Rosenthal, 2019).
- Keep instructions clear and simple and provide written materials in large print (Burchum & Rosenthal, 2019).
- Teach the complications and interactions of all over-the-counter medications (Accreditation Canada, 2021).
- Teach the older person to set up a daily or weekly schedule for medications using memory aids such as a calendar (Boscart et al., 2023). Have a caregiver help with medication administration, as needed. Include patient's support person or caregiver in any type of instruction.
- Reduce the chance of errors by colour-coding or labelling medication bottles (Verloo et al., 2017).
- Evaluate teaching by having patient teach back instructions.

two most common methods of calculating pediatric dosages are based on the child's weight or body surface area (BSA). Refer to a pediatric pharmacology resource, a pharmacist, or the health care provider if you have to calculate a medication based on BSA. Most of the time, medication dose is calculated based on the child's weight.

Older Person Doses. Older persons also require special consideration during medication administration (Box 20.8). Changes associated with aging alter pharmacokinetics. In addition to physiological changes of aging, behavioural and social and economic issues influence the older person's use of medications.

A common problem for older persons is polypharmacy. There is no consensus definition for *polypharmacy,* although the common definitions include five or more concurrent medications or the mixing of nutritional or herbal supplements with medications (Burchum & Rosenthal, 2019). Older persons experience polypharmacy when they seek relief from a variety of symptoms (e.g., constipation, insomnia, pain) and see multiple health care providers. When determining polypharmacy, the nurse must review all the prescribed medications that an older person is taking as well as all other supplements and OTC medications. Polypharmacy increases the risk for patient safety incidents and interactions with other medications.

The entire health care team shares the responsibility of reducing or eliminating the risk factors associated with the medication regimens that older persons receive. Safety precautions include assessing a patient's health status, current medication regimen (including OTC medications and herbal products), the reason for existing and proposed medications, and any environmental factors that influence accurate and safe medication administration by the patient and caregiver(s). Refer to ISMP Canada's Beers List (https://www.ismp-canada.org/beers_list/#l=qone) for a list of potentially inappropriate medications for older persons.

EVIDENCE-INFORMED PRACTICE

Many medication errors occur when nurses become distracted or lose focus during medication administration or fail to follow best-practice protocols and procedures related to medication administration (Accreditation Canada, 2021). Research reveals that $397 million is spent every year in Canada as a result of preventable ADEs (Healthcare Excellence Canada, 2015). Nurses become interrupted while accessing dispensing systems, depositing medications into delivery containers, and confirming prescriptions on computer screens. The majority of distractions have been identified as a result of interruptions by patients, family and friends of the patient, or other factors in the clinical environment such as noise, chaotic environments, or heavy workloads (Schroers et al., 2021). The following systems help nurses to avoid distractions and prevent medication errors:

- Wearing a medication safety vest, sash, or red apron
- Using visible medication preparation signs
- Using medication administration checklists
- Providing staff and patient education
- Establishing no-interruption zones (NIZs), defined by a red tape outline around the medication ADS

NURSING PROCESS

Application of the nursing process ensures that critical thinking and clinical judgement are integrated into patient care. As a nurse, your role extends beyond simply giving medications to a patient. You are responsible for understanding why your patient is receiving the medication; monitoring patients' responses to medications; providing education to patients and caregivers; and informing health care providers when medications are effective, ineffective, or no longer necessary.

Assessment

As a nurse, before administering medications, you will first perform a physical assessment. Doing so will reveal physical findings for any indications or contraindications for medication therapy (e.g., inability to swallow because of mucositis). Be sure to also assess the patient's sensory, motor, and cognitive functions to determine whether the patient can prepare and administer medications at home. Continue your assessment by determining whether the patient has a history of medication allergies. When assessing for medication allergies, you must differentiate between actual allergic reactions, which can be life threatening, and medication sensitivities, which are uncomfortable side effects. In an acute care setting, patients with allergies wear identification bands that list each medication allergy. All allergies and types of reactions are noted on the patient's admission notes, medication records, and history and physical examination. *Never give a patient a medication when there is a known allergy.*

Your assessment also involves identifying medications that a patient takes every day at home, including prescriptions, OTC preparations, and herbal supplements. Determine how long the patient has taken each medication, current dosage schedule, and whether the patient has experienced any adverse effects to any of the medications. The patient should know the name, purpose, dosage, route, and side effects of medications and supplements that are being taken. Often, patients take many medications and carry a list that includes this information. Patients have different levels of understanding. One patient may describe a diuretic as a "water pill," whereas another describes it as a medication to minimize swelling and lower blood pressure. Practise person-centred care and assess the patient's level of knowledge to determine the need for teaching. If a patient is unable to understand or remember pertinent information, it may be necessary to involve a caregiver.

Once you have completed the appropriate assessments, which may include vital signs, laboratory data, and the nature and severity of symptoms, you must evaluate the data. If the data contraindicate medication administration, withhold the medication and notify the health care provider. When in doubt about medication information, check available medication references or the pharmacy.

Planning

During planning, organize nursing activities to ensure the safe administration of medications. Current evidence shows that distractions or interruptions during preparation for medication administration increase the risk of medication errors (Schroers et al., 2021). The following are general goals of medication administration:

- Patient achieves therapeutic effect of the prescribed medication.
- There are no patient complications related to the prescribed medication.
- Patient and caregiver understand medication therapy.
- Patient and caregiver self-administer medication safely (when appropriate).

Implementation

Nursing interventions focus on safe and effective medication administration. This includes careful medication preparation, accurate and timely administration, and patient education.

Preadministration Activities

1. Identify the medication action, purpose, and side effects as well as nursing implications of administering and monitoring. Ensure that the medication prescription has not expired. Follow employer policy for prescription renewal.
2. Minimize distractions during medication preparation (e.g., discussion with staff, phone call, pager): close the door of the medication room or post "Do Not Disturb" signage, and do not perform other tasks while preparing a medication. Do not allow interruptions.
3. Make sure that the information on the medication computer sheet or MAR exactly matches the health care provider's written prescription and the medication container label. Do not interpret illegible handwriting; clarify with the health care provider.
4. Read the label on the medication container and compare it with the MAR **at least 3 times:** before removing the container from the supply drawer, when preparing the medication, and just before administering the medication to the patient.
5. Double-check all calculations and other high-risk medication administration processes (e.g., insulin, patient-controlled analgesia) and verify with another nurse.
6. Review any preadministration assessments (e.g., vital signs, review of laboratory results).
7. Use proper hand hygiene. Avoid touching tablets and capsules. Use sterile technique for parenteral medications. Wear clean gloves when administering parenteral medications and certain topical medications.
8. Administer only those medications that you personally prepare. Do not ask another person to administer medications that you prepare. Keep medications secure.
9. When preparing medications, be sure that the label is clear and legible and that the medication is mixed properly; has not changed in colour, clarity, or consistency; and has not expired.
10. Keep tablets and capsules in their wrappers and open them at the patient's bedside. This allows you to review each medication with the patient. If a patient refuses medication, there will be no question as to which one was withheld.
11. Health Canada (2019a) has a standard for labelling prescription medications. Before a procedure, all medicines that are not labelled should be labelled (e.g., medicines in syringes and basins), the ink used should be resistant to isopropyl or ethyl alcohol. This task should be done in the area where medicines and supplies are set up.

Medication Administration

1. Follow the 10 rights of medication administration.
2. Educate the patient about the name, purpose, action, and common side effects of each medication. Evaluate their knowledge of the medication and provide appropriate teaching using teach-back technique.
3. Stay with the patient until the medication is taken. Provide help as necessary. Do not leave medication at the bedside without a health care provider's prescription. For example, some patients may take their own vitamins while in the hospital.
4. Respect the patient's right to refuse a medication. If the medication wrapper remains intact, refer to employer policy to determine whether medication can be returned to the drawer or should be disposed of. When medication is refused, determine the reason and take action accordingly.

Postadministration Activities

1. Record medications immediately after administration (see employer policy). Include the medication name, dose, route, time, and your signature.
2. Document preassessment as required (e.g., measuring blood pressure before administering antihypertensives).
3. Document postassessment data pertinent to patient's response. This step is especially important when giving prn medications.
4. If a patient refuses a medication, document that it was not given, the reason for the refusal, the patient education that was provided, and that you notified the health care provider.

Evaluation

After you administer a medication, consider how the medication is expected to affect the patient and evaluate their condition and response to it. Look for therapeutic and adverse effects. If adverse effects develop, you need to recognize the clinical signs and respond quickly:

1. Monitor for evidence of therapeutic effects, side effects, and ADEs. This includes monitoring physical response (e.g., heart rhythm, blood pressure, urine output, or laboratory results).
2. When a medication is given for relief of symptoms, ask the patient to report if symptoms have diminished or been relieved. For example, complete a pain assessment after medication is administered (e.g., 30 minutes after medicating for pain).
3. Observe injection sites for bruises, inflammation, localized pain, numbness, or bleeding.
4. Evaluate patient's and caregiver's understanding of purpose of medication therapy, dose regimens, and ability to self-administer medication by using teach-back techniques.

PATIENT AND CAREGIVER TEACHING

A well-informed patient is more likely to take medications correctly. However, many patients have limited health literacy, meaning that they do not understand how to read medication labels and calculate doses. Thus, any education requires a person-centred approach to assess a patient's learning needs and abilities.

Nurses need to provide person-centred teaching according to patient preference, using visual aids, instructional booklets written in simple language or the patient's language, video recordings, or online resources. When teaching patients about their medications, include people identified as being significant to the patient's recovery (e.g., family members, caregivers, or home care providers).

Begin providing patient teaching as soon as possible so you have time for several teaching sessions. It is ideal to use instructional materials written no higher than a Grade 6 reading level. Provide instructions written in the patient's language, if available. When providing instruction, have the patient or caregiver repeat the name and use for each medication plus the dosing instructions. Current recommendations suggest the use of teach-back as a method to confirm patient learning and improve health care provider education (Shersher et al.,

2021). Have the patient explain the topic you taught them so you can confirm their understanding, and have the patient demonstrate preparation of each medication. Provide time to discuss problem scenarios (e.g., side effects develop or a syringe becomes contaminated) to ensure that the patient is aware of what to do should something go wrong. Determine whether the patient requires an adherence aid or memory cue. This is especially important among older persons. If the patient speaks another language, have a professional interpreter available during instruction. Do not use a family member as an interpreter. Medication dose containers organized by the hours and days of the week are very useful. In the event that patients miss a dose of medication, they need to know how to safely adjust their medication schedule.

Evaluating the effectiveness of teaching ensures that a patient can administer medications in a safe manner. One method of evaluating patient understanding is to create medication cards with the generic and trade names of the medication on the front of the card and all pertinent medication information on the back of the card. Another method is to have patients read labels on prepared medications. Remember that medication bottles often have fine print and are difficult to read for patients with impaired vision. Have the pharmacy prepare large-print labels when appropriate. If the patient correctly identifies the name of the medication, ask the following questions:

- Why are you taking this medication?
- How often do you take this medication and at what time of day?
- What side effects can occur with this medication?
- If this side effect occurs, what are you going to do about it?

Be sure to also assess the patient's sensory, motor, and cognitive functions (e.g., ability to open medication bottles). Impairments may affect the patient's ability to safely self-administer medications, and caregivers or community health workers may need to help with medication administration. Many self-help devices are also available for purchase (e.g., pill boxes with times displayed and electronic dispensers).

Care in the Community: Home Management

Nurses practising in hospital or in the community may support patients and/or caregivers in learning safe medication self-administration (see Skill 20.1).

✦ SKILL 20.1 Teaching Medication Self-Administration

A patient's medication regime can undergo various changes, either during a hospital stay or following a visit to the doctor (ISMP Canada, 2017). The nurse can find resources and address issues that may influence a patient's adherence to their medication regimen (e.g., ability to purchase medications, transportation to pharmacy, adverse effects). Teaching patients how to correctly administer medications is very important, but first the nurse needs to identify and address any issues that are of concern.

The word *compliance* was used in the past to describe whether patients' behaviours matched that of health care providers' recommendations when it came to taking prescribed medications or adhering to prescribed treatments. Recent literature supports the term *adherence*, since this term emphasizes a patient's active role in decision making (Scialli et al., 2021). One method that increases adherence involves understanding and then supporting patients' decisions in how they take their medications. Nurses need to use teaching methods that incorporate active listening so that they can adapt patients' needs and concerns into the medication regimen.

Some barriers to medication adherence include fear of adverse reactions from medications, belief that a medication does not help, inconvenience of taking medication, cost of medication, inadequate knowledge, forgetfulness, and relationship with the health care provider (Scialli et al., 2021). Considering these potential barriers, nurses can provide information and support to ensure that a patient or caregiver is making a well-informed decision when it comes to whether to take a medication. Once a patient has mastered the skill of administering medications, the nurse must continue to validate that the skill is being performed correctly and assess for new issues and concerns.

Delegation and Collaboration

Interprofessional collaboration (e.g., pharmacist) is required to explore methods of administration such as dosettes and blister packs that would aid in self-administration and adherence. The skill of teaching patients how to self-administer medication cannot be delegated to an unregulated care provider (UCP). The nurse directs the UCP to do the following:

- Communicate to the nurse problems that the patient reports with medication self-administration

Equipment

- Medication
- Liquid to take with medication
- Medication administration record or other up-to-date list of current medications from health care provider
- Medication log
- Container for daily or weekly preparation
- Measuring devices, as needed (e.g., medicine cup, teaspoon)
- Teaching tools (e.g., charts, written instructions, colour codes for medicine containers)

STEP	RATIONALE
ASSESSMENT	
1. Identify patient using at least two person-specific identifiers (e.g., name and date of birth, or name and medical record number), according to employer policy, during the first home visit. Facial recognition can be used as one of two identifiers for ongoing subsequent home visits.	Ensures correct patient. Complies with Accreditation Canada's standards and improves patient safety (Accreditation Canada, 2020).
2. Throughout the procedure, the 4 moments for hand hygiene are to be implemented; hand hygiene should occur before initial patient (or patient environment) contact, before an aseptic procedure, after body fluid exposure risk, and after patient (or patient environment) contact. Additional hand hygiene should be performed when hands are visibly soiled.	Proper hand hygiene helps prevent the spread of infectious agents to health care providers.

STEP	RATIONALE
ASSESSMENT	
3. Assess patient's cognitive, sensory, and motor function: level of consciousness, sight, hearing, touch, health literacy level, swallowing ability, mobility, activity tolerance, social support, and willingness to cooperate.	Cognitive, sensory, and motor deficits frequently affect a patient's ability to take or prepare prescribed medication correctly and participate in instruction.
4. Assess patient and caregiver resources for obtaining medications when needed (e.g., finances, social support, and transportation).	Lack of resources is a major factor that negatively affects adherence to medication self-administration regimen (Scialli et al., 2021).
5. Assess patient's learning readiness and ability to concentrate (consider presence of pain, nausea, or fatigue and patient interest in instruction) and preferred learning style.	Presence of significant illness, frailty, or confusion affects a person's ability to attend to a teaching plan. Indicates need to rely on caregiver for learning and implementation (if available) on a short- or long-term basis. Learning style affects the choice of teaching resources.
6. Assess patient's and caregiver's knowledge of medication therapy: names of medications, how to administer them, purpose or action, daily doses and times to be taken, adverse effects to expect, and what to do if problems occur.	Patients may be unintentionally nonadherent with medications when they lack understanding of medication purpose (Scialli et al., 2021). Caregiver's confidence in administering medication influences their ability to manage medication for the patient.
7. Assess patient's belief in need for medication therapy. Consider prior experiences, cultural values, religious beliefs, personal experiences with medications, and caregiver's values about medications.	Many factors influence a patient's willingness to follow a medication regimen.
8. Assess patient's prescribed and OTC medications, including use of herbal supplements: Has more than one health care provider prescribed medications? Are labels clearly marked? Are time schedules confusing? Do different medications look alike? Does patient store medications together or out of original containers? Are expiration dates on bottles still current?	Determines sources of confusion affecting patient's adherence. Adherence to medication therapy (especially in older persons) is often complicated by polypharmacy (multiple chronic conditions are often treated with multiple medications, sometimes prescribed by more than one health care provider). Adherence is more complicated when medication regimens are complex.
9. Be sure that caregiver knows patient's medication allergies.	As new medications are prescribed, the caregiver often becomes the one to monitor for inappropriate medication prescription.
10. Consult with health care provider to review medications that patient is receiving and simplify regimen if possible.	Review of medications helps minimize risk for interactions from multiple medications and ensures accuracy of medication regimen. Simplification of regimen improves adherence, particularly with regard to daily frequency of prescribed doses.

NURSING DIAGNOSES

- Anxiety
- Insufficient knowledge regarding medication self-administration
- Inadequate health maintenance
- Readiness for enhanced knowledge

Related factors and risk factors are individualized on the basis of patient's condition or needs.

PLANNING

STEP	RATIONALE
1. Expected outcomes following completion of procedure:	
• Patient or caregiver can state the purpose of each medication and why it is beneficial. If a medication has been discontinued, patient or caregiver correctly explains why this was done.	Demonstrates cognitive learning.
• Patient or caregiver identifies common adverse effects and relief measures.	Encourages adherence to medication therapy.
• Patient or caregiver can state when to notify health care provider about medication problems.	Empowers patient to participate in care.
• Patient or caregiver reads each label and explains when each medication should be taken.	Prevents medication administration errors.
• Patient or caregiver demonstrates self-administration of medication by prescribed route.	Demonstrates skill achieved.
2. Prepare environment for teaching session:	Increases likelihood that patient and caregiver will be attentive to instruction.

STEP	RATIONALE

PLANNING

STEP	RATIONALE
• Select a room that is well lit and offers comfortable seating. • Be sure that the patient is close and can see the nurse clearly. • Control sources of noise and distractions.	Room environment needs to minimize existing sensory alterations. A comfortable environment free of distractions increases patient's attention.
3. Prepare teaching materials. **a.** Plan an approach that matches the patient's learning preference (visual, auditory, read/write, kinesthetic): **(1)** Written materials printed in large, bold letters (set in 14-point or larger type) **(2)** DVD or online instructional programs **(3)** Illustrations of medication safety guidelines **(4)** Handling equipment and supplies	Person-centred care focuses on working in partnership with patients. Using an instructional approach tailored to the patient's learning style is a person-centred approach that maximizes patient learning. Assists patients with visual limitations.
4. Ensure that patient is wearing glasses or hearing aids if needed during teaching session.	Use of glasses or hearing aids increases the patient's sensory perception and likelihood of attending to teaching session and understanding content.
5. Arrange teaching time to ensure participation of caregiver (see Step 5 illustration).	Caregivers can serve as a positive resource to patients and often reinforce information provided.

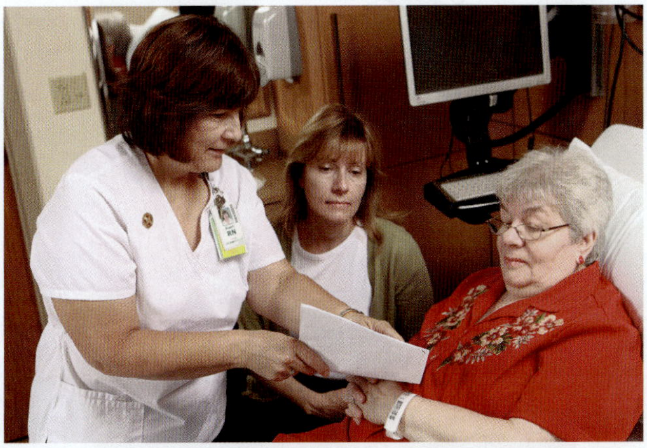

STEP 5 Patient and caregiver participate in medication self-administration teaching program.

IMPLEMENTATION

STEP	RATIONALE
1. Instruct patient or caregiver about the importance of performing hand hygiene before medication self-administration.	Reduces transmission of microorganisms.
2. Present information clearly and concisely.	Improves patient's ability to attend to and understand instruction (Scialli et al., 2021).
a. Face learner in a well-lit room.	Allows visualization of patient's nonverbal responses to education. A patient with hearing loss or visual impairment is able to see your expressions, read written information, and hear your voice more clearly.
b. Use short sentences and speak slowly in a low-pitched voice.	Enhances understanding of information.
c. Provide descriptions in understandable terms.	Prevents confusion of terminology. Patients learn more quickly when you present information at the level of the learner (Coskun & Bagcivan, 2021).
3. Provide frequent pauses so patient or caregiver can ask questions and express understanding of content.	Increases learner participation. Ongoing feedback ensures that patient is acquiring information.
4. Instruct patient or caregiver on the following content: purpose of regularly scheduled and prn (as needed) medications and their desired effects, how medication works and why it helps, dosage schedules and rationale, common adverse effects, what to do to relieve adverse effects, what to do if a dose is missed, when to call the health care provider with problems, who to call with problems, medication safety guidelines, and implications when medications are not taken.	Provides patient or caregiver with sufficient information to understand medications and their effects and to take them safely at home.

STEP	RATIONALE
IMPLEMENTATION	
5. Instruct patient or caregiver on the appropriate route of medication delivery, including oral, subcutaneous, intramuscular, inhalation, and topical.	Patients need to be proficient in all routes of medication administration. Adverse effects often occur if medications are administered incorrectly.
6. Provide frequent, short teaching sessions. Plan to have several teaching sessions, especially if patient needs to take multiple medications.	Frequent sessions improve patient's attention to and retention of information discussed.
7. Provide teaching about OTC medications and herbal supplements.	Patients may not understand the effects of OTC and herbal supplements (Health Canada, 2017).
8. Provide patient with written schedules or individualized instruction sheets for review. Offer special charts, diagrams, learning aids, written information, weekly pill organizers, and online resources (see Step 8 illustration).	Clearly written information, charts, and other resources such as websites enhance patient learning and allow for reinforcement of information (Coskun & Bagcivan, 2021).

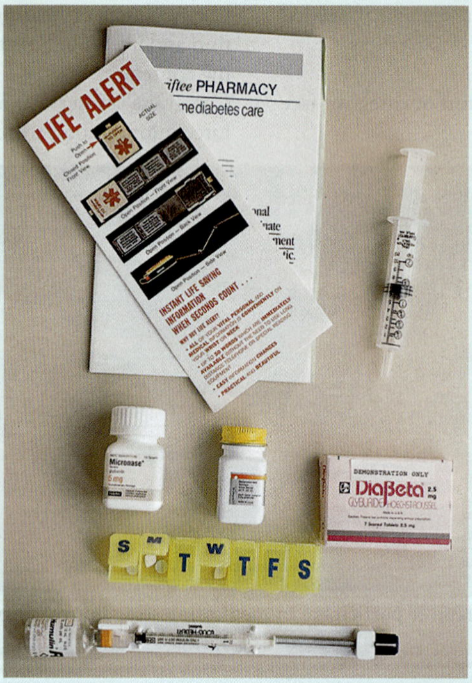

STEP 8 Examples of aids for patient self-administration of medication.

STEP	RATIONALE
9. Offer help as the patient practises preparing medication (e.g., "Let's prepare the medications you will take with your meals or the medicines you take first in the morning").	Allows for observation of patient's ability to read labels correctly and prepare all medications for prescribed times.
10. Have pharmacy provide clear, large-print labels for medication bottles and medication teaching handouts, if appropriate.	Improves patient's ability to read and follow directions.
11. Have pharmacy provide containers that patient can open independently if manual dexterity is limited.	Most pharmacies dispense pills in childproof containers, which patients with limited manual dexterity often find difficult to manipulate or open.

Critical Decision Point *If there are pets or small children in the home or children who frequently visit the home, help the patient establish a safe place for medication storage to reduce risk of accidental ingestion by pets or children.*

STEP	RATIONALE
12. Facilitate arrangements for pharmacy to receive written prescriptions in a timely fashion if required for dispensing. Arrange for pharmacy to deliver medications to the home if patient is unable to arrange for transportation to the pharmacy.	Availability of medications influences adherence.
13. Discuss with patient or caregiver how to dispose of discontinued or expired medications.	Ensures safe disposal.

STEP	RATIONALE
EVALUATION	
1. Ask patient or caregiver to explain information about each medication: its purpose, actions, and routes; timing of medications and maximum frequency of use of either prescribed or OTC medications; adverse effects and interactions; and foods, herbals, or OTC medications to avoid.	Patients and caregivers need to be able to understand and remember the information they are given (Coskun & Bagcivan, 2021).
2. Ask patient or caregiver to describe when to call the health care provider or refer to printed information for resources.	Developing techniques to gain information and solve problems can increase patient adherence and reduces potential problems with carrying out the medication regimen.
3. Have patient or caregiver prepare and administer doses for all prescribed medications.	Indicates understanding of medication dosages and schedules. Provides an objective evaluation of the information the patient has learned.
4. Use teach-back: "I want to be sure I explained how to safely dispose of medicines you are no longer taking. Tell me in your own words the correct way to dispose of your tablets here in the home." Develop a revised teaching plan if patient or caregiver is unable to teach back correctly.	Determines patient's and caregiver's level of understanding of instructional topic.

Unexpected Outcomes	Related Interventions
1. Patient or caregiver makes errors in preparing medications or is unable to recall or explain information discussed in teaching sessions.	• Provide additional instruction and teaching materials for consultation when information is forgotten or unclear. • Ensure that written instructions are at the patient's level of understanding. Some commercially prepared booklets contain instructions that are too complex or contain medical jargon that is difficult to understand. • Consider use of different pictures, colour-coding, diagrams, and recorded instructions for patients with visual impairment or a reading disability. • Consider use of weekly pill organizers. • Periodically observe how patient or caregiver prepares and administers medications.
2. Medication self-administration plan is not possible because of patient's self-care deficits. This issue is very common when the patient develops cognitive changes.	• Develop an alternative plan, which often relies on caregivers to provide safe administration of home medication regimen.
3. Patient refuses to take medications as prescribed.	• Explore and identify reasons for nonadherence, which often include the following: cost, adverse effects, complexity of regimen, problems with swallowing or other adverse effects, and cultural preferences. • Box 20.9 lists nursing interventions to improve medication adherence.

Communication and Documentation

- Document instruction provided and learning outcomes achieved by patient and caregiver in the home care record.
- Develop a system of recording (patient diary/log) for patient or caregiver to use to document adherence to dosage schedules and self-monitoring of any problems.
- Always leave a phone number and instructions on how to reach a home care nurse if needed.

Special Considerations

Dosing

- It is recommended that the patient or caregiver be provided with an oral syringe or dosing cup to accurately measure medication.
- Determine whether patient has the manual dexterity or visual acuity to split tablets. If possible, arrange for pharmacy to split the pills or encourage the health care provider to order medications that do not require splitting.

Teaching

- See Chapter 42 for guidelines on maintaining medication safety in the home.
- If it is difficult to plan a separate teaching session, teach patient while administering medications.

BOX 20.9

Evidence-Informed Nursing Interventions That Enhance Adherence to Medication Therapy

- Involve patients as partners in collaboration. Encourage them to express their views and share in the decision making with you.
- Provide education about diagnosis and treatment to engage patients and caregivers in care.
- Use motivational interviewing strategies to encourage patients to take their medications.
- Use medication reminders and devices such as smartphone alarms and pill boxes.
- Collaborate with caregivers and family to provide support.
- Utilize supportive methods to increase the patient's motivation to take their medications and their willingness to work with health care providers to adhere to treatments.

Adapted from Simon, S., Kini, V., Levy, A., et al. (2021). Medication adherence in cardiovascular medicine. *BMJ, 374*(1493), 1–19. https://doi.org/10.1136/bmj.n1493

- Examples of learning aids include homemade calendars for each week that contain plastic bags with medications to take at specific times, egg cartons divided into colour-coded sections with medications for the day, clock faces for patients who cannot read or see clearly, colour-coding for medication types (e.g., blue for sedative, red for pain pill), and pill boxes that identify days of the week and times of day.

Pediatric

- Instruct adults to keep all medications locked and securely out of reach of children.
- Encourage caregivers not to tell children that medications are treats because this increases the likelihood that children will mistake medicine for candy, thus increasing risk of overdose.
- Successful medication teaching involves the child's parents or other caregivers and the child and siblings whenever possible. To provide effective medication teaching to children, take the child's developmental and cognitive abilities into consideration when planning teaching sessions (Hockenberry et al., 2024).
- Caregivers need to supervise older children as they begin taking responsibility for their own treatment.

Gerontological

- The capacity to learn new information remains as people age (in the absence of dementia); however, older patients often need additional time to accomplish learning. Allow adequate time and number of teaching sessions to support successful learning. Effective teaching strategies for older persons include memory aids, information written in large letters, involvement of a caregiver, follow-up teaching sessions either over the telephone or in person, and computer-assisted teaching guides (Boscart et al., 2023).
- Cognition problems coupled with complexity of medication regimens have a negative effect on older persons' ability to self-administer medication safely. Try to decrease the complexity of medication regimens in patients with cognitive deficits whenever possible to promote safe medication self-administration practices.
- Older persons often must take medications via multiple routes (e.g., oral, inhaled, injections). Many times, problems with physical dexterity, eyesight, cognitive skills, and memory negatively affect adherence to medication schedules. Establish a therapeutic nurse–patient relationship as part of person-centred care to help patients overcome these barriers to adherence and explore adaptive devices that may support patient's self-care.

✦ REVIEW QUESTIONS

A 72-year-old patient (he/him) visits the medical clinic 1 month after a myocardial infarction (heart attack). He denies any chest pain since his angioplasty, which involved insertion of a stent into one of his coronary arteries to dilate the artery and improve blood flow to the heart. He is currently taking an antidepressant, a thyroid supplement, a stool softener, and a cardiac medication (beta-adrenergic blocker). In addition, he takes an herbal preparation for sleep that contains melatonin. The health care provider has recently revised the cardiac medication to metoprolol. The patient is now instructed to take 75 mg of metoprolol by mouth twice daily. The nurse notes that the medication is available in 150-mg tablets. The patient tells the clinic nurse that he has experienced some weakness and dizziness over the past week. Review Questions 1 to 4 relate to the case study presented here.

1. Which of the medications taken by the patient are likely to cause weakness and dizziness? Which nursing interventions should be included if he is experiencing these issues?
2. What might the health care provider who prescribed the medication do after receiving the nurse's report of the patient's weakness and dizziness? Use one of the methods discussed in this chapter to calculate the number of tablets of medication to administer.
3. As the nurse, which factors would be important for you to assess so the patient may take the 75-mg dose safely? Using SBAR (situation–background–assessment–recommendation), show how you would communicate with the health care team about this patient.
4. The health care provider has written the following prescriptions. Which prescriptions do you need to clarify before administering the medication? (*Select all that apply.*) Provide rationale for your answers, and rewrite the prescription so it follows the ISMP current medication prescription safety guidelines.
   1. Timoptic .25% solution 1 drop OD bid
   2. Metoprolol 12.50 mg qd
   3. Insulin glargine 6 u SC twice a day
   4. Enalapril 2.5 mg. PO three times a day; hold for systolic blood pressure <100
5. An older person states that they cannot see the medication bottles clearly to determine when to take their prescription. What should the nurse do? (*Select all that apply.*)
   1. Provide a pill-dispensing system that allows the patient or caregiver to prepare medications for each day of the week.
   2. Provide large-print, easier-to-read labels on medication bottles.
   3. Tell the patient what is in each container of medication.
   4. Have a caregiver administer the medication.
   5. Use teach-back to ensure that patient knows what medication to take and when.
6. The nurse must take a verbal order during an emergency on the unit. Which of the following guidelines can be used for taking verbal or telephone orders? (*Select all that apply.*)
   1. Only authorized staff receive and record verbal or telephone orders. Facility identifies in writing the staff who are authorized.
   2. Clearly identify patient's name, room number, and diagnosis.
   3. Read back all orders to health care provider.
   4. Use clarification questions to avoid misunderstandings.
   5. Write "verbal order" or "telephone order," including date and time, name of patient, and complete prescription; write the name of the health care provider and sign the entry.

Visit the Evolve site for a complete list of answers to the Review Questions.

✦ NEXT GENERATION NCLEX® (NGN)

For practice with answering exam questions related to unfolding NGN case studies, please consult the Next Generation NCLEX® (NGN)-Style Case Studies for Skills and Techniques on the Evolve website: http://evolve.elsevier.com/Canada/Perry/clinicalskills/

REFERENCES

Accreditation Canada. (2020). *Required organizational practices–2020 handbook.* https://physicians.nshealth.ca/resources/required-organizational-practices-2020-handbook

Accreditation Canada. (2021). *Medication management standards.* https://store.accreditation.ca/products/medication-management-standards

Blumenthal, K. G., Peter, J. G., Trubiano, J. A., et al. (2019). Antibiotic allergy. *Lancet*, 393(10167), 183–198. https://doi.org/10.1016/S0140-6736(18)32218-9

Boscart, V., McCleary, L., Sheiban Taucar, L., et al. (2023). *Ebersole and Hess' gerontological nursing and health aging in Canada* (3rd ed.). Elsevier.

British Columbia College of Nurses and Midwives. (2020). *Medication: Practice standard for registered nurses.* https://www.bccnm.ca/RN/PracticeStan dards/Pages/medication.aspx

Burchum, J., & Rosenthal, L. (2019). *Lehne's pharmacology for nursing care* (10th ed.). Saunders.

Canadian Association of Nurses in Oncology (CANO). (2017). *Standards and competencies for cancer chemotherapy nursing practice.* https://cdn.ymaws.com/www.cano-acio.ca/resource/resmgr/Resources/EN_CANO_Chemotherapy_Standar.pdf [Seminal Reference]

Canadian Association of Provincial Cancer Agencies. (2015). *Oral cancer drug therapy safe use and safe handling guidelines.* https://capca.ca/wp-content/uploads/2020/10/En-Oral-Chemotherapy-Guideline-Final-11-May-2015.pdf [Seminal Reference]

Canadian Nurses Protective Society (CNPS). (2021). *InfoLaw: Medication errors.* https://cnps.ca/article/medication-errors/

College of Registered Nurses of Alberta. (2018). *Guideline for medication and vaccine injectables.* https://nurses.ab.ca/media/q5gn52kz/guidelines-for-medication-and-vaccine-injection-safety-acp-crna-cpsa-2018.pdf

Coskun, S., & Bagcivan, G. (2021). Associated factors with treatment adherence of patients diagnosed with chronic disease: Relationship with health literacy. *Applied Nursing Research, 57*, 1–6. https://doi.org/10.1016/j.apnr.2020.151368

Dykstra, J., Sendelbach, D., & Steege, L. M. (2016). Fatigue in float nurses: Patient, nurse, task, and environmental factors across unit work systems. *Proceedings of the Human Factors and Ergonomics Society - Annual Meeting, 60*(1), 623–627. https://doi.org/10.1177/1541931213601142 [Seminal Reference]

Elshayib, M., & Pawola, L. (2020). Computerized provider order entry–related medication errors among hospitalized patients: An integrative review. *Health Informatics Journal, 26*(4), 2834–2859. https://doi.org/10.1177/1460458220941750

Goodman, C., & Brett, A. (2021). Race and pharmacogenomics—Personalized medicine or misguided practice? *JAMA, 325*(7), 625–626. https://doi.org/10.1001/jama.2020.25473

Health Canada. (2017). *Using medications safely.* https://www.canada.ca/en/health-canada/services/drugs-medical-devices/using-medications-safely.html

Health Canada. (2018). *Access to generic drugs in Canada.* https://www.canada.ca/en/health-canada/services/drugs-health-products/drug-products/fact-sheets/access-to-generic-drugs.html

Health Canada. (2019a). *Good label and package practices guide for prescription drugs.* https://www.canada.ca/en/health-canada/services/drugs-health-products/reports-publications/medeffect-canada/good-label-package-practices-guide-prescription-drugs-profile/guidance-document.html

Health Canada. (2019b). *Mandatory reporting of serious adverse drug reactions and medical device incidents by hospitals–Guidance document.* https://www.canada.ca/en/health-canada/services/drugs-health-products/medeffect-canada/adverse-reaction-reporting/mandatory-hospital-reporting/drugs-devices/guidance.html

Health Canada. (2022). *Canada vigilance program.* https://www.canada.ca/en/health-canada/services/drugs-health-products/medeffect-canada/canada-vigilance-program.html

Healthcare Excellence Canada. (n.d.). *Medication safety.* https://www.patientsafetyinstitute.ca/en/About/PatientSafetyForwardWith4/pages/medication-safety.aspx

Healthcare Excellence Canada. (2011). *Canadian disclosure guidelines: Being open with patients and families.* https://www.patientsafetyinstitute.ca/en/toolsResources/disclosure/Documents/CPSI%20Canadian%20Disclosure%20Guidelines.pdf [Seminal Reference]

Healthcare Excellence Canada. (2015). *The economics of patient safety in acute care. A technical report.* https://www.patientsafetyinstitute.ca/en/toolsResources/Research/commissionedResearch/EconomicsofPatientSafety/Documents/Economics%20of%20Patient%20Safety%20-%20Acute%20Care%20-%20Final%20Report.pdf.[Seminal Reference]

Hockenberry, M. J., Duffy, E. A., & Gibbs, K. (2024). *Wong's nursing care of infants and children* (12th ed.). Elsevier.

Institute for Safe Medication Practices (ISMP). (2006). *Tablet splitting: Do it only if you "half" to, and then do it safely.* https://www.ismp.org/resources/tablet-splitting-do-it-only-if-you-half-and-then-do-it-safely [Seminal Reference]

Institute for Safe Medication Practices (ISMP). (2011). *Guidelines for timely administration of scheduled medications (acute).* https://www.ismp.org/guidelines/timely-administration-scheduled-medications-acute [Seminal Reference]

Institute for Safe Medication Practices (ISMP). (2018). *High-alert medications in acute care.* https://www.ismp.org/recommendations/high-alert-medications-acute-list

Institute for Safe Medication Practices (ISMP). (2020). *Oral dosage forms that should not be crushed.* https://www.ismp.org/recommendations/do-not-crush

Institute for Safe Medication Practices (ISMP). (2022a). *2020–2021 ISMP targeted medication safety best practices for hospitals.* https://www.ismp.org/sites/default/files/attachments/2020-02/2020-2021%20TMSBP-%20FINAL_1.pdf

Institute for Safe Medication Practices (ISMP). (2022b). *Key elements of safe medication use.* https://www.ismp.org/ten-key-elements

Institute for Safe Medication Practices Canada. (n.d.). *ISMP Canada activities for the CMIRPS.* https://www.ismp-canada.org/cmirps/

Institute for Safe Medication Practices Canada (ISMP Canada). (2014). *Preventable medication errors–Look-alike/sound-alike drug names.* https://www.ismp-canada.org/download/PharmacyConnection/PC2014-02-Spring_LookalikeSoundalike.pdf [Seminal Reference]

Institute for Safe Medication Practices Canada (ISMP Canada). (2016). *Drug labelling and the application of TALLman lettering project report.* https://www.ismp-canada.org/download/TALLman/TALLmanLettering-ProjectReport.pdf [Seminal Reference]

Institute for Safe Medication Practices Canada (ISMP Canada). (2017). *Errors associated with hospital discharge prescriptions: A multi-incident analysis.* https://www.ismp-canada.org/download/safetyBulletins/2017/ISMPCSB2017-01-HospitalDischargePrescriptions.pdf [Seminal Reference]

Institute for Safe Medication Practices Canada (ISMP Canada). (2018). *Do not use. Dangerous abbreviations, symbols, and dose designations.* https://www.ismp-canada.org/download/ISMPCanadaListOfDangerousAbbreviations.pdf

Lee, S., & Kang, J. (2021). Unintended consequences and workarounds of electronic medical record implementation in clinical nursing practice. *Computers, Informatics, Nursing, 39*(12), 898–908. https://doi.org/10.1097/CIN.0000000000000785

Lin, K., Chan, K., Mohindra, R., et al. (2017). SGEM hot off the press: Computer provider order entry (CPOE) and emergency department flow. *Canadian Journal of Emergency Medicine, 19*(2), 147–153. https://doi.org/10.1017/cem.2017.7 [Seminal Reference]

MacDonald, N., & Attaran, A. (2009). Medical errors, apologies and apology laws. *Canadian Medical Association Journal, 180*(1), Article 11. https://doi.org/10.1503/cmaj.081997 [Seminal Reference]

Nova Scotia College of Nursing. (2022). *Medication guidelines for nurses.* https://cdn1.nscn.ca/sites/default/files/documents/resources/MedicationGuidelines.pdf

Rohde, E., & Domm, E. (2017). Nurses' clinical reasoning practices that support safe medication administration: An integrative review of the literature. *Journal of Clinical Nursing, 17*(3–4), e402–e412. https://doi.org/10.1111/jocn.14077 [Seminal Reference]

Schroers, G., Gunberg Ross, J., & Moriarty, H. (2021). Nurses' perceived causes of medication administration errors: A qualitative systematic review. *Joint Commission Journal on Quality and Patient Safety, 47*, 38–53. https://doi.org/10.1016/j.jcjq.2020.09.010

Scialli, A., Saavedra, K., & Fugh-Berman, A. (2021). The benefits and risks of adherence to medical therapy. *Journal of Scientific Practice and Integrity, 3*(1). https://doi.org/10.35122/001c.21386

Shersher, V., Haines, T. P., Sturgiss, L., et al. (2021). Definitions and use of the teach back method in healthcare consultations with patients: A systematic review and thematic synthesis. *Patient Education and Counseling, 104*, 118–129. https://doi.org/10.1016/j.pec.2020.07.026

Strudwick, G., Reisdorfer, E., Warnock, C., et al. (2018). Factors associated with barcode medication administration technology that contribute to patient safety: An integrative review. *Journal of Nursing Care Quality, 33*(1), 79–85. https://doi.org/10.1097/NCQ.0000000000000270

Verloo, H., Chiolero, A., Kiszio, B., et al. (2017). Nurse interventions to improve medication adherence among discharged older adults: A systematic review. *Age and Ageing, 46*(5), 747–754. https://doi.org/10.1093/ageing/afx076

Walker, K., Migneault, D., Lindsay, H. C., et al. (2019). Use of personal mobile devices to record patient data by Canadian emergency physicians and residents. *Canadian Journal of Emergency Medicine, 21*(4), 455–460. https://doi.org/10.1017/cem.2019.29

Zheng, W., Lichtner, V., Van Dort, B. A., et al. (2020). The impact of introducing automated dispensing cabinets, barcode medication administration, and closed-loop electronic medication management systems on work processes and safety of controlled medications in hospitals: A systematic review. *Research in Social and Administrative Pharmacy, 17*(5), 832–841. https://doi.org/10.1016/j.sapharm.2020.08.001

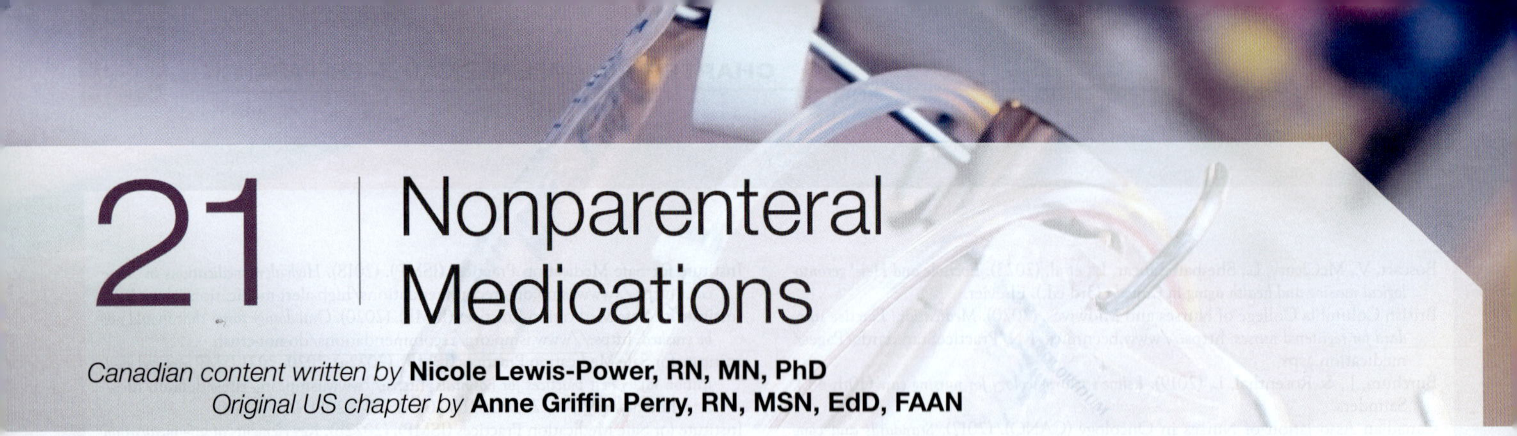

21 Nonparenteral Medications

Canadian content written by **Nicole Lewis-Power, RN, MN, PhD**
Original US chapter by **Anne Griffin Perry, RN, MSN, EdD, FAAN**

SKILLS AND PROCEDURES

OBJECTIVES

Mastery of content in this chapter will enable the nurse to:

- Describe common principles to follow in the administration of medications.
- Explain patient-centred practices to use to improve a patient's medication adherence.
- Safely and correctly administer a medication by oral, enteral, and topical routes.
- Identify guidelines for administering oral, enteral, and topical medications.
- Describe factors to assess before administering medications.
- Differentiate types of topical administrations that require sterile technique and those that require clean medical aseptic technique.
- Instruct patients in the proper use of a metered-dose inhaler, a dry powder inhaler, and a small-volume nebulizer.
- Identify conditions contraindicating the administration of medications by various oral and topical routes.
- Prepare a teaching plan regarding medication use for a selected patient.

MEDIA RESOURCES

- http://evolve.elsevier.com/Canada/Perry/clinicalskills/

PURPOSE

Nonparenteral medications include those that are administered orally, enterally, or topically. Nonparenteral medications exclude any medication administered via an injection or intravenous infusion. The nonparenteral route chosen depends on the properties and desired effects of the medication and the physical and mental condition of a patient. There are many reasons why it may be necessary to change from one route to another. When this situation arises, the nurse is responsible for consulting with a health care provider for a prescription or conferring with the pharmacist to safely meet a patient's needs.

STANDARDS OF CARE

- Accreditation Canada (2019)—*Required Organizational Practices Handbook, Version 14* (https://physicians.nshealth.ca/resources/required-organizational-practices-2020-handbook)
- Accreditation Canada (2020)—*Required Organizational Practices–2020 Handbook* (https://physicians.nshealth.ca/resources/required-organizational-practices-2020-handbook)
- Institute for Safe Medication Practices (ISMP) and ISMP Canada:

- ISMP (2011)–*Guidelines for Timely Administration of Scheduled Medications (Acute)* (https://www.ismp.org/guidelines/timely-administration-scheduled-medications-acute)
- ISMP Canada (2018)–*Do Not Use. Dangerous Abbreviations, Symbols, and Dose Designations* (https://www.ismp-canada.org/download/ISMPCanadaListOfDangerousAbbreviations.pdf)
- ISMP (2019b)–*List of Confused Drug Names* (https://www.ismp.org/recommendations/confused-drug-names-list)
- ISMP (2020)–*Oral Dosage Forms That Should Not Be Crushed** (https://www.ismp.org/recommendations/do-not-crush)
- ISMP (2022)–*2022–2023 Targeted Medication Safety Best Practices for Hospitals* (https://www.ismp.org/guidelines/best-practices-hospitals)

PRINCIPLES FOR PRACTICE

- The major principle for practice regarding nonparenteral medication administration is patient safety (see Safety Guidelines).
- The oral route (by mouth) is the easiest and most desirable way to administer medications.
- Topical administration of medications involves applying medications directly to skin or mucous or tissue membranes. Box 21.1 provides examples of topical medication routes.
- Medications are applied to the skin by spraying, painting, or spreading medication over a localized area. Transdermal patches (adhesive-backed medicated discs) applied to the skin provide a continuous release of medication over several hours or days.
- Medications applied to membranes such as the cornea of the eye or the rectal mucosa are absorbed quickly because of the vascularity of the membrane; they can also have systemic effects. In addition, nurses can experience systemic effects of a topical medication if they do not wear clean gloves.

PERSON-CENTRED CARE

- An excellent time to provide patient education is during medication administration. The nurse must assess the patient's and caregiver's health literacy, health beliefs, and cultural practices.
- The goal of patient education is to improve patient adherence to medication regimens. Patients fail to adhere to medication regimens because of patient, medication, and health care provider issues. Patient issues include medication knowledge, health literacy, and financial limitations. Clear, concise, and, at times, one-on-one patient education can improve adherence to medication, which in turn improves patient outcomes (Ampofo et al., 2020; Lilley et al., 2020).
- Print materials used for instruction should be written at an appropriate reading level (e.g., Grade 6) and delivered in a manner that meets individual patient needs such as visual impairment or hearing or cognitive impairments. Involve caregivers in the education sessions because they may be the ones administering medications.
- Cognitive impairment and depression have an effect on health literacy. Individualized patient education techniques that simplify tasks and patient roles may help to overcome cognitive load and suboptimal performance in self-administration of medication (Dineen-Griffin et al., 2019).
- Medication issues related to medication nonadherence include complex medication regimens and medication discrepancies. Health care provider issues include poor instruction, inappropriate prescriptions, and lack of provider knowledge about adherence. Patients need explanations about the purpose of medications, benefits, expected effects, and how to plan a daily schedule.
- Health beliefs vary by culture and influence how patients manage and respond to medication therapy. Differences in values, attitudes, and beliefs affect a patient's adherence to medication therapy. For example, herbal remedies and alternative therapies may be common practice in some cultures and interfere with prescribed medications. It is also important to consider cultural influences on medication response, metabolism, and adverse effects if a patient is not responding to medication therapy as expected. For example, certain cultural food preferences may have food–medication interactions.
- Vegetarian diets can affect warfarin or medications for glycemic control. The prescriber may need to make a change in the medication, or the patient may need counselling about how to change their dietary patterns.

*The ISMP removed the "do not crush" list from its website on November 17, 2022. The organization encourages health care providers and institutions to maintain, update, and periodically review oral dosage forms that may require alteration.

BOX 21.1

Examples of Topical Medication Routes

1. *Sublingual:* Medication placed under the tongue; is dissolvable
2. *Buccal:* Medication placed between the cheek area and either upper or lower molars; is dissolvable
3. *Direct application to skin or mucosa:* Lotion, ointment, cream, powder, foam, spray, patch, and disc
4. *Direct application to mucous membrane:* Eyedrops, gargling, swabbing the throat
5. *Spraying:* Instillation into nose or throat
6. *Inhalation of medicated aerosol spray:* Distributes medication throughout the nasal passages and the tracheobronchial airway; two types of devices designed for this purpose: metered-dose inhalers (MDIs) and small-volume nebulizers
7. *Inhalation of dry powder medication:* Distributes medication in powder form throughout the tracheobronchial airway; device designed for this purpose: dry powder inhaler (DPI)
8. *Inserting medication into a body cavity:* Rectal or vaginal suppositories, vaginal creams, or foams

EVIDENCE-INFORMED PRACTICE

- Medication competency is a skill that all nurses must possess to improve the quality and safety of medication administration. When nurses follow the 10 rights of medication administration (see Chapter 20) and the ISMP Canada guidelines (i.e., timely administration, correct crushing and splitting of pills, avoiding confusing abbreviations, and double-checking for sound-alike/look-alike medications), medication errors are reduced (ISMP, 2011, 2019b, 2020; 2022; ISMP Canada, 2018).
- Knowledge of technology and nurse competencies is essential to increase patient safety and promote best practices (Astier et al., 2020; Cho & Choi, 2018).
- Use of medication administration technology, such as bar code medication administration (BCMA) or automated dispensing medication cabinets (e.g., Pyxis), helps to verify that the right patient receives the right medication in the right dose via the right route at the right time and also reduces medication errors (Metsämuuronen et al., 2020; Risør et al., 2018).
- Evidence suggests that a quiet environment free of distractions and interruptions allows the nurse to focus when preparing medications. Thus, having a medication zone free of distractions, clutter, and interruptions helps reduce the risk for medication errors (Kavanagh & Donnelly, 2020).

- Nurses need to follow best practices for calculating medication doses, double-check the calculations, and *not* administer medication if the dosage appears incorrect (Douglass et al., 2018). They should follow employer policy for medication calculations for the very young or when preparing high-risk medications (e.g., cardiotonics, insulin, and some opioid medications).
- Best practice guidelines for safe medication administration require critical thinking, clinical decision-making competency, and theoretical and clinical practice competency. Medication administration is not a routine nursing action; nurses must adhere to the 10 rights of medication administration at all times to ensure patient safety. As a nurse, you must think critically about the medications you are giving. For instance, you might ask yourself, "Is the medication still appropriate for the patient's condition or do I need to contact the health care provider?" Or you might pause and think, "This pill looks different. I need to verify with pharmacy" (Hanson & Haddad, 2021; Martyn et al., 2019).

SAFETY GUIDELINES

- Safe medication administration requires that nurses follow the 10 rights of medication administration for all nonparenteral medications. Nurses should also know the ISMP (2022) guidelines, medication actions and interactions, and potential side effects and adverse effects and how to safely administer medication through various nonparenteral routes. When the 10 rights (see Chapter 20) are not followed, negative and sometimes harmful effects can occur. For example, administering medications to the wrong patient can result in major health consequences (e.g., the patient could develop hypoglycemia if insulin is administered), as can giving a patient an incorrect dose (e.g., too much morphine could cause respiratory depression).
- Assess a patient's sensory function, including sight, hearing, touch, and physical coordination and dexterity. Sensory function and coordination deficits impair a patient's ability to see medications, read labels at home, and discriminate one medication from another. Coordination and dexterity impairments reduce a patient's ability to open prescription bottles and dispense the correct dosage.
- Patients often receive more than one oral medication at a time. It is important to evaluate each medication for potential medication–medication or medication–food interactions. When unsure, consult with a pharmacist to clarify the risk of an interaction and determine the measure to reduce it.
- Some medications require double-checks by two nurses to ensure that the right medication and right dose are given (always check employer policy as to which medications require double-checks by two nurses). Double-checks are carried out for high-risk medications (e.g., insulin), in pediatric settings, and for chemotherapy medications (Washburn et al., 2021; Westbrook et al., 2021).
- Nurses must always assess for medication allergies. If the patient reports having an allergy, ask about the type of reaction that occurred.
- Evaluate whether the patient can take medication with food. In most cases, the presence of food in the stomach delays medication absorption. However, some medications must be taken before meals, and others may need to be taken with meals. Some medications irritate the stomach lining and need to be taken with food.
- For all medications administered, review the prescription for the patient's name, medication, dosage, route, and time of administration.
- Use the correct equipment for administering all medications. For example, when delivering liquid medications, use only unit-dose containers dispensed by the pharmacy (ISMP, 2022).
- For all medications administered, gather information pertinent to the medication(s) prescribed: purpose, normal dosage and route, common side effects, time of onset and peak, contraindications, and nursing implications.
- Determine whether any of the medications require specific nursing actions (e.g., obtaining vital signs, medication levels, or electrolytes) before administration.
- Prepare the patient for discharge by instructing them in self-administration techniques, as appropriate. Include caregivers if possible.
- Check the expiration date on all medications.

✦ SKILL 21.1 Administering Oral Medications

Video Clip NSO Nursing Skills Online Nonparenteral Medication Administration Module 6 / Lesson 1

Patients are usually able to ingest or self-administer oral medications with few problems. If oral medications are contraindicated (e.g., inability to swallow, gastric suction), it is important to take precautions to protect patients from aspiration (see Skill 31.3). Nurses usually prepare medications in areas designed for medication preparation or at unit-dose carts.

The form or preparation of an oral medication affects how well it is absorbed after being ingested. Liquids are absorbed faster than tablets or capsules and are usually absorbed in the stomach. Give an oral medication with a meal if its absorption is enhanced by the presence of food in the stomach. Some medications must be taken between meals, 2 to 3 hours after eating (Lilley et al., 2020). When administering multiple oral medications, give oral medications before sublingual and buccal medications. Use interprofessional collaboration (e.g., pharmacist) for further guidance as required.

Other oral medications are absorbed in the intestinal tract. Enteric-coated preparations resist being dissolved by gastric juices. The enteric coating protects the stomach lining from being irritated by the medication. These preparations are absorbed in the small intestine. Never crush or split an enteric-coated medication. Crushing or splitting these preparations causes the medication to be released too early; the medication may become inactive in the stomach or fail to reach the intended site of action (ISMP, 2020).

Delegation and Collaboration

The skill of administering oral medications may be delegated to an unregulated care provider (UCP) in some jurisdictions (e.g., in the home setting). Always check employer policy. The nurse instructs the UCP about the following:

- Potential adverse effects of medications and reporting their occurrence
- Informing the nurse if the patient's condition changes or worsens (e.g., pain, itching, or rash) after medication administration

Equipment

- Medication administration record (MAR) (electronic or printed)
- Automated, computer-controlled medication dispensing system (i.e., ADS) or unit-dose medication cart
- Oral syringes marked "oral use only"
- Glass of water, juice, or preferred liquid and drinking straw
- Device for crushing or splitting tablets *(optional)*
- Paper towels
- Clean gloves (if handling an oral medication). NOTE: Gloves must be worn when administering an oral chemotherapy medication.
- Medication cup

STEP	RATIONALE
ASSESSMENT	
1. Identify patient using at least two person-specific identifiers (e.g., name and date of birth or name and medical record number) according to employer policy.	Ensures correct patient. Complies with Accreditation Canada's standards and improves patient safety (Accreditation Canada, 2020).
2. Throughout the procedure, the 4 moments for hand hygiene are to be implemented; hand hygiene should occur before initial patient (or patient environment) contact, before an aseptic procedure, after body fluid exposure risk, and after patient (or patient environment) contact. Additional hand hygiene should be performed when hands are visibly soiled.	Proper hand hygiene helps prevent the spread of infectious agents to health care providers.
3. Check accuracy and completeness of each MAR by comparing with health care provider's medication prescription. Check patient's name and medication name, dosage, and route and time of administration. Clarify incomplete or unclear prescriptions with health care provider before administration.	The prescription sheet is the most reliable source and only legal record of medications that patient is to receive. It ensures that patient receives correct medication (College of Physicians and Surgeons of Ontario, 2019; Pharmacy Association of Nova Scotia, n.d.). Handwritten MARs are a source of medication errors (Parthasarathi et al., 2021; Tariq et al., 2022).
4. Review pertinent information related to medication, including action, purpose, normal dose and route, adverse effects, time of onset and peak action, and nursing implications.	Allows you to anticipate effects of medication and observe patient's response.
5. Assess for any contraindications to patient receiving oral medication, including being on NPO (nothing by mouth) status, inability to swallow, nausea/vomiting, bowel inflammation, reduced peristalsis, recent gastrointestinal (GI) surgery, gastric suction, and decreased level of consciousness (LOC). Notify health care provider if any contraindications are present.	Alterations in GI function can interfere with medication absorption, distribution, and excretion. Giving oral medications to patients with impaired swallowing or decreased LOC increases their risk of aspiration (Zuercher et al., 2019). Patients with GI suction do not receive actions of oral medications because the medications are suctioned from the GI tract before they can be absorbed.
6. Assess risk for aspiration using a dysphagia screening tool if available (see Skill 31.3). Protect patient from aspiration by assessing swallowing ability (Box 21.2).	Aspiration occurs when food, fluid, or medication intended for GI administration is inadvertently administered into the respiratory tract. Patients with altered ability to swallow are at higher risk of aspiration (Zuercher et al., 2019).
7. Assess patient's medical, medication, and diet history and history of allergies. List any medication allergies on each page of MAR (in red ink) and prominently display on patient's medical record. When allergies are present, patient should wear an allergy bracelet.	Information reflects patient's need for and potential responses to medication. Information reveals potential food and medication interactions. Communication of allergies is essential for safe, effective patient care.
8. Gather and review physical assessment findings and laboratory data that influence medication administration, such as vital signs and results of renal and liver function studies.	Data may reveal need to contraindicate medication administration. Renal and liver function status affects metabolism and excretion of medications (Lilley et al., 2020).
9. Assess patient's knowledge regarding health and medication use, medication schedule, and ability to prepare medications.	Determines patient's need for medication education and guidance needed to achieve medication adherence (e.g., involvement of caregiver).
10. Assess patient's preference for fluids and determine whether medications can be given with these fluids. Maintain fluid restrictions as prescribed.	Some fluids interfere with medication absorption (e.g., dairy products affect tetracycline). Offering fluids during medication administration is an excellent way to increase patient's fluid intake. Fluids ease swallowing and facilitate absorption from the GI tract. However, fluid restrictions exist; skillful planning of fluid intake must be coordinated with medication administration times and type of medications.

NURSING DIAGNOSES

- Inadequate swallowing
- Inadequate knowledge regarding medications and medication administration
- Readiness for enhanced self-health management
- Potential for nonadherence
- Potential for aspiration

Related factors and risk factors are individualized on the basis of patient's condition or needs.

BOX 21.2

Protecting the Patient From Aspiration

- Assess patient's ability to swallow and cough and check for presence of gag reflex.
- Prepare oral medication in form that is easiest to swallow.
- Allow patient to self-administer medications if possible.
- If patient has unilateral (one-sided) weakness, place medication on stronger side of mouth.
- Administer pills one at a time, ensuring that each medication is properly swallowed before next one is introduced.
- Thicken regular liquids or offer fruit nectars if patient cannot tolerate thin liquids.
- Avoid straws because they decrease control patient has over volume intake, which increases risk of aspiration.
- Have patient hold and drink from a cup if possible.
- Time medications to coincide with meals or when patient is well rested and awake, if possible.
- Administer medications using another route if risk of aspiration is severe.

STEP	RATIONALE
PLANNING	
1. Expected outcomes following completion of procedure:	
• Patient responds appropriately to desired medication effect within period of onset of medication action.	Medication has exerted its therapeutic action.
• Patient denies any GI discomfort or symptoms of alterations.	Oral medications can irritate GI mucosa.
• Patient explains purpose of medication and medication dosage schedule.	Demonstrates understanding of medication therapy.
2. Explain procedure to patient. Be specific if patient wishes to self-administer medications.	Makes patient a participant in care, which minimizes anxiety. Begins patient teaching regarding medications. Prepares patient to self-administer medication, which increases feelings of independence.
3. Collect appropriate equipment and MAR.	Promotes time management and efficiency when preparing medications for all patients.
4. Plan preparation of medication to avoid interruptions and distractions. Do not take phone calls or talk with others (see employer policy).	Interruptions contribute to occurrence of medication administration errors (Kavanagh & Donnelly, 2020).
IMPLEMENTATION	
1. Prepare medications.	
a. Arrange medication tray and cups in medication preparation area or move medication cart to position outside patient's room.	Organization of equipment saves time and reduces error.
b. Log on to ADS or unlock medicine drawer or cart.	Medications are safeguarded when locked in cabinet, cart, or ADS.
c. Prepare medications for *one patient at a time.* Follow the 10 rights of medication administration. Keep all pages of MARs or computer printouts for one patient together or look at only one patient's medication administration computer screen.	Prevents preparation errors.
d. Select correct medication from ADS, unit-dose drawer, or stock supply. Compare name of medication on label with MAR or computer printout (see Step 1d illustration). Exit ADS after removing medication(s).	Reading label and comparing it against transcribed prescription reduces errors. Exiting ADS ensures that no one else can remove medications using your identity. *This is the first check for accuracy.*

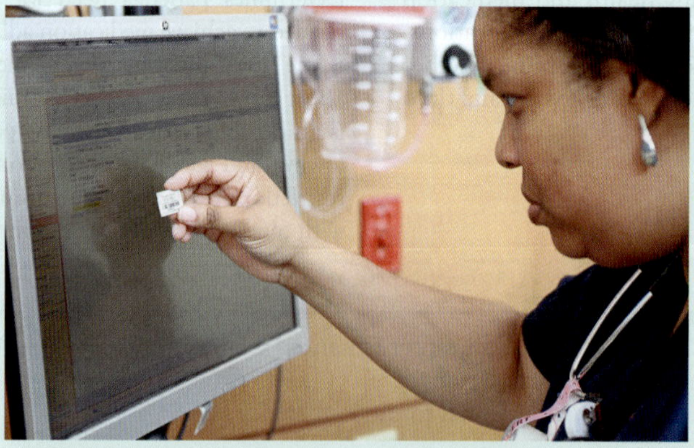

STEP 1D Nurse compares label of medication with transcribed medication prescription on computerized MAR.

STEP	RATIONALE

IMPLEMENTATION

STEP	RATIONALE
e. Check or calculate medication dose as necessary. Double-check any calculation. Check expiration date on all medications and return outdated medication to pharmacy.	Double-checking pharmacy calculations reduces risk for error. Employer policy may require you to check calculations of certain medications (e.g., insulin) with another nurse (ISMP, 2019a; Lilley et al., 2020). Expired medications may be inactive or harm patient.
f. If preparing a controlled substance, check record for previous medication count and compare current count with available supply. Controlled medications may be stored in a computerized locked cart (see Chapter 20).	Controlled substance laws require nurses to carefully monitor and count dispensed narcotics.
g. Prepare solid forms of oral medications.	
(1) To prepare unit-dose tablets or capsules, place packaged tablet or capsule directly into medication cup without removing wrapper. Administer medications only from containers with labels that are clearly marked. Double-check medication label with patient MAR.	Wrappers maintain cleanliness and identify medication name and dose, which can facilitate teaching. *This is the second check for accuracy.*
(2) When using a blister pack, "pop" medications through foil or paper backing into a medication cup.	Packs provide a 1-month supply, with each "blister" usually containing a single dose.
(3) If it is necessary to give half the dose of medication, pharmacy should split, label, package, and send medication to unit. If you need to split a medication, cut with a clean pillating device. Tablets that can be cut in half must be prescored (i.e., have a manufactured line that traverses the centre of the tablet).	Reduces contamination of tablet.
(4) Place all tablets or capsules that patient will receive in one medicine cup, except for medications requiring preadministration assessments (e.g., pulse rate or blood pressure). Place those medications in separate, additional cup with wrapper intact.	Keeping medications that require preadministration assessments separate from others serves as reminder and makes it easier to withhold medications as necessary.
(5) If patient has difficulty swallowing and liquid medications are not an option, use a pill-crushing device. Clean device before using. Place medicine between two cups, and grind and crush (see Step 1g[5] illustration). Mix ground tablet in small amount (teaspoon) of soft food (custard or applesauce).	Large tablets are often difficult to swallow. Ground tablet mixed with palatable, soft food is usually easier to swallow.

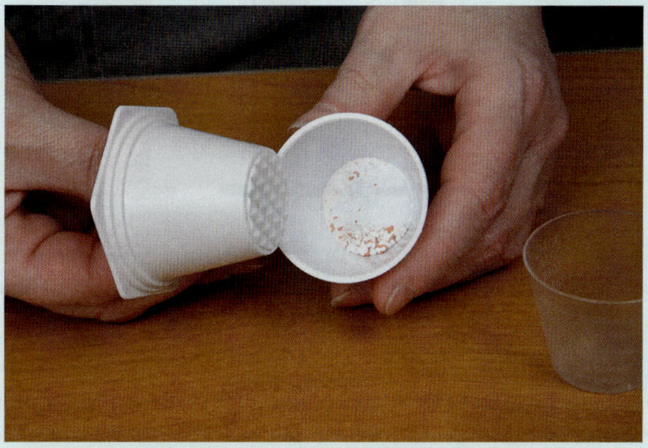

STEP 1G(5) Crushing tablet with pill-crushing device.

Critical Decision Point *Not all medications can be crushed safely (e.g., capsules, enteric-coated pills). Use interprofessional collaboration (e.g., pharmacist) or the* ISMP's (2020) *"do not crush" list when unsure whether it is safe to crush a medication.*

STEP	RATIONALE

IMPLEMENTATION

h. Prepare liquids.

(1) Use unit-dose container with correct amount of medication. Gently shake container. Administer medication packaged in a single-dose cup directly from the single-dose cup. Double-check medication label with patient MAR. Do not pour medicine into another cup. Check expiration date.	Using unit-dose container with correct dosage of medication provides most accurate dose of medication (ISMP, 2022). Shaking container ensures that medication is mixed before administration. *This is the second check for accuracy.*

Critical Decision Point *On the basis of current best practice* (ISMP, 2022), *liquid medications that are not available or are not in correct dose in a unit-dose container should be dispensed by the pharmacy in special oral syringes marked "Oral Use Only." These syringes do not connect to any type of parenteral (e.g., intravenous [IV]) tubing. In addition, current evidence shows that use of liquid measuring devices on patient care units leads to inaccurate dosing. Having oral medications prepared in the pharmacy ensures that you give the most accurate dose possible of a medication and prevents parenteral administration of oral medications.*

(2) Administer medications in "oral use only" syringes prepared by pharmacy (see Step 2h[2] illustration). *Do not* use hypodermic syringe or syringe with needle or syringe cap (see Chapter 20).	Only use syringes specifically designed for oral use when administering liquid medications. If using hypodermic syringes, the medication may be administered parenterally accidently; or the syringe cap or needle, if not removed from the syringe before administration, may become dislodged and accidently aspirated during administration of oral medications (ISMP, 2022).
(3) Gently shake container. If medication is in a multidose bottle, remove bottle cap from container and place cap upside down on work surface.	
(4) Hold bottle with label against palm of hand while pouring.	Allows more accurate measurement of small amounts.
(5) Hold medication cup at eye level and fill to desired level on scale. Scale should be even with fluid level at its surface or base of meniscus.	
(6) Discard any excess liquid into sink. Wipe lip and neck of bottle with paper towel and recap bottle.	
(7) For doses of liquid medications less than 10 mL, draw liquid into a calibrated oral syringe.	

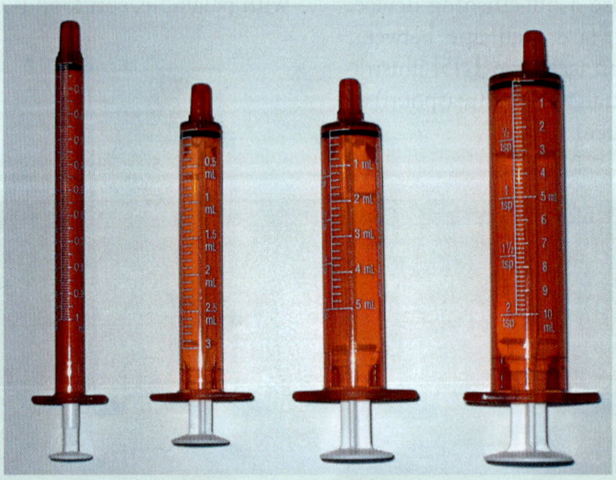

STEP 1H(2) Use special oral medication syringes to prepare small amounts of liquid medications.

i. Check the medication label one more time before returning stock containers or unused unit-dose medications to shelf or drawer. Label medication cups and poured medications with patient's name before leaving medication preparation area. Never leave medications unattended.	Ensures that correct medications are prepared for correct patient. *This is the third check for accuracy.*
2. Identify patient using at least two person-specific identifiers (e.g., name and date of birth, or name and medical record number) according to employer policy.	Ensures correct patient. Complies with Accreditation Canada's standards and improves patient safety (Accreditation Canada, 2020).

STEP	RATIONALE

IMPLEMENTATION

STEP	RATIONALE
3. Administer medications.	
a. Take medication(s) to patient at correct time (see employer policy). Medications that require exact timing include stat, first-time or loading doses, and one-time doses. Give time-critical scheduled medications (e.g., antibiotics, anticoagulants, insulin, anticonvulsants, immunosuppressive medications) at exact time prescribed (no later than 30 minutes before or after scheduled dose). Give non–time-critical scheduled medications within a range of 1 or 2 hours of scheduled dose, according to employer policy (ISMP, 2011). During administration, apply 10 rights of medication administration.	Employers must adopt medication administration policy and procedure for timing of medication administration that considers nature of the prescribed medication, specific clinical application, and patient needs. Time-critical scheduled medications are those for which early or delayed administration of maintenance doses of greater than 30 minutes before or after the scheduled dose may cause harm or result in substantially suboptimal therapy or pharmacological effect. Non–time-critical medications are those for which early or delayed administration within a specified range of either 1 or 2 hours should not cause harm or result in substantially suboptimal therapy or pharmacological effect (ISMP, 2011).
b. At patient's bedside, again compare MAR or computer printout with names of medications on medication labels and patient name. Ask patient whether they have allergies.	Ensures that right patient receives right medication. Confirms patient's allergy history.
c. Explain the purpose, action, and most common possible adverse effects of each medication. Allow sufficient time for patient to ask questions.	Patient has right to be informed, and their understanding of each medication improves adherence to medication therapy.
d. Perform necessary preadministration assessment (e.g., blood pressure, pulse) for specific medications. Ask patient whether they have allergies.	Determines whether specific medications should be withheld at that time. Confirms patient's allergy history.

Critical Decision Point *If patient expresses concern regarding accuracy of a medication, do not give the medication. Explore patient's concern and verify health care provider's prescription before administering. Listening to patient's concerns may prevent a medication error.*

STEP	RATIONALE
e. Help patient to sitting or Fowler's position. Use side-lying position if they are unable to sit. Have patient stay in this position for 30 minutes after administration.	Decreases risk of aspiration during swallowing.
f. *For tablets:* Patient may wish to hold solid medications in hand or cup before placing in mouth. Offer water or preferred liquid to help patient swallow medications.	Patient can become familiar with medications by seeing each medication. Choice of fluid can improve fluid intake.

Critical Decision Point *If administering an oral chemotherapy medication, administer it from the cup directly into the patient's mouth or apply gloves before handling pill or tablet. Never use bare hands to touch a chemotherapy medication, as residue can be absorbed through your skin* (Kennedy et al., 2022; Lilley et al., 2020).

STEP	RATIONALE
g. *For orally disintegrating formulations (tablets or strips):* Remove medication from packet just before use. Do not push tablet through foil. Place medication on top of patient's tongue. Caution against chewing it.	Orally disintegrating formulations begin to dissolve when placed on tongue. Water is not needed. Careful removal from packaging is necessary because tablets and strips are thin and fragile.
h. *For sublingual medications:* Have patient place medication under tongue and allow it to dissolve completely (see Step 3h illustration). Caution patient against swallowing tablet.	Medication is absorbed through blood vessels in undersurface of tongue. If swallowed, medication is destroyed by gastric juices or rapidly detoxified by the liver, preventing therapeutic blood level.
i. *For buccal medications:* Have patient place medication in mouth against mucous membranes of cheek and gums until it dissolves (see Step 3i illustration).	Buccal medications act locally or systemically as they are swallowed in saliva.

STEP	RATIONALE

IMPLEMENTATION

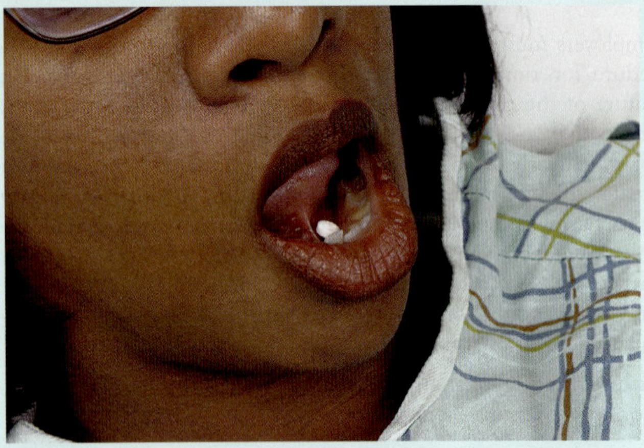

STEP 3H Proper placement of sublingual tablet in sublingual pocket.

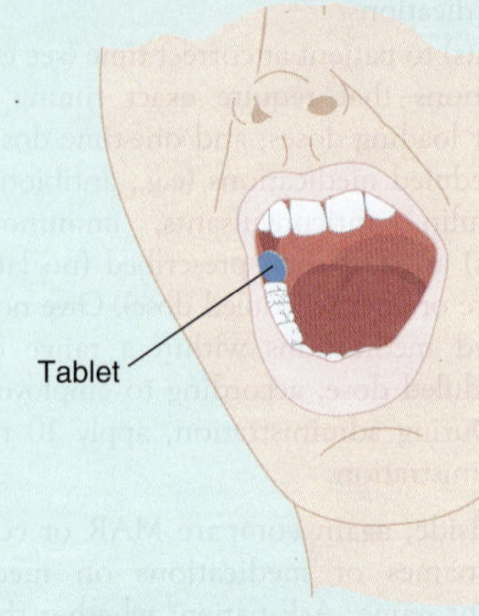

STEP 3I Buccal administration of tablet.

Critical Decision Point *Avoid administering anything by mouth until orally disintegrating buccal or sublingual medication is completely dissolved.*

STEP	RATIONALE
j. *For powdered medications:* Mix with liquids at bedside and give to patient to drink.	When prepared in advance, powdered medications thicken; some even harden, making swallowing difficult.
k. *For crushed medications mixed with food:* Give each medication separately in teaspoon of food.	Ensures that patient swallows all of medicine.
l. *For lozenge:* Caution patient against chewing or swallowing lozenges.	Lozenges act through slow absorption through oral mucosa, not gastric mucosa.
m. *For effervescent medication:* Add tablet or powder to glass of water. Administer immediately after dissolving.	Effervescence improves unpleasant taste and often relieves GI problems.
n. If patient is unable to hold medications, place medication cup to lips and gently introduce each medication into mouth one at a time. A spoon can also be used to place pill in patient's mouth. Do not rush or force medications.	Administering a single tablet or capsule eases swallowing and decreases risk of aspiration.

Critical Decision Point *If tablet or capsule falls to the floor, discard it and repeat preparation. Medication is contaminated.*

STEP	RATIONALE
o. Stay until patient swallows each medication completely or takes it by the prescribed route. Ask patient to open mouth if uncertain whether medication has been swallowed.	Ensures that patient receives prescribed dose. If left unattended, patient may not take dose or may save medications, causing health risks.
p. For highly acidic medications (e.g., Aspirin), offer patient a nonfat snack (e.g., crackers) if not contraindicated by their condition.	Reduces gastric irritation. Fat content of foods may delay medication absorption.
5. Help patient return to position of comfort.	Maintains patient's comfort.
6. Dispose of soiled supplies. Return cart to medication room if used. Clean work area.	Reduces spread of microorganisms.
7. Replenish stock such as cups and straws, return cart to medication room, and clean work area.	Enhances efficiency and reduces transfer of microorganisms.

STEP	RATIONALE
EVALUATION	
1. Return to bedside to evaluate patient's response to medications at times that correlate with onset, peak, and duration of medication action.	Evaluates therapeutic benefit of medication and helps detect onset of adverse effects or allergic reactions. Sublingual medications act in 15 minutes; most oral medications act in 30–60 minutes.
2. Ask patient or caregiver to identify medication name and explain purpose, action, dose schedule, and potential side effects.	Determines level of knowledge gained by patient and caregiver.
3. Use **teach-back:** "I want to be sure I showed you how to use your sublingual nitroglycerine. Show me where you will place your pill in your mouth." Develop a revised teaching plan if patient or caregiver is unable to teach back correctly.	Determines patient's and caregiver's level of understanding of instructional topic.

Unexpected Outcomes	Related Interventions
1. Patient exhibits adverse effects (e.g., side effect, toxic effect, allergic reaction).	• Notify health care provider and pharmacy. • Withhold further doses. • Assess vital signs. • Symptoms such as urticaria, rash, pruritus, rhinitis, and wheezing may indicate an allergic reaction and need for emergency medications. • Add allergy information to patient's medical record.
2. Patient refuses medication.	• Assess why patient is refusing medication. • Provide further instruction. • Do not force patient to take medications. • Notify health care provider.
3. Patient is unable to explain medication information.	• Further assess patient's or caregiver's knowledge of medications and guidelines for medication safety. • Further instruction or different approach to instruction is necessary.

Communication and Documentation

- Document medication, dose, route, and time administered on patient's MAR immediately after administration, not before. Include initials or signature.
- Document patient's response to medication, patient teaching, and validation of patient's understanding on flow sheet or in progress notes in electronic health record (EHR) or chart.
- If medication is withheld or refused, document reason on flow sheet or in progress notes in EHR or chart and follow employer policy for noting withheld doses.
- Report adverse effects, patient response, and/or withheld medications to nurse in charge or health care provider. Depending on medication, immediate notification of health care provider may be required.

DOCUMENTATION EXAMPLE

Patient administered digoxin 0.125 mg PO as prescribed. Heart rate 75 beats per minute. Patient verbalized understanding of why they are taking this medication and why their heart rate was checked prior to administration.

Special Considerations

Teaching

- Instruct patient and caregiver about specific information pertaining to medication regimen (purpose, action, dose, dosage intervals, adverse effects, foods to avoid or take with medications).
- If patient is taking multiple medications, consider recommending a dose organizer. Use interprofessional collaboration (e.g., pharmacist) to assist patients with organizing their medications, and consider the use of blister packs with the times for administration highlighted.
- All patients should learn the basic guidelines for medication safety in the home (see Skill 42.3).

Pediatric

- Liquid forms of medication are safer for children to swallow; avoid small pills, as these can be aspirated.
- Children refuse bitter or unpleasant-tasting oral preparations. Mix the medication with a small amount (about 5 mL) of a sweet-tasting substance such as jam, applesauce, sherbet, ice cream, or fruit puree. Do not use honey for infants because of the risk of botulism. Offer the child juice or a flavoured ice pop after medication administration. Do not place medication in an essential food item such as milk or formula; the child may refuse the food at a later time.
- Measure liquid medications with a plastic calibrated oral dosing syringe or a spoon. Using interprofessional collaboration, nurses and pharmacists can teach parents how to draw up liquid medications prior to discharge.

Gerontological

- Physiological changes of aging influence how oral medications are distributed, absorbed, and excreted. Common changes include loss of elasticity in oral mucosa; reduction in parotid gland secretion, causing dry mouth; delayed esophageal clearance; impaired swallowing; reduction in gastric acidity and stomach peristalsis; increased susceptibility to highly acidic medications; reduced liver function, resulting in altered medication metabolism; and reduced renal function and colon motility, slowing medication excretion (Boscart et al., 2023). Both altered medication metabolism and excretion may lead to medication toxicity (Boscart et al., 2023; Lilley et al., 2020).

- Give medications with a full glass of water (unless restricted) to aid passage of the medication. Give patient time to swallow.
- Patients may have several health problems or chronic conditions requiring the use of multiple medications often prescribed by different health care providers. Polypharmacy creates a high risk for medication interactions and adverse reactions (National Institute on Aging, 2021).

Care in the Community: Home Management

- Instruct patients and caregivers on how to accurately use a dosing cup to administer liquid medications at home (see Chapter 20).
- See Skills 42.3 and 43.6.

SKILL 21.2 Administering Medications Through a Feeding Tube

NSO *Nursing Skills Online Nonparenteral Medication Administration Module 6 / Lesson 2*

Patients who have enteral feeding tubes are unable to receive food or medications by mouth. Nasogastric (NG) feeding tubes generally are small-bore tubes that are inserted into the stomach via one of the nares (see Chapter 32). For long-term enteral feedings, a percutaneous endoscopic gastrostomy (PEG) tube or a jejunostomy tube may be inserted surgically. *Do not administer medications into NG tubes that are inserted for decompression.*

In addition to administering the correct medication, it is important that the enteral access connector be appropriate for the type of enteral tube (Lord, 2018). These devices are not compatible with Luer or needleless connectors. They are designed for specific enteral feeding tubes. The goal of these new access connectors is to reduce enteral tube misconnections and medication errors (Lord, 2018; US FDA, 2023).

Preferably, medications administered by enteral tubes should be in liquid form. However, when the liquid form of the medication is not available, you need to prepare an oral medication tablet or capsule by crushing or dissolving it. Facility pharmacies may be able to provide the prescribed medication in a liquid suspension, which does not affect its effectiveness (Health Canada, 2009; US FDA, 2022). However, *do not crush* sublingual, sustained-release, chewable, long-acting, capsule, or enteric-coated medications. Use interprofessional collaboration (e.g., pharmacist) to confirm whether you may crush or dissolve a medication. Always verify correct placement of an NG tube before administering medications (see Skill 32.2).

Delegation and Collaboration

The skill of administering medications by enteral feeding tubes cannot be delegated to a UCP. The nurse instructs the UCP to do the following:

- Keep the head of the bed elevated a minimum of 30 degrees (preferably 45 degrees) for 1 hour after medication administration (follow employer policy)
- Report immediately to the nurse coughing, choking, gagging, or drooling of liquid or dissolved pills
- Report to the nurse occurrence of possible medication adverse effects (specific to medication)

Equipment

- MAR (electronic or printed)
- Appropriate medication syringe or 60-mL Asepto syringe for large-bore tubes only
- Enteral-only connector (ENFit) designed to fit the specific enteral tube (Fig. 21.1)
- Gastric pH test strip (scale of 1 to 11)
- Graduated container
- Medication to be administered
- Pill crusher (for medication in tablet form)
- Water or sterile water for immunocompromised patients
- Tongue blade or straw to stir dissolved medication
- Clean gloves
- Stethoscope and pulse oximeter (for evaluation)

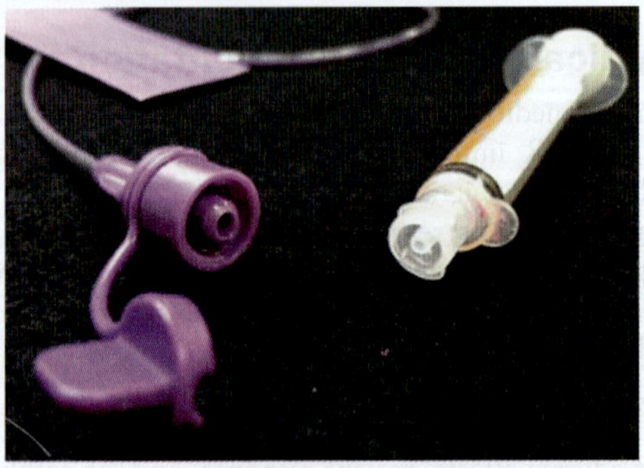

FIG 21.1 Enteral connector.

STEP	RATIONALE
ASSESSMENT	
1. Identify patient using at least two person-specific identifiers (e.g., name and date of birth or name and medical record number) according to employer policy.	Ensures correct patient. Complies with Accreditation Canada's standards and improves patient safety (Accreditation Canada, 2020).
2. Throughout the procedure, the 4 moments for hand hygiene are to be implemented; hand hygiene should occur before initial patient (or patient environment) contact, before an aseptic procedure, after body fluid exposure risk, and after patient (or patient environment) contact. Additional hand hygiene should be performed when hands are visibly soiled.	Proper hand hygiene helps prevent the spread of infectious agents to health care providers.

STEP	RATIONALE

ASSESSMENT

STEP	RATIONALE
3. Check accuracy and completeness of each MAR by comparing with health care provider's medication prescription. Check patient's name, medication name and dosage, route of administration, and time for administration. Clarify incomplete or unclear prescriptions with health care provider before administration.	The prescription sheet is the most reliable source and only legal record of medications that patient is to receive. Ensures that patient receives correct medication (College of Physicians and Surgeons of Ontario, 2019; Pharmacy Association of Nova Scotia, n.d.). Handwritten MARs are a source of medication errors (Parthasarathi et al., 2021; Tariq et al., 2022).
4. Review pertinent information related to medication, including action, purpose, normal dose and route, adverse effects, time of onset and peak action, and nursing implications.	Allows you to anticipate effects of medication and observe patient's response.
5. Assess for any contraindications to receiving enteral medications, including presence of bowel inflammation, reduced peristalsis, recent GI surgery, and gastric suction that cannot be turned off.	Alterations in GI function can interfere with medication absorption, distribution, and excretion. Patients with GI suction do not benefit from medication because it may be suctioned from the GI tract before it can be absorbed.
6. Assess patient's medical, medication, and diet history and history of allergies. List patient's food and medication allergies on each page of the MAR and prominently display it on the patient's medical record per employer policy. When patient has allergy, provide allergy bracelet. If you identify contraindications, withhold medication and inform health care provider.	Information reflects patient's need for and potential responses to medications. Information also indicates potential food and medication interactions. Some medications may require tube feeding to be stopped for an hour before and 2 hours after dose (Lilley et al., 2020). Communication of allergies is essential for safe, effective care.
7. For postoperative patient, review postoperative prescriptions for type of enteral tube care.	Manipulation and irrigation of tube or instillation of medications may be contraindicated.
8. Gather and review physical assessment data (e.g., bowel sounds, abdominal distension) and laboratory data (e.g., renal and liver function) that may influence medication administration.	Physical examination findings or laboratory data may contraindicate medication administration.
9. Check with pharmacy for availability of liquid preparation of patient's medications. Prescriber may need to change dosage form.	When possible, liquid formulation of the medication is the best option. The employer pharmacy may have the ability to provide a liquid preparation that is compatible with the enteral nutrition formula. Reduces risk of aspiration.
10. Before administration of enteral medications, verify placement of feeding tube (see Skill 32.2) and confirm that tube is placed in the stomach or small intestine correctly.	Ensures that point of medication absorption is not bypassed by feeding tube. For example, some medications (e.g., antacids) are absorbed in the stomach. If the patient's tube is placed in the intestines, these medications are not absorbed because the stomach is bypassed by the tube (Bandy et al., 2019).

NURSING DIAGNOSES

- Inadequate swallowing
- Inadequate feeding and/or self-care
- Potential for aspiration

Related factors and risk factors are individualized on the basis of patient's condition or needs.

PLANNING

STEP	RATIONALE
1. Expected outcomes following completion of procedure:	
• Patient experiences desired medication effect within period of onset of medication.	Medication has exerted its therapeutic action.
• Patient's feeding tube remains patent after administration of medication.	Patent enteral tube indicates passage of medication into stomach, ensuring proper absorption. If tube becomes blocked, administration of other medications and feedings is not possible.
• Patient does not aspirate during or after medication administration.	Patient safety in medication administration is maintained.
2. Collect appropriate equipment and MAR.	Ensures time management and efficiency.

IMPLEMENTATION

STEP	RATIONALE
1. Prepare medications for instillation into feeding tube (see Skill 21.1). Check medication label against MAR two times (when removing medication from drawer/cabinet and prior to preparing medication for administration). Fill graduated container with 50–100 mL of tepid water. Use sterile water for immunocompromised or critically ill patients (Doley, 2022).	*These are the first two checks for accuracy.* Preparation process ensures that right patient receives right medication. Tepid water prevents abdominal cramping, which can occur with cold water.

STEP	RATIONALE

IMPLEMENTATION

Critical Decision Point *Whenever possible, use liquid medications instead of crushed tablets. If you have to crush tablets, flush the tubing before and after medication administration to prevent the medication from adhering to the inside of the tube. In addition, make sure that concentrated medications are thoroughly diluted. Never add crushed medications directly to a tube feeding* (Anderson, 2019; Doley, 2022).

STEP	RATIONALE
a. *Tablets:* Crush each tablet into a fine powder using pill-crushing device or two medication cups (see Skill 21.1). Dissolve each tablet in separate cup of 30 mL of warm water.	Fine powder dissolves more easily, reducing chance of occluding feeding tube.
b. *Capsules:* Ensure that contents of capsule (granules or gelatin) can be expressed from covering (consult with pharmacist). Apply gloves and open capsule or pierce gel cap with sterile needle, then empty contents into 30 mL of warm water (or solution designated by manufacturer). Gel caps dissolve in warm water, but this may take 15–20 minutes.	Ensures that contents of capsules are in solution to prevent occlusion of tube.
c. Prepare liquid medication according to Skill 21.1.	
2. Identify patient using at least two person-specific identifiers (e.g., name and date of birth, or name and medical record number) according to employer policy. Compare identifiers with information on patient's MAR or medical record and identification (ID) band. Replace missing or faded ID bands.	Ensures correct patient. Complies with Accreditation Canada's standards and improves patient safety (Accreditation Canada, 2020).
3. Take medication(s) to patient at correct time (see employer policy). Medications that require exact timing include stat, first-time or loading doses, and one-time doses. Give time-critical scheduled medications (e.g., antibiotics, anticoagulants, insulin, anticonvulsants, immunosuppressive) at exact time prescribed (no later than 30 minutes before or after scheduled dose). Give non–time-critical scheduled medications within a range of 1 or 2 hours of scheduled dose, according to employer policy (ISMP, 2011). During administration, apply 10 rights of medication administration.	Hospitals must adopt medication administration policy and procedure for timing of medication administration that considers nature of the prescribed medication, specific clinical application, and patient needs. Time-critical scheduled medications are those for which early or delayed administration of maintenance doses of greater than 30 minutes before or after the scheduled dose may cause harm or result in substantially suboptimal therapy or pharmacological effect. Non–time-critical medications are those for which early or delayed administration within a specified range of either 1 or 2 hours should not cause harm or result in substantially suboptimal therapy or pharmacological effect (ISMP, 2011).
4. At patient's bedside, again compare MAR or computer printout with names of medications on medication labels and patient name. Ask patient whether they have allergies.	Ensures that right patient receives right medication. Confirms patient's allergy history.
5. Explain procedure to patient and discuss purpose, action, and possible adverse effects of each medication. Allow patient to ask any questions about the medications.	Helps patient be a participant in care, which minimizes anxiety. Patient has right to be informed, and their understanding of each medication improves adherence to medication therapy. Begins patient teaching regarding medications.
6. Assist patient to sitting position. Elevate head of bed to minimum of 30 degrees and preferably 45 degrees (unless contraindicated), or sit patient up in a chair (Doley, 2022; Tatsumi, 2019).	Keeping head above stomach reduces risk of aspiration.
7. If continuous enteral tube feeding is infusing, adjust infusion pump setting to hold tube feeding. If the patient needs to take the medication on an empty stomach or if the medication is not compatible with the feeding solution, stop the feeding 15–30 minutes before medication administration.	Feeding solution should not infuse while residuals are checked or while medications are administered. The presence of a feeding solution may impede medication absorption (Doley, 2022; Tatsumi, 2019).
8. Apply clean gloves. Check placement of feeding tube (see Skill 32.2) by observing gastric contents and checking pH of aspirate contents. *Gastric pH <5.0 is a good indicator that tip of tube is correctly placed in stomach* (Anderson 2019; Doley, 2022).	Reduces transmission of microorganisms. Ensures proper tube placement and reduces risk of introducing fluids into respiratory tract.
9. Check for gastric residual volume (GRV). Draw up 10–30 mL of air into a 60-mL syringe and connect syringe to feeding tube. Flush tube with air and pull back slowly to aspirate gastric contents (see Step 9 illustration). Determine GRV using either scale on syringe or a graduated container. Return aspirated contents to stomach unless a single GRV exceeds 250 mL (see employer policy). When GRV is excessive, hold medication and contact health care provider. The frequency of determining GRV may vary; check your employer's policy.	Large residuals indicate delayed gastric emptying and put patient at increased risk of aspiration (Metheny, 2021).

STEP	RATIONALE

IMPLEMENTATION

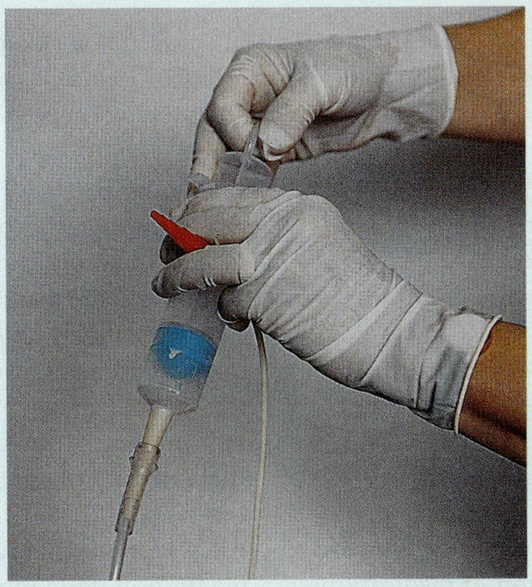

STEP 9 Aspirate stomach contents for residual volume.

10. Irrigate the tubing.

a. Pinch or clamp enteral tube and remove syringe. Draw up 30 mL of water into syringe. Reinsert tip of syringe into tube, release clamp, and flush tubing. Clamp tube again and remove syringe.

Pinching or clamping tubing prevents leakage or spillage of stomach contents. Flushing ensures that tube is patent.

b. Using the appropriate enteral connector (see Fig. 21.1), attach to enteral tube.

Standardization of connector tubing improves patient safety. Tubing standards are designed to reduce tubing misconnections, which can result in patient injury (Lord, 2018).

Critical Decision Point *Verify that the connector meets the ISO tubing connector standards. Do not attach the enteral tubing to a standardized Luer syringe or needleless device* (Lord, 2018).

11. Remove bulb or plunger of syringe and reinsert syringe into tip of feeding tube.

Removal of bulb or plunger prepares syringe for delivery of medications.

12. Administer dose of first liquid or dissolved medication by pouring into syringe (see Step 12 illustration). Allow to flow by gravity.

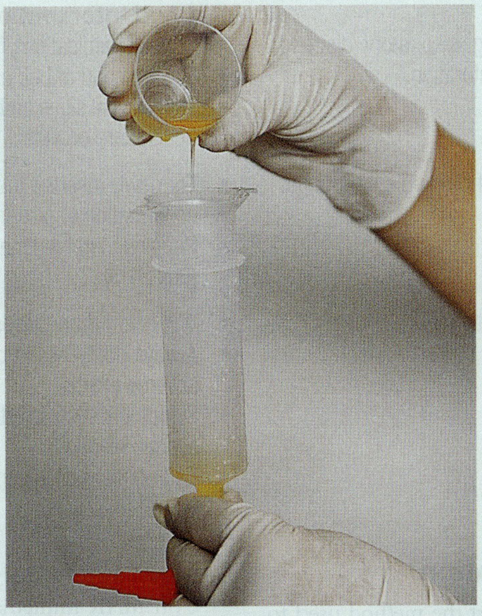

STEP 12 Pour liquid medication into syringe.

STEP	RATIONALE

IMPLEMENTATION

Critical Decision Point *Sometimes it is necessary to transfer oral medications into a medication cup for enteral administration. If medication does not flow freely, raise the height of the syringe to increase the rate of flow or try having the patient change position slightly because the end of the feeding tube may be against the gastric mucosa. If these measures do not improve the flow, a gentle push with bulb of Asepto syringe or plunger of the syringe may facilitate flow of fluid.*

STEP	RATIONALE
a. If giving only one dose of medication, flush tubing with 30–60 mL of water after administration.	Maintains patency of enteral tube and ensures that medication passes through tube to stomach (Anderson, 2019; Doley, 2022).
b. To administer more than one medication, give each separately and flush between medications with 15–30 mL of water.	Allows for accurate identification of medication if dose is spilled. In addition, some medications may be incompatible, and giving medication separately followed by a flush solution decreases the risk for medication incompatibilities (Alhashemi et al., 2019).
c. Follow last dose of medication with 30–60 mL of water.	Maintains patency of enteral tube and ensures passage of medication into stomach (Alhashemi et al., 2019).
13. Clamp proximal end of feeding tube if tube feeding is not being administered, then cap end of tube.	Prevents air from entering stomach between medication doses.
14. When continuous tube feeding is being administered by infusion pump, follow medication administration. If medications are not compatible with feeding solution, hold feeding for additional 30–60 minutes (Anderson, 2019; Doley, 2022).	Allows for adequate absorption of medication and avoids potential medication–food interaction between medication and enteral feeding (Anderson, 2019; Doley, 2022).
15. Help patient to comfortable position and keep head of bed elevated for 1 hour (see employer policy).	Reduces risk of aspiration.
16. Dispose of soiled supplies, rinse graduated container and syringe with tap water, and remove and dispose of gloves.	Reduces spread of microorganisms.

EVALUATION

STEP	RATIONALE
1. Observe patient for signs of aspiration, such as choking, gurgling, gurgling speech, breath sounds, and difficulty breathing.	Provides for prompt intervention if aspiration has occurred.
2. Return within 30 minutes to evaluate patient's response to medications.	Monitoring patient's response evaluates therapeutic benefit of medication and helps detect onset of adverse effects or allergic reactions.
3. **Use teach-back:** "I want to be sure I explained clearly why your father must take his medications through his feeding tube. Tell me why he is receiving his medications through his feeding tube." Develop a revised teaching plan if caregiver is unable to teach back correctly.	Determines caregiver's level of understanding of instructional topic.

Unexpected Outcomes	Related Interventions
1. Patient exhibits signs of aspiration, including respiratory distress, changes in vital signs, or changes in oxygen saturation.	• Stop all medications/fluids being administered through feeding tube. • Elevate head of bed and stay with patient. • Assess vital signs and breath sounds while another staff member notifies health care provider.
2. Patient does not receive medication because of blocked enteral tube.	• For newly inserted tube, notify health care provider and obtain X-ray film confirmation of placement. • Requires interventions to unclog tube to ensure medication delivery (Box 21.3).
3. Patient exhibits adverse effects or allergic reaction.	• Withhold further doses. • Always notify health care provider and pharmacy when patient exhibits adverse effects. • Symptoms such as urticaria, rash, pruritus, rhinitis, and wheezing indicate allergic reaction. • Enter patient allergy in medical record.

Communication and Documentation

- Document in progress notes in EHR or chart the method used to check placement of enteral tube, GRV, and pH of stomach aspirate.
- Document actual time that each medication was administered on MAR immediately after administration, not before. Include initials or signature.

BOX 21.3

Unclogging a Blocked Feeding Tube

- Prevent tube from becoming blocked by flushing it with at least 15–30 mL of tepid water before and after administering each dose of medication, and at least 30–60 mL after last dose of medication; flushing before and after checking gastric residual volumes; and flushing every 4–12 hours around the clock (refer to employer policies).
- Gently flush tube with large-bore syringe and warm water. Do not use small-bore syringe because it exerts too much pressure and may rupture tube.
- If irrigation with water is not effective, obtain a prescription for a pancrelipase tablet and follow manufacturer guidelines for tube irrigation. In addition, a declogging stylus may be used (see employer policy).
- The tube may have to be removed and a new one inserted if the medication is urgent.

Adapted from Hayes, K. D., & Hayes, D. D. (2018). Best practices for unclogging feeding tubes in adults. *Nursing*, *48*(6), 66–72. https://doi.org/10.1097/01.NURSE.0000532744.80506.5e

- Document patient's response to medication, patient teaching, and validation of patient understanding on flow sheet or in progress notes in EHR or chart.
- Document total amount of water used for medication administration on proper intake and output (I&O) form.
- Report and document adverse effects, patient response, and/or withheld medications to nurse in charge or health care provider.

DOCUMENTATION EXAMPLE

NG tube medications administered as prescribed and tolerated well. NG tube placement checked prior to administration, pH of stomach aspirate 5. Gastric residual volume 20 mL. Continuous feeds of Nutren with fibre administering at a rate of 100 mL/hr as prescribed. Patient sitting in chair visiting with family.

Special Considerations

Teaching

- Teach patient or caregiver how to store medications and tube-feeding supplements (see Chapter 32).
- Demonstrate to patient or caregiver how to prepare medications, including crushing them if appropriate.
- Demonstrate to patient or caregiver how to verify correct placement of tube.
- Teach patient or caregiver the importance of consistent flushing of feeding tube before and after medication administration.

Pediatric

- Volumes for instillation of medications or for irrigation of enteral tubes should be small enough to clear tubing (Keenan-Lindsay et al., 2022).

✦ SKILL 21.3 Applying Topical Medications to the Skin

Video Clip NSO *Nursing Skills Online Nonparenteral Medication Administration Module 6 / Lesson 3*

Topical administration of medication involves applying medications locally to the skin, mucous membranes, or tissues. Topical medications such as lotions, transdermal patches, pastes, and ointments primarily produce local effects; but they can create systemic effects if absorbed through the skin. Systemic effects are more likely to occur if the skin is thin, the medication concentration is high, contact with the skin is prolonged, or the medication is applied to skin that is not intact. In addition, skin hydration and environmental humidity affect percutaneous absorption of a medication. An increase in skin hydration increases absorption (Yu et al., 2021). Apply topical medications using gloves and applicators to protect from accidental exposure. Skin encrustations and dead tissue harbour microorganisms and block contact of medications with the affected tissue or membrane.

Never apply new medication over a previously applied medication because it will decrease the therapeutic benefit to a patient. Always clean the skin or wound thoroughly before applying a new dose of a topical medication. Apply each type of medication, whether an ointment, lotion, powder, or patch, in the correct way to ensure proper penetration and absorption (Lilley et al., 2020).

Delegation and Collaboration

The skill of administering most topical medications, including skin patches, cannot be delegated to a UCP. However, some facilities (e.g., long-term care) may allow UCPs to apply some forms of topical medications (e.g., skin barriers) to irritated skin or for the protection of the perineum during morning or perineal care. Check employer policies. The nurse instructs the UCP to do the following:

- Report immediately to the nurse any patient skin irritation, burning, blistering, or increased itching
- Not apply any dressing over the topical medication unless instructed to do so

Equipment

- MAR (electronic or printed)
- Clean gloves (for intact skin) or sterile gloves (for nonintact skin)
- Cotton-tipped applicators or tongue blades *(optional)*
- Prescribed medication (powder, cream, lotion, ointment, spray, patch)
- Basin of warm water, washcloth, towel, nondrying soap
- Sterile dressing, tape (if needed)
- Felt-tip pen *(optional)*
- Plastic wrap, transparent dressing (if prescribed) *(optional)*

STEP	RATIONALE
ASSESSMENT	
1. Identify patient using at least two person-specific identifiers (e.g., name and date of birth or name and medical record number) according to employer policy.	

STEP	RATIONALE
ASSESSMENT	
2. Throughout the procedure, the 4 moments for hand hygiene are to be implemented; hand hygiene should occur before initial patient (or patient environment) contact, before an aseptic procedure, after body fluid exposure risk, and after patient (or patient environment) contact. Additional hand hygiene should be performed when hands are visibly soiled.	
3. Check accuracy and completeness of each MAR by comparing with health care provider's medication prescription. Check patient's name, medication name and dosage, route of administration, and time for administration. Clarify incomplete or unclear prescriptions with health care provider before administration.	The prescription sheet is the most reliable source and only legal record of medications that patient is to receive. It ensures that patient receives correct medications (College of Physicians and Surgeons of Ontario, 2019; Pharmacy Association of Nova Scotia, n.d.). Handwritten MARs are a source of medication errors (Parthasarathi et al., 2021; Tariq et al., 2022).
4. Review pertinent information related to medication, including action, purpose, normal dose and route, adverse effects, time of onset and peak action, and nursing implications.	Allows you to anticipate effects of medication and observe patient's response.
5. Assess condition of skin or membrane where medication is to be applied (see Chapter 8). Apply clean gloves. First, wash site thoroughly with mild, nondrying soap and warm water, rinse, and dry. Be sure to remove any previously applied medication or debris. Also remove any blood, body fluids, secretions, or excretions. Assess for symptoms of skin irritation such as pruritus or burning. Remove gloves when finished.	Cleaning site thoroughly promotes proper assessment of skin surface. Assessment provides baseline to determine change in condition of skin after therapy. Application of certain topical medications can lessen or aggravate these symptoms. Cleaning removes any residual medication from the previous dose, which reduces potential adverse medication reactions or skin irritation (Brunaugh et al., 2019; Yu et al., 2021).
6. Assess patient's medical and medication history and history of allergies (including latex and topical medication). Ask if patient has had reaction to a cream or lotion applied to skin. List medication allergies on each page of the MAR and display it prominently on the patient's medical record per employer policy. When patient has allergy, provide allergy bracelet.	Information reflects patient's need for and potential responses to medications. Allergic contact dermatitis is relatively common and can worsen dermatological (skin) condition. In addition, some patients may be allergic to preservatives or fragrances in topical medications. Latex allergy requires use of nonlatex gloves. Communication of allergies is essential for safe and effective care.
7. Determine amount of topical medication required for application by assessing skin site, reviewing health care provider's prescription, and reading application directions carefully (a thin, even layer is usually adequate).	An excessive amount of topical medication can irritate skin chemically, negate effectiveness of medication, and/or cause adverse systemic effects such as decreased white blood cell (WBC) counts.
8. Assess patient's knowledge of action and purpose of medication being given, application schedule, and willingness to adhere to medication regimen.	Determines patient's level of understanding and whether instruction is necessary.
9. Determine whether patient or caregiver is physically able to apply medication by assessing grasp, hand strength, reach, and coordination.	Necessary if patient is to self-administer medication at home.

NURSING DIAGNOSES

- Inadequate knowledge regarding medication and medication application
- Pain (acute or chronic)
- Reduced physical mobility
- Reduced skin integrity
- Readiness for enhanced self-management of health
- Potential for infection

Related factors and risk factors are individualized on the basis of patient's condition or needs.

PLANNING

STEP	RATIONALE
1. Expected outcomes following completion of procedure:	
• Patient is able to identify medication and describe action, purpose, dose, adverse effects, and schedule of medication.	Demonstrates learning.
• Patient is able to apply medication without help on prescribed schedule.	Demonstrates learning and adherence.
• With repeated applications, skin becomes clear, without inflammation or drainage from lesions.	Existing lesions heal and/or disappear as result of therapeutic action of medication.
2. Collect appropriate equipment and MAR.	Ensures time management and efficiency.

STEP	RATIONALE
IMPLEMENTATION	
1. Prepare medications for application. Check label of medication against MAR two times (when removing medication from drawer/cabinet and prior to preparing medication for administration; see Skill 21.1). Preparation usually involves taking bottle or tube of lotion, cream, ointment, or patch out of storage and to patient's room. Check expiration date on container.	Reduces transmission of infection. *These are the first two checks for accuracy.* Process ensures that right patient receives right medication.
2. Identify patient using at least two person-specific identifiers (e.g., name and date of birth, or name and medical record number) according to employer policy. Compare identifiers with information on patient's MAR or medical record and ID band. Replace missing or faded ID bands.	Ensures correct patient. Complies with Accreditation Canada's standards and improves patient safety (Accreditation Canada, 2020).
3. Take medication(s) to patient at correct time (see employer policy). Medications that require exact timing include stat, first-time or loading doses, and one-time doses. Give time-critical scheduled medications (e.g., antibiotics, anticoagulants, insulin, anticonvulsants, immunosuppressive medications) at exact time prescribed (no later than 30 minutes before or after scheduled dose). Give non–time-critical scheduled medications within a range of 1 or 2 hours of scheduled dose, according to employer policy (ISMP, 2011). During administration, apply 10 rights of medication administration. Close room curtain or door.	Agencies must adopt medication administration policies for timing of medication administration that considers nature of the prescribed medication, specific clinical application, and patient needs. Time-critical scheduled medications are those for which early or delayed administration of maintenance doses of greater than 30 minutes before or after the scheduled dose may cause harm or result in substantially suboptimal therapy or pharmacological effect. Non–time-critical medications are those for which early or delayed administration within a specified range of either 1 or 2 hours should not cause harm or result in substantially suboptimal therapy or pharmacological effect (ISMP, 2011).
4. Help patient to comfortable position. Arrange supplies at bedside.	Allows easy access to application site.
5. At patient's bedside, again compare MAR or computer printout with names of medications on medication labels and patient name. Ask patient whether they have allergies.	Ensures that right patient receives right medication. Confirms patient's allergy history.
6. Explain procedure to patient and discuss purpose, action, and possible adverse effects of each medication. Allow patient to ask any questions about the medications.	Demonstrates person-centred care, which minimizes anxiety. Patient has right to be informed, and their understanding of each medication improves adherence to medication therapy. Begins patient teaching regarding medications.
7. If skin is broken, apply sterile gloves. Otherwise, apply clean gloves.	Reduces transmission of microorganisms.
8. Apply topical creams, ointments, and oil-based lotions.	
a. Expose affected area while keeping unaffected areas covered.	Provides visualization for application and protects privacy.
b. Wash, rinse, and dry affected area before applying medication if not done earlier (see Assessment, Step 3).	Cleaning removes microorganisms from remaining debris and any surface medication.
c. If skin is excessively dry and flaking, apply topical medication while skin is still damp.	Increased skin hydration and surface humidity enhance absorption of topical medication (Yu et al., 2021).
d. After washing, remove gloves. Apply new clean or sterile gloves.	Sterile gloves are used when applying medications to open, noninfectious skin lesions. Changing gloves prevents cross-contamination of infected or contagious lesions. Gloves also protect you from topical absorption of the medication and subsequent medication effects (Lilley et al., 2020).
e. Place required amount of medication in palm of gloved hand and soften by rubbing briskly between hands.	Softening topical medications makes it easier to spread on skin.
f. Tell patient that initial application of medications may feel cold. Once medication is softened, spread it evenly over skin surface, using long, even strokes that follow direction of hair growth. Do not vigorously rub skin. Apply to thickness specified by manufacturer instructions.	Ensures even distribution and sufficient dosage of medication. Technique prevents irritation of hair follicles.
g. Explain to patient that skin may feel greasy after application.	Ointments often contain oils.
9. Technique for applying antianginal (nitroglycerine) ointment.	
a. Remove previous dose paper. Fold used paper containing any residual medication with used sides together and dispose of it in biohazard garbage container. Wipe off residual medication with tissue.	Prevents overdose that can occur with multiple-dose papers left in place. Proper disposal protects you and others from accidental exposure to medication.

STEP	RATIONALE
IMPLEMENTATION	
b. Write date, time, and your initials on new application paper.	Label provides reference to prevent missing doses.
c. Antianginal (nitroglycerine) ointments are usually prescribed in inches and can be measured on small sheets of paper marked off in 1.25-cm (0.5-inch) markings. Unit-dose packages are available. Apply desired number of inches of ointment to paper-measuring guide (see Step 9c illustration).	Ensures correct dose of medication.

Critical Decision Point *Unit-dose packages are available.* N*OTE: One package equals 2.5 cm (1 inch); smaller amounts should not be measured from this package.*

STEP	RATIONALE
d. Select new application site, rotating sites: apply nitroglycerine to chest area, back, abdomen, or anterior thigh (Lilley et al., 2020). Do not apply on nonintact skin or hairy surfaces or over scar tissue.	Application sites are rotated to reduce skin irritation. Application on nonintact skin may result in increased absorption of medication. Application on hairy surfaces or scar tissue may decrease absorption (Lilley et al., 2020).

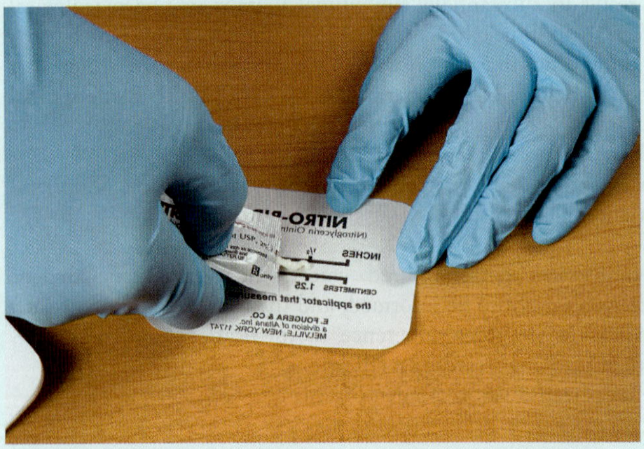

STEP 9C Ointment spread in centimetres (inches) over measuring guide.

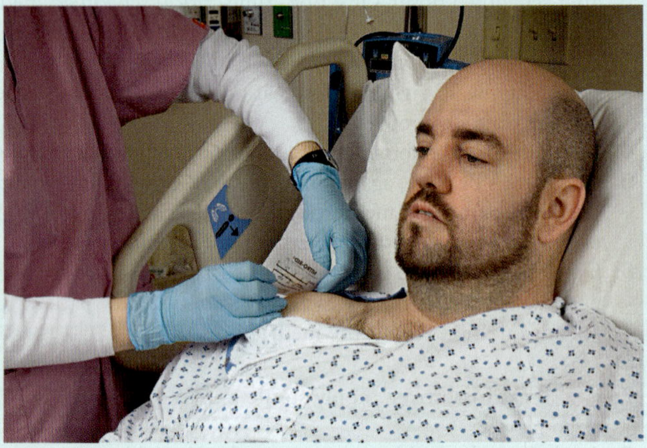

STEP 9E Nurse applies wrapper with medication to patient's skin.

STEP	RATIONALE
e. Apply ointment to skin surface by holding edge or back of paper-measuring guide and placing ointment and wrapper directly on skin (see Step 10e illustration). Do not rub or massage ointment into skin.	Minimizes chance of ointment covering gloves and later touching nurse's hands. Medication is designed to absorb slowly over several hours; massaging increases absorption rate.
f. Secure ointment and paper with transparent dressing or strip of tape. Apply dressing or plastic wrap only when instructed by pharmacy (Lilley et al., 2020; US FDA, 2021).	Prevents staining of clothing or inadvertent removal of medication. Covering topical medications with dressing or plastic wrap increases heat and skin humidity and rate of absorption of medication (Lilley et al., 2020; US FDA, 2023).
10. Technique for applying transdermal patches (e.g., analgesic, nicotine, nitroglycerine, estrogen).	
a. If old patch is present, remove it and clean area. Be sure to check between skinfolds for patch.	Failure to remove old patch can result in overdose. Many patches are small, clear, or flesh coloured and can be easily hidden between skinfolds. Cleaning removes residual medication traces of previous patch.
b. Dispose of old patch by folding in half with sticky sides together. Some facilities require patch to be cut before disposal (see employer policy). Dispose of it in biohazard garbage bag.	Proper disposal prevents accidental exposure to medication.
c. Date and initial outer side of new patch before applying it and note time of administration. Use soft-tip or felt-tip pen.	Visual reminder prevents missing or extra doses. Ballpoint pen damages patch and alters medication delivery.

STEP	RATIONALE
IMPLEMENTATION	
d. Choose a new site that is clean, intact, dry, and free of hair. Some patches have specific instructions for placement locations (e.g., Testoderm patches are placed on scrotum; a scopolamine patch is placed behind the ear; *never apply* an estrogen patch to breast tissue or waistline). Do not apply patch on skin that is oily, burned, cut, or irritated in any way.	Ensures complete medication absorption. Estrogen patches should never be placed on the breast, genitals, or other reproductive organs. There is a risk for systemic absorption of the hormone, which can increase patient's risk for breast, testicular, or ovarian cancer (Lilley et al., 2020; Medline Plus, 2022a).
e. Carefully remove patch from its protective covering by pulling off liner. Hold patch by edge without touching adhesive edges.	Touching only edges ensures that patch will adhere to the skin and that medication dose has not changed. Removing protective covering allows medication to be absorbed through skin.
f. Apply patch. Hold palm of one hand firmly over patch for 10 seconds. Make sure that it sticks well, especially around edges. Apply overlay if provided with patch.	Adequate adhesion prevents loss of patch, which results in decreased dose and effectiveness.

Critical Decision Point *Never apply heat, such as with a heating pad, over a transdermal patch because this results in an increased rate of absorption with potentially serious adverse effects* (Lilley et al., 2020; US FDA, 2021).

STEP	RATIONALE
g. Do not apply patch to previously used sites for at least 1 week.	Rotation of application site reduces skin irritation from medication and adhesive (Medline Plus, 2015).
h. Instruct patient that transdermal patches are never to be cut in half; a change in dose would require prescription for new strength of transdermal medication.	Cutting transdermal patch in half would alter intended medication delivery of transdermal system, resulting in inadequate or altered medication levels.

Critical Decision Point *It is recommended to have a daily "patch-free" interval of 10–12 hours because tolerance develops if patches are used 24 hours a day, every day* (Lilley et al., 2020; US FDA, 2021). *Apply a new patch each morning, leave in place for 12–14 hours, and remove in the evening. This applies only to certain types of patches; for example, pain patches should not have a "patch-free" break to ensure consistent pain management.*

STEP	RATIONALE
i. Instruct patient to always remove old patch and clean skin before applying new one. Patients should not use alternative forms of medication when using patches. For example, patients should not apply nitroglycerine ointment in addition to patch unless specifically prescribed to do so by their health care provider.	Use of patch with additional or alternative medication preparation can result in toxicity or other adverse effects.
11. Technique for administering aerosol sprays (e.g., local anaesthetic sprays).	
a. Shake container vigorously. Read container label for distance recommended to hold spray away from area, usually 15–30 cm (6–12 inches).	Mixing ensures delivery of fine, even spray. Proper distance ensures that fine spray hits skin surface. Holding container too close results in thin, watery distribution.
b. Ask patient to turn face away from spray or briefly cover face with towel while spraying neck or chest.	Prevents inhalation of spray.
c. Spray medication evenly over affected site (in some cases, time spray for a period of seconds).	Ensures that affected area of skin is covered with thin spray.
12. Technique for applying suspension-based lotion.	
a. Shake container vigorously.	Mixes powder throughout liquid to form well-mixed suspension.
b. Apply small amount of lotion to small gauze dressing or pad and apply to skin by stroking evenly in direction of hair growth.	Method of application leaves protective film of powder on skin after water base of suspension dries. Technique prevents irritation to hair follicles.
c. Explain to patient that area will feel cool and dry.	Water evaporates to leave thin layer of powder.
13. Technique for applying powder.	
a. Be sure that skin surface is thoroughly dry. With your nondominant hand, fully spread apart any skinfolds such as between toes or under axilla and dry with towel.	Minimizes caking and crusting of powder. Fully exposes skin surface for application.
b. If area of application is near face, ask patient to turn face away from powder or briefly cover face with towel.	Prevents inhalation of powder.
c. Dust skin site lightly with dispenser so area is covered with fine, thin layer of powder. *Option:* Cover skin area with dressing if prescribed by health care provider.	Thin layer of powder has slight lubricating properties, which reduces friction and promotes drying (Mitchell & Hill, 2020).

STEP	RATIONALE

IMPLEMENTATION

14. Help patient to comfortable position, reapply gown, and cover with bed linen as desired.	Provides for patient's sense of well-being.
15. Dispose of soiled supplies in receptacle especially designated for such articles. Remove and dispose of gloves.	Keeps patient's environment neat, and reduces spread of infection and residual medication to others.

EVALUATION

1. Inspect condition of skin between applications.	Determines whether skin condition is improving, and verifies that skin is intact and not irritated.
2. Have patient keep diary of doses taken.	Confirms adherence to prescribed therapy.
3. Observe patient or caregiver apply topical medication.	Return demonstration measures learning.
4. Use **teach-back:** "I want to be sure I explained the action of the dose of medicine you are taking and the side effects of cortisone cream medication. In your own words, tell me how the medication works, your correct dose, and any side effects." Develop a revised teaching plan if patient or caregiver is unable to teach back correctly.	Determines patient's and caregiver's level of understanding of instructional topic.

Unexpected Outcomes	Related Interventions
1. Skin site appears inflamed and edematous with blistering and oozing of fluid from lesions. These signs indicate subacute inflammation or eczema that can develop if skin lesions are getting worse.	• Withhold medication. • Notify health care provider; alternative therapies may be needed.
2. Patient is unable to explain information about medication or does not administer as prescribed.	• Identify possible reasons for nonadherence and explore alternative approaches or options.
3. Patient continues to report tenderness and/or pruritus. These signs may indicate slow or impaired healing.	• Notify health care provider; alternative therapies may be needed.

Communication and Documentation

- Document actual time that each medication was administered, type of medication applied, strength, and site of application in MAR immediately after administration, not before. Include initials or signature.
- Document patient's response to medication, patient teaching, and validation of patient's understanding on flow sheet or in progress notes in EHR or chart.
- Document condition of skin before each application on flow sheet or in progress notes in EHR or chart.
- Report adverse effects, patient response, and/or withheld medications to nurse in charge or health care provider. Depending on medication, immediate notification of health care provider may be required.

DOCUMENTATION EXAMPLE

Patient correctly applied corticosteroid cream to their arms as prescribed. Patient able to state why the cream was prescribed, how to apply the cream (including how often), and side effects.

Special Considerations

Teaching

- Instruct patient and caregiver to:
  - Not apply to irritated or damaged skin.
  - Not use heating pads, hot water bottle, or warm compresses over medication.
  - Only use a bandage or plastic wrap if instructed by a pharmacist.
  - Use medication exactly as prescribed.
  - Contact health care provider if medication comes in contact with eyes or other mucous membranes such as the mouth.
- Instruct patients to use only warm-water rinse without soap for cleaning inflamed skin.
- If a transdermal patch loosens or falls off before the next scheduled dose, refer to your health care provider's instructions or the manufacturer's instructions, according to the drug that is being administered transdermally. In general, for a loose patch, use the palm of your hand to press the patch back onto the skin (Murrell, 2018). If one edge of the patch becomes loose, use tape of a sticky adhesive film to secure the loose edge (Murrell, 2018). If the patch

falls off, do not reapply it but apply a new one, either immediately or at the next scheduled dose, depending on the medication.

Gerontological

- Changes in the skin of an older person include increased fragility, wrinkling, dryness, flaking, and increased tendency to bruise. Be aware of these changes when applying topical medications to ensure proper application.

Care in the Community: Home Management

- Instruct patient to wrap applicators, used patches, and similar materials and dispose of them into cardboard or plastic disposable containers. Careful disposal is necessary to ensure the safety of patient, other adults, children, and pets.

✦ SKILL 21.4 Administering Ophthalmic Medications

Video Clip **NSO** *Nursing Skills Online Nonparenteral Medication Administration Module 6 / Lesson 4*

Common eye (ophthalmic) medications are delivered in the form of drops and ointments, including over-the-counter (OTC) preparations such as artificial tears and vasoconstrictors. However, many patients receive prescribed ophthalmic medications for eye conditions such as glaucoma and infection and following cataract extraction. In addition, there is a third type of delivery system, the intraocular disc. Medications delivered via disc resemble a contact lens; however, the disc is placed in the conjunctival sac, not on the cornea, and it remains in place for up to 1 week.

The eye is the most sensitive organ to which medications are applied. The cornea is richly supplied with sensitive nerve fibres. Care must be taken to prevent instilling medication directly onto the cornea. The conjunctival sac is much less sensitive and thus a more appropriate site for medication instillation.

Any patient receiving topical eye medications should learn correct self-administration of the medication, especially patients with glaucoma, who must often undergo lifelong medication administration for control of their disease. The nurse can easily instruct patients while administering medications. Caregivers often administer eye medications when patients are unable to manipulate applicators (e.g., arthritis or neurological condition), immediately after eye surgery, and when a patient's vision is so impaired that it is difficult to assemble needed supplies and handle applicators correctly.

Delegation and Collaboration

The skill of administering ophthalmic medications cannot be delegated to a UCP. The nurse instructs the UCP about the following:

- The specific potential adverse effects of medications and to report their occurrence.
- The potential for temporary burning or blurring of vision after administration of eye medications.

Equipment

- MAR (electronic or printed)
- Appropriate medication (e.g., eyedrops with sterile eyedropper, ointment tube, or medicated intraocular disc)
- Clean gloves

Eyedrops/Ointment

- Cotton ball or tissue
- Wash basin filled with warm water and washcloth
- Eye patch and tape (*optional*)

STEP	RATIONALE
ASSESSMENT	
1. Identify patient using at least two person-specific identifiers (e.g., name and date of birth or name and medical record number) according to employer policy.	
2. Throughout the procedure, the 4 moments for hand hygiene are to be implemented; hand hygiene should occur before initial patient (or patient environment) contact, before an aseptic procedure, after body fluid exposure risk, and after patient (or patient environment) contact. Additional hand hygiene should be performed when hands are visibly soiled.	
3. Check accuracy and completeness of each MAR by comparing with health care provider's medication prescription. Check patient's name, medication name and dosage, route (one or both eyes), and time for administration. Clarify incomplete or unclear prescriptions with health care provider before administration.	The prescription sheet is the most reliable source and only legal record of medications that patient is to receive. Ensures that patient receives correct medications (College of Physicians and Surgeons of Ontario, 2019; Pharmacy Association of Nova Scotia, n.d.). Handwritten MARs are a source of medication errors (Parthasarathi et al., 2021; Tariq et al., 2022).
4. Review pertinent information related to medication, including action, purpose, normal dose and route, adverse effects, time of onset and peak action, and nursing implications.	Allows you to anticipate effects of medication and observe patient's response.
5. Assess condition of external eye structures (see Chapter 8). This may be done just before medication instillation (if drainage is present, apply clean gloves).	Provides baseline to determine whether local response to medications occurs. Also indicates need to clean eye before medication application.
6. Determine whether patient has any symptoms of eye discomfort or visual impairment.	Certain eye medications act to either lessen or increase these symptoms.

ASSESSMENT

STEP	RATIONALE
7. Assess patient's medical and medication history and history of allergies (including latex). List medication allergies on each page of the MAR and prominently display it on the patient's medical record per employer policy. When patient has allergy, provide allergy bracelet.	These factors influence how certain medications act. Reveals patient's need for and likely response to medication. Communication of allergies is essential for safe and effective care.
8. Assess patient's LOC and ability to follow directions.	If patient becomes restless or combative during procedure, greater risk of accidental eye injury exists.
9. Assess patient's knowledge regarding medication therapy and desire to self-administer medication.	Indicates need for health teaching. Motivation influences teaching approach.
10. Assess patient's ability to manipulate and hold dropper or ocular disc.	Reflects patient's ability to learn to self-administer medication.

NURSING DIAGNOSES

- Inadequate knowledge regarding medication and self-administration
- Pain (acute or chronic)
- Reduced physical mobility
- Readiness for enhanced self-management of health
- Potential for injury

Related factors and risk factors are individualized on the basis of patient's condition or needs.

PLANNING

STEP	RATIONALE
1. Expected outcomes following completion of procedure:	
• Patient experiences desired effect of medication.	Medication is administered correctly without injury to patient.
• Patient denies discomfort.	Medication is administered correctly without injury to patient.
• Patient experiences no adverse effects, and symptoms (e.g., irritation) are relieved.	Medication is distributed and absorbed properly.
• Patient can discuss information about medication and technique correctly.	Demonstrates learning.
• Patient demonstrates self-instillation of eyedrops.	Demonstrates learning.
2. Collect appropriate equipment and MAR.	Ensures time management and efficiency.

IMPLEMENTATION

STEP	RATIONALE
1. Prepare medications for instillation. Check label of medication against MAR two times (when removing medication from drawer/cabinet and prior to preparing medication for administration; see Skill 21.1). Preparation usually involves taking eyedrops out of refrigerator and rewarming to room temperature before administering to patient. Check expiration date on container.	Warming eyedrops reduces eye irritation. *These are the first two checks for accuracy.* Process ensures that right patient receives right medication.
2. Identify patient using at least two person-specific identifiers (e.g., name and date of birth, or name and medical record number) according to employer policy. Compare identifiers with information on patient's MAR or medical record and ID band. Replace missing or faded ID bands.	Ensures correct patient. Complies with Accreditation Canada's standards and improves patient safety (Accreditation Canada, 2020).
3. Take medication(s) to patient at correct time (see employer policy). Medications that require exact timing include stat, first-time or loading doses, and one-time doses. Give time-critical scheduled medications (e.g., antibiotics, anticoagulants, insulin, anticonvulsants, immunosuppressive medications) at exact time prescribed (no later than 30 minutes before or after scheduled dose). Give non–time-critical scheduled medications within a range of 1 or 2 hours of scheduled dose, according to employer policy (ISMP, 2011). During administration, apply 10 rights of medication administration.	Employers must adopt medication administration policy and procedure for timing of medication administration that considers nature of the prescribed medication, specific clinical application, and patient needs. Time-critical scheduled medications are those for which early or delayed administration of maintenance doses of greater than 30 minutes before or after the scheduled dose may cause harm or result in substantially suboptimal therapy or pharmacological effect. Non–time-critical medications are those for which early or delayed administration within a specified range of either 1 or 2 hours should not cause harm or result in substantially suboptimal therapy or pharmacological effect (ISMP, 2011).
4. Help patient to comfortable sitting position. Arrange supplies at bedside.	Ensures an organized procedure.

STEP	RATIONALE

IMPLEMENTATION

5. At patient's bedside, again compare MAR or computer printout with names of medications on medication labels and patient name. Ask patient whether they have allergies.	Ensures that right patient receives right medication. Confirms patient's allergy history.
6. Explain procedure to patient and sensations to expect. Discuss purpose, action, and possible adverse effects of each medication. Allow patient to ask any questions about the medications. Patients who self-instill medications may be allowed to give drops under nurse's supervision (check employer policy). Tell patients receiving eyedrops (mydriatics) that vision will be blurred temporarily and sensitivity to light may occur.	Helps patient be a participant in care, which minimizes anxiety. Patient has right to be informed, and their understanding of each medication improves adherence to medication therapy. Begins patient teaching regarding medications.

Critical Decision Point *Instruct and reinforce that patient should not drive or operate machinery or perform any activity that requires clear vision until vision and sensitivity to light return to normal.*

7. Instill eye medications.	If administering more than one eye medication, wait 10 minutes in between medications to ensure that the first medication has had time to absorb and that the second medication does not wash out the first one. Eye ointments should be applied last.
a. Apply clean gloves. Ask patient to lie supine or sit back in chair with head slightly hyperextended, looking up.	Reduces transmission of microorganisms. Position provides easy access to eye for medication instillation and minimizes drainage of medication into tear duct.

Critical Decision Point *Do not hyperextend the neck of a patient with cervical spine injury.*

b. If drainage or crusting is present along eyelid margins or inner canthus, gently wash away. Soak any dried crusts with warm, damp washcloth or cotton ball over eye for several minutes. Always wipe clean from inner to outer canthus (see Step 7b illustration). Remove gloves.	Soaking allows easy removal of crusts without applying pressure to eye. Cleaning from inner to outer canthus avoids entrance of microorganisms into lacrimal duct (American Academy of Ophthalmology, 2021; Lampert et al., 2019).

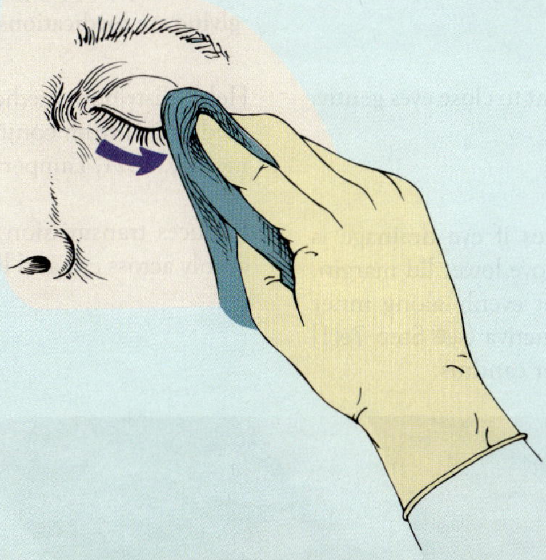

STEP 7B Clean patient's eye, washing from inner to outer canthus, before administering drops or ointment.

c. Explain that there might be temporary burning sensation from drops.	Corneas are highly sensitive.
d. Instill eyedrops.	
(1) *Option:* Apply clean gloves if eye drainage present. Hold clean cotton ball or tissue in nondominant hand on patient's cheekbone just below lower eyelid.	Prevents transmission of microorganisms. Cotton or tissue absorbs medication that escapes eye.
(2) With tissue or cotton ball resting below lower lid, gently press downward with thumb or forefinger against bony orbit, exposing conjunctival sac. Never press directly against patient's eyeball.	Prevents pressure and trauma to eyeball and prevents fingers from touching eye.

STEP	RATIONALE

IMPLEMENTATION

STEP	RATIONALE
(3) Ask patient to look at ceiling. Rest dominant hand on patient's forehead; hold filled medication eyedropper approximately 1–2 cm (approximately 0.25–0.5 inches) above conjunctival sac.	Action moves cornea up and away from conjunctival sac and reduces blink reflex. Prevents accidental contact of eyedropper with eye and reduces risk of injury and transfer of microorganisms to dropper (ophthalmic medications are sterile).
(4) Drop prescribed number of drops into conjunctival sac (see Step 7d[4] illustration).	Conjunctival sac normally holds 1 or 2 drops. Provides even distribution of medication across eye.
(5) If patient blinks or closes eye, causing drops to land on outer lid margins, repeat procedure.	Therapeutic effect of medication is obtained only when drops enter conjunctival sac.
(6) When administering drops that may cause systemic effects, apply gentle pressure to patient's nasolacrimal duct with clean tissue for 30–60 seconds over each eye, one at a time (see Step 7d[6] illustration). Avoid placing pressure directly against patient's eyeball.	Prevents overflow of medication into nasal and pharyngeal passages. Prevents absorption into systemic circulation (American Academy of Ophthalmology, 2021; Lilley et al., 2020).

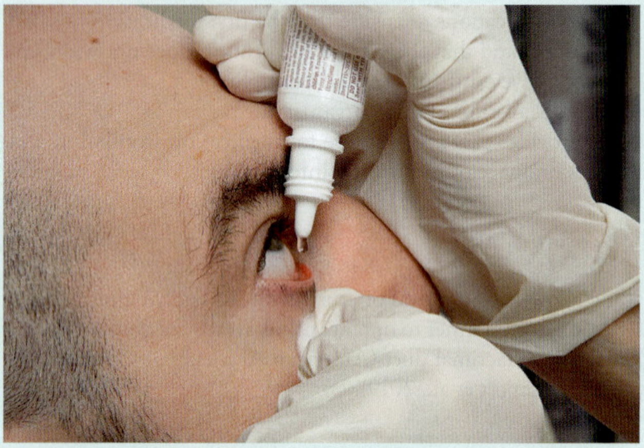

STEP 7D(4) Hold eyedropper over lower conjunctival sac.

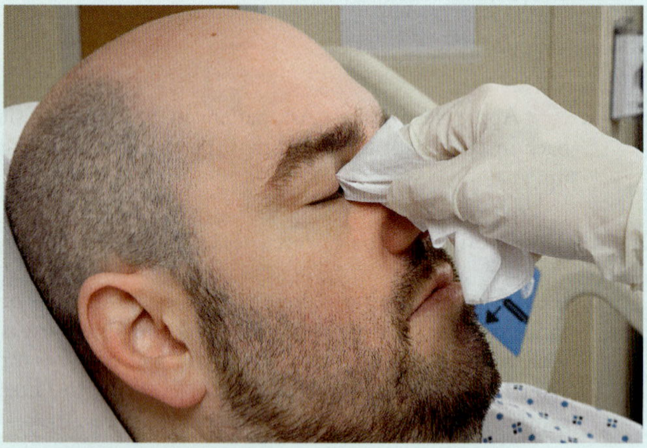

STEP 7D(6) Apply gentle pressure against nasolacrimal duct after giving eye medications.

STEP	RATIONALE
(7) After instilling drops, ask patient to close eyes gently.	Helps distribute medication. Squinting or squeezing eyelids forces medication from conjunctival sac (American Academy of Ophthalmology, 2021; Lampert et al., 2019).
e. Instill ophthalmic ointment.	
(1) *Option:* Apply clean gloves if eye drainage is present. Holding applicator above lower lid margin, apply thin ribbon of ointment evenly along inner edge of lower eyelid on conjunctiva (see Step 7e[1] illustration) from inner to outer canthus.	Reduces transmission of microorganisms. Distributes medication evenly across eye and lid margin.

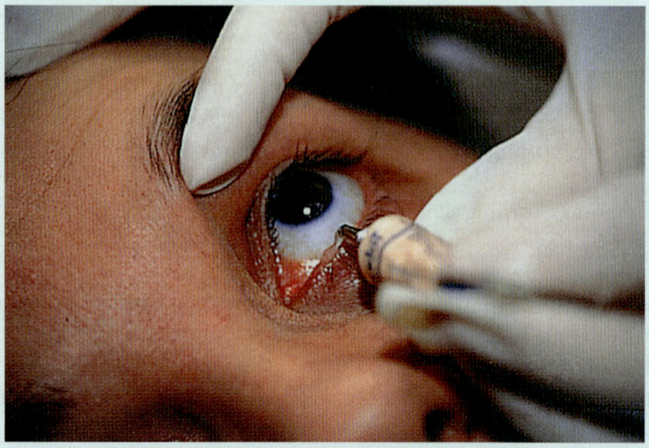

STEP 7E(1) Nurse applies ointment along inner edge of lower eyelid from inner to outer canthus.

STEP	RATIONALE

IMPLEMENTATION

STEP	RATIONALE
(2) Have patient close eye and rub lid lightly in circular motion with cotton ball if not contraindicated. Avoid placing pressure directly against patient's eyeball.	Further distributes medication without traumatizing eye.
(3) If excess medication is on eyelid, gently wipe it from inner to outer canthus.	Promotes comfort and prevents trauma to eye.
(4) If patient needs an eye patch, apply clean one by placing it over affected eye so entire eye is covered. Tape securely without applying pressure to eye.	Clean eye patch reduces risk of infection.
f. Insert intraocular disc.	
(1) Apply clean gloves. Open package containing disc. Gently press your fingertip against disc so it adheres to your finger. It may be necessary to moisten gloved finger with sterile saline. Position convex side of disc on your fingertip.	Reduces transmission of microorganisms. Allows you to inspect disc for damage or deformity.
(2) With your other hand, gently pull patient's lower eyelid away from eye. Ask patient to look up.	Prepares conjunctival sac for receiving medicated disc and moves sensitive cornea away.
(3) Place disc in conjunctival sac so it floats on sclera between iris and lower eyelid (see Step 7f[3] illustration).	Ensures delivery of medication.
(4) Pull patient's lower eyelid out and over disc (see Step 7f[4] illustration). You should not be able to see disc at this time. Repeat if you can see disc.	Ensures accurate medication delivery.

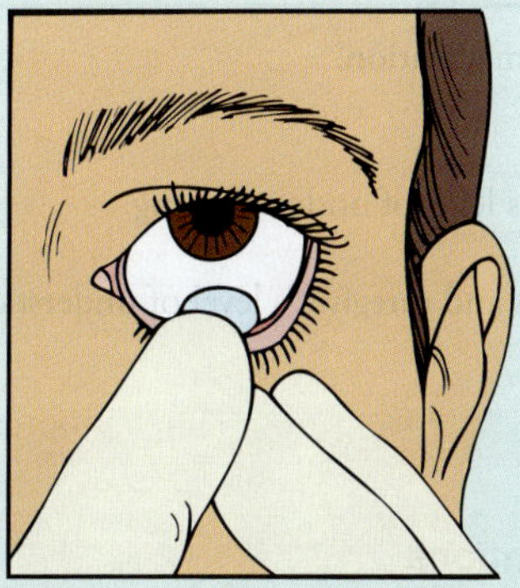

STEP 7F(3) Place intraocular disc in conjunctival sac between iris and lower eyelid.

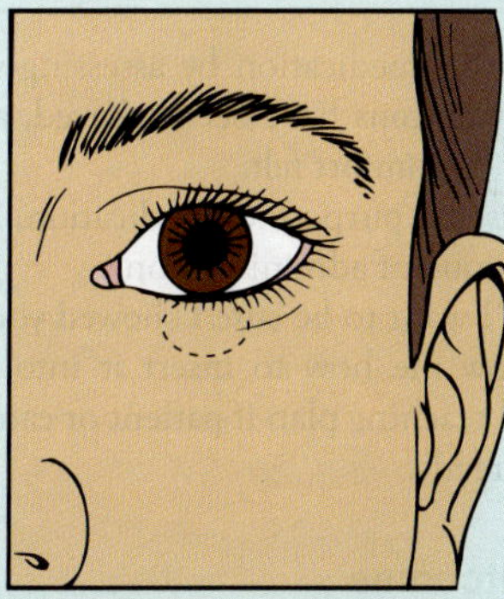

STEP 7F(4) Gently pull patient's lower eyelid over disc.

STEP	RATIONALE
8. After administering eye medications, remove and dispose of gloves and soiled supplies in appropriate receptacle.	Reduces spread of microorganisms.
9. Remove intraocular disc.	
a. Apply clean gloves. Gently pull downward on lower eyelid using your nondominant hand.	Reduces transmission of microorganisms. Exposes disc.
b. Using forefinger and thumb of your dominant hand, pinch disc and lift it out of patient's eye (see Step 9b illustration).	

STEP	RATIONALE

IMPLEMENTATION

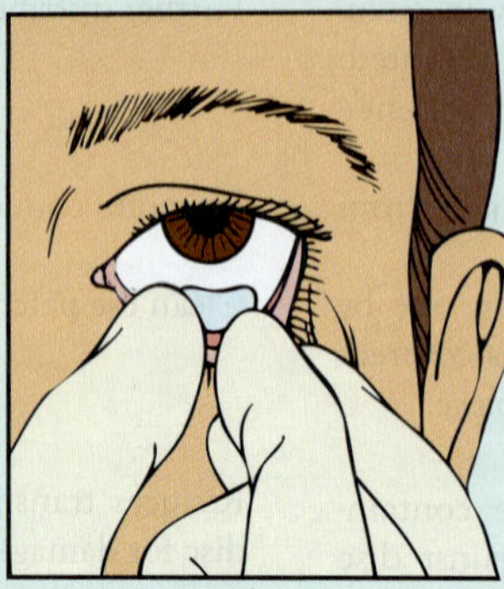

STEP 9B Carefully pinch disc to remove it from patient's eye.

EVALUATION

1. Observe response to medication by assessing visual changes, asking whether symptoms have been relieved, and noting any adverse effects or discomfort felt.	Evaluates effects of medication.
2. Ask patient to discuss purpose of medication, action, adverse effects, and technique of administration.	Determines patient's level of understanding.
3. Use teach-back: "I want to be sure I showed you how to insert the eye disc. Show me how to insert it into your left eye." Develop a revised teaching plan if patient or caregiver is unable to teach back correctly.	Determines patient's and caregiver's level of understanding of instructional topic.

Unexpected Outcomes	Related Interventions
1. Patient reports burning or pain or experiences local adverse effects (e.g., headache, bloodshot eyes, local eye irritation). Medication concentration and patient's sensitivity both influence chances of adverse effects developing.	• Eyedrops may have been instilled onto cornea, or dropper touched surface of eye. • Notify health care provider for possible adjustment in medication type and dosage.
2. Patient experiences systemic effects from drops (e.g., increased heart rate and blood pressure from epinephrine, decreased heart rate and blood pressure from timolol).	• Notify health care provider immediately. • Remain with patient. Assess vital signs. • Withhold further doses.
3. Patient is unable to explain medication information or steps for taking eyedrops and/or has trouble manipulating dropper.	• Repeat instructions and include caregiver as appropriate. Include return demonstration.

Communication and Documentation

- Document medication, concentration, dose or strength, number of drops, site of application (left, right, or both eyes), and time of administration on MAR immediately after administration, not before. Include initials or signature.
- Document patient teaching and validation of patient's understanding on flow sheet or in progress notes in EHR or chart.
- Document objective data related to tissues involved (e.g., redness, drainage, irritation), any subjective data (e.g., pain, itching, altered vision), and patient's response to medications. Note any adverse effects experienced on flow sheet or in progress notes in EHR or chart.
- Report adverse effects, patient response, and/or withheld medications to nurse in charge or health care provider. Depending on

medication, immediate notification of health care provider may be required.

DOCUMENTATION EXAMPLE

Patient safely administered their prescribed eye drops at 1000 hours. Patient understood why the drops were prescribed and how to self-administer the drops. No side effects noted. Patient stated they feel comfortable administering the drops at home.

Special Considerations

Teaching

- Warn patients that mydriatics (medication used to dilate the pupils) temporarily blur vision. Wearing sunglasses reduces photophobia. If necessary, have patient make arrangements for transportation home from an office or clinic visit.
- Patients who receive medications that paralyze the ciliary muscles of the eye (e.g., scopolamine, atropine, and cycloplegics) should not drive or attempt to perform any activity that requires acute vision after receiving medication.

Pediatric

- Infants often clench the eyes tightly to avoid eyedrops. Place the drops at the nasal corner where the lids meet while the infant is supine. When the infant opens their eyes, the medication will flow into it.
- If the eye ointment is to be given once a day, administer at bedtime because it will blur the child's vision (Keenan-Lindsay et al., 2022).
- When parents are present, have them gently hold the child's head with the child in their lap, when appropriate. Keep the child's hands away from the eyes.

Gerontological

- Before discharging an older person, evaluate patient's ability to perform all the necessary steps for the administration of eyedrops and ointments.

Care in the Community: Home Management

- When using OTC eyedrops, patients should not share medications with other caregivers. Risk for infection transmission is high. In addition, instruct patients to carefully follow manufacturer instructions for dosing.

✦ SKILL 21.5 Administering Ear Medications

Video Clip *NSO Nursing Skills Online Nonparenteral Medication Administration Module 6 / Lesson 5*

Ear (otic) medications are usually delivered in a solution and instilled as drops. When administering ear medications, be aware of certain safety precautions. Internal ear structures are very sensitive to temperature extremes; administer eardrops at room temperature. Instilling cold drops can cause vertigo (severe dizziness) or nausea and debilitate a patient for several minutes. Although the structures of the outer ear are not sterile, use sterile drops and solutions in case the eardrum is ruptured. A final safety precaution is to avoid forcing any solution into the ear. Do not occlude the ear canal with a medicine dropper because this can cause pressure within the canal during instillation and subsequent injury to the eardrum. If you follow these precautions, instillation of eardrops is a safe and effective therapy.

Equipment

- MAR (electronic or printed)
- Medication bottle with dropper
- Cotton-tipped applicator, cotton balls
- Clean gloves if drainage is present

Delegation and Collaboration

The skill of administering ear medications cannot be delegated to a UCP. The nurse instructs the UCP about the following:

- Potential adverse effects of medications and to report their occurrence
- The potential for dizziness or irritation after administration of ear medications

STEP	RATIONALE
ASSESSMENT	
1. Identify patient using at least two person-specific identifiers (e.g., name and date of birth or name and medical record number) according to employer policy.	Ensures correct patient. Complies with Accreditation Canada's standards and improves patient safety (Accreditation Canada, 2020).
2. Throughout the procedure, the 4 moments for hand hygiene are to be implemented; hand hygiene should occur before initial patient (or patient environment) contact, before an aseptic procedure, after body fluid exposure risk, and after patient (or patient environment) contact. Additional hand hygiene should be performed when hands are visibly soiled.	Proper hand hygiene helps prevent the spread of infectious agents to health care providers.
3. Check accuracy and completeness of each MAR by comparing with health care provider's medication prescription. Check patient's name, medication name and dosage, route, and time for administration. Clarify incomplete or unclear prescriptions with health care provider before administration.	The prescription sheet is the most reliable source and only legal record of medications that patient is to receive. It ensures that patient receives correct medications (College of Physicians and Surgeons of Ontario, 2019; Pharmacy Association of Nova Scotia, n.d.). Handwritten MARs are a source of medication errors (Parthasarathi et al., 2021; Tariq et al., 2022).
4. Review pertinent information related to medication, including action, purpose, normal dose and route (one or both ears), adverse effects, time of onset and peak action, and nursing implications.	Allows you to anticipate effects of medication and observe patient's response.

STEP	RATIONALE
ASSESSMENT	
5. Assess condition of external ear structures (see Chapter 8). This may be done just before medication instillation (if drainage is present, apply clean gloves).	Provides baseline to determine whether local response to medications occurs. Also indicates need to clean ear before medication application.
6. Determine whether patient has any symptoms of ear discomfort or hearing impairment.	Certain ear medications act to either lessen or increase these symptoms. Occlusion of external ear canal by swelling, drainage, or cerumen can impair hearing acuity and cause pain.
7. Assess patient's medical and medication history and history of allergies (including latex). List medication allergies on each page of the MAR and prominently display it on the patient's medical record per employer policy. When patient has allergy, provide allergy bracelet.	The factors influence how certain medications act. Reveals patient's need for medication. Communication of allergies is essential for safe and effective care.
8. Assess patient's LOC and ability to follow directions.	If patient becomes restless or combative during procedure, greater risk for accidental ear injury exists.
9. Assess patient's knowledge regarding medication therapy and desire to self-administer medication.	Indicates need for health teaching. Motivation influences teaching approach.
10. Assess patient's ability to manipulate and hold ear dropper.	Reflects patient's ability to learn to self-administer medication.

NURSING DIAGNOSES

- Insufficient knowledge regarding medication and self-administration
- Pain (acute or chronic)
- Reduced physical mobility
- Readiness for enhanced self-management of health
- Potential for injury

Related factors and risk factors are individualized on the basis of patient's condition or needs.

STEP	RATIONALE
PLANNING	
1. Expected outcomes following completion of procedure:	
• Patient experiences desired effect of medication.	Medication is administered correctly without injury to patient.
• Patient denies discomfort.	Medication is administered correctly without injury to patient.
• Patient experiences no adverse effects, and symptoms (e.g., dizziness, ear irritation) are relieved.	Medication is distributed and absorbed properly.
• Patient can discuss information about medication and technique correctly.	Demonstrates learning.
• Patient demonstrates self-instillation of eardrops.	Demonstrates learning.
2. Collect appropriate equipment and MAR.	Ensures time management and efficiency.
IMPLEMENTATION	
1. Prepare medications for instillation. Check label of medication against MAR two times (when removing medication from drawer/cabinet and prior to preparing medication for administration; see Skill 21.1). Preparation usually involves taking eardrops out of refrigerator and rewarming to room temperature before administering to patient. Check expiration date on container.	Ear structures are very sensitive to temperature extremes. Cold may cause vertigo and nausea. *These are the first two checks for accuracy.* Process ensures that right patient receives right medication at right time.
2. Identify patient using at least two person-specific identifiers (e.g., name and date of birth, or name and medical record number) according to employer policy. Compare identifiers with information on patient's MAR or medical record and ID band. Replace missing or faded ID bands.	Ensures correct patient. Complies with Accreditation Canada's standards and improves patient safety (Accreditation Canada, 2020).
3. Take medication(s) to patient at correct time (see employer policy). Medications that require exact timing include stat, first-time or loading doses, and one-time doses. Give time-critical scheduled medications (e.g., antibiotics, anticoagulants, insulin, anticonvulsants, immunosuppressive medications) at exact time prescribed (no later than 30 minutes before or after scheduled dose). Give non-time-critical scheduled medications within a range of 1 or 2 hours of scheduled dose, according to employer policy (ISMP, 2011). During administration, apply 10 rights of medication administration.	Hospitals must adopt medication administration policy and procedure for timing of medication administration that considers nature of the prescribed medication, specific clinical application, and patient needs. Time-critical scheduled medications are those for which early or delayed administration of maintenance doses of greater than 30 minutes before or after the scheduled dose may cause harm or result in substantially suboptimal therapy or pharmacological effect. Non-time-critical medications are those for which early or delayed administration within a specified range of either 1 or 2 hours should not cause harm or result in substantially suboptimal therapy or pharmacological effect (ISMP, 2011).

STEP	RATIONALE

IMPLEMENTATION

STEP	RATIONALE
4. Arrange supplies at bedside.	Ensures an organized procedure.
5. At patient's bedside, again compare MAR or computer printout with names of medications on medication labels and patient name. Ask patient whether they have allergies.	Ensures that right patient receives right medication. Confirms patient's allergy history.
6. Explain procedure to patient and sensations to expect. Discuss purpose, action, and possible adverse effects of each medication. Allow patient to ask any questions about the medications. Patients who self-instill medications may be allowed to give drops under nurse's supervision (check employer policy).	Helps patient be a participant in care, which minimizes anxiety. Patient has right to be informed, and their understanding of each medication improves adherence to medication therapy. Begins patient teaching regarding medications.
7. Position patient on side (if not contraindicated) with ear to be treated facing up, or patient may sit in chair or at bedside. Stabilize patient's head with their own hand. *Option:* Apply clean gloves if ear drainage is present.	Facilitates distribution of medication into ear.
8. Straighten ear canal by pulling pinna up and back to 10 o'clock position (for adults and for children older than age 3) (see Step 8 illustration) or down and back to 6 to 9 o'clock position (children under age 3).	Straightening ear canal provides direct access to deeper ear structures. Anatomical differences in younger children and infants necessitate the use of different methods of positioning ear canal (Keenan-Lindsay et al., 2022).
9. If cerumen or drainage occludes outermost part of ear canal, wipe out gently with cotton-tipped applicator (see Step 9 illustration). Take care not to force cerumen into canal.	Cerumen and drainage harbour microorganisms and can block distribution of medication into canal. Occlusion blocks sound transmission.
10. Instill prescribed drops holding dropper 1 cm (about 0.5 inches) above ear canal.	Avoiding contact with external ear canal prevents contamination of dropper, which could contaminate medication in container.

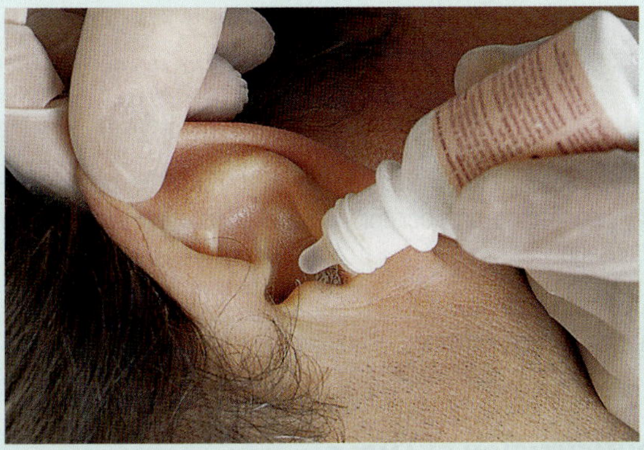

STEP 8 Pull pinna up and back for adults and for children older than 3 years. (*From Astle, B. J., & Duggleby, W. [Eds.]. [2024]. Potter and Perry's Canadian fundamentals of nursing [7th ed.]. Elsevier.*)

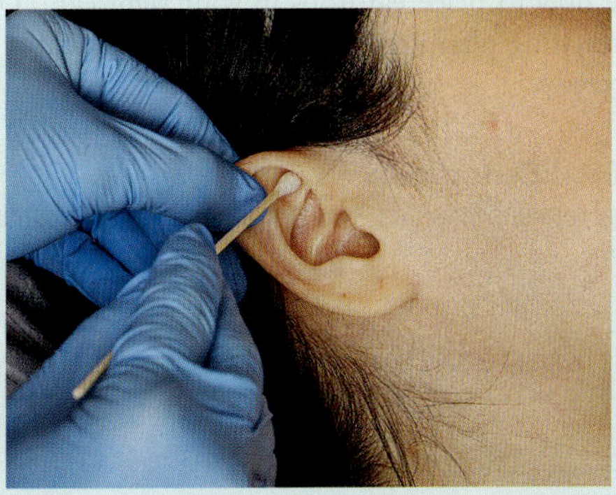

STEP 9 Always clean outer canal only. Do not push cerumen or secretions into ear.

STEP	RATIONALE
11. Ask patient to remain in side-lying position for a few minutes. Apply gentle massage or pressure to tragus of ear with finger (see Step 11 illustration).	Allows complete distribution of medication. Pressure and massage move medication inward.

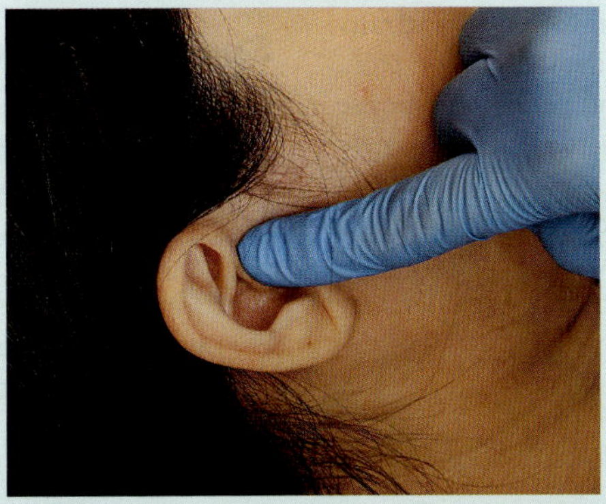

STEP 11 Nurse applies gentle pressure to tragus of ear after instilling drops.

STEP	RATIONALE
IMPLEMENTATION	
12. If prescribed, gently insert part of cotton ball into outermost part of canal. Do not press cotton into canal.	Prevents escape of medication when patient sits or stands.
13. Remove cotton after 15 minutes. Help patient to comfortable position after drops are absorbed.	Allows time for medication distribution and absorption.
14. Dispose of soiled supplies in proper receptacle. Remove and dispose of gloves.	Reduces spread of microorganisms.
EVALUATION	
1. Observe response to medication by assessing hearing changes, asking whether symptoms have been relieved, and noting any adverse effects or discomfort felt.	Evaluates effects of medication.
2. Ask patient to discuss purpose of medication, action, adverse effects, and technique of administration.	Determines patient's level of understanding.
3. **Use teach-back:** "I want to be sure I clearly showed you how to administer eardrops. Let's take this time we have so you can show me how to place eardrops in your right ear." Develop a revised teaching plan if patient or caregiver is unable to teach back correctly.	Determines patient's and caregiver's level of understanding of instructional topic.

Unexpected Outcomes	Related Interventions
1. Ear canal remains inflamed, swollen, and tender to palpation. Drainage is present.	• Hold next dose. • Notify health care provider for possible adjustment in medication type and dosage.
2. Patient's hearing acuity does not improve.	• Notify health care provider. • Cerumen may be impacted, requiring ear irrigation.

Communication and Documentation

- Document medication, concentration, dose or strength, number of drops, site of application (left, right, or both ears), and time of administration on MAR immediately after administration, not before. Include initials or signature.
- Document patient teaching and validation of patient's understanding on flow sheet or in progress notes in EHR or chart.
- Document objective data related to tissues involved (e.g., drainage, tenderness, irritation), any subjective data (e.g., ear pain, ringing in ears, change in hearing acuity), and patient's response to medications. Note any adverse effects experienced in progress notes in EHR or chart.
- Report adverse effects, patient response, and/or withheld medications to nurse in charge or health care provider. Depending on medication, immediate notification of health care provider may be required.

DOCUMENTATION EXAMPLE

Patient's ear drops administered as prescribed. Patient stated that their right ear hurt after the drops were placed. The pain was rated as a 3 out of 10 and lasted for approximately 15 minutes. There was no change noted in their hearing on that side. The health care provider was notified and stated they will assess the patient on rounds.

Special Considerations

Pediatric

- Insert cotton pledgets (small wads of absorbent cotton) loosely into ear canal to prevent medication from flowing out. To prevent cotton from absorbing medication, premoisten it with a few drops of medication (Keenan-Lindsay et al., 2022).
- Ensure that parents are taught how to correctly administer the eardrops (e.g., for children under age 3, gently pull the pinna downward and straight back).
- Teach parents of children with frequent otitis media the signs of hearing loss and the need for follow-up care.

✦ SKILL 21.6 Administering Nasal Instillations

Patients with nasal sinus problems may receive medications by spray, drops, or tampons. The most commonly administered form of nasal instillation is a decongestant spray or drops used to relieve sinus congestion and cold symptoms. Many OTC nasal preparations contain sympathomimetic medications (e.g., Neo-Synephrine). These medications are relatively safe when administered nasally because only small doses are needed. However, the medications can enter the systemic circulation by way of the nasal mucosa or by the GI tract if an excess amount is swallowed, causing restlessness, nervousness, tremors, or insomnia in some patients. Long-term use of decongestant nasal spray can worsen nasal congestion because of a rebound effect. Nasal sprays are easy for a patient to self-administer. Health care providers treat severe nosebleeds by placing nasal packing or tampons and administering epinephrine to slow bleeding.

Delegation and Collaboration

The skill of administering nasal instillations cannot be delegated to a UCP. The nurse directs the UCP about the following:

- Potential adverse effects of medications and to report their occurrence to the nurse.
- Reporting any bloody nasal drainage to the nurse.

Equipment

- MAR (electronic or printed)
- Prepared medication with clean dropper or spray container
- Facial tissue
- Small pillow *(optional)*
- Washcloth *(optional)*
- Clean gloves

STEP	RATIONALE
ASSESSMENT	
1. Identify patient using at least two person-specific identifiers (e.g., name and date of birth or name and medical record number) according to employer policy.	Ensures correct patient. Complies with Accreditation Canada's standards and improves patient safety (Accreditation Canada, 2020).
2. Throughout the procedure, the 4 moments for hand hygiene are to be implemented; hand hygiene should occur before initial patient (or patient environment) contact, before an aseptic procedure, after body fluid exposure risk, and after patient (or patient environment) contact. Additional hand hygiene should be performed when hands are visibly soiled.	Proper hand hygiene helps prevent the spread of infectious agents to health care providers.
3. Check accuracy and completeness of each MAR by comparing with health care provider's medication prescription. Check patient's name, medication name and dosage, route (which sinus), and time for administration. Clarify incomplete or unclear prescriptions with health care provider before administration.	The prescription sheet is the most reliable source and only legal record of medications that patient is to receive. It ensures that patient receives the correct medications (College of Physicians and Surgeons of Ontario, 2019; Pharmacy Association of Nova Scotia, n.d.). Handwritten MARs are a source of medication errors (Parthasarathi et al., 2021; Tariq et al., 2022).
4. Review pertinent information related to medication, including action, purpose, normal dose and route, adverse effects, time of onset and peak action, and nursing implications.	Allows you to anticipate effects of medication and observe patient's response.
5. Assess patient's medical history (e.g., hypertension, heart disease, diabetes, and hyperthyroidism), medication history, and history of allergies. List medication allergies on each page of the MAR and prominently display it on the patient's medical record per employer policy. When patient has allergy, provide allergy bracelet.	These conditions contraindicate use of decongestants that stimulate central nervous system. Communication of allergies is essential for safe and effective care.
6. Use penlight and inspect condition of nose and sinuses (see Chapter 8). Palpate sinuses for pain or tenderness. Note type of drainage if present.	Provides baseline to monitor effects of medication. Presence of discharge interferes with medication absorption. Clear nasal discharge indicates sinus problem. Yellow or greenish discharge indicates infection.
7. Assess patient's knowledge regarding use of nasal instillations, technique for instillation, and willingness to learn self-administration.	Requires health teaching regarding use of medications. Motivation influences teaching approach.

NURSING DIAGNOSES

- Insufficient knowledge regarding medication action and purpose
- Pain (acute or chronic)
- Readiness for enhanced self-management of health
- Potential for injury

Related factors and risk factors are individualized on the basis of patient's condition or needs.

STEP	RATIONALE

PLANNING

1. Expected outcomes following completion of procedure:	
• Patient can breathe without difficulty through nose.	Nasal congestion has been relieved.
• Patient's nasal sinuses are clear, moist, pink, and without drainage after repeated instillations (applies to anti-infective medications).	Inflammation of mucosa has been relieved.
• Patient can explain purpose of medication and administers nasal instillations correctly.	Feedback reflects patient's learning.
2. Collect appropriate equipment and MAR.	Ensures time management and efficiency.

IMPLEMENTATION

1. Prepare medications for instillation. Check label of medication against MAR two times (when removing medication from drawer/cabinet and prior to preparing medication for administration; see Skill 21.1). Preparation usually involves taking nasal drops or sprays out of storage and into patient's room. Check expiration date on container.	*These are the first two checks for accuracy.* Process ensures that right patient receives right medication at right time.
2. Identify patient using at least two person-specific identifiers (e.g., name and date of birth, or name and medical record number) according to employer policy.	Ensures correct patient. Complies with Accreditation Canada's standards and improves patient safety (Accreditation Canada, 2020).
3. Take medication(s) to patient at correct time (see employer policy). Medications that require exact timing include stat, first-time or loading doses, and one-time doses. Give time-critical scheduled medications (e.g., antibiotics, anticoagulants, insulin, anticonvulsants, immunosuppressive medications) at exact time prescribed (no later than 30 minutes before or after scheduled dose). Give non–time-critical scheduled medications within a range of 1 or 2 hours of scheduled dose, according to employer policy (ISMP, 2011). During administration, apply 10 rights of medication administration.	Hospitals must adopt medication administration policy and procedure for timing of medication administration that considers nature of the prescribed medication, specific clinical application, and patient needs. Time-critical scheduled medications are those for which early or delayed administration of maintenance doses of greater than 30 minutes before or after the scheduled dose may cause harm or result in substantially suboptimal therapy or pharmacological effect. Non–time-critical medications are those for which early or delayed administration within a specified range of either 1 or 2 hours should not cause harm or result in substantially suboptimal therapy or pharmacological effect (ISMP, 2011).
4. At patient's bedside, again compare MAR or computer printout with names of medications on medication labels and patient name. Ask patient whether they have allergies.	Ensures that right patient receives right medication. Confirms patient's allergy history.
5. Explain procedure to patient and sensations to expect. Discuss purpose, action, and possible adverse effects of each medication. Allow patient to ask any questions about medications. Patients who self-instill medications may be allowed to give drops under nurse's supervision (check employer policy). Tell patients receiving nasal instillation that they may experience burning or stinging of mucosa or choking sensation as medication trickles into throat.	Helps patient be a participant in care, which minimizes anxiety. Patient has right to be informed, and their understanding of each medication improves adherence to medication therapy. Begins patient teaching regarding medications.
6. Arrange supplies and medications at bedside. Apply clean gloves (if drainage is present).	Reduces transmission of microorganisms; ensures smooth, orderly procedure.
7. Gently roll or shake container. Instruct patient to clear or blow nose gently unless contraindicated (e.g., risk of increased intracranial pressure or nosebleed).	Ensures distribution of medication. Allows medication to reach sinuses.
8. Administer nose drops.	
a. Help patient to upright position (Binita et al., 2020; Smith & Hasham, 2021).	Proper positioning provides access to specific nasal passages.

STEP	RATIONALE

IMPLEMENTATION

(1) For access to posterior pharynx, tilt patient's head backward.

(2) For access to ethmoid or sphenoid sinus, tilt head back over edge of bed or place small pillow under patient's shoulder and tilt head back (see Step 8a[2] illustration).

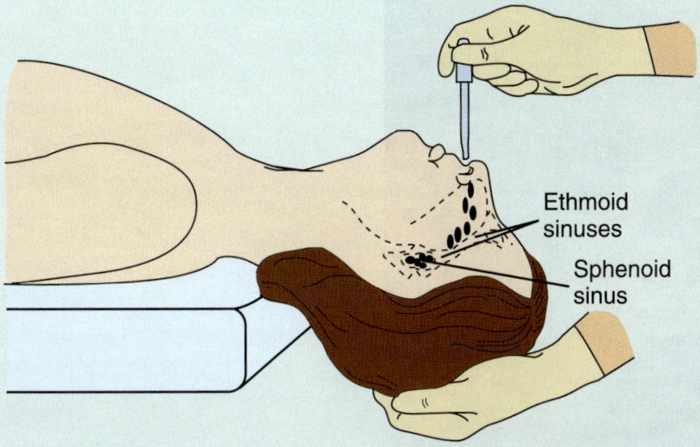

STEP 8A(2) Position for instilling nose drops into ethmoid or sphenoid sinus.

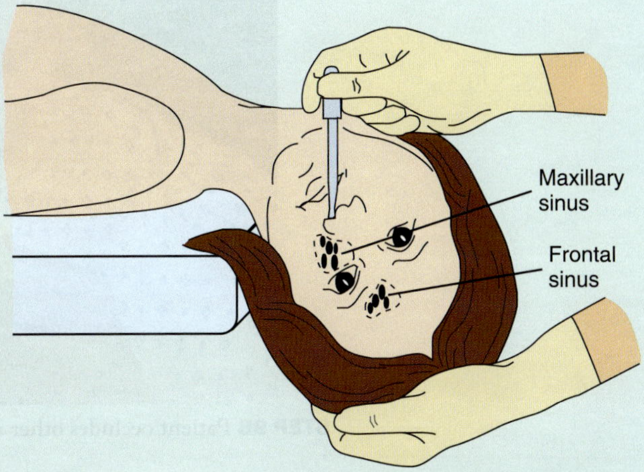

STEP 8A(3) Position for instilling nose drops into frontal and maxillary sinus.

STEP	RATIONALE
(3) For access to frontal and maxillary sinus, tilt head back over edge of bed or pillow with head turned toward side to be treated (see Step 8a[3] illustration).	Position allows medication to drain into affected sinus.
b. Support patient's head with nondominant hand.	Prevents straining neck muscles.
c. Instruct patient to breathe through mouth.	Mouth breathing reduces chance of aspirating nasal drops into trachea and lungs.
d. Hold dropper 1 cm (about 0.5 inches) above nares and instill prescribed number of drops toward midline of ethmoid bone.	Avoids contamination of dropper. Instilling toward ethmoid bone facilitates distribution of medication over nasal mucosa.
e. Have patient remain in supine position for 5 minutes.	Prevents premature loss of medication through nares.
f. Offer facial tissue to blot runny nose but caution patient against blowing nose for several minutes.	Provides comfort but allows for absorption of medication.
9. Administer nasal spray.	
a. Help patient into upright position with head tilted slightly forward.	Proper positioning permits medication spray to reach nasal passages.
b. Instruct (or assist) patient to insert tip of nasal spray into appropriate nares and occlude other nostril with finger (see Step 9b illustration). Point spray tip toward side and away from centre of nose (Binita et al., 2020; Smith & Hasham, 2021).	Allows for proper administration of medication.

STEP	RATIONALE

IMPLEMENTATION

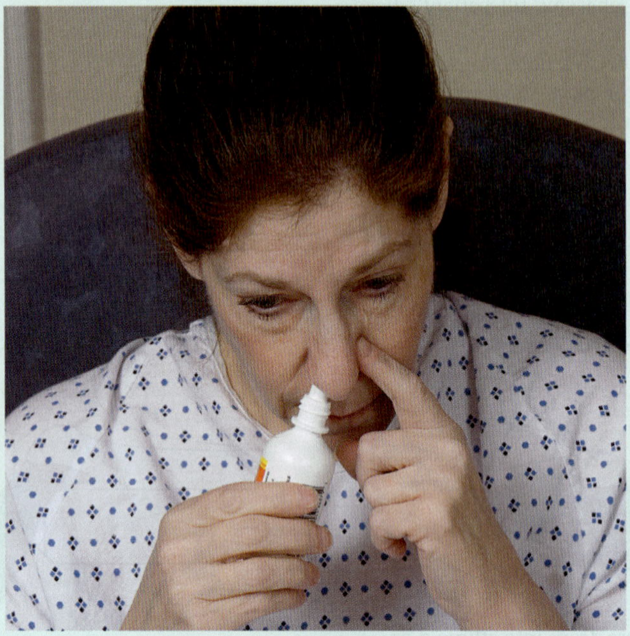

STEP 9B Patient occludes other nostril before self-administering nasal spray.

c. Have patient spray medication into nose while inhaling. Help them remove nozzle from nose and instruct them to breathe out through mouth.	Allows for proper administration and distribution of nasal medication as high into nasal passages as possible.
d. Offer facial tissue to blot runny nose but caution patient against blowing nose for several minutes.	Provides comfort but allows for absorption of medication.

Critical Decision Point *Some medications are designed for one spray per dose. Examples include calcitonin, desmopressin, and sumatriptan. It is essential to ensure that the patient understands the correct number of sprays to use per dose to prevent overdosing.*

10. Help patient to a comfortable position after medication is absorbed.	Restores comfort.
11. Dispose of soiled supplies, and remove and dispose of gloves.	Reduces spread of microorganisms.

EVALUATION

1. Observe patient for onset of adverse effects for 15–30 minutes after administration.	Medications absorbed through mucosa can cause systemic reaction.
2. Ask patient whether they can breathe through nose after decongestant administration. It may be necessary to have patient occlude one nostril at a time and breathe deeply.	Determines effectiveness of decongestant medication.
3. Reinspect condition of nasal passages between instillations.	Condition of mucosa reveals response to medication.
4. Ask patient to describe risks of overusing decongestants and methods for administration.	Feedback ensures that patient can self-administer medications properly.
5. Have patient demonstrate self-medication.	Feedback demonstrates learning.
6. **Use teach-back:** "I want to be sure I explained the importance of not overusing your nasal spray. Explain to me why it is important not to overuse nasal sprays." Develop a revised teaching plan if patient or caregiver is unable to teach back correctly.	Determines patient's and caregiver's level of understanding of instructional topic.

Unexpected Outcomes	Related Interventions
1. Patient is unable to breathe easily through nasal passages. Mucosa appears swollen, and congestion is unrelieved, possibly because of rebound effect.	• Stop medication use. • Notify health care provider and consider alternative therapy.
2. Nasal mucosa remains inflamed and tender, with discharge from nares.	• Consider alternative therapy.
3. Patient indicates sinus headache. Sinuses remain congested.	• Consider alternative therapy.

Communication and Documentation

- Document medication name, concentration, number of drops, nare into which medication was instilled, and actual time of administration on MAR immediately after administration, not before. Include initials or signature.
- Document patient's response to medication, patient teaching, and validation of patient's understanding on flow sheet or in progress notes in her or chart.
- Report any unusual systemic or adverse effects and patient response and/or withheld medications to nurse in charge or health care provider.

DOCUMENTATION EXAMPLE

Patient correctly self-administered their nasal spray as prescribed. Patient tolerated the spray well and stated they were comfortable self-administering the nasal spray.

Special Considerations

Teaching

- Instruct patients that each medication should have a different dropper or spray applicator. Instruct patients to wash or rinse applicators after each use.
- Use OTC nasal sprays or nose drops for only one illness; bottles easily become contaminated with bacteria.
- Overuse of nasal sprays and drops can cause rebound sinus congestion, resulting in sinus pain and headache.

Pediatric

- Infants are nose breathers, and the possible congestion caused by nasal medications may inhibit their sucking. Administer nose drops if prescribed 20 to 30 minutes before feedings (Keenan-Lindsay et al., 2022).

✦ SKILL 21.7 Using Metered-Dose Inhalers

NSO *Nursing Skills Online Nonparenteral Medication Administration Module 6 / Lesson 6*

Medications administered with handheld metered-dose inhalers (MDIs) are dispersed through an aerosol spray, mist, or powder that penetrates the airways. For aerosol medication administration, some aerosols are administered by connecting to the wall outlet–either medical air or oxygen. Whether to use medical air or oxygen will depend on employer policy and the patient population (e.g., a patient with chronic obstructive pulmonary disease [COPD] would require medical air, whereas a pediatric patient would require oxygen). Pressurized metered-dose inhalers (pMDIs), breath-actuated metered-dose inhalers (BAIs), and dry powder inhalers (DPIs) deliver medications that produce local effects such as bronchodilation. Some of these medications are absorbed rapidly through the pulmonary circulation and create systemic side effects (e.g., albuterol may cause palpitations, tremors, and tachycardia). Patients who receive medications by inhalation frequently suffer from asthma and chronic respiratory disease. Medications administered by inhalation provide control of airway hyperactivity or bronchial constriction. Because patients depend on these medications for disease control, patient education is vital for correct use of inhalers and to ensure effectiveness of inhaled medications.

An MDI is a small, handheld device that disperses medication into the airways through an aerosol spray or mist by activation of a propellant. Dosing is usually achieved with 1 or 2 puffs. DPIs deliver inhaled medication in a fine powder formulation to the respiratory tract (see Procedural Guideline 21.1). The deeper passages of the respiratory tract provide a large surface area for medication absorption, and the alveolar-capillary network absorbs medication rapidly.

An MDI delivers a measured dose of the medication with each depression of a canister. Approximately 2.3 to 4.5 kg (5 to 10 lb) of pressure is needed to activate the aerosol. This action is difficult for some older patients because hand strength diminishes with age. Because use of an MDI requires coordination with the breathing cycle, many patients spray only the back of their throats and fail to receive a full dose. The inhaler must be depressed to expel medication just as the patient inhales. This ensures that the medication reaches the lower airways. A patient with poor coordination may need to use a spacer device or a BAI to administer the medication properly. A spacer device decreases the amount of medication deposited into the oropharyngeal mucosa. Some spacers have a one-way valve that activates on inhalation, thereby removing the need for good hand-breath coordination (Keeley & Partridge, 2019). Box 21.4 summarizes common problems that occur when using an inhaler.

Delegation and Collaboration

The skill of administering MDIs cannot be delegated to a UCP. The nurse instructs the UCP about the following:

- Potential adverse effects of medications and reporting their occurrence to the nurse
- Reporting breathing difficulty (e.g., paroxysmal or sustained coughing, audible wheezing) to the nurse

Equipment

- MAR (electronic or printed)
- Inhaler device with medication canister (MDI or DPI) (Fig. 21.2, A–C)
- Spacer device such as AeroChamber or InspirEase *(optional)*
- Facial tissues *(optional)*
- Stethoscope
- Peak flowmeter *(optional)*

BOX 21.4

Common Problems With Using an Inhaler

- *Not taking the medication as prescribed:* Taking either too much or too little.
- *Incorrect activation:* This problem usually occurs when the canister is depressed before taking a breath. These actions should be done simultaneously so that the medication can be carried down to the lungs with the breath.
- *Forgetting to shake the inhaler:* The medication is in a suspension; therefore, particles may settle. If the inhaler is not shaken, it may not deliver the correct dose of the medication.
- *Not waiting long enough between puffs:* A delay between puffs is needed before taking a second puff; otherwise, an incorrect dose may be delivered, or the medication may not penetrate into the lungs.
- *Failure to clean the valve:* Particles may jam the valve in the mouthpiece unless it is cleaned occasionally. This problem is a frequent cause of failure to get 200 puffs from one inhaler.
- *Failure to observe whether the inhaler is actually releasing a spray:* If it is not, the inhaler should be checked by the pharmacist.
- *Failure to recognize when the canister is empty:* This occurs when the metered-dose inhaler has no built-in dose counter or instructions for dose counting.

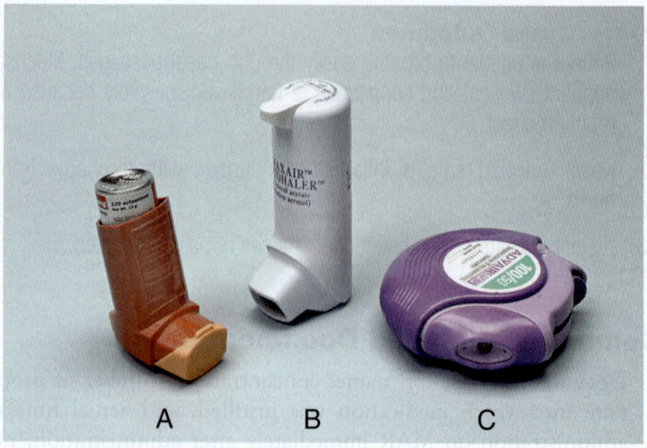

FIG 21.2 Types of inhalers. A, Metered-dose inhaler (MDI). B, Breath-actuated metered-dose inhaler (BAI). C, Dry powder inhaler (DPI).

STEP	RATIONALE
ASSESSMENT	
1. Identify patient using at least two person-specific identifiers (e.g., name and date of birth or name and medical record number) according to employer policy.	Ensures correct patient. Complies with Accreditation Canada's standards and improves patient safety (Accreditation Canada, 2020).
2. Throughout the procedure, the 4 moments for hand hygiene are to be implemented; hand hygiene should occur before initial patient (or patient environment) contact, before an aseptic procedure, after body fluid exposure risk, and after patient (or patient environment) contact. Additional hand hygiene should be performed when hands are visibly soiled.	Proper hand hygiene helps prevent the spread of infectious agents to health care providers.
3. Check accuracy and completeness of each MAR by comparing with health care provider's medication prescription. Check patient's name, medication name and dosage, route, and time for administration. Clarify incomplete or unclear prescriptions with health care provider before administration.	The prescription sheet is the most reliable source and only legal record of medications that patient is to receive. It ensures that patient receives correct medications (College of Physicians and Surgeons of Ontario, 2019; Pharmacy Association of Nova Scotia, n.d.). Handwritten MARs are a source of medication errors (Parthasarathi et al., 2021; Tariq et al., 2022).
4. Review pertinent information related to medication, including action, purpose, normal dose and route, adverse effects, time of onset and peak action, and nursing implications.	Allows you to anticipate effects of medication and observe patient's response.
5. Assess patient's medical and medication history and history of allergies. List medication allergies on each page of the MAR and prominently display it on the patient's medical record per employer policy. When patient has allergy, provide allergy bracelet.	These factors influence how certain medications act. Reveals patient's need for medication. Communication of allergies is essential for safe and effective care.
6. Assess respiratory pattern and auscultate breath sounds (see Chapter 8). Also assess exercise tolerance; does patient develop shortness of breath easily?	Establishes baseline of airway status for comparison during and after treatment.
7. Assess patient's ability to hold, manipulate, and depress canister and inhaler.	Any impairment of grasp or presence of hand tremors interferes with patient's ability to depress canister within inhaler. Spacer device is often necessary.
8. If patient was previously instructed in self-administration, have them demonstrate how to use the device.	Patients who have adequate understanding of how to use an inhaler often forget the procedure. Ongoing assessment of inhaler technique identifies areas for further education and reinforcement (Asmare et al., 2021; Kim at al., 2021).
9. Assess patient's readiness and ability to learn (e.g., asks questions about medication; is alert; participates in own care; is not fatigued, in pain, or in respiratory distress).	One-on-one patient assessment prepares patient for self-management and greater adherence to inhaler use (Asmare et al., 2021; Kim et al., 2021). In some situations, mental or physical limitations affect the patient's ability to learn and the methods used for instruction.
10. Assess patient's knowledge and understanding of their condition and purpose and action of prescribed medications.	Knowledge of condition is essential for patient to understand how to correctly use inhaler.

STEP	RATIONALE

NURSING DIAGNOSES

- Inadequate breathing pattern
- Reduced gas exchange
- Reduced stamina
- Anxiety
- Insufficient knowledge regarding use of MDI
- Ready for enhanced self-management of health
- Potential for injury

Related factors and risk factors are individualized on the basis of patient's condition or needs.

PLANNING

STEP	RATIONALE
1. Expected outcomes following completion of procedure:	
• Patient correctly self-administers a metered dose.	Demonstrates learning.
• Patient describes proper time during respiratory cycle to inhale and spray and number of inhalations for each administration.	Demonstrates learning and ensures correct administration of medication.
• Patient's breathing pattern improves, and lung sounds indicate that airways are less restrictive.	Demonstrates therapeutic effect of medication in improving gas exchange.
2. Collect appropriate equipment and MAR.	Ensures time management and efficiency.

IMPLEMENTATION

STEP	RATIONALE
1. Prepare medications for inhalation. Check label of medication against MAR two times (when removing medication from drawer/cabinet and prior to preparing medication for administration; see Skill 21.1). Preparation usually involves taking inhaler device out of storage and into patient's room. Check expiration date on container.	*These are the first two checks for accuracy.* Process ensures that right patient receives right medication at right time.
2. Identify patient using at least two person-specific identifiers (e.g., name and date of birth, or name and medical record number) according to employer policy.	Ensures correct patient. Complies with Accreditation Canada's standards and improves patient safety (Accreditation Canada, 2020).
3. Take medication(s) to patient at correct time (see employer policy). Medications that require exact timing include stat, first-time or loading doses, and one-time doses. Give time-critical scheduled medications (e.g., antibiotics, anticoagulants, insulin, anticonvulsants, immunosuppressive medications) at exact time prescribed (no later than 30 minutes before or after scheduled dose). Give non–time-critical scheduled medications within a range of 1 or 2 hours of scheduled dose, according to employer policy (ISMP, 2011). During administration, apply 10 rights of medication administration.	Hospitals must adopt medication administration policy and procedure for timing of medication administration that considers nature of the prescribed medication, specific clinical application, and patient needs. Time-critical scheduled medications are those for which early or delayed administration of maintenance doses of greater than 30 minutes before or after the scheduled dose may cause harm or result in substantially suboptimal therapy or pharmacological effect. Non–time-critical medications are those for which early or delayed administration within a specified range of either 1 or 2 hours should not cause harm or result in substantially suboptimal therapy or pharmacological effect (ISMP, 2011).
4. At patient's bedside, again compare MAR or computer printout with names of medications on medication labels and patient name. Ask patient whether they have allergies.	Ensures that right patient receives right medication. Confirms patient's allergy history.
5. Explain procedure to patient. Be specific if patient wishes to self-administer medication. Explain where and how to set up at home. Discuss purpose, action, and possible adverse effects of each medication. Allow patient to ask any questions about the medications. Explain what a metered dose is and how to administer. Warn about overuse of inhaler and side effects.	Helps patient be a participant in care, which minimizes anxiety. Patient has right to be informed, and their understanding of each medication improves adherence to medication therapy. Begins patient teaching regarding medications.
6. Allow adequate time for patient to manipulate inhaler, canister, and spacer device (if provided). Explain and demonstrate how canister fits into inhaler.	Patient must be familiar with how to use equipment.

STEP	RATIONALE

IMPLEMENTATION

Critical Decision Point *If using an MDI that is new or has not been used for several days, push a "test spray" into the air to prime the device before using. This step ensures that the MDI is patent and the metal canister is positioned properly.*

STEP	RATIONALE
7. Explain and demonstrate steps for administering MDI without spacer.	Simple one-on-one instruction and demonstration of step-by-step administration allows patient to ask questions at any point during procedure and increases patient adherence to inhaler use (Asmare et al., 2021).
a. Remove mouthpiece cover from inhaler after inserting MDI canister into holder.	
b. Shake inhaler well for 2–5 seconds (five or six shakes).	Ensures mixing of medication in canister.
c. Hold inhaler in dominant hand.	
d. Have patient stand or sit and instruct them to position inhaler in one of two ways:	
(1) Have patient place the mouthpiece in the mouth between the teeth and over the tongue, aimed toward back of throat, with lips closed tightly around it. Do not block the mouthpiece with the teeth or tongue (see Step 7d[1] illustration).	Ensures proper fit to inhale medication.
(2) Position mouthpiece 2.5–5 cm (1–2 inches) in front of wide-open mouth (see Step 7d[2] illustration), with opening of inhaler aimed toward back of throat. Lips should not touch inhaler.	Directs aerosol spray toward airway. This is best way to deliver medication without a spacer.

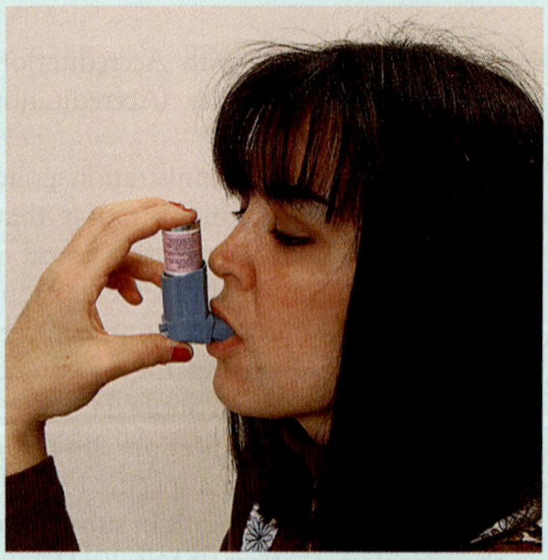

STEP 7D(1) Patient opens lips and places inhaler mouthpiece in mouth with opening aimed toward back of throat.

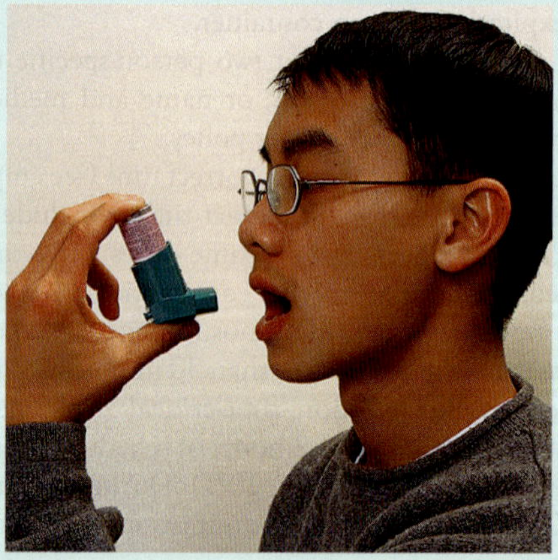

STEP 7D(2) Patient positions inhaler mouthpiece 2 to 4 cm (1 to 2 inches) from wide-open mouth. This position is considered the best way to deliver medication without a spacer.

STEP	RATIONALE
e. While holding the mouthpiece away from the mouth, have patient take deep breath and exhale completely.	Empties lung volume and prepares airway to receive medication.
f. With inhaler positioned, have patient hold it with thumb at mouthpiece and index and middle fingers at top. This is a three-point or bilateral hand position.	Hand position ensures proper activation of MDI and distribution of dosage (Asmare et al., 2021).
g. Instruct patient to tilt head back slightly and inhale slowly and deeply through mouth for 3–5 seconds while depressing canister fully.	Medication is distributed to airways during inhalation.
h. Have patient hold breath for about 10 seconds.	Allows tiny drops of aerosol spray to reach deeper branches of airways.
i. Remove MDI from mouth before exhaling and exhale slowly through nose or pursed lips.	Keeps small airways open during exhalation.
8. Explain and demonstrate steps to administer MDI using spacer device.	Simple one-on-one instruction and demonstration of step-by-step administration allows patient to ask questions at any point during procedure and increases patient adherence to inhaler use (Keeley & Partridge, 2019).

STEP	RATIONALE
IMPLEMENTATION	
a. Remove mouthpiece cover from MDI and mouthpiece of spacer device.	Inhaler fits into end of spacer device.
b. Shake inhaler well for 2–5 seconds (five or six shakes).	Ensures mixing of medication in canister.
c. Insert MDI into end of spacer device.	Spacer device traps medication released from MDI; patient then inhales medication from device. These devices improve delivery of correct dose of inhaled medication (Keeley & Partridge, 2019).
d. Instruct patient to place spacer device mouthpiece in mouth and close lips. Do not insert beyond raised lip on mouthpiece. Avoid covering small exhalation slots with lips.	Medication should not escape through mouth.
e. Have patient breathe normally through spacer device mouthpiece (see Step 8e illustration).	Allows patient to relax before delivering medication.

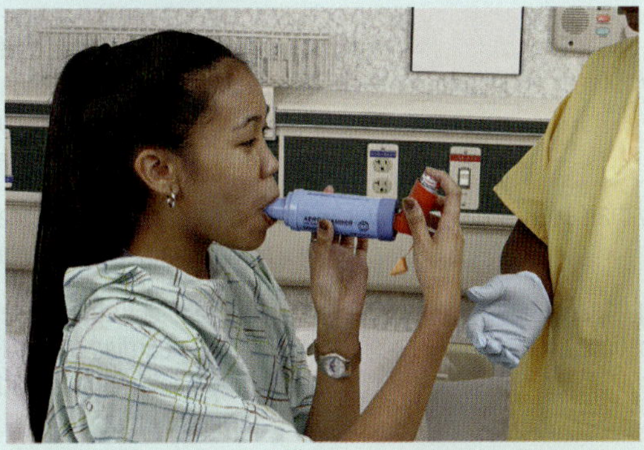

STEP 8E Using spacer device with an MDI.

STEP	RATIONALE
f. Instruct patient to depress medication canister, spraying 1 puff into spacer device.	Device contains fine spray and allows patient to inhale more medication. The spacer increases medication delivery and deposition of the medication on the oropharyngeal mucosa (Asmare et al., 2021).
g. Patient breathes in slowly and fully (for 5 seconds).	Ensures that particles of medication are distributed to deeper airways.
h. Instruct patient to hold full breath for 10 seconds.	Ensures full medication distribution.
9. Instruct patient to wait 20–30 seconds between inhalations (if same medication) or 2–5 minutes between inhalations (if different medications).	Medications must be inhaled sequentially. Always administer bronchodilators before steroids so dilators can open airway passages (Asthma Canada, n.d.-a; Lilley et al., 2020).
10. Instruct patient not to repeat inhalations before next scheduled dose.	Medications are prescribed to be delivered at intervals during the day to provide constant medication levels and minimize adverse effects. Beta-adrenergic MDIs are used either on an "as needed" basis or regularly every 4–6 hours.
11. Warn patients that they may feel gagging sensation in throat caused by droplets of medication on pharynx or tongue.	This occurs when medication is sprayed and inhaled incorrectly.
12. Instruct patient to rinse mouth with warm water about 2 minutes after last dose and then spit water out.	Steroids may alter normal flora of oral mucosa and lead to development of fungal infection. Rinsing the mouth reduces risk of fungal infection (Asmare et al., 2021; Lilley et al., 2020).
13. Clean the MDI.	Removes residual medication and reduces spread of microorganisms.
a. For daily cleaning, instruct patient to remove medication canister, rinse inhaler and cap with warm running water, and be sure that inhaler is completely dry before reuse. Patient should not get valve mechanism of canister wet.	Water damages valve mechanism of canister.
b. Instruct patient to clean mouthpiece twice a week with a mild dishwashing soap, rinse it thoroughly, and dry it completely before storage.	
14. Ask if patient has any questions.	Clarifies misconceptions or misunderstanding and provides opportunity for further patient education (Kim et al., 2021).
15. Help patient to comfortable position.	Reduces spread of microorganisms and promotes patient comfort.

STEP	RATIONALE
EVALUATION	
1. Auscultate patient lungs, listen for abnormal breath sounds, and obtain peak flow measures if prescribed.	Determines patient response to medication.
2. Have patient explain and demonstrate steps in use and cleaning of inhaler.	Return demonstration provides feedback for measuring patient's learning.
3. Ask patient to explain medication schedule and dose of medication.	Improves likelihood of adherence to therapy.
4. Ask patient to describe adverse effects of medication and criteria for calling health care provider.	Allows patient to recognize signs of overuse and need to seek medical support when medications are ineffective.
5. **Use teach-back:** "I want to be sure I clearly showed you how to use your inhaler. Show me how you will use the inhaler to take your medicine." Develop a revised teaching plan if patient or caregiver is unable to teach back correctly.	Determines patient's and caregiver's level of understanding of instructional topic.

Unexpected Outcomes	Related Interventions
1. Patient's respirations are rapid and shallow; breath sounds indicate wheezing.	• Evaluate vital signs and respiratory status. • Notify health care provider. • Reassess type of medication and/or delivery method.
2. Patient needs bronchodilator more frequently than every 4 hours (may indicate respiratory problem).	• Reassess type of medication and delivery methods needed. • Notify health care provider.
3. Patient experiences cardiac dysrhythmias (lightheadedness, syncope), especially if receiving beta-adrenergic medications.	• Withhold all further doses of medication. • Evaluate cardiac and pulmonary status (see Chapter 8). • Notify health care provider for reassessment of type of medication and delivery method.

Communication and Documentation

- Document medication administered, dose or strength, route, number of inhalations, and actual time administered on MAR immediately after administration, not before. Include initials or signature.
- Document patient teaching and validation of patient's understanding on flow sheet or in progress notes in EHR or chart.
- Document on flow sheet or in progress notes in EHR or chart patient's response to MDI (e.g., breath sounds), evidence of adverse effects (e.g., arrhythmia, feelings of anxiety), and ability to use MDI.
- Report adverse effects, patient response, and/or withheld medications to nurse in charge or health care provider.

DOCUMENTATION EXAMPLE

Patient self-administered MDI PRN dose of Ventolin due to an increase in respiratory rate to 24 breaths/min and wheezes noted on auscultation. Post Ventolin, respiratory rate decreased to 18 breaths/min and chest sounds clear bilateral. Will reassess patient in 1 hour.

Special Considerations

Teaching

- Allow for one-on-one supervised practice of the procedures. Patients may have difficulty timing an inhalation with activation of the medication canister without repeated instruction (Asmare et al., 2021; Kim et al., 2021).
- Teach patient to keep track of the number of inhalations in the MDI (Box 21.5).
- Teach patients to use small, handheld peak flowmeters to monitor response to therapy when inhalers are prescribed (Adeniyi et al., 2018; Asthma Canada, n.d.-b). A peak flowmeter measures the peak expiratory flow rate (PEFR), which is a person's maximum speed of expiration (Box 21.6).
- Teach patient to rinse their mouth with water after the use of inhalers.

Pediatric

- A spacer is of benefit to young children because they have difficulty coordinating inhaler activation and inhaling (Keenan-Lindsay et al., 2022).
- Educate child and parent about the need to use the inhaler during school hours. Help family find resources within the school

BOX 21.5

Counting Doses of a Metered-Dose Inhaler

Most metered-dose inhalers (MDIs) currently do not have automatic dose counters. Patients need to keep careful track of the number of inhalations used in their MDIs. Failure to do so may result in patients using an empty inhaler during an acute exacerbation of a respiratory problem. The following steps should be used to track the number of doses:

- Note first day of use on a calendar.
- Note number of inhalations in the canister (e.g., 200 inhalations per MDI).
- Note number of inhalations used per day (e.g., 2 inhalations/day × 3 times/day = 6 inhalations/day).
- Divide the total number of inhalations in the canister by the number of inhalations needed per day to determine the number of days that the inhaler should last (e.g., 200 inhalations divided by 6 inhalations/day = approximately 33 days of dosing at a rate of 3 times/day).
- Mark on a calendar the date the inhaler will be empty and obtain a refill of the inhaler a few days before this target date.

BOX 21.6

How to Use a Peak Flowmeter

1. Move the marker to the bottom of the numbered scale and connect the mouthpiece to the peak flowmeter.
2. Have patient stand up if they are able.
3. Have patient take a deep breath, filling the lungs completely.
4. Have the patient place their lips tightly around the mouthpiece of the flowmeter and then blow as hard and as fast as possible with a single breath.
5. Note the final position of the marker. This is the patient's peak flow rate.
6. Have the patient repeat Steps 1–5 two more times. Record the highest reading of the three.

or day care facility. Many school systems do not permit self-administration of MDIs. Follow school policy regarding having the MDI available for use during school hours. A health care provider's prescription may be necessary.

Gerontological

- Older persons may be unable to depress medication canisters because of weakened grasp or inability to coordinate actuation of the canister with inhalation. The use of a spacer device may be helpful.

Care in the Community: Home Management

- Remind patients to carry prescribed inhalers to use as immediate treatment in case of an acute asthma attack.

PROCEDURAL GUIDELINE 21.1 *Using Dry Powder–Inhaled Medications*

Dry powder inhalers (DPIs) hold dry powder medication and create an aerosol when the patient inhales through a reservoir that contains the medication. In contrast with the metered-dose inhaler (MDI), a DPI has no propellant. DPIs require less manual dexterity, and because the device is breath activated, there is no need to coordinate puffs with inhalation. Compared with MDIs, DPIs deliver more medication to the lungs (Chrystyn & Lavorini, 2020). A DPI does not require a spacer. Medication inside a DPI can clump if the patient lives in a humid climate. Some patients cannot inhale fast enough to administer the entire dose of medication.

Delegation and Collaboration

The skill of administering DPI medications cannot be delegated to a UCP. The nurse directs the UCP about the following:

- Potential adverse effects of medications and reporting their occurrence to the nurse
- Reporting to the nurse paroxysmal coughing, audible wheezing, and patient's report of breathlessness or difficulty breathing

Equipment

- MAR (electronic or printed)
- DPI (see Fig. 21.2, C)
- Stethoscope
- Wash basin or sink with warm water
- Facial tissues *(optional)*

Procedural Steps

1. Identify patient using at least two person-specific identifiers (e.g., name and date of birth or name and medical record number) according to employer policy.
2. Throughout the procedure, the 4 moments for hand hygiene are to be implemented; hand hygiene should occur before initial patient (or patient environment) contact, before an aseptic procedure, after body fluid exposure risk, and after patient (or patient environment) contact. Additional hand hygiene should be performed when hands are visibly soiled.
3. Check accuracy and completeness of each MAR by comparing with health care provider's medication prescription. Check patient's name, medication name and dosage, route (which sinus), and time for administration. Clarify incomplete or unclear prescriptions with health care provider before administration.
4. Review pertinent information related to medication, including action, purpose, normal dose and route, adverse effects, time of onset and peak action, and nursing implications.
5. Assess patient's medical and medication history and history of allergies. List medication allergies on each page of the MAR and prominently display it on the patient's medical record per employer policy. When patient has allergy, provide allergy bracelet.
6. Assess respiratory pattern and auscultate breath sounds (see Chapter 8).
7. Assess patient's knowledge of medication and readiness to learn (e.g., asks questions about medication, requests education in use of DPI, is mentally alert, participates in own care).
8. Assess patient's ability to learn; patient should not be fatigued, in pain, or in respiratory distress. Assess level of understanding of technical vocabulary terms.
9. Determine patient's ability to hold, manipulate, and activate DPI.
10. If previously instructed in self-administration of DPI, assess patient's technique in using it.
11. Prepare medication for inhalation, and check label on inhaler against MAR three times (when removing medication from drawer/cabinet, prior to preparing medication for administration, and prior to returning medication container to drawer or discarding one-time use vial; see Skill 21.1). Preparation usually involves taking inhaler device out of storage and into patient's room. *These are the three checks for accuracy. Check expiration date on container.*
12. Take medication to patient at correct time (see employer policy). Give medications that require exact or precise timing when prescribed, give time-critical medications at time prescribed (no later than 30 minutes before or after), and give non–time-critical medications within 1 or 2 hours of scheduled dose (see employer policy) (ISMP, 2011). During administration, apply 10 rights of medication administration.
13. At patient's bedside, again compare MAR or computer printout with names of medications on medication labels and patient name. Ensures that right patient receives right medication. Ask patient whether they have allergies.
14. Explain procedure and discuss purpose, action, and possible adverse effects of each medication. Allow patient to ask any

PROCEDURAL GUIDELINE 21.1 *Using Dry Powder–Inhaled Medications—cont'd*

questions about the medications. Explain what a DPI is and how to use it. Warn about overuse of inhaler and adverse effects.

15. If DPI has an external counter, note number indicated to determine doses remaining. Otherwise, use technique in Box 21.5 for counting doses.
16. Prepare DPI for administration. Some DPIs require loading medication before administration; some require rotation of a lever to load medication or insert a capsule; and some require insertion of a disc into inhaler device. Follow manufacturer-specific instructions.

Critical Decision Point *The patient's inhaled breath pulls the medication into the airway. DPIs may differ as to how fast the patient should inhale the medication; consult specific instructions of manufacturer. In addition, do not shake DPI because powdered medication may spill out of device.*

17. Have patient exhale fully and then place lips over mouthpiece of DPI and inhale quickly and as deeply as possible. Instruct patient to remove inhaler from mouth as soon as inhalation is complete.
18. Have patient hold breath for 10 seconds or as long as possible and then exhale. Instruct patient not to exhale into DPI.
19. Inform patient that, unlike with other inhaled medications, they may not taste or feel the dry powder or there may be a slight sweet taste.
20. After using DPI, have patient rinse mouth with warm water and spit it out to reduce throat irritation and prevent oral candidiasis.
21. Return DPI to closed position or remove loaded capsule or disc if necessary. If an external counter is present, note number, which should be one less than the number in Step 15.
22. Have patient demonstrate use of DPI at next scheduled dose. Ask them to discuss purpose, action, and adverse effects of medication.
23. Auscultate breath sounds, evaluate respiratory rate, and ask patient about their ease of breathing.
24. Record medication, dose or strength, route, number of inhalations, and time administered on MAR immediately after administration, not before. Include initials or signature.
25. Record patient teaching and validation of patient's understanding in progress notes in EHR or chart.
26. **Use teach-back:** "I want to be sure I explained how often you need to use this DPI medication. Tell me when you will use this medication." Develop a revised teaching plan if patient or caregiver is unable to teach back correctly.

✦ SKILL 21.8 Using Small-Volume Nebulizers

Nebulization is the process of adding medications or moisture to inspired air by mixing particles of various sizes with air. Adding moisture to the respiratory system through nebulization improves clearance of pulmonary secretions. Medications such as bronchodilators, mucolytics, and corticosteroids are often administered by nebulization.

Small-volume nebulizers convert a medication solution into a mist that is then inhaled by a patient into their tracheobronchial tree. The droplets in the mist are much finer than those created by metered-dose inhalers (MDIs) or dry powder inhalers (DPIs). A face mask or a mouthpiece held between the teeth delivers a nebulized mist. A nebulized medication is designed to create a local effect, but it can be absorbed into the bloodstream through the alveoli. As a result, systemic effects from the medication may occur.

Delegation and Collaboration

In many health care facilities, a respiratory therapist performs the skill of administering medications by nebulizer. The nurse must be aware of the type and actions of the inhaled medication that the patient is receiving. The skill of administering medications by nebulizer cannot be delegated to a UCP. The nurse instructs the UCP about the following:

- Potential adverse effects of medications and reporting their occurrence to the nurse.
- Reporting paroxysmal coughing, ineffective breathing patterns, and other respiratory difficulties to the nurse.

Equipment

- MAR (electronic or printed)
- Medication prescribed and diluent (if needed)
- Medicine dropper or syringe
- Nebulizer bottle and tubing assembly
- Small-volume nebulizer machine (often called *handheld nebulizer* or *nebulizer*)
- Pulse oximeter and peak flow device
- Stethoscope
- Nose clip *(optional)*

STEP	RATIONALE
ASSESSMENT	
1. Identify patient using at least two person-specific identifiers (e.g., name and date of birth or name and medical record number) according to employer policy.	Ensures correct patient. Complies with Accreditation Canada's standards and improves patient safety (Accreditation Canada, 2020).
2. Throughout the procedure, the 4 moments for hand hygiene are to be implemented; hand hygiene should occur before initial patient (or patient environment) contact, before an aseptic procedure, after body fluid exposure risk, and after patient (or patient environment) contact. Additional hand hygiene should be performed when hands are visibly soiled.	Proper hand hygiene helps prevent the spread of infectious agents to health care providers.

STEP	RATIONALE

ASSESSMENT

STEP	RATIONALE
3. Check accuracy and completeness of each MAR by comparing with health care provider's medication prescription. Check patient's name, medication name and dosage, route, and time for administration. Clarify incomplete or unclear prescriptions with health care provider before administration.	The prescription sheet is the most reliable source and only legal record of medications that patient is to receive. It ensures that patient receives correct medications (College of Physicians and Surgeons of Ontario, 2019; Pharmacy Association of Nova Scotia, n.d.). Handwritten MARs are a source of medication errors (Parthasarathi et al., 2021; Tariq et al., 2022).
4. Review pertinent information related to medication, including action, purpose, normal dose and route, adverse effects, time of onset and peak action, and nursing implications.	Allows you to anticipate effects of medication and observe patient's response.
5. Assess patient's medical and medication history and history of allergies. List medication allergies on each page of the MAR and prominently display it on the patient's medical record per employer policy. When patient has allergy, provide allergy bracelet.	These factors influence how certain medications act. Information also reflects patient's need for medications and risk for adverse effects. Communication of allergies is essential for safe and effective care.
6. Assess patient's grasp and ability to assemble, hold, and manipulate nebulizer equipment.	Any impairment of cognition or grasp or the presence of hand tremors affects patient's ability to use equipment.
7. Assess pulse, respirations, breath sounds, pulse oximetry, and peak flow measurement (if prescribed) before beginning treatment.	Establishes baseline for comparison during and after treatment.
8. Assess patient's knowledge of medication and readiness to learn (e.g., patient asks questions about medication, requests education in use of nebulizer, is mentally alert, participates in own care).	Determines level of instruction needed to assume self-administration.
9. Assess patient's ability to learn; patient should not be fatigued, in pain, or in respiratory distress. Assess level of understanding of technical vocabulary terms.	Determines best time to provide instruction and techniques to use.
10. Assess patient's ability to manipulate nebulizer mouthpiece and tubing.	Presence of mobility restrictions indicates need for assistance.

NURSING DIAGNOSES

- Reduced gas exchange
- Inadequate breathing pattern
- Reduced stamina
- Anxiety
- Insufficient knowledge regarding use of nebulizers
- Readiness for enhanced self-management of health
- Potential for injury

Related factors and risk factors are individualized on the basis of patient's condition or needs.

PLANNING

STEP	RATIONALE
1. Expected outcomes following completion of procedure:	
• Patient's breathing pattern is effective.	Demonstrates therapeutic effect of medication.
• Patient's oxygen saturation level is adequate.	Demonstrates therapeutic effect of medication.
• Patient describes adverse effects of medication and criteria for calling health care provider (e.g., low peak flow rate).	Increases likelihood of adherence to therapeutic regimen.
• Patient demonstrates self-administration of nebulized dose of medication correctly.	Demonstrates learning and ensures correct administration of medication.
2. Collect appropriate equipment and MAR.	Ensures time management and efficiency.

IMPLEMENTATION

STEP	RATIONALE
1. Prepare medications for inhalation. Check label of medication against MAR two times (when removing medication from drawer/cabinet and prior to preparing medication for administration; see Skill 21.1). Preparation usually involves taking medication vial out of storage and taking to patient's room. Check expiration date on container.	*These are the first two checks for accuracy.* Process ensures that right patient receives right medication at right time.

STEP	RATIONALE
IMPLEMENTATION	
2. Identify patient using at least two person-specific identifiers (e.g., name and date of birth, or name and medical record number) according to employer policy.	Ensures correct patient. Complies with Accreditation Canada's standards and improves patient safety (Accreditation Canada, 2020).
3. Take medication(s) to patient at correct time (see employer policy). Medications that require exact timing include stat, first-time or loading doses, and one-time doses. Give time-critical scheduled medications (e.g., antibiotics, anticoagulants, insulin, anticonvulsants, immunosuppressive medications) at exact time prescribed (no later than 30 minutes before or after scheduled dose). Give non–time-critical scheduled medications within a range of 1 or 2 hours of scheduled dose, according to employer policy (ISMP, 2011). During administration, apply 10 rights of medication administration.	Hospitals must adopt medication administration policy and procedure for timing of medication administration that considers nature of the prescribed medication, specific clinical application, and patient needs. Time-critical scheduled medications are those for which early or delayed administration of maintenance doses of greater than 30 minutes before or after the scheduled dose may cause harm or result in substantially suboptimal therapy or pharmacological effect. Non–time-critical medications are those for which early or delayed administration within a specified range of either 1 or 2 hours should not cause harm or result in substantially suboptimal therapy or pharmacological effect (ISMP, 2011).
4. At patient's bedside, again compare MAR or computer printout with names of medications on medication labels and patient name. Ask patient whether they have allergies.	Ensures that right patient receives right medication. Confirms patient's allergy history.
5. Explain procedure to patient. Be specific if patient wishes to self-administer medication. Discuss purpose, action, and possible adverse effects of each medication. Allow patient to ask any questions about the medications. Explain how to assemble and use nebulizer.	Helps patient be a participant in care, which minimizes anxiety. Patient has right to be informed, and their understanding of each medication improves adherence to medication therapy. Begins patient teaching regarding medications (Lilley et al., 2020).
6. Assemble nebulizer equipment per manufacturer directions.	Assembly may vary slightly between different manufacturers. Proper assembly ensures safe delivery of medication.
7. Add prescribed medication by pouring medicine into nebulizer cup. (*Option:* You may use a medicine dropper or syringe to instill medication.)	Ensures proper dose and delivery of prescribed medication.
8. Attach top to nebulizer cup and be sure that it is secure. Then connect cup to mouthpiece or face mask.	Prevents loss of medication.
9. Connect tubing to both aerosol compressor and nebulizer cup.	Ensures aerosol delivery to mouthpiece.
10. Have patient hold mouthpiece between lips with gentle pressure, but be sure lips are sealed (see Step 10 illustration).	Prevents escape of nebulized medication.

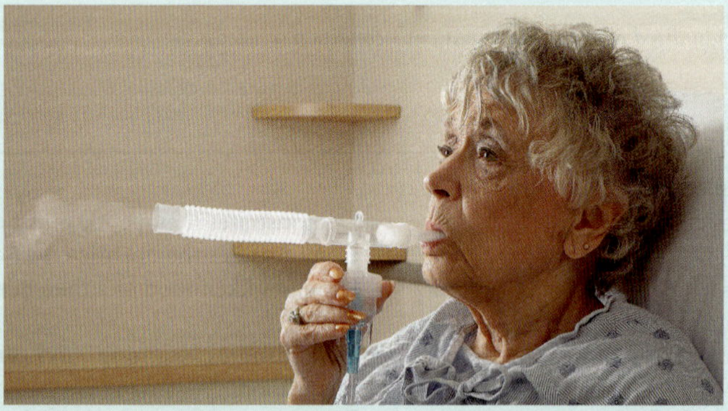

STEP 10 Nebulizer mouthpiece placed between patient's lips.

STEP	RATIONALE
a. If patient is an infant, child, or tired adult or unable to follow instructions, use face mask.	Use of face mask does not require patient to remember to hold mouthpiece correctly. Correct delivery ensures sufficient deposition of medication.
b. Use special adapters for patients with tracheostomy.	Promotes greater deposition of medication in airways.
11. Turn on small-volume nebulizer machine and ensure that a sufficient mist begins to flow.	Verifies that equipment is working properly during delivery of medication.
12. Instruct patient to take slow, deep breath to a volume slightly greater than normal. Encourage brief, end-inspiratory pause for about 2–3 seconds; then have patient exhale passively. *Option:* If needed, use a nose clip so patient breathes only through the mouth (Medline Plus, 2022b).	Improves effectiveness of medication.

STEP	RATIONALE
IMPLEMENTATION	
a. If patient is dyspneic, encourage them to hold every fourth or fifth breath for 5–10 seconds.	Maximizes effectiveness of medication.
b. Remind patient to repeat breathing pattern until medication is completely nebulized. This usually takes about 10–15 minutes (Medline Plus, 2022b).	Maximizes effectiveness of medication.
(1) Some health care providers prescribe time limit as length of treatment rather than waiting for medication to completely nebulize.	
c. Tap nebulizer cup occasionally during and toward end of treatment.	Releases droplets that are clinging to side of cup, thus allowing for renebulization of solution.
d. Monitor patient's pulse during procedure, especially if beta-adrenergic bronchodilators are used.	Enables you to observe potential adverse effects of medications.
13. When medication is completely nebulized, turn off machine. Rinse nebulizer cup per employer policy. Dry completely and store tubing assembly per employer policy.	Proper storage reduces transfer of microorganisms.
14. If steroids are nebulized, instruct patient to rinse mouth and gargle with warm water after nebulizer treatment. Have patient spit out solution.	Removes medication residue from oral cavity and helps prevent oral candidiasis, a possible adverse effect of inhaled steroid therapy.
15. After nebulizer treatment is complete, have patient take several deep breaths and cough to expectorate mucus.	Nebulized medication is often prescribed to open airways and promote expectoration of mucus.
16. Help patient to comfortable position.	Promotes patient comfort.

EVALUATION

1. Assess patient's respirations, breath sounds, cough effort, sputum production, pulse oximetry, and peak flow measures if prescribed.	Determines status of breathing pattern and adequacy of ventilation/gas exchange. Allows comparison with baseline data and evaluation of effectiveness of procedure.
2. Ask patient to explain medication schedule.	Improves likelihood of adherence to therapy.
3. Ask patient to describe adverse effects of medication and criteria for calling health care provider.	Allows patient to recognize signs of overuse and need to seek medical support when medications are ineffective.
4. **Use teach-back:** "I want to be sure I was clear about how to put together the nebulizer and add medications. Show me the steps for assembling the nebulizer and adding medications." Develop a revised teaching plan if patient or caregiver is unable to teach back correctly.	Determines patient's and caregiver's level of understanding of instructional topic.

Unexpected Outcomes	Related Interventions
1. Patient's breathing pattern is ineffective; respirations are rapid and shallow; breath sounds indicate wheezing.	• Reassess type of medication and/or delivery method. • Notify health care provider.
2. Patient experiences paroxysms of coughing. Aerosolized particles can irritate posterior pharynx.	• Reassess type of medication and/or delivery method. • Notify health care provider.
3. Patient experiences cardiac dysrhythmias (lightheadedness, syncope), especially if receiving beta-adrenergic medications.	• Withhold all further doses of medication. Assess vital signs. • Notify health care provider for reassessment of type of medication and delivery method.

Communication and Documentation

- Document medication, dose and strength, route, length of treatment, and time administered on MAR immediately after administration, not before. Include initials or signature.
- Document patient teaching and validation of patient's understanding on flow sheet or in progress notes in EHR or chart.
- Document patient's response to treatment on flow sheet or in progress notes in EHR or chart.
- Report adverse effects, patient response, and/or withheld medications to nurse in charge or health care provider.

DOCUMENTATION EXAMPLE

Patient administered steroid medication as prescribed. Patient education regarding the medication completed, including rinsing of the mouth after the medication. Patient verbalized understanding of rationale requiring them to rinse their mouth after medication administration.

Special Considerations

Teaching

- Teach patient not to store medication in nebulizer for later use.
- Advise patients who are taking long-acting beta-agonists about possible adverse effects, including nervousness, restlessness, tremor, headache, nausea, rapid or pounding heart rate, and dizziness.
- Teach patients how to use small handheld peak flowmeters to monitor response to therapy when inhaled medications are prescribed (Adeniyi et al., 2018; Asthma Canada, n.d.-b) (see Box 21.6).

Pediatric

- Use a mask for the nebulizer treatment if child is too young to hold mouthpiece correctly for the duration of the treatment (Keenan-Lindsay et al., 2022).
- Instruct child to breathe normally with mouth open to provide a direct route to the airways for the medication.
- Educate child and parent about the need to use the nebulizer during school or daycare hours. Help family find resources within the school or day care facility. Follow school policy regarding having the nebulizer and medication available for use during school hours. A health care provider's prescription may be necessary.

Gerontological

- Older persons with a weak grasp, hand tremors, or coordination problems may not be able to manipulate or hold a nebulizer. In some situations, an aerosol mask would be more beneficial (e.g., for an older patient with Parkinson's disease).

Care in the Community: Home Management

- When patient is using treatment at home, nebulizer parts should be rinsed after each use with clear water and air-dried (Medline Plus, 2022b). Do not store nebulizer parts until completely dry.

✦ SKILL 21.9 Administering Vaginal Instillations

NSO *Nursing Skills Online Nonparenteral Medication Administration Module 6 / Lesson 7*

Patients who develop vaginal infections often require topical application of anti-infective medications. Vaginal medications are available in foam, jelly, cream, or suppository form. Medicated irrigations or douches can also be given. However, their excessive use can lead to vaginal irritation.

Vaginal suppositories are oval shaped and come individually packaged in foil wrappers. They are larger and more oval than rectal suppositories (Fig. 21.3). Storage in a refrigerator prevents the solid suppositories from melting. A suppository is inserted into the vagina with an applicator or a gloved hand. After insertion, body temperature causes the suppository to melt, enabling effective medication distribution. Foam, jellies, and creams can be inserted using an inserter or applicator. Patients often prefer administering their own vaginal medications, and they should be given privacy to do so. Offer the patient a perineal pad to wear after medication instillation to collect excess drainage. Because vaginal medications are frequently given to treat infection, any discharge is often foul smelling. Follow good aseptic technique and offer the patient frequent opportunities for perineal hygiene (see Procedural Guideline 18.1).

Delegation and Collaboration

The skill of administering vaginal medications cannot be delegated to a UCP. The nurse instructs the UCP about the following:

- Potential adverse effects of medications and reporting their occurrence to the nurse
- Reporting any change in comfort level or new or increased vaginal discharge or bleeding to the nurse

Equipment

- MAR (electronic or printed)
- Vaginal cream, foam, jelly, tablet, suppository, or irrigating solution
- Applicators (if needed) (Fig. 21.4)
- Clean gloves
- Tissues
- Towels, washcloths, or both
- Perineal pad; drape or sheet
- Water-soluble lubricants
- Bedpan
- Irrigation or douche container (if needed)
- Gooseneck lamp *(optional)*

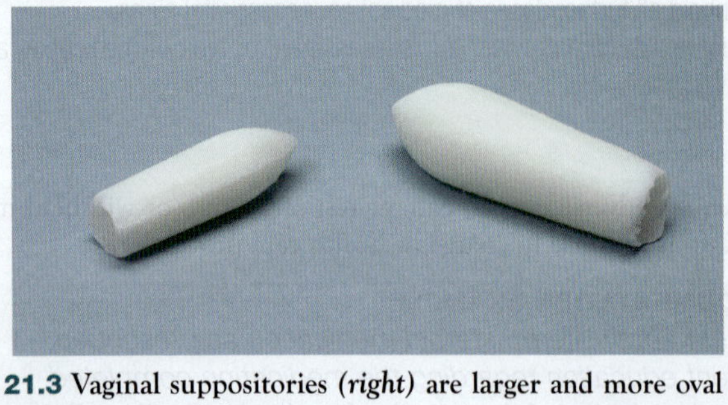

FIG 21.3 Vaginal suppositories *(right)* are larger and more oval than rectal suppositories *(left)*.

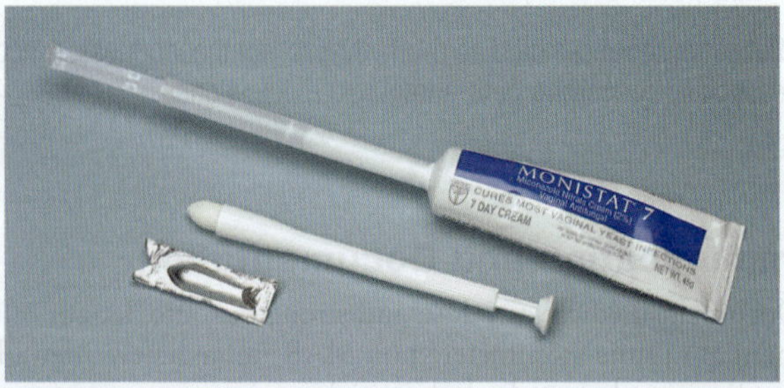

FIG 21.4 From top to bottom: Vaginal cream with applicator; applicator; and vaginal suppository. (*From Lilley, L. L., Collins, S. R., & Snyder, J. S. [2011]. Pharmacology and the nursing process [6th ed.]. Mosby.*)

STEP	RATIONALE

ASSESSMENT

STEP	RATIONALE
1. Identify patient using at least two person-specific identifiers (e.g., name and date of birth or name and medical record number) according to employer policy.	Ensures correct patient. Complies with Accreditation Canada's standards and improves patient safety (Accreditation Canada, 2020).
2. Throughout the procedure, the 4 moments for hand hygiene are to be implemented; hand hygiene should occur before initial patient (or patient environment) contact, before an aseptic procedure, after body fluid exposure risk, and after patient (or patient environment) contact. Additional hand hygiene should be performed when hands are visibly soiled.	Proper hand hygiene helps prevent the spread of infectious agents to health care providers.
3. Check accuracy and completeness of each MAR by comparing with health care provider's medication prescription. Check patient's name, medication name and dosage, route, and time for administration. Clarify incomplete or unclear prescriptions with health care provider before administration.	The prescription sheet is the most reliable source and only legal record of medications that patient is to receive. It ensures that patient receives correct medications (College of Physicians and Surgeons of Ontario, 2019; Pharmacy Association of Nova Scotia, n.d.). Handwritten MARs are a source of medication errors (Parthasarathi et al., 2021; Tariq et al., 2022).
4. Review pertinent information related to medication, including action, purpose, normal dose and route, adverse effects, time of onset and peak action, and nursing implications.	Allows you to anticipate effects of medication and observe patient's response.
5. Assess patient's medical and medication history and history of allergies. List medication allergies on each page of the MAR and prominently display it on the patient's medical record per employer policy. When patient has allergy, provide allergy bracelet.	These factors influence how certain medications act. Information also reflects patient's need for medications and risk for adverse effects. Communication of allergies is essential for safe and effective care.
6. Apply clean gloves. During perineal care, inspect condition of vaginal tissues; note whether drainage is present. Remove gloves and perform hand hygiene.	Reduces transmission of microorganisms. Identifies symptoms of vaginal irritation or infection.
7. Ask if patient is experiencing any symptoms of pruritus, burning, or discomfort.	Identifies symptoms of vaginal irritation or infection.
8. Review patient's knowledge of medication and readiness to learn (e.g., asks questions about medication, requests education in use of suppository).	Indicates need for health teaching. Understanding influences adherence to therapy.
9. Assess patient's ability to manipulate applicator, suppository, or irrigation equipment and to properly position self to insert medication (may be done just before insertion).	Presence of mobility restrictions indicates need for help.

NURSING DIAGNOSES

- Insufficient knowledge regarding vaginal medication administration
- Pain (acute or chronic)
- Reduced functional mobility
- Potential sexual dysfunction

Related factors and risk factors are individualized on the basis of patient's condition or needs.

PLANNING

STEP	RATIONALE
1. Expected outcomes following completion of procedure:	
• Vaginal tissues are pink and smooth. Genitalia are clear and without discharge.	Tissues take on normal characteristics.
• Patient denies symptoms of discomfort and expresses relief from symptoms of infection or inflammation. Small amount of discharge the colour of medication is present.	Inflammation or infection has resolved. When suppository or cream becomes distributed, small amount may escape from vaginal orifice.
• Patient can discuss information about prescribed medication.	Feedback reflects patient's learning.
• Patient demonstrates self-administration of suppository, medication, or irrigation.	Demonstrates learning.
2. Collect appropriate equipment and MAR.	Ensures time management and efficiency.

IMPLEMENTATION

STEP	RATIONALE
1. Prepare suppository for administration. Check label of medication against MAR two times (when removing medication from drawer/cabinet and prior to preparing medication for administration; see Skill 21.1). Preparation usually involves taking suppository out of refrigerator and taking to patient's room. Check expiration date on container.	*These are the first two checks for accuracy.* Process ensures that right patient receives right medication.

STEP	RATIONALE
IMPLEMENTATION	
2. Identify patient using at least two person-specific identifiers (e.g., name and date of birth, or name and medical record number) according to employer policy.	Ensures correct patient. Complies with Accreditation Canada's standards and improves patient safety (Accreditation Canada, 2020).
3. Take medication(s) to patient at correct time (see employer policy). Medications that require exact timing include stat, first-time or loading doses, and one-time doses. Give time-critical scheduled medications (e.g., antibiotics, anticoagulants, insulin, anticonvulsants, immunosuppressive medications) at exact time prescribed (no later than 30 minutes before or after scheduled dose). Give non–time-critical scheduled medications within a range of 1 or 2 hours of scheduled dose, according to employer policy (ISMP, 2011). During administration, apply 10 rights of medication administration.	Hospitals must adopt medication administration policy and procedure for timing of medication administration that considers nature of the prescribed medication, specific clinical application, and patient needs. Time-critical scheduled medications are those for which early or delayed administration of maintenance doses of greater than 30 minutes before or after the scheduled dose may cause harm or result in substantially suboptimal therapy or pharmacological effect. Non–time-critical medications are those for which early or delayed administration within a specified range of either 1 or 2 hours should not cause harm or result in substantially suboptimal therapy or pharmacological effect (ISMP, 2011).
4. At patient's bedside, again compare MAR or computer printout with names of medications on medication labels and patient name. Ask patient whether they have allergies.	Ensures that right patient receives right medication. Confirms patient's allergy history.
5. Explain procedure to patient. Be specific if patient plans to self-administer medication. Discuss purpose, action, and possible adverse effects of each medication. Allow patient to ask any questions about the medications. Explain procedure if patient plans to self-administer medication.	Helps patient be a participant in care, which minimizes anxiety. Patient has right to be informed, and their understanding of each medication improves adherence to medication therapy. Begins patient teaching regarding medications.
6. Arrange supplies at bedside and apply clean gloves. Close door or pull curtain.	Reduces transmission of microorganisms.
7. Have patient void (using bathroom facilities or bedpan). Help patient lie in dorsal recumbent position. Patients with restricted mobility in knees or hips may lie supine with legs abducted.	Voiding prevents passing of urine during insertion of suppository. Position provides easy access to and good exposure of vaginal canal. Dependent position also allows suppository to completely dissolve in vagina.
8. Keep abdomen and lower extremities draped.	Minimizes patient's embarrassment by limiting exposure.
9. Be sure that vaginal orifice is well illuminated by room light. Otherwise, position portable gooseneck lamp.	Proper insertion requires visualization of external genitalia if medication is not self-administered.
10. Insert vaginal suppository.	
a. Remove suppository from wrapper and apply liberal amount of water-soluble lubricant to smooth or rounded end (see Step 10a illustration). Be sure that suppository is at room temperature. Lubricate gloved index finger of dominant hand.	Lubrication reduces friction against mucosal surfaces during insertion. Use of petroleum jelly may leave residue that harbours bacteria and fungi (e.g., yeast).
b. With nondominant gloved hand, gently separate labial folds in front-to-back direction.	Exposes vaginal orifice.

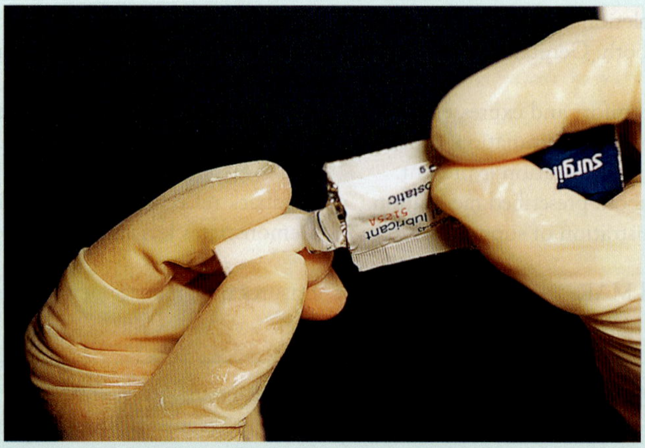

STEP 10A Lubricate tip of suppository.

STEP	RATIONALE

IMPLEMENTATION

STEP	RATIONALE
c. With dominant gloved hand, insert rounded end of suppository along posterior wall of vaginal canal the entire length of finger (7.5–10 cm [3–4 inches]) (see Step 10c illustration).	Proper placement of suppository ensures equal distribution of medication along walls of vaginal cavity.

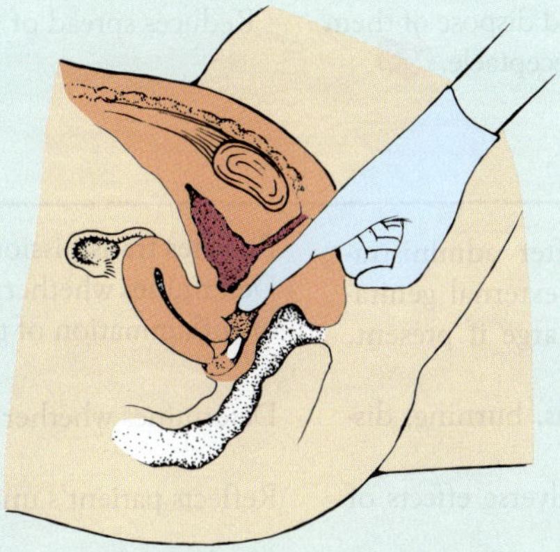

STEP 10C Angle of vaginal suppository insertion.

STEP	RATIONALE
d. Withdraw finger and use tissue or cloth to wipe away remaining lubricant from around orifice and labia.	Maintains comfort.
11. Apply cream or foam.	
a. Fill cream or foam applicator following package directions.	Dose is based on volume in applicator.
b. With nondominant gloved hand, gently separate labial folds.	Exposes vaginal orifice.
c. With dominant gloved hand, gently insert applicator approximately 5–7.5 cm (2–3 inches). Push applicator plunger to deposit medication into vagina (see Step 11c illustration).	Allows equal distribution of medication along vaginal walls.

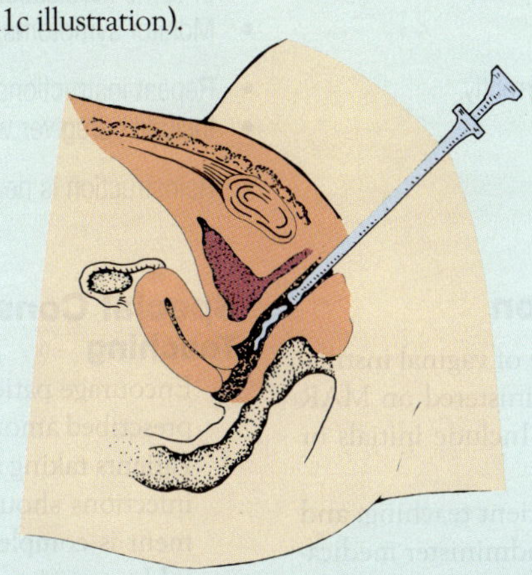

STEP 11C Applicator inserted into vaginal canal. Plunger pushed to instill medication.

STEP	RATIONALE
d. Withdraw applicator and place on paper towel. Use tissue or cloth to wipe off residual cream from labia or vaginal orifice.	Maintains patient comfort.
12. Administer irrigation or douche, if prescribed.	
a. Place patient on bedpan with absorbent pad underneath.	Allows hips to be higher than shoulders and solution to reach posterior wall of vagina. Bedpan collects solution.
b. Be sure that irrigation or douche fluid is at body temperature. Run fluid through container nozzle (priming the tubing).	Body temperature promotes patient comfort. Priming tubing removes air and moistens nozzle tip.
c. Gently separate labial folds and direct nozzle toward sacrum, following floor of vagina.	Correct angle allows nozzle access into vagina.
d. Raise container approximately 30–50 cm (12–20 inches) above level of vagina. Insert nozzle 7–10 cm (3–4 inches). Allow solution to flow while rotating nozzle. Administer all irrigating solution.	Rotating nozzle allows irrigation of all areas in vagina.
e. Withdraw nozzle and help patient to comfortable sitting position.	Remaining solution drains by gravity.
f. Allow patient to remain on bedpan for a few minutes. Clean perineum with soap and water.	Ensures that all solution drains from vagina. Provides comfort for patient.
g. Help patient off bedpan. Dry perineal area.	Provides comfort.

STEP	RATIONALE
13. Instruct patient who received suppository, cream, or tablet to remain on their back for at least 10 minutes.	Allows melting and spreading of medication throughout vaginal cavity and prevents loss through vaginal orifice.
14. If using an applicator, wash with soap and warm water, rinse, air dry, and then store for future use.	Vaginal cavity is not sterile. Soap and water help to remove bacteria and residual cream from applicator.
15. Offer perineal pad when patient resumes ambulation.	Provides patient comfort.
16. Discard gloves by turning them inside out and dispose of them and other soiled equipment in appropriate receptacle.	Reduces spread of microorganisms.

EVALUATION

1. Apply clean gloves. Thirty minutes after administration, inspect condition of vaginal canal and external genitalia between applications. Assess vaginal discharge if present. Remove gloves and perform hand hygiene.	Reduces transmission of microorganisms. Determines whether vaginal medication effectively reduced irritation or inflammation of tissues.
2. Question patient regarding continued pruritus, burning, discomfort, or discharge.	Determines whether symptoms are relieved.
3. Ask patient to discuss purpose, action, and adverse effects of medication.	Reflects patient's understanding of medication therapy.
4. **Use teach-back:** "I want to be sure I explained how to use the vaginal cream applicator. Tell me how you will draw the correct amount of cream into the applicator." Develop a revised teaching plan if patient or caregiver is unable to teach back correctly.	Determines patient's and caregiver's level of understanding of instructional topic.

Unexpected Outcomes	Related Interventions
1. Patient reports localized pruritus and burning.	• Results of infection or inflammation but may be possible adverse effects of some medications (e.g., miconazole). • Monitor symptoms; report to health care provider.
2. Patient is unable to discuss medication therapy correctly.	• Repeat instructions or assess whether patient can learn. • Include caregiver when appropriate.
3. Patient is unable to self-administer medications.	• Reinstruction is necessary.

Communication and Documentation

- Document medication (or solution, in the case of vaginal instillation), dose, type of instillation, and time administered on MAR immediately after administration, not before. Include initials or signature.
- Document patient response to medication, patient teaching, and validation of understanding and ability to self-administer medication on flow sheet or in progress notes in EHR or chart.
- Report to health care provider if patient states that symptoms have not disappeared or symptoms have worsened.
- Report adverse effects, patient response, and/or withheld medications to supervisor or health care provider.

DOCUMENTATION EXAMPLE

Patient self-administered vaginal cream correctly. Stated their understanding of why the medication is prescribed and stated they had no questions or concerns at this time.

Special Considerations

Teaching

- Encourage patient to take *all* the medication as prescribed, for the prescribed amount of time, to ensure effectiveness of the treatment.
- Patients taking antifungal medications for the treatment of vaginal infections should abstain from sexual intercourse until the treatment is completed and the infection is resolved. They should be told to continue to take the medication even if actively menstruating. Patients should notify the health care provider if symptoms persist past the prescribed treatment period (Lilley et al., 2020).
- Many patients prefer to self-administer vaginal irrigations and medications. These procedures may be self-administered while patient is sitting on the toilet. Ensure that patient is able to perform the procedure correctly.

Gerontological

- Older persons may have difficulty manipulating suppository, applicator, or irrigating equipment. If so, a caregiver may need instruction on how to administer the medication.

✦ SKILL 21.10 Administering Rectal Suppositories

NSO Nursing Skills Online Nonparenteral Medication Administration Module 6 / Lesson 8

A rectal suppository is a type of medication delivery system designed to be inserted into the rectum, where it melts and releases the medication it contains. The medication is then absorbed into the rectal mucosa and enters the bloodstream. Rectal medications exert either local effects on GI mucosa (e.g., promoting defecation) or systemic effects (e.g., relieving nausea or providing analgesia). The rectal route is not as reliable as oral or parenteral routes in terms of medication absorption and distribution. However, the medications are relatively safe because they rarely cause local irritation or adverse effects. Rectal medications are contraindicated in patients with recent surgery on the rectum, bowel, or prostate gland; rectal bleeding or prolapse; and very low platelet counts (Lilley et al., 2020).

Rectal suppositories are thinner and more bullet-shaped than vaginal suppositories (see Fig. 21.3). The rounded end prevents anal trauma during insertion. When administering a rectal suppository, placing it past the internal anal sphincter and against the rectal mucosa is important. Improper placement can result in expulsion of the suppository before the medication dissolves and is absorbed into the mucosa. If a patient prefers to self-administer a suppository, give specific instructions to ensure that the medication is deposited correctly. Do not cut the suppository into sections to divide the dosage; the active medication may not be distributed evenly within the suppository, and the result may be an inaccurate dose (Lilley et al., 2020; Mitchell, 2019).

Delegation and Collaboration

The skill of administering rectal medication cannot be delegated to a UCP. The nurse instructs the UCP about the following:

- Reporting expected fecal discharge or bowel movement to the nurse
- Potential adverse effects of medications and reporting their occurrence to the nurse
- Informing the nurse of any rectal pain or bleeding

Equipment

- MAR (electronic or printed)
- Rectal suppository
- Water-soluble lubricating jelly
- Clean gloves
- Tissue
- Drape

STEP	RATIONALE
ASSESSMENT	
1. Identify patient using at least two person-specific identifiers (e.g., name and date of birth or name and medical record number) according to employer policy.	Ensures correct patient. Complies with Accreditation Canada's standards and improves patient safety (Accreditation Canada, 2020).
2. Throughout the procedure, the 4 moments for hand hygiene are to be implemented; hand hygiene should occur before initial patient (or patient environment) contact, before an aseptic procedure, after body fluid exposure risk, and after patient (or patient environment) contact. Additional hand hygiene should be performed when hands are visibly soiled.	Proper hand hygiene helps prevent the spread of infectious agents to health care providers.
3. Check accuracy and completeness of each MAR by comparing with health care provider's medication prescription. Check patient's name, medication name and dosage, route, and time for administration. Clarify incomplete or unclear prescriptions with health care provider before administration.	The prescription sheet is the most reliable source and only legal record of medications that patient is to receive. It ensures that patient receives correct medications (College of Physicians and Surgeons of Ontario, 2019; Pharmacy Association of Nova Scotia, n.d.). Handwritten MARs are a source of medication errors (Parthasarathi et al., 2021; Tariq et al., 2022).
4. Review pertinent information related to medication, including action, purpose, normal dose and route, adverse effects, time of onset and peak action, and nursing implications.	Allows you to anticipate effects of medication and observe patient's response.
5. Review patient's medical history for history of rectal surgery or bleeding, cardiac problems, history of allergies, and medication history. List medication allergies on each page of the MAR and prominently display it on the patient's medical record per employer policy. When patient has allergy, provide allergy bracelet.	Conditions may contraindicate use of suppository. Communication of allergies is essential for safe and effective care.
6. Review any presenting signs and symptoms of GI alterations (e.g., constipation or diarrhea).	Conditions indicate use of suppository.
7. Assess patient's ability to hold suppository and position self to insert medication.	Mobility restriction indicates need for nurse to help with medication administration.
8. Review patient's knowledge of purpose of medication therapy and interest in self-administering suppository.	Indicates need for health teaching. Level of motivation influences teaching approach.

NURSING DIAGNOSES

- Pain (acute or chronic)
- Reduced functional ability
- Constipation
- Insufficient knowledge regarding suppository administration
- Ready for enhanced self-management of health

Related factors and risk factors are individualized on the basis of patient's condition or needs.

PLANNING

1. Expected outcomes following completion of the procedure:	
• Patient reports relief or reduction in symptoms for which medication is prescribed.	Medication acts effectively.

STEP	RATIONALE
• Patient describes purpose of medication.	Feedback reflects patient's learning.
• Patient demonstrates self-administration of rectal suppository.	Demonstrates learning.
2. Collect appropriate equipment and MAR.	Ensures time management and efficiency.

IMPLEMENTATION

STEP	RATIONALE
1. Prepare suppository for administration. Check label of medication against MAR two times (when removing medication from drawer/cabinet and prior to preparing medication for administration; see Skill 21.1). Check expiration date on container.	*These are the first two checks for accuracy.* Process ensures that right patient receives right medication at right time.
2. Identify patient using at least two person-specific identifiers (e.g., name and date of birth, or name and medical record number) according to employer policy.	Ensures correct patient. Complies with Accreditation Canada's standards and improves patient safety (Accreditation Canada, 2020).
3. Take medication(s) to patient at correct time (see employer policy). Medications that require exact timing include stat, first-time or loading doses, and one-time doses. Give time-critical scheduled medications (e.g., antibiotics, anticoagulants, insulin, anticonvulsants, immunosuppressive medications) at exact time prescribed (no later than 30 minutes before or after scheduled dose). Give non–time-critical scheduled medications within a range of 1 or 2 hours of scheduled dose, according to employer policy (ISMP, 2011). During administration, apply 10 rights of medication administration.	Hospitals must adopt medication administration policy and procedure for timing of medication administration that considers nature of the prescribed medication, specific clinical application, and patient needs. Time-critical scheduled medications are those for which early or delayed administration of maintenance doses of greater than 30 minutes before or after the scheduled dose may cause harm or result in substantially suboptimal therapy or pharmacological effect. Non–time-critical medications are those for which early or delayed administration within a specified range of either 1 or 2 hours should not cause harm or result in substantially suboptimal therapy or pharmacological effect (ISMP, 2011).
4. At patient's bedside, again compare MAR or computer printout with names of medications on medication labels and patient name. Ask patient whether they have allergies.	Ensures that right patient receives right medication. Confirms patient's allergy history.
5. Explain procedure to patient and sensations to expect; provide additional detail if patient plans to self-administer medication. Discuss purpose, action, and possible adverse effects of each medication. Allow patient to ask any questions about the medications.	Helps patient be a participant in care, which minimizes anxiety. Patient has right to be informed, and their understanding of each medication improves adherence to medication therapy. Begins patient teaching regarding medications.
6. Arrange supplies at bedside and apply clean gloves. Close room curtain or door.	Reduces transmission of microorganisms. Maintains privacy and minimizes embarrassment.
7. Help patient assume modified left lateral recumbent position with upper leg flexed upward.	Position exposes anus and relaxes external anal sphincter. Modified left lateral recumbent position lessens likelihood that suppository or feces will be expelled.
8. If patient has mobility impairment, help into lateral position. Obtain help to turn patient, and use pillows under upper arm and leg.	Provides support during procedure and patient comfort.
9. Keep patient draped with only anal area exposed.	Maintains privacy and facilitates relaxation.
10. Examine condition of anus externally. *Option:* Palpate rectal walls as needed (e.g., if impaction is suspected) (see Chapter 8). If you palpate rectal walls, dispose of gloves by turning them inside out and placing them in proper receptacle if they become soiled. Otherwise, keep gloves on your hands and proceed to Step 12.	Determines presence of active rectal bleeding. Palpation determines whether rectum is filled with feces, which interferes with suppository placement. Reduces spread of infection.

Critical Decision Point *Do not palpate patient's rectum if there is a recent history of rectal surgery. A suppository is contraindicated in the presence of active rectal bleeding and diarrhea* (Mitchell, 2019).

STEP	RATIONALE
11. Apply new pair of clean gloves (if previous gloves were soiled and discarded).	Minimizes contact with fecal material to reduce transmission of infection.
12. Remove suppository from foil wrapper and lubricate rounded end with water-soluble lubricant. Lubricate gloved index finger of dominant hand. If patient has hemorrhoids, use liberal amount of lubricant and touch area gently.	Lubrication reduces friction as suppository enters rectal canal.

STEP	RATIONALE

IMPLEMENTATION

STEP	RATIONALE
13. Ask patient to take slow, deep breaths through mouth and relax anal sphincter.	Forcing suppository through constricted sphincter causes pain.
14. Retract patient's buttocks with nondominant hand. With gloved index finger of dominant hand, insert suppository gently through anus, past internal sphincter, and against rectal wall, 10 cm (4 inches) in adults (see Step 14 illustration) or 5 cm (2 inches) in infants and children. You should feel rectal sphincter close around your finger.	Suppository needs to be against rectal mucosa for eventual absorption and therapeutic action.

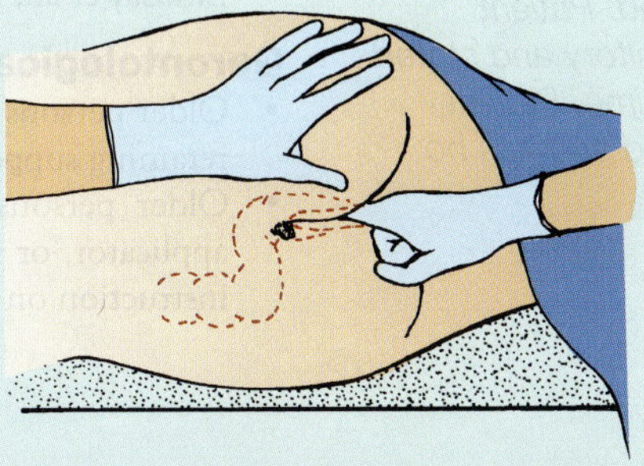

STEP 14 Insert rectal suppository past sphincter and against rectal wall.

Critical Decision Point *Do not insert suppository into a mass of fecal material; this will reduce effectiveness of medication.*

STEP	RATIONALE
15. *Option:* A suppository may be given through a colostomy (not ileostomy) if prescribed. Patient should lie supine. Use small amount of water-soluble lubricant for insertion.	
16. Withdraw finger and wipe patient's anal area.	Provides comfort.
17. Ask patient to remain flat or on side for 5 minutes.	Prevents expulsion of suppository.
18. Discard gloves by turning them inside out and dispose of them and used supplies in appropriate receptacle.	Reduces transfer of microorganisms.
19. If suppository contains laxative or fecal softener, place call light within reach so patient can obtain help to reach bedpan or toilet.	Ability to call for help provides patient with sense of control over elimination.
20. If suppository was given for constipation, remind patient *not* to flush commode after bowel movement.	Allows staff to evaluate results of suppository.

EVALUATION

STEP	RATIONALE
1. Return to bedside within 5 minutes to determine whether suppository was expelled.	Determines whether medication is distributed properly. Reinsertion may be necessary.
2. Ask if patient experienced localized anal or rectal discomfort during insertion.	Determines whether insertion of suppository was irritating.
3. Evaluate patient at time of peak medication effect for relief of symptoms for which medication was prescribed.	Determines effectiveness of medication.
4. **Use teach-back:** "I want to be sure I explained clearly to you how to insert a rectal suppository. Describe the steps you take to insert the suppository." Develop a revised teaching plan if patient or caregiver is unable to teach back correctly.	Determines patient's and caregiver's level of understanding of instructional topic.

Unexpected Outcomes	Related Interventions
1. Patient's symptoms are unrelieved.	• Explore alternative therapy.
2. Patient experiences decreased heart rate during rectal suppository insertion.	• Unintended vagal stimulation may occur, resulting in bradycardia in some patients. • Monitor heart rate of patient. Rectal route may not be suitable for certain cardiac conditions.
3. Patient reports rectal pain during insertion.	• Suppository may need more lubrication. • Rectal route may not be suitable; assess and notify health care provider.

Communication and Documentation

- Document the medication, dosage, route, and actual time and date of administration on MAR immediately after administration, not before. Include initials or signature.
- Document patient response to medication, patient teaching, and validation of patient understanding and self-administration of suppository on flow sheet or in progress notes in EHR or chart.
- Report adverse effects, patient response, and/or withheld medication to nurse in charge or health care provider.

DOCUMENTATION EXAMPLE

Rectal suppository administered as prescribed. Patient taught how to self-administer a rectal suppository and stated they would like to try to self-administer next time. Patient understands why the medication is prescribed and has no questions at this time.

Special Considerations

Teaching

- Be certain that patient is aware that the foil wrapper must be removed before insertion and that the suppository is to be inserted rectally and not taken orally. If patient chooses to self-administer suppositories or if a caregiver plans to administer, teach principles and techniques of infection control to prevent contact with and spread of fecal material.

Pediatric

- With children, it is often necessary to gently hold the buttocks together for 5 to 10 minutes to relieve pressure on the anal sphincter until the urge to expel the suppository is gone (Keenan-Lindsay et al., 2022).

Gerontological

- Older persons with loss of sphincter control may have difficulty retaining suppository.
- Older persons may have difficulty manipulating suppository, applicator, or irrigating equipment. If so, a caregiver may need instruction on how to insert the medication.

✦ REVIEW QUESTIONS

A 75-year-old patient (she/her) is hospitalized for 3 days with a diagnosis of dehydration, following a week of gastroenteritis. Patient has a history of hypertension, asthma, angina (heart pain), and osteoarthritis in her hands. Patient also has an abscess on her right calf that was caused by an infected bug bite. She is taking the following medications:

- *Hydrochlorothiazide, 25 mg every morning by mouth (PO) (diuretic)*
- *Diltiazem SR capsule, 60 mg twice a day PO (calcium channel blocker)*
- *Salbutamol MDI, 2 puffs four times a day (inhaled bronchodilator)*
- *Bacitracin topical ointment (500 units/g) applied topically to wound twice a day (antibiotic)*
- *Nitroglycerine transdermal patch, 0.2 mg/hr, one each morning topically (nitrate)*
- *Nitroglycerine sublingual tablets, 400 mcg, as needed for chest pain (nitrate)*

Review Questions 1 to 3 relate to the case study presented here.

1. The patient is discharged and has a community nurse follow-up appointment. On initial history, she tells the nurse that she sometimes feels dizzy when she changes position. She also has a cough. The nurse decides to do a cardiopulmonary assessment first. While listening to her breath sounds, the nurse notes that she has three nitroglycerine transdermal patches on her chest. What should the nurse do first?
2. While inspecting the patient's abscess, the nurse finds that there is a thick crust of old medication on the wound. The patients states, "I don't like to waste the medication that is already there, so I just put the new medicine on top of it." How should the nurse intervene?
3. The nurse returns to the home 2 days later and notices that the patient is still not cleaning the wound and that the wound is now larger (3 cm × 5 cm [1.25 inches × 2 inches]), is blistered, and has yellow, foul-smelling drainage. Using SBAR (situation–background–assessment–recommendation), show how to communicate about this patient with other community care nurses.
4. A patient is to receive medications through a small-bore nasogastric (NG) feeding tube. Which nursing actions are appropriate? (*Select all that apply.*)
   1. Verifying tube placement after medications are given
   2. Mixing all medications together and giving all at once
   3. Using an enteral tube syringe to administer medications
   4. Flushing the tube with 30 to 60 mL of water after the last dose of medication
   5. Checking for gastric residual before giving the medications
   6. Keeping the head of the bed elevated for 30 to 60 minutes after the medications are given
5. The nurse is caring for a patient who is receiving nitroglycerine ointment. Which nursing interventions are most appropriate to protect the nurse against accidental exposure? (*Select all that apply.*)
   1. Cleaning skin thoroughly before applying the next dose of medication
   2. Wearing gloves when applying the ointment
   3. Using the appropriate applicator to apply the medication
   4. Drawing blood to test for therapeutic medication values
   5. Wearing gloves to discard used ointment wrappers
   6. Performing hand hygiene immediately after medication application
6. A nurse is administering a metered-dose inhaler (MDI) with a spacer to a patient with chronic obstructive pulmonary disease (COPD). Place the steps of the procedure in the correct order:
   1. Insert MDI into end of spacer.
   2. Perform a respiratory assessment.
   3. Remove mouthpiece from MDI and spacer device.
   4. Place spacer mouthpiece into patient's mouth and instruct patient to close lips around it.
   5. Depress medication canister, spraying 1 puff into spacer device.
   6. Shake inhaler for 2 to 5 seconds.
   7. Instruct patient to hold breath for 10 seconds.
   8. Instruct patient to breathe in slowly through mouth for 3 to 5 seconds.

Visit the Evolve site for a complete list of answers to the Review Questions.

NEXT GENERATION NCLEX® (NGN)

For practice with answering exam questions related to unfolding NGN case studies, please consult the Next Generation NCLEX® (NGN)-Style Case Studies for Skills and Techniques on the Evolve website: http://evolve.elsevier.com/Canada/Perry/clinicalskills/

REFERENCES

Accreditation Canada. (2019). *Required organizational practices handbook, Version 14*. http://www.wrha.mb.ca/quality/files/201 9ROPHandbook.pdf

Accreditation Canada. (2020). *Required organizational practices–2020 handbook*. https://physicians.nshealth.ca/resources/required-organizational-practices-2020-handbook.

Adeniyi, B. O., Adebayo, A. M., Ilesanmi, O. S., et al. (2018). Knowledge of spacer device, peak flow meter and inhaler technique (MDIs) among health care providers: An evaluation of doctors and nurses. *Ghana Medical Journal*, *52*(1), 15–21. https://doi.org/10.4314/gmj.v52i1.4

Alhashemi, S. H., Ghorbani, R., & Vazin, A. (2019). Improving knowledge, attitudes, and practice of nurses in medication administration through enteral feeding tubes by clinical pharmacists: A case-control study. *Advances in Medical Education and Practice*, *10*, 493–500. https://doi.org/10.2147/AMEP.S203680

American Academy of Ophthalmology. (2021). *How to put in eye drops*. https://www.aao.org/eye-health/treatments/how-to-put-in-eye-drops

Ampofo, A. G., Khan, E., & Ibitoye, M. B. (2020). Understanding the role of educational interventions on medication adherence in hypertension: A systematic review and meta-analysis. *Heart & Lung*, *49*(5), 537–547. https://doi.org/10.1016/j.hrtlng.2020.02.039

Anderson, L. (2019). Enteral feeding tubes: An overview of nursing care. *British Journal of Nursing*, *28*(12), 748–754. https://doi.org/10.12968/bjon.2019.28.12.748

Asmare, T., Belayneh, A., & Dessie, B. (2021). Practice on metered dose inhaler techniques and its associated factors among asthmatic patients at debre markos comprehensive specialized hospital, east gojjam, Ethiopia: A prospective study. *The Scientific World Journal*, *2021*. https://doi.org/10.1155/2021/6615727

Asthma Canada. (n.d.-a). *Controller medications*. https://asthma.ca/get-help/treatment/controllers/

Asthma Canada. (n.d.-b). *How to monitor your asthma*. https://asthma.ca/get-help/living-with-asthma/peak-flow-meters/

Astier, A., Carlet, J., Hoppe-Tichy, T., et al. (2020). What is the role of technology in improving patient safety? A French, German and UK healthcare professional perspective. *Journal of Patient Safety and Risk Management*, *25*(6), 219–224. https://doi.org/10.1177/2516043520975661

Bandy, K. S., Albrecht, S., Parag, B., et al. (2019). Practices involved in the enteral delivery of drugs. *Current Nutrition Reports*, *8*(4), 356–362. https://doi.org/10.1007/s13668-019-00290-4

Binita, K. C., Khan, G. M., & Shrestha, N. (2020). Nasal spray use technique among patients attending the out-patient department of a tertiary care hospital, Gandaki Province, Nepal. *Integrated Pharmacy Research and Practice*, *9*, 155. https://doi.org/10.2147/IPRP.S266191

Boscart, V., McCleary, L., Sheiban Taucar, L., et al. (2023). *Ebersole and Hess' gerontological nursing and healthy aging in Canada* (3rd ed.). Elsevier.

Brunaugh, A. D., Smyth, H. D. C., & Williams, R. O., III. (2019). Topical and transdermal drug delivery. In *Essential pharmaceutics: AAPS introductions in the pharmaceutical sciences* (pp. 131–147). Springer. https://doi.org/10.1007/978-3-030-31745-4_9

Cho, S. M., & Choi, J. (2018). Patient safety culture associated with patient safety competencies among registered nurses. *Journal of Nursing Scholarship*, *50*(5), 549–557. https://doi.org/10.1111/jnu.12413

Chrystyn, H., & Lavorini, F. (2020). The dry powder inhaler features of the Easyhaler that benefit the management of patients. *Expert Review of Respiratory Medicine*, *14*(4), 345–351. https://doi.org/10.1080/17476348.2020.1721286

College of Physicians and Surgeons of Ontario. (2019). *Prescribing drugs*. https://www.cpso.on.ca/Physicians/Policies-Guidance/Policies/Prescribing-Drugs

Dineen-Griffin, S., Garcia-Cardenas, V., Williams, K., et al. (2019). Helping patients help themselves: A systematic review of self-management support strategies in primary health care practice. *PLOS ONE*, *14*(8), e0220116. https://doi.org/10.1371/journal.pone.0220116

Doley, J. (2022). Enteral nutrition overview. *Nutrients*, *14*(11), 2180. https://doi.org/10.3390/nu14112180

Douglass, A. M., Elder, J., Watsons, R., et al. (2018). A randomized controlled trial on the effect of a double check on the detection of medication errors. *Annals of Emergency Medicine*, *71*(1), 74–82. https://doi.org/10.1016/j.annemergmed.2017.03.022

Hanson, A., & Haddad, L. M. (2021). *Nursing rights of medication administration*. StatPearls. https://pubmed.ncbi.nlm.nih.gov/32809489/

Hayes, K. D., & Hayes, D. D. (2018). Best practices for unclogging feeding tubes in adults. Nursing, 48(6), 66–72. https://doi.org/10.1097/01.NURSE.0000532744.80506.5e

Health Canada. (2009). *Policy on manufacturing and compounding drug products in Canada (POL-0051)*. https://www.canada.ca/en/health-canada/services/drugs-health-products/compliance-enforcement/good-manufacturing-practices/guidance-documents/policy-manufacturing-compounding-drug-products.html

Institute for Safe Medication Practices Canada. (2018). *Do not use. Dangerous abbreviations, symbols, and dose designations*. https://www.ismp-canada.org/download/ISMPCanadaListOfDangerousAbbreviations.pdf

Institute for Safe Medication Practices. (2011). *Guidelines for timely administration of scheduled medications (acute)*. https://www.ismp.org/guidelines/timely-administration-scheduled-medications-acute

Institute for Safe Medication Practices Canada. (2018). *Do not use. Dangerous abbreviations, symbols, and dose designations*. https://www.ismp-canada.org/ download/ISMPCanadaListOfDangerousAbbreviations.pdf

Institute for Safe Medication Practices. (2019a). Independent double checks: Worth the effort if used judiciously and properly. *ISMP Medication Safety Alert*, *18*(12). https://www.ismp.org/resources/independent-double-checks-worth-effort-if-used-judiciously-and-properly

Institute for Safe Medication Practices. (2019b). *List of confused drug names*. https://www.ismp.org/recommendations/confused-drug-names-list

Institute for Safe Medication Practices. (2020). *Oral dosage forms that should not be crushed*. https://www.ismp.org/recommendations/do-not-crush

Institute for Safe Medication Practices. (2022). *2022–2023 targeted medication safety best practices for hospitals*. https://www.ismp.org/guidelines/best-practices-hospitals.

Kavanagh, A., & Donnelly, J. (2020). A Lean approach to improve medication administration safety by reducing distractions and interruptions. *Journal of Nursing Care Quality*, *35*(4), E58–E62. https://doi.org/10.1097/NCQ.0000000000000473

Keeley, D., & Partridge, M. R. (2019). Emergency MDI and spacer packs for asthma and COPD. *Lancet Respiratory Medicine*, *7*(5), 380–382. https://doi.org/10.1016/S2213-2600(19)30046-3

Keenan-Lindsay, L., Sams, C. A., & O'Connor, C. L. (2022). *Perry's maternal child nursing care in Canada* (3rd ed.). Elsevier.

Kennedy, K., Vu, K., Coakley, N., et al. (2022). *Safe handling of hazardous drugs*. Cancer Care Ontario (Ontario Health). https://www.cancercareontario.ca/en/guidelines-advice/types-of-cancer/2161

Kim, J. S., Hashweh, N., Li, H., et al. (2021). Effectiveness of one-on-one coaching in improving pressurized metered dose inhaler (pMDI) technique among COPD patients: A prospective clinical study. BMC *Pulmonary Medicine*, 21, Article 266. https://doi.org/10.1186/s12890-021-01627-y

Lampert, A., Bruckner, T., Haefeli, W. E., et al. (2019). Improving eye-drop administration skills of patients—A multicenter parallel-group cluster-randomized controlled trial. *PLoS One*, *14*(2), e0212007. https://doi.org/10.1371/journal.pone.0212007

Lilley, L. L., Collins, S. R., & Snyder, J. S. (2020). *Pharmacology and the nursing process* (9th ed.). Mosby.

Lord, L. M. (2018). Enteral access devices: Types, function, care and challenges. *Nutrition in Clinical Practice*, *33*(1), 16–38. https://doi.org/10.1002/ncp.10019

Martyn, J. A., Paliadelis, P., & Perry, C. (2019). The safe administration of medication: Nursing behaviours beyond the five-rights. *Nurse Education in Practice*, *37*, 109–114. https://doi.org/10.1016/j.nepr.2019.05.006

Medline Plus. (2015). *Nitroglycerin transdermal patch*. US National Library of Medicine. https://medlineplus.gov/druginfo/meds/a601085.html

Medline Plus. (2022a). *Estradiol transdermal patch*. US National Library of Medicine. https://medlineplus.gov/druginfo/meds/a605042.html

Medline Plus. (2022b). *How to use a nebulizer*. US National Library of Medicine. https://medlineplus.gov/ency/patientinstructions/000006.htm

Metheny, N. A. (2021). CE: Monitoring adult patients for intolerance to gastric tube feedings. *American Journal of Nursing*, *121*(8), 36–43. https://doi.org/10.1097/01.NAJ.0000767356.16777.f1

Metsämuuronen, R., Kokki, H., Naaranlahti, T., et al. (2020). Nurses' perceptions of automated dispensing cabinets—an observational study and an online survey. *BMC Nursing*, *19*(27), 1–9. https://doi.org/10.1186/s12912-020-00420-2

Mitchell, A. (2019). Administering a suppository: Types, considerations and procedure. *British Journal of Nursing*, *28*(5), 288–289. https://doi.org/10.12968/bjon.2019.28.5.288

Mitchell, A., & Hill, B. (2020). Moisture-associated skin damage: An overview of its diagnosis and management. *British Journal of Community Nursing*, *25*(3), S12–S18. https://doi.org/10.12968/bjcn.2020.25.Sup3.S12

Murrell, D. (2018). *How to apply a transdermal patch*. Healthline. https://www.healthline.com/health/general-use/how-to-use-transdermal-patch

National Institute on Aging. (2021). *The dangers of polypharmacy and the case for deprescribing in older adults.* https://www.nia.nih.gov/news/dangers-polypharmacy-and-case-deprescribing-older-adults

Parthasarathi, A., Puvvada, R., Patel, H., et al. (2021). Evaluation of medication errors in a tertiary care hospital of a low- to middle-income country. *Curēus, 13*(7), e16769. https://doi.org/10.7759/cureus.16769

Pharmacy Association of Nova Scotia. (n.d.). *Filling a prescription (dispensing).* https://pans.ns.ca/public/pharmacy-services/filling-prescription-dispensing

Risør, B. W., Lisby, M., & Sørensen, J. (2018). Complex automated medication systems reduce medication administration errors in a Danish acute medical unit. *International Journal for Quality in Health Care, 30*(6), 457–465. https://doi.org/10.1093/intqhc/mzy042

Smith, W. K., & Hasham, A. M. Z. (2021). How to counsel patients on the administration of nasal sprays, drops and ointments and performing nasal irrigation. *The Pharmaceutical Journal, 307*, Article 7954. https://doi.org/10.1211/PJ.2021.1.105205

Tariq, R. A., Vashisht, R., Sinha, A., et al. (2022). Medication dispensing errors and prevention. *StatPearls.* https://www.ncbi.nlm.nih.gov/books/NBK519065/

Tatsumi, H. (2019). Enteral tolerance in critically ill patients. *Journal of Intensive Care, 7*, Article 30. https://doi.org/10.1186/s40560-019-0378-0

US Food and Drug Administration. (2021). *2017 GDUFA science and research report: Transdermal drug products.* https://www.fda.gov/industry/generic-drug-user-fee-amendments/fys-2013-2017-gdufa-science-and-research-report-transdermal-drug-products

US Food and Drug Administration. (2022). *Compounding and the FDA: Questions and answers.* https://www.fda.gov/drugs/human-drug-compounding/compounding-and-fda-questions-and-answers

US Food and Drug Administration. (2023). *Examples of medical device misconnections.* https://www.fda.gov/medical-devices/medical-device-connectors/examples-medical-device-misconnections

Washburn, N. C., Dossett, H. A., Fritschle, A. C., et al. (2021). High-alert medication stratification tool-revised: An exploratory study of an objective, standardized medication safety tool. *Journal of Patient Safety, 17*(7), e672–e683. https://doi.org/10.1097/PTS.0000000000000445

Westbrook, J. I., Li, L., Raban, M. Z., et al. (2021). Associations between double-checking and medication administration errors: A direct observational study of paediatric inpatients. *BMJ Quality and Safety, 30*(4), 320–330. https://doi.org/10.1136/bmjqs-2020-011473

Yu, Y. Q., Yang, X., Wu, X.-F., et al. (2021). Enhancing permeation of drug molecules across the skin via delivery in nanocarriers: Novel strategies for effective transdermal applications. *Frontiers in Bioengineering and Biotechnology, 9*, Article 646554. https://doi.org/10.3389/fbioe.2021.646554

Zuercher, P., Moret, C. S., Dziewas, R., et al. (2019). Dysphagia in the intensive care unit: Epidemiology, mechanisms, and clinical management. *Critical Care, 23*, Article 103. https://doi.org/10.1186/s13054-019-2400-2

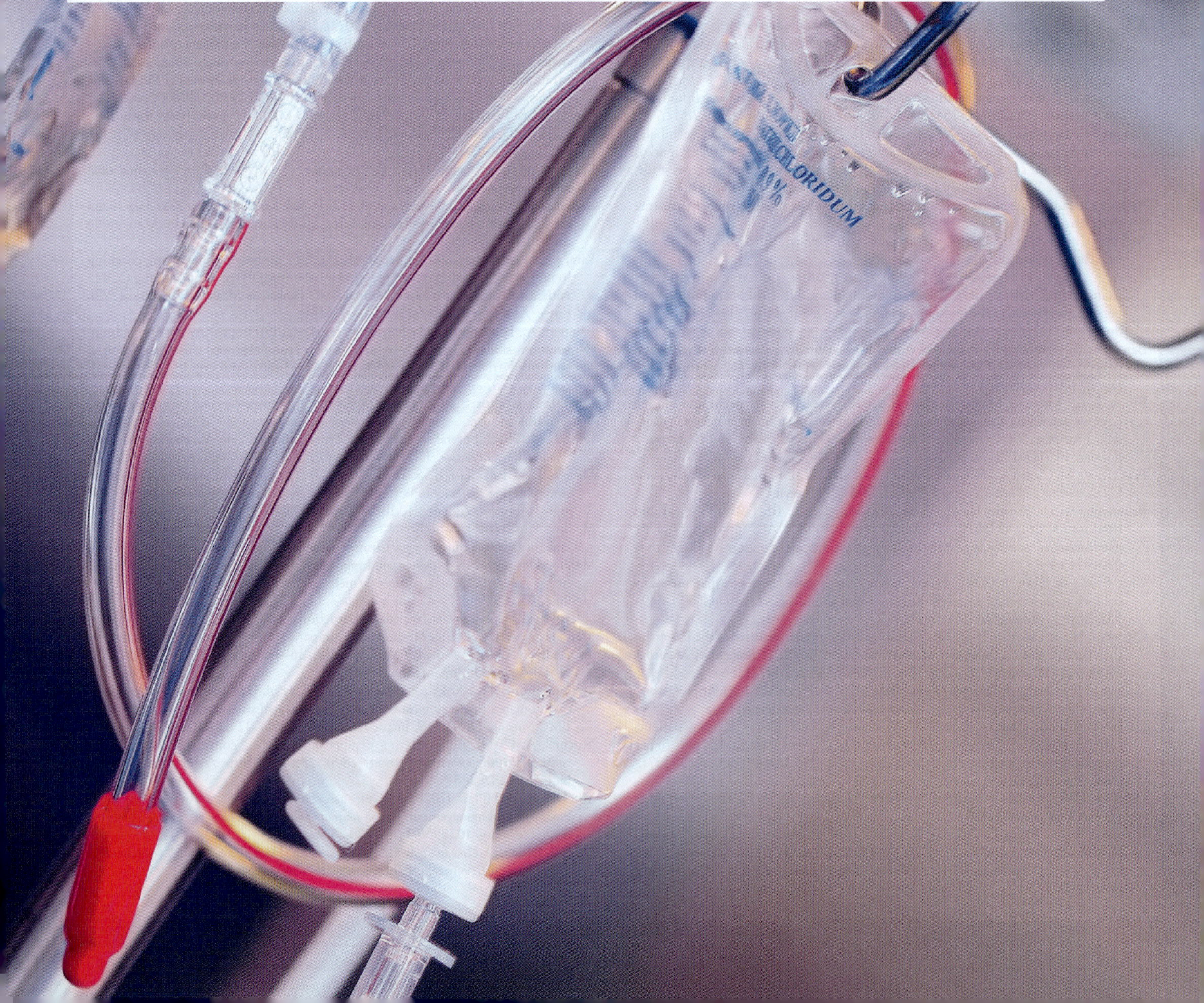

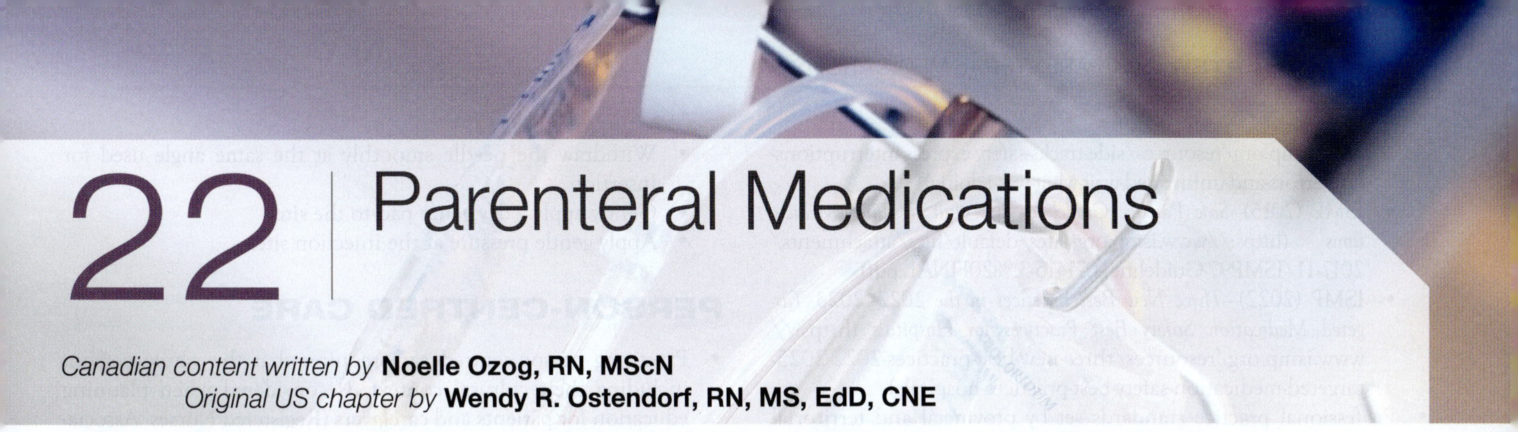

22 Parenteral Medications

Canadian content written by **Noelle Ozog, RN, MScN**

Original US chapter by **Wendy R. Ostendorf, RN, MS, EdD, CNE**

SKILLS AND PROCEDURES

OBJECTIVES

Mastery of content in this chapter will enable the nurse to:

- Correctly prepare injectable medications from a vial and an ampoule.
- Identify advantages, disadvantages, and risks of administering medications by each type of parenteral route.
- Evaluate the effectiveness and outcomes of administering medications by each type of parenteral route.
- Explain the importance of selecting an appropriately sized syringe and needle for an injection into tissue (intradermal, subcutaneous, and intramuscular).
- Describe factors to consider when selecting tissue injection sites.
- Identify the anatomical landmarks used to locate each tissue injection site.
- Describe ways to promote patient comfort while administering an injection into tissue.
- Correctly administer intradermal, subcutaneous, and intramuscular injections.
- Initiate, maintain, and discontinue a continuous subcutaneous infusion.
- Compare the risks of three different intravenous routes.
- Correctly administer an intravenous medication by intermittent intravenous infusion or intravenous direct.

MEDIA RESOURCES

- http://evolve.elsevier.com/Canada/Perry/clinicalskills/

PURPOSE

Medications administered by the *parenteral* route enter body tissues and the circulatory system by injection. Injected medications are more quickly absorbed than oral medications. Parenteral routes are used when patients are vomiting, cannot swallow, or are NPO (nothing by mouth) or when rapid onset of a medication is needed. These medication administration procedures are invasive and thus pose greater risks than those associated with administering nonparenteral medications (see Chapter 21).

The four most common routes for parenteral administration are described in this chapter:

- *Subcutaneous (SUBCUT) injection:* Injection into subcutaneous tissue, the layer of skin just under the dermis
- *Intramuscular (IM) injection:* Injection deep into a muscle
- *Intradermal (ID) injection:* Injection into the dermis, the layer of skin just under the epidermis
- *Intravenous (IV) injection or infusion:* Injection into a vein

STANDARDS OF CARE

- Accreditation Canada (2020)—*Required Organizational Practices—2020 Handbook* (https://physicians.nshealth.ca/resources/required-organizational-practices-2020-handbook)
- Canadian Nurses Association (CNA, 2017)—*Code of Ethics for Registered Nurses* (https://www.cna-aiic.ca/en/nursing/regulated-nursing-in-canada/nursing-ethics)
- Canadian Vascular Access Association (CVAA, 2019)—*Canadian Vascular Access and Infusion Therapy Guidelines* (https://cvaa.info/en/education/national-guidelines-2019)
- Institute for Safe Medication Practices (ISMP):
  - ISMP (2011)—*Guidelines for Timely Administration of Scheduled Medications (Acute)* (https://www.ismp.org/guidelines/timely-administration-scheduled-medications-acute)
  - ISMP (2012)—*Side Tracks on the Safety Express. Interruptions Lead to Errors and Unfinished . . . Wait, What Was I Doing?* (https://

www.ismp.org/resources/side-tracks-safety-express-interruptions-lead-errors-and-unfinished-wait-what-was-i-doing)

- ISMP (2015)—*Safe Practice Guidelines for Adult IV Push Medications* (https://www.ismp.org/sites/default/files/attachments/2017-11/ISMP97-Guidelines-071415-3.%20FINAL.pdf)
- ISMP (2022)—*Three New Best Practices in the 2022–2023 Targeted Medication Safety Best Practices for Hospitals* (https://www.ismp.org/resources/three-new-best-practices-2022-2023-targeted-medication-safety-best-practices-hospitals)
- Professional practice standards set by provincial and territorial colleges and associations of nursing

PRINCIPLES FOR PRACTICE

- When managing a patient's medications, incorporate the patient's priorities of care and preferences, as much as is feasible.
- Follow employer policy for technology (e.g., bar scanning, electronic medication administration record [MAR]) that is available in the facility when preparing and giving medications (ISMP, 2022). **Note:** MAR refers to both paper and electronic MARs. Follow employer policy.
- Provide information to patients and their caregivers about each medication the patient is receiving while you are administering medications. Make sure that you answer all questions before administering medications. Patients often can identify inappropriate medications.
- Minimize a patient's discomfort when giving an injection:
  - Use age-appropriate distraction techniques such as playing with a toy, watching an Internet video, wearing a virtual reality headset (Addab et al., 2022; Cho & Choi, 2021), breathing for relaxation (Birnie et al., 2018), or blowing bubbles (Yilmaz & Alemdar, 2019).
  - Use nonpharmacological, tactile strategies such as cold/vibration devices (Su et al., 2021; Yilmaz & Alemdar, 2019).
  - Use employer policy as a guide to determine when it may be appropriate to apply a vapocoolant spray (e.g., Fluori-Methane spray) or topical anaesthetic (e.g., EMLA [eutectic mixture of local anaesthetics] cream) to an injection site.
- In general, when injecting a medication into tissue:
  - Insert the needle at the proper angle, smoothly, and quickly (Fig. 22.1). Do not hesitate.
  - Inject the medication slowly (1 mL/10 seconds), but smoothly.
  - Hold the syringe steady once the needle is in the tissue to prevent tissue damage.
  - Withdraw the needle smoothly at the same angle used for insertion.
  - Gently apply a dry gauze pad to the site.
  - Apply gentle pressure at the injection site.

PERSON-CENTRED CARE

- Practising person-centred care requires that the whole person, including their cultural context, is considered when planning education for patients and caregivers (Registered Nurses' Association of Ontario, 2015).
- Dietary preferences, tobacco and alcohol use, and use of herbal remedies may affect medication action and response.
- Most clinical trials of medication are completed with homogeneous groups of subjects, who are typically White and male-identified (Clark et al., 2019). As a result, patients may experience a therapeutic response at a different dosage than is recommended. Knowledge about adverse effects, dosing variation, and careful monitoring is essential in administering medications.
- As a nurse, you need to be able to communicate with diverse patient populations about their medications. Effective therapeutic communication is not about memorizing "rules" you can apply to communicating with a patient whose background differs from your own. Rather, it is about active listening, building trust, and being open to providing information in a way that is understandable to each individual patient.

EVIDENCE-INFORMED PRACTICE

- The rectus femorus (anterior thigh) is *not* a safe location for IM injection owing to its proximity to the lateral circumflex femoral artery and femoral nerve (Nakajima et al., 2020). Similarly, the dorsalgluteal site (buttocks) is *not* a safe location for IM injection owing to the risk of sciatic nerve injury (Rodger & King, 2000). Do not use these sites for IM injections.
- The historical practice of aspiration during IM injections was based on expert opinion (Paull, 2018). Aspiration before giving an IM injection is painful and not recommended (Paull, 2018; Sisson, 2015), particularly as currently recommended IM injection sites are situated away from major blood vessels. Always follow employer policy, and be alert if any specific medications indicate that aspiration must be done before an IM injection.

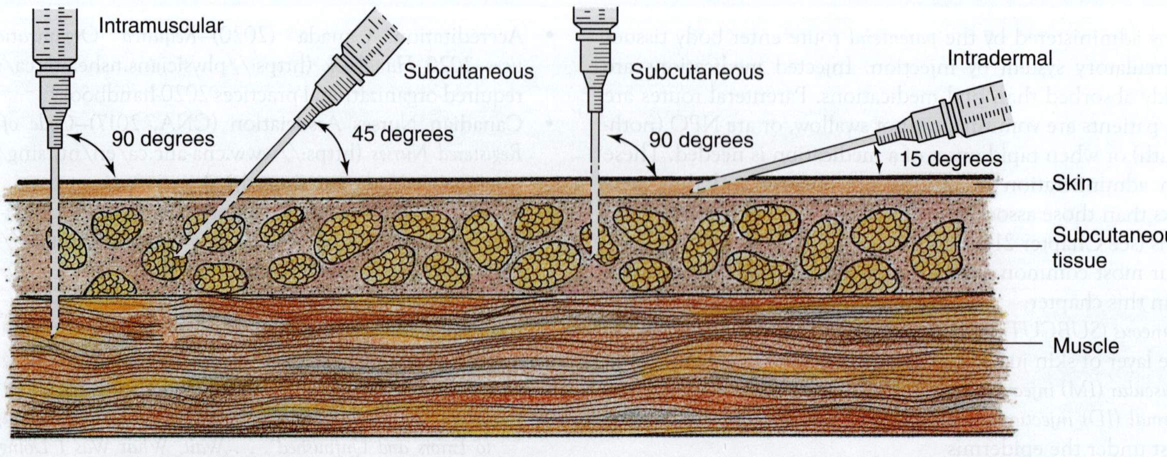

FIG 22.1 Comparison of angles of insertion of intramuscular (90 degrees), subcutaneous (45 or 90 degrees), and intradermal (15 degrees) injections.

- The SUBCUT fat covering the deltoid muscle varies based on age, assigned sex at birth, and body mass index (BMI) (Sebro, 2022). For example, cisgender women tend to have a thicker SUBCUT fat pad over the deltoid than cisgender men at the same BMI (Sebro, 2022). For people receiving hormones as part of gender-affirming hormone care, hormones such as estradiol will increase overall body fat, whereas testosterone will decrease it (Klaver et al., 2018). When choosing a needle, ensure that you consider the individual patient's distribution of body fat to make certain that the needle enters the intended tissue.

SAFETY GUIDELINES

- Patient safety in administering medication involves following the 10 rights of medication administration (see Chapter 20).
- The "three checks," whereby a nurse compares the information on the medication packaging with that in the MAR, occur at specific times during the medication preparation process to ensure accuracy (College of Registered Nurses of Saskatchewan, 2021):
  1. Before removing the medication vial/container from storage (drawer, medication cupboard, etc.).
  2. When the prescribed amount of the medication is removed from the original packaging ("drawn up").
  3. Prior to giving medication to the patient.
- Create no-interruption zones (NIZs) by placing red tape or tile borders on the floor around medication carts. Support your colleagues by not interrupting nurses working in these zones (ISMP, 2012).
- Minimize distractions during medication preparation and administration:
  - Prepare medications for one patient at a time.
  - Prepare one medication at a time.
  - Keep all pages of the paper MAR for one patient together.
  - Look at only one patient's MAR at a time.
  - Verify that the medications have not expired.
- It is normal for newer nurses and students to require more time to prepare medications than experienced colleagues. If the time to prepare a medication was extensive, verify that medication orders have not been changed or discontinued during the preparation stage before you go to administer the medication to your patient.
- Follow best practice guidelines for timing of medication administration:
  - Medications that require exact timing include stat, first-time or loading doses, and one-time doses.
  - *Time-critical medications* are drugs that may cause harm or result in substantially suboptimal therapy or pharmacological effect if not administered at the scheduled time (must be given no later than 30 minutes before or after the scheduled dose; e.g., antibiotics, insulin, anticoagulants, anticonvulsants, immunosuppressive medications).
  - *Non–time-critical medications* are drugs that should not cause harm or result in substantially suboptimal therapy or pharmacological effect if given within a range of 1 or 2 hours of the scheduled time (ISMP, 2011).
- Staff nurses are under extreme pressure to work efficiently. When technology failures, missing supplies, staffing ratios, or other situational factors make it hard to meet patient needs in a timely manner and to follow employer policy, many nurses feel compelled to use "workaround" behaviours to bypass policy (Bianchi & Ghirotto, 2021; Heron & Bruk-Lee, 2020). An example of a workaround is not checking the patient's identification band; in this case, the time taken to check the identification band is viewed as a barrier to accomplishing the goal of administering the medication. Unfortunately, workaround behaviours can contribute to adverse events (Bianchi & Ghirotto, 2021). Use workplace reporting systems to notify policymakers of policies that are incompatible with workplace reality.
- Clarify unclear medication prescriptions and ask for help whenever you are uncertain about a prescription or calculation. Consult with other health care team members, and be sure that you have resolved all concerns related to medication administration before preparing and giving medications.
- Some commonly administered parenteral medications (e.g., insulin, heparin) can cause significant harm if an error is made; for these medications, an independent double-check by a second nurse is often required (ISMP, 2018). Follow your employer policy.
- Use strict aseptic technique during medication preparation and administration (Table 22.1).
- Rotate injection sites (and document this rotation) to prevent the formation of indurations and abscesses.
- The nurse usually cannot delegate medication administration. Ensure that you follow standards set by the legislation in your province/territory and employer policy.

Selecting a Syringe

Syringes are single use, disposable, and either Luer-Lok or non–Luer-Lok. The design of the syringe tip influences the name. Figure 22.2 shows the parts of a syringe. Luer-Lok syringes (Fig. 22.3, A) use standard needles or needleless devices that are twisted onto the tip and lock themselves in place. The Luer-Lok

TABLE 22.1
Preventing Infection During an Injection Into Tissue

Principle	Technique
Prevent contamination of solution	Ampoules should not sit open, and medication should be removed quickly.
Prevent needle contamination	Avoid letting needle touch contaminated surface (e.g., outer edges of ampoule or vial, outer surface of needle cap, your hands, countertop, or table surface). A second layer of prevention is added by drawing up medications with a blunt fill needle, then switching to a patient- and injection site–appropriate needle after medication has been drawn up. The new needle will be sterile and have had no opportunity to touch a contaminated surface prior to injection. Avoid touching length of plunger or inner part of barrel. Keep tip of syringe covered with cap or needle.
Prepare skin	Wash skin soiled with dirt, drainage, or feces using soap and water. Use friction and a circular motion while cleaning with an antiseptic swab. Swab from centre of site and move outward in a 5-cm (2-inch) radius.
Reduce transfer of microorganisms	Perform hand hygiene for a minimum of 20 seconds.

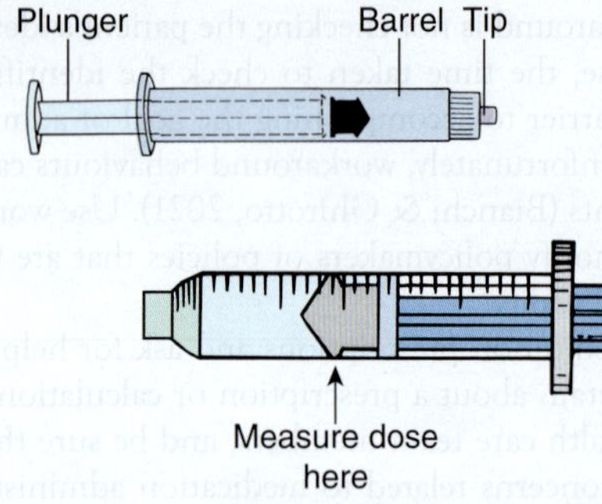

FIG 22.2 Parts of a syringe.

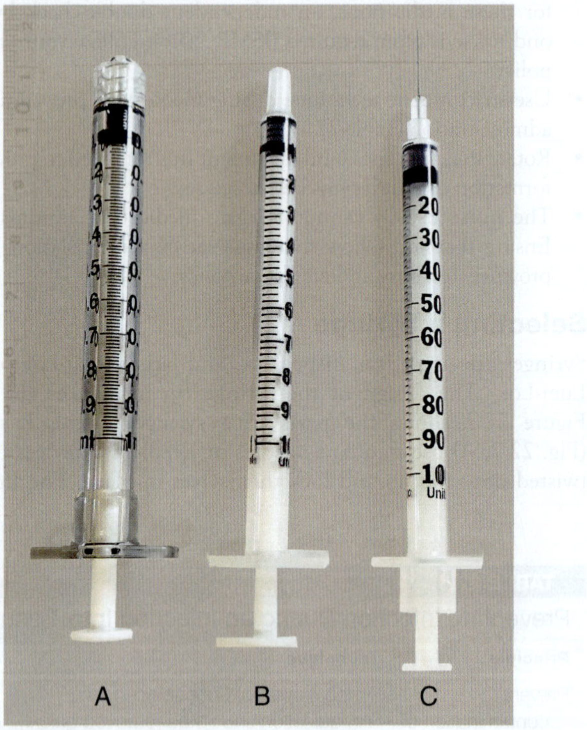

FIG 22.3 Examples of 1-mL syringes. A, Luer-Lok. B, Non–Luer-Lok. C, Insulin syringe marked in units (100). (*Courtesy Noelle Ozog.*)

design, in addition to preventing the accidental removal of a needle from the syringe, allows the syringe to be connected to a needleless connector on an IV line or SUBCUT butterfly; this design avoids the use of a needle and thereby reduces the risk of needle-stick injury. Non–Luer-Lok syringes use needles or needleless devices that slip onto the tip (Fig. 22.3, *B*). Some non–Luer-Lok syringes are manufactured with the needle attached (Fig. 22.3, C).

Syringes come in a variety of sizes, ranging in capacity from 0.5 to 60 mL (Fig. 22.4). The increments marked on the side of a syringe vary with size; 1-mL syringes are typically marked in increments of hundredths of a millilitre (i.e., every 0.01 mL; Fig. 22.3, A), whereas 50-mL syringes might only be marked in increments of millilitres (i.e., every 1 mL). When selecting a syringe, choose the smallest syringe size possible to improve the accuracy of medication preparation. Insulin syringes (see Fig. 22.3, *B–C*) are typically designed for use with U-100–strength insulin. Each millilitre of solution contains 100 units of insulin.

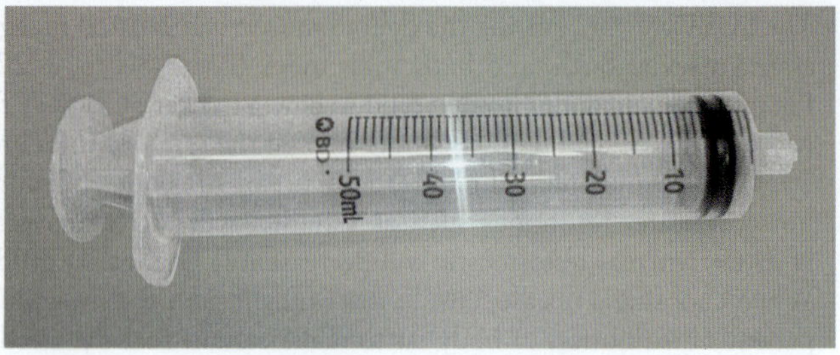

FIG 22.4 Example of a 50-mL syringe. (*Courtesy Noelle Ozog.*)

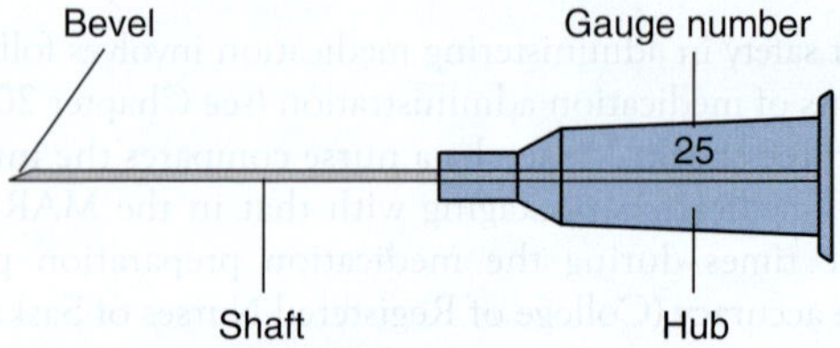

FIG 22.5 Parts of a needle.

Selecting a Needle

Some needles come attached to syringes, while others come packaged individually to allow flexibility in selecting the right needle for a patient. Needles are disposable, and most are made of stainless steel. A needle has three parts: the hub, which fits onto the tip of a syringe; the shaft, which connects to the hub; and the bevel, or slanted tip (Fig. 22.5). Note that colour of the needle hub corresponds to the needle gauge; these colours are standardized internationally.

The needle hub, shaft, and bevel must remain sterile at all times. To prevent contamination, use gentle force to twist a Luer-Lok needle onto the syringe with the cap intact (Fig. 22.6, *A–B*). Needles intended for injection into a patient's tissue have a sharp tip (Fig. 22.7, *A–B*); needles intended to allow nurses to draw up and reconstitute medications have a blunt tip ("blunt fill needles"; Fig. 22.7, *C–D*). Some blunt fill needles contain filters for drawing up medication from a glass ampoule to avoid any glass particles (CVAA, 2019). Do not use the filtered blunt fill needle to administer or transfer the medication because the filter has a one-way flow; once used to withdraw a medication and trap glass particles, it should not be "pushed" in the other direction during injection (CVAA, 2019).

The tip of a needle, or the bevel, is always slanted. The bevel creates a narrow slit when injected into tissue that quickly closes after the needle is removed to prevent leakage of medication, blood, or serum. Longer bevelled tips are sharper and narrower, which minimizes tissue discomfort during a SUBCUT or IM injection.

Most needles vary in length from 6.4 mm (0.25 inches) to 76 mm (3 inches). Choose the needle length according to the type of tissue into which the medication will be injected, injection site, and the patient's individual distribution of body fat (Klaver et al., 2018; Larkin et al., 2018; Sebro, 2022). Use longer needles (25 mm [1 inch] to 40 mm [1.5 inches] for IM injections and a shorter needle (9 mm [0.375 inches] to 16 mm [0.625 inches]) for SUBCUT injections. Figure 22.8 shows 25-gauge needles at three different lengths. As the needle gauge becomes smaller, the needle diameter becomes larger (Fig. 22.9). The selection of a gauge depends on the viscosity of fluid to be injected or infused; the greater the viscosity, the larger

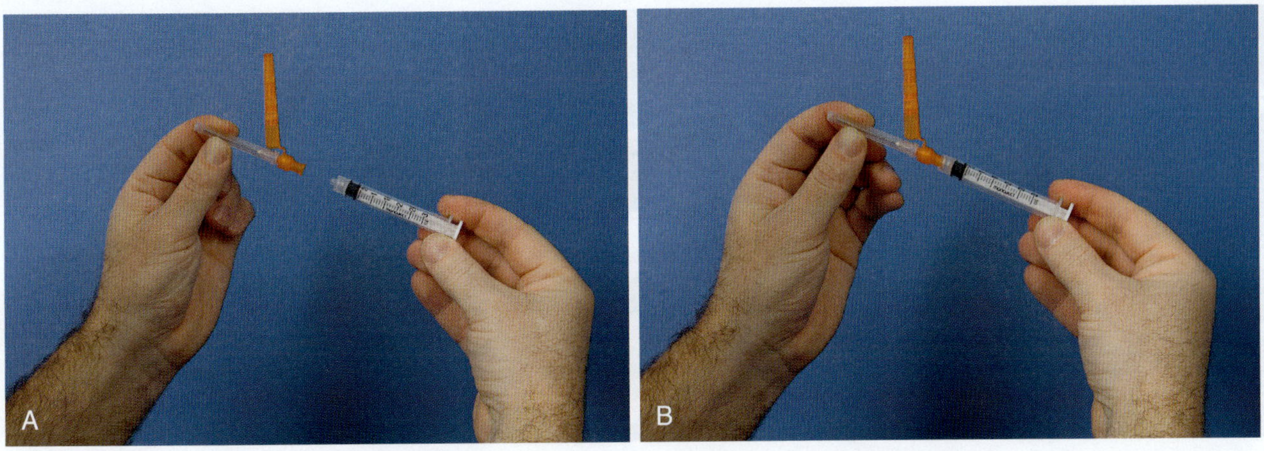

FIG 22.6 A, Capped needle placed on syringe tip. B, Needle secured.

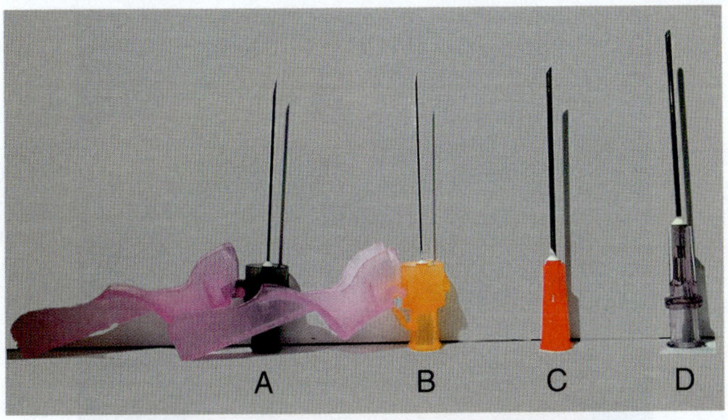

FIG 22.7 A, 22-gauge, 40-mm needle. B, 25-gauge, 40-mm needle. C, 18-gauge blunt fill needle. D, 18-gauge filtered blunt fill needle. (*Courtesy Noelle Ozog.*)

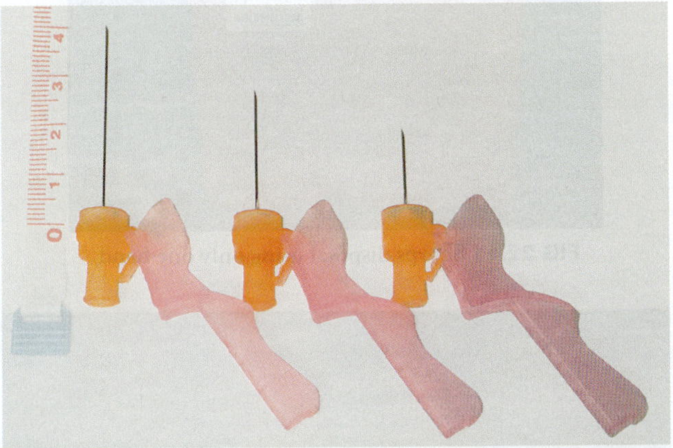

FIG 22.8 Comparison of length in 25-gauge needles (from left to right): 40 mm, 25 mm, 16 mm. (*Courtesy Noelle Ozog.*)

the gauge. For example, testosterone and Ativan are viscous medications that need to be drawn up and administered using a larger-bore needle.

Needle-Stick Prevention

The most frequent route of exposure to bloodborne disease for health care workers is from needle-stick injuries (Canadian Centre

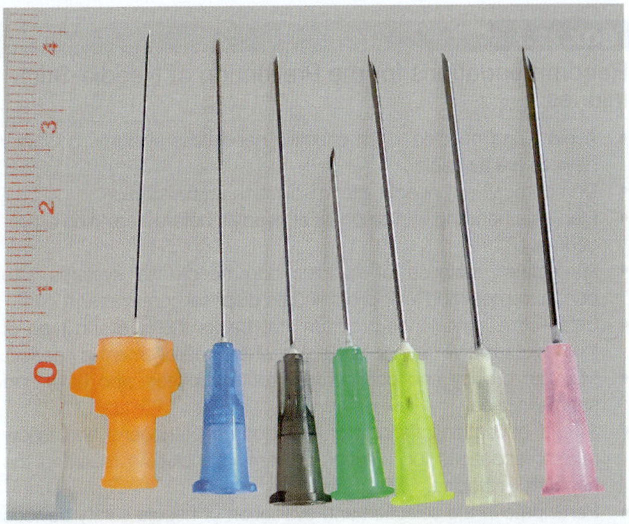

FIG 22.9 Comparison of gauge in 40-mm (1.5-inch) needles (from left to right): 25 gauge, 23 gauge, 22 gauge, 21 gauge (25 mm length), 20 gauge, 19 gauge, 18 gauge. (*Courtesy Noelle Ozog.*)

for Occupational Health and Safety [CCOHS], 2018). These injuries occur when health care workers recap needles or leave needles at a patient's bedside. Replacing needles with needleless connection devices (Fig. 22.10, *A*), when possible, is one way the employer can support nurse safety.

When it is not possible to eliminate sharps, safety-engineered devices can prevent needle-stick injuries (CCOHS, 2018). These include plastic guards that can be manually slipped over the needle as it is withdrawn from the skin (Fig. 22.10, *B–C*), and needles that automatically retract after injection. Box 22.1 lists recommendations to reduce the risk of needle-stick injuries.

Special puncture- and leak-proof containers are available for the disposal of sharps. The design of the containers enables nurses to use only one hand when disposing of an uncapped needle (Fig. 22.11). In addition, containers must stand upright, not be allowed to overfill, and be labelled with a biohazard symbol (Fig. 22.12). They are often yellow, but may also be other colours.

Disposable Injection Units

Single-dose, prefilled, disposable syringes are available for some medications. They can reduce preparation time for nurses when a

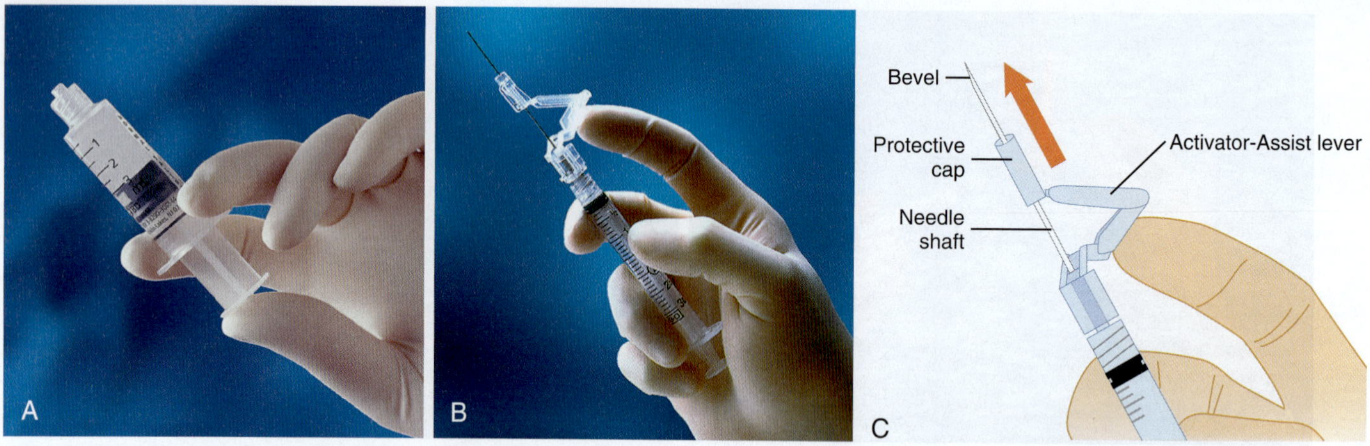

FIG 22.10 A, Syringe with Luer-Lok needleless connection system. B, Safety needle system. C, Detail of safety needle system. (*A and B, Courtesy and copyright © Becton, Dickinson and Company.*)

BOX 22.1

Recommendations for the Prevention of Needle-Stick Injuries

- Avoid using needles when effective needleless systems or safety devices are available.
- Do not recap any needle after medication administration.
- Plan safe handling and disposal of needles before beginning a procedure.
- Immediately dispose of needles and needleless systems into puncture-proof and leak-proof sharps disposal containers.
- Establish a surveillance program that tracks the rate and type of injuries, causative factors, and areas where improvement is needed.
- Maintain privacy and confidentiality of employees who have had sharps injuries.
- Attend education offerings on bloodborne pathogens and follow recommendations for infection prevention, including receiving the hepatitis B vaccine.
- Participate in the selection and evaluation of needle safety devices with safety features within your facility whenever possible.

Data from Public Health Agency of Canada. (2016). *Routine practices and additional precautions for preventing the transmission of infection in healthcare settings*. https://www.canada.ca/content/dam/phac-aspc/documents/services/publications/diseases-conditions/routine-practices-precautions-healthcare-associated-infections/routine-practices-precautions-healthcare-associated-infections-2016-FINAL-eng.pdf

medication has a standard dose (e.g., dalteparin for deep vein thrombosis [DVT] prophylaxis in hospital inpatients of average weight), but are typically more expensive and thus not always available. Before expelling air from a prefilled syringe, always check the manufacturer's recommendation, because the air bubble is *not* to be removed prior to administration of some medications. Prefilled unit-dose systems (e.g., the Imitrex prefilled syringe system [Fig. 22.13]) include a reusable syringe holder and disposable, prefilled, sterile cartridge units. This design reduces the risk of needle-stick injury.

! SAFETY ALERT It is important to check the medication and concentration in a prefilled syringe very carefully, because prefilled syringes look very similar.

Pumps and Smart Pumps

To ensure a constant and accurate delivery of medication, use electronic infusion pumps to deliver IV or continuous subcutaneous infusions (CSCI). Pumps that have preprogrammed medication libraries with appropriate dose limits ("smart pumps") should be used to reduce the risk of errors (CVAA, 2019; ISMP, 2022).

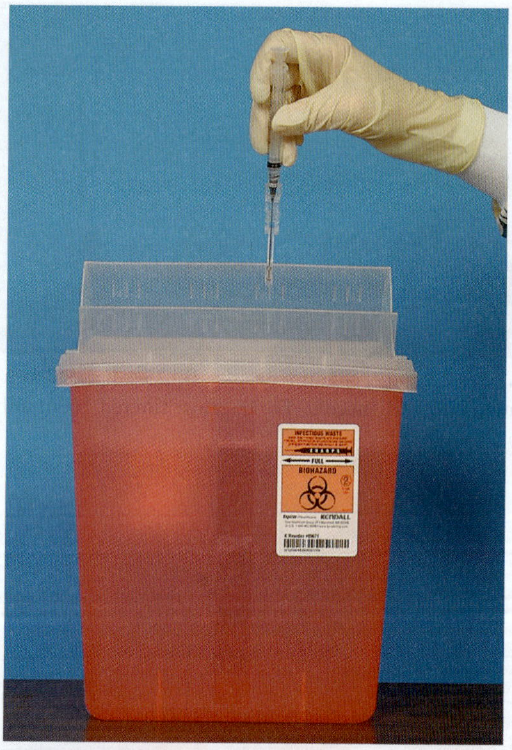

FIG 22.11 Sharps disposal using only one hand.

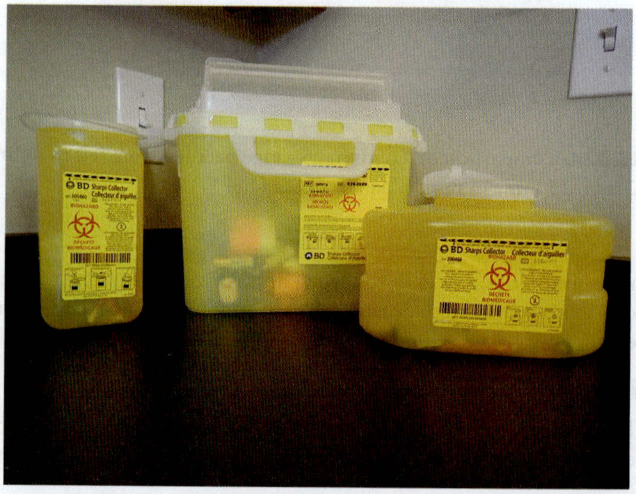

FIG 22.12 Sharps containers come in many shapes and sizes. (*Courtesy Noelle Ozog.*)

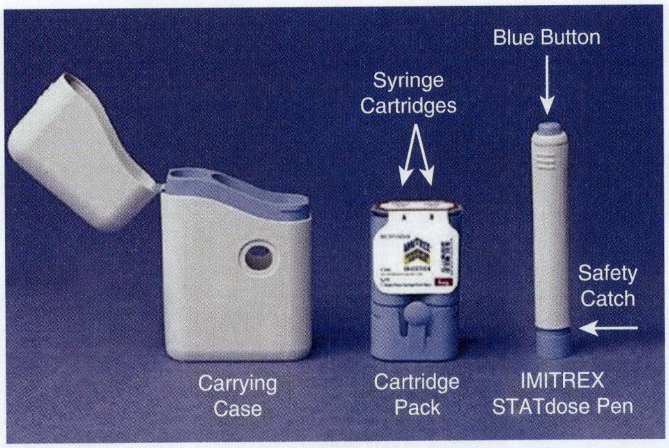

FIG 22.13 **Prefilled syringe system: sumatriptan (Imitrex).** (*From GlaxoSmithKline Canada.*)

✦ SKILL 22.1 Preparing Injections From Ampoules and Vials

NSO *Nursing Skills Online Administration of Parenteral Medications: Injections Module 7 / Lesson 2*

Ampoules contain single doses of injectable medication in a liquid form. An ampoule is made of glass (Fig. 22.14, *A*) or plastic (Fig. 22.14, *B*) with a constricted, prescored neck that is snapped off to allow access to a medication. A coloured ring around the neck of a glass ampoule indicates where the ampoule is prescored to be broken easily, and a coloured dot indicates where to place your thumb while opening it. Once the neck is snapped off, an ampoule becomes an *open system*, meaning that the inside of the ampoule is open to the rest of the room and air can move freely in and out. As a result, the pressure inside the ampoule is the same as the air outside. The shape of the ampoule neck and the surface tension of the liquid allow an opened ampoule to be inverted without spilling the medication. Medication is easily withdrawn from the ampoule by aspirating with a blunt fill needle (Fig. 22.7, *C–D*) and syringe.

A vial is a single- or multi-dose plastic or glass container with a rubber seal at the top (see Fig. 22.14, *C*). After you open a single-dose vial, discard it, regardless of the amount of medication used. A multi-dose vial contains several doses of a medication and thus can be used several times. When using a multi-dose vial, write the date the vial was opened on the vial label. Verify employer policy as to how long you are permitted to use an opened multi-dose vial. Properly discard a multi-dose vial when the allowed time for being open has expired.

It is best practice to only use a multi-dose vial with the same patient (College of Physicians and Surgeons of British Columbia, 2018). However, some multi-dose vials are intended by the manufacturer to be used with different patients (e.g., Pfizer and Moderna COVID-19 vaccines). Furthermore, some hospitals may not have the resources to supply individual vials for each patient (e.g., multi-dose insulin vials are still used with different patients in many hospitals). Nurses should advocate for the adoption of best practices in their workplace whenever possible. Nurses must also follow employer policy when resource limitations beyond the control of the individual nurse necessitate deviations from best practice.

A metal or plastic cap protects the rubber seal of the vial from physical damage, but not all drug manufacturers guarantee that rubber seals of unused vials are sterile. This rubber seal separates the medication and air inside the vial from the air in the rest of the room. Vials may contain liquid or dry forms of medications; medications that are unstable in solution are packaged in dry form. When the medication is supplied in this form, the product monograph or employer policy specifies the solvent or diluent used to dissolve or reconstitute the medication and the amount needed to prepare a desired medication concentration. Normal saline and sterile water are the most common solutions. Some vials have two chambers separated by a rubber stopper (Fig. 22.15). One chamber contains the diluent solution, while the other contains the dry medication. Before preparing the medication, the nurse pushes on the upper chamber to dislodge the rubber stopper, allowing the powder and the diluent to mix.

Unlike an ampoule, a vial is a *closed system*, meaning that the fluids inside (air and liquid medication) are separated from the air in the room by the rubber seal. Additionally, the hard plastic or glass container of an ampoule cannot change size in response to volume changes. If you try to remove the liquid medication without injecting the same volume of air to replace it, you will decrease the pressure inside the vial and create a vacuum. Doing so makes it very hard to withdraw the medication. You must inject air into the vial to replace the volume of medication being removed in order to permit easy withdrawal of the solution.

Delegation and Collaboration

The skill of preparing injections from ampoules and vials cannot be delegated to an unregulated care provider (UCP).

Equipment

- Medication administration record (MAR)
- Filtered blunt fill needle, if aspirating medication from a glass ampoule
- Blunt fill needle or needleless vial access adapter (Fig. 22.16)
- Syringe for aspirating dose of medication
- If medication requires reconstitution:
  - Second syringe for aspirating diluent
  - Diluent
- If planning to inject medication into patient tissue:
  - Appropriately sized safety needle
  - Gauze pad
- If planning to administer medication as an infusion:
  - IV mini-bag or cassette specific to pump
- Medication in vial or ampoule
- Puncture-proof container for disposal of syringes, needles, and glass
- Alcohol swabs

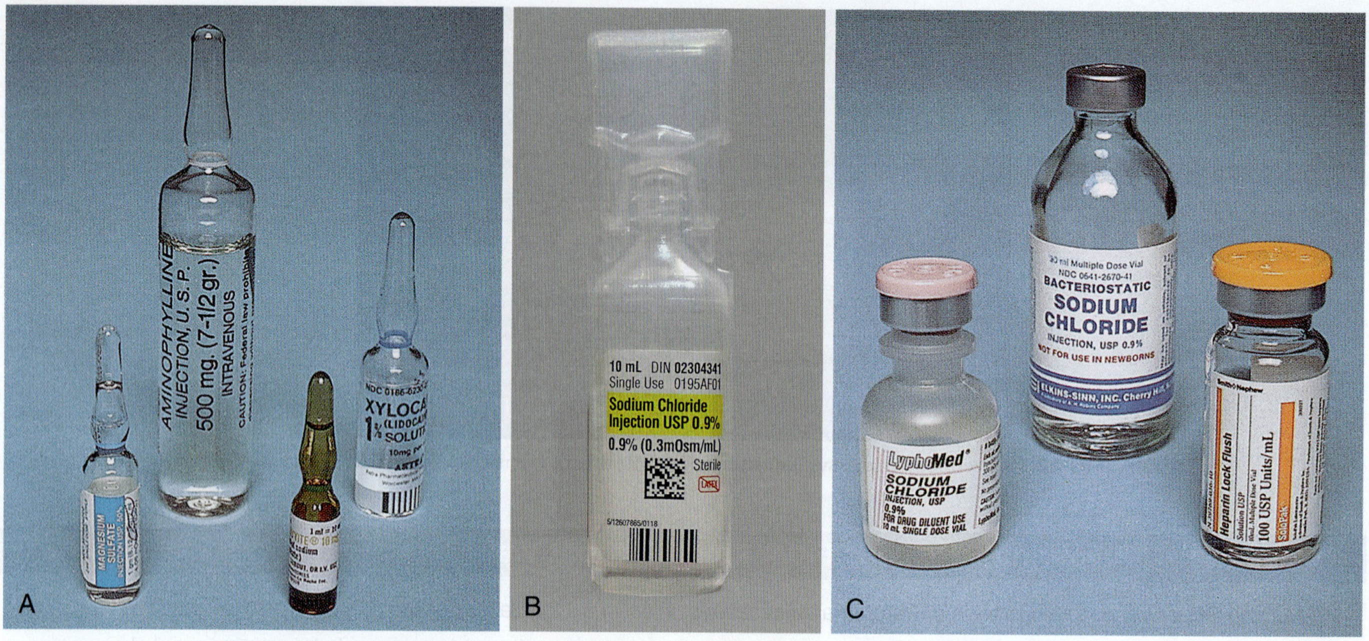

FIG 22.14 A, Medication in glass ampoules. B, Medication in a plastic ampoule. C, Medication in vials. (*B, Courtesy Noelle Ozog.*)

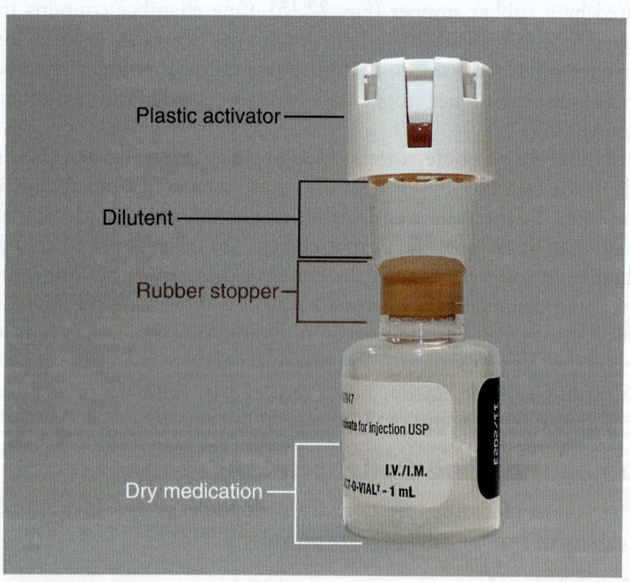

FIG 22.15 Two-chambered vial with dry powder medication and diluent solution. (*Courtesy Noelle Ozog.*)

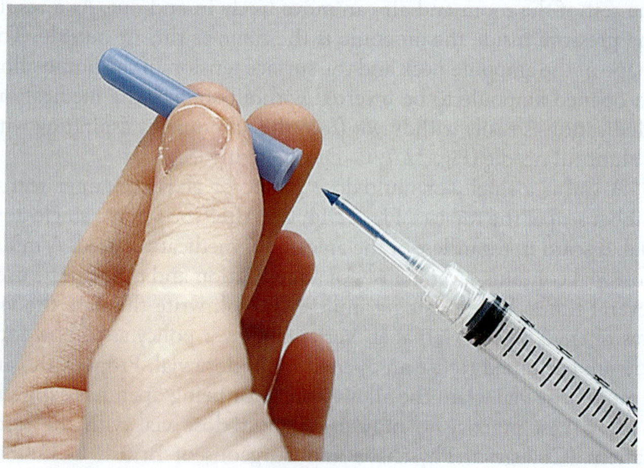

FIG 22.16 Syringe with needleless vial access adapter.

STEP	RATIONALE

ASSESSMENT

1. Identify patient using at least two person-specific identifiers (e.g., name and date of birth or name and medical record number) according to employer policy.
2. Throughout the procedure, the 4 moments for hand hygiene are to be implemented; hand hygiene should occur before initial patient (or patient environment) contact, before an aseptic procedure, after body fluid exposure risk, and after patient (or patient environment) contact. Additional hand hygiene should be performed when hands are visibly soiled.

STEP	RATIONALE
ASSESSMENT	
3. Check accuracy and completeness of each MAR by comparing with health care provider prescription. Check patient's name, medication name and dosage, route of administration, and time of administration. Recopy or reprint any part of the MAR that is difficult to read.	The health care provider prescription is the most reliable source and only legal record of medications that the patient is to receive.
4. Assess patient's medical and medication history.	Determines need for medication or possible contraindications for medication administration.
5. Assess patient's history of allergies: known type of allergies and normal allergic response.	Do not prepare medication if there is a known patient allergy to the medication.
6. Review medication reference information for action, purpose, adverse effects, and nursing implications.	Allows you to administer medication properly and monitor patient's response. Also ensures you are giving medication for the right reason and are prepared to provide the right education for the patient.
7. Review employer parenteral medication administration manual for information about recommended type and volume of diluent (if reconstitution required or medication intended to be given as a primary or secondary IV infusion).	Allows you to prepare medication properly.
8. Assess patient's age, body fat distribution, and muscle tone if giving SUBCUT or IM medication.	Determines type and size of syringe and needle for injection into tissue.
PLANNING	
1. Expected outcomes following completion of procedure: • Proper dose is prepared. • No air bubbles are in the syringe barrel.	Air bubbles displace medication. Elimination of air ensures accuracy of dose.
IMPLEMENTATION	
1. Prepare medications	
a. If using a medication cart, move it outside patient's room.	Organization of equipment saves time and reduces chance of error.
b. Unlock medication drawer or cart or log onto automated dispensing system (ADS).	Medications are safeguarded when locked in the cabinet, cart, or ADS.
c. Follow employer's NIZ policy and avoid distraction.	Interruptions are a common impediment to safe, timely medication administration (Alteren et al., 2021).
d. Select correct medication from stock supply or unit-dose drawer. Compare label of medication with MAR.	Reading label and comparing it with transcribed prescription reduce errors. *This is the first check of three checks for accuracy.*
e. Check expiration date on each medication, one at a time.	Expired medications are sometimes inactive, less effective, or harmful to patients.
f. Calculate medication dose as necessary. Double-check calculation. Ask another nurse to check calculations if needed.	Double-checking reduces occurrence of errors.
g. If preparing a controlled substance (e.g., morphine, lorazepam), count available supply and compare with previous medication count. Follow employer policy for management of any wasted medication.	The *Controlled Drugs and Substances Act, 1996* requires careful monitoring of dispensed narcotics.
h. Do not leave medications unattended.	The nurse is responsible for safekeeping of medications.
2. Compare medication label with MAR.	*This is the second of three checks for accuracy.*
3. Remove medication from ampoule or vial and reconstitute as necessary.	
a. Medication from an ampoule	
(1) Tap top of ampoule lightly and quickly with finger until fluid moves from its neck (see Step 3a[1] illustration). Alternatively, you can hold the top of the ampoule and swirl it or quickly flip it to dislodge fluid from the neck.	Dislodges any fluid that collects above neck of ampoule. All solution moves into lower chamber. In nursing there is often more than one technique to achieve something.
(2) Cleanse the neck of the ampoule with antiseptic swab and allow it to dry (see Step 3a[2] illustration).	Disinfects the neck of the ampoule and reduces risk of contamination (Boom et al., 2021).
(3) Place commercial ampoule breaker (if available) or small gauze pad around neck of ampoule.	Protects fingers from trauma as glass tip is broken off. Do not use opened alcohol swab to wrap around top of ampoule because alcohol may leak into ampoule.
(4) Snap neck of ampoule quickly and firmly away from hands (see Step 3a[4] illustration).	Protects your fingers and face from shattering glass.

STEP	RATIONALE

IMPLEMENTATION

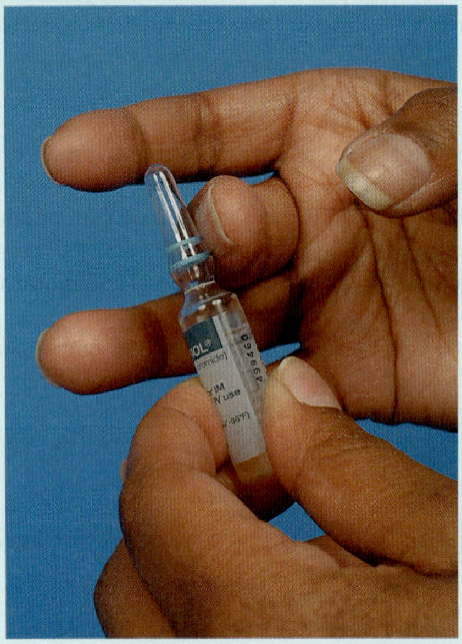

STEP 3A(1) Tapping ampoule moves fluid down neck.

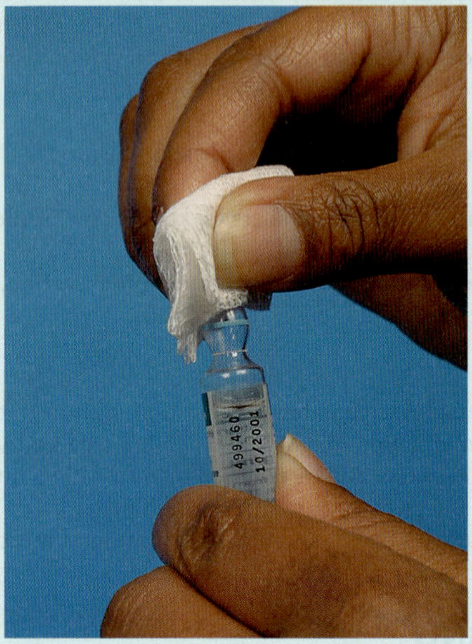

STEP 3A(2) Gauze pad placed around neck of ampoule.

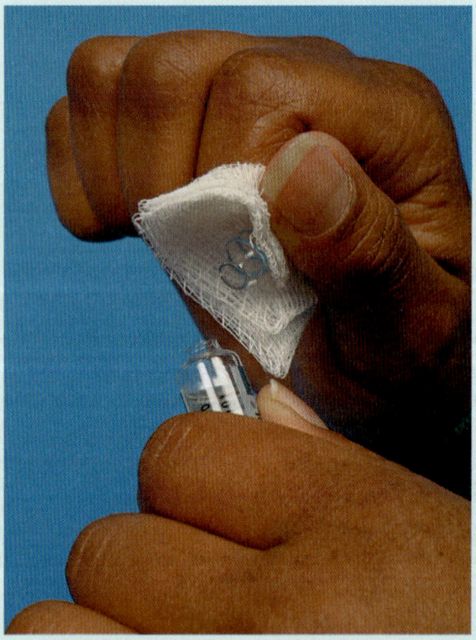

STEP 3A(4) Neck snapped away from hands.

STEP	RATIONALE
(5) Using a blunt fill needle long enough to reach the bottom of the ampoule, either hold ampoule upside down or set it on flat surface and insert needle into centre of ampoule opening. Do not allow needle tip or shaft to touch the rim of the ampoule. NOTE: Use a filtered blunt fill needle if ampoule is made of glass.	Broken rim of ampoule is considered contaminated. When ampoule is inverted, solution dribbles out if needle tip or shaft touches rim of ampoule. System is open to airborne contaminants. Filter needles filter out any fragments of glass (CVAA, 2019).
(6) Aspirate medication into syringe by gently pulling back on plunger (see Step 3a[6] illustration).	Withdrawal of plunger creates negative pressure within syringe barrel, which pulls fluid into syringe.

STEP	RATIONALE

IMPLEMENTATION

STEP	RATIONALE
(7) Keep needle tip under surface of liquid. Tip ampoule to bring all fluid within reach of needle.	Prevents aspiration of air bubbles. Troubleshooting tips for air bubbles are included with later steps.
(8) If you aspirate air bubbles, do not expel air into ampoule.	Air pressure forces fluid out of ampoule, and medication will be lost.
b. Medication solution from a vial	
(1) Remove cap covering top of unused vial to expose rubber seal. If a multi-dose vial has been used before, cap is already removed.	Vial comes packaged with cap that cannot be replaced after seal removal.
(2) For an unused multi-dose vial, make label that includes date of opening and your initials. For a used multi-dose vial, ensure vial opening date is within employer time frame for use. Discard multi-use vials with no opening date.	Ensures that nurses will prepare future doses correctly. You discard some medications within a certain time frame after mixing. There is no way to tell when an unlabelled open multi-use vial has been in use.
(3) Scrub rubber seal with disinfectant swab and allow it to dry.	Not all drug manufacturers guarantee that rubber seals of unused vials are sterile. Swabbing with disinfectant reduces transmission of microorganisms. Allowing disinfectant to dry prevents it from coating needle and mixing with medication.
(4) Pick up syringe and remove needle cap or cap covering needleless access device. Pull back on plunger to draw amount of air into syringe equivalent to volume of medication to be aspirated from vial.	Injecting air into vial prevents buildup of negative pressure in vial when aspirating medication.
(5) With vial on flat surface, use firm pressure to insert tip of needle or needleless device through centre of rubber seal (see Step 3b[5] illustration).	Centre of seal is thinner and easier to penetrate. Using firm pressure prevents dislodging of rubber particles that could enter vial or needle.
(6) Inject air into air space of vial and firmly hold plunger down.	Injecting into air space of vial prevents formation of bubbles and an inaccurate dose. Injection of air into vial creates a vacuum in the syringe barrel that will allow flow into syringe in the next step. If not held firmly, the plunger is sometimes forced backward by air pressure within vial.

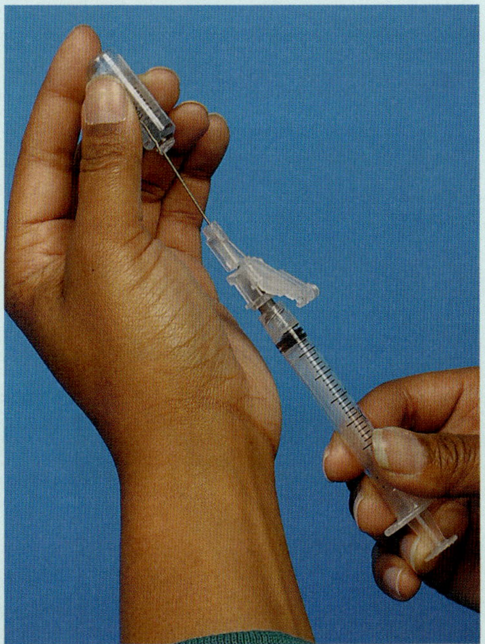

STEP 3A(6) Medication aspirated with ampoule inverted.

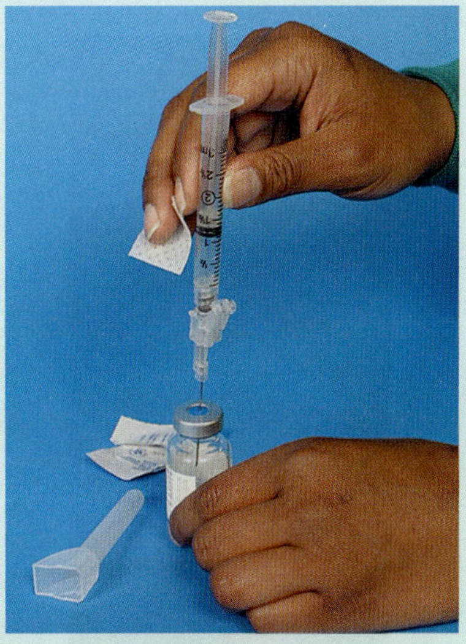

STEP 3B(5) Insert safety needle through centre of vial diaphragm (with vial flat on table).

STEP	RATIONALE

IMPLEMENTATION

STEP	RATIONALE
(7) Invert vial while keeping firm hold on syringe and plunger. Hold vial between thumb and middle fingers of nondominant hand (see Step 3b[7] illustration) and lift it up to eye level. Ensure you can see the tip of the needle inside. At the same time, grasp end of syringe barrel and plunger with thumb and forefinger of dominant hand to counteract pressure in vial.	Inverting vial allows fluid to settle above the rubber stopper. Holding the vial at eye level with the tip below the medication line prevents aspiration of air. Position of hands prevents forceful movement of plunger and permits easy manipulation of syringe.
(8) Allow increased pressure from inside vial to fill syringe gradually with medication. If necessary, pull back slightly on plunger to obtain correct amount of medication.	Positive pressure within vial forces fluid into syringe.
(9) When you obtain desired volume, position needle or needleless device into air space of vial; tap side of syringe barrel gently to dislodge any air bubbles (see Step 3b[9] illustration). Eject any air remaining at top of syringe into vial.	Forcefully striking barrel while needle is inserted in vial may bend needle. Accumulation of air displaces medication and causes dose errors.
(10) Remove needle or needleless access device from vial by pulling back on barrel of syringe.	Pulling plunger rather than barrel causes plunger to separate from barrel, resulting in loss of medication.

Critical Decision Point *When preparing medication from a vial containing medication solution, draw up a volume based on the listed concentration. Do not assume that volume listed on the label is the actual total volume in vial. Some manufacturers provide a small amount of extra liquid, expecting loss during preparation.*

STEP	RATIONALE
c. Dry medication from a vial (reconstitution)	
(1) Draw up recommended volume of diluent into syringe following Step 3a if in an ampoule or Step 3b if in a vial.	Prepares diluent for injection into vial containing powdered medication.
(2) Remove cap covering top of vial containing dry medication to expose rubber seal.	Vial comes packaged with cap that cannot be replaced after seal removal.
(3) Scrub rubber seal with disinfectant swab and allow it to dry.	Not all drug manufacturers guarantee that rubber seals of unused vials are sterile. Swabbing with disinfectant reduces transmission of microorganisms. Allowing disinfectant to dry prevents it from coating needle and mixing with medication.
(4) With vial on flat surface, use firm pressure to insert tip of needle or needleless device through centre of rubber seal.	This is the thinnest part of the rubber seal and easiest place to puncture.

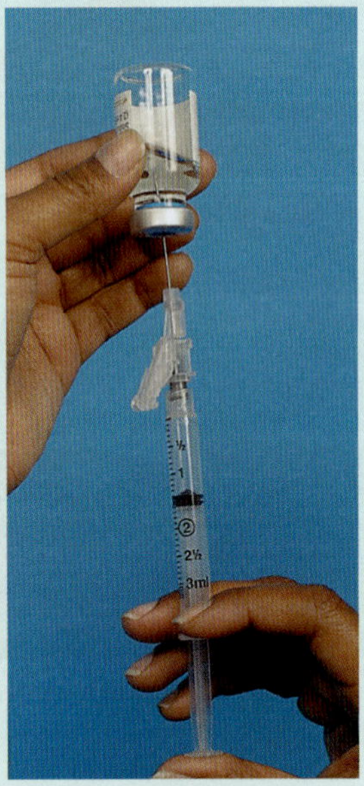

STEP 3B(7) Withdraw fluid with vial inverted.

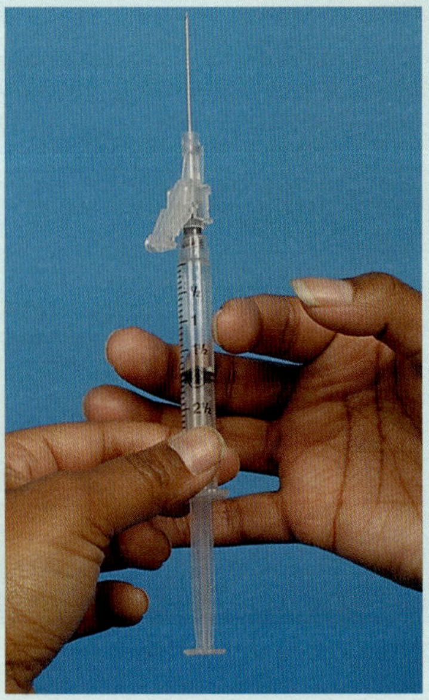

STEP 3B(9) Hold syringe upright; tap barrel to dislodge air bubbles.

STEP	RATIONALE
IMPLEMENTATION	
(5) Inject diluent into vial airspace in vial. Allow air to aspirate into syringe, if needed.	Some manufacturers seal dry powder vials with a vacuum that will draw diluent into the vial, but others do not. If there is already air pressure in the vial equal to the air pressure in the room, the pressure in the vial will be increased when you inject the diluent, and allowing it to enter the syringe will prevent medication from leaking out during needle withdrawal.
(6) Remove blunt fill needle from vial and recap.	Prevents needle-stick injury.
(7) Mix medication in vial thoroughly per drug monograph/employer policy.	Ensures proper dispersal of medication throughout solution. Note that some medications cannot be shaken vigorously; refer to employer policy.
d. Reconstituted medication in vial is ready to be drawn into new syringe. Read label carefully to determine concentration after reconstitution.	Once you add diluent, concentration of medication (mg/mL) determines dose to administer. Reading medication label carefully decreases medication errors.
e. Draw up reconstituted medication into syringe following Step 3b.	Prepares medication for administration.

Critical Decision Point *Some employers require that you verify the dose of certain "high-alert" medications (e.g., insulin and heparin) for accuracy with another nurse* (ISMP, 2022).

STEP	RATIONALE
4. Cover blunt fill needle with its safety sheath or cap if you have not already done so.	Minimizes needle-sticks.
5. Special considerations for tissue injection and glass ampoules:	
a. ***Tissue injections:*** Draw back on the plunger of the syringe to remove any medication within the blunt fill needle. Disconnect the blunt fill needle from the syringe and replace with a safety needle with appropriate gauge and length according to route of medication administration.	Blunt fill needles are large, dull, and cannot be used for injection. Inserting needle through rubber stopper dulls the bevelled tip. The large bore of the needle holds a lot of medication. The new needle is sharper and, because no fluid is along shaft, does not track medication through tissues.
b. ***IV injections:*** If the medication was drawn from a glass ampoule, draw back on the plunger of the syringe to remove any medication within the filtered blunt fill needle. Disconnect the blunt fill needle from the syringe and replace with a regular blunt fill needle.	The filter has a one-way flow and—once used to withdraw a medication and trap glass particles—it should not be "pushed" in the other direction (CVAA, 2019) because this could, theoretically, transfer glass particles.
6. Hold syringe at eye level at a 90-degree angle with the needle end pointing upward. Force remaining bubbles to rise to the top of the syringe and dissipate by tapping barrel with a firm object.	Holding syringe vertically allows fluid to settle in bottom of barrel. Tapping dislodges air to top of barrel.
7. Draw back slightly on plunger, then push it upward to eject air.	Pulling back on plunger allows fluid within needle to enter barrel so you do not expel fluid. You then expel air at top of barrel and within needle.
8. Visually confirm a small drop at the tip of needle. Do not eject fluid.	Visual indicator that medication has filled needle. Syringe measurement markings account for dead space within the needle.
9. Recheck volume of medication.	Confirms that no part of dose has been lost while removing air bubbles or changing needles.
10. If medication needs to be diluted in an IV mini-bag:	
a. Scrub medication port with disinfectant swab.	Prevents transmission of microorganisms.
b. Lay mini-bag on a flat surface and puncture the medication port with the blunt fill needle that is attached to the syringe containing the prepared dose of medication. Depress plunger of syringe to inject medication into mini-bag.	Transfers medication to mini-bag. Mini-bags are made of flexible material and will expand and contract with volume changes within the bag, so air does not need to be removed.
11. Label syringes that will be used for injection into tissue (Skills 22.2, 22.3, 22.4, 22.5) or that will be used to give IV direct medication (Skill 22.6) per employer policy. Label IV mini-bags for intermittent IV infusion (Skill 22.6) per employer policy. Check the label you have created against the medication's original label, *not* against the MAR.	Checking against the manufacturer's original medication label ensures that the medication in the syringe is identified accurately during the next check.
12. Check your labelled syringe or mini-bag against the MAR.	*This is your third of three checks for accuracy.*
13. Place broken ampoule and/or used vials and used needle or needleless device in puncture- and leak-proof container.	Proper disposal of glass and needle prevents accidental injury to staff.
14. Dispose of soiled supplies in appropriate receptacle. Clean work area.	Controls transmission of infection.

Unexpected Outcomes	Related Interventions
1. Air bubbles remain in syringe (unless contraindicated by type of medication).	• Expel air from syringe and add medication to it until you prepare correct dose. • If air bubbles were introduced to medication during the reconstitution process, allow them to dissipate before aspirating medication. • Ensure the fill needle is securely connected via the Luer-Lok to barrel of syringe; loose connections can entrain ("suck in") air. • Slow your rate of aspiration. • Ensure you are holding needle vertically during aspiration from vial or ampoule, checking dose and removing air bubbles. Tilted needles increase adherence of bubbles to the inside surface of syringe, especially for narrow diameter syringes.
2. Incorrect dose is prepared.	• Discard prepared dose. • Prepare correct new dose.

PROCEDURAL GUIDELINE 22.1 *Mixing Parenteral Medications in One Syringe*

Some medications need to be mixed from two vials or from a vial and an ampoule. Mixing compatible medications avoids the need to give a patient more than one injection. First, as the nurse, you must check that the medications are compatible and can be mixed in one syringe. Compatibility charts are found in drug reference guides, posted within patient care units, or available electronically. If you are uncertain about medication compatibilities, consult a pharmacist. When mixing medications, you must correctly aspirate fluid from each type of container, especially a multi-dose vial, without contaminating the medication with the contents from another vial or ampoule.

When mixing medications from a vial and an ampoule, prepare medications from the vial first. Then withdraw medication from the ampoule using the same syringe and a filter needle. When mixing medications from two vials, avoid contaminating one medication with another, ensure that the final dose is accurate, and maintain aseptic technique.

Give special consideration to the proper preparation of insulin, the hormone used to treat diabetes mellitus. Insulin is supplied in vials or cartridges for injection pens and is classified by onset, peak effect, and duration of action (Table 22.2). Patients with diabetes mellitus often receive a combination of different types of insulin to control their blood glucose levels. Before preparing the insulin, ensure that you check the patient's blood glucose. Some insulin preparations contain a protein that needs to be resuspended before administration: gently roll intermediate-acting ("cloudy") insulin preparations (e.g., Humulin N) 10 times between the palms of your hands, then tip it 10 times to resuspend the insulin (Forum for Injection Technique Canada [FIT Canada], 2020; Novo Nordisk Canada Inc., 2021).

If more than one type of insulin is required to manage a patient's diabetes, you can mix them into one syringe if they are compatible. Intermediate-acting insulin looks "cloudy" because of the protein attached to the insulin, which slows its rate of absorption into cells (Saleem & Sharma, 2022). Always prepare the short- or rapid-acting insulin first to prevent it from being contaminated with the long-acting insulin (Novo Nordisk Canada Inc., 2021). In some settings, insulin is not mixed. Box 22.2 lists recommendations for mixing different types of insulin.

Delegation and Collaboration

The skill of mixing medications in one syringe cannot be delegated to a UCP. The nurse directs the UCP about the following:

- Potential adverse effects of medications and immediately reporting their occurrence to the nurse.

Equipment

- Single- or multi-dose vials and ampoules containing medication
- Syringe
- Two needles:
  - Blunt-tip needleless vial access cannula or needle for drawing up medication
  - Filter needle, if indicated
  - Safety needle for injection
- Alcohol swab
- Puncture-proof container for disposing of syringes, needles, and glass
- MAR

Procedural Steps

1. Identify patient using at least two person-specific identifiers (e.g., name and date of birth or name and medical record number) according to employer policy.
2. Throughout the procedure, the 4 moments for hand hygiene are to be implemented; hand hygiene should occur before initial patient (or patient environment) contact, before an aseptic procedure, after body fluid exposure risk, and after patient (or patient environment) contact. Additional hand hygiene should be performed when hands are visibly soiled.
3. Check accuracy and completeness of MAR by comparing with health care provider's prescription. Check patient's name, medication name and dosage, route of administration, and time of administration. Recopy or reprint any part of MAR that is difficult to read.
4. Review pertinent information related to medication, including action, purpose, adverse effects, and nursing implications.
   If mixing insulin: Check patient blood glucose and follow employer policy (or health care provider prescription) if it is outside of the expected range for the patient.
5. Confirm compatibility and stability of medications per employer policy.
6. Check expiration date of medication printed on vial or ampoule.
7. Prepare medication for one patient at a time following the 10 rights of medication administration (see Chapter 20). Select an ampoule or vial from the unit-dose drawer or ADS. Compare the label of each medication with the MAR. In the case of insulin, ensure that the correct type or types of insulin are prepared. *This is the first check for accuracy.*
8. Mix medications
   a. Option A: Mixing medications from two vials (see Step 8a illustration):

PROCEDURAL GUIDELINE 22.1 *Mixing Parenteral Medications in One Syringe—cont'd*

TABLE 22.2

Comparison of Insulin Preparations

Insulin Type* (Trade Name)	Onset	Peak Effect (Hours)	Duration of Action (Hours)
Bolus Insulins (Mealtime or Preprandial)			
Rapid-Acting (Clear)			
Insulin lispro (Humalog)	10–15 min	1–2	3–4.75
Insulin aspart (NovoRapid)	9–20 min	1–1.5	3–5
Insulin glulisine (Apidra)	10–15 min	1–1.5	3.5–5
Fast-acting insulin aspart (Fiasp)	4 min	0.5–1.5	3–5
Short-Acting (Clear)			
Regular insulin† (e.g., Humulin R, Novolin ge Toronto)	30 min	2–3	6.5
Basal Insulins			
Intermediate-Acting (Cloudy)			
Isophane insulin suspension (Novolin ge NPH, Humulin N)	1–3 hours	5–8	Up to 18
Long-Acting (Clear)			
Insulin detemir (Levemir)†	1.5 hours	Not applicable	16–24
Insulin glargine U-100 (Lantus)†	1.5 hours	Not applicable	24
Insulin glargine U-300 (Toujeo)†	1.5 hours	Not applicable	>30
Insulin glargine biosumular (Basaglar)	1.5 hours	Not applicable	
Degludec (Tresiba)	1.5 hours	Not applicable	42

*All insulins are available in 100-unit strengths.

†Cannot be mixed with other insulins.

Data from Gillespie, J. D. (2018). Types of insulin. *Canadian Journal of Diabetes, 42*(Suppl. 1), S314. https://doi.org/10.1016/j.jcjd.2017.12.006

BOX 22.2

Recommendations for Mixing Insulins

- Patients whose blood glucose levels are well controlled on a mixed-insulin dose need to maintain their individual routine when preparing and administering their insulin.
- Do not mix insulin with any other medications.
- Do not mix insulin for subcutaneous injection with diluents.
- Never mix insulin glargine (Lantus, Toujeo, Basaglar) or insulin detemir (Levemir) with other types of insulin.
- Inject rapid-acting insulins mixed with NPH insulin within 15 minutes before a meal.
- Verify insulin doses by asking another nurse to perform an independent double-check while you are preparing the injection (ISMP, 2022).

(1) Take syringe with needleless device or filter needle and aspirate volume of air equivalent to first medication dose (vial A).

(2) Calculate medication dose as necessary. Double-check calculation.

(3) Compare the medication label of both vials with MAR. ***This is the second check for accuracy.*** Inject air into vial A, making sure that needle or needleless device does not touch solution (see Step 8a, illustration A).

(4) Holding onto plunger, withdraw needle or needleless device and syringe from vial A. Aspirate air equivalent to second medication dose (vial B) into syringe.

(5) Insert needle or needleless device into vial B, inject volume of air into vial B, and withdraw medication from vial B into syringe (see Step 8a, illustration B).

(6) Withdraw needle or needleless device and syringe from vial B. Ensure that proper volume has been obtained.

(7) Insert needle or needleless device into vial A, being careful not to push plunger and expel medication within syringe into vial. Invert vial and carefully withdraw the desired amount of medication from vial A into syringe (see Step 8a, illustration C).

(8) Withdraw needle or needleless device and expel any excess air from syringe. Check fluid level in syringe for proper dose. Medications are now mixed.

Critical Decision Point *If too much medication is withdrawn from second vial, discard syringe and start over. Do not push medication back into either vial.*

(9) Change needle or needleless device for appropriately sized needle if medication is being injected into tissue. Keep needle or needleless device capped until administration time.

b. Option B: Mixing insulin:

Continued

PROCEDURAL GUIDELINE 22.1 *Mixing Parenteral Medications in One Syringe—cont'd*

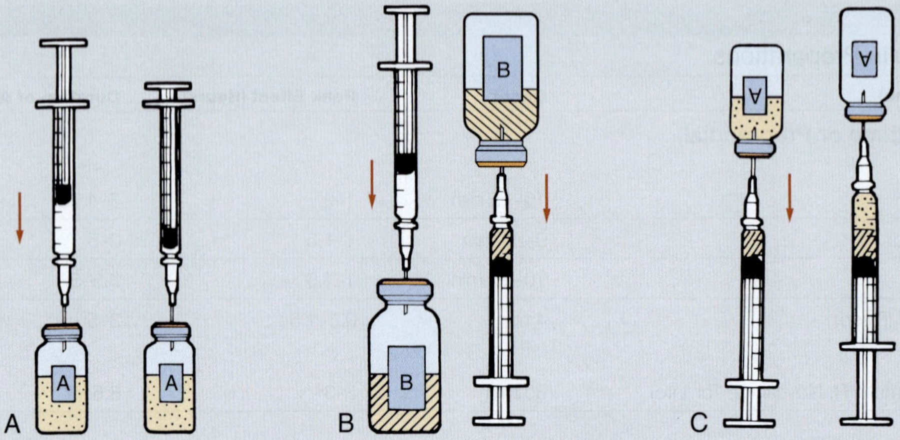

STEP 8A A, Inject air into vial A. B, Inject air into vial B and withdraw dose. C, Withdraw medication from vial A; medications are now mixed.

(1) If patient takes insulin that is cloudy, roll bottle of insulin between hands to resuspend insulin preparation.
(2) Scrub tops of both insulin vials with disinfectant swab.
(3) Verify insulin dose by comparing with MAR.

Critical Decision Point *If long-acting insulin glargine (Lantus) or insulin detemir (Levemir) is prescribed, it should not be mixed with other insulin preparations in the same syringe.*

(4) If mixing rapid- or short-acting insulin with intermediate- or long-acting insulin, take insulin syringe and aspirate volume of air equivalent to dose to be withdrawn from intermediate- or long-acting insulin first (see Step 8b[4] illustration). If two intermediate- or long-acting insulins are mixed, it makes no difference which vial is prepared first.
(5) Insert needle and inject air into vial of intermediate- or long-acting insulin. Do not let tip of needle touch solution.
(6) Remove syringe from vial of insulin without aspirating medication.
(7) With the same syringe, inject air equal to the dose of rapid- or short-acting insulin into vial and withdraw correct dose into syringe (see Step 8b[7] illustration).
(8) Remove syringe from rapid- or short-acting insulin and remove any air bubbles to ensure accurate dose.
(9) Verify short-acting insulin dosage by comparing with MAR, and show insulin prepared in syringe to another nurse to verify that correct dosage of insulin was prepared. Add the number of units of both insulins together (e.g., 4 units Regular + 10 units NPH) to determine which marking on the syringe scale is expected to represent the final dose of insulin (14 units total). Verify combined dose.

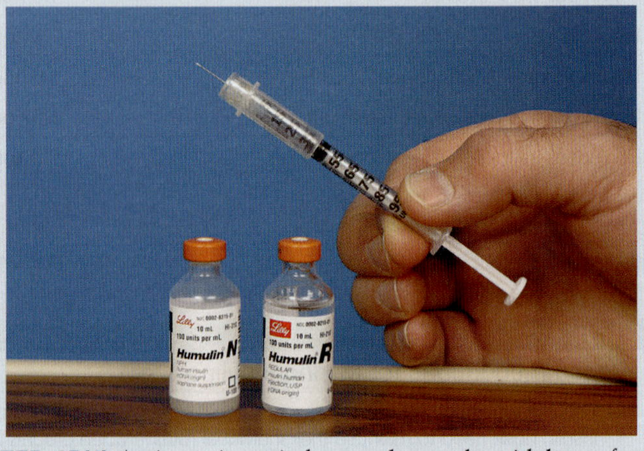

STEP 8B(4) Aspirate air equivalent to dose to be withdrawn from intermediate insulin.

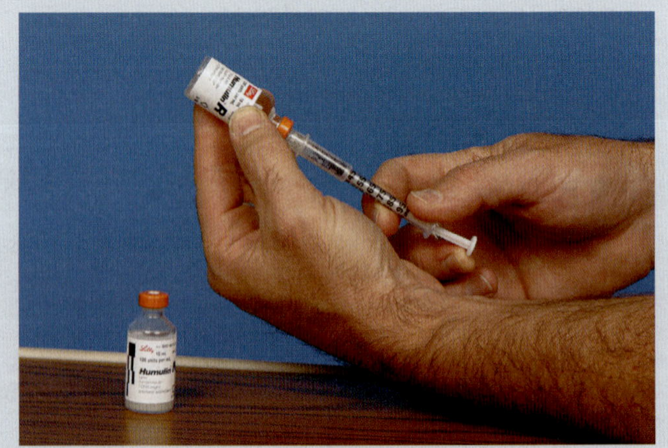

STEP 8B(7) Withdraw short-acting insulin.

PROCEDURAL GUIDELINE 22.1 *Mixing Parenteral Medications in One Syringe—cont'd*

(10) Place needle of syringe back into vial of intermediate- or long-acting insulin. Be careful not to push plunger of syringe (i.e., do not inject insulin from syringe into vial).

(11) Invert vial and carefully withdraw desired amount of insulin into syringe (see Step 8b[11] illustration).

(12) Withdraw needle and check fluid level in syringe. Verify with another nurse that correct total dose was prepared. Keep needle of prepared syringe sheathed or capped until ready to administer medication.

c. Mixing medications from a vial and an ampoule:

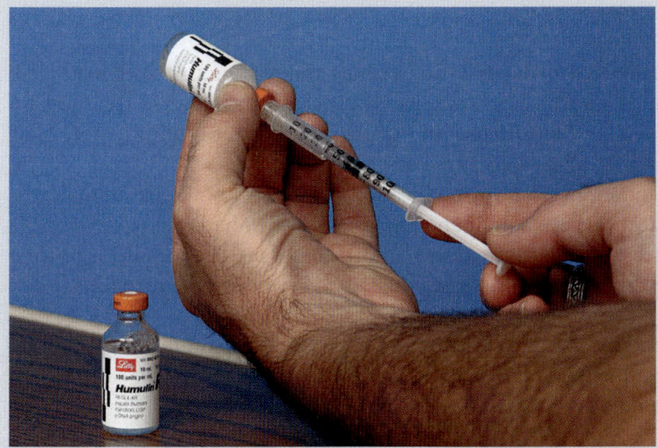

STEP 8B(11) Withdraw intermediate insulin.

(1) Prepare medication from vial first, following Skill 22.1, Step 3b.

(2) Determine which marking on the syringe scale is expected to represent the combined volume of medications.

Critical Decision Point *If needleless access device was used in preparing medication from vial, change needleless system to a filter needle to remove medication from ampoule.*

(3) Next, using the same syringe, prepare second medication from ampoule, following Step 3a in Skill 22.1.

(4) Withdraw filter needle from ampoule and verify fluid level in syringe. Change filter needle to appropriate safety needle. Keep device or needle sheathed or capped until ready to administer medication.

(5) Check syringe carefully for total combined dose of medications.

9. Compare MAR with prepared medication and labels on vials/ampoules. ***This is the third check for accuracy.***

10. Dispose of soiled supplies in appropriate receptacle. Place used ampoules and/or vials and needle or needleless device in puncture- and leak-proof container.

11. Clean work area.

12. Check syringe again carefully for total combined dose of medications.

✦ SKILL 22.2 Administering Intradermal Injections

Video Clip NSO *Nursing Skills Online Administration of Parenteral Medications: Injections Module 7 / Lesson 4*

ID injections are typically used for skin testing (e.g., tuberculosis [TB] screening, allergy tests). For patients with a history of multiple allergies, the health care provider may perform skin testing. Skin testing often requires you to visually inspect the test site; therefore, make sure that the ID sites are free of lesions and injuries and relatively hairless. The inner forearm and upper back are ideal locations.

Use a tuberculin or small syringe with a short (3.2 mm [0.125 inches] to 16 mm [0.625 inches]), fine-gauge (25 or 27) needle to administer an ID injection. The angle of insertion for an ID injection is 5 to 15 degrees (see Fig. 22.1). Inject only small amounts of medication (0.01 to 0.1 mL) intradermally. If a bleb does not appear or if the site bleeds after needle withdrawal, the medication may have entered SUBCUT tissues. In this situation, skin test results will not be valid.

Delegation and Collaboration

The skill of administering ID injections cannot be delegated to a UCP. The nurse directs the UCP about the following:

- Potential medication adverse effects or allergic response signs and reporting their occurrence to the nurse
- Reporting any change in the patient's vital signs or condition to the nurse

Equipment

- Syringe: 1-mL tuberculin syringe with preattached 25- or 27-gauge needle, 3.2 mm (0.125 inches) to 16 mm (0.625 inches)
- Small gauze pad
- Alcohol swab
- Vial or ampoule of medication
- Clean gloves
- MAR
- Puncture-proof container
- Anaphylaxis kit

ASSESSMENT

STEP	RATIONALE
1. Identify patient using at least two person-specific identifiers (e.g., name and date of birth or name and medical record number) according to employer policy.	
2. Throughout the procedure, the 4 moments for hand hygiene are to be implemented; hand hygiene should occur before initial patient (or patient environment) contact, before an aseptic procedure, after body fluid exposure risk, and after patient (or patient environment) contact. Additional hand hygiene should be performed when hands are visibly soiled.	
3. Check accuracy and completeness of MAR by comparing with health care provider prescription. Check patient's name, medication name and dosage, route of administration, and time of administration. Recopy or reprint any part of MAR that is difficult to read.	The prescription sheet is the most reliable source and only legal record of medications that the patient is to receive.
4. Review medication reference information about expected reaction or anticipated effects when testing skin with specific allergen or when giving medication and appropriate time to read site.	Type of reaction depends on patient's ability to mount a cell-mediated immune response. Knowledge of expected and adverse reactions to skin testing helps determine which symptoms to monitor for, how frequently, and when to reassess the patient.
5. Assess patient's history of allergies: known type of allergens and normal allergic reaction.	Do not administer any medication if there is known patient allergy. Medications are potent and can cause severe anaphylaxis.
6. Assess for contraindication to ID injections such as reduced local tissue perfusion. Assess for history of severe adverse reactions or necrosis from previous ID injection.	Decreased perfusion reduces absorption of medication. Prior history of severe reactions increases the risk for future severe reactions.
7. Assess patient's knowledge of purpose of and response to skin testing.	Patients need to know when to return for follow-up reading of a skin test and when and how to report any reaction.
8. Check date of expiration on medication.	Dose potency increases or decreases when outdated.

NURSING DIAGNOSES

- Anxiety
- Fear
- Insufficient knowledge regarding skin testing

Related factors are individualized on the basis of patient's condition or needs.

PLANNING

STEP	RATIONALE
1. Expected outcomes following completion of procedure:	
• Patient experiences very mild burning sensation during injection but no discomfort after injection.	Normal reaction to medication deposited in dermis.
• Small, light-coloured bleb approximately 6 mm (0.25 inches) in diameter forms at site and gradually disappears. Minimal bruising may be present.	Medication is in dermis and eventually absorbed. Bruising is result of minor bleeding from capillaries.
• Patient can identify signs of skin reaction and their significance.	Demonstrates learning.

IMPLEMENTATION

STEP	RATIONALE
1. Prepare medications for one patient at a time using aseptic technique, as described in Skill 22.1 (starting at "Implementation" steps) and/or Procedural Guideline 22.1, when preparing medication.	Ensures that medication is sterile. Interruptions are a common impediment to safe, timely medication administration (Alteren et al., 2021).
2. Identify patient using at least two person-specific identifiers (e.g., name and date of birth, or name and medical record number) according to employer policy.	Ensures correct patient. Complies with Accreditation Canada's standards and improves patient safety (Accreditation Canada, 2020).
3. Take medication(s) to patient at correct time (see employer policy). During administration, apply 10 rights of medication administration and complete three checks for accuracy. Close room curtain or door.	Employer policies regarding timing of medications must consider the nature of the prescribed medication, specific clinical application, and patient needs (ISMP, 2011).

Critical Decision Point *Before administering an ID injection, ensure an emergency anaphylaxis kit is on site and easily accessible. Medications given via the ID route, such as allergens for allergy testing, carry a risk of anaphylaxis* (Gordon et al., 2013).

STEP	RATIONALE
IMPLEMENTATION	
4. Ask patient if they have any allergies.	Confirms patient's identity and allergy history.
5. Discuss purpose, action, and possible adverse effects of each medication. Allow patient to ask any questions. Tell them that the injection will cause a slight burning or stinging sensation.	It is an ethical responsibility of nurses to provide education to patients to support informed decision making (CNA, 2017).
6. Apply clean gloves. Keep sheet or gown draped over body parts not requiring exposure.	Reduces transmission of infection.
7. Select appropriate site. Note lesions or discolorations of skin. If possible, select site three to four finger widths below antecubital space and one hand width above wrist. If you cannot use forearm, inspect upper back. If necessary, use sites appropriate for SUBCUT injections.	An ID injection site free of discoloration, moles, scars, and hair enables clear viewing and interpretation of results of skin test (Doyle & McCutcheon, 2021).
8. Help patient to comfortable position. Have them extend the elbow, and support it and forearm on flat surface.	Stabilizes injection site for easy accessibility.
9. Clean site with antiseptic swab. Apply swab at centre of site and rotate outward in circular direction for about 5 cm (2 inches). *Option:* Use vapocoolant spray (e.g., ethyl chloride) before injection.	Mechanical action of swab removes secretions containing microorganisms. Decreases pain at injection site.
10. Hold swab or gauze between third and fourth fingers of nondominant hand.	Gauze or swab remains readily accessible when withdrawing needle.
11. Remove needle cap from needle by pulling it straight off.	Preventing needle from touching sides of cap prevents contamination.
12. Hold syringe between thumb and forefinger of dominant hand, with bevel of needle pointing up.	Smooth injection requires proper manipulation of syringe parts. With bevel up, you are less likely to deposit medication into tissues below dermis.
13. Administer injection.	
a. With nondominant hand, stretch skin over site with forefinger or thumb.	Needle pierces tight skin more easily.
b. With needle bevel up, almost against patient's skin, insert it slowly at 5- to 15-degree angle until resistance is felt. Advance needle through epidermis to approximately 3.2 mm (0.125 inches) below skin surface. You will see bulge of needle tip through skin (see Step 13b illustration).	Ensures that needle tip is in dermis. You will not obtain accurate results if you do not inject needle at correct angle and depth (Doyle & McCutcheon, 2021).
c. Inject medication slowly. Normally, you should feel resistance. If not, needle is too deep; remove and begin again with a new needle.	Slow injection minimizes discomfort at site. Dermal layer is tight and does not expand easily when you inject solution. It is difficult (and potentially painful) to change the angle of insertion when the needle is already inside the patient.
d. While injecting medication, note that small bleb (approximately 6.4 mm [0.25 inches]) resembling mosquito bite appears on skin surface (see Step 13d illustration).	Bleb indicates that you deposited medication in dermis.

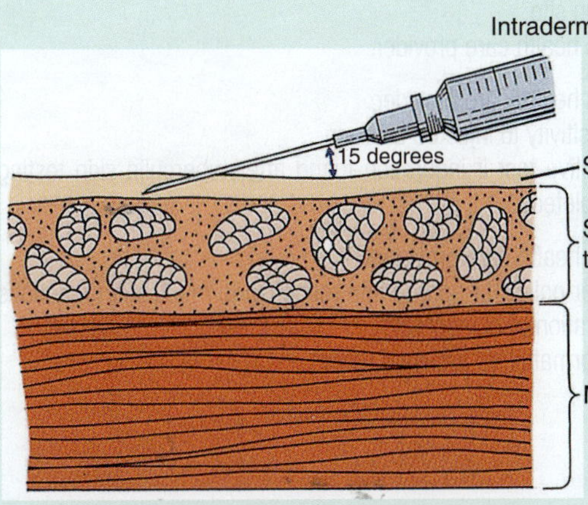

STEP 13B Intradermal needle tip inserted into dermis.

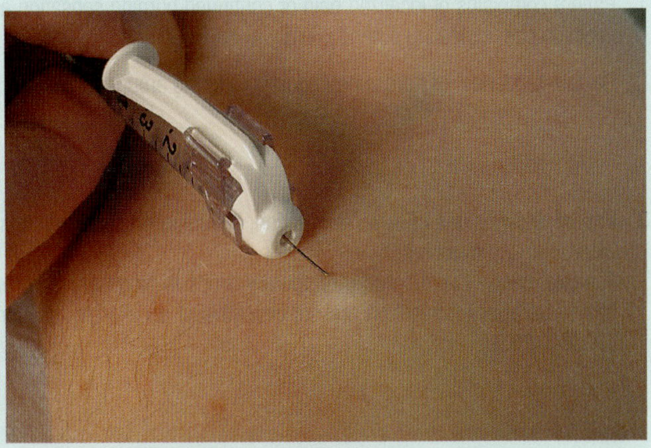

STEP 13D Injection creates small bleb.

STEP	RATIONALE
IMPLEMENTATION	
e. After withdrawing needle, engage safety shield and apply gauze gently over site.	Do not massage site. Apply bandage if needed.
14. Help patient to comfortable position.	Gives patient sense of well-being.
15. Discard uncapped needle or needle enclosed in safety shield and attached syringe in puncture- and leak-proof receptacle.	Prevents injury to patients and health care personnel. Recapping needles increases risk of needle-stick injury (Elmi et al., 2018).
16. Remove gloves.	Reduces transmission of microorganisms.
17. Stay with patient for several minutes and observe for any allergic reactions. If the patient received allergy immunotherapy, instruct them to stay for 30 minutes following the injection.	Dyspnea, wheezing, and circulatory collapse are signs of severe anaphylactic reaction and are likely to occur immediately after injection, or within 30 minutes of the injection.
EVALUATION	
1. Return to room in 15–30 minutes and ask patient whether they feel any acute pain, burning, numbness, or tingling at injection site.	Continued discomfort could indicate injury to underlying tissues.
2. Ask patient to discuss implications of skin testing and signs of hypersensitivity.	Patient's ability to recognize signs of skin testing helps ensure timely reporting of results.
3. Inspect bleb. *Option:* Use skin pencil and draw circle around perimeter of injection site. Read TB test site using employer or public health guidelines at 48–72 hours; look for induration (hard, dense, raised area) of skin around injection site (British Columbia Centre for Disease Control [BCCDC], 2019). Do not mistake erythema as a sign of a positive TB skin test (BCCDC, 2019).	Determines whether reaction to antigen has occurred; indication positive for TB or tested allergens. Site must be read at various intervals to determine test results. Pencil marks make site easy to find. Results of skin testing are determined at various times, based on type of medication used or type of skin testing completed. Manufacturer directions determine when to read test results.
4. Use teach-back: "I want to be sure I explained to you the purpose of tuberculin skin testing and what you might see after the test. Explain to me what the injection site might look like in 2 to 3 days." Develop a revised teaching plan if patient or caregiver is unable to teach back correctly.	Determines patient's and caregiver's level of understanding of topic (Yen & Leasure, 2019).

Unexpected Outcomes	**Related Interventions**
1. Patient complains of localized pain or continued burning sensation at injection site, indicating potential injury to nerve or vessels.	• Assess injection site. • Notify patient's health care provider.
2. Raised, reddened, or hard zone (induration) forms around ID test site.	• Notify patient's health care provider. • Document sensitivity to injected allergen. • Document positive test if induration found after tuberculin skin testing has been completed.
3. Patient shows signs of adverse reaction, including urticaria, pruritus, wheezing, and dyspnea. Fainting, pallor, sweating, and temporary drops in blood pressure or heart rate after an injection are not indicative of an allergic reaction (BCCDC, 2019).	• Notify patient's health care provider. • Follow employer policy for appropriate response to medication reactions (e.g., administration of epinephrine). • Add allergy information to patient's record.

Communication and Documentation

- Document medication, dose, route, site, time, and date on MAR in progress notes in electronic health record (EHR) or chart immediately after administration, not before. Correctly sign MAR according to employer policy.
- Document area of ID injection and appearance of skin.
- Document any undesirable or adverse effects from medication and report these to patient's health care provider.
- Document patient teaching, validation of understanding, and patient's response to medication.

Special Considerations

Teaching

- Instruct patient not to squeeze medication out of injection site.
- Teach patient that negative allergy skin tests may not rule out allergies, especially when low concentrations of medication are used.
- Patient should wear medical identification band listing all allergies.
- Caution patient not to wash off pencil markings around injection site.
- Explain to patient how to observe for skin reactions.
- Ensure that patient knows when follow-up appointment is booked (e.g., 48–72 hours for tuberculin skin test; BCCDC, 2016).

Pediatric

- Up to 30% of children with TB infection will have a negative tuberculin skin test (Dwilow et al., 2022).
- Interpret test per local public health guidelines in the context of the child's symptoms, previous contact with someone who has TB, and chest X-ray findings of TB infection (Dwilow et al., 2022).
- If a child is diagnosed with TB, it is essential to search for the source case to prevent further spread of infection (Dwilow et al., 2022).

Gerontological

- The skin of older persons is less elastic and must be held taut to ensure that ID injection is administered correctly.
- Older persons may have had TB at a younger age, or may have been vaccinated against TB (no longer common practice in Canada); ensure you assess patient TB and vaccination history to avoid false positives in test interpretation (Campbell et al., 2022).

✦ SKILL 22.3 Administering Subcutaneous Injections

Video Clip NSO *Nursing Skills Online Administration of Parenteral Medications: Injections Module 7 / Lesson 3*

SUBCUT injections involve depositing medication into the loose connective tissue underlying the dermis. Because SUBCUT tissue does not contain as many blood vessels as muscles, medications are absorbed more slowly than with IM injections (Usach et al., 2019). Physical exercise or application of hot or cold compresses influences the rate of medication absorption by altering local blood flow to tissues. Any condition that impairs blood flow (e.g., hypothermia, peripheral neuropathy) is a contraindication for SUBCUT injections.

SUBCUT tissue contains pain receptors, so patients often experience discomfort with injection. The tissue is sensitive to viscous solutions and large volumes of medications. As a result, current practice is to limit SUBCUT injections to 1.5 mL in adults (McCartan et al., 2021). A recent review found that SUBCUT injection pain is reduced by use of volumes less than 0.8 mL, room-temperature solution, and abdominal injection site (Usach et al., 2019). In children, practice is to give smaller volumes, up to 0.5 mL. Examples of medications administered by SUBCUT injection include insulin, allergen desensitization therapy, opioids, and heparin.

The best SUBCUT injection sites include the outer aspect of the upper arms; the abdomen, from below the costal margins to the iliac crests; and the anterior aspects of the thighs (Fig. 22.17). These areas are easily accessible and are large enough to allow multiple injections to be rotated within each anatomical area.

Choose an injection site that is free of skin lesions, bony prominences, and large underlying muscles or nerves. Patients who are lean often do not have sufficient tissue for SUBCUT injections; the upper abdomen is usually the best site in such cases. Site rotation prevents the formation of lipohypertrophy (increased growth in fatty tissue) or lipoatrophy (loss of fat tissue) in the skin. Estimate the amount of SUBCUT tissue at a particular site based on patient age, assigned sex at birth, use of hormone therapy, observed distribution of body fat, and BMI (Klaver et al., 2018; Larkin et al., 2018; Sebro, 2022). Choose the needle length and angle of insertion accordingly. Nurses typically use a 25-gauge, 16-mm (0.625-inch) needle inserted at a 45-degree angle or a 13-mm (0.5-inch) needle inserted at a 90-degree angle to administer SUBCUT medications to an adult patient. Some children require only a 13-mm (0.5-inch) needle. To ensure that a SUBCUT medication reaches the SUBCUT tissue, follow this rule: If you can grasp 5 cm (2 inches) of SUBCUT tissue, insert the needle at a 90-degree angle; if you can grasp only 2.5 cm (1 inch) of SUBCUT tissue, insert the needle at a 45-degree angle.

Another option for SUBCUT injections is use of in-dwelling SUBCUT needles or catheters. In-dwelling devices reduce the frequency of puncturing the skin barrier and thereby contribute to patient comfort. Two examples of such devices are the *subcutaneous injection device* (e.g., Insuflon; Fig. 22.18) and the *subcutaneous butterfly* (Fig. 22.19). In both these examples, the device is inserted into the SUBCUT tissue; the needle is then removed, leaving the cannula in the tissue to provide an avenue for administering medications. Follow manufacturer instructions or employer policy to determine how the long device can be left in situ.

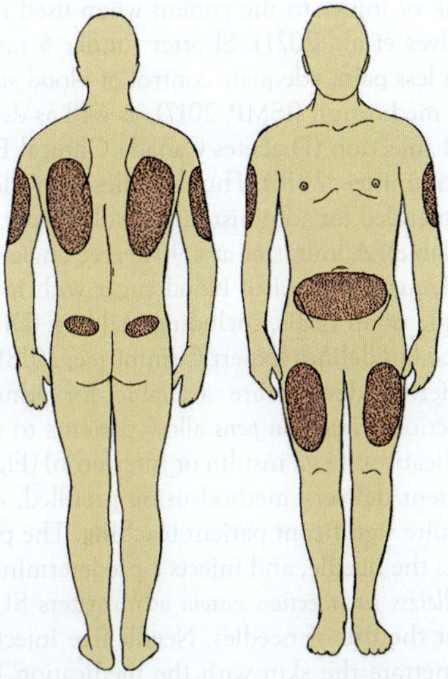

FIG 22.17 Common sites for subcutaneous injections.

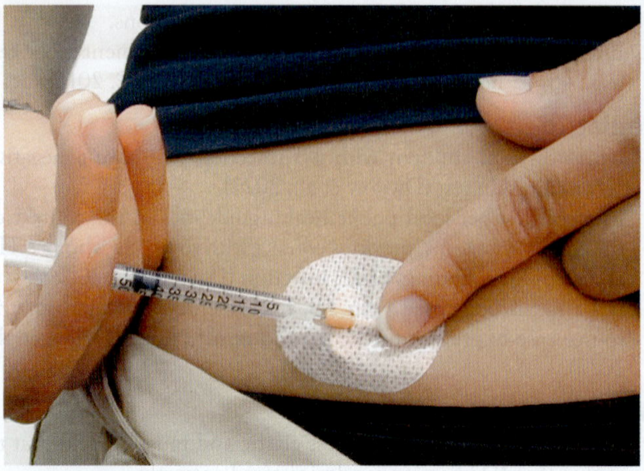

FIG 22.18 **Subcutaneous device.** (*Image courtesy IntraPump Infusion Systems. All rights reserved.*)

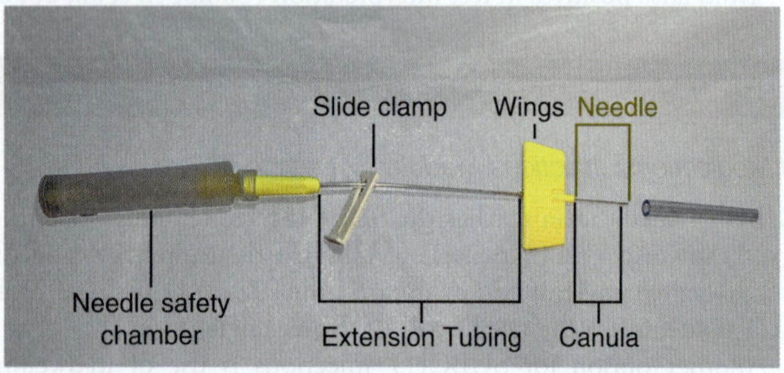

FIG 22.19 **Subcutaneous butterfly.** (*Courtesy Noelle Ozog.*)

! SAFETY ALERT It is essential to check a patient's blood glucose prior to administering any dose of insulin.

Special Considerations for Administration of Insulin

To manage type 1 diabetes mellitus, most patients take insulin injections. Nurses need to be knowledgeable and vigilant when preparing insulin because it is a "high-alert" medication, one that is associated with a high risk of injury to the patient when used in error (ISMP, 2017; Sodré Alves et al., 2021). Shorter (under 5 mm) needles are associated with less pain, adequate control of blood sugar, and minimal leakage of medication (ISMP, 2017), as well as decreased risk of inadvertent IM injection (Diabetes Canada Clinical Practice Guidelines Expert Committee, 2018). Thus, needles with a length of 4 to 8 mm are recommended for administering insulin (start with the shortest needle available). Administer at a 90-degree angle to reduce pain and achieve adequate control of blood sugar with minimal adverse effects for people of all BMIs, including children (Diabetes Canada Clinical Practice Guidelines Expert Committee, 2018).

Several different devices are available for administration of SUBCUT injections. *Injection pens* allow patients to self-administer SUBCUT medications (e.g., insulin or interferon) (Fig. 22.20). They offer a convenient delivery method using prefilled, disposable cartridges but require significant patient teaching. The patient pinches the skin, inserts the needle, and injects a predetermined medication dose. The *needleless jet injection system* administers SUBCUT medications without the use of needles. Needle-free injections use high pressure to penetrate the skin with the medication into the SUBCUT tissue (Fig. 22.21).

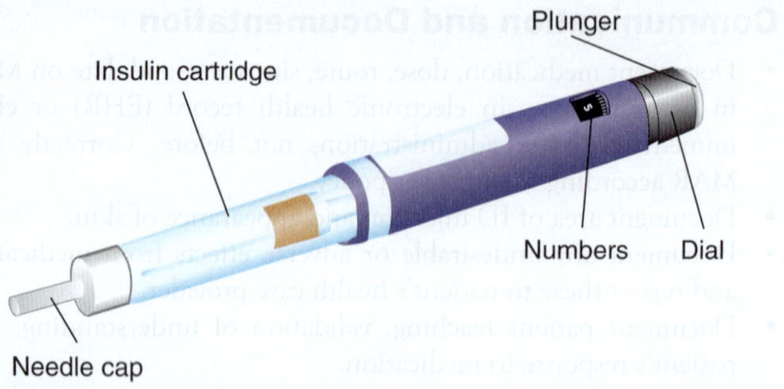

FIG 22.20 **Insulin injection pen.** (*From Lewis, S. L., Bucher, L., Heitkemper, M. M., et al. [2017]. Medical-surgical nursing: Assessment and management of clinical problems [10th ed.]. Mosby.*)

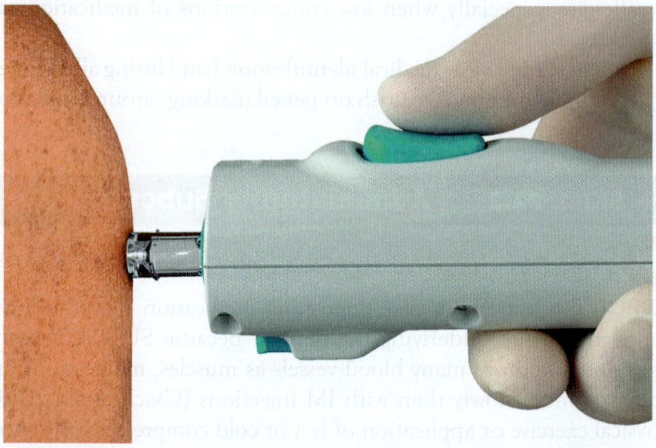

FIG 22.21 **Jet injection system is held perpendicular to skin.** (*Image courtesy PharmaJet. All rights reserved.*)

To prevent lipohypertrophy, patients and nurses choose one anatomical area (e.g., the abdomen) and systematically rotate sites within that region. Doing so maintains consistent insulin absorption from day to day (FIT Canada, 2020). Insulin is most quickly absorbed in the abdomen and most slowly in the thighs (FIT Canada, 2020).

The timing of insulin injections is critical. Health care providers plan insulin injection times based on blood glucose levels; when a patient will eat; and the onset, peak, and duration of the insulin to be administered. Knowing the peak action and duration of the insulin is essential when developing an effective diabetes management plan. See Table 22.2 for a comparison of a variety of insulin preparations. Box 22.3 provides general guidelines for insulin administration.

Special Considerations for Administration of Heparin

Heparin therapy provides therapeutic anticoagulation to reduce the risk of thrombus formation by suppressing clot formation. Therefore, patients receiving heparin are at risk of bleeding, including bleeding gums, hematemesis, hematuria, or melena. Results from coagulation blood tests (e.g., activated partial thromboplastin time [aPTT] and partial thromboplastin time [PTT]) allow the nurse to monitor the desired therapeutic range for heparin therapy.

Before administering heparin, which is also identified as a high-alert medication, assess for pre-existing conditions that contraindicate its use, including cerebral or aortic aneurysm, cerebrovascular hemorrhage, severe hypertension, and blood dyscrasias. In addition, assess for conditions in which increased risk of hemorrhage is present: recent childbirth; severe diabetes and renal disease; liver disease;

BOX 22.3
General Guidelines for Insulin Administration

- Store vials of insulin in the refrigerator, not the freezer. Keep vials currently being used at room temperature for up to 1 month. Do not inject cold insulin.
- Inspect vials before each use for changes in appearance (e.g., clumping, frosting, precipitation, change in clarity or colour) that indicate lack of potency.
- Do not interchange insulin types unless approved by the patient's health care provider.
- Preferred injection sites include the abdomen (avoiding a 5-cm [2-inch] radius around the umbilicus) and the outer aspect of the thighs.
- Have patient self-administer insulin whenever possible.
- Patients who take insulin need to self-monitor their blood glucose.
- Insulin syringes with needles attached and insulin pen needles should be used only once.
- All patients who take insulin should carry at least 15 g carbohydrate (e.g., glucose tablets—preferred choice, 15 mL table sugar dissolved in water, 175 mL juice or regular soft drink) in the event of a hypoglycemic reaction.

Adapted from Diabetes Canada Clinical Practice Guidelines Expert Committee. (2018). 2018 Diabetes Canada clinical practice guidelines for the prevention and management of diabetes in Canada. *Canadian Journal of Diabetes, 42*(Suppl. 1), S1–S325. https://guidelines.diabetes.ca/docs/CPG-2018-full-EN.pdf

severe trauma; and active ulcers or lesions of the gastrointestinal (GI), genitourinary (GU), or respiratory tract. Assess the patient's current medication regimen, including use of over-the-counter (OTC) and herbal medications (e.g., garlic, ginger, ginkgo, horse chestnut, or feverfew), for possible interaction with heparin. Other medications that interact with heparin include Aspirin, nonsteroidal anti-inflammatory drugs (NSAIDs), cephalosporins, antithyroid medications, probenecid, and thrombolytics.

Low-molecular-weight heparins (LMWHs) (e.g., enoxaparin) are as effective as heparin but are more predictable, have a longer half-life, and require less laboratory monitoring (Adams et al., 2021). To minimize the pain and bruising associated with LMWH, it is given subcutaneously on the right or left side of the abdomen, at least 5 cm (2 inches) away from the umbilicus. Administer LMWH in its prefilled syringe with the attached needle, and do not expel the air bubble in the syringe before giving the medication. There is some evidence to support a slower injection rate of 30 seconds to reduce bruising and pain (Mohammady et al., 2021; Sanofi-Aventis Canada, 2018).

Delegation and Collaboration

The skill of administering SUBCUT injections cannot be delegated to a UCP. The nurse instructs the UCP about the following:

- Potential medication adverse effects and immediately reporting their occurrence to the nurse

Equipment

- MAR
- Commercial prefilled syringe *or* medication prepared by nurse from an ampoule or vial into a syringe (Skill 22.1)
- Safety needle:
  - Most medications: 25- to 27-gauge needle, 3.2- to 16-mm (0.125 to 0.625 inches) length
  - Immunizations: 23- to 25-gauge needle, 16-mm (0.625-inch) length (Beirne et al., 2015)
  - U-100 insulin: Insulin syringes often come with a preattached needle (30 to 32 gauge, 4- to 8-mm length).
  - U-500 insulin: 25- to 31-gauge needle, 6-mm length preferred. Follow manufacturer instructions.

! SAFETY ALERT Do not draw insulin from insulin pen cartridges using a conventional or insulin needle and syringe.

- Small gauze pad
- Alcohol swab
- Clean gloves
- Puncture-proof container

STEP	RATIONALE
ASSESSMENT	
1. Identify patient using at least two person-specific identifiers (e.g., name and date of birth or name and medical record number) according to employer policy.	
2. Throughout the procedure, the 4 moments for hand hygiene are to be implemented; hand hygiene should occur before initial patient (or patient environment) contact, before an aseptic procedure, after body fluid exposure risk, and after patient (or patient environment) contact. Additional hand hygiene should be performed when hands are visibly soiled.	
3. Check accuracy and completeness of each MAR by comparing with health care provider prescription. Check patient's name, medication name and dosage, route of administration, time of administration, and recent administration site selection. Recopy or reprint any part of MAR that is difficult to read.	The prescription is the most reliable source and only legal record of medications that the patient is to receive.
4. Assess patient's medical and medication history.	Determines need for medication or possible contraindications for medication administration.
5. Assess patient's history of allergies: known type of allergies and normal allergic reaction.	Do not prepare medication if there is known patient allergy.
6. Review medication reference information for medication action, purpose, normal dose, adverse effects, time and peak of onset, and nursing implications.	Allows you to administer medication safely and monitor patient's response to therapy.

STEP	RATIONALE

ASSESSMENT

STEP	RATIONALE
7. Check date of expiration on medication.	Dose potency increases or decreases when outdated.
8. Observe patient's previous verbal and nonverbal responses regarding injection and review progress notes for information about needle fear/syncope.	Anticipating patient's anxiety allows you to use distraction to reduce pain awareness.
9. Assess for contraindication to SUBCUT injections, such as circulatory shock or reduced local tissue perfusion.	Reduced tissue perfusion interferes with drug absorption and distribution.
10. Assess patient's symptoms before initiating medication therapy.	Provides information to evaluate desired effect of medication.
11. Assess adequacy of patient's adipose tissue.	Adipose tissue influences methods for administering injections.
12. Assess relevant laboratory results (e.g., point-of-care [POC] blood glucose, PTT).	Provides baseline for measuring medication response.
13. Assess patient's knowledge of medication.	Poses implications for patient education.

NURSING DIAGNOSES

- Acute pain
- Anxiety
- Insufficient knowledge regarding medication administration or medication therapy
- Fear
- Reduced health maintenance

Related factors and risk factors are individualized on the basis of patient's condition or needs.

PLANNING

STEP	RATIONALE
1. Expected outcomes following completion of procedure:	
• Patient experiences no pain or mild burning at injection site.	Medications may cause minor tissue irritation.
• Patient achieves desired effect of medication with no signs of allergies or undesired effects.	Medication administered without patient injury.
• Patient explains purpose, dosage, and effects of medication.	Demonstrates learning.

IMPLEMENTATION

STEP	RATIONALE
1. Prepare medication using aseptic technique. Check label of medication carefully by comparing with MAR three times (see Skill 22.1 or Procedural Guideline 22.1) when preparing medication.	Ensures that medication is sterile.
2. Identify patient using at least two person-specific identifiers (e.g., name and date of birth, or name and medical record number) according to employer policy. Compare identifiers with information on patient's MAR.	Ensures correct patient. Complies with Accreditation Canada's standards and improves patient safety (Accreditation Canada, 2020).
3. Take medication(s) to patient at correct time (see employer policy). During administration, apply 10 rights of medication administration and complete three checks for accuracy. Close room curtain or door.	Hospitals must adopt medication administration policy and procedure for timing of medication administration that considers nature of the prescribed medication, specific clinical application, and patient needs (ISMP, 2011).
4. Ask patient if they have allergies.	Confirms patient's allergy history.
5. Discuss purpose, action, and possible adverse effects of each medication. Allow patient to ask any questions. Tell patient that injection will cause slight burning or stinging sensation.	It is an ethical responsibility of nurses to provide education to patients to support informed decision making (CNA, 2017).
6. Apply clean gloves. Keep sheet or gown draped over body parts not requiring exposure.	Reduces transmission of infection. Respects patient's dignity while injection area is exposed.
7. Select appropriate injection site. Inspect skin surface over sites for bruises, inflammation, or edema. Do not use an area that is bruised or has signs associated with infection.	Injection sites are free of abnormalities that interfere with drug absorption. Sites used repeatedly become hardened from lipohypertrophy.

Critical Decision Point *Use nonpharmacological pain management techniques (e.g., vibration, pressure) and psychological pain management techniques (e.g., distraction, bubble blowing) as appropriate. Use pharmacological strategies per employer policy.*

STEP	RATIONALE

IMPLEMENTATION

8. Palpate sites and avoid those with masses, bruising, or tenderness. Be sure that needle is correct size by grasping skinfold at site with thumb and forefinger. Measure fold from top to bottom. Make sure that needle is one-half length of fold.	You can mistakenly give SUBCUT injections in muscle, especially in abdomen and thigh sites. Appropriate size of needle ensures that you inject medication into SUBCUT tissue (Larkin et al., 2018).
a. When administering insulin or heparin, use abdominal injection sites first, then posterior arms, and lastly, thigh injection site.	Risk of bruising is not affected by site.
b. When administering LMWH subcutaneously, choose site on right or left side of abdomen, at least 5 cm (2 inches) away from umbilicus.	Injecting LMWH on side of abdomen helps decrease pain and bruising at injection site (Sanofi-Aventis Canada, 2018).
c. Rotate insulin injection site within an anatomical area (e.g., abdomen), and systematically rotate sites within that area.	Rotating injection sites within same anatomical site maintains consistency in day-to-day insulin absorption.
9. Help patient into comfortable position. Have them relax arm, leg, or abdomen, depending on site selection.	Relaxation of site minimizes discomfort.
10. Locate site using anatomical landmarks.	Injection into correct anatomical site prevents injury to nerves, bone, and blood vessels.
11. Clean site with antiseptic swab. Apply swab at centre of site and rotate outward in circular direction for about 5 cm (2 inches) (see Step 11 illustration).	Mechanical action of swab removes secretions containing microorganisms.
12. Hold swab or gauze between third and fourth fingers of nondominant hand.	Swab or gauze remains readily accessible for use when withdrawing needle after the injection.
13. Remove needle cap or protective sheath by pulling it straight off.	Preventing needle from touching sides of cap prevents contamination.
14. Hold syringe between thumb and forefinger of dominant hand; hold as dart (see Step 14 illustration).	Quick, smooth injection requires proper manipulation of syringe parts.
15. Administer injection:	
a. For average-sized patient, hold skin across injection site or pinch skin with nondominant hand.	Needle penetrates tight skin more easily than loose skin. Pinching elevates SUBCUT tissue and desensitizes area.
b. Inject needle quickly and firmly at 45- to 90-degree angle (see Step 15b illustration). Release skin if pinched. *Option:* When using injection pen or giving heparin, continue to pinch skin while injecting medicine.	Quick, firm insertion minimizes discomfort. (Injecting medication into compressed tissue irritates nerve). Correct angle prevents accidental injection into muscle.
c. After needle enters site, grasp lower end of syringe barrel with nondominant hand to stabilize it. Move dominant hand to end of plunger and slowly inject medication over several seconds (see Step 15c illustration). When giving heparin, inject over 30 seconds (Mohammady et al., 2021; Sanofi-Aventis Canada, 2018). Avoid moving syringe.	Movement of syringe may displace needle and cause discomfort. Slow injection (over 30 seconds) of heparin may reduce pain and bruising intensity (Mohammady et al., 2021).

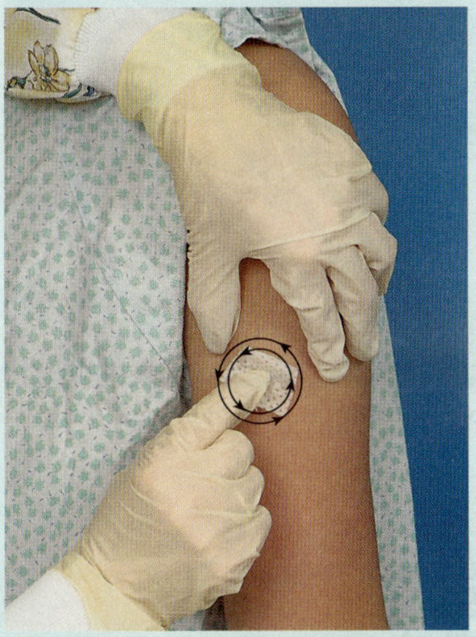

STEP 11 Subcutaneous site: Posterior aspect of upper arm. Clean site with circular motion.

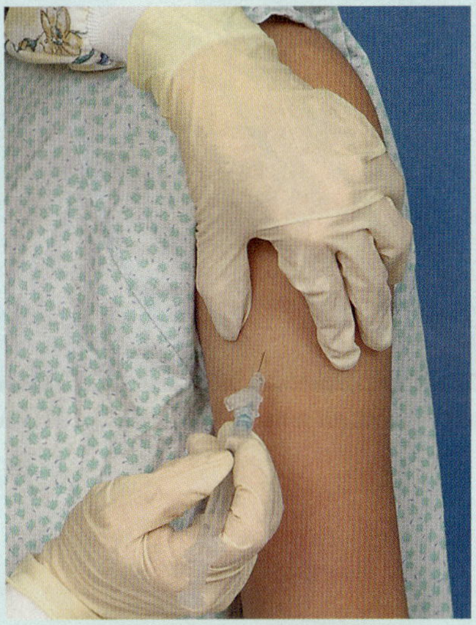

STEP 14 Subcutaneous injection in the posterior aspect of the upper arm. Hold syringe as if grasping a dart.

STEP	RATIONALE

IMPLEMENTATION

Step	Rationale
d. Withdraw needle quickly while placing gauze gently over site.	Supporting tissues around injection site minimizes discomfort during needle withdrawal. Dry gauze may minimize patient discomfort associated with alcohol on nonintact skin.
16. Apply gentle pressure to site. *Do not massage site.* (If heparin is given, hold gauze to site for 30–60 seconds.)	Aids absorption. Massage can damage underlying tissue. Time interval prevents bleeding at site.
17. Help patient to comfortable position.	Gives patient sense of well-being.
18. Discard uncapped needle or needle enclosed in safety shield (see Step 18 illustrations) and attached syringe into puncture- and leak-proof receptacle.	Prevents injury to patients and health care personnel. Recapping needles increases risk of needle-stick injury (Elmi et al., 2018).
19. Remove gloves.	Reduces transmission of microorganisms.
20. Stay with patient for several minutes and observe for any allergic reactions.	Dyspnea, wheezing, and circulatory collapse are signs of severe anaphylactic reaction.

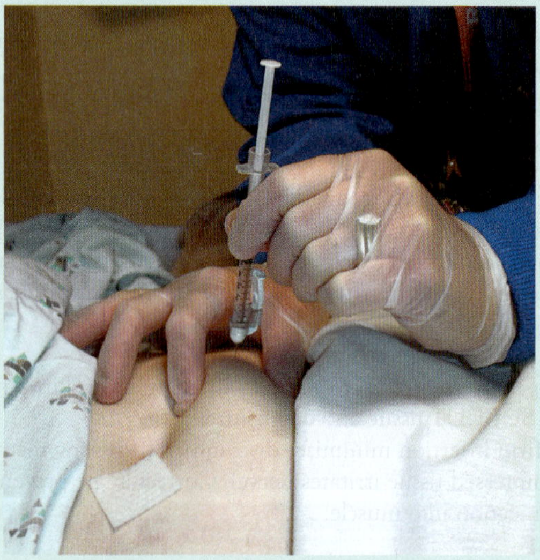

STEP 15B Subcutaneous injection. Angle and needle length depend on thickness of skinfold.

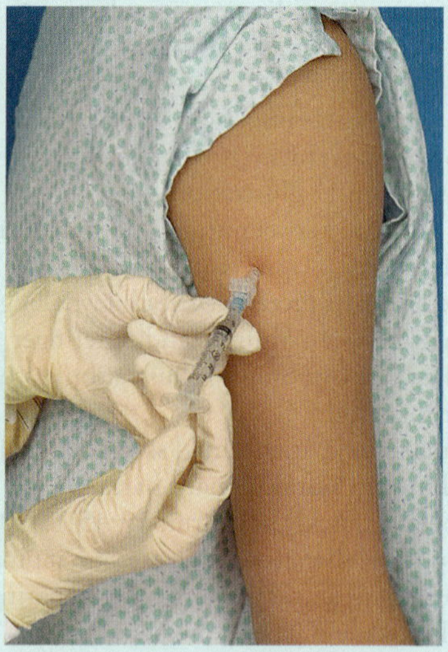

STEP 15C Inject medication slowly.

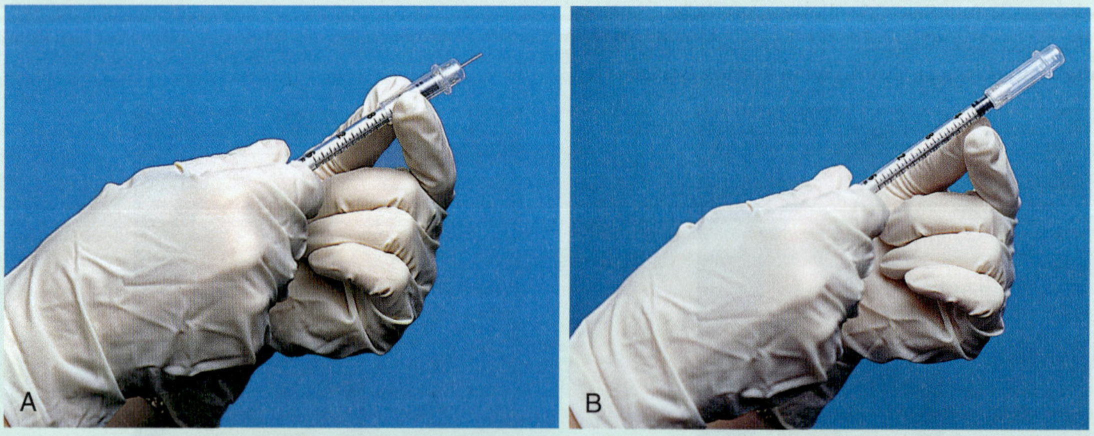

STEP 18 Needle with plastic guard prevents needle-sticks. A, Position of guard before injection. B, After injection, guard locks in place, covering needle.

STEP	RATIONALE
EVALUATION	
1. Return to room in 15–30 minutes and ask patient whether they feel any acute pain, burning, numbness, or tingling at injection site.	Continued discomfort may indicate injury to underlying bones or nerves.
2. Inspect site, noting bruising or induration. Provide warm compress to site.	Bruising or induration indicates complication associated with injection. NOTE: Bruising can be expected with heparin (Mohammady et al., 2021).
3. Observe patient's response to medication at times that correlate with onset, peak, and duration of action. Review laboratory results as appropriate (e.g., blood glucose, PTT).	Adverse effects of parenteral medications develop rapidly. Evaluate effect of medication on basis of onset, peak, and duration of action.
4. Use **teach-back:** "I want to be sure I explained to you the reason for this subcutaneous injection. Tell me why you are receiving this injection." Develop a revised teaching plan if patient or caregiver is unable to teach back correctly.	Determines patient's and caregiver's level of understanding of topic (Yen & Leasure, 2019).

Unexpected Outcomes	Related Interventions
1. Patient experiences postinjection localized pain, numbness, tingling, or burning at injection site.	• Assess injection site; may indicate potential injury to nerve or tissues. • Notify patient's health care provider and do not reuse site.
2. Patient displays adverse reaction with signs of urticaria, eczema, pruritus, wheezing, and dyspnea.	• Monitor patient's vital signs. • Follow employer policy for appropriate response to allergic reactions or anaphylaxis (e.g., IM epinephrine). • Notify patient's health care provider immediately. • Add allergy information to patient's record.
3. Lipohypertrophy of skin develops from repeated SUBCUT injection.	• Do not use site for future injections. • Instruct patient not to use site for 6 months.

Communication and Documentation

- Immediately after administration, document medication, dose, route, site, time, and date given on MAR in progress notes in EHR or chart. Correctly sign MAR according to employer policy.
- Document patient teaching, validation of understanding, and patient's response to medication.
- Document any undesirable or adverse effects from medication and report to patient's health care provider.

Special Considerations

Teaching

- Instruct patient to wear medical identification bracelet indicating important medical information, including bleeding tendencies, chronic conditions (e.g., diabetes mellitus), and allergies.
- Patients who require daily injections need to learn techniques of self-administration to ensure that they deliver the correct dose of medication; this learning is often provided as part of an intensive diabetes education program.
- For insulin pens, teach patients the importance of priming the pen before use. Priming involves pointing the pen needle up in the air, dialling one or two units (see package directions) on the pen, and then pressing the plunger fully with the thumb, repeating until a drop appears. This clears the needle of air and ensures that a full dose is ready (FIT Canada, 2020).
- Support patient independence and evaluate technique by encouraging patients to prepare and inject their own insulin in hospital, if allowed by employer policy.
- Teach injection techniques to a caregiver if the patient is unable to understand the instructions themselves or if the caregiver will be giving the injections.

Pediatric

- The maximum volume to be used when administering a SUBCUT injection to a small infant is 0.5 mL. (Hockenberry et al., 2024).
- Adolescence is a time of transition. Adolescent patients with type 1 diabetes mellitus are at an increased risk of skipping their insulin injections owing to mental health issues, weight concerns, and "diabetes burnout" (FIT Canada, 2020).

Gerontological

- Older persons have loss of skin elasticity and reduced SUBCUT skinfold thickness. The upper abdominal region is the best site to use when the patient has little SUBCUT tissue.

Care in the Community: Home Management

- Ideally, medication pumps are individualized on the basis of the medication being delivered and patient needs. Nurses also need to consider the availability and cost of the pump and supplies. When possible, patients should select the pump that fits their individual and home needs and is easiest to use.
- Improper disposal of used needles and sharps in the home setting poses a health risk to the public and to waste management employees. Several options for safe sharps disposal at home exist, including allowing patients to transport their own sharps containers from home to collection sites (e.g., hospital or pharmacy); syringe exchange programs; or special devices that destroy the

needle on the syringe, rendering it safe for disposal. If the patient cannot implement any of these options, have them dispose of needles and other sharps in a hard plastic or metal container with a tightly sealed lid (e.g., empty detergent bottle or coffee can). Pamphlets for safe home disposal of sharps are available from provincial public health services and most pharmacies, as are numerous online sites such as https://www.pshsa.ca/resources/safe-handling-disposal-of-sharps-medical-supplies-in-home-health-settings.

- Instruct patients that each insulin pen needle and insulin syringe should be used only once (Diabetes Canada Clinical Practice Guidelines Expert Committee, 2018).
- Teach patient and caregiver about injection techniques that minimize patient discomfort.

SKILL 22.4 Administering Continuous Subcutaneous Infusions

NSO Nursing Skills Online Administration of Parenteral Medications: Intravenous Medications Module 7 / Lesson 3

The continuous subcutaneous infusion (CSCI) route of medication administration allows selected medications (e.g., opioids, insulin) and infusion of fluids for hydration or nutrition (Caccialanza et al., 2018) to an in-dwelling SUBCUT needle or catheter (see Figs. 22.18 and 22.19). The route is also effective for use with medications to stop preterm labour (e.g., terbutaline) and to treat pulmonary hypertension (e.g., treprostinil sodium). One factor that determines the infusion rate of CSCI is the rate of medication absorption. Most medications can be absorbed at a rate of 1 to 2 mL/hr, but the rate of absorption depends more on osmotic pressure than on the rate of administration (Caccialanza et al., 2018). The procedure to initiate and discontinue CSCI therapy is similar, regardless of the type of medication being delivered. However, nursing assessment and interventions vary depending on the type of medication administered.

With CSCI, patients are able to manage their illness and pain without the risks associated with IV medication administration (Caccialanza et al., 2018). The route is relatively easy for patients and families to learn and understand in the home setting. Box 22.4 summarizes the benefits associated with the use of CSCI for pain management.

The recommended anatomical sites for CSCI are the same as those for SUBCUT injection, namely the upper arm, thigh, abdomen, as well as the upper chest. Site selection depends on a patient's activity level and the type of medication to be delivered. For example, pain medications given to ambulatory patients are best delivered in the upper chest, which allows a patient to move freely. Insulin is absorbed most consistently in the abdomen; thus, choose a site in the abdomen away from the waistline. Always avoid sites where the tubing of the pump could be disturbed. Rotate sites used for medication administration at least every 7 days or whenever complications such as leaking, bruising, erythema, or pain occur (CVAA, 2019).

The CSCI route requires a computerized pump with safety features, including lockout intervals and warning alarms (Fig. 22.22).

BOX 22.4

Pain Management Benefits With Use of Continuous Subcutaneous Infusion

- Benefits patients with poor venous access
- Provides pain relief to patients who are unable to tolerate oral pain medications
- Allows patients greater mobility
- Rapid onset of action, about 20 minutes
- Better pain control than intramuscular injections
- Lower rates of infection

Adapted from Arthur, A. (2015). Innovations in subcutaneous infusions. *Journal of Infusion Nursing, 38*(3), 179; Bartz, L., Klein, C., Seifert, A., et al. (2014). Subcutaneous administration of drugs in palliative care: Result of a systematic observational study. *Journal of Pain Symptom Management, 48*(4), 540.

Delegation and Collaboration

The skill of administering CSCI medications cannot be delegated to a UCP. The nurse instructs the UCP about the following:

- Potential medication adverse effects or reactions and immediately reporting their occurrence to the nurse.
- Reporting complications (e.g., leaking, redness, discomfort) at the CSCI needle insertion site to the nurse.
- Obtaining any required vital signs and reporting them to the nurse.

Equipment

Initiating CSCI

- Clean gloves
- Alcohol swab
- Antibacterial skin preparation such as chlorhexidine gluconate (CHG)
- Small (25- to 27-gauge) winged catheter with attached tubing or CSCI-designed catheter (e.g., Sof-Set)
- Infusion pump
- Occlusive, transparent dressing
- Label, if required by employer policy
- Medication in appropriate syringe or container
- MAR

Discontinuing CSCI

- Clean gloves
- Small gauze dressing
- Tape or adhesive bandage
- Alcohol swab and CHG *(optional)*
- Puncture-proof container

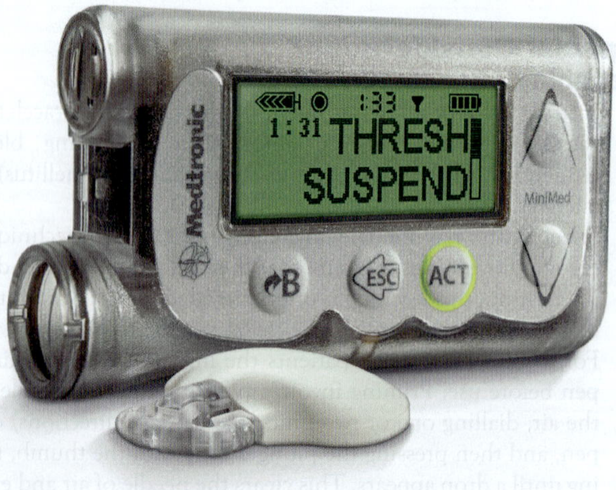

FIG 22.22 MiniMed Paradigm REAL-Time insulin pump and continuous glucose monitoring system. (*Courtesy Medtronic, Inc., Northridge, CA.*)

STEP	RATIONALE

ASSESSMENT

STEP	RATIONALE
1. Identify patient using at least two person-specific identifiers (e.g., name and date of birth or name and medical record number) according to employer policy.	
2. Throughout the procedure, the 4 moments for hand hygiene are to be implemented; hand hygiene should occur before initial patient (or patient environment) contact, before an aseptic procedure, after body fluid exposure risk, and after patient (or patient environment) contact. Additional hand hygiene should be performed when hands are visibly soiled.	
3. Check accuracy and completeness of each MAR by comparing with health care provider prescription. Check patient's name, medication name and dosage, route of administration, and time of administration. Recopy or reprint any part of MAR that is difficult to read.	The prescription sheet is the most reliable source and only legal record of medications that the patient is to receive.
4. Assess patient's medical and medication history.	Determines need for medication or possible contraindications for medication administration.
5. Assess patient's history of allergies: known type of allergens and normal allergic reaction.	CSCI administration of medications may cause a rapid response. Allergic response is immediate.
6. Collect medication reference information necessary to administer medication safely, including action, purpose, adverse effects, normal dose, time of peak onset, how slowly to give medication, and nursing implications.	Knowledge of medication allows you to give medication safely and monitor patient's response to therapy.
7. Assess patient's previous verbal and nonverbal responses to needle insertion.	Anticipating patient's anxiety allows you to use distraction to reduce pain awareness.
8. If an analgesic is being administered, assess patient's pain severity using an appropriate pain rating scale or tool.	Provides an objective measure of pain severity.
9. Assess for contraindications to CSCI (e.g., thrombocytopenia or reduced local tissue perfusion).	Any existing coagulation disorder contraindicates heparin infusion. Reduced tissue perfusion interferes with medication absorption and distribution.
10. Assess adequacy of patient's adipose tissue to determine appropriate infusion site.	Physiological changes of aging or patient illness influence amount of SUBCUT tissue, which affects choice of catheter insertion site.
11. Assess patient's knowledge regarding medication to be received and use of medication pump.	Provides background to determine need for patient education.
12. Assess patient's symptoms before initiating medication therapy. Determine severity of pain (if using analgesia) or measure blood glucose level (if using insulin).	Provides information to evaluate desired effects of CSCI medication.
13. Review manufacturer directions for pump.	Ensures proper use of equipment.

NURSING DIAGNOSES

- Pain (acute, chronic)
- Anxiety
- Fear
- Insufficient knowledge regarding CSCI therapy
- Inadequate health maintenance
- Potential for infection
- Potential for injury

Related factors and risk factors are individualized on the basis of patient's condition or needs.

PLANNING

STEP	RATIONALE
1. Expected outcomes following completion of procedure:	
• Insertion site remains free from infection.	Risk for infection at needle insertion site is potential complication of CSCI therapy.
• Patient achieves desired effect of medication with no signs of adverse reactions.	Medication is delivered safely, with desired therapeutic effect achieved.
• Patient explains purpose, dosage, and effects of medication and verbalizes understanding of CSCI therapy.	Demonstrates learning.

STEP	RATIONALE

IMPLEMENTATION

STEP	RATIONALE
1. *If medication is packaged in a vial or ampoule*: Prepare medication following the steps in Skill 22.1. *If medication is packaged in a prefilled syringe or pump-specific cassette:* Complete three checks for accuracy by comparing with MAR.	Ensures that medication is sterile. Checking label of medication against transcribed prescription reduces occurrence of error.
2. Identify patient using at least two person-specific identifiers (e.g., name and date of birth, or name and medical record number) according to employer policy. Compare identifiers with information on patient's MAR.	Ensures correct patient. Complies with Accreditation Canada's standards and improves patient safety (Accreditation Canada, 2020).
3. Load medication into pump and prime tubing per manufacturer instructions. Program medication administration pump.	Ensures that medication dose administered is accurate.
4. Ask patient if they have allergies.	Confirms patient's allergy history.
5. Discuss purpose, action, and possible adverse effects of each medication. Allow patient to ask any questions. Tell patient that needle insertion will cause slight burning or stinging sensation.	It is an ethical responsibility of nurses to provide education to patients to support informed decision making (CNA, 2017).
6. Position patient supine, drape, and provide for privacy.	Respects patient's dignity.
7. Initiate CSCI:	
a. Be sure that patient is comfortable, either sitting or lying down.	Eases pain associated with insertion of needle.
b. Select appropriate injection site (i.e., free of irritation and away from bony prominences and waistline). Most common sites used are subclavicular region and abdomen.	Ensures proper medication absorption.
c. Apply clean gloves. Clean injection site with alcohol using circular motion, then apply antiseptic using straight cleaning strokes. Allow both agents to dry.	Reduces risk for infection at insertion site.
d. Hold needle in dominant hand and remove needle guard.	Prepares needle for insertion.
e. Gently pinch or lift up skin with nondominant hand.	Ensures that needle will enter SUBCUT tissue.
f. Gently and firmly insert needle at 45- to 90-degree angle (see Step 7f illustration), based on manufacturer directions.	Decreases pain related to insertion of needle.
g. If inserting a cannula with a sharp needle covered with a plastic catheter, remove the needle according to manufacturer directions and leave the plastic catheter in the skin.	
h. Place occlusive, transparent dressing over insertion site (see Step 7h illustration). Label line if employer policy indicates.	Protects site from infection and allows you to assess site during medication infusion.
i. Attach tubing from needle to tubing from infusion pump and turn pump on.	Allows you to administer medication.
j. Dispose of any sharps in appropriate leak- and puncture-proof container. Discard used supplies and remove gloves.	Prevents accidental needle-stick injuries and follow employer guidelines for disposal of sharps.
k. Inspect site before leaving patient and instruct patient to inform you if site becomes red or begins to leak.	Initiate new site with new needle whenever erythema or leaking occurs. If site is free from complications, rotate site every 7 days for medication doses or infusions or every 1–2 days for hydration infusions (CVAA, 2019).

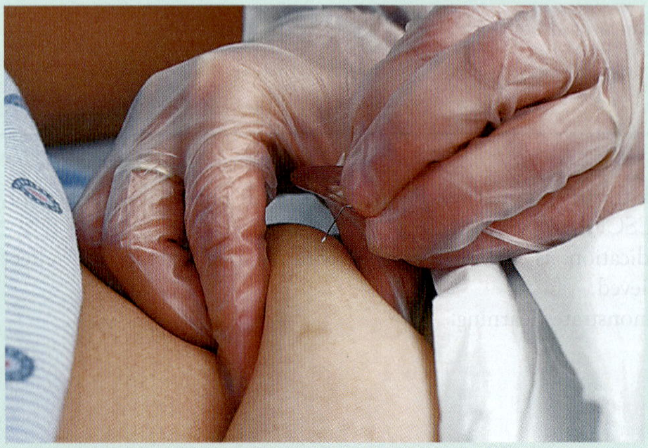

STEP 7F Insert butterfly needle into subcutaneous tissue of abdomen.

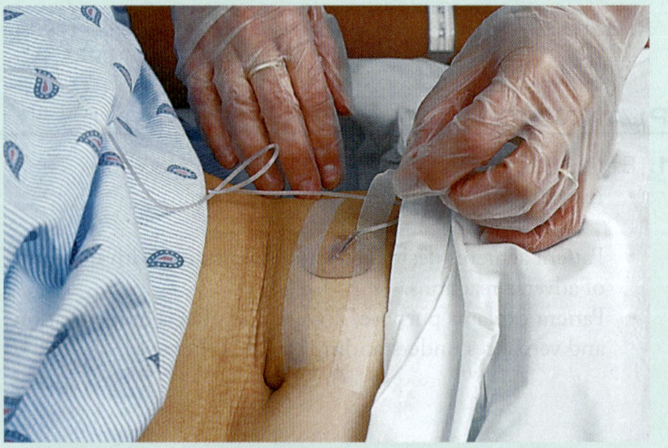

STEP 7H Place transparent dressing over insertion site.

STEP	RATIONALE
IMPLEMENTATION	
l. Stay with patient for several minutes and observe for any allergic reactions.	Dyspnea, wheezing, and circulatory collapse are signs of severe anaphylactic reaction.
8. Discontinue CSCI:	
a. Verify prescription and establish alternative method for medication administration if applicable.	If medication will be required after discontinuing CSCI, a different medication and/or route is often necessary to continue to manage patient's illness or pain.
b. Stop infusion pump.	Prevents medication from spilling.
c. Apply clean gloves.	Hand hygiene reduces risk of contamination of equipment. Gloves provide barrier in event of exposure to blood or body fluids (Infection Prevention and Control Canada, 2017).
d. Remove dressing without dislodging or removing needle/in-dwelling catheter. Discard properly.	Exposes needle.

Critical Decision Point *If site is infected, clean it with alcohol and antiseptic. Apply triple antibiotic cream to site if it is excoriated (abraded).*

STEP	RATIONALE
e. Pull needle out at same angle at which it was inserted.	Minimizes patient discomfort.
f. Apply gentle pressure at site until no fluid leaks out of skin.	Dressing adheres to site if skin remains dry.
g. Apply small sterile gauze dressing or adhesive bandage to site.	Prevents bacterial entry into puncture site.
9. Dispose of uncapped needles and syringes in puncture- and leak-proof container.	Prevents accidental needle-stick injuries and follows guidelines for disposal of sharps (CCOHS, 2018).
10. Remove and dispose of gloves.	Reduces transmission of microorganisms.
EVALUATION	
1. Evaluate patient's response to medication.	Determines effect of therapy. Decreased or absent response to medication may indicate that patient is not receiving medication into SUBCUT tissue (e.g., pump malfunction, medication leaking at site).
2. Assess site at least every 4 hours for redness, pain, drainage, or swelling.	Indicates infection at insertion site.
3. **Use teach-back:** "I want to be sure you understand your continuous infusion into your skin and the medication you are receiving. Tell me in your own words why you have a continuous infusion to receive your medication." Develop a revised teaching plan if patient or caregiver is unable to teach back correctly.	Determines patient's and caregiver's level of understanding of topic (Yen & Leasure, 2019).

Unexpected Outcomes	Related Interventions
1. Patient indicates localized pain or burning sensation at insertion site; or site appears red or swollen or is leaking, indicating potential infection or needle dislodgement.	• Remove needle and place new needle at different site. • Continue to monitor original site for signs of infection and notify health care provider if you suspect infection.
2. Patient displays signs of allergic reaction to medication.	• Stop delivering medication immediately and follow employer policy or guidelines for appropriate response to allergic reaction (e.g., administration of antihistamine such as diphenhydramine or epinephrine) and reporting of adverse medication reactions. • Notify patient's health care provider of adverse effects immediately. • Add allergy information to medical record.
3. CSCI becomes dislodged.	• Stop infusion, apply pressure at site until no fluid leaks out of skin, cover site with gauze dressing or adhesive bandage, and initiate infusion at new site. • Assess patient to determine effects of not receiving medication (e.g., assess patient's pain level using age-appropriate pain scale, obtain blood glucose level).

Communication and Documentation

- After initiating CSCI, immediately chart medication, dose, route, site, time, date, and type of medication pump on MAR in progress notes in EHR or chart.
- If medication is an opioid, follow employer policy to document waste.
- Document patient's response to medication and appearance of site according to employer policy.
- Document patient teaching, validation of understanding, and patient's response to medication.
- Document any undesirable or adverse effects from medication and report these to patient's health care provider.

Special Considerations

Teaching

- Instruct patient to wear medical alert bracelet along with medical information, including chronic health condition (e.g., diabetes mellitus), allergies, and a contact phone number for the pump manufacturer for technical support.
- Instruct patients to carry backup batteries and extra medication if they are going to be away from home.
- Patients receiving insulin require intensive diabetes management education (Box 22.5).
- Patients with diabetes mellitus who use CSCI for management of blood glucose levels are carefully selected and receive intense diabetes self-management education from qualified diabetes educators and insulin pump trainers. Adults and children living with diabetes mellitus who use insulin pumps require less insulin, have superior glycemic control, and have better health-related quality of life (Pozzilli et al., 2016). Insulin pumps are becoming the treatment of choice for children living with type 1 diabetes. The Medtronic MiniMed integrates an insulin pump with real-time continuous glucose monitoring (see Fig. 22.22). Age-appropriate education for the child and the entire family, and ideally, school personnel, is essential. Education should include psychosocial support and nutritional information, including how to count carbohydrates.
- Never immerse pumps in water or expose them to X-ray films or magnetic resonance imaging.

BOX 22.5

Education Topics for Patients Receiving Insulin With Continuous Subcutaneous Infusion

- Blood glucose monitoring
- Meal planning and food choices
- Incorporating exercise into daily routine
- How to program and use an insulin pump
- Illness guidelines and management
- Management of hypoglycemia
- Prevention and management of hyperglycemia
- Prevention of infection, especially at continuous subcutaneous infusion (CSCI) site
- Problem-solving and decision-making skills when pump malfunctions
- Special considerations and precautions (e.g., what to do with pump when showering and sleeping)

Adapted from Diabetes Canada Clinical Practice Guidelines Expert Committee. (2018). Diabetes Canada 2018 clinical practice guidelines for the prevention and management of diabetes in Canada. *Canadian Journal of Diabetes, 42*(Suppl. 1), S1–S325. https://guidelines.diabetes.ca/docs/CPG-2018-full-EN.pdf

Pediatric

- CSCI improves glycemic control in children and adolescents. There is a decreased rate of severe hypoglycemia, catheter-site infection, and weight gain (Hockenberry et al., 2024).
- Insulin pumps offer adolescents more flexibility and give them the responsibility of managing their own diabetes. Extensive child and family education is needed to use CSCI (Hockenberry et al., 2024).
- Clean and change CSCI sites in children every 48 to 72 hours or at the first signs of inflammation (Hockenberry et al., 2024).

Gerontological

- CSCI delivers isotonic IV solutions to older persons who are dehydrated; this is known as *hypodermoclysis therapy*. This method of providing hydration avoids the need to transfer a patient from home or a long-term care facility to an acute care hospital.
- Up to 1 500 mL can be given over 24 hours to one site (CVAA, 2019). The rate and volume of isotonic infusion should be prescribed by a health care provider and should not exceed those used for IV infusion (CVAA, 2019). A health care provider may prescribe use of hyaluronidase to facilitate dispersion and absorption of solutions (CVAA, 2019). Hypodermoclysis is an easy-to-use, safe, and cost-effective alternative to IV hydration for older persons (Caccialanza et al., 2018).

Care in the Community: Home Management

- Patients in the home using CSCI need a responsible caregiver, if available.
- Teach the patient and caregiver about the desired effect of the medication, adverse effects, operation of the pump, how to evaluate the effectiveness of the medication, when and how to assess and rotate injection sites, and when to call a health care provider because of problems.
- Patients need to know where and how to obtain and dispose of all required supplies.
- Patients managing CSCI at home may use an antibacterial soap (e.g., Hibiclens) instead of alcohol and CHG to clean the insertion site.

✦ SKILL 22.5 Administering Intramuscular Injections

Video Clip NSO Nursing Skills Online Administration of Parenteral Medications Module 7 / Lesson 5

The IM injection route deposits medication into deep muscle tissue, which has a rich blood supply, allowing medication to absorb faster than by the SUBCUT route. Any factor that interferes with local tissue blood flow affects the rate and extent of drug absorption. There is an increased risk of injecting medications directly into blood vessels using the IM route. Therefore, whenever administering a medication by the IM route, first verify that the injection is justified (Nicoll & Hesby, 2002; World Health Organization, 2022).

Needle size selection is influenced by the viscosity of the medication, injection site, and patient factors (BMI, gender, and amount of adipose tissue). Determine the appropriate needle gauge according to the medication to be administered. For example, vaccines for hepatitis B and Tdap (tetanus, diphtheria, pertussis) may only be administered by IM injection. Use a longer needle to pass through SUBCUT tissue and penetrate deep muscle tissue (see Fig. 22.1). Because most facilities have needles that range in length from only 9.5 mm (0.375 inches) to 40 mm (1.5 inches), investigate different medication routes, especially when IM injections are prescribed for patients who are obese. Table 22.3 summarizes recommendations based on the length and gauges of needles typically available in Canadian health care settings.

The angle of insertion for an IM injection is 90 degrees. Muscle is less sensitive to irritating and viscous medications. A normal, well-developed adult patient tolerates injection of 2 to 5 mL of medication into a larger muscle without severe muscle discomfort (Nicoll & Hesby, 2002). However, larger volumes of medication (4 to 5 mL) are unlikely to be absorbed properly. Children, older persons, and thin patients tolerate only 2 mL of an IM injection. Do not give more than 1 mL to small children and older infants, and do not give more than 0.5 mL to smaller infants (Hockenberry et al., 2024).

Rotate IM injection sites to decrease the risk of hypertrophy. Emaciated or atrophied muscles absorb medication poorly, thus avoid their use when possible. The Z-track method, a technique for pulling the skin during an injection, is recommended for IM injections (Nicoll & Hesby, 2002). It prevents leakage of medication into SUBCUT tissues, seals medication in the muscle, and minimizes irritation. To use the Z-track method, apply the appropriately sized needle to the syringe and clean and select an IM site, preferably in a large, deep muscle such as the ventrogluteal muscle. Pull the overlying skin and SUBCUT tissues approximately 2.5 to 3.5 cm (1 to 1.5 inches) laterally using the ulnar side of the nondominant hand. Hold the skin in this position until you have administered the injection (Fig. 22.23, *A*). Inject the needle deeply into the muscle. Keep the needle inserted for 10 seconds to allow the medication to disperse evenly. Release the skin after withdrawing the needle. This leaves a zigzag path that seals the needle track wherever tissue planes slide across one another (see Fig. 22.23, *B*). The medication is sealed in the muscle tissue.

Injection Sites

When selecting an IM site, verify that the site is free of pain, infection, necrosis, bruising, and abrasions. Also consider the location of underlying bones, nerves, and blood vessels and the volume of medication to be administered.

> **! SAFETY ALERT** Owing to the location of the sciatic nerve, the dorsogluteal muscle is not recommended as an injection site.

Ventrogluteal Site

The ventrogluteal muscle involves the gluteus medius; it is a deep muscle situated away from major nerves and blood vessels. This site is the preferred and safest site for all adults, children, and infants, especially for administering medications that have larger volumes and are more viscous and irritating (Hockenberry et al., 2024). Vaccines administered to infants and children are an exception; in this case, the vastus lateralis is the preferred site (Hockenberry et al., 2024). Research shows that injuries such as fibrosis, nerve damage, abscess, tissue necrosis, muscle contraction, gangrene, and pain are associated with all the common IM sites *except* the ventrogluteal site (Hopkins & Arias, 2013). However, because this part of the body is almost always covered by patient clothing, it is not always a feasible choice, especially in the outpatient setting or when privacy is not possible.

To locate the ventrogluteal muscle, have the patient lie in either the supine or lateral position; place the heel of your hand over the greater trochanter of the patient's hip with the wrist almost perpendicular to the femur. Use your right hand for the left hip and the left hand for the right

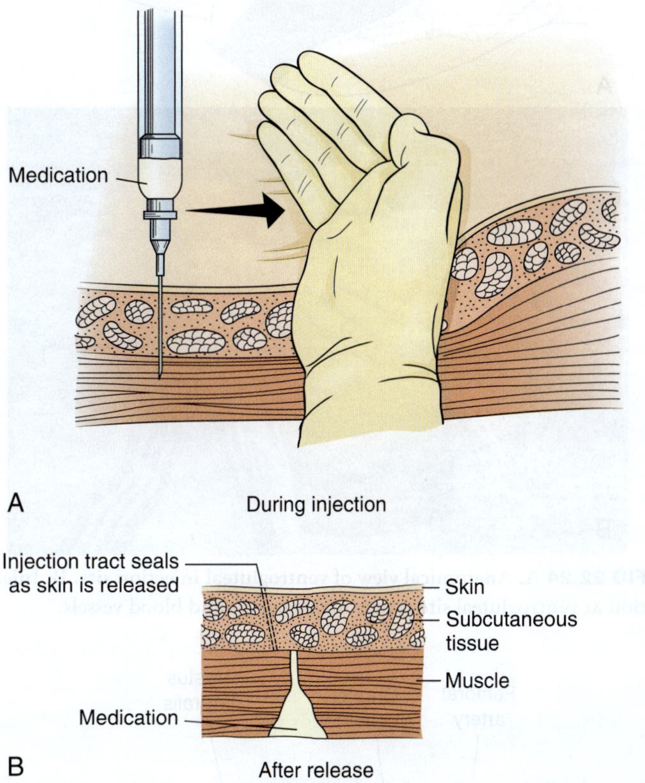

FIG 22.23 **A, Pulling on overlying skin with dorsum of hand during intramuscular injection moves tissue to prevent later tracking. B, Z-track left after injection prevents deposit of medication through sensitive tissue.**

TABLE 22.3

Summary of Needle Choices for Intramuscular Injections

Needle	Length	16 mm (0.625 inches)	25 mm (1 inch)	38 mm (1.5 inches)
	Gauge	25 gauge	23 gauge 25 gauge	22 gauge 23 gauge 25 gauge
Site	Deltoid	1 month–12 years 12 years+, under 60 kg	1–12 years Men 18 years+, up to 118 kg Women 18 years+, up to 90 kg	Men 18 years+, 118 kg+ Women 18 years+, 90 kg+
	Vastus lateralis	Preterm <28 days	1 month+	Not recommended
	Ventral gluteal	Not recommended	Not recommended	18+ years

Note: "Men" refers to people assigned "male" at birth or taking testosterone as part of gender-affirming care; "women" refers to people assigned "female" at birth or taking estradiol as part of gender-affirming care.

Adapted from Nicoll, L., & Hesby, A. (2002). Intramuscular injection: An integrative research review and guideline for evidence-based practice. Applied Nursing Research, 16(2), 159. https://doi.org/10.1053/apnr.2002.34142; Public Health Agency of Canada. (2017). Table 3: Needle selection guidelines. In Vaccine administration practices: Canadian immunization guide. https://www.canada.ca/en/public-health/services/publications/healthy-living/canadian-immunization-guide-part-1-key-immunization-information/page-8-vaccine-administration-practices.html#t3; and Sebro, R. (2022). Statistical estimation of deltoid subcutaneous fat pad thickness: Implications for needle length for vaccination. Scientific Reports, 12(1). Article 1069. https://doi.org/10.1038/s41598-022-05020-5.

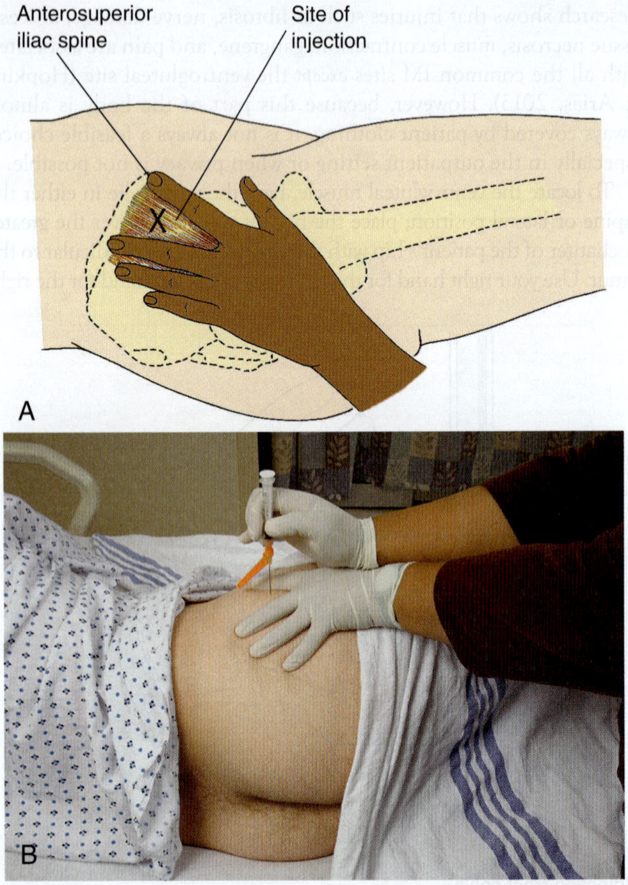

FIG 22.24 A, Anatomical view of ventrogluteal injection site. B, Injection at ventrogluteal site avoids major nerves and blood vessels.

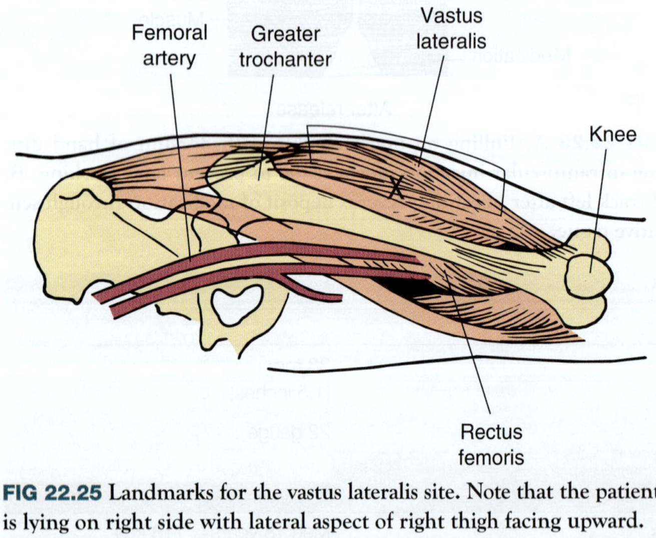

FIG 22.25 Landmarks for the vastus lateralis site. Note that the patient is lying on right side with lateral aspect of right thigh facing upward.

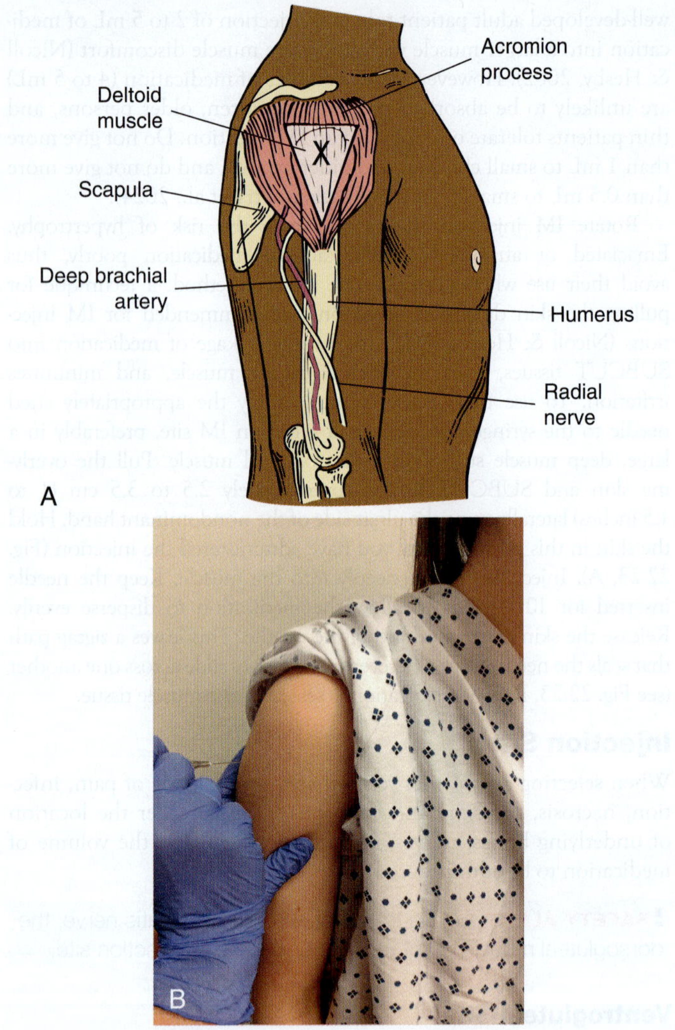

FIG 22.26 A, Landmarks for deltoid site. B, Giving intramuscular injection in deltoid site. (*B, Courtesy Maureen MacInnis-Wheatley.*)

hip. Point the thumb toward the patient's groin; point the index finger to the anterior superior iliac spine; and extend the middle finger back along the iliac crest toward the buttock. The index finger, the middle finger, and the iliac crest form a V-shaped triangle. The injection site is at the centre of the triangle (Fig. 22.24, *A*). To relax this muscle, the patient lies on their side or back, flexing the knee and hip (see Fig. 22.24, *B*).

Vastus Lateralis Muscle

The vastus lateralis muscle is another injection site used in adults and is the preferred site for administration of biologics (e.g., vaccines) in infants, toddlers, and children (Hockenberry et al., 2024). The muscle is thick and well developed and located a safe distance from important blood vessels and nerves (Nakajima et al., 2020). It is located on the anterior lateral aspect of the thigh. In an adult, it extends from a hand breadth above the knee to a hand breadth below the greater trochanter of the femur (Fig. 22.25). Use the middle third of the muscle for injection. The width of the muscle usually extends from the midline of the thigh to the midline of the outer side of the thigh. With young children or cachectic patients, it helps to grasp the body of the muscle during injection to be sure that the medication is deposited in muscle tissue. To help relax the muscle, ask the patient to lie flat with the knee slightly flexed and the foot externally rotated, or have them assume a sitting position (see Fig. 22.25).

Deltoid Muscle

Although the deltoid site is easily accessible, it is not well developed in many adults. There is potential for injury because the axillary, radial, brachial, and ulnar nerves and the brachial artery lie within the upper arm under the triceps and along the humerus. *Carefully assess the condition of the deltoid muscle; consult medication references for suitability of medication; and carefully locate the injection site using anatomical landmarks.* Use this site for small medication volumes (2 mL or less) (Hopkins & Arias, 2013; Nicoll & Hesby, 2002); for administration of routine vaccines in toddlers, older children, and adults; or when other sites are inaccessible because of dressings or casts.

Locate the deltoid muscle by fully exposing the patient's upper arm and shoulder and asking them to relax the arm at the side or by supporting the patient's arm and flexing the elbow. Do not roll up any tight-fitting sleeves. Allow the patient to sit, stand, or lie down. Palpate the lower edge of the acromion process, which forms the base

TABLE 22.3

Summary of Needle Choices for Intramuscular Injections

Needle		Site		
Length	**Size (G)**	**Deltoid**	**Vastus lateralis**	**Ventral gluteal**
16 mm (0.625 inches)	25	1 month–12 years 12 years+, under 60 kg	Preterm <28 days	Not recommended
25 mm (1 inch)	23 or 25	1–12 years Men 18 years+, up to 118 kg Women 18 years+, up to 90 kg	1 month+	Not recommended
38 mm (1.5 inches)	22 or 25	Men 18 years+, 118 kg+ Women 18 years+, 90 kg+	Not recommended	18+ years

Note: "Men" refers to people assigned "male" at birth or taking testosterone as part of gender-affirming care; "women" refers to people assigned "female" at birth or taking estradiol as part of gender-affirming care.

Adapted from Nicoll, L., & Hesby, A. (2002). Intramuscular injection: An integrative research review and guideline for evidence-based practice. *Applied Nursing Research, 16(2)*, 159. https://doi.org/10.1053/apnr.2002.34142; Public Health Agency of Canada. (2017). Table 3: Needle selection guidelines. In Vaccine administration practices: Canadian immunization guide. https://www.canada.ca/en/public-health/services/publications/healthy-living/canadian-immunization-guide-part-1-key-immunization-information/page-8-vaccine-administration-practices.html#t3; andSebro, R. (2022). Statistical estimation of deltoid subcutaneous fat pad thickness: Implications for needle length for vaccination. Scientific Reports, 12(1). Article 1069. https://doi.org/10.1038/s41598-022-05020-5

of a triangle in line with the midpoint of the lateral aspect of the upper arm. The injection site is in the centre of the triangle, about 3 to 5 cm (1.2 to 2 inches) below the acromion process (Fig. 22.26, *A*). Locate the apex of the triangle by placing four fingers across the deltoid muscle, with the top finger along the acromion process. The injection site is three finger widths below the acromion process (see Fig. 22.26, *B*).

Delegation and Collaboration

The skill of administering IM injections cannot be delegated to a UCP. The nurse instructs the UCP about the following:

- Potential medication adverse effects and immediately reporting their occurrence to the nurse
- Reporting any change in the patient's condition to the nurse

Equipment

- MAR
- Commercial prefilled syringe *or* medication prepared by nurse from an ampoule or vial into a syringe (Skill 22.1)
- 20- to 25-gauge safety needle (Public Health Agency of Canada [PHAC], 2017); length based on the injection site and the BMI, age, and body composition of the patient (see Table 22.3)
- Small gauze pad
- Alcohol swab
- Clean gloves
- Puncture-proof container

STEP	RATIONALE
ASSESSMENT	
1. Identify patient using at least two person-specific identifiers (e.g., name and date of birth or name and medical record number) according to employer policy.	
2. Throughout the procedure, the 4 moments for hand hygiene are to be implemented; hand hygiene should occur before initial patient (or patient environment) contact, before an aseptic procedure, after body fluid exposure risk, and after patient (or patient environment) contact. Additional hand hygiene should be performed when hands are visibly soiled.	
3. Check accuracy and completeness of each MAR by comparing with health care provider's prescription. Check patient's name, medication name and dosage, route of administration, and time of administration. Recopy or reprint any part of MAR that is difficult to read.	The prescription sheet is the most reliable source and only legal record of medications that the patient is to receive.
4. Assess patient's medical and medication history.	Determines need for medication or possible contraindications for medication administration.
5. Assess patient's history of allergies: known type of allergies and normal allergic reaction.	Do not prepare medication if there is a known patient allergy.
6. Review medication reference information for medication action, purpose, normal dose, adverse effects, time of peak onset, and nursing implications.	Allows you to administer medication safely and monitor patient's response to therapy.
7. Check date of expiration on medication.	Dose potency increases or decreases when outdated.
8. Observe patient's previous verbal and nonverbal responses to injection and review progress notes for information about needle fear/syncope.	Anticipating patient's anxiety allows you to use distraction to reduce pain awareness.

STEP	RATIONALE
9. Assess for contraindication to IM injections, such as muscle atrophy, reduced blood flow, or circulatory shock. Assess adequacy of adipose tissue.	Atrophied muscle absorbs medication poorly. Factors interfering with blood flow to muscles impair medication absorption.
10. Assess patient's symptoms before initiating medication therapy.	Provides information to evaluate desired effects of medication.

Critical Decision Point *Because of the documented adverse effects of IM injections, other routes of medication injection are preferred. Consider contacting health care provider for alternative route of medication administration.*

11. Assess patient's knowledge regarding medication to be received.	Provides background to determine need for patient education.

NURSING DIAGNOSES

- Acute pain
- Anxiety
- Fear
- Insufficient knowledge regarding medication administration or medication therapy

Related factors and risk factors are individualized on the basis of patient's condition or needs.

PLANNING

1. Expected outcomes following completion of procedure:	
• Patient experiences no pain or mild burning sensation at injection site.	Medications may cause minor tissue irritation.
• Patient achieves desired effect of medication with no signs of allergies or undesired effects.	Medication administered without patient injury.
• Patient explains purpose, dosage, and effects of medication.	Demonstrates learning.

IMPLEMENTATION

1. Prepare medications for one patient at a time using aseptic technique, as described in Skill 22.1 (starting at "Implementation" steps) and/or Procedural Guideline 22.1, when preparing medication.	Ensures that medication is sterile. Interruptions are a common impediment to safe, timely medication administration (Alteren et al., 2021).
2. Identify patient using at least two person-specific identifiers (e.g., name and date of birth, or name and medical record number) according to employer policy.	Ensures correct patient. Complies with Accreditation Canada's standards and improves patient safety (Accreditation Canada, 2020).
3. Take medication(s) to patient at correct time (see employer policy). During administration apply 10 rights of medication administration and complete three checks for accuracy. Close room curtain or door.	Hospital policies regarding timing of medications must consider the nature of the prescribed medication, specific clinical application, and patient needs. Provides privacy.
4. Ask patient if they have allergies.	Confirms patient's allergy history.
5. Discuss purpose, action, and possible adverse effects of each medication. Allow patient to ask any questions. Tell patient that injection will cause a slight burning or stinging sensation.	It is an ethical responsibility of nurses to provide education to patients to support informed decision making (CNA, 2017)
6. Apply clean gloves. Keep sheet or gown draped over body parts not requiring exposure.	Reduces transmission of infection. Respects patient's dignity while injection site is exposed.
7. Select appropriate site. Note integrity and size of muscle. Palpate for tenderness or hardness; avoid these areas. If patient receives frequent injections, rotate sites. Use ventrogluteal muscle if possible.	Ventrogluteal muscle is preferred injection site for adults. It is also preferred site for children of all ages (Hockenberry et al., 2024).
8. Help patient to comfortable position. Position patient depending on chosen site (e.g., sitting, or lying flat, on side, or prone).	Reduces strain on muscle and minimizes injection discomfort.

Critical Decision Point *Ensure that medical condition (e.g., circulatory shock, orthopedic surgery) does not contraindicate patient's position for injection.*

9. Relocate site using anatomical landmarks.	Injection into correct anatomical site prevents injury to nerves, bone, and blood vessels.
10. Clean site with antiseptic swab. Apply swab at centre of site and rotate outward in circular direction for about 5 cm (2 inches).	Mechanical action of swab removes secretions containing microorganisms.
11. Hold swab or gauze between third and fourth fingers of nondominant hand.	Swab or gauze remains readily accessible for use when withdrawing needle after injection.
12. Remove needle cap or sheath by pulling it straight off.	Preventing needle from touching sides of cap prevents contamination.
13. Hold syringe between thumb and forefinger of dominant hand; hold as dart, palm down.	Quick, smooth injection requires proper manipulation of syringe parts.

STEP	RATIONALE
IMPLEMENTATION	
14. Administer injection:	
a. Position ulnar side of nondominant hand just below site and pull skin laterally approximately 2.5–3.5 cm (1–1.5 inches). Hold position until medication is injected. With dominant hand, inject needle quickly at 90-degree angle into muscle (see Fig. 22.23, A).	Z-track creates zigzag path through tissues that seals needle track, avoiding leakage or tracking of medication. A quick dartlike injection reduces discomfort. Use Z-track for all IM injections (Strohfus et al., 2018).
b. *Option:* If patient's muscle mass is small, grasp body of muscle between thumb and forefingers.	Ensures that medication reaches muscle mass (Hockenberry et al., 2024).
c. After needle pierces skin, while still pulling on skin with nondominant hand, grasp lower end of syringe barrel with fingers of nondominant hand to stabilize it. Move dominant hand to end of plunger. Avoid moving syringe.	Smooth manipulation of syringe reduces discomfort from needle movement. Skin remains pulled until after medication is injected to ensure Z-track administration.
d. Inject medication slowly at rate of 10 sec/mL (Nicoll & Hesby, 2002).	Slow injection rate reduces pain and tissue trauma and reduces chance of leakage of medication back through needle track (Hockenberry et al., 2024; Nicoll & Hesby, 2002).
e. Once medication is injected, wait 10 seconds, then smoothly and steadily withdraw needle, release skin, and apply gauze gently over site (see Fig. 22.23, B).	Allows time for medication to absorb into muscle before removing syringe. Dry gauze minimizes discomfort associated with alcohol on nonintact skin.
15. Apply gentle pressure to site. *Do not massage site.* Apply bandage if needed.	Massage damages underlying tissue.
16. Help patient to comfortable position.	Gives patient sense of well-being.
17. Discard uncapped needle or needle enclosed in safety shield and attached syringe into puncture- and leak-proof receptacle.	Prevents injury to patients and health care personnel. Recapping needles increases risk of needle-stick injury (Elmi et al., 2018).
18. Remove gloves.	Reduces transmission of microorganisms.
19. Stay with patient for several minutes and observe for any allergic reactions.	Dyspnea, wheezing, and circulatory collapse are signs of severe anaphylactic reaction.
EVALUATION	
1. Return to room in 15–30 minutes and ask patient whether they feel any acute pain, burning, numbness, or tingling at injection site.	Continued discomfort may indicate injury to underlying bones or nerves.
2. Inspect site; note any bruising or induration. Apply warm compress to site.	Bruising or induration indicates complication associated with injection. Document findings and notify health care provider.
3. Observe patient's response to medication at times that correlate with onset, peak, and duration of action.	IM medications are absorbed rapidly. Adverse effects of parenteral medications develop rapidly.
4. Use **teach-back:** "I want to be sure I explained to you the purpose of this intramuscular injection. Explain to me why you are receiving the injection and what you might expect to feel during the injection." Develop a revised teaching plan if patient or caregiver is unable to teach back correctly.	Determines patient's and caregiver's level of understanding of topic (Yen & Leasure, 2019).

Unexpected Outcomes	Related Interventions
1. Patient indicates localized pain or continued burning sensation at injection site, indicating potential injury to nerve or vessels.	• Assess injection site. • Notify patient's health care provider.
2. Patient displays adverse reaction with signs of urticaria, eczema, pruritus, wheezing, and dyspnea.	• Follow employer policy or guidelines for appropriate response to allergic reactions (e.g., administration of antihistamine such as diphenhydramine or epinephrine). • Notify patient's health care provider immediately. • Add allergy information to patient's record.

Communication and Documentation

- Immediately after administration, record medication, dose, route, site, time, and date given on MAR in progress notes in EHR or chart. Correctly sign MAR according to employer policy.
- Document patient teaching, validation of understanding, and patient's response to medication in progress notes.
- Document any undesirable or adverse effects from medication and report these to the health care provider.

DOCUMENTATION EXAMPLE

Patient presented ambulatory to clinic for once-monthly vitamin B12 injection. Denies acute concerns, denies needle fear. Patient accurately able to explain purpose of B12 to this writer; 1000 mcg B12 administered IM to L deltoid. No bleeding noted to injection site. No SOB, hives, or other sign of allergic reaction after 20 minutes monitoring post-injection. Patient left ambulatory with plan to return on June 15, 2024, at 0900 hours for next B12 injection.

Special Considerations

Teaching

- Patients who require regular injections (e.g., vitamin B12) need to learn techniques of self-administration. Teach a family member or caregiver injection techniques and the importance of rotating sites to decrease the risk of hypertrophy.
- Instruct patient and caregiver to observe injection sites for complications and immediately report complications to the health care provider.
- Instruct patient and caregiver to observe for effectiveness of medication and adverse reactions and report ineffectiveness of medication and adverse reactions to the health care provider.
- Have patient perform several return demonstrations of medication preparation to validate that learning has taken place.

Pediatric

- Children can be very anxious about or fearful of needles. Help with proper positioning and holding the child is sometimes necessary. Distraction such as blowing bubbles and pressure at the injection site before giving the injection can help alleviate anxiety (Hockenberry et al., 2024).

Gerontological

- Older persons may have decreased muscle mass, which reduces medication absorption from IM injections. In addition, older persons may have loss of muscle tone and strength, which impairs mobility and places them at high risk for falls from guarding an injection site.

Care in the Community: Home Management

- Self-administration of an IM injection is difficult, especially at the ventrogluteal site. Teach a caregiver to identify and administer injections at this site.
- Instruct adult patients who require frequent injections to apply EMLA (eutectic mixture of local anaesthetics) cream to the injection site before administration.
- Instruct patients about the need for safe disposal of syringes and needles (see Skill 22.3, "Care in the Community: Home Management" section).
- See Skill 42.1 for information about modifying safety risks in the home.

✦ SKILL 22.6 Administering Intravenous Medications by Direct Route

NSO *Nursing Skills Online Administration of Parenteral Medications: Intravenous Medications Module 8 / Lesson 3*

In the past, nurses often mixed medications into large volumes of IV fluids (500 to 1 000 mL). However, today's safety standards and evidence-informed practice no longer support this practice on a routine basis (ISMP, 2011). Many patient safety risks, such as incorrect calculation, poor aseptic technique, incorrect labelling, pump programming errors, lack of medication knowledge, and mix-up with another medication, occur when nurses have to prepare medications in IV containers on patient care units. There are a number of current best practices for preparation and administration of IV medication (Box 22.6).

IV direct (formerly called IV push) is one method of administering medication that is becoming more common on patient care units. It introduces a concentrated dose of a medication directly into a vein by way of existing IV access. IV direct usually requires small volumes of fluid, which is an advantage for patients who are at risk for fluid overload. Administering IV direct medications is common in emergencies when nurses need to deliver a fast-acting medication quickly. Because these medications act quickly, it is essential to monitor patients closely for adverse reactions. Employer policies identify specific medications that nurses can administer via IV direct and other IV routes. These policies are based on the medication, compatibility and availability of staff, and type of monitoring equipment available. There are advantages and disadvantages to administering IV direct medications (Box 22.7).

IV direct is a dangerous method of administering medications because it allows no time to correct errors. Administering an IV direct medication too quickly can cause death. Therefore, be very careful in calculating the correct amount of the medication to give and the rate of administration (see employer policy or manufacturer directions). Always ensure the reversal medication is on hand for the medication you are about to administer via IV direct (ISMP, 2022). In addition, IV direct administration may cause direct irritation to the lining of blood vessels; thus, always confirm placement of the IV catheter or needle. Never give IV direct if the insertion site appears edematous or reddened or if the IV fluids do not flow at the prescribed rate. Accidental injection of some medications into tissues surrounding a vein can cause pain, abscesses, and tissue necrosis.

Verify the rate of administration of IV direct medication using the employer parenteral administration manual or a medication reference manual. The Canadian Vascular Access Association (CVAA, 2019) has identified the following strategies to reduce harm from IV direct medications:

- Do NOT dilute IV direct medications unless recommended by the manufacturer or by pharmacist.
- Use appropriately sized syringe to administer dose.
- Administer at the rate recommended by the manufacturer, employer policy, or reference literature.
- Flush with saline before and after medication administration. The saline flush after medication administration should be at the same rate as the medication administration rate, since the flush is moving medication that was left in the patient's IV catheter into the patient's blood stream.
- Appropriately label syringes containing prepared medication.
- Do not use unlabelled syringes unless medication was prepared and given immediately at the bedside.

Verify the rate of administration of IV direct medication and compatibility using employer guidelines or a medication reference

BOX 22.6

Best Practices for Administration of Intravenous Solutions and Medications

- Use standardized concentrations and dosages of medication.
- Use standardized procedures for prescribing, preparing, and administering intravenous (IV) medications.
- Administer solutions and medications prepared and dispensed from the pharmacy or commercially prepared when possible.
- Never prepare high-alert medications (e.g., heparin, dopamine, dobutamine, nitroglycerin, potassium, antibiotics, or magnesium) on a patient care unit.*
- Use standardized infusion concentrations of "high-alert" medications.
- Limit the use of add-on devices to reduce risk of contamination and accidental disconnection.
- Standardize the storage of IV medications.
- Do not add medications to infusing containers of IV solutions.
- Use the mnemonic CATS PRRR to help remember safety checks for administering IV medications: *C*, compatibilities; *A*, allergies; *T*, tubing correct; *S*, site checked; *P*, pump safety checked; *R*, right rate; *R*, release clamps; *R*, return and reassess the patient.
- Use standardized label practices. Bold patient name, generic medication name, and patient-specific dose. Remember to include the date and time the medication was prepared, who prepared it, and how long it will remain stable.
- Perform a medication reconciliation at each care transition (e.g., transfer, discharge) and when a new medication is prescribed.
- Correctly use technology such as intelligent-infusion devices, bar code–assisted medication administration, and electronic medication administration record (MAR).

***Note:** While this is best practice, it may not be feasible in some settings for medications to be prepared in the pharmacy (e.g., antibiotics are usually prepared on unit in the emergency department or when the patient has been prescribed a STAT dose on an inpatient unit).

Adapted from Infusion Nurses Society. (2016). Infusion therapy standards of practice. *Journal of Intravenous Nursing, 39*(1S); Institute for Safe Medication Practices. (2010). *Guidelines for standard order sets*. https://www.ismp.org/guidelines/standard-order-sets; Institute for Safe Medication Practices. (2019). *Guidelines for safe electronic communication of medication information*. https://www.ismp.org/resources/guidelines-safe-electronic-communication-medication-information

BOX 22.7

Advantages and Disadvantages of the Intravenous Direct Route

Advantages

- Rapid onset of medication effects (useful in patients experiencing critical or emergent health problems).
- Medications can be prepared quickly and given over a shorter time than by secondary IV line infusion.
- Doses of short-acting medications can be titrated on the basis of a patient's needs and responses to the medication therapy; this is important for infants, children, and older patients.
- Method provides a more accurate dose of medication delivered because no medication is left in the IV line.

Disadvantages

- Not all medications can be delivered IV direct.
- Higher risk of infusion reactions; some are mild to severe because the medication action peaks quickly.
- When giving medication quickly (e.g., less than 1 minute), there is very little opportunity to stop the injection if an adverse reaction occurs.
- Increased risk of infiltration and phlebitis, especially if using a highly concentrated medication, a small peripheral vein, or a short venous access device.
- Hypersensitivity reaction can cause an immediate or delayed systemic reaction to a medication, requiring supportive measures.

manual. Typically, the rate will be given as the dose of medication that can be given per *minute*. It can be very difficult to mentally estimate how fast that is in practical terms. However, converting this rate to a smaller unit of volume (e.g., *tenths of a millilitre*) and shorter unit of time (i.e., *seconds*) allows accurate control of the push rate and avoids the most common error of pushing too fast. For example, if the reference manual states the medication must be given over 1 minute, and the medication is supplied as 20 mg/2 mL, calculate the rate as follows:

$$\frac{\text{mL}}{\text{second (sec)}} = \frac{2\text{ mL}}{1} \times \frac{1}{60\text{ sec}} = \frac{2\text{ mL}}{60\text{ sec}} = \frac{1\text{ mL}}{30\text{ sec}} = \frac{0.5\text{ mL}}{15\text{ sec}} = \frac{0.1\text{ mL}}{3\text{ sec}}$$

Now you know that only 0.1 mL of medication should be going in every 3 seconds, and it will be easier to control the rate and notice whether you are injecting the medication too quickly.

Understand the purpose of the medication and any potential adverse reactions related to the rate and route of administration. Some IV medications can only be given by IV direct safely when a patient is being monitored continuously for dysrhythmias, blood pressure changes, or other adverse effects. Therefore, you can administer some medications via IV direct only in specific areas within a health care facility (e.g., critical care unit). Confirm employer policy regarding requirements for special monitoring.

IV direct medications are given through either an existing continuous IV infusion or an intermittent venous access (commonly called a *saline lock*). A saline lock is an IV catheter with a small "well" or chamber covered by a rubber cap. An IV catheter can be converted into a lock by inserting a special rubber-seal injection cap into the end of the catheter (see Chapter 29). Use of a lock saves time by eliminating constant monitoring of an IV line. It also offers better mobility, safety, and comfort for patients by eliminating the need for a continuous IV line. After you administer a medication by IV direct through an intermittent venous access, flush with a normal saline solution at *the same rate you administered the medication* to keep the IV line patent and ensure the full dose of medication was received.

Delegation and Collaboration

The skill of administering medications by IV direct cannot be delegated to a UCP. The nurse instructs the UCP about the following:

- Potential medication actions and adverse effects of the medications and immediately reporting their occurrence to the nurse.
- Reporting any patient complaints of moisture or discomfort around IV insertion site.
- Obtaining any required vital signs and reporting them to the nurse.

Equipment

- Watch with second hand
- Clean gloves
- Antiseptic swab
- Medication in vial or ampoule
- Properly sized syringes for medication and saline flush with needleless device or safety needle (21 to 25 gauge)
- IV lock: Prefilled normal saline flush or vial of normal saline flush solution (CVAA, 2019). If employer continues to use heparin flush, use the lowest concentration available (usually 10 units/mL; CVAA, 2019); follow employer policy.
- MAR
- Puncture-proof container

STEP	RATIONALE
ASSESSMENT	
1. Identify patient using at least two person-specific identifiers (e.g., name and date of birth or name and medical record number) according to employer policy.	
2. Throughout the procedure, the 4 moments for hand hygiene are to be implemented; hand hygiene should occur before initial patient (or patient environment) contact, before an aseptic procedure, after body fluid exposure risk, and after patient (or patient environment) contact. Additional hand hygiene should be performed when hands are visibly soiled.	
3. Check accuracy and completeness of each MAR by comparing with health care provider's prescription. Check patient's name, medication name and dosage, route of administration, and time of administration. Recopy or reprint any part of MAR that is difficult to read.	The prescription sheet is the most reliable source and only legal record of medications that the patient is to receive.
4. Assess patient's medical and medication history.	Identifies need for medication.
5. Review medication reference information for medication action, purpose, adverse effects, normal dose, time of peak onset, how slowly to give medication, and nursing implications, such as need to dilute medication or administer it through a filter. a. Calculate the IV direct rate in mL/sec.	Knowledge of medication allows you to give it safely and monitor patient's response to therapy.
6. If giving medication through an existing IV line, determine compatibility of medication with IV fluids and any additives within IV solution.	IV medication is not always compatible with IV solution and/or additives, and a new site may need to be initiated.
7. Assess condition of IV needle insertion site for signs of infiltration or phlebitis.	Do not administer medication if site is edematous or inflamed.
8. Assess patency of patient's existing IV infusion line or saline lock (see Chapter 29).	For medication to reach venous circulation effectively, IV line must be patent and fluids must infuse easily.
9. Check patient's history of medication allergies: known allergens and normal allergic response.	IV direct administration delivers medication rapidly. Allergic response is immediate.
10. Assess patient's symptoms before initiating medication therapy.	Provides information to evaluate desired effects of medication.
11. Assess patient's understanding of purpose of medication therapy.	Provides background to determine need for patient education.

NURSING DIAGNOSES

- Acute pain
- Insufficient knowledge regarding medication administration or medication therapy

Related factors and risk factors are individualized on the basis of the patient's condition or needs.

PLANNING

STEP	RATIONALE
1. Expected outcomes following completion of procedure:	
• Patient experiences no medication adverse effects or allergic reactions.	Medication administered safely with desired therapeutic effect achieved.
• IV site remains intact without signs of swelling or inflammation or symptoms of tenderness at site.	Medication infuses without complications to IV site and surrounding tissues.
• Patient explains purpose and adverse effects of medication.	Demonstrates learning.

IMPLEMENTATION

STEP	RATIONALE
1. Prepare medications for one patient at a time using aseptic technique, as described in Skill 22.1 (starting at "Implementation" steps) and/or Procedural Guideline 22.1, when preparing medication.	Ensures that medication is sterile. Preventing distractions reduces medication preparation errors. Use NIZ when possible (McMahon, 2017).

Critical Decision Point *Current guidelines recommend that medications NOT be diluted unless specified by the manufacturer and peer-reviewed literature* (CVAA, 2019). *Diluting medications when it is not required adds to the complexity of administering the medication and increases the risk of error* (ISMP, 2015).

STEP	RATIONALE
2. Identify patient using at least two person-specific identifiers (e.g., name and date of birth, or name and medical record number) according to employer policy.	Ensures correct patient. Complies with Accreditation Canada's standards and improves patient safety (Accreditation Canada, 2020).

STEP	RATIONALE

IMPLEMENTATION

STEP	RATIONALE
3. Take medication(s) to patient at correct time (see employer policy). During administration, apply 10 rights of medication administration and complete three checks for accuracy. Close room curtain or door.	Hospital policies regarding timing of medications must consider the nature of the prescribed medication, specific clinical application, and patient needs (ISMP, 2011). Provides privacy.
4. Ask patient if they have allergies.	Confirms patient's allergy history.
5. Discuss purpose, action, and possible adverse effects of each medication. Allow patient to ask any questions. Explain that you will give medication through existing IV line. Encourage patient to report symptoms of discomfort at IV site.	Keeping patient informed of planned therapies minimizes anxiety. Patients who verbalize pain at IV site help in detecting IV infiltrations early, lessening damage to surrounding tissues.
6. Apply clean gloves.	Reduces transmission of infection.
7. Set up IV direct (*existing IV line*):	
a. Select injection port of IV tubing closest to patient. Use needleless injection port.	Administering IV direct medications by the closest port to the patient is current best practice (CVAA, 2019). Needleless systems reduce the risk of needle-stick injury, ensure a secure connection, and decrease risk of bacterial contamination (CVAA, 2019).

Critical Decision Point *Never administer IV medications through tubing that is infusing blood, blood products, or parenteral nutrition solutions.*

STEP	RATIONALE
b. Vigorously scrub injection port with disinfectant swab, such as 70% alcohol (CVAA, 2019). Allow to dry.	Prevents transfer of microorganisms during blunt cannula insertion.
c. Connect syringe to IV line: Insert needleless tip of syringe containing medication through centre of port (see Step 7c illustration).	Prevents introduction of microorganisms. Prevents damage to port diaphragm and possible leakage from site.
d. Occlude IV line by pinching tubing just above injection port (see Step 7d illustration).	Final check ensures that medication is being delivered into bloodstream.

Critical Decision Point *If IV site does not show signs of infiltration and IV fluid is infusing without difficulty, give IV direct.*

STEP	RATIONALE
e. Keep the tubing above the injection port occluded and inject medication within the recommended amount of time. Use watch to time administrations (see Step 7e illustration).	Ensures safe medication infusion. Rapid injection of IV medication can be fatal.

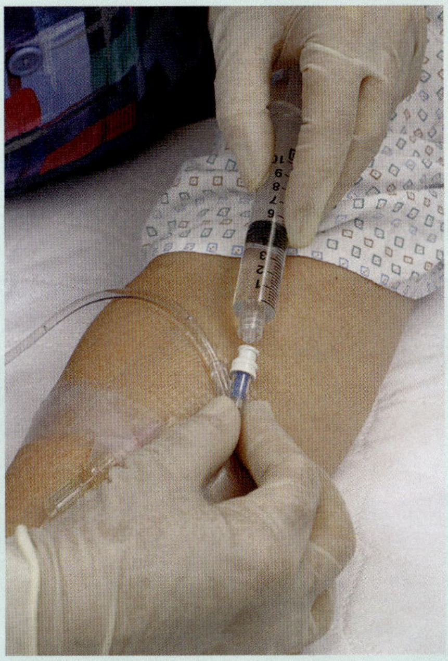

STEP 7C Connect syringe to IV line with needleless blunt cannula tip.

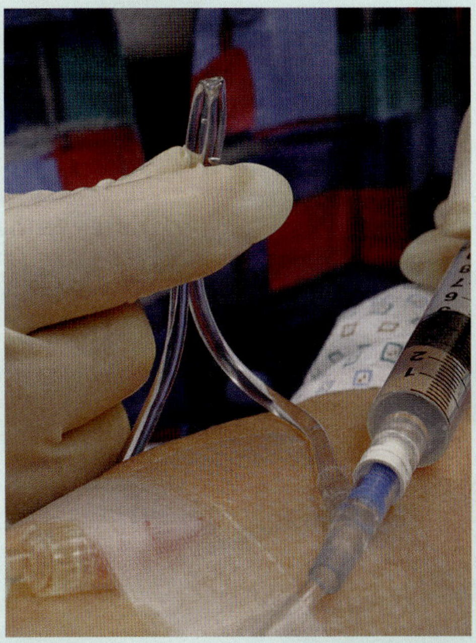

STEP 7D Occlude IV tubing above injection port.

STEP	RATIONALE

IMPLEMENTATION

STEP	RATIONALE
f. After injecting medication, disconnect syringe, flush with another 10 mL of normal saline at *same rate* as medication was administered, and recheck IV fluid infusion rate.	IV direct administration may alter rate of fluid infusion. Rapid fluid infusion can cause circulatory fluid overload.
g. If IV medication is incompatible with IV fluids, stop IV fluids, clamp IV line, and flush with 10 mL of normal saline or sterile water (see employer policy). Then give IV direct medication over appropriate amount of time and flush with another 10 mL of normal saline at *same rate* as medication was administered.	Allows medication to be administered without risks associated with IV incompatibilities. Ensure that employer guidelines permit flushing lines with incompatible medications. A new site may need to be initiated.
h. If IV line currently hanging is a medication, disconnect it and administer IV direct medication as outlined in Step 9. Verify employer policy for stopping IV fluids or continuous IV medications. If unable to stop IV infusion, start new IV site (see Chapter 29) and administer medication using IV direct (IV lock) method.	Avoids giving patient a sudden bolus of medication in existing IV line.
8. Set up IV direct (*saline lock*):	
a. Prepare flush solutions according to employer policy.	
(1) *Saline flush method (preferred method)*: Prepare two 10-mL barrel syringes filled with 2–3 mL of normal saline (0.9%) or use prefilled normal saline syringes if available.	Normal saline is effective in keeping IV locks patent and is compatible with wide range of medications.
(2) Heparin flush method (refer to employer policy).	
b. Administer medication:	
(1) Scrub needleless port of main IV line vigorously with disinfectant swab for at least 15 seconds, then allow to dry (CVAA, 2019).	Prevents transfer of microorganisms during needle insertion.

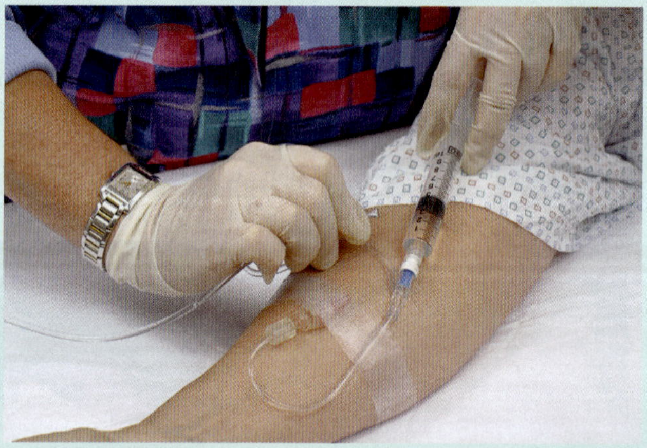

STEP 7E Use watch to time IV direct medication.

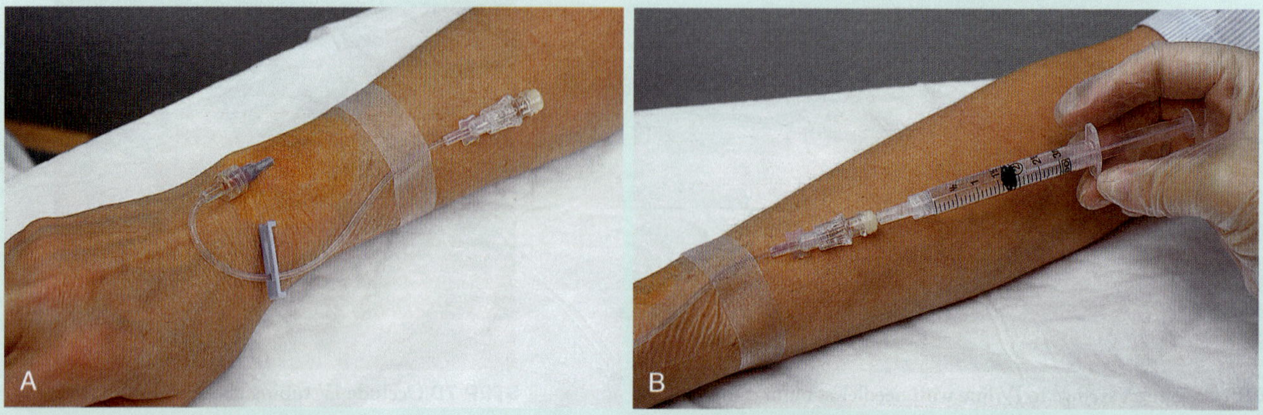

STEP 8B(2) A, IV catheter with saline lock adapter. B, Syringe inserted into injection port.

STEP	RATIONALE
IMPLEMENTATION	
(2) Insert needleless tip of syringe with 0.9% normal saline through centre of injection port of IV lock (see Step 8b[2] illustrations).	
(3) Pull back gently on syringe plunger and check for blood return.	Indicates whether catheter is in vein and is patent.
(4) Flush IV catheter with normal saline using a pulsatile technique (stop–start) to create turbulence (CVAA, 2019).	Clears needle and reservoir of blood. Flushing without difficulty indicates patent IV line.

Critical Decision Point *Carefully observe the area of skin above the IV catheter. Note any puffiness or swelling as the IV site is flushed, which could indicate infiltration, requiring removal of catheter. Note that in the case of smaller-gauge IV needles, blood return sometimes is not aspirated even if IV line is patent.*

STEP	RATIONALE
(5) Remove saline-filled syringe.	
(6) Scrub injection port vigorously with disinfectant swab for at least 15 seconds, then allow to dry (CVAA, 2019).	Prevents transmission of microorganisms.
(7) Insert needleless tip of syringe containing prepared medication through injection port of IV lock.	Allows administration of medication.
(8) Inject medication within recommended amount of time (calculate rate in mL per 10- or 15-second blocks). Use watch to time administration.	Many medication errors are associated with IV direct medications being administered too quickly. Following guidelines for IV direct rates helps promote patient safety.
(9) After administering medication, disconnect syringe.	
(10) Scrub injection port vigorously with disinfectant swab for at least 15 seconds, then allow to dry (CVAA, 2019).	Prevents transmission of microorganisms.
(11) Flush injection port.	
(a) Attach syringe with normal saline and inject flush at same rate that medication was delivered.	Flushing IV line with saline prevents occlusion of IV access device and ensures that all medication is delivered. Flushing IV catheter at same rate as medication ensures that any medication remaining within IV needle is delivered at the correct rate.
9. Dispose of needles and syringes in puncture- and leak-proof container.	Prevents needle-stick injuries.
10. Stay with patient for several minutes and observe for any allergic reactions.	Dyspnea, wheezing, and circulatory collapse are signs of anaphylactic reaction.
11. Remove gloves.	Reduces transmission of microorganisms.
EVALUATION	
1. Observe patient closely for adverse reactions during administration and for several minutes thereafter.	IV medications act rapidly.
2. Observe IV site during injection for sudden swelling and for 48 hours after IV direct.	Swelling indicates infiltration into tissues surrounding vein. Signs of infiltration may not occur for 48 hours.
3. Assess patient's status after giving medication to evaluate effectiveness of the medication.	Some IV direct medications can cause rapid changes in patient's physiological status. Some medications require careful monitoring and assessment and possibly future laboratory testing (e.g., vasopressors and antiarrhythmics require blood pressure and heart rate monitoring, and heparin requires laboratory studies after administration to determine therapeutic levels).
4. Use **teach-back**: "I want to be sure I explained to you why you are receiving this IV medication. Can you explain to me what the medication is for and when to call the nurse?" Develop a revised teaching plan if patient or caregiver is unable to teach back correctly.	Determines patient's and caregiver's level of understanding of topic (Yen & Leasure, 2019).

Unexpected Outcomes	Related Interventions
1. Patient develops adverse reaction to medication.	• Stop delivering medication immediately and follow employer policy or guidelines for appropriate response to allergic reaction (e.g., administration of antihistamine such as diphenhydramine or epinephrine) and reporting of adverse drug reactions. • Notify health care provider of adverse effects immediately. • Add allergy information to patient's record.
2. IV medication is incompatible with IV fluids (e.g., IV fluid becomes cloudy in tubing) (see employer policy).	• Stop IV fluids and clamp IV line. • Flush IV line with 10 mL of 0.9% sodium chloride or sterile water. • Give IV direct medications over appropriate amount of time. • Flush with another 10 mL of 0.9% sodium chloride or sterile water at same rate as medication was administered. • Restart IV fluids with new tubing at prescribed rate. • If unable to stop IV infusion, initiate IV access at a new site (see Chapter 29) and administer medication using IV direct (IV lock) method.
3. IV site shows symptoms of infiltration or phlebitis (see Chapter 29).	• Stop IV infusion immediately or discontinue access device and restart at another site. • Determine how much damage IV medication can produce in SUBCUT tissue. • Provide IV extravasation care as indicated by employer policy. Use a medication reference, and consult pharmacist to determine appropriate follow-up care.

Communication and Documentation

- Immediately document medication administration, including medication, dose, route, time instilled, and date and time administered, on MAR in progress notes in EHR or chart. Include initials or signature.
- Document patient teaching, validation of understanding, and patient's response to medication in progress notes.
- Report any adverse reactions to patient's health care provider. Patient's response sometimes indicates need for additional medical therapy.
- Document patient's medication response.

Special Considerations

Teaching

- Teach patient and caregiver that effects of IV direct medications occur rapidly. Explain reasons for giving medication slowly and teach signs of adverse effects.

Pediatric

- The therapeutic dosage of IV direct medications for infants and children is often small and difficult to prepare accurately, even with a tuberculin syringe. These medications need to be infused slowly and in small volumes because of the risk for fluid volume overload (Hockenberry et al., 2024). Carefully follow employer policy when administering medications via IV direct to pediatric patients.

Gerontological

- The renal and metabolic systems in older persons do not function as efficiently because of the aging process. Older persons may tolerate IV direct medications if they are given over longer periods of time.

Care in the Community: Home Management

- IV direct medications are frequently given in the home. Use interprofessional collaboration (e.g., nurses, pharmacists, physicians) in the care of these patients. Patients and caregivers who are responsible for managing IV medications need to understand all aspects of administration safety. Adequate eyesight and manual dexterity are necessary to manipulate the syringe. Patients need to understand their venous access device, rate at which to give medications, and how to flush their access device. Patients need to store their medications safely and dispose of their IV supplies, and they should know whom to contact in case of an emergency.

SKILL 22.7 Administering Intravenous Medications by Intermittent Infusion

NSO Nursing Skills Online Administration of Parenteral Medications: Intravenous Medications Module 8 / Lesson 2

One method of administering IV medications uses small volumes (25 to 250 mL) of compatible IV fluids infused over a desired period of time. This method reduces the risk of rapid dose infusion and provides independence for patients. Patients must have an established IV line that is kept patent by either a continuous infusion or intermittent flushes of normal saline. Nurses can administer intermittent infusion of medication using any of the following methods:

- *Secondary IV line ("piggyback"), controlled by gravity:* A small (25- to 250-mL) IV bag (mini-bag) is connected to a short tubing line that connects to the *upper* Y-port of a primary infusion line. This setup is sometimes called a *piggyback* because the small bag or bottle is set *higher* than the primary infusion bag. In the secondary line setup, the primary line does not infuse when a compatible secondary line medication is infusing. The port of the primary IV line contains a back-check valve that automatically stops the flow of the primary infusion once the secondary infusion flows. After the secondary solution infuses and the solution within the tubing falls below the level of the primary infusion drip chamber, the back-check valve opens, and the primary infusion starts to flow again. For this method to be used safely, the nurse must calculate the rate of infusion using the drip rate formula as follows:

$$\frac{\text{Volume to be infused (mL)}}{\text{Time required for infusion (min)}} \times \text{Drop factor (gtt/min)}$$

The drip rate formula converts the volume of medication being administered from *millilitres* to *drops*; note that time must be measured in minutes. The drop factor is printed on the IV tubing package and refers to the size of the drops created by the catheter inside the IV spike that fall into the drip chamber. If the primary and secondary line tubing have different drop factors, use the drop factor from the tubing directly connected to the medication (i.e., the secondary line tubing).

- *Secondary IV line ("piggyback"), volumetric infusion pump*: Similar to the secondary IV line that is controlled by gravity, but here the primary IV line is loaded into a battery-operated pump, which controls the rate.
- *Syringe (also called mini-infusion) pump*: The syringe pump is battery operated and delivers medication in very small amounts of fluid (5 to 60 mL) within controlled infusion times using standard syringes (Fig. 22.27).
- *Volume-control administration:* These administration sets (e.g., Volutrol, Buretrol) are small (50- to 150-mL) containers that attach just below the primary infusion bag to prevent overdoses of medication. With advancements in volumetric pump technology, these have become less common in Canada. Follow manufacturer directions for setup and priming sets.

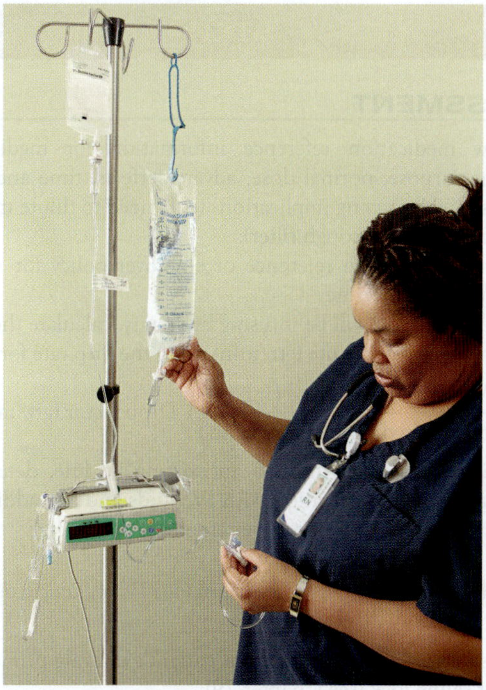

FIG 22.27 Syringe pump.

Delegation and Collaboration

The skill of administering IV medications by intermittent infusion cannot be delegated to a UCP. The nurse instructs the UCP about the following:

- Potential medication actions and adverse effects and immediately reporting their occurrence to the nurse.
- Reporting any patient indications of moisture or discomfort around IV insertion site.
- Reporting any change in patient's condition or vital signs to the nurse.

Equipment

- Adhesive tape *(optional)*
- Disinfectant swab (e.g., 70% alcohol)
- Clean gloves
- IV pole
- MAR
- Puncture-proof container
- Medication prepared in a mini-bag or syringe (Skill 22.1)
- Prefilled syringe of normal saline flush solution (for saline lock only)
- Secondary line IV tubing set with blunt-end (needleless) cannula attachment
- Primary IV line
- Infusion pump, if available

STEP	RATIONALE
ASSESSMENT	
1. Identify patient using at least two person-specific identifiers (e.g., name and date of birth or name and medical record number) according to employer policy.	
2. Throughout the procedure, the 4 moments for hand hygiene are to be implemented; hand hygiene should occur before initial patient (or patient environment) contact, before an aseptic procedure, after body fluid exposure risk, and after patient (or patient environment) contact. Additional hand hygiene should be performed when hands are visibly soiled.	
3. Check accuracy and completeness of each MAR by comparing with health care provider prescription. Check patient's name, medication name and dosage, route of administration, and time of administration. Recopy or reprint any part of MAR that is difficult to read.	The prescription sheet is the most reliable source and only legal record of medications that the patient is to receive.
4. Assess patient's medical and medication history.	Determines need for medication or possible contraindications for medication administration.
5. Assess patient's history of allergies: known type of allergens and normal allergic reaction.	IV administration of medication may cause rapid response. Allergic response is immediate.

STEP	RATIONALE

ASSESSMENT

STEP	RATIONALE
6. Review medication reference information for medication action, purpose, normal dose, adverse effects, time and peak of onset, and nursing implications (e.g., need to dilute medication, administer through filter).	Allows you to administer medication safely and monitor patient's response to therapy.
7. Refer to medication reference or employer policy for recommended infusion time. If the medication will be infusing by gravity, calculate the drip rate in drops per minute (gtt/min) using the drip rate formula: $$\frac{\text{Volume to be infused (mL)}}{\text{Time required for infusion (min)}} \times \text{Drop factor (gtt/min)}$$	Allows medication to be safely administered.
8. If giving medication through an existing IV line, determine compatibility of medication with IV fluids and any additional additives within IV solution per employer policy.	IV medication is sometimes not compatible with IV solution and/or additives.

Critical Decision Point *Never administer IV medications through tubing that is infusing blood, blood products, or parenteral nutrition solutions.*

STEP	RATIONALE
9. Assess patency and placement of patient's existing primary IV line or saline lock (see Chapter 29).	Do not administer medication if site is edematous or inflamed.

Critical Decision Point *If patient's IV catheter is saline locked, scrub injection port vigorously with disinfectant swab for at least 15 seconds, then allow to dry. Assess the patency of the IV catheter by attempting to aspirate blood, then flush with 2–3 mL of sterile sodium chloride and again attempt to aspirate blood* (CVAA, 2019).

STEP	RATIONALE
10. Assess patient's symptoms before initiating medication therapy.	Provides information to evaluate desired effects of medication.
11. Assess patient's knowledge of medication.	Provides background to determine need for patient education.

NURSING DIAGNOSES

- Insufficient knowledge regarding medication administration or medication therapy
- Potential for imbalanced fluid volume
- Potential for ineffective health maintenance

Related factors and risk factors are individualized on the basis of patient's condition or needs.

PLANNING

STEP	RATIONALE
1. Expected outcomes following completion of procedure:	
• Patient experiences no adverse reactions.	Medication was administered safely with desired therapeutic effect.
• Medication infuses within desired time frame.	IV line remains patent.
• IV site remains intact without signs of swelling or inflammation or symptoms of tenderness at site.	Fluid infuses into vein, not tissues.
• Patient explains medication purposes, action, adverse effects, and dosage.	Demonstrates learning.

IMPLEMENTATION

STEP	RATIONALE
1. Prepare medications for one patient at a time using aseptic technique, as described in Skill 22.1 (starting at "Implementation" steps) and/or Procedural Guideline 22.1, when preparing medication.	Ensures that medication is sterile. Preventing distractions reduces medication preparation errors.
2. Identify patient using at least two person-specific identifiers (e.g., name and date of birth, or name and medical record number) according to employer policy.	Ensures correct patient. Complies with Accreditation Canada's standards and improves patient safety (Accreditation Canada, 2020).
3. Take medication(s) to patient at correct time (see employer policy). During preparation and administration apply 10 rights of medication administration and complete three checks for accuracy. Close room curtain or door.	Hospital policies regarding timing of medications must consider the nature of the prescribed medication, specific clinical application, and patient needs (ISMP, 2011). Closing curtain/door provides privacy.
4. Ask patient if they have allergies.	Confirms patient's allergy history.

STEP	RATIONALE

IMPLEMENTATION

STEP	RATIONALE
5. Discuss purpose, action, and possible adverse effects of each medication. Allow patient to ask any questions. Explain that you will give medication through existing IV line. Encourage patient to report symptoms of discomfort at site.	Keeping patient informed of planned therapies minimizes anxiety. Patients who verbalize pain at IV site help in detecting IV infiltrations early, lessening damage to surrounding tissues.
6. Ensure patient has a primary line ("backup bag") hanging (see Chapter 29) for the duration of medication administration.	Allows tubing to be flushed of medication to prevent patient missing part of dose.
7. Administer medication by IV infusion.	
a. Option A: Secondary line:	
(1) Connect infusion tubing to medication bag (see Chapter 29).	Allows priming of tubing.
(2) Squeeze the drip chamber to fill it, and prime the tubing by opening regulator flow clamp. Once tubing is primed (all the air is removed by fluid), close clamp and cap end of tubing.	Filling infusion tubing with solution and freeing air bubbles prevent air embolus.
(3) Hang medication bag (see Step 7a[3] illustration) above level of primary fluid bag. (Use hook to lower main bag.)	Height of fluid bag affects rate of flow to patient, even when using an infusion pump (depending on manufacturer).
(4) Scrub needleless port of upper Y-port of primary infusion line vigorously with disinfectant swab for at least 15 seconds (CVAA, 2019), allow to dry, and insert cannula tip of secondary line infusion tubing (see Step 7a[4] illustrations).	Vigorous scrubbing to decrease bacterial contamination is the current recommended best practice (CVAA, 2019). Use needleless connections to prevent needle-stick injuries, ensure a secure connection, and decrease risk of bacterial contamination by maintaining a closed system (CVAA, 2019).

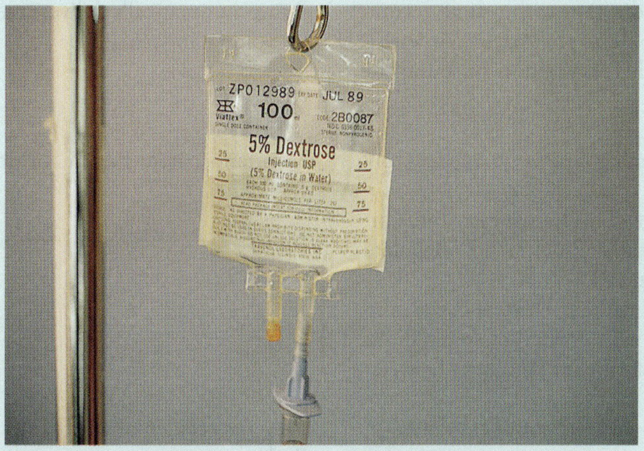

STEP 7A(3) Small-volume mini-bag for secondary IV line infusion.

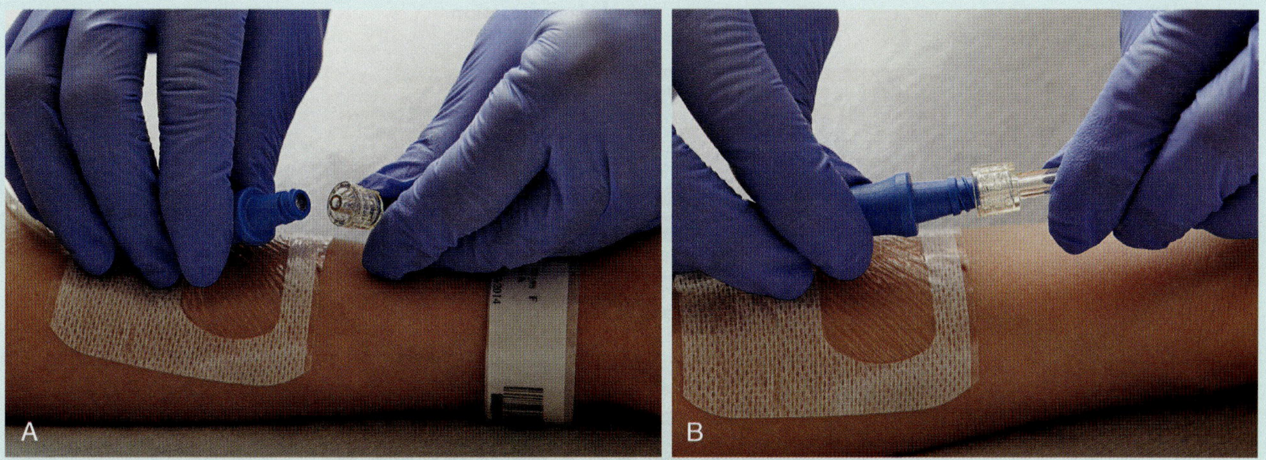

STEP 7A(4) A, Needleless lock cannula system. B, Blunt-ended cannula inserts into port and locks.

STEP	RATIONALE
IMPLEMENTATION	
(5) Regulate the flow rate by adjusting the regulator clamp on the primary IV line (the regulator clamp on the secondary line should be open all the way) to ensure the rate matches what you calculated earlier. If infusing by IV pump, set the rate advised by the medication manual or employer policy (mL/hr) *or* use the smart pump medication library to program the rate.	Provides slow, safe, intermittent infusion of medication and maintains therapeutic blood levels.
b. Option B: Syringe-pump administration:	
(1) Connect syringe to syringe-pump tubing; remove end cap of tubing.	Special tubing designed to fit syringe delivers medication to main IV line.
(2) Carefully apply pressure to syringe plunger, allowing tubing to fill with medication.	Ensures that tubing is free of air bubbles to prevent air embolus.
(3) Place syringe into syringe pump (see Step 7b[3] illustration) (follow product directions).	Secure placement is needed for proper infusion.
(4) Connect end of mini-infusion tubing to primary IV line or saline lock:	Establishes route for IV medication to enter main IV line.
(i) *Existing IV line:* Scrub needleless port on main IV line with disinfectant swab, allow to dry, and insert tip of mini-infusion tubing through centre of port.	Needleless connections reduce risk of accidental needle-stick injuries.
(ii) *Normal saline lock:* Follow Steps 8a(1) through 8b(6) in Skill 22.6 to flush and prepare lock. Scrub port with disinfectant swab, allow to dry, and insert tip of tubing.	
(5) Set pump to deliver medication within time recommended by employer policy, pharmacist, or medication reference manual. Press button on pump to begin infusion.	Pump automatically delivers medication at safe, constant rate based on volume in syringe.
8. Once medication has infused:	
a. Disconnect and discard secondary line or syringe and tubing as per employer policy.	Maintains patent IV line for primary IV fluids.
b. *If a primary infusion is running:* Check flow rate. Infusion automatically begins to flow once pump stops. Regulate infusion to desired rate as needed.	
c. *Normal saline lock:* Disconnect tubing, clean port with disinfectant, and flush IV line with 2–3 mL of sterile 0.9% sodium chloride. Maintain sterility of IV tubing between intermittent infusions.	
9. Dispose of supplies in puncture- and leak-proof container.	Prevents accidental needle-sticks.
10. Remove gloves.	Reduces transmission of microorganisms.
11. Stay with patient for several minutes and observe for any allergic reactions.	Dyspnea, wheezing, and circulatory collapse are signs of severe anaphylactic reaction.

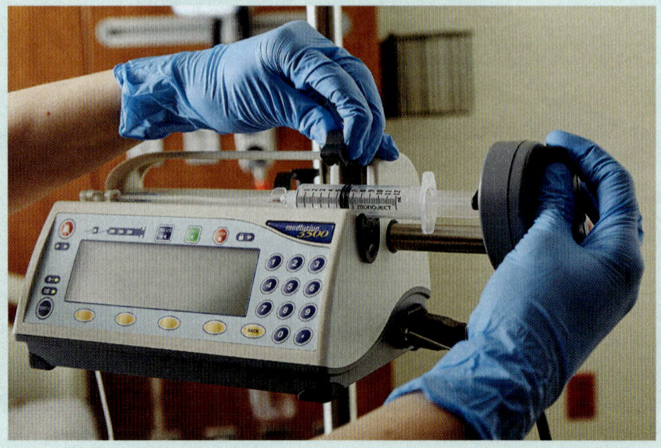

STEP 7B(3) Ensure that syringe is secure after placing it into syringe pump.

STEP	RATIONALE

EVALUATION

1. Observe patient for signs or symptoms of adverse reaction.	IV medications act rapidly.
2. During infusion, periodically check infusion rate and condition of IV site.	IV line must remain patent for proper medication administration. Infiltration of IV site requires discontinuing infusion.
3. Ask patient to explain purpose and adverse effects of medication.	Evaluates patient's understanding of instruction.
4. **Use teach-back:** "I want to be sure I explained to you the reason for this IV medication. Can you explain to me why you are receiving the medication and what to report to the nurse?" Develop a revised teaching plan if patient or caregiver is unable to teach back correctly.	Determines patient's and caregiver's level of understanding of topic (Yen & Leasure, 2019).

Unexpected Outcomes	Related Interventions
1. Patient develops adverse or allergic reaction to medication.	• Stop medication infusion immediately. • Follow employer policy for appropriate response to allergic reaction (e.g., administration of antihistamine such as diphenhydramine or epinephrine) and reporting of adverse medication reactions. • Notify patient's health care provider of adverse effects immediately. • Add allergy information to patient record per employer policy.
2. Medication does not infuse over established time frame.	• Determine reason (e.g., improper calculation of flow rate, poor positioning of IV needle at insertion site, infiltration). • Take corrective action as indicated.
3. IV site shows signs of infiltration or phlebitis (see Chapter 29).	• Stop IV infusion and discontinue access device. • Treat IV site as indicated by employer policy. • Insert new IV catheter if therapy continues. • For infiltration, determine how harmful IV medication is to SUBCUT tissue. Provide IV extravasation care (e.g., injecting phentolamine around IV infiltration site) as indicated by employer policy or consult pharmacist to determine appropriate follow-up care.

Communication and Documentation

- Immediately document medication, dose, route, infusion rate, and date and time administered on MAR in progress notes in EHR or chart.
- Document volume of fluid given on intake and output (I&O) form.
- Document patient teaching, validation of understanding, and patient's response to medication.
- Report any adverse reactions to patient's health care provider.

Special Considerations

Teaching

- Review all IV medications with patient and caregivers, including why patient is receiving the medication and potential adverse effects, and explain signs of allergic responses to watch for.
- Teach patient and caregiver not to alter the prescribed rate of infusion without consulting the health care provider. IV medications need to be infused at a specified rate to achieve their desired effect and to avoid adverse effects.
- Teach patient and caregiver to report any adverse effects immediately.

Pediatric

- Infants and young children are more vulnerable to alterations in fluid balance and do not adjust quickly to changes in it. Therefore, to assess fluid balance, monitor I&O carefully when infusing IV medications (Hockenberry et al., 2024).

Gerontological

- Altered pharmacokinetics of medications and the effects of polypharmacy place older persons at risk for medication toxicity. Carefully monitor the response of older persons to IV medications (Boscart et al., 2023).
- Older persons are at risk of developing fluid volume overload and require careful assessment for signs of overload and heart failure.

Care in the Community: Home Management

- Patients or caregivers who administer IV medications at home require education about the steps of medication administration. The patient or caregiver needs to perform several return demonstrations of IV medication administration before performing this skill independently. In addition, patients and caregivers need to know signs of IV medication administration complications such as phlebitis and infiltration and what to do for any problems.

✦ REVIEW QUESTIONS

The nurse is developing a plan of care for an alert and oriented patient with thrombophlebitis of the left leg who received heparin 5000 units subcutaneously on admission to the unit and every 8 hours; this is the fourth day after admission. The pharmacy provides heparin in a 1-mL single-dose vial of 5000 units/mL.

Review Questions 1 to 4 relate to the case study presented here.

1. Which information does the nurse need to know about the medication and the vial before administration?
2. Which information does the nurse need to know about the patient before administration of the heparin?
3. Which aspects of the patient's care related to the administration of heparin can the nurse delegate to the unregulated care provider (UCP)?
4. The patient weighs 100 kg (220 lb). Using a medication calculation, the nurse has determined that 1 mL of heparin needs to be administered. Which size syringe and needle will be used to administer the injection?
5. The patient reports soreness and tenderness at the heparin injection site. They deny other concerns or pain, shortness of breath, chest pain, or hemoptysis. When you review the patient's bloodwork, partial thromboplastin time (PTT) is 70 seconds (target is 60 to 80 seconds, per physician prescription). Using SBAR (situation–background–assessment–recommendation), show how you would communicate with the health care team about this patient.
6. Place the steps of administering an intradermal injection in the correct order.
   1. Inject medication slowly.
   2. Note the presence of a bleb.
   3. Advance needle through epidermis to 3 mm.
   4. Using nondominant hand, stretch skin over site with forefinger.
   5. Insert needle at a 5- to 15-degree angle into skin until resistance is felt.
   6. Clean site with antiseptic swab.
7. A patient with diabetes mellitus is receiving insulin using a continuous subcutaneous infusion (CSCI) pump. Place the steps of discontinuing the insulin pump in the correct order.
   1. Apply clean gloves.
   2. Stop infusion pump.
   3. Remove dressing and discard properly.
   4. Apply gentle pressure to site until no fluid is leaking from skin.
   5. Verify prescription and establish an alternate route for medication if applicable.
   6. Apply small sterile gauze dressing to site.
   7. Remove needle securement device and pull needle out. Inspect tip of needle and confirm it is still intact.
8. The nurse is administering an intravenous (IV) direct medication to a patient who has a compatible IV fluid running through IV tubing. The IV site is free of redness, pain, swelling, and other complications. Place the steps of this process in the appropriate order.
   1. Keep tubing pinched and inject medication within amount of time recommended by employer policy, pharmacist, or medication reference manual. Use watch to time administration.
   2. Select injection port of IV tubing closest to patient. Whenever possible, injection port should accept a needleless syringe. Use IV filter if required by medication reference or employer policy.
   3. After injecting medication, release tubing, disconnect syringe, and recheck fluid infusion rate.
   4. Connect syringe to port of IV line. Insert needleless tip of syringe containing prepared medication through centre of injection port.
   5. Clean injection port with antiseptic swab. Allow to dry.
   6. Occlude IV line by pinching tubing just above injection port.

Visit the Evolve site for a complete list of answers to the Review Questions.

✦ NEXT GENERATION NCLEX® (NGN)

For practice with answering exam questions related to unfolding NGN case studies, please consult the Next Generation NCLEX® (NGN)-Style Case Studies for Skills and Techniques on the Evolve website: http://evolve.elsevier.com/Canada/Perry/clinicalskills/

REFERENCES

Accreditation Canada. (2020). *Required organizational practices–2020 handbook.* https://physicians.nshealth.ca/resources/required-organizational-practices-2020-handbook

Adams, M. P., Urban, C. Q., El-Hussein, M., et al. (2021). Pharmacotherapy of coagulation disorders. In *Pharmacology for nurses: A pathophysiological approach* (3rd Cdn. ed., Chapter 56). Pearson Canada.

Addab, S., Hamdy, R., Thorstad, K., et al. (2022). Use of virtual reality in managing paediatric procedural pain and anxiety: An integrative literature review. *Journal of Clinical Nursing, 31*(21–22), 3032–3059. https://doi.org/10.1111/jocn.16217

Alteren, J., Hermstad, M., Nerdal, L., et al. (2021). Working in a minefield; Nurses' strategies for handling medicine administration interruptions in hospitals—a qualitative interview study. *BMC Health Services Research, 21.* Article 1094. https://doi.org/10.1186/s12913-021-07122-8

Arthur, A. (2015). Innovations in subcutaneous infusions. *Journal of Infusion Nursing, 38*(3), 179.

Bartz, L., Klein, C., Seifert, A., et al. (2014). Subcutaneous administration of drugs in palliative care: Result of a systematic observational study. *Journal of Pain Symptom Management, 48*(4), 540.

Beirne, P. V., Hennessy, S., Cadogan, S. L., et al. (2015). Needle size for vaccination procedures in children and adolescents. *Cochrane Database of Systematic Reviews, 2015*(6). Article CD010720. https://doi.org/10.1002/14651858.CD010720.pub2

Bianchi, M., & Ghirotto, L. (2021). Nurses' perspectives on workarounds in clinical practice: A phenomenological analysis. *Journal of Clinical Nursing, 31*(19–20), 2850–2859. https://doi.org/10.1111/jocn.16110

Birnie, K. A., Noel, M., Chambers, C. T., et al. (2018). Psychological interventions for needle-related procedural pain and distress in children and adolescents. *Cochrane Database of Systematic Reviews, 2018*(10), 74–75. https://doi.org/10.1002/14651858.CD005179.pub4

Boom, F. A., Le Brun, P. P. H., Boehringer, S., et al. (2021). Improving the aseptic transfer procedures in hospital pharmacies. Part B: Evaluation of disinfection methods for materials with a non-sterile surface. *European Journal of Hospital Pharmacy, 28*(5), 271–275. https://doi.org/10.1136/ejhpharm-2018-001673

Boscart, V., McCleary, L., Sheiban Taucar, L., et al. (2023). *Ebersole and Hess' gerontological nursing and healthy aging in Canada* (3rd ed.). Elsevier.

British Columbia Centre for Disease Control. (2016). *Tuberculin skin test (TST)–quick reference guide for health care providers.* http://www.bccdc.ca/resource-gallery/Documents/Communicable-Disease-Manual/Chapter 4 - TB/TST Quick Reference Guide.pdf. [Seminal Reference].

British Columbia Centre for Disease Control. (2019). *Communicable disease control manual, Chapter 2: Immunization, Part 3–management of anaphylaxis in the non-hospital setting.* http://www.bccdc.ca/resource-gallery/Documents/Guidelines and Forms/Guidelines and Manuals/Epid/CD Manual/Chapter 2 - Imms/Part_3_Anaphylaxis.pdf

Caccialanza, R., Constans, T., Cotogni, P., et al. (2018). Subcutaneous infusion of fluids for hydration or nutrition: A review. *Journal of Parenteral and Enteral Nutrition, 42*(2), 296–307. https://doi.org/10.1177/0148607116676593

Campbell, J. R., Pease, C., Daley, P., et al. (2022). Canadian tuberculosis standards (8th ed.), Chapter 4: Diagnosis of tuberculosis infection. *Canadian Journal of Respiratory, Critical Care, and Sleep Medicine, 6*(Suppl. 1), 49–65. https://doi.org/10.1080/24745332.2022.2036503

Canadian Centre for Occupational Health and Safety. (2018). *Needlestick and sharps injury.* http://www.ccohs.ca/oshanswers/diseases/needlestick_injuries.html

Canadian Nurses Association. (2017). *Code of ethics for registered nurses.* https://www.cna-aiic.ca/en/nursing/regulated-nursing-in-canada/nursing-ethics. [Seminal Reference].

Canadian Vascular Access Association. (2019). *Canadian vascular access and infusion therapy guidelines.* https://cvaa.info/en/education/national-guidelines-2019

Cho, M. K., & Choi, M. Y. (2021). Effect of distraction intervention for needle-related pain and distress in children: A systematic review and meta-analysis. *International Journal of Environmental Research and Public Health, 18*(17). Article 9159. https://doi.org/10.3390/ijerph18179159

Clark, L. T., Watkins, L., Piña, I. L., et al. (2019). Increasing diversity in clinical trials: Overcoming critical barriers. *Current Problems in Cardiology*, *44*(5), 148–172. https://doi.org/10.1016/j.cpcardiol.2018.11.002

College of Physicians and Surgeons of British Columbia. (2018). *Non-hospital medical and surgical facilities accreditation program accreditation standards: Single-use devices and multi-dose vials*. https://www.cpsbc.ca/files/pdf/NHMSFAP-AS-Single-Use-Devices.pdf

College of Registered Nurses of Saskatchewan. (2021). *Medication management guideline*. https://www.srna.org/wp-content/uploads/2021/09/Medication-Management-Guideline-SRNA-2021.pdf

Diabetes Canada Clinical Practice Guidelines Expert Committee. (2018). Diabetes Canada 2018 clinical practice guidelines for the prevention and management of diabetes in Canada. *Canadian Journal of Diabetes*, *42*(Suppl. 1), S1–S325. https://guidelines.diabetes.ca/docs/CPG-2018-full-EN.pdf

Doyle, G. R., & McCutcheon, J. A. (2021). Parenteral medication administration. In *Clinical procedures for safer patient care* (version 1.08, Chapter 7). BCcampus. https://opentextbc.ca/clinicalskills/chapter/7-1-introduction/

Dwilow, Hui, C., Kakkar, F., & Kitai, I. (2022). Canadian tuberculosis standards (8th ed.), Chapter 9: Pediatric tuberculosis. *Canadian Journal of Respiratory, Critical Care, and Sleep Medicine*, 6(Suppl. 1), 129–148. https://doi.org/10.1080/24745332.2022.2043055

Elmi, S., Babaie, J., Malek, M., et al. (2018). Occupational exposures to needle stick injuries among health care staff: A review study. *Journal of Analytical Research in Clinical Medicine*, 6(1). https://doi.org/10.15171/jarcm.2018.001

Forum for Injection Technique Canada. (2020). *Recommendations for best practice in injection technique* (4th ed.). http://fit4diabetes.com/files/7816/0803/3133/FIT_Recommendations_2020.pdf

Gillespie, J. D. (2018). Types of insulin. *Canadian Journal of Diabetes*, 42(Suppl. 1), S314. https://doi.org/10.1016/j.jcjd.2017.12.006

Gordon, B. R., Hurst, D. S., Fornadley, J. A., et al. (2013). Safety of intradermal skin tests for inhalants and foods: A prospective study. *International Forum of Allergy and Rhinology*, 3(3), 171–176. https://doi.org/10.1002/alr.21091. [Seminal Reference].

Heron, L., & Bruk-Lee, V. (2020). When empowered nurses are under stress: Understanding the impact on attitudes and behaviours. *Stress and Health*, *36*(2), 147–159. https://doi.org/10.1002/smi.2905

Hockenberry, M. J., Duffy, E. A., & Gibbs, K. (2024). *Wong's nursing care of infants and children* (12th ed.). Elsevier.

Hopkins, U., & Arias, C. (2013, January/February). Large-volume IM injections: A review of best practices. *Oncology Nurse Advisor*, 32–37. https://www.oncologynurseadvisor.com/wp-content/uploads/sites/13/2019/01/ona_feature0213_injections_10767.pdf. [Seminal Reference].

Infection Prevention and Control Canada. (2017). *IPAC Canada practice recommendations: Hand hygiene in health care settings*. https://ipac-canada.org/photos/custom/Members/pdf/17JulHand%20Hygiene%20Practice%20Recommendations_final.pdf. [Seminal Reference].

Infusion Nurses Society. (2016). Infusion therapy standards of practice. *Journal of Intravenous Nursing*, 39(1S).

Institute for Safe Medication Practices. (2010). *Guidelines for standard order sets*. https://www.ismp.org/guidelines/standard-order-sets

Institute for Safe Medication Practices. (2011). *Guidelines for timely administration of scheduled medications (acute)*. https://www.ismp.org/guidelines/timely-administration-scheduled-medications-acute. [Seminal Reference].

Institute for Safe Medication Practices. (2012). *Side tracks on the safety express. Interruptions lead to errors and unfinished . . . Wait, what was I doing?* https://www.ismp.org/resources/side-tracks-safety-express-interruptions-lead-errors-and-unfinished-wait-what-was-i-doing?id=37. [Seminal Reference].

Institute for Safe Medication Practices. (2015). *Safe practice guidelines for adult IV push medications*. https://www.ismp.org/sites/default/files/attachments/2017-11/ISMP97-Guidelines-071415-3.%20FINAL.pdf. [Seminal Reference].

Institute for Safe Medication Practices. (2017). *Guidelines for optimizing safe subcutaneous insulin use in adults*. https://www.ismp.org/guidelines/subcutaneous-insulin. [Seminal Reference].

Institute for Safe Medication Practices. (2018). *ISMP list of high-alert medications in acute care settings*. https://www.ismp.org/sites/default/files/attachments/2018-08/highAlert2018-Acute-Final.pdf

Institute for Safe Medication Practices. (2019). *Guidelines for safe electronic communication of medication information*. https://www.ismp.org/resources/guidelines-safe-electronic-communication-medication-information

Institute for Safe Medication Practices. (2022). *Three new best practices in the 2022–2023 targeted medication safety best practices for hospitals*. https://www.ismp.org/resources/three-new-best-practices-2022-2023-targeted-medication-safety-best-practices-hospitals

Klaver, M., de Blok, C. J. M., Wiepjes, C. M., et al. (2018). Changes in regional body fat, lean body mass and body shape in trans persons using cross-sex hormonal therapy: Results from a multicenter prospective study. *European Journal of Endocrinology*, 178(2), 163–171. https://doi.org/10.1530/EJE-17-0496

Larkin, T. A., Ashcroft, E., Hickey, B. A., et al. (2018). Influence of gender, BMI and body shape on theoretical injection outcome at the ventrogluteal and dorsogluteal sites. *Journal of Clinical Nursing*, *27*(1–2), e242–e250. https://doi.org/10.1111/jocn.13923

McCartan, A. J. S., Curran, D. W., & Mrsny, R. J. (2021). Evaluating parameters affecting drug fate at the intramuscular injection site. *Journal of Controlled Release*, *336*, 322–335. https://doi.org/10.1016/j.jconrel.2021.06.023

McMahon, J. T. (2017). Improving medication administration safety in the clinical environment. *Medsurg Nursing*, *26*(6), 374–409.

Mohammady, M., Radmehr, M., & Janani, L. (2021). Slow versus fast subcutaneous heparin injections for prevention of bruising and site pain intensity. *Cochrane Database of Systematic Reviews*, *2021*(6). Article CD008077. https://doi.org/10.1002/14651858.CD008077.pub6

Nakajima, Y., Fujii, T., Mukai, K., et al. (2020). Anatomically safe sites for intramuscular injections: A cross-sectional study on young adults and cadavers with a focus on the thigh. *Human Vaccines & Immunotherapeutics*, *16*(1), 189–196. https://doi.org/10.1080/21645515.2019.1646576

Nicoll, L., & Hesby, A. (2002). Intramuscular injection: An integrative research review and guideline for evidence-based practice. *Applied Nursing Research*, *16*(2), 159. https://doi.org/10.1053/apnr.2002.34142. [Seminal Reference].

Novo Nordisk Canada Inc. (2021). *NOVOLIN®GE insulin, human biosynthetic*. https://www.novonordisk.ca/content/dam/nncorp/ca/en/products/novolin-product-monograph1.pdf

Paull, T. (2018). *Intramuscular injection: Aspiration [evidence summary]. JBI EBP Database*. https://www.wolterskluwer.com/en/know/jbi-resources

Pozzilli, P., Battelino, T., Danne, T., et al. (2016). Continuous subcutaneous insulin infusion in diabetes: Patient populations, safety, efficacy, and pharmacoeconomics. *Diabetes*, *32*(1), 21–39. https://doi.org/10.1002/dmrr.2653. [Seminal Reference].

Public Health Agency of Canada. (2016). *Routine practices and additional precautions for preventing the transmission of infection in healthcare settings*. https://www.canada.ca/content/dam/phac-aspc/documents /services/publications/diseases-conditions/routine-practices-precautions-healthcare-associated-infections/routine-practices-precautions-healthcare-associated-infections-2016-FINAL-eng.pdf

Public Health Agency of Canada. (2017). Table 3: Needle selection guidelines. In *Vaccine administration practices: Canadian immunization guide*. https://www.canada.ca/en/public-health/services/publications/healthy-living/canadian-immunization-guide-part-1-key-immunization-information/page-8-vaccine-administration-practices.html#t3. [Seminal Reference].

Registered Nurses' Association of Ontario. (2015). *Person- and family-centered care*. https://rnao.ca/bpg/guidelines/person-and-family-centred-care. [Seminal Reference].

Rodger, M. A., & King, L. (2000). Drawing up and administering intramuscular injections: A review of the literature. *Journal of Advanced Nursing*, *31*(3), 574–582. https://doi.org/10.1046/j.1365-2648.2000.01312.x. [Seminal Reference].

Saleem, F., & Sharma, A. (2022). *NPH insulin*. StatPearls. https://www.ncbi.nlm.nih.gov/books/NBK549860/

Sanofi-Aventis Canada. (2018). *Lovenox and Lovenox HP product monograph*. http://products.sanofi.ca/en/lovenox.pdf

Sebro, R. (2022). Statistical estimation of deltoid subcutaneous fat pad thickness: Implications for needle length for vaccination. *Scientific Reports*, *12*(1). Article 1069. https://doi.org/10.1038/s41598-022-05020-5

Sisson, H. (2015). Aspirating during the intramuscular injection procedure: A systematic literature review. *Journal of Clinical Nursing*, *24*, 2368–2375. https://doi.org/10.1111/jocn.12824. [Seminal Reference].

Sodré Alves, B. M. C., de Andrade, T. N. G., Cerqueira Santos, S., et al. (2021). Harm prevalence due to medication errors involving high-alert medications: A systematic review. *Journal of Patient Safety*, *17*(1), e1–e9. https://doi.org/10.1097/PTS.0000000000000649

Strohfus, P., Paugh, O., Tindell, C., et al. (2018). Evidence calls for practice change in intramuscular injection techniques. *Journal of Nursing Education and Practice*, *8*(2), 83–92. https://doi.org/10.5430/jnep.v8n2p83

Su, H.-C., Hsieh, C.-W., Lai, N. M., et al. (2021). Using vibrating and cold device for pain relievers in children: A systematic review and meta-analysis of randomized controlled trials. *Journal of Pediatric Nursing*, *61*, 23–33. https://doi.org/10.1016/j.pedn.2021.02.027

Usach, I., Martinez, R., Festini, T., et al. (2019). Subcutaneous injection of drugs: Literature review of factors influencing pain sensation at the injection site. *Advances in Therapy*, 36(11), 2986–2996. https://doi.org/10.1007/s12325-019-01101-6

World Health Organization. (2022). *Tuberculosis*. https://www.who.int/en/news-room/fact-sheets/detail/tuberculosis

Yen, P. H., & Leasure, A. R. (2019). Use and effectiveness of the teach-back method in patient education and health outcomes. *Federal Practitioner*, *36*(6), 284–289. https://cdn.mdedge.com/files/s3fs-public/issues/articles/fdp03606284.pdf

Yilmaz, G., & Alemdar, D. K. (2019). Using buzzy, shotblocker, and bubble blowing in a pediatric emergency department to reduce the pain and fear caused by intramuscular injection: A randomized controlled trial. *Journal of Emergency Nursing*, 45(5), 502–511. https://doi.org/10.1016/j.jen.2019.04.003

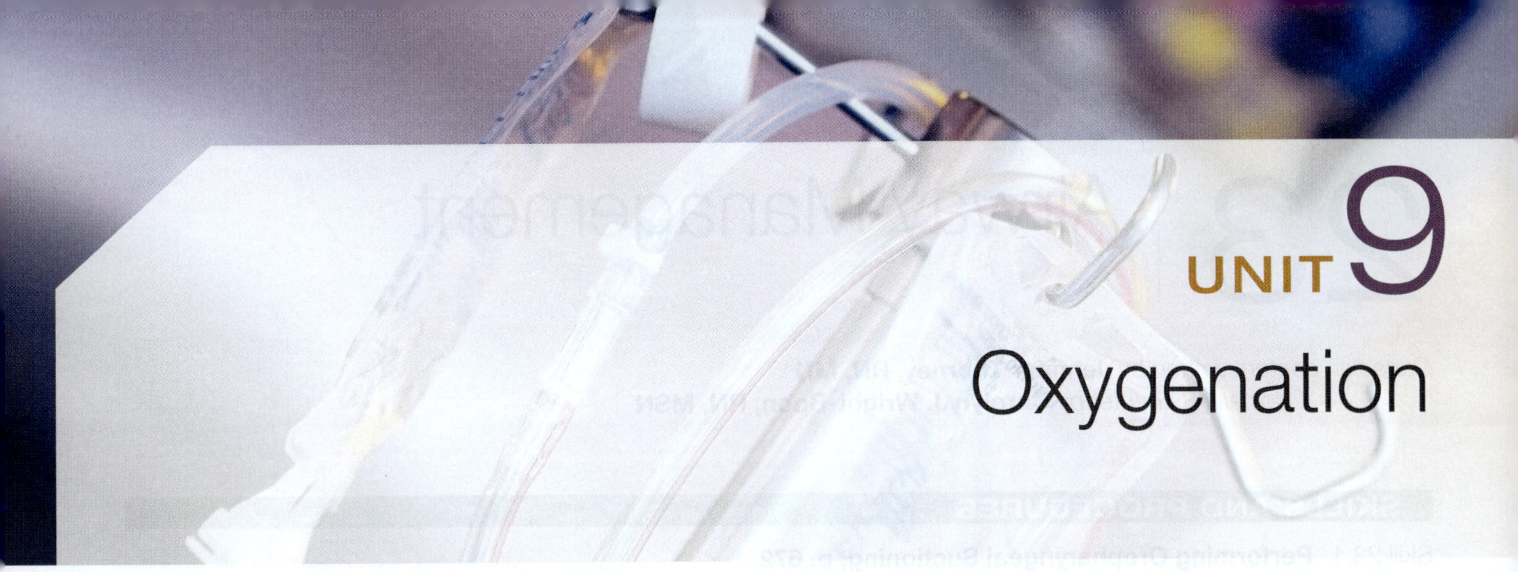

UNIT 9 Oxygenation

The skills commonly used to support oxygenation do so by improving either ventilation or respiratory gas exchange. Clinical judgement in the care of patients with impaired oxygenation involves assessing patient data, analyzing clinical cues, diagnosing the patients' problems, and making clinical decisions on the appropriate skills to use. Knowledge of a patient's clinical condition, the physiology of gas exchange and ventilation, and experience caring for patients with similar alterations will assist not only in knowing what to assess but also in selecting appropriate interventions. Experience is vital in knowing how to adapt skills to meet a patient's unique needs. When conditions such as abdominal surgery or traumatic rib fracture occur, you will learn that the associated pain of these conditions reduces ventilation. With less air moving through airways, oxygenation is also reduced. Interventions for maximizing ventilation (e.g., positioning) and pain control (analgesia) become care priorities. When a condition directly affects gas exchange (e.g., pneumonia, bronchitis, flu), potential interventions for maximizing oxygenation include administration of oxygen therapy, airway management (e.g., suctioning, coughing exercises, chest physiotherapy), and fluid hydration to thin secretions.

The following are two examples that illustrate impaired oxygenation from different pathologies. In one example, a patient has pneumonia, and you are told that the patient is diaphoretic and tachycardic; has a fever and thick sputum; and has difficulty coughing. Reflect on your knowledge about normal lung function and the pathology of pneumonia. You focus data collection to confirm the reported findings and look for additional cues such as temperature (38.9°C [102°F]), respiratory rate (26 breaths/min), pulse (110 beats/min), oxygen saturation (85%), blood pressure (100/80 mm Hg), pallor, inability to clear airway with coughing, and abnormal lung sounds. Analysis of these cues indicates that the patient has poor oxygenation and is unable to clear airway secretions, and therefore needs interventions to improve oxygenation (e.g., oxygen therapy) and airway management (e.g., suctioning).

In a second example, a patient has heart failure, a form of cardiovascular disease. You are told that the patient is on oxygen therapy but short of breath all the time, has difficulty moving from bed to chair, is confused, and has a weak pulse and cold extremities. Use clinical judgement to conduct a focused cardiovascular assessment, including vital signs, auscultation of heart sounds, palpation of peripheral pulses, mental status, and activity tolerance. Once you complete data collection, look for cues such as respiratory rate (30 breaths/min), pulse (120 beats/min and thready), oxygen saturation (83%), blood pressure (90/70 mm Hg), pallor, poor peripheral pulses, cold extremities, somewhat confused but oriented, short of breath when moving from bed to chair, and unable to ambulate at this time. Analysis of these cues indicates that this patient, like the patient in the first example, has poor oxygenation, but this case is due to failure of the heart to perfuse blood, not an inflammatory condition affecting the patient's airways. The patient needs interventions to improve oxygenation (e.g., oxygen therapy and medications that will strengthen heart contractility).

Patients with oxygenation alterations can change very quickly clinically. Thorough ongoing assessment is critical, and as a nurse you need to monitor a patient closely by knowing the physiological changes to expect in order to conduct correct and timely assessments. In addition, any respiratory problem can have consequences that affect a patient's cardiac status. Sometimes the consequence can threaten life, necessitating knowledge and skill in implementing emergency life-support measures.

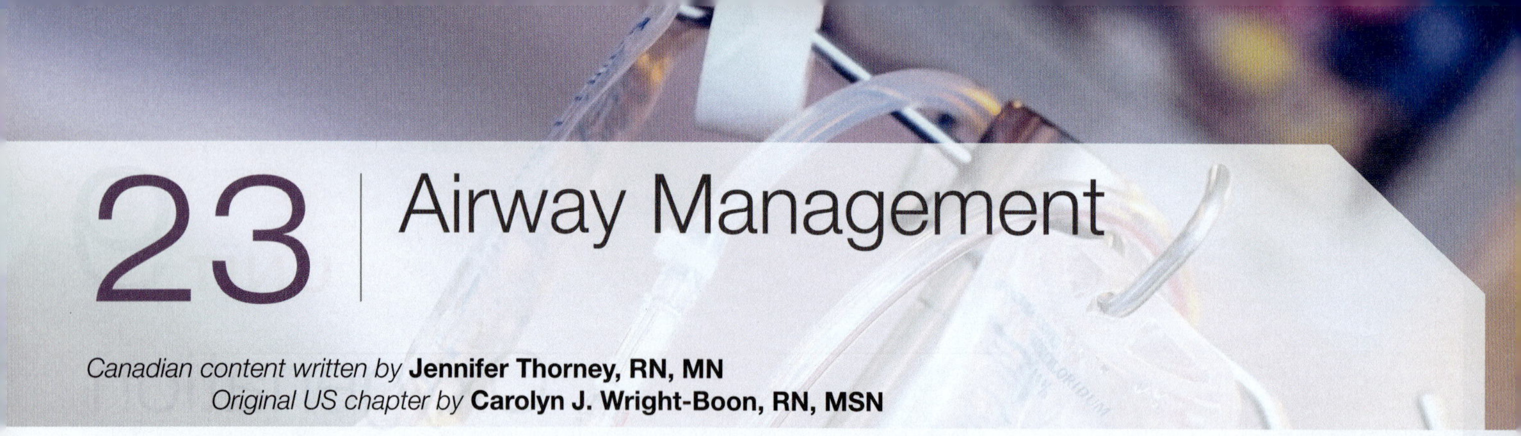

23 | Airway Management

Canadian content written by **Jennifer Thorney, RN, MN**
Original US chapter by **Carolyn J. Wright-Boon, RN, MSN**

SKILLS AND PROCEDURES

OBJECTIVES

Mastery of content in this chapter will enable the nurse to:

- Identify safety guidelines for managing a patient's airway.
- Describe person-centred approaches to airway management.
- Describe the nursing interventions for airway management.
- Explain the indications for airway suctioning.
- Explain the indications for tracheostomy care.
- Correctly perform oropharyngeal, nasopharyngeal, nasotracheal, and tracheal suctioning; endotracheal care; and tracheostomy tube care.
- Correctly inflate a cuff on an endotracheal or tracheostomy tube.
- Change a tracheostomy tube or inner cannula.

MEDIA RESOURCES

- http://evolve.elsevier.com/Canada/Perry/clinicalskills/

PURPOSE

Airway management involves nursing interventions to maintain the patency of a patient's nose, mouth, upper airway, trachea, and lower airway of the respiratory system. The primary goal of airway management is to protect the airway, which helps promote and maintain adequate tissue oxygenation.

STANDARDS OF CARE

- Accreditation Canada (2020)—*Required Organizational Practices–2020 Handbook* (https://physicians.nshealth.ca/resources/required-organizational-practices-2020-handbook)
- American Association of Respiratory Care (AARC)*
  - AARC (2004)—*AARC Clinical Practice Guideline: Nasotracheal Suctioning–2004 Revision and Update* (https://www.aarc.org/wp-content/uploads/2014/08/09.04.1080.pdf)
  - AARC (2010)—*AARC Clinical Practice Guideline: Endotracheal Suctioning of Mechanically Ventilated Patients With Artificial Airways 2010* (https://www.aarc.org/wp-content/uploads/2014/08/06.10.0758.pdf)
  - AARC (2011)—*AARC Clinical Practice Guideline: Capnography/Capnometry During Mechanical Ventilation: 2011* (https://www.aarc.org/wp-content/uploads/2014/08/04.11.0503.pdf)
  - AARC (2012)—*AARC Clinical Practice Guideline: Humidification During Invasive and Noninvasive Mechanical Ventilation: 2012* (https://www.aarc.org/wp-content/uploads/2014/08/12.05.0782.pdf)
- Healthcare Excellence Canada (2009)—*The Safety Competencies* (https://www.healthcareexcellence.ca/media/115mbc4z/cpsi-safetycompetencies_en_digital-final-ua.pdf)
- Healthcare Excellence Canada (2020)—*Hospital Harm Improvement Resource: Pneumonia* (https://www.patientsafetyinstitute.ca/en/toolsResources/Hospital-Harm-Measure/Improvement-Resources/Pneumonia/Documents/HHIR-Pneumonia-B16.pdf)
- Institute for Healthcare Improvement (2012)—*How-To Guide: Prevent Ventilator-Associated Pneumonia* (https://www.ihi.org/resources/Pages/Tools/HowtoGuidePreventVAP.aspx)
- Intensive Care Society (Hellyer et al., 2016)—*The Intensive Care Society Recommended Bundle of Interventions for the Prevention of Ventilator-Associated Pneumonia* (https://doi.org/10.1177/1751143716644461)

*AARC clinical practice guidelines are used in Canada and are seminal publications. Some of the most up-to-date guidelines and practices are US resources. Each employer follows the direction of their chosen resource guideline.

PRINCIPLES FOR PRACTICE

- Various techniques for airway management are available to promote an open or patent airway, which has the potential to become blocked by mucus, a mechanical obstruction (i.e., soft tissue in upper airway), or a foreign body.
- Hydration, positioning, nutrition, chest physiotherapy techniques, deep breathing, coughing, humidity, incentive spirometry, and aerosol therapy are noninvasive techniques that are helpful in maintaining a patent airway.
- When patients are unable to protect their own airway or clear airway secretions with coughing, chest physiotherapy, or other noninvasive techniques, more invasive measures such as suctioning or inserting an artificial airway are needed.
- An artificial airway is a plastic or rubber device (such as a tracheostomy or endotracheal tube) that is inserted into the upper or lower respiratory tract to facilitate ventilation or the removal of secretions.
- An oral airway is not used in a conscious, cooperative patient because it causes excessive gagging and pressure areas to the mouth and tongue.
- Mechanical assistance may be needed to maintain airway patency.
- Indications for mechanical ventilation include upper airway obstructions (e.g., secondary to burns, tumour, bleeding), apnea, high risk of aspiration, inability to clear secretions, and respiratory distress.

PERSON-CENTRED CARE

- Artificial airways alter patients' ability to communicate, possibly causing feelings of fear, frustration, anxiety, and vulnerability.
- The nurse must understand the possible feelings of the patient on a ventilator and be competent in using alternate methods of communication to accurately assess them. Family members and nurses both play a key role in assessing the frustration and anger of the patient and in facilitating communication between the patient and the interprofessional health care team (Khan & Nishi, 2021).
- Nurses need to thoroughly educate patients and caregivers using plain language that is culturally sensitive and verify their understanding of any procedures or tests.
- Collaboration with caregivers is essential when providing alternative means of communication for patients. Once communication is established, a patient and caregiver will have more trust in the care provided, which will promote cooperation and rapport.
- Use interprofessional collaboration when caring for patients who do not speak one of Canada's official languages in order to prevent misunderstanding of treatment options.
- Obtain professional translators or other communication aids to ensure that patients and caregivers understand the need for an artificial airway and subsequent treatments.
- Assess the dysfunction of body movement in intubated patients to determine whether any communication device such as picture boards or pen and paper for writing would be appropriate. Ensure that functioning hearing aids and glasses are in place and working to make communication easier and less frustrating for patients with these needs (Khan & Nishi, 2021).

EVIDENCE-INFORMED PRACTICE

- There are significant concerns regarding the definition of ventilator-associated pneumonia (VAP) and ventilator-associated event (VAE). The Centers for Disease Control and Prevention (CDC, 2023) developed a lengthy algorithm to help health care providers accurately diagnose these complications through interprofessional collaboration.
  - The key points in the definition of VAE are "deterioration in respiratory status after a period of stability or improvement on the ventilator, evidence of infection or inflammation, and laboratory evidence of respiratory infection" (CDC, 2023, pp. 10–4).
  - The patient must be mechanically ventilated for more than 2 calendar days to be eligible for VAE (CDC, 2023).
- VAP/VAE bundles are available to help guide nursing practice (see also Skill 25.5). The following key interventions are included in these bundles:
  - Elevation of the head of bed (HOB) to between 30 and 45 degrees
  - Daily interruption of sedation and daily assessment of a patient's readiness to extubate
  - Peptic ulcer disease prophylaxis
  - Deep venous thrombosis prophylaxis (unless contraindicated)
  - Daily oral care with chlorhexidine gluconate (CHG)
  - Delirium monitoring and management
  - Early exercise and mobility
- Endotracheal tubes (ETs) meant for subglottic suctioning have a port for suction above the cuff. The subglottic port above the cuff is meant to drain secretions above the cuff. Various studies have used continuous subglottic suctioning (CSS) and intermittent subglottic suctioning, but current research concludes that closed endotracheal suctioning techniques are preferred over open endotracheal suctioning. During closed suctioning, the patient remains on a ventilator and suctioning is performed through an ET, a procedure that has fewer traumatic effects on the patient (Dhawan, 2018).
- Closed endotracheal suctioning techniques have many benefits compared with open endotracheal suctioning: They prevent the loss of positive end-expiratory pressure (PEEP) and lung volume, prevent hypoxia and changes in mean arterial blood pressure, and decrease caregiver exposure to infection (Dhawan, 2018).
- New products are being developed to decrease the risk of biofilm formation on ETs. Biofilms are associated with increased risks of developing VAP.
  - These new products include systems that scrape the inside of the ET to remove the secretions. Polyamide- or silver nanoparticle-coated ETs are also being investigated for their use in the prevention of biofilm formation (Lethongkam et al., 2020).
  - Manual cuff pressure measurements are the standard of care. It is recommended that these pressure values not be checked overly often, as doing so can decrease the required seal (Lethongkam et al., 2020).

SAFETY GUIDELINES

- Know a patient's baseline range of vital signs and oxygen saturation levels. Baseline physiological measures aid in identifying individual abnormalities and recognizing signs that a patient's condition is deteriorating.
- Know a patient's medical history. Smoking alters normal mucociliary clearance. Certain disorders, such as chronic obstructive pulmonary disease (COPD), asthma, cystic fibrosis (CF), pneumonia, thoracic surgery, chest trauma, and abdominal surgery, place patients at increased risk of developing an obstructed airway.
- Identify factors that increase a patient's risk of aspirating gastric contents into the lungs, which can result in airway obstruction.

These factors include the presence of enteral feeding tubes or nasal and oral gastric tubes, a decreased level of consciousness, and a decreased swallowing ability.

- Caution must be used when suctioning patients who have head injuries, as suctioning causes increased intracranial pressure (ICP) (Harrois et al., 2020). Reduce the risk of ICP by promoting vasoconstriction, therapeutic hyperventilation before suctioning, and hypocarbia.
- Determine whether a patient has a history of nasal problems such as nasal trauma, nasal polyps, deviated nasal septum, or chronic sinusitis. Allergy problems may cause mucosal swelling that narrows nasal passages, which affects the ability to easily pass a suction catheter.
- Review a patient's respiratory assessments from the past 12 or 24 hours. These are relative baseline measurements that help distinguish between gradual and acute changes in a patient's status.
- Perform a systematic pulmonary assessment of upper and lower airways, including respiratory rate, respiratory pattern, accessory muscle use, breath sounds, ability to cough effectively, integrity of the rib cage, and the characteristics of sputum production.
- Identify and become familiar with the use of equipment available at the facility. Many types of artificial airways, suction catheters, and suction machines are available. Knowing how to operate the equipment before use helps lead to positive outcomes.
- Test all equipment before use. Have adequate supplies on hand at the bedside. Equipment must work properly to provide safe nursing care. Confirm that the suction machine is generating adequate negative suction pressure and that suction catheters and appropriate equipment are available at the bedside.
- Know the adverse effects of medications and other therapies. Some medications, such as beta-adrenergic blockers, cause the adverse effect of bronchospasm. An adverse effect of opioids and sedatives is respiratory depression. Similarly, too much oxygen reduces the drive to breathe in patients with chronic hypercapnia (elevated arterial carbon dioxide [CO_2] tension). Some position changes can also affect a patient adversely. For example, in patients with impaired spinal cord innervations of the respiratory muscles, supine positions place the diaphragm at a mechanical disadvantage and increase the risk of aspiration.

✦ SKILL 23.1 Performing Oropharyngeal Suctioning

Video Clip NSO *Nursing Skills Online Airway Management Module 9 / Lesson 2*

Prior to initiating oropharyngeal suctioning, ensure that supplemental oxygen with appropriate delivery devices is readily available at the bedside. A Yankauer, or tonsillar tip, suction device is used for oropharyngeal suctioning (i.e., the removal of pharyngeal secretions through the mouth) (Fig. 23.1). A Yankauer suction catheter is made of rigid, minimally flexible plastic. The tip of this suction catheter usually has one large and several small openings through which the mucus enters with the application of negative pressure. The Yankauer suction catheter is angled to facilitate removal of secretions through a patient's mouth. Oropharyngeal suctioning only removes secretions from the back of the throat. Perform oral suctioning when a patient is able to cough effectively but is unable to clear secretions, such as for patients with a neuromuscular injury who cannot manage their own oral secretions. The Yankauer suction device is also used to provide oral hygiene to patients with artificial airways and impaired swallowing.

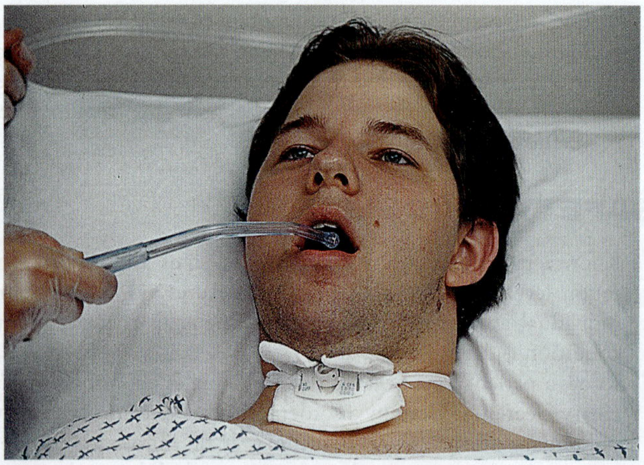

FIG 23.1 Oropharyngeal suctioning.

Delegation and Collaboration

The skill of performing oropharyngeal suctioning may be delegated to an unregulated care provider (UCP), depending on employer policy. Do not delegate this skill for patients with oral or neck surgery in the immediate postoperative period. The nurse is responsible for assessing the patient's respiratory status. The nurse instructs the UCP about the following:

- Appropriate suction limits for oropharyngeal suctioning for a particular patient (e.g., the appropriate suction pressure, expected frequency of suctioning, and expected colour and volume of secretions)
- The risks of applying excessive or inadequate suction pressure
- Avoiding mouth sutures, applying suction against sensitive tissues, and dislodging tubes in the patient's nose or mouth
- Avoiding stimulation of the gag reflex
- Immediately reporting to the nurse any change in vital signs, pulse oximetry (SpO_2), sputum (i.e., bloody), difficulty breathing, or discomfort during or after the procedure

Equipment

- Yankauer (or tonsillar tip) suction catheter
- Clean gloves
- Towel, cloth, or disposable paper drape
- Personal protective equipment (PPE), as indicated
- Disposable cup or nonsterile basin
- Tap water or normal saline (about 100 mL)
- Suction machine or wall suction device with regulator
- Connecting tubing (1.8 metres [6 feet])
- Oral airway (if indicated)
- Washcloth (if indicated)
- Pulse oximeter, stethoscope
- Manual self-inflating resuscitation bag (bag-valve mask) with oxygen-connecting tubing

STEP	RATIONALE

ASSESSMENT

STEP	RATIONALE
1. Identify patient using at least two person-specific identifiers (e.g., name and date of birth, or name and medical record number) according to employer policy.	Ensures correct patient. Complies with Accreditation Canada's standards and improves patient safety (Accreditation Canada, 2020).
2. Throughout the procedure, the 4 moments for hand hygiene are to be implemented; hand hygiene should occur before initial patient (or patient environment) contact, before an aseptic procedure, after body fluid exposure risk, and after patient (or patient environment) contact. Additional hand hygiene should be performed when hands are visibly soiled.	Proper hand hygiene helps prevent the spread of infectious agents to health care providers.
3. Identify risk factors for airway obstruction: impaired cough or gag reflex, weakened respiratory muscles, impaired swallowing, and decreased level of consciousness.	Risk factors prevent patient from protecting airway from aspiration or clearing secretions safely.
4. Assess for signs and symptoms of hypoxia: anxiety, change in level of consciousness, change in vital signs, decreased SpO_2, adventitious sounds (see also Box 25.1).	Suctioning of oropharyngeal airway is indicated with alterations in oxygenation associated with secretion accumulation.
5. Obtain patient's oxygen saturation level via SpO_2 (see Chapter 7). Keep pulse oximeter in place.	Provides an objective baseline measure of oxygen saturation and an early indication of changes in oxygenation status. Aids in assessment of patient during and after oropharyngeal suctioning.
6. Determine patient's ability to hold or manipulate catheter and their knowledge about use of suction catheter and procedure.	Encourages cooperation; minimizes risks and anxiety. Identifies teaching needs. Physical factors such as impaired mobility of upper extremities prevent patient from using catheter to help control oral secretions.
7. Assess for signs and symptoms of upper airway obstruction: gurgling on inspiration or expiration, restlessness, obvious excessive oral secretions, drooling, gastric secretions or vomitus in mouth, or coughing without clearing secretions from upper airway.	Secretions pool in the upper airway, which can cause total airway obstruction and hypoxia. The risk for aspiration of gastric contents and airway obstruction is increased in patients with vomiting; delayed gastric emptying; impairment in esophageal sphincter control, cough, swallowing, or gag reflex; or receiving enteral feedings.
8. Auscultate for presence of adventitious sounds (see Chapter 8 and Skill 23.2).	Determines whether lower airway secretions are present and establishes baseline.

NURSING DIAGNOSES

- Reduced airway clearance
- Inadequate breathing pattern
- Reduced gas exchange
- Inadequate swallowing
- Insufficient knowledge regarding use of suction
- Potential for aspiration
- Potential for infection

Related factors and risk factors are individualized on the basis of patient's condition or needs.

PLANNING

STEP	RATIONALE
1. Expected outcomes following completion of procedure:	
• No gurgling sounds are heard in patient's pharynx on inspiration and expiration.	Suctioning is effective. Secretions are removed from large upper airway.
• Drooling is diminished or absent.	Excessive drooling indicates that patient is unable to handle oral secretions.
• Vomitus or gastric secretions are absent from mouth.	Gastric secretions retained in oral cavity increase patient's risk of aspiration pneumonia.
• SpO_2 improves or remains at patient's normal baseline.	Removal of secretions helps improve oxygen saturation level.

Critical Decision Point *In patients living with chronic pulmonary disease, the SpO_2 value may remain the same after oropharyngeal suctioning. This baseline value may be lower than the typical normal values of greater than 95%.*

STEP	RATIONALE
2. Gather equipment and supplies. Close room door or curtain.	Ensures well-organized procedure. Provides patient privacy as part of person-centred care.
3. Explain to patient how procedure helps clear airway secretions and relieves some breathing problems. Explain that coughing, gagging, or (less commonly) sneezing is normal and lasts only a few seconds. Encourage patient to cough out secretions and show how to splint painful areas during procedure. Have patient practise coughing, if able.	Gagging or coughing occurs when the posterior pharynx is suctioned or because of excess secretions. Coughing secretions out of lower airway or the posterior pharynx decreases the amount of suctioning required. Splinting reduces abdominal incision discomfort during coughing or gagging.
4. Position patient in semi-Fowler's or sitting position. Place towel, cloth, or paper drape across patient's neck and chest.	Promotes patient comfort and removal of airway secretions. Towel protects gown and bed linen from contamination by secretions.

IMPLEMENTATION

STEP	RATIONALE
1. Apply clean gloves and appropriate PPE (see Box 5.1).	Reduces transmission of microorganisms.
2. Fill cup or basin with approximately 100 mL of water or normal saline.	Helps to clean catheter after suctioning and verifies that equipment functions.
3. Connect one end of connecting tubing to suction machine and other to Yankauer suction catheter. Turn on suction machine; set vacuum regulator to appropriate setting (infants, 80–100 mm Hg; children, 100–120 mm Hg; adults, 100–150 mm Hg) (AARC, 2010).	Prepares suction apparatus. Pressures should not exceed 150 mm Hg because elevated pressure settings increase risk of trauma to oral mucosa (AARC, 2010).
4. Check that suction machine is functioning properly by placing tip of catheter in water or normal saline and suctioning small amount from cup or basin.	Ensures that equipment functions and lubricates catheter.
5. Remove patient's oxygen mask if present. Nasal cannula may remain in place. Keep oxygen mask near patient's face.	Allows access to mouth. Reduces chance of hypoxia.

Critical Decision Point *Be prepared to quickly reapply supplemental oxygen if SpO_2 value falls below 90% or respiratory distress develops during or at the end of oropharyngeal suctioning. Be prepared to use the bag-valve mask if patient has serious acute respiratory distress or decline in SpO_2.*

STEP	RATIONALE
6. Insert catheter into mouth along gum line to pharynx. Move catheter around mouth until secretions have cleared. Encourage patient to cough. Replace oxygen mask.	Movement of catheter prevents suction tip from invaginating oral mucosal surfaces and causing trauma. Coughing moves secretions from lower airway into mouth and upper airway.

Critical Decision Point *Be careful when using a Yankauer suction catheter in a patient who has had recent oral or head and neck surgery. Aggressive suctioning and excessive coughing should not be used or encouraged in patients who have undergone throat surgery such as a tonsillectomy. These acts can aggravate the operative site, increasing the risk of infection or bleeding* (Hockenberry et al., 2024).

STEP	RATIONALE
7. Rinse catheter with water or normal saline in cup or basin until connecting tubing is cleared of secretions. Turn off suction. Place catheter in clean, dry area or in labelled bag with date on which product was opened, and ensure all equipment is readily available.	Rinses catheter and reduces probability of transmission of microorganisms. Clean suction tubing enhances delivery of set suction pressure.
8. Wash face if secretions are present on patient's skin.	Prevents skin breakdown.
9. Observe respiratory status. Repeat procedure if indicated. A standard suction catheter may need to be used to reach into the trachea if respiratory status is not improved (see Skill 23.2).	Directs nurse to continue, cease intervention, or choose another intervention.
10. Remove towel, cloth, or disposable drape and place in garbage or in laundry. Reposition patient; side-lying position encourages drainage and should be used if patient has decreased level of consciousness.	Reduces transmission of microorganisms. Facilitates drainage of oral secretions.
11. Discard remaining water or normal saline into appropriate receptacle. Rinse basin in warm, soapy water and dry with paper towels (check employer policy). Discard disposable cup into appropriate receptacle.	Reduces transmission of microorganisms and maintains medical asepsis. Moist environment encourages microorganism growth.

Critical Decision Point *Keep catheter in non-airtight container such as a brown paper or plastic bag attached to bedrail or in suction canister area. Do not store the catheter where it will come in contact with secretions or excretions, as these fluids promote bacterial growth.*

STEP	RATIONALE
12. Remove PPE and dispose of in appropriate receptacle.	Reduces transmission of microorganisms to other patients and equipment.
13. Position patient and provide oral hygiene as needed.	Promotes patient's comfort.

STEP	RATIONALE
EVALUATION	
1. Compare assessment findings before and after procedure.	Identifies physiological response to suction procedure.
2. Auscultate chest and airways for adventitious sounds.	Presence of lower airway adventitious sounds suggests need for lower airway suctioning.
3. Inspect mouth for any vomitus or remaining secretions.	A clear oral airway is necessary to prevent aspiration.
4. Obtain and record postsuction SpO_2 value. Compare with presuction level.	Provides objective measure of effectiveness of suction procedure (AARC, 2004).
5. Use **teach-back:** "I want to ensure that you understand why I need to suction your mouth. Can you tell me why I need to do this?" Develop a revised teaching plan if patient or caregiver is unable to teach back correctly.	Determines patient's and caregiver's level of understanding of instructional topic.

Unexpected Outcomes	Related Interventions
1. Patient's respiratory distress increases.	• Suction further or implement nasal or tracheal suctioning (Skill 23.2). • Evaluate need for other means to protect airway (e.g., oral intubation, oral airway, positioning). • Provide supplemental oxygen. • Notify health care provider.
2. Bloody secretions are suctioned.	• Assess oral cavity for trauma or lesions. • Reduce amount of suction pressure used. • Observe catheter tip for nicks, which cause mucosal trauma. • Increase frequency of oral hygiene.

Communication and Documentation

- Document the amount, consistency, colour, and odour of secretions; number of times suctioned; patient's response to suctioning; and presuction and postsuction cardiopulmonary assessment findings on flow sheet or progress notes in electronic health record (EHR) or chart.
- Document patient's and caregiver's understanding through teach-back of reasons for safe oral suctioning.
- Interprofessional collaboration should be prioritized by promptly notifying the health care provider of any unresolved outcomes, such as worsening respiratory distress.

DOCUMENTATION EXAMPLE

Patient was having trouble clearing lung secretions and oxygen saturation dropped from 98% to 92%, with coughing noted. Patient HR 132 beats/min during this time. Nurse suctioned via tracheostomy with size 14 French catheter twice and obtained moderate amount of clear, thick, secretions with foul odour. Postsuctioning, the patient no longer had a cough, HR decreased to 80 beats/min, chest sounded clear to all lung fields, and no secretions noted postsuctioning. Catheter was cleaned with NS and placed in non-airtight labelled bag.

Special Considerations

Teaching

- Instruct patient and caregiver not to allow catheter to fall to the floor. If this occurs, teach patient and caregiver how to clean or obtain a clean catheter (see Care in the Community: Home Management).
- Provide information regarding signs and symptoms of worsening respiratory status.

Pediatric

- Airways of infants and children are smaller than those of adults; even small amounts of mucus cause airway obstruction. Smaller suction catheters may need to be used (Hockenberry et al., 2024).
- Bulb syringes may be used to suction the oral cavity in newborns and infants. To properly use a bulb syringe, compress the bulb before inserting into mouth to decrease the risk of forcing the secretions into lower airways. If the bulb syringe cannot remove the secretions, use appropriately sized mechanical suction equipment (Hockenberry et al., 2024).
- Use lower suction pressures with infants and children than with adults (Hockenberry et al., 2024).
- Position infants with breathing problems or excessive vomitus in side-lying position to decrease risk of aspiration (Hockenberry et al., 2024).
- Suctioning, particularly for young infants, should be performed for only 5 seconds because of risk for deoxygenation. Allow 30 to 60 seconds for patient to reoxygenate (Hockenberry et al., 2024).
- Perform oral suctioning first and then nasal suctioning to decrease the risk of aspiration, particularly for newborn infants (Hockenberry et al., 2024).

Gerontological

- Patients with dysphagia may benefit from oral suctioning before, during, and after meals.
- The oral mucosa in older persons is fragile (Boscart et al., 2023). Use a lower suction pressure if bleeding starts to occur. Be particularly alert for bleeding when performing suctioning in older persons who are taking anticoagulant medications.
- Older persons are prone to aspiration of oral secretions because of decreased cough and gag reflexes and increased incidence of dysphagia (Boscart et al., 2023).

Patients With Physical or Cognitive Challenges

- Patients with neuromuscular conditions, such as muscular dystrophy or amyotrophic lateral sclerosis (ALS), have weak and ineffective swallowing and have weak respiratory muscles and need oropharyngeal suctioning to assist in airway clearance (Hockenberry et al., 2024).
- Patients with dysphagia may benefit from oral suctioning before, during, and after meals. Ensure that dysphagia screens are performed for all patients and that properly functioning equipment is available (Boscart et al., 2023).

Care in the Community: Home Management

- Make sure that patient and caregiver know how to clean and disinfect or change the secretion collection container every 24 hours according to home care protocol. Many facilities seal and dispose of the entire disposable secretion collection canister as biohazardous material.
- Assess knowledge level of patient and caregiver to determine amount of instruction required and frequency of home health visits necessary to reach goals.
- Assess home for the presence of respiratory irritants, including cigarette smoke, dust, pollen, animal dander, mould, and chemicals.

✦ SKILL 23.2 Performing Airway Suctioning

NSO *Nursing Skills Online Airway Management Module 9 / Lessons 1, 2, and 3*

Airway suctioning is necessary when patients are unable to clear respiratory secretions. If the secretions are limited to the nose and mouth, then only the pharynx requires suctioning. However, in most instances both the pharynx and the trachea will need to be suctioned. Suction secretions from the pharynx as often as necessary using oropharyngeal suctioning (see Skill 23.1). Secretions that are not removed are more likely to be aspirated into the lungs, increasing the risk of infection, VAP, and respiratory failure. Retained lower airway secretions require the use of tracheal suctioning to remove them. If frequent nasotracheal suctioning is indicated, consider application of a nasopharyngeal airway to prevent trauma.

Prior to initiating airway suctioning, ensure that supplemental oxygen with appropriate delivery devices is readily available at the bedside.

Tracheal airway suctioning is a sterile procedure. It extends into the lower airway and is indicated to remove respiratory secretions and maintain optimum ventilation and oxygenation in patients who are unable to remove these secretions independently. This skill can be performed in people with or without an artificial airway.

Tracheal suctioning has many complications, including hypoxemia, cardiac dysrhythmias, changes in blood pressure (either hypertensive or hypotensive), laryngeal or bronchospasm, pain, infection, and bradycardia. Bradycardia is associated with stimulation of the vagus nerve. Respiratory or cardiac arrest can even occur as a result of tracheal suctioning. Nasal trauma and bleeding can develop from a suction catheter being introduced through the nares (Urden et al., 2020; Wiegand, 2017).

Patient assessment, not routine suctioning, guides the frequency of airway suctioning (Urden et al., 2020). Patient assessment factors indicating the need for suctioning include oxygen saturation below 90%; visible secretions in the airway; patient's inability to produce an effective, productive cough; auscultation of coarse crackles over the trachea; and acute respiratory distress. If the patient has an artificial airway in place or is mechanically ventilated, other indications for suctioning include the presence of a saw-tooth pattern on the flow-volume loop on the ventilator monitor, increased peak inspiratory pressure or decreased tidal volumes noted on the ventilator monitor, abnormal capnography waveforms, and suspected aspiration (Urden et al., 2020; Wiegand, 2017).

Artificial Airway Suctioning

Endotracheal tubes (ETs) and tracheostomy tubes (TTs) are artificial airways inserted to maintain respiratory flow and prevent airway obstruction, provide a route for mechanical ventilation, permit easy access for secretion removal, and protect the airway from gross aspiration in patients with impaired cough or gag reflexes.

Endotracheal Tubes

NSO *Nursing Skills Online Airway Management Module 9 / Lesson 4*

ET intubation is a procedure performed by a health care provider or other specially trained personnel (e.g., certified registered nurse anaesthesiologist, respiratory therapist, or rescue personnel). An ET is inserted through the nares (nasotracheal tube) or most commonly through the mouth (oral ET), past the epiglottis and vocal cords, and into the trachea (Fig. 23.2, A–B). Oral ETs are usually made of plastic or rubber. Adult (and some pediatric) sizes of ETs have a cuff moulded onto the tube. When the cuff is inflated, it seals the airway around the tube to prevent the aspiration of oral secretions or gastric contents into the lungs and to obstruct the escape of air from mechanical ventilator breaths through the upper airway. Some newer ETs also contain a port that can be connected for continuous subglottic suctioning (CSS).

The length of time that an ET should remain in place is disputed. Complications from long-term intubation include laryngeal and tracheal stenosis or a cricoid abscess (Urden et al., 2020). Sources differ on when a patient should be changed from an ET to a TT. The recommended length of time to be intubated ranges from 7 to 10 days (Urden et al., 2020; Wang et al., 2019). It is appropriate to consult with a health care provider if a patient begins to show signs of complications from the airways themselves, such as erosion of the oral mucosa. Known benefits of having a TT versus an ET include less need for deeper sedation, shorter ventilator weaning time (time it takes to get a patient off a ventilator), and shorter critical care unit (CCU) and hospital stay (Wang et al., 2019).

Tracheostomy Tubes

NSO *Nursing Skills Online Airway Management Module 9/ Lesson 5*

A TT can be temporary or permanent, depending on a patient's condition. It is inserted either surgically or percutaneously directly into the trachea through a small incision made in a patient's neck. Reasons for using a TT include the need for prolonged mechanical ventilation, upper airway obstruction secondary to trauma or tumour, and difficulties with airway clearance that occur in conditions such as spinal cord injury or neuromuscular disease (Urden et al., 2020). TTs are made of several different materials, including polyvinyl chloride or silicone-based plastics and stainless steel or metallic compounds. Metal TTs are thermally sensitive and must be protected from extreme heat and cold to prevent tissue injury in a patient. Most metal and plastic TTs contain an inner cannula that is withdrawn temporarily for cleaning airway-occluding mucus without removing the entire TT. The inner cannula can be cleaned and reused or may be a disposable plastic device (see Skill 23.4) (Urden et al., 2020).

The use of closed-system suction catheters for suctioning artificial airways has increased in recent years and is used with patients that are on a ventilator. Use of a closed-system catheter (in-line) allows

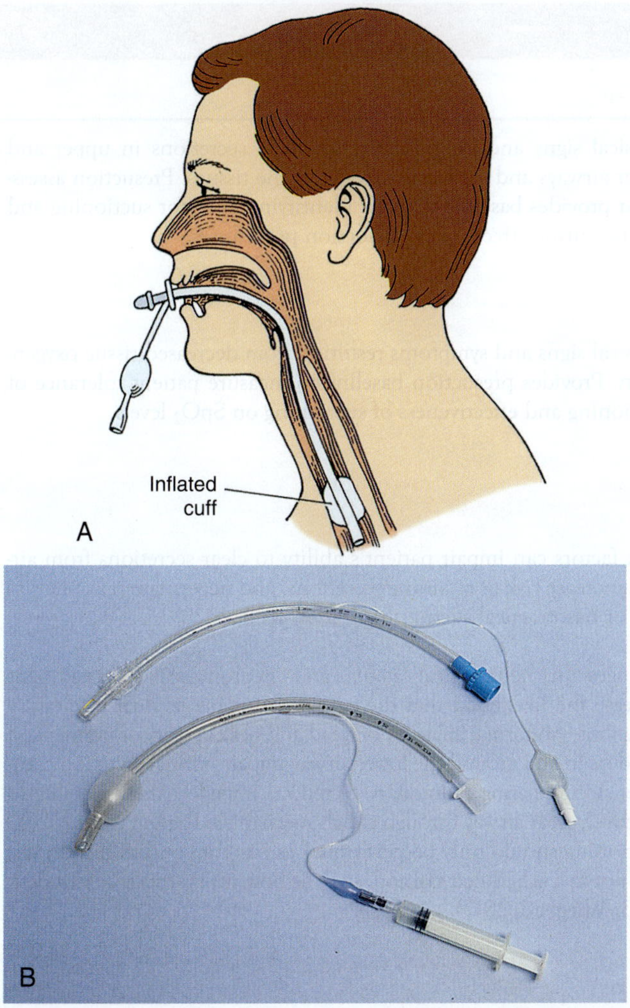

FIG 23.2 A, Endotracheal tube with inflated cuff. B, Endotracheal tubes with uninflated and inflated cuffs and syringe for inflation.

quicker lower airway suctioning without application of sterile gloves or a mask, and it does not interrupt ventilation and oxygenation in critically ill patients (see Procedural Guideline 23.1). With a closed-system method, the patient's artificial airway is not disconnected from the mechanical ventilator; therefore, there is no loss of PEEP. Another advantage of this system includes quicker, more efficient performance of the suctioning procedure. When comparing closed versus open suctioning, the incidence of VAP is unchanged. However, with a closed system, a health care provider faces decreased risk of infection from exposure to patient secretions (Letchford & Bench, 2018; Urden et al., 2020). The recommended frequency for replacing closed-system suction catheters is every 24 to 48 hours, or according to employer policy.

Delegation and Collaboration

The skill of performing airway suctioning of newly inserted artificial airways cannot be delegated to a UCP. The nurse instructs the UCP about the following:

- Any modifications of the skill, such as the need for supplemental oxygen or the use of a clean versus sterile suction technique
- Appropriate suction limits for suctioning ETs and TTs and risks of applying excessive or inadequate suction pressure
- Reporting any changes in the patient's respiratory status, level of consciousness, restlessness, secretion colour and amount, and unresolved coughing or gagging
- Reporting any change in the patient's colour, vital signs, or indications of pain

Collaborate with the interprofessional team (e.g., respiratory therapist, physiotherapist, occupational therapist) to determine whether there are any needed alterations to the suctioning procedure, such as not increasing oxygen before suctioning or not changing patient position. Communicate frequency of suctioning and patient response to suctioning.

Equipment

- Stethoscope
- Pulse oximeter
- Portable or wall suction machine
- Connecting tubing (1.8 metres [6 feet])
- Bedside table
- PPE, as indicated (see Box 5.1)

Endotracheal or Tracheostomy Suctioning

- Appropriately sized suction catheter, usually 12–16 French (Fr). It should be the smallest diameter that will remove secretions effectively, preferably one that is no more than half the internal diameter of the artificial airway, to minimize decrease in partial pressure of oxygen (PaO_2) (Billington & Luckett, 2019).
- Two sterile gloves, or one sterile and one clean glove
- Clean towel or paper drape
- Small Y-adapter (if catheter does not have a suction control port)
- Sterile basin or solution container
- Sterile normal saline solution or water, about 100 mL
- Pulse oximeter, stethoscope, and end-tidal CO_2 detector
- Manual self-inflating manual resuscitation bag-valve device with appropriately sized mask
- PEEP valve for resuscitation bag

STEP	RATIONALE
ASSESSMENT	
1. Identify patient using at least two person-specific identifiers (e.g., name and date of birth, or name and medical record number) according to employer policy.	Ensures correct patient. Complies with Accreditation Canada's standards and improves patient safety (Accreditation Canada, 2020).
2. Throughout the procedure, the 4 moments for hand hygiene are to be implemented; hand hygiene should occur before initial patient (or patient environment) contact, before an aseptic procedure, after body fluid exposure risk, and after patient (or patient environment) contact. Additional hand hygiene should be performed when hands are visibly soiled.	Proper hand hygiene helps prevent spread of infectious agents to health care providers.

STEP	RATIONALE
ASSESSMENT	
3. Apply gloves if there is risk of exposing self to secretions. Assess for signs and symptoms of upper and lower airway obstruction that indicate suctioning is required: abnormal respiratory rate, adventitious lung sounds, nasal secretions, gurgling, drooling, restlessness, gastric secretions or vomitus in mouth, and coughing without clearing airway secretions or improving adventitious lung sounds.	Physical signs and symptoms result from secretions in upper and lower airways and decreased oxygen to the tissues. Presuction assessment provides baseline data for identifying need for suctioning and for measuring effectiveness of suction procedures.
4. Assess vital signs and signs and symptoms associated with hypoxia and hypercapnia: decreased SpO_2, increased pulse and blood pressure, apprehension, anxiety, lack of concentration, lethargy, decreased level of consciousness, confusion, dizziness, behavioural changes (e.g., irritability), irregular heartbeat, pallor, and cyanosis (a very late sign of hypoxia). Keep pulse oximeter on patient.	Physical signs and symptoms resulting from decreased tissue oxygenation. Provides presuction baseline to measure patient tolerance of suctioning and effectiveness of suctioning on SpO_2 levels.
5. Assess for risk factors for upper and lower airway obstruction, including COPD, impaired mobility, decreased level of consciousness, nasal feeding tube, decreased cough or gag reflex, and decreased swallowing ability.	Risk factors can impair patient's ability to clear secretions from airway, increase risk of retaining secretions, and necessitate nasopharyngeal or nasotracheal suctioning (Urden et al., 2020).
6. Identify patients with an increased risk of inadequate airway clearance (e.g., patients with decreased level of consciousness, neuromuscular or neurological impairment, or anatomical factors that influence upper or lower airway function, such as recent head or neck surgery or neck tumours).	Changes in neurological status and neuromuscular impairment increase the likelihood that the patient is unable to clear respiratory secretions. Abnormal anatomy or head and neck surgery or trauma and tumours in and around the lower airway impair normal secretion clearance. Accumulating pulmonary secretions impede patient's ability to effectively clear airway through cough mechanism (Urden et al., 2020).
7. Assess for excessive amounts of secretions or secretions visible in the artificial airway, signs of respiratory distress (increased work of breathing, increased respiratory rate), presence of rhonchi on auscultation, excessive coughing, or decrease in patient pulse oximeter; if patient is on mechanical ventilation, also assess for increased peak inspiratory pressures, saw-tooth pattern on ventilator monitor, or changes in capnography waveform.	Suctioning should only be performed as patient condition indicates and not in a scheduled fashion, such as hourly (Tyerman & Cobbett, 2023; Wiegand, 2017).
8. Assess patency of ET with capnography/end-tidal CO_2 detector.	ET may become displaced or blocked by secretions. CO_2 detector is pH sensitive and can be used to identify changes in CO_2 levels caused by retained secretions.
9. Assess factors that may affect volume and consistency of secretions.	Thickened or copious secretions increase risk of airway obstruction.
a. Fluid balance	Fluid overload increases amount of secretions. Dehydration promotes thicker secretions.
b. Lack of humidity	Environment influences secretion formation and gas exchange. Airway suctioning is needed when patient cannot clear secretions effectively.
c. Infection (e.g., pneumonia)	Patients with respiratory infections are prone to increased secretions that are thicker and sometimes more difficult to expectorate.
10. For endotracheal suctioning, assess patient's peak inspiratory pressure (when on volume-controlled ventilation) or tidal volume (when on pressure-controlled ventilation).	Increased peak inspiratory pressure or decreased tidal volume may indicate airway obstruction (Urden et al., 2020).

Critical Decision Point *The patient's vital signs, pulse oximetry, end-tidal CO_2, and respiratory status will be assessed before and continuously throughout the procedure* (Wiegand, 2017).

STEP	RATIONALE
11. Identify contraindications to nasotracheal suctioning: occluded nasal passages; nasal bleeding; epiglottis or croup; acute head, facial, or neck injury or surgery; coagulopathy or bleeding disorder; irritable airway; laryngospasm or bronchospasm; gastric surgery with high anastomosis; and myocardial infarction (AARC, 2004; Hockenberry et al., 2024; Wiegand, 2017).	These conditions are contraindicated because passage of a suction catheter through the nasal route causes trauma to existing facial trauma or surgery, increases nasal bleeding, or causes severe bleeding in presence of coagulopathy or bleeding disorders. In presence of epiglottis or croup, laryngospasm, or irritable airway, passage of a suction catheter through the nose causes intractable coughing, hypoxemia, and severe bronchospasm, necessitating emergency intubation or tracheostomy. Hypoxemia could worsen cardiac damage in myocardial infarction (AARC, 2004).

ASSESSMENT

STEP	RATIONALE
12. Review sputum microbiology data in laboratory report.	Certain bacteria are easier to transmit or require isolation because of virulence or antibiotic resistance.
13. Determine presence of apprehension, anxiety, decreased ability to concentrate, lethargy, decreased level of consciousness (especially acute), increased fatigue, dizziness, behavioural changes (especially irritability), pallor, cyanosis, dyspnea, or use of accessory muscles.	These are signs and symptoms of hypoxia and/or hypercapnia, which can indicate need for suction. These signs can also help in identifying patient's ability to cooperate with procedure.
14. Assess for patient's understanding of procedure and presence of any apprehension.	Reveals need for instruction or psychosocial support.

NURSING DIAGNOSES

- Inadequate spontaneous ventilation
- Inadequate breathing pattern
- Inadequate gas exchange
- Inadequate swallowing
- Reduced airway clearance
- Anxiety
- Insufficient knowledge regarding suctioning
- Fatigue
- Reduced comfort
- Potential for aspiration
- Potential for infection

Related factors and risk factors are individualized on the basis of patient's condition or needs.

PLANNING

STEP	RATIONALE
1. Expected outcomes following completion of procedure:	
• Upper and lower airways demonstrate absent or diminished gurgles, crackles, rhonchi, and wheezes on inspiration and expiration.	Absent or diminished adventitious sounds indicate that airways are cleared of secretions and are patent.
• Heart rate, blood pressure, respiratory rate, and effort are within normal range for patient.	When airway secretions are removed and oxygenation improves, patient's vital signs and respiratory assessment findings improve.
• Patient's SpO_2 is at or above baseline, whereas end-tidal CO_2 concentration, if being monitored, is at or below baseline.	Demonstrates improvement in gas exchange (Wiegand, 2017).

Critical Decision Point *While normal end-tidal CO_2 ranges from 35 to 45 mm Hg, it is important to ensure that the patient's value is below the normal baseline. Persons with pulmonary diseases often have abnormal CO_2 values.*

STEP	RATIONALE
• Patient's peak inspiratory pressure decreases back to baseline, and exhaled tidal volume increases back to baseline.	Demonstrates removal of secretions (Wiegand, 2017).
2. Help patient to comfortable position, typically semi-Fowler's or high Fowler's.	Reduces stimulation of gag reflex, promotes patient comfort and secretion drainage, and prevents aspiration.
3. If not already present, place pulse oximeter on patient's finger. Take reading and leave oximeter in place.	Provides continuous SpO_2 value to determine patient's response to suctioning.
4. Explain to patient how procedure will help clear airway and relieve breathing difficulty. Explain that temporary coughing, sneezing, gagging, or shortness of breath is normal during procedure.	Encourages cooperation and minimizes risks, anxiety, and pain of procedure.

IMPLEMENTATION

STEP	RATIONALE
1. Apply appropriate PPE, as indicated.	Reduces transmission of microorganisms.
2. Adjust bed to appropriate height (if not already done) and lower side rail on side nearest you. Check locks on bed wheel.	Minimizes caregiver's muscle strain and prevents injury. Prevents bed from moving.
3. Connect one end of connecting tubing to suction device and place other end in convenient location near patient. Turn suction device on and set suction pressure to a level as low as possible and yet able to effectively clear secretions. This value is typically between 100 and 150 mm Hg in adults (between 60 and 100 mm Hg in neonates) (American Association of Critical-Care Nurses [AACN], 2010; AARC, 2010). Occlude end of suction tubing to check pressure.	Ensures equipment function. Excessive negative pressure damages tracheal mucosa and induces greater hypoxia (Weigand, 2017).

STEP	RATIONALE
IMPLEMENTATION	
4. Prepare suction catheter for all types of open suctioning.	
a. Using aseptic technique, open suction kit or catheter package. If sterile drape is available, place it across patient's chest or on bedside table. Do not allow suction catheter to touch any nonsterile surfaces.	Prepares catheter, maintains asepsis, and reduces transmission of microorganisms. Provides sterile surface on which to lay catheter between passes.
b. Unwrap or open sterile basin and place on bedside table. Be careful not to touch inside of basin. Fill with about 100 mL sterile normal saline solution or water (see Step 4b illustration).	Saline or water is used to clean tubing after each suction pass.
c. If performing nasotracheal suctioning, open packet of water-soluble lubricant and apply small amount to catheter. NOTE: Lubricant is not necessary for artificial airway suctioning.	Water-soluble lubricant helps prevent lipid aspiration pneumonia. An excessive amount of lubricant occludes catheter.
5. Apply sterile gloves to each hand, or nonsterile glove to nondominant hand and sterile glove to dominant hand.	Reduces transmission of microorganisms and maintains sterility of suction catheter.
6. Pick up suction catheter with dominant hand without touching nonsterile surfaces. Pick up connecting tubing with nondominant hand. Secure catheter to tubing (see Step 6 illustration).	Maintains catheter sterility. Connects catheter to suction.

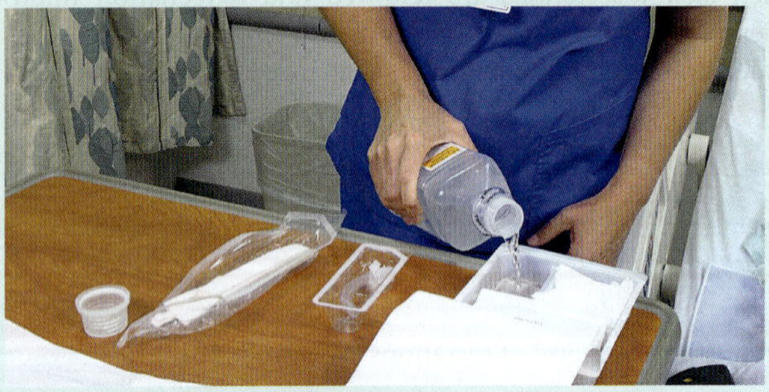

STEP 4B Pouring sterile saline into tray.

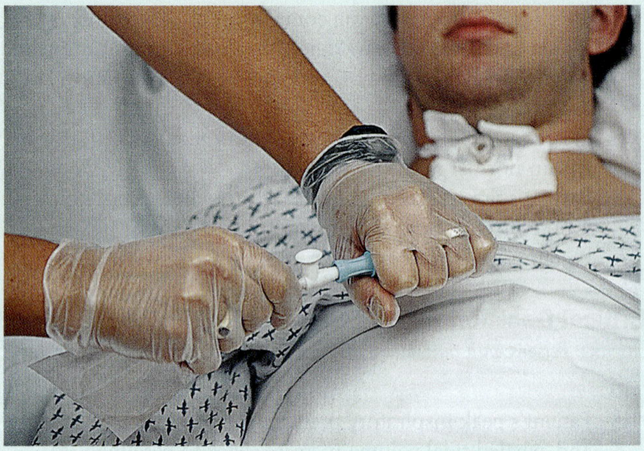

STEP 6 Attaching suction catheter to suction tubing.

STEP	RATIONALE
7. Place tip of catheter into sterile basin and suction small amount of normal saline solution from basin by occluding suction vent.	Ensures equipment function. Lubricates internal catheter and tubing.
8. Suction airway.	
a. Nasopharyngeal and nasotracheal suctioning:	
(1) Have patient take deep breaths, if able, or increase oxygen flow rate with delivery device through cannula or mask (if prescribed).	May help decrease risk of hypoxemia.
(2) Lightly coat distal 5–8 cm (2–3 inches) of catheter with water-soluble lubricant.	Lubricates catheter for easier insertion.
(3) Remove oxygen delivery device, if applicable, with nondominant hand.	Allows access to nares and catheter.

Critical Decision Point *Be sure to insert the catheter during patient inhalation, especially if inserting it into the trachea, because the epiglottis is open. Do not insert during swallowing or the catheter will most likely enter the esophagus.* ***Never apply suction during insertion.*** *The patient should cough. If patient gags or becomes nauseated, the catheter is most likely in the esophagus and you need to remove it.*

STEP	RATIONALE

IMPLEMENTATION

(a) *Nasopharyngeal (without applying suction):* As patient takes a deep breath, insert catheter following natural course of naris; slightly slant catheter downward and advance to back of pharynx. Do not force through naris. In adults, insert catheter approximately 16 cm (6.5 inches); in older children, 8–12 cm (3–5 inches); in infants and young children, 4–7.5 cm (1.5–3 inches). The rule of thumb is to insert catheter the distance from tip of nose (or mouth) to angle of mandible.	Ensures that catheter tip reaches pharynx for suctioning.

Critical Decision Point *If resistance is met during insertion, you may need to try the other naris. Do not force the catheter up the nares because this will cause mucosal damage.*

(i) Apply intermittent suctioning for no more than 10 seconds by placing and releasing nondominant thumb over catheter vent. Slowly withdraw catheter while rotating it back and forth between the thumb and forefinger.	Intermittent suctioning for up to 10 seconds safely removes pharyngeal secretions. Suction time greater than 10 seconds increases risk of suction-induced hypoxemia (AARC, 2010; Urden et al., 2020; Wiegand, 2017).
(b) *Nasotracheal (without applying suction):* As patient takes a deep breath, advance catheter following natural course of naris. Advance catheter slightly slanted and downward to just above entrance into larynx and then trachea. While patient takes a deep breath, quickly insert catheter: for adults, insert approximately 15–20 cm (6–8 inches) into trachea (see Step 8a[3][b] illustration). Patient will begin to cough; then pull back catheter 1–2 cm (0.4–0.8 inches) before applying suction. NOTE: In older children, insert catheter 15–20 cm (6–8 inches); in infants and young children, insert 8–14 cm (3–5.5 inches).	Ensures that catheter tip reaches trachea for suctioning.

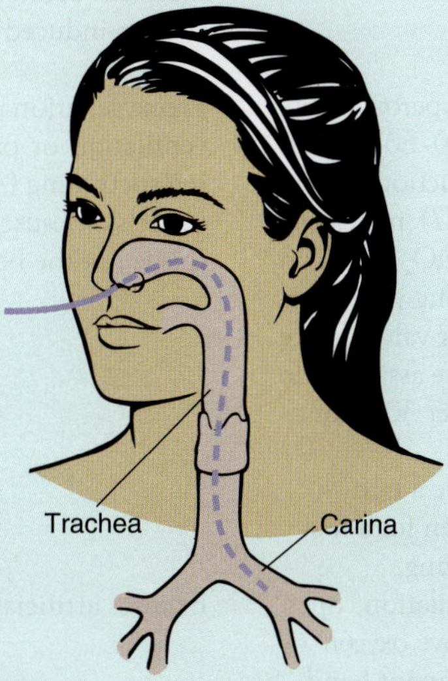

STEP 8A(3)(B) Distance of insertion of nasotracheal catheter.

STEP	RATIONALE

IMPLEMENTATION

Critical Decision Point *When using the nasal approach, perform tracheal suctioning before pharyngeal suctioning whenever possible. The mouth and pharynx contain more bacteria than the trachea. If copious oral secretions are present before beginning the procedure, suction mouth with oral suction device first.*

Critical Decision Point *When there is difficulty in passing the catheter, ask patient to cough or say "ahh," or try to advance the catheter during inspiration. Both measures help open the glottis to permit passage of the catheter into the trachea.*

(i) *Positioning option:* In some instances, turning patient's head helps increase effectiveness of suctioning. If resistance is felt after insertion of the catheter, use caution; catheter has probably hit the carina. Pull catheter back 1–2 cm (0.4–0.8 inches) before applying suction (AARC, 2004; Wiegand, 2017).

Turning patient's head to side elevates bronchial passage on opposite side. Turning head to right helps with suctioning of left main-stem bronchus; turning head to left helps with suctioning right main-stem bronchus. Suctioning too deeply may cause tracheal mucosa trauma.

(ii) Apply intermittent suctioning for no more than 10 seconds by placing and releasing nondominant thumb over catheter vent. Slowly withdraw catheter while rotating it back and forth between thumb and forefinger.

Suction time greater than 10 seconds increases risk of suction-induced hypoxemia (AACN, 2010; AARC, 2010; Urden et al., 2020). Suctioning too frequently or for a prolonged time can cause an increase in secretions. Intermittent suctioning and rotation of catheter prevents injury to tracheal mucosa. If catheter "grabs" mucosa, remove thumb to release suction.

Critical Decision Point *Monitor patient's vital signs and oxygen saturation throughout suctioning process. Stop suctioning if there is a 20 beats/min change (increase or decrease) in pulse rate or if SpO_2 falls below 90% or deviates 5% from baseline.*

(4) Reapply oxygen delivery device and encourage patient to take some deep breaths, if able.

Helps decrease risk of hypoxia. Increases patient comfort.

(5) Rinse catheter and connecting tubing with normal saline or water until cleared.

Secretions that remain in suction catheter or connecting tubing decrease suctioning efficiency.

(6) Assess for need to repeat suctioning. Do not perform more than two passes with catheter. Allow patient to rest at least 1 minute (AACN, 2010; AARC, 2010). Ask patient to breathe deeply and cough.

Observe for alterations in cardiopulmonary status. Suctioning induces hypoxemia, irregular pulse, laryngospasm, and bronchospasm (AACN, 2010; AARC, 2010). Hyperoxygenation is recommended before, during, and after open suctioning to reduce suction-induced hypoxemia (Urden et al., 2020; Wiegand, 2017).

b. Artificial airway:

(1) When patient has an artificial airway, hyperoxygenate patient with 100% oxygen for at least 30–60 seconds before suctioning by (1) pressing suction hyperoxygenation button on ventilator *or* (2) increasing baseline fraction of inspired oxygen (FiO_2) level on mechanical ventilator *or* (3) disconnecting ventilator, attaching self-inflating resuscitation bag-valve device to tube with nondominant hand (or have assistant do this), and administering 5–6 breaths over 30 seconds (or have assistant do this).

NOTE: Some mechanical ventilators have a button that, when pushed, delivers 100% oxygen for a few minutes and then resets to previous setting.

Preoxygenation reduces risk of decreased arterial oxygen levels while ventilation or oxygenation is interrupted and volume is lost during suctioning (AACN, 2010; AARC, 2010; Wiegand, 2017). Some models of resuscitation bags do not deliver 100% oxygen; therefore, this is not the best way to oxygenate patient (Wiegand, 2017).

(2) If patient is receiving mechanical ventilation, open the swivel adapter or, if necessary, remove oxygen- or humidity-delivery device using nondominant hand.

Exposes artificial airway.

Critical Decision Point *Suctioning can cause elevation in ICP in patients with head injuries. Reduce this risk by using presuction hyperoxygenation, which results in hypocarbia, which in turn induces vasoconstriction. Vasoconstriction reduces the potential for an increase in ICP* (Urden et al., 2020).

STEP	RATIONALE

IMPLEMENTATION

(3) Advise patient that you are about to begin suctioning. Without applying suction, gently but quickly insert catheter into artificial airway using dominant thumb and forefinger (it is best to try to time catheter insertion into artificial airway with inspiration) (see Step 8b[3] illustration). Advance catheter until you meet resistance or patient coughs; then, pull back 1 cm (0.4 inches) (Billington & Luckett, 2019).

Application of suction pressure while introducing catheter into trachea increases risk of damage to tracheal mucosa and increased hypoxia. Pulling back stimulates cough and removes catheter from mucosal wall so catheter is not resting against tracheal mucosa during suctioning. Shallow suctioning is recommended to prevent tracheal mucosa trauma (AACN, 2010; Wiegand, 2017).

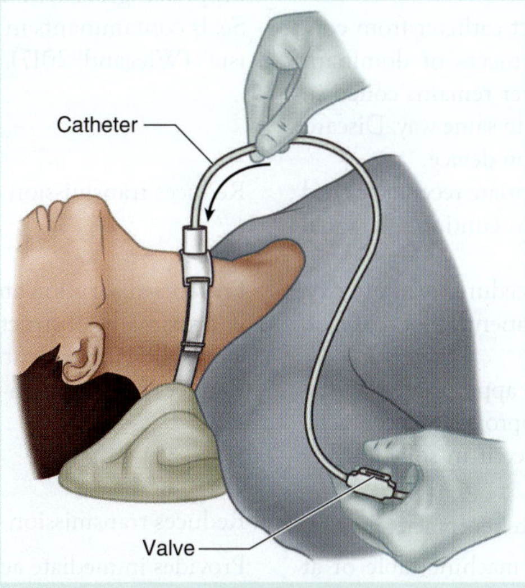

STEP 8B(3) Suctioning tracheostomy.

Critical Decision Point *If you are unable to insert the catheter past the end of the ET, the catheter is probably caught in the Murphy eye (i.e., side hole at the distal end of the ET that allows for collateral airflow in the event of tracheal main-stem intubation). If this happens, rotate the catheter to reposition it away from the Murphy eye or withdraw it slightly and reinsert with the next inhalation. Usually, the catheter meets resistance at the carina. One indication that the catheter is at the carina is acute onset of coughing, because the carina contains many cough receptors. Pull the catheter back 1 cm (0.4 inches)* (Billington & Luckett, 2019).

(4) Apply intermittent suctioning for 10 seconds (AACN, 2010; AARC, 2010; Wiegand, 2017) by placing and releasing nondominant thumb over vent of catheter; slowly withdraw catheter while rotating it back and forth between dominant thumb and forefinger. Do not use suction for greater than 15 seconds. Encourage patient to cough. Watch for respiratory distress.

Suction time greater than 10 seconds increases risk of suction-induced hypoxemia (AACN, 2010; AARC, 2010; Urden at al., 2020; Wiegand, 2017). Intermittent suctioning and rotation of catheter prevent injury to tracheal mucosa. If catheter "grabs" mucosa, remove thumb to release suction.

Critical Decision Point *If patient develops respiratory distress during the suctioning procedure, immediately withdraw catheter and supply additional oxygen and breaths as needed. In an emergency, administer oxygen directly through the catheter. Disconnect suction and attach oxygen at prescribed flow rate through the catheter. If the patient does not tolerate the suctioning procedure, you may need to consider switching to closed (in-line) suctioning or allowing longer recovery times. Notify health care provider if patient develops significant cardiopulmonary compromise during suctioning* (Urden et al., 2020; Wiegand, 2017).

(5) If patient is receiving mechanical ventilation, close swivel adapter or replace oxygen delivery device. Hyperoxygenate patient for 30–60 seconds.

Re-establishes artificial airway. Helps decrease risk of hypoxia.

(6) Rinse catheter and connecting tubing with normal saline until clear. Use continuous suction.

Removes catheter secretions. Secretions left in tubing decrease suctioning efficiency and provide environment for microorganism growth.

(7) Assess patient's vital signs, cardiopulmonary status, and ventilator measures for secretion clearance. Repeat Steps 1–6 once or twice more to clear secretions. Allow adequate time (at least 1 full minute) between suction passes.

Suctioning can induce dysrhythmias, hypoxia, and bronchospasm and impair cerebral circulation or adversely affect hemodynamic stability (Wiegand, 2017).

STEP	RATIONALE

IMPLEMENTATION

Critical Decision Point *The number of suction passes should be based on patient assessment and presence of secretions. If secretions persist after two passes, allow patient more time to rest and recover from these procedures* (Wiegand, 2017).

STEP	RATIONALE
(8) When pharynx and trachea are sufficiently cleared of secretions, perform oropharyngeal suctioning (Skill 23.1) to clear mouth of secretions. Do not suction nose again after suctioning mouth.	Removes upper airway secretions. More microorganisms generally are present in mouth. Upper airway is considered "clean," and lower airway is considered "sterile." You can use the same catheter to suction from sterile to clean areas (e.g., tracheal suctioning to oropharyngeal suctioning) but not from clean to sterile areas.
9. When suctioning is complete, disconnect catheter from connecting tubing. Roll catheter around fingers of dominant hand. Pull glove off inside out so catheter remains coiled in glove. Pull off other glove over first glove in same way. Discard in appropriate receptacle. Turn off suction device.	Seals contaminants in gloves. Reduces transmission of microorganisms (Wiegand, 2017).
10. Remove towel, place in laundry or appropriate receptacle, and reposition patient. (Apply clean gloves to continue personal care.)	Reduces transmission of microorganisms. Promotes comfort.
11. If oxygen level was changed during procedure, readjust oxygen to original prescribed level because patient's blood oxygen level should have returned to baseline.	Prevents absorption atelectasis (i.e., tendency for airways to collapse if proximally obstructed by secretions). Prevents oxygen toxicity while allowing patient time to reoxygenate blood.
12. Discard remainder of normal saline into appropriate receptacle. If basin is disposable, discard into appropriate receptacle. If basin is reusable, rinse it out and place it in soiled utility room.	Reduces transmission of microorganisms.
13. Remove PPE and discard into appropriate receptacle.	Reduces transmission of microorganisms.
14. Place unopened suction kit on suction machine table or at HOB.	Provides immediate access to suction catheter for next procedure.
15. Help patient to comfortable position and provide oral hygiene as needed.	

EVALUATION

STEP	RATIONALE
1. Compare patient's vital signs, cardiopulmonary assessments, and end-tidal CO_2 and SpO_2 values before and after suctioning. If patient is on ventilator, compare FiO_2 and tidal volumes and peak inspiratory pressures.	Identifies physiological effects of suction procedure to restore airway patency.
2. Ask patient whether breathing is easier and congestion is decreased.	Provides subjective confirmation that suctioning procedure has relieved airway.
3. Auscultate lungs and compare patient's respiratory assessment before and after suctioning.	Provides objective information about any change in lung sounds.
4. Observe character of airway secretions.	Provides data to document presence or absence of respiratory tract infection or thickened secretions.
5. Use teach-back: "I need to perform airway suctioning on your father. I want to be sure that I explained the suctioning procedure and when I need to do it. Please tell me in your own words why he needs suctioning." Develop a revised teaching plan if patient or caregiver is unable to teach back correctly.	Determines patient's and caregiver's level of understanding of instructional topic.

Unexpected Outcomes	Related Interventions
1. Patient has decrease in overall cardiopulmonary status as evidenced by decreased SpO_2, increased end-tidal CO_2, continued tachypnea, continued increased work of breathing, and cardiac dysrhythmias.	• Limit length of suctioning. • Determine need for more frequent suctioning, possibly of shorter duration. • Determine need for supplemental oxygen or increase in supplemental oxygen. Supply oxygen between suctioning passes. • Notify health care provider.
2. Bloody secretions are returned after suctioning.	• Determine amount of suction pressure used. It may need to be decreased. • Ensure that suction is completed correctly using intermittent suctioning and catheter rotation. Do not apply suction until after catheter has been pulled back 1 cm (0.4 inches) to prevent application of suction while catheter is touching carina. • Evaluate suctioning frequency. • Provide more frequent oral hygiene.
3. Patient has paroxysms of coughing or bronchospasm.	• Administer supplemental oxygen. • Allow patient to rest between passes of suction catheter. • Consult with health care provider regarding need for inhaled bronchodilators or topical anaesthetics.
4. Inability to obtain secretions during suction procedure.	• Evaluate patient's fluid status and adequacy of humidification on oxygen delivery device. • Assess for signs of infection. • Determine need for chest physiotherapy (see Chapter 24).

Communication and Documentation

- Document the amount, consistency, colour, and odour of secretions; size of catheter; route of suctioning; and patient's response to suctioning on flow sheet in progress notes in EHR or chart.
- Document need for hyperoxygenation, type of hyperoxygenation, and percent of oxygenation used.
- Document patient's and caregiver's understanding through teach-back.
- Document patient's presuctioning and postsuctioning vital signs, cardiopulmonary status, and ventilation measures on flow sheet in progress notes in EHR or chart.
- Report patient's intolerance to procedure or unexpected physiological changes to health care provider.

Special Considerations

Teaching

- Instruct patient that coughing increases and that there will be some discomfort during the procedure.
- Explain why supplemental oxygen is given before and after suctioning if indicated.

Pediatric

- The size of the suction catheter should occlude less than 70% of the artificial airway in infants and less than 50% of the artificial airway in children (AACN, 2010; AARC, 2010).
- Hyperoxygenate with 100% oxygen in pediatric patients and 10% increase of baseline in neonates before suctioning (Hockenberry et al., 2024).
- Perform ET suctioning only when clinically indicated in infants and neonates. Clinical signs are notable changes in respiratory rate and breath sounds, increased secretions, bradycardia, or restlessness (Hockenberry et al., 2024).
- Thick secretions are more difficult to remove because of the small diameter of the suction catheter. Normal saline should not be instilled in the airway in an attempt to thin the secretions (AACN, 2010; AARC, 2010).
- Make sure that distance suctioned is not greater than 0.5 cm (0.2 inches) beyond the tip of the artificial airway. To determine distance, place catheter near a sample artificial airway (Hockenberry et al., 2024).
- Infant airways have less cartilage and may collapse easily, especially in premature infants or those with reactive airways.
- Suctioning should not last beyond 5 seconds, and negative pressure should not exceed 100 mm Hg (Hockenberry et al., 2024).

Gerontological

- Older persons lose some properties of elastic recoil and gas exchange.
- Capillaries of older persons are often fragile, predisposing patients to bleeding problems.
- Patients with coronary artery disease are at greater risk of cardiopulmonary compromise.

Care in the Community: Home Management

- Most patients with airway clearance problems at home have a tracheostomy.
- Instruct patient and caregiver to clean and disinfect or change the secretion collection container every 24 hours according to employer policy.
- In the home setting, stress the importance of brief intervals of applying suction pressure. Instruct those performing suctioning to hold their breath during the application of negative suction pressure to help them remember to not suction for too long.

Procedural Guideline 23.1 *Closed (In-Line) Suctioning*

NSO Nursing Skills Online Airway Management Module 9 / Lesson 4

Closed (or in-line) suctioning is another method of suctioning an artificial airway. It involves the use of a multi-use suction catheter that is housed within a plastic sleeve and attached to a patient's artificial airway (Fig. 23.3, *A–B*). This method of suctioning is associated with decreased risk of hypoxia and cardiovascular complications compared with open suctioning. It is also the recommended method of suctioning for patients who cannot tolerate loss of PEEP, such as those with severe respiratory disorders who require high amounts of PEEP or oxygen (Dhawan, 2018).

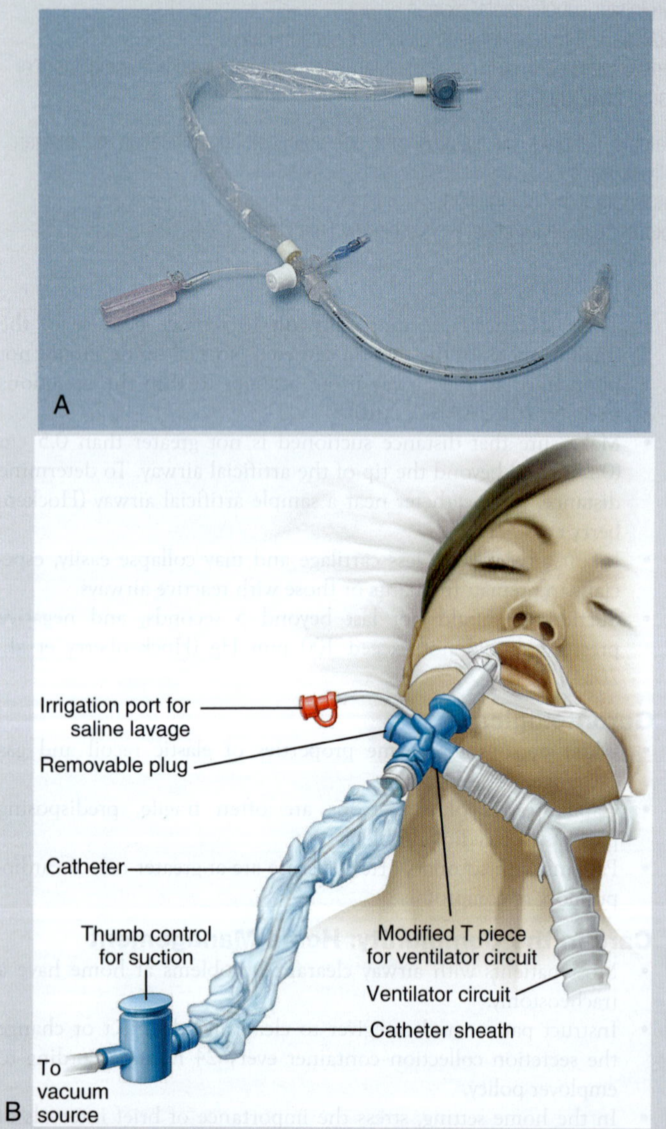

FIG 23.3 A, Closed-system suction catheter attached to endotracheal tube. B, Closed suction system attached to an endotracheal tube. *(B from Blanchard, B. [2011]. Thoracic surgery. In Rothrock, J. C., & McEwen, D. R. [Eds.], Alexander's care of the patient in surgery [14th ed.]. Mosby.)*

Delegation and Collaboration

The skill of performing airway suctioning with a closed (in-line) suction catheter cannot be delegated to a UCP. In special situations, such as suctioning a well-established permanent tracheostomy, this procedure may be delegated to a UCP (refer to employer policy). The nurse is responsible for cardiopulmonary assessment and evaluation of the patient. The nurse instructs the UCP about the following:

- Any individualized aspects of patient care that pertain to suctioning (e.g., position, duration of suction, pressure settings)
- Expected quality, quantity, and colour of secretions and informing the nurse immediately if there are changes
- Patient's anticipated response to suction and reporting immediately to the nurse changes in vital signs, indications of pain, shortness of breath, confusion, or increased restlessness

The nurse often uses interprofessional collaboration (e.g., respiratory therapist) when assessing the patient and performing the suctioning procedure.

Equipment

- Closed-system (or in-line) suction catheter
- Sterile saline solution lavage containers (5–10 mL)
- Suction machine/source with regulator
- Connecting tubing (1.8 metres [6 feet])
- Two clean gloves
- Oral suction kit/supplies for oropharyngeal suctioning
- Mask, goggles, or face shield; gown if isolation precautions indicate
- Oral mucus trap for specimen collection (if prescribed)
- Pulse oximeter and stethoscope
- Manual self-inflating resuscitation bag (bag-valve mask) with appropriately sized mask, while not necessary for the procedure, is safe to have on hand

Procedural Steps

1. Identify patient using at least two person-specific identifiers (e.g., name and date of birth, or name and medical record number) according to employer policy (Accreditation Canada, 2020).
2. Throughout the procedure, the 4 moments for hand hygiene are to be implemented; hand hygiene should occur before initial patient (or patient environment) contact, before an aseptic procedure, after body fluid exposure risk, and after patient (or patient environment) contact. Additional hand hygiene should be performed when hands are visibly soiled.
3. Gather equipment and supplies and close room door or curtain.
4. Explain procedure to patient and the importance of coughing during the suctioning procedure. Even if patients cannot speak, they have the right to be informed about the procedure.
5. Adjust the bed to an appropriate height and lower side rail on the side nearest you. Check locks on the bed.

Procedural Guideline 23.1 *Closed (In-Line) Suctioning—cont'd*

6. Help patient assume a position of comfort for both patient and nurse, usually semi-Fowler's or high Fowler's position. Place towel across patient's chest.
7. Apply clean gloves and face shield and attach suction:
   a. In many facilities, a respiratory therapist attaches the catheter to the mechanical ventilator circuit. If the catheter is not already in place, open suction catheter package using aseptic technique, then attach closed suction catheter to ventilator circuit by removing swivel adapter and placing closed suction catheter apparatus on ET or TT. Connect Y on mechanical ventilator circuit to closed suction catheter with flex tubing (see Fig. 23.3, *A*).
   b. Connect one end of connecting tubing to suction machine; connect other end to the end of a closed-system (or in-line) suction catheter. Turn suction device on, set vacuum regulator to appropriate negative pressure, and check pressure. Many closed-system suction catheters require slightly higher suction pressures (consult manufacturer guidelines).
8. Hyperoxygenate patient (usually 100% oxygen) by adjusting the FiO_2 setting on the ventilator or by using a temporary oxygen enrichment program available on microprocessor ventilators according to employer policy. (Manual ventilation is not recommended.)
9. Unlock suction control mechanism if required by manufacturer. Open saline port and attach saline syringe or vial.
10. Pick up suction catheter enclosed in plastic sleeve with dominant hand.
11. Wait until patient inhales to insert catheter. Then, insert catheter using a repeating manoeuvre of pushing catheter and sliding (or pulling) plastic sleeve back between thumb and forefinger until resistance is felt or patient coughs. Pull back 1 cm (0.4 inches) before applying suction to avoid tissue damage to tracheal carina.
12. Encourage patient to cough, and apply suction by squeezing on suction control mechanism while withdrawing catheter. NOTE: It is difficult to apply intermittent pulses of suction and nearly impossible to rotate the catheter compared with a standard catheter. Apply continuous suction for 10 seconds as you remove the suction catheter (AACN, 2010; AARC, 2010; Wiegand, 2017). Be sure to withdraw the catheter completely into the plastic sheath and past the tip of the airway so it does not obstruct airflow.
13. If specimen collection is prescribed, connect the long, soft end of the mucous specimen trap (Fig. 23.4) to the output for suction vacuum (Fig. 23.4, *B*) and the suction catheter to collection port (Fig. 23.4, *D*). Follow Steps 11 and 12. Mucus will then be collected into the collection bottle (Fig. 23.4, *A*). Label and send sample to laboratory immediately.
14. Reassess cardiopulmonary status, including SpO_2 and ventilator measures, to determine need for subsequent suctioning or complications. Repeat Steps 8–12 one more time to clear secretions if patient condition indicates. Allow adequate time (at least 1 full minute) between suction passes for ventilation and reoxygenation.
15. When airway is clear, withdraw catheter completely into sheath. Be sure that coloured indicator line on catheter is visible in the sheath. Attach sterile solution lavage container or sterile saline or water syringe to side port of suction catheter. Squeeze vial or push syringe while applying suction to rinse inner lumen of catheter. Use at least 5–10 mL of saline to rinse the catheter until it is clear of retained secretions, as these fluids can cause bacterial growth and increase the risk of infection (AARC, 2010; Wiegand, 2017). Lock suction mechanism if applicable and turn off suction.

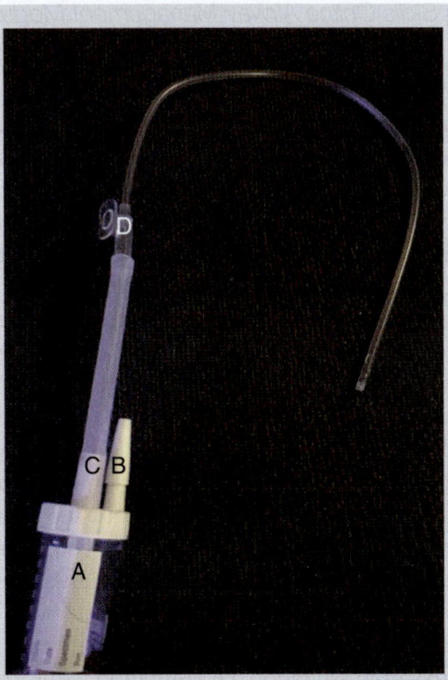

FIG 23.4 Arrangement of device used in the collection of mucus. A, Collection bottle. B, Output for suction vacuum. C, Entry of secretions. D, Suction catheter. *(Courtesy Jane Tyerman.)*

16. Hyperoxygenate for at least 1 minute by following the same technique used to preoxygenate (Wiegand, 2017).
17. If patient requires oral or nasal suctioning, perform Skill 23.1 or 23.2 with separate standard suction catheter.
18. Place the Yankauer suction catheter on a clean, dry area for reuse with suction turned off, or place within patient's reach with suction on if patient is capable of suctioning their own mouth.
19. Reposition patient. Remove gloves, face shield, and other PPE; discard into appropriate receptacle.
20. Compare patient's vital signs and SpO_2 before and after suctioning.
21. Auscultate lung fields and compare with baseline.
22. Observe airway secretions.
23. Ask patient whether breathing is easier and congestion is decreased.
24. **Use teach-back:** "I want to be sure I explained this suctioning procedure correctly. Please squeeze my hand if you understand these steps. Each time I suction, I will explain these steps again." Develop a revised teaching plan as indicated if patient is not squeezing hand in response.

✦ SKILL 23.3 Performing Endotracheal Tube Care

NSO Nursing Skills Online Airway Management Module 9 / Lesson 4

Endotracheal tubes (ETs) are flexible, plastic tubes placed in the mouth or through the nose and advanced down into the trachea to establish short-term artificial airways to administer mechanical ventilation, relieve upper airway obstruction, protect against aspiration, and clear secretions (see Fig. 23.2). Routine care maintains the correct position of the tube and good hygiene. Prior to performing ET care, it is crucial that supplemental oxygen with appropriate delivery devices be readily available at the bedside.

After insertion of an ET, the cuff is inflated, and the tube is secured with tape or a commercially available device. A cuff on an ET prevents the escape of air between the tube and the walls of the trachea and reduces the risk of aspiration when a patient is receiving mechanical ventilation (Box 23.1). The amount of air or water inserted in a cuff is based on two factors: the size of the patient's trachea and the external diameter of the artificial airway. If the cuff pressures are too high, permanent damage to the tracheal mucosa occurs, leading to complications such as tracheomalacia; tracheoesophageal fistula; or erosion of the innominate artery, which can be fatal. If the cuff pressure is too low, the mechanical ventilation will not be effective, and the patient will be at increased risk of developing VAP from aspiration (i.e., aspiration is due to the space left between the cuff and the trachea) (Nwosu et al., 2022).

Preventing tube-related complications is a critical component of care and depends on securing the tube and inflating the cuff properly. In many facilities, these functions are the responsibility of respiratory therapists. However, the nurse is responsible for assessing the patient's respiratory status, ventilator settings and functioning, and integrity of the airway cuff.

Properly securing an ET prevents inadvertent extubation from coughing, gagging, or accidental pulling on the tube. Additional risks associated with movement of an artificial airway are tracheal stenosis (narrowing of windpipe); tracheomalacia (flaccidity of supporting tracheal cartilage); barotrauma (excess alveolar air during mechanical ventilation); erosion of the innominate artery; and tracheoesophageal fistula, particularly when the cuff is overinflated (Landsperger et al., 2019). In addition, the risk for medical device–related pressure injuries increases because of pressure from the artificial airway on adjacent tissues (e.g., lips, oral mucosa) (Wiegand, 2017).

Once a tube is inserted, confirmation of placement is achieved using a chest X-ray film and a disposable end-tidal CO_2 detector (Fig. 23.5) (Wiegand, 2017). Capnography, the noninvasive measurement of the partial pressure of CO_2 ($PaCO_2$) in exhaled breath, expressed as the CO_2 concentration over time, is used to continuously monitor CO_2 once the patient is placed on mechanical ventilation. It is recommended as a reliable way to validate the correct placement of an ET (AARC, 2011). The CO_2 monitor measures CO_2 directly from the airway, with the sensor located on the airway adapter at the hub of the ET.

After a tube is inserted and secured and the cuff is inflated, the nurse's chief concern is to maintain patency of the ET and prevent a VAE (see Chapter 25 for more information regarding VAE). In patients who cannot clear their secretions, periodic suctioning of the artificial airway achieves airway patency.

BOX 23.1

Indications for Cuff Inflation

Mechanical Ventilation

- Continuous positive airway pressure
- Positive end-expiratory pressure (PEEP)
- Inability to meet ventilatory requirements with cuff down
- Inability to meet oxygen requirements with cuff down

Risk of Aspirating Gastric Contents

- Feeding tube, especially large bore, in stomach
- Gastroesophageal reflux disease
- Hiatal hernia
- During and after meals
- Impaired gastric emptying
- Decreased gag reflex
- Impaired swallowing

Delegation and Collaboration

This skill of performing ET care cannot be delegated a UCP. The UCP may assist the nurse with ET care. The nurse directs the UCP to immediately do the following:

- Report any signs of respiratory problems or increased airway secretions
- Report if the ET appears to have moved or become obstructed or dislodged
- Report changes in the patient's mood, level of consciousness, irritability, vital signs, decreased pulse oximetry value, or changes in end-tidal CO_2 values

Often, the nurse uses interprofessional collaboration (e.g., respiratory therapist) in performing tube care. This skill usually requires two people (either a nurse and respiratory therapist, or two nurses) in order to be safely completed without risk for extubation.

Equipment

- Towel
- ET and oropharyngeal suction equipment
- Adhesive or waterproof tape (do not use paper or silk tape) with a width of 1.3 cm (0.5 inches) or 2.5 cm (1 inch) or commercial ET holder and mouth guard (follow manufacturer instructions for securing)
- Oral airway and bite block (bite block is optional and only used if patient is biting ET)
- Suction equipment
- Clean gloves
- Adhesive remover swab or acetone on cotton ball
- Oral hygiene supplies: pediatric toothbrush (or suction toothbrush), toothette for edentulous patients
- Cleaning solution: 0.12 to 0.20% CHG mouthwash, rinse, or gel

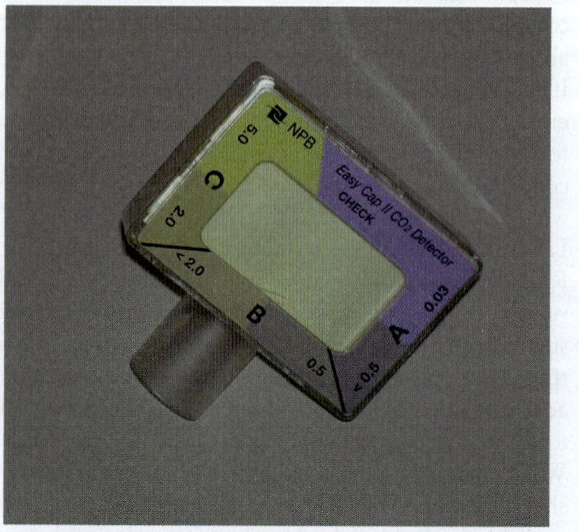

FIG 23.5 End-tidal carbon dioxide detector. *(Used by permission from Nellcor Puritan Bennett LLC, Boulder, CO, doing business as Covidien.)*

- Face cleaner (e.g., wet washcloth, towel, soap, shaving supplies)
- Clean 5 cm × 5 cm (2 inch × 2 inch) gauze pad
- Tincture of benzoin, liquid adhesive, or skin preparation swabs
- Tongue blade (optional)
- Mask, goggles, face shield (if indicated); gown if isolation procedures indicate
- Stethoscope
- Pulse oximeter, end-tidal CO_2 detector
- Another interprofessional team member (two people are needed to perform some of the steps)
- Communication device (letter or picture board, tablet, paper and pen)

STEP	RATIONALE
ASSESSMENT	
1. Identify patient using at least two person-specific identifiers (e.g., name and date of birth, or name and medical record number) according to employer policy.	Ensures correct patient. Complies with Accreditation Canada's standards and improves patient safety (Accreditation Canada, 2020).
2. Throughout the procedure, the 4 moments for hand hygiene are to be implemented; hand hygiene should occur before initial patient (or patient environment) contact, before an aseptic procedure, after body fluid exposure risk, and after patient (or patient environment) contact. Additional hand hygiene should be performed when hands are visibly soiled.	Proper hand hygiene helps prevent spread of infectious agents to health care providers.
3. Auscultate lungs and observe respiratory rate and depth.	Provides baseline measure of ventilation.
4. Apply gloves. Observe condition of tissues surrounding ET for impaired skin integrity (e.g., blistering, abrasions, pressure injuries) on nares, lips, cheeks, or corners of mouth; excess nasal or oral secretions; patient moving tube with tongue, biting tube or tongue, and foul-smelling mouth.	Presence of ET impairs ability of patient to swallow oral secretions. Patient is at increased risk of developing pressure areas from impaired circulation as tube is pulled or pressed against mucosal tissues (Dhawan, 2018).
5. Observe patency of airway: excess intratracheal or endotracheal secretions, diminished airflow, and sign and symptoms of airway obstruction.	Buildup of secretions in ET impairs oxygen delivery and subsequent tissue oxygenation.
6. Observe for signs and symptoms of gurgling on expiration, decreased exhaled tidal volume (mechanically ventilated patient), signs and symptoms of inadequate ventilation (rising end-tidal CO_2 concentration, patient–ventilator dyssynchrony, or dyspnea), spasmodic coughing, tense test balloon on tube, flaccid test balloon on tube, and ability to speak or vocalize.	The risk for aspiration increases when the cuff is underinflated because it allows room for secretions to pass by and allows for vocalization. Cuff overinflation may cause ischemia or necrosis of tracheal tissue from obstruction of capillary bed, resulting in tracheomalacia or tracheoesophageal fistula (Harrois et al., 2020).
7. Observe for factors that increase risk of complications from ET: type and size of tube, movement of tube up and down trachea (in and out), duration of tube placement, presence of facial trauma, malnutrition, and neck or thoracic radiation.	Tube rotating from side to side can cause medical device–related pressure injuries (MDRPIs). Tube can become dislodged from lower airway (incidental extubation), or it can enter right main-stem bronchus. Longer duration of intubation is associated with increased risk of lower airway complications such as VAE or VAP (Lewis et al., 2018).
8. Assess for patient's ability to verbalize around ET or for presence of audible air leak.	Underinflated cuff allows passage of air through patient's vocal cords and increases patient's risk of aspiration (Harrois et al., 2020).

Critical Decision Point *When assessment indicates possible overinflation or underinflation of ET cuff, notify respiratory therapy and follow employer policy for correcting cuff pressures. Most sources agree that 20 cm H_2O is the lowest acceptable pressure, but some sources recommend that the highest pressure to maintain the cuff is 25 cm H_2O* (AACN, 2018; Letvin et al., 2018; Wiegand, 2017).

STEP	RATIONALE
9. Determine proper ET depth as noted by centimetres at lip or gum line. This line is marked on tube and recorded in patient's record at time of intubation and every shift.	Ensures that tube is at proper depth to adequately ventilate both lungs and that it is not too high, which causes vocal cord damage, or too low, which results in right main-stem intubation, whereby only the right lung is ventilated.
10. Remove gloves and disgard	Gloves were put on during the assessment phase so they need to be removed.
11. Assess patient's knowledge of procedure.	Encourages cooperation, minimizes risks and anxiety. Identifies teaching needs.

NURSING DIAGNOSES

- Reduced airway clearance
- Insufficient breathing pattern
- Reduced gas exchange
- Fatigue
- Inadequate verbal communication
- Reduced skin integrity (or potential for)
- Potential for aspiration
- Potential for impaired oral mucous membrane
- Potential for infection

Related factors and risk factors are individualized on the basis of patient's condition or needs.

STEP	RATIONALE
PLANNING	
1. Expected outcomes following completion of procedure:	
• ET remains in correct position in patient's trachea as evidenced by depth of tube being same as when started or as prescribed (same centimetre marking at gums or lips); bilateral breath sounds are equal; and end-tidal CO_2 values remain at patient baseline.	Maintaining ET position promotes adequate ventilation of lungs. Complications of lower airway and vocal cord trauma are prevented.
• Patient's skin around mouth and oral mucous membranes remains intact without evidence of pressure or other injury from biting or from ET itself.	ET does not place undue pressure against corners of mouth, which could cause pressure injury. ET may be repositioned from side to side. Patient is unable to bite inner cheeks or tongue.
2. Gather equipment and supplies and arrange at bedside. Close room curtain or door.	Ensures that nurse has necessary equipment to implement all interventions that should be completed for patient. Ensures patient privacy.
3. Obtain assistance from available staff for this procedure.	Reduces risk of accidental extubation of ET.
4. Assist patient in assuming comfortable position for both patient and you. Elevate patient's HOB to at least 30 degrees, unless patient is at risk for pressure injury.	Having HOB at 30 degrees helps reduce risk of aspiration; if patient is conscious, this position is also more comfortable (Dhawan, 2018).
5. Explain procedure and patient's need to participate, including not biting or moving ET with tongue, trying not to cough when tape is off ET, keeping hands down, and not pulling on tubing.	Reduces anxiety, encourages cooperation, and reduces risk of accidental extubation.
IMPLEMENTATION	
1. Apply clean gloves and mask, goggles, or face shield if indicated. Have assistant do so as well.	Reduces transmission of microorganisms.
2. Place clean towel across patient's chest.	Reduces soiling of bed clothes and linen.
3. Perform endotracheal or oropharyngeal suctioning if indicated (see Skills 23.1 and 23.2 and Procedural Guideline 23.1).	Removes secretions. Diminishes patient's need to cough during procedure.
4. Connect Yankauer suction catheter to suction source and have it ready to use. Ensure that suction source/machine for oral suctioning is on and functioning properly.	Functioning equipment needed to perform oral care appropriately. Prepares suction apparatus.
5. Remove oral airway or bite block, if present, and place on towel.	Provides access to and completes observation of patient's oral cavity.

Critical Decision Point *If patient is biting the tube, do not remove bite block until absolutely necessary. This prevents obstruction of the ET and occlusion of the airway.*

STEP	RATIONALE
6. Brush teeth with soft toothbrush, using solution or toothpaste that helps to break down plaque buildup on teeth. Suction oropharyngeal secretions as necessary.	Pediatric toothbrush may be needed, depending on size of patient's oral cavity. There are no definitive guidelines to support the frequency of oral brushing.
7. Use CHG solution and oral swabs to clean mouth. Suction oropharyngeal secretions as necessary. Apply mouth moisturizer to oral mucosa and lips after each cleaning.	The swabs, solution, and moisturizer may come in a prepackaged kit from the manufacturer. CHG mouthwash has been proven effective in reducing VAP; oral care should be completed every 2–4 hours or more frequently if an increase in secretions is noted (Reese et al., 2021).

Critical Decision Point *Rates of VAP and length of CCU stay are significantly lower among patients intubated with ETs with the subglottic suction port above the cuff, closed endotracheal suctioning, and diligent oral care* (Dhawan, 2018).

STEP	RATIONALE
8. Prepare ET securement options:	
a. *Tape method:* Prepare tape by cutting a piece of tape long enough to go completely around patient's head from naris to naris plus 15 cm (6 inches). This is typically 30–60 cm (12–24 inches) in total length. Lay tape with adhesive side up on bedside table. Cut and lay 8–15 cm (3–6 inches) of second piece of tape, adhesive sides together, in centre of the long strip to prevent tape from sticking to hair. A smaller strip of tape should cover area between the ears, around the back of the head.	Preparing tape ahead of time decreases amount of time one has to manually hold ET throughout procedure, therefore decreasing risk of tube dislodgement. Adhesive tape needs to encircle head below ears, with sufficient tape left over to wrap around tube.

STEP	RATIONALE

IMPLEMENTATION

STEP	RATIONALE
b. *Commercially available ET holder:* Open package per manufacturer instructions. Set device aside with head guard in place. If using Velcro strips instead of cloth ties, ensure strips are in the open position.	Commercial devices are latex-free, fast, convenient, and disposable.

Critical Decision Point *Use the devices that your facility provides and collaborate with the respiratory therapist to understand which device is better based on patient's treatment plan (e.g., prone or supine, size, skin turgor).*

STEP	RATIONALE
9. Remove old tape or device.	
a. *Tape:* While one person is holding and stabilizing ET, the other person removes tape from patient using adhesive tape remover. The tape will also need to be removed from ET itself.	Provides access to skin under tape for assessment and hygiene. Adhesive tape remover ensures easier, less traumatic removal of the tape.

Critical Decision Point *Clean ET with soap and water as needed. Do not apply adhesive tape remover to the ET itself. This action will make it nearly impossible for the new tape to appropriately stick to the ET, which increases risk of tube dislodgement.*

STEP	RATIONALE
b. *Commercially available device:* Remove Velcro strips from ET and remove ET holder from patient.	Velcro adhesive strips hold ET in place and provide marker to measure distance to patient's lips or gums. These devices all permit access to patient's mouth and lips for ease of oropharyngeal suctioning and oral hygiene.

Critical Decision Point *Do not allow assistant to hold the tube away from the lips or nares. Doing so allows too much movement in the tube and increases the risk of tube movement and accidental extubation. Never let go of the ET because it could become dislodged.*

STEP	RATIONALE
10. Remove excess secretions or adhesive from patient's face. Clean face with mild soap and water and dry thoroughly. Apply tape adherence product such as tincture of benzoin to face.	Tape adherence products helps the tape stick to the patient's face; some brands also have a skin barrier protectant in them, promoting skin integrity.

Critical Decision Point *Do not remove oral airway or bite block if patient is actively biting. Wait until new tape or commercial device is partially or completely secured to ET.*

STEP	RATIONALE
11. Note level of ET by looking at mark or noting centimetre value on tube itself. Move oral ET to other side of mouth and ensure that tube marking at lip is unchanged. Perform oral care as needed on side where tube was initially positioned. Clean oral airway or bite block with warm, soapy water and rinse well. Reinsert as necessary.	Moving the ET from side to side at specified intervals helps prevent skin breakdown in one place and allows the nurse to complete total mouth care in all areas (Wiegand, 2017).

Critical Decision Point *The patient may cough excessively when the tube is being moved. The person holding the ET in place should be prepared for this and take extra caution while holding the tube. The assistant needs to continue holding the ET in place until oral care (and shaving, if necessary) is completed and the commercial ET holder is stabilized and secured. In some cases, the patient may need to receive a dose of antianxiety or sedating medication.*

If a nasotracheal tube is in place, take special care in removing and reapplying tape to secure the tube. The nasotracheal tube is not moved or repositioned. It is outside the nurse's scope of practice to move the nasotracheal tube from one naris to another and could cause great harm to the patient.

STEP	RATIONALE
12. Secure tube (assistant continues to hold ET).	
a. Tape method:	
(1) Slip tape under patient's head and neck, adhesive side up. Take care not to twist tape or catch hair. Do not allow tape to stick to itself. It helps to gently stick end of tape to tongue blade, which serves as guide. Then, slide tongue blade under patient's neck. Centre tape so double-faced tape extends around back of neck from ear to ear (Step 12a[2], illustration *A–B*).	Positions tape to secure ET in proper position. Do not allow tape to go over earlobe.

STEP	RATIONALE

IMPLEMENTATION

STEP	RATIONALE
(2) On one side of face, secure tape from ear to naris (nasal ET) or over lip to ET (oral ET). Tear remaining tape in half lengthwise, forming two pieces that are 1–1.5 cm (0.4–0.6 inches) wide. Secure bottom half of tape across upper lip (oral ET) or across top of nose (nasal ET) to opposite ear (see Step 12a[2], illustration *B*). Wrap top half of tape around tube and up from bottom (see Step 12a[2], illustration C). Tape should encircle tube at least two times for security.	Secures tape to face. Using top tape to wrap prevents downward drag on ET.
(3) Gently pull other side of tape firmly to pick up slack, and secure to opposite side of face and ET, same as first piece (see Step 12a[2] illustration *D*). Note: ET is secured. Assistant can release hold. Check depth mark at lips or gum line.	Secures tape to face and tube. ET should be at same depth at lips or gum line. Check earlier assessment for verification of tube depth in centimetres.

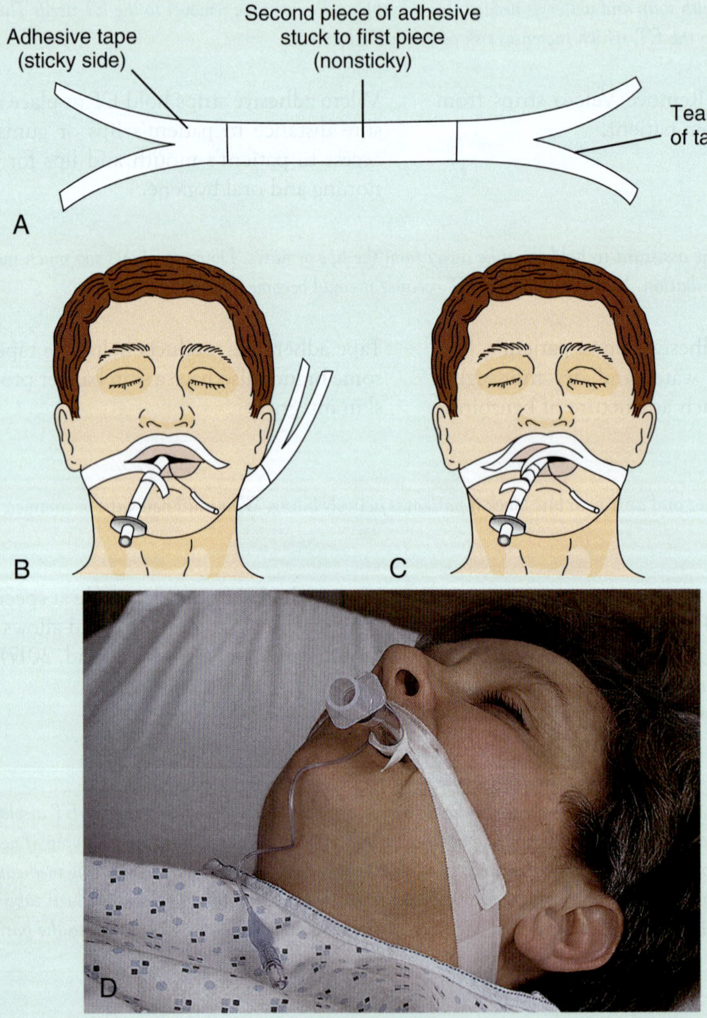

STEP 12A(2) A, Positioning for adhesive tape. B, Securing bottom half of tape across patient's upper lip and top half of tape around tube. C–D, Tape securing endotracheal tube. *(Images from Wiegand, D. L. [Ed.]. [2017]. AACN procedure manual for high acuity, progressive, and critical care [7th ed.]. Elsevier.)*

STEP	RATIONALE

IMPLEMENTATION

b. Commercially available ET securement device:

Critical Decision Point *This step will only need to be completed if the device is visibly soiled and cannot be cleaned or if it is no longer adhering to the face and keeping the ET secure.*

Step	Rationale
(1) Thread ET through opening designed to secure it. Be sure that pilot balloon is accessible.	Commercially available holders have a slit in front of holder designed to secure ET; specific designs and samples provided to facilities may vary.
(2) Place strips of ET holder under patient at occipital region of head.	
(3) Verify that ET is at established depth, using lip or gum line marker as guide.	Ensures that ET remains at correct depth as determined during assessment.
(4) Attach Velcro strips at base of patient's head. Leave 1 cm (0.4 inch) slack in strips.	
(5) Verify that tube is secure, that tube does not move forward from patient's mouth or back down into patient's throat, and that there are no pressure areas on oral mucosa or occipital region of head (see Step 12b[5] illustration).	Tube must be secure so it remains at correct depth. It can be secured without being tight and causing pressure.

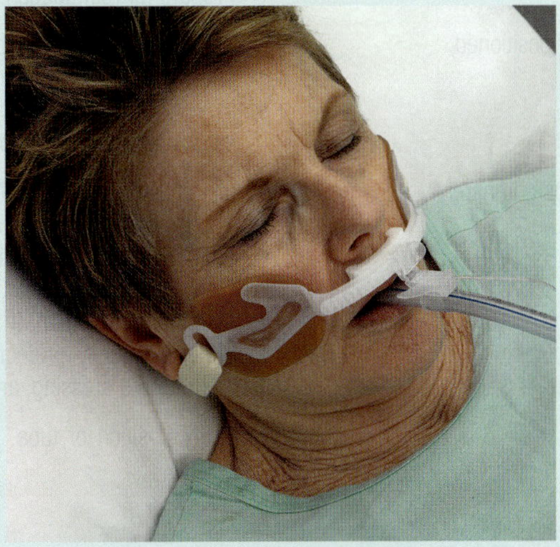

STEP 12B(5) Commercial endotracheal tube holder. *(Adapted from Sills, J. R. [2000]. Entry-level respiratory therapist exam guide [3rd ed.]. Mosby.)*

Step	Rationale
13. For unconscious patient, reinsert oral airway without pushing tongue into oropharynx and secure with tape.	Prevents patient from biting ET and allows access for oropharyngeal suctioning.
14. Clean rest of face and neck using soapy washcloth, rinse, and dry. Shave male patient as necessary.	Moisture and beard growth prevent adhesion of adhesive tape.

Critical Decision Point *When shaving patients, take great care to keep the cuff inflation port away from the razor. The razor can inadvertently cut or nick the tubing, causing air loss from the cuff and the possible need for reintubation.*

Critical Decision Point *If a nasotracheal tube is in place, all of the preceding steps will be completed, except that the tube will not be moved nor its position changed. It is outside the nurse's scope of practice to move the ET from one naris to another and could cause great harm to the patient. For more information, see the* Regulated Health Professions Act, 1991, *available at* https://www.ontario.ca/laws/statute/91r18.

Step	Rationale
15. Discard soiled items in appropriate receptacle. Remove towel and place in laundry.	Reduces transmission of microorganisms.
16. Reposition patient and ask them what else they need.	Promotes comfort; gives patient opportunity to communicate their needs.
17. Remove gloves and mask, goggles, or face shield or gown; discard in receptacle. (Assistant performs same steps.) Place clean items (e.g., tincture of benzoin, oral care solution, excess swabs) in storage area.	Reduces transmission of microorganisms. Ensures that contaminated gloves and hands do not touch clean items.

STEP	RATIONALE
EVALUATION	
1. Compare respiratory assessments before and after ET care.	Identifies any physiological changes, including presence and quality of breath sounds after procedure.
2. Observe depth and position of ET according to health care provider recommendation.	Position of ET should not be altered.
3. Assess security of tape by *gently* tugging at tube.	Tape should remain attached to face. Patient may cough during tugging.
4. Assess skin around mouth and oral mucous membranes for intactness and pressure sores.	Tape should not tear skin. Pressure areas should be absent.
5. Compare end-tidal CO_2 values from before and after ET care.	Changes in end-tidal CO_2 can help identify displacement or dislodgement of ET.
6. Observe for excessive phonation, presence of gastric secretions in airway secretions, or tracheoesophageal fistula.	Occurs with inadequate or excessive cuff inflation.

Unexpected Outcomes	Related Interventions
1. Patient is extubated accidently.	• Remain with patient while calling for help. • Ventilate with bag-valve mask as needed. • Assess patient for airway patency, spontaneous breathing, and vital signs. • Prepare for reintubation.
2. ET moves in airway and becomes incorrectly positioned.	• Call for help and repeat taping or securing procedure. Be prepared for chest X-ray film to confirm placement. • In very active patients without facial injury who are at risk for self-extubation, consider applying second piece of tape around back of head.
3. Patient has pressure injury in mouth or on lips and nares.	• Increase frequency of ET care. • Apply antimicrobial ointment per employer policy. • Align oxygen and humidity supply tubing so they do not pull ET and thus create pressure sores. • Monitor for infection. If skin tear is present on cheeks or over nose or upper lip, apply protective barrier, such as stoma adhesive patch or hydrocolloid dressing, and apply tape to it.
4. Cuff leak develops.	• Verify position of tube, notify respiratory therapy, and follow employer policy.

Communication and Documentation

- Document respiratory assessments before and after care, patient's tolerance of procedure, prescribed and actual depth of ET, frequency of ET care, integrity of oral and nasal mucosa, pressure sore care (if performed), and frequency and extent of ET care on flow sheet in progress notes in EHR or chart.
- Document repositioning of ET, side on which it is placed, and the securement technique used.
- Report unequal breath sounds, accidental extubation, cuff leak, or respiratory distress to the health care provider.

Special Considerations

Teaching

- Instruct patient and caregivers not to manipulate the ET, tape, or ET holder. If patient is complaining or appears uncomfortable, instruct caregiver to ask for the nurse.
- Instruct patient and caregiver to inform the nurse if the tube causes gagging. Repositioning of the tube, sedation, or both are options for reducing gagging.

Pediatric

- Neonatal and pediatric procedures for securing ETs and suctioning airways vary. Refer to employer policy for specific procedures (Hockenberry et al., 2024).
- Infant skin is more prone to tearing when removing tape (Hockenberry et al., 2024).
- Because of infants' delicate skin, you will not always use adhesive tape remover to remove the tape or skin preparation before securing the ET. ET holders are best used in this population, as long as appropriately sized holders are available for the child.

Gerontological

- Older persons' skin is more prone to tearing when removing tape.
- Older persons with a tendency toward inadequate nutrition are more prone to complications (e.g., infection, breakdown of oral mucosa).

SKILL 23.4 Performing Tracheostomy Care

Video Clip NSO Nursing Skills Online Airway Management Module 9 / Lesson 5

A tracheostomy is a surgical or percutaneous creation of a stoma through the neck and into the trachea that allows for the insertion of an artificial airway called a *tracheostomy tube (TT)*. TTs are placed in patients who require long-term airway management because of airway obstruction, airway clearance needs, or long-term need for mechanical ventilation (Bolsega & Sole, 2018). A TT offers several advantages over long-term ET placement, including decreased risk of laryngeal and tracheal injury, less sedation, shorter ventilator weaning time (the time it takes to get a patient off a ventilator), and improved comfort for the patient. Some TTs even allow more patient freedom in the performance of activities of daily living such as feeding, speaking, and mobility (Wang et al., 2019).

TTs can be fenestrated and nonfenestrated. A fenestrated tube has an opening in the side of the shaft, while a nonfenestrated tube does not. This opening allows air to enter so that the patient can speak with the tube in place. TTs in adults are generally between 7.0 and 8.5 mm in diameter (Karmali & Rose, 2020). TTs consist of several components (Fig. 23.6). The shaft is the main component of the tube and is what sits inside the trachea, keeping the airway open. Flanges rest against the patient's neck and prevent the TT from migrating into the trachea. The 15-mm connector/adaptor, located on the shaft or the inner cannula, is where the ventilator tubing or resuscitation bag attaches to the TT. The obturator is placed inside the TT and used during the TT insertion process, then replaced with an inner cannula (if necessary) once inserted. The inner cannula is located inside the shaft of the TT and is a safety feature because it can be quickly removed and replaced if obstructed; these can be disposable or reusable and are commonly made of silicone or polyurethane. The curve in the inner cannula mimics the natural shape of the trachea. Inner cannulas can be disposable or reusable. Metal inner cannulas are rarely used at this time (Aeppli et al., 2019).

A TT is cuffed or uncuffed. A cuff on a TT serves the same purpose as the cuff on an ET. Cuffs are made of a balloon-like inflatable plastic typically inflated with air, although there are brands that are inflated with liquid such as water or saline. Uncuffed tubes allow patients to clear their airway, but they provide no protection from aspiration. It is also more difficult to use positive-pressure ventilation in patients with these types of TTs (Wiegand, 2017).

Some TTs allow a patient to speak. This ability to verbalize needs and wants provides psychological benefits to the patient. The openings in fenestrated tubes allow air to flow from the lungs over the vocal cords. However, these tubes must be used with caution; only patients who can swallow without aspiration should use them. There are speaking valves that can be used with TTs. The patient must have a cuffless TT in place or be able to tolerate deflation of the cuff without risk for respiratory distress or aspiration. Patients may not tolerate the speaking valves when first placed; therefore, patients will need to be carefully monitored for signs of intolerance or respiratory distress.

Nurses also need to monitor for emergency events, such as tube obstruction or dislodgement. Box 23.2 provides a list of equipment that should be kept in the room or at the bedside of any patient who has a tracheostomy. Table 23.1 describes the signs of TT obstruction or dislodgement and the interventions that should be performed.

Delegation and Collaboration

The skill of performing tracheostomy care is not routinely delegated to a UCP. In some settings, patients who have well-established TTs may have the care delegated to a UCP (refer to employer policy). The nurse is responsible for assessing a patient and evaluating for proper artificial airway care, often using interprofessional collaboration (e.g., respiratory therapist). The nurse is also responsible for educating the patient and caregiver regarding care of an established tracheostomy in the home. The nurse directs the UCP to immediately do the following:

- Report any changes in the patient's respiratory status, level of consciousness, confusion, restlessness or irritability, or level of comfort

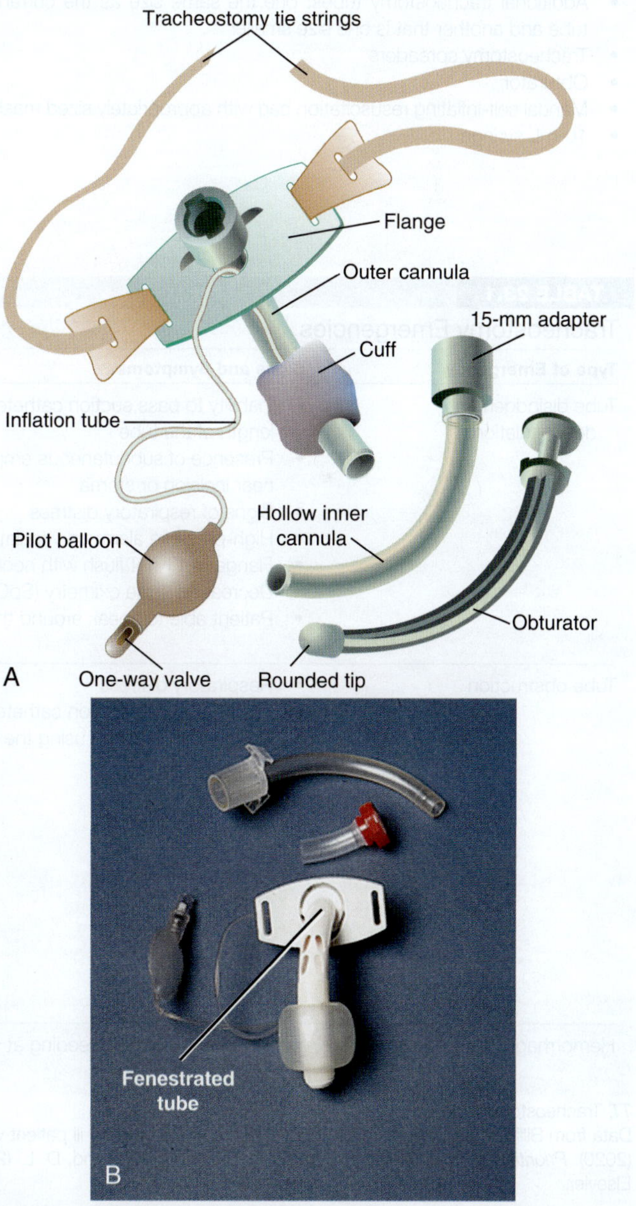

FIG 23.6 A, Parts of tracheostomy tube. B, Fenestrated tracheostomy tube with cuff, inner cannula, decannulation plug, and pilot balloon. (From Harding, M. M., Kwong, J., Roberts, D., et al. [2020]. *Lewis's medical-surgical nursing: Assessment and management of clinical problems* [11th ed.]. Mosby.)

- Report any dislodgement or excessive movement of the TT
- Report abnormal colour of the tracheal stoma and drainage

Equipment

- Bedside table
- Person to help change the tracheostomy tie/holder
- Towel
- Artificial airway suction supplies (see Skill 23.2)
- Oropharyngeal suction supplies (see Skill 23.1)
- Sterile tracheostomy care kit, if available (be sure to collect supplies listed that are not available in kit), or two sterile 10 cm × 10 cm (4 inch × 4 inch) gauze pads
    - Sterile cotton-tipped applicators
    - Sterile tracheostomy dressing (precut and sewn surgical dressing)
    - Sterile basin
    - Sterile normal saline or water
    - Small sterile brush (pipe cleaner) (or disposable inner cannula)
    - Roll of twill tape, tracheostomy ties, or commercial tracheostomy holder
    - Scissors
- Inner cannula that fits the patient's TT
- Pulse oximeter, end-tidal CO_2 detector
- Clean gloves (two pairs)
- PPE, as indicated (e.g., goggles, if there is concern regarding contact with secretions)
- Self-inflating manual resuscitation bag-valve device and appropriately sized mask
- Extra sterile tracheostomy kit

BOX 23.2

Bedside Equipment for a Tracheostomy Patient

- Oxygen administration equipment with appropriate delivery devices
- Suction machine and equipment
- Suction tubing
- Suction catheters (Yankauer and tracheal)
- Sterile saline
- Additional tracheostomy tubes, one the same size as the current tube and another that is one size smaller
- Tracheostomy spreaders
- Obturator
- Manual self-inflating resuscitation bag with appropriately sized mask
- 10-mL syringe

TABLE 23.1

Tracheostomy Emergencies

Type of Emergency	Signs and Symptoms	Interventions

Tube dislodgement/ decannulation	• Inability to pass suction catheter past the length of the tube
	• Presence of subcutaneous emphysema near incision or stoma
	• Signs of respiratory distress
	• High-pressure alarm on ventilator
	• Flange of TT not flush with neck
	• Decreased pulse oximetry (SpO_2)
	• Patient able to speak around the TT
		• Call for help
		• Ensure tracheostomy spreader is available at the bedside
		• If stoma is <1 week old:
		  • Notify surgeon
		  • Bag-valve mask ventilation
		  • Prepare for intubation or surgical reinsertion of new TT
		• If stoma is well established (typically >1 week old):
		  • Replace with a new TT, inserting at a 90-degree angle into the trachea, then angling downward another 90 degrees

Tube obstruction	• Respiratory distress
	• Inability to pass suction catheter
	• Resistance felt when using the self-inflating resuscitation bag
		• Call for help
		• Remove and inspect the inner cannula (if one present); clean or replace with a new one
		• Mature site (>1 week):
		  • Replace the TT (if changing inner cannula did not relieve the obstruction)
		  • Patient may need more invasive intervention, such as bronchoscopy
		• Immature site (<1 week):
		  • Ensure TT is in correct position
		  • Prepare for more invasive intervention, such as oral endotracheal intubation, tracheostomy revision, or placement of a longer TT

Hemorrhage	• More than minimal bleeding at stoma site	• Notify health care provider • Provide oxygen, if not already in place

TT, Tracheostomy tube.

Data from Billington, J., & Luckett, A. (2019). Care of the critically ill patient with a tracheostomy. *Nursing Standard, 34*(2), 59–65; Urden, L., Stacy, K., & Lough, M. (2020). *Priorities in critical care nursing* (8th ed). Elsevier; Wiegand, D. L. (2017). *AACN procedure manual for high acuity, progressive, and critical care* (7th ed.). Elsevier.

STEP	RATIONALE
ASSESSMENT	
1. Identify patient using at least two person-specific identifiers (e.g., name and date of birth, or name and medical record number) according to employer policy.	Ensures correct patient. Complies with Accreditation Canada's standards and improves patient safety (Accreditation Canada, 2020).
2. Throughout the procedure, the 4 moments for hand hygiene are to be implemented; hand hygiene should occur before initial patient (or patient environment) contact, before an aseptic procedure, after body fluid exposure risk, and after patient (or patient environment) contact. Additional hand hygiene should be performed when hands are visibly soiled.	Proper hand hygiene helps prevent spread of infectious agents to health care providers.
3. Observe for signs and symptoms of gurgling on expiration, decreased exhaled tidal volume (mechanically ventilated patient), signs and symptoms of inadequate ventilation (rising end-tidal CO_2 concentration, patient–ventilator dyssynchrony, or dyspnea), spasmodic coughing, tense test balloon on tube, flaccid test balloon on tube, and ability to speak or vocalize (see Box 23.1).	Reduces contact with infectious microorganisms. Cuff underinflation increases risk of aspiration by allowing secretions to enter trachea and permits vocalization. Cuff overinflation may cause ischemia or necrosis of tracheal tissue from obstruction of capillary bed, resulting in tracheomalacia or tracheoesophageal fistula (Wiegand, 2017).
4. Observe for excess peristomal secretions, excess intratracheal secretions, soiled or damp tracheostomy ties, soiled or damp tracheostomy dressing, diminished airflow through TT, or signs and symptoms of airway obstruction that indicate suctioning is required.	These signs indicate the need for tracheostomy care caused by presence of secretions at stoma site or within TT. Irritation of mucosa caused by tube itself can also cause increase in secretions (Aeppli et al., 2019).
5. Observe skin around tracheal stoma, under TT, and under tracheal ties for signs of skin breakdown such as blistering, erythema, drainage, or other discoloration.	Observing the skin frequently could prevent pressure-related injuries or prompt early intervention to a potential device-related injury.
6. Assess patient's hydration status, humidity delivered to airway, status of any existing infection, patient's nutritional status, and ability to cough.	Determines factors that affect amount and consistency of secretions in tracheostomy and patient's ability to clear airway.
7. Assess patient's cardiopulmonary status, including SpO_2, end-tidal CO_2, vital signs, respiratory effort, lung sounds, and level of consciousness. Keep pulse oximeter in place.	Provides baseline for determining patient response to and tolerance of therapy.
8. Assess patient's or caregiver's understanding of and ability to perform tracheostomy care.	Determines patient's and caregiver's level of understanding of instructional topic potential need for additional instruction.
9. Check when tracheostomy care was last performed.	Tracheostomy care is provided at least every 4–8 hours and more often if indicated.

NURSING DIAGNOSES

- Inadequate airway clearance
- Inadequate breathing pattern
- Reduced gas exchange
- Insufficient knowledge regarding tracheostomy care
- Reduced comfort
- Reduced verbal communication
- Potential for aspiration
- Potential for infection

Related factors and risk factors are individualized on the basis of patient's condition or needs.

STEP	RATIONALE
PLANNING	
1. Expected outcomes following completion of procedure:	
• Inner and outer cannulas of TT are free of secretions; ties are clean, secured snugly, and tied in double square knot.	TT is patent and secure, optimizing amount of oxygen delivered to patient and limiting risk for infection from retained secretions.
• Stoma site is pink; does not bleed; and is free of secretions, signs of infection, skin breakdown and pressure areas, and signs of granuloma formation.	Indicates absence of infection at stoma site. Dry, intact tracheostomy stoma reduces risk of subsequent systemic infection.
• No evidence of skin breakdown under tracheostomy ties or commercial tube holder.	Patients with excessive secretions or diaphoresis are at risk for skin breakdown under TT stabilizer.
2. Have an available colleague stabilize the device while you complete the procedure.	Prevents accidental extubation of TT.
3. Gather supplies and arrange at bedside. Close room door or curtain.	Ensures a well-organized procedure. Demonstrates person-centred care by ensuring patient privacy.
4. Assist patient to comfortable position, raise HOB to level of comfort.	Comfort measures can help reduce anxiety and fear.

STEP	RATIONALE

PLANNING

5. Explain procedure and patient's participation.	Encourages cooperation, minimizes risks, and reduces anxiety.

Critical Decision Point *Ensure that one or two extra TTs (one size above and one size below patient's current size) are available at HOB in case patient's TT dislodges and must be replaced in an emergency* (Billington & Luckett, 2019). *Follow your facility's protocols for setting up the safety features of the room for a patient on a ventilator or with a tracheostomy.*

IMPLEMENTATION

1. Apply PPE as indicated.	Reduces transmission of microorganisms.
2. Adjust bed to appropriate height and lower side rail on side nearest you. Check locks on bed wheel.	Minimizes caregiver's muscle strain and prevents injury. Prevents bed from moving.
3. Preoxygenate patient for 30 seconds or ask patient to take five to six deep breaths. Then, perform suctioning on tracheostomy (see Skill 23.2). Before removing gloves, remove soiled tracheostomy dressing and discard in glove with coiled catheter.	Removes secretions to avoid occluding outer cannula while inner cannula is removed. Reduces need for patient to cough.
4. Prepare equipment on bedside table.	Prepares equipment and allows for smooth, organized completion of tracheostomy care. Tracheostomy care should be performed every 4–8 hours or per employer policy (Wiegand, 2017).
a. Open sterile tracheostomy kit. Open two 10 cm × 10 cm (4 inch × 4 inch) gauze packages using aseptic technique and pour normal saline on one package. Leave second package dry. Open two cotton-tipped swab packages and pour normal saline on one package. Do not recap normal saline.	
b. Open sterile tracheostomy dressing package.	
c. Unwrap sterile basin and pour about 0.5–2 cm (0.2–0.8 inches) of normal saline into it.	
d. Open small, sterile brush package and place aseptically into sterile basin.	
e. Prepare TT fixation device.	
(1) *If using twill tape:* Prepare length of twill tape long enough to go around patient's neck two times, about 60–75 cm (24–30 inches) for an adult. Cut ends on diagonal. Lay aside in dry area.	Cutting ends of tie on a diagonal aids in insertion of tie through eyelet.
(2) *If using commercially available TT holder:* Open package according to manufacturer directions.	
f. Open inner cannula package (if new one is to be inserted, such as with disposable inner cannulas or if patient does not tolerate being disconnected from oxygen source while cleaning reusable inner cannula).	
5. Apply sterile gloves. Keep dominant hand sterile throughout procedure.	Reduces transmission of microorganisms.
6. Remove oxygen source if present.	

Critical Decision Point *It is important to stabilize the TT at all times during tracheostomy care to prevent injury, unnecessary discomfort, or accidental extubation. Have an assistant such as a UCP help during the procedure. Instruct the UCP to stabilize the tube using gloved hands.*

7. Care of tracheostomy with reusable inner cannula:	
a. While touching only outer aspect of tube, unlock and remove inner cannula with nondominant hand, following line of tracheostomy. Drop inner cannula into normal saline basin.	Removes inner cannula for cleaning. Normal saline loosens secretions from inner cannula.

Critical Decision Point *If the patient is receiving mechanical ventilation, you may want the person assisting you to hold the TT stable and remove the ventilator tube from the connection while you remove the inner cannula. This action helps to ensure that the TT itself is not removed accidently if there are difficulties removing the ventilator from the TT or the inner cannula from the TT.*

STEP	RATIONALE

IMPLEMENTATION

STEP	RATIONALE
b. Place tracheostomy collar, TT, or ventilator oxygen source over outer cannula. (NOTE: You may not be able to attach TT and ventilator oxygen devices to all outer cannulas when inner cannula is removed.)	Maintains supply of oxygen to patient as needed.

Critical Decision Point *If the patient is unable to tolerate being disconnected from the ventilator, replace the inner cannula with a clean new one and reattach the ventilator to the tracheostomy. Then proceed with cleaning the original inner cannula as described in the next steps and store it in a sterile container until the next inner cannula change* (Wiegand, 2017).

STEP	RATIONALE
c. To prevent oxygen desaturation in affected patients, quickly pick up the inner cannula and use a small brush to remove secretions inside and outside the inner cannula (see Step 7c illustration).	A tracheostomy brush provides mechanical force to remove thick or dried secretions.
d. Hold inner cannula over basin and rinse with sterile normal saline, using nondominant (clean) hand to pour normal saline. Dry with sterile gauze.	Removes secretions and normal saline from inner cannula.
e. Remove oxygen source, replace inner cannula (see Step 7e illustration), and secure "locking" mechanism. Reapply ventilator, tracheostomy collar, or TT. Hyperoxygenate patient if needed.	Secures inner cannula and re-establishes oxygen supply.

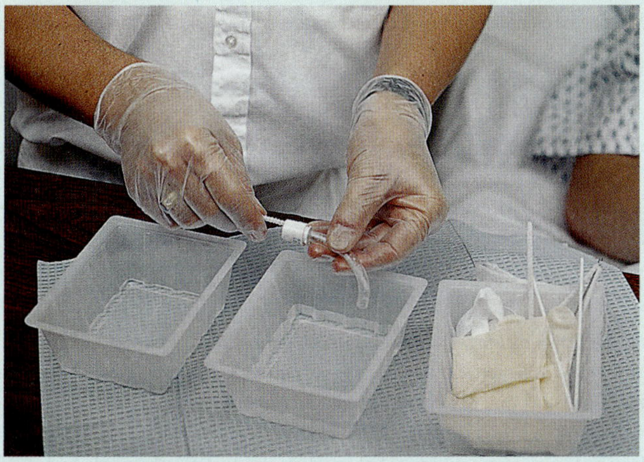

STEP 7C Cleaning tracheostomy inner cannula.

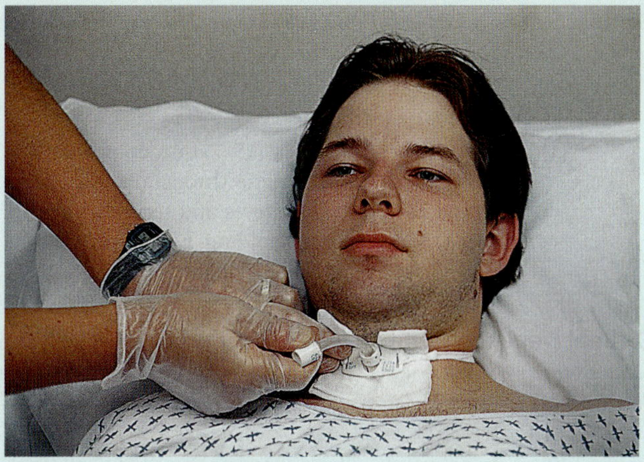

STEP 7E Reinserting inner cannula.

STEP	RATIONALE
8. Care of tracheostomy with disposable inner cannula:	
a. Remove new cannula from manufacturer packaging.	Prepares for change of inner cannula.
b. While touching only outer aspect of tube, withdraw inner cannula and replace with a new cannula. Lock it into position.	Provides clean, sterile inner cannula for patient.

Critical Decision Point *If the patient is receiving mechanical ventilation, you may want the person assisting you to hold the TT stable and remove the ventilator tube from the connection while you remove the inner cannula. This action helps to ensure that the TT itself is not accidently removed if there are difficulties removing the ventilator or the inner cannula from the TT.*

STEP	RATIONALE
c. Dispose of contaminated cannula in appropriate receptacle and reconnect to ventilator or oxygen supply.	Prevents transmission of infection. Restores oxygen delivery.
9. Using normal saline-saturated cotton-tipped swabs and 10 cm × 10 cm (4 inch × 4 inch) gauze, clean exposed outer cannula surfaces and stoma under faceplate extending 5–10 cm (2–4 inches) in all directions from stoma (see Step 9 illustration). Clean in circular motion from stoma site outward with dominant hand to handle sterile supplies. Do not go over previously cleaned area.	Aseptically removes secretions from stoma site. Moving in outward circle pulls mucus and other contaminants from stoma to periphery.

STEP	RATIONALE

IMPLEMENTATION

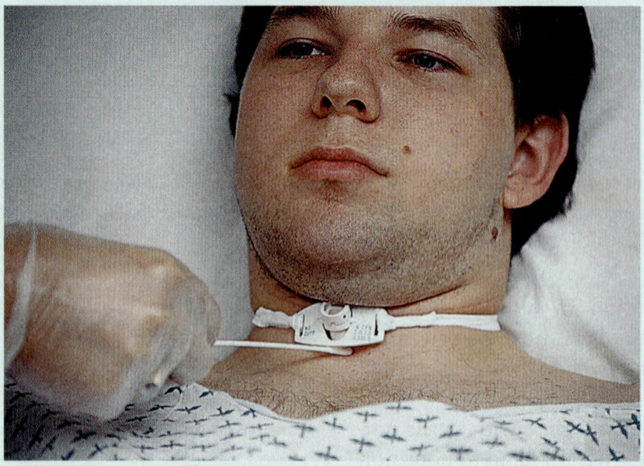

STEP 9 Cleaning around stoma.

STEP	RATIONALE
10. Using dry 10 cm × 10 cm (4 inch × 4 inch) gauze, pat lightly at skin and exposed outer cannula surfaces.	Drying the skin can prevent skin breakdown, excoriation, and growth of microorganisms.
11. Secure tracheostomy.	

Critical Decision Point *Follow your facility policies and protocols concerning when to first complete stoma and tracheostomy care in order to prevent accidental harm to the new site.*

STEP	RATIONALE
a. Tracheostomy tie method:	
(1) Instruct assistant to also complete the 4 moments of hand hygiene throughout the procedure and to apply clean gloves and securely hold TT in place. With assistant holding TT, cut old ties. Be sure not to cut pilot balloon of cuff.	Proper hand hygiene helps prevent the spread of infectious agents to health care providers. Secures TT to prevent accidental dislodgement. Ensures that balloon remains safe, as it is the only way to inflate the cuff.

Critical Decision Point *Assistant must not release hold on the TT until new ties are firmly secured. If working without an assistant, do not cut old ties until new ties are in place and secured* (Tyerman & Cobbett, 2023). *When ties are off, this is a good time to clean the back of the patient's neck and assess the patient's skin under the TT flange and under the ties or tube holder: ensure that skin is intact, free of pressure, and dry before applying securement device.*

STEP	RATIONALE
(2) Take prepared twill tape, insert one end of tie through faceplate eyelet, and pull ends even (see Step 11a[2] illustration).	Diagonal cuts ensure ease of threading end of tie through holes of eyelet (Wiegand, 2017).

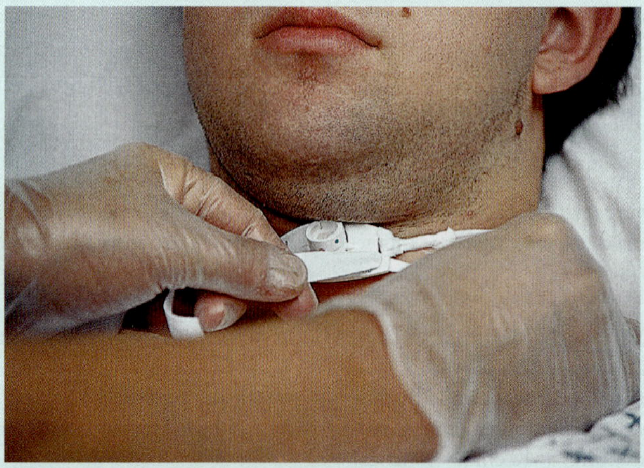

STEP 11A(2) Replacing tracheostomy ties. Do not remove old tracheostomy ties until new ones are secure.

STEP	RATIONALE
(3) Slide both ends of tie behind head and around neck to other eyelet, and insert one tie through second eyelet.	
(4) Pull snugly.	Secures TT.

STEP	RATIONALE

IMPLEMENTATION

STEP	RATIONALE
(5) Tie ends securely in double square knot, allowing space for insertion of only one loose or two snug finger widths between tie and neck (see Step 11a[5] illustration).	One finger width of slack prevents ties from being too tight when tracheostomy dressing is in place and also prevents movement of TT into lower airway (Wiegand, 2017).
(6) Insert new 10 cm × 10 cm (4 inch × 4 inch) tracheostomy dressing under clean ties and faceplate (see Step 11a[6] illustration).	Absorbs drainage. Dressing prevents pressure on clavicle heads (Wiegand, 2017).

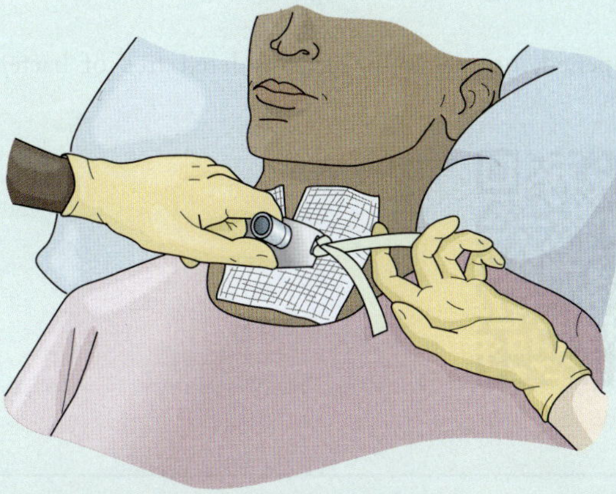

STEP 11A(5) Tracheostomy ties properly placed. *(From Sorrentino, S. A. [2013]. Mosby's textbook for nursing assistants [8th ed.]. Mosby.)*

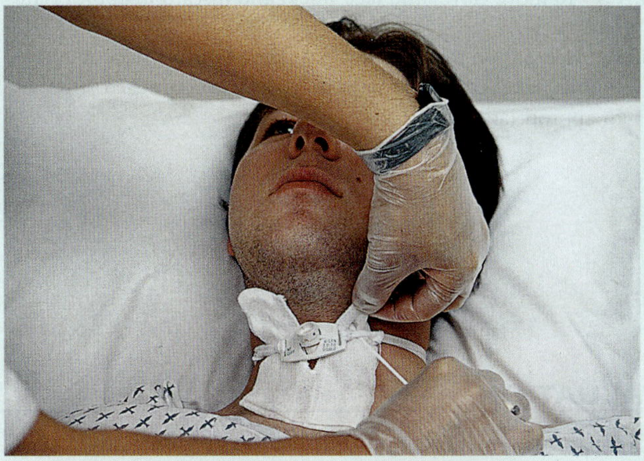

STEP 11A(6) Applying tracheostomy dressing.

STEP	RATIONALE
b. TT holder method:	
(1) Instruct assistant, if available, to apply clean gloves and securely hold TT in place. When an assistant is not available, leave old TT holder in place until new device is secure.	Reduces transmission of microorganisms. Prevents accidental dislodgement of tube. Ensures that TT stays in correct position.
(2) Align strap under patient's neck. Be sure that Velcro attachments are on either side of TT.	
(3) Place narrow end of ties under and through faceplate eyelets. Pull ends even and secure with Velcro closures (see Step 11b[3] illustration).	Ensures proper securement of TT.
(4) Verify that there is space for only one loose or two snug finger widths to be inserted under neck strap.	Ensures proper securement of TT without securement device being too tight.

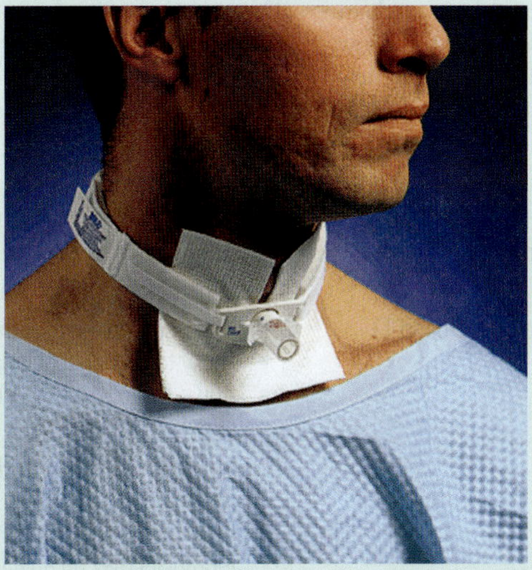

STEP 11B(3) Tracheostomy tube holder in place. *(Courtesy Dale Medical Products, Plainville, MA.)*

Critical Decision Point *Never cut a gauze pad to fit around TT. The cut fibres from the gauze pad may shed fibres that could be inhaled by patient and lead to pulmonary damage or infection. Use a pad manufactured for this purpose* (Wiegand, 2017).

STEP	RATIONALE
12. Perform oral care with toothbrush or oral swabs and CHG rinse.	Use of CHG may decrease patient risk of developing a VAE or VAP and promotes patient comfort.

STEP	RATIONALE
IMPLEMENTATION	
13. Reposition patient comfortably, with HOB elevated to at least 30 degrees (unless at risk for pressure injury) and assess respiratory status.	Promotes comfort. Some patients require post-tracheostomy care suctioning.
14. Be sure that oxygen or humidification delivery sources are in place and set at correct levels.	Humidification provides moisture for airway, makes it easier to suction secretions, and decreases risk of mucous plugs (AARC, 2012; Wiegand, 2017).
15. Remove gloves and face shield and discard in appropriate receptacle.	Reduces transmission of microorganisms.
16. Replace cap on reusable normal saline bottles. Store reusable liquids, label container with date, and store unused supplies in appropriate place.	Once opened, normal saline is considered free of bacteria for 24 hours.
EVALUATION	
1. Compare assessments before and after tracheostomy care.	Determines effectiveness of tracheostomy care and patient's tolerance of procedure.
2. Assess fit of new tracheostomy ties and ask patient whether tube feels comfortable. Palpate tube for pulsation and for air under skin.	Tracheostomy ties are uncomfortable and place patient at risk for tissue injury when they are too loose or too tight. A pulsating feeling in a TT can indicate early signs of innominate artery erosion. Air under skin suggests presence of subcutaneous emphysema.
3. Inspect inner and outer cannulas for secretions.	Presence of secretions on cannulas indicates need for more frequent tracheostomy care.
4. Assess stoma, surrounding skin, and skin under ties for inflammation, edema, bleeding, or discoloured secretions.	Broken skin places patient at risk for infection. Stoma infection requires change in tracheostomy skin care plan. Stomas located below second and third cartilage rings are at risk of causing innominate artery erosion (Wiegand, 2017).
5. Observe for excessive phonation, presence of gastric secretions in airway secretions, or tracheoesophageal fistula.	Occurs with inadequate or excessive cuff inflation.
6. Use teach-back: "I want to be sure I explained how to clean your tracheostomy tube and place new ties. Let's take time now and you can show me how to clean the tubing and place new ties." Develop a revised teaching plan if patient or caregiver is unable to teach back correctly.	Determines patient's and caregiver's level of understanding of instructional topic.

Unexpected Outcomes	Related Interventions
1. Excessively loose or tight tracheostomy ties or tracheostomy holder.	• Adjust ties or apply new ties or tracheostomy holder.
2. Cuff leak develops.	• Verify position of tube, notify respiratory therapy, and follow employer policy.
3. Inflammation of tracheostomy stoma or pressure area around TT.	• Increase frequency of tracheostomy care. • Apply topical antibacterial solution; apply bacterial barrier if prescribed. • Apply hydrocolloid or transparent dressing just under stoma to protect skin from breakdown. • Consult with skin care specialist.
4. Accidental decannulation or dislodgement	• Call for help. • Replace old TT with new tube. Some experienced nurses or respiratory therapists may be able to reinsert TT quickly. • Same-size ET can be inserted in stoma in an emergency. • Insert suction catheter to confirm that new tube is in trachea. • Be prepared to manually ventilate patients in whom respiratory distress develops using self-inflating resuscitation bag until tracheostomy is replaced. • Notify health care provider.
5. Respiratory distress from mucous plugs in cannula.	• Remove inner cannula if applicable for cleaning or suction cannula. • Notify health care provider if TT requires replacement.

Communication and Documentation

- Document respiratory assessments before and after care; type and size of TT and inner cannula; frequency and extent of care, including inner cannula, dressing, and securement device changes; type, colour, and amount of secretions; patient tolerance and understanding of procedure; and special care in event of unexpected outcomes in progress notes in EHR or chart.
- Document condition of stoma and skin around stoma site and under dressing.
- Document any interventions that were performed to address patient complications.
- Document patient's and caregiver's understanding through teach-back.
- Report accidental decannulation or respiratory distress to the health care provider.

DOCUMENTATION EXAMPLE

Nurse proceeded with morning tracheostomy assessment per protocol. Old drain sponges were removed and skin around the #6 XLT tracheostomy was observed. Inner cannula was removed and disposed of, and new # 6 disposable inner cannula applied with no concerns. The skin at the stoma site was intact, but was noted to be reddened, and health care provider was informed of this. No drainage noted to the site. Area was cleansed with sterile cotton swabs and normal saline, dried with sterile gauze and new drain sponges applied to site. Patient tolerated procedure well and did not have any pain, restlessness, or change in vital signs during this task.

Special Considerations

Teaching

- Different types of TTs have different faceplates. Some are rigid; others are not. Instruct caregivers not to lift up rigid faceplates or they will dislodge the tube.
- Some commercial TT holders require removal of excess tie material to fit properly.
- If you anticipate long-term placement of tracheostomy, then plan to teach patient and caregiver tracheostomy care.
- Patients with new tracheostomy frequently have bloody secretions for 2 or 3 days after tubing change (Wiegand, 2017).

Pediatric

- Children generally have shorter necks, making the stoma more difficult to clean.
- Pediatric TTs (smaller than size 4) do not contain an inner cannula.
- Nurses perform routine TT changes weekly after a tract has formed, which generally takes 5 days (Hockenberry et al., 2024).

Gerontological

- Some older persons may have more fragile skin and are more prone to skin breakdown from secretions or pressure (Boscart et al., 2023).
- Some older persons with impaired nutrition do not heal well.

Patients With Physical or Cognitive Challenges

- Patients with physical or cognitive challenges may not understand the procedure, leading to increase anxiety and less cooperation. Try to perform the procedure at a time when a trusted caregiver is available and able to help calm and soothe the patient.

Care in the Community: Home Management

- Coordinate with patient, caregiver, and community care facility to ensure ability to secure appropriate supplies for use at home.
- Coordinate with community care services to ensure that home has appropriate electricity to support the equipment, particularly if patient is receiving mechanical ventilation or requires suctioning (see Skill 25.5, Care in the Community).

✦ SKILL 23.5 Teaching Home Tracheostomy Care and Suctioning

Performing tracheostomy care and suctioning in the home is similar to performing these skills in the hospital except for one key variable: the use of *medical asepsis*, or *clean technique*. The home environment has fewer germs than hospitals; therefore, clean technique can be used. Aseptic technique is used in hospital because the patient is more susceptible to infection and more virulent or pathogenic microorganisms are usually present. In the home setting, the majority of patients use clean technique. Nurses need to use judgement in choosing the correct technique for each patient (e.g., use aseptic technique with patients who are immunocompromised; are infected [not colonized]; or have caregivers infected with viral, bacterial, or fungal microorganisms). Patients who live in unclean conditions also need to be suctioned with aseptic technique whenever possible to try to prevent infection. All caregivers need to use routine practices when suctioning with either clean or aseptic technique.

Caring for a tracheostomy at home begins in the hospital with teaching and return demonstration. The patient or caregiver usually learns better when instruction in less invasive techniques (e.g., tracheal stoma care) precedes that for more invasive techniques (e.g., inner cannula care and suctioning). The nurse needs to continually develop, implement, and evaluate the teaching plan based on patient performance. It is imperative that patients and their caregivers have the ability to practise suctioning frequently before discharge to develop confidence with skill performance; otherwise, arrangements to provide 24-hour care are necessary before discharge.

Delegation and Collaboration

The skill of teaching home tracheostomy care and suctioning cannot be delegated to a UCP. In some community settings, the skill of suctioning a patient with an established tracheostomy can be performed by a UCP (check employer policy). The nurse instructs the UCP to do the following:

- Document changes in the patient's level of consciousness, irritability, or vital signs or a decrease in pulse oximetry
- Report increased airway secretions

Equipment

- Suction machine with connecting tube
- Clean or sterile gloves
- Three small basins
- Hydrogen peroxide
- Normal saline
- Appropriately sized sterile or clean and disinfected suction catheter (diameter no greater than half the diameter of the TT [e.g., if TT is 8 mm (0.3 inches), use 16-Fr or smaller suction catheter])
- Tracheostomy care kit or clean 10 cm × 10 cm (4 inch × 4 inch) gauze pads (nonshredding)
    - Small nylon bottle brush or pipe cleaners
    - Replacement inner cannula if patient has disposable inner cannulas
- Cotton-tipped applicators

- Tracheostomy ties (twill tape [0.125-inch width preferably] or Velcro-type tie holders)
- Mirror
- Wet washcloth or paper towel *(optional)*
- Dry cloth, towel, or paper towel *(optional)*
- Protective eyewear *(optional)*
- Garbage bag (plastic, leak-proof preferred)
- Disposable apron *(optional)*
- Bag-valve mask with oxygen supply *(optional)*

STEP	RATIONALE
ASSESSMENT	
1. Identify patient using at least two person-specific identifiers during first home visit. Facial recognition can be used as one of two identifiers for ongoing subsequent home visits.	Ensures correct patient. Complies with Accreditation Canada's standards and improves patient safety (Accreditation Canada, 2020).
2. Throughout the procedure, the 4 moments for hand hygiene are to be implemented; hand hygiene should occur before initial patient (or patient environment) contact, before an aseptic procedure, after body fluid exposure risk, and after patient (or patient environment) contact. Additional hand hygiene should be performed when hands are visibly soiled.	Proper hand hygiene helps prevent the spread of infectious agents to health care providers.
3. Assess patient's and caregiver's vision and fine motor function for the ability to perform tracheostomy care and suctioning properly. Also assess patient's level of consciousness and ability to attend to care and problem solve.	Instructing the caregiver is essential if the patient's physical and cognitive impairment prevents them from performing tracheostomy care and suctioning. Emergency situations usually require a caregiver to suction.
4. Assess patient's and caregiver's knowledge of indications for the need to perform the following:	
a. Tracheostomy care, including presence of excess peristomal secretions, excess intratracheal secretions, soiled or damp tracheostomy dressing and ties, and diminished airway through the TT.	Knowledge needed for patient or caregiver to accurately assess need to provide tracheostomy care. Signs and symptoms are related to presence of secretions at the stoma site or within the TT.
b. Suctioning, including patient's perceived need for suctioning, presence of gurgling, wheezes on inspiration or expiration, restlessness, ineffective coughing, tachypnea, cyanosis, acutely decreased level of consciousness, tachycardia or bradycardia, acutely shallow respirations, or acute dyspnea.	Knowledge allows patient or caregiver to accurately determine the need to perform TT suctioning. Physical signs and symptoms result from lower airway obstruction and tissue hypoxia.
5. Assess patient's or caregiver's ability to assess pulse rate and respirations.	Necessary for appropriate monitoring in the home.
6. Assess patient's learning readiness and ability to concentrate; consider presence of pain, nausea, or fatigue and patient interest in instruction.	Presence of significant illness, frailty, or confusion affects a patient's ability to attend to a teaching plan. Indicates need to rely on a caregiver for learning and implementation (if available) on a short- or long-term basis.

NURSING DIAGNOSES

- Inadequate breathing pattern
- Insufficient knowledge regarding tracheostomy care
- Inadequate health maintenance
- Potential for caregiver role strain
- Potential for infection

Related factors and risk factors are individualized on the basis of patient's condition or needs.

PLANNING

STEP	RATIONALE
1. Expected outcomes following completion of procedure:	
• Patient or caregiver identifies signs and symptoms indicating need for tracheostomy care and suctioning.	Patient or caregiver can institute preventive means to maintain airway.
• Patient or caregiver states factors that influence tracheostomy airway functioning.	Tracheostomy often impairs normal airway clearance, humidification, and gas exchange.
• Patient or caregiver correctly demonstrates complete TT care and suctioning in a controlled setting.	Provides validation of ability to perform procedure.
• Patient or caregiver identifies signs of stoma inflammation or respiratory tract infection and when to notify health care provider.	Measures cognitive learning.
• Lower and upper airways are cleared of secretions as evidenced by absent or diminished wheezes and gurgles in large airways, normalization of pulse and respiratory rate, increased depth of respirations, absence of cyanosis, improved colour, and decreased dyspnea.	Suctioning by patient or caregiver is successful.

STEP	RATIONALE

PLANNING

- Stoma site is clean and free of an infection and transesophageal fistula. Signs of transesophageal fistula include frequent coughing when eating, aspiration, or fever.
- Inner cannula is free of secretions.

Tracheostomy care is successful.

2. Select a setting in the home where the patient or caregiver is most likely to perform TT care:

Practising skill in the same setting where skill will be routinely performed facilitates comprehension and learning.

- Select a room that is well lit with comfortable seating.
- Be sure that the patient is close and can see the nurse clearly.
- Control sources of noise and distractions.

Room environment needs to minimize existing sensory alterations. A comfortable environment free of distractions increases patient's attention.

3. Discuss and demonstrate with patient or caregiver proper position for procedure (high Fowler's position in front of mirror).

Promotes understanding of comfort and safety principles and facilitates visibility.

IMPLEMENTATION

1. Suctioning:

a. Verify health care provider's prescriptions for suctioning. Ensure that patient and caregiver understand suctioning prescription.

Invasive procedure requires prescription. Prescription may be written for as-needed suctioning; ensures that patient and caregiver understand what this means.

b. Teach patient or caregiver techniques for hand hygiene and application of clean gloves.

Reduces transmission of microorganisms.

c. Explain and demonstrate step-by-step preparation and completion of TT suctioning using either open or closed suctioning (see Step 1c illustration).

Demonstration is a reliable technique for teaching psychomotor skill and enables the patient or caregiver to ask questions throughout the procedure. Steps used to suction patients in the hospital are also used in the home.

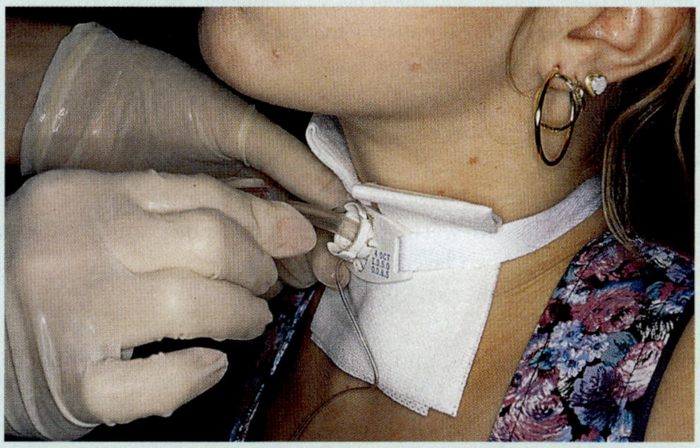

STEP 1C Insertion of suction catheter into tracheostomy tube.

d. After the patient or caregiver suctions tracheostomy, teach them how to suction the nasal and oral pharynx and perform mouth care. Encourage patient or caregiver to brush teeth with a small, soft toothbrush two times a day and use mouth moisturizer to moisturize the lips every 2–4 hours.

Suctioning removes secretions from trachea and lower airway that patients are unable to clear by coughing. Dental plaque harbours microorganisms.

e. At conclusion of the procedure, have patient take two to three deep breaths; reassess status of breathing.

Deep breathing reduces oxygen loss and prevents hypoxia. Expect patient's respiratory status to improve following suctioning.

f. Demonstrate how to disconnect suction catheter; coil and discard catheter in appropriate receptacle. If catheter is to be cleaned and disinfected, put in labelled bag. Have patient or caregiver remove soiled gloves and dispose of them in appropriate container; teach them to perform hand hygiene.

Prevents transmission of microorganisms.

STEP	RATIONALE

IMPLEMENTATION

2. Tracheostomy care:

   a. Have patient sit at a table with a mirror. Instruct patient or caregiver how to perform hand hygiene and apply clean gloves with you. Teach skills of tracheostomy care, including cleaning stoma and TT and changing tracheostomy ties and dressing (see Step 2a illustrations). EXCEPTION: Clean inner cannula with hydrogen peroxide and a small brush (Cleveland Clinic, 2022).

   Rationale: Prevents transmission of microorganisms. Steps used to provide tracheostomy care in the hospital are also used in the home.

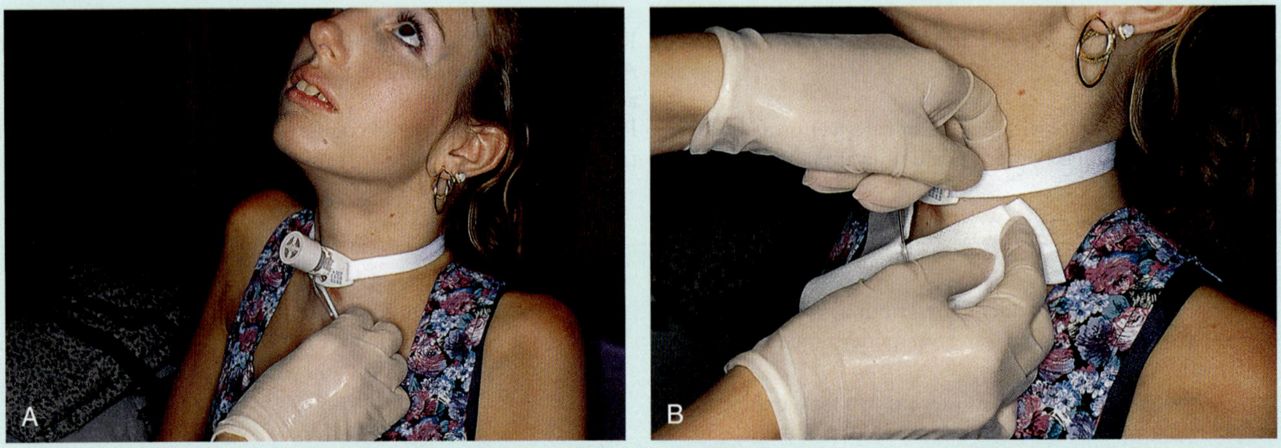

STEP 2A A, Cleaning area around tracheal stoma. B, Applying clean tracheostomy dressing.

Critical Decision Point *During tracheostomy care, a patient is at risk of the TT coming out. Instruct patient or caregiver to never remove the old TT ties until the new ties are secured properly. Keep two TTs, one the same size as the patient's and one a size smaller, accessible to the patient so a new TT can be inserted if the tube comes out. If the patient has a disposable inner cannula, they need to have replacement cannulas available.*

   b. Have patient or caregiver remove and dispose of gloves, and direct them to perform hand hygiene.

   Rationale: Reduces transmission of microorganisms.

   c. Instruct patient or caregiver to apply clean gloves. Demonstrate technique for cleaning reusable supplies in warm, soapy water. Rinse thoroughly and dry between two layers of clean paper towels. Store supplies in a loosely closed clear plastic bag; label the bag.

   Rationale: Reduces transmission of microorganisms. Air must circulate, as humidity in bag can promote microorganism growth.

   d. Have patient or caregiver remove and discard gloves, and direct them to perform hand hygiene.

   Rationale: Reduces transmission of microorganisms.

3. Disinfecting supplies:

   a. Explain procedure for disinfecting reusable supplies. Disinfection needs to be done at least weekly. To disinfect supplies, use one of following methods:

   Rationale: Removes microorganisms and reduces risk of infection.

      (1) *Method 1*: Boil reusable (boilable) supplies for 15 minutes. Allow to cool and dry.

      (2) *Method 2*: Soak reusable supplies in equal parts of vinegar and water for 30 minutes. Remove, rinse thoroughly, and dry.

      (3) *Method 3*: Soak reusable supplies in prepared solutions of quaternary ammonium chloride compounds according to manufacturer instructions. Rinse and dry.

4. Have patient or caregiver perform each step with guidance from you.

   Rationale: Adults learn psychomotor skills best by active participation, and you can correct any errors in technique as they occur and discuss their implications.

STEP	RATIONALE
IMPLEMENTATION	
5. Teach patient or caregiver signs and symptoms of the following: **a.** Stoma infection (redness, tenderness, drainage) **b.** Respiratory tract infection (fever, increased sputum, change in colour of sputum, foul sputum odour, increased cough, chills, night sweats) **c.** Transesophageal fistula (air leaking through stoma, nose, or mouth with cuff properly inflated; more air needed to inflate cuff; aspiration of food or liquid during suctioning; excessive belching; coughing when swallowing)	Patient or caregiver must be able to recognize the onset of complications associated with long-term tracheostomy use early so that medical treatment can begin; doing so reduces risk of more serious negative outcomes. Emphasize the importance of notifying the health care provider when signs and symptoms of complications occur.
EVALUATION	
1. Observe patient or caregiver demonstrate technique for TT care and suctioning.	Feedback through independent demonstration of psychomotor skill is a reliable method to evaluate learning.
2. Ask patient or caregiver to describe signs and symptoms indicating need for tracheostomy care and suctioning and the factors that influence tracheostomy airway functioning.	Demonstrates learning and patient's and caregiver's ability to respond when airway problems develop.
3. Have patient and caregiver explain the problems that need to be reported to their health care provider.	Demonstrates patient's and caregiver's ability to take steps for emergent care.
4. Use **teach-back:** "I want to be sure I explained how you will feel and what you may see if you develop problems or complications with your tracheostomy. Tell me the signs and symptoms for needing to suction your tracheostomy." Develop a revised teaching plan if patient or caregiver is unable to teach back correctly.	Determines patient's and caregiver's level of understanding of instructional topic.

Unexpected Outcomes	Related Interventions
1. Stoma site is reddened or hard, with or without drainage.	• Evaluate patient's or caregiver's technique. • Increase frequency of tracheostomy care.
2. Copious coloured secretions are present around stoma or when patient or caregiver suctions tracheostomy.	• Have patient use sterile technique for suctioning and tracheostomy care. • Secretions may be pink, rust-coloured, or blood-tinged, depending on problem; documenting colour helps health care provider diagnose the problem. • Evaluate for adequate humidity (use room humidifier or tracheostomy collar, if needed). • Notify health care provider.
3. Bloody secretions are suctioned.	• Evaluate suctioning technique, suctioning frequency, and size of catheter used. • Usual length to insert catheter is length of TT plus 64 mm (0.25 inches). • Assess for signs of infection. • Assess patient for use of anticoagulant medications.
4. No secretions are suctioned.	• Evaluate patient's fluid status, need for increased humidity. • Determine whether appropriately size suction catheter is used. • Reassess need to suction.
5. Skin breakdown is present at stoma site.	• Assess site for pressure areas or site infection. • Remove pressure source.

Communication and Documentation

- Document patient instruction and patient's and caregiver's ability to demonstrate tracheostomy care, suctioning skills, and disinfecting skills in the home health record.
- Develop a system for patient or caregiver to document and keep track of tracheostomy care provided.

Special Considerations

Teaching

- The nose and mouth normally provide warmth, filtering, and moisture for the air we breathe. A TT bypasses these mechanisms. Humidification must be provided to keep secretions thin and to avoid mucous plugs.

- Caution patients and caregivers against using alcohol-based products to clean supplies because they can cause the materials to become hard and brittle. Do not place equipment or supplies in the dishwasher.
- Always leave a phone number and instructions on how to reach a home care nurse if needed.

Pediatric

- Encourage parents to give tracheostomy care as soon as the child is stable in the hospital. The more time they have to practise these skills, the more comfortable they will be in caring for the child at home.
- Children with tracheostomies need to socialize and play with other children who are close to their own age. Encourage caregivers to take the child out of the home. However, an additional adult needs to travel with the child to help if problems arise while in the car (Hockenberry et al., 2024).
- To prevent hypoxia, teach caregivers that suctioning needs to last no more than 5 seconds. Allow the child to rest for at least 30 to 60 seconds between suctioning passes and to not suction more than three times (Hockenberry et al., 2024).
- Teach caregivers pediatric cardiopulmonary resuscitation (CPR), including use of bag-valve mask or mouth-to-tracheostomy technique. They also need to notify the local paramedics of the child's condition and the presence of a tracheostomy and provide paramedics with a list of equipment in the home (Hockenberry et al., 2024).
- Encourage caregivers to have a cool-mist humidifier in the same room as the child; humidity helps keep secretions thin and decreases the likelihood of mucous plugging (Hockenberry et al., 2024).
- Caring for a child with a tracheostomy often disrupts caregivers' ability to socialize and can cause sleep deprivation. Develop a plan that includes respite care to allow caregivers time to meet their own needs (Hockenberry et al., 2024).
- Teach caregivers to avoid dressing the child in clothes that could cover the tracheostomy opening, such as turtlenecks and clothes that have a tight-fitting collar. Avoid clothing, toys, and pets that shed fine hair or lint because it could get into the tracheostomy and cause breathing problems (Hockenberry et al., 2024).

Gerontological

- Older persons lose some properties of elastic recoil and often have greater difficulty clearing airway secretions through cough. As a result, they require more suctioning and airway care and have increased risk of infection (Boscart et al., 2023).
- Assess for cognitive, mobility, or sensory impairments that decrease ability to manage an artificial airway at home, and teach the caregiver if the patient is unable to manage the airway independently.
- Anxiety accompanies decreased ability to breathe and may cause the older person to become too nervous to perform suctioning independently.

✦ REVIEW QUESTIONS

A 65-year-old patient (he/him) experienced a severe stroke 2 days ago and at this time cannot communicate verbally. The interprofessional team is monitoring him for the ability to control his secretions and maintain an airway. The nurse walks into his room and notices cyanotic oral mucous membranes, pulse oximeter reading of 78%, and a large amount of oral secretions. The patient is gasping for air and tachypneic.

Review Questions 1 to 3 relate to the case study presented here.

1. What action should the nurse take first?
   1. Apply oxygen via nasal cannula.
   2. Perform oropharyngeal suctioning.
   3. Call respiratory therapy.
   4. Place the patient in supine position.
2. The nurse has used oropharyngeal suctioning in an attempt to clear the patient's airway, but the patient continues to gasp for air, and the pulse oximeter has improved only to 82%, even with the addition of 10 L oxygen via nonrebreather face mask. Rhonchi are noted on auscultation of breath sounds and trachea. The patient also continues to present with a large amount of oral secretions. The nurse recognizes that the health care provider needs to be notified. Using SBAR (situation–background–assessment–recommendation) format, how should the nurse communicate the patient's status to the provider?
3. The patient was intubated; however, because of an inability to control secretions and maintain an airway, he was unable to be weaned off the ventilator. The decision was made to perform a tracheostomy. The nurse is teaching the patient's spouse about how the nurses will manage the tracheostomy tube. What should be included in the teaching plan, and why are these interventions performed?
4. The nurse is assessing a patient with an endotracheal tube (ET) and receiving positive-pressure mechanical ventilation. Which assessment findings should alert the nurse to the need to perform endotracheal suctioning? (*Select all that apply.*)
   1. Increased exhaled tidal volume above patient baseline
   2. Auscultation of rhonchi in the lungs
   3. Elevated exhaled carbon dioxide levels
   4. Decreased peak inspiratory pressures noted on the ventilator
   5. Presence of yellow fluid within the ET
   6. Patient speaking around the ET
5. A patient who is receiving mechanical ventilation via tracheostomy tube is preparing for discharge home. Which statements, made by the patient's primary caregiver, indicate an understanding of the care needed for this patient? (*Select all that apply.*)
   1. "We should suction the tracheostomy tube every 4 hours during the day."
   2. "We will need to rinse the nondisposable inner cannula with sterile saline to clean it."
   3. "We should make sure that the tracheostomy holder is tight against the skin."
   4. "We should check the pressure in the cuff at least three times a day."
   5. "We will need to clean the stoma site at least every 8 hours and more frequently if there are secretions or signs of infection."
6. Put the steps for performing tracheal suctioning in the correct order:
   1. Hyperoxygenate the patient.
   2. Assess for the need for suctioning.
   3. Perform oropharyngeal suctioning.
   4. Withdraw catheter while applying suction.
   5. Insert catheter into endotracheal or tracheostomy tube.

Visit the Evolve site for a complete list of answers to the Review Questions.

✦ NEXT GENERATION NCLEX® (NGN)

For practice with answering exam questions related to unfolding NGN case studies, please consult the Next Generation NCLEX® (NGN)-Style Case Studies for Skills and Techniques on the Evolve website: http://evolve.elsevier.com/Canada/Perry/clinicalskills/

REFERENCES

Accreditation Canada. (2020). *Required organizational practices–2020 handbook.* https://physicians.nshealth.ca/resources/required-organizational-practices-2020-handbook

Aeppli, B., Lindauer, B., Steurer, M. P., et al. (2019). Endotracheal tube cuff pressure changes during manual cuff pressure control manoeuvres: An in–vitro assessment. *Acta Anaesthesiologica Scandinavica, 63*(1), 55–60. https://doi.org/10.1111/aas.13249

American Association of Critical-Care Nurses (AACN). (2010). *AACN practice alert: Oral care for patients at risk for ventilator-associated pneumonia.* https://www.aacn.org/docs/EventPlanning/WB0011/oral-care-patients-at-risk-vap-r44spvmp.pdf [Seminal Reference]

American Association of Critical-Care Nurses (AACN). (2018). *AACN practice alert: Prevention of aspiration in adults.* https://www.aacn.org/clinical-resources/practice-alerts/prevention-of-aspiration [Seminal Reference]

American Association of Respiratory Care (AARC). (2004). AARC clinical practice guideline: Nasotracheal suctioning–2004 revision and update. *Respiratory Care, 49*(9), 1080–1084. https://www.aarc.org/wp-content/uploads/2014/08/09.04.1080.pdf [Seminal Reference]

American Association of Respiratory Care (AARC). (2010). AARC clinical practice guideline: Endotracheal suctioning of mechanically ventilated patients with artificial airways 2010. *Respiratory Care, 55*(6), 758–764. https://www.aarc.org/wp-content/uploads/2014/08/06.10.0758.pdf [Seminal Reference]

American Association of Respiratory Care (AARC). (2011). AARC clinical practice guideline: Capnography/capnometry during mechanical ventilation: 2011. *Respiratory Care, 56*(4), 503–509. https://www.aarc.org/wp-content/uploads/2014/08/04.11.0503.pdf [Seminal Reference]

American Association of Respiratory Care (AARC). (2012). AARC clinical practice guideline: Humidification during invasive and noninvasive mechanical ventilation: 2012. *Respiratory Care, 57*(5), 782–788. https://www.aarc.org/wp-content/uploads/2014/08/12.05.0782.pdf [Seminal Reference]

Billington, J., & Luckett, A. (2019). Care of the critically ill patient with a tracheostomy. *Nursing Standard, 34*(2), 59–65. https://doi.org/10.7748/ns.2019.e11297

Bolsega, T., & Sole, M. (2018). Tracheostomy care practices in a simulated setting: An exploratory study. *Clinical Nurse Specialist, 32*(4), 182–188. https://doi.org/10.1097/nur.0000000000000385

Boscart, V., McCleary, L., Sheiban Taucar, L., et al. (2023). *Ebersole and Hess' gerontological nursing and healthy aging in Canada* (3rd ed.). Elsevier.

Centers for Disease Control and Prevention (CDC). (2023). *Ventilator-associated event (VAE).* http://www.cdc.gov/nhsn/PDFs/pscManual/10-VAE_FINAL.pdf

Cleveland Clinic. (2022). *Tracheostomy care.* https://my.clevelandclinic.org/health/treatments/23231-tracheostomy

Dhawan, G. (2018). Subglottic and closed endotracheal suctioning versus open endotracheal suctioning–effect on ventilator-associated pneumonia rates and length of intensive care stay. *Journal of Evolution of Medical and Dental Sciences, 7*(34), 3730–3733. https://doi.org/10.14260/jemds/2018/838

Harrois, A., Anstey, J., Deane, A. M., et al. (2020). Effects of routine position changes and tracheal suctioning on intracranial pressure in traumatic brain injury patients. *Journal of Neurotrauma, 37*(20), 2227–2233. https://doi.org/10.1089/neu.2019.6873

Healthcare Excellence Canada. (2009). *The safety competencies.* https://www.healthcareexcellence.ca/media/115mbc4z/cpsi-safetycompetencies_en_digital-final-ua.pdfhttp://www.patientsafetyinstitute.ca/en/toolsResources/safetyCompetencies/Documents/SafetyCompetencies.pdf [Seminal Reference]

Healthcare Excellence Canada. (2020). *Hospital harm improvement resource: Pneumonia.* https://www.patientsafetyinstitute.ca/en/toolsResources/Hospital-Harm-Measure/Improvement-Resources/Pneumonia/Documents/HHIR-Pneumonia-B16.pdf

Hellyer, T. P., Ewan, V., Wilson, P., et al. (2016). The Intensive Care Society recommended bundle of interventions for the prevention of ventilator-associated pneumonia. *Journal of the Intensive Care Society, 17*(3), 238–243.

Hockenberry, M., Duffy, E. A., & Gibbs, K. (2024). *Wong's nursing care of infants and children* (12th ed.). Elsevier.

Institute for Healthcare Improvement. (2012). *How-to guide: Prevent ventilator-associated pneumonia.* https://www.ihi.org/resources/Pages/Tools/HowtoGuidePreventVAP.aspx [Seminal Reference]

Karmali, S., & Rose, P. (2020). Tracheal tube size in adults undergoing elective surgery–A narrative review. *Anaesthesia, 75*(11), 1529–1539. https://doi.org/10.1111/anae.15041

Khan, M., & Nishi, S. E. (2021). Mechanically ventilated patients experience stress and feelings of vulnerability. *Evidence-Based Nursing, 25*(2), Article 51. https://doi.org/10.1136/ebnurs-2020-103364

Landsperger, J., Byram, J. M., Lloyd, B. D., et al. (2019). The effect of adhesive tape versus endotracheal tube fastener in critically ill adults: The endotracheal tube securement (ETTS) randomized controlled trial. *Critical Care, 23*(161), 1–7. https://doi.org/10.1186/s13054-019-2440-7

Letchford, E., & Bench, S. (2018). Ventilator-associated pneumonia and suction: A review of the literature. *British Journal of Nursing, 27*(1), 13–18. https://doi.org/10.12968/bjon.2018.27.1.13

Lethongkam, S., Daengngam, C., Tansakul, C., et al. (2020). Prolonged inhibitory effects against planktonic growth, adherence, and biofilm formation of pathogens causing ventilator-associated pneumonia using a novel polyamide/silver nanoparticle composite-coated endotracheal tube. *Biofouling, 36*(3), 292–307. https://doi.org/10.1080/08927014.2020.1759041

Letvin, A., Kremer, P., Silver, P. C., et al. (2018). Frequent versus infrequent monitoring of endotracheal tube cuff pressures. *Respiratory Care, 63*(5), 495–501. https://doi.org/10.4187/respcare.05926

Lewis, T. D., Dehne, K. A., Morbitzer, K., et al. (2018). Influence of single-dose antibiotic prophylaxis for early-onset pneumonia in high-risk intubated patients. *Neurocritical Care, 28*(3), 362–369. https://doi.org/10.1007/s12028-017-0490-8

Nwosu, A. D. G., Ossai, E. N., Onyekwulu, F. A., et al. (2022). Knowledge and practice of tracheal tube cuff pressure monitoring: A multicenter survey of anaesthesia and critical care providers in a developing country. *Patient Safety in Surgery, 16*(1), Article 4. https://doi.org/10.1186/s13037-021-00311-8

Reese, S., Kielty, A., Schleicher, L., et al. (2021). Development and implementation of a ventilator-associated pneumonia prevention oral care. *American Journal of Infection Control, 49*(6), S11–S12. https://doi.org/10.1016/j.ajic.2021.04.045

Tyerman, J., & Cobbett, S. (Eds.). (2023). *Lewis's medical-surgical nursing in Canada: Assessment and management of clinical problems* (5th ed.). Elsevier.

Urden, L., Stacy, K., & Lough, M. (2020). *Priorities in critical care nursing* (8th ed.). Elsevier.

Wang, R., Changkun, P., Xiaokun, W., et al. (2019). The impact of tracheotomy timing in critically ill patients undergoing mechanical ventilation: A meta-analysis of randomized controlled clinical trials with trial sequential analysis. *Heart & Lung, 48*(1), 46–54. https://doi.org/10.1016/j.hrtlng.2018.09.005

Wiegand, D. L. (2017). *AACN procedure manual for high acuity, progressive, and critical care* (7th ed.). Elsevier.

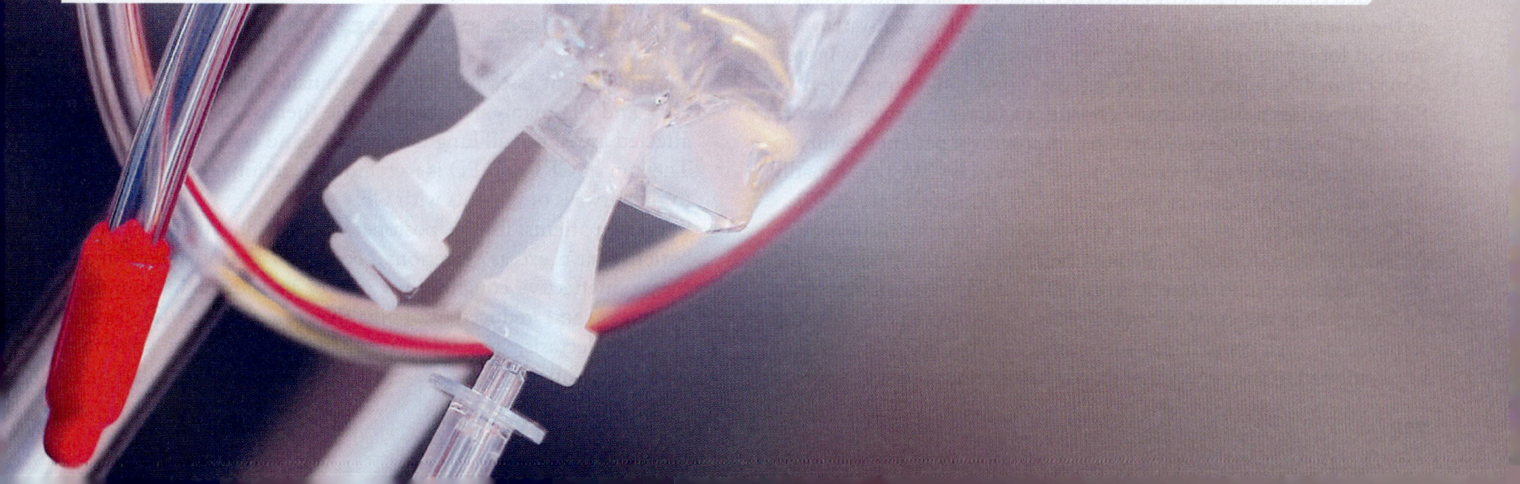

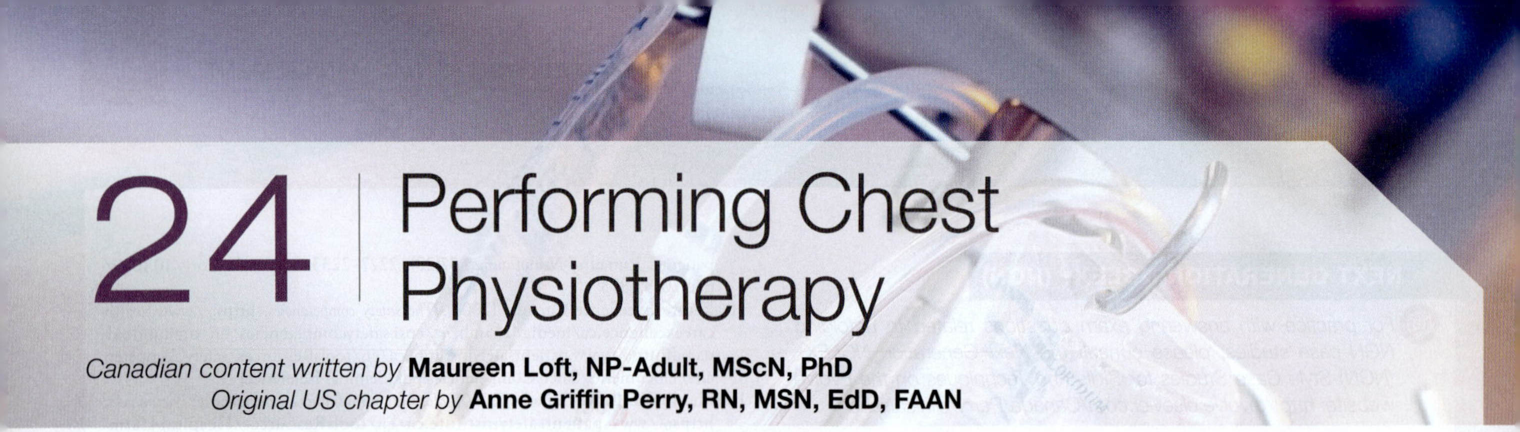

24 Performing Chest Physiotherapy

Canadian content written by **Maureen Loft, NP-Adult, MScN, PhD**
Original US chapter by **Anne Griffin Perry, RN, MSN, EdD, FAAN**

SKILLS AND PROCEDURES

OBJECTIVES

Mastery of content in this chapter will enable the nurse to:

- Assess for the need to perform chest physiotherapy (CPT) manoeuvres.
- Determine the need to modify or discontinue CPT manoeuvres.
- Explain how to prepare a patient and caregiver for the performance of each CPT manoeuvre.
- Perform the outlined CPT manoeuvres, including standard and modified versions.
- Describe the use of a positive expiratory pressure device and high-frequency chest wall oscillation vest airway clearance system.
- Describe expected and unexpected outcomes of each CPT manoeuvre.
- Describe discharge teaching and planning related to the use of each CPT manoeuvre in the home setting.

MEDIA RESOURCES

- http://evolve.elsevier.com/Canada/Perry/clinicalskills/

PURPOSE

Chest physiotherapy (CPT) is a treatment involving manipulation of the external chest wall, including percussion, vibration, and postural drainage (PD) therapy—alone or in combination—to loosen and remove secretions from patients' airways. CPT is usually followed by productive coughing or suctioning to remove secretions. The effectiveness of traditional CPT is strongly influenced by the patient population to which it is applied (Sereearuno et al., 2020). CPT has been shown to benefit patients with chronic obstructive pulmonary disease (COPD) (Pakpahan et al., 2021) and is an essential therapy for patients with cystic fibrosis (CF). For these patients, the use of manual percussion and vibration, positive expiratory pressure (PEP), and high-frequency chest wall oscillation (HFCWO) device modalities is determined by patient preference and varies at different stages of the disease (Morrison & Milroy, 2018). An HFCWO system is a method for delivering CPT using high-frequency chest wall compressions created by bursts of air for external chest wall compression. A PEP device uses positive airway pressure to increase airway pressure and oscillations to loosen secretions, improving a patient's ability to clear secretions. PD and percussion, PEP, and HFCWO are broadly classified as *airway clearance techniques (ACTs)* (Phillips et al., 2020).

Careful patient assessment is a prerequisite for administering any ACTs. The auscultation of all lung fields is essential to determine which regions would benefit from CPT. CPT manoeuvres move secretions into the large central airways; these secretions are then removed through coughing or suctioning. PD requires that a patient be positioned in such a way that gravity helps remove secretions from the targeted lung segment. PEP and HFCWO devices are more commonly used by CF patients in the community, but may also be used by patients with COPD or neuromuscular diseases.

STANDARDS OF CARE

- Accreditation Canada (2020)—*Required Organizational Practices–2020 Handbook* (https://physicians.nshealth.ca/resources/required-organizational-practices-2020-handbook)
- American Association for Respiratory Care (Strickland et al., 2015)—*AARC Clinical Practice Guideline: Effectiveness of Pharmacologic Airway Clearance Therapies in Hospitalized Patients* (https://www.aarc.org/wp-content/uploads/2014/08/pharm_cpg.pdf)

PRINCIPLES FOR PRACTICE

- Careful patient assessment is a prerequisite for administering any CPT and PD manoeuvre because the therapy usually targets the affected areas, not all lung fields (Strickland et al., 2015).
- The aim of CPT and PD is to remove secretions that accumulate in the airways of patients with CF.
- Surgical patients in the postoperative period and critically ill patients have excess secretions because of the effects of anaesthesia, ineffective coughing because of incision pain or muscle weakness, and reduced mobility (Naswa et al., 2017). Mucus plugs, atelectasis, and lobular collapse occur when secretions accumulate in the airways. Early mobility and ambulation in

combination with chest physiotherapy are essential to reduce postoperative pulmonary complications (Villeneuve, 2018).

- CPT and PD are often used in combination with other therapies, including antibiotics, bronchodilators, mucolytic agents, and inhaled and nebulized medications, in patients with CF (Chaudary & Balasa, 2021). These other therapies reduce mucus production and promote airway clearance. The goals of these therapies are (1) to clear the airways of excessive secretions to reduce the work of breathing and (2) to improve a patient's ability to cough up secretions (Morrison & Milroy, 2018).
- In the normal lung, the mucociliary transport system clears the airways of excessive mucus and inhaled particles. Airways normally remain clear, and mucus is constantly being cleared almost as fast as it is made. Normal mucus remains thin, white, and watery.
- In various disease states of the lungs, mucus clearance slows down or the cilia become overwhelmed by production of large quantities of mucus. The lungs no longer clear the mucus as fast as it is produced, which allows for bacterial colonization, ultimately leading to infection. Altered ion clearance causes an overwhelming inflammatory response (Boucher, 2019).

PERSON-CENTRED CARE

- When patients' physiological capacities are weakened, they are often anxious because of their illness or surgery, and they may be in pain. It is important to complete a pain assessment and administer prescribed analgesics 20 to 30 minutes before initiating any CPT manoeuvres. Premedication ensures that the patient is comfortable and as pain-free as possible.
- Assess the patient's activity tolerance. Patients with cardiopulmonary disease, severe arthritis, and certain musculoskeletal diseases often have diminished activity tolerance and cannot tolerate a complete CPT session. Plan CPT during short periods interspersed with rest periods, at a time when the patient is rested, and not immediately after a meal.
- Encourage mobility and ambulation to reduce pulmonary complications and promote airway clearance (Larsen et al., 2019).
- Patients with chronic pulmonary illnesses such as CF pose different challenges. These patients must devote several hours of their day to activities that assist in airway clearance. It is important that CPT and other airway clearance techniques do not impact a patient's quality of life (QOL). To maintain this QOL, try to integrate CPT and other airway clearing techniques into their routine, personal goals, and social activities (Chaudary & Balasa, 2021; Wilson, 2018).
- Because CPT skills involve considerable physical contact with the patient, it is important to be mindful of cultural differences and practise trauma-informed care. For example, some cultures consider it inappropriate to touch in public. In addition, CPT may sometimes involve gentle percussion or vibration of a patient's rib cage. Patients and families who have encountered culture- and gender-based violence need detailed information about the procedure to reassure them about the intent and objective of CPT and to prevent misunderstandings. Always explain what type of physical contact is involved and what a patient may feel during the treatment. Provide an opportunity for the patient to temporarily stop and rest during the procedure (Giger & Haddad, 2021).

EVIDENCE-INFORMED PRACTICE

- ACTs such as CPT and PD manoeuvres are effective only in selected patients, such as those with CF, bronchiectasis, and other chronic pulmonary diseases, and following some surgeries. When disease processes alter the body's normal mechanisms for clearing the lungs, therapies must be instituted to ensure that the airways remain free of secretions. Doing so reduces the risk for pulmonary infection and ensures that the oxygen demands of the body are met (Powner et al., 2019). When secretions are stagnant, they obstruct the airways, are conduits for bacterial colonization and infections, stimulate an inflammatory response, and contribute to airway and tissue damage (Boucher, 2019).
- ACT is not recommended as routine therapy for patients with COPD unless secretion retention is present (Strickland et al., 2015).
- In selected intubated patients in the critical care unit (CCU), early and routine CPT benefits patients by improving airway patency, secretion clearance, and oxygen delivery to the tissues. In addition, early CPT reduces some CCU complications, such as health care–acquired infections (HAIs).
- HFCWO devices such as the vest airway clearance system (see Procedural Guideline 24.2) are effective in aiding sputum clearance for a variety of adult and pediatric lung diseases (Chaudary & Balasa, 2021).

SAFETY GUIDELINES

- Assess the patient's normal range of vital signs. Conditions such as CF and complicated pneumonia requiring CPT can affect a patient's vital signs. The degree of change is related to the level of hypoxia, overall cardiopulmonary status, and tolerance of the procedure.
- Assess the patient's current medications. Some medications, particularly diuretics and antihypertensives, cause fluid and hemodynamic changes. These changes affect a patient's tolerance of positional changes. Steroid medications, age, and malnutrition increase a patient's risk for pathological rib fractures and often contraindicate rib vibration.
- Review the patient's medical and surgical history. Certain conditions, such as increased intracranial pressure, spinal cord injuries, abdominal aneurysm resection, bone metastases, and severe osteoporosis, contraindicate the positional changes required for PD (Box 24.1). Thoracic trauma contraindicates percussion and vibration.

BOX 24.1

Contraindications for Postural Drainage

- Increased intracranial pressure
- Head and neck injury, until stabilized
- Active hemorrhage with hemodynamic instability
- Recent spinal surgery (e.g., laminectomy) or acute spinal injury
- Active hemoptysis
- Empyema
- Bronchopleural fistula
- Pulmonary edema associated with heart failure
- Large pleural effusions
- Pulmonary embolism
- Older, confused, or anxious patients who are unable to tolerate position change
- Rib fracture, with or without flail chest
- Surgical wound or healing tissue

Trendelenburg position is contraindicated for the following conditions:

- Uncontrolled hypertension
- Distended abdomen
- Esophageal surgery
- Recent gross hemoptysis
- Uncontrolled airway at risk for aspiration

Adapted from White, G. C. (2013). *Basic clinical lab competencies for respiratory care: An integrated approach* (5th ed.). Cengage Learning.

- Assess the patient's level of cognitive function. Alteration in mental status often makes it difficult or impossible for a patient to understand the procedure and participate in coughing and expectorating secretions.
- Have suction machine equipment available to help clear airway secretions (see Chapter 23).
- Patients who receive long-term steroid therapy are at risk for pathological fractures. Physical manoeuvres such as chest percussion and vibration may be contraindicated because of the risk for rib fractures. These patients benefit from individualized airway clearance measures such as use of a PEP device (Strickland et al., 2015).

✦ SKILL 24.1 Performing Postural Drainage

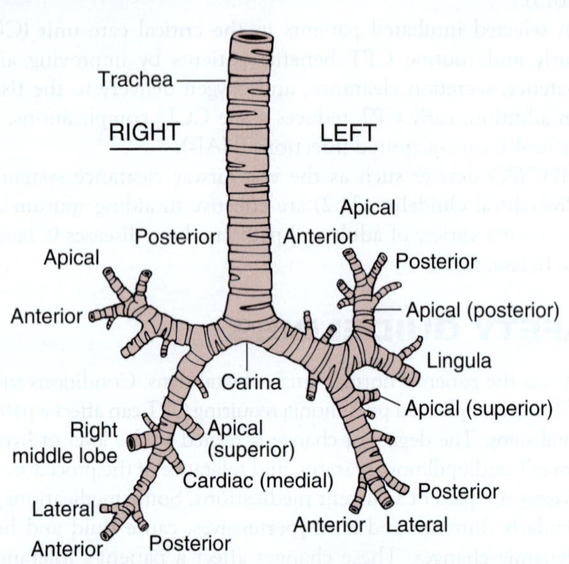

FIG 24.1 Tracheobronchial tree. *(Adapted from Frownfelter, D. L., & Dean, E. [2006]. Principles and practice of cardiopulmonary therapy [43rd ed.]. Mosby.)*

Postural drainage (PD) is the use of positioning techniques to drain secretions from specific segments of the lungs and bronchi into the trachea (Fig. 24.1). Each position drains a specific corresponding section of the tracheobronchial tree, from the upper, middle, or lower lung field into the trachea (Table 24.1). Additional coughing or airway suctioning helps remove secretions from the trachea.

Use physical assessment findings and a review of the chest X-ray to determine which lung segments require PD. Patients needing PD usually have chronic conditions that affect their activity tolerance. Knowing which lung segments require PD promotes patient cooperation, adherence to therapy, and prevention of excessive fatigue. In addition, use knowledge of a patient's condition and disease process and the extent of the pathological condition to individualize PD therapy.

Delegation and Collaboration

The skill of performing PD can be delegated to an unregulated care provider (UCP). It is the nurse's responsibility to assess the patient, review laboratory and chest X-ray results, and determine whether the patient is stable and able to tolerate the procedure. The nurse instructs the UCP to do the following:

- Immediately report to the nurse changes in the patient's comfort level, changes in breathing pattern, and tolerance of the procedure

TABLE 24.1

Positions and Procedures for Drainage, Percussion, and Vibration

Area and Procedure	Anatomical Area	Position of Patient
Left and Right Upper Lobe Anterior Apical Bronchi		
Position patient in chair, or high Fowler's, leaning back. Percuss and vibrate with heel of hands at shoulders and fingers over collarbones (clavicles) in front; do both sides at same time. Note body posture and arm position of nurse. Nurse's back is kept straight, and elbows and knees are slightly flexed.	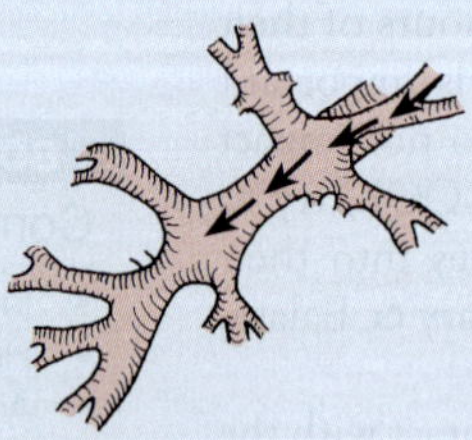	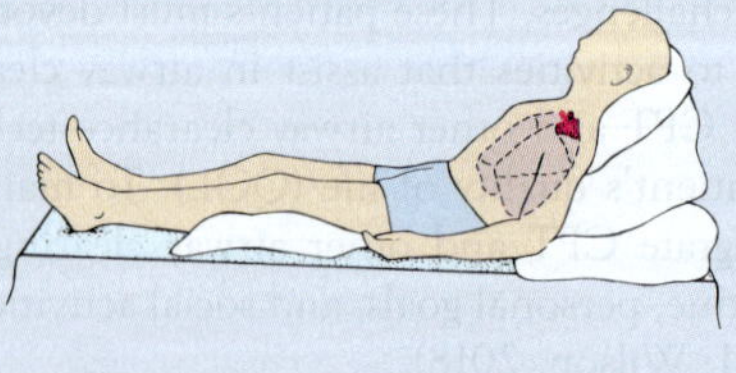 Anterior apical segments
Direction of mucus flow through upper lobe anterior apical bronchi.	Position hands for chest physiotherapy over left and right upper anterior apical bronchi.	
Left and Right Upper Lobe Posterior Apical Bronchi		
Position patient in chair, leaning forward on pillow or table. Percuss and vibrate with hands on either side of upper spine. Do both sides at same time.	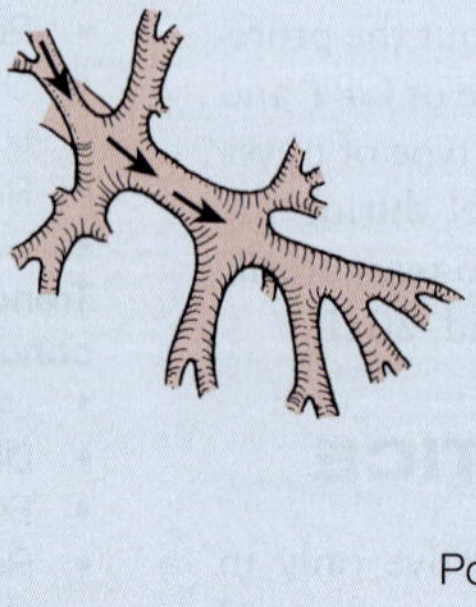	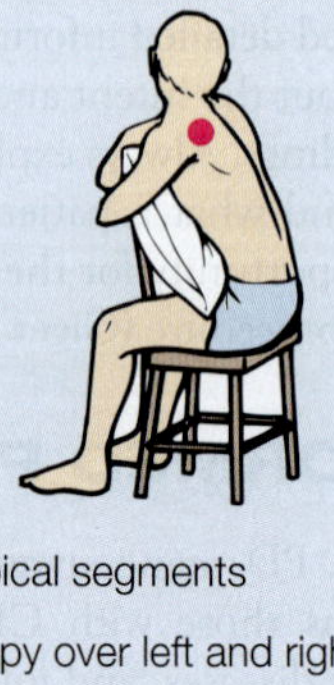 Posterior apical segments
Direction of mucus flow through upper lobe posterior apical bronchi.	Position hands for chest physiotherapy over left and right upper lobe posterior apical bronchi.	

Continued

TABLE 24.1

Positions and Procedures for Drainage, Percussion, and Vibration—cont'd

Area and Procedure	Anatomical Area	Position of Patient
Left and Right Upper Lobe Anterior Bronchi Position patient flat on back with small pillow under knees. Percuss and vibrate just below clavicle on either side of sternum.	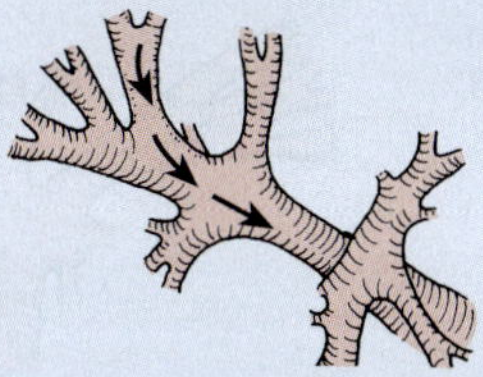	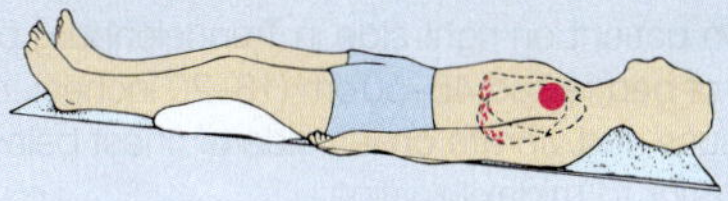 Anterior upper lobe segments
Direction of mucus flow through anterior upper bronchi.	Position hands for chest physiotherapy over right and left anterior upper lobe bronchi.	
Left Upper Lobe Lingular Bronchus Position patient on right side with arm overhead in Trendelenburg position, with foot of bed raised 30 cm (12 inches), as tolerated.* Place pillow behind back, and roll patient one-quarter turn onto pillow. Percuss and vibrate lateral to left nipple below axilla.	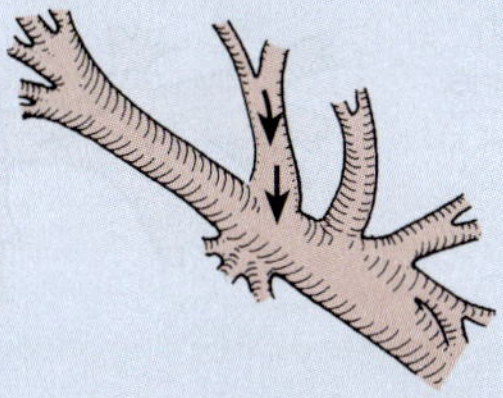	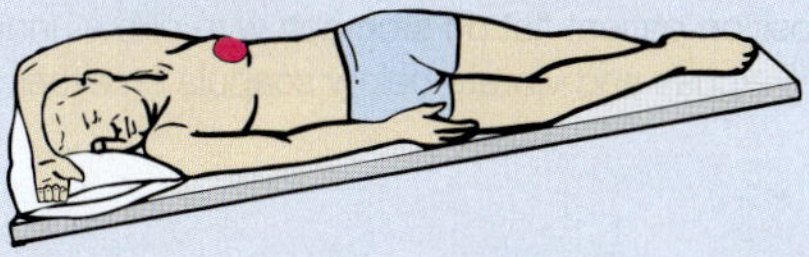 Left upper lobe lingular segment
Direction of mucus flow through left upper lobe lingular bronchus.	Position hands for chest physiotherapy over left upper lobe lingular bronchus.	
Right Middle Lobe Bronchus Position patient on left side or abdomen. Place pillow behind back and roll patient one-quarter turn onto pillow. Percuss and vibrate to right nipple below axilla.	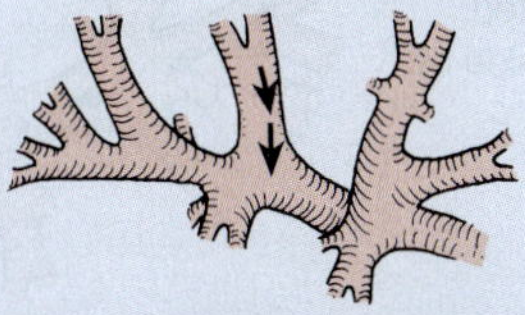	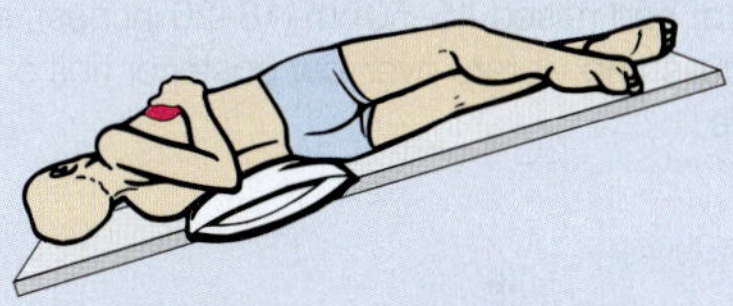 Right middle lobe segment
Direction of mucus flow through right middle lobe bronchus.	Position hands for chest physiotherapy over right middle lobe bronchus.	
Left and Right Lower Lobe Anterior Bronchi Position patient on back, with foot of bed elevated 45–50 cm (18–20 inches). Have knees bent on pillow. Percuss and vibrate over lower anterior ribs on both sides.	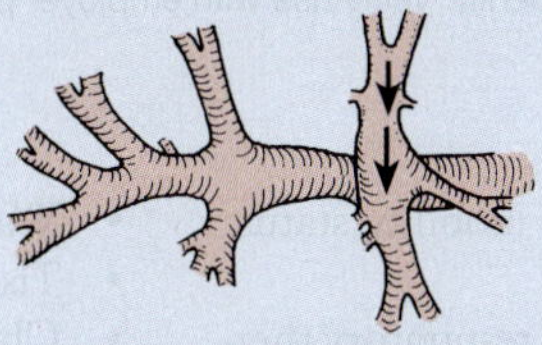	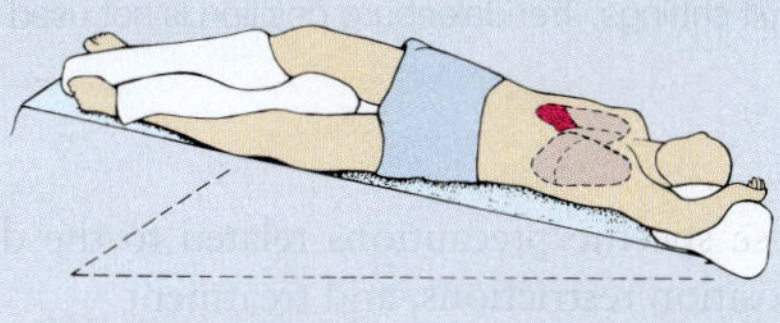 Anterior lower lobe segments
Direction of mucus flow through anterior lower lobe bronchi.	Position hands for chest physiotherapy over left and right anterior lower lobe bronchi.	
Right Lower Lobe Lateral Bronchus Position patient on abdomen in Trendelenburg position with foot of bed raised 45–50 cm (18–20 inches), as tolerated. Percuss and vibrate on left and right sides of chest below shoulder blades (scapulae) posterior to midaxillary line.	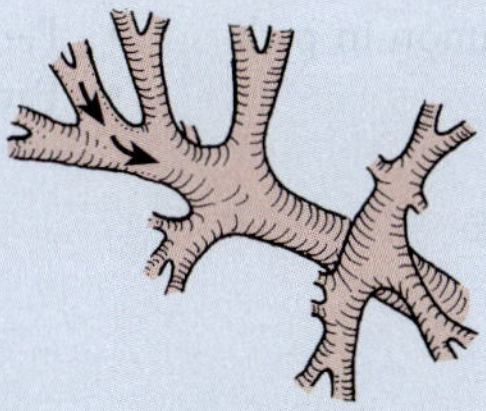	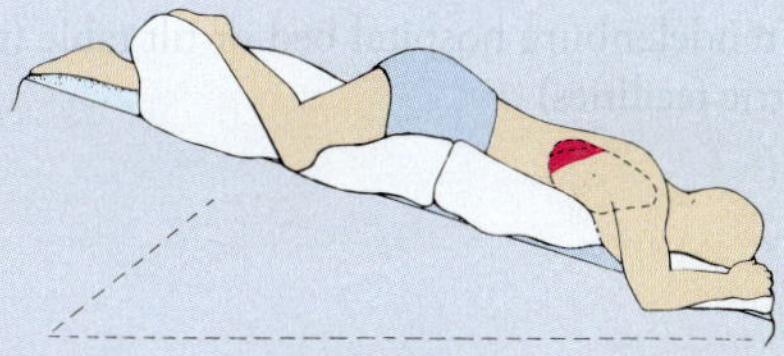 Right lower lateral lobe segment
Direction of mucus flow through right lower lobe lateral bronchus.	Position hands for chest physiotherapy over right lower lobe lateral bronchus.	

TABLE 24.1
Positions and Procedures for Drainage, Percussion, and Vibration—cont'd

Area and Procedure	Anatomical Area	Position of Patient
Left Lower Lobe Lateral Bronchus		
Position patient on right side in Trendelenburg position with foot of bed raised 45–50 cm (18–20 inches), as tolerated. Percuss and vibrate on left side of chest below scapulae posterior to midaxillary line.	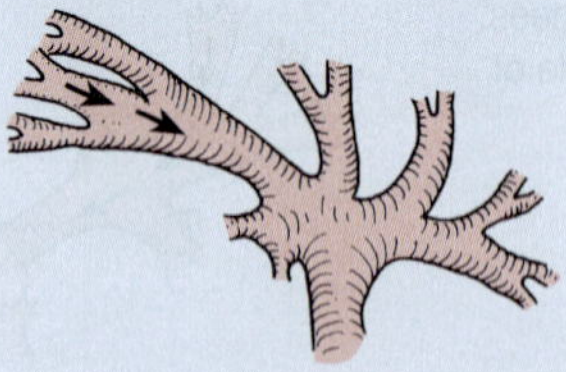	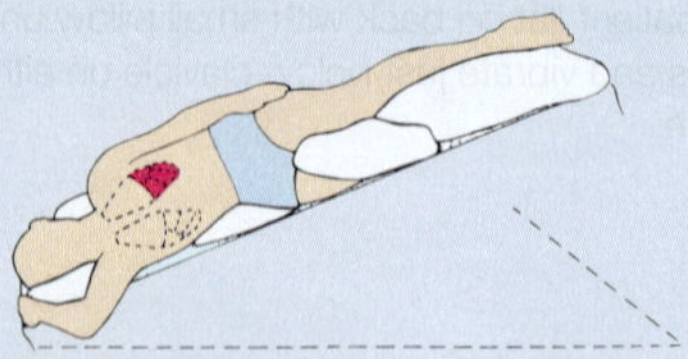 Left lower lobe lateral segment
Direction of mucus flow through left lower lobe lateral bronchus.	Position hands for chest physiotherapy over left lower lobe lateral bronchus.	
Right and Left Lower Lobe Superior Bronchi		
Position patient flat on stomach with pillow under stomach. Percuss and vibrate below scapula on either side of spine.	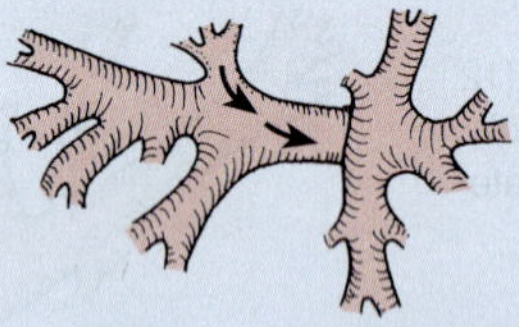	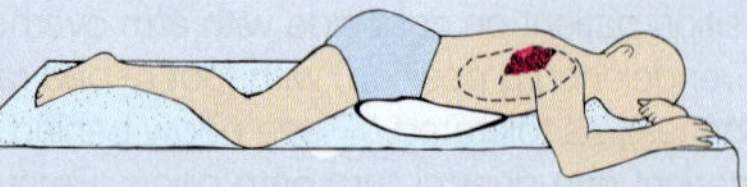 Lower lobe superior segments
Direction of mucus flow through lower lobe superior bronchi.	Position hands for chest physiotherapy over right and left lower lobe superior bronchi.	
Right and Left Posterior Basal Bronchi		
Position patient on stomach in Trendelenburg position with foot of bed raised 45–50 cm (18–20 inches), as tolerated. Percuss and vibrate over low posterior ribs on either side of spine.	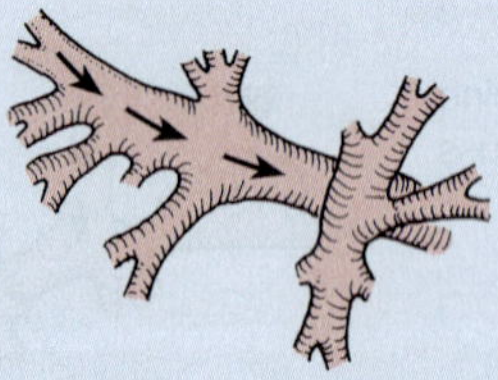	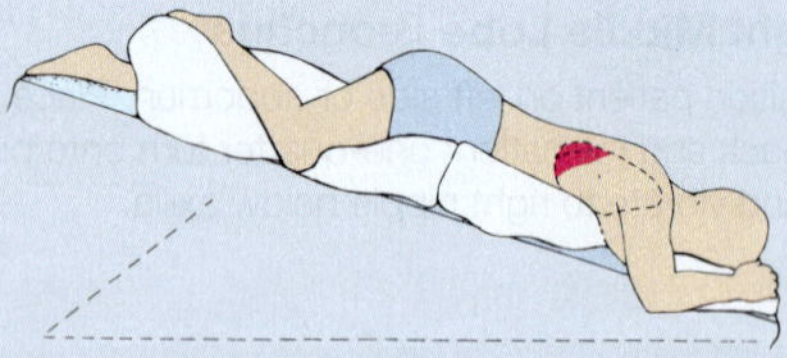 Posterior segments
Direction of mucus flow through posterior basal bronchi.	Position hands for chest physiotherapy over right and left posterior lower lobe bronchi.	

*In adult settings, Trendelenburg position is not used as frequently. Verify use with employer policy and health care provider's prescription.

- Use specific precautions related to the disease, mobility status, position restrictions, and treatment

Collaborate with the interprofessional team (e.g., respiratory therapist) to facilitate PD schedules.

Equipment

- Stethoscope
- Pulse oximeter
- Trendelenburg hospital bed or tilt table (more common in pediatric facilities)
- Water in pitcher and glass
- Tissues and paper bag
- Chair (for draining upper lobes)
- Extra pillows
- Clear graduated screw-top container for sputum collection *(optional)*
- Oral hygiene products
- Suction equipment (if patient is unable to cough and clear own secretions)
- Personal protective equipment (PPE), as required
- Patient education materials

STEP	RATIONALE
ASSESSMENT	
1. Identify patient using at least two person-specific identifiers (e.g., name and date of birth, or name and medical record number) according to employer policy.	Proper hand hygiene helps prevent the spread of infectious agents to health care providers.
2. Throughout the procedure, the 4 moments for hand hygiene are to be implemented; hand hygiene should occur before initial patient (or patient environment) contact, before an aseptic procedure, after body fluid exposure risk, and after patient (or patient environment) contact. Additional hand hygiene should be performed when hands are visibly soiled.	Ensures correct patient. Complies with Accreditation Canada's standards and improves patient safety (Accreditation Canada, 2020).
3. Assess patient for history of decreased level of consciousness, decreased activity tolerance, and muscle weakness or chronic disease processes such as complicated pneumonia and COPD (see Box 24.1).	Conditions that pose risk for impaired airway clearance require PD.

Critical Decision Point *If the use of Trendelenburg position or other postures causes severe hypertension, severe hypoxemia, or severe shortness of breath, therapy is contraindicated* (see Box 24.1). *In addition, when patients have a risk for or a history of gastroesophageal reflux disease (GERD), which is regurgitation of stomach contents into the esophagus, head-down positions should not be used.*

STEP	RATIONALE
4. Review medical record and assess patient for signs and symptoms, including X-ray film changes consistent with atelectasis, lobar collapse pneumonia, or bronchiectasis; ineffective coughing; and thick, sticky, tenacious, and discoloured secretions that are difficult to cough up.	Indicates need to perform PD. Chest X-ray and signs and symptoms indicate accumulation of pulmonary secretions and ineffective airway clearance. Airway clearance techniques are additional therapies to improve removal of airway secretions (O'Neill et al., 2019).
5. Auscultate all lung fields for decreased breath sounds and adventitious lung sounds.	Findings identify specific lung segments needing drainage.
6. Obtain vital signs and pulse oximetry (SpO_2) before PD treatment.	Provides baseline to evaluate patient's response and tolerance to therapy.
7. Determine patient's and caregiver's understanding of and ability to perform home PD.	Identifies potential areas for instruction for discharge planning. Home PD treatment is essential for airway secretion management in patients with CF (Morrison & Milroy, 2018).
8. Use a pain rating scale from 0 to 10 (0 = no pain, 10 = the worst pain ever) to determine patient's level of comfort.	Determines patient's level of pain and if preprocedure analgesia is needed.

NURSING DIAGNOSES

- Insufficient airway clearance
- Inadequate breathing pattern
- Reduced gas exchange
- Acute pain
- Insufficient knowledge regarding PD and airway clearance

Related factors and risk factors are individualized on the basis of patient's condition or needs.

STEP	RATIONALE
PLANNING	
1. Expected outcomes following completion of procedure:	
• Lung sounds improve or become clear to auscultation.	Clearing of airways confirms effectiveness of procedure.
• Sputum is more easily expectorated or suctioned out.	PD manoeuvres loosen airway secretions, facilitating secretion removal.
• Secretions appear more normal in colour and consistency.	When infection is present, returning to normal secretion characteristics indicates resolving infection.
• SpO_2 levels increase and dyspnea decreases.	As secretions are removed, exchange of respiratory gases improves and dyspnea gradually declines.
• Chest X-ray shows improvements: lobar collapse and atelectasis are decreased or eliminated.	PD drains secretions into major airways, facilitating removal during coughing and CPT. As a result, there is visual improvement on chest X-ray.
2. Prepare patient for procedure:	
a. If patient has an increased pain rating on assessment, administer analgesia 20 minutes before CPT manoeuvres.	Pain control is essential for patient to actively participate in PD manoeuvres and cough forcefully to clear airways.

STEP	RATIONALE

PLANNING

STEP	RATIONALE
c. Unless contraindicated, encourage high fluid intake (minimum of 1500 mL) daily. Maintain record of fluid intake and output.	Fluids may thin secretions and make them easier to cough up. Patients need close monitoring and encouragement when first starting a high-fluid intake program.
d. Plan treatments so they do not overlap with meals or tube feeding. Avoid PD 1–2 hours before or 1–2 hours after meals or bolus tube feedings. Stop all continuous gastric tube feedings for 30–45 minutes before PD. Check for residual feeding in patient's stomach; if >100 mL, hold treatment.	Performing PD when patient's stomach is empty helps avoid gastric reflux or vomiting and aspiration of stomach contents.
e. Schedule treatments at appropriate times during the day.	Scheduling of PD avoids conflict with other interventions and diagnostic testing.

Critical Decision Point *If patient is receiving inhaled medication through bronchodilator, nebulizer, or aerosol treatment, provide PD 20 minutes after such therapy. PD following bronchodilator therapy enhances patient oxygenation during procedure* (Barker, 2022).

STEP	RATIONALE
f. Have patient remove any tight or restrictive clothing.	Helps patient relax and promotes deep breathing.

IMPLEMENTATION

STEP	RATIONALE
1. Close room door or pull curtains around patient's bed. Apply clean gloves as indicated.	Maintains privacy. Reduces transmission of microorganisms.
2. Use findings from physical assessment and chest X-ray to select congested areas for draining. Consult with primary health care provider as needed.	Individualized treatment helps relieve specific areas of congestion identified during patient assessment.
3. Help patient to desired position to drain congested areas (see Table 24.1). Place pillows for support and comfort. Drape patient appropriately.	Proper patient positioning assists gravity in helping movement of secretions from peripheral airways to larger bronchi, where they can be cleared.
4. Have patient maintain position for 10–15 minutes.	In adults, draining each area takes time.
5. After 10–15 minutes of drainage in selected postures, perform chest percussion and vibration (see Procedural Guideline 24.2) over affected lung region. Table 24.1 shows all postures and hand placement for percussion and vibration.	Provides mechanical forces to help move airway secretions.
6. After 10–15 minutes of drainage in first posture, have patient sit up and cough. If indicated, save expectorated secretions in clear container. If patient cannot cough, suctioning is necessary (see Chapter 23).	Any secretions moved to central airways are removed by coughing or suctioning before patient assumes next drainage position. Coughing is most effective when patient is sitting up and leaning forward.

Critical Decision Point *Sometimes patients experience transient dyspnea and fatigue because of airway irritation and bronchospasm from secretions. These patients often benefit from an oscillating or vibrating PEP device* (see Procedural Guideline 24.1).

STEP	RATIONALE
7. Have patient rest briefly, if necessary, between positions. Note pulse oximeter readings.	Short rest periods between postures prevent fatigue and increase tolerance. SpO_2 values may fall slightly.
8. Have patient take sips of water.	Keeping mouth moist aids in expectoration of secretions.
9. Repeat Steps 4–9 until all affected areas selected are drained. Make sure that each treatment does not exceed 30–60 minutes.	Drainage is used to drain selected areas only and is based on individual assessment.
10. Offer to help patient with oral hygiene.	Promotes comfort and reduces foul-smelling breath.
11. Remove gloves.	Reduces transmission of microorganisms.

STEP	RATIONALE
EVALUATION	
1. Auscultate lung fields.	Clearance of secretions usually relieves gurgling, early inspiratory crackles, and palpable crepitus.
2. Inspect character and amount of sputum.	Determines whether more secretions are coughed up and whether they are thinned adequately.
3. Review diagnostic reports, including sputum collections and cultures, chest X-rays, and arterial blood gas (ABG) levels.	Provides objective data on improvements in lung function.
4. Obtain vital signs and SpO_2.	Procedure can result in dysrhythmias and decreases in oxygen saturation <90% in some patients.
5. **Use teach-back:** "I want to be sure I explained why you need to position yourself over the back of a chair with a pillow supporting your chest. Tell me why this position is important." Develop a revised teaching plan if patient or caregiver is unable to teach back correctly.	Determines patient's and caregiver's level of understanding of instructional topic.

Unexpected Outcomes	Related Interventions
1. Patient experiences severe dyspnea, bronchospasm, hypoxemia, or hypercarbia and/or is unable to tolerate treatment.	• Discontinue, modify, or shorten treatments. • Administer bronchodilator or nebulizer therapy 20 minutes before CPT. • Suction and ventilate with bag-valve mask to improve patient oxygenation. Closely monitor ABG levels, oxygen saturation, and vital signs.
2. No improvement in chest assessment or chest X-ray examination results.	• Initially, increase treatments and encourage and teach coughing exercises. • Increase hydration (if medically appropriate). • Notify health care provider because patient may need sputum culture, change in antibiotics, mucolytics, or a bronchoscopy to remove thick mucus plugs.
3. Hemoptysis occurs; or patient develops acute hypotension, severe chest pain, vomiting, aspiration, and/or dysrhythmias.	• Stop therapy, place patient in high Fowler's position, and obtain vital signs. • Call for help and notify health care provider. • Remain with patient; keep patient comfortable, calm, warm, and quiet. • If patient vomits or aspirates, suction airway and place them on their side. • Reapply patient's oxygen device if prescribed.

Communication and Documentation

- Document pretherapy and post-therapy assessment findings, SpO_2 readings, and chest X-ray results; frequency and duration of treatment; postures used and bronchial segments drained; cough effectiveness; need for suctioning; colour, amount, and consistency of sputum; hemoptysis or other unexpected outcomes; and patient's tolerance and reaction in the progress notes in electronic health record (EHR) or chart.
- Document your evaluation of patient and caregiver learning.

DOCUMENTATION EXAMPLE

Patient agreed to receive percussion and vibration prior to bedtime to facilitate postural drainage of left lower lobe bronchus. Chest X-ray today demonstrated pneumonia. Vital signs within patient's normal limits before and after treatment (see vital signs record). Oxygen saturation was 92% on 2 litres of oxygen via nasal prongs before treatment and 94% following treatment. Patient tolerated right side-lying Trendelenburg position well for 30 minutes of treatment with foot of bed elevated to 50 cm. Moderate quantity of thick, greenish-yellow mucus expectorated by patient during the treatment after strong cough effort. Patient reported no pain or shortness of breath throughout the procedure.

Special Considerations

Teaching

- Instruct patient and caregiver that the best times for treatments are (1) in the morning before breakfast, when patient can clear secretions that accumulate overnight, and (2) about 1 hour before bedtime, so that lungs are clear before sleeping and patient has time after treatment to cough up any mobilized secretions. Frequency depends on need and patient's tolerance and varies from once daily to every 2 to 4 hours in an acute situation.
- Instruct caregiver how to recognize when patient's respiratory status requires breathing exercises or PD.

Pediatric

- In a child with CF, PD is a cornerstone therapy and is usually performed at least twice daily, on rising in the morning and in the evening (Hockenberry et al., 2024).
- Many patients with CF benefit from the use of the vest airway clearance system (see Procedural Guideline 24.2) (Chaudary & Balasa, 2021; Morrison & Milroy, 2018).
- CPT is not beneficial in the treatment of bronchiolitis in children younger than 2 years of age (Hockenberry et al., 2024).
- Children with pneumonia, bronchiolitis, and asthma receive limited benefits from administration of CPT (Morrow, 2019).

Gerontological

- Take extra care and thoroughly assess patient when using PD in older persons. Certain medications such as antihypertensive and cardiac medications may increase the risk for dizziness when positions are changed rapidly (Salvo, 2018). Therefore, change positions more slowly, and closely assess for any changes in oxygen saturation or vital signs with position changes.
- Older persons with chronic cardiac and pulmonary conditions do not always tolerate a supine or side-lying position for PD. If a patient experiences a decrease in oxygen saturation (decreased SpO_2) or increased breathlessness in these positions, reposition them to a semi-Fowler's position and perform CPT.

Patients With Physical or Cognitive Challenges

- The techniques of percussion and drainage may elicit different responses for patients who are confused or have cognitive challenges. Assess the patient's cognitive functioning in order to individualize preparation according to the patient's needs and help the patient remain calm during the procedure (Sullivan et al., 2018).

Care in the Community: Home Management

- Teach patient and caregiver how to assume PD positions at home. Some positions need modification to meet patient needs. For example, if the patient is very short of breath, place them in a side-lying semi-Fowler's or side-lying Trendelenburg position to drain lateral lower lobes.
- Obtain foam wedge or multiple pillows for correct positioning.
- If eligible, refer patient to a pulmonary rehabilitation program.

Procedural Guideline 24.1 *Using a Positive Expiratory Pressure Device*

A positive expiratory pressure (PEP) device is a handheld airway clearance device (Fig. 24.2). The device has a control that can adjust the frequency of oscillations and resistance to expiratory flow. PEP treatment stabilizes airways and improves aeration of the distal lung areas. During exhalation, pressure from the airways is transmitted to the PEP device, which helps mucus dislodge from the airway walls and as a result prevents airway collapse, accelerates expiratory flow, and moves mucus toward the trachea (Strickland et al., 2015). Some patients living with CF may benefit more from this device than from standard CPT (Chapman et al., 2021). However, patients with CF must receive some type of routine airway clearance therapy daily.

Delegation and Collaboration

The skill of using a PEP device can be delegated to a UCP. The nurse is responsible for performing respiratory assessment, determining whether the procedure is appropriate and whether a patient can tolerate it, and evaluating a patient's response to it. Interprofessional collaboration is required when preparing to use a PEP device (e.g., respiratory therapist). When delegating to an UCP, the nurse instructs the UCP to do the following:

- Be alert for patient's tolerance of the procedure, such as comfort level and changes in breathing pattern, and immediately report changes to the nurse.
- Use specific patient precautions, such as positioning restrictions related to disease or treatment.

Equipment

- Stethoscope
- Pulse oximeter
- Water in pitcher and glass
- Chair
- Tissues and paper bag
- Clear graduated screw-top container
- Suction equipment (if patient is unable to cough and clear own secretions)
- PEP device (see Fig. 24.2)
- PPE
- Patient education materials

Procedural Steps

1. Identify patient using at least two person-specific identifiers (e.g., name and date of birth, or name and medical record number) according to employer policy (Accreditation Canada, 2020).
2. Throughout the procedure, the 4 moments for hand hygiene are to be implemented; hand hygiene should occur before initial patient (or patient environment) contact, before an aseptic procedure, after body fluid exposure risk, and after patient (or patient environment) contact. Additional hand hygiene should be performed when hands are visibly soiled.
3. Verify the need for a health care provider's prescription per employer policy.

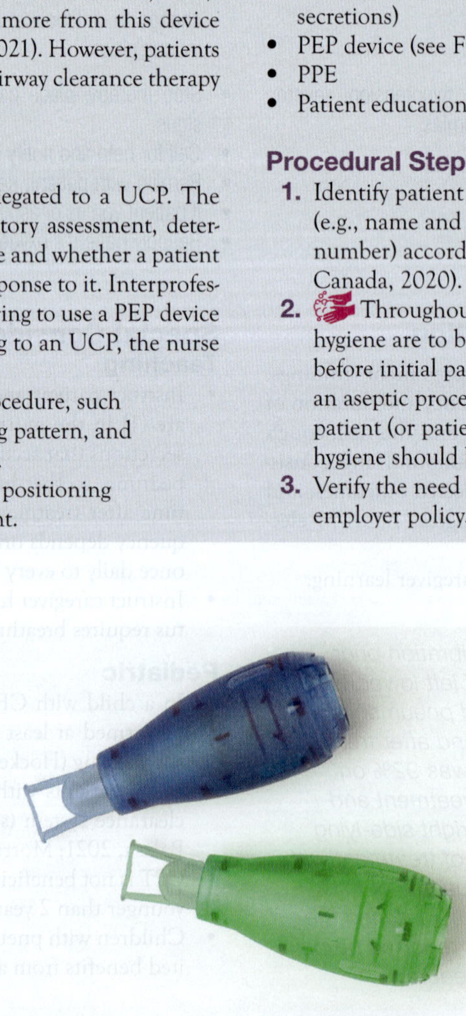

FIG 24.2 Positive expiratory pressure (PEP) device example—Acapella device. *(Used with permission from Smithsmedical.com.)*

Procedural Guideline 24.1 *Using a Positive Expiratory Pressure Device—cont'd*

4. Perform respiratory assessment to determine lung segments requiring percussion and/or vibration.
5. Assess patient's and caregiver's understanding of the device and procedure, and explain and clarify procedure as needed.
6. Prepare prescribed PEP device per manufacturer's recommendations

Critical Decision Point *Verify that the correct device is used to match patient's expiratory flow rate. Refer to manufacturer's instructions and health care provider's prescription.*

   a. Initial setting: As prescribed by health care provider.
   b. As patient improves or is more proficient, adjust the proper resistance level upward as prescribed by health care provider.

Critical Decision Point *Determine whether aerosol medication therapy is prescribed, and if so, attach a nebulizer to the end of the PEP valve.*

7. Instruct patient to:
   a. Sit comfortably.
   b. Take in a breath that is larger than normal but does not fill lungs completely. Instruct patient to inhale to about 75% of inspiratory capacity.
   c. Place mouthpiece into mouth, maintaining a tight seal.
   d. Hold breath for 2–3 seconds.
   e. Try not to cough, and exhale slowly for 3–4 seconds through the device while it vibrates.

Critical Decision Point *If patient cannot maintain an exhalation for this length of time, adjust the PEP device as indicated by the manufacturer to allow the patient to exhale at a lower flow rate.*

   f. Repeat cycle for 5–10 breaths as tolerated.
   g. Remove mouthpiece and perform one or two forceful exhalations and "huff" coughs.
   h. Repeat Steps 7a–7g, as required.
8. Auscultate lung fields.
9. Obtain vital signs and SpO_2.
10. Inspect colour, character, and amount of sputum.
11. Help patient with oral hygiene and cleaning of the PEP device.
12. **Use teach-back:** "I want to be sure that you can use this device safely. Show me how you use the PEP device during this airway treatment." Develop a revised teaching plan if patient or caregiver is unable to teach back correctly.
13. Review Unexpected Outcomes for Skill 24.1.
14. Document procedure and patient's tolerance. Document your evaluation of patient learning.

Procedural Guideline 24.2 *Performing Percussion and Vibration*

During PD, a nurse, respiratory therapist, or trained caregiver sometimes uses physical manoeuvres such as percussion and vibration on the rib cage over the lung tissue. The clinician uses techniques on specific parts of the rib cage over each affected lung region. Normally, the mucociliary escalator and cough transport of the body can clear airway secretions effectively. However, when a patient's ability to clear the airways is reduced, the techniques of percussion and vibration are combined with PD (see Skill 24.1).

Percussion is the manual external clapping of a patient's chest wall with cupped hands or with a mechanical device in a rhythmic fashion to loosen secretions from the bronchial walls. To apply vibration to a patient's external chest wall, place both hands (one over the other) over the areas to be vibrated. Then tense and contract the shoulder and arm muscles to create a vibration while the patient exhales to mobilize secretions (Strickland et al., 2015). Vibration augments the natural movement of the rib cage during exhalation and helps with secretion clearance. Never use the clavicles, breast tissue, sternum, spine, waist, or abdomen for percussion and vibration; only perform these manoeuvres over the ribs.

High-Frequency Chest Wall Oscillation

High-frequency chest wall oscillation (HFCWO) consists of an inflatable vest linked to an air-pulse generator. One HFCWO device is the vest airway clearance system, which helps to loosen and remove secretions from the airways (Fig. 24.3). HFCWO systems deliver high-frequency, small-volume expiratory pulses to a patient's external chest wall. This mechanical action helps to loosen and mobilize airway secretions (Wilson, 2018). It is beneficial for

Continued

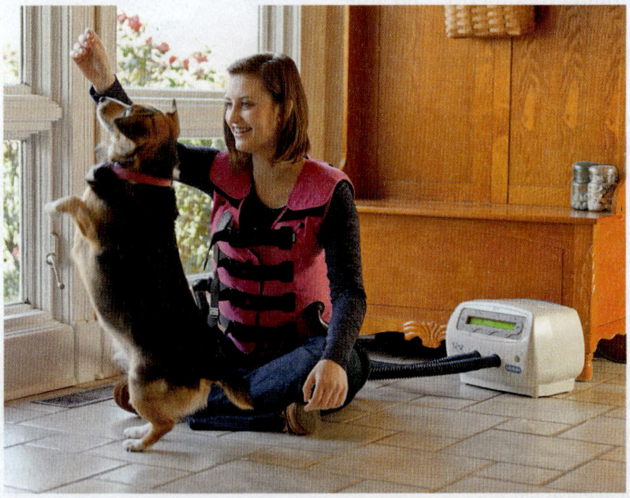

FIG 24.3 High-frequency chest wall oscillation (HFCWO) vest for home use. *(Copyright © 2012 Hill-Rom Services, Inc. Reprinted with permission. All rights reserved.)*

Procedural Guideline 24.2 *Performing Percussion and Vibration—cont'd*

selected patients, including those with neuromuscular diseases, CF, and ineffective coughing and airway clearance. In addition, patients with sputum production of 25–30 mL/day also benefit from this device because HFCWO decreases the viscosity of mucus, making it easier to cough productively (Leemans et al., 2020).

Delegation and Collaboration

The skill of performing percussion and vibration can be delegated to a UCP (refer to employer policy). The nurse is responsible for the respiratory assessment and review of the patient's chest X-ray (in collaboration with a health care provider) to determine patient stability, which areas of the lungs are affected, and specific positions for the patient to assume. The nurse instructs the UCP about the following:

- Any patient precautions related to disease or treatment.
- Reporting to the nurse any problems the patient has with tolerance of the procedure, pain, or dyspnea, or changes in vital signs.

Equipment

- Stethoscope
- Hospital bed (tilt table placed in Trendelenburg position [*optional*]; check employer policy)
- Chair (for upper lobes)
- One to four pillows
- Water in pitcher and glass
- Tissues and paper bag
- Clear graduated screw-top container
- Mechanical vibrator or percussor *(optional)*
- HFCWO device, such as the vest airway clearance system
- Single layer of clothing
- PPE
- Oral hygiene products: toothbrush, toothpaste, mouthwash, or chlorhexidine gluconate (CHG) oral rinse (if prescribed)
- Suction equipment *(optional)*
- Stethoscope, pulse oximeter

Procedural Steps

1. Identify patient using at least two person-specific identifiers (e.g., name and date of birth, or name and medical record number) according to employer policy (Accreditation Canada, 2020).
2. Throughout the procedure, the 4 moments for hand hygiene are to be implemented; hand hygiene should occur before initial patient (or patient environment) contact, before an aseptic procedure, after body fluid exposure risk, and after patient (or patient environment) contact. Additional hand hygiene should be performed when hands are visibly soiled.
3. Assess patient and review medical record for signs, symptoms, and conditions that indicate need to perform percussion and vibration (see Skill 24.1, Assessment).
4. Perform respiratory assessment (including vital signs, SpO_2, inspection, and palpation) to assess breathing pattern, including muscles used for breathing, respiratory rate and depth, extent of excursion, chest wall movement, and oxygen saturation.
5. Auscultate lung sounds over lung segments drained during PD (see Skill 24.1).

Critical Decision Point *Percussion and vibration are contraindicated with rib fracture, fracture of other rib cage structures such as the clavicle or sternum, pain, severe dyspnea, and severe osteoporosis. Thin, weak patients with osteoporosis are most susceptible to injury and are taught other secretion-control measures (e.g., forceful coughing, humidification).*

6. Inspect and gently palpate rib cage over affected bronchial segment(s) for pain, tenderness, abnormal configuration, abnormal excursion or chest wall movement during breathing, and muscle tension. Percussion or vibration is contraindicated if one of these assessment findings is present, because the treatment has the potential to cause further injury and impair chest wall motion.
7. Determine patient's understanding and assess ability to cooperate with therapy, both in hospital and at home.
8. Explain procedure in detail: patient's positioning, sensations, how it will be done, how long it will take, use of vest (if applicable), and any discomforts or side effects.
9. Help patient relax and breathe deeply during procedure. Have them practise exhaling slowly through pursed lips while relaxing chest wall muscles. They should blow out air using their abdominal muscles, not rib cage muscles.
10. Apply clean gloves as appropriate.
11. Elevate bed to comfortable working height and stand close to bed with arms directly in front and knees slightly bent.
12. Use findings from physical assessment and chest X-ray to select congested areas of lung. Position patient in appropriate drainage position (see Table 24.1) and place pillows for support and comfort.
13. Perform percussion and vibration.
    a. Percussion and vibration with hands:
    (1) Perform percussion for 3–5 minutes in each position as tolerated. Begin on appropriate part of chest wall over draining area (see Table 24.1). Always ask if patient is experiencing any discomfort such as undue pressure or stinging of the skin.
    (2) Place hands side by side on chest wall over area to be drained. Cup hands, with fingers and thumbs held tightly together. Make sure that entire outer part of hand makes contact with chest wall to avoid air leaks (see Step 13a[2] illustration).

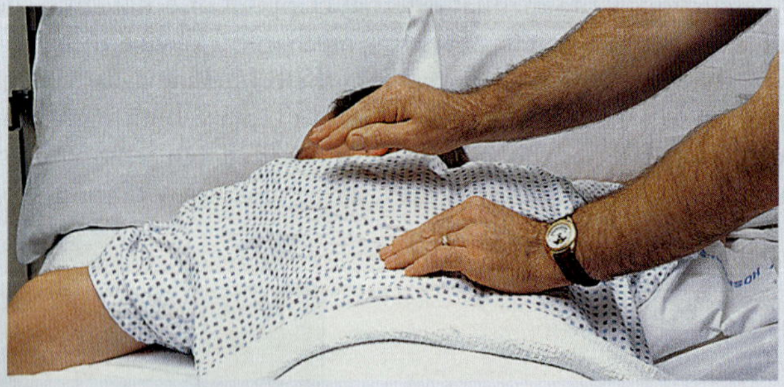

STEP 13A(2) Chest wall percussion, alternating hand clapping against patient's chest wall.

    (3) When clapping, most arm movement comes from the elbow and wrist joints. Clapping is often done for 5 minutes without stopping or for 2–3 minutes, alternating with vibration.
    (4) Alternately, clap chest with cupped hands to create rhythmic popping sound resembling galloping horse. Perform clapping at moderate or fast speed, whichever is most comfortable and effective.
    (5) Perform chest wall vibration over each affected area (see Table 24.1). Perform vibrations in sets of three followed by coughing so that any loosened secretions are expectorated.

Procedural Guideline 24.2 *Performing Percussion and Vibration—cont'd*

(a) Place flat part of hand over area and have patient take slow, deep breath through nose.
(b) Gently resist chest wall as it rises during inhalation.
(c) Have patient hold breath for 2–3 seconds and exhale through pursed lips while contracting abdominal muscles and relaxing chest wall muscles. Chest wall relaxes and falls.
(d) While patient is exhaling, gently push down and vibrate chest wall with flat part of hand.
(e) Repeat vibration three times, and instruct patient to cascade cough by taking a deep breath and doing a series of small coughs until end of breath. Instruct patient not to inhale between coughs. Vibrate chest wall as patient coughs. When applying pressure to ribs, always follow natural movement of the rib cage. Allow patient to sit up and cough as needed.

Critical Decision Point *When excessive pulmonary secretions are present, such as in patients with CF, mechanical vibration is more effective than manual vibration at removing secretions.*

(f) Monitor patient's tolerance of vibration and ability to relax chest wall and breathe properly as instructed.
(g) Perform a total of three or four sets of three vibrations, with vibration followed by coughing over each lung segment as tolerated. Strength and frequency of vibration will vary.

b. HFCWO device:
(1) Apply PPE.
(2) Place vest on patient and assess for proper fit.
(a) With vest deflated, adjust closures so the vest fits comfortably.
(b) Vest should rest on shoulder and extend to top of hip bone.
(3) Assess chest wall motion. Breathing should not be restricted when vest is deflated.
(4) Connect tubing to the generator and ports of the vest. Turn on power.
(5) Adjust pressure control as prescribed; usually pressure is between 5 and 6.
(6) Adjust frequency; usually it is set between 10 and 15 Hz.
(7) Administer any aerosol therapy as prescribed.
(8) Depress and maintain pressure on the hand or foot control to initiate vest therapy.
(9) After 5–10 minutes, release hand or foot control.

14. Instruct patient to cough, or suction if they are unable to cough up mucus (see Chapter 23).
15. Continue with treatment, usually 15–30 minutes.
16. Help patient with oral hygiene.
17. Remove PPE.
18. If long-term therapy is needed, teach patient and caregivers the procedure for home use of PEP or HFCWO devices. If they are unable to learn, use interprofessional collaboration to determine outpatient or community care follow-up requirements.
19. Auscultate lung fields.
20. Obtain vital signs and SpO_2.
21. Inspect colour, character, and amount of sputum.
22. **Use teach-back:** "We discussed the importance of using this vest to manage your respiratory secretions. Tell me why it is important to keep your airways clear of secretions." Develop a revised teaching plan if patient or caregiver is unable to teach back correctly.
23. Document procedure and patient's response. Document your evaluation of patient learning.

✦ REVIEW QUESTIONS

A 29-year-old university student (he/him) has a 22-year history of cystic fibrosis (CF). He is on the lung transplant list and adheres to his chest physiotherapy (CPT) and medication regimen. One week ago, he developed a cold, which continued to worsen, and his respiratory secretions were difficult to clear with his usual treatments. He was admitted to the hospital 3 days ago for complicated pneumonia, with a temperature of 40°C, pulse of 100 beats/min, respiratory rate of 34 breaths/min, BP of 130/80 mm Hg, and 85% saturation (SaO_2) on 2 L/min of oxygen via nasal cannula. Chest X-ray showed bilateral lower lobe pneumonia and lobar collapse of his right middle lobe.

Review Questions 1 to 3 relate to the case study presented here.

1. Based on the chest X-ray findings, what should the nurse expect to find on physical examination of the chest, and which additional signs and symptoms should the nurse expect to see?
2. CPT was prescribed. Which positions should the nurse use for postural drainage (PD)?
3. After 24 hours of aggressive CPT and PD, a chest X-ray examination was repeated. It showed no improvement. Using SBAR (situation–background–assessment–recommendation), show how the nurse should communicate with the health care team about this patient.
4. The nurse is caring for a patient who requires postural drainage three times a day. Which of the following are necessary to prepare the patient for postural drainage? (*Select all that apply.*)
   1. Encourage adequate fluid intake.
   2. Provide a light meal 30 minutes beforehand.
   3. Explain the procedure and positioning techniques.
   4. Review any chest X-rays and auscultate all lung fields.
   5. Coordinate treatments with other respiratory or medical therapies.
   6. Plan on performing CPT on all lung regions.
5. The nurse is implementing PD on a patient. Place the following steps in the correct order:
   1. Obtain vital signs and pulse oximetry.
   2. Position patient in proper position to drain selected lung segment.
   3. Maintain position for 10 to 15 minutes.
   4. Perform CPT manoeuvres.

5. Perform respiratory assessment.
6. Provide a rest period between positions.

6. Which of the following are contraindications for Trendelenburg positioning during postural drainage? (*Select all that apply.*)
1. Risk for aspiration
2. Left hip repair
3. Increased intracranial pressure
4. Lower lobe infiltrates
5. Distended abdomen

7. Your patient is being discharged with an Acapella device. Which of the following indicate that the patient needs further patient education? (*Select all that apply.*)
1. Patient takes a normal breath.
2. Patient maintains a tight seal around mouth.
3. Patient holds breath for 2 to 4 seconds.
4. Patient coughs while device is vibrating.
5. Patient performs forceful exhalations and huffing or other coughing technique.

Visit the Evolve site for a complete list of answers to the Review Questions.

NEXT GENERATION NCLEX® (NGN)

For practice with answering exam questions related to unfolding NGN case studies, please consult the Next Generation NCLEX® (NGN)-Style Case Studies for Skills and Techniques on the Evolve website: http://evolve.elsevier.com/Canada/Perry/clinicalskills/

REFERENCES

Accreditation Canada. (2020). *Required organizational practices handbook.* https://physicians.nshealth.ca/resources/required-organizational-practices-2020-handbook

Barker, A. F. (2022). Treatment of bronchiectasis in adults. *UpToDate.* https://www.uptodate.com/contents/treatment-of-bronchiectasis-in-adults

Boucher, R. C. (2019). Muco-obstructive lung diseases. *New England Journal of Medicine, 380*(20), 1941–1953. https://doi.org/10.1056/nejmra1813799

Chapman, N., Watson, K., Hatton, T., et al. (2021). Methods used to evaluate the immediate effects of airway clearance techniques in adults with cystic fibrosis: A systematic review and meta-analysis. *Journal of Clinical Medicine, 10*(5280), 1–22. https://doi.org/10.3390/jcm10225280

Chaudary, N., & Balasa, G. (2021). Airway clearance therapy in cystic fibrosis patients insights from a clinician providing cystic fibrosis care. *International Journal of General Medicine, 14*, 2513–2521. https://doi.org/10.2147/ijgm.s274196

Giger, J. N., & Haddad, L. (2021). *Transcultural nursing* (8th ed.). Mosby.

Hockenberry, M. J., Duffy, E. A., & Gibbs, K. (2024). *Wong's nursing care of infants and children* (12th ed.). Elsevier.

Larsen, T., Lee, A., Brooks, D., et al. (2019). Effect of early mobility as a physiotherapy treatment for pneumonia: A systematic review and meta-analysis. *Physiotherapy Canada, 71*(1), 82–89. https://doi.org/10.3138/ptc.2017-51.ep

Leemans, G., Belmans, D., Van Holsbeke, C., et al. (2020). The effectiveness of a mobile high-frequency chest wall oscillation (HFCWO) device for airway clearance. *Pediatric Pulmonology, 55*(8), 1984–1992. https://doi.org/10.1002/ppul.24784

Morrison, L., & Milroy, S. (2018). Oscillating devices for airway clearance in people with cystic fibrosis. *Paediatric Respiratory Reviews, 25*, 30–32. https://doi.org/10.1016/j.prrv.2017.07.001

Morrow, B. M. (2019). Airway clearance therapy in acute paediatric respiratory illness: A state-of-the-art review. *South African Journal of Physiotherapy, 75*(1), Article A1295. https://doi.org/10.4102/sajp.v75i1.1295

Naswa, S., Tuteja, R., Gupta, V., et al. (2017). Comparison of Acapella® versus active cycle of breathing technique in post-operative pulmonary complications after valve replacement surgeries. *Indian Journal of Physiotherapy & Occupational Therapy, 11*(2), 24–29.

O'Neill, K., O'Donnell, A. E., & Bradley, J. M. (2019). Airway clearance, mucoactive therapies and pulmonary rehabilitation in bronchiectasis. *Respirology, 24*, 227–237. https://doi.org/10.1111/resp.13459

Pakpahan, R., Permatasari Tarigan, A., & Sitohang, N. A. (2021). The effect of the combination of chest physiotherapy and active cycle breathing technique on respiratory rate and ability to expend sputum in chronic exacerbation obstructive lung disease patients at Haji Adam Malik Hospital Medan. *European Journal of Molecular & Clinical Medicine, 8*(3), 616–623.

Phillips, J., Lee, A., Pope, R., et al. (2020). Effect of airway clearance techniques in patients experiencing an acute exacerbation of bronchiectasis: A systematic review. *Physiotherapy Theory and Practice, 36*(12), 1300–1315. https://doi.org/10.1080/09593985.2019.1579286

Powner, J., Nesmith, A., Kirkpatrick, D. P., et al. (2019). Employment of an algorithm of care including chest physiotherapy results in reduced hospitalizations and stability of lung function in bronchiectasis. *BMC Pulmonary Medicine, 19*(1), Article 82. https://doi.org/10.1186/s12890-019-0844-4

Salvo, S. (2018). *Mosby's pathology for massage therapists* (4th ed.). Elsevier.

Sereearuno, T., Rittayamai, N., Lawansil, S., et al. (2020). Effectiveness of a chest physiotherapy care map on hospitalized patients. *Heart & Lung, 49*(5), 616–621. https://doi.org/10.1016/j.hrtlng.2020.03.014

Strickland, S. L., Rubin, B. K., Haas, C. F., et al. (2015). AARC clinical practice guideline: Effectiveness of pharmacologic airway clearance therapies in hospitalized patients. *Respiratory Care, 60*(7), 1071–1077. https://doi.org/10.4187/respcare.04165 [Seminal Reference]

Sullivan, W. F., Diepstra, H., Heng, J., et al. (2018). Primary care of adults with intellectual and developmental disabilities: 2018 Canadian consensus guidelines. *Canadian Family Physician, 64*(4), 254–279. https://www.cfp.ca/content/cfp/64/4/254.full.pdf

Villeneuve, P. (2018). Interventions to avoid pulmonary complications after lung cancer resection. *Journal of Thoracic Disease, 10*(S32), S3781–S3788. https://doi.org/10.21037/jtd.2018.09.26

Wilson, A. (2018). Oscillating devices for airway clearance in people with cystic fibrosis: A cochrane review summary. *International Journal of Nursing Studies, 88*, 165–166. https://doi.org/10.1016/j.ijnurstu.2018.02.007

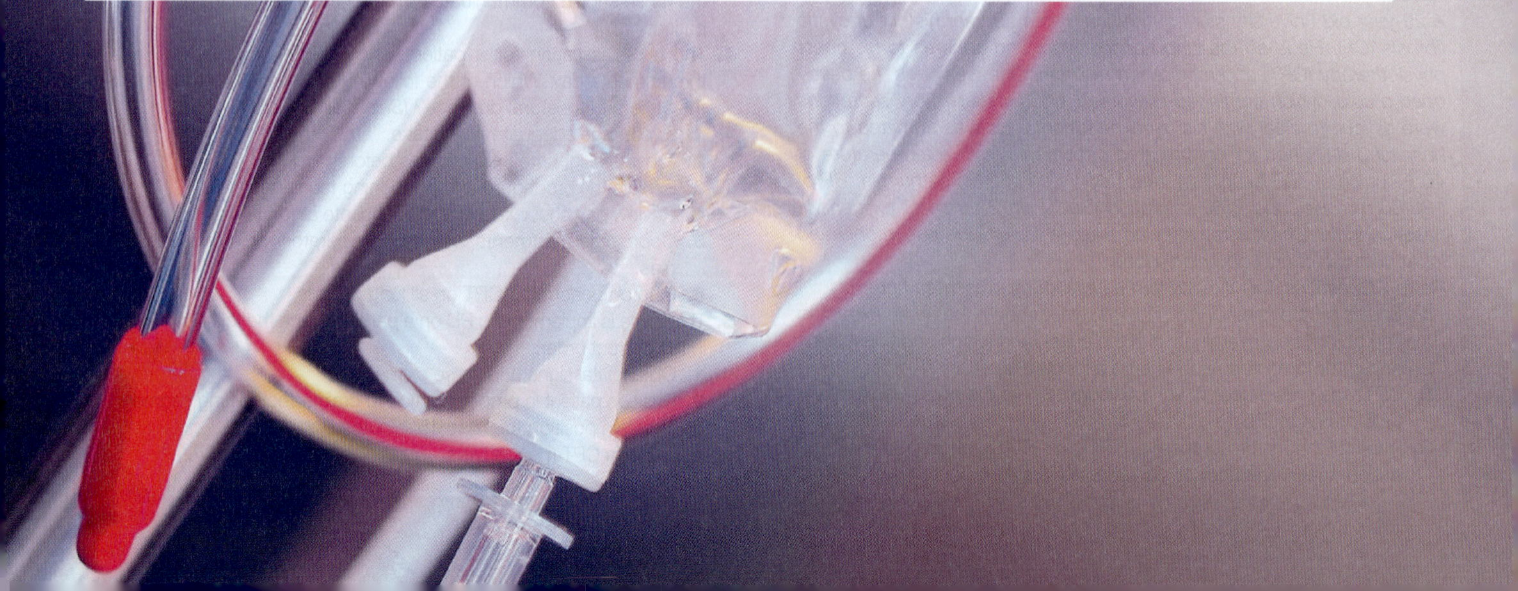

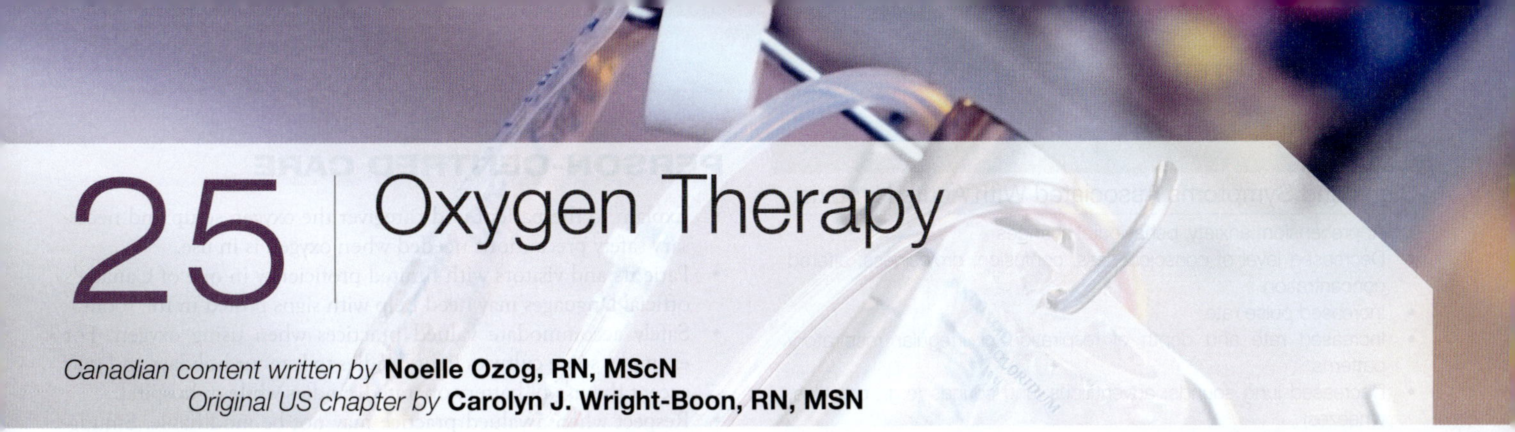

25 Oxygen Therapy

Canadian content written by **Noelle Ozog, RN, MScN**
Original US chapter by **Carolyn J. Wright-Boon, RN, MSN**

SKILLS AND PROCEDURES

OBJECTIVES

Mastery of content in this chapter will enable the nurse to:

- Describe indications and precautions for oxygen therapy.
- Describe methods for administering oxygen therapy.
- Demonstrate application of a conventional oxygen delivery device.
- Demonstrate application of a conventional oxygen delivery device to a patient with an artificial airway.
- Demonstrate proper use of incentive spirometry.
- Describe the use of noninvasive positive-pressure ventilation using continuous positive airway pressure (CPAP) or bi-level positive airway pressure (BiPAP).
- Demonstrate how to obtain peak expiratory flow rate (PEFR) measurements.
- Demonstrate care of a patient receiving mechanical ventilation.
- Choose evidence-informed teaching strategies to support patients' use of home oxygen equipment.

MEDIA RESOURCES

- https://booksite.elsevier.com/Perry-Potter/Clinicalskills2e/video25.php

PURPOSE

Oxygen therapy is the administration of supplemental oxygen to prevent or treat hypoxia and hypoxemia in a patient. Routes of administration include conventional oxygen therapy (e.g., nasal cannula, masks), noninvasive positive-pressure ventilation (NIPPV), and positive-pressure ventilators. Special care is required for each delivery device.

STANDARDS OF CARE

- Accreditation Canada (2020)—*Required Organizational Practices–2020 Handbook* (https://physicians.nshealth.ca/resources/required-organizational-practices-2020-handbook)
- Napolitano et al. (2021)—*AARC Clinical Practice Guideline: Management of Pediatric Patients With Oxygen in the Acute Care Setting* (https://doi.org/10.4187/RESPCARE.09006)
- Norton et al. (2021)—*Best Practice Recommendations for the Prevention and Management of Pressure Injuries* (https://doi.org/10.1142/9789814354912_0082)
- Piraino et al. (2022)—*AARC Clinical Practice Guideline: Management of Adult Patients With Oxygen in the Acute Care Setting: Respiratory Care* (https://doi.org/10.4187/respcare.09294)
- Rochwerg et al. (2017)—*Official European Respiratory Society (ERS)/American Thoracic Society (ATS) Clinical Practice Guidelines: Noninvasive Ventilation for Acute Respiratory Failure* (https://www.thoracic.org/statements/resources/cc/niv-guidelines.pdf)

PRINCIPLES FOR PRACTICE

- *Oxygenation* describes the diffusion of oxygen gas from the lungs (more specifically, the alveoli) into the blood stream (Theodore, 2022).
- Oxygen can dissolve in the bloodstream or bind to *hemoglobin*, the protein that brings respiratory gases to and from the tissues and cells. Hemoglobin contains four binding sites where molecules of oxygen or carbon dioxide (CO_2) typically bind (Benner et al., 2022).
- Hemoglobin is less attracted to oxygen when blood pH is low (acidemia) or the partial pressure of CO_2 ($PaCO_2$) is high (Benner et al., 2022). This is called the *Bohr effect*, and the result is that oxygen is "unloaded" by the hemoglobin to meet the oxygen needs of those tissues (Benner et al., 2022).
- If oxygenation is inadequate, a patient becomes *hypoxemic* (insufficient oxygen in the blood). Persistent hypoxemia will lead to *hypoxia* (Box 25.1), a condition in which there is insufficient oxygen to meet the metabolic demands of the tissues and cells (Theodore, 2022).

BOX 25.1

Signs and Symptoms Associated With Acute Hypoxia

- Apprehension, anxiety, behavioural changes
- Decreased level of consciousness, confusion, drowsiness, altered concentration
- Increased pulse rate
- Increased rate and depth of respiration or irregular respiratory patterns
- Decreased lung sounds, adventitious lung sounds (e.g., crackles, wheezes)
- Elevated blood pressure evolving to decreased blood pressure
- Pulse oximetry (SpO_2) <90%, or <88% in a patient at risk for hypercapnia (Piraino et al., 2022)
- Reported dyspnea
- Use of accessory muscles of respiration, rib retractions
- Cardiac dysrhythmias
- Pallor, cyanosis
- Increased fatigue
- Dizziness

- Various diseases can lead to inadequate oxygenation. For example, in pneumonia, the increased fluid in the lungs impairs diffusion of oxygen to the blood (Torres et al., 2021). In chronic obstructive pulmonary disease (COPD), a patient's airway is chronically inflamed owing to exposure to noxious elements (i.e., tobacco smoke). Over time, this condition decreases lung elasticity and destroys structural elements of the lung, chronically disrupting oxygenation (GOLD Science Committee, 2023).
- Oxygen therapy is an inexpensive and widely available therapy used to prevent and treat hypoxia.
- Managing oxygen therapy requires the nurse to assess the patient's oxygenation status in the context of the patient's history, vital signs, physical exam findings, and laboratory values (i.e., hemoglobin, acid–base balance).
- Pulse oximetry (SpO_2; Chapter 7) is a noninvasive measure of oxygenation that is taken as part of the patient's vital signs and is one of the primary tools used to measure oxygenation. SpO_2 uses light to measure the proportion of hemoglobin molecules that are fully saturated (i.e., all four binding sites are full) compared with the total amount of hemoglobin in the bloodstream (Hafen & Sharma, 2022).
- Nurses should treat oxygen therapy as a medication and collaborate with the respiratory therapist and health care provider to ensure that the patient meets the prescribed oxygenation target. Follow the 10 rights of medication administration (see Chapter 20).
- Precautions for oxygen therapy:
  - *Congenital heart defect (CHD)*: Some babies are born with structural differences in their hearts that affect blood flow and oxygenation. In CHD patients, too much oxygen is thought to increase blood flow to the lungs at the expense of adequate oxygenation to the rest of the body (Khalil et al., 2019). Depending on the individual patient, their target SpO_2 may be 75 to 85% (Khalil et al., 2019). Follow employer policy and health care provider direction.
  - *Chronic pulmonary diseases:* In COPD patients, *uncontrolled* oxygen therapy increases the patient's risk for elevated CO_2 in the blood (*hypercapnia* [also called *hypercarbia* or CO_2 *retention*]). This hypercapnia is thought to be mainly due to an inhibition of pulmonary vasoconstriction, the body's mechanism of reducing perfusion to poorly ventilated alveoli, resulting in further mismatch between ventilation and perfusion (Branson, 2018). These patients should receive oxygen sparingly; target an SpO_2 of 88 to 92% (Piraino et al., 2022).

PERSON-CENTRED CARE

- Explain to the patient and caregiver the oxygen setup and necessary safety precautions needed when oxygen is in use.
- Patients and visitors with limited proficiency in one of Canada's official languages may need help with signs posted in the room.
- Safely accommodate valued practices when using oxygen. For example, some cultures light candles to honour holidays and may accept the use of battery-operated candles while in hospital.
- Respect when a valued practice may not be modifiable. Smudging, a ceremony involving the burning of sweetgrass, sage, cedar, or tobacco, is a part of some Indigenous cultures and requires the sacred element of fire. Collaborate with the patient, caregivers, Elders, and employer to determine how to safely accommodate cultural healing practices.

EVIDENCE-INFORMED PRACTICE

- The accuracy of SpO_2 can be affected by poor perfusion, movement of the patient, or the colour of the patient's skin (Louie et al., 2018; Sjoding et al., 2020). Misleading readings can also be caused by carbon monoxide poisoning, nail polish or artificial nails, and anemia (Hafen & Sharma, 2022).
- Good lighting is essential for a proper physical assessment of patient skin. Use the palmar surface of a patient's fingertips, a location where it is easier to notice colour changes in any skin tone, to assess for cyanosis (Baranoski et al., 2017). Note that cyanosis is not generally detectable in patients until arterial oxygen saturation (SaO_2) is as low as 73 to 78% (Martin & Khalil, 1990), a range much lower than the target of 94 to 98% that is appropriate for most patients (Piraino et al., 2022).
- Relative to other oxygen delivery systems, use of a high-flow nasal cannula (HFNC) reduces the likelihood that a patient will require intubation (Ferreyro et al., 2020). An HFNC has not been associated with increased infection risk when compared with conventional oxygen therapy (Piraino et al., 2022; Rochwerg et al., 2019).
- NIPPV is an effective intervention in patients with COPD who are experiencing an acute episode of respiratory failure with hypercapnia or who have disordered sleep breathing (Shah et al., 2018).
- There is no evidence to support use of incentive spirometry (IS) alone to prevent pulmonary complications in patients who have undergone upper abdominal or chest surgery (Sullivan et al., 2021).
- Oxygen tents for pediatric patents are no longer recommended (Napolitano et al., 2021).

SAFETY GUIDELINES

- Know a patient's normal range of vital signs, including SpO_2 targets.
- Be aware of environmental conditions. Patients with chronic respiratory diseases have difficulty maintaining optimal oxygen levels in polluted environments.
- Document a patient's smoking history in pack-years (average number of cigarette packs smoked per day multiplied by number of years smoking; Lung Cancer Canada, 2018). Smoking damages the mucociliary clearance mechanism of the lungs and paralyzes the ciliary action, resulting in a decreased ability to clear mucus from the airways. Cigarette smoking is the leading environmental risk factor for COPD (GOLD Science Commitee, 2023).
- Know a patient's past and current hemoglobin and arterial blood gas (ABG) values.

BOX 25.2

General Oxygen Safety Guidelines

- Remind patients that oxygen is a medication and is not to be adjusted without a prescription from a health care provider.
- Keep oxygen delivery systems at least 3 metres (10 feet) from any heat source.
- Oxygen supports combustion; however, it will not explode.
- No smoking while on oxygen or near someone on oxygen.
- When using oxygen cylinders, secure them so they will not fall over.
- Verify that all electrical equipment in the room is functioning correctly and properly grounded (see Chapter 14). An electrical spark in the presence of oxygen will result in a serious fire.
- Avoid using items that create a spark (e.g., electric razor) while nasal cannula is in use; avoid placing electrical or mechanical toy inside oxygen tent; avoid using objects made of synthetic fabrics that cause static electricity.
- Check the oxygen level of portable tanks before transporting a patient to ensure ample oxygen supply. Do not remove patient oxygen to allow the patient to use the washroom; use extension tubing or a wheeled portable oxygen cylinder as appropriate in the setting.

- Have suction equipment available to help clear airway secretions, particularly in patients with artificial airways such as an endotracheal tube or a tracheostomy.
- Have a self-inflating resuscitation bag and appropriately sized mask (i.e., a bag-valve mask) available in the rooms of patients requiring mechanical ventilation.
- Provide education to the patient and caregiver about oxygen therapy to ensure they understand proper use of the equipment and safety measures (Box 25.2).
- An aerosol-generating medical procedure (AGMP) is any activity that can produce small suspended droplets containing viral or bacterial particles from the patient's body and thus is more likely to cause transmission of respiratory illnesses (Public Health Agency of Canada [PHAC], 2022). Examples of AGMPs include open endotracheal suctioning and NIPPV (PHAC, 2022). Some settings consider any form of oxygen delivered at greater than 15 L/min to be an AGMP (Nova Scotia Health & IWK Infection Prevention and Control, 2021). Typically, airborne precautions are required for these procedures; follow your employer's policy.

✦ SKILL 25.1 Applying an Oxygen Delivery Device

Video Clip

Selection of an oxygen delivery system is made according to an assessment of the patient's health history (including age and developmental level), current level of orientation, respiratory status, severity of hypoxia, and disease process. The presence of an artificial airway, the setting (acute, community or home), and available support need to be considered as well.

Oxygen Delivery Devices

Oxygen delivery devices are categorized as high flow or low flow, depending on their ability to provide enough *flow* to match the patient's *spontaneous minute volume*; this matching is imperative for patient comfort and adequate oxygen delivery. High-flow devices provide a higher flow of oxygen to meet the higher minute volume of patients in respiratory distress or failure. Both types of devices can deliver a range of fraction of inspired oxygen (FiO_2) to patients. High-flow devices control the FiO_2 with less dependence on the patient's breathing pattern and include Venturi masks (Fig. 25.1), large-volume nebulizers, and HFNCs (Fig. 25.2). Low-flow devices include low-flow nasal cannulae (Fig. 25.3), oxygen-conserving nasal cannulae (Fig. 25.4), simple face masks (Fig. 25.5), partial rebreather masks, and nonrebreather masks (Fig. 25.6). Advantages and disadvantages of each are listed in Table 25.1.

An oxygen flowmeter regulates the flow rate of oxygen being delivered in litres per minute (L/min). Figure 25.7 shows a float ball oxygen flowmeter set to 1 L/min. The flow rate is read from the middle of the ball (Amico Patient Care Corporation, 2022). Oxygen cylinders include large H cylinders and smaller E cylinders (Fig. 25.8).

Nasal Cannula

Several types of nasal cannulae are used to deliver oxygen to the patient (see Table 25.1). A low-flow nasal cannula is a simple and effective device for delivering oxygen to a patient (see Fig. 25.3). The two prongs of the cannula (about 1.5-cm [0.5-inches] long) protrude from the centre of a disposable tube and are inserted into the nostrils. Oxygen is delivered via the prongs and does not require humidification at low-flow rates (Piraino et al., 2022). An oxygen-conserving cannula can be used by patients who require higher oxygen concentrations than what can be provided via traditional nasal cannulae (see Fig. 25.4). The oxygen-conserving cannula possesses a built-in reservoir that allows for an increase in oxygen concentration at a lower flow rate. For example, the Oxymizer oxygen-conserving cannula delivers a 2:1 ratio (e.g., 6 L/min nasal cannula is approximately equivalent to 3.5 L/min with the Oxymizer device).

An HFNC has larger-diameter prongs than low-flow cannulae and is connected to an air–oxygen blender that has an adjustable FiO_2 and flow rate (Fig. 25.9). This system can deliver a heated and humidified air–oxygen mixture at up to 60 L/min (Adhikari et al., 2021). It is used with alert, spontaneously breathing patients whose inspiratory demand is greater than the flows delivered by traditional oxygen therapy (Adhikari et al., 2021) and with patients in hypoxemic respiratory failure (Piraino et al., 2022). An HFNC is thought to reopen collapsed alveoli by delivering a small amount of positive end-expiratory pressure (PEEP; pressure remaining in the alveoli at the end of expiration) to the lungs (Adhikari et al., 2021).

Oxygen Masks

The simple face mask (see Fig. 25.5) is for short-term, low-flow oxygen therapy. A face mask with a reservoir bag (including partial rebreather, partial nonrebreather, and full nonrebreather masks; see Fig. 25.6) is another low-flow device that maintains a high-concentration oxygen supply in the reservoir bag. The nurse should frequently inspect the bag to make sure that it is fully inflated; if not, the patient may breathe in large amounts of exhaled CO_2 (Herren et al., 2017). In partial rebreathers, there is a two-way valve between the mask and the reservoir bag. In nonrebreathers, a one-way valve allows oxygen into the mask but not exhaled CO_2 into the reservoir on either one (partial nonrebreathers) or both (full nonrebreathers) exhalation ports. (Herren et al., 2017).

A Venturi mask is a high-flow device with interchangeable Venturi jet attachments inserted into the base of the mask tubing to control the FiO_2 delivered (see Fig. 25.1). There is ongoing

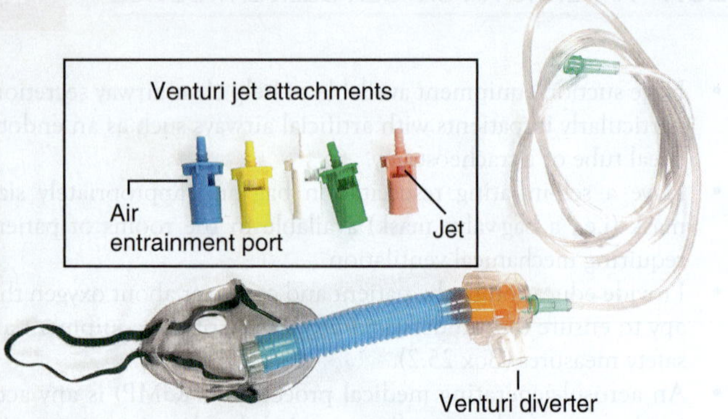

FIG 25.1 Ventimask (Venturi mask) with interchangeable jet ports. *(Courtesy Noelle Ozog.)*

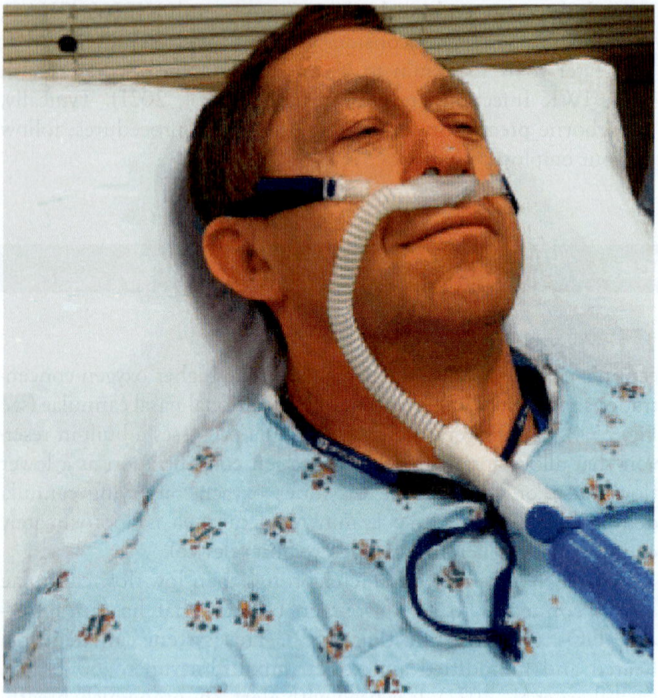

FIG 25.2 High-flow nasal cannula. *(Courtesy Fisher & Paykel Healthcare.)*

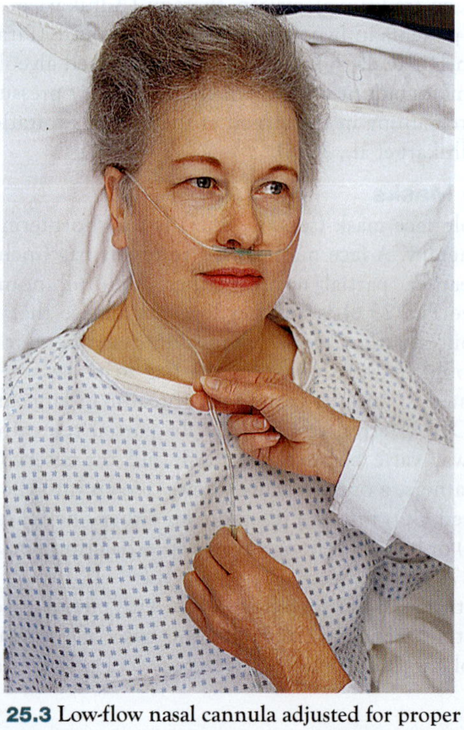

FIG 25.3 Low-flow nasal cannula adjusted for proper fit.

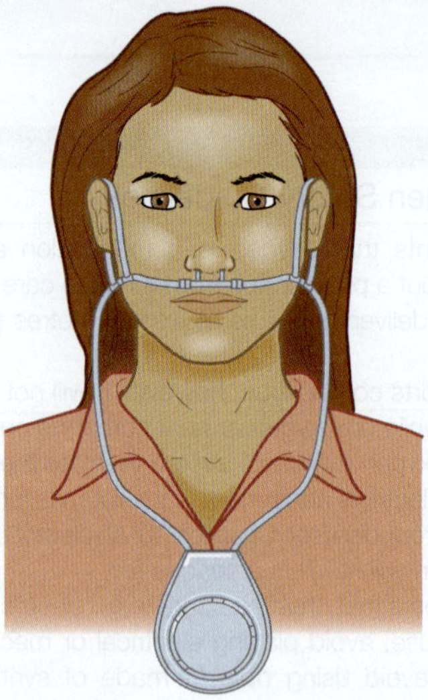

FIG 25.4 Oxygen-conserving nasal cannula. *(From Lewis, S. L., Dirksen, S. R., Heitkemper, M. M., & Bucher, L. [2014]. Medical-surgical nursing: Assessment and management of clinical problems [9th ed.]. Mosby.)*

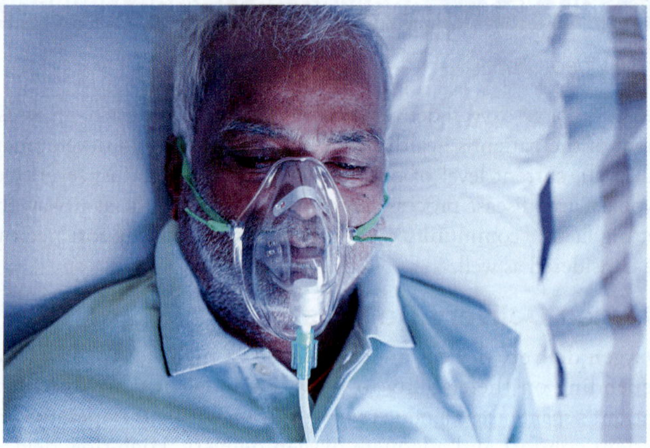

FIG 25.5 Simple face mask. *(iStockphoto/lakshmiprasad)*

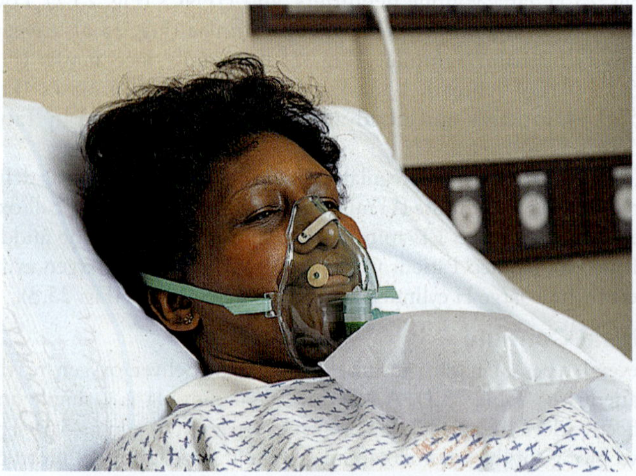

FIG 25.6 Plastic face mask with reservoir bag being used as a nonrebreather (note one-way valve on exhalation port).

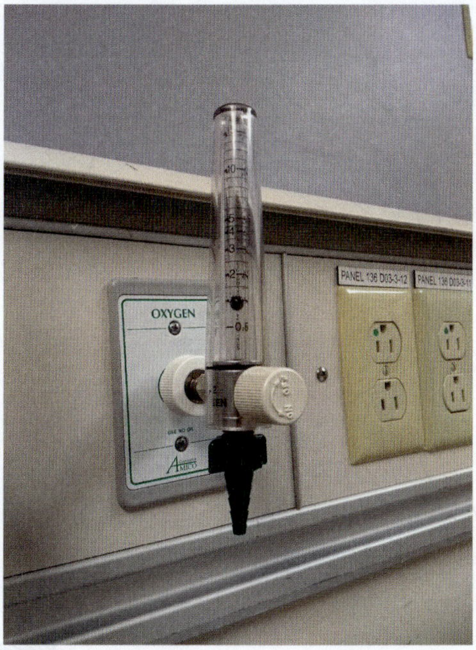

FIG 25.7 Oxygen flowmeter set to 1 L/min. *(Courtesy Noelle Ozog.)*

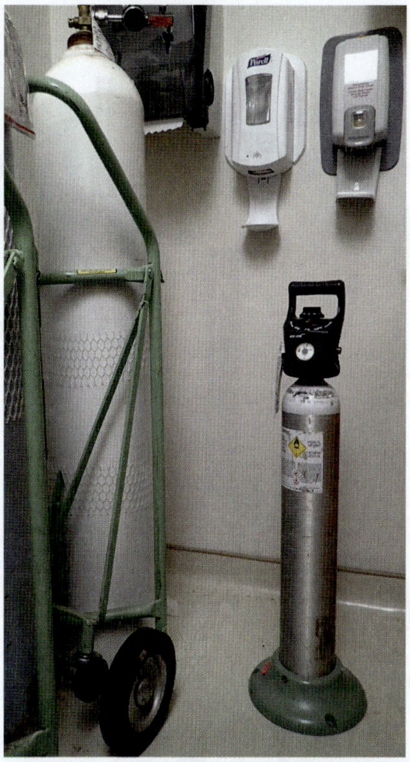

FIG 25.8 Large H tank and smaller E tank for portability. *(Courtesy Noelle Ozog.)*

TABLE 25.1

Common Oxygen Delivery Systems

Delivery System	Flow and Delivered FiO_2	Advantages	Disadvantages
High-Flow Delivery Devices			
Venturi mask (see Fig. 25.1)	24–50% 40 L	Wide range of FiO_2 FiO_2 independent of patient respiratory pattern (Sun et al., 2019)	Increased risk of aspiration May induce feelings of claustrophobia Interferes with eating and drinking Potential AGMP (Novia Scotia Health & IWK Infection Prevention and Control, 2021)
High-flow nasal cannula (see Fig. 25.2)	21–100% Flow adjustable independent of O_2 (2–60 L/min)	Wide range of FiO_2 FiO_2 independent of patient respiratory pattern (Adhikari et al., 2021; Sun et al., 2019) Can be used on adults, children, and infants Does not impede eating, drinking, or talking	Unable to use with nasal obstruction High risk of patient fatigue; must have a defined time frame in which the nurse will reassess the patient and a plan for initiation of positive-pressure ventilation if not improving (Rochwerg et al., 2019) Potential AGMP (Nova Scotia Health & IWK Infection Prevention and Control, 2021)
Low-Flow Delivery Devices			
Low-flow nasal cannula (see Fig. 25.3)	1–6 L/min: 22–40% (Sorg & Chatburn, 2022)	Simple Effective for low concentrations Does not impede eating, drinking, or talking Inexpensive, disposable	Unable to use with nasal obstruction Dries mucous membranes Can dislodge easily Patient's breathing pattern affects exact FiO_2
Oxygen-conserving nasal cannula (Oxymizer) (see Fig. 25.4)	8 L/min: up to 30–60%	Allows increased oxygen concentration at lower total flow Does not impede eating, drinking, or talking	Same as for low-flow nasal cannula More expensive than standard cannula
Simple face mask (see Fig. 25.5)	5–10 L/min: 55–70% (Sorg & Chatburn, 2022)	Useful for short periods of time Useful for patients who primarily breathe through their mouths	Increased risk of aspiration May induce feelings of claustrophobia Impedes eating and drinking Patient's breathing pattern affects exact FiO_2
Partial rebreather Partial nonrebreather Full nonrebreather (see Fig. 25.6)	10–15 L/min; 70–86% (Sorg & Chatburn, 2022)	Useful for immediate care of acute hypoxia Delivers increased FiO_2 Easily humidifies oxygen Does not dry mucous membranes	Increased risk of aspiration May induce feelings of claustrophobia Impedes eating, drinking, and talking Patient's breathing pattern affects exact FiO_2 Bag may twist and deflate

AGMP, Aerosol-generating medical procedure; *FiO_2,* fraction of inspired oxygen.

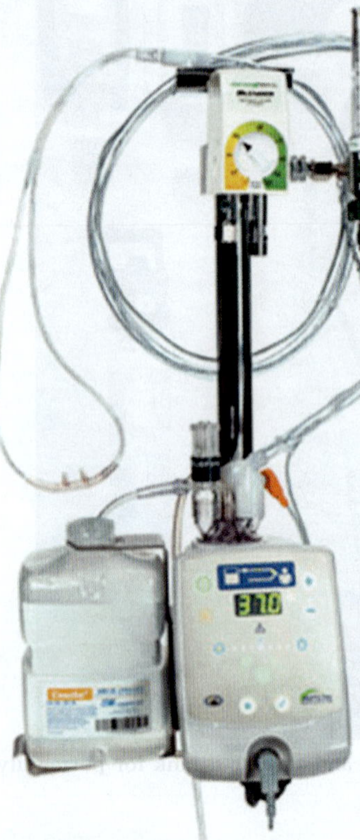

FIG 25.9 High-flow nasal cannula blender. *(Comfort Flo® Humidification System courtesy Teleflex Medical.)*

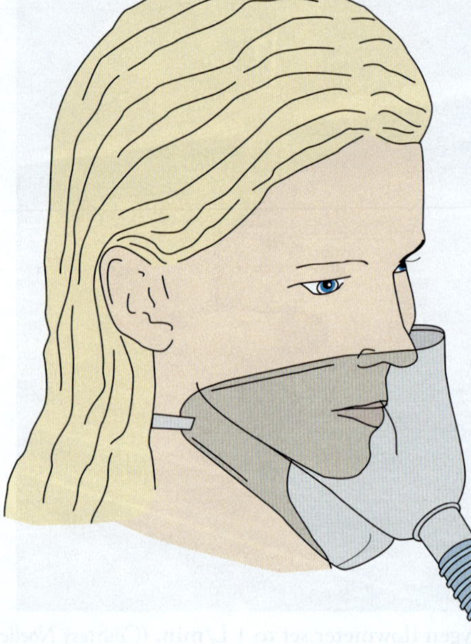

FIG 25.10 Face tent for oxygen delivery. *(From Hockenberry, M. J., Duffy, E. A., & Gibbs, K. [2024]. Wong's nursing care of infants and children [12th ed.]. Elsevier.)*

discussion as to the mechanism that allows this to occur, but simply put, the narrow tube (jet) within the attachments controls the FiO_2 delivered to the patient (Soto-Ruiz et al., 2011). The air entrainment ports additionally take in room air, and together this increases the flow delivered to the patient (Soto-Ruiz et al., 2011). The bottom of each attachment will indicate what value to set the oxygen flowmeter to in order to deliver a specific FiO_2 with a total flow of approximately 40 L/min to the patient (Intersurgical Limited, 2011).

Oxygen Tents

Tents are less commonly used delivery devices than nasal cannulae or masks. The face tent is a shield-like device that fits under a patient's chin and sweeps around the face (Fig. 25.10). It is loosely placed, and a mist is always present. Face tents are sometimes used for patients with facial trauma (e.g., burns), oral or nasal surgery, and those who experience claustrophobia with a regular aerosol mask (Saskatoon Health Region, 2020). There is no way to estimate how much oxygen is delivered to the patient. Oxygen tents (Fig. 25.11) can be used in the pediatric setting to provide high concentrations of humidified oxygen, but this is no longer recommended practice (Napolitano et al., 2021).

T-Tubes and Tracheostomy Masks

An artificial airway bypasses the normal filtering and humidification process of the nose and mouth. An artificial airway inserted through the mouth or nose into the trachea is called an endotracheal tube (ET). An artificial airway inserted directly through a surgically created opening in the neck to the trachea is called a tracheostomy tube (TT). The T-tube, also called a *Briggs adaptor*, is a T-shaped device with a 15-mm (0.33-inch) connection that connects an oxygen source to an artificial airway such as an ET or a TT (Fig. 25.12). A tracheostomy mask is a curved device with an adjustable strap that fits around a patient's neck (Fig. 25.13). Note that patients with an artificial airway require constant humidification to the airway because the body's natural humidification systems are being bypassed (see Chapter 23).

Delegation and Collaboration

The skill of applying a nasal cannula or oxygen mask to most patients can be delegated to an unregulated care provider (UCP), depending on the competence of the UCP to perform this skill in a particular situation and on employer policy. The exception is administering oxygen therapy to a patient with an artificial airway, which can be delegated to a UCP.

The nurse is responsible for assessing the patient's respiratory system, implementing oxygen therapy, including adjustment of oxygen flow rate, and evaluating patient response to oxygen therapy. The nurse directs the UCP about the following:

- How to safely adjust the device (e.g., loosening the strap on the oxygen cannula or mask), and clarifying its correct placement and positioning
- For patients with artificial airways: Teaching about patient-specific variations for application or adjustment of the T-tube or tracheostomy collar (e.g., methods to avoid device-related pressure areas or pulling on the artificial airway, methods for handling accumulated secretions in devices based on a particular patient's needs)
- Informing the nurse immediately about any changes in vital signs; changes in level of consciousness (LOC); increase in secretions; skin irritation from the cannula, mask, or straps; or patient reports of pain or breathlessness
- How to reapply the oxygen therapy device, and notifying nurse if patient is pulling it off or not tolerating its use
- Instructing personnel to provide extra skin care around the patient's ears and nose

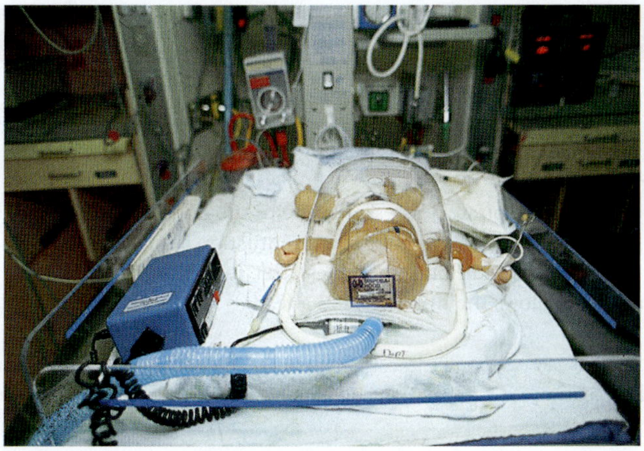

FIG 25.11 Oxygen tent.

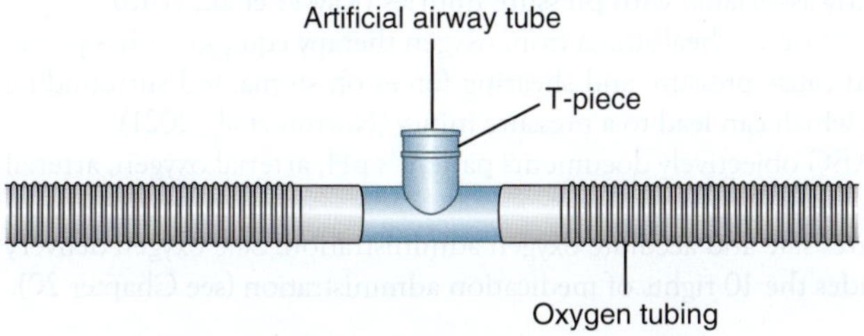

FIG 25.12 T-tube (also called a Briggs adaptor).

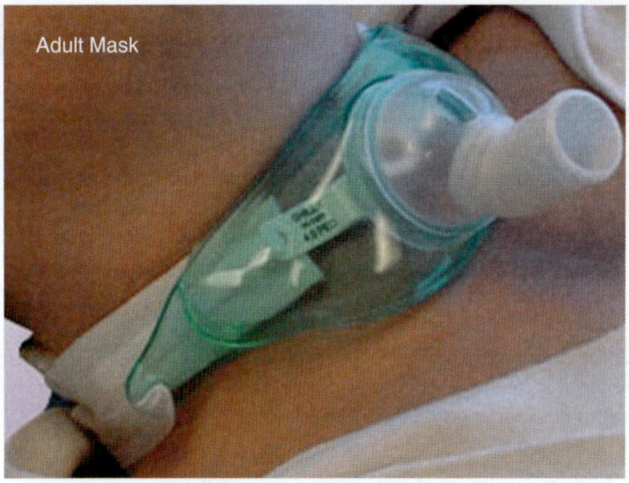

FIG 25.13 Tracheostomy mask. *(Courtesy Marpac Company.)*

The nurse collaborates with the health care provider to ensure that the prescribed oxygen targets are appropriate for the patient and to facilitate transfer to a higher level of care when oxygen needs cannot be met in the current setting.

Interprofessional collaboration with a respiratory therapist, when available, is essential in situations in which the patient suddenly needs a higher flow or FiO_2 to maintain their SpO_2 within the target range or is having difficulty breathing despite normal SpO_2 levels.

Equipment

- Oxygen delivery device, as appropriate, based on nursing assessment
- Oxygen tubing (consider extension tubing)
- Humidifier (required for artificial airways; consider for patient comfort a flow over 4 L/min [Piraino et al., 2022])
- Sterile water for humidifier, if using
- Suction device (wall or portable)
- Suction catheter
- Oxygen source
- Oxygen flowmeter
- Pulse oximeter
- Stethoscope
- Personal protective equipment (PPE), per employer policy

STEP	RATIONALE
ASSESSMENT	
1. Identify patient using at least two person-specific identifiers (e.g., name and date of birth, or name and medical record number) according to employer policy.	Ensures correct patient. Complies with Accreditation Canada's standards and improves patient safety (Accreditation Canada, 2020).
2. Throughout the procedure, the 4 moments for hand hygiene are to be implemented; hand hygiene should occur before initial patient (or patient environment) contact, before an aseptic procedure, after body fluid exposure risk, and after patient (or patient environment) contact. Additional hand hygiene should be performed when hands are visibly soiled.	Proper hand hygiene helps prevent the spread of infectious agents to health care providers.
3. Assess airway patency and remove airway secretions by having patient cough and expectorate mucus or by suctioning (see Chapter 23). Note: Apply PPE per employer policy and/or point-of-care risk assessment.	Secretions plug the airway, decreasing amount of oxygen available for gas exchange in lungs. Secretions also occlude the T-tube or tracheostomy collar, impeding oxygen delivery.

Critical Decision Point *Excessive amounts of secretions, signs of respiratory distress (increased work of breathing, increased respiratory rate), rhonchi on auscultation, excessive coughing, or decrease in patient SpO_2 can indicate need for suctioning* (Chapter 23). *If these signs occur suddenly, especially in patients with artificial airways, the patient may be experiencing hypoxia secondary to airway obstruction. The airway must be determined to be patent before oxygen is administered. If patients continue to show signs of hypoxia once obstruction is removed or ruled out, oxygen should be applied.*

STEP	RATIONALE

ASSESSMENT

STEP	RATIONALE
4. Perform respiratory assessment, including vital signs, auscultation of lungs, inspection for symmetrical chest wall expansion, chest wall abnormalities, temporary conditions affecting ventilation (e.g., pregnancy, trauma), sputum production (amount, characteristics), and signs and symptoms associated with hypoxia (see Box 25.1).	Changes in ventilation and gas exchange resulting in hypoxia require oxygen therapy. The rest of the respiratory assessment helps the nurse identify potential underlying causes of changes in ventilation and gas exchange that may require additional therapies after the initiation of oxygen therapy, and allows the nurse to plan ahead.

Critical Decision Point *Patients with sudden changes in their vital signs, LOC, or behaviour may be experiencing profound hypoxia and acutely require oxygen therapy. Patients with crackles or wheezes to their lungs on auscultation may additionally require a pharmacological intervention prescribed by a health care provider to treat the cause of these adventitious sounds.*

STEP	RATIONALE
5. Inspect condition of skin around nose and ears. For patients with an artificial airway, assess condition of lips around ET or condition of tracheal stoma.	Provides baseline for monitoring development of skin breakdown from medical device irritation. Nasal oxygen delivery devices are frequently associated with pressure injuries (Kayser et al., 2018). Tension on tracheal stoma from oxygen therapy equipment has potential to cause pressure and shearing forces on stoma and surrounding skin, which can lead to a pressure injury (Norton et al., 2021).
6. If available, note patient's most recent ABG results and/or SpO_2 values.	An ABG objectively documents patient's pH, arterial oxygen, arterial CO_2, or SaO_2.
7. Review patient's medical record for prescription for oxygen, noting delivery method (if indicated) and parameters for titration of oxygen (i.e., SpO_2 >94% *or* 88–92% for a patient at risk for hypercapnia).	Ensures safe and accurate oxygen administration. Safe oxygen delivery includes the 10 rights of medication administration (see Chapter 20).
8. Assess patient's and caregiver's understanding of oxygen therapy.	Determines level of instruction required.
9. Remove gloves if donned and discard.	

NURSING DIAGNOSES

- Reduced airway clearance
- Inadequate breathing pattern
- Reduced gas exchange
- Fatigue
- Anxiety
- Potential for impaired skin integrity
- Insufficient knowledge regarding purpose of oxygen therapy

Related factors and risk factors are individualized on the basis of patient's condition or needs.

PLANNING

STEP	RATIONALE
1. Expected outcomes following completion of procedure:	
• Patient's SpO_2 and/or ABG values return to or remain within normal limits or baseline levels.	Objective determinants of stable or improved oxygenation.
• Patient's heart rate and blood pressure remain stable or return to baseline.	When there is no underlying cardiovascular disease, patients adapt to decreased oxygen levels by increasing pulse and blood pressure; this is a short-term adaptive response. Once signs of hypoxia are reduced or controlled, patient's vital signs usually return to normal.
• Patient's work of breathing decreases (i.e., respiratory rate returns to baseline, absence of accessory muscle use, patient able to speak in longer sentences).	Pulmonary conditions such as pneumonia or asthma cause varying degrees of airway narrowing. HFNC is thought to reopen collapsed alveoli to the lungs (Adhikari et al., 2021), improving oxygenation and decreasing the work of breathing.
• Patient's LOC returns to baseline.	Improvement in oxygenation relieves hypoxia and improves patient's mental status.
• Patient verbalizes improved levels of comfort, and subjective sensations of anxiety, fatigue, and breathlessness decrease.	Increased oxygen levels in the blood reduce patient's anxiety, fatigue, and breathlessness.
• Patient's ears, nares, and nasal mucosa remain intact and free of nonblanchable erythema.	Intact skin indicates no device-related pressure injury to underlying skin and mucous membrane (Norton et al., 2021).
• Patient demonstrates understanding of purpose of oxygen therapy and oxygen delivery device.	It is an ethical responsibility of nurses to provide education to patients to support informed decision making (Canadian Nurses Association [CNA], 2017).
2. Gather equipment and supplies according to employer policy.	Provides organized implementation of the oxygen delivery device.

STEP	RATIONALE
IMPLEMENTATION	
1. Explain procedure to patient and caregiver.	It is an ethical responsibility of nurses to provide education to patients to support informed decision making (CNA, 2017).
2. Adjust bed to appropriate height and lower side rail on side nearest you. Check locks on bed wheel.	Minimizes caregiver's muscle strain and prevents injury. Prevents bed from moving.
3. *If patient has artificial airway* **or** *is having difficulty clearing own secretions:* Set up suction equipment at patient's bedside.	Humidification increases airway secretions.
4. Attach oxygen delivery device (e.g., cannula, mask, T-tube) to oxygen tubing, then attach end of tubing to oxygen source adjusted to prescribed flow rate (see Fig. 25.7), with humidification if appropriate.	Humidity has not been found to have a clinical benefit, but it improves patient comfort and therefore tolerability of masks and nasal cannulae (Pirano et al., 2022). Artificial airways bypass the body's natural humidification systems and thus require added humidity.
5. Apply oxygen device:	
a. *Nasal cannula:* Place tips of the cannula into patient's nares. If tips are curved, they should point downward inside nostrils. Then loop cannula tubing up and over patient's ears. Adjust lanyard against patient's chin so cannula fits snugly but does not put pressure on patient nares and ears (see Fig. 25.3).	Tips of cannula direct flow of oxygen into patient's upper respiratory tract.
b. *Masks:* Apply a mask by placing it over patient's mouth and nose. Then bring straps over patient's head and adjust to form a comfortable but tight seal (see Fig. 25.5).	A properly fitting device that does not create pressure on nares or ears is comfortable, and patient is more likely to keep it in place; reduces risk of skin breakdown (Norton et al., 2021).
c. Attach T-tube to artificial airway.	
d. Place tracheostomy mask over TT and adjust straps so it fits snugly.	
6. Maintain sufficient slack on oxygen tubing and secure to patient's clothes.	Allows patient to move without causing oxygen device to shift or disconnect. Shearing forces/friction increase patient's discomfort and risk of device-related pressure injuries (Norton et al., 2021).
7. Cushion high-risk areas (e.g., bridge of nose) with protective dressings.	Current recommended practice to reduce medical device–related pressure injuries (MDRPIs) (Norton et al., 2021).
8. Observe for proper function of oxygen delivery device (e.g., delivery device sitting appropriately on patient, all tubing connected securely).	Ensures patency of delivery device and accuracy of prescribed oxygen flow rate.
9. Verify setting on flowmeter and oxygen source for proper setup and appropriate flow rate to meet prescribed SpO_2 target.	Ensures delivery of prescribed oxygen therapy in conjunction with specific delivery device.
10. Check cannula/mask with every set of vital signs or per employer policy.	Ensures patency of cannula and oxygen flow.
11. Assess adequacy of oxygen flow with every set of vital signs or per employer policy.	Ensures patency of oxygen delivery device.
12. *If using humidification:* Keep container filled at all times. Observe oxygen tubing frequently for accumulation of fluid caused by condensation. If fluid is present, drain tube away from patient, disconnect from collar or T-tube, and discard fluid in proper receptacle.	Excess water is medium for bacterial growth. Draining contaminated water into proper receptacle prevents contamination of entire humidifying unit.
13. Post "Oxygen in Use" signs on wall behind bed and at entrance to room.	Alerts visitors and care providers that oxygen is in use.
14. Properly dispose of gloves (if used).	Reduces transmission of microorganisms.
EVALUATION	
1. Monitor patient's response to oxygen therapy with SpO_2. NOTE: Monitor ABGs when prescribed; however, obtaining ABG measurement is an invasive procedure and therefore ABGs are not measured frequently.	Regular monitoring with SpO_2 is required for patients on oxygen therapy. Continual monitoring may be necessary for patients with unstable oxygenation status. Base changes in supplemental oxygen on individual patient's oxygen saturation levels.

STEP	RATIONALE
EVALUATION	
2. Repeat respiratory assessment, including vital signs, inspection for symmetrical chest wall expansion, chest wall abnormalities, temporary conditions affecting ventilation (e.g., pregnancy, trauma), sputum production (amount, characteristics), and signs and symptoms associated with hypoxia.	Part of evaluation of patient's response to supplemental oxygen. As patient's oxygen level improves, expect physical signs and symptoms to improve. If they do not, the nurse's assessment findings can help direct what other interventions may be appropriate (e.g., incentive spirometry, administration of prescribed medications, NIPPV, etc.)
3. Inspect patient's external ears, bridge of nose, nares, and nasal mucous membranes *or* tracheal stoma *or* oral mucous membranes, as appropriate, for evidence of skin breakdown.	The delivery device can cause skin breakdown (Kayser et al., 2018).
4. Use teach-back: "I want to be sure I explained how oxygen will help you. Explain to me why oxygen is beneficial for you to use right now." Develop a revised teaching plan if patient or caregiver is unable to teach back correctly.	Determines patient's and caregiver's level of understanding of topic (Yen & Leasure, 2019).

Unexpected Outcomes	Related Interventions
1. Patient experiences continued hypoxia.	• Notify health care provider. • Obtain prescription for follow-up ABG. • Consider measures to improve airway patency, including, but not limited to, deep breathing and coughing techniques, positioning patient with head of bed (HOB) elevated 45–90 degrees (unless contraindicated), and oropharyngeal or orotracheal suctioning (Chapter 23). • Collaborate with health care provider to determine appropriateness of pharmacological therapy to treat cause of hypoxia (e.g., antibiotics, bronchodilators, diuretics, etc.).
2. Patient experiences skin irritation or breakdown (e.g., at ears, bridge of nose, nares, other pressure areas), sinus pain, or epistaxis.	• Provide appropriate skin care. Do not use petroleum-based gel around oxygen because it is flammable (Davidson et al., 2016).
3. Patient experiences nasal and upper airway mucosal dryness.	• Oxygen is a dry gas; consider adding a humidifier to oxygen if flow rate is >4 L/min (Piraino et al., 2022). • Assess patient's fluid status and increase fluids if appropriate. • Provide frequent oral care.

Communication and Documentation

- Document the initial respiratory assessment findings, method of oxygen delivery, FiO_2, flow rate, patient's response to intervention, any adverse reactions or side effects, and which providers were notified of patient's change in respiratory status in progress notes in electronic health record (EHR) or chart.
- Document your health teaching and evaluation of patient and caregiver learning.
- Communicate any unexpected outcome to health care provider or nurse in charge.

DOCUMENTATION EXAMPLE

Patient called nurse to the bedside and reported dyspnea after independent ambulation to washroom. Patient reported removing nasal prongs because they would not reach to the washroom. This writer observed increased work of breathing (speaking 5-word sentences, respirations heavy). RR = 24 breaths/min, SpO_2 = 87%. Nasal prongs applied with 2 L/min O_2 and patient SpO_2 increased to 94%, respiratory rate decreased to 20 breaths/min within 5 minutes of oxygen application. Patient respirations are now deep and easy, patient speaking full sentences. This writer provided health teaching to patient re: purpose of nasal cannula and connected patient nasal prongs to extension tubing of sufficient length to reach washroom. Patient confirms understanding of health teaching and need to keep nasal cannula in nose. Will reassess patient every 2 hours (current frequency of voiding) to confirm patient is using oxygen at all times.

Special Considerations

Teaching

- If oxygen therapy continues after discharge, see teaching points for Skill 25.2.
- Discuss safety precautions for oxygen use (see Box 25.2) with patient and caregiver.
- Discuss signs of hypercapnia (e.g., confusion, headache, decreased LOC, somnolence, CO_2 narcosis, respiratory arrest) that patient or caregiver needs to report to the health care provider.

Pediatric

- Some infants and small children are able to tolerate a nasal cannula. Secure the prongs of the cannula with transparent tape or strips of transparent dressing over the child's cheek.
- Provide comfort and reassurance to the child. Make sure that they are able to see someone nearby. Children may still be held by their parents while receiving oxygen via nasal cannula or face mask (Hockenberry et al., 2024).

Gerontological

- Because of the fragility of older persons' skin and mucous membranes, offer oral hygiene and skin care more frequently. Do not use petroleum-based gel around oxygen because it is flammable (Davidson et al., 2016). Water-based gels such as Biotène are useful but also dry quickly and need more frequent application.
- Confused patients may not be able to understand why the oxygen device needs to remain in place. Consider the need for a

securement device (e.g., a transparent tape over straps) or increased monitoring (e.g., on centrally monitored SpO_2, position near nursing station, constant supervision by staff or family member, etc.).

Care in the Community: Home Management

- Obtain appropriate referrals to determine whether patient meets the standards for long-term oxygen therapy before discharge. See Skill 25.2 for more details.

✦ SKILL 25.2 Teaching Patients to Use Home Oxygen Equipment

Home oxygen requires a patient to meet eligibility criteria and have a prescription from a health care provider. Eligibility for home oxygen prescription is assessed by measuring ABGs. Generally, criteria include a partial pressure of oxygen (PaO_2) of 55 mm Hg or less when the patient is clinically stable (Lacasse et al., 2015). When patients have peripheral edema (cor pulmonale); hematocrit greater than or equal to 55% (polycythemia); or right ventricular hypertrophy, pulmonary hypertension, or erythrocytosis, they are often eligible with a PaO_2 of 56 to 59 mm Hg (Lacasse et al., 2015). However, each province and territory has its own eligibility and reimbursement criteria for long-term oxygen use. Funding may be different for people whose health care is delivered through Veterans Affairs Canada (https://www.veterans.gc.ca/eng/services) or the Non-Insured Health Benefits Program (https://www.sac-isc.gc.ca/eng/1572537161086/1572537234517).

The health care provider oxygen prescription needs to include three pieces of information: the dose, route of administration, and duration. Choice of home oxygen equipment should support as much patient independence as possible (Carter & Nwasuruba, 2022). The oxygen delivery device may be a low-flow device (see Table 25.1) or an oxygen-conserving devices. Oxygen-conserving devices were introduced to reduce the weight of portable oxygen systems and extend operating time by not wasting oxygen through continuous flow. There are three types:

- *Reservoir nasal cannula*: Stores oxygen in a small chamber during exhalation for subsequent delivery during early-phase inhalation (see Fig. 25.4).
- *Demand pulsing oxygen delivery system*: Delivers a burst of oxygen at the onset of inspiration; small oxygen pulses are very effective in oxygenating a patient.
- *Transtracheal oxygen catheter*: Delivers oxygen directly through a small catheter placed directly into the trachea (Christopher et al., 2011).

Home Oxygen Storage

Oxygen sources in the home include liquid oxygen systems, compressed oxygen in tanks, and oxygen concentrators (Fig. 25.14, *A*) (Tyerman & Cobbett, 2023). Some oxygen tanks (e.g., for compressed oxygen) are large and stationary (see Fig 25.8). Portable tanks weighing more than 4.5 kg (10 lb) are not designed to be carried; they deliver oxygen for about 5 hours at 2 L/min. Ambulatory tanks weigh less than 4.5 kg (10 lb), are designed to be carried (Fig. 25.14, *B*), and deliver oxygen for at least 4 hours at 2 L/min. Table 25.2 compares the different types of home oxygen delivery systems.

Compressed oxygen requires a regulator and flowmeter. The patient receives delivery of several large oxygen tanks to the home. The size of the tank and flow rate determine how long compressed oxygen tanks will last. Box 25.3 describes how to calculate how long a liquid oxygen system will last, depending on the prescribed flow rate. Liquid systems take up less space because oxygen is stored in a liquid state. Liquid oxygen is stored at or below −183°C (−297°F) and requires the use of a small ambulatory tank that is filled from a reservoir in the home (Fig. 25.15). The oxygen concentrator method extracts oxygen from room air and supplies oxygen to the patient at prescribed flow rates. Oxygen concentrators deliver a lower

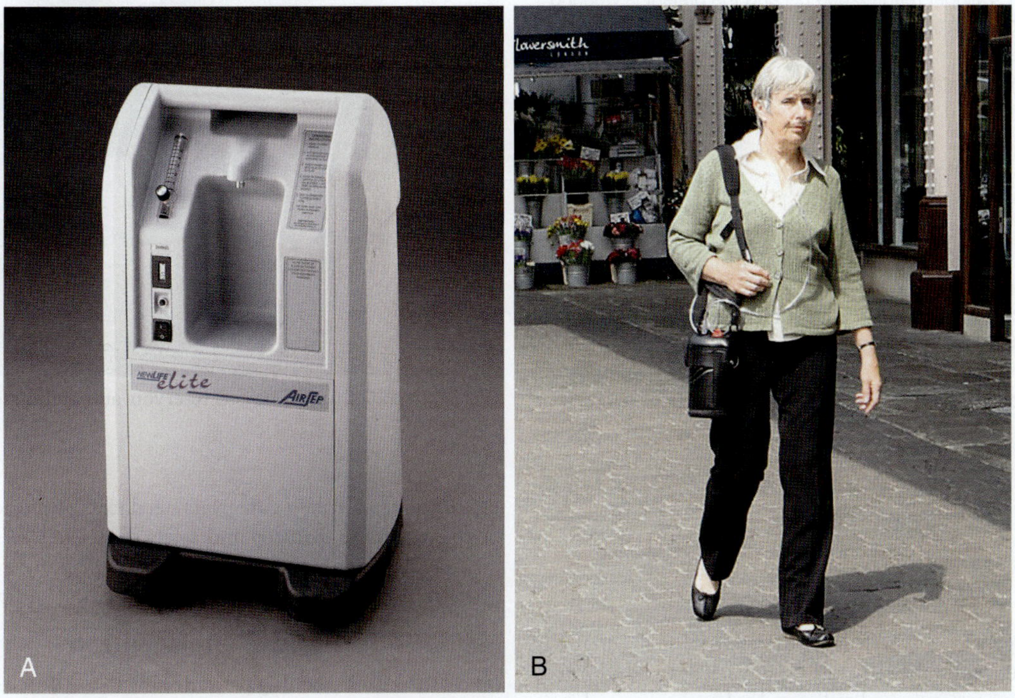

FIG 25.14 A, Portable oxygen concentrator for home use. B, Ambulatory tank is small enough to be carried easily. (*Courtesy AirSep Corporation.*)

TABLE 25.2

Home Oxygen Delivery Systems

	Advantages	Disadvantages
Compressed Oxygen		
Oxygen is stored under pressure in a cylinder equipped with a regulator that controls the flow rate.	An oxygen-conserving device may be attached to the system to avoid waste; the device releases gas only on inhalation and cuts it off with exhalation; it does not require an electrical source; smaller tanks are available.	Large tanks are heavy and only suitable for stationary use. Patient must know how to read the regulator and understand when to call the medical supplier for a replacement cylinder.
Liquid Oxygen System		
Oxygen is stored as a very cold liquid in a vessel similar to a thermos. When released, the liquid converts to a gas and is breathed in just like compressed gas.	Storage method takes up less space than the compressed gas cylinder; it can transfer the liquid to a small, portable vessel at home.	More expensive than compressed gas, and the vessel vents when it is not in use. An oxygen-conserving device may be built into the vessel to conserve the oxygen.
Oxygen Concentrator		
Separates the oxygen out of the air, concentrates it, and stores it.	It does not have to be resupplied, and it is not as costly as liquid oxygen. Extra tubing permits the user to move around with minimal difficulty. Small, portable systems have been developed that afford even greater mobility.	Must have a cylinder of oxygen as a backup in the event of a power failure.

BOX 25.3

How Long Will an Oxygen Cylinder Last?

Oxygen manufacturers provide tables that can be used as a reference to determine how long a particular size of oxygen tank will last at a particular flow rate.

The following formula can be used to approximate the length of time a tank will last (in minutes):

$$[\text{Pressure on cylinder gauge (psi)} - 500 \text{ psi (safety factor)}] \times \text{Cylinder factor} \div \text{L/min}$$

The cylinder factor for an E cylinder is **0.3**; for an H cylinder, the cylinder factor is **3.1**.

Example 1: An E cylinder reads 2 000 psi and the patient is wearing nasal prongs set to 2 L/min:

$$\text{Length of time tank will last} = (2\,000 - 500) \times 0.3 \div 2$$
$$= 1\,500 \times 0.15$$
$$= 450 \div 2$$
$$= 225 \text{ minutes (3 hours 45 min)}$$

Example 2: An E cylinder reads 2 000 psi and the patient is wearing a nonrebreather mask set to 15 L/min:

$$\text{Length of time tank will last} = (2\,000 - 500) \times 0.3 \div 15$$
$$= 1\,500 \times 0.02$$
$$= 450 \div 15$$
$$= 30 \text{ minutes}$$

percentage of oxygen to the flowmeter. Therefore, if a patient is switched to a concentrator, the flow rate usually needs to be adjusted. Patients using a concentrator need to have a backup system such as a portable oxygen tank in case of power failure.

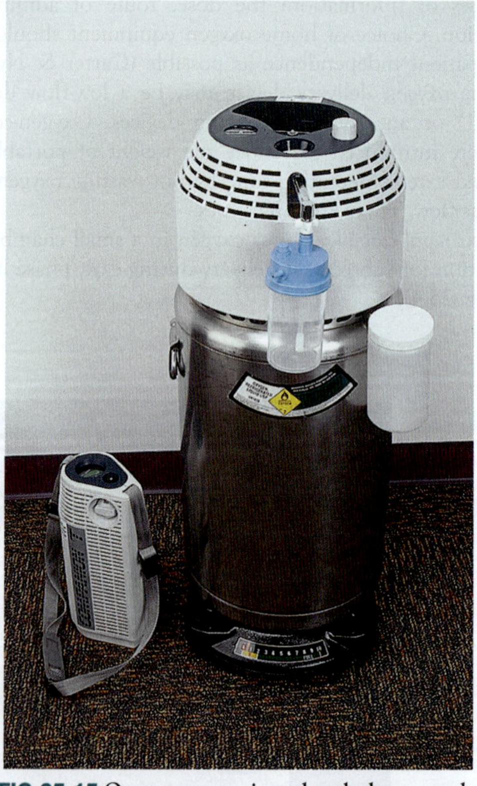

FIG 25.15 Oxygen reservoir and ambulatory tank.

Patients and their caregivers need extensive teaching to use home oxygen therapy correctly and safely (Box 25.4). When initiating and managing ongoing oxygen therapy, collaborate with the patient, health care provider, caregivers, and medical equipment provider.

Delegation and Collaboration

- The skill of teaching patients how to use home oxygen equipment cannot be delegated to a UCP.

BOX 25.4

Teaching Points for Safe Home Oxygen Therapy

Although oxygen is not flammable, it will burn if it comes in contact with fire. Therefore, patients should take the following precautions.

Fire Safety

- Use and store oxygen in a well-ventilated area.
- Do not use open flames (e.g., matches, fireplaces, stoves, space heaters, candles) when oxygen is in use.
- No smoking on the premises. Those who smoke while on home oxygen are at a higher risk of starting a fire than nonsmokers (Moslander et al., 2020).
- Install smoke detectors and have a fire extinguisher available in the home. Test smoke detectors twice a month.
- Help patient or caregiver plan a fire evacuation route. Have two routes out of every room and an outside meeting place.

Oxygen Storage and Handling

- In the home setting, place an "Oxygen in Use" sign on the door of the residence.
- Store oxygen tanks upright in carts or stands to prevent tipping or falling, or place tanks flat on the floor when not in use.
- Do not store oxygen tanks in the trunk of a car.
- When transporting oxygen in a vehicle, ensure that tanks are secured properly in the passenger area with the windows opened 5–7.5 cm (2–3 inches) to allow adequate ventilation.

Concentrator Safety

- Plug concentrators into properly grounded outlets.
- Do not use extension cords, power strips, or multioutlet adapters with concentrators.
- Ensure that the power supply or circuit meets or exceeds the amperage requirements of the concentrator.

Liquid Oxygen Safety

- Avoid direct contact with liquid oxygen because it can cause frostbite. The vapours are also extremely cold; they can damage delicate tissues such as the eyes.
- Do not touch connectors that are frosted or icy.
- Keep ambulatory tanks upright; do not lay them down or place them on their side.

Adapted from National Fire Protection Association. (2015). *Safety tip sheets—Medical oxygen*. https://www.nfpa.org/Public-Education/Teaching-tools/Safety-tip-sheets; Tyerman, J., & Cobbett, S. (Eds.). (2023). *Lewis's medical-surgical nursing in Canada: Assessment and management of clinical problems* (5th ed.). Elsevier.

Equipment

- Oxygen delivery device
- Oxygen tubing
- Home oxygen delivery system (compressed oxygen, oxygen concentrator, or liquid oxygen) with all required equipment (varies with supplier and system used)
- "No Smoking/Oxygen in Use" sign for each entrance to the home

STEP	RATIONALE
ASSESSMENT	
1. Identify patient using at least two person-specific identifiers during hospital and first home visit. Facial recognition can be used as one of two identifiers for ongoing subsequent home visits.	Ensures correct patient. Complies with Accreditation Canada's standards and improves patient safety (Accreditation Canada, 2020).
2. Throughout the procedure, the 4 moments for hand hygiene are to be implemented; hand hygiene should occur before initial patient (or patient environment) contact, before an aseptic procedure, after body fluid exposure risk, and after patient (or patient environment) contact. Additional hand hygiene should be performed when hands are visibly soiled.	Proper hand hygiene helps prevent the spread of infectious agents to health care providers.
3. While patient is still in hospital, determine patient's or caregiver's ability to apply and regulate oxygen equipment correctly. In home setting, reassess for appropriate use of equipment.	Physical or cognitive impairments indicate need to teach caregiver how to operate home oxygen equipment. Determines specific components of skill that patient and caregiver are able to complete easily. Smoking while on oxygen increases patient risk for major burns and death (Moore, 2019; Moslander et al., 2020; Singer et al., 2020).
4. Determine appropriate resources in community for equipment and assistance, including maintenance and repair services and medical equipment supplier.	Adults using home oxygen often experience equipment issues and require ongoing support (Jacobs, 2019).
5. Determine appropriate backup systems for compressor in event of power failure (e.g., notify local emergency medical services [EMS]). Have a spare oxygen tank available for emergency use.	Prepares for an emergency to reduce likelihood of patient losing access to oxygen.
6. Assess patient's learning readiness and ability to concentrate; consider presence of pain, nausea, or fatigue and patient interest in instruction.	Presence of significant illness, frailty, or confusion affects patient's ability to attend to teaching plan. Indicates need to rely on caregiver for learning and implementation (if available) on a short- or long-term basis.

NURSING DIAGNOSES

- Anxiety
- Insufficient knowledge regarding oxygen therapy
- Inadequate health maintenance

Related factors and risk factors are individualized on the basis of patient's condition or needs.

STEP	RATIONALE
PLANNING	
1. Expected outcomes following completion of procedure:	
• Patient receives oxygen at prescribed rate.	Oxygen system is set up correctly.
• Patient or caregiver verbalizes purpose and correct use of home oxygen.	Provides measurable criteria to determine level of understanding.
• Patient or caregiver demonstrates how to apply, regulate, and maintain oxygen system.	Indicates learning has occurred.
• Patient or caregiver states indications for calling medical equipment provider to replenish oxygen supply and reorder oxygen delivery supplies.	Patient needs a constant supply of oxygen at home.
• Patient or caregiver verbalizes safety guidelines for oxygen use (see Box 25.4).	Provides measure of understanding of oxygen use.
• Patient or caregiver verbalizes emergency plan of care.	Ensures safe, continuous delivery of home oxygen.
2. Select a setting in the home where patient is most likely to use oxygen equipment and that is conducive to a teaching session:	Practising in the same environment where skill is routinely performed facilitates comprehension and learning.
• Select a room that is well lit with comfortable seating. • Be sure that patient is close and can see the nurse clearly. • Control sources of noise and distractions.	Minimizes existing sensory alterations. A comfortable environment free of distractions increases patient's attention.
IMPLEMENTATION	
1. Teach patient or caregiver how to perform hand hygiene before handling oxygen equipment.	Reduces transmission of microorganisms.
2. Place oxygen delivery system in a clutter-free environment that is well ventilated; away from walls, drapes, curtains, bedding, and combustible materials; and at least 2.4 metres (8 feet) from heat sources.	Keeps system balanced and prevents injury.
Critical Decision Point *Do not place oxygen delivery system in a closet.*	
3. Demonstrate steps for preparation and maintenance of oxygen therapy:	Demonstration is a reliable technique for teaching psychomotor skills and enables the patient to ask questions.
a. Compressed oxygen system:	
(1) Turn cylinder valve counterclockwise two to three turns with a wrench.	Turns on oxygen.
(2) Check cylinders by reading amount on pressure gauge.	Verifies adequate oxygen supply for patient use.
(3) Store wrench with oxygen tank or in another safe place.	Storing wrench in a safe place ensures that it is available whenever needed.
b. Oxygen concentrator system:	
(1) Plug concentrator into appropriate outlet.	Provides power safely to concentrator.
(2) Turn on power switch.	Starts concentrator motor.
(3) Alarm will sound for a few seconds.	Alarm shuts off when desired pressure inside concentrator is reached.
c. Liquid oxygen system:	
(1) Check liquid system by depressing button at lower right corner and reading dial on stationary oxygen reservoir or ambulatory tank.	Verifies adequate oxygen supply for patient use.
(2) Collaborate with medical equipment provider to provide instruction in refilling ambulatory tank when it becomes empty.	Ensures that continuous oxygen therapy is not interrupted.
Critical Decision Point *Ambulatory tanks are filled only when they are empty. Liquid oxygen is stored at or below −183°C (−297°F) inside the reservoir, and the temperature inside the ambulatory tank is warmer. If cold oxygen from the reservoir mixes with warmer oxygen left in the ambulatory tank, the ambulatory tank malfunctions. Keep the medical equipment supplier contact number in a visible location for asking questions about the equipment.*	

STEP	RATIONALE
IMPLEMENTATION	
(3) To refill liquid oxygen tank:	
(a) Wipe both filling connectors with a clean, dry, lint-free cloth.	Removes dust and moisture from system.
(b) Turn off flow selector of ambulatory unit.	
(c) Attach ambulatory unit to stationary reservoir by inserting female adapter from ambulatory tank into male adapter of stationary reservoir (see Step 3c[3][c] illustration).	Secures connection between oxygen reservoir and ambulatory tank.
(d) Open fill valve on ambulatory tank (e.g., lever, button, key) and apply firm pressure to top of stationary reservoir (see Step 3c[3][d] illustration). Stay with unit while it is filling. You will hear a loud hissing noise. The tank should be filled in about 2 minutes.	Prevents leakage of oxygen during filling process. If oxygen leaks during filling process, the connection between the ambulatory tank and reservoir will potentially ice up, and ambulatory and reservoir tanks will stick together.
(e) Disconnect ambulatory unit from stationary reservoir when hissing noise changes and vapour cloud begins to form from stationary unit.	Overfilling causes ambulatory unit to malfunction as a result of high pressure in the tank.

Critical Decision Point *If the ambulatory unit does not separate easily, valves from the reservoir and ambulatory unit are frozen together. Wait until valves warm to disengage (about 5–10 minutes). Do not touch any frosted areas because contact with skin causes skin damage from frostbite.*

STEP	RATIONALE
(f) Wipe both filling connectors with a clean, dry, lint-free cloth.	Ice often forms during the filling process. Removes moisture from oxygen system.
4. Connect oxygen delivery device (e.g., nasal cannula) to oxygen delivery system (see Skill 25.1) (see Step 4 illustration).	Connects oxygen source to delivery method.
5. Adjust oxygen flow rate (L/min) to prescribed rate.	Ensures that prescribed oxygen dose is delivered.
6. Have patient or caregiver apply oxygen delivery device (e.g., nasal cannula) correctly (see Skill 25.1). Ensure that patient has two sets of oxygen delivery devices and tubing.	Ensures understanding of use of equipment and troubleshooting ability. Extra set of equipment is used when equipment is cleaned or in case of equipment malfunction.

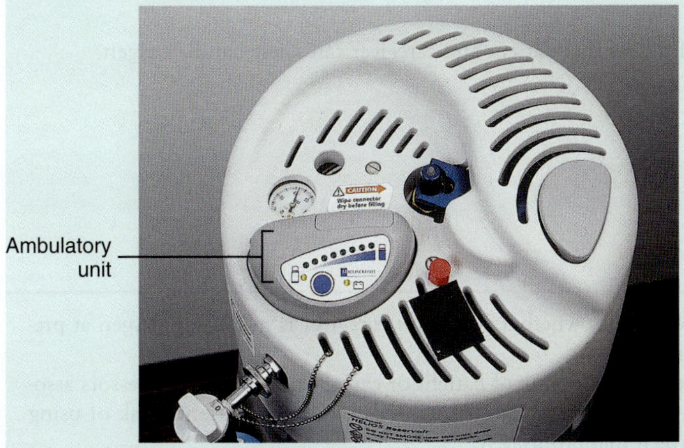

STEP 3C(3)(C) Top view of stationary reservoir.

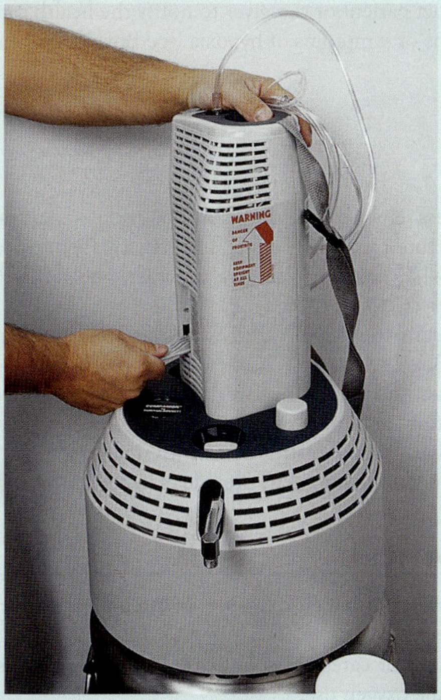

STEP 3C(3)(D) Fill valve on ambulatory tank is opened while applying firm pressure to top of ambulatory tank.

STEP	RATIONALE

IMPLEMENTATION

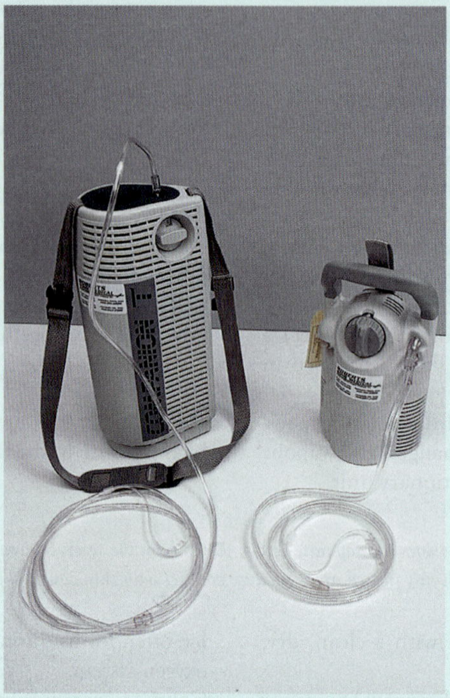

STEP 4 Oxygen delivery device (nasal cannulae) and tubing attached to ambulatory oxygen tanks.

STEP	RATIONALE
7. Instruct patient and caregiver to treat oxygen as a medication and not change oxygen flow rate.	Exceeding the prescribed amount of oxygen is sometimes harmful (Khalil et al., 2019; Piraino et al., 2022)
8. Have patient or caregiver perform each step with guidance. Provide written material for reinforcement and review.	Allows for correction of any errors in technique and discussion of their implications.
9. Instruct patient or caregiver to notify the health care provider if signs or symptoms of hypoxia (see Box 25.1) occur.	Hypoxia sometimes occurs at home when the patient uses oxygen. Possible causes of hypoxia include poor tubing connections; use of long oxygen tubing; or worsening of patient's physical problem, with change in respiratory status. Respiratory tract infections increase oxygen demand and often affect oxygen transfer from the lungs to blood, creating exacerbation of the patient's pulmonary disease.
10. Discuss emergency plans for power loss, natural disaster, and acute respiratory distress. Instruct patient or caregiver to call 9-1-1, notify health care provider, and notify home care employer.	Ensures appropriate response and can prevent worsening of patient's condition.
11. Instruct patient and caregiver in safe home oxygen practices (see Box 25.4).	Ensures that patient and caregiver can safely handle oxygen.
12. Instruct the patient or caregiver in appropriate cleaning, disinfection, and maintenance of all oxygen delivery systems and supplies. Verify instructions with manufacturer guidelines and medical equipment provider's instructions.	

EVALUATION

STEP	RATIONALE
1. Monitor rate at which oxygen is being delivered during each home visit.	Determines whether patient or caregiver is regulating oxygen at prescribed rate.
2. Ask patient or caregiver about ease of or problems associated with home oxygen use.	Determines ability of patient or caregiver to deal with stressors associated with home oxygen use. Also indicates patient's risk of using oxygen inappropriately.

STEP	RATIONALE
EVALUATION	
3. Use teach-back: Ask patient or caregiver to state safety guidelines, emergency precautions, and emergency plan. "I want to be sure you understand what to do in an emergency. Tell me in your own words what you would do if the power went out or your oxygen stopped working." "Tell me in your own words what you would do if you (or your loved one) suddenly had trouble breathing." Develop a revised teaching plan if patient or caregiver is unable to teach back correctly.	Determines patient's or caregiver's knowledge of what to do if power fails, there is a failure in equipment, or patient's status worsens. Teach-back is an effective way to determine patient's and caregiver's level of understanding of topic.
4. Use teach-back: "I want to be sure I explained how to use your home oxygen system correctly. Tell me in your own words (or show me) how to set up and apply your oxygen."	Teach-back is an effective way to determine patient's and caregiver's level of understanding of topic (Yen & Leasure, 2019).

Unexpected Outcomes	Related Interventions
1. Patient has signs and symptoms associated with hypoxia.	• Determine whether oxygen delivery device and oxygen source are delivering oxygen properly. • Determine whether prescribed oxygen flow rate is set properly. • Assess patient for change in respiratory status, such as airway plugging, respiratory tract infection, or bronchospasm. • Teach patient or caregiver when to notify health care provider or activate EMS because of signs of hypoxia.
2. Patient uses unsafe practices with oxygen therapy, uses oxygen around fire or cigarette smoking, or sets incorrect flow rate.	• Reinforce patient education (see Box 25.4) and perform follow-up reassessment. • Include caregiver in instruction and set up problem-solving exercises with patient.
3. Patient is unable to fill ambulatory system.	• Identify and instruct caregiver who can help patient fill tank.

Communication and Documentation

- Document teaching plan, information provided to patient, and patient's and caregiver's ability to discuss information in the home care record.
- Communicate patient's or caregiver's learning progress to other health care providers involved in the patient's care.
- Document oxygen delivery system, related supplies, and prescribed oxygen flow rate in home care record.
- Report respiratory complications or concerns to the health care provider.

Special Considerations

Teaching

- Potential for oxygen desaturation and decreased oxygen delivery to the brain impairs the patient's ability to remember previous learning. Provide frequent teaching sessions on the points in Implementation Steps 7 through 12 as well as written or pictorial instructions to reinforce previous learning of teaching plan.
- Always leave a phone number and instructions on how to reach a home care nurse if needed and how to contact the medical equipment supplier.
- Some patients who are at home have both a permanent tracheostomy and a T-tube or a tracheostomy collar. The patient or caregiver needs to be physically able to perform tracheostomy care and suctioning techniques and must understand how to manage oxygen (see Chapter 23). Community-based care providers of these services may be expensive or of limited availability.

Pediatric

- Keep equipment out of reach of any children in the home. Do not allow children to handle or operate home oxygen equipment.
- Keep children away from fire and flames at all times; explain dangers of oxygen coming into contact with fire in a cognitively and age-appropriate manner.

Gerontological

- Older persons have less efficient respiratory systems and less surface area for gas exchange; thus, they are at greater risk for cerebral anoxia and confusion when they experience decreased oxygen levels. They may be unable to recognize respiratory problems or problems with their oxygen delivery system. Therefore, they need frequent contact with a designated caregiver.

✦ SKILL 25.3 Using Incentive Spirometry

Incentive spirometry (IS) helps a patient to breathe deeply. It works by providing visual feedback that helps encourage the patient to take long, deep, slow breaths (Smetana, 2022). The use of IS alone is not recommended to prevent postoperative pulmonary complications. It should be used in combination with other pulmonary manoeuvres such as deep breathing and coughing (see Chapter 37), early mobilization of the patient, and directed coughing (do Nascimento et al., 2014; Smetana, 2022).

There are two types of IS devices: flow oriented and volume oriented. Flow-oriented IS devices have one or more plastic chambers with freely moving coloured balls. The advantage of a flow-oriented IS device is the slow, steady expansion of the lung. As a patient inhales

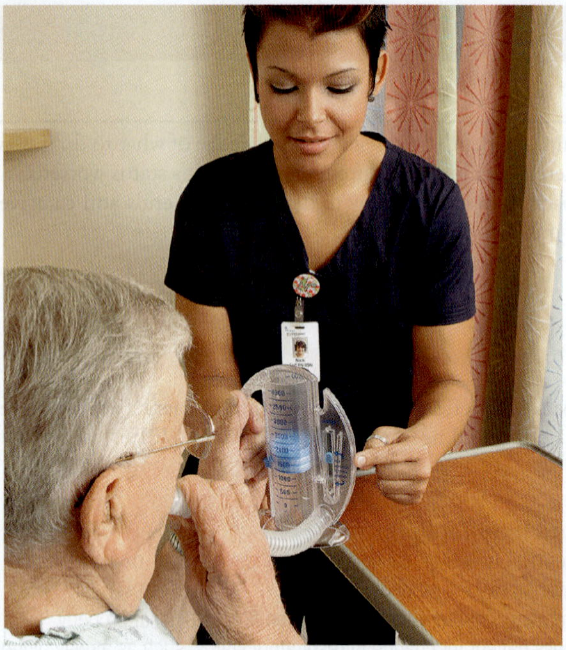

FIG 25.16 Flow-oriented incentive spirometer.

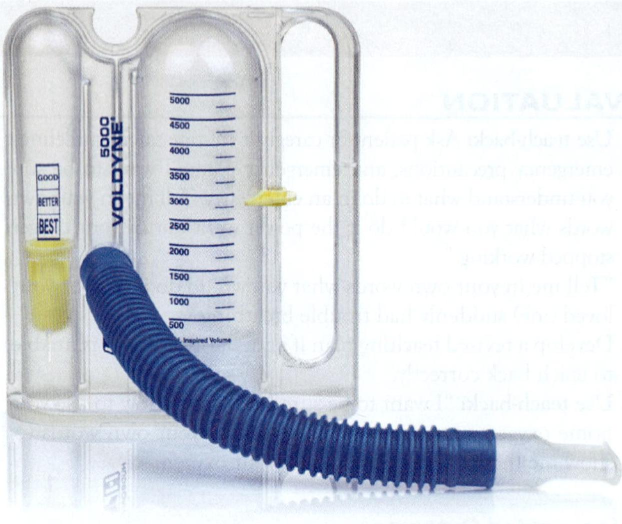

FIG 25.17 Volume-oriented incentive spirometer.

slowly, the balls elevate to a premarked area (Fig. 25.16). A patient's goal is to keep the balls elevated for as long as possible to ensure maximal sustained inhalation. Even if a very slow inspiration does not elevate the balls, this pattern helps a patient improve lung expansion.

Volume-oriented devices use a bellows that a patient must raise to a predetermined volume by inhaling slowly (Fig. 25.17). The advantage of the volume-oriented IS device is that a patient can achieve a known inspiratory volume and measure it with each breath.

Delegation and Collaboration

The skill of helping a patient to use IS can be delegated to a UCP, depending on the competence of the UCP to perform this skill in a particular situation and on employer policy. The nurse is responsible for assessing and monitoring the patient, evaluating the patient response, educating the patient about the proper use of the IS device, and evaluating the patient education provided. The nurse instructs the UCP about the following:

- The patient's target goal for IS
- Immediately notifying the nurse about any unexpected outcomes, such as chest pain, excessive sputum production, and fever

Equipment

- Flow- or volume-oriented IS device
- Stethoscope
- Pulse oximeter monitor

STEP	RATIONALE
ASSESSMENT	
1. Identify patient using at least two person-specific identifiers (e.g., name and date of birth, or name and medical record number) according to employer policy.	Ensures correct patient. Complies with Accreditation Canada's standards and improves patient safety (Accreditation Canada, 2020).
2. Throughout the procedure, the 4 moments for hand hygiene are to be implemented; hand hygiene should occur before initial patient (or patient environment) contact, before an aseptic procedure, after body fluid exposure risk, and after patient (or patient environment) contact. Additional hand hygiene should be performed when hands are visibly soiled.	Proper hand hygiene helps prevent the spread of infectious agents to health care providers.
3. Review medical record to identify patients who will benefit from the use of an IS device (e.g., existing pulmonary disease, obesity, debilitating chronic illness, heavy smokers, neuromuscular disease, or sickle cell disease with acute chest syndrome; Smetana, 2022).	Alerts health care personnel to patients at risk for respiratory complications during illness or after surgery.
4. Assess patient for confusion, cognitive impairment, ability to follow directions, age, developmental level, LOC, and decreased necessary motor skills (Smetana, 2022).	Determines risks for difficulty performing IS.

Critical Decision Point *Patients who are unable to follow directions or who are not developmentally or physically able to perform the actions associated with this skill are not candidates for this intervention. This assessment helps the nurse determine whether to use the flow-oriented or volume-oriented IS device.*

STEP	RATIONALE
ASSESSMENT	
5. Perform respiratory assessment, including vital signs, auscultation of lungs, inspection for symmetrical chest wall expansion, chest wall abnormalities, temporary conditions affecting ventilation (e.g., pregnancy, trauma), sputum production (amount, characteristics), and signs and symptoms associated with hypoxia (see Box 25.1).	Decreased chest wall movement, crackles or decreased lung sounds, increased respiratory rate, and increased sputum production can indicate a need for IS to improve lung expansion.
6. Assess level of pain at rest and during activity (e.g., coughing) using appropriate pain rating scale (e.g., rate your pain on a scale of 0–10, with 0 = no pain and 10 = the worst pain ever).	Pain decreases effectiveness of IS by restricting chest expansion. Assessing pain scale allows the nurse to know when to administer prescribed analgesia for the patient and is part of assessing its efficacy.
7. Review interprofessional team recommendations and prescriptions for IS.	Ensures appropriate use of IS.

NURSING DIAGNOSES

- Impaired breathing pattern
- Ineffective airway clearance
- Acute pain
- Impaired gas exchange

Related factors and risk factors are individualized on the basis of patient's condition or needs.

STEP	RATIONALE
PLANNING	
1. Expected outcomes following completion of procedure:	
• Patient demonstrates correct use of IS.	Demonstrates learning.
• Patient achieves target volume and number of repetitions per hour.	Demonstrates increased lung expansion.
• Patient has improved breath sounds and increased pulse oximeter reading.	Incentive spirometry helps patient breathe deeply and manage airway secretions.
2. Explain procedure to patient and caregiver.	It is an ethical responsibility of nurses to provide education to patients to support informed decision making (CNA, 2017).
3. Indicate to patient where target volume is on IS device. NOTE: If possible, demonstrate use of IS device.	Encourages patients to "do better" with each breath and meet or exceed target volume. When patients have a visual target, they can gauge their improvement.
IMPLEMENTATION	
1. Gather equipment and supplies according to employer policy.	Ensures that you have the necessary equipment.
2. Position patient in most erect position (e.g., high Fowler's, if tolerated) in bed or chair.	Promotes optimal lung expansion during respiratory manoeuvre.
3. Instruct patient to hold IS device upright, exhale normally and completely through mouth, and place lips tightly around mouthpiece (Fig. 25.18).	Allows for proper functioning of IS device (Smetana, 2022). Showing patient how to correctly place mouthpiece is reliable technique for teaching psychomotor skill and enables patient to ask questions.
4. Instruct patient to take a slow, deep breath and maintain constant flow, like drinking water through a straw. If flow-oriented IS device is used, inhalation should raise the ball. If volume-oriented IS device is used, inhalation should raise the piston. Remove mouthpiece at point of maximal inhalation; then have patient hold their breath for 3 seconds and exhale normally.	Maintains maximal inspiration; reduces risk of progressive collapse of individual alveoli.

Critical Decision Point *Some patients are unable to hold their breath for 3 seconds. Encourage them to do their best and try to extend the duration of breath holding. Allow patients to rest between IS breaths to prevent hyperventilation and fatigue.*

STEP	RATIONALE
5. Have patient repeat manoeuvre, encouraging them to reach prescribed goal.	Ensures correct use of IS device and patient's understanding of use.
6. Encourage patient to independently use IS device at prescribed frequency. Frequently prescribed timing schedules of IS use are up to 30 deep breaths with 30- to 60-second rests between sets of 10 (Smetana, 2022).	Repeated use of IS improves lung expansion and promotes clearing of airways. Encouraging patients to perform IS independently gives them a sense of control over their care.

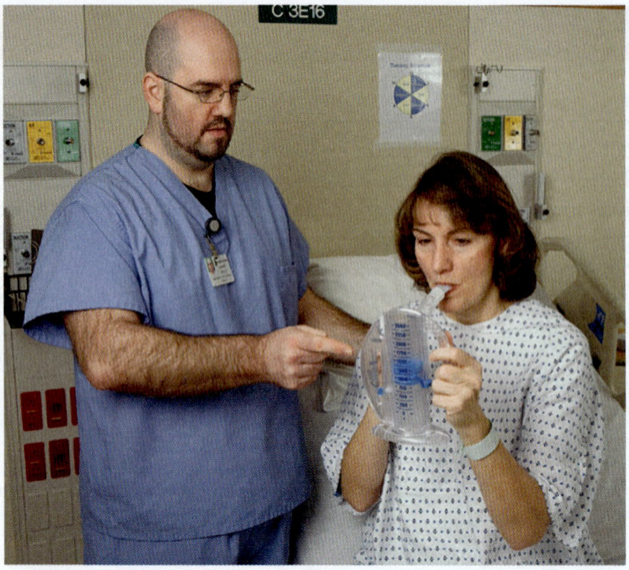

FIG 25.18 Proper placement of lips around incentive spirometer.

STEP	RATIONALE

EVALUATION

1. Observe patient's ability to use IS by return demonstration.	Determines patient's ability to perform breathing exercise correctly.
2. Assess whether patient is able to achieve target volume or frequency.	Measures adherence to therapy and lung expansion.
3. Auscultate chest during respiratory cycle and obtain pulse oximeter reading (Smetana, 2022).	Documents lung expansion, identifies any abnormal lung sounds, and determines whether airways are clear. Identifies improvement in pulse oximeter readings.
4. Use teach-back: "I want to be sure I explained how and when to use the IS device. Show me how to use your IS device, and tell me how frequently you should use it." Develop a revised teaching plan if patient is unable to teach back correctly.	Effective way to determine patient's and caregiver's level of understanding of topic (Yen & Leasure, 2019).

Unexpected Outcomes	Related Interventions
1. Patient is unable to achieve IS target volume.	• Encourage patient to attempt IS more frequently, followed by rest periods. • Teach cough-control exercises. • Teach patient how to splint and protect incision sites during deep breathing (see Chapter 37). • Administer prescribed analgesic if acute pain is inhibiting use of IS.
2. Patient has decreased lung expansion and/or abnormal breath sounds or decreased pulse oximeter readings.	• Teach patient cough-control exercises. • Provide help with suctioning if patient cannot cough up secretions effectively.
3. Patient develops hyperventilation.	• Encourage longer rest periods between breaths.

Communication and Documentation

- Document lung sounds, respiratory rate, and pulse oximeter readings before and after IS; frequency of use; volumes achieved; and any adverse effects in progress notes in EHR or chart.
- Document your evaluation of patient learning.

Special Considerations

Teaching

- Teach patient to examine sputum for consistency, amount, and colour changes. Sputum should become clearer over time and decrease in volume.

Pediatric

- IS is not typically used in pediatrics except for school-age children; a pediatric patient needs the fine motor skills and ability to follow instructions to use an IS device effectively (Hockenberry et al., 2024).
- Allowing a child to play with and try out the IS device helps to decrease their anxiety and encourages participation in care.
- Use games or bubbles and pinwheels to encourage small children to take deep breaths. These activities help achieve the same goals as IS in some children.

Gerontological

- Older persons with chronic illnesses or arthritis may have difficulty coordinating the use of the IS device. They may require additional time to demonstrate the procedure (Boscart et al., 2023).
- Weakened respiratory muscles and decreased elastic recoil properties of the lungs affect a patient's ability to cough and deep breathe. Therefore, it takes an older person longer to achieve the target volume (Boscart et al., 2023).

✦ SKILL 25.4 Care of a Patient Receiving Noninvasive Positive-Pressure Ventilation

Noninvasive positive-pressure ventilation (NIPPV or NPPV), or noninvasive ventilation (NIV), maintains positive airway pressure and improves alveolar ventilation in the spontaneously breathing patient without the need for an artificial airway. There are two types of NIPPV: continuous positive airway pressure (CPAP) and bi-level positive airway pressure (BiPAP). BiPAP and CPAP are usually applied via a mask covering the nose (Fig. 25.19) or both the mouth and nose, but those who require home CPAP may wear nasal pillows instead (Fig. 25.20) (Hill & Kramer, 2022; Pooboni & Markowitz, 2022).

NIPPV is increasingly used in care settings in the community to treat a variety of conditions, including obstructive sleep apnea (OSA), COPD, and neuromuscular disorders. In the Canadian acute care setting, it is used in patients with acute respiratory failure due to cardiogenic pulmonary edema or COPD exacerbation (Digby et al., 2015; Keenan et al., 2011). NIPPV is only appropriate if these patients are cooperative, able to protect their own airway, and not acutely deteriorating (Rochwerg et al., 2017).

The advantages of NIPPV over invasive ventilation include an increased ability to communicate with caregivers, better ability to cough and clear secretions, and allowance for eating and drinking. NIPPV can also decrease the risk of invasive ventilation complications such as pneumonia, and in some cases can decrease the need for sedation and the length of a patient's hospital stay (Rochwerg et al., 2017). This type of ventilation also has disadvantages (Table 25.3). The mask should be moulded against the patient's face and have a good seal to prevent air from leaking. This can cause feelings of claustrophobia and intolerance in patients, which can lead to issues with adherence to therapy. Wearing an overly tight mask can also lead to skin breakdown, particularly on the bridge of the nose (Davidson et al., 2016).

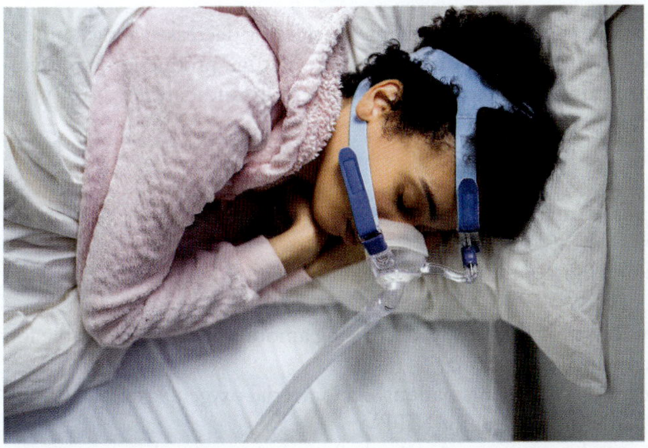

FIG 25.19 Nasal continuous positive airway pressure (CPAP) mask. *(iStockphoto/Andrey Popov)*

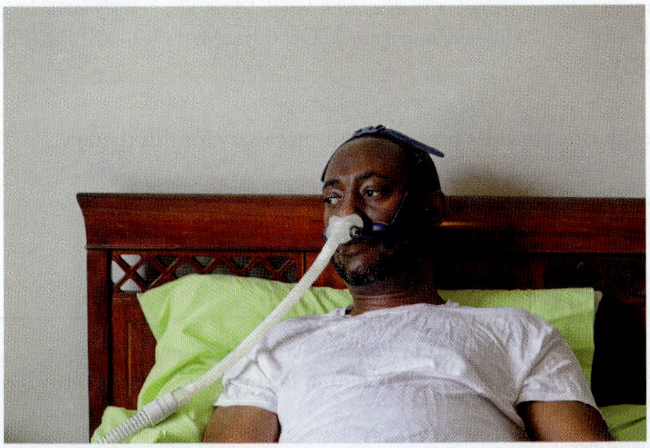

FIG 25.20 Nasal pillow continuous positive airway pressure (CPAP). *(iStockphoto/Robin Gentry)*

Delegation and Collaboration

The skill of caring for a patient receiving noninvasive ventilation cannot be delegated to a UCP. However, the skills of patient positioning, deep breathing and coughing, and CPAP/BiPAP mask application can be delegated to a UCP, depending on the competence of the UCP to perform this skill in a particular situation and on employer policy. The nurse directs the UCP to immediately do the following:

- Report to the nurse any changes in patient's vital signs; oxygen saturation; mental status; skin colour; or skin abrasions, bruising, or blistering around mask area
- Report to the nurse any ventilator or CPAP/BiPAP machine alarms or patient monitor alarms
- Report to the nurse any change in settings or patient comfort

TABLE 25.3 Problems Associated With Continuous Positive Airway Pressure and Bi-Level Positive Airway Pressure

Problem	Cause
Discomfort	Mask that fits over patient's nose is tight fitting. Oxygen flow rate causes dry mucous membranes, which may cause eye irritation in full face masks.
Psychosocial	Relationship with sleep partner is difficult. There are possible sensations of claustrophobia.
Risks to skin integrity	Fit of mask causes pressure and increased risk of skin breakdown. Patients may need to remove mask to relieve pressure.
Hypercapnia	Although CPAP improves alveolar function, which increases CO_2 clearance from the blood, it also causes air trapping. In some patients, this causes a rise in CO_2 levels. Initially, the nurse needs to monitor patient's ABG levels.
Gastric distension	CPAP/BiPAP forces more air into the stomach, which causes distension and discomfort.
Noise	Some patients find the older machines very noisy, which interferes with sleep and leisure activities such as watching television or listening to music.

ABG, Arterial blood gas; *BiPAP*, bi-level positive airway pressure; CO_2, carbon dioxide; *CPAP*, continuous positive airway pressure.

Data from Pooboni, S. K., & Markowitz, J. E. (2022). *Noninvasive ventilation procedures*. https://emedicine.medscape.com/article/1417959-overview

Interprofessional collaboration is essential when providing care for the patient. When available, respiratory therapists are an essential part of code blue and critical response teams. They can be consulted directly by the nurse to assist with a patient who has a declining or complicated respiratory status. In some settings, the respiratory therapist may be responsible for managing the CPAP/BiPAP machine, but the nurse retains primary responsibility for the patient. Nurses must communicate their assessment of the patient's respiratory status in response to NIPPV, as well as any concerns, to all team members to optimize patient care and safety.

Equipment

NOTE: When device is used in the community setting, the equipment vendor provides the equipment.

- Nasal mask/full face mask (with quick-release straps), or nasal pillows
- Oxygen source and tubing
- CPAP/BiPAP health care provider prescription
- Humidification source, if indicated
- BiPAP and/or CPAP ventilator
- Delivery tubing
- Pulse oximetry (SpO_2)
- Clean gloves
- PPE as appropriate
- Stethoscope
- Suction equipment
- Self-inflating manual resuscitation bag-valve mask

STEP	RATIONALE
ASSESSMENT	
1. Identify patient using at least two person-specific identifiers (e.g., name and date of birth, or name and medical record number) according to employer policy.	Ensures correct patient. Complies with Accreditation Canada's standards and improves patient safety (Accreditation Canada, 2020).
2. Throughout the procedure, the 4 moments for hand hygiene are to be implemented; hand hygiene should occur before initial patient (or patient environment) contact, before an aseptic procedure, after body fluid exposure risk, and after patient (or patient environment) contact. Additional hand hygiene should be performed when hands are visibly soiled.	Proper hand hygiene helps prevent the spread of infectious agents to health care providers.
3. Assess patient's respiratory status, including symmetry of chest wall expansion, respiratory rate and depth, oxygen saturation, sputum production (amount, characteristics), and lung sounds (see Chapter 8). When possible, ask patient about dyspnea and observe for signs and symptoms associated with hypoxia (see Box 25.1).	Decreased chest wall movement, crackles or decreased lung sounds, increased respiratory rate, increased sputum production, or signs of worsening hypoxia may make patient a candidate for NIPPV or changes in NIPPV settings.
4. Observe patient's skin where it is in contact with the mask or straps, especially over bridge of nose and around external part of ears.	The mask can place pressure on skin and increase risk of skin breakdown (Norton et al., 2021). Ears and nose are the most common location for MDRPIs (Kayser et al., 2018).
5. Observe patient's ability to clear and remove airway secretions via deep breathing and coughing.	Secretions plug the airway, decreasing amount of oxygen available for gas exchange in the lung.
6. Assess patient's vital signs and SpO_2; when available, note patient's most recent ABG results.	Objectively documents patient's pH, arterial oxygen, arterial CO_2, or SaO_2. Identifies need for NIPPV.
7. Assess patient's LOC, behaviours, and ability to maintain and protect airway.	Patients who cannot maintain their own airway or who are uncooperative are not candidates for NIPPV.

Critical Decision Point *NIPPV is contraindicated in patients who are in cardiac or respiratory arrest or in those with facial deformities, hemodynamic instability, airway patency issues (including blood, emesis, secretions, or inability to protect airway), severe agitation, or impaired LOC* (DynaMed Plus, 2018). *NIPPV may be used in palliative and end-of-life care for dyspneic patients* (Rochwerg et al., 2017).

STEP	RATIONALE
8. Review patient's medical record for prescription for CPAP/BiPAP and appropriate settings.	A health care provider prescription is necessary for this therapy.
9. Assess patient's and caregiver's understanding of purpose of CPAP and ongoing maintenance.	Determines level of instruction required.

NURSING DIAGNOSES

- Impaired gas exchange
- Reduced stamina
- Impaired comfort
- Sleep deprivation
- Deficient knowledge regarding purpose of CPAP/BiPAP
- Potential for aspiration
- Potential for impaired skin integrity

Related factors and risk factors are individualized on the basis of patient's condition or needs.

PLANNING

STEP	RATIONALE
1. Expected outcomes following completion of procedure:	
• Patient has increased lung expansion.	Patient experiences improved gas exchange when lungs are expanded.
• Patient maintains ABG levels and/or SpO_2 readings improve or remain normal.	NIPPV delivered appropriately based on patient assessment data.

Critical Decision Point *When first initiating CPAP/BiPAP, it is important to monitor gas exchange, especially in patients with COPD, cardiogenic pulmonary edema, or acute respiratory failure. You do this to observe for hypercapnia. If patient has "do not resuscitate/allow natural death" directives, has a resuscitation care plan, or is receiving palliative care services, noninvasive ventilation may reduce breathlessness* (Rochwerg et al., 2017), *but careful consideration should be given to patient comfort and goals of care.*

STEP	RATIONALE
• Patient experiences reduction in feelings of dyspnea and work of breathing.	In patients with acute conditions, dyspnea usually improves. Patients with chronic pulmonary diseases may require nocturnal CPAP/BiPAP indefinitely to achieve long-term benefits.
• Patient's vital signs and respiratory assessment parameters improve.	Reduced pulse and respiratory rate, improved mental status, improved skin colour, and decreased use of accessory and abdominal muscles occur because patient's work of breathing decreases as level of oxygenation improves.
• Patient's skin around bridge of nose, ears, and back of head remains clear without breakdown.	Mask is applied properly and monitored for pressure occurrence.
• Patient is able to describe how to use CPAP in the home setting.	Demonstrates learning.
2. Explain to patient and caregiver the purpose of and reasons for CPAP/BiPAP.	It is an ethical responsibility of nurses to provide education to patients to support informed decision making (CNA, 2017).

IMPLEMENTATION

STEP	RATIONALE
1. Use interprofessional collaboration (e.g., respiratory therapist) to gather correct equipment and supplies according to employer policy.	Ensures that you have necessary equipment to apply the NIPPV system.
2. Apply clean gloves. Use appropriate PPE (goggles, mask, gown) if secretions are projectile or if patient is on additional precautions (see Box 5.1).	Reduces transmission of microorganisms. Reduces exposure to pulmonary secretions.
3. Adjust bed to appropriate height and lower side rail on side nearest you. Check locks on bed wheels.	Minimizes caregiver's muscle strain and prevents injury. Prevents bed from moving.
4. Determine correct mask size. Use masking chart to determine correct size (S, M, L, XL). NOTE: It is imperative that mask have quick-release straps.	Mask should fit snugly over patient's nose (CPAP) or nose and/or mouth (BiPAP) to create a tight seal for delivering positive pressure. In case of emergency (e.g., vomiting, respiratory arrest), quick-release straps allow mask to be removed quickly. This system also allows patient to remove mask quickly as needed (Urden et al., 2016).

Critical Decision Point *A patient receiving NIPPV via a full face mask should* ***never*** *be restrained. The patient must be able to remove the mask if they begin to vomit, need to remove excess secretions, or need to reposition a mask that has moved. A displaced mask can force the patient's jaw inward, which can obstruct the patient's airway* (Urden et al., 2016).

STEP	RATIONALE
5. Connect CPAP/BiPAP device delivery tubing to pressure generator.	Ensures that patient is receiving proper NIPPV as prescribed.
6. Connect patient to pulse oximetry (SpO_2).	It is important to continually monitor patient's level of oxygenation when initiating NIPPV.
7. Set CPAP/BiPAP initial settings per prescription or employer policy.	Interprofessional collaboration is required after initiation to determine initial patient response.
a. *CPAP*: 5–15 cm H_2O is the typically prescribed pressure range (Pooboni & Markowitz, 2022).	CPAP provides single positive pressure throughout breathing cycle, which helps to keep alveoli open at end expiration.
b. *BiPAP*: Inspiratory pressure is usually set to 10–12 cm H_2O initially and can be titrated up to 15–20 cm H_2O as patient condition dictates; expiratory pressure is usually set to 5–7 cm H_2O initially and can be titrated up as patient condition warrants (Pooboni & Markowitz, 2022).	BiPAP supplies pressure at both inhalation and exhalation. The inhalation pressure is set according to health care provider's prescription and helps prevent airway closure. Expiratory pressure is set according to health care provider's prescription and keeps alveoli open at end expiration (Davidson et al., 2016).

STEP	RATIONALE
IMPLEMENTATION	
8. Select FiO_2 level as indicated.	Patients on NIPPV may also need supplemental oxygen to decrease signs and symptoms of hypoxia (Hill & Kramer, 2022).
9. If using humidification, ensure that humidification and heating appliances are connected and on.	Humidification is not required but can be used if patient is experiencing dryness or thick secretions (Davidson et al., 2016).
10. Ensure that mask is fitted according to manufacturer instructions, no air leak is present, and there are no excessive pressure points.	An ill-fitting mask leads to loss of pressure getting into airways, dyssynchrony with ventilator, and patient discomfort (Davidson et al., 2016). Pressure points around mask area can cause MDRPIs (Norton et al., 2021).
11. If patient is to use CPAP at home, have patient or caregiver demonstrate mask placement and adjustment of settings.	Return demonstration indicates learning.
12. Dispose of supplies as appropriate, remove gloves and other PPE.	Reduces transmission of microorganisms.
13. Continuous care of patient	
a. Ensure that all alarms are on and active and that ventilator circuit is intact and properly functioning.	Ensures patient safety.
b. Ensure that emergency resuscitation equipment is at bedside.	Allows for quick resuscitation in case of worsening patient condition.
c. Investigate any and all alarms that come with ventilator/CPAP machine and/or patient monitor.	Alarms can alert the interprofessional team to problems with patient or with circuit that adversely affects patient status.
d. Change patient's position every 2 hours or encourage patient to change position every 2 hours.	Reduces incidence of atelectasis or pneumonia secondary to stasis of secretions.
EVALUATION	
1. Observe for decreased anxiety, improved LOC and cognitive abilities, decreased fatigue, and absence of dizziness.	Determines patient's response to NIPPV. As hypoxia and hypercapnia are reduced or corrected, patient's behavioural assessment parameters improve.
2. Measure vital signs, perform respiratory assessment and observe skin colour, and ask patient to describe sense of dyspnea.	Physical assessment parameters reveal oxygenation status.
3. Monitor pulse oximetry (SpO_2).	Documents patient's level of oxygenation. When first initiating NIPPV, it is important to obtain ABG levels in patients in whom abnormal gas exchange is suspected, after the first hour, and per employer protocol.
4. Observe skin integrity over bridge of patient's nose every 2 hours. Ask patient about level of comfort (Hill & Kramer, 2022).	Pressure points around mask area can cause pressure injuries (Norton et al., 2021). Studies have found that ischemic damage can occur in skeletal muscle after only 2 hours of sustained pressure (Gefen et al., 2022).
5. If NIPPV is planned for use in home, observe and monitor patient's and caregiver's ability to manipulate CPAP or BiPAP machine/ventilator and face mask.	Determines patient's ability to use CPAP/BiPAP machine and allows patient/caregiver to troubleshoot problems with health care provider. Support for solving machine problems and collaborative troubleshooting may increase adherence (Mehrtash et al., 2019).
6. Use **teach-back:** "I want to be sure I explained how NIPPV works and why you are receiving this therapy. Explain to me why this therapy is necessary." Develop a revised teaching plan if patient or caregiver is unable to teach back correctly.	Determines patient's and caregiver's level of understanding of topic (Yen & Leasure, 2019).

Unexpected Outcomes	Related Interventions
1. Patient experiences hypoxia, hypercapnia, or other signs of worsening respiratory function.	• Notify health care provider. • Reassess patient vital signs, ABGs, and respiratory status. • Consider measures to improve airway patency, including, but not limited to, deep breathing and coughing techniques, positioning patient with HOB elevated 45–90 degrees (unless contraindicated), and oropharyngeal or orotracheal suctioning (Chapter 23). • Determine correct settings and integrity of NIPPV.
2. Patient develops skin breakdown at mask sites or sites where mask straps are located, such as bridge of nose, nasal septum, or ears.	• Notify health care provider. • Place protective synthetic coverings on nasal bridge or areas of irritation (or possible irritation) to protect skin. • Fit mask appropriately to patient's face—mask should be tight enough to prevent air leaks but not so tight as to cause skin breakdown or irritation. • Reassess patient (Davidson et al., 2016).

Unexpected Outcomes	Related Interventions
3. Patient reports sense of being smothered or claustrophobia.	• Explain system to patient again. • Demonstrate use of quick-release straps. • Have patient demonstrate use of quick-release straps. • Consider alternate mask style, if available.
4. Stomach distension secondary to positive-pressure air being forced into esophagus and trachea (Pooboni & Markowitz, 2022).	• Notify health care provider. • Be prepared for possible insertion of nasogastric tube (see Chapter 35).
5. CPAP/BiPAP machine alarms go off.	• First, assess patient's respiratory status and vital signs. • If patient is hemodynamically stable, start at the patient mask and move toward the machine, looking for air leaks in mask/tubing, kinks, built-up condensation, disconnections, etc. • For further troubleshooting, check the user manual for the brand of machine used by your employer.

Communication and Documentation

- Document respiratory assessment findings, CPAP/BiPAP settings, vital signs and SpO_2, patient response, and skin assessment in progress notes in EHR or chart.
- Document your patient teaching and evaluation of patient and caregiver learning.
- Communicate sudden changes in patient's behaviour or respiratory status and any decline in ABG levels or SpO_2 values to nurse in charge or health care provider.

DOCUMENTATION EXAMPLE

Patient arrived ambulatory to room. Lips blue, indrawing of ribs noted, speaking 1-word sentences, GCS15. Initial SpO_2 = 68% on room air, RR = 40 breaths/min, HR = 120 beats/min, BP 140/68 mm Hg, T = 36.6°C orally. As per verbal prescription from Dr. C Ligoure, BiPAP initiated at 10/5 and 0.4 FiO_2. Patient SpO_2 now 89%, RR = 32 breaths/min, HR = 120 beats/min, BP 138/70 mm Hg, T = 36.6°C orally. Lips pink, indrawing still present, speaking 3-word sentences. As per health care provider prescription: (1) Target SpO_2 = 88–92% because pt has history of hypercapnia. (2) ABGs collected and sent to lab. (3) Will continue to repeat vital signs q5 minutes. (4) Will reassess patient respiratory status collaboratively in 30 minutes (sooner if deterioration); if no marked improvement, health care provider plans to intubate.

Special Considerations

Teaching

- Teach patient and caregiver the prescribed hours to use the machine. If machine is not in use 24 hours/day, work with the patient and/or caregiver to identify the ideal time for use (e.g., bedtime, watching television).
- Teach patient and caregiver how to apply the mask, connect it to the machine, and add oxygen if prescribed.
- Instruct caregiver to bring the machine, along with a list of correct settings, to the hospital any time patient is admitted.

Care in the Community: Home Management

- Using interprofessional collaboration, develop a teaching plan to ensure that the patient and caregiver have working knowledge of the system before discharge.
- When patients require home NIPPV, instruct in complete care of the CPAP/BiPAP system. Skills include assembling the system, cleaning it, and maintaining the equipment daily.
- Teach patient and caregiver what to do in case of respiratory distress or power failure.
- Notify appropriate power company to ensure that they prioritize the home in the event of a power outage.
- Remind patient that they must bring their own CPAP machine with them if they require an overnight hospital stay in future.
- Follow the safety precautions for oxygen use (see Box 25.4).

Procedural Guideline 25.1 *Use of a Peak Flowmeter*

For patients who have measurable changes in the flow of their airways, such as patients with asthma or reactive airway disease, peak expiratory flow rate (PEFR) measurements are useful. The PEFR is the maximum flow of air that a patient forces out during one quick, forced expiration and is measured in litres per minute. These measurements are used as an objective indicator of a patient's current status or the effectiveness of treatment. Patients with asthma perform PEFR measures in the home to monitor the status of their airways. Asthma Canada (n.d.) recommends that patients measure their PEFR three times in succession, and then record the best reading. This can be done once or twice daily, before and after taking asthma medicines, and at other times recommended by their health care provider.

Decreased PEFR may indicate the need for further interventions, such as increased doses of bronchodilators, anti-inflammatory medications, or even seeking emergency medical attention. Normal PEFR values vary according to a person's age, gender, and size. In collaboration with a health care provider, patients should measure PEFR when they are not having an exacerbation of respiratory symptoms to help determine their own target (Asthma Canada, n.d.). Once an initial measurement is set, the goal is a PEFR of at least 80% of the target value (Asthma Canada, n.d.).

Delegation and Collaboration

Initial assessment of the patient's condition is a nursing responsibility and cannot be delegated. The skills of follow-up PEFR measurements in a stable patient can be delegated to a UCP, depending on the competence of the UCP to perform this skill in a particular

Continued

Procedural Guideline 25.1 *Use of a Peak Flowmeter—cont'd*

situation and on employer policy. The nurse instructs the UCP to do the following:

- Report immediately to the nurse the patient's difficulty breathing or decrease in PEFR measurement

Equipment

- Peak flowmeter (Fig. 25.21)
- Patient diary/action plan (if appropriate)

Procedural Steps

1. Identify patient using at least two person-specific identifiers (e.g., name and date of birth, or name and medical record number) according to employer policy (Accreditation Canada, 2020).
2. Throughout the procedure, the 4 moments for hand hygiene are to be implemented; hand hygiene should occur before initial patient (or patient environment) contact, before an aseptic procedure, after body fluid exposure risk, and after patient (or patient environment) contact. Additional hand hygiene should be performed when hands are visibly soiled.
3. Review medical record for patient's baseline PEFR (if available).
4. Assess previous PEFR readings and the target set by patient's health care provider.
5. Help patient to stand or to assume high Fowler's position or any other position that promotes optimum lung expansion.
6. Assess patient's baseline knowledge of when and how to use PEFR and correct response to results.
7. Slide clean mouthpiece into base of the numbered scale.
8. Instruct patient to take a deep breath through the nose and slowly blow out through the mouth. Have patient take a second deep breath.
9. Have patient place meter mouthpiece in the mouth and close lips, making a firm seal.
10. Have patient blow out as hard and fast as possible through the mouth only.
11. Monitor PEFR results and assess whether patient is in expected range.
12. Inform patient of their individualized acceptable range and mark the value on meter.
13. If patient is to record PEFR at home, have them demonstrate how to record it accurately on chart using a "traffic light" pattern. A system of asthma zones–green, yellow, and red–is commonly used. Green indicates that the PEFR is 80 to 100% of the patient's personal best value and means that they should continue with the currently prescribed treatment regimen. Yellow indicates that the PEFR is 60 to 80% of the personal best and that the person should add the prescribed quick-relief medication to the treatment regimen and continue with their daily long-term control medications. Red indicates that the PEFR is less than 60% of the patient's personal best and that the person should take the prescribed quick-relief medication and seek medical attention (Fig. 25.22).
14. **Use teach-back:** "I want to make sure that I showed you how to correctly measure your PEFR. Show me how you would use this PEFR device." Develop a revised teaching plan if patient or caregiver is unable to teach back correctly.
15. Compare patient's PEFR with their personal best.
16. Record PEFR measurement before and after therapy and patient's ability and effort to perform PEFR in progress notes in EHR or chart.
17. Instruct patient to clean unit weekly following manufacturer instructions.

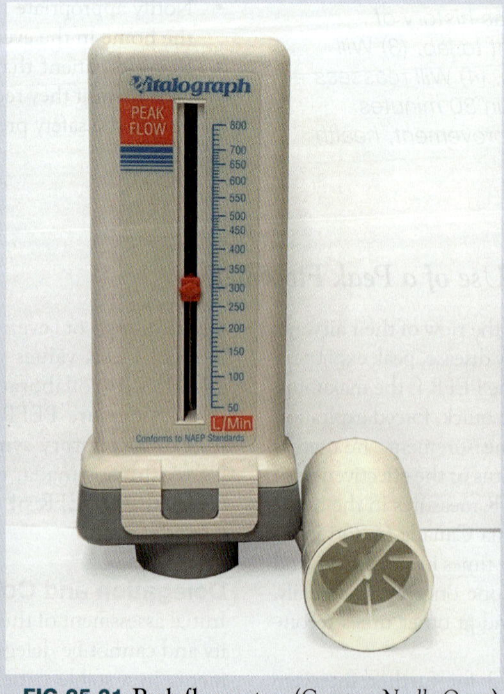

FIG 25.21 Peak flowmeter. (*Courtesy Noelle Ozog.*)

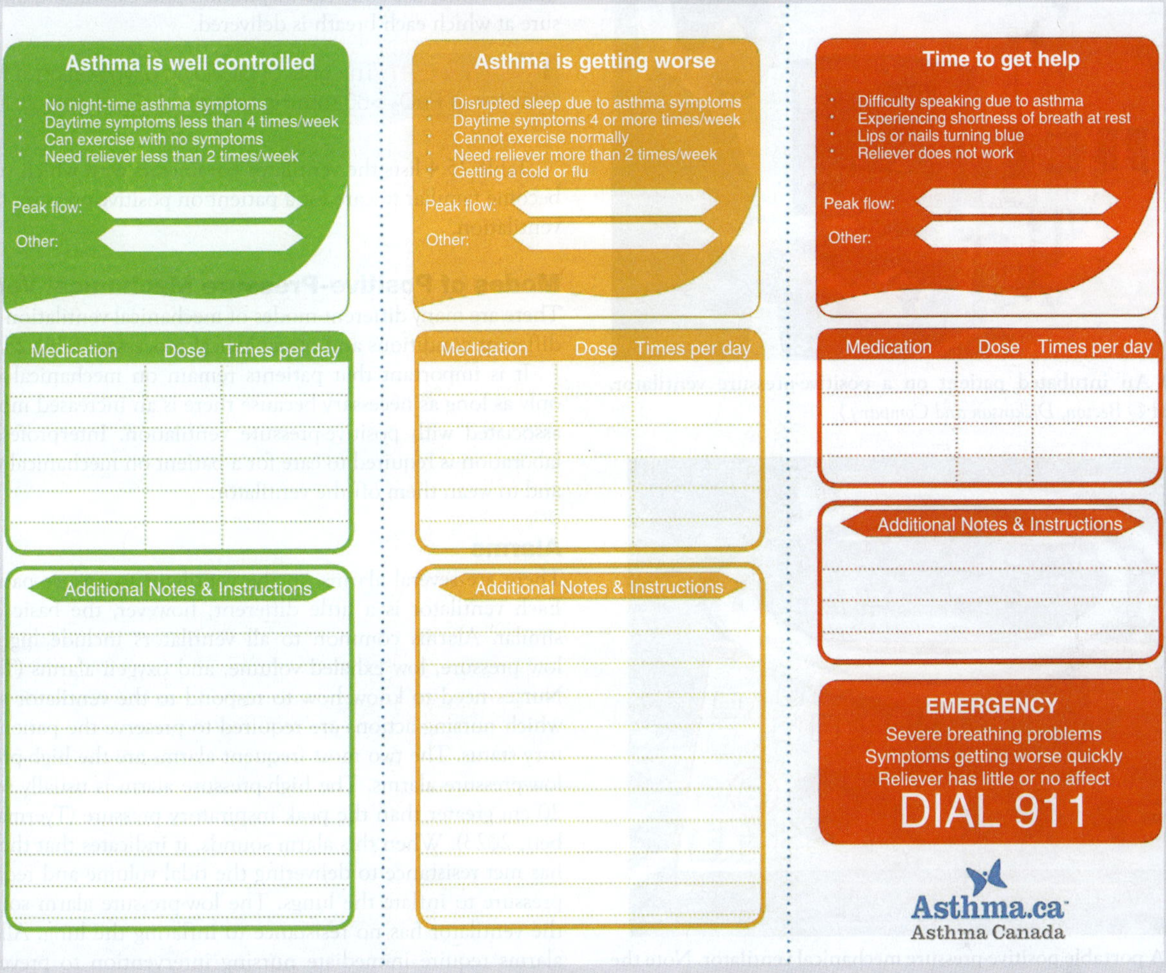
Asthma is well controlled
No night-time asthma symptoms
Daytime symptoms less than 4 times/week
Can exercise with no symptoms
Need reliever less than 2 times/week
Peak flow:
Other:
Medication Dose Times per day
Additional Notes & Instructions
Asthma is getting worse
Disrupted sleep due to asthma symptoms
Daytime symptoms 4 or more times/week
Cannot exercise normally
Need reliever more than 2 times/week
Getting a cold or flu
Peak flow:
Other:
Medication Dose Times per day
Additional Notes & Instructions
Time to get help
Difficulty speaking due to asthma
Experiencing shortness of breath at rest
Lips or nails turning blue
Reliever does not work
Peak flow:
Other:
Medication Dose Times per day
Additional Notes & Instructions
EMERGENCY
Severe breathing problems
Symptoms getting worse quickly
Reliever has little or no affect
DIAL 911
Asthma.ca
Asthma Canada

FIG 25.22 Asthma action plan. (*From Asthma Canada,* https://asthma.ca/wp-content/uploads/2020/06/Asthma-Action-Plan_optimized.pdf. *Reprinted with permission.*)

✦ SKILL 25.5 Care of a Patient on a Mechanical Ventilator

Mechanical ventilation is a life-saving therapy used in patients who have an inability to protect their airway or an illness that leads to respiratory failure. There are two types of mechanical ventilation: negative pressure and positive pressure.

Negative-pressure ventilation is a noninvasive technique that mimics normal physiological ventilation. It is used in the chronic management of patients with primary neuromuscular illnesses that interfere with normal respiratory muscle function (e.g., multiple sclerosis and muscular dystrophy). It is generally not used during acute illness and is therefore not discussed further in this skill.

Positive-pressure ventilation is a common method of ventilation where air is pushed into the lungs through an artificial airway such as an ET or TT (Fig. 25.23). Multiple complications are associated with positive-pressure ventilation, including decreased cardiac output, aspiration, barotrauma, and ventilator-associated events (VAEs) such as ventilator-associated pneumonia (VAP) (see Chapter 23). Be alert for these side effects. The skill described here focuses on positive-pressure mechanical ventilation.

Patients receiving mechanical ventilation are most often in a critical care unit (CCU), but may be seen in long-term care or other community settings (Fig. 25.24). The nurse must collaborate with the respiratory therapist when caring for patients receiving mechanical ventilation. At many institutions, the respiratory therapist is charged with caring for and monitoring the ventilator.

! SAFETY ALERT Do not let the ventilator intimidate you! If the ventilator is not functioning properly, disconnect the patient and ventilate them manually with a bag-valve mask until help arrives. As well, ventilators have a "100% O_2" button that provides 60 seconds of 100% FiO_2, which provides additional time to get help.

Using the Mechanical Ventilator

Mechanical ventilation controls or helps a patient's respirations when they are unable to maintain adequate gas exchange because of respiratory or ventilatory failure. The ventilator takes over the physical work of moving air into and out of the lungs, but it does not replace or alter the physiological function of the lung. Mechanical ventilation maintains or improves ventilation, oxygenation, and breathing pattern.

Ventilator Settings

The mechanical ventilator has a number of settings to adjust the amount of oxygen delivered, the number of breaths per minute, the

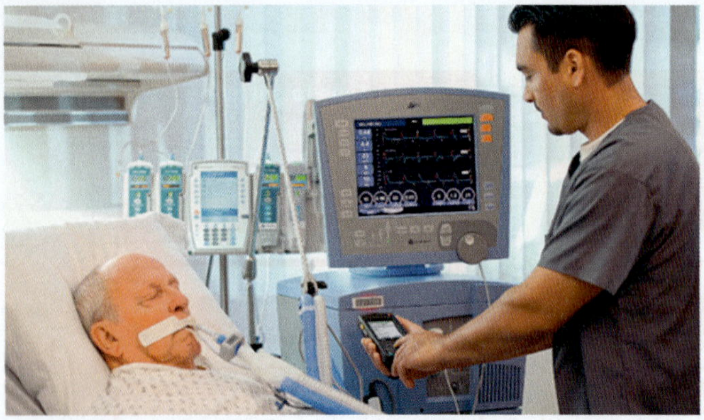

FIG 25.23 An intubated patient on a positive-pressure ventilator. *(Courtesy and © Becton, Dickinson and Company.)*

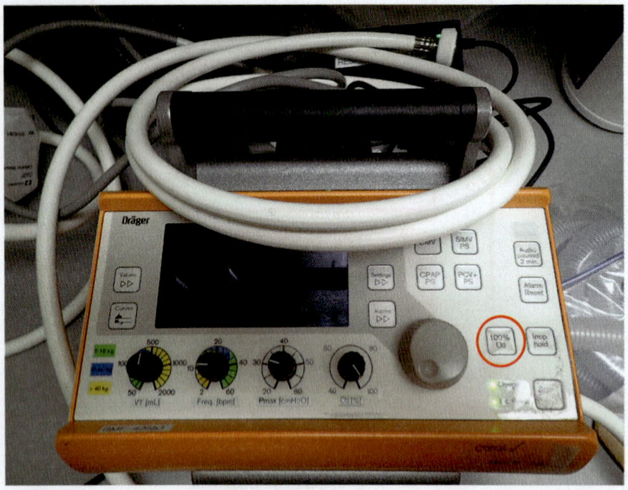

FIG 25.24 A portable positive-pressure mechanical ventilator. Note the 100% O_2 button. *(Courtesy Noelle Ozog.)*

tidal volume, the time for inspiration and expiration, and the pressure at which each breath is delivered.

> **! SAFEY ALERT** The goal of providing oxygenation is to maintain a PaO_2 >60 mm Hg using an FiO_2 of 40% or less.

Table 25.4 lists the ventilator parameters with which you need to become familiar to care for a patient on positive-pressure mechanical ventilation.

Modes of Positive-Pressure Mechanical Ventilation

There are many different modes of mechanical ventilation to support different conditions and physiological processes (Table 25.5).

It is important that patients remain on mechanical ventilation only as long as necessary because there is an increased mortality risk associated with positive-pressure ventilation. Interprofessional collaboration is required to care for a patient on mechanical ventilation and to wean them off the ventilator.

Alarms

There are several alarms on the ventilator to ensure patient safety. Each ventilator is a little different; however, the basic alarms are similar. Alarms common to all ventilators include high pressure, low pressure, low exhaled volume, and oxygen alarms (Table 25.6). Nurses need to know how to respond to the ventilator alarms and which nursing actions are required to preserve the patient's respiratory status. The two most frequent alarms are the high-pressure and low-pressure alarms. The high-pressure alarm is usually set to 10 to 20 cm greater than the peak inspiratory pressure (Tyerman & Cobbett, 2023). When this alarm sounds, it indicates that the ventilator has met resistance to delivering the tidal volume and requires more pressure to inflate the lungs. The low-pressure alarm sounds when the ventilator has no resistance to inflating the lung. All ventilator alarms require immediate nursing intervention to prevent patient harm.

TABLE 25.4

Ventilator Parameters

Parameter	Definition	Ventilator Setting
Tidal volume (V_t)	Amount of air inspired and expired with each breath; can be set by ventilator or can measure patient's own spontaneous breaths	<10 mL/kg of patient body weight 4–6 mL/kg in patients with ARDS to avoid lung injury
Respiratory rate (R or RR)	Number of breaths delivered by ventilator per minute	Usually 10–20 breaths/min Usually adjusted with a set V_t to maintain specific $PaCO_2$, and depending on clinical goals (rest versus weaning)
Fraction of inspired oxygen (FiO_2)	Amount of oxygen that patient receives	Ideally less than 50% to maintain PaO_2 >60 mm Hg and SpO_2 >90%
Positive end-expiratory pressure (PEEP)	Positive pressure applied at end expiration of ventilator breaths to open alveoli and improve oxygenation	5 cm H_2O approximates physiological PEEP. May require higher levels (10–20 cm H_2O) in respiratory failure (e.g., refractory hypoxemia). If patient has a PEEP >10 cm H_2O, the circuit should not be interrupted.
Sensitivity	Determines patient's inspiratory effort required to trigger the ventilator	A breath can be triggered by a change in either flow or pressure. Pressure trigger is usually 0.5–1.5 cm H_{20} below baseline. Flow trigger is usually 1–3 L/min below baseline.
I:E ratio	Comparison of inspiratory (I) to expiratory (E) time	**Example:** Inspiration 0.5 seconds, expiration 1 second, then I:E = 1:2. Usually set to 1:2 to 1:3 because expiration is typically longer than inspiration. Can use inverse ratios for certain disease states such as ARDS in attempt to open alveoli.
Exhaled minute ventilation (V_E)	Measures exhaled minute ventilations in litres	Alarm set to 15% greater than patient's average V_E

ARDS, Acute respiratory distress syndrome; *$PaCO_2$*, partial pressure of carbon dioxide; *PaO_2*, partial pressure of oxygen; *SpO_2*, pulse oximetry.

Data from Gallagher, J. (2017). Invasive mechanical ventilation through an artificial airway). In D. L. Wiegand (Ed.), *AACN procedure manual for high acuity, progressive, and critical care* (7th ed., pp. 226–248). Elsevier; Urden, L., Stacy, K. M., & Lough, M. E. (2016). *Priorities in critical care nursing* (7th ed.). Mosby.

TABLE 25.5

Modes of Mechanical Ventilation

Mode	Ventilator Controls	Patient Controls	Indications	Nursing Considerations
Low Frequency				
Continuous positive airway pressure (CPAP)	Positive pressure during entire respiratory cycle	Spontaneous breathing	Hypoxemic respiratory failure Weaning	Helps open alveoli at end expiration, thereby improving oxygenation. Patients with COPD may tire after long hours of CPAP and require increased pressure support. Used in both invasive and noninvasive ventilation modes.
Pressure support ventilation (PSV)	Preset amount of positive pressure	Patient determines rate and tidal volume	Augmenting a spontaneously breathing patient's inspiratory efforts	Helps overcome resistance of airway and ventilator tubing. Reduces patient work of breathing and improves ventilator-patient synchrony.
Assist-control (AC) or continuous mandatory ventilation (CMV)	Backup control delivers preset number of breaths at set volume	Initiation of breathing	*Volume-controlled CMV:* patients with weak respiratory muscles *Pressure-controlled CMV:* Patients with increased airway resistance or decreased lung compliance	Watch for volutrauma in volume-controlled CMV. Watch for hypercapnia in pressure-controlled CMV. Sedation may be needed to control respiratory rate.
Synchronized intermittent mandatory ventilation (SIMV)	Set number of breaths at specified volume	Some patients breathe spontaneously between SIMV breaths at volumes differing from those set	Primary method of ventilation in many settings	Requires frequent monitoring during weaning from mechanical ventilation. May increase patient's work of breathing.
Pressure-regulated volume-control ventilation (PRVCV or PRVC)	A preset tidal volume at the lowest possible airway pressure (pressure will not exceed preset maximum limit)		Patient with changing pulmonary mechanics and dynamics	Variation of CMV combining the feature of both volume- and pressure-control settings. Potential complications are limited when compared with AC or pressure controlled–intermittent mandatory ventilation (PC-IMV) modes.
Airway pressure release ventilation (APRV)	Inspiratory and expiratory levels of CPAP are applied for predetermined periods of time	Spontaneous breathing mode, spontaneous breathing can occur at both levels	Recruits alveoli with decreased risk of high peak pressures, decreasing risk of barotrauma	Patient should be monitored for hypercapnia.
High Frequency				
High-frequency jet ventilation (HFJV)	Delivers gas rapidly under low pressure via special injector cannula Delivers 100–600 cycles/min with lower-than-normal tidal volumes		Uncommon in adults; more commonly used in neonates	Patient on any mode of high-frequency ventilation requires continuous sedation and neuromuscular blocking medication administration. Requires intensive monitoring and care.
High-frequency oscillatory ventilation (HFOV)	Delivers 900–3000 cycles/min with very small tidal volumes. Airway pressure controlled		Most common high-frequency type. Uncommon in adults; more commonly used in infants and children.	Maintains alveolar ventilation with low airway pressure; useful for treating esophageal or bronchopleural fistulas; helps avert barotraumas in high-risk patients if used early in treatment. Requires use of continuous sedation and neuromuscular blocking medication. Requires intensive monitoring and care.

COPD, Chronic obstructive pulmonary disease.

Data from Urden, L. D., Stacy, K. M., & Lough, M. E. (2016). *Priorities in critical care nursing* (7th ed.). Mosby.

TABLE 25.6

Troubleshooting Mechanical Ventilation

Ventilator Alarm	Possible Causes	Nursing Interventions
Sudden increase in peak airway pressure (high-pressure alarm)	Coughing Airway plugging/excess secretions Changes in patient position Pneumothorax Incorrect ET position Kinked ventilator circuit Excessive water in ventilator circuit Patient biting tube Patient not in synchrony with ventilator Ventilator malfunction	Clear secretions by suctioning. Reposition patient. Assess breath sounds and chest wall movement. Verify placement of ET. Verify centimetre level of ET. Check circuit; unkink tubing. Drain ventilator tubing. Insert bite block. Sedate patient. Notify health care provider if interventions are not effective.
Gradual increase in peak airway pressure	Decreasing lung compliance Exacerbation of acute process	Evaluate breath sounds; suction. Check for reversible causes: airway plugging, bronchospasm. Notify health care provider if interventions are not effective.
Decrease in peak airway pressure (low-pressure alarm)	Patient disconnected from ventilator Leak in ventilator circuit ET displaced into pharynx Cuff not inflated properly Improved lung compliance Decrease in amount of secretions	Check for disconnection. Evaluate circuit connections; tighten loose connections. Assess cuff for appropriate pressure (see Skill 25.4).
Change in minute ventilation or tidal volume	Leak in ET cuff Patient stops spontaneously breathing Other conditions that trigger low- or high-pressure alarms	Check cuff seal (see Skill 25.4). Evaluate patient.
Increase in respiratory rate	Patient anxiety Increased metabolic demand Hypoxia	Reassure patient. Evaluate body temperature, heart rate, and rhythm. Monitor pulse oximetry.
Apnea	Respiratory arrest Oversedation Incidental extubation	Reverse/discontinue sedating medications. Provide breaths via self-inflating resuscitation bag. Prepare for reintubation if tube is dislodged and patient requires it.
Ventilator inoperative or low battery	Equipment malfunction Machine not plugged in	Plug in machine. Notify respiratory therapist. Provide breaths via self-inflating resuscitation bag if necessary.

ET, Endotracheal tube.

Data from Gallagher, J. (2017). Invasive mechanical ventilation through an artificial airway). In D. L. Wiegand (Ed.), *AACN procedure manual for high acuity, progressive, and critical care* (7th ed., pp. 226–248). Elsevier; Urden, L. D., Stacy, K. M., & Lough, M. E. (2016). *Priorities in critical care nursing* (7th ed.). Mosby.

Ventilator-Associated Events

VAP, a type of VAE, has an estimated 5.8% mortality rate in patients receiving mechanical ventilation and costs the Canadian health care system an estimated $46 million each year (Muscedere et al., 2008), although more recent Canadian estimates are limited. The simplified way to identify VAP includes observing deterioration in the patient's respiratory status after a period of stability while on the ventilator, objective evidence of inflammation or infection, and laboratory evidence of respiratory infection. A patient can be considered to have acquired VAP only after they have received mechanical ventilation for more than 2 calendar days (Centers for Disease Control and Prevention, 2023).

In an attempt to decrease the incidence of VAEs, practice bundles have been developed and implemented at health care facilities across the country (see Chapter 23). Other interventions exist, although they are not listed specifically within the care bundles being used to decrease the risk of VAEs. One of these interventions is to maintain continuous ET cuff pressure between 20 and 30 cm H_2O pressure to decrease the risk of microaspiration of oral secretions and gastric contents or tracheal ischemic lesions (Klompas, 2023). Refer to Skill 23.4 for directions for this procedure. Using ETs that allow for drainage of subglottic secretions has been shown to decrease VAP risk but not mortality or length of CCU stay (Klompas, 2023).

Delegation and Collaboration

The skill of caring for a patient on a mechanical ventilator cannot be delegated to a UCP. The nurse directs the UCP to do the following:

- Report immediately to the nurse any change in the patient's respiratory status, vital signs, or oxygen saturation and if patient indicates breathlessness
- Inform the nurse immediately if any of the ventilator alarms sound.
- Help in daily care, such as bathing and repositioning the patient

Interprofessional collaboration is essential in optimizing care and ensuring patient safety. In some settings, the respiratory therapist may be responsible for managing the ventilator, but the nurse retains primary responsibility for the patient. In some settings, the health care provider may prescribe the ventilator settings, whereas in other facilities employer policy dictates these settings. Using interprofessional collaboration, the nurse must continually communicate assessment findings about the patient's respiratory status in response to mechanical ventilation, and any concerns, to maintain patient safety and provide the best care possible.

Equipment

- Artificial airway
- Appropriate mechanical ventilator
- Heater and humidifier for circuit
- Oxygen source
- Pulse oximetry (SpO_2) probe and monitor
- Electrocardiogram (ECG) monitoring (if in a CCU or per institutional policy)
- Capnography (end-tidal CO_2 [$EtCO_2$]) window and monitor (if available)
- Heat and moisture exchange (HME) filter
- Stethoscope
- 5- or 10-mL syringe
- Oral airway or bite block, as needed
- Manual self-inflating resuscitation bag (bag-valve mask) with oxygen-connecting tubing and flowmeter
- Appropriately sized resuscitation face mask
- Cuff pressure monitoring device
- Sedation monitoring scale (e.g., Richmond Agitation Sedation Scale) if patient is receiving sedation
- PPE per employer policy
- Suction equipment at bedside (in-line/individual catheters)
- Suction equipment for subglottic and oral suctioning
- Chlorhexidine gluconate (CHG) solution (0.12%), oral swab, and toothbrush for oral care
- Method for patient communication (e.g., letter/picture board, common word lists)
- Ventilator flow sheet to document ventilator changes and settings (may be a paper flow sheet or part of the EHR)

STEP	RATIONALE

ASSESSMENT

STEP	RATIONALE
1. Identify patient using at least two person-specific identifiers (e.g., name and date of birth, or name and medical record number) according to employer policy.	Ensures correct patient. Complies with Accreditation Canada's standards and improves patient safety (Accreditation Canada, 2020).
2. Throughout the procedure, the 4 moments for hand hygiene are to be implemented; hand hygiene should occur before initial patient (or patient environment) contact, before an aseptic procedure, after body fluid exposure risk, and after patient (or patient environment) contact. Additional hand hygiene should be performed when hands are visibly soiled.	Proper hand hygiene helps prevent the spread of infectious agents to health care providers
3. Assess patient's LOC and ability to cooperate with mechanical ventilation and tolerate special positioning, such as HOB at 30 degrees.	Determines patient's ability to cooperate and understand aspects of care. Anxious and combative patients may require sedation to tolerate mechanical ventilation.
4. Assess patient's need for sedation (check employer policy).	Sedation is often used to improve patient tolerance of the ventilator (Davidson et al., 2016).

Critical Decision Point *When patients on mechanical ventilation become excessively anxious or combative or try to override the ventilator, sedation is often used. Be aware that sedation is associated with increased length of time on the ventilator, increased risk of delirium, and increased mortality* (Davidson et al., 2016). *Follow employer policy for administering sedation medication and monitoring sedation levels.*

STEP	RATIONALE
5. Assess patient's respiratory status, including symmetry of chest wall expansion, respiratory rate and depth, sputum production (amount, characteristics), and lung sounds (see Chapter 8), and assess for signs and symptoms associated with hypoxia (see Box 25.1).	Decreased chest wall movement; crackles or decreased or absent lung sounds; increased respiratory rate; increased sputum production; or signs of worsening hypoxia indicate need for mechanical ventilation or changes in current ventilator settings to improve oxygenation and ventilation.
6. Assess patient's cardiovascular condition, including blood pressure, heart rate, regularity of heart rate, and quality of peripheral pulses (see Chapter 8).	Positive-pressure mechanical ventilation can increase patient's intrathoracic pressure. This can cause a decrease in cardiac output and cardiovascular function (Davidson et al., 2016).
7. Assess for signs and symptoms of inadvertent extubation (able to vocalize, low-pressure ventilator alarms, decreased or absent breath sounds, gastric distension, changes in ET depth according to markings, changes in $EtCO_2$ waveform and values, patient holding tube with hand).	Inadvertent extubation can lead to a decrease in patient oxygenation and cardiopulmonary status.

Critical Decision Point *Sometimes patients tolerate inadvertent extubation. The nurse needs to carefully assess the patient and be prepared to apply a different type of oxygen delivery device (nasal cannula, face mask, or NIPPV) or to reintubate the patient* (Hill & Kramer, 2022). *The nurse may need to perform ventilation with a bag-valve mask until a health care provider who can reintubate the patient arrives in the room.*

STEP	RATIONALE
8. Check ventilator, $EtCO_2$ (if available), SpO_2, and ventilator and cardiac alarms at beginning of each shift and periodically throughout care and compare with health care provider prescription.	Verifies that ventilator settings are as prescribed. Ensures patient safety.

STEP	RATIONALE

ASSESSMENT

9. Apply clean gloves and verify placement of artificial airway through auscultation of lung sounds, verification of distal tip marking on ET, and/or $EtCO_2$ value. Verify that tube is secure and stable (see Chapter 23).	Reduces transmission of microorganisms. Prevents migration of tube into right or left bronchus and accidental extubation.

Critical Decision Point *When patients have periodic chest X-ray film examinations, verify placement of the artificial airway.*

a. Auscultate over trachea for presence of air leak. When air leak is present, you will hear movement of air over trachea. Assess and compare inhaled and exhaled tidal volumes as measured by ventilator.	Cuff of artificial airway needs to be inflated to create a seal in order for positive-pressure ventilation to occur.
b. Use cuff pressure monitoring device.	Cuff pressure of ET should be between 20 and 30 cm H_2O (Klompas, 2023). Use 10-mL syringe to inflate or deflate cuff to achieve desired pressure.

Critical Decision Point *ET cuff pressures need to be monitored carefully. Pressures that are too low lead to microaspiration of oral and subglottic secretions, increasing the patient's risk of developing VAP. If the cuff pressures are too high, the patient is at risk of developing tracheal mucosal damage* (Santiago-Rosado et al., 2022). *Hypopharyngeal suctioning should be performed before a cuff is deflated to decrease risk of aspiration of secretions* (Hyzy, 2023).

10. Ensure that suction system is functioning properly.	It is important to know that the emergency equipment is functioning before it is needed.
11. Observe for patent airway and, if necessary, remove airway secretions by suctioning (see Chapter 23). Remove and dispose of gloves.	Secretions plug airway, decreasing amount of oxygen available for gas exchange in lung. Secretions also occlude T-tube or tracheostomy collar, impeding oxygen delivery to patient.

Critical Decision Point *Routine suctioning of the patient should be avoided* (Blakeman et al., 2022). *Indications for suctioning include coarse crackles auscultated over trachea, the presence of a saw-tooth pattern in the pressure and flow curves on the ventilator, acutely increased peak inspiratory pressures or decreased tidal volumes, and visible secretions in the airway* (Blakeman et al., 2022).

12. Assess integrity of patient's oral mucous membrane and skin around tube stabilization device.	Provides baseline to recognize signs of oral mucous membrane or skin breakdown.
13. If available, note patient's most recent ABG results or SpO_2. Determine whether any factors have changed during mechanical ventilation.	Objectively documents patient's pH, arterial oxygen, arterial CO_2, or SaO_2.
14. Determine method for communication with patient. If possible, review previous communication techniques with patient and caregiver.	Patients with an artificial airway and mechanical ventilation cannot communicate verbally. Practise person-centred care and choose a communication tool based on patient preference; reassess and document its effectiveness regularly.
15. Review patient's medical record for prescription for mechanical ventilation, noting mode of ventilation, respiratory rate, oxygen setting, pressure support, PEEP, and tidal volume.	Mechanical ventilation and changes in ventilator settings require health care provider prescription. Knowing mode of ventilation should inform nurse about priority values to monitor.

NURSING DIAGNOSES

- Ineffective airway clearance
- Impaired spontaneous ventilation
- Ineffective breathing pattern
- Impaired gas exchange
- Dysfunctional ventilatory weaning response
- Impaired verbal communication
- Potential for infection
- Potential for impaired oral mucous membrane

Related factors and risk factors are individualized on the basis of patient's condition or needs.

PLANNING

1. Expected outcomes following completion of procedure:	
• Patient has improved lung expansion.	As patient's lungs and lung mechanics improve, lung expansion increases.
• Patient maintains or has improving PaO_2 and $PaCO_2$, as well as pH levels and oxygen saturation within normal range or at patient baseline.	Verifies that ventilator settings are effective in improving or maintaining patient's level of oxygenation and ventilation.

STEP	RATIONALE
PLANNING	
• Patient's vital signs and respiratory assessment parameters improve.	Reduced pulse and respiratory rate, improved mental status, improved skin colour, and decreased use of accessory and abdominal muscles occur because patient's work of breathing decreases as level of oxygenation improves.
• Patient experiences reduction in feelings of dyspnea and work of breathing. NOTE: Dyspnea scales, such as the Medical Research Council Dyspnea Scale, are available to provide more objective data.	Indicates effectiveness of therapy.
• Patient uses communication board, paper and pencil, mobile device, or computer to state needs.	Selected communication system matches patient's abilities. Helps patient express their needs and wishes.
2. Explain ventilator system to patient and caregiver and be sure to include purpose of and reasons for initiation of mechanical ventilation.	Reinforces need for ventilation to improve patient condition.
3. Position patient with HOB elevated 45 degrees (unless contraindicated).	Positioning patients with HOB elevated 45 degrees (semirecumbent position) prevents clinical VAP better than positioning in the supine position (Klompas, 2023).
IMPLEMENTATION	
1. Apply clean gloves and appropriate PPE (mask, gown, and goggles if secretions are projectile or if patient is on additional precautions).	Reduces transmission of microorganisms and exposure to pulmonary secretions.
2. Attach mechanical ventilator to ET or TT if not already attached or connected to patient. Observe for proper functioning of mechanical ventilator.	Connects artificial airway to ventilator and ensures closed system, which enables ventilator to exert appropriate pressure or volume to meet patient's oxygen and ventilation demands.

Critical Decision Point *The mechanical ventilator must be programmed with accurate settings before being attached to the patient. This step is most often the responsibility of the respiratory therapist; it requires interprofessional collaboration and is a nursing responsibility.*

STEP	RATIONALE
3. Verify that ET or TT is properly positioned during an inspiratory and expiratory cycle by listening to both lungs and assessing chest wall symmetry. Capnography can also be used to verify proper placement (Hyzy, 2023). When chest X-ray film is available, observe tube placement.	Properly placed artificial airway ensures that both lungs are ventilated equally. Improper airway placement leads to unilateral lung ventilation or inadequate oxygenation.
4. Observe patient for synchronization with mechanical ventilation and response to therapy.	Ensures that patient is comfortable using ventilator and has not experienced any adverse hemodynamic effects.
5. Monitor heart rate, blood pressure, respiratory rate, temperature, and cardiac rhythm routinely (see employer policy).	Implementation of mechanical ventilation results in decreased venous return and associated hemodynamic changes. The patient is also at increased risk of developing an infection (Klompas, 2023), and thus temperature needs to be monitored.
6. Reassess and mark level of ET at lips or nares (see Chapter 23). Ensure that ET is secured.	Provides measure to compare with baseline for depth of tube placement. ET must be placed through vocal cords into trachea. Helps to ensure that tube is not too close to carina or in right main-stem bronchus. ET may be secured with use of tape or commercial tube holder.
7. Ensure that suction equipment is set up and functioning, including oral suctioning (see Chapter 23).	The nurse needs to provide airway care and suctioning of ET or TT as needed to prevent plugging of airway and to reduce risk of infection.
8. Reposition patient regularly (minimum of every 2 hours), maintaining an HOB elevation of 45 degrees. In some instances, patient may even be placed in prone position. Monitor SpO_2 levels during and after positioning.	Elevated HOB positioning improves oxygenation and ventilation. In addition, HOB elevation reduces risk of VAP (Coppadoro et al., 2019). SpO_2 drops during position change, but should recover once patient has been repositioned. A sustained drop in SpO_2 indicates that patient is unable to tolerate that particular position at that time. Regular turning reduces risk of pressure injury development involving the skin. Some patients cannot safely have the HOB elevated. Prone positioning requires assistance of four or five staff members or a specialty bed; it is not associated with a difference in VAP rates when compared with patients placed in semirecumbent position (Coppadoro et al., 2019).

Critical Decision Point *Assess oral cavity for need for suctioning before repositioning patient. After repositioning, check cuff pressures and level of ET.*

STEP	RATIONALE
IMPLEMENTATION	
9. Collaborate with health care provider frequently about status of patient, response to therapy, and ongoing monitoring.	Assesses oxygenation status and continued need for mechanical ventilation.
a. Monitor SpO_2 continuously.	Provides ability to continually assess oxygenation levels.
b. Monitor $EtCO_2$ continually (if available and indicated) and serial ABG levels to detect possible overventilation or inadequate alveolar ventilation.	Overventilation causes respiratory alkalosis from decreased CO_2. Inadequate alveolar ventilation causes respiratory acidosis from increased hypercapnia.
c. Obtain ABG levels with changes in patient's condition or ventilator changes per provider prescription.	Provides more accurate measure of oxygen saturation and PaO_2 and $PaCO_2$.
10. Perform hourly safety checks on patient and ventilator system:	
a. Make sure that patient can reach call light.	Provides mechanism for patient to contact health care personnel.
b. Check security of all ventilator connections; make sure that alarms are all turned on, including both high- and low-pressure alarms and volume alarms.	Ensures continuous safe and proper functioning of ventilator system. Enables identification and correction of problems in a timely manner.
c. Verify that all ventilator settings are correct and correspond to health care provider prescription.	Maintains integrity of system and ensures that all settings are consistent with health care provider prescription.
d. Check and refill humidifier as needed. Check corrugated tubing for condensation; drain away from patient but not into humidifier, and appropriately discard liquid.	Ensures continuous humidification. Condensation that returns to humidifier can potentially cause bacterial contamination. Condensation that drains into patient can cause pneumonia or severe coughing episode that can lead to increased patient distress (Vargas et al., 2017).
e. When present, observe temperature gauges on panel of mechanical ventilator, making sure that gas is delivered at correct temperature. Desired temperature of inspired gas is 35–37°C (95–98.6°F).	The temperature of inspired gas artificially alters patient's body temperature.
11. Perform mouth care at least every 12 hours (can be every 1–2 hours, depending on patent status) with CHG (Healthcare Excellence Canada, 2016) to brush teeth, gums, and tongue with soft toothbrush. Water-based moisturizer should be applied every 2–4 hours (see Chapter 18).	VAP is common and is associated with microaspiration of oropharyngeal secretions. Frequent mouth care reduces patient's risk for VAP. Oral care helps reduce risk of pneumonias (Hess, 2022).
12. Insert bite block if patient bites ET.	Prevents patient from occluding airway. Oral mucous membranes and tongue need to be monitored for any signs of breakdown.
13. Administer sedating medications only as prescribed.	Sedating medications help to keep patient comfortable and breathing in synchrony with ventilator, but in excess, they can increase length of CCU stay (Davidson et al., 2016).
14. Perform daily interruption in sedation; assess readiness to extubate.	Sometimes patients need to be sedated to keep them comfortable or to increase synchrony with ventilator (Davidson et al., 2016). Providing daily interruptions of sedation allows assessment for weaning, delirium, and readiness to extubate (Sharma et al., 2022).
15. Institute venous thromboembolism (VTE) prophylaxis as prescribed. This includes use of anticoagulants (if no contraindications such as bleeding are present) and sequential compression devices.	VTE prevention protocols reduce patient's risk (Tang et al., 2022).
16. Perform nursing activities to prevent hazards of immobility (e.g., help patient change position, perform range-of-motion exercises, and encourage independence and early mobility as tolerated) (see Chapter 12).	Maintaining activity and promoting early mobility avoids complications associated with decreased mobility, such as pressure injuries, pneumonia, VTE, and activity intolerance. Patients receiving mechanical ventilation need help with activity but can ambulate.
17. Ensure that communication method is in place for patient. Practise person-centred care and use methods that the patient prefers (e.g., letter/picture boards, common word and phrase lists, writing utensil and paper, or a computer, tablet, or smartphone).	Patients unable to communicate report feeling increased fear compared with patients who are able to communicate while receiving mechanical ventilation (Roberts et al., 2019).
18. Keep patient and caregiver informed about progress and plan for weaning off mechanical ventilator.	Apprehension and anxiety occur when patient and caregiver are not properly informed about progress, changes in care, or changes in ventilator setting.
19. Remove and dispose of PPE.	Reduces transmission of microorganisms and exposure to pulmonary secretions.

STEP	RATIONALE
EVALUATION	
1. Monitor and evaluate patient's response to mechanical ventilation every 1–4 hours:	Patients requiring mechanical ventilation have unstable physiological status. It is important to perform key focused evaluation measures frequently as patient's condition warrants.
a. *Neurological assessment:* LOC, orientation, sleepiness, changes in anxiety, sedation levels	
b. *Pulmonary assessment:* Lung sounds, airway clearance, work of breathing, breathing pattern, rate of respirations, SpO_2, $EtCO_2$	
c. *Cardiovascular assessment:* Vital signs, heart rhythm, heart sounds, lower-extremity edema, pulse quality	
2. Observe SpO_2 and $EtCO_2$ and monitor gas exchange.	Documents patient's level of oxygenation and ventilation.
3. Observe integrity of patient's ventilator system.	Ensures adequate delivery of mechanical ventilation.
4. Observe and evaluate effectiveness of person-centred communication methods:	Communication, or lack of it, increases patient's frustration, anxiety, and depression during mechanical ventilation and weaning process.
a. Ask patient if needs and concerns are addressed.	
b. Observe for signs of frustration (e.g., patient shaking head in irritation, crying, withdrawal).	
c. Observe patient and caregiver and health care personnel use of communication methods.	
5. Use **teach-back:** "I want to be sure I explained how the ventilator works and why we are using it to treat your partner. Explain to me why mechanical ventilation is necessary." Develop a revised teaching plan if caregiver is unable to teach back correctly.	Allow caregiver opportunity to ask questions and for clarification about ventilator use. Determines patient's and caregiver's level of understanding of topic (Yen & Leasure, 2019).

Unexpected Outcomes	Related Interventions
1. Patient experiences a VAE such as VAP.	• Notify health care provider. • Conduct complete cardiac and pulmonary assessment. • Be prepared for initiation of antibiotic therapy.
2. Patient experiences no improvement in or worsening of respiratory status.	• Notify health care provider. • Reassess patient. • Consider measures to improve airway patency, including, but not limited to, deep breathing and coughing techniques, positioning patient with HOB elevated (unless contraindicated), and oropharyngeal or orotracheal suctioning (Chapter 23). • Assess integrity of ventilator system. • Expect ventilator change (increased PEEP, increase in respiratory rate or tidal volume).
3. Patient experiences self-extubation.	• Remain with patient and call for help. • Maintain patent airway by suctioning and inserting oral airway. • Provide oxygen. • Assess patient's respiratory status and level of oxygenation and ventilation. • Notify health care provider. • Patient may need sedation and/or use of restraints to prevent this complication from occurring in the future (see Chapter 14).
4. Patient experiences barotrauma such as tension pneumothorax (an emergency situation).	• Remain with patient and call for help. • Remove patient from ventilator and ventilate patient with bag-valve mask (see Chapter 28). • Notify health care provider. • Ask additional personnel to obtain patient's vital signs and obtain chest tube insertion kit.
5. Patient develops hemodynamic instability.	• Remain with patient and call for help. • Notify health care provider. • Be prepared to change ventilator settings or initiate intravenous inotropes or vasopressors.

Communication and Documentation

- Document the following in progress notes in EHR or chart: respiratory assessment findings, mode of mechanical ventilation, oxygen level, actual patient tidal volume, actual patient respiratory rate, peak inspiratory pressure, vital signs, size and level of ET, ABG results (if performed as a point-of-care test), patient level of comfort, sedation-level scores (if sedation is used), and degree of HOB elevation.
- Document any nursing interventions that are performed, including oral care, repositioning, range-of-motion exercises, medications that were administered, and suctioning.
- Document your evaluation of patient and caregiver learning.
- Communicate sudden change in patient's respiratory status, ventilator-associated problems, or adverse reactions to nurse in charge or health care provider.

Special Considerations

Teaching

- Teach patient and caregiver about the rationale for mechanical ventilation and the alarms and what they mean.
- Teach patient and caregiver preferred alternative communication techniques to reduce frustration and fear.
- Teach patient about rationale for all interventions, including oral care and frequent repositioning.

Pediatric

- Increasing numbers of children are on home mechanical ventilation. For this reason, it is important to include the parent in the child's care as appropriate. Parents also need to be prepared that, in the event readmission to hospital occurs, the child may not be readmitted to a CCU but rather may remain on the general medical or surgical area owing to the chronic nature of the illness (Hockenberry et al., 2024).
- Once the child is stable on the mechanical ventilator, promote normal or near-normal activities as the child's condition warrants (e.g., promote play, resume school activities, and encourage mobility).

Gerontological

- Presence of comorbidities increases patient's risk for longer stays in CCU, hospital.
- Older persons do not usually tolerate sedative or antianxiety medications prescribed. The prescribed dose is based on the patient's baseline kidney and liver functions (Boscart et al., 2023).

Care in the Community: Home Management

- Planning for home ventilation is performed by an interprofessional team.
- Patients need to be assessed for acceptance of ventilator dependence and the ability to understand and demonstrate daily care of the artificial airway, ventilator, and ventilator circuit.
- Patients also need their home environment, personal/monetary resources, and availability of community care resources assessed. Family caregiving costs for children who need home ventilation are substantial: median \$9 929 monthly (Nonoyama et al., 2020).
- Evaluate the following areas during each visit: environmental safety assessment, oxygen flow, alarm system, inspiratory pressure, high-pressure alarm, tidal volume setting, humidifier, respiratory rate, tubing, temperature, resuscitation bag, tracheostomy care, breath sounds, suctioning, and tubing changes.
- Teach patient and caregiver what to do in case of respiratory distress or power failure. Check to determine availability of emergency batteries and instruct caregiver in use of the bag-valve mask (see Chapter 28).

✦ REVIEW QUESTIONS

A 59-year-old patient (he/him) with a history of well-controlled chronic obstructive pulmonary disease (COPD) developed an upper respiratory tract infection 2 weeks ago and was treated with antibiotics. He completed his full course of antibiotics, but his symptoms continued. He has a 4-day history of fever above 39.4°C, fatigue, productive cough with yellow sputum, worsening dyspnea, and decreased activity tolerance. His health care provider does a complete examination, prescribes a chest X-ray, and obtains blood work, including cultures. Preliminary chest X-ray results indicate pneumonia in right lower lobe; white blood cell count is 17. He is admitted to a general medicine floor for treatment with intravenous (IV) antibiotics, supplemental oxygen at 2 L/min via nasal cannula, and pulmonary hygiene measures.

Review Questions 1 to 3 relate to the case study presented here.

1. The nurse observes the patient and notices that he is fatigued, has difficulty speaking, and in general looks very uncomfortable. The nurse decides to do a focused assessment. Which system(s) will the nurse assess, and what information does the nurse expect to find?

2. The patient's condition continues to worsen, and the nurse pages the health care provider. The health care provider, who is in the room, tells the unregulated care provider (UCP) to place the patient on a simple face mask at 50% fraction of inspired oxygen (FiO_2) with a flow rate of 10 L/min and to encourage the patient to use an incentive spirometer. Why should the nurse question this prescription?

3. The patient is placed on a Venturi mask at 45% FiO_2, the first dose of IV antibiotic is administered, and the patient continues to be in distress. Patient now has SpO_2 of 85%, respiratory rate of 32 breaths/min, heart rate of 110 beats/min, blood pressure of 144/76 mm Hg, and temperature of 38.7°C. Crackles persist in the right lower lobe. In all other lobes, lung sounds are clear but diminished. The patient is using accessory muscles to breathe, and his cough is no longer productive. The patient states, "I can't breathe, I am going to die." The nurse recognizes that the health care provider needs to be notified. Using SBAR (situation–background–assessment–recommendation) format, how should the nurse communicate the patient's status to the health care provider?

4. The nurse is caring for a patient receiving bi-level positive airway pressure (BiPAP) ventilation via face mask for treatment of respiratory distress. Which interventions can usually be delegated to an unregulated care provider (UCP)? (*Select all that apply.*)

   1. Educating the patient and caregiver about the use of BiPAP
   2. Repositioning patient in bed or chair
   3. Titrating patient's FiO_2
   4. Adjusting mask if it becomes displaced
   5. Recording patient's SpO_2 value
   6. Assessing patient's respiratory status

5. The nurse is assessing a patient with no history of chronic lung disease who is experiencing respiratory distress. Which findings would best indicate the need for supplemental oxygen therapy? (*Select all that apply.*)

   1. Shortness of breath
   2. PaO_2 58 mm Hg
   3. SpO_2 89%

4. Diminished breath sounds in all lobes
5. Cyanosis of oral mucous membranes
6. The nurse is teaching the patient how to use the peak flowmeter. The nurse asks the patient to demonstrate the procedure. Place the steps of using a peak flowmeter in the correct order.
   1. Have patient take a deep breath and hold it.
   2. Place marker of meter at bottom of scale.
   3. Have patient place mouthpiece in the mouth.
   4. Have patient blow out as hard and fast as possible.
   5. Have patient stand up, if able.
   6. Record the value.

Visit the Evolve site for a complete list of answers to the Review Questions.

NEXT GENERATION NCLEX® (NGN)

For practice with answering exam questions related to unfolding NGN case studies, please consult the Next Generation NCLEX® (NGN)-Style Case Studies for Skills and Techniques on the Evolve website: http://evolve.elsevier.com/Canada/Perry/clinicalskills/

REFERENCES

Accreditation Canada. (2020). *Required organizational practices–2020 handbook*. https://physicians.nshealth.ca/resources/required-organizational-practices-2020-handbook

Adhikari, P., Bhattarai, S., Gupta, A., et al. (2021). Physiological effects of high-flow nasal cannula therapy and its use in acute cardiogenic pulmonary edema. *Cureus, 13*(2), Article e13372. https://doi.org/10.7759/cureus.13372

Amico Patient Care Corporation. (2022). *Operating and maintenance manual*. https://www.amico.com/sites/default/files/product/downloads/amico-sot-flowmeters-manual.pdf

Asthma Canada. (n.d.). *Peak flow meters*. https://asthma.ca/get-help/living-with-asthma/peak-flow-meters/

Baranoski, G. V. G., Van Leeuwen, S. R., & Chen, T. F. (2017). On the detection of peripheral cyanosis in individuals with distinct levels of cutaneous pigmentation. In *2017 39th Annual International Conference of the IEEE Engineering in Medicine and Biology Society (EMBC)* (pp. 4260–4264). Institute of Electrical and Electronics Engineers (IEEE). https://doi.org/10.1109/EMBC.2017.8037797 [Seminal Reference]

Benner, A., Patel, A. K., Singh, K., et al. (2022). Physiology, Bohr effect. *StatPearls*. http://www.ncbi.nlm.nih.gov/pubmed/30252284

Blakeman, T. C., Scott, J. B., Yoder, M. A., et al. (2022). AARC clinical practice guidelines: Artificial airway suctioning. *Respiratory Care, 67*(2), 258–271. https://doi.org/10.4187/respcare.09548

Boscart, V., McCleary, L., Sheiban Taucar, L., et al. (2023). *Ebersole and Hess' gerontological nursing and healthy aging in Canada* (3rd ed.). Elsevier.

Branson, R. D. (2018). Oxygen therapy in COPD. *Respiratory Care, 63*(6), 734–748. https://doi.org/10.4187/respcare.06312

Canadian Nurses Association (CNA). (2017). *Code of ethics for registered nurses*. https://www.cna-aiic.ca/en/nursing/regulated-nursing-in-canada/nursing-ethics [Seminal Reference]

Carter, R., & Nwasuruba, C. (2022). Long-term supplemental oxygen therapy. *UpToDate*. https://www.uptodate.com/contents/long-term-supplemental-oxygen-therapy

Centers for Disease Control and Prevention. (2023). *Ventilator-associated event*. https://www.cdc.gov/nhsn/PDFs/pscManual/10-VAE_FINAL.pdf

Coppadoro, A., Bellani, G., & Foti, G. (2019). Non-pharmacological interventions to prevent ventilator-associated pneumonia: A literature review. *Respiratory Care, 64*(12), 1586–1595. https://doi.org/10.4187/RESPCARE.07127

Davidson, A. C., Banham, S., Elliott, M., et al. (2016). BTS/ICS guideline for the ventilatory management of acute hypercapnic respiratory failure in adults. *Thorax, 71*(Suppl. 2), ii1–ii35. https://doi.org/10.1136/thoraxjnl-2015-208209 [Seminal Reference]

Digby, G. C., Keenan, S. P., Parker, C. M., et al. (2015). Noninvasive ventilation practice patterns for acute respiratory failure in Canadian tertiary care centres: A descriptive analysis. *Canadian Respiratory Journal, 22*(6), 331–340. https://doi.org/10.1155/2015/971218 [Seminal Reference]

do Nascimento, P., Módolo, N. S. P., Andrade, S., et al. (2014). Incentive spirometry for prevention of postoperative pulmonary complication in upper abdominal surgery. Article No. CD006058. *Cochrane Database of Systematic Reviews, 2014*(2). https://doi.org/10.1002/14651858.CD006058.pub3 [Seminal Reference]

DynaMed Plus. (2018). *Noninvasive positive pressure ventilation (NPPV) in adults*. https://www.dynamed.com/procedure/noninvasive-positive-pressure-ventilation-nppv-in-adults

Ferreyro, B. L., Angriman, F., Munshi, L., et al. (2020). Association of noninvasive oxygenation strategies with all-cause mortality in adults with acute hypoxemic respiratory failure: A systematic review and meta-analysis. *JAMA, 324*(1), 57–67. https://doi.org/10.1001/jama.2020.9524

Gefen, A., Brienza, D. M., Cuddigan, J., et al. (2022). Our contemporary understanding of the aetiology of pressure ulcers/pressure injuries. *International Wound Journal, 19*(3), 692–704. https://doi.org/10.1111/iwj.13667

GOLD Science Committee. (2023). 2023 report: Global strategy for the diagnosis, management, and prevention of chronic obstructive pulmonary disease. *Global Initiative for Chronic Obstructive Lung Disease (GOLD)*. https://goldcopd.org/2023-gold-report-2/

Hafen, B. B., & Sharma, S. (2022). Oxygen saturation. *StatPearls*. https://www.ncbi.nlm.nih.gov/books/NBK525974/?report=reader

Healthcare Excellence Canada. (2016). *Hospital harm improvement resource: Pneumonia*. https://www.patientsafetyinstitute.ca/en/toolsResources/Hospital-Harm-Measure/Documents/Resource-Library/HHIR%20Pneumonia.pdf [Seminal Reference]

Herren, T., Achermann, E., Hegi, T., et al. (2017). Carbon dioxide narcosis due to inappropriate oxygen delivery: A case report. *Journal of Medical Case Reports, 11* Article 204. https://doi.org/10.1186/s13256-017-1363-7 [Seminal Reference]

Hess, D. (2022). The ventilator circuit. *UpToDate*. https://www.uptodate.com/contents/the-ventilator-circuit

Hill, N., & Kramer, N. (2022). Noninvasive ventilation in adults with chronic respiratory failure from neuromuscular and chest wall diseases: Adaptation and follow-up after initiation. *UpToDate*. https://www.uptodate.com/contents/noninvasive-ventilation-in-adults-with-chronic-respiratory-failure-from-neuromuscular-and-chest-wall-diseases-adaptation-and-follow-up-after-initiation

Hockenberry, M. J., Duffy, E. A., & Gibbs, K. (2024). *Wong's nursing care of infants and children* (12th ed.). Elsevier.

Hyzy, R. C. (2023). Complications of the endotracheal tube following initial placement: Prevention and management in adult intensive care patients. *UpToDate*. https://www.uptodate.com/contents/complications-of-the-endotracheal-tube-following-initial-placement-prevention-and-management-in-adult-intensive-care-unit-patients

Intersurgical Limited. (2011). *Venturi valves and Eco mask kits*. https://media.intersurgical.com/global/documents/info_sheets/IS1022_Venturi.pdf [Seminal Reference]

Jacobs, S. S. (2019). Clinician strategies to improve the care of patients using supplemental oxygen. *Chest, 156*(3), 619–628. https://doi.org/10.1016/j.chest.2019.06.011

Kayser, S. A., VanGilder, C. A., Ayello, E. A., et al. (2018). Prevalence and analysis of medical device-related pressure injuries: Results from the International pressure Pressure Ulcer Prevalence survey. *Advances in Skin & Wound Care, 31*(6), 276–285. https://doi.org/10.1097/01.ASW.0000532475.11971.aa

Keenan, S. P., Sinuff, T., Burns, K. E. A., et al. (2011). Clinical practice guidelines for the use of noninvasive positive-pressure ventilation and noninvasive continuous positive airway pressure in the acute care setting. *Canadian Medical Association Journal, 183*(3), E195–E214. https://doi.org/10.1503/cmaj.100071 [Seminal Reference]

Khalil, M., Jux, C., Rueblinger, L., et al. (2019). Acute therapy of newborns with critical congenital heart disease. *Translational Pediatrics, 8*(2), 114–126. https://doi.org/10.21037/tp.2019.04.06

Klompas, M. (2023). Risk factors and prevention of hospital-aquired and ventilator-associated pneumonia in adults. *UpToDate*. https://www.uptodate.com/contents/risk-factors-and-prevention-of-hospital-acquired-and-ventilator-associated-pneumonia-in-adults

Lacasse, Y., Bernard, S., & Maltais, F. (2015). Eligibility for home oxygen programs and funding across Canada. *Canadian Respiratory Journal, 22*(6), 324–330. https://doi.org/10.1155/2015/280604 [Seminal Reference]

Louie, A., Feiner, J. R., Bickler, P. E., et al. (2018). Four types of pulse oximeters accurately detect hypoxia during low perfusion and motion. *Anesthesiology, 128*(3), 520–530. https://doi.org/10.1097/ALN.0000000000002002

Lung Cancer Canada. (2018). *Lung cancer screening in Canada*. https://www.lungcancercanada.ca/en-CA/Lung-Cancer/Screening.aspx

Martin, L., & Khalil, H. (1990). How much reduced hemoglobin is necessary to generate central cyanosis? *Chest, 97*(1), 182–185. https://doi.org/10.1378/chest.97.1.182 [Seminal Reference]

Mehrtash, M., Bakker, J. P., & Ayas, N. (2019). Predictors of continuous positive airway pressure adherence in patients with obstructive sleep apnea. *Lung, 197*(2), 115–121. https://doi.org/10.1007/s00408-018-00193-1

Moore, D. (2019). Home oxygen therapy in patients with COPD: Safety issues for nurse prescribers. *British Journal of Nursing, 28*(14), 912–917. https://doi.org/10.12968/bjon.2019.28.14.912

Moslander, C., Lat, T., Giri, B., et al. (2020). Long-term oxygen therapy and risk of fire-related events. *Federal Practitioner*, *37*(10), 442–446. https://doi.org/10.12788/fp.0048

Muscedere, J. G., Martin, C. M., & Heyland, D. K. (2008). The impact of ventilator-associated pneumonia on the Canadian health care system. *Journal of Critical Care*, *23*(1), 5–10. https://doi.org/10.1016/j.jcrc.2007.11.012 [Seminal Reference]

Napolitano, N., Berlinski, A., Walsh, B. K., et al. (2021). AARC Clinical Practice Guideline: Management of pediatric patients with oxygen in the acute care setting. *Respiratory Care*, *66*(7), 1214–1223. https://doi.org/10.4187/RESPCARE.09006

Nonoyama, M. L., Katz, S. L., Amin, R., et al. (2020). Healthcare utilization and costs of pediatric home mechanical ventilation in Canada. *Pediatric Pulmonology*, *55*(9), 2368–2376. https://doi.org/10.1002/ppul.24923

Norton, L., Parslow, N., Johnston, D., et al. (2021). *Best practice recommendations for the prevention and management of pressure injuries. In Foundations of best practice for skin and wound management: A supplement of Wound Care Canada.* Wounds Canada. https://www.woundscanada.ca/docman/public/health-care-professional/bpr-workshop/172-bpr-prevention-and-management-of-pressure-injuries-2/file

Nova Scotia Health & IWK Infection Prevention and Control. (2021). *COVID-19: Aerosol generating medical procedures (AGMP) in healthcare settings*. https://policy.nshealth.ca/Site_Published/covid19/document_render.aspx?documentRender.IdType=6&documentRender.GenericField=&documentRender.Id=76545

Piraino, T., Madden, M., Roberts, K. J., et al. (2022). AARC Clinical Practice Guideline: Management of adult patients with oxygen in the acute care setting. *Respiratory Care*, *67*(1), 115–128. https://doi.org/10.4187/respcare.09294

Pooboni, S. K., & Markowitz, J. E. (2022). *Noninvasive ventilation procedures*. https://emedicine.medscape.com/article/1417959-overview

Public Health Agency of Canada (PHAC). (2022). *Infection prevention and control for COVID-19: Second interim guidance for acute healthcare settings*. https://www.canada.ca/en/public-health/services/diseases/2019-novel-coronavirus-infection/health-professionals/infection-prevention-control-covid-19-second-interim-guidance.html

Roberts, M., Bortolotto, S. J., Weyant, R. A., et al. (2019). The experience of acute mechanical ventilation from the patient's perspective. *Dimensions of Critical Care Nursing*, *38*(4), 201–202. https://doi.org/10.1097/DCC.0000000000000361

Rochwerg, B., Brochard, L., Elliott, M. W., et al. (2017). Official *European Respiratory Society (ERS)/American Thoracic Society (ATS)* clinical practice guidelines: Noninvasive ventilation for acute respiratory failure. *European Respiratory Journal*, *50*(2), Article 1602426. https://doi.org/10.1183/13993003.02426-2016 [Seminal Reference]

Rochwerg, B., Granton, D., Wang, D. X., et al. (2019). High flow nasal cannula compared with conventional oxygen therapy for acute hypoxemic respiratory failure: A systematic review and meta-analysis. *Intensive Care Medicine*, *45*(5), 563–572. https://doi.org/10.1007/s00134-019-05590-5

Santiago-Rosado, L. M., Sigmon, D. F., & Lewison, C. S. (2022). Tracheal trauma. *StatPearls*. https://www.ncbi.nlm.nih.gov/books/NBK500015/

Saskatoon Health Region. (2020). *Oxygen administration*. https://www.saskatoonhealthregion.ca/about/NursingManual/1115.pdf

Christopher, K. L., & Schwartz, M. D. (2011). Transtracheal oxygen therapy. *CHEST*, *139*(2), 435–440. https://doi.org/10.1378/chest.10-1373

Shah, N. M., D'Cruz, R. F., & Murphy, P. B. (2018). Update: Non-invasive ventilation in chronic obstructive pulmonary disease. *Journal of Thoracic Disease*, *10*(Suppl. 1), S71–S79. https://doi.org/10.21037/jtd.2017.10.44

Singer, K. E., Harvey, J. A., Heh, V., et al. (2020). Mortality from burns sustained on home oxygen therapy exceeds predicted mortality. *Journal of Burn Care and Research*, *41*(5), 976–980. https://doi.org/10.1093/jbcr/iraa097

Sjoding, M. W., Dickson, R. P., Iwashyna, T. J., et al. (2020). Racial bias in pulse oximetry measurement. *New England Journal of Medicine*, *383*(25), 2477–2478. https://doi.org/10.1056/nejmc2029240

Smetana, G. W. (2022). Strategies to reduce postoperative complications in adults. *UpToDate*. https://www.uptodate.com/contents/strategies-to-reduce-postoperative-pulmonary-complications-in-adults

Sorg, M. E., & Chatburn, R. L. (2022). Oxygen delivery with an open oxygen mask and other conventional masks: A simulation-based study. *Respiratory Care*, *67*(3), 316–321. https://doi.org/10.4187/respcare.09399

Soto-Ruiz, K. M., Peacock, W. F., & Varon, J. (2011). The men and history behind the Venturi mask. *Resuscitation*, *82*(3), 244–246. https://doi.org/10.1016/j.resuscitation.2010.11.016 [Seminal Reference]

Sullivan, K. A., Churchill, I. F., Hylton, D. A., et al. (2021). Use of incentive spirometry in adults following cardiac, thoracic, and upper abdominal surgery to prevent post-operative pulmonary complications: A systematic review and meta-analysis. *Respiration*, *100*(11), 1114–1127. https://doi.org/10.1159/000517012

Sun, Y. H., Dai, B., Peng, Y., et al. (2019). Factors affecting FiO_2 and PEEP during high-flow nasal cannula oxygen therapy: A bench study. *Clinical Respiratory Journal*, *13*(12), 758–764. https://doi.org/10.1111/crj.13087

Tang, X., Lyu, W.-R., Wang, R., et al. (2022). Modern thromboprophylaxis protocol based on guidelines applied in a respiratory intensive care unit: A single-center prospective cohort study. *Thrombosis Journal*, 20, Article 76. https://doi.org/10.1186/s12959-022-00439-2.

Theodore, A. C. (2022). Measures of oxygenation and mechanisms of hypoxemia. *UpToDate*. https://www.uptodate.com/contents/measures-of-oxygenation-and-mechanisms-of-hypoxemia

Torres, A., Cilloniz, C., Niederman, M. S., et al. (2021). Pneumonia. *Nature Reviews Disease Primers*, 7, Article 25. https://doi.org/10.1038/s41572-021-00259-0

Torres, C., & Schwartz, M. (2017). *Transtracheal oxygen therapy*. National Jewish Health. https://www.nationaljewish.org/conditions/medications/on-the-go-with-oxygen [Seminal Reference]

Tyerman, J., & Cobbett, S. (Eds.). (2023). *Lewis's medical-surgical nursing in Canada: Assessment and management of clinical problems* (5th ed.). Elsevier.

Vargas, M., Chiumello, D., Sutherasan, Y., et al. (2017). Heat and moisture exchangers (HMEs) and heated humidifiers (HHs) in adult critically ill patients: A systematic review, meta-analysis and meta-regression of randomized controlled trials. *Critical Care*, *21*, 123. https://doi.org/10.1186/s13054-017-1710-5

Yen, P. H., & Leasure, A. R. (2019). Use and effectiveness of the teach-back method in patient education and health outcomes. *Federal Practitioner*, *36*(6), 284–289. https://www.ncbi.nlm.nih.gov/pmc/articles/PMC6590951

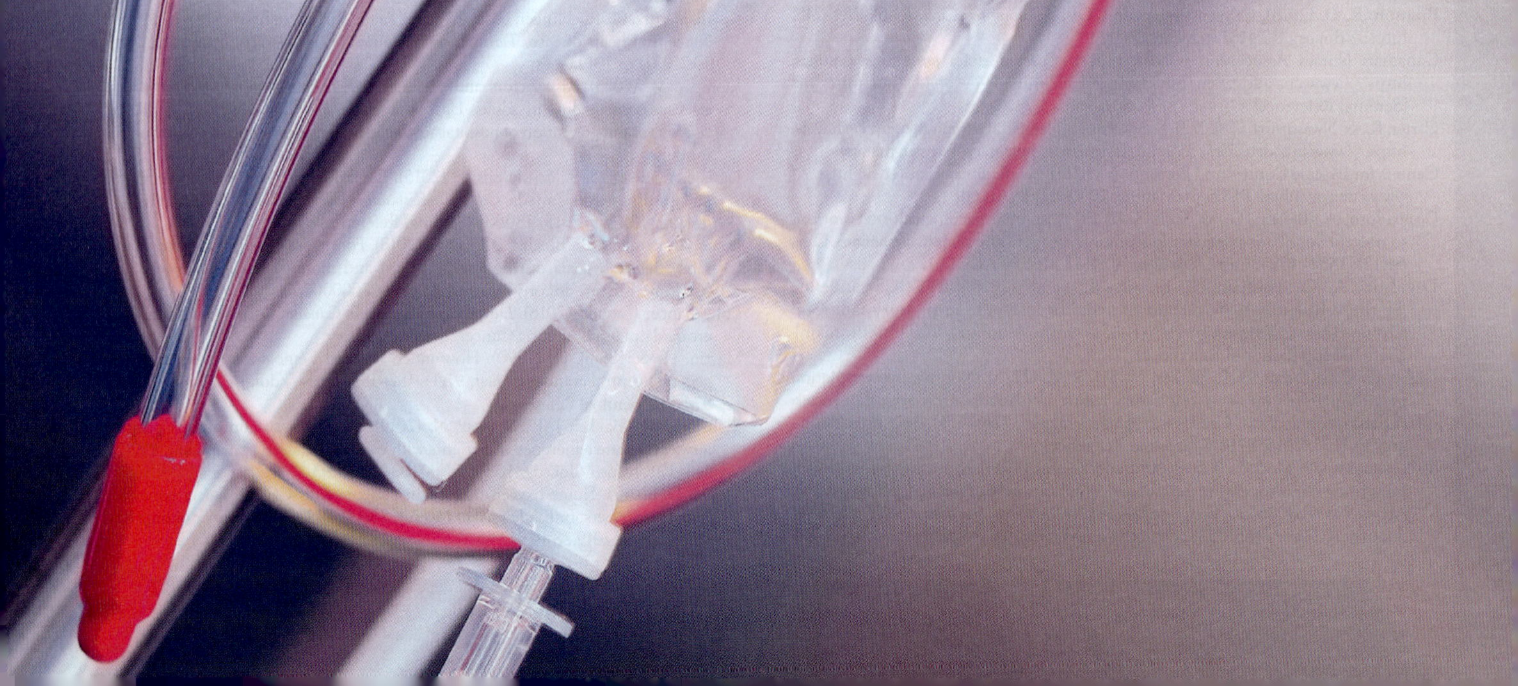

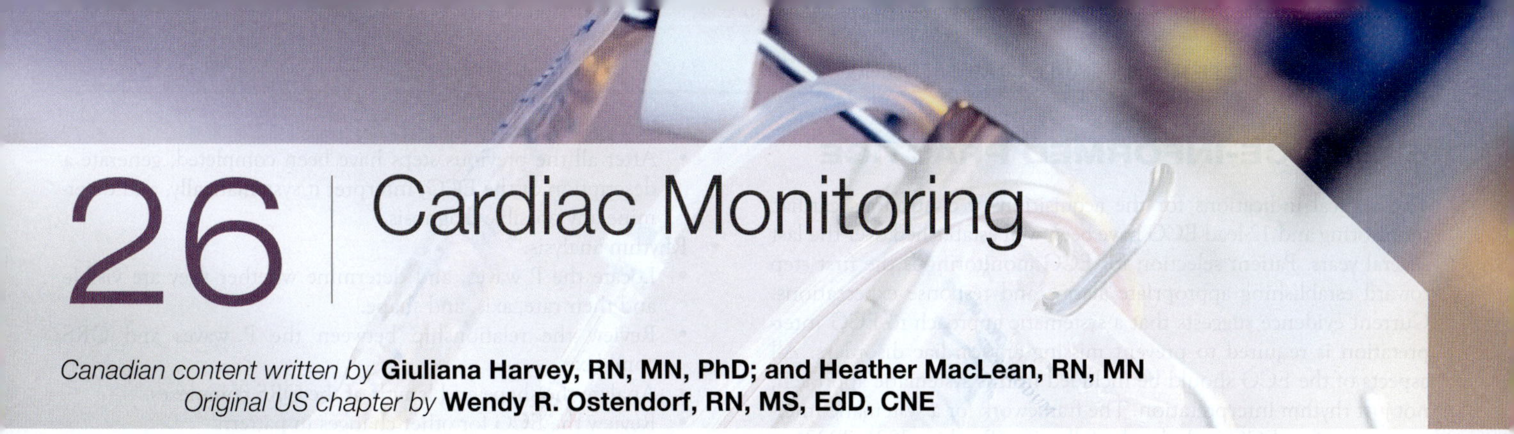

26 | Cardiac Monitoring

Canadian content written by **Giuliana Harvey, RN, MN, PhD; and Heather MacLean, RN, MN**
Original US chapter by **Wendy R. Ostendorf, RN, MS, EdD, CNE**

SKILLS AND PROCEDURES

OBJECTIVES

Mastery of content in this chapter will enable the nurse to:

- Identify the indications to perform a 12-lead electrocardiogram and cardiac monitor application.
- Determine correct electrode placement to obtain an accurate electrocardiogram tracing.
- Describe measures to reduce false alarms.

MEDIA RESOURCES

- http://evolve.elsevier.com/Canada/Perry/clinicalskills/

PURPOSE

The electrocardiogram (ECG) is the graphic representation of the electrical activities, or conduction system, of the heart used for diagnostic and treatment purposes. The accuracy of these waveforms depends on the correct placement and clean application of electrodes to the skin. Monitoring of the ECG can be done at one point in time or on a continuous basis.

STANDARDS OF CARE

- Accreditation Canada (2020)—*Required Organizational Practices–2020 Handbook* (https://physicians.nshealth.ca/resources/required-organizational-practices-2020-handbook)
- American Association of Critical-Care Nurses (AACN, 2018b)—*AACN Practice Alert: Ensuring Accurate ST-Segment Monitoring* (https://www.aacn.org/clinical-resources/practice-alerts/st-segment-monitoring)
- American Association of Critical-Care Nurses (AACN, 2018c)—*Managing Alarms in Acute Care Across the Life Span: Electrocardiography and Pulse Oximetry* (https://www.aacn.org/clinical-resources/practice-alerts/managing-alarms-in-acute-care-across-the-life-span)
- Sandau et al. (2017)—*Update to Practice Standards for Electrocardiographic Monitoring in Hospital Settings: A Scientific Statement from the American Heart Association* (https://doi.org/10.1161/CIR.0000000000000527)

PRINCIPLES FOR PRACTICE

- Cardiac monitoring provides continuous ECG observation of the acutely ill patient. Proper placement of ECG electrodes is essential to ensure real-time detection of arrhythmias (Sandau et al., 2017).
- A 12-lead ECG records 12 different angles of the heart with a 2.5-second view of each lead. It is a diagnostic tool used to determine emergency treatment of patients with acute coronary syndrome or acute onset of potentially life-threatening dysrhythmias. Accuracy and timeliness are the key principles of acquisition (Sandau et al., 2017).
- The normal sequence through the conduction system of the heart is called normal sinus rhythm (NSR) (Fig. 26.1). NSR implies that the cardiac impulses originate from the sinoatrial (SA) node and follow the normal conduction system. The P wave represents the electrical conduction through both atria, and the PR interval represents the impulse travel time through the atrioventricular (AV) node and bundle of His (120–200 msec). The QRS complex refers to the electrical impulse moving through the ventricles (60–100 msec) via the left or right bundle branches to the Purkinje fibres. The time needed for ventricular depolarization and repolarization is called the QT interval (120–240 msec); it is heart rate dependent (Fig. 26.2).
- Common cardiac dysrhythmias are presented in Table 26.1.

PERSON-CENTRED CARE

- Placement of the electrodes requires exposure of a patient's chest. Measures to maintain the person's privacy and modesty are essential.
- Cisgender women and nonoperative transgender men require special consideration: electrodes should be placed as close to the chest wall as possible, avoiding the breast tissue.
- Patients and caregivers, especially those with a cultural need for modesty, may need detailed information about the procedure so they do not misunderstand the intent and objective of cardiac monitoring.
- Always explain to the patient what you are doing so they understand the purpose of the interaction.

EVIDENCE-INFORMED PRACTICE

The clinical indications for the acquisition of continuous cardiac monitoring and 12-lead ECG have been well established over the last several years. Patient selection for ECG monitoring is the first step toward establishing appropriate alarms and response expectations. Current evidence suggests that a systematic approach to ECG interpretation is required to prevent missing any cardiac disorders. All aspects of the ECG should be included in this systematic approach, not just rhythm interpretation. The framework for a systematic interpretation of an ECG includes the following (Prutkin, 2021, 2022):

- Approach to interpretation:
  - Determine the rate first.
  - Identify the underlying rhythm.
  - Review the axis and identify whether there is a right or left axis deviation.
  - Review the P wave, including its morphology, amplitude, and duration.
  - Examine the QRS complex for widening, voltage, and presence of a Q wave.
  - Examine the ST segment and T wave for abnormalities such as elevation or depression.
  - After all the previous steps have been completed, generate a description of the ECG, interpret it systematically, and determine any possible diagnosis.
- Rhythm analysis:
  - Locate the P waves, and determine whether they are visible and their rate, axis, and shape.
  - Review the relationship between the P waves and QRS complexes.
  - Analyze the shape and length of the QRS complexes.
  - Review the ECG for other changes in pattern.
  - Finally, interpret the ECG.

Indications and contraindications for 12-lead ECG acquisitions follow.

Indications

- Suspected acute coronary syndrome, including myocardial infarction
- Evaluation of implanted defibrillators and pacemakers
- Disorders of the cardiac rhythm
- Evaluation of syncope
- Evaluation of metabolic disorders
- Effects and adverse effects of pharmacotherapy
- Evaluation of primary and secondary cardiomyopathic processes

Contraindications

- There are no absolute contraindications to performing an ECG other than patient refusal.
- Some patients may have allergies or, more commonly, sensitivities to the adhesive used to affix the leads. In these cases, hypoallergenic alternatives are available from various manufacturers.

SAFETY GUIDELINES

- Know the indications for a 12-lead ECG. Patients experiencing chest pain need to have their 12-lead ECG within 10 minutes of the assessment and onset of pain. A 12-lead ECG will determine the next step in their treatment plan.

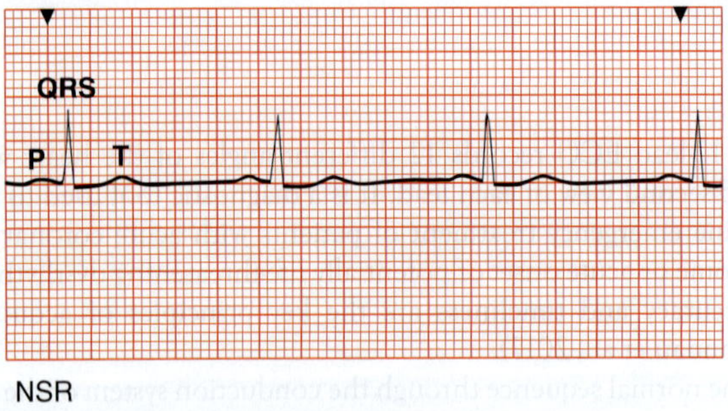

FIG 26.1 Normal sinus rhythm. *(From Wesley, K. [2017]. Huszar's ECG and 12-lead ECG interpretation [5th ed.]. Elsevier.)*

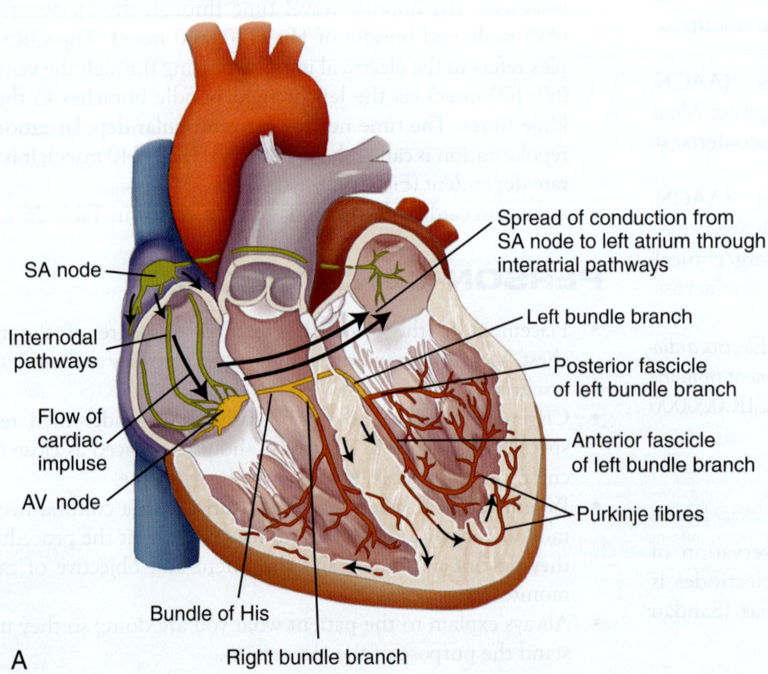

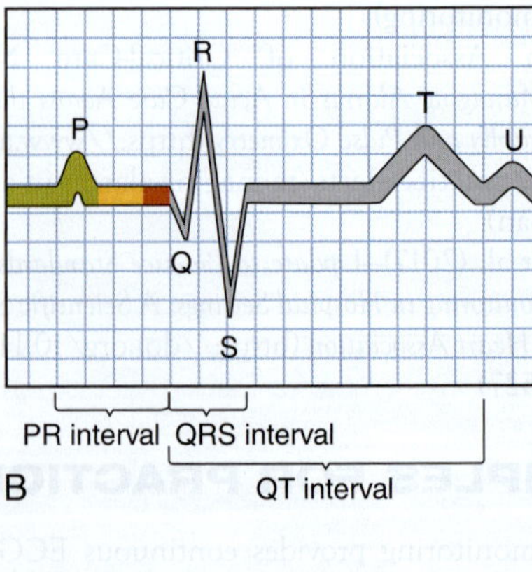

FIG 26.2 A, Conduction system of the heart. B, The normal electrocardiogram pattern. *(From Tyerman, J., & Cobbett S. [Eds.]. [2023]. Lewis's medical-surgical nursing in Canada: Assessment and management of clinical problems [5th ed.]. Elsevier Inc.)*

TABLE 26.1

Common Cardiac Dysrhythmias*

Rhythm Characteristics and Etiology	Clinical Significance and Management
Sinus Tachycardia	
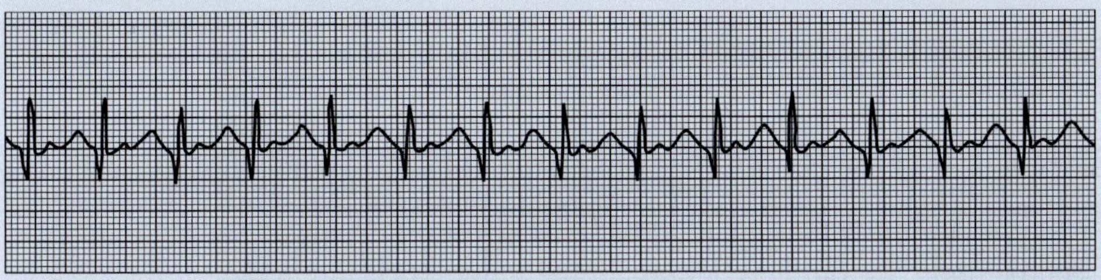	
Regular rhythm, rate 100–180 beats/min (higher in infants), normal P wave, normal QRS complex.	Some patients with heart disease are unable to increase their heart rate to meet increased oxygen demands.
Rate increase is often a normal response to exercise; emotion; or stressors such as pain, fever, pump failure, hyperthyroidism, and certain medications (e.g., caffeine, nitrates, epinephrine, nicotine).	Correct underlying factors; discontinue medications producing the adverse effect.
Sinus Bradycardia	
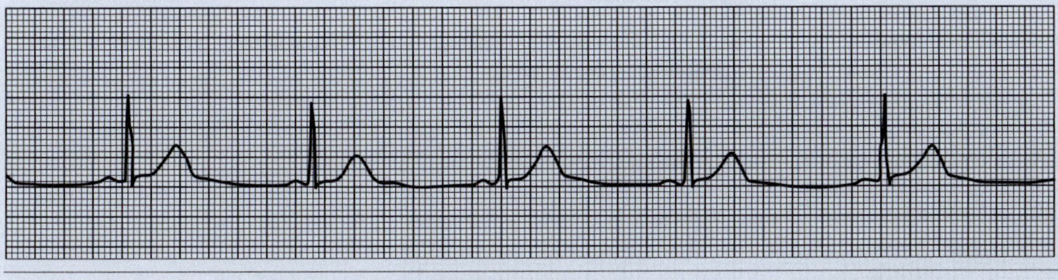	
Regular rhythm, rate less than 60 beats/min, normal P wave, normal PR interval, normal QRS complex.	No clinical significance unless associated with signs and symptoms of reduced cardiac output, such as dizziness or syncope, or presence of chest pain.
Rate decrease is a normal response to sleep or in a well-conditioned athlete; diminished blood flow to sinoatrial (SA) node, vagal stimulation, hypothyroidism, increased intracranial pressure, or medications (e.g., digoxin, propranolol, quinidine, procainamide) sometimes cause abnormal drops in rate.	Bradycardia with hypotension and decreased cardiac output is treated with atropine; pacemaker is sometimes necessary.
Atrial Fibrillation (A-fib)	
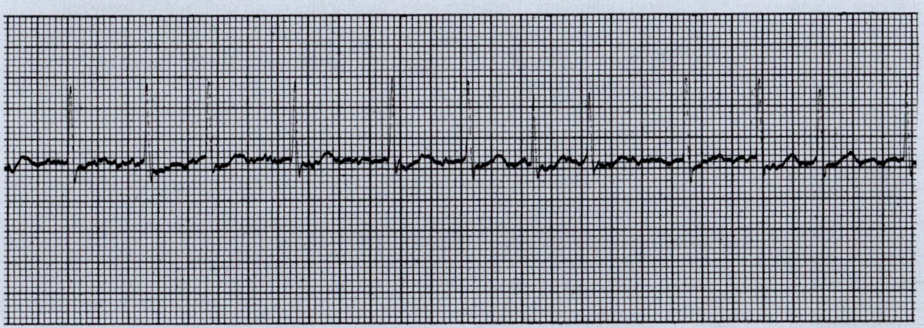	
Chaotic, irregular atrial activity resulting in an irregular ventricular response. No identifiable P waves. Irregular ventricular response resulting in an irregular cardiac rate and rhythm. The conduction of the multiple atrial impulses across the atrioventricular (AV) node determines the rate. Caused by aging, calcification of the SA node, or changes in myocardial blood supply.	There is loss of the atrial kick (part of the cardiac output squeezed in the ventricles with a coordinated atrial contraction), pooling of blood in the atria, and development of microemboli. Anticoagulants such as warfarin (Coumadin) may be used to reduce the risk of stroke. The patient often complains of fatigue, a fluttering in the chest, or shortness of breath if the ventricular response is rapid. Dysrhythmia occurs commonly in the aging and older person.

Continued

TABLE 26.1

Common Cardiac Dysrhythmias*—cont'd

Rhythm Characteristics and Etiology	Clinical Significance and Management
Ventricular Tachycardia	
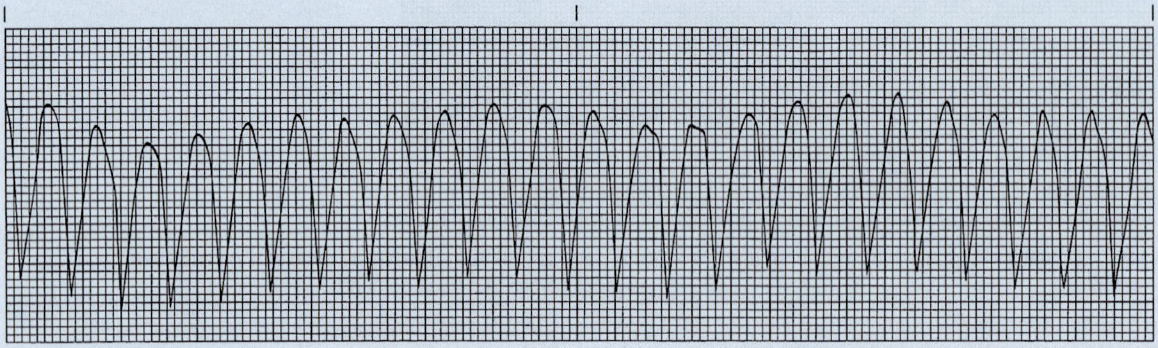	
Rhythm slightly irregular, rate 100–200 beats/min, P wave absent, PR interval absent, QRS complex wide and bizarre, >0.12 seconds.	Results in decreased cardiac output caused by decreased ventricular filling time; often leads to severe hypotension and loss of pulse and consciousness.
Caused by changes in the normal pacemaker of the heart, such as decrease in blood flow, ischemia, or embolus.	Acute loss of pulse and respiration. Immediate chest compressions and defibrillation are required.
Ventricular Fibrillation	
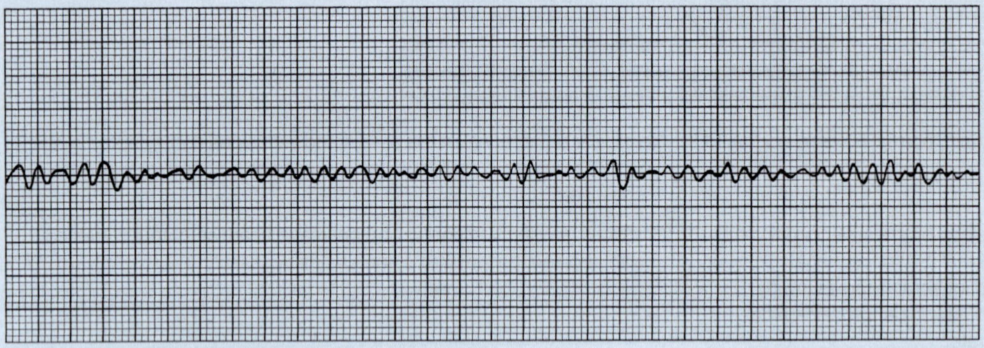	
Uncoordinated electrical activity. No identifiable P, QRS, or T wave. Causes include sudden cardiac death, electrical shock, acute myocardial infarction, drowning, or trauma.	Acute loss of pulse and respiration. Immediate chest compressions and defibrillation are required. Availability of an automated external defibrillator (AED) is recommended in public and private places where large numbers of people gather or where people who are at high risk for heart attack live.
Asystole	
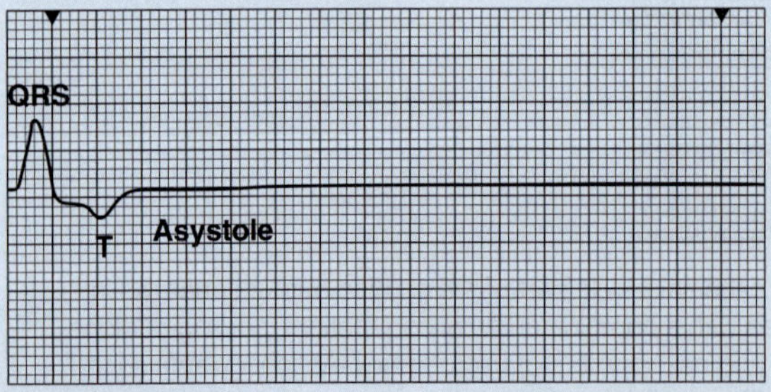 Asystole	
Usually a flat line, no waves.	Lethal arrhythmia; no pulse; requires immediate cardiopulmonary resuscitation (CPR) unless patient has a "do not resuscitate (DNR)" or "allow natural death (AND)" prescription (see employer policy); some facilities may use an interprofessional approach to develop a resuscitation care plan with the patient.

*Graph adapted from Wesley, K. [2017]. *Huszar's ECG and 12-lead ECG interpretation* [5th ed.]. Elsevier.

Adapted from Panchal, A. R., Bartos, J. A., Cabañas, J. G., et al. (2020). 2020 American Heart Association guidelines for cardiopulmonary resuscitation and emergency cardiovascular care. Part 3: Adult basic and advanced life support. *Circulation, 142*(Suppl. 2), S366–S468. https://doi.org/10.1161/CIR.0000000000000916

- Women of South Asian, Chinese, and Afro-Caribbean descent experience higher rates of heart disease than White Canadians (Heart and Stroke Foundation of Canada, 2018). This is significant difference given that only 29% of women receive an ECG within 10 minutes, compared with 38% of men (Heart and Stroke Foundation of Canada, 2018).
- Inquire on admission whether the patient has taken nitroglycerin, because this may alter the ECG.
- Know a patient's current medications. Some medications, particularly beta blockers, and some calcium channel blockers and other antiarrhythmics can cause dysrhythmias.
- Patients who are being continuously monitored via ECG are at risk for medical adhesive-related skin injury (MARSI) because the skin surface stays in contact with the adhesive around the electrodes (Fumarola et al., 2020). Regular skin inspection for redness, edema, blisters, or tearing is important.

✦ SKILL 26.1 Obtaining a 12-Lead Electrocardiogram

NSO Nursing Skills Online Cardiac Care Module 10 / Lesson 2

Electrical impulses of the heart are conducted to the surface of the body and are detected by electrodes placed on the skin of the limbs and torso. The electrodes carry these impulses to either a continuous monitor or a 12-lead ECG machine. The appearance of the ECG pattern or waveform helps to diagnose whether there are any abnormalities in the electrical conduction through the heart. A 12-lead ECG provides a snapshot of the waveforms from 12 different angles or views of the heart. One electrode is placed on each of the 4 extremities, and 6 electrodes are placed at specific sites on the chest, for a total of 10 electrodes on the patient's skin. The sites of the electrodes are bipolar limb leads I, II, III; augmented limb leads aV_R, aV_L, aV_F; and precordial chest leads V_1 to V_6. The leads view a specific part of the surface of the heart and can help determine which part of the heart has sustained damage and the origin and flow of the impulse.

Delegation and Collaboration

The skill of obtaining a 12-lead ECG is restricted to health care providers who are specifically trained in this skill (see employer policy) and cannot be delegated to an unregulated care provider (UCP). The nurse directs the UCP to do the following:

- Immediately report to the nurse changes in the patient's cardiac status, such as indications of chest pain
- Immediately deliver the completed 12-lead ECG recording to a health care provider for interpretation
- Use specific patient precautions related to disease, mobility status, or position restrictions

Collaborate with the interprofessional team (e.g., code team, cardiac clinical nurse specialist, health care provider) for possible emergency needs.

Equipment

- 12-lead ECG machine
- 10 ECG leads with alligator clip, suction cup, or snap-on attachments
- 10 ECG electrodes (disposable, self-adhesive) or electrode paste
- Clean, dry towel or sponge wipes
- Hair clippers (optional depending on hair at electrode sites)

STEP	RATIONALE
ASSESSMENT	
1. Identify patient using at least two person-specific identifiers (e.g., name and date of birth, or name and medical record number) according to employer policy.	Ensures correct patient. Complies with Accreditation Canada's standards and improves patient safety (Accreditation Canada, 2020).
2. Throughout the procedure, the 4 moments for hand hygiene are to be implemented; hand hygiene should occur before initial patient (or patient environment) contact, before an aseptic procedure, after body fluid exposure risk, and after patient (or patient environment) contact. Additional hand hygiene should be performed when hands are visibly soiled.	Proper hand hygiene helps prevent the spread of infectious agents to health care providers.
3. Determine indications for obtaining ECG. Assess patient's history and cardiopulmonary status (e.g., heart rate and rhythm, blood pressure, respirations).	If 12-lead ECG is prescribed for chest pain or other ischemic signs and symptoms, obtain ECG within 10 minutes of patient's pain report.
4. Assess for chest pain using an appropriate symptom assessment tool (e.g., COLDSPAA, OPQRST); rate acuity on appropriate pain rating scale.	Determines level of chest discomfort, which may be warning for cardiac ischemia.
5. Ask if patient has history of contact dermatitis from use of adhesives.	Dermatitis results from severity to chemicals in adhesive. Hypoallergenic electrodes may be considered.
6. Assess patient's ability to follow directions and remain still in supine position if there are no patient-specific contraindications to this position (e.g., certain surgical procedures, continuous tube feedings).	Provides clear, accurate recording without artifact; however, patient's position may need to be altered based on patient health status (e.g., semi-Fowler's position).
7. Assess patient's knowledge, prior experience with ECG, and expectations of the procedure.	Allows for individualized patient care.

STEP	RATIONALE

NURSING DIAGNOSES

- Acute pain
- Anxiety
- Insufficient knowledge regarding purpose and steps of procedure
- Fear

Related factors and risk factors are individualized on the basis of patient's condition or needs.

PLANNING

STEP	RATIONALE
1. Expected outcomes following completion of procedure: • Patient tolerates procedure without anxiety or discomfort. • Clear, accurate recording of ECG waveform is obtained.	Appropriate preparation and education decrease anxiety.
2. Explain procedure to patient.	Reduces anxiety and promotes cooperation.
3. Close room door or bedside curtains.	Provides privacy.
4. Gather equipment for ECG.	Allows for increased efficiency of procedure.

IMPLEMENTATION

STEP	RATIONALE
1.	Reduces transmission of microorganisms.
2. Prepare patient for procedure:	
a. Remove or reposition patient's clothing to expose only patient's chest and arms. Keep abdomen and thighs covered.	Facilitates correct placement of cardiac leads and maintains patient's modesty. Improper lead placement produces artifact, which necessitates repeating test or interpretation errors.
b. Place patient in supine position with head of bed no higher than 30 degrees.	Electrodes must be placed on anterior chest for standard 12-lead ECG (Prutkin, 2020).
c. Instruct patient to lie still without talking and to keep their legs uncrossed.	Body movement or talking produces artifact, which may necessitate repeating the test.
3. Turn on machine; enter required demographic information.	Turning machine on first helps you identify electrode and lead issues on application.
4. Clean and prepare skin with soap and water for isolated electrode placement. Wipe area with a dry washcloth. Clip excessive hair from electrode area. Where possible, avoid the use of products that dry skin, such as alcohol-based skin preps (Fumarola et al., 2020).	The skin should be prepared before ECG electrodes are placed (Sandau et al., 2017). Proper skin preparation decreases skin impedance signal noise, thereby producing a clean, accurate recording. Do not use alcohol to clean area because it will dry the skin and increase the risk for MARSI. Clipping hair in the electrode area is preferred, as shaving leaves nicks that predispose the area to infection (Anderson & Sexton, 2021).
5. Apply electrodes in correct positions. If using leads with suction cups, apply electrode paste to areas before attaching leads. **a.** Chest (precordial) leads (Fig. 26.3) • V_1–Fourth intercostal space (ICS) at right sternal angle • V_2–Fourth ICS at left sternal border • V_3–Midway between V_2 and V_4 • V_4–Fifth ICS at midclavicular line • V_5–Left anterior axillary line at level of V_4 horizontally • V_6–Left midaxillary line at level of V_4 horizontally	Proper placement of leads is essential for accurate interpretation of a 12-lead ECG. Ensure that the correct lead is in the correct location. If any leads are misplaced, the ECG reading will be inaccurate and can result in misdiagnosis and inappropriate treatment (Prutkin, 2021, 2022).
b. Extremities: One lead on each extremity (Fig. 26.4); right wrist, left wrist, left ankle, right ankle.	
c. Right precordial leads placement for right ventricular infarct used without standard lead placement (Fig. 26.5).	
d. Standard lead placement for diagnosing posterior wall infarcts requires adding posterior precordial leads, specifically leads V7, V8, and V9; thus, it is also referred to as a 15-lead ECD (Fig. 26.6).	
6. Check 12-lead ECG machine for messages to correct electrode or lead issues. If no messages occur, press button to obtain 12-lead ECG.	
7. If you obtain ECG tracing without artifact, disconnect leads and wipe off excess electrode paste from patient's chest.	Promotes comfort and hygiene.
8. If STAT, immediately deliver ECG tracing (if not computerized) to appropriate health care provider for interpretation (Fig. 26.7 shows an example of a 12-lead ECG).	If non-STAT, place 12-lead ECG tracing in patient's chart or designated area.

STEP	RATIONALE

IMPLEMENTATION

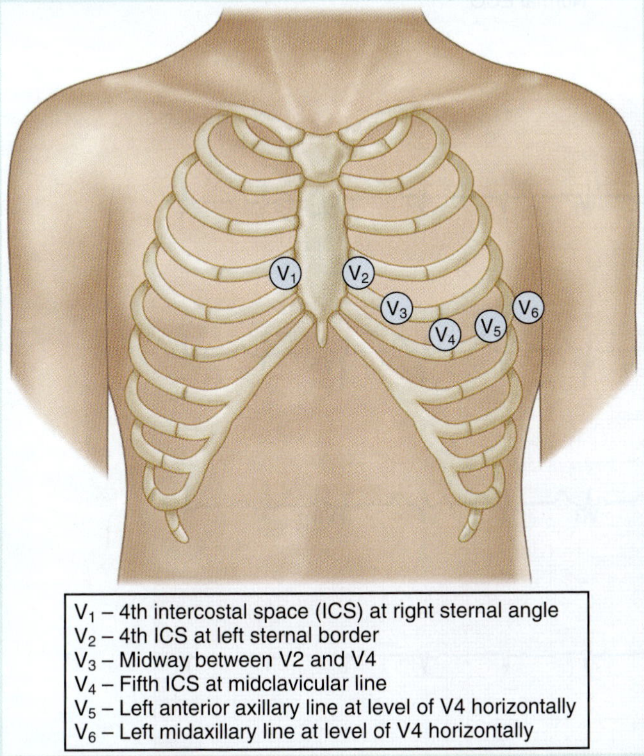

FIG 26.3 Precordial (chest) lead placement for a standard 12-lead electrocardiogram (ECG).

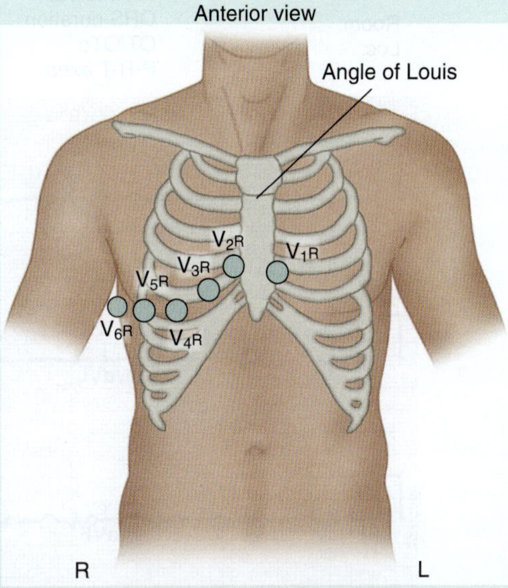

FIG 26.5 Right precordial leads placement for right ventricular infarct. *(From Urden, L., Stacy, K., & Lough, M. [2022]. Critical care nursing: Diagnosis and management [9th ed.]. Elsevier.)*

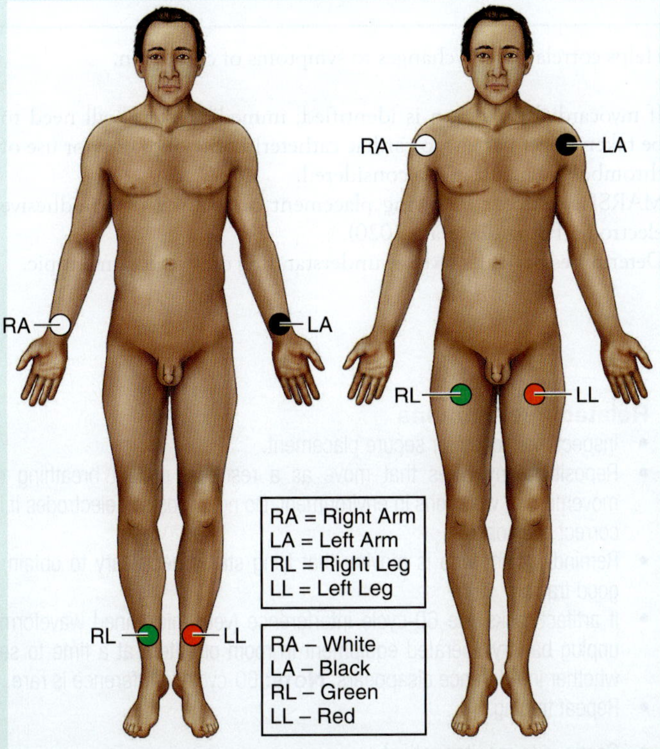

FIG 26.4 Limb lead placement for a standard 12-lead electrocardiogram (ECG).

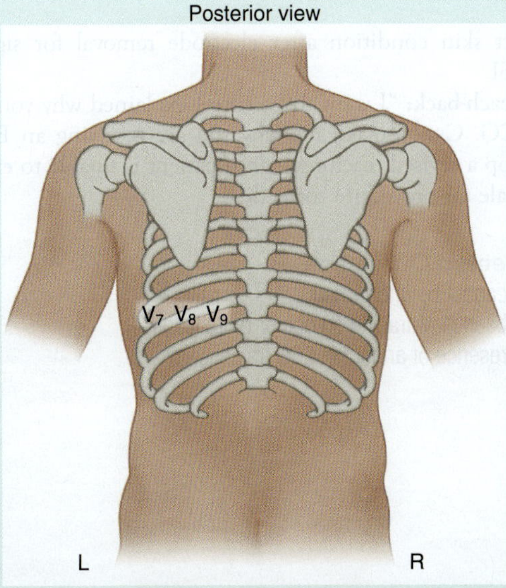

FIG 26.6 Posterior precordial leads for posterior wall infarct. *(From Urden, L., Stacy, K., & Lough, M. [2022]. Critical care nursing: Diagnosis and management [9th ed.]. Elsevier.)*

STEP	RATIONALE

IMPLEMENTATION

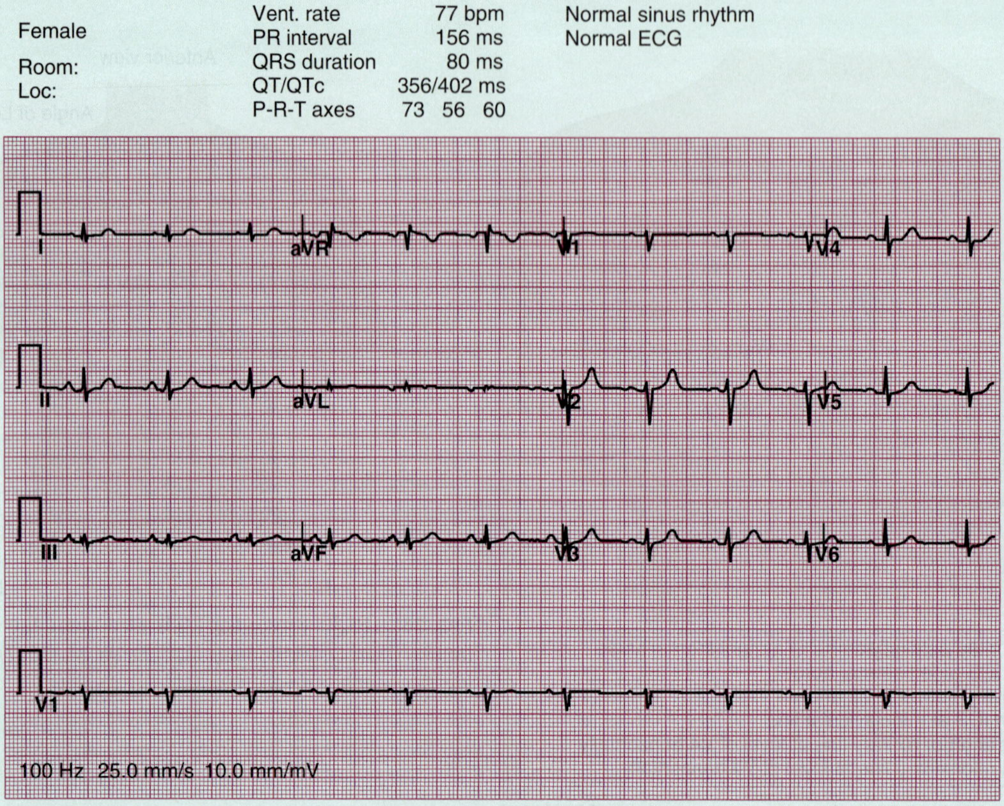

FIG 26.7 **A 12-lead electrocardiogram (ECG).** *(From Aehlert, B. [2018]. ECGs made easy [6th ed.]. Elsevier.)*

EVALUATION

STEP	RATIONALE
1. Note and document whether patient is experiencing any chest discomfort during procedure.	Helps correlate ECG changes to symptoms of chest pain.
2. Discuss findings and results of 12-lead ECG with health care provider to determine next steps in patient's treatment plan.	If myocardial infarction is identified, immediate steps will need to be taken to get patient to cardiac catheterization laboratory or use of thrombolytic medications considered.
3. Inspect skin condition after electrode removal for signs of MARSI.	MARSI can occur following placement or removal of an adhesive electrode (Fumarola et al., 2020).
4. **Use teach-back:** "I want to be sure I explained why you need an ECG. Can you tell me why you are receiving an ECG?" Develop a revised teaching plan if patient is unable to explain rationale for procedure correctly.	Determines patient's level of understanding of instructional topic.

Unexpected Outcomes	Related Interventions
1. ECG cannot be interpreted: • Absence of tracing on one or more leads • Presence of artifact in ECG tracings	• Inspect electrodes for secure placement. • Reposition any wires that move as a result of patient breathing or movement or vibrations in environment. Do not reposition electrodes if in correct position. • Remind patient who is moving that lying still is necessary to obtain a good tracing. • If artifact looks like 60-cycle interference (very thick–lined waveform), unplug battery-operated equipment in room one item at a time to see whether interference disappears. **NOTE:** 60-cycle interference is rare. • Repeat tracing.
2. Patient has chest pain or anxiety.	• Continue to monitor patient. • Reassess factors contributing to anxiety or distress. • Follow specific prescriptions related to findings. • Notify health care provider.

Communication and Documentation

- Document date and time ECG was obtained, reason for obtaining ECG, and to whom ECG was given for interpretation in progress notes in electronic health record (EHR) or chart.
- Report any unexpected outcomes immediately.
- Document your evaluation of patient learning.

DOCUMENTATION EXAMPLE

A prescription was received for a routine 12-lead ECG. The procedure was explained, and the patient demonstrated understanding of the topic. The 12-lead ECG was then completed by the health care provider. The patient tolerated the procedure well, and the 12-lead ECG report was given to the health care provider for interpretation.

Special Considerations

Teaching

- Be aware that medications such as digitalis and amiodarone can affect ECG results.
- For patients with breast tissue, ensure that electrodes are placed directly on the chest wall and not the breast tissue. The breast may need to be lifted to accommodate chest leads V_4, V_5, and V_6.
- Lead placement for patients with a permanent pacemaker may require an augmented position if there is interference between the pacemaker and intrinsic signals.

Pediatric

- Most children with chest pain will be stable, but an ECG may be warranted if there are additional symptoms of cardiac disease (Geggel & Endom, 2022).
- Keeping a child still while completing an ECG may be difficult; thus, if appropriate, having the parent hold the child in their arms may be helpful.

Gerontological

- First-degree heart block can be a normal finding in an older person with no history of cardiac disease (Prutkin, 2020).

Care in the Community: Home Management

- Electronic textile ECG systems may be used for home-based patients, thus minimizing patient disruption (Teferra et al., 2018). New wearable ECG systems may be used for patients at home for early diagnosis of atrial fibrillation (Steinhubl et al., 2018).
- A Holter monitor is a device that may be worn for 24 to 48 hours to obtain an ambulatory ECG during daily activity. Holter monitors may be used when there is an inconclusive ECG.

✦ SKILL 26.2 Applying a Continuous (Telemetry) Cardiac Monitor

NSO *Nursing Skills Online Cardiac Care Module 10 / Lesson 3*

The use of continuous cardiac monitors is common inside hospitals, clinics, and outpatient settings. The cardiac monitor can be a bedside, hard-wired monitor or a wireless transmitter used with telemetry systems. A continuous ECG rhythm is obtained using three or five electrodes and leads on the patient. Cardiac monitors are attached to patients for immediate dysrhythmia detection; some dysrhythmias can be life threatening. They can also monitor a decrease or increase in heart rate. Most cardiac monitor systems have dysrhythmia detection software and provide alarms when dysrhythmias appear or when heart rate limits are exceeded.

It is important to monitor only patients with clinical indications for cardiac monitoring. This can significantly decrease the number of false alarms (McGuffin & Ortiz, 2019). The American Heart Association updated existing standards for ECG monitoring in hospitalized patients (Sandau et al., 2017) (Box 26.1). These standards are also used in Canada. Alarm fatigue occurs when a person is exposed to an excessive number of false alarms, leading to sensory overload (McGuffin & Ortiz, 2019). This may cause the person to become desensitized to the alarms and potentially influence their response time (McGuffin & Ortiz, 2019). Patient safety may be jeopardized if the alarms are silenced or ignored (AACN, 2018c). The American Association of Critical-Care Nurses (AACN, 2018c) has provided strategies for alarm management to enhance patient safety (Box 26.2). These strategies are applicable in the Canadian health care environment.

Delegation and Collaboration

The skill of applying a cardiac monitor is restricted to health care providers who are specifically trained in ECG monitoring (see employer policy), and it cannot be performed by a UCP. The nurse directs the UCP to do the following:

- Immediately report alarms or patient statements of pain or evidence of shortness of breath or hypotension
- Ensure that the parameters for alarms and heart rate are set per health care provider prescription

BOX 26.1

Class I Indications for Continuous Cardiac Monitoring

- Post-resuscitation patients
- Chest pain/coronary artery disease (e.g., early phase acute coronary syndrome)
- Major cardiac interventions (e.g., cardiac surgery)
- Arrhythmias (e.g., atrioventricular block, long QT syndrome, accessory pathway conduction, symptomatic bradycardia, atrial tachyarrhythmias)
- Syncope of suspected cardiac origin
- After electrophysiology procedure or ablations
- After pacemaker or implantable cardioverter–defibrillator implantation procedure
- Temporary or transcutaneous pacing
- Noncardiac conditions (e.g., after moderate sedation)
- Medical conditions (e.g., moderate to severe imbalance of potassium or magnesium; drug overdose)

Data from Sandau, K., Funk, M., Auerback, A., et al. (2017). Update to practice standards for electrocardiographic monitoring in hospital settings: A scientific statement from the American Heart Association. *Circulation, 136*(19), e1–e72. https://doi.org/10.1161/CIR.0000000000000527

BOX 26.2

Reducing Alarm Fatigue

- Provide proper skin preparation for ECG electrodes.
- Change ECG electrodes daily.
- Check alarm settings at the start of every shift, with any change in patient condition, and with any change in caregiver.
- Customize alarm parameters and levels of ECG monitors.
- Provide initial and ongoing education about devices with alarms.
- Establish interprofessional teams to address issues related to alarms, such as through development of policies and procedures.
- Monitor only patients with clinical indications for monitoring.
- Alarm settings set for appropriate patient population.

ECG, Electrocardiogram.
Adapted from American Association of Critical-Care Nurses. (2018a). *AACN Practice Alert: Alarm management.*

Equipment

- Bedside cardiac monitor or telemetry transmitter
- Three or five ECG electrodes (disposable, self-adhesive)
- Three or five ECG leads with snap-on attachments
- Clean, dry towel, washcloth, or gauze
- Hair clippers (*optional;* depends on amount of hair at electrode sites)

STEP	RATIONALE
ASSESSMENT	
1. Identify patient using at least two person-specific identifiers (e.g., name and date of birth, or name and medical record number) according to employer policy.	Ensures correct patient. Complies with Accreditation Canada's standards and improves patient safety (Accreditation Canada, 2020).
2. Throughout the procedure, the 4 moments for hand hygiene are to be implemented; hand hygiene should occur before initial patient (or patient environment) contact, before an aseptic procedure, after body fluid exposure risk, and after patient (or patient environment) contact. Additional hand hygiene should be performed when hands are visibly soiled.	Proper hand hygiene helps prevent the spread of infectious agents to health care providers.
3. Determine reason for continuous cardiac monitoring. Assess patient's history and cardiopulmonary status.	Knowing reason for monitoring allows for focused, improved response to an alarm.
4. Assess patient's level of understanding of procedure, including any concerns. Also assess for chest pain.	Determines extent of instruction and level of support required.
5. Check skin for excess oil or moisture. If present, wipe chest or limbs with clean, dry towel.	Provides clear, accurate recording without artifact.
6. Assess the need to secure or reapply electrodes.	Electrodes should be replaced on a routine basis according to facility policy (AACN, 2018b).

NURSING DIAGNOSES

- Acute pain
- Anxiety
- Insufficient knowledge regarding purpose and steps of procedure
- Fear

Related factors and risk factors are individualized on the basis of patient's condition or needs.

STEP	RATIONALE
PLANNING	
1. Expected outcomes following completion of procedure:	
• Patient tolerates procedure without anxiety or discomfort.	Appropriate preparation decreases anxiety.
• Clear, accurate, ongoing recording of ECG rhythm is obtained.	
2. Explain procedure to patient. If applicable, teach patient how to report chest pain.	Reduces anxiety and promotes cooperation. Reporting of chest pain by patient may promote early intervention.
3. Close room door or bedside curtains.	Provides privacy.
4. Gather equipment for ECG monitoring.	Allows for increased efficiency of procedure.
IMPLEMENTATION	
1.	Reduces transmission of microorganisms.
2. Prepare patient for procedure:	
a. Remove or reposition patient's gown to expose only patient's chest. Keep abdomen and thighs covered.	Facilitates correct placement of cardiac leads and maintains patient's modesty.
b. Place patient in supine position.	Electrodes must be placed on anterior chest.
3. Clean and prepare chest area with soap and water for electrode placement. Wipe area with a dry washcloth (Sandau et al., 2017). Where possible, avoid the use of products that dry skin, such as alcohol-based skin preps (Fumarola et al., 2020). Clip excessive hair from electrode area rather than shaving.	Proper skin preparation decreases skin impedance and signal noise, thus providing an accurate recording. Do not use alcohol to clean area because it will dry the skin and increase the risk for MARSI. Clipping excessive hair rather than shaving reduces the risk for infection.
4. Apply electrodes in correct positions for either a three- or five-electrode system (Fig. 26.8).	Proper placement of leads is essential for accurate dysrhythmia interpretation.
a. For cisgender women and nonoperative trans men, the precordial leads (V_3–V_6) should be placed under the left breast.	Reduces interference with ECG reading (Prutkin, 2021).

STEP	RATIONALE

IMPLEMENTATION

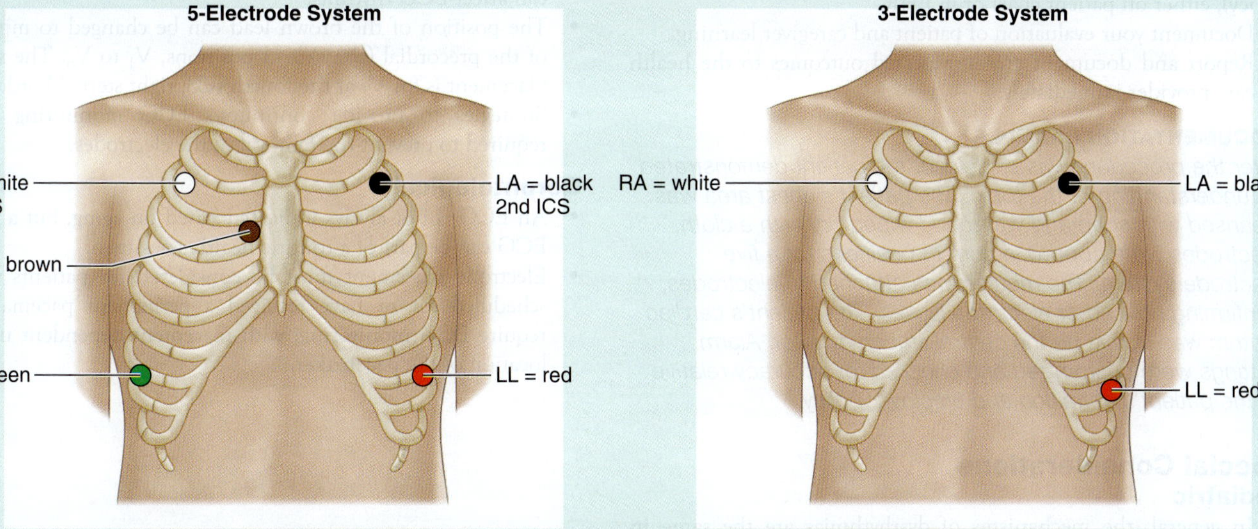

FIG 26.8 **Cardiac monitor lead placement for three- and five-electrode systems.** *ICS*, Intercostal space; *LA*, left arm; *LL*, left leg; *RA*, right arm; *RL*, right leg.

STEP	RATIONALE
5. Attach monitor leads to electrodes. Colours of leads represent their polarity. White is negative. Black is positive. Red is ground or neutral. Two additional leads on a five-lead system would include a green lead (positive or negative) and a brown lead (positive), which can be placed at V lead locations on the precordial chest.	Colouring system (labelling) allows for consistent application of leads.
6. Check bedside monitor or telemetry station for any messages indicating electrode or lead issues. Troubleshoot as needed.	Monitoring system itself may detect bad electrode contact with skin or loose connection.
7. Check that the ECG rhythm can be visualized on bedside monitor, central station, or remote viewing station.	If staff are watching monitor remotely, communicate with them before you leave the room so you can correct any issues while on the phone with viewers. This call can also serve as notification that monitoring has started.
8. Change ECG electrodes daily or more often if electrode contact to skin is loose. Inspect condition of skin.	Changing ECG electrodes decreases the number of false alarms (McGuffin & Ortiz, 2019). Monitors for development of MARSI.
9. Customize alarm limits within 1 hour of assuming care of patient and on condition changes. Changes made should be in accordance with employer policies and health care provider prescription.	Alarm settings need to be individualized, checked for accuracy, and detectable (McGuffin & Ortiz, 2019).

EVALUATION

STEP	RATIONALE
1. Although procedure is painless, it is important to note and document whether patient experiences any distress.	
2. Ensure that all appropriate alarms are on.	Ensures accurate monitoring. Refer to employer policies.
3. Inspect condition of skin after electrode removal for signs of MARSI.	Continual electrode placement and removal can lead to development of MARSI.
4. **Use teach-back:** "I want to be sure I explained to you why you need this monitoring. Can you tell me why monitoring your heart is important?" Develop a revised teaching plan if patient or caregiver is unable to explain rationale for procedure correctly.	Determines patient's and caregiver's level of understanding of instructional topic.

Unexpected Outcomes	Related Interventions
1. Monitor tracing cannot be interpreted: • Absence of tracing on one or more leads • Presence of artifact in ECG tracings	• Inspect electrodes for secure placement. Replace as needed and provide new skin preparation. • Reposition any wires that move as a result of patient breathing or movement or vibrations in environment. Do not reposition electrodes if in correct position. • If artifact looks like 60-cycle interference (very thick–lined waveform), unplug battery-operated equipment in room one item at a time to see whether interference disappears. **Note:** 60-cycle interference is rare.

Communication and Documentation

- Review alarm trends and waveforms at least once a shift and on report of an alarm.
- Document at least one rhythm strip per shift (see employer policy), either on patient chart or in EHR.
- Document your evaluation of patient and caregiver learning.
- Report and document any unexpected outcomes to the health care provider immediately.

DOCUMENTATION EXAMPLE

After the procedure was explained, the patient demonstrated an understanding of the topic. The patient's chest area was cleansed with soap and water and wiped dry with a cloth. Electrodes were applied in correct positions for a five-electrode system. The monitor was attached to electrodes, confirming no lead or electrode issues. The patient's cardiac rhythm was visible on the central station monitor. Alarm settings were customized and checked for accuracy relative to the patient's condition and employer policy.

Special Considerations

Pediatric

- In general, the mechanisms of dysrhythmias are the same in children as they are in adults; however, the appearance of the dysrhythmias on the ECG may differ because of developmental issues such as heart size, baseline heart rate, SA and AV node function, and autonomic innervation.
- Be aware that medications such as digitalis and antiarrhythmics can affect ECG rhythms.
- The position of the brown lead can be changed to mirror one of the precordial (chest) lead positions, V_1 to V_6. The standard placement is for V_1 at the fourth ICS, right sternal border.
- Strategies to provide continuous ECG monitoring may be required to prevent the removal of the electrodes.

Gerontological

- An ECG is not always indicated based on aging, but a baseline ECG can be part of a routine health assessment.
- Electrode placement must be considered for patients who are scheduled for or have received a permanent pacemaker and require ECG monitoring, with placement dependent upon the location of the pacemaker.

✦ REVIEW QUESTIONS

1. A 25-year-old person was recently admitted to a medical unit for continuous cardiac monitoring related to tachycardia, shortness of breath, and agitation. The cardiologist believes that the symptoms are related to the ingestion of too many energy beverages. The nurse hears the alarms beeping in this patient's room. As the nurse enters the room, they notice a significant change in the cardiac rhythm.
   1. What should the nurse do next?
   2. What nursing actions should be considered relative to alarm safety?
   3. If the cardiac rhythm is an artifact, what nursing interventions should the nurse consider?

2. A 55-year-old patient (she/her) is postoperative day 4 following a total hip replacement. She has a history of a previous non-ST segment myocardial infarction (MI); thus, continuous cardiac monitoring has been ordered. The patient informs the nurse that they are experiencing chest pain, nausea, and shortness of breath. Vital signs are as follows: BP, 100/50 mm Hg (previous BP 128/70); pulse, 150 beats/min and regular (previous pulse 95); respiratory rate, 28 breaths/min; pulse oximetry (SpO_2), 90% on room air; and temperature, 37.5°C. The current telemetry rhythm reveals sinus tachycardia with a heart rate of 150. The nurse decides to call the health care provider.
   1. What does the nurse suspect is the primary physical concern for this patient? Based on the current patient findings (listed above), what further assessments would be required before contacting the health care provider?
   2. Based on the patient's signs and symptoms, which prescription should the nurse anticipate?
   3. Using SBAR (situation–background–assessment–recommendation), how would the nurse communicate with the health care provider about this patient?

3. The nurse has initiated cardiac monitoring via telemetry and notices an artifact on the patient's electrocardiogram (ECG) rhythm. How should the nurse troubleshoot this artifact problem? (*Select all that apply.*)
   1. Move electrodes to different locations on the chest.
   2. Wipe electrode skin areas with alcohol.
   3. Prepare skin by washing with soap and water and drying with a washcloth.
   4. Not change electrodes for 2 days.
   5. Inspect electrodes for secure placement.
   6. Consider the patient's activity level.

4. What are the indications for a 12-lead electrocardiogram (ECG)? (*Select all that apply.*)
   1. Suspected acute coronary syndromes, including myocardial infarction
   2. Evaluation of implanted defibrillators and pacemakers
   3. Disorders of the cardiac rhythm
   4. Evaluation of shortness of breath
   5. Evaluation of metabolic disorders
   6. Suspected posterior myocardial infarction

5. When preparing a patient for a 12-lead electrocardiogram (ECG), it is necessary to apply six precordial chest leads. Match the lead with the correct anatomical position on the patient's chest.

1. V_1	1. Fifth intercostal space (ICS) at midclavicular line
2. V_2	2. Left midaxillary line at level of V_4 horizontally
3. V_3	3. Left anterior axillary line at level of V_4 horizontally
4. V_4	4. Fourth ICS at right sternal border
5. V_5	5. Midway between V_2 and V_4
6. V_6	6. Fourth ICS at left sternal border

6. Indications for completing a 12-lead ECG monitoring patients include (a) ________, ________, and ________. The advantages of continuous monitoring include (b) ________ and ________.

Answer options for (a):
- Acute coronary syndrome
- Potentially life-threatening dysthymias
- Change in patient status
- Order for continuous cardiac monitoring

Answer options for (b):
- Wireless transmitter
- Monitor during ambulation
- "Snapshot" of cardiac electrical activity
- Reduce risk of alarm fatigue

Visit the Evolve site for a complete list of answers to the Review Questions.

NEXT GENERATION NCLEX® (NGN)

For practice with answering exam questions related to unfolding NGN case studies, please consult the Next Generation NCLEX® (NGN)-Style Case Studies for Skills and Techniques on the Evolve website: http://evolve.elsevier.com/Canada/Perry/clinicalskills/

REFERENCES

Accreditation Canada. (2020). *Required organizational practices handbook*. https://physicians.nshealth.ca/resources/required-organizational-practices-2020-handbook

American Association of Critical-Care Nurses (AACN). (2018a). *AACN practice alert: Alarm management*

American Association of Critical-Care Nurses (AACN). (2018b). *AACN practice Alert: Ensuring accurate ST-segment monitoring*. https://www.aacn.org/clinical-resources/practice-alerts/st-segment-monitoring

American Association of Critical-Care Nurses (AACN). (2018c). *Managing alarms in acute care across the life span: Electrocardiography and pulse oximetry*. https://www.aacn.org/clinical-resources/practice-alerts/managing-alarms-in-acute-care-across-the-life-span

Anderson, D., & Sexton, D. J. (2021). Overview of control measures for prevention of surgical site infection in adults. *UpToDate*. https://www.uptodate.com/contents/overview-of-control-measures-for-prevention-of-surgical-site-infection-in-adults

Fumarola, S., Allaway, R., Callaghan, R., et al. (2020). Overlooked and underestimated: Medical adhesive-related skin injuries. Best practice consensus document on prevention. *Journal of Wound Care, 29*(Suppl. 3c), S1–S4. https://doi.10.12968/jowc.2020.29.Sup3c.S1

Geggel, R., & Endom, E. (2022). Nontraumatic chest pain in children and adolescents: Approach and initial management. *UpToDate*. https://www.uptodate.com/contents/nontraumatic-chest-pain-in-children-and-adolescents-approach-and-initial-management/

Heart and Stroke Foundation of Canada. (2018). *Ms. Understood: Women's hearts are victim of a system that is ill-equipped to diagnose, treat and support them*. https://www.heartandstroke.ca/-/media/pdf-files/canada/2018-heart-month/hs_2018-heart-report_en.ashx

McGuffin, K. S., & Ortiz, S. (2019). Daily electrocardiogram electrode change and the effect on frequency of nuisance alarms. *Dimensions of Critical Care Nursing, 38*(4), 187–191. https://doi.10.1097/DCC.0000000000000362

Panchal, A. R., Bartos, J. A., Cabañas, J. G., et al. (2020). 2020 American Heart Association guidelines for cardiopulmonary resuscitation and emergency cardiovascular care. Part 3: Adult basic and advanced life support. *Circulation, 142*(Suppl. 2), S366–S468. https://doi.org/10.1161/CIR.0000000000000916

Prutkin, J. M. (2020). ECG tutorial: Chamber enlargement and hypertrophy. *UpToDate*. https://www.uptodate.com/contents/ecg-tutorial-chamber-enlargement-and-hypertrophy

Prutkin, J. M. (2021). ECG tutorial: Electrical components of the ECG. *UpToDate*. https://www.uptodate.com/contents/ecg-tutorial-electrical-components-of-the-ecg/print

Prutkin, J. M. (2022). ECG tutorial: Basic principles of ECG analysis. *UpToDate*. https://www.uptodate.com/contents/ecg-tutorial-basic-principles-of-ecg-analysis

Sandau, K., Funk, M., Auerback, A., et al. (2017). Update to practice standards for electrocardiographic monitoring in hospital settings: A scientific statement from the American Heart Association. *Circulation, 136*(19), e1–e71. https://doi.org/10.1161/CIR.0000000000000527

Steinhubl, S. R., Wallen, J., Edwards, A. M., et al. (2018). Effect of home-based wearable continuous ECG monitoring patch on detection of undiagnosed atrial fibrillation: The mSToPS randomized clinical trial. *JAMA, 320*(2), 146–155. https://doi.10.1001/jama.2018.8102

Teferra, M. N., Kourbelis, C., Newman, P., et al. (2018). Electronic textile electrocardiogram monitoring in cardiac patients: A scoping review protocol. *JBI Database of Systemic Reviews and Implementation Reports, 17*(2), 147–156. https://doi.org/10.11124/JBISRIR-2017-003630

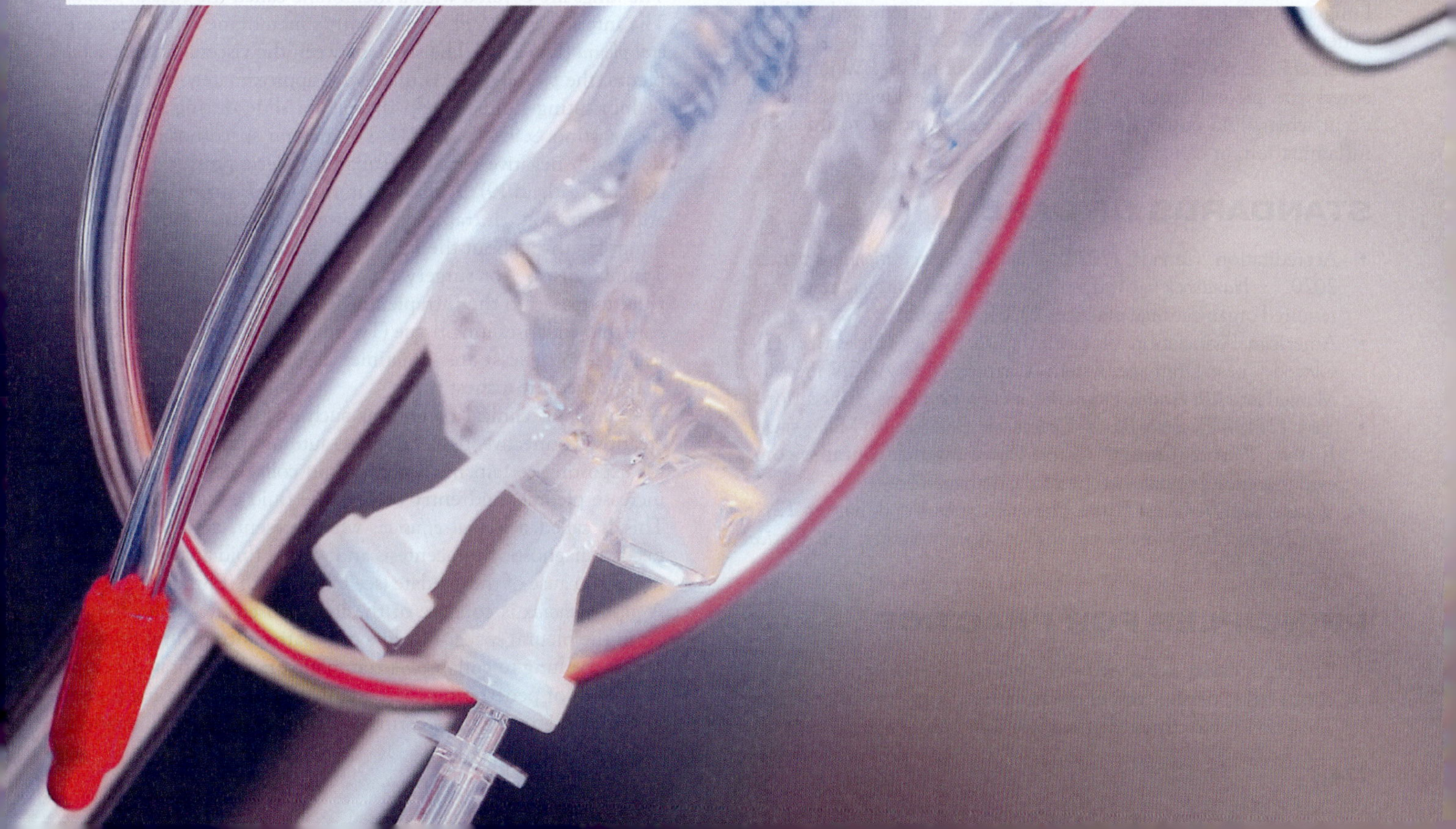

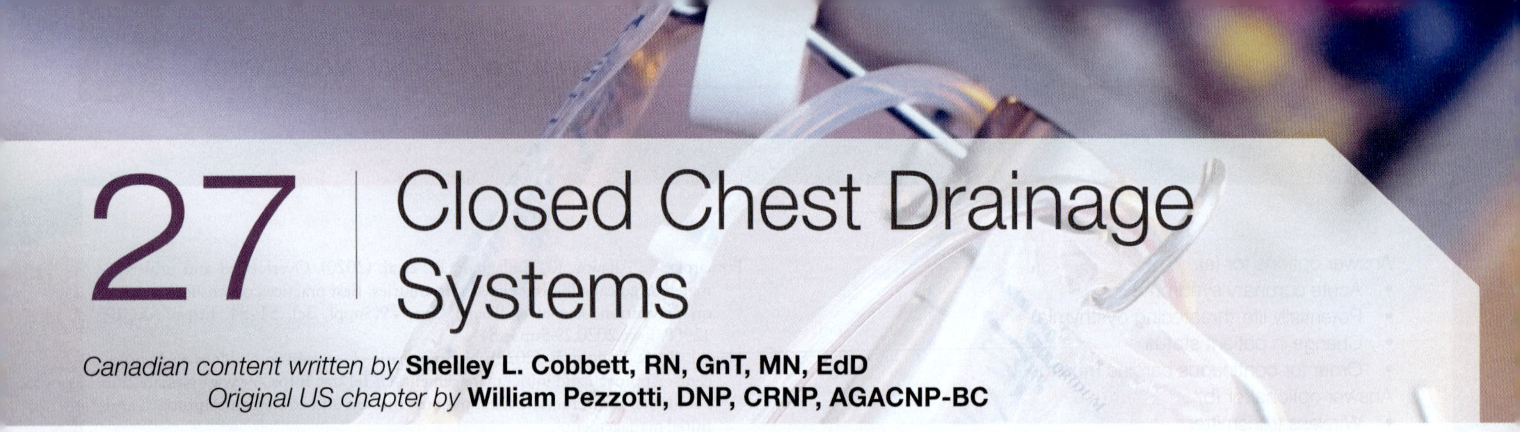

27 | Closed Chest Drainage Systems

Canadian content written by **Shelley L. Cobbett, RN, GnT, MN, EdD**
Original US chapter by **William Pezzotti, DNP, CRNP, AGACNP-BC**

SKILLS AND PROCEDURES

OBJECTIVES

Mastery of content in this chapter will enable the nurse to:

- Explain the physiology of normal respiration.
- List three common sites for chest tube placement.
- List three conditions requiring chest tube insertion.
- Explain closed chest drainage systems: water-seal and waterless systems.
- Explain the principles and mechanisms of chest tube suction.
- Describe measures to maintain patient safety during chest tube insertion, maintenance, and removal.
- Describe methods of troubleshooting chest tube systems.
- Explain the nursing principles for managing patients with chest tubes.
- Describe autotransfusion.

MEDIA RESOURCES

- http://evolve.elsevier.com/Canada/Perry/clinicalskills/

PURPOSE

The purpose of a closed chest drainage system, with or without suction, is to promote drainage of air and fluid from the pleural space. Lung re-expansion occurs as the fluid or air is removed and the patient's oxygenation improves (Tyerman & Cobbett, 2023). When air enters the pleural space, a pneumothorax occurs. When blood enters the pleural space, a hemothorax occurs. Pleural effusions occur when fluid enters the pleural space in response to infection, inflammation, or cancer.

STANDARDS OF CARE

- Accreditation Canada (2020)—*Required Organizational Practices–2020 Handbook* (https://physicians.nshealth.ca/resources/required-organizational-practices-2020-handbook)
- American Association of Critical-Care Nurses (Pickett, 2017)—Closed Chest Drainage System (Chapter 25 in *AACN Procedure Manual for High Acuity, Progressive, and Critical Care*, 7th edition)
- Sasa (2019)—*Evidence-Based Update on Chest Tube Management: Is Your Practice Current?* (https://www.myamericannurse.com/evidence-based-update-on-chest-tube-management/)
- Waters (2017)—Chest Tube Placement (Assist) (Chapter 22 in *AACN Procedure Manual for High Acuity, Progressive, and Critical Care*, 7th edition)

PRINCIPLES FOR PRACTICE

- The chest cavity is a closed structure bounded by muscle, bone, connective tissue, vascular structures, and the diaphragm. This cavity has three distinct sections, each sealed from the others: one section for each lung and a third section for the mediastinum, which surrounds the heart, esophagus, trachea, and great vessels.
- The lungs are covered with a membrane called the *visceral pleura*. The interior chest wall is lined with a membrane called the *parietal pleura* (Fig. 27.1). The space between the visceral and parietal pleura, the *pleural space*, is filled with approximately 10 to 20 mL of lubricating fluid to help the pleura slide during respiration (D'Agostino & Edens, 2021). The pleural space normally functions with negative pressure (subatmospheric pressure) (Banasik & Copstead, 2019). Although it fluctuates during inspiration and expiration, intrapleural pressure remains approximately 4 mm Hg throughout the breathing cycle.
- Trauma, disease, or surgery can cause air, blood, pus, or lymph fluid to leak into the intrapleural space, creating a positive pressure that collapses lung tissue (Tyerman & Cobbett, 2023). Small leaks (24% or less) are sometimes absorbed spontaneously and may not require a chest tube.
- A number of clinical conditions such as cancer, infection, pancreatitis, connective tissue disease, autoimmune diseases, asbestos exposure, certain medications, and collagen vascular diseases increase pleural fluid entry or decrease fluid exit from the lung. This is called a *pleural effusion*; when present, a patient usually needs a diagnostic thoracentesis and pleural fluid analysis to determine the cause of the exudate (see Chapter 10) (Ehrhardt, 2017).
- A *pneumothorax* is collapse of the lung caused by a collection of air in the pleural space. The loss of negative intrapleural pressure causes the lung to collapse. A traumatic pneumothorax develops as a result of penetrating chest trauma such as a stabbing (open) or the chest striking the steering wheel in an automobile accident

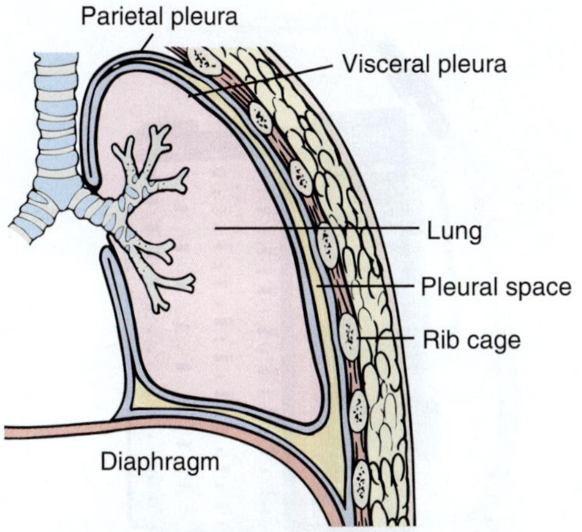

FIG 27.1 Partial structures of lungs.

(closed). A spontaneous or primary pneumothorax sometimes occurs from the rupture of a small bleb (blister) on the surface of the lung or an invasive procedure, such as insertion of a subclavian intravenous (IV) line. Secondary pneumothorax occurs from an underlying disease, such as emphysema. A patient with a pneumothorax usually feels sharp chest pain that worsens on inspiration or coughing because atmospheric air irritates the parietal pleura (Banasik & Copstead, 2019).

- A tension pneumothorax, a life-threatening situation, occurs from rupture in the pleura when air accumulates in the pleural space more rapidly than it is removed. If left untreated, the lung on the affected side collapses, and the mediastinum shifts to the opposite (unaffected side), leading to tracheal deviation, reduced venous return, and subsequent decrease in cardiac output. Tracheal deviation is a late sign and may be absent in some cases (Huggins et al., 2022; Waters, 2017). Sudden chest pain, a fall in blood pressure, tachycardia, acute pleuritic pain, diaphoresis, dry cough, and cardiopulmonary arrest can occur.
- If emergent treatment is required, a needle decompression is achieved with a large-gauge needle (14 or 16 gauge) inserted into the second intercostal space, midclavicular line. A "hissing" sound is noted, followed by a rapid stabilization of the patient's vital signs and respiratory status (Huggins et al., 2022).
- A *hemothorax* is collapse of the lung caused by an accumulation of blood and fluid in the pleural cavity between the chest wall and the lung, usually as a result of trauma. It produces a counterpressure and prevents the full expansion of the lung. A hemothorax is also caused by rupture of small blood vessels from inflammatory processes such as pneumonia or tuberculosis. In addition to pain and dyspnea, signs and symptoms of shock can develop if blood loss is severe (Mancini, 2022).
- Chest tube insertion is the treatment for most types of effusions, pneumothorax, hemothorax, and postoperative chest surgery or trauma. A *chest tube* is a large catheter inserted through the thorax to remove fluid (effusions), blood (hemothorax), and/or air (pneumothorax).
- A pleural chest tube (Fig. 27.2) is inserted when air or fluid enters the pleural space, compromising oxygenation or ventilation.
- The location of the chest tube indicates the type of drainage expected. Apical (second or third intercostal space) and anterior chest tube placement promotes removal of air. Because air rises, these chest tubes are placed high, allowing evacuation of air from the intrapleural space and lung re-expansion (Fig. 27.3). The air is discharged into the atmosphere, and there is little or no drainage in the collection chamber.

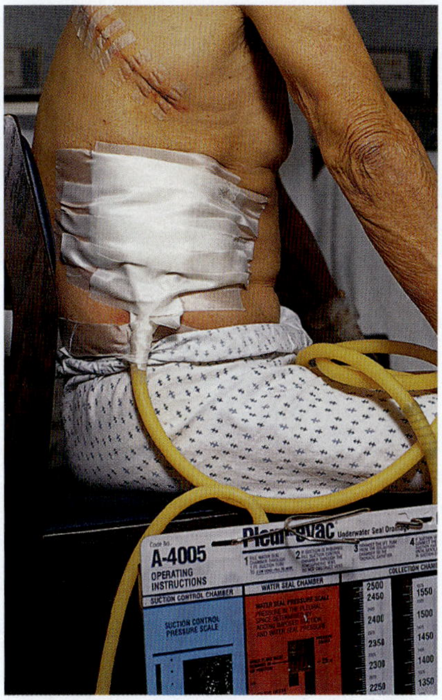

FIG 27.2 Pleural chest tube in place following thoracic surgery.

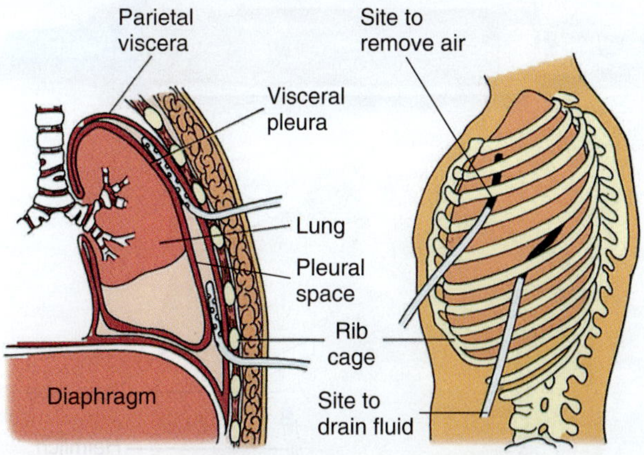

FIG 27.3 Diagram of sites for chest tube placement.

- Chest tubes placed low (usually in the fifth or sixth intercostal space) and posteriorly or laterally drain fluid (see Fig. 27.3). Fluid in the intrapleural space is affected by gravity and localizes in the lower part of the lung cavity. Tubes placed in these positions drain blood and fluid. Fluid drainage is expected after open-chest surgery and with some chest trauma.
- A mediastinal chest tube is placed in the mediastinum, just below the sternum (Fig. 27.4), and is connected to a drainage system. This tube drains blood or fluid, preventing its accumulation around the heart. A mediastinal tube is commonly used after open-heart surgery.
- In emergent situations, a small pneumothorax catheter is inserted through the chest wall, and a rubber flutter one-way valve (e.g., a Heimlich valve) is attached to the catheter (Fig. 27.5, *A–B*). As a patient exhales, the positive pressure generated by the air leaving the chest enters the tubing, causing the valve to open so air is released. During inspiration, the tube collapses on itself, preventing air from re-entering the chest. This type of valve is not used when patients need fluid drained, such as from a hemothorax or a pleural effusion (Tyerman & Cobbett, 2023).

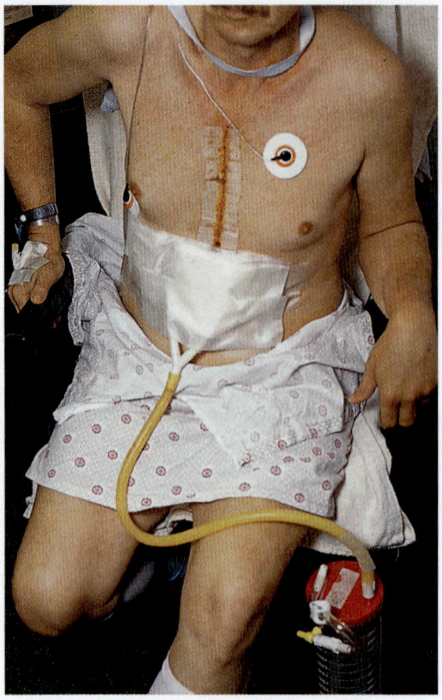

FIG 27.4 Mediastinal chest tube.

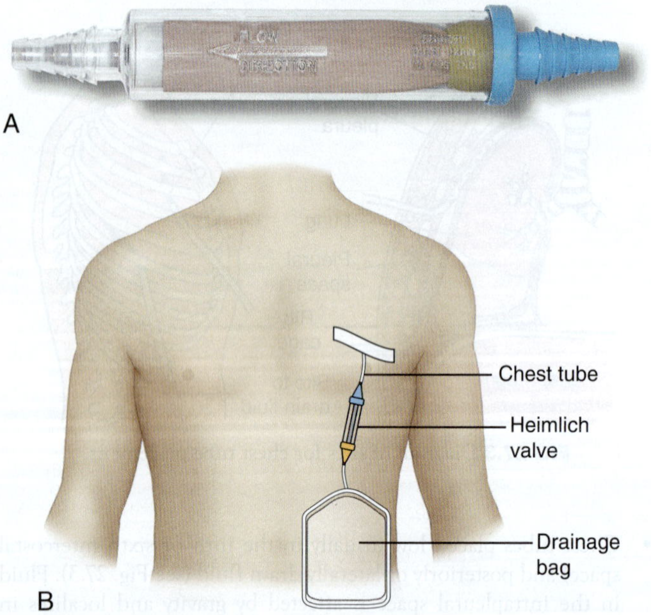

FIG 27.5 **A, The Heimlich chest drain valve is a specially designed flutter valve that is used in place of a chest drainage unit for a small, uncomplicated pneumothorax with little or no drainage and no need for suction. The valve allows for escape of air but prevents re-entry of air into the pleural space. B, Placement of valve between chest tube and drainage bag; this device can be worn under clothing.** (*A, Image courtesy Becton, Dickenson and Company, Franklin Lakes, New Jersey. All rights reserved.*)

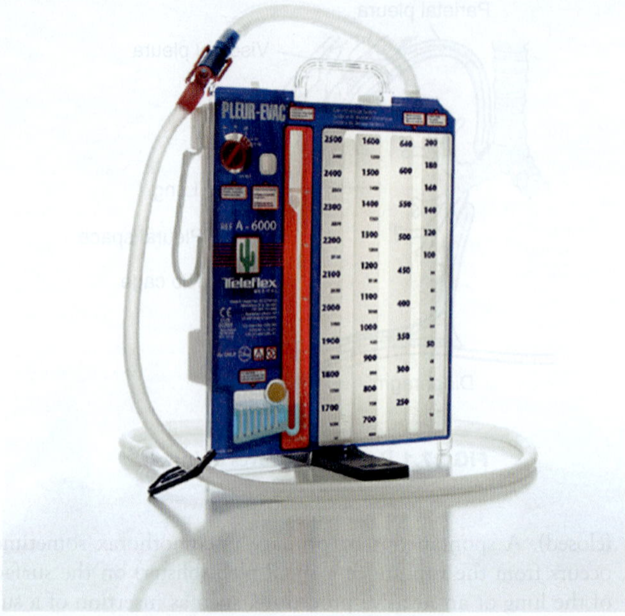

FIG 27.6 **Disposable chest drainage systems.** (*Multiple-chamber Pleur-Evac image courtesy Teleflex Medical, Research Triangle Park, NC.*)

- Smaller "pigtail catheters" are also used and are less traumatic than the large-bore tubes. Ambulatory management with pigtail catheters is reasonable first-line treatment for spontaneous pneumothoraxes (Tyerman & Cobbett, 2023).
- Mobile chest drains are devices that are lighter and self-contained; they allow patients to move with less restriction and cause less discomfort. These mobile systems rely on gravity or dry suction for drainage. They are ideal for home use for patients with persistent drainage or air leaks requiring prolonged use of a chest tube.
- Disposable chest drainage systems, such as Atrium or Pleur-Evac, are one-piece moulded plastic units that consist of a single- or multiple-chamber closed drainage system (Fig. 27.6). A single-chamber system allows air from a pneumothorax to bubble out of the water seal and escape through the air outlet while preventing it from re-entering the intrapleural space. The drawback of a single-chamber system is that any chest drainage present collects in the same chamber that provides the water seal. If the single-chamber system fills with chest fluid, the water-seal level would rise, making it more difficult for the patient to expel any air. Thus, single-chamber systems are not recommended for the evacuation of fluid. An increased height of fluid in the water seal increases the resistance to drainage on expiration and eventually stops drainage entirely.
- A two- or three-chamber system drains both a hemothorax and a pneumothorax effectively. The two-chamber system permits liquid to flow into the collection chamber and air to flow into the water-seal chamber. A three-chamber system promotes the drainage of fluid and air with controlled suction. In both systems, the first chamber provides a compartment for fluid or blood drainage and the second compartment has either a water seal or a one-way valve. In the three-chamber system, the third compartment is used for suction control, which may or may not be required. Disposable units appear to be the system of choice because they are cost effective and some facilitate autotransfusion; they are occasionally used in open-heart surgeries.

PERSON-CENTRED CARE

- Infections, though rare with chest tubes, can include skin infections at the insertion site; *empyema*, a collection of pus in the pleural cavity; and even necrotizing infections (Rajan, 2022).
- Nurses must be vigilant when patient assessment findings indicate the need for a chest tube. Nurses should encourage patients to practise deep-breathing exercises and early mobility, and the use of appropriate analgesia to promote activity, as well as patient education regarding these activities (Tyerman & Cobbett, 2023).

- Autotransfusion may pose a challenge to nurses caring for patients with certain religious beliefs (e.g., Jehovah's Witness faith). A patient may wish to discuss options with elders of their church before consenting to any blood transfusions.

EVIDENCE-INFORMED PRACTICE

- Small chest tubes often become blocked by blood clots and fibrin. Large-bore catheters (such as 28F) safely remove secretions (Waters, 2017).
- Milking and stripping a chest tube to clear the clots are controversial practices and when done on a routine basis can do more harm than good (Huggins et al., 2022; Sasa, 2019). Stripping causes a dangerous increase in intrathoracic pressure, which damages the lung tissue (Sasa, 2019; Tyerman & Cobbett, 2023). Chest drainage stripping or milking demonstrates no safety or efficacy benefits, slightly increases intrathoracic pressure, and risks tissue damage (Sasa, 2019).
- Careful management of chest tube drainage prevents chest tube occlusion (Bauman & Handley, 2018):
  - Avoid having dependent loops of the drainage tube; or, when these loops cannot be avoided (such as when the patient is sitting), lift and clear the tube every 15 to 30 minutes.
  - Keep the chest drainage tubing and the collection system below the level of the patient's chest. Keep the tubing above the collection system to allow drainage by gravity.
  - Tailor the length of the drainage tube to a patient. The tubing must be long enough to allow a patient to move but not so long that dependent loops hang down the side of the bed. If the tubing is coiled, looped, or clotted, the drainage is impeded and can result in a tension pneumothorax (Huggins et al., 2022; Tyerman & Cobbett, 2023).

SAFETY GUIDELINES

- Document patient's baseline vital signs, oxygen saturation, lung sounds, and respiratory status. Changes in vital signs or respiratory status often indicate a malfunction of a chest drainage system.
- Observe the water seal for intermittent bubbling or a rise and fall of fluid that is synchronous with respirations (Tyerman & Cobbett, 2023; Waters, 2017). For example, in a spontaneously breathing patient, the fluid level rises during inspiration and falls during expiration. When a patient is on a mechanical ventilator, the opposite occurs.
  - Constant bubbling in the water seal or a sudden, unexpected stoppage of water-seal activity is considered abnormal and requires immediate attention (Sasa, 2019; Waters, 2017).
  - Unexpected stoppage of chest tube activity may indicate a blockage or lung re-expansion. In these situations, immediate attention and correction are indicated. After 2 or 3 days, tidalling or bubbling on expiration is expected to stop, indicating that the lung has re-expanded and that the chest tube can be removed (Sasa, 2019).
- In a waterless system, look for a rise and fall of fluid in the diagnostic air-leak indicator, synchronous with respirations. Constant left-to-right bubbling (when facing the indicator) or violent rocking is considered abnormal and indicates an air leak.
- Note the expected amount of chest tube drainage and monitor drainage on a regular basis (e.g., every hour initially and then every 4 hours). At the end of the shift, make a mark to indicate the fluid level with the date and time on the side of the drainage collection chamber. Note the drainage amount as output.
  - A sudden decrease in the amount of chest tube drainage can indicate a possible clot or obstruction in the chest tube (Quinte Health Care [QHC], 2020; Sasa, 2019).
  - Notify a health care provider when there is a sudden increase of more than 250 mL of drainage over 1 hour, which can indicate fresh bleeding from the thorax (QHC, 2020; Sasa, 2019).
  - Drainage from a pneumothorax is generally limited. Any fluid buildup is caused by chest tube insertion trauma. The chest tubes promote the removal of air from the intrapleural space.
- Know the expected colour of the drainage. Drainage from recent open-chest surgery initially is bright red and gradually becomes serous as the postoperative course continues. Blood-tinged fluid usually indicates malignancy, pulmonary infarction, or severe inflammation. Frank blood indicates a hemothorax. Pus indicates an empyema (Tyerman & Cobbett, 2023).
- In the water-seal system, observe for constant, gentle bubbling in the suction-control chamber when it is connected to suction. In the waterless system, a designated amount of suction is maintained by setting the suction source and dialling the prescribed suction level in the float ball column.
- Assess both types of systems for air leaks. If an air leak exists, determine whether it is in the patient (patient-centred air leak) or in the chest tube system (system-centred air leak). To rule out an air leak as patient centred, assess the patient's respiratory status. Document and report any changes in lung sounds, pulse oximetry, respiratory rate, or mentation. Remember that continuous bubbling in the water-seal chamber with an absence of bubbles in the suction-control chamber indicates that there is a leak in the system (Sasa, 2019). Ensure that all tubing connections are tight.
- Be sure that the drainage system is stable. Most chest drainage units have attached adjustable hangers that allow the device to hang on the side or end of the patient's bed. Many have a swing-out floor stand to reduce the chance of accidently knocking over the chest drainage system if it is placed on the floor. Some manufacturers make a reusable drain caddy that allows the chest drainage system to be connected to an IV pole to facilitate patient movement and eliminate the possibility of knocking over the system.
- Do not attempt to empty a chest tube drainage system.
- Chest tube drainage systems are replaced only when the collection chamber is full or if the system is contaminated.
- Never clamp a chest tube without a health care provider's prescription.
- Only clamp a chest tube if (1) changing the drainage system, (2) assessing for an air leak, (3) the chest tube becomes disconnected from the chest drainage system (short time only), or (4) removing the chest tube.

✦ SKILL 27.1 Managing Closed Chest Drainage Systems

NSO Nursing Skills Online Chest Tubes Module 11 / Lessons 2 and 3

There are two types of commercial drainage systems: water-seal and waterless systems (Table 27.1). This procedure involves interprofessional collaboration, although only the health care provider may insert the chest tube. This skill reviews the nursing responsibilities and interventions related to safe management of chest tubes. Review the actions, roles, and responsibilities of the health care provider for chest tube placement (Table 27.2).

TABLE 27.1

Comparison of Chest Tube Drainage Systems

Drainage System Type	Function	Advantage	Disadvantage
Water-seal system (Fig. 27.7)	Two-chamber system provides one-way valve for chest drainage. Water seal prevents re-entry of air into lung. Three-chamber system adds a chamber to aid evacuation of chest drainage.	Easy setup and use Cost effective	System must be kept upright to maintain seal. Drainage chamber may fill up quickly if patient has large amount of drainage. Sterile water must be added several times a day to maintain suction and water seal because of evaporation.
Waterless system (Fig. 27.8)	Also provides three chambers, but no water is required to establish a seal.	Seal maintained by one-way valve Accidental tipping of system does not compromise patient's condition More space provided for drainage	Water must be added to an air-leak indicator if patient requires evaluation for an air leak.
Dry suction system (Fig. 27.9)	Also provides three chambers, but suction is controlled by an integrated valve.	Easy setup Quiet operation Can be used when higher levels of suction are required	Sterile water must be added to system to provide a water seal.

TABLE 27.2

Process for Insertion of Chest Tubes

Action	Purpose and Roles
Explain purpose, procedure, and possible complications to patient and ensure patient has signed the consent form.	The health care provider provides information and obtains informed consent.
Have pain medication available to administer before or immediately after chest tube insertion as appropriate according to patient's condition.	The nurse obtains the medication prescription prior to the procedure. Analgesia improves patient comfort throughout procedure and helps patient take appropriate deep breaths to promote lung expansion and drainage of fluid in pleural space.
Unless an emergent situation exists, perform "time-out" step before initiating procedure (see Chapter 38).	This interprofessional collaborative protocol is performed immediately prior to a planned procedure as a universal patient safety initiative. During this procedure, the team confirms patient identity, surgical site, and planned procedure.
Clean chest wall with antiseptic.	All team members ensure aseptic technique is performed. Reduces transmission of microorganisms.
Apply mask and gloves.	All team members don appropriate personal protective equipment (PPE). Maintains surgical asepsis.
Drape area of chest tube insertion with sterile towels. Health care provider injects local anaesthetic and allows time for it to take effect.	Health care provider maintains surgical asepsis. Decreases pain during procedure.
Health care provider makes a small incision over the rib space where tube is to be inserted. Health care provider threads a clamped chest tube through the incision. Health care provider clamps chest tube until system is connected to water seal.	Inserts chest tube into intrapleural space. Clamping prevents entry of atmospheric air into chest and worsening of pneumothorax.
Health care provider sutures chest tube in place if suturing is policy or health care provider preference.	Secures chest tube in place.
Nurse covers chest tube insertion site with sterile 10 cm × 10 cm (4 inch × 4 inch) gauze and large dressing to form an occlusive dressing. Sterile petrolatum-impregnated gauze is used around the tube.	Holds chest tube in place and occludes site around it. Helps stabilize chest tube and holds dressing tightly in place. Sterile petrolatum-impregnated gauze helps prevent air leak.
Water-Seal System	
Remove connector cover from patient's end of chest drainage tubing with sterile technique. Secure drainage tubing to chest tube and drainage system.	Health care provider is responsible for making certain that system is set up properly, proper amount of water is in the water seal, dressing is secure, and chest tube is connected to drainage system securely.
Water-Seal Suction	
Connect system to suction or supervise a nurse connecting it to suction if suction is to be used.	Health care provider is responsible for determining and checking amount of fluid that is to be added to suction-control chamber and prescribing suction setting.
Waterless System	
Remove connector cover from patient's end of chest drainage tubing with sterile technique. Secure drainage tubing to chest tube and drainage system.	Health care provider is responsible for making certain that system is set up properly and chest tube is securely connected to drainage system.

TABLE 27.2

Process for Insertion of Chest Tubes—cont'd

Action	Purpose and Roles
Waterless Suction	
Turn on suction source. Set suction indicator (float ball or bellows) to prescribed setting.	Health care provider is responsible for prescribing suction level.
Health care provider or nurse adds sterile water or normal saline (NS) to diagnostic indicator on waterless system.	Allows quick assurance that system is functioning properly. Connects chest tube to drainage.
Health care provider or nurse unclamps chest tube.	Verifies correct chest tube placement.
Health care provider prescribes and assesses chest radiographic studies.	

Water-Seal Systems

NSO *Nursing Skills Online Chest Tubes Module 11 / Lessons 1 and 2*

Two-Chamber Water-Seal System

On expiration, fluid or air is forced out of the intrapleural space. Suction pulls air or fluid through the chest tube into the drainage collection chamber. On entering the drainage collection chamber, this fluid or air displaces the air present in the chamber by pushing it through the water seal and out of the system into the atmosphere. The water-seal chamber is left open to air to drain. If the tubing is clamped, there is no mechanism for air to vent. To maintain the water-seal system, the chest tube system must remain upright. When it is tipped or overturned, the water seal is disrupted.

Three-Chamber Water-Seal System

If suction is used, the three-chamber water-seal system (see Fig. 27.7) is set up with the suction-control chamber added. A prescribed amount of sterile fluid (e.g., 20 cm of water) is poured into the suction-control chamber, which is then attached to a suction source by tubing. The amount of sterile water added depends on manufacturer recommendations. The chamber is filled to the set volume for the prescribed amount of suction. It is the height of the water in the suction-control chamber that determines the amount of suction. Sterile water is added several times a day because of evaporation. As the fluid level decreases, the amount of suction also declines.

If the suction source delivers more negative pressure than the suction-control chamber water level allows, the extra air pulled into the chamber causes vigorous bubbling. If this occurs, lower the suction source setting to reduce noise and evaporation of the fluid. The absence of bubbling indicates that no suction is being exerted into the system. Raise the suction setting to restore gentle bubbling.

The middle chamber is the water seal. The water seal allows air to exit from the pleural space on exhalation and prevents it from entering the pleural cavity or mediastinum on inhalation. When the appropriate amount of sterile water is added, a 2-cm water seal is established. To maintain an effective water seal, the chest drainage unit must remain upright; also, monitor the water level in the water-seal chamber to check for evaporation. Bubbling in the water-seal chamber indicates an air leak.

Waterless Systems

Two-Chamber Waterless System

The principles of the waterless system are similar to those of the water-seal system except that fluid is not required for setup. Because water is not used, accidently tipping the system does not compromise the patient's condition.

The water seal is replaced by a one-way valve (see Fig. 27.8) located near the top of the system. Most of the container serves as the drainage chamber. The suction chamber does not depend on water. Instead, it contains a float ball, which is set by a suction-control dial after the suction source is turned on. A diagnostic air-leak indicator is located on the face of the unit. It requires the addition of 15 mL of fluid for visualization. The function of the indicator is to identify one of the following:

1. The lung is expanding normally. This is indicated by a gentle tidalling of the fluid in the diagnostic indicator.
2. The lung is probably re-expanded if after 2 or 3 days the tidalling has stopped.
3. There is an air leak in the system if, when facing the system, the observer sees the fluid bubbling left to right. Locate and correct the source of the air leak.

Three-Chamber Waterless System

When suction is prescribed, attach the suction chamber port to the suction source by tubing, turn the suction on, and set the suction indicator (float ball or bellows) to the prescribed setting. If the suction indicator does not move to the prescribed level, increase the suction source setting until it does. The system is now functioning with suction.

There are usually two suction settings: one at either the suction-control chamber or the indicator setting and the other at the suction source. The settings are safety factors to reduce the possibility that the intrapleural tissues receive too much suction, causing injury.

Dry Suction System

Dry suction-control systems provide many advantages (see Fig. 27.9), including higher suction pressure levels if needed, easy setup, no water in the suction-control chamber, and the absence of continuous bubbling, which provides for quiet operation. A self-compensating regulator controls the dry suction unit. A dial is set to the prescribed suction-control setting. These units are preset to −20 cm of water pressure, but they are adjustable from −10 to −40 cm. However, the dry suction-control systems require or have presealed sterile water to use in the water-seal chamber (Pickett, 2017).

Delegation and Collaboration

The skill of managing a closed chest drainage system cannot be delegated to an unregulated care provider (UCP). The nurse instructs the UCP about the following:

- Proper positioning of the patient with chest tubes to facilitate chest tube drainage and optimal functioning of the system
- Ambulating and transferring the patient with chest drainage
- Reporting changes in vital signs, symptoms of chest pain or sudden shortness of breath, or excessive bubbling in the water-seal chamber to the nurse immediately

- Danger of any disconnection of drainage system, change in type and amount of drainage, sudden bleeding, or sudden cessation of bubbling or tidalling

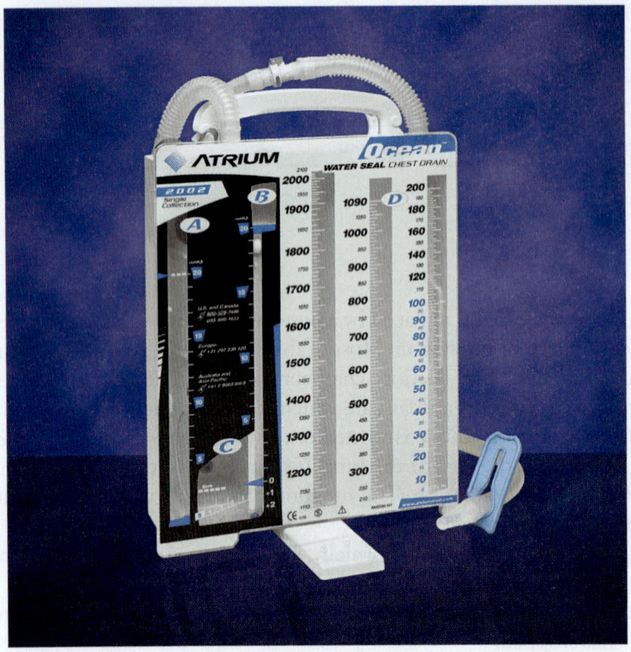

FIG 27.7 Disposable water-seal chest drainage system with suction. (*Used with permission, Atrium Medical Corp.*)

Equipment

- Prescribed chest drainage system
- Suction source and setup (wall canister or portable)
  - *Water-seal system:* Add sterile water or normal saline (NS) solution to cover the lower 2 cm of the water-seal chamber. Pour sterile water or NS into the suction-control chamber if suction is to be used (see manufacturer's directions).
  - *Waterless system:* Add vial of 30- to 45-mL sterile sodium chloride or water (for diagnostic air-leak indicator), 20-mL syringe, 21-gauge needle, and antiseptic swab
  - Dry suction system
- Clean gloves
- Sterile gauze sponges
- Local anaesthetic, if not an emergent procedure
- Chest tube tray (all items are sterile): knife handle (1), knife blade No. 10 or disposable safety scalpel No. 10, chest tube clamp, small sponge forceps, needle holder, size 3-0 silk sutures, tray liner (sterile field), curved 8-inch Kelly clamps (2), 10 cm × 10 cm (4 inch × 4 inch) sponges (10), suture scissors, hand towels (3), sterile gloves
- Dressings: Petrolatum or Xeroform gauze, split chest-tube dressings, several 10 cm × 10 cm (4 inch × 4 inch) gauze dressings, large gauze dressings (2), and 10-cm (4-inch) tape
- Head cover
- Face mask/face shield
- Sterile gloves
- Two rubber-tipped hemostats (shodded) for each chest tube
- 2.5-cm (1-inch) waterproof adhesive tape or plastic zip ties for securing connections
- Stethoscope, sphygmomanometer, and pulse oximeter

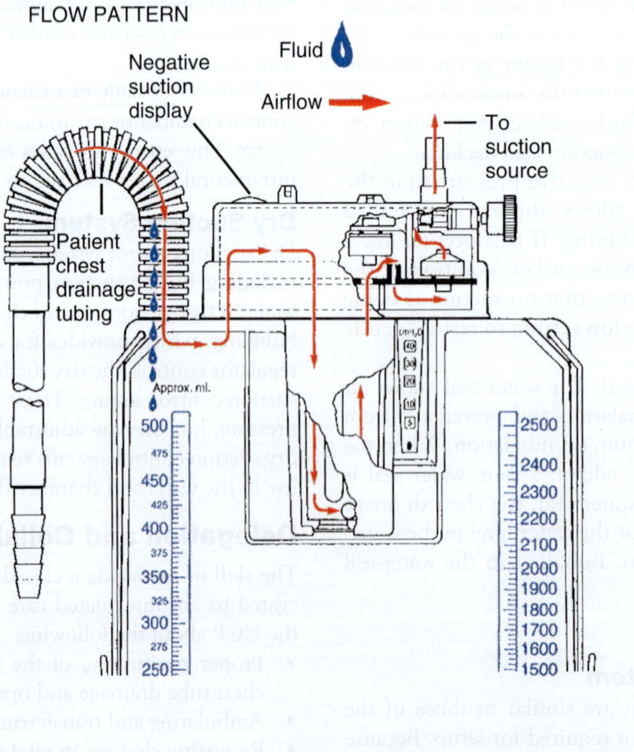

FIG 27.8 Disposable waterless chest drainage system with suction.

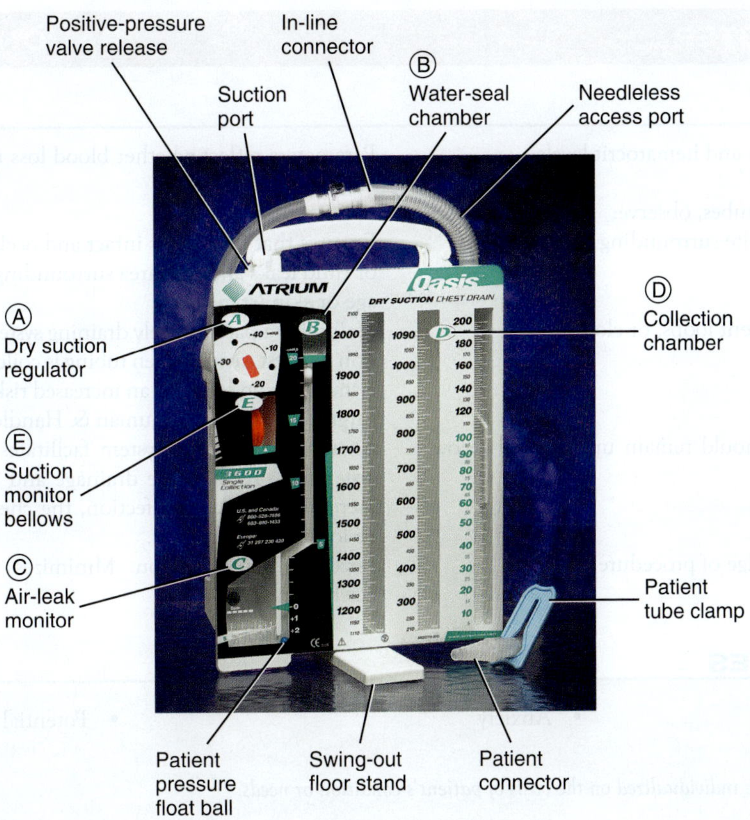

FIG 27.9 **Dry suction chest drainage system.** (*Used with permission, Atrium Medical Corp.*)

STEP	RATIONALE
ASSESSMENT	
1. Assess patient for known allergies. Ask patient whether they have had a problem with medications, latex, or anything applied to the skin.	Povidone-iodine or chlorhexidine gluconate (CHG) are antiseptic solutions used to clean skin before tube insertion (Huggins et al., 2022; Porcel, 2018). Lidocaine is a local anaesthetic administered to reduce pain. The chest tube will be held in place with tape and sutures.
2. Identify patient using at least two person-specific identifiers (e.g., name and date of birth, or name and medical record number) according to employer policy.	Ensures correct patient. Complies with Accreditation Canada's standards and improves patient safety (Accreditation Canada, 2020).
3. Throughout the procedure, the 4 moments for hand hygiene are to be implemented; hand hygiene should occur before initial patient (or patient environment) contact, before an aseptic procedure, after body fluid exposure risk, and after patient (or patient environment) contact. Additional hand hygiene should be performed when hands are visibly soiled.	Proper hand hygiene helps prevent the spread of infectious agents to health care providers.
4. Perform a complete respiratory assessment, including baseline vital signs and pulse oximetry (SpO_2).	Baseline assessment and vital signs are essential for any invasive procedure. Chest tube insertion often causes respiratory distress.
a. Assess for signs and symptoms of increased respiratory distress and hypoxia (e.g., decreased breath sounds over affected and unaffected lungs, marked cyanosis, asymmetrical chest movements, displaced trachea, shortness of breath, and confusion).	Signs and symptoms associated with respiratory distress are related to the type and size of pneumothorax, hemothorax, or pre-existing illness. Signs of hypoxia are related to inadequate oxygen to tissues.
b. Assess for sharp, stabbing chest pain or chest pain on inspiration, hypotension, and tachycardia. If possible, ask patient to rate level of comfort, using an appropriate pain rating scale.	Sharp stabbing chest pain, with or without decreased blood pressure and increased heart rate, may indicate tension pneumothorax. Presence of pneumothorax or hemothorax is painful, frequently causing sharp inspiratory pain. In addition, discomfort is associated with presence of a chest tube, not just with its insertion. As a result, patients tend not to cough or change position in an effort to minimize this pain (Chotai, 2022).
5. Review patient's medication record for anticoagulant therapy, including aspirin, warfarin, heparin, or platelet aggregation inhibitors such as ticlopidine or dipyridamole.	Anticoagulation therapy can increase procedure-related blood loss.

STEP	RATIONALE

ASSESSMENT

STEP	RATIONALE
6. Review patient's hemoglobin and hematocrit levels.	Parameters reflect whether blood loss is occurring, which may affect oxygenation.
7. For patients who have chest tubes, observe:	
a. Chest tube dressing and site surrounding tube insertion.	Ensures that dressing is intact and occlusive seal remains without air or fluid leaks and that area surrounding insertion site is free of drainage or skin irritation.
b. Tubing for kinks, dependent loops, or clots.	Maintains a patent, freely draining system, preventing fluid accumulation in chest cavity. When tubing is coiled, looped, or clotted, drainage is impeded, and there is an increased risk for tension pneumothorax or surgical emphysema (Bauman & Handley, 2018; Pickett, 2017).
c. Chest drainage system should remain upright and below level of tube insertion.	An upright drainage system facilitates drainage and maintains the water seal. To facilitate drainage and prevent backflow that would increase the risk for infection, the chest tube drainage system must be lower than the chest.
8. Determine patient's knowledge of procedure.	Encourages cooperation. Minimizes risks and anxiety. Identifies teaching needs.

NURSING DIAGNOSES

- Reduced gas exchange
- Acute pain
- Anxiety
- Potential for infection

Related factors and risk factors are individualized on the basis of patient's condition or needs.

PLANNING

STEP	RATIONALE
1. Expected outcomes following completion of procedure:	
• Patient is oriented and less anxious.	Hypoxia is relieved.
• Vital signs are stable.	Decreased hypoxia improves vital sign measures.
• Patient reports no chest pain.	Re-expansion of lung reduces chest pain.
• Breath sounds are auscultated in all lobes. Lung expansion is symmetrical, SpO_2 is stable or improved, and respirations are unlaboured.	Re-expansion of lung promotes normal respirations.
• Chest tube remains in place, and chest drainage system remains airtight.	Indicates correct placement and patency of chest tube drainage system.
• Gentle tidalling (fluctuations or rocking) is evident in water-seal or diagnostic indicator.	Indicates that system is functioning normally. Reflects changes in intrapleural pressure.

IMPLEMENTATION

STEP	RATIONALE
1. Check employer policy and determine whether informed consent is needed. Complete "time-out" procedure.	Invasive medical procedures typically require informed consent. "Time-out" step is completed to determine right patient, procedure, and location of insertion or incision site (Operating Room Nurses Association of Canada [ORNAC], 2023).
2. Review health care provider's prescription for chest tube placement.	Insertion of chest tube requires health care provider prescription.
3. Apply clean gloves. Set up water-seal system (or dry system with suction); see manufacturer's guidelines.	
a. Obtain chest drainage system. Remove wrappers and prepare to set up two- or three-chamber system.	Maintains sterility of system for use under sterile operating room conditions.
b. While maintaining sterility of drainage tubing, stand system upright and add sterile water or NS to appropriate compartments.	Reduces possibility of contamination.
(1) *Two-chamber system (without suction)*: Add sterile solution to water-seal chamber (second chamber), bringing fluid to required level as indicated.	Water-seal chamber acts as one-way valve so air cannot enter pleural space (Sasa, 2019).

STEP	RATIONALE

IMPLEMENTATION

(2) *Three-chamber system (with suction):* Add sterile solution to water-seal chamber (second chamber). Add amount of sterile solution prescribed by health care provider to suction-control chamber (third chamber), usually 20 cm of water pressure. Connect tubing from suction-control chamber to suction source. Tailor length of drainage tube to patient. NOTE: Suction-control chamber vent must not be occluded when using suction (see Step 3b[2] illustration).

Depth of fluid level dictates highest amount of negative pressure that can be present within system. For example, 20 cm of water is approximately 20 cm of water pressure. Any additional negative pressure applied to the system is vented into the atmosphere through the suction-control vent. This safety device prevents damage to pleural tissues from an unexpected surge of negative pressure from the suction source.

After chest tube is inserted, turn up the wall or portable suction device until water in suction-control bottle exhibits continuous, gentle bubbling.

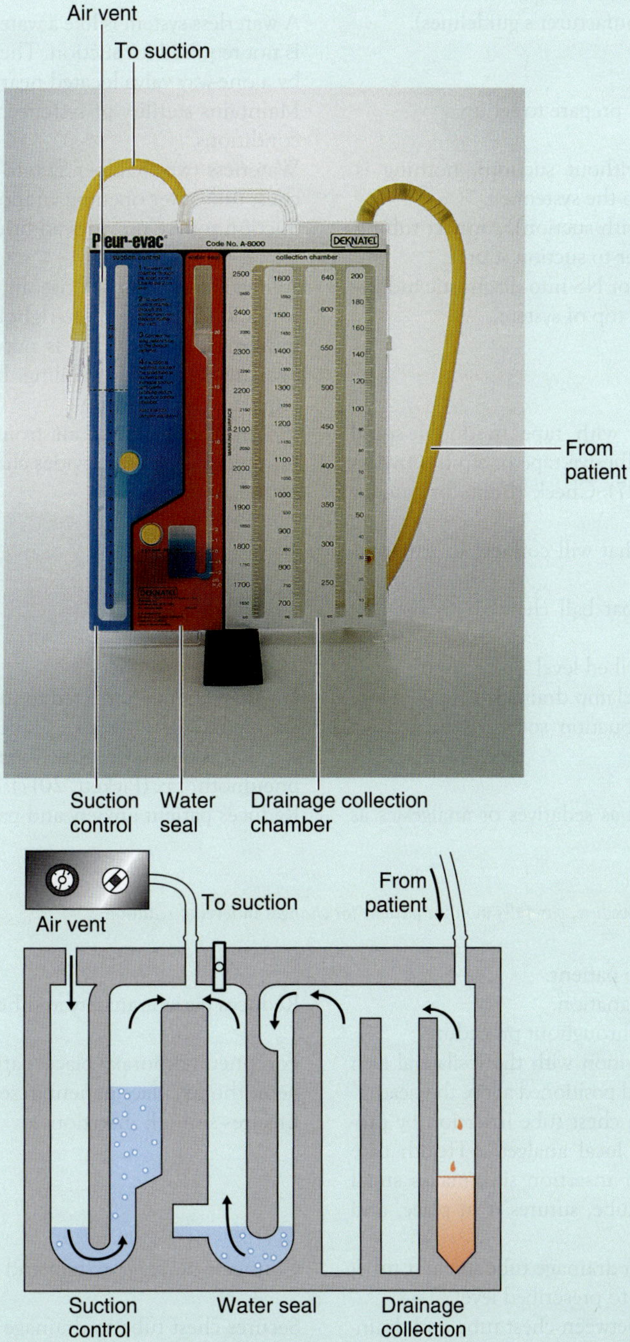

STEP 3B(2) Top, Pleur-Evac drainage system, a commercial three-chamber chest drainage device. Bottom, Schematic of drainage device.

STEP	RATIONALE

IMPLEMENTATION

Critical Decision Point *When increasing suction, remember that increased bubbling does not result in more suction to the chest cavity, but rather serves to evaporate the water more quickly.*

STEP	RATIONALE
(3) *Dry suction system:* Fill water-seal chamber with sterile solution. Adjust suction-control dial to prescribed level of suction; suction ranges from −10 to −40 cm of water pressure. Suction-control chamber vent is never occluded when suction is used. NOTE: On dry suction system, DO NOT obstruct positive-pressure relief valve. This allows air to escape.	Automatic control valve on dry suction-control device adjusts to changes in patient air leaks and fluctuation in suction source and vacuum to deliver prescribed amount of suction.
4. Set up waterless system (see manufacturer's guidelines).	A waterless system is like a water-seal system except that sterile water is not required for suction. The suction-control chamber is replaced by a one-way valve located near the top of the system.
a. Remove sterile wrappers and prepare to set up.	Maintains sterility of system for use under sterile operating room conditions.
b. For two-chamber system (without suction), nothing is added or needs to be done to the system.	Waterless two-chamber system is ready for connecting to patient's chest tube after opening wrappers.
c. For three-chamber system (with suction), connect tubing from suction-control chamber to suction source.	Suction source provides additional negative pressure to system.
d. Instill 15 mL of sterile water or NS into diagnostic indicator injection port located on top of system.	Allows observation of rise and fall of water in diagnostic air-leak window. Constant left-to-right bubbling or rocking is abnormal and indicates air leak. This is not necessary for mediastinal drainage because there is no tidalling. In an emergency, the system *does not* require water for setup.
5. Secure all tubing connections with tape in double-spiral fashion using 2.5-cm (1-inch) adhesive tape or zip ties (nylon cable) with a clamp (Pickett, 2017). Check system for patency by: **a.** Clamping drainage tubing that will connect to patient's chest tube **b.** Connecting tubing from float ball chamber to suction source **c.** Turning on suction to prescribed level	Prevents atmospheric air from leaking into system and patient's intrapleural space. Provides chance to ensure airtight system before connection to patient.
6. Turn off suction source and unclamp drainage tubing before connecting patient to system. Suction source is turned on again after patient is connected.	Having patient connected to suction when it is initiated could damage pleural tissues from a sudden increase in negative pressure. Tubing that is coiled or looped may become clotted and cause tension pneumothorax (Pickett, 2017).
7. Administer premedication such as sedatives or analgesics as prescribed.	Reduces patient anxiety and pain during procedure.

Critical Decision Point *During procedure, carefully monitor patient for changes in level of sedation.*

STEP	RATIONALE
8. Provide psychological support to patient. **a.** Reinforce preprocedure explanation. **b.** Coach and support patient throughout procedure.	Reduces patient anxiety and helps complete procedure efficiently.
9. Position patient in a supine position with the ipsilateral arm abducted, elbow flexed, and hand positioned above the head.	For pneumothorax, place patient in lateral supine position; for hemothorax, place patient in semi-Fowler's position (Chotai, 2022).
10. Assist health care provider with chest tube insertion by providing needed equipment and local analgesic. Health care provider anaesthetizes skin over insertion site, makes small skin incision, inserts clamped tube, sutures it in place, and applies occlusive dressing.	Ensures smooth insertion.
11. Help health care provider attach drainage tube to chest tube; remove clamp. Turn on suction to prescribed level.	Connects drainage system and suction (if prescribed) to chest tube.
12. Tape or zip-tie all connections between chest tube and drainage tube. (NOTE: Chest tube is usually taped by health care provider at time of tube placement; check employer policy).	Secures chest tube to drainage system and reduces risk for air leak that causes breaks in airtight system (Chotai, 2022).

STEP	RATIONALE

IMPLEMENTATION

STEP	RATIONALE
13. Check systems for proper functioning. Health care provider prescribes chest radiography.	Verifies intrapleural placement of tube.
14. After tube placement, position patient:	Permits optimum drainage of fluid and/or air.
a. Use semi-Fowler's or high Fowler's position to evacuate air (pneumothorax) (Chotai, 2022).	
b. Use high Fowler's position to drain fluid (hemothorax) (Chotai, 2022).	
15. Check patency of air vents in system.	
a. Water-seal vent must have no occlusion.	Permits displaced air to pass into atmosphere.
b. Suction-control chamber vent is not occluded when suction is used.	Provides safety factor of releasing excess negative pressure into atmosphere.
c. Waterless systems have relief valves without caps.	Provides safety factor of releasing excess negative pressure.
16. Position excess tubing horizontally on mattress next to patient. Secure with clamp provided so it does not obstruct tubing.	Prevents excess tubing from hanging over edge of mattress in dependent loop. Drainage collected in loop can occlude drainage system, which predisposes patient to tension pneumothorax (Pickett, 2017; Tyerman & Cobbett, 2023).
17. Adjust tubing to hang in straight line from chest tube to drainage chamber.	Promotes drainage and prevents fluid or blood from accumulating in pleural cavity.

Critical Decision Point *Frequent gentle lifting of the drain allows gravity to help blood and other viscous material to move to the drainage bottle. Patients with recent chest surgery or trauma need to have the chest drain lifted on the basis of assessment of the amount of drainage; some patients might need chest tube drains lifted every 5–10 minutes until drainage volume decreases. However, when coiled or dependent looping of tubing is unavoidable, lift the tubing every 15 minutes at a minimum to promote drainage* (Pickett, 2017).

STEP	RATIONALE
18. Place two rubber-tipped hemostats (for each chest tube) in easily accessible position (e.g., taped to top of patient's headboard). These should remain with patient when ambulating.	Chest tubes are double clamped under specific circumstances: (1) to assess for air leak (Table 27.3), (2) to empty or quickly change disposable systems, or (3) to assess whether patient is ready for tube removal.

TABLE 27.3

Problem Solving With Chest Tubes

Assessment	Intervention
Air leak can occur at insertion site, at connection between tube and drainage device, or within drainage device itself. Determine when air leak occurs during respiratory cycle (e.g., inspiration or expiration). Continuous bubbling is noted in water-seal chamber that is attached to suction (Pickett, 2017).	Check all connections between chest tube and drainage system to make sure they are tight. When in doubt, remove tape without disconnecting the tube to inspect connections. Inspect the chest drainage unit for cracks or breaks that can allow air into the system. Leaks are corrected when constant bubbling stops.
Assess for location of leak by squeezing the chest drainage tubing between your hands. If the bubbling stops, the air leak is inside patient's thorax or at chest insertion site.	Release the pressure on the drainage tube, reinforce chest dressing, and notify the health care provider immediately. Leaving the chest tube clamped can cause collapse of the lung, mediastinal shift, and eventual collapse of the other lung from buildup of air pressure within the pleural cavity.
If bubbling continues, it indicates that the leak is in the drainage system.	Change the drainage system. Notify the health care provider, as a chest X-ray may be required.
Assess for tension pneumothorax: • Severe respiratory distress • Low oxygen saturation • Chest pain • Absence of breath sounds on affected side • Tracheal shift to unaffected side (seen on inspection or palpated) • Hypotension and signs of shock • Tachycardia	Make sure that chest tubes are patent: Remove clamps, eliminate kinks, or eliminate occlusion. Notify health care provider immediately and prepare for another chest tube insertion. A one-way flutter (Heimlich) valve or large-gauge needle may be used for short-term emergency release of pressure in the intrapleural space. Have emergency equipment, oxygen, and code cart available because condition is life-threatening.
Water-seal tube is no longer submerged in sterile fluid because of evaporation.	Add sterile water to water-seal chamber until distal tip is 2 cm under surface level. Most chest drainage units are marked at the 2 cm level to indicate the fill line.

STEP	RATIONALE

IMPLEMENTATION

Critical Decision Point *In the event of a chest tube disconnection, which increases risk for contamination, immediately re-establish the water-seal system and attach a new drainage system as soon as possible. Depending on employer policy, consider submerging the tube 2.5–5 cm (1–2 inches) below the surface of a 250-mL bottle of sterile water or NS until a new chest tube unit can be set up* (Tyerman & Cobbett, 2023).

STEP	RATIONALE
19. Dispose of all equipment in appropriate receptacles and remove gloves.	
20. Perform care of patient after chest tube insertion:	
a. Assess vital signs, oxygen saturation; skin colour; breath sounds; rate, depth, and ease of respirations; and insertion site every 15 minutes for first 2 hours, and then at least every shift (see employer policy).	Reduces transmission of microorganisms. Provides immediate information about procedure-related complications such as respiratory distress and leakage.
b. Monitor colour, consistency, and amount of chest tube drainage every 15 minutes for first 2 hours. Indicate level of drainage fluid, date, and time on write-on surface of chamber.	Provides baseline for continuous assessment of type and quantity of drainage. Ensures early detection of complications.
(1) From mediastinal tube, expect less than 100 mL/hr immediately after surgery and no more than 500 mL in first 24 hours.	Sudden gush of drainage may result from coughing or change in patient's position (i.e., releasing pooled/collected blood rather than indicating active bleeding).
(2) Report sudden fluctuations or changes in chest tube output (especially a sudden increase from previous drainage) or changes in colour (especially bright red blood, which could indicate hemorrhage) (Tyerman & Cobbett, 2023).	Acute bleeding indicates hemorrhage. Health care provider should be notified if there is >100 mL of bloody drainage in an hour, or according to health care provider prescription (Pickett, 2017; Tyerman & Cobbett, 2023).
(3) Expect little or no output from anterior chest tube that is inserted for a pneumothorax.	
c. Observe chest dressing for drainage.	Drainage around tube may indicate blockage. Reduces transmission of microorganisms.
d. Apply clean gloves. Palpate around tube for swelling and crepitus (subcutaneous emphysema) as noted by crackling.	Indicates presence of air trapping in subcutaneous tissues. Most occurrences of crepitus are minor as small amounts are absorbed. Large amounts are potentially dangerous and the health care provider should be notified (Pickett, 2017; Sasa, 2019).

Critical Decision Point *Some patients may develop subcutaneous emphysema (i.e., a collection of air under the skin after chest tube placement), which can occur if tubing is blocked or kinked. Symptoms include crepitus on palpation; distension or bloating in the abdomen, chest, neck or face; visual distortion; and phonation* (Kukuruza & Aboeed, 2022).

STEP	RATIONALE
e. Check tubing to ensure that it is free of kinks and dependent loops.	Promotes drainage.
f. Observe for fluctuation of drainage in tubing and water-seal chamber during inspiration and expiration. Observe for clots or debris in tubing.	If fluctuation or tidalling stops, it means that either the lung is fully expanded or the system is obstructed (Pickett, 2017). In a spontaneously breathing patient, fluid rises in water-seal or diagnostic indicator (waterless system) with inspiration and falls with expiration. The opposite occurs in a patient who is mechanically ventilated. This indicates that the system is functioning properly (Tyerman & Cobbett, 2023).
g. Keep drainage system upright and below level of patient's chest.	Promotes gravity drainage and prevents backflow of fluid and air into pleural space.
h. Check for air leaks by monitoring bubbling in water-seal chamber. Intermittent bubbling is normal during expiration when air is being evacuated from pleural cavity, but continuous bubbling during both inspiration and expiration indicates leak in system.	Absence of bubbling may indicate that lung is fully expanded in patient with pneumothorax. Check all connections and locate sources of air leak (see description in Table 27.3).
i. Dispose of all equipment in appropriate receptacles and remove gloves.	Prevents accidents involving contaminated equipment.

STEP	RATIONALE
EVALUATION	
1. Evaluate patient for decreased respiratory distress and chest pain. Auscultate patient's lungs and observe chest expansion.	Determines status of lung expansion.
2. Monitor vital signs and SpO_2.	Determines whether level of oxygenation has improved.
3. Reassess patient's level of comfort using an appropriate pain rating scale, comparing level with patient's comfort before chest tube insertion.	Indicates need for analgesia. Patient with chest tube discomfort hesitates to take deep breaths and as a result is at risk for pneumonia and atelectasis.
4. Evaluate patient's ability to use deep-breathing exercises while maintaining comfort.	Indicates patient's ability to promote lung expansion and prevent complications.
5. Monitor continued functioning of system as indicated by reduction in amount of drainage, resolution of air leak, and complete re-expansion of the lung.	Detects early signs of system complications or indicates possible removal of chest tube.
6. Use teach-back: "I want to be sure I explained why you have a chest tube. Tell me the reason why you have it." Develop a revised teaching plan if patient or caregiver is unable to teach back correctly.	Determines patient's and caregiver's level of understanding of instructional topic.

Unexpected Outcomes	Related Interventions
1. Patient develops respiratory distress. Chest pain, decrease in breath sounds over affected and unaffected lungs, marked cyanosis, asymmetrical chest movements, presence of subcutaneous emphysema around tube insertion site or neck, hypotension, tachycardia, and mediastinal shift are critical and indicate severe change in patient status, such as excessive blood loss or tension pneumothorax.	• Notify health care provider immediately. • Assess vital signs and SpO_2. • Prepare for chest radiography. • Provide oxygen as prescribed.
2. Air leak is unrelated to patient's respirations.	• See Table 27.3 for determining source of an air leak and for problem solving. • Notify health care provider.
3. There is no chest tube drainage.	• Observe for kink in chest drainage system. • Observe for possible clot in chest drainage system. • Observe for mediastinal shift or respiratory distress (medical emergency). • Notify health care provider.
4. Chest tube is dislodged.	• Immediately apply pressure over chest tube insertion site. • Have assistant obtain sterile petroleum gauze dressing. Apply as patient exhales. Secure dressing with tight seal. Dressing with tape over three of four sides may allow for escape of air if there is residual pneumothorax. • Notify health care provider.
5. Substantial increase in bright red drainage is observed.	• Obtain vital signs. • Monitor drainage. • Assess patient's cardiopulmonary status. • Notify health care provider.

Communication and Documentation

- Document respiratory assessment, type of drainage device, amount of suction if used, amount of drainage in chamber, and presence or absence of air leak in progress notes in electronic health record (EHR) or chart.
- Document the integrity of the dressing and the colour and type of drainage for comparison between shifts.
- Document patient teaching and validation of understanding on flow sheet or progress notes in EHR or chart.
- Document level of patient comfort and baseline vital signs, including oxygen saturation. For a postoperative patient, record vital signs and oxygen saturation every 15 minutes for at least 2 hours after surgery on flow sheet or progress notes in EHR or chart.
- Document and report any unexpected outcomes immediately to the nurse in charge or health care provider.

DOCUMENTATION EXAMPLE

Patient has chest tube present in right lower portion of rib cage at the axillary line and connected to a two-chamber drainage system. Respirations 22 breaths/min, regular; O_2 sat increased to 94% from baseline of 88%. Breath sounds auscultated in all lobes and lung expansion is symmetrical. Draining moderate amount of serosanguineous fluid. Suction at 20 cm H_2O; gentle bubbling noted in suction chamber. Tidalling was present in water-seal chamber, no air leak noted. No evidence of swelling or crepitus noted around tube and no signs of abdominal distension. Patient rates pain as a 1 on a 1 to 10 pain scale; states, "It is uncomfortable, but not hurting"; occlusive dressing remains intact. Patient indicated to writer rationale for chest tube. Patient resting with bed in semi-Fowler's position and call bell within reach.

Special Considerations

Teaching

- Instruct patient and caregiver on proper functioning of chest tube and drainage system.
- Instruct patient to remain in bed if chest tube is attached to suction.
- Instruct patient to not lie on tubing or allow it to get kinked, to promote drainage.
- Instruct patient to immediately report any changes in chest comfort.
- Instruct patient to call immediately for help if the chest tube becomes dislodged.

Pediatric

- If possible, using pictures and special dolls, familiarize child and family with equipment before inserting chest drainage system (Hockenberry et al., 2024).
- Chest tube drainage greater than 3 mL/kg/hr for more than 3 consecutive hours is excessive and may indicate postoperative hemorrhage. Notify the health care provider immediately (Hockenberry et al., 2024).

Gerontological

- Fragility of the older person's skin requires special care and planning for management of chest tube dressing. Frequently assess skin surrounding chest tube for signs of skin breakdown.

Patients With Physical or Cognitive Challenges

- Patients with cognitive or physical challenges may have limited understanding and may be unable to tolerate their chest tube devices. Consider the need for use of soft restraints to ensure patient safety and prevent removal of chest tube by patient. Restraints will require health care provider order.
- Frequent nursing assessments should be done to assess for dyspnea and sputum retention due to ineffective cough (Porcel, 2018). Bronchoscopic suctioning may be required.

Care in the Community: Home Management

- Patients living with chronic conditions (e.g., uncomplicated pneumothorax, effusions, empyema) that require use of a long-term chest tube may be discharged with smaller mobile drains.
- Teach patient how to ambulate and remain active with a mobile chest tube drainage system.
- Instruct patient and caregiver about when to contact the health care provider regarding changes in the drainage system (e.g., chest pain, breathlessness, change in colour or amount of drainage, leakage on dressing around the chest tube).
- Provide patient and caregiver information specific to the type of drain; when possible, have patient demonstrate proper maintenance of the mobile drainage system. Most of these systems do not have a suction-control chamber and use a mechanical one-way valve instead of a water-seal chamber.
- Although rare, a patient may be discharged home with a Heimlich valve. The health care provider should arrange for home care to assist with changing the bandage, emptying the drainage bag (if there is one), and assessing for infection. Patients should be instructed on the following:
  - Avoid tub baths; a waterproof dressing should be applied prior to showering.
  - If the valve becomes disconnected from the chest tube, reconnect immediately by inserting the blue end of the valve into the chest tube; then contact your health care provider. If unable to reconnect, turn stopcock off or use tape to cover the end of the chest tube and immediately go to the emergency department.
  - Contact health care provider if temperature is more than 38°C (100.4°F); amount of drainage from chest tube increases; bandage becomes loose or wet; fluid leaks from the drainage site; or skin around the bandage is red, swollen, painful, or warm to touch (Regina Qu'Appelle Health Region, 2017).
- Small-bore chest tubes and Heimlich valves should be used with caution in patients on mechanical ventilators owing to the potential for rapid accumulation of air and a tension pneumothorax (Tyerman & Cobbett, 2023).

✦ SKILL 27.2 Assisting With Removal of Chest Tubes

NSO Nursing Skills Online Chest Tubes Module 11/ Lesson 4

Actual removal of a chest tube is most often the responsibility of a physician or health care provider such as a physician's assistant or nurse practitioner (verify employer policy). Prepare a patient for chest tube removal by assessing the need for preremoval analgesia, obtaining the required medication prescriptions, and instructing the patient about the process and what will be requested of them.

There has been debate about the optimal timing of chest tube removal in relation to the respiratory cycle. The primary goal of chest tube removal is removal of the tubes without introducing air into the pleural space. Studies have shown that removal either at the end of inspiration or at the end of expiration does not affect the outcome (Huggins et al., 2022). Some pain on chest tube removal is expected, and it is essential that the patient practise how to exhale during removal so that they do not accidently gasp during removal (Huggins et al., 2022). Instruct the patient to perform a Valsalva's manoeuvre at either end inspiration or end expiration. The Valsalva's manoeuvre is needed to provide positive pressure in the pleural cavity and prevent the patient from gasping when the tube is removed. An occlusive dressing is applied immediately after tube removal to maintain a tight seal.

Delegation and Collaboration

The skill of assisting with removal of chest tubes cannot be delegated to a UCP. The nurse directs the UCP to do the following:

- Immediately report to the nurse if patient experiences sensations of shortness of breath, increased chest pain, dizziness, or increased anxiety
- Report to the nurse any drainage on the dressing placed over the chest tube site

Equipment

- Suture removal set
- Sterile scissors
- Sterile forceps
- Clean gloves
- Sterile gloves
- Face mask/face shield
- Prepared sterile dressing: petrolatum-impregnated gauze, 10 cm × 10 cm (4 inch × 4 inch) gauze dressings, and large dressings (two to four)
- Rubber-tipped Kelly clamps
- 10-cm (4-inch) adhesive tape or elastic bandage (Elastoplast) cut into strips
- Stethoscope, sphygmomanometer, pulse oximeter
- Disposable bed pad

STEP	RATIONALE

ASSESSMENT

STEP	RATIONALE
1. Identify patient using at least two person-specific identifiers (e.g., name and date of birth, or name and medical record number) according to employer policy.	Ensures correct patient. Complies with Accreditation Canada's standards and improves patient safety (Accreditation Canada, 2020).
2. Throughout the procedure, the 4 moments for hand hygiene are to be implemented; hand hygiene should occur before initial patient (or patient environment) contact, before an aseptic procedure, after body fluid exposure risk, and after patient (or patient environment) contact. Additional hand hygiene should be performed when hands are visibly soiled.	Proper hand hygiene helps prevent the spread of infectious agents to health care providers.
3. Perform respiratory assessment and assess for lung re-expansion.	
a. Provide health care provider with results of chest radiography.	Reveals position of lung tissue in chest cavity and whether sufficient lung re-expansion has occurred (Huggins et al., 2022).
b. Note trend in water-seal fluctuation over last 24 hours. Determine whether bubbling is present.	Pleura of expanded lung seals holes on internal tip of chest tube, halting fluctuation in water seal. Halt in fluctuation for 24 hours indicates that lung is expanded. Presence of bubbling usually indicates that lung has not fully expanded (Huggins et al., 2022).
c. Confirm that drainage has decreased to 100–250 mL in the prior 24 hours if the tube was placed for a hemothorax, empyema, or pleural effusion or <100 mL in 8 hours after cardiac surgery (QHC, 2020).	Pleural drainage was removed, allowing lung to re-expand.
d. Percuss lung for resonance (see Chapter 8).	Normal resonance occurs with re-expansion.
e. Auscultate lung sounds.	Normal breath sounds are heard bilaterally with re-expansion.
4. Assess patient's level of comfort using an appropriate pain rating scale and determine when the last analgesic medication was given.	Chest tube removal is often painful; additional analgesia or breathing exercises are often necessary (Huggins et al., 2022; Tyerman & Cobbett, 2023).
5. Determine patient's understanding of chest tube removal procedure.	Encourages cooperation and minimizes risks and anxiety. Identifies teaching needs.
6. Do not clamp chest tube before removal. Assess for changes in vital signs, oxygen saturation, chest pain, apprehension, and symptoms of tension pneumothorax.	Clamping chest tube before removal to assess patient's tolerance is no longer recommended because there is no benefit to the practice. If a chest tube that was continuing to bubble is clamped, tension pneumothorax may occur (Wiegand, 2017).

NURSING DIAGNOSES

- Acute pain
- Anxiety
- Potential for inadequate gas exchange

Related factors and risk factors are individualized on the basis of patient's condition or needs.

PLANNING

STEP	RATIONALE
1. Expected outcomes following completion of procedure:	
• Lung re-expansion is maintained.	Source of air or fluid loss is sealed or has healed.
• Patient does not experience discomfort.	Pain management is achieved.
• Spontaneous healing of chest tube insertion site occurs after removal of tube without infection or other complications.	Large, nonporous occlusive dressing at puncture site promotes uncomplicated healing.
2. Explain procedure to patient.	Reduces anxiety and promotes patient cooperation.

IMPLEMENTATION

STEP	RATIONALE
1. Administer prescribed medication for pain relief about 30 minutes before procedure.	Reduces discomfort and relaxes patient. Medication reaches peak effect at time of tube removal. Patients report sensations ranging from pain to pulling when chest tube is removed (Chotai, 2022).
2. Perform "time-out" procedure with health care provider to verify patient identification, planned procedure, correct tube(s), and that chest tube is visible and patient position is correct.	The "time-out" step reliably identifies patient as the individual for whom the procedure is intended and matches the procedure to the patient (ORNAC, 2023).
3. Assist patient to sitting position on edge of bed, lying supine, or lying on side without chest tubes. Place pad under chest tube site.	Health care provider prescribes patient's position to facilitate tube removal. Pad absorbs any drainage associated with tube removal.

STEP	RATIONALE

IMPLEMENTATION

STEP	RATIONALE
4. Health care provider prepares an occlusive dressing of petrolatum-impregnated gauze on pressure dressing, sets it aside on sterile field, and applies sterile gloves.	Essential to prepare in advance for quick application to wound on tube withdrawal.
5. Support patient physically and emotionally while health care provider removes dressing and clips sutures.	Patients state that when they know the tube is being pulled, they can mentally prepare themselves for the procedure. Support from the health care team reduces anxiety and promotes cooperation.
6. Health care provider asks patient to exhale completely and hold breath while bearing down (Valsalva's manoeuvre).	Prevents accidental entrance of air into the pleural space (Huggins et al., 2022).
7. Health care provider rapidly and smoothly pulls out chest tube and tightens and ties purse-string suture if present, after which patient is instructed to breathe normally.	This procedure forms an airtight seal and prevents entry of air through the chest wound. Sutures decrease the possibility that air will enter pleural space and aid in skin closure.
8. Health care provider applies sterile occlusive dressing over wound and firmly secures it in position with wide tape.	Keeps wound aseptic. Prevents entry of air into chest. Wound closure occurs spontaneously.
9. Health care provider inspects end of chest tube(s) before disposal to ensure complete removal.	Inspection of end of chest tube helps to verify that all of the tube was removed.
10. Help patient to upright position supported by pillows.	Restores patient's comfort. Patients report that proper positioning following chest tube removal helps relieve procedure-related sensations of pain and pulling (Chotai, 2022).
11. Dispose of all equipment in appropriate receptacles and remove gloves.	

EVALUATION

STEP	RATIONALE
1. Auscultate lung sounds.	Helps confirm that lung remains expanded.
2. Palpate skin over area where tube was inserted for subcutaneous emphysema and inspect for redness, inflammation, and blistering.	Subcutaneous emphysema results from entrance of air into the subcutaneous space. It is usually minor and resolves independent of interventions. If extensive, subcutaneous emphysema may be painful, preventing full lung expansion.
3. Evaluate for signs of respiratory distress immediately after tube removal and during first few hours after removal.	Provides for early notification of health care provider if adverse symptoms occur. Chest tubes may need reinsertion.

Critical Decision Point *If air is heard escaping from the chest tube site, reinforce the occlusive dressing and immediately notify the health care provider.*

STEP	RATIONALE
4. Evaluate patient's vital signs, oxygen saturation, pulmonary status, and psychological status.	Detects early signs and symptoms of complications.
5. Review chest radiography, if prescribed.	Evidence does not support routine postremoval X-ray films in either adults or pediatric or neonatal patients (Huggins et al., 2022). If complications are noted, bedside ultrasound imaging or computed tomography (CT), which is better at identifying the chest cavity, may be prescribed.
6. Ask about patient's level of pain or comfort. Observe for nonverbal cues of pain, and assess level of discomfort using an appropriate pain rating scale.	Indicates that wound did not close well. Determines patient's tolerance of procedure.
7. Check chest dressing for drainage and patency. When changing dressing, note wound for signs of healing.	Ensures occlusion and proper healing of chest wound.
8. **Use teach-back:** "I want to be sure I explained what happens after your chest tube is removed. Tell me what you know about what we did." Revise your instruction now or develop a plan for revised patient or family caregiver teaching if the patient or family caregiver is unable to teach back correctly.	Determines patient's and caregiver's level of understanding of instructional topic.

Unexpected Outcomes	Related Interventions
1. Dyspnea and laboured respirations noted after chest tube removal; potential recurrence of pneumothorax, hemothorax, or effusion.	• Notify health care provider. • Obtain vital signs and oxygen saturation. • Stay with patient.
2. Infection is noted at insertion site.	• Prepare for possible chest tube reinsertion. • Assess patient's vital signs for elevated temperature, tachypnea, and tachycardia. Assess wound for drainage, odour, erythema, or increased pain.

Communication and Documentation

- Document removal of tube, amount and appearance of drainage in the collection bottle, appearance of wound and dressing, and patient's response and understanding of the procedure on flow sheet or in progress notes in EHR or chart.
- Document vital signs and respiratory assessment on flow sheet or progress notes in EHR or chart.
- Document patient learning.
- Document and report unexpected outcomes to the nurse in charge or health care provider.

DOCUMENTATION EXAMPLE

No bubbling noted in water seal drainage ×4 hours; 20 mL serosanguinous drainage in collection bottle over the last 8 hours. Patient taught reason for chest tube removal and relaxation breathing techniques. Morphine 4 mg administered IV 20 minutes prior to chest tube removal by health care provider. Chest tube removed intact and patient tolerated procedure well. Chest tube insertion site clean with no redness or edema noted; site covered with a sterile occlusive dressing. Vital signs normal as documented on patient flow sheet, normal breath sounds heard bilaterally, and no dyspnea noted. Patient reported pain to be a 2 on a 1 to 10 pain scale. Patient was assisted to upright position with pillows for support.

Special Considerations

Teaching

- Instruct patient and caregiver to immediately report signs of chest pain, shortness of breath, or sensations of chest discomfort.

Pediatric

- Pediatric patients usually require analgesia (e.g., morphine sulphate 0.1 mg/kg in combination with midazolam) before chest tube removal (Hockenberry et al., 2024).
- EMLA cream (locally applied lidocaine/prilocaine anaesthetic patch) placed under the occlusive dressing at the chest tube insertion site 1 hour before tube removal reduces pain of the procedure. However, the child may still feel the "pulling" sensation (Hockenberry et al., 2024).

Care in the Community: Home Management

- Teach patient the importance of ambulating and remaining active once the chest tube has been removed.
- Instruct patient and caregivers to contact health care provider if one of the following occurs: changes to patient's skin around chest tube removal site (e.g., change in colour or amount of drainage, leakage on the dressing from chest tube removal site), chest pain, or breathlessness.
- Provide patient and caregiver with information specific to the type of wound care needed; when possible, have patient demonstrate proper wound care (Sasa, 2019).

✦ SKILL 27.3 Autotransfusion of Chest Tube Drainage

NSO Nursing Skills Online Chest Tubes Module 11 / Lesson 5

In autotransfusion, blood lost from trauma, injury, or surgery is infused back into a patient's circulatory system. When reinfusion is linked with chest drainage, it is a relatively risk-free, inexpensive, and easy method of replacing blood. Benefits of autotransfusion include an immediate blood supply, little risk of transfusion reaction and disease transmission, and more oxygen supplied to vital organs (Wiegand, 2017). Patients must also have a patent IV line in place (see Chapter 29). Autotransfusion is contraindicated in patients with coagulation disorders, septicemia, cancer, and renal or hepatic insufficiency. However, any of these contraindications can be overruled if the patient is exsanguinating and there is not an adequate supply of banked blood available (Wiegand, 2017).

Delegation and Collaboration

The skill of managing autotransfusion of chest tube drainage cannot be delegated to a UCP. The nurse directs the UCP to do the following immediately:

- Inform the nurse of changes in patient's vital signs or SpO_2 levels
- Inform the nurse about increased or decreased drainage from the chest tube

The nurse may need to collaborate with the interprofessional health care team members about the following:

- Any change in the patient's baseline assessment, including respiratory status
- Blood accumulation >200 mL/hr
- New onset of clots
- Concern for infection or septicemia

Equipment

- Adult/pediatric single-use chest drainage and autotransfusion unit (Fig. 27.10)
- *Optional:* Continuous autotransfusion system (ATS) with a blood-compatible infusion pump (check employer policy)
- Microaggregate blood filter (40-micron filter; see manufacturer's instructions)
- Nonvented blood-compatible IV administration set
- Antiseptic swab
- Infusion pump (see manufacturer's instructions)
- Replacement bag
- Personal protective equipment (PPE), as needed

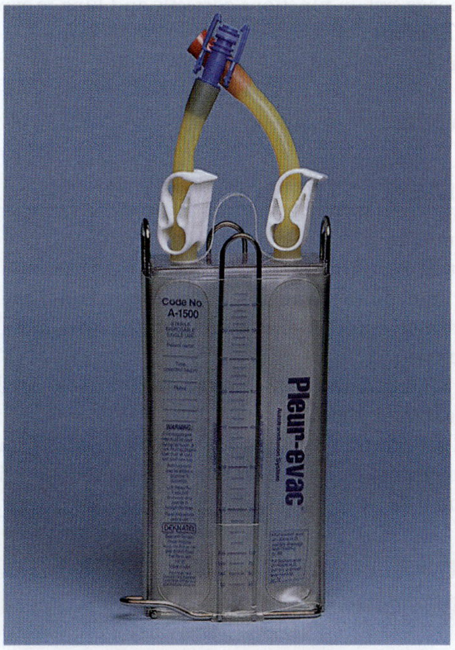

FIG 27.10 Example of autotransfusion unit.

STEP	RATIONALE
ASSESSMENT	
1. Identify patient using at least two person-specific identifiers (e.g., name and date of birth, or name and medical record number) according to employer policy.	Ensures correct patient. Complies with Accreditation Canada's standards and improves patient safety (Accreditation Canada, 2020).
2. Throughout the procedure, the 4 moments for hand hygiene are to be implemented; hand hygiene should occur before initial patient (or patient environment) contact, before an aseptic procedure, after body fluid exposure risk, and after patient (or patient environment) contact. Additional hand hygiene should be performed when hands are visibly soiled.	Proper hand hygiene helps prevent the spread of infectious agents to health care providers.
3. See Assessment for Skill 27.1.	
4. Determine presence of active bleeding (at least 50–100 mL/hr) through chest tube.	Indicates need for possible reinfusion of chest tube drainage.

Critical Decision Point *Reinfuse blood within 6 hours of collection and ensure that the transfusion is complete within 4 hours of initiation* (Wiegand, 2017).

STEP	RATIONALE
5. Assess IV site (see Chapter 29); note size of IV catheter. An 18-gauge angiocatheter is preferred.	Determines presence of adequate and patent IV site for administration of blood products.
6. Obtain baseline laboratory data (e.g., hemoglobin and hematocrit).	Provides data to measure effectiveness of reinfusion of chest drainage on patient's circulating blood volume.
7. Assess patient's knowledge, prior experience with autotransfusion, and feelings about the procedure.	Reveals need for patient teaching and/or support.

NURSING DIAGNOSES

- Reduced cardiac output
- Insufficient peripheral tissue perfusion
- Potential for infection

Related factors and risk factors are individualized on the basis of patient's condition or needs.

PLANNING

STEP	RATIONALE
1. Expected outcomes following completion of procedure:	
• Vital signs, hematocrit, and hemoglobin stabilize.	Reinfusion reduces significant blood loss associated with closed chest drainage.
• Drainage system functions correctly and lung re-expands in 48–72 hours.	Negative pressure is re-established in intrapleural space.
• IV line remains patent.	Patent IV is necessary for reinfusion of cleansed mediastinal tube drainage.
2. Explain procedure to patient.	Reduces anxiety and promotes patient cooperation.

IMPLEMENTATION

STEP	RATIONALE
1. System setup:	
a. Set up ATS according to technique that maintains sterility of unit and following three steps printed on front of unit.	Contamination of unit provides ready source of infection to patient.
b. Make certain that all connections are tight and all clamps are open.	Tight connections ensure airtight system, and open clamps allow chest drainage to enter ATS bag.
c. A 200-micron double-sided mesh filter is located in ATS bag to filter drainage.	Filtering drainage removes extraneous materials and microemboli.
d. ATS collection bag has capacity of 1000 mL marked in increments of 25 mL and an area for marking times and amounts.	Dark red drainage is expected only during immediate postoperative period. This drainage turns serous over time.

Critical Decision Point *Continuous ATS may be prescribed following cardiac surgery. This is a closed system with a specific infusion pump and IV circuit. This system requires specific education and is used in selected situations. Check employer policy.*

STEP	RATIONALE
IMPLEMENTATION	
2. Prepare chest drainage for reinfusion.	
a. Following manufacturer directions, open replacement bag, and close two white clamps.	Contamination of unit provides ready source of contamination to patient. Closed clamps maintain closed system during replacement.
b. Use high-negativity relief valve to reduce excessive negativity.	Eases removal of initial collection bag from metal support stand.
c. Bag transfer:	
(1) Close clamp on chest drainage tubing.	Prevents air from entering chest cavity through tube and collapsing lung.
(2) Close clamps on top of initial ATS collection bag.	Maintains closed system for reinfusion, preventing contamination of blood.
(3) Connect chest drainage tube to new ATS bag.	Establishes new ATS.
(4) Make certain that all connections are tight.	Ensures airtight system.
(5) Open all clamps on chest drainage tube and replacement bag.	Re-establishes ATS.
d. Connect connectors on top of initial collection bag and remove bag by lifting it from side hook and then from foot hook.	Maintains closed system within bag and removes it for use in autotransfusion.
e. Secure replacement bag by connecting foot hook, replacing metal frame into side hook of chest drainage unit, and pushing down to secure frame onto hook.	Provides safe attachment of replacement bag to chest drainage unit.
f. Place thumbs on top of metal frame and push up with fingers to slide bag out; remove replacement bag.	
3. Reinfuse chest drainage.	
a. Use new microaggregate filter to reinfuse each autotransfusion bag.	Prevents infusion of microemboli and provides maximal filtration for each bag.
b. Access bag by inverting it, wiping off port with antiseptic swab, and spiking through port with microaggregate filter and twisting.	Connects autotransfusion bag to transfusion tubing.
c. With bag upside down, gently squeeze it to remove air and prime filter with blood.	Gentle pressure is used to prevent hemolysis.
d. Hang bag on IV pole and continue to prime tubing until all air is gone. Clamp tubing, attach it to patient's IV access, and adjust clamp to deliver reinfusion at appropriate rate.	Removes all air from transfusion tubing. Reinfusion is delivered by gravity, application of a blood cuff (pressure not to exceed 150 mm Hg), or blood-compatible IV pump (see Chapter 29).
e. If prescribed, anticoagulants (anticoagulant citrate dextrose solution A or citrate phosphate dextrose solution, USP) are added to reinfusion through self-sealing port in autotransfusion connector.	Prevents clotting in autotransfusion. Reversing heparin with protamine to preoperative levels or collection of nonheparinized blood following emergency chest trauma may require a citrate anticoagulant (Wiegand, 2017).
f. Monitor patient's vital signs and SpO_2 according to patient condition and employer policy. For some patients, this may be as frequently as every 15 minutes; for other patients, it may be every hour.	Patients who require autotransfusion usually have complex physiological needs, and their vital signs change quite rapidly. Consistent, frequent monitoring allows for timely identification of changes and initiation of appropriate interventions to restore physiological stability.
4. Discontinue autotransfusion.	
a. Clamp chest drainage tube only briefly and only if prescribed by a health care provider and connect it directly to chest drainage unit with red and blue connectors.	Clamping chest tube for any length of time can cause tension pneumothorax (Tyerman & Cobbett, 2023; Wiegand, 2017).
b. Open chest drainage tube clamp.	All drainage will be collected directly in drainage unit and discarded appropriately.
5. Dispose of all equipment in appropriate receptacles and remove gloves.	
EVALUATION	
1. Monitor vital signs, hematocrit, and hemoglobin.	Helps determine effects of treatment.
2. Monitor chest drainage system and patient's lung sounds.	Helps determine proper functioning of system and its effectiveness.
3. Evaluate IV infusion site for infiltration and phlebitis.	Patent IV infusion site is maintained.
4. **Use teach-back:** "I want to be sure I explained why you needed this procedure. Tell me why this procedure was important." Develop a revised teaching plan if patient or caregiver is unable to teach back correctly.	Determines patient's and caregiver's level of understanding of instructional topic.

Unexpected Outcomes	Related Interventions
1. Chest tube is dislodged.	• Immediately apply pressure over chest tube insertion site. • Have assistant apply sterile petrolatum-impregnated occlusive dressing. • Notify health care provider.
2. Patient has dyspnea, chest pain, and laboured respirations.	• Verify that chest tube is patent and draining. • Obtain vital signs. • Notify health care provider.
3. Patient has signs of infection, fever, and chills.	• Obtain wound cultures as prescribed. • Obtain vital signs.

Communication and Documentation

- Document drainage and reinfusion with times and amounts of each; include patient's response to reinfusion in progress notes in EHR or chart. Describe condition of IV infusion site.
- Document patient teaching and validation of understanding on flow sheet or in progress notes in EHR or chart.

DOCUMENTATION EXAMPLE

100 mL sanguineous drainage from chest tube noted during last 45 minutes, with 280 mL total over last 2 hours. Explained to patient need for autotransfusion and procedure; patient repeated rationale for procedure back to writer. Reinfused 280 mL sanguineous drainage with an 18-gauge angiocatheter via blood-compatible IV pump per health care provider prescription. No redness or edema noted at IV site. Vital signs are within normal limits; SpO_2 95% on room air; no dyspnea noted. Patient denies pain and is resting with ongoing vital sign assessment every 15 minutes.

Special Considerations

Teaching

- Prepare patient and caregiver for the procedure so they will understand when the patient's blood is reinfused. Patients and their caregivers may have had this instruction before surgery but need reinforcement.

Gerontological

- Pulmonary edema due to transfusion-associated circulatory or volume overload may occur, especially in patients with compromised cardiac function.

✦ REVIEW QUESTIONS

A patient (he/him) is in the critical care unit following open-heart surgery. He has a chest tube in the right pleural cavity and another in the mediastinal area to allow for drainage. Last vital signs were BP of 110/64 mm Hg, pulse of 86 beats/min, respirations on mechanical ventilator of 16 breaths/min; SpO_2 of 96%; and temperature of 37.2°C (axillary). The last hourly chest tube drainage was 75 mL from the pleural tube and 100 mL from the mediastinal tube.

Review Questions 1 to 3 relate to the case study presented here.

1. Why is it important to check vital signs, check for air leaks, and note the amount of chest drainage every 15 to 30 minutes for at least 2 hours after the patient returns from surgery?
2. The patient is 12 hours postoperative and is no longer on mechanical ventilation. He is transferred from the bed to a chair. Immediately following this transfer, the nurse notes drainage of 50 mL of dark red fluid. What should the nurse do?
3. Using SBAR (situation–background–assessment–recommendation), how should the nurse document this episode with the patient's chest drainage noted in Review Question 2?
4. Patients with chest tubes that remove bloody drainage from the chest cavity usually are at risk for respiratory problems. These patients have many care priorities. What are two important priorities related to management of the chest tube system?
   1. Monitoring chest tube drainage
   2. Promoting activity
   3. Promoting airway clearance
   4. Maintaining chest tube patency
   5. Observing dressing
5. The nurse is caring for a patient with a chest tube. Which activities can a nurse delegate to an unregulated care provider (UCP)? (*Select all that apply.*)
   1. Proper positioning of the patient to facilitate chest tube drainage
   2. Helping to remove a chest tube
   3. Helping to ambulate and transfer a patient with chest drainage
   4. Reporting any abnormal vital signs or symptoms of chest pain or shortness of breath
   5. Reinfusion of chest tube drainage
   6. Reporting any change in the amount of drainage or sudden bleeding
6. Correctly organize the following steps to manage autotransfusion of chest tube drainage:
   1. Hang the bag on an intravenous (IV) pole and continue to prime the tubing until all air is gone.
   2. Access the bag by inverting it and spiking it through the spike port with the microaggregate filter and twisting.
   3. Use a new microaggregate filter to reinfuse each autotransfusion bag.
   4. If prescribed, add anticoagulants to the reinfusion through the self-sealing port in the autotransfusion connector.

5. With the bag upside down, gently squeeze it to remove the air and prime the filter with blood.
6. Monitor patient's vital signs and pulse oximetry (SpO_2) according to patient condition and employer policy.

7. A patient is about to have a chest tube removed by the health care provider. As the nurse assisting with the removal, which of the following actions will you perform? (*Select all that apply.*)
   1. Teach the patient how to take a deep breath out and inhale rapidly while the tube is being removed.
   2. Gather supplies needed, which will include a petrolatum-impregnated gauze dressing per provider preference.
   3. Place the patient in semi-Fowler's position.
   4. Have the patient take a deep breath, exhale, and bear down during the removal of the tube.
   5. Premedicate the patient with pain medicine prior to the tube removal, as prescribed by the health care provider.
   6. Place the patient in prone position after removal of chest tube.

Visit the Evolve site for a complete list of answers to the Review Questions.

NEXT GENERATION NCLEX® (NGN)

For practice with answering exam questions related to unfolding NGN case studies, please consult the Next Generation NCLEX® (NGN)-Style Case Studies for Skills and Techniques on the Evolve website: http://evolve.elsevier.com/Canada/Perry/clinicalskills/

REFERENCES

Accreditation Canada. (2020). *Required organizational practices–2020 handbook.* https://physicians.nshealth.ca/resources/required-organizational-practices-2020-handbook

Banasik, J., & Copstead, L. (2019). *Pathophysiology* (6th ed.). Elsevier Inc.

Bauman, M., & Handley, C. (2018). *Best practices: Chest tube management.* American Nurse Today. https://www.myamericannurse.com/wp-content/uploads/2018/02/ANT_ChestTube_Management.pdf

Chotai, P. (2022). Tube thoracostomy management. *Medscape.* https://emedicine.medscape.com/article/1503275-overview

D'Agostino, H. P., & Edens, M. A. (2021). *Physiology, pleural fluid. StatPearls.* https://www.ncbi.nlm.nih.gov/books/NBK513353/

Ehrhardt, P. (2017). Anatomy of the chest wall and pleura. In T. Kiefer (Ed.), *Chest drains in daily clinical practice* (1st ed., pp. 1–15). Springer. [Seminal Reference]

Hockenberry, M. J., Duffy, E. A., & Gibbs, K. (2024). *Wong's nursing care of infants and children* (12th ed.). Elsevier.

Huggins, J. T., Carr, S. R., & Woodward, G. A. (2022). *Thoracostomy tubes and catheters: Indications and tube selection in adults and children.* UpToDate. https://www.uptodate.com/contents/thoracostomy-tubes-and-catheters-indications-and-tube-selection-in-adults-and-children

Kukuruza, K., & Aboeed, A. (2022). Subcutaneous emphysema. *StatPearls.* https://www.ncbi.nlm.nih.gov/books/NBK542192/

Mancini, M. C. (2022). Hemothorax clinical presentation. *Medscape.* https://emedicine.medscape.com/article/2047916-clinical

Operating Room Nurses Association of Canada. (2023). *The ORNAC standards, guidelines, and position statements for perioperative registered nurses* (16th ed.). https://www.ornac.ca/en/standards

Pickett, J. (2017). Closed chest drainage system. In D. Weigand (Ed.), *AACN procedure manual for high acuity, progressive, and critical care* (7th ed., pp. 195–205). Elsevier. [Seminal Reference]

Porcel, J. M. (2018). Chest tube drainage of the pleural space: A concise review for pulmonologists. *Tuberculosis and Respiratory Diseases, 81*(2), 106–115. https://doi.org/10.4046/trd.2017.0107

Quinte Health Care. (2020). *Chest tube insertion, maintenance, and removal–resource manual.* https://ppno.ca/wp-content/uploads/2021/02/Chest-Tube-Insertion-Maintenance-and-Removal-August-2020-revised.pdf

Rajan, C. (2022). Tube thoracostomy management. *Medscape.* http://emedicine.medscape.com/article/1503275-overview

Regina Qu'Appelle Health Region. (2017). *Heimlich valve and chest tube–discharge instructions.* https://rqhealth.ca/rqhr-central/.files/1339.pdf. [Seminal Reference]

Sasa, R. I. (2019). Evidence-based update on chest tube management: Is your practice current? *American Nurse Today, 14*(4), 10–15. https://www.myamericannurse.com/evidence-based-update-on-chest-tube-management/

Tyerman, J., & Cobbett, S. (Eds.). (2023). *Lewis's medical-surgical nursing in Canada: Assessment and management of clinical problems* (5th ed.). Elsevier Inc.

Waters, J. (2017). Chest tube placement (assist). In D. Wiegand (Ed.), *AACN procedure manual for high acuity, progressive, and critical care* (7th ed., pp. 178–183). Elsevier. [Seminal Reference]

Wiegand, D. (Ed.). (2017). *AACN procedure manual for high acuity, progressive, and critical care* (7th ed.). Elsevier. [Seminal Reference]

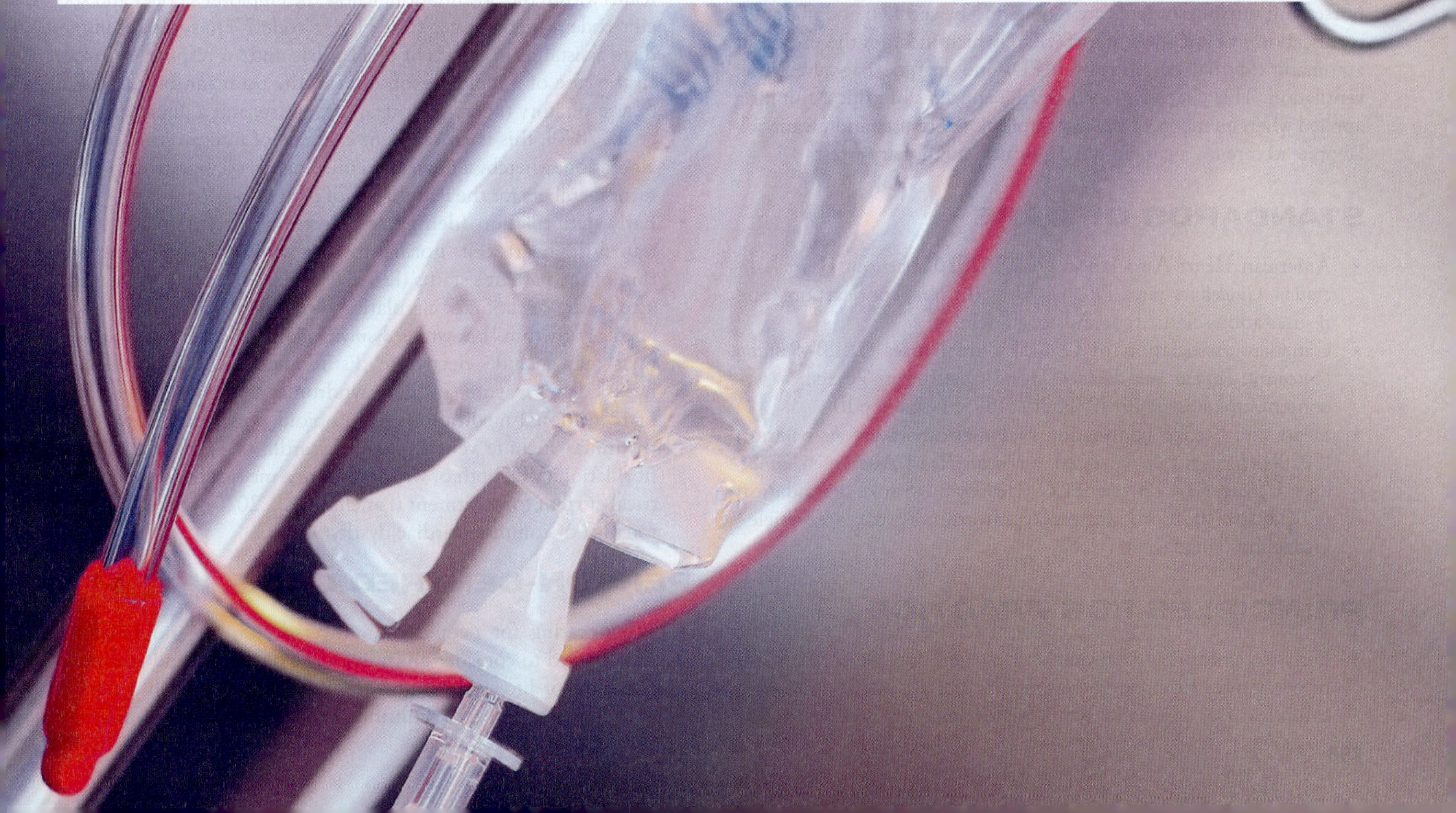

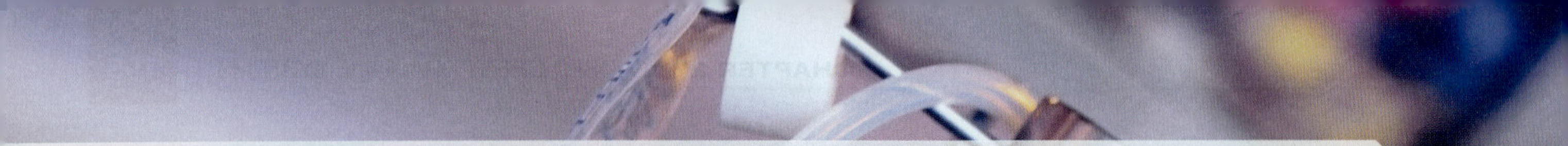

28 Emergency Measures for Life Support

Canadian content written by **Danielle Byrne, RN, MN, CCSNE**
Original US chapter by **Nelda K. Martin, RN, ANP-BC, CCNS**

SKILLS AND PROCEDURES

OBJECTIVES

Mastery of content in this chapter will enable the nurse to:

- Describe indications for basic airway adjunct insertion.
- State indications for cardiopulmonary resuscitation.
- Identify indications for use of an external defibrillator (automated or manual).
- Describe the nurse's role during a cardiac arrest.

MEDIA RESOURCES

http://evolve.elsevier.com/Canada/Perry/clinicalskills/

PURPOSE

Cardiopulmonary arrests are emergency situations that nurses must be prepared to handle at any time, whether the arrest occurs in the community or in the hospital setting. Nurses are expected to follow current resuscitation guidelines in a systematic and organized manner. The goal is to provide resuscitation in a timely manner to restore cardiopulmonary function and avoid poor neurological outcomes. All nurses and nursing students are required to be certified and maintain certification in basic life support (BLS), which includes the use of an automatic external defibrillator (AED) and manual bag-valve mask ventilation. This chapter focuses on the concepts of critical thinking applied when members of the interprofessional resuscitation team collaborate to care for a patient during a cardiopulmonary arrest.

STANDARDS OF CARE

- American Heart Association (2020)—*2020 American Heart Association Guidelines for CPR and ECC* (https://cpr.heart.org/en/resuscitation-science/cpr-and-ecc-guidelines)
- Canadian Association of Critical Care Nurses (2018)—*Position Statement: Patient- and Family-Centred Care* (https://caccn.ca/wp-content/uploads/2019/10/PS062018PSPFCCare.pdf)
- Heart and Stroke Foundation & American Heart Association (2020)—*Highlights of the 2020 American Heart Association Guidelines Update for CPR and ECC* (Heart and Stroke Foundation of Canada Edition) (https://cpr.heartandstroke.ca/s/article/Guidelines?language=en_US)

PRINCIPLES FOR PRACTICE

- Early recognition and prevention strategies improve survival and recovery rates from cardiac events (Hall et al., 2020). Prior to a cardiac arrest, signs and symptoms of impending deterioration include tachycardia, hypotension, tachypnea, decreasing oxygen saturation below 90% despite provision of supplemental oxygen, and a decreasing urine output of less than 50 mL in 4 hours. These are reasons for activating an emergency or rapid response team (Agency for Healthcare Research and Quality, 2019).
- Activation of emergency response varies depending on setting (e.g., community versus hospital), policies, and availability of response teams within the organization. Know the employer's policy and specific code or signal (e.g., "code blue," "code 7") to summon immediate assistance in the event of a cardiac and/or respiratory arrest. In the case of a rapid response team, the team can be composed of a respiratory therapist, critical care nurse, and a physician (Hall et al., 2020); this is an excellent example of interprofessional collaboration, whereby a nurse can consult and collaborate with other team members for the betterment of patient care.
- Early defibrillation (delivery of electrical current) may quickly return the heart to its normal rhythm without further deterioration of the patient's status (Panchal et al., 2020). In some cardiac arrests, the cessation of circulating blood flow is caused by irregular heart rhythms known as *dysrhythmias.* The causes of dysrhythmias may include electrolyte disturbances (e.g., hypokalemia/hyperkalemia), acute coronary syndrome, and certain prescribed or recreational medications (e.g., opioid poisoning). Lethal dysrhythmias include ventricular tachycardia (VT) and ventricular fibrillation (VF), both of which require a medically delivered electrical current for treatment (Panchal et al., 2020). (See Table 26.1 for a list of common cardiac dysrhythmias.)

PERSON-CENTRED CARE

- When caring for people from diverse cultures and religions, nurses need to consider an individual's beliefs around and interpretation of life support and resuscitation. Although a person may be part of a specific cultural or religious group, they may not follow all aspects of that culture or religion. Therefore, it is essential that nurses consider each person's interpretation and wishes to ensure the right of self-determination and implementation of culturally appropriate, person-centred nursing care (Canadian Association of Critical Care Nurses [CACCN], 2018).

- When necessary, use a professional language interpreter to explain the patient's health status to the patient and their caregiver. In addition, use cultural and religious support personnel (e.g., Indigenous Elders) to facilitate the patient's and caregiver's understanding of events.
- Advance directives and resuscitation care plans offer valuable information concerning a person's plan related to resuscitation status and decisions regarding resuscitation efforts. Although advance directives are often addressed before or during a person's hospitalization, nurses play an important role in advocating for and encouraging the person to discuss their wishes with the health care team. Whenever a person requires resuscitation, a member of the interprofessional team (e.g., social worker, pastoral care worker) can support family presence at the bedside during the event.
- Follow employer policy related to communicating and flagging a person's electronic health record (EHR) or chart when a decision is made concerning do not resuscitate (DNR), do not attempt resuscitation (DNaR), and allow natural death (AND) orders.
- Nurses need to be prepared for a large number of visitors to remain at the bedside to provide support for the family or pray for the person. Nurses should collaborate with the family decision maker and leader to plan rotating visits at the bedside. When visitation is restricted or limited (e.g., pandemic, isolation), nurses can support connections through audio and video technological devices. Review employer policies related to visitation practices and electronic devices (Munshi et al., 2021).

EVIDENCE-INFORMED PRACTICE

The International Liaison Committee on Resuscitation (ILCOR) promotes, disseminates, and advocates for the international implementation of evidence-informed resuscitation for both initial care (BLS) and ongoing measures (advanced life support [ALS]). The Heart and Stroke Foundation (HSF) is an active member of this consensus-building organization. The HSF and American Heart Association (AHA) work collaboratively to develop North American guidelines (HSF & AHA, 2020). The 2020 AHA guidelines for in-hospital cardiac arrest chain of survival focus on the following aspects (Panchal et al., 2020):

- Early recognition and prevention
- Activation of emergency response
- Immediate, high-quality cardiopulmonary resuscitation (CPR)
- Early defibrillation with advanced cardiac life support interventions
- Post–cardiac arrest care
- Recovery

There is increased emphasis on providing high-quality CPR, ensuring that chest compressions are performed at an adequate rate and depth, while allowing for full chest recoil between compressions. Interprofessional resuscitation teams should work collaboratively to minimize interruptions in chest compressions and avoid excessive ventilation, aiming for early defibrillation (if indicated) (Panchal et al., 2020).

Family members might be at the bedside of the patient when a cardiac arrest occurs. Family presence during resuscitation (FPDR) should be considered an important part of person-centred care by the interprofessional resuscitation team. Through interprofessional collaboration, a team member may be designated to help prepare the family for what they might see, hear, and smell prior to an event occurring. This team member can also be there to support the family during the event (CACCN, 2018). Development of policies and education for designated family members can support the safe and effective implementation of FPDR (Meghani, 2021).

SAFETY GUIDELINES

- Know a patient's baseline vital signs, noting any irregularities in cardiac rhythm. Dysrhythmias can precipitate a cardiopulmonary arrest. Conditions that place a patient at risk for dysrhythmias include coronary artery disease, myocardial infarction, open-heart surgeries, acid–base imbalances, and toxicities.
- Know a patient's most recent serum electrolyte values. Electrolyte imbalances (e.g., potassium, magnesium, and calcium) can precipitate cardiopulmonary arrest.
- When a patient has been exposed to a chemical, prescription medication, or drug, attempt to determine the type and amount of the substance involved. Certain chemicals (e.g., ethanol, tranquilizers, opiates) depress the respiratory centre, resulting in respiratory arrest. Oversedation involving the use of patient-controlled analgesia (PCA) pumps or epidural administration can also contribute to respiratory depression. Overdoses of some medications can cause ventricular dysrhythmias and cardiopulmonary arrest.
- Clear communication with all others in the room is essential at the time of defibrillation so that everyone is aware and does not touch the patient or the bed upon delivery of the electrical current. Verbalization using loud and clear speech assists in closing the loop of communication once the prescribed interventions have been stated by the resuscitation leader and creates a shared mental model of the current situation. Verbalization of completed interventions assists the recorder/timekeeper with documentation (Lauridsen et al., 2021).
- Resuscitation situations involve many aerosol-generating procedures (AGPs), including chest compressions, positive-pressure ventilation, and establishment of an advanced airway. Balancing the emergent need of the patient and the safety of health care personnel is essential when responding to situations where contagious viral particles (e.g., SARS-CoV-2) can remain suspended in air. Therefore, strategies to reduce exposure need to be followed (Atkins et al., 2022). Box 28.1 lists general principles to follow when airborne or droplet isolation precautions are required.

✦ SKILL 28.1 Inserting an Oropharyngeal Airway

An *oropharyngeal airway (OPA)* is a semicircular, minimally flexible, curved piece of hard plastic (Fig. 28.1). When inserted, it extends from just outside the lips, over the tongue, and to the pharynx (Fig. 28.2). Oral airways allow nurses to suction through a central core or along the side of the airway and maintain airway patency in an unconscious patient by displacing the tongue forward and toward the oral cavity floor. Choose the correct size of an OPA based on a patient's age and the width and length of their mouth (Table 28.1). Size is correct if, when the flange is held parallel to the front teeth with the airway against the patient's cheek, the end of the curve reaches the angle of the jaw (Fig. 28.3).

BOX 28.1

General Principles for Resuscitation in Patients on Airborne or Droplet Isolation Precautions

- Before entrance to the room, all rescuers must don appropriate PPE to guard against contact with both airborne and droplet particles.
- Limit personnel in the room to only those essential for patient care.
- Relieve personnel who are not wearing appropriate PPE for aerosol-generating procedures.
- Clearly communicate isolation precautions to any new health care provider.
- Use a HEPA filter for all ventilation (bag-valve mask with tight seal or mechanical ventilator). If mechanically ventilated, maintain patient on closed circuit with oxygen level at 100%.
- Until bag-valve mask ventilation with HEPA filter is available, consider passive oxygenation with a nonbreathing face mask covered by a surgical mask for a short duration.
- Consider early intubation with cuffed endotracheal tube after initial defibrillation or consider supraglottic airway.
- Engage the intubator with the highest chance of first-pass success and consider use of video laryngoscopy (if available); may pause chest compression to facilitate intubation if needed.
- Minimize endotracheal administration of medications to avoid aerosol generation.

HEPA, High-efficiency particulate air; *PPE*, personal protective equipment.

Atkins, D., Sasson, C., Hsu, A., et al. (2022). 2022 interim guidance to health care providers for basic and advanced cardiac life support in adults, children, and neonates with suspected or confirmed COVID-19: From the Emergency Cardiovascular Care Committee and Get With The Guidelines-Resuscitation Adult and Pediatric Task Forces of the American Heart Association in collaboration with the American Academy of Pediatrics, American Association for Respiratory Care, the Society of Critical Care Anesthesiologists, and American Society of Anesthesiologists. *Circulation: Cardiovascular Quality and Outcomes, 15*(4), e008900. https://doi.org/10.1161/CIRCOUTCOMES.122.008900

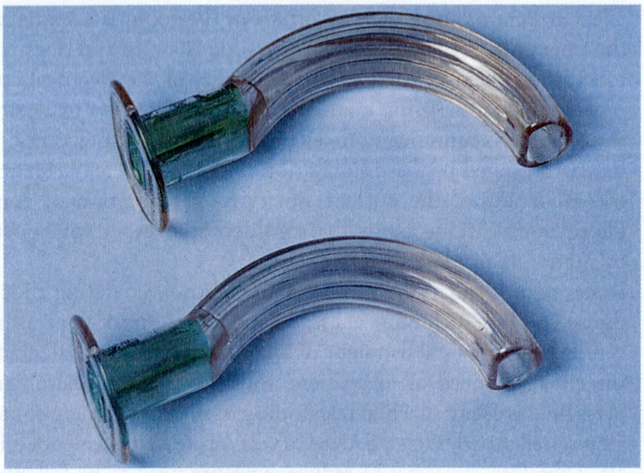

FIG 28.1 Oral airways.

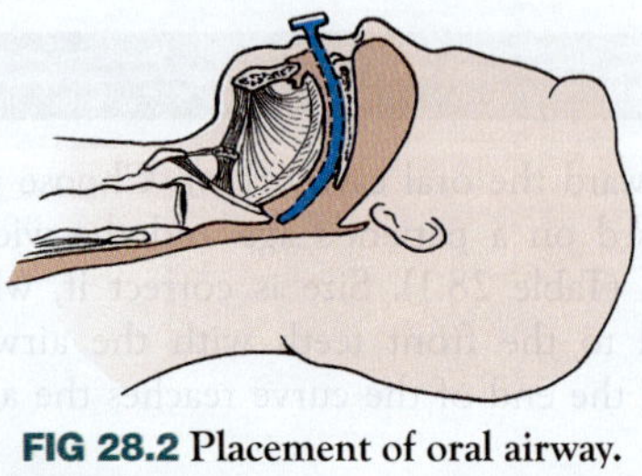

FIG 28.2 Placement of oral airway.

TABLE 28.1

Oral Airway Guidelines for Size* by Age

Size	Age
30 mm or size 000	Premature neonates
45 mm or size 00	Newborn
55 mm or size 0	Newborn to 1 year
60 mm or size 1	1–2 years
70 mm or size 2	2–6 years
80 mm or size 3	6–18 years
90 mm or size 4	Adult medium
100 mm or size 5	Adult large
110 mm or size 6	Adult extra large

*Measure from the corner of the mouth to the angle of the jaw just below the ear for size estimation (Castro & Freeman, 2021).

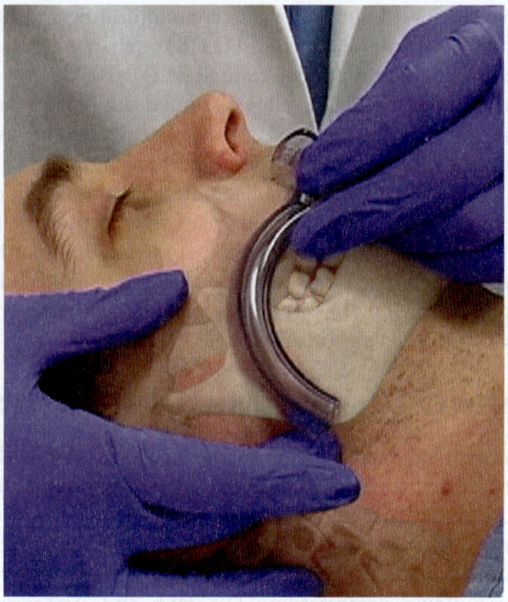

FIG 28.3 Measuring for an oral airway. (*From Roberts, J. R. [2019]. Roberts and Hedges' clinical procedures in emergency medicine and acute care [7th ed.]. Elsevier.*)

Delegation and Collaboration

The skill of inserting an OPA cannot be delegated to an unregulated care provider (UCP). The nurse directs the UCP to do the following:

- Immediately report to the nurse any signs of airway distress, vomiting, or change in level of consciousness

The nurse needs to use interprofessional collaboration (e.g., respiratory therapist) for safe OPA insertion.

Equipment

- Appropriately sized oral airway (see Table 28.1 and Fig. 28.3)
- Tongue blade
- Stethoscope
- Pulse oximeter
- Tissues or washcloths
- Clean gloves
- Face shield
- Mask and gown appropriate for level of isolation
- Suction equipment, if indicated
- Nonallergenic tape (*optional*)

STEP	RATIONALE
ASSESSMENT	
1. Identify patient using at least two person-specific identifiers (e.g., name and date of birth, or name and medical record number) according to employer policy.	Ensures correct patient. Complies with Accreditation Canada's standards and improves patient safety (Accreditation Canada, 2020).
2. Throughout the procedure, the 4 moments for hand hygiene are to be implemented; hand hygiene should occur before initial patient (or patient environment) contact, before an aseptic procedure, after body fluid exposure risk, and after patient (or patient environment) contact. Additional hand hygiene should be performed when hands are visibly soiled.	Proper hand hygiene helps prevent the spread of infectious agents to health care providers.
3. Don appropriate level of personal protective equipment (PPE) prior to entering the room (See Box 5.1 and Skill 5.2).	Prevents exposure to, or contamination from, body fluid or aerosol-generating procedures (Atkins et al., 2022).
4. Identify need to insert an OPA. Signs and symptoms include upper airway gurgling with breathing, absent cough or gag reflex, increased oral secretions, excessive drooling, grinding teeth, clenched teeth, biting endotracheal or gastric tubes, decline in oxygen saturation, laboured respirations, or difficulty in maintaining airway during manual ventilation with bag-valve mask.	These conditions place patient at risk for obstruction of the upper airway. Use OPAs only in unconscious patients. It may stimulate vomiting or laryngospasm if inserted in a semiconscious or conscious patient with a gag reflex.
5. Determine factors that may contribute to upper airway obstruction, such as age (children have a proportionally larger tongue) or presence of a nasal or oral airway and drainage tubes (swallowing is more difficult with tubes in place).	Allows accurate assessment of need for OPA placement. Patients at greater risk for upper airway obstruction are infants; children; and adults with upper airway congestion, loss of consciousness, seizure disorders, neuromuscular diseases, or increased oral secretions.
6. Ensure that patient does not have dentures in place before attempting an OPA insertion.	Removal of dentures or partial plates prior to insertion can prevent dislodgement and airway obstruction.
7. Measure for correct size of OPA (see Table 28.1 and Fig. 28.3).	Inappropriate size may cause or worsen airway obstruction (Castro & Freeman, 2021).

Critical Decision Point *Never insert an OPA in a conscious patient with a gag reflex or a patient with recent oral or facial trauma, oral surgery, or loose teeth. Never force an airway into place.*

STEP	RATIONALE
8. Assess caregiver's knowledge of procedure.	Identifies learning needs of caregiver. Patient will be unconscious.

NURSING DIAGNOSES

- Inadequate airway clearance
- Potential for aspiration

Related factors and risk factors are individualized on the basis of patient's condition or needs.

PLANNING

STEP	RATIONALE
1. Expected outcomes following completion of procedure:	
• Patient's respiratory status improves, as evidenced by respirations with normal rate, easier removal of secretions, and lack of gurgling noise in throat with respirations.	Airway is clear of secretions.
• Patient is unable to grind teeth or bite tubes.	Oral airway prevents tooth contact with other teeth or with tubes.
• Patient's tongue does not obstruct airway, allowing for adequate ventilation.	Oral airway keeps tongue in correct position to maintain patent airway.
2. Caregiver can verbalize understanding of need for OPA.	Teaching was successful.
3. Close room door and bedside curtain.	Provides for patient privacy.
4. Obtain and organize equipment for airway insertion at bedside.	Ensures more efficient procedure.

IMPLEMENTATION

STEP	RATIONALE
1. Apply clean gloves and face shield if required.	Reduces transmission of microorganisms.
2. Position unconscious patient in semi-Fowler's position if possible.	Provides easy access to oral cavity.

STEP	RATIONALE

IMPLEMENTATION

STEP	RATIONALE
3. Whenever possible, use padded tongue blade to open patient's mouth; if necessary, use thumb and forefinger of nondominant hand to open jaws and teeth.	Provides access to oral cavity. To avoid a bite, do not insert your fingers into the patient's mouth. Use extreme caution if manually opening patient's jaw and teeth.
4. Insert OPA.	When inserting airway, take care not to push patient's tongue into pharynx.
a. Hold OPA with curved end up toward the hard palate and insert distal end until airway reaches back of throat; then turn airway over 180 degrees and follow natural curve of tongue. *Option:* Hold airway sideways, insert halfway, and rotate 90 degrees while gliding it over natural curvature of the tongue (preferred technique for infants and small children).	Proper insertion of airway prevents displacement of patient's tongue into posterior oropharynx. Secure OPA with tape on upper and lower flange.
b. Make sure that outer flange is just outside the patient's lips.	

Critical Decision Point *In a pediatric patient, DO NOT rotate the oral airway on insertion because the airway tip will damage the soft palate.*

STEP	RATIONALE
5. Suction secretions as needed (see Skill 23.1).	Removes secretions; maintains patent airway.
6. Clean patient's face with soft tissue or washcloth.	Promotes hygiene.
7. Place nurse call system in accessible location; raise side rails (as appropriate) and lower bed to lowest position.	Promotes patient safety in case patient regains consciousness or caregiver needs assistance.
8. Discard equipment and used supplies into appropriate receptacles. Remove PPE (see Skill 5.3 and Box 5.1) and discard in appropriate receptacle.	Reduces transmission of microorganisms.

Critical Decision Point *Oral airways will need to be removed, cleaned or discarded, and replaced in patients with excessive oral secretions. Frequent mouth care and suctioning of the oral cavity may be required. Oral airways are not a long-term solution. They can create pressure on underlying tissue and cause significant lip and tongue erosion, which can result in a medical device–related pressure injury (MDRPI)* (Norton et al., 2021).

EVALUATION

STEP	RATIONALE
1. Reassess patient's respiratory status by auscultating lung sounds and measuring oxygen saturation, then compare respiratory assessments before and after insertion of the OPA.	Identifies patient's response to insertion of airway, patency of airway.
2. Verify that airway is patent and that patient's tongue does not obstruct it.	Ensures route for oxygen delivery to patient.
3. Observe adjacent and underlying tissue for signs of redness, abrasion, or bruising.	Identifies early signs of MDRPI.
4. Observe for patient pushing airway out with tongue or coughing.	Patient's ability to clear own airway may have returned. Indicates reassessment of need for oral airway.
5. Use teach-back: "I know this information can be overwhelming. In your words, tell me what is going to happen during this procedure." Develop a revised teaching plan if caregiver is unable to repeat explanation correctly.	Determines caregiver's level of understanding of instructional topic.

Unexpected Outcomes	Related Interventions
1. Patient continually coughs and gags when airway is inserted.	• Do not continue inserting airway if patient begins to gag. Stimulation of gag reflex can cause vomiting and aspiration. • Remove oral airway and position patient on side. • Reassess need for artificial airway prn (as needed).
2. Airway obstruction is not relieved.	• Obtain immediate assistance. • Reinsert airway or determine from health care provider whether another form of airway is needed. • Assess for other causes of obstruction.
3. Patient pushes airway out of place or out of mouth.	• Reassess patient's need for an OPA.
4. Unable to insert OPA; patient is combative or you are unable to open the patient's mouth.	• Get help. • Reassess patient's need for an OPA. • Provide sedation as prescribed.

Communication and Documentation

- Document assessment findings indicating need for insertion and the patient's response while inserting the OPA; size of OPA; other interventions performed at the same time, especially positioning and suctioning; and patient's response to procedure on flow sheet or in progress notes in EHR or chart.
- Document your evaluation of caregiver learning.

DOCUMENTATION EXAMPLE

Patient's Glasgow Coma Scale score = 6: no eye opening (1), no verbal response (1), and only withdraws to painful stimuli (4). Unable to elicit gag reflex, snoring respirations = 18 breaths per minute with oxygen saturation = 85% on non-rebreather mask. Mouth is clear of secretions and no loose teeth or partial plates noted. Measured for OPA size 4. Inserted OPA without difficulty. Postinsertion, patient's neurological assessment remains unchanged. Breath sounds are clear bilaterally to the bases = 20 breaths per minute and oxygen saturation increased to 92% on non-rebreather mask. Followed up with respiratory therapist and caregiver to update them on the patient's status.

Special Considerations

Pediatric

- Oral airways are seldom used in the treatment of airway obstruction in infants and children. Because the airway is narrow, OPAs are often more occlusive than beneficial (Hockenberry et al., 2024). Children may better tolerate a nasopharyngeal airway than an OPA (Ralston, 2022).

✦ SKILL 28.2 Inserting a Nasopharyngeal Airway

A *nasopharyngeal airway (NPA)* is a soft, flexible rubber tube. The uncuffed tube is inserted nasally along the floor of the nasopharynx past the base of the tongue (Fig. 28.4). An NPA allows nurses to suction through a central core and maintain airway patency in conscious, semiconscious, or unconscious patients. It is important to choose the correct length by measuring from the tip of the patient's nose to the tragus of the ear (Fig. 28.5). The external diameter of the NPA should be slightly smaller than the patient's external nares opening but not be too large to blanch the nares on insertion (Wittels, 2022).

Delegation and Collaboration

The skill of inserting an NPA cannot be delegated to a UCP. The nurse directs the UCP to do the following:

- Immediately report to the nurse any signs of airway distress, vomiting, or change in level of consciousness

Nurses need to use interprofessional collaboration (e.g., respiratory therapist) for safe NPA insertion.

Equipment

- Appropriately sized nasopharyngeal airway (see Fig 28.5)
- Stethoscope
- Pulse oximeter
- Water-soluble lubricant
- Tissues or washcloths
- Face shield
- Mask and gown appropriate for level of isolation
- Suction equipment, if indicated
- Nonallergenic tape *(optional)*

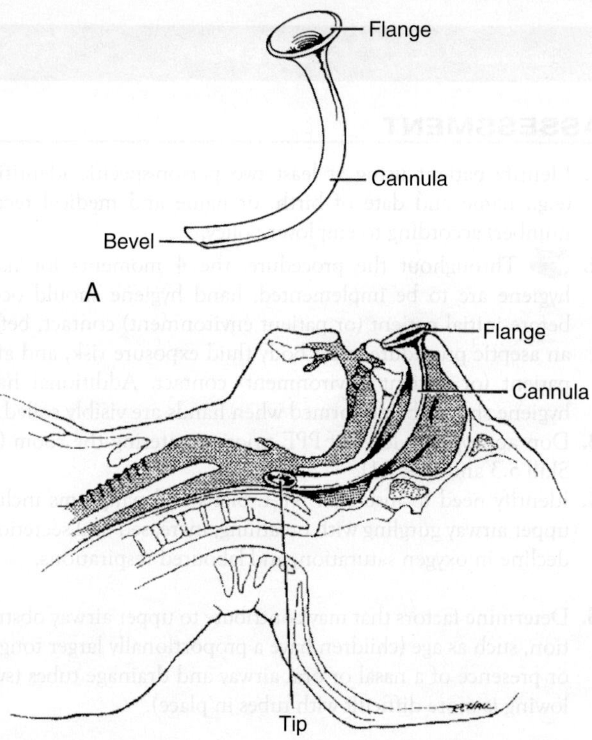

FIG 28.4 Nasopharyngeal airway. A, Airway parts. B, Proper placement. (From Weigand, D. [2011]. *AACN procedure manual for critical care* [6th ed., Figure 10.1, p. 69]. Image originally from Eubanks, D. H., & Bone, R. C. [1990]. *Comprehensive respiratory care: A learning system* [p. 518]. Mosby.)

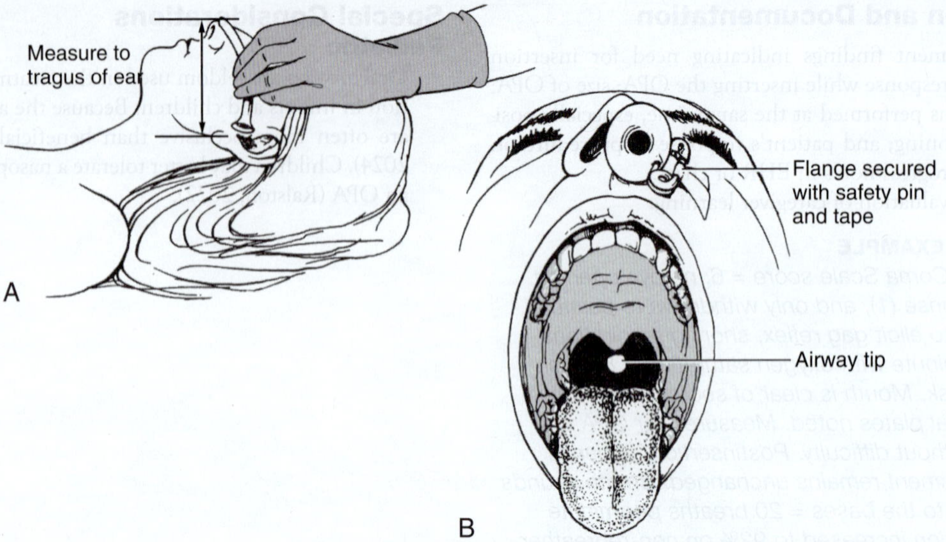

FIG 28.5 **A, Estimating nasopharyngeal airway size. B, Nasopharyngeal position after insertion.** (*From Weigand, D. [2011]. AACN procedure manual for critical care [6th ed., Figure 10.2, p. 70]. Image originally from Eubanks, D. H., & Bone, R. C. [1990]. Comprehensive respiratory care: A learning system [p. 552]. Mosby.*)

STEP	RATIONALE
ASSESSMENT	
1. Identify patient using at least two person-specific identifiers (e.g., name and date of birth, or name and medical record number) according to employer policy.	Ensures correct patient. Complies with Accreditation Canada's standards and improves patient safety (Accreditation Canada, 2020).
2. Throughout the procedure, the 4 moments for hand hygiene are to be implemented; hand hygiene should occur before initial patient (or patient environment) contact, before an aseptic procedure, after body fluid exposure risk, and after patient (or patient environment) contact. Additional hand hygiene should be performed when hands are visibly soiled.	Proper hand hygiene helps prevent the spread of infectious agents to health care providers.
3. Don appropriate level of PPE prior to entering the room (see Skill 5.3 and Box 5.1).	Prevents exposure to, or contamination from, body fluid or aerosol-generating procedures (Atkins et al., 2022).
4. Identify need to insert an NPA. Signs and symptoms include upper airway gurgling with breathing, increased oral secretions, decline in oxygen saturation, and laboured respirations.	These conditions place patient at risk for obstruction of the upper airway. Use an NPA on conscious, semiconscious, or unconscious patients. NPAs may stimulate vomiting or laryngospasm if measured incorrectly (i.e., NPA is too long) (Wittels, 2022).
5. Determine factors that may contribute to upper airway obstruction, such as age (children have a proportionally larger tongue) or presence of a nasal or oral airway and drainage tubes (swallowing is more difficult with tubes in place).	Allows accurate assessment of need for NPA placement. Patients at greater risk for upper airway obstruction are infants; children; and adults with upper airway congestion, loss of consciousness, seizure disorders, neuromuscular disease, or increased oral secretions.

Critical Decision Point *Never insert an NPA in a patient who has obstructed nasal passages, is prone to epistaxis, or has facial or head trauma when basilar skull fracture or cranial vault communication is suspected. Never force an airway into place.*

STEP	RATIONALE
6. Assess patient or caregiver's knowledge of procedure.	Identifies learning needs of patient and caregiver. Patient may be unconscious.
7. Measure for correct size of NPA (see Fig. 28.5).	Inappropriate size may cause or worsen airway obstruction.

NURSING DIAGNOSES

- Inadequate airway clearance
- Potential for aspiration

Related factors and risk factors are individualized on the basis of patient's condition or needs.

STEP	RATIONALE

PLANNING

STEP	RATIONALE
1. Expected outcomes following completion of procedure:	
• Patient's respiratory status improves, as evidenced by respirations with normal rate, easier removal of secretions, and lack of gurgling noise in throat with respirations.	Airway is clear of secretions.
• Patient's tongue does not obstruct airway, allowing for adequate ventilation.	NPA keeps tongue in correct position to maintain patent airway.
2. Patient or caregiver can verbalize understanding of the need for an NPA.	Teaching was successful.
3. Close room door and/or bedside curtain.	Provides for patient privacy.

IMPLEMENTATION

STEP	RATIONALE
1. Position patient in semi-Fowler's position if possible.	Provides easy access to oral cavity.
2. Apply clean gloves and face shield.	Reduces transmission of microorganisms.
3. Insert NPA:	
a. Generously lubricate the tip and outer tube with water-soluble lubricant.	When inserting an NPA, take care not to push the patient's tongue into the pharynx.
b. With the bevel facing toward the septum, slide tube gently into the selected nostril with the dominant hand. Once the tip is beyond the septum, rotate the tube 180 degrees so curve faces downward. Advance until flange rests external to the nares.	Proper insertion of airway prevents displacement of patient's tongue into posterior oropharynx. Secure airway with tape on flange.
4. Suction secretions as needed (see Skill 23.2).	Removes secretions; maintains patent airway.
5. Clean patient's face with soft tissue or washcloth.	Promotes hygiene.
6. Place nurse call system in accessible location; raise side rails (as appropriate) and lower bed to lowest position.	Promotes patient safety in case patient or caregiver needs assistance.
7. Discard equipment and used supplies into appropriate receptacles. Remove PPE (see Skill 5.3) and discard in appropriate receptacle.	Reduces transmission of microorganisms.

Critical Decision Point *An NPA will need to be removed, cleaned or discarded, and replaced in patients with excessive secretions. An NPA can create pressure on underlying tissue and pressure necrosis of the nasal ala, which can result in MDRPI* (Norton et al., 2021).

EVALUATION

STEP	RATIONALE
1. Reassess patient's respiratory status by auscultating lung sounds and measuring oxygen saturation, then compare respiratory assessments before and after insertion of NPA.	Identifies patient's response to insertion of airway, patency of airway.
2. Verify that airway is patent.	Ensures route for oxygen delivery to patient.
3. Observe adjacent and underlying tissue for signs of redness, abrasion, or bruising.	Identifies early signs of MDRPI.
4. Observe for patient pulling airway out.	Patient's ability to clear own airway may have returned. Indicates reassessment of need for airway.
5. Use **teach-back:** "I want to be sure I explained why the nasal airway is needed. In your own words, tell me why it is important." Provide repeat explanation or develop a revised teaching plan if patient or caregiver is unable to teach back correctly.	Determines patient's and caregiver's level of understanding of instructional topic.

Unexpected Outcomes	Related Interventions
1. Patient continually coughs and gags when airway is inserted.	• Do not continue inserting airway if patient begins to gag. Stimulation of gag reflex can cause vomiting and aspiration. • Remove airway and position patient on side. • Reassess need for artificial airway prn.
2. Airway obstruction not relieved.	• Obtain immediate assistance. • Reinsert airway or determine from health care provider whether another form of airway is needed. • Assess for other causes of obstruction.
3. Patient pushes or pulls airway out of place.	• Reassess patient's need for an NPA.
4. Unable to insert airway; patient is combative, or you meet resistance when inserting airway.	• Get help. • Reassess patient's need for an NPA. • Provide sedation as prescribed.

Communication and Documentation

- Document assessment findings indicating need for insertion and those while inserting NPA; size of airway; other interventions performed at same time, especially positioning and suctioning; and patient's response to procedure on flow sheet or in progress notes in EHR or chart.
- Document your evaluation of patient and caregiver learning.

DOCUMENTATION EXAMPLE

Patient requiring frequent nasopharyngeal suctioning for thick yellow secretions because of very weak cough and inability to expectorate. Patient is reporting that nasal passage is becoming "sore." Redness noted, but no bleeding. Explained the purpose of an NPA. Patient is agreeable to try. Measured for NPA #6 Portex. Water-soluble lubricant used to ease insertion into left naris. Coached patient through procedure; no coughing or gagging noted, oxygen saturation maintained at 95% throughout procedure. Cleaned face of extra lubricant. Secured NPA with tape to cheek. No bleeding noted at naris. Patient denies any difficulty breathing and stated, "I think that will help when I have to be suctioned."

✦ SKILL 28.3 Resuscitation Management

Responding to cardiopulmonary arrests efficiently means that the interprofessional team needs to follow a standardized, straightforward approach to optimize interventions by all resuscitation team members. Training for team members can involve either BLS or advanced ALS skills. For an in-hospital resuscitation response, health care providers with two levels of training merge to care for the patient.

BLS certification with an AED and manual bag-valve mask training is a requirement for nurses and nursing students. Therefore, the specific skills included in BLS training will not be covered in detail within this chapter. Table 28.2 summarizes basic points regarding BLS skills, highlighting differences in adult, child, and infant techniques. The ALS response team usually includes a physician, critical care nurse, respiratory therapist, anaesthesiology personnel, and possibly radiology and laboratory technologists who have been trained in cardiac rhythm interpretation, manual defibrillation, timing of pharmacological interventions, and advanced airway management. A pastoral care representative or social worker is often available to be with the family. This skill outlines the initial response followed by the advanced response once ALS-trained health care team members have arrived to assist within the hospital setting.

Regardless of the level of training, the in-hospital initial response begins with rapid recognition of a resuscitation event, activation of the emergency response (rapid response) system, prompt initiation of high-quality chest compressions, and early defibrillation of shockable cardiac rhythm (e.g., VT or VF) (Panchal et al., 2020). Equipment may be readily available at the bedside or in a designated area of the hospital unit. It is the nurse's responsibility to know how to use this equipment and to know its location and the contents of the resuscitation or crash cart.

Delegation and Collaboration

The skill of managing resuscitation cannot be delegated to a UCP. However, a UCP who is certified in BLS techniques can perform the basic skills of CPR. Most UCPs are certified in BLS and can use an AED. Most facilities reserve the skill of performing manual defibrillation for licensed personnel who are ALS certified or have received competency validation to perform manual defibrillation. All other skills performed during the resuscitation situation are directed by the resuscitation team leader and implemented by nurses, respiratory therapists, and other health care providers.

Equipment

- Emergency resuscitation cart (Fig. 28.6)—Most adult carts have the following equipment:
  - Clean and sterile gloves, gown, protective eyewear, masks, face shield
  - Oxygen source
  - Bag-valve mask or resuscitation bag
  - Oral and nasopharyngeal airways
  - Laryngoscope, handle, and laryngoscope straight and curved blades

TABLE 28.2

Adult, Child, and Infant Cardiopulmonary Resuscitation Techniques (Health Care Providers)

Technique	Adult	Child (1–8 Years Old)	Infant (Under 1 Year), Excluding Newborn Period
Chest compressions: Push hard and fast to allow complete recoil. If available, change compressors every 2 minutes.	Begin compressions if no pulse felt within 10 seconds. Compression rate: 100–120/min Lower half of sternum, between nipples Heel of one hand, other hand on top Compression depth: 5 cm (2 inches) One or two rescuers: 30 compressions to 2 breaths (30:2) Continue until AED is available and ready to analyze rhythm.	Begin compressions if no pulse or pulse <60 beats/min. Compression rate: 100–120/min Lower half of sternum, between nipples Heel of one hand or as for adults At least one-third depth of chest diameter One rescuer: 30 compressions, 2 breaths (30:2) Two rescuers: 15 compressions, 2 breaths (15:2)	Begin compressions if no pulse or pulse <60 beats/min. Compression rate: 100–120/min Just below nipple line (lower half of sternum) Two fingers or two thumbs (encircling hands) At least one-third depth of chest diameter One rescuer: 30 compressions, 2 breaths (30:2) Two rescuers: 15 compressions, 2 breaths (15:2)
Defibrillation using AED: Follow machine prompts.	Use adult pads. AED should be applied as soon as available, and shock as soon as advised. Resume compressions immediately after shock.	Use child pads whenever possible. If none, use adult pads, but do not overlap them. Apply AED as soon as available, and shock as soon as advised.	If there is a shockable rhythm, manual defibrillation is used.
Airway	Head tilt–chin lift Suspected trauma, use jaw thrust	Head tilt–chin lift Suspected trauma, use jaw thrust	Head tilt–chin lift Suspected trauma, use jaw thrust
Rescue breathing: Mouth-to-mask or bag-valve mask with pulse	10 breaths/min (1 breath every 6 seconds) Give each breath over 1 second	20–30 breaths/min (approximately 1 breath every 2–3 seconds)	20–30 breaths/min (approximately 1 breath every 2–3 seconds)
Rescue breaths with advanced airway in place (supraglottic or tracheal tube) during continuous CPR	10 breaths/min (1 breath every 6 seconds)	20–30 breaths/min (approximately 1 breath every 2–3 seconds)	20–30 breaths/min (approximately 1 breath every 2–3 seconds)

AED, Automatic external defibrillator; *CPR,* cardiopulmonary resuscitation

Data from Panchal, A. R., Bartos, J. A., Cabañas, J. G., et al. (2020). Part 3: Adult basic and advanced life support: 2020 American Heart Association guidelines for cardiopulmonary resuscitation and emergency cardiovascular care. *Circulation, 142*(16, Suppl. 2), S366–S468. https://doi.org/10.1161/CIR.0000000000000916; Topjian, A. A., Raymond, T. T., Atkins, D., et al. (2020). Part 4: Pediatric basic and advanced life support: 2020 American Heart Association guidelines for cardiopulmonary resuscitation and emergency cardiovascular care. *Circulation, 142*(16, Suppl. 2), S469–S523. https://doi.org/10.1161/CIR.0000000000000901

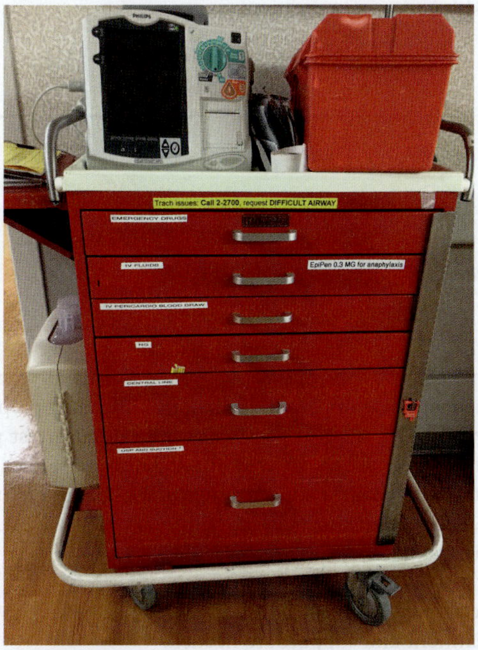

FIG 28.6 Emergency resuscitation cart.

- Endotracheal (ET) tubes, various sizes (5–9 mm for adults; 0–4 mm for pediatrics)
- Supraglottic airways of various sizes *(optional)*
- Carbon dioxide detector to confirm advanced airway tube placement
- Tape or commercial ET tube holder
- Suction source and suction equipment if not with crash cart
- Backboard
- AED and/or manual defibrillator with "hands-off" defibrillator pads
- Intravenous (IV) needles (sizes for adults and pediatrics)
- Central vascular access kit
- IV tubing and fluids (normal saline [NS] and 5% dextrose in water [D_5W])
- Syringes
- Laboratory specimen tubes
- Arterial blood gas kit
- Emergency medications (e.g., epinephrine, amiodarone, lidocaine)
- ALS guidelines or algorithms

Follow employer's policy related to routine checks of emergency equipment functioning and supplies located on the crash cart.

STEP	RATIONALE

ASSESSMENT

1. Identify patient using at least two person-specific identifiers (e.g., name and date of birth, or name and medical record number) according to employer policy.	Ensures correct patient. Complies with Accreditation Canada's standards and improves patient safety (Accreditation Canada, 2020).
2. Throughout the procedure, the 4 moments for hand hygiene are to be implemented; hand hygiene should occur before initial patient (or patient environment) contact, before an aseptic procedure, after body fluid exposure risk, and after patient (or patient environment) contact. Additional hand hygiene should be performed when hands are visibly soiled.	Proper hand hygiene helps prevent the spread of infectious agents to health care providers.
3. Don appropriate level of PPE prior to entering the room (see Box 5.1 and Skill 5.3).	Prevents exposure to, or contamination from, body fluid or aerosol-generating procedures. See Box 28.1 (Atkins et al., 2022).
4. Determine whether patient is unconscious by gently shaking them and shouting, "Are you okay?" Assess patient unresponsiveness and call for help.	Confirms that patient is unresponsive rather than intoxicated, sleeping, or hearing impaired. Substance misuse, hypoglycemia, toxicities, seizures, trauma, ketoacidosis, and shock also can cause unconsciousness.
5. Establish absence of respirations and lack of circulation within 10 seconds: no pulse, no respirations, no movement (Panchal et al., 2020). Check carotid pulse in adult or child; check brachial or femoral pulse in infant.	Indicates need for emergency measures, including AED. Carotid pulse is the easiest to locate in adults and children. Femoral pulse may also be palpated in a child or an infant.

Critical Decision Point *If an unresponsive person has adequate respirations and pulse, remain with the person until further help arrives. Place the patient in a modified lateral recovery position (see Step 5 illustration). Continue to assess for the presence of respirations and pulse because a recurrent arrest may develop. Determine whether there is a resuscitation care plan on the patient's EHR or chart, and proceed per the employer's policy for DNR, DNaR, and AND prescriptions.*

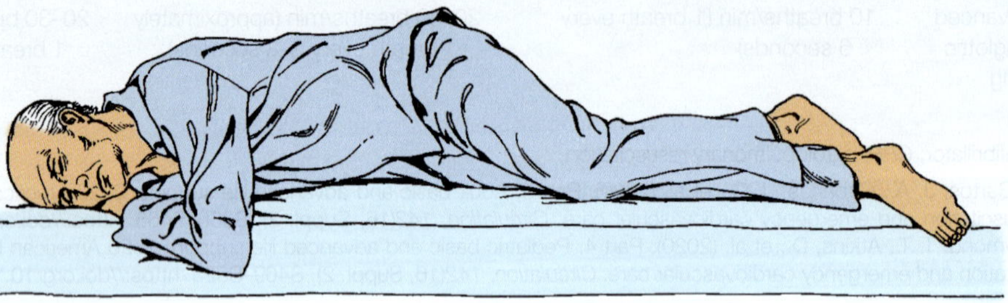

STEP 5 Modified recovery position.

NURSING DIAGNOSES

- Inadequate spontaneous ventilation
- Inadequate breathing pattern
- Reduced cardiac output
- Inadequate gas exchange

Related factors and risk factors are individualized on the basis of patient's condition or needs

PLANNING

1. Immediately activate the emergency response team. Tell co-workers to bring AED (if available) and resuscitation cart to bedside.	Ensures timely application of defibrillation, CPR, and preparation for the arrival of ALS team to assist with the cardiac arrest patient. Some hospitals have AEDs located throughout the building; the accompanying defibrillator pads are designed for "hands-off" use and can later be connected to a manual defibrillator by the ALS team upon their arrival.
2. Expected outcomes following completion of procedure:	
• Patient regains pulse and respirations.	CPR was successful.
• Patient receives postresuscitation care.	Ongoing treatment and support are needed.
• Patient is transported to critical care unit (CCU) for ongoing care.	Resuscitation was successful.

STEP	RATIONALE

IMPLEMENTATION

1. Place patient on hard surface such as floor, ground, or backboard. Patient must be flat. Logroll patient to flat, supine position using spine precautions if trauma is suspected.

   External compression of heart is facilitated. Heart is compressed between sternum and spinal vertebrae, which must take place on a hard surface. DO NOT delay the start of CPR. Positioning patient on hard surface may take more than one or two rescuers. May need to wait to safely move patient. Place patient on backboard or position them as soon as appropriate help arrives.

2. Start high-quality CPR.

   As personnel arrive at the bedside, assign an immediate task (compression, ventilation, or apply AED). To minimize interruption time of chest compressions, continue CPR while AED pads are being applied and turned on.

   a. Perform cycles of 30 compressions and 2 breaths using the correct hand position (see Table 28.2) (see Step 2a illustrations).

   Specific hand position, compression depth, and ratio are different for adults, children, and infants to prevent injury to the heart, lungs, and liver (see Table 28.2).

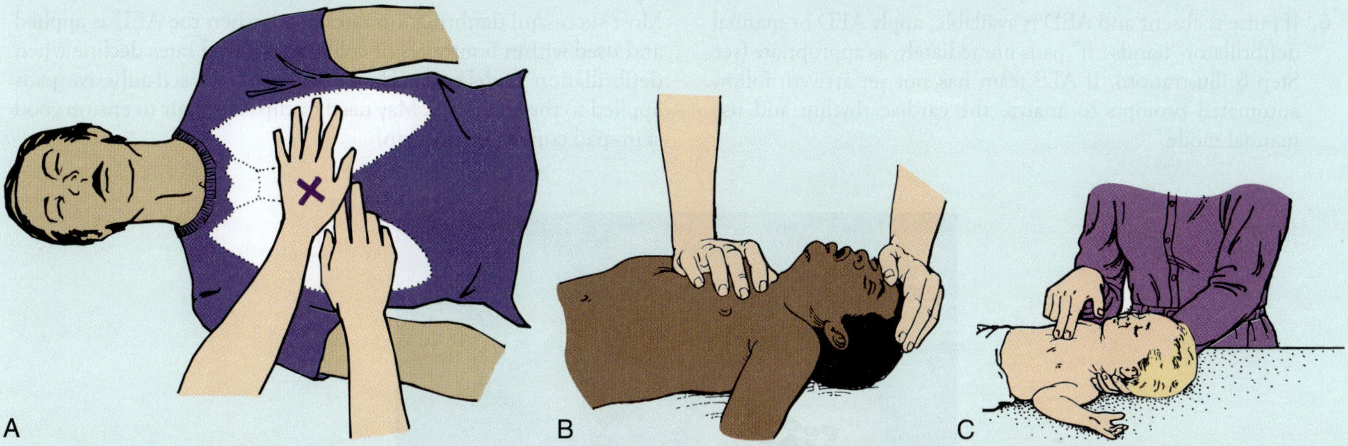

STEP 2A A, Proper hand position—adult. B, Proper hand position—child. C, Proper hand position—infant.

Critical Decision Point *Ensure that fingers are off the ribs and lowermost part of the xiphoid process. This position minimizes the chance of rib fracture, which could result in a punctured lung or liver laceration, further compromising cardiopulmonary status. Continue chest compressions, ventilation, and AED use.*

   b. Open airway using head-tilt/chin-lift manoeuvre or jaw thrust (cervical trauma). Deliver breaths by mouth to mask or bag-valve mask device or wait until second rescuer can assist with ventilation, as in the case of droplet or airborne isolation precautions (see Box 28.1; see Step 2b illustrations).

   The tongue is the most common cause of a blocked airway in an unresponsive patient. Suspect spinal cord injury in patients with trauma. Jaw-thrust manoeuvre prevents head extension and neck movement and further paralysis or spinal cord injury. Apply rigid cervical collar and immobilize patient as soon as possible to reduce cervical spine motion.

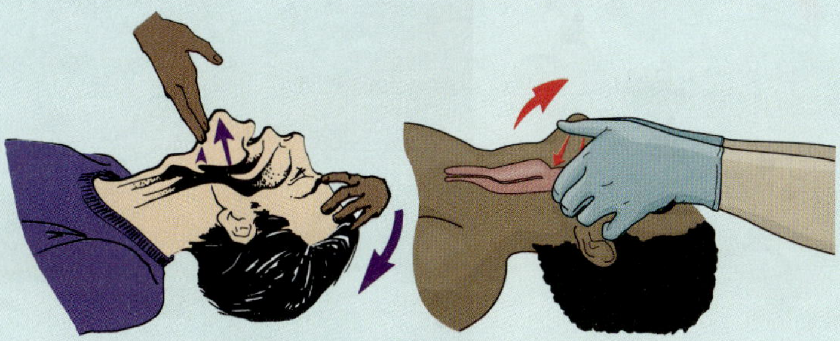

STEP 2B A, Head-tilt/chin-lift manoeuvre. B, Jaw thrust without head tilt. (*A, From Sorrentino, S. [2008]. Mosby's textbook for nursing assistants [7th ed.]. Mosby.*)

STEP	RATIONALE
IMPLEMENTATION	
3. Attempt to ventilate patient with slow breaths using one of the following methods:	Deliver each breath over 1 second (adult) at low pressure to reduce risk of gastric distension.
a. Mouth-to-mouth using barrier device.	Forms airtight seal to prevent air from escaping through nose.
b. Mouth-to-mask using pocket mask (see Step 3b illustration).	Provides secure seal and permits use of supplemental oxygen.
c. Bag-valve mask device (see Step 3c illustrations). Preferred method of ventilation.	Gives breaths with enough force to make chest rise (500–600 mL for adult) at 100% oxygen. Ensure adequate seal with either a one-hand or two-hand technique. Two-hand technique requires two rescuers (one to ventilate and another to use two hands to maintain the mask's seal) (Wittels, 2022).
4. If available, insert appropriate airway adjunct (see Skill 28.1 and Skill 28.2).	Maintains tongue on anterior floor of mouth and prevents obstruction of posterior airway by tongue.
5. Suction secretions if necessary or turn patient's head to one side unless trauma is suspected (see Skill 23.2).	Suctioning prevents airway obstruction. Turning patient's head to one side allows gravity to drain any secretions, decreasing risk for aspiration.
6. If pulse is absent and AED is available, apply AED or manual defibrillator "hands-off" pads immediately, as appropriate (see Step 6 illustration). If ALS team has not yet arrived, follow automated prompts to analyze the cardiac rhythm and use manual mode.	Most successful defibrillation rates occur when the AED is applied and used within 5 minutes of collapse. Survival rates decline when defibrillation is delayed. "Hands-off" pads are self-adhesive pads applied to the chest wall. May need to clip chest hair to ensure good skin–pad contact or dry skin.

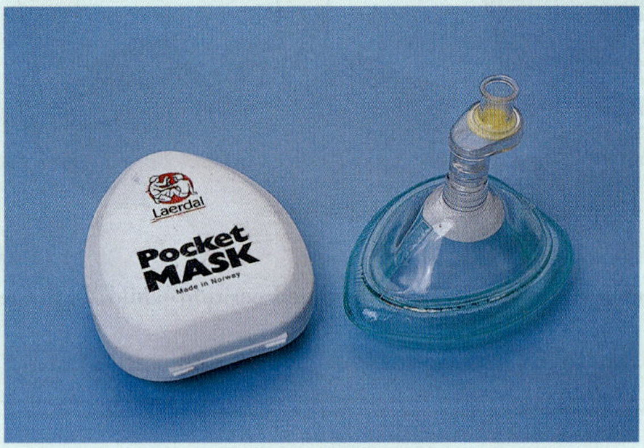

STEP 3B Pocket mask.

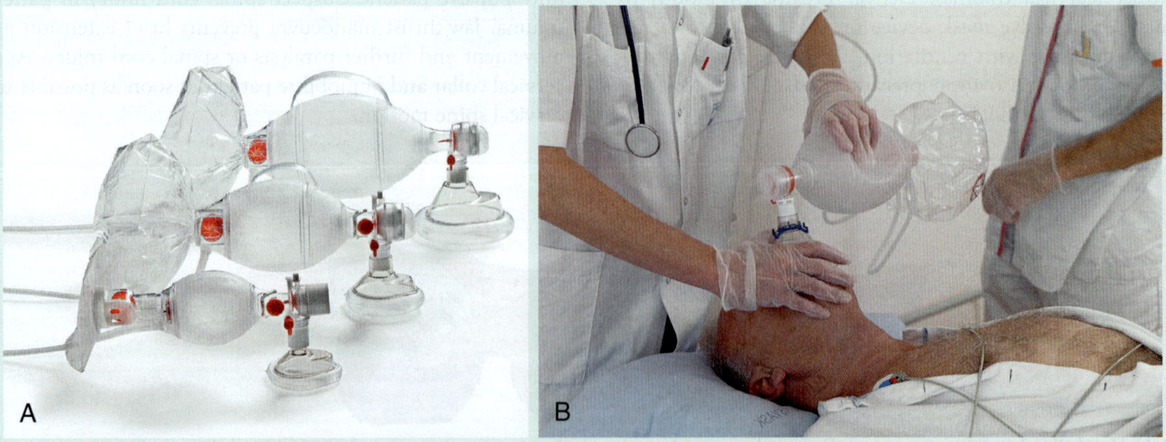

STEP 3C **A, Bag-valve mask device. B, Two-rescuer breathing with bag-valve mask device.** (*Courtesy Ambu USA.*)

STEP	RATIONALE

IMPLEMENTATION

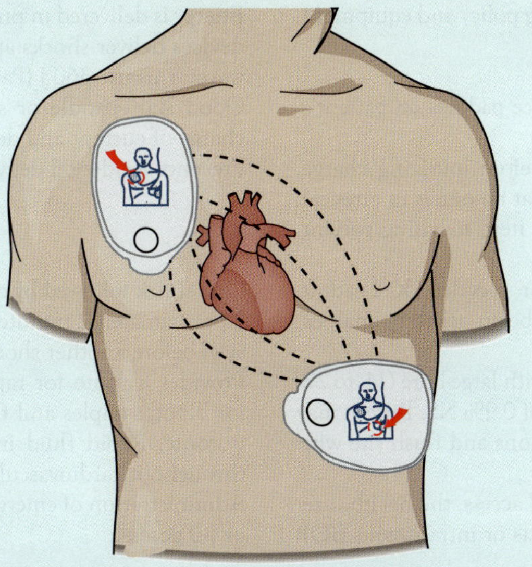

STEP 6 "Hands-off" pad placement for defibrillation.

STEP	RATIONALE
a. After one shock, resume CPR for 5 cycles (30:2, adult compressions/breath ratio) and begin rhythm analysis and shock sequence again.	One shock followed by chest compressions for 5 cycles of 30:2 ratio (approximately 2 minutes) provides sufficient blood flow and perfusion before another set of shocks is delivered.

Critical Decision Point *As the ALS team arrives, identify specific roles: resuscitation leader, compressor, airway management, medications, defibrillator, recorder. Minimize disruption of CPR to maintain high-quality compressions. As more members arrive, consider changing the compressor role every 2 minutes. As more members arrive, the following steps can occur simultaneously.*

STEP	RATIONALE
7. Without disrupting CPR, provide resuscitation leader with hand-off report describing events performed before the team's arrival (i.e., goals of care, vital signs, medical diagnosis, and emergency interventions).	This information is critical in selecting appropriate treatment for patient.
8. On arrival of sufficient personnel, assign the following tasks as appropriate while core group continues with resuscitation efforts:	Assignment of roles/tasks is essential to meeting critical needs of patient and their family in a timely matter.
a. Assist patient's roommate and visitors away from code scene. Assign pastoral care or other nurses to communicate with patient's family. Consider allowing family to witness resuscitation (see policy).	Family members allowed to witness resuscitation efforts have been found to have a significant reduction in anxiety and self-reports of a greater sense of resolution and fulfillment (Tennyson, 2019).
b. Remove excess furniture or equipment from room (see employer policy).	Provides room for emergency equipment and responders.
c. Bring patient's chart or access patient's electronic chart at the bedside.	Clarifies patient's medical condition, code status, and presence of any allergies.
d. *Recorder nurse:* Documents events of the emergency.	Ensures accurate documentation of events, team members, medications, and treatments administered.
e. *Cart nurse:* Prepares medications and supplies from resuscitation cart to hand off to team members.	Provides team members with appropriate medication and equipment in a timely fashion.
f. *Bedside nurse:* Provides direct patient care by administering medications, obtaining vitals, and assisting with procedures.	Positioned at side of bed to obtain easy access to the arm with IV access (if available).
9. Switch defibrillator from automatic to manual mode or switch machines to manual defibrillator. Attach electrocardiogram (ECG) electrodes to visualize cardiac rhythm (see Skill 26.2).	A defibrillator/monitor provides immediate rhythm display for analysis without disruption of rescue breathing and chest compression. This type of device can provide multiple leads to view the cardiac rhythms and enable functions of synchronized cardioversion or external pacemaker.
10. If cardiac rhythm is "shockable," continue CPR and assist resuscitation team with manual defibrillation.	Manual defibrillation is performed by ALS-certified personnel.

STEP	RATIONALE
IMPLEMENTATION	
a. Select proper energy level following policy and equipment directions.	Energy is delivered in prescribed doses. For adults: Manual biphasic devices deliver shocks at a lower level (200 joules [J]); monophasic waveforms use 360 J (Panchal et al., 2020).
b. If using paddles with gel pads, place paddles on patient's chest wall.	Good skin-paddle or skin-pad contact ensures appropriate discharge of current and decreases chance of skin burns.
c. A warning must be called out before initiating charge (e.g., announce "Clear"). Verify that no one is in physical contact with patient, bed, or any item touching patient during defibrillation.	Prevents accidental delivery of shock or injury to personnel.
d. After one shock, resume CPR for 5 cycles (30:2, adult compressions/breath ratio) and begin rhythm analysis and shock sequence again.	One shock followed by chest compressions for 5 cycles of 30:2 ratio (approximately 2 minutes) provides sufficient blood flow and perfusion before another shock is delivered.
11. Establish IV access (see Chapter 29) with large-bore (14- to 22-gauge) IV needle and begin infusion of 0.9% NS. Patient may already have IV access. Stop all infusions and flush site with 0.9% NS to ensure patency.	Provides a route for rapid medication administration and access for blood samples and fluid administration. Physiological saline is isotonic. Rapid fluid infusion facilitates dispersal of medication throughout cardiovascular system.
a. If you cannot obtain peripheral IV access, the health care provider may pursue central venous or intraosseous (IO) access.	Administration of emergency medications is dependent on vascular or IO access.
12. Administer IV medications as prescribed. Some emergency medications are packaged as prefilled syringes for ease of use.	Medication used for treatment of VF and VT (adult) (Panchal et al., 2020): • Epinephrine: 1 mg every 3–5 minutes IV/IO (recommended every 4 minutes) • Amiodarone: First dose—300 mg bolus IV/IO; second dose—150 mg bolus IV/IO, or • Lidocaine: First dose—1–1.5 mg/kg IV/IO; second dose—0.5–0.75 mg/kg IV/IO. *Recorder nurse* needs to keep track of time intervals to prompt team for repeat doses when time has elapsed.
13. Help with procedures as needed (e.g., intubation, IO insertion, central venous access).	Most equipment needed for special procedures during code is on the resuscitation cart. Knowledge of cart contents is essential to providing personnel with appropriate equipment during code.
14. Continue CPR until relieved (i.e., until patient regains spontaneous pulse and respiration, rescuer is exhausted and unable to perform CPR effectively, or health care provider prescribes discontinuation of CPR).	Interruptions in CPR are planned and organized. They usually occur during change of CPR personnel, defibrillation, and intubation. An interruption should not exceed 10 seconds (Panchal et al., 2020).
15. If respirations are absent, assist resuscitation team with advanced airway placement.	ET intubation provides a patent airway and facilitates pulmonary ventilation. Supraglottic airways (e.g., laryngeal mask, laryngeal tube, or esophageal-tracheal Combitube) can also be used to provide advanced airway support without interrupting chest compressions (Panchal et al., 2020).
a. Have available laryngoscope handle, laryngoscope blades, curved and straight blades, ET tubes, stylet, suction, and tape or ET tube holder. Ensure that light source on laryngoscope is functional.	Light is necessary on laryngoscope to visualize vocal cords and intubate trachea. Batteries may need to be changed. Preference for type of tube depends on the training of the ALS team member (see Box 28.1).
b. Help to confirm correct placement of ET tube or advanced airway support by auscultating lungs for bilateral breath sounds and monitoring the carbon dioxide (CO_2) detector.	Auscultation of lungs and monitoring of exhaled CO_2 or esophageal detector device further verify correct airway placement and adequacy of ventilation and gas exchange (Panchal et al., 2020). Chest X-ray film is usually obtained after patient has been stabilized to confirm placement of ET tube and central venous catheters.
c. Ventilate using bag device on intubation. **Avoid hyperventilation.**	Increased intrathoracic pressure caused by incomplete exhalation results in reduced cardiac output (Panchal et al., 2020).
16. Obtain prescribed laboratory and diagnostic studies.	Aids in determination of cause of arrest.
17. Dispose of all equipment in appropriate receptacles.	

STEP	RATIONALE

EVALUATION

STEP	RATIONALE
1. Observe for spontaneous return of respirations or heart rate every 2 minutes.	Assessment of pulse, respiration, heart rate, and cardiac rhythm can occur after chest compressions and ventilation have been interrupted briefly every 2 minutes.
2. Ensure that interruptions in CPR are minimized (i.e., no longer than 10 seconds).	Interruptions are associated with reduced coronary artery perfusion pressure and lower mean coronary perfusion pressure (Panchal et al., 2020).
3. Use teach-back: "I want to be sure I clearly explained what has happened to your loved one and why we performed cardiopulmonary resuscitation, known as CPR. In your own words, tell me why we had to perform CPR." Develop a revised teaching plan if caregiver is unable to repeat back correctly.	Determines caregiver's level of understanding and the needed psychological supports.

Unexpected Outcomes	Related Interventions
1. Patient develops skeletal injury such as fractured ribs or sternum or internal organ injury such as lacerated lung or liver as result of chest compressions.	• Obtain appropriate diagnostic tests to document injuries. • Assess patient's postarrest breathing for symmetry and pain. • Assess for intrathoracic or intra-abdominal bleeding (hematomas, increasing abdominal girth).
2. Patient's CPR is unsuccessful.	• Contact chaplain services, if appropriate. • Consult social worker. • Complete postmortem care on patient (see Chapter 17). • Notify coroner and organ and tissue donation organization in accordance with employer policy and provincial/territorial law. • Provide for privacy for patient's family to grieve and mourn loss of loved one.
3. Rescuer is unassisted, tires, and is unable to continue.	• Get help.

Communication and Documentation

- Immediately report arrest via the organization-wide communication system, indicating exact location of patient.
- Cardiopulmonary arrest requires precise documentation. Most employers use a form designed specifically for documenting patient arrests and subsequent care.
- Document in progress notes in EHR or chart or on designated CPR worksheet: onset of arrest, time and number of AED shocks (if initiated), time and energy level of manual defibrillations, medications given, procedures performed, cardiac rhythm, use of CPR, patient's response, and education and interventions provided to family.

Special Considerations

Teaching

- While in hospital, offer the opportunity (if appropriate) to be present during a resuscitation by reviewing what may occur and clarifying expectations with designated family. Refer to employer policies related to family presence during resuscitation (Tennyson, 2019).
- If patient is at risk for cardiopulmonary arrest, encourage the caregiver(s) to obtain BLS certification through a certified instructor.

Pediatric

- All people involved in administering CPR must understand different breathing/compression ratios, hand (fingers) placement, and depth of compression in children and infants compared with that in adults.
- Infants and children experience respiratory arrest much more frequently than full cardiopulmonary arrest.
- Colour-coded quick reference guides are frequently used in pediatric codes to quickly determine appropriate medication doses and equipment sizes.
- Most AEDs are specifically designed for adult use only and are therefore not recommended for use with children younger than 8 years of age or weighing less than 25 kg (Topjian et al., 2020). Adult pads can be used if child pads are not available; place one pad on the front chest and the other on the back. Manual defibrillation performed by a health care provider using lower-energy settings (2–4 J/kg) is the most common method of pediatric defibrillation (Topjian et al., 2020).

Gerontological

- In older persons, compressions often result in rib or cartilage fractures.
- Remove loose-fitting dentures to avoid obstructing the airway. If dentures fit securely, leave them in to provide a tight seal when providing ventilations.

Care in the Community: Home Management

- Cardiopulmonary arrest in the community setting requires activation of the emergency response system (call 9-1-1). BLS- and ALS-trained paramedics can begin resuscitation management in the community before bringing patient to the emergency department.
- In the community and in long-term care facilities, patients may have implanted cardioverter defibrillators (ICDs), pacemakers, or both. For these patients, families need to know how to administer CPR and the specific capabilities of the patient's ICD or pacemaker. Placement of defibrillator or AED pads/paddles may need to be altered to avoid placement directly on top of an ICD or pacemaker generator. Remove medication patches from chest.
- Soft surfaces such as a mattress or car seat decrease efficiency of external cardiac compressions.
- AEDs are available for use in the community and home setting.

✦ REVIEW QUESTIONS

You are the charge nurse for the night shift on a general medical floor. Your next patient is 85 years old and admitted with heart failure. On your rounds, you find the patient lying on the floor of the bathroom. You gently shake them and call their name. The patient is unresponsive and pulseless. An automatic external defibrillator (AED) is available down the hall. Review Questions 1 to 4 relate to the case study presented here.

1. What should you do first? Explain your choice.
    1. Apply the AED.
    2. Call for help.
    3. Start high-quality cardiopulmonary resuscitation (CPR).
    4. Open the airway and provide two breaths.
2. Your co-worker arrives to the room with the AED. You've started chest compressions already. What is your next step? Explain your choice.
    1. Check for a pulse.
    2. Call for help.
    3. Tell your co-worker to apply the AED.
    4. Continue with 10 breaths/min.
3. The nurse is performing CPR during a cardiac arrest. Which of the following techniques ensures the highest-quality chest compressions? (*Select all that apply.*)
    1. Minimizing interruption in chest compressions
    2. Avoiding full chest recoil
    3. Providing excessive ventilations
    4. Adequate depth and rate of compression
    5. Ensuring the AED is in place
4. The advanced life support (ALS) resuscitation team has arrived to continue resuscitation attempts on the patient. Using SBAR (situation–background–assessment–recommendation), how would you communicate to the arriving team?
5. Place the following steps for using an external defibrillator (manual) in the correct order:
    1. Select the proper energy level as indicated by the resuscitation leader.
    2. Resume chest compressions.
    3. Perform a visual check to ensure that no one is in contact with the patient.
    4. Apply "hands-off" pads to the patient and turn on defibrillator power.
    5. Assess for unresponsiveness, pulselessness, and breathlessness.
    6. Announce "Clear."
    7. Start chest compressions.
    8. Press the shock button.

Visit the Evolve site for a complete list of answers to the Review Questions.

✦ NEXT GENERATION NCLEX® (NGN)

For practice with answering exam questions related to unfolding NGN case studies, please consult the Next Generation NCLEX® (NGN)-Style Case Studies for Skills and Techniques on the Evolve website: http://evolve.elsevier.com/Canada/Perry/clinicalskills/

REFERENCES

Accreditation Canada. (2020). *Required organizational practices–2020 handbook.* https://physicians.nshealth.ca/resources/required-organizational-practices-2020-handbook

Agency for Healthcare Research and Quality. (2019). *Rapid response systems.* https://psnet.ahrq.gov/primer/rapid-response-systems

American Heart Association (AHA). (2020). *2020 American Heart Association guidelines for CPR and ECC.* https://cpr.heart.org/en/resuscitation-science/cpr-and-ecc-guidelines

Atkins, D., Sasson, C., Hsu, A., et al. (2022). 2022 interim guidance to health care providers for basic and advanced cardiac life support in adults, children, and neonates with suspected or confirmed COVID-19: From the Emergency Cardiovascular Care Committee and Get with the Guidelines-Resuscitation Adult and Pediatric Task Forces of the American Heart Association in collaboration with the American Academy of Pediatrics, American Association for Respiratory Care, the Society of Critical Care Anesthesiologists, and American Society of Anesthesiologists. *Circulation: Cardiovascular Quality and Outcomes, 15*(4), Article e008900. https://doi.org/10.1161/CIRCOUTCOMES.122.008900

Canadian Association of Critical Care Nurses (CACCN). (2018). *Position statement: Patient- and family-centred care.* https://caccn.ca/wp-content/uploads/2019/10/PS062018PSPFCCare.pdf

Castro, D., & Freeman, L. A. (2021). *Oropharyngeal airway.* StatPearls. https://www.ncbi.nlm.nih.gov/books/NBK470198/

Hall, K. K., Lim, A., & Gale, B. (2020). The use of rapid response teams to reduce failure to rescue events: A systematic review. *Journal of Patient Safety, 16*(3), S3–S7. https://doi.org/10.1097/PTS.0000000000000748

Heart and Stroke Foundation & American Heart Association (HSF & AHA). (2020). *Highlights of the 2020 American Heart Association guidelines update for CPR and ECC (Heart and Stroke Foundation of Canada edition).* https://cpr.heartandstroke.ca/s/article/Guidelines?language=en_US

Hockenberry, M. J., Duffy, E. A., & Gibbs, K. (2024). *Wong's nursing care of infants and children* (12th ed.). Elsevier.

Lauridsen, K. G., Krogh, K., Müller, S. D., et al. (2021). Barriers and facilitators for in-hospital resuscitation: A prospective clinical study. *Resuscitation, 164*, 70–78. https://doi.org/10.1016/j.resuscitation.2021.05.007

Meghani, S. (2021). Witnessed resuscitation: A concept analysis. *Intensive and Critical Care Nursing, 64*, 1–6. https://doi.org/10.1016/j.iccn.2020.103003

Munshi, L., Evans, G., & Razak, F. (2021). The case for relaxing no-visitor policies in hospitals during the ongoing COVID-19 pandemic. *Canadian Medical Association Journal, 193*(4), E135–E137. https://doi.org/10.1503/cmaj.202636

Norton, L., Parslow, N., Johnston, D., et al. (2021). Best practice recommendations for the prevention and management of pressure injuries. In *Foundations of best practice for skin and wound management: A supplement of Wound Care Canada.* Wounds Canada. https://www.woundscanada.ca/docman/public/health-care-professional/bpr-workshop/172-bpr-prevention-and-management-of-pressure-injuries-2/file

Panchal, A. R., Bartos, J. A., Cabañas, J. G., et al. (2020). Part 3: Adult basic and advanced life support: 2020 American Heart Association guidelines for cardiopulmonary resuscitation and emergency cardiovascular care. *Circulation, 142*(16, Suppl. 2), S366–S468. https://doi.org/10.1161/CIR.0000000000000916

Ralston, M. E. (2022). Basic airway management in children. *UpToDate.* https://www.uptodate.com/contents/basic-airway-management-in-children

Tennyson, C. D. (2019). Family presence during resuscitation: Updated review and clinical pearls. *Geriatric Nursing, 40*(6), 645–647. https://doi.org/10.1016/j.gerinurse.2019.11.004

Topjian, A. A., Raymond, T. T., Atkins, D., et al. (2020). Part 4: Pediatric basic and advanced life support: 2020 American Heart Association guidelines for cardiopulmonary resuscitation and emergency cardiovascular care. *Circulation, 142*(16, Suppl. 2), S469–S523. https://doi.org/10.1161/CIR.0000000000000901

Wittels, K. A. (2022). Basic airway management in adults. *UpToDate.* https://www.uptodate.com/contents/basic-airway-management-in-adults

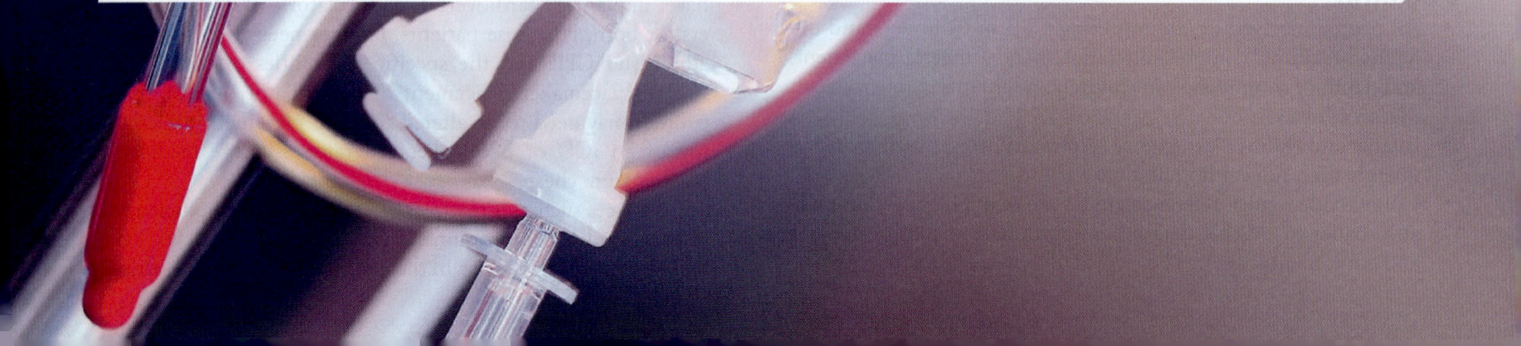

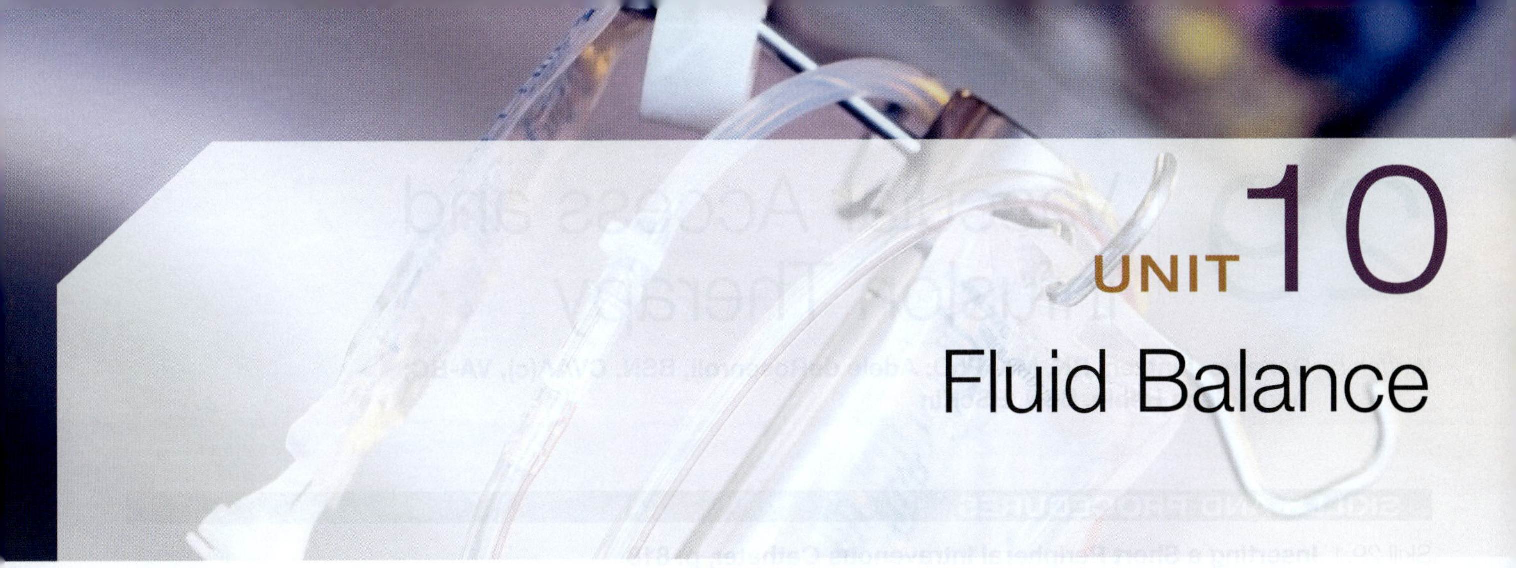

UNIT 10 Fluid Balance

The skills used to support a patient's fluid balance involve applying the principles of surgical asepsis and infection control, safe medication practices, patient safety and comfort, and protection of skin integrity. Your knowledge base and experience in applying these principles aid in directing your patient assessments, identifying patient problems, and making decisions about applying the skills correctly.

Administration of intravenous and vascular access therapy is a complex, time-sensitive, and time-pressured nursing action. For safe therapy, remove any distractions as you apply all the principles of safe medication practices by knowing the action, purpose, side effects, and nursing implication of each fluid or additive medication. Apply knowledge about a patient's clinical condition or physical risks in the event that there are factors that might affect the rate of infusion. Cross-check the label on an intravenous fluid container to compare with the health care provider's prescription. Prior to bringing the fluid container to the patient's bedside, accurately calculate and double-check the infusion rate.

Inserting an intravenous catheter is an invasive procedure. Use your knowledge about infection control, surgical asepsis, and anatomical location of large peripheral veins and arteries when you select an insertion site. The preparation of the site requires measures to reduce the risk of central line–associated bloodstream infection (CLABSI). Apply the Infusion Nurses Society's infusion therapy standards and routine practices for infection control. Your experience in vein selection is invaluable in being able to choose a site that is less likely to be compromised by patient positioning or physical care activities.

A thorough patient assessment is necessary when initiating, regulating, or maintaining any fluid therapy. Use clinical judgement in assessing for signs and symptoms of dehydration or fluid overload, signs of catheter site inflammation or CLABSI, and any signs associated with pressure injuries under catheter tubing or catheter-stabilization devices. Your assessment can identify cues that indicate fluid overload or deficit, infection, or early pressure injury. If these problems arise, you may need to contact the health care provider to change a fluid prescription. When a site infection is noted, remove the catheter and select a new site. If CLABSI is present, remove the catheter, have it cultured for microorganisms, collect other specimens per employer protocol, and, in most cases, prepare the patient for a new insertion. If a patient has a medical device–related pressure injury (MDRPI) from the infusion port, you may need to remove the catheter and select a new insertion site, as well as provide appropriate skin and wound care to the pressure injury site.

Central vascular access devices (CVADs) are implanted devices inserted by a health care provider. The location of the device in the central circulation creates significant patient risks, particularly infection, thrombus, and dislodgement, among others. Thorough ongoing patient assessments are necessary to detect any complications early. Site care is particularly important in preventing CLABSI; follow current practice standards rigorously.

A patient who requires a CVAD has serious health problems that require ongoing fluid therapy, frequent blood sampling, and long-term intravenous medications, such as chemotherapy, antibiotics, or cardiac support medications. Safe use of a CVAD and administration of any fluid or medication requires critical thinking when you assess the integrity and function of the vascular access device and patient tolerance of the vascular access device and prescribed therapies, including medications and blood products.

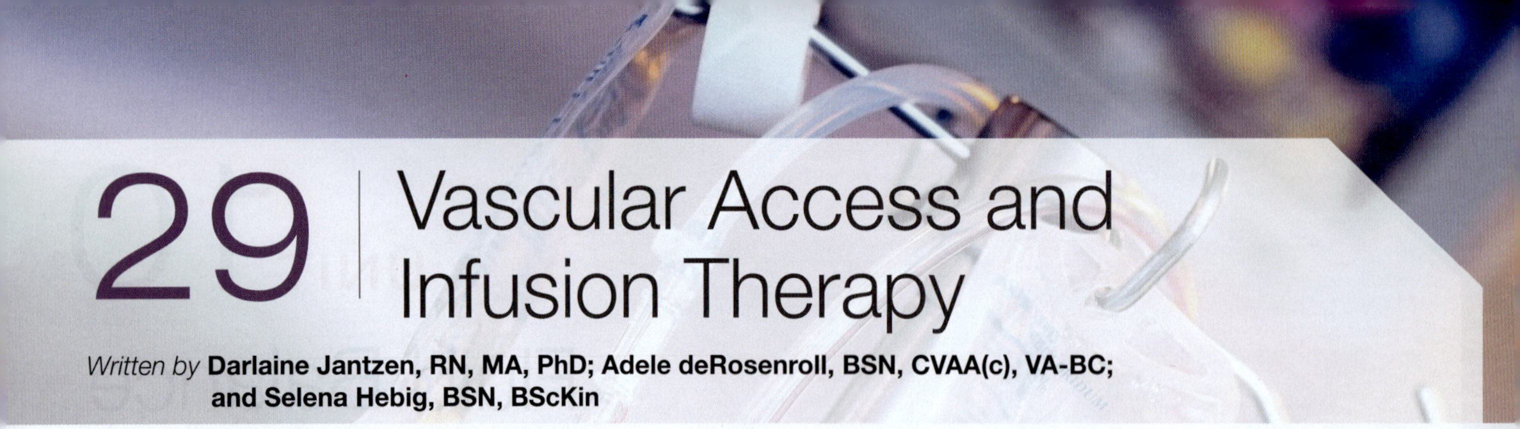

29 Vascular Access and Infusion Therapy

Written by **Darlaine Jantzen, RN, MA, PhD; Adele deRosenroll, BSN, CVAA(c), VA-BC; and Selena Hebig, BSN, BScKin**

SKILLS AND PROCEDURES

OBJECTIVES

Mastery of content in this chapter will enable the nurse to:

- Describe current evidence-informed practices for infusion therapy.
- Describe common indications for intravenous (IV) therapy.
- Identify safety guidelines for IV fluid administration.
- Explain how to prepare a patient and caregiver for infusion therapy.
- Recognize complications of infusion therapy.
- Identify strategies to promote person-centred care when providing infusion therapy, including cultural considerations, diversity, and personal beliefs and values.
- Identify the educational needs of patients with vascular access devices (VADs) and those receiving infusion therapy.
- Explain techniques for preventing transmission of infection when caring for a patient with a VAD and receiving infusion therapy.
- Demonstrate initiating infusion therapy, regulating IV flow rate, changing IV solutions, changing IV administration sets, changing peripheral intravenous catheter (PIVC) dressings, and discontinuing a PIVC.
- Identify common types of central vascular access devices (CVADs).
- Demonstrate assessment and maintenance of CVADs and discontinuation of a CVAD.

MEDIA RESOURCES

- http://evolve.elsevier.com/Canada/Perry/clinicalskills/

PURPOSE

Vascular access is established when patients require infusion therapy or hemodynamic monitoring. Infusion therapy is used to correct or maintain fluid and electrolyte balance; to administer continuous or intermittent medications, blood or blood products, and diagnostic agents and anaesthesia; and to correct or maintain nutritional status. Vascular access, one of the most common invasive procedures performed by health care providers worldwide, poses risks to patients; therefore, competence and dexterity are essential to safe patient care.

STANDARDS OF CARE

- Accreditation Canada (2020)—*Required Organizational Practices–2020 Handbook* (https://physicians.nshealth.ca/resources/required-organizational-practices-2020-handbook)
- Canadian Vascular Access Association (CVAA, 2019)—*Occlusion Management Guideline for Central Venous Access* (2nd ed.) (http://cvaa.info/publications/occlusion-management-guideline-omg)
- Infusion Nurses Society (Gorski et al., 2021)—*Infusion Therapy Standards of Practice*, 8th edition (https://www.ins1.org/publications/infusion-therapy-standards-of-practice/)
- Public Health Agency of Canada (PHAC, 2016)—*Routine Practices and Additional Precautions for Preventing the Transmission of Infection in Healthcare Settings* (https://www.canada.ca/en/public-health/services/publications/diseases-conditions/routine-practices-precautions-healthcare-associated-infections.html)

PRINCIPLES FOR PRACTICE

- Evidence-informed practices guide the safe, efficient, high-quality care necessary to provide vascular access and infusion therapy.

- Successful vascular access depends on thorough patient assessment, correct device and site selection, and proper catheter insertion technique.
- Indications and protocols for all aspects of vascular access and infusion therapy are established in practice guidelines and employer policies, informed by the best evidence, and carried out according to manufacturer directions for use (Gorski et al., 2021).
- Assessments of a patient's circulatory system anatomy and physiology, fluid and electrolyte balance, disease pathophysiology, allergies, and response to illness are essential for safe infusion therapy.
- It is essential to practise the 10 rights of medication administration when administering parenteral solutions or medications (see Chapters 20 and 22).
- Knowledge of the following is required to ensure safe infusion therapy: most appropriate vascular access device (VAD) required for the plan of care; medications or solutions to be infused; how to initiate and regulate the infusion; care and maintenance of the VAD and how to identify complications; and use of infusion-related devices.

Intravenous Catheters

- To administer intravenous (IV) infusates and medications, a VAD is inserted into a vein. VADs can be located peripherally (i.e., short peripheral intravenous catheter [PIVC],* midline [Fig. 29.1]) or centrally (i.e., tunnelled, nontunnelled, peripherally inserted central catheter [PICC], implanted port [intravenous access device, or IVAD]).
- When selecting the appropriate VAD, consider a patient's prescribed therapy, anticipated duration of treatment, and vascular characteristics, as well as the patient's age, comorbidities, history of infusion therapy, preference for VAD location, and resources available to care for the device (Gorski et al., 2021).

Intravenous Solutions

- Many prepared IV solutions are available for use (Table 29.1).
- IV solutions fall into three categories: isotonic, hypotonic, and hypertonic. Isotonic solutions have the same osmolality as body fluids.
- Administer IV solutions as prescribed.
- Isotonic solutions can cause increased risk of fluid overload in patients with renal or cardiac disease; hypotonic solutions can exacerbate a hypotensive state; and hypertonic solutions are irritating to the vein and can cause increased risk of heart failure and pulmonary edema.
- PIVCs are *not* recommended for continuous vesicant therapy, parenteral nutrition, or infusates with an osmolarity greater than 600 mOsm/L or extreme pH (<5 or >9). PIVCs should only be used if there is an accessible peripheral vein and for short-term therapy. To prevent complications and vein depletion, a central venous access device (CVAD) is recommended (CVAA, 2019).
- Commercially prepared solutions are recommended for use in order to reduce risks of infection and reconstitution errors.

*The term *peripheral intravenous catheter* (PIVC) is used throughout this chapter. Please note that terms vary across geography and areas of practice. Other common terms include *peripheral venous access device* or *peripheral vascular access device (PVAD)* and *venous access device* or *vascular access device (VAD)*. PIVC must be understood as ***being both inserted and dwelling in the peripheral vasculature***, while some central lines are inserted peripherally, such as a peripherally inserted central catheter (PICC).

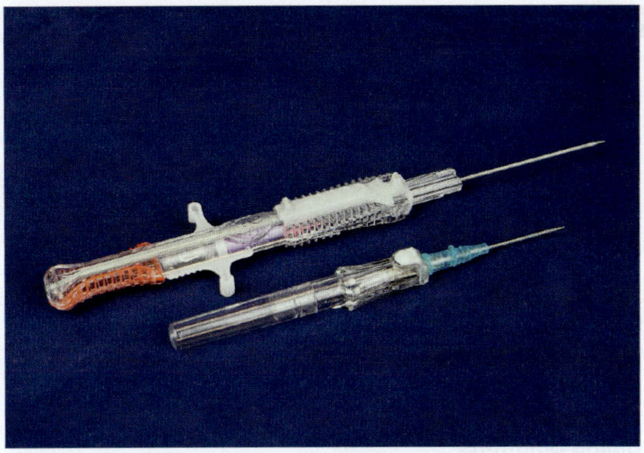

FIG 29.1 Peripheral intravenous access devices (PIVCs): Midline (top) and short (bottom). *(Courtesy Burl Jantzen.)*

- A patient's specific fluid and electrolyte imbalance and serum electrolyte values guide selection of the appropriate IV fluid (Jantzen & Hebig, 2024).

PERSON-CENTRED CARE

- Communication, comfort, and education are essential components of person-centred care.
- Person-centred nursing practice should be implemented by engaging patients in the decision-making process and collaborating on the plan of care. This process includes soliciting and responding to patient preferences regarding their active involvement and the involvement of their caregivers.
- Preparing the patient prior to initiation of VAD or infusion therapy reduces their anxiety. Become familiar with the patient's past experience and current concerns and expectations. Speak directly to patients and answer questions as honestly as possible.
- Provide privacy throughout the procedure–during assessment, initiation of the VAD, and patient education.
- Place patients in a comfortable position and use techniques to minimize discomfort. Consider using local anaesthetic medications (see employer policy) based on patient condition, needs, risks, benefits, and anticipated discomfort of the procedure (Gorski et al., 2021).
- Effective education for patients and caregivers includes assessment of their learning needs, capabilities, and preferences. This includes attending to patients' cultural and linguistic needs and recognizing diversity and cultural sensitivities (Foster et al., 2016; Gorski et al., 2021).
- Consider the environment and context for treatment and education. Minimize distractions and interruptions during education, upon initiation of VAD, and while initiating therapy.
- Patient teaching should also include information regarding care of the VAD, infection prevention, and potential VAD complications and the signs and symptoms to report (Gorski et al., 2021).
- Pain is an individual experience. Perception and expressions of pain vary with individuals and may be informed by cultural or personal beliefs and values as well as past experience.

EVIDENCE-INFORMED PRACTICE

Nurses must incorporate evidence-informed practice and clinical expertise when providing vascular access and infusion therapy (Gorski et al., 2021):

TABLE 29.1

Intravenous Solutions

Solution	Concentration	General Information, Uses, and Risks
Dextrose in Water Solutions*		
Dextrose 5% in water (D_5W)	Isotonic	Isotonic when first enters vein; dextrose enters cells rapidly, leaving free water, which dilutes ECF; most of water then enters cells by osmosis. Commonly used to rehydrate, provide calories (nutrients), and assist with administering some medications. Risk of hyponatremia and fluid overload.
Dextrose 10% in water ($D_{10}W$)	Hypertonic	Hypertonic when first enters vein; dextrose enters cells rapidly, leaving free water, which dilutes ECF; most of water then enters cells by osmosis. Used in treatment of diabetic ketoacidosis and provides calories. Higher risk of fluid overload, electrolyte shifts.
Saline Solutions		
0.225% NaCl (one-quarter normal saline, 0.25 NS)	Hypotonic	Saline is NaCl in water. Expands ECV (vascular and interstitial) and rehydrates cells. Rarely used, except in some hyperosmolar conditions.
0.45% NaCl (one-half normal saline, 1/2 NS)	Hypotonic	Expands ECV (vascular and interstitial) and rehydrates cells. Used to replace intracellular fluid, treat hypernatremia, hyperosmolarity. Risk of fluid shift from extracellular to intracellular space.
0.9% NaCl (normal saline, NS)	Isotonic	Expands ECV (vascular and interstitial); does not enter cells. Used to treat ECV deficit, replace or maintain fluid, treat metabolic alkalosis, large sodium losses (burns), and assist with administering some medications. Does not replace electrolyte or calories, therefore should not be used if patient not taking nutrition by mouth or alternate means. Caution with patients who have heart or renal conditions.
3% or 5% NaCl (hypertonic saline)	Hypertonic	Draws water from cells into ECF by osmosis. Used only in severe hyponatremia, cerebral edema. Severe risk of fluid overload, heart failure.
Dextrose in Saline Solutions		
Dextrose 5% in 0.45% NaCl (D_5 1/2 NS)	Hypertonic	Dextrose enters cells rapidly, leaving 0.45% NaCl. Rehydration and replacement of calories and sodium. Risk of fluid overload and heart failure.
Dextrose 5% in 0.9% NaCl (D_5NS)	Hypertonic	Dextrose enters cells rapidly, leaving 0.9% NaCl. Rehydration and replacement of calories and sodium. Risk of fluid overload and heart failure.
Balanced Electrolyte Solutions		
Lactated Ringer's (LR)	Isotonic	Contains Na^+, K^+, Ca^{2+}, Cl^-, and lactate, which liver metabolizes to HCO_3^-. Expands ECV (vascular and interstitial); does not enter cells. Provides fluid and electrolyte replacement. May be used to treat metabolic acidosis.
Dextrose 5% in lactated Ringer's (D_5LR)	Hypertonic	Dextrose enters cells rapidly, leaving lactated Ringer's. Used for hydration, calories, and electrolytes. Risk of electrolyte imbalances.

ECF, Extracellular fluid; *ECV,* extracellular fluid volume; *LR,* lactated Ringer's; *NaCl,* sodium chloride; *NS,* normal saline.

*Dextrose is the name used for glucose in intravenous solutions.

- Current best practice standards, current research, and expert knowledge are applied in all aspects of vascular access and infusion therapy.
- Clinical quality indicators for quality improvement may include surveillance and analysis of infection rates (e.g., catheter-associated bloodstream infections [CABSIs]), VAD insertion attempts).
- Utilization of benchmarks develops a culture of accountability (Gorski et al., 2021).
- Commercially prepared 10-mL barrel 0.9% sodium chloride (normal saline [NS]) syringes are recommended to decrease risks of infection and aid optimal and safe flushing technique. Alternate locking solutions may be used according to manufacturer instructions for use or organizational policy (e.g., sodium citrate, ethanol, taurolidine, or tetrasodium EDTA (ethylenediaminetetraacetic acid) may be considered for certain populations). Heparin is derived from animal products (e.g., porcine, bovine) and its use may be in conflict with some patients' religious beliefs. (CVAA, 2019; Gorski et al., 2021).
- PIVCs and midline catheters required for intermittent therapy must be locked with a minimum of 3 mL of preservative-free 0.9% sodium chloride (NS). (CVAA, 2019; Gorski et al., 2021).
- CVADs required for intermittent therapy must be locked with a minimum of 10 mL of preservative-free 0.9% sodium chloride (NS) (CVAA, 2019).
- Remove VADs for unresolved complication and when no longer necessary for the plan of care (Gorski et al., 2021).

- Disinfect VAD needle-free connectors prior to every access with active or passive disinfection agent to reduce the introduction of intraluminal microbes (CVAA, 2019; Gorski et al., 2021).
- Disinfection caps that contain a sponge saturated with 70% alcohol placed on the end of the needle-free connector between intermittent infusions provide active disinfection of the needle-free connector. These disinfection caps or antiseptic barrier caps have been shown to reduce intraluminal contamination, peripheral catheter bloodstream infections, and CABSI rates (Voor in 't holt et al., 2017).
- Primary and secondary administration sets that are used to administer solutions other than lipid, blood, or blood products should be changed with the initiation of new VAD, if contamination is suspected and based on the type of infusion. Change administration sets for continuous infusions every 4 to 7 days and intermittent infusions every 24 hours or according to employer policy (CVAA, 2019; Gorski et al., 2021).

SAFETY GUIDELINES

- Conduct a complete history and physical, including vital signs, and review laboratory findings before initiating any solutions or medications. Consider prolonged environmental conditions that affect a patient's fluid status (e.g., exposure to hot, humid weather) and lead to fluid and electrolyte imbalances, particularly in infant, older persons, and those with chronic illness.
- Know the indications for prescribed therapy before initiating infusion therapy. Obtain and review the health care provider's prescription to ensure the appropriateness of the prescribed solution or medication for the patient's age, health status, medical diagnosis, allergy status, and acuity, and the VAD type and tip location, dose, frequency, and route of administration.
- Assess all VADs for patency and functioning before initiating infusion therapy. Observe site for signs and symptoms of complications (see Tables 29.3 and 29.4). Always use a commercially prepared 10-mL barrel prefilled 0.9% NS syringe, assess for patency by slowly aspirating the VAD for blood return, and flush to test for resistance. Do not force if resistance is evident. Palpate the site and ask patient if they are experiencing any discomfort (Gorski et al., 2021).
- Reduce the risk of disconnection and medication errors by tracing the path between infusion and patient, labelling administration sets near patient connection and solution container, and routing tubings with different purposes in different directions. Use Luer-Lok whenever possible. Inform the patient, caregivers, and unregulated care providers (UCPs) to seek help if administration set and PIVC become disconnected.
- Use aseptic non-touch technique (ANTT®) for all VAD access and infusion therapy. Add-on devices and administration sets should be discarded if contamination is suspected (Box 29.1).
- Know and implement routine practices and additional precautions (e.g., *Routine Practices and Additional Precautions for Preventing the Transmission of Infection in Healthcare Settings* [PHAC, 2016]) to prevent transmission of health care–associated infections (HAIs) or occupational exposure to bloodborne pathogens (Box 29.2).

BOX 29.1

Infusion Nurses Society Standards to Decrease Intravascular Infection Related to Intravenous Therapy

- Perform hand hygiene before providing any assessment or care and maintenance of a vascular access device (VAD). Implement the 4 moments of hand hygiene with any vascular access care.
- Practise aseptic non-touch technique (ANTT®) for all VADs and proper hand hygiene when implementing *all* infusion and vascular access procedures. Refer to clinical guidelines on ANTT for intravenous therapy and hand hygiene (ANTT, 2018; Gorski et al., 2021).
- Use an approved antiseptic solution to cleanse the skin prior to VAD insertion and care and maintenance of the site. A combination of 2% chlorhexidine gluconate (CHG) with 70% isopropyl alcohol is preferred for use on adult patients and on children older than 2 months of age. This solution has an immediate action to reduce bacteria found on the skin and is also persistent. If an alternative antiseptic is required because of patient sensitivity, consider the use of povidone–iodine, 70% alcohol, or tincture of iodine.
- Apply 2% CHG and 70% alcohol solution using a single-use applicator in a back-and-forth and side-to-side motion. This provides maximal contact between the skin and antiseptic and helps the solution reach and disinfect deeper cell layers of the skin, thereby improving efficacy.
- Allow antiseptic solutions to completely dry for a minimum of 30 seconds prior to insertion of peripheral intravenous catheter (PIVC) and before applying a dressing. Do not blot or fan solution or wipe it away to dry. Dry time varies with solutions, therefore follow manufacturer instructions.
- Assess PIVC insertion site and surrounding tissue a minimum of every 4 hours for patients in the hospital and daily when in the community (Gorski et al., 2021). Central venous access devices (CVADs) should be assessed at least once per day in acute care patients and with every scheduled community care visit.
- Assess VAD site for signs and symptoms of complication. Visually inspect for redness, swelling, drainage, or leaking; palpate through an intact dressing for any pain, discomfort, or cording along the vein pathway.
- Transparent dressings are recommended to allow for insertion site assessment. Change transparent semipermeable dressing every 5–7 days or according to institutional policy (Gorski et al., 2021).
- Ensure that the dressing is dry and occlusive. If dressing is loose, wet, or soiled, change it immediately. The site must be cleaned with appropriate antiseptic before a new sterile dressing is applied.
- If a gauze dressing is required, the dressing should be changed every 2 days (Gorski et al., 2021).
- Change needle-free connectors using ANTT, a minimum of every 7 days, if removed for any reason, if contamination is suspected, or if it cannot be flushed clear of blood.
- Use an antiseptic swab (alcohol or 2% CHG and 70% alcohol) to scrub the hub of the needle-free connector before each access.
- Change administration sets, including add-on devices, according to type of infusion (intermittent or continuous) and with placement of a new VAD. Always change immediately if contamination is suspected.
- Always attach a sterile end cap to the male end of intermittent tubing when not in use.

Adapted from Aseptic Non Touch Technique. (2018). *ANTT core clinical guidelines, 2018*. https://www.antt.org/antt-procedure-guidelines.html; Gorski, L. A., Hadaway, L., Hagle, M. E., et al. (2021). Infusion Therapy Standards of Practice, 8th edition. *Journal of Infusion Nursing, 44*(1S), S1–S224. https://www.aspirus.org/Uploads/Public/Documents/Library/Infusion_Therapy_Standards_of_Practice,_8th.1.pdf

BOX 29.2

Standards for Reducing Occupational Exposure to Bloodborne Pathogens

1. Wear gloves when performing procedures if there is a reasonable expectation of contact with blood or body fluids (e.g., short peripheral intravenous catheter [PIVC] initiation, dressing changes, blood draws).
2. Use safety-engineered equipment according to instructions for use in order to reduce risk of needle-stick injury.
3. Always place medical sharps in a puncture-resistant, leakproof container identified for biohazard use immediately after their use. Do not overfill sharps container over observer-recommended fill line, close the container securely, and discard appropriately according to employer policy.
4. Do not bend, shear, recap, or remove contaminated needles before disposing in sharps container.
5. Follow employer and Public Health Agency of Canada (2016) standards for safe handling of all medical sharps and hazardous substances.
6. Report and document all exposure to potentially infectious material, including sharps injuries, according to employer procedure.
7. Facilities must have engineering and work practice controls to eliminate or minimize employee exposure.

Adapted from Public Health Agency of Canada. (2016). *Routine practices and additional precautions for preventing the transmission of infection in healthcare settings.* https://www.canada.ca/en/public-health/services/publications/diseases-conditions/routine-practices-precautions-healthcare-associated-infections.html

✦ SKILL 29.1 Inserting a Short Peripheral Intravenous Catheter

Video Clip **NSO** *Nursing Skills Online Intravenous Fluid Therapy Management Module 14 / Lessons 1 and 2*

A vascular access device (VAD) provides access to the venous system to deliver solutions and medications or blood and blood products. Assessment and selection of the most appropriate VAD are essential for safe, effective delivery of infusates. A variety of short peripheral intravenous catheters (PIVCs) are available in a range of gauge sizes and lengths (see Fig. 29.1, Fig. 29.2, and Table 29.2). The most commonly used PIVC is an over-the-needle catheter. This type includes a metal stylet to pierce the skin and a flexible catheter that is threaded into the vein. PIVCs can be used to deliver continuous and intermittent infusion therapy; however, they are not recommended for continuous vesicant infusates nor for solutions or medications with an osmolarity greater than 600 mOsm/L or an extreme pH (CVAA, 2019).

Delegation and Collaboration

The skill of inserting a PIVC may be completed by other members of the health care team who have appropriate education and if the skill is within their governing body's scope of practice. Assessment and care of PIVCs require effective communication and a collaborative interprofessional health care team. Always refer to employer policy.

The skill of inserting a PIVC cannot be performed by a UCP or by those who have not demonstrated competence in initiating IV therapy (Gorski et al., 2021). However, it is important for UCPs to report to the nurse the following immediately:

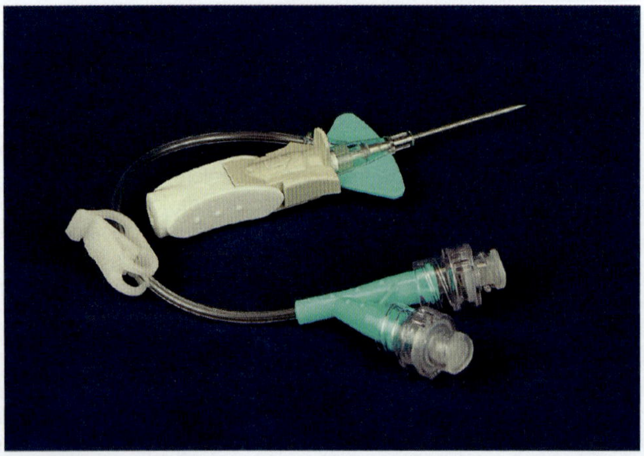

FIG 29.2 Short peripheral intravenous catheter (PIVC) with integrated extension set and stabilization platform. *(Courtesy Burl Jantzen.)*

- Signs and symptoms of complications (redness, swelling, leaking, bleeding, or drainage under the dressing, or patient expression of pain or discomfort)
- A loose, wet, or soiled dressing
- Low volume in an IV solution bag
- Triggering of electronic infusion device (EID) alarms

Equipment

- Use a commercially prepared IV start kit or collect the following:
  - Single-use tourniquet, transparent semipermeable membrane (TSM) dressing with securement properties (preferred)
  - Appropriate PIVC with integrated extension set and safety engineered mechanical sharps (see Fig. 29.2)
  - Short extension set with needle-free connector if not using PIVC with integrated extension set
  - Single-use antiseptic swab or wipe (2% chlorhexidine gluconate [CHG] and 70% alcohol preferred; alternates include 2% CHG, povidone–iodine, or 70% alcohol)

TABLE 29.2

Recommendations for Short Peripheral Catheter Selection

Catheter Size (Gauge)	Clinical Indication
14, 16, 18	Trauma; surgery; rapid blood transfusions; rapid fluid replacement
20	Continuous or intermittent infusions in adults; administration of blood transfusions in adults
22	Continuous or intermittent infusions in adults, children, neonates, and older persons; administration of blood or blood products in adults, children, neonates, and older persons
24	Continuous or intermittent infusions in adults, children, neonates, and older persons; administration of blood or blood products in adults, children, neonates, and older persons

Adapted from Gorski, L. A., Hadaway, L., Hagle, M. E., et al. (2021). Infusion Therapy Standards of Practice, 8th edition. *Journal of Infusion Nursing, 44*(1S), S1–S224. https://www.aspirus.org/Uploads/Public/Documents/Library/Infusion_Therapy_Standards_of_Practice,_8th.1.pdf

- 5 cm × 5 cm (2 inch × 2 inch) gauze pads
- Tape
- Clean gloves (or sterile gloves if re-palpation of the vein is required after skin antiseptics)
- Commercially prepared 10-mL barrel prefilled 0.9% NS syringe
- Single-use hair clippers or scissors for hair removal, if indicated
- Skin barrier swab, for sensitive skin
- Vein visualization device, as needed
- Patient gown with snaps at shoulder seams, if available (makes removal during infusion therapy easier)
- Biomedical container for disposal of medical sharps

STEP	RATIONALE
ASSESSMENT	
1. Identify patient using at least two person-specific identifiers (e.g., name and date of birth, or name and medical record number) according to employer policy.	Ensures correct patient. Complies with Accreditation Canada's standards and improves patient safety (Accreditation Canada, 2020).
2. Throughout the procedure, the 4 moments for hand hygiene are to be implemented; hand hygiene should occur before initial patient (or patient environment) contact, before an aseptic procedure, after body fluid exposure risk, and after patient (or patient environment) contact. Additional hand hygiene should be performed when hands are visibly soiled.	Proper hand hygiene helps prevent spread of infectious agents to health care providers.
3. Confirm prescription for PIVC in patient's record. Assess clinical need for PIVC.	A prescription for IV medications is sufficient for PIVC insertion. Verification that prescription is complete prevents medication errors.
4. Review patient allergies or skin sensitivities related to equipment required for insertion (e.g., latex, antiseptics, dressing adhesives, skin barrier solution).	Prevents unnecessary complications or discomfort. Equipment used during PIVC insertion may contain substances to which patient is allergic.
5. Review prescribed therapy, anticipated length of treatment, and patient characteristics to ensure that the most appropriate VAD is selected (e.g., PIVC or CVAD).	Infusions of continuous vesicants or solution with osmolarity >600 mOsm/L or extreme pH (<5 or >9) are not recommended for PIVC (CVAA, 2019). Patient assessment must include vascular characteristics, age, history of vascular access, comorbidities, and patient preferences (Fiorini et al., 2019; Piredda et al., 2017).
6. Select the most appropriate gauge of catheter required for infusion therapy or diagnostics.	Use of the smallest-gauge PIVC appropriate promotes vein preservation, reduces risk of phlebitis, and causes the least discomfort. Selection of the best gauge and device is critical to vessel health and preservation (Hallam et al., 2021).
7. Assess patient's knowledge of procedure, understanding of reason for prescribed therapy, arm placement preference, knowledge of risks related to PIVC, and awareness of signs and symptoms of complications and the need to report these immediately.	Demonstrates learning and conforms with informed consent (Gorski et al., 2021), as it ensures safe delivery of care using a person-centred approach.
8. Conduct a complete assessment, including clinical status, allergies, and past health history (see Skill 29.2).	Provides baseline to determine effectiveness or adverse effects of prescribed therapy. A systems approach is recommended to assess for fluid and electrolyte imbalances (Jantzen & Hebig, 2024).

NURSING DIAGNOSES

- Anxiety
- Insufficient knowledge regarding infusion therapy
- Potential for pain related to vascular catheter insertion
- Potential for infection
- Potential for complications of vascular access
- Potential for electrolyte imbalance

Related factors and risk factors are individualized on the basis of patient's condition or needs.

PLANNING

STEP	RATIONALE
1. Expected outcomes following completion of procedure:	
• PIVC selection is the most appropriate for prescribed therapy and vessel size.	Ensures patient safety, reinforces the importance of vein preservation, and improves patient's experience and satisfaction.
• PIVC remains patent for delivery of infusion therapy and site is free of complications.	Ensures safe and effective delivery of required therapy without delays or complications (CVAA, 2019).
• Patient is able to explain purpose and risks of PIVC placement and is aware of signs and symptoms of complications and need to report these immediately.	Demonstrates learning and conforms with informed consent (Gorski et al., 2021), as it ensures safe delivery of care using a person-centred approach.

STEP	RATIONALE
IMPLEMENTATION	
1. Provide patient education about rationale for infusion, including solution and medications prescribed; procedure for initiating PIVC; and signs and symptoms of complications (e.g., redness, pain tenderness, swelling, bleeding, drainage, or leaking at insertion site). Include rationale for device selection (e.g., short-term therapy, comfort). Obtain informed consent.	Promotes person-centred care and patient safety.
2. Change patient's gown or clothing to allow for easy removal. A gown with snaps at the shoulder may be used, if available.	Reduces risk of inadvertently dislodging VAD or administration set when changing.
3. Ensure patient is sitting or lying in a comfortable position that provides adequate light and positioning for vein assessment and PIVC insertion.	Promotes comfort, relaxation, and vasodilation for the patient. Also enables good body mechanics to prevent injury and increases likelihood of successful insertion.
4. Collect and organize equipment on clean, clutter-free bedside stand or over-bed table. Wipe surface with an antiseptic wipe prior to use.	Having easy access to equipment improves efficiency.
5. Apply single-use tourniquet on upper arm or at least 10 cm (4 inches) above intended insertion site (see Step 5 illustration). Do not apply too tightly. Assess patient comfort and confirm presence of pulse distal to the tourniquet.	The tourniquet provides dilation of the vein for ease of visualization or palpation; it should impede venous flow while maintaining arterial circulation. Caution should be used with older persons or patients who have fragile skin. Apply over patient gown to prevent skin impairments or pulling of arm hair. Consider use of a blood pressure cuff for patient comfort. Inflate to approximately 50 mm Hg to apply appropriate amount of pressure.
6. Select the most appropriate vein and location through visual inspection and palpation (see Step 6 illustration), using the following guidelines: • Veins should feel soft and bouncy and be adequate in size to accommodate the selected catheter gauge. • Use the most distal site above the wrist (nondominant side preferred). • Do not use areas of flexion (e.g., antecubital fossa) unless required for <48 hours or in an emergency situation. • Avoid veins located in the hands unless for short-term use. • Do not use a site below a failed insertion attempt, unless completely healed. • Skin must be intact and free of signs of infection. • Ensure a minimum of 8 cm (3.2 inches) or three fingers above the wrist. • Do not use an arm that has a fistula or a graft for dialysis. • Avoid the use of veins in the upper extremity on the affected side following breast surgery with axillary node dissection or lymphedema, after radiation, or with arteriovenous (AV) fistulas or grafts, or in an affected extremity from a cerebrovascular accident (CVA) (Gorski et al., 2021). • Consider use of dry heat (warm blanket or compress).	• Using smallest-gauge peripheral catheter that will accommodate prescribed therapy and patient needs (Gorski et al., 2021) promotes insertion success and vein preservation and decreases risk of phlebitis. • Site selection with varying skin tones and in the presence of tattoos or scarring may require visualization device to assist in locating veins (Gorski et al., 2021, p. 63). • Use of the hands can be very painful, limiting the patient's activities of daily living (ADLs) and ability to perform hand hygiene. • Areas of flexion cause patients discomfort and disrupt infusions. These areas have significantly higher risks of infiltration and developing mechanical or bacterial phlebitis owing to movement of the catheter and inability to maintain an occlusive dressing. • Venipuncture below a failed PIVC may lead to infiltration or extravasation of infusates. • Insertion attempt in an area of skin impairment increases the risk of infection and patient discomfort. • Insertion sites at the wrist are associated with increased risks of nerve damage. • Using vein sites that may have impaired circulation or decreased sensation may increase risk of complications. • Heat promotes comfort, decreases anxiety, and prevents vasoconstriction. Moist heat application increases risk of burns and also cools more rapidly. • Heat enhances vasodilation, improving visualization and palpation of the vein. Moist heat may cause maceration of skin, increasing risk of infection.

STEP	RATIONALE

IMPLEMENTATION

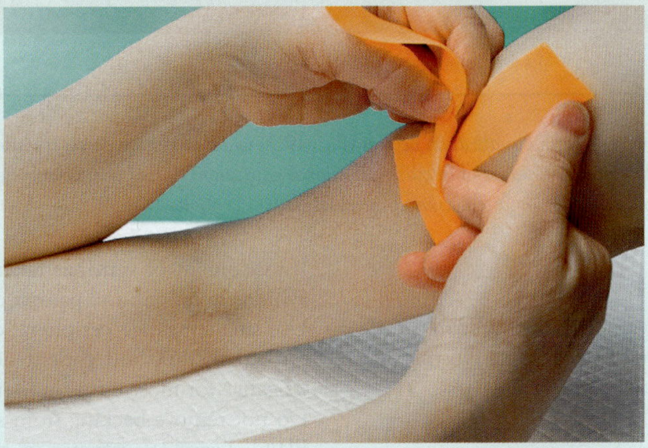

STEP 5 Application of tourniquet. *(Courtesy Patrick Coble.)*

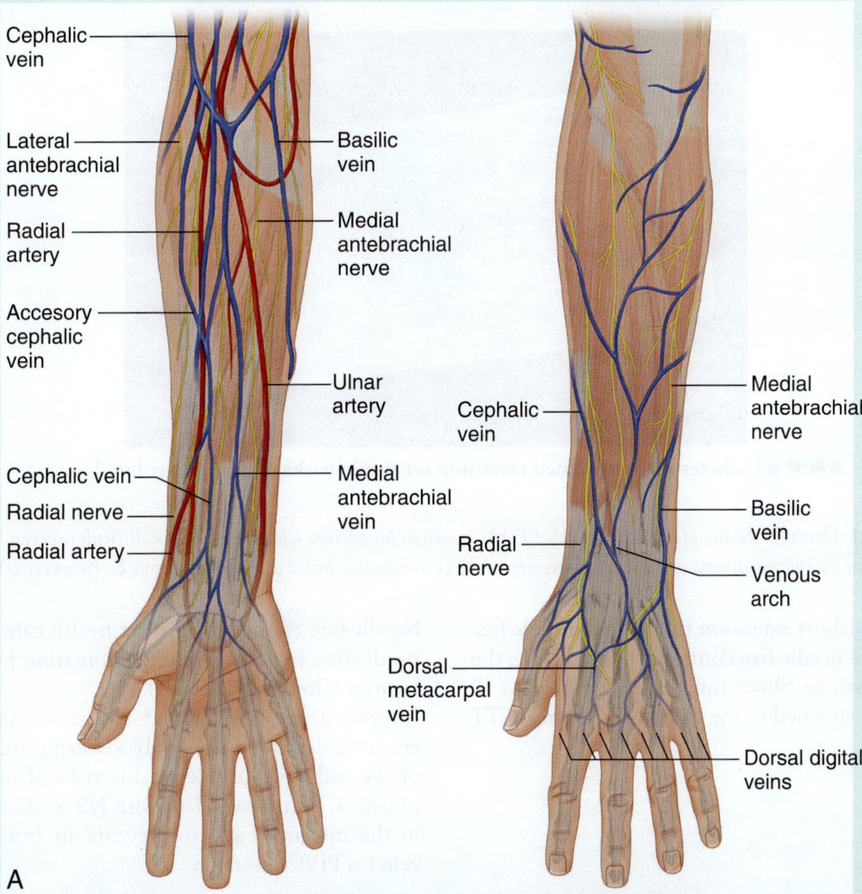

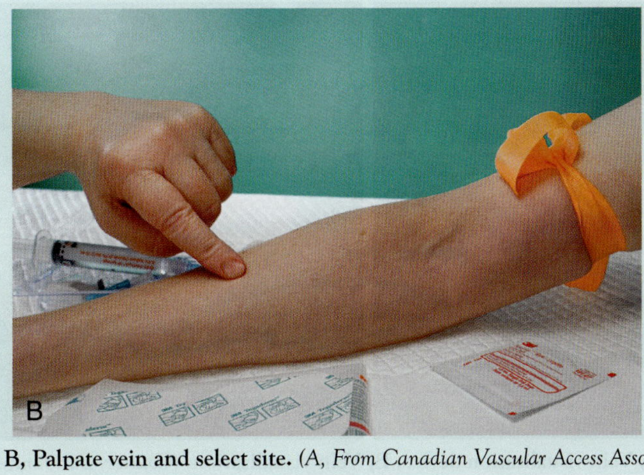

STEP 6 A, Vein map. B, Palpate vein and select site. *(A, From Canadian Vascular Access Association. B, Courtesy Patrick Coble.)*

STEP	RATIONALE

IMPLEMENTATION

Critical Decision Point *Consider the use of vein visualization devices* (Fig. 29.3) *when no venous access is visible or easily palpated (if available in the facility). Options may include near-infrared light devices or ultrasound (requires additional education). Using vein visualization devices improves success of cannulation, decreases risks associated with traumatic or missed insertion attempts, and increases patient comfort.*

STEP	RATIONALE
7. Remove tourniquet.	If assessment of vein has taken >1 minute, remove tourniquet to avoid vein fatigue and patient discomfort.
8. Select appropriately sized catheter. Open and prepare sterile packages using ANTT (see Chapter 6) (see Step 8 illustration).	Use smallest-gauge peripheral catheter that will accommodate prescribed therapy and patient need (Gorski et al., 2021). Consider 22-gauge for most infusion therapy (CVAA, 2019). Do not remove backing from sterile dressing until ready to secure PIVC. Leave IV catheter in the sterile packaging until ready to insert, to maintain asepsis.

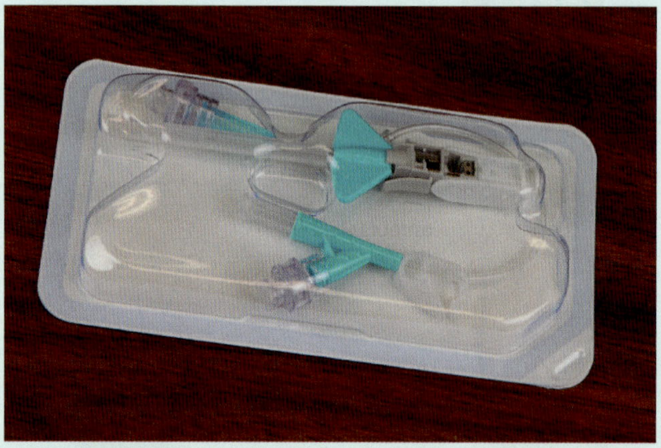

STEP 8 **Catheter with integrated extension set sterile packaging.** *(Courtesy Burl Jantzen.)*

Critical Decision Point *Consider the use of ultrasound-guided PIVC insertion for persons who are at risk for difficult-to-access vasculature, including persons with obesity, vascular disease, or chronic conditions or those who have been subject to repeated failed attempts* (Morata & Bowers, 2020).

STEP	RATIONALE
9. Prime add-on device (short extension tubing with needle-free connector or separate needle-free connector) by attaching the prefilled 10 mL NS syringe. Slowly infuse the NS to remove all air and leave syringe attached to the device. Maintain ANTT at all times.	Needle-free connectors protect health care workers by providing a needle-free system therefore eliminating potential for needle-stick injuries (Gorski et al., 2021). Integrated IV catheter and extensions provide a closed system ensuring decreased risks of blood exposure, and less manipulation of the catheter hub, decreasing risks of mechanical and bacterial phlebitis. Removing all air with NS or allowing blood to flow back in the integrated system prevents air from entering the patient's vein on PIVC insertion.

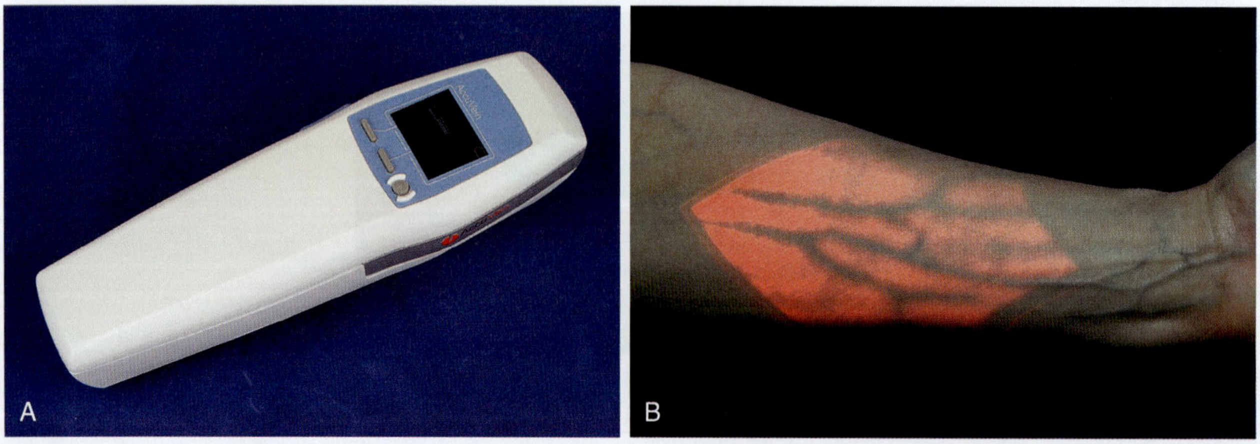

FIG 29.3 **A, Vein visualization device. B, Vein visualization.** *(Courtesy Burl Jantzen.)*

STEP	RATIONALE

IMPLEMENTATION

Critical Decision Point *If an integrated IV extension set is not in use in the facility, short extension sets are recommended for use with PIVCs for continuous and intermittent infusions. This reduces catheter manipulation and improves ease of IV administration set change, decreasing risks of contamination at catheter hub. All connections should be of Luer-Lok type* (Gorski et al., 2021).

STEP	RATIONALE
10. Prepare insertion site. If hair removal is required, use surgical clipper or scissors to trim hair. If site is visibly soiled, clean with soap and water prior to application of antiseptic solution.	Razors should not be used because they cause microscopic cuts in the skin, leading to increased risk of infection (Gorski et al., 2021). Removal of hair is essential, as it ensures adequate skin antisepsis as well as maintenance of an occlusive dressing to prevent infection. Cleaning the skin prior to application of antiseptic solutions improves efficacy.
11. Apply gloves.	Decreases potential risk of microbial contamination and cross-contamination (Gorski et al., 2021).

Critical Decision Point *Gloves are not necessary to locate the vein but must be applied for PIVC insertion using ANTT where the site is not palpated after skin antisepsis* (Gorski et al., 2021).

STEP	RATIONALE
12. Reapply single-use tourniquet using the same technique for vein assessment.	Assessment and insertion may be completed at the same application of the tourniquet by more experienced inserters. Always be aware of the length of time the tourniquet is in place and avoid applying too tightly. It should not exceed 1 minute (CVAA, 2019).
13. With your fingertip, palpate selected vein at intended insertion site by pressing downward. Note resilient, soft, bouncy feeling while releasing pressure. Have patient open and close hand to increase blood flow.	Fingertip is more sensitive and better for assessing vein location and condition.

Critical Decision Point *Vigorous friction, slapping, or hard tapping of a vein, especially in older persons, can cause venous constriction and bruising and hematoma* (CVAA, 2019; Gorski et al., 2021).

Critical Decision Point *If vein palpation is necessary after performing skin antisepsis, use sterile gloves for palpation or perform skin antisepsis again, as touching a cleaned area introduces microorganisms from your finger to the site* (Gorski et al., 2021).

STEP	RATIONALE
14. Clean insertion site with a single-use applicator or swab with preferred antiseptic (2% CHG and 70% alcohol), using a friction scrub in a side-to-side and up-and-down motion for a minimum of 30 seconds, then allow to fully dry (see Step 14 illustration).	A combination of 2% CHG and 70% alcohol is preferred (CVAA, 2019) because this solution is a broad-spectrum biocide effective against Gram-positive and Gram-negative bacteria and fungi. It has a quicker kill rate than other antimicrobials and has been shown to inhibit growth for at least 48 hours. The addition of alcohol decreases drying time on the skin. All antiseptic solutions must be applied according to instructions for use to ensure adequate antisepsis in order to reduce risk of insertion-site and systemic infections. Mechanical friction enables penetration of the solution to the epidermal layers of skin. Antiseptics must be allowed to fully dry to assure efficacy. Do not wipe, blot, fan, or blow on the skin to speed up dry time (see Box 29.1).
15. Stabilize the vein with nondominant hand by placing fingers above and below intended insertion site, pulling skin taut (see Step 15 illustration).	Stabilization of the vein for needle insertion is key to preventing rolling of the vein. Stretching the skin taut decreases drag and discomfort during insertion.
16. Perform venipuncture with bevel up, align catheter on top of intended insertion site at no more than a 30-degree angle, and puncture the skin and anterior vein wall (Gorski et al., 2021). Observe for blood return in catheter (flashback) (see Step 16 illustration). If patient experiences any paresthesia-like pain, including electrical shock, tingling, burning, or numbness, remove device immediately to prevent potential nerve damage.	Ensures patient knows to anticipate needle stick and to remain as still as possible. Some manufacturers require loosening of the catheter from the needle prior to insertion (follow manufacturer's instruction for use and employer policy). Insert a short PIVC at no more than a 30-degree angle (Gorski et al., 2021).

STEP	RATIONALE

IMPLEMENTATION

Critical Decision Point *Use a new sterile VAD for each insertion attempt* (CVAA, 2019).

17. Once blood return is observed in the catheter or flashback chamber, lower the angle so the needle is parallel with the skin. Keeping skin taut, advance the needle slightly farther into the vein. Advance or thread catheter into the vein using the push-off tab and then release the tourniquet (see Step 17 illustrations). If catheter does not thread, do not reinsert the needle into the catheter.

Lowering the angle after blood return decreases risk of puncturing the posterior vein wall.
Advancing with skin taut will ensure the catheter and needle tip are inside the vein wall.
Do not push using the catheter hub, as this contaminates the lumen. Using an integrated catheter/extension closed system eliminates this potential risk.
Reinsertion of the needle into the catheter can cause the catheter to shear off and embolize into the vein.
Advancing entire stylet into vein may penetrate wall of vein, resulting in hematoma.
Advancing catheter with finger on the open hub causes contamination (Gorski et al., 2021).

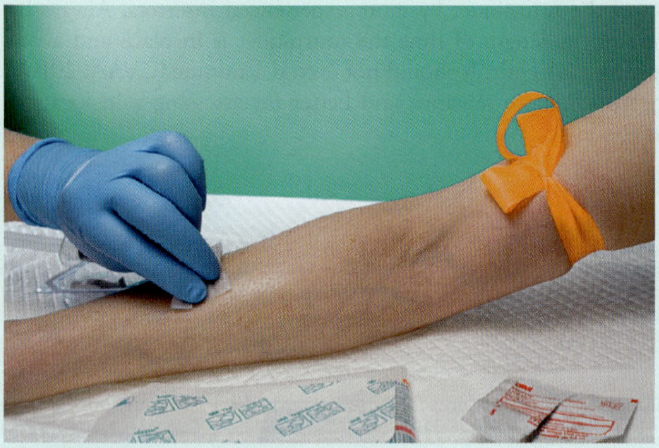

STEP 14 Clean venipuncture site. *(Courtesy Patrick Coble.)*

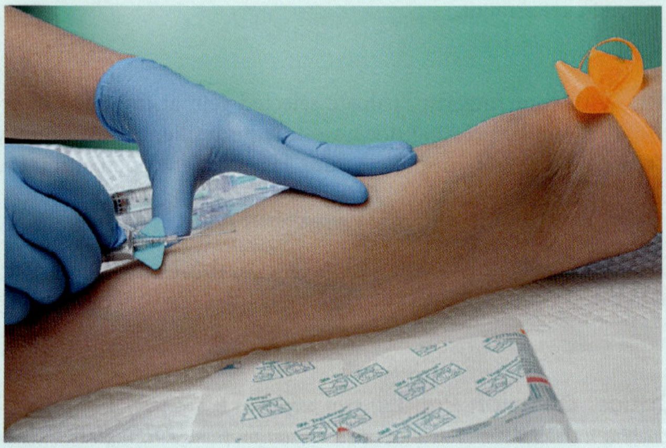

STEP 15 Stabilize vein. *(Courtesy Patrick Coble.)*

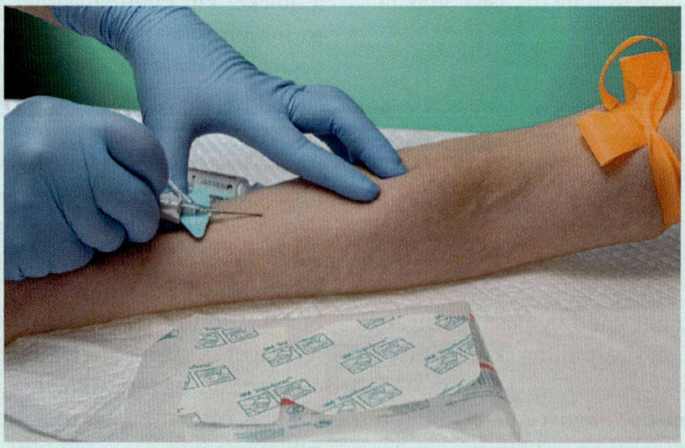

STEP 16 Perform venipuncture and observe for flashback. *(Courtesy Patrick Coble.)*

STEP	RATIONALE

IMPLEMENTATION

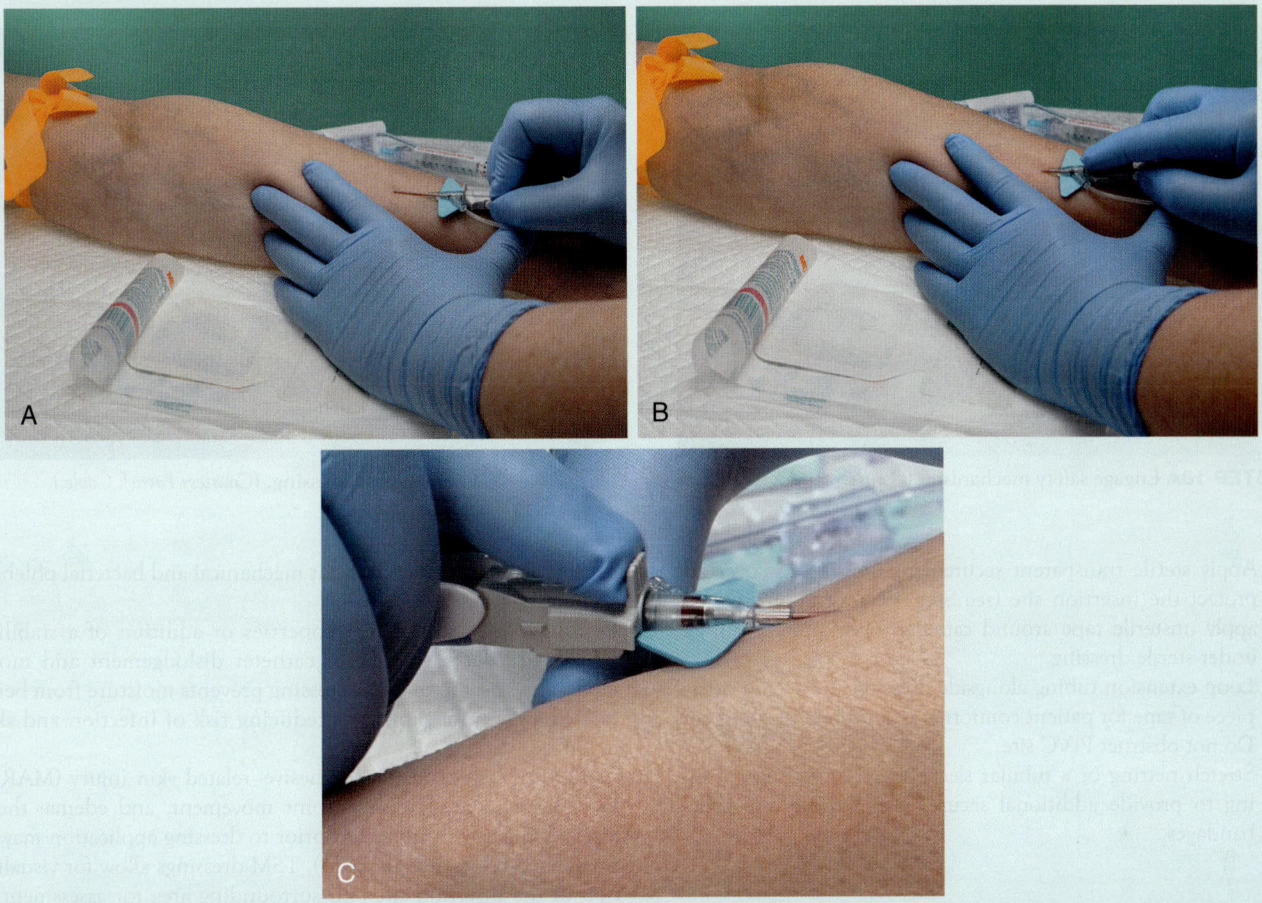

STEP 17 **A, Lower catheter. B, Advance and thread. C, Thread catheter into vein using push tab.** *(Courtesy Patrick Coble.)*

Critical Decision Point *Attempts at initiating a PIVC are limited. A single clinician may have only two unsuccessful attempts, after which a clinician with higher-level skills is requested. There is a limit of four attempts in total. The location and number of unsuccessful attempts must be documented* (CVAA, 2019; Gorski et al., 2021).

STEP	RATIONALE
18. After successful insertion of the catheter into the vein, engage safety mechanism to cover needle per manufacturer's instructions, and engage clamp if present (see Step 18a illustration).	Safety-engineered PIVCs are designed to prevent needle-stick injuries by covering or enclosing the sharp on removal.
a. If the PIVC has a blood control mechanism (e.g., clamp on integrated extension or filter in hub), this will stop blood flow until add-on extension or needle-free connector is attached. When using a straight catheter (nonintegrated), attach primed add-on device (extension set or needle-free connector) with attached syringe to catheter (disengaging clamp, if present). Use ANTT when securing extension or needle-free connectors to catheter hub.	Blood control PIVC significantly decreases risk of blood exposure and enables attachment of add-on devices without risk of hub contamination.
b. If PIVC does not have blood control, apply gentle but firm pressure above the insertion site to occlude blood flow, then attach add-on device. Avoid touching sterile connection ends. Dispose of sharps in biohazard container immediately after PIVC is secured.	Digital pressure minimizes blood loss and allows attachment of extension set or needle-free connector. Prompt connection maintains patency of vein and reduces backflow of blood if catheter does not have blood control (Gorski et al., 2021).

STEP	RATIONALE

IMPLEMENTATION

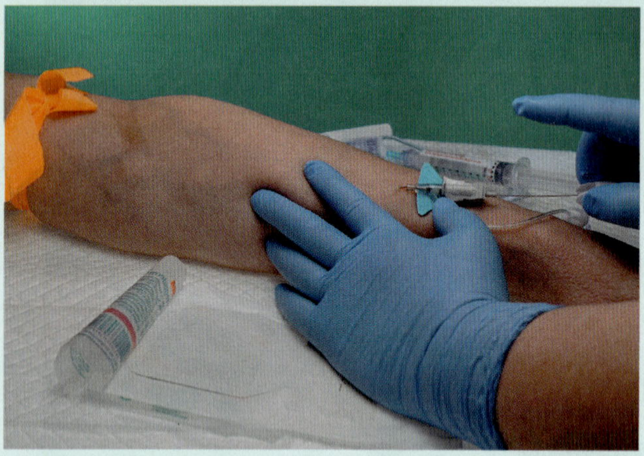

STEP 18A Engage safety mechanism. *(Courtesy Patrick Coble.)*

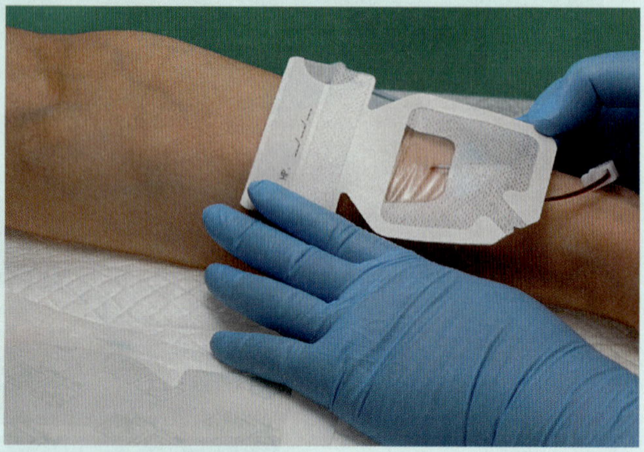

STEP 19 Apply dressing. *(Courtesy Patrick Coble.)*

STEP	RATIONALE
19. Apply sterile transparent securement dressing to cover and protect the insertion site (see Step 19 illustration). Do not apply unsterile tape around catheter, over catheter hub, or under sterile dressing.	Occlusive, dry dressings prevent mechanical and bacterial phlebitis and loss of access.
Loop extension tubing alongside dressing and secure with a piece of tape for patient comfort and additional securement. Do not obstruct PIVC site.	Dressing with securement properties or addition of a stabilization device decreases risk of catheter dislodgement and movement. Tape on top of TSM dressing prevents moisture from being carried away from skin, thus reducing risk of infection and skin irritation.
Stretch netting or a tubular sleeve may be used over dressing to provide additional securement. Do not use rolled bandages.	OPTIONAL: Risk of medical adhesive–related skin injury (MARSI) increases as a result of age, joint movement, and edema; therefore, adding a skin protectant prior to dressing application may be considered (Gorski et al., 2021). TSM dressings allow for visualization of the insertion site and surrounding area for assessment of complications. Removal of tape from TSM dressing can tear dressing and cause catheter dislodgement. If a gauze dressing is required owing to patient sensitivities to TSM dressing, assessment must be performed by palpation over the dressing, observing for any drainage and patient assessment of discomfort. Rolls of nonsterile tape can become contaminated with pathogenic bacteria, increasing risk of PIVC contamination if applied under the sterile dressing. Rolled bandages can impair circulation or flow of infusion and obscure visualization for site assessment of complications.
20. Flush catheter using a push–pause or pulsatile technique to clear all visible blood from extension set and needle-free connector. Observe insertion site for swelling during flushing. If not using a commercially prepared prefilled syringe, leave 0.5–1.0 mL of NS in the flush syringe to prevent syringe-induced blood reflux in the catheter (see Step 20 illustration).	Pulsatile flushing helps remove buildup of residue from mediations or fibrin. It creates a turbulent flush that helps clear sides and centre of catheter. Clearing blood reduces risk of catheter occlusion and infection. If patient experiences discomfort or if swelling or leaking of fluid is observed during flushing, this indicates that the catheter is no longer in the vein and must be removed immediately.
21. Remove flush syringe from needle-free connector using the appropriate clamping technique) (see Step 21a illustration). **a.** Refer to Skill 41.2 if initiating infusion.	Needle-free connectors come in many types and styles. Identifying connector properties (i.e., neutral, negative, or positive displacement) determines whether a specific clamping sequence is required to prevent reflux of blood into the PIVC on removal of syringe.

STEP	RATIONALE

IMPLEMENTATION

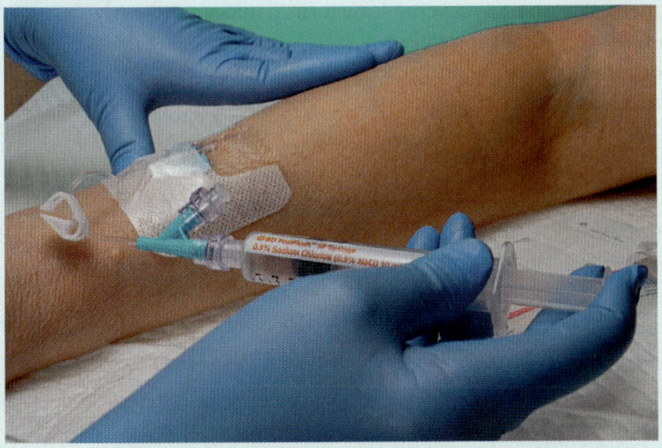

STEP 20 Flush PIVC. *(Courtesy Patrick Coble.)*

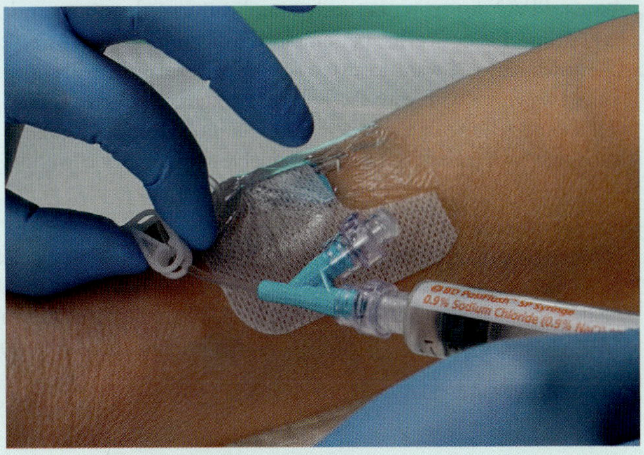

STEP 21A Close clamp. *(Courtesy Patrick Coble.)*

Critical Decision Point *Needle-free connectors protect health care workers and decrease risk of needle-stick injuries. Connectors have different internal mechanisms for fluid displacement and vary in the flush–clamp–disconnect sequence used to prevent reflux of blood into catheter upon disconnection* (Gorski et al., 2021). *The sequence depends on the type of internal mechanism:*

- *Neutral displacement devices do not have a specified flush–clamp–disconnect sequence.*
- *For negative-pressure displacement devices, flush, clamp catheter, then disconnect syringe.*
- *For positive-pressure displacement devices, flush, disconnect syringe, then clamp catheter.*

22. Label dressing according to employer policy (see Step 22 illustration). Include date of insertion and initials.

PIVCs are changed on the basis of clinical assessment. It is important to know the insertion date to determine the length of time the PIVC has been in place and to alert the need for dressing change (see Box 29.1). Monitor for MARSI.

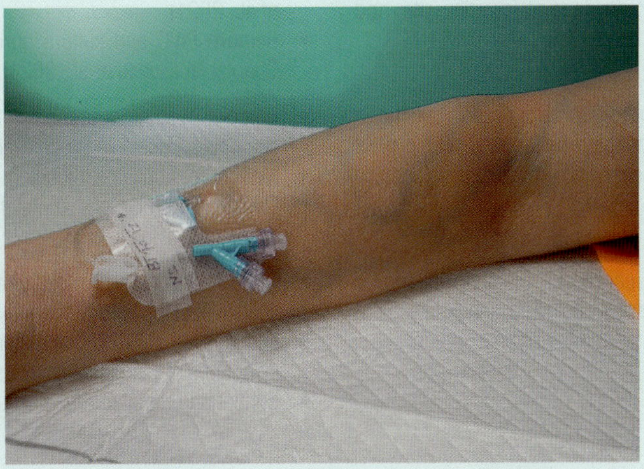

STEP 22 Label dressing. *(Courtesy Patrick Coble.)*

23. Dispose of any sharps in appropriate container. Discard supplies, and remove and discard gloves.

Reduces transmission of microorganisms; prevents accidental needle-stick injuries (PHAC, 2016).

24. Review with patient the care and maintenance of PIVC, and report any signs and symptoms of complications immediately to a health care provider.

Promotes patient engagement in care of PIVC.

Determines patient's and caregiver's level of understanding of instructional topic.

STEP	RATIONALE

EVALUATION

1. Assess PIVC for patency and complications, dressing, and patient-specific concerns, per employer policy and procedure.	Frequent assessment prevents long-term damage, and early recognition leads to prompt treatment.
2. Use teach-back: "I want to make sure that I explained what you should watch for with your IV. Tell me the signs or symptoms that you should tell me or the other nurses about." Develop a revised teaching plan if patient or caregiver is unable to teach back correctly.	Determines patient's and caregiver's level of understanding of instructional topic.

Unexpected Outcomes	Related Interventions
1. Catheter occlusion can occur from a kinked catheter, positional catheter (catheter resting against catheter wall), kink or knot in extension tubing, clot formation, or precipitate formation from administration of incompatible medications or solutions. Do not flush against resistance.	• Determine cause and consider catheter removal. • Positional catheters can be repositioned to improve IV flow. • Remove occluded PIVC immediately. Occluded catheters should not be flushed because an embolus can result from dislodging a clot.
2. Medical adhesive–related skin injury (MARSI)	• Monitor site for signs of injury and change dressing, using a different type of dressing, if indicated.

3. Phlebitis (i.e., vein inflammation): pain, redness, warmth, swelling, induration, or presence of palpable cord along course of vein pathway (Gorski et al., 2021) (see Table 29.3 and Table 29.4).	• Consider that infusate may be irritating the vein wall.
	• Assess whether vascular access is still required for plan of care.
	• Determine cause (e.g., chemical, mechanical, bacterial):
	  • *Chemical phlebitis:* Apply warm compress, elevate limb, consider slowing infusion rate, and determine whether catheter removal is necessary (Gorski et al., 2021).
	  • *Mechanical phlebitis:* Stabilize catheter, apply heat, elevate limb, continue to monitor, consider catheter removal if signs and symptoms persist (Gorski et al., 2021).
	  • *Bacterial phlebitis:* Remove short PIVC (Gorski et al., 2021).
	• Document phlebitis using a standardized scale, including nursing interventions per employer policy and procedure (Tables 29.3 and 29.4).

4. Catheter-related infection can present as redness, swelling around or above short PIVC site, pain, purulent drainage at insertion site, and elevated body temperature (Gorski et al., 2021).	• Notify health care provider. Obtain prescription to culture drainage (Gorski et al., 2021). • Remove PIVC and culture purulent drainage from around IV site (see Chapter 9) (Gorski et al., 2021).
5. Hematoma bleeding under skin owing to trauma to vessel wall. It can occur during PIVC insertion if needle punctures either adjacent vessels or posterior vein wall or can be seen with multiple venipuncture attempts.	• Remove IV catheter immediately and apply digital pressure to puncture site until hemostasis is achieved (CVAA, 2019). • Monitor for additional bleeding. • Elevate extremity and monitor for circulatory, neurological, or motor dysfunction (Gorski et al., 2021).
6. Nerve injuries during PIVC insertion can occur. Observe patient for signs of pain or reports of paresthesias, including shock-like pain, tingling or pins and needles, burning, or numbness on insertion.	• Notify health care provider of any signs and symptoms of nerve injury (Gorski et al., 2021). • Immediately stop PIVC insertion and remove device if patient indicates symptoms of paresthesias (Gorski et al., 2021). • Continue to monitor neurovascular status (Gorski et al., 2021).

Communication and Documentation

- Document PIVC insertion and unsuccessful attempts in progress notes in patient's electronic health record (EHR) or chart, including the following information, or per employer policy:
  - Date and time
  - Indication for use
  - Location of PIVC insertion (e.g., cephalic vein on dorsal surface of right lower arm)
  - Gauge, length, and type of PIVC (e.g., 22 g × 2.5 cm [1.0 inch], brand name)
  - Number of attempts
  - Functionality of PIVC (i.e., flushes without resistance, no signs of complications)
  - Local anaesthetic, if used
  - Use of visualization technology, if used
  - Patient response to procedure
  - Education provided to patient and caregiver, including level of understanding, ability to follow instructions, awareness of reporting of signs and symptoms of complications
  - Signs and symptoms of IV-related complications, including interventions and patient response to treatment
- Document ongoing assessment of device according to employer policy.
- Document patient's status, IV fluid, amount infused, and integrity and patency of system according to employer policy.
- Report the following for patient handover:

TABLE 29.3

Phlebitis Scale

Grade	Clinical Criteria
0	No symptoms
1	Erythema at access site with or without pain
2	Pain at access site with erythema and/or edema
3	Pain at access site with erythema and/or edema Streak formation Palpable venous cord
4	Pain at access site with erythema and/or edema Streak formation Palpable venous cord >2.5 cm (1 inch) in length Purulent drainage

Adapted from Gorski, L. A., Hadaway, L., Hagle, M. E., et al. (2021). Infusion Therapy Standards of Practice, 8th edition. *Journal of Infusion Nursing, 44*(1S), S1–S224. https://www.aspirus.org/Uploads/Public/Documents/Library/Infusion_Therapy_Standards_of_Practice,_8th.1.pdf

TABLE 29.4

Visual Infusion Phlebitis Scale

Score	Observation
1	IV site appears healthy
2	One of the following is evident: Slight pain near IV site *or* slight redness near IV site
3	Two of the following signs are evident: • Pain at IV site • Erythema • Swelling
4	All of the following signs are evident: • Pain along the path of cannula • Induration
5	All of the following signs are evident and extensive: • Pain along the path of cannula • Erythema • Induration • Palpable venous cord
6	All of the following signs are evident and extensive: • Pain along the path of cannula • Erythema • Induration • Palpable venous cord • Pyrexia

IV, Intravenous.

Adapted from Gorski, L. A., Hadaway, L., Hagle, M. E., et al. (2021). Infusion Therapy Standards of Practice. *Journal of Infusion Nursing, 44*(1S), S1–S224. https://www.aspirus.org/Uploads/Public/Documents/Library/Infusion_Therapy_Standards_of_Practice,_8th.1.pdf

- Location and gauge of PIVC, site assessment, IV-related complications, and status of PIVC (e.g., saline lock or continuous infusion running)
- For any infusions, include type of fluid, flow rate, status of VAD, amount of fluid remaining in present solution, expected time to hang subsequent IV container, and patient condition.

DOCUMENTATION EXAMPLE

Patient requiring IV fluid for rehydration. #22 2.5-cm catheter inserted cephalic vein, left lower arm, left forearm, [brand name] on first attempt. Patient tolerated procedure well with no reports of pain.

Special Considerations

Teaching

- Educate patient to report any signs or symptoms of complications (e.g., redness, pain, tenderness, swelling, bleeding, drainage, or loose or soiled dressing), if flow rate slows or stops, or if patient sees blood in the IV administration set or on the dressing.

Pediatric

- Consider performing venipuncture in a neutral space to allow the child's room to remain a safe place (Gorski et al., 2021).
- In addition to the usual venipuncture sites, other site selections may include the four scalp veins used in infants and toddlers and, if the child is not walking, the dorsum of the foot (Gorski et al., 2021).
- Needle selection is based on vein assessment and potential use. A typical gauge for PIVC is 26 to 24 gauge for neonates, and 24 to 22 gauge for children.
- Use local anaesthetic and distraction strategies to minimize distress associated with venipuncture (Gorski et al., 2021).
- Apply latex-free tubing or use a blood pressure cuff inflated to just below diastolic blood pressure.
- Allow older children to select PIVC site so they believe that they have some control over their treatment; doing so may increase their cooperation (Gorski et al., 2021).
- To increase success rate and improve safety for PIVC insertion, have assistance available to support and position the child. Use therapeutic holding, usually in a sitting position, to provide close contact and decrease movement that may result in unsuccessful initiation or dislodgement (Keenan-Lindsay et al., 2022).
- Consider the use of securement devices to help prevent PIVC from dislodging during daily activities and play, ensuring the device does not impede circulation or ability to assess site.
- Choose age-appropriate activities compatible with maintenance of the IV infusion to support normal growth and development.

Gerontological

- Older persons may have fragile veins and skin. They have less subcutaneous support tissue, and their skin is thinning (Jantzen & Hebig, 2024). Consider use of a barrier film before dressing application to protect fragile skin.
- Avoid sites that are easily moved or bumped (e.g., the hand) and areas that may affect mobility and independence. For example, avoid using the back of the older person's hand or the dominant arm, when feasible.
- Use a commercial protective device to protect the site and reduce manipulation.
- Appropriate gauge selection is a key factor in successful insertion and maintaining access (e.g., 22- or 24-gauge catheter). Smaller-gauge catheters are less traumatizing to the vein and allow better blood flow, increasing hemodilution of infusates.

Care in the Community: Home Management

- Ensure that patient is able and willing to self-administer infusion therapy or that there is a reliable caregiver to provide infusion therapy care at home.
- Teach patient or caregiver to assess PIVC site at least once per day or every 4 hours while awake during continuous infusions (Gorski et al., 2021).
- Teach patient or caregiver to report the following to their home care or other health care provider: any signs or symptoms of complications (e.g., redness, pain, tenderness, swelling, bleeding, drainage, or loose or soiled dressing), if flow rate slows or stops, or if patient sees blood in the IV administration set or on the dressing.

- Teach patient and caregiver about hand hygiene and ANTT for all care related to PIVC site and equipment.
- Teach caregiver to apply pressure with sterile gauze if catheter falls out and, if patient is on anticoagulant therapy, to tape sterile gauze in place for at least 20 minutes with pressure or until bleeding stops.
- Ensure that all sharps and equipment contaminated by blood are disposed of appropriately based on their community's standards. Some suppliers provide sharps containers for needle disposal. Teach patient and caregiver appropriate sharps disposal.
- Teach patient about activity restrictions (e.g., avoiding strenuous exercise of the arm with the IV line, protecting site while bathing/showering).

✦ SKILL 29.2 Initiating, Regulating, and Discontinuing Intravenous Infusions

Video Clip NSO Nursing Skills Online Maintenance of Intravenous Fluid Therapy Management Module 14 / Lesson 2

Accurate infusion rates in IV therapy are essential in the safe delivery of solutions and medications (see Chapter 22). Appropriate regulation of infusion rates reduces complications (e.g., phlebitis, infiltration, fluid overload, or clotting of the VAD) associated with infusion therapy (Gorski et al., 2021). Infusion rates can be affected by changes in patient position, flexion of the IV site extremity, occlusion of the VAD, venospasm, venous trauma, or manipulation of the VAD. A patient achieves therapeutic outcomes and fewer complications when an IV system and flow rates are assessed systematically (Gorski et al., 2021).

Infusion or flow-control devices are used for regulating infusion rates for the safe delivery of prescribed IV therapies. The type of flow-control device selected should be based on clinical assessment and may include type of VAD, type of medications or solutions, dosing, medication stability, age, mobility, condition, patient preferences, and options available for use.

There are both manual and electronic device options for regulating infusion rates. Manual devices use gravity and a mechanical method to regulate the rate of infusion (e.g., roller clamps, dials, spring-based pumps, and elastomeric balloon pumps). Manual devices are recommended for low-risk infusions where some variation in the rate of infusion is not considered critical to patient safety. Patients in alternative care settings (e.g., long-term care) can receive infusion therapy with ambulatory pumps, which promote independence and improved quality of life.

Electronic infusion devices (EIDs) are recommended for use with CVADs and when precise volume of infusions is required. An EID should include anti-free-flow protection, air in line detection, and occlusion alarms. This device delivers a measured amount of fluid over a period of time (e.g., 100 mL/hr) using positive pressure and records the volume.

Smart pumps or dose-error reduction technology should be considered whenever possible to reduce the risk of infusion-related medication errors. Smart pumps have an integrated medication library to ensure that appropriate rates are used for specific doses and volumes. The pump has an audible and visual alert when its setting does not match the preselected dose or volume limits. The use of this technology reduces the risk of medication errors and improves patient outcomes.

The reduction of infusion errors is critical to patient safety; however, the use of EIDs does not replace the need for ongoing assessment and monitoring of the rate of infusion and signs and symptoms of VAD complications (e.g., phlebitis, occlusion, infiltration, extravasation).

Determining when to discontinue an infusion and when to discontinue a PIVC involves clinical judgement, knowledge of organizational policies, and use of best practice evidence. When phlebitis or infiltration occurs, the infusion must be discontinued. However, as Hallam and colleagues (2021) describe, PIVC assessment and the related clinical decisions for device removal are critical for maintaining vessel health and preservation and should continually be at the forefront of all nurses' minds.

Delegation and Collaboration

The skills of initiating, regulating, and discontinuing IV infusions cannot be delegated to a UCP. The scope of practice of a licensed practical nurse (LPN) or registered practical nurse (RPN) varies by province/territory and health authority. The skill of initiating and regulating IV infusions may be delegated to other health care team members—always check employer policy. Caring for patients with IV infusions requires effective communication and a collaborative interprofessional health care team. The nurse instructs the UCP to immediately report the following:

- IV solution bag is low and a new bag is required.
- EID alarm triggered.
- Patient indicates any discomfort related to infusion, such as pain, burning, bleeding, or swelling at the VAD site.

Equipment

Initiating and regulating infusion:

- Prescribed IV solution
- Single-use antiseptic swab or wipe(s)
- Commercially prepared 10-mL barrel prefilled 0.9% NS syringe(s)
- Clean gloves
- IV administration set (IV tubing), either macrodrip or microdrip, depending on prescribed rate; if using EID, administration set must be compatible with the electronic device
- 0.2-micron filter, if recommended for type of infusion
- EID and IV pole
- Watch with second hand to calculate drip rate (if using gravity infusion)
- Calculator, paper, and pencil
- Tape
- Label
- Biomedical sharps container
- Stethoscope
- Patient gown with shoulder snaps for easy removal with continuous infusion therapy (if available)

Discontinuing infusion (converting to saline lock):

- Antiseptic swab(s)
- Commercially prepared 10-mL barrel prefilled 0.9% NS syringe(s)
- Clean gloves
- Sterile cap for end of IV tubing

STEP	RATIONALE
ASSESSMENT	
1. Identify patient using at least two person-specific identifiers (e.g., name and date of birth, or name and medical record number) according to employer policy.	Ensures correct patient. Complies with Accreditation Canada's standards and improves patient safety (Accreditation Canada, 2020).
2. Throughout the procedure, the 4 moments for hand hygiene are to be implemented; hand hygiene should occur before initial patient (or patient environment) contact, before an aseptic procedure, after body fluid exposure risk, and after patient (or patient environment) contact. Additional hand hygiene should be performed when hands are visibly soiled.	Proper hand hygiene helps prevent spread of infectious agents to health care providers.
3. Review accuracy and completeness of health care provider's prescription for patient name and correct solution: type, volume, additives, infusion rate, and duration of infusion therapy. Follow the 10 rights of medication administration (see Chapter 20).	Ensures delivery of correct IV solution and prescribed volume over prescribed time. Prevents catheter clotting, thus preserving venous access while infusing a minimal amount of fluid.
a. If keep vein open (KVO) rate is prescribed, check employer policy regarding flow rate of KVO.	A prescription for KVO rate must specify an infusion rate, as required by the rights of medication administration. Rates may vary from 0.5 to 30 mL/h based on type of VAD, patient-specific therapy, and method of infusion (gravity or EID).
4. Assess for clinical factors and conditions that will be affected by infusion therapy, including laboratory values, clinical markers of volume, allergies, and behaviour and cognition.	Knowledge of infusion therapy modalities (e.g., PVAD, CVAD, solution, medication, volume) is necessary to identify key assessments and treatment evaluation.
a. *Body weight*	Changes in body weight can be an indication of fluid loss or gain.
b. *Clinical markers of vascular volume:*	
(1) Urine output (decreased, dark yellow)	Kidneys respond to extracellular fluid volume (ECV) deficit by reducing urine production and concentrating urine. Kidney disease can also cause oliguria.
(2) Vital signs: blood pressure, respirations, pulse, temperature	Changes in blood pressure may be associated with fluid volume status (fluid volume deficit [FVD]) seen in postural hypotension. Respirations can be altered in presence of acid–base imbalances. Temperature elevations increase need for fluid requirements (Jantzen & Hebig, 2024).
(3) Distended neck veins (normally, veins are full when person is supine and flat when person is upright)	Indicator of fluid volume status: flat or collapsing with inhalation when supine with ECV deficit; full when upright or semi-upright with ECV excess.
(4) Auscultation of lungs	Crackles or rhonchi in dependent parts of lung may signal fluid buildup caused by ECV excess.
(5) Capillary refill	Indirect measure of tissue perfusion (sluggish with ECV deficit).
c. *Clinical markers of interstitial volume:*	
(1) Skin turgor (pinch skin over sternum or inside of forearm)	Failure of skin to return to normal position after several seconds indicates FVD.
(2) Dependent edema (pitting or nonpitting) (see Chapter 8)	Edema is not usually apparent until 2–4 kg (4.4–8.8 lb) of fluid is retained. A weight gain of 1 kg (2.2 lb) is equivalent to the retention of 1 L of body water (Holroyd, 2020).
(3) Oral mucous membrane between cheek and gum (see Chapter 8)	More reliable indicator than dry lips or skin. Dryness between cheek and gums indicates ECV deficit.
d. *Thirst*	Occurs with hypernatremia and severe ECV deficit. Not a reliable indicator for older persons (Arai et al., 2014; El-Sharkawy et al., 2020).
e. *Behaviour and level of consciousness:*	
(1) Restlessness and mild confusion	Occurs with FVD or acid–base imbalance.
(2) Decreased level of consciousness (lethargy, confusion, coma)	Occurs with severe ECV deficit. May occur with osmolality, fluid and electrolyte, and acid–base imbalances.
5. Identify patient risk for fluid and electrolyte imbalance given type of IV solution (e.g., neonate, history of cardiac or renal disease).	Helps prioritize assessments. Volume control needs to be strict. Guides choice of infusion device.
6. Assess VAD function and patency just prior to administration (Gorski et al., 2021).	Identifies complications that compromise integrity of VAD and may necessitate replacement of VAD. Reduces transmission of infection. Reduces risk of infiltration or extravasation (Gorski et al., 2021).

STEP	RATIONALE
ASSESSMENT	
7. Assess IV system for patency from catheter insertion site to solution container.	Ensures delivery of prescribed volume over prescribed time.
8. Assess infusate for vesicant or irritant properties.	The presence of a vesicant or irritant would prompt more frequent assessments and may require changing the VAD to a more suitable type to prevent vessel damage (see Gorski et al., 2021).
9. Assess patient's knowledge related to prescribed treatment, signs and symptoms of infusion-related complications, and how to report complications.	Decreases patient anxiety and promotes cooperation with and adherence to therapy. Prepares patient and caregiver by explaining procedure, its purpose, and what is expected of patient.

NURSING DIAGNOSES

- Insufficient fluid volume
- Excessive fluid volume
- Insufficient knowledge regarding infusion therapy
- Potential for infection

Related factors and risk factors are individualized on the basis of patient's condition or needs.

STEP	RATIONALE
PLANNING	
1. Expected outcomes following completion of procedure:	
• Fluid and electrolyte balance returns to, or remains within, normal range.	Proper solution is infused at proper rate and monitored, resolving fluid and electrolyte imbalance (Jantzen & Hebig, 2024).
• Patient's VAD remains patent, and site is free from signs and symptoms of IV-related complications.	Ensures that patient receives prescribed infusion therapy and that VAD is without complications (Gorski et al., 2021).
• Patient is able to explain how positioning of IV site affects rate and describe complications related to inaccurate flow rate.	Demonstrates learning (Gorski et al., 2021).
2. Have paper and pencil or calculator to calculate flow rate.	Use mathematical calculations to obtain correct rate. Refer to medication math resources for assistance with calculations.
3. Check prescription to see how long each litre of fluid should infuse. If hourly rate (mL/hr) is not provided in prescription, calculate it by dividing volume by hours. For example, if 1 L is prescribed for 8 hours, the infusion rate is calculated as follows: $\text{Infusion rate} = \frac{\text{Total infusion (mL)}}{\text{Length of infusion (hr)}}$ $= 1\,000\text{ mL}/8\text{ hr} = 125\text{ mL/hr}$ Alternatively, if 3 L is prescribed for 24 hours, the infusion rate is: $3\,000\text{ mL}/24\text{ hr} = 125\text{ mL/hr}$	Basis of calculation to ensure infusion of solution over prescribed hourly rate.
4. *Infusion via EID*—Use hourly rate (mL/hr) to program pump.	EID automatically delivers correct minute flow rate (gtt/mL).
5. *Infusion via gravity*—Use hourly rate to calculate minute flow rate (gtt/min). Know calibration (drop factor), in drops per millilitre (gtt/mL), of infusion set used by employer:	Gravity infusion requires calculation of minute flow rate (gtt/mL).
a. Microdrip: 60 gtt/mL. Used to deliver rates <100 mL/hr.	Microdrip tubing universally delivers 60 gtt/mL. Used when small or very precise volumes are to be infused.
b. Macrodrip: 10–15 gtt/mL (depending on manufacturer). Used to deliver rates >100 mL/hr.	There are different commercial parenteral administration sets for macrodrip tubing. Used when large volumes or fast rates are necessary. Know drip factor for tubing being used.
6. Select one of the following formulas to calculate minute flow rate (drops per minute) based on the drop factor of the infusion set: **a.** $\frac{\text{mL/hr}}{60\text{ min}} = \text{mL/min}$ $\text{Drop factor} \times \text{mL/min} = \text{Drops/min}$ or **b.** $\text{mL/hr} \times \frac{\text{Drop factor}}{60\text{ min}} = \text{Drops/min}$	Once hourly rate is determined, these formulas compute the correct flow rate.

STEP	RATIONALE
PLANNING	
c. EXAMPLE: Calculate minute flow rate for a 1 000 mL bag of dextrose 5% in water (D_5W) at 125 mL/hr.	
Microdrip: $$125\,mL/hr \times 60\,gtt/mL = 7\,500\,gtt/hr$$ $$7500\,gtt \div 60\,min = 125\,gtt/min$$	When using microdrip, millilitres per hour (mL/hr) always equals drops per minute (gtt/min).
Macrodrip: $$125\,mL/hr \times 15\,gtt/mL = 1875\,gtt/hr$$ $$1\,875\,gtt \div 60\,min = 31 - 32\,gtt/min$$	Multiply volume by drop factor and divide product by time (in minutes).
IMPLEMENTATION	
1. Preparing IV administration set and solution for continuous or intermittent infusion:	
a. Confirm IV solution using the 10 rights of medication administration (see Chapters 20 and 22). Verify that label information is accurate by reviewing name of medication or solution, dosage and concentration, beyond-use and expiration dates, and sterility state. Prepare all infusions just prior to administration.	IV administration sets are changed at established intervals, when a VAD is changed, or if contamination is suspected. Administration set changes should be planned to coincide with initiation of a new solution container or medication. For continuous infusions, change every 4–7 days or per organizational policy. For intermittent infusions, administration sets are changed every 24 hours or per organizational policy (CVAA, 2019). Reviewing label for accuracy reduces risk of medication errors (Gorski et al., 2021).
b. Check solution for colour and clarity. Check bag for leaks.	Sterility may be compromised if any of the following are observed: • Leaking of the container or bag • Discoloration of solution • Precipitate is visible • Solution is beyond-use date or expiration has passed. *Do not use if contamination is suspected.*
c. Open administration set (IV tubing), maintaining sterility. NOTE: EIDs sometimes have a dedicated administration set; follow manufacturer instructions.	Prevent touch contamination, which allows microorganisms to enter infusion equipment and bloodstream.
d. Place roller clamp about 2–5 cm below drip chamber, and move roller clamp to "off" or "closed" position.	Maintaining proximity of roller clamp to drip chamber allows more accurate regulation of flow rate. Moving clamp to "off" prevents accidental spillage of IV solution during priming.
e. Remove protective cap over spike port on IV container or bag.	
f. Remove protective cover from spike of administration set (IV tubing) and insert into port of IV bag using a twisting motion and adhering to ANTT (see Step 1f illustration). If solution container is a glass bottle, clean rubber stopper on glass-bottled solution with antiseptic swab and insert spike into rubber stopper of IV bottle. Bottles require vented tubing. If sterility of spike is compromised, discard IV administration set and open a new set.	Provides access for insertion of IV administration set spike into solution using sterile technique.
g. Compress drip chamber and release, allowing it to fill one-third to one-half full.	Creates suction effect; fluid enters drip chamber to prevent air from entering tubing.

STEP	RATIONALE

IMPLEMENTATION

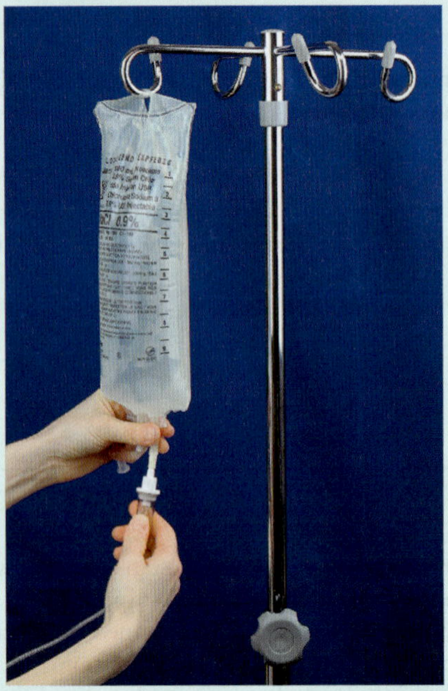

STEP 1F **Prepare infusate container and administration set.** *(Courtesy Burl Jantzen.)*

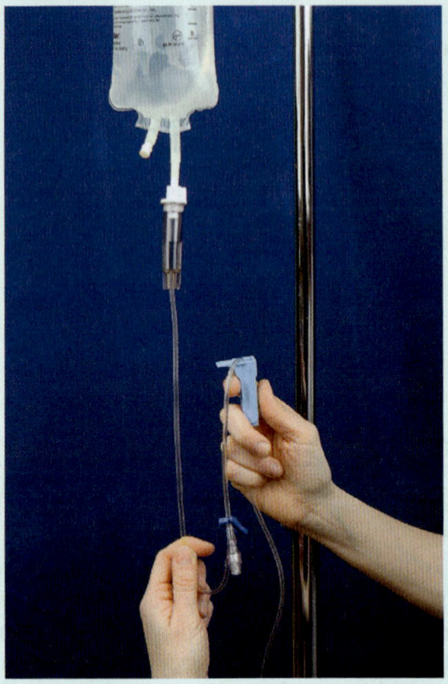

STEP 1H **Purge air from administration set using roller clamp.** *(Courtesy Burl Jantzen.)*

STEP	RATIONALE
h. Purge air from administration set by slowly opening the roller clamp (see Step 1h illustration). This will allow the IV solution to flow from the drip chamber to fill the tubing. If the administration set has in-line access ports, invert the port as the solution fills the tubing; this will ensure complete removal of air. When solution reaches the distal end of tubing, close clamp. Label administration set with time and date, according to employer policy and procedure.	Priming ensures that IV administration set is clear of air and filled with IV solution before connecting to VAD. Slowly filling tubing decreases turbulence and chance of bubble formation. Closing clamp prevents loss of solution. Labelling IV administration set identifies when administration set needs to be changed.
i. Confirm by visual inspection that tubing is clear of air and air bubbles. To remove small air bubbles, firmly tap tubing where they are located.	Large air bubbles may act as emboli (Gorski et al., 2021, p. S60).
2. Initiating and regulating infusion:	
a. Apply clean gloves	Reduces transmission of microorganisms.
b. Assess VAD function and patency.	Assessing just prior to initiating infusion reduces risk of infiltration and extravasation.
c. Scrub VAD needle-free connector with employer-approved antiseptic swab for at least 15 seconds and let dry. Remove protective cap from administration set and connect via Luer-Lok to needle-free connector (see Step 2c illustration). Maintain ANTT at all times.	

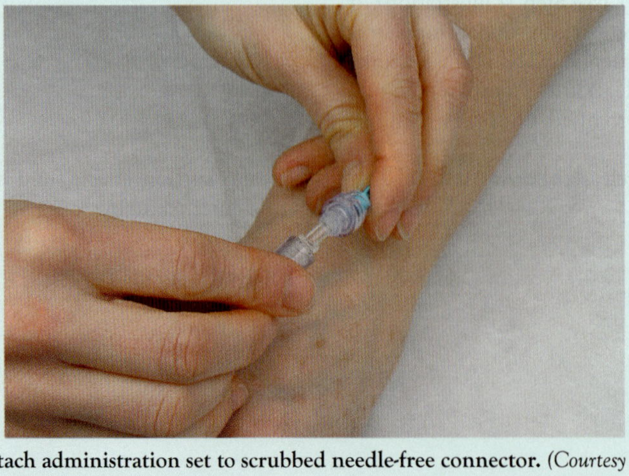

STEP 2C **Attach administration set to scrubbed needle-free connector.** *(Courtesy Patrick Coble.)*

STEP	RATIONALE

IMPLEMENTATION

STEP	RATIONALE
d. Regulate infusion. **(1)** *Regulate infusion via gravity infusion:* **(a)** Place adhesive or fluid indicator tape on IV bag next to volume markings.	Tape provides a visual cue as to whether fluids are being administered over correct time period.
(b) Ensure that IV container is at least 76.2 cm (30 inches) above IV site for adults, and increase height for viscous fluids (Gorski et al., 2021).	Pressure caused by gravity is necessary to overcome venous pressure and resistance from tubing and catheter.
(c) Slowly open roller clamp on tubing until drops are visible in the drip chamber. Hold a watch with a second hand at the same level as the drip chamber and count drip rate for 1 minute. Adjust roller clamp to increase or decrease rate of infusion.	Regulates flow to prescribed rate.

Critical Decision Point *An anti–free flow safeguard (preventing bolus infusion in the event of machine malfunction or when tubing is removed from machine) is an important element of an EID and is required. Always check and follow manufacturer recommendations for specific device features.*

STEP	RATIONALE
(2) *Regulate infusion via EID:* **(a)** Load primed administration into EID (see Step 2d[2][a] illustration). Check manufacturer recommendations for correct IV container height. **(b)** Program EID to regulate infusion at prescribed rate.	To ensure accuracy. Manufacturers may vary as to the optimal distance between EID and IV solution container.

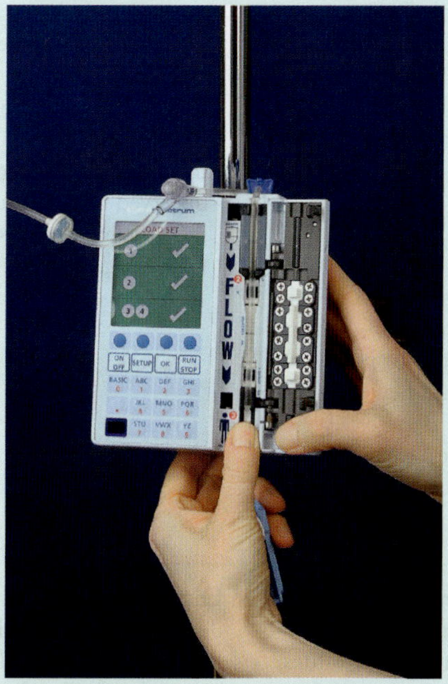

STEP 2D(2)(A) Insert administration set into EID. *(Courtesy Patrick Coble.)*

STEP	RATIONALE
e. Monitor infusion rate and IV site for complications at least hourly. Use watch to verify rate of infusion, even when using EID. Assess IV system from container to VAD insertion site when alarm is triggered.	Many factors influence drip rate; frequent monitoring ensures IV fluid administration as prescribed. Flow controllers and pumps do not replace frequent, accurate nursing evaluation. EIDs can continue to infuse IV solutions after a complication has developed (Gorski et al., 2021). Alarm indicates a situation that requires attention. EID alarm may be triggered by empty solution container, tubing kinks, closed clamp, infiltration, clotted catheter, air in tubing, or low battery.
f. Teach patient purpose of EID if infusion therapy is delivered by EID, purpose of alarms, to avoid raising hand or arm because it affects flow rate, and to avoid touching control clamp.	Information enables patient to protect IV site and informs them about rationale for not altering flow rate.

STEP	RATIONALE
IMPLEMENTATION	
3. Discontinuing infusion (converting to saline lock):	
a. Check health care provider's prescription for discontinuation of IV therapy. For intermittent medications, ensure patient has received entire dose.	Prescription is required for discontinuation of fluids or medication.
b. Apply clean gloves.	Reduces transmission of microorganisms.
c. Stop EID and move roller clamp to "off" position.	Prevents fluid spillage.
d. Disconnect administration set from VAD needle-free connector. If clamp present on VAD extension, engage before disconnecting IV tubing or follow appropriate clamping sequence according to type of needle-free connector. Attach a new sterile cap to end of administration set (Gorski et al., 2021). Maintain ANTT.	Specific clamping sequence is required to prevent reflux of blood into VAD catheter. Maintains sterility of administration set if required for intermittent use.
e. Scrub needle-free connector with antiseptic swab and attach commercially prepared 10-mL barrel prefilled 0.9% NS flush syringe (disengage clamp on VAD if present). Maintain ANTT.	Reduces risk of drip chamber emptying and maintains sterility.
f. Flush catheter using a push–pause or pulsatile technique. Observe insertion site for swelling, with flush. If not using a commercially prepared prefilled syringe, leave 0.5–1.0 mL of NS in flush syringe to prevent syringe-induced blood reflux in the catheter.	Pulsatile flushing helps remove buildup of residue from mediations or fibrin. It creates a turbulent flush that helps clear the sides as well as the centre of the catheter. Clearing blood prevents risk of catheter occlusion and infection. If patient experiences discomfort or swelling, or if leaking of fluid is observed during flush, this indicates that the catheter is no longer in the vein and must be removed immediately.
g. Remove flush syringe from needle-free connector using the appropriate clamping sequence. Flush and lock with appropriate volume according to type of VAD, number of lumens, type of infusion, and per employer policy and procedure. Scrub needle-free connector with new antiseptic swab before each access (see Skill 29.6).	Clamping sequence prevents blood reflux into catheter.
h. Discard of used supplies and remove gloves.	
EVALUATION	
1. Observe patient every 1–2 hours (see employer policy), noting volume of IV fluid infused and rate of infusion.	Ensures delivery of prescribed volume over prescribed time and decreases risk of fluid and electrolyte imbalance.
2. Evaluate patient's response to therapy (e.g., laboratory values, input and output [I&O], weights, vital signs, postprocedure assessments).	Provides ongoing evaluation of patient's fluid status, including monitoring for fluid volume excess (FVE) or FVD. Early recognition of complications leads to prompt treatment.
3. Evaluate patient at established intervals per employer policy for signs and symptoms of IV-related complications.	Prevents complications that compromise integrity of VAD or cause inaccurate IV solution flow rate.
4. **Use teach-back:** "I want to be sure that I explained the importance of running your IV fluids at the correct rate. Tell me what you think may cause the pump's alarm to go off and what you would do." Develop a revised teaching plan if patient or caregiver is unable to teach back correctly.	Determines patient's and caregiver's level of understanding of instructional topic.

Unexpected Outcomes	Related Interventions
1. Solution does not infuse at prescribed rate. a. Sudden infusion of large volume of solution occurs; patient develops dyspnea, crackles in lung, dependent edema (edema in legs), and increased urine output, indicating FVE.	• Slow infusion rate: KVO rates must have specific rate prescribed by health care provider. • Notify health care provider immediately. • Place patient in high Fowler's position. • Anticipate new IV prescriptions. • Anticipate administration of oxygen per prescription. • Administer diuretics if prescribed.
b. IV solution runs slower than prescribed.	• Check for positional change that affects rate, height of IV container, kinking of tubing, or obstruction. • Check VAD site for complications. • Consult health care provider for new prescription to provide necessary fluid volume.
2. IV patency is lost subsequent to emptying of IV solution container.	• Discontinue present IV infusion and restart new PIVC in new site.

Communication and Documentation

- Document IV solution and rate of infusion in drops per minute (gtt/min) for infusions via gravity or millilitres per hour (mL/hr) in progress notes in EHR or chart.
- Document integrity and patency of system including VAD according to employer policy.
- Document use of any EID or control device and identification number on that device, if required by employer policy.
- Document patient response (e.g., laboratory values, I&O, weights, vital signs, postprocedure assessments) to therapy and unexpected outcomes (e.g., signs and symptoms of FVE, FVD, or IV-related complications).
- Document patient's and caregiver's level of understanding following instruction.
- At change of shift or when leaving on break, report rate of infusion and volume of solution remaining to nurse in charge or next nurse assigned to care for patient.

DOCUMENTATION EXAMPLE

D_5W infusion started at 125 mL/hr with EID and infusing well. Patient provided with education regarding signs or symptoms to report. Intake and output record initiated.

Special Considerations

Teaching

- Instruct patient to notify nurse if any signs or symptoms of IV complications are noted (e.g., redness, pain, tenderness, swelling, bleeding, drainage, or leakage from under dressing).
- Patient using an EID should know the significance of alarms and when to notify nursing staff.
- Teach patient about factors affecting flow rate, how to protect IV site, and about importance of not altering rate control.

Pediatric

- Do not use IV bags or containers exceeding 150 mL in children younger than 2 years of age, exceeding 250 mL in children younger than 5 years of age, or exceeding 500 mL in children younger than 10 years of age. Always use tamper-resistant volume-controlled EIDs to ensure accurate fluid delivery (Gorski et al., 2021).

Gerontological

- Use an EID and microdrip tubing to administer IV solutions to older persons. Monitor vital signs, electrolyte levels, blood urea nitrogen (BUN), creatinine, urine output, and body weight (Jantzen & Hebig, 2024).

Care in the Community: Home Management

- Ensure that patient is able and willing to operate an EID and administer infusion therapy. If patient is unable to provide self-care, be sure that a reliable caregiver is available in the home.
- Discuss proper EID function with patient. Consider use of an ambulatory-type device. Observe patient operating infusion EID and administering infusion therapy.
- Teach patient and caregiver what EID alarms mean, methods to troubleshoot them, and how to disconnect the IV administration set from the EID pump in the event of a pump failure.
- Ensure that patient's electrical outlets are properly grounded.
- Provide patient with a contact phone number to access 24 hours a day for addressing problems, if resources are available in the patient's setting.

✦ SKILL 29.3 Changing Intravenous Solution Containers

NSO *Nursing Skills Online Maintenance of Intravenous Fluid Therapy Management Module 14 / Lesson 3*

Patients receiving IV therapy require periodic changes of IV solutions. IV containers include plastic bags and glass bottles. The nurse changes a container when there is a prescription for a new solution or when it is time to add a sequential container. As patients respond to therapy, a new solution may be prescribed. The maximum hang time for routine replacement of IV containers is established by employer policy (Gorski et al., 2021). Maximum hang time is based on assumptions that strict aseptic technique (ANTT) has been followed throughout and that the system remains closed. Stability of the solution or medication being infused also determines hang time. Organizational skills are necessary to manage the changing of IV containers or solutions in a manner that decreases the risk of infusion-related complications such as the emptying of an infusion container or the clotting of a VAD.

Delegation and Collaboration

The skill of changing IV solutions may be delegated to other health care team members if they have had appropriate education, the skill is within their governing body scope of practice, and it is approved by employer policy. Caring for patients with IV infusions requires interprofessional collaboration for effective communication and patient safety.

The skill of changing IV solutions cannot be delegated to a UCP. The nurse instructs the UCP to report the following to the nurse immediately:

- IV container is nearing completion
- Any cloudiness or precipitate in the IV solution
- Alarm triggered on EID
- Any patient indications of discomfort related to infusion, such as pain, burning, bleeding, or swelling

Equipment

- Clean gloves
- IV solution as prescribed by health care provider
- Label

STEP	RATIONALE
ASSESSMENT	
1. Identify patient using at least two person-specific identifiers (e.g., name and date of birth, or name and medical record number) according to employer policy.	Ensures correct patient. Complies with Accreditation Canada's standards and improves patient safety (Accreditation Canada, 2020).
2. Throughout the procedure, the 4 moments for hand hygiene are to be implemented; hand hygiene should occur before initial patient (or patient environment) contact, before an aseptic procedure, after body fluid exposure risk, and after patient (or patient environment) contact. Additional hand hygiene should be performed when hands are visibly soiled.	Proper hand hygiene helps prevent spread of infectious agents to health care providers.
3. Review accuracy and completeness of health care provider's prescription in patient's medical record for patient name and correct solution type, volume, additives, rate, and duration of infusion therapy. Follow the 10 rights of medication administration (see Chapter 20).	Ensures delivery of correct IV solution and prescribed volume over prescribed time (Gorski et al., 2021).
4. Note date and time when IV administration set and solution were last changed.	Ensures correct timing of tubing changes.
5. Determine patient understanding of need for continued infusion therapy.	Indicates need for any patient education and ensures informed consent.
6. Apply clean gloves; inspect and gently palpate skin around and above VAD site over dressing. Assess VAD for patency and signs and symptoms of IV-related complications (e.g., infiltration, occlusion of VAD, phlebitis, infection, patient indication of pain, or leakage under dressing). Discard gloves.	Reduces transmission of microorganisms. Identifies complications that compromise integrity of VAD and necessitate replacement of VAD.
7. Check infusion system from solution container down to VAD insertion site for integrity, including, but not limited to, discoloration, cloudiness, leakage, and expiration date. Determine compatibility of all IV solutions and additives by consulting approved online database, drug reference, or pharmacist.	If there has been a break in integrity of solution container, a new bag is needed (Gorski et al., 2021). May indicate need for IV administration set change. Incompatibilities cause physical, chemical, and therapeutic changes with adverse patient outcomes.
8. Check pertinent laboratory data.	Compare data with baseline to determine ongoing response to IV solution administration.

NURSING DIAGNOSES

- Insufficient fluid volume
- Insufficient knowledge regarding IV infusion
- Potential for infection

Related factors and risk factors are individualized on the basis of patient's condition or needs.

STEP	RATIONALE
PLANNING	
1. Expected outcomes following completion of procedure:	
• IV solution is correct.	Patient receives solution prescribed for treatment of diagnosis.
• Fluid and electrolyte levels return to normal.	IV solution helps maintain fluid and electrolyte levels.
• Patient's VAD remains patent, and site is free from signs and symptoms of IV-related complications.	Ensures access for delivery of prescribed infusion therapy (Gorski et al., 2021).
• Patient and caregiver can explain purpose of IV solution change.	Demonstrates learning (Gorski et al., 2021).

STEP	RATIONALE
PLANNING	
2. Collect equipment. Have next solution prepared at least 1 hour before needed. If solution is prepared in pharmacy, ensure that it has been delivered to patient care unit. Allow solution to warm to room temperature if it has been refrigerated. Check that solution is correct and properly labelled. Check solution expiration date. Ensure that any light sensitivity restrictions are followed.	Reduces transmission of infection and contamination of equipment (Gorski et al., 2021). Proper handling of solutions prevents IV-related complications such as occlusion. Checking that solution is correct prevents medication error.
3. Prepare patient and caregiver by explaining procedure, its purpose, and what is expected of patient.	Promotes person-centred care and decreases anxiety.
IMPLEMENTATION	
1. Change solution when prescription changes or when a small amount, about 50 mL, remains.	Prevents waste of solution. Employer policy will specify maximum hang time for IV solution containers.
2. Prepare new solution for changing. If using plastic bag, hang on IV pole and remove protective cover from IV administration set port. If using glass bottle, remove metal cap and metal and rubber discs.	Permits quick, smooth, and organized change from old to new container.
3. Close roller clamp on existing solution to stop flow rate. Remove IV administration set from EID if necessary to prevent contamination of the new solution port or tubing spike (if used). Then remove old IV solution container from IV pole. Invert solution container.	Prevents drip chamber from emptying while changing solutions. Prevents solution in bag from spilling.
4. Quickly remove spike from old solution container and, without touching tip, insert spike into new container.	Reduces risk of drip chamber emptying and maintains sterility.
Critical Decision Point *If spike becomes contaminated by coming into contact with an unsterile object, discard and open a new administration set.*	
5. Hang new container of solution on IV pole.	Gravity helps with delivery of fluid into drip chamber.
6. Check for air in IV administration set. If air bubbles have formed, remove them by closing roller clamp, stretching tubing downward, and tapping tubing with finger (bubbles rise in fluid to drip chamber).	Reduces risk of air entering tubing. Use of an air-eliminating filter also reduces risk.
7. Make sure that drip chamber is one-third to one-half full. If drip chamber is too full, level can be decreased by removing bag from IV pole, pinching off IV administration set below drip chamber, inverting container, squeezing drip chamber, releasing and turning solution container upright, and releasing pinch on tubing.	Reduces risk of air entering IV administration set. If chamber is completely filled, you cannot observe or regulate drip rate.
8. If infusing with gravity, place time label on side of container and label with time hung, time of completion, and appropriate hourly intervals. If using plastic bags, mark only on label, not on container.	Provides visual comparison of volume infused compared with prescribed rate of infusion.
9. Where relevant, reinstruct patient on purpose of new IV solution, additives, flow rate, potential adverse effects, how to avoid occluding tubing, and what to report.	Information educates patient about purpose of continued infusion therapy, what to report, and how to maintain VAD patency.
10. Discard used supplies.	
EVALUATION	
1. Observe patient every 1–2 hours or at established intervals per employer policy for function, intactness, and patency of IV system; correct infusion rate; and type and amount of IV solution infused.	Ensures delivery of prescribed volume over prescribed time and decreases risk of fluid and electrolyte imbalance.
2. Evaluate patient to determine response to therapy (e.g., laboratory values, I&O, weights, vital signs, postprocedure assessments).	Provides ongoing evaluation of patient's fluid status.

STEP	RATIONALE
EVALUATION	
3. Monitor patient for signs of FVE, FVD, or signs and symptoms of electrolyte imbalances.	Early recognition of complications leads to prompt treatment.
4. Evaluate patient at established intervals per employer policy for signs and symptoms of IV-related complications.	Prevents complications that compromise integrity of VAD or cause inaccurate IV solution flow rate.
5. Use teach-back: "We talked about the importance of running your IV solutions continuously. I want to be sure I explained this clearly. Tell me in your own words what you should do if you notice that the IV is not dripping." Develop a revised teaching plan if patient or caregiver is unable to teach back correctly.	Determines patient's and caregiver's level of understanding of instructional topic.

Unexpected Outcomes	Related Interventions
1. Flow rate is incorrect; patient receives too little or too much solution.	• Notify health care provider if patient's anticipated infusion is 100–200 mL less than or greater than anticipated (per employer policy). • Evaluate patient for signs and symptoms of adverse effects of infusion (e.g., FVD or FVE). • Determine and correct cause of incorrect flow rate (e.g., change in position, tubing kink, loss of IV patency or intactness). • Use EID when accurate flow rate is critical.
2. Patient experiences fluid and/or electrolyte imbalances.	• Notify health care provider. • Anticipate prescriptions for changes in IV solution or additives.

Communication and Documentation

- Document in progress notes or on appropriate flow sheet in EHR or chart the IV solution, rate of infusion, and integrity and patency of system.
- Document IV solution and rate of infusion in drops per minute (gtt/min) for infusions via gravity or millilitres per hour (mL/hr).
- Document integrity and patency of system including VAD according to employer policy.
- Document use of any EID or control device and identification number on that device, if required by employer policy.
- Document patient response (e.g., laboratory values, I&O, weights, vital signs, postprocedure assessments) to therapy and unexpected outcomes (e.g., signs and symptoms of FVE, FVD, or IV-related complications).
- Document patient's and caregiver's level of understanding following instruction.
- At change of shift or when leaving on break, report rate of infusion and volume of solution remaining to nurse in charge or next nurse assigned to care for patient.

Special Considerations

Teaching

- Inform patient of new solution, additives, and potential side effects, including those to report to the nurse.
- Instruct patient to notify nurse or UCP if flow rate slows or IV container is empty.

Care in the Community: Home Management

- Ensure that patient and caregiver are willing and able to perform an IV solution change.
- Teach patient and caregiver how to perform an IV solution change. Observe them as they perform the procedure.

✦ SKILL 29.4 Changing Administration Sets (Infusion Tubing)

NSO *Nursing Skills Online Maintenance of Intravenous Fluid Therapy Management Module 14 / Lesson 3*

Maintaining the integrity of the IV system through the conscientious use of infection prevention principles is critical to achieving positive patient outcomes. To prevent entry of bacteria into the bloodstream, sterility must be maintained during tubing and solution changes. In addition to the main tubing, the IV system may also include add-on devices (e.g., filters, extension sets) that connect to the primary administration set. Secondary administration sets may be used as a method to administer medications in conjunction with the primary infusion (e.g., antibiotics). Luer-Lok needleless connectors are recommended to prevent accidental tubing disconnection (Gorski et al., 2021). Administration sets are replaced whenever a vascular access site change occurs (Gorski et al., 2021) or if the IV solution or tubing becomes damaged. Factors that determine administration set changes include suspected contamination, type of solution infusing, and frequency of the infusion. Follow employer policy for specific requirements (Table 29.5).

Administration sets used for parenteral nutrition (see Chapter 33) and blood or blood products (see Chapter 30) have specific criteria with which nurses need to be familiar (see employer policy). Whenever possible, schedule IV administration set changes when it is time to hang a new IV container (see Skill 29.3).

Delegation and Collaboration

The skill of changing IV administration sets may be delegated to other health care team members if they have had appropriate education, the skill is within their governing body scope of practice, and it is approved by employer policy.

TABLE 29.5

Intravenous Administration Set Changes

Primary and Secondary Continuous Infusions	Primary Intermittent Infusions	Use of Add-on Devices
• Change no more frequently than every 96 hours for solutions *other* than lipid, blood, or blood products. • In addition to routine changes, change the administration set whenever the short peripheral IV site is changed or a new CVAD is placed. • If the secondary set is removed from the primary set, the secondary set is now an intermittent set and should be changed every 24 hours.	• Should be changed every 24 hours because of increased risk of infection with repeated disconnecting and reconnecting of administration set. • Aseptically attach a new, sterile covering device to the Luer end of the administration set after each intermittent use. *Avoid* attaching the exposed end of the administration set to the port on the same set (e.g., looping).	• Should be minimized because each is a potential source of contamination and disconnection. • Use of administration sets with devices as part of the set is preferred. • Aseptically change with insertion of new VAD or with each administration set replacement. • Change if the integrity of the product is compromised or suspected of being compromised.

CVAD, Central vascular access device; *IV,* intravenous; *VAD,* vascular access device.
Adapted from Gorski, L. A., Hadaway, L., Hagle, M. E., et al. (2021). Infusion Therapy Standards of Practice, 8th edition. *Journal of Infusion Nursing, 44*(1S), S1–S224. https://www.aspirus.org/Uploads/Public/Documents/Library/Infusion_Therapy_Standards_of_Practice,_8th.1.pdf

The skill of changing IV administration sets cannot be delegated to a UCP. The nurse instructs the UCP to report the following to the nurse immediately:

- Any leakage from or around the IV administration set
- If tubing has become contaminated (e.g., lying on the floor)

Equipment

- Clean gloves
- Microdrip or macrodrip IV administration set as appropriate
- Single-use antiseptic swab(s), according to employer policy
- Commercially prepared 10-mL barrel prefilled 0.9% NS syringe(s)
- Add-on device as necessary (e.g., filters, extension set, needle-free connector)
- Tubing label

STEP	RATIONALE
ASSESSMENT	
1. Identify patient using at least two person-specific identifiers (e.g., name and date of birth, or name and medical record number) according to employer policy.	Ensures correct patient. Complies with Accreditation Canada's standards and improves patient safety (Accreditation Canada, 2020).
2. Throughout the procedure, the 4 moments for hand hygiene are to be implemented; hand hygiene should occur before initial patient (or patient environment) contact, before an aseptic procedure, after body fluid exposure risk, and after patient (or patient environment) contact. Additional hand hygiene should be performed when hands are visibly soiled.	Proper hand hygiene helps prevent spread of infectious agents to health care providers.
3. Note date and time when IV administration set was last changed (see Table 29.5 for recommendations on administration set changes).	Decreases risk of infection.
4. Assess IV administration set for puncture, contamination, or occlusion, which requires immediate change.	Compromised tubing results in fluid leakage and bacterial contamination.
5. Determine patient understanding of need for continued infusion therapy.	Reinforces need for further instruction.

NURSING DIAGNOSES

- Insufficient knowledge regarding infusion therapy
- Potential for infection

Related factors and risk factors are individualized on the basis of patient's condition or needs.

PLANNING

STEP	RATIONALE
1. Expected outcomes following completion of procedure:	
• Patient experiences no leakage of solution from or around IV administration set.	Intact system decreases risk of microbial contamination.
• Patient's IV administration set is patent, and patient receives infusion therapy as prescribed.	Brief interruption of IV infusion does not result in occlusion of VAD.

STEP	RATIONALE
PLANNING	
• Patient's VAD remains patent, and site is free from signs and symptoms of IV-related complications.	Adherence to administration set changes decreases risk of complications.
• Patient and caregiver are able to explain purpose of tubing change and how patient can avoid occlusion of tubing.	Demonstrates learning.
2. Prepare patient by explaining procedure, its purpose, and what is expected of them.	Decreases anxiety, promotes cooperation, and prevents sudden movement of extremity, which could dislodge IV catheter.
3. Coordinate IV administration set changes with solution changes when possible.	Decreases number of times system is open.
4. Collect equipment.	Provides easy access to equipment for efficient procedure.
IMPLEMENTATION	
1. Open new infusion set and connect add-on pieces (e.g., filters, extension tubing) using ANTT. Keep protective coverings over infusion spike and distal adapter. Place roller clamp about 2–2.5 cm (1–2 inches) below drip chamber, and move roller clamp to "off" position. Secure all connections.	Maintaining proximity of roller clamp to drip chamber allows more accurate regulation of flow rate. Securing connections reduces risk of air emboli and infection developing later on. Protective covers reduce entrance of microorganisms. All connections should be of Luer-Lok type (Gorski et al., 2021).
2. Apply clean gloves.	Reduces transmission of microorganisms.
3. Prepare IV administration set with new IV container. (See Skill 29.2.)	When possible, coordinate IV administration set changes with solution changes or when new VAD inserted.
4. Preparing IV administration set (tubing) with existing continuous IV infusion bag:	When solution change is not required.
a. Move roller clamp on new IV administration set to "off" position.	Prevents fluid spillage.
b. Slow rate of infusion through old tubing to KVO rate using EID or roller clamp.	Prevents occlusion of VAD.
c. Compress and fill drip chamber of old tubing.	Ensures that drip chamber remains full until new tubing is changed.
d. Invert container and remove old tubing by pulling out the spike. Hold previously used spike to retain pressure of gravity while keeping the new spike sterile and upright.	Solution in drip chamber will continue to run and maintain catheter patency.
e. Insert spike of new infusion tubing into solution container. Hang solution bag on IV pole, then compress drip chamber on new tubing and release, allowing it to fill one-third to one-half full.	Permits drip chamber to fill and promotes rapid, smooth flow of solution through tubing.
f. Prime air out of IV administration set by filling with IV solution per Skill 29.2. Return roller clamp to "off" position after priming tubing (filled with IV solution). Replace protective cover on end of IV administration set. Place end of adapter near patient's IV site.	Priming ensures that IV administration set is clear of air before connection with VAD and filled with IV solution. Closing clamp prevents accidental loss of fluid. Maintains sterility. Equipment is positioned for quick connection of new tubing.
g. Stop EID or turn roller clamp on old tubing to "off" position.	Prevents fluid spillage.
5. Re-establish infusion.	
a. Gently disconnect old tubing from extension tubing (or from IV catheter hub) and quickly insert Luer-Lok end of new tubing or saline lock into extension tubing connection or IV catheter hub.	Allows smooth transition from old to new tubing, minimizing time that system is open.
b. For continuous infusion, open roller clamp on new administration set and regulate drip rate using roller clamp *or* insert tubing into EID, program according to prescribed rate, and initiate infusion.	Ensures catheter patency and prevents occlusion.
c. Attach piece of tape or preprinted label with date and time of IV administration set change onto tubing below drip chamber.	Provides reference to determine next time for tubing change.
d. Form loop of tubing and secure it to patient's arm with strip of tape.	Avoids accidental pulling against site and stabilizes catheter.
6. Remove spike and discard in sharps container. Discard old administration set. Remove and dispose of gloves.	Reduces transmission of microorganisms.

STEP	RATIONALE
EVALUATION	
1. Observe patient every 1–2 hours or at established intervals per employer policy for function, intactness, and patency of IV system and leaking at connection sites.	Ensures that IV system is functioning appropriately and minimizes risk of infection caused by breach in system integrity.
2. Evaluate patient at established intervals per employer policy for signs and symptoms of IV-related complications.	Prevents complications that compromise integrity of VAD or cause inaccurate IV solution flow rate.

Unexpected Outcomes	Related Interventions
1. IV solution infuses more slowly than prescribed.	• Check for positional change that affects rate, height of IV container, kinking of tubing, or obstruction. • Check for patency by opening roller clamp. • Check VAD site for complications. • Consult health care provider for new prescription to provide necessary fluid volume.

Communication and Documentation

- Document tubing change, type of solution, volume, and rate of infusion in progress notes in EHR or chart. Use a special infusion therapy flow sheet for parenteral solutions per employer policy.
- Document patient's and caregiver's understanding of what IV problems they should report.

Special Considerations

Teaching

- Instruct patient to notify nurse if fluid leaks from or around IV site or tubing or if tubing separates from catheter.

Care in the Community: Home Management

- Ensure that patient is able and willing to perform IV administration set change and maintain access site or that there is a reliable person at home to provide this infusion therapy care.
- Instruct patient or caregiver in procedure for performing a sterile tubing change. Observe them as they perform the procedure.

✦ SKILL 29.5 Changing a Short Peripheral Intravenous Catheter Dressing

NSO *Nursing Skills Online Maintenance of Intravenous Fluid Therapy Management Module 14 / Lesson 4*

VAD insertion and maintenance require strict adherence to infection prevention measures to prevent complications (e.g., CABSI, phlebitis, loss of access). TSM dressing changes should be performed every 5 to 7 days, while gauze dressing changes should be performed every 2 days; when dressing is loose, wet, or visibly soiled; or when integrity is compromised (Gorski et al., 2021). If a gauze dressing is underneath a TSM, it should be changed every 2 days (Gorski et al., 2021). Gauze dressing is no longer recommended, except when required for patient care. Stabilization of short PIVCs decreases the risk of catheter-related complications (mechanical and bacterial phlebitis) and premature loss of access caused by catheter movement. Preferred options for stabilization include a securement TSM dressing with a border or a TSM film dressing with an additional engineered stabilization device (ESD). Use of sterile tape or surgical strips should be avoided because they are not an effective substitute for securement dressings or an ESD (Gorski et al., 2021).

Delegation and Collaboration

The skill of changing a short PIVC dressing may be delegated to other health care providers if they have had appropriate education, the skill is within their governing body scope of practice, and it is approved by employer policy. Assessment and care of PIVCs require effective communication and a collaborative team approach.

The skill of changing a PIVC dressing cannot be delegated to a UCP. The nurse instructs the UCP about the following:

- Reporting to the nurse immediately if dressing is visibly soiled, loose, or wet or if patient reports that dressing is moist or loose
- Protecting PIVC dressing during hygiene and ADLs

Equipment

- Single-use antiseptic swabs (2% CHG in 70% alcohol solution [preferred], povidone–iodine, or 70% alcohol)
- Sterile TSM dressing (with border preferred), or TSM dressing and added ESD
- Clean gloves

STEP	RATIONALE
ASSESSMENT	
1. Identify patient using at least two person-specific identifiers (e.g., name and date of birth, or name and medical record number) according to employer policy.	Ensures correct patient. Complies with Accreditation Canada's standards and improves patient safety (Accreditation Canada, 2020).

STEP	RATIONALE
ASSESSMENT	
2. Throughout the procedure, the 4 moments for hand hygiene are to be implemented; hand hygiene should occur before initial patient (or patient environment) contact, before an aseptic procedure, after body fluid exposure risk, and after patient (or patient environment) contact. Additional hand hygiene should be performed when hands are visibly soiled.	Proper hand hygiene helps prevent spread of infectious agents to health care providers.
3. Review patient chart to determine type of dressing and when last changed. Dressing should be labelled with date and time applied and insertion date of PIVC.	TSM dressings are changed at least every 7 days or immediately if dressing integrity is compromised. Gauze dressings are used only for patients with sensitivities; they are no longer recommended because they prevent assessment of the site (Gorski et al., 2021, p. S119). If dressing integrity is compromised, there is increased risk of infection or PIVC dislodgement.
4. Assess continuing need for device and remove if indicated.	
5. Assess patient's understanding of the procedure, including the need to hold affected extremity still during dressing change.	Promotes cooperation and active participation in person-centred care.

NURSING DIAGNOSES

- Pain or discomfort
- Insufficient knowledge regarding infusion therapy
- Potential for infection
- Potential for loss of venous access

Related factors and risk factors are individualized on the basis of patient's condition or needs.

STEP	RATIONALE
PLANNING	
1. Expected outcomes following completion of procedure:	
• Patient's PIVC remains patent and site is free from signs and symptoms of infusion-related complications.	Proper care maintains IV site.
• Patient and caregiver can explain procedure and purpose of PIVC dressing change.	Demonstrates learning.
2. Explain procedure and purpose to patient and caregiver. Explain that patient will need to hold affected extremity still. Explain how long procedure will take.	Decreases anxiety, encourages cooperation, and promotes active participation in person-centred care.
IMPLEMENTATION	
1. Organize equipment on a clean, clutter-free bedside stand or over-bed table. Wipe surface with antiseptic wipe prior to use.	Reduces transmission of infection and contamination of equipment (Gorski et al., 2021).
2. Apply clean gloves.	Reduces transmission of microorganisms.
3. Assess PIVC insertion site for signs and symptoms of infusion-related complications. If complication exists, determine whether PIVC requires removal.	Identifies complications that compromise integrity of PVAD and may necessitate its replacement. Presence of the following complications indicate the need for PIVC removal: redness, swelling, leakage, drainage, or pain or discomfort.
4. Remove existing dressing. Stabilize catheter with nondominant hand (see Step 4 illustration). Remove dressing by pulling dressing away from the skin from proximal edge toward insertion site (Gorski et al., 2021). Repeat on all sides until dressing has been removed. Use alcohol swab on TSM dressing next to patient's skin to loosen dressing.	Technique minimizes discomfort and injury to skin during removal. Stabilization of the catheter prevents loss of access. Removing dressing parallel and close to the skin in slow motion helps prevent MARSI.

STEP	RATIONALE

IMPLEMENTATION

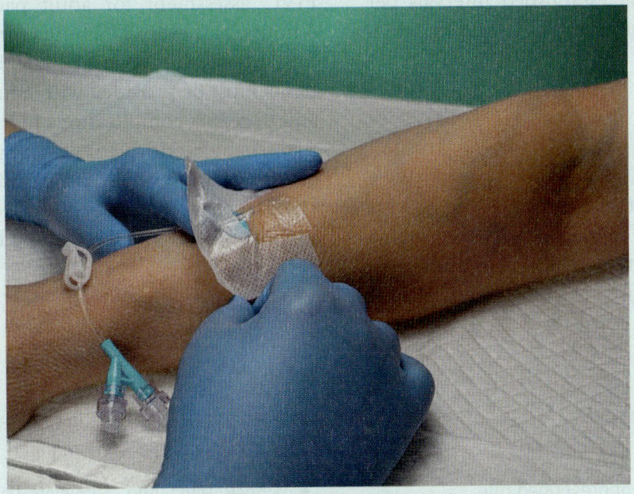

STEP 4 Remove TSM dressing. *(Courtesy Patrick Coble.)*

Critical Decision Point *Stabilize catheter throughout process while maintaining asepsis. If patient is restless or uncooperative, it is helpful to have another staff member help with the procedure.*

STEP	RATIONALE
5. Perform skin antisepsis at insertion site with 2% CHG and 70% alcohol swab using friction in back-and-forth motion for at least 30 seconds, and allow to dry completely (minimum of 30 seconds). Alternative antiseptic solutions may be used for patient sensitivities (alcohol, povidone–iodine, CHG).	Reduces incidence of catheter-related infections. Allow any skin antiseptic agent to fully dry for complete antisepsis and to prevent MARSI (Gorski et al., 2021).
6. Optional: Apply skin protectant to areas where an adhesive will attach to skin. Avoid area directly around insertion site. Allow to dry.	Apply skin barrier solution to help protect skin integrity, prevent irritation from adhesive, and promote adhesion of dressing.
7. Apply sterile dressing over site (procedures differ; follow employer policy and procedures and manufacturer guidelines) (see Skill 29.1).	Protects catheter insertion site and minimizes risk of infection. TSM dressing allows visualization of insertion site and surrounding area for assessment of complications (Gorski et al., 2021).
8. Remove and discard gloves and used equipment.	Prevents transmission of microorganisms.
9. Secure extension tubing with tape. Do not tape over dressing.	Prevents accidental dislodgement of PIVC. Provides safety and comfort for patient.
10. Label dressing per employer policy and procedure. Information on label includes date of dressing change and initials.	Communicates type of device and time interval for dressing change and site rotation.

EVALUATION

STEP	RATIONALE
1. Evaluate function and patency of PIVC after dressing change by doing the following: **a.** Swab the needle-free connector, then flush with a commercially prepared 10-mL barrel prefilled 0.9% NS syringe. Assess the site for signs and symptoms of complications and ask if patient is experiencing any discomfort. **b.** Observe flow rate for continuous infusion; check for alarms if using an EID. Assess site for signs and symptoms of complications and ask if patient is experiencing any discomfort.	Validates that the PIVC is patent and functioning correctly. Manipulation of catheter and tubing may cause PIVC dislodgement.

STEP	RATIONALE
EVALUATION	
2. Assess patient and insertion site at established intervals per employer policy for signs and symptoms of PIVC- and infusion-related complications.	PIVC assessment for adult patients is required minimally every 4 hours, and every 1–2 hours for critically ill or sedated patients and for patients with cognitive impairment (Gorski et al., 2021). Outpatients must be provided with education to perform daily assessments and to report complications to a health care provider. Assessment is critical for detecting early signs of infection, infiltration, or extravasation or inaccurate infusion of solutions or medications.
3. Use teach-back: "I want to be sure that I explained the reasons why we change the IV dressing. Tell me in your own words the problems that you would report that would require us to change the dressing." Develop a revised teaching plan if patient or caregiver is unable to teach back correctly.	Determines whether additional education is required to promote and support patient safety regarding IV dressing care and maintenance.

Unexpected Outcomes	Related Interventions
1. PIVC is removed or dislodged accidentally.	• Restart new PIVC site in other extremity or above previous insertion site if continued therapy is required.
2. Solution or medication is not infusing at prescribed rate.	• Check PIVC and administration set tubing for bending, kinking, or dislodgement. • Check if infusion is dependent on patient's arm position. • Check and adjust height of infusion container. • Ensure that there are no signs and symptoms of infiltration or extravasation at insertion site or surrounding PIVC location.

Communication and Documentation

- Document in progress notes in patient's EHR or chart the time and date the PIVC dressing was changed, reason for the change, type of dressing material used, patency of system, description of PIVC site, and patient tolerance.

DOCUMENTATION EXAMPLE

PIVC dressing changed following shower. TSM (transparent semipermeable membrane) dressing applied. PIVC remains intact and patent. Site clean, dry, and pain-free. Patient tolerated procedure well.

Special Considerations

Pediatric

- More frequent assessment of the PIVC site and infusion therapy is required for neonatal and pediatric patients (hourly at a minimum) (Gorski et al., 2021).
- Pediatric patients are not always able to understand explanations fully. Presence of a parent or security toy during the procedure helps decrease fear and increase patient cooperation. Performing the procedure on patient's toy or doll first may help with understanding and cooperation.
- Help from a second health care provider or parent is often required to keep patient still and prevent PIVC dislodgement.
- Use CHG with care in premature infants and those under 2 months of age because of the risks of skin irritation and chemical burns (Gorski et al., 2021).
- Dried povidone–iodine should be removed with sodium chloride or sterile water for neonates with compromised skin integrity (Gorski et al., 2021).

Gerontological

- Many older persons have fragile skin; prevent skin tears by minimizing the use of tape directly on the skin. Use a skin barrier solution prior to applying dressing to decrease risks associated with MARSI.
- Site assessment by palpation is very important for detecting fluid infiltration. Visual assessment alone may not be adequate to detect accumulating fluid in the tissue because older persons tend to have decreased elasticity of skin and loose skinfolds. Patients may not experience discomfort before there is a large amount of fluid infiltration owing to their decreased tactile sensations.

Care in the Community: Home Management

- Educate patient and caregiver about the signs and symptoms of PIVC- and infusion-related complications.
- Acknowledge to patient and caregiver that dressing change procedures in the community setting may be different from those used in health care facilities, and provide them with a rationale and reassurance.
- Observe patient and caregiver as they perform hand hygiene.
- Ensure that patient and caregiver are aware of the need to protect PIVC site during bathing or showering and that the site cannot be submerged in water. Instruct patient and caregiver to cover the site with an occlusive plastic wrap or bag to keep the dressing dry and intact.
- Teach patient and caregiver what to do if dressing becomes compromised. If PIVC falls out or becomes dislodged, instruct them to apply gauze with enough pressure to stop any bleeding and to notify the health care provider.

PROCEDURAL GUIDELINE 29.1 *Removing a Short Peripheral Intravenous Catheter*

NSO *Nursing Skills Online Intravenous Fluid Administration Module 13 / Lesson 4*

A short PIVC is removed by the health care provider when the prescribed therapy is completed or no longer needed for the plan of care, or if removal is clinically indicated because of a complication (e.g., phlebitis, infiltration, or catheter occlusion). The technique for removing a PIVC follows infection prevention guidelines to minimize the likelihood of the patient's acquiring an infection.

Delegation and Collaboration

The skill of removing a PIVC may be delegated to other health care team members if they have had appropriate education, the skill is within their governing body scope of practice, and it is approved by employer policy. The skill of removing a PIVC cannot be carried out by a UCP. The nurse instructs the UCP to report the following to the nurse immediately:

- Any bleeding at the site after the catheter has been removed
- Any indications of pain by the patient or observation of redness at the site by the patient postremoval

Equipment

- Clean gloves
- Sterile 5 cm × 5 cm (2 inch × 2 inch) or 10 cm × 10 cm (4 inch × 4 inch) gauze sponge or small adhesive dressing
- Tape

Procedural Steps

1. Identify patient using at least two person-specific identifiers (e.g., name and date of birth, or name and medical record number) according to employer policy.
2. Throughout the procedure, the 4 moments of hand hygiene are to be implemented; hand hygiene should occur before initial patient (or patient environment) contact, before an aseptic procedure, after body fluid exposure risk, and after patient (or patient environment) contact. Additional hand hygiene should be performed when hands are visibly soiled.
3. Key assessments prior to removal of PIVC include identifying whether the patient is on any anticoagulant or antiplatelet therapy or has a disorder that causes slow clotting (*Rationale:* Such therapies can prolong clotting time and delay hemostasis). If required, review accuracy and completeness of health care provider's prescription for discontinuation of PIVC, if required.
4. Apply clean gloves. Palpate catheter site through intact dressing.
5. Assess patient's understanding of the reason for PIVC removal.
6. Explain procedure to patient before removing catheter.
7. If PIVC connected to administration set, turn administration set roller clamp to "off" position, or turn EID off and turn roller clamp to "off" position.
8. Carefully remove PIVC dressing per Skill 29.5.

Critical Decision Point *Never use scissors to remove tape or dressing because you may accidentally cut the catheter.*

9. Place clean, sterile gauze above insertion site and, using dominant hand, withdraw catheter using a slow, steady motion while keeping the hub parallel to the skin (see Step 9 illustration).

Critical Decision Point *Do not raise or lift catheter before it is completely out of the vein to avoid trauma or hematoma formation.*

10. Apply pressure to site for a minimum of 30 seconds, until bleeding has stopped. If patient has increased clotting time, maintain pressure until hemostasis occurs.
11. Apply clean, folded gauze dressing over insertion site and secure with tape or a small adhesive dressing.
12. Inspect catheter for intactness after removal; note tip integrity and length.
13. Discard used supplies; remove and discard gloves.
14. Document procedure in patient's medical record in EHR or chart.
15. Ensure patient understands purpose of PIVC dressing, that dressing should remain in place for a minimum of 24 hours, and need to report any signs and symptoms of insertion site complications to health care provider.

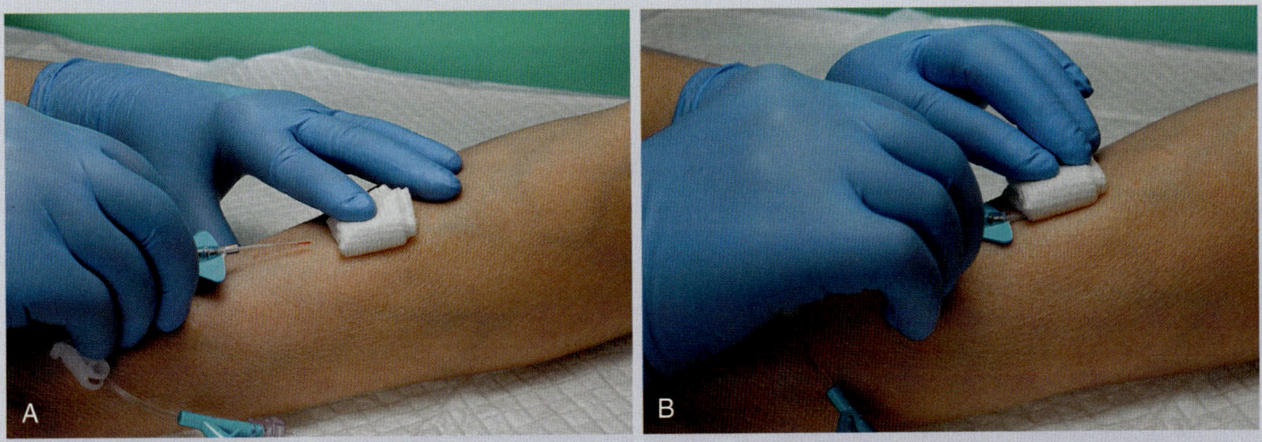

STEP 9 PIVC removal. A, Apply pressure to site. B, Cover site and remove catheter. *(Courtesy Patrick Coble.)*

✦ SKILL 29.6 Caring for Patients With Central Vascular Access Devices

The selection of the most appropriate CVAD for infusion therapy must be based on patient assessments, which may include intended length of treatment (greater than 7 days); type of infusion; patient characteristics such as age, vascular history, and comorbidities; and the care environment. Selecting the most appropriate device is critical to patient clinical outcomes, safety, and patient satisfaction.

CVAD selection requires critical thinking and assessment, along with interprofessional collaboration. The following are evidence-informed indications for use of a CVAD:

- Continuous vesicant therapy
- Solutions with an osmolarity greater than 900 mOsm/L
- History of poor peripheral access
- Clinical instability
- Complex care with multiple infusion needs, total parenteral nutrition (TPN), and for long-term infusion therapy

A CVAD differs from a peripheral VAD (PIVC) or midline in terms of where the tip of the catheter is located. PIVCs and midlines terminate in peripheral veins, while CVADs terminate in a centrally located vein. The ideal CVAD tip location for upper-body catheter insertion is in the distal superior vena cava at the cavoatrial junction. Catheters inserted from the femoral vein should terminate in the inferior vena cava above the level of the diaphragm (CVAA, 2019).

CVADs are categorized as nontunnelled, tunnelled, implanted (IVAD), and peripherally inserted (PICC) (Fig. 29.4). A tunnelled catheter is shown in Fig. 29.5. They may be designed for power injection and are made of different materials (e.g., polyurethane, silicone, or coated with antimicrobial or antithrombotic materials). Nurses must be able to identify each type of catheter and be educated about appropriate access, use, care, and maintenance of the device.

CVADs can be nonvalved (clamps present) or have a valve located either distally or proximally. Distally located valves are referred to as Groshong catheters and have a rounded catheter tip (see Fig. 29.4, *B*). The valve is distally located on the side of the catheter and is pressure activated by infusion or aspiration. When the catheter is not in use, the valve remains closed. The valve helps prevent reflux of blood into the catheter, reducing the risk of occlusion, and also prevents air embolism or blood loss if the needle-free connector is removed. Proximal valves are located close to the catheter hub and provide the same benefits (e.g., PASV or Solo valve). Valved catheters are locked with 0.9% NS when not in use to prevent occlusion and maintain patency.

Nonvalved CVADs, similar to a straw, are open and thus require clamps on the external segments to remain closed when the catheter is not in use, to prevent reflux of blood into the catheter tip, and to prevent the risk of air embolism or blood loss if the needle-free connector or administration set is removed. There is insufficient clinical evidence to recommend only locking with heparin lock solution. Randomized controlled trials have shown equivalent outcomes with heparin lock and preservative-free 0.9% NS (Gorski et al., 2021).

CVADs have single or multiple lumens. The choice of the number of lumens depends on the patient's condition and prescribed therapy. Evidence-informed practice recommends selecting the smallest gauge and the fewest number of lumens suitable for the patient's prescribed therapy (CVAA, 2019). Patients who require numerous infusions and blood samplings may have a device placed with more than one lumen, allowing simultaneous administration of solutions and medications. (For blood sampling from a CVAD, see Skill 9.8.) In addition, the use of multiple lumens allows for the administration of incompatible solutions or medications at the same time. Access to each lumen occurs via the needle-free connector attached to the catheter hub.

An IVAD has a reservoir (port body) placed in a pocket under the skin, with the catheter tip placed at the cavoatrial junction (Fig. 29.6). IVADs have no external lumen or hub. They are accessed using a noncoring needle of the appropriate gauge and length. The noncoring needle is inserted using sterile technique at a 90-degree

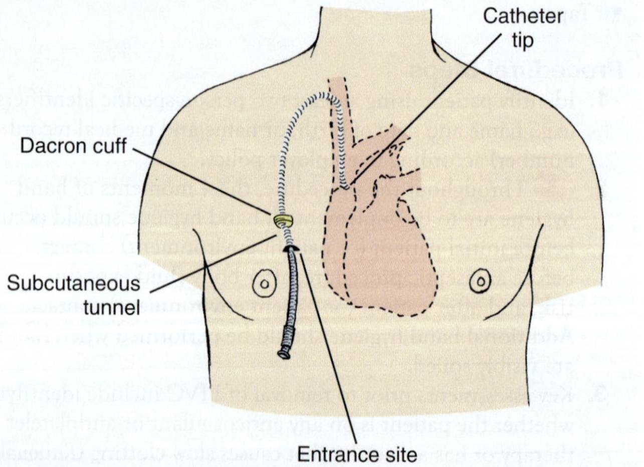

FIG 29.5 **Tunnelled catheter placement, with terminal tip location at the cavoatrial junction.**

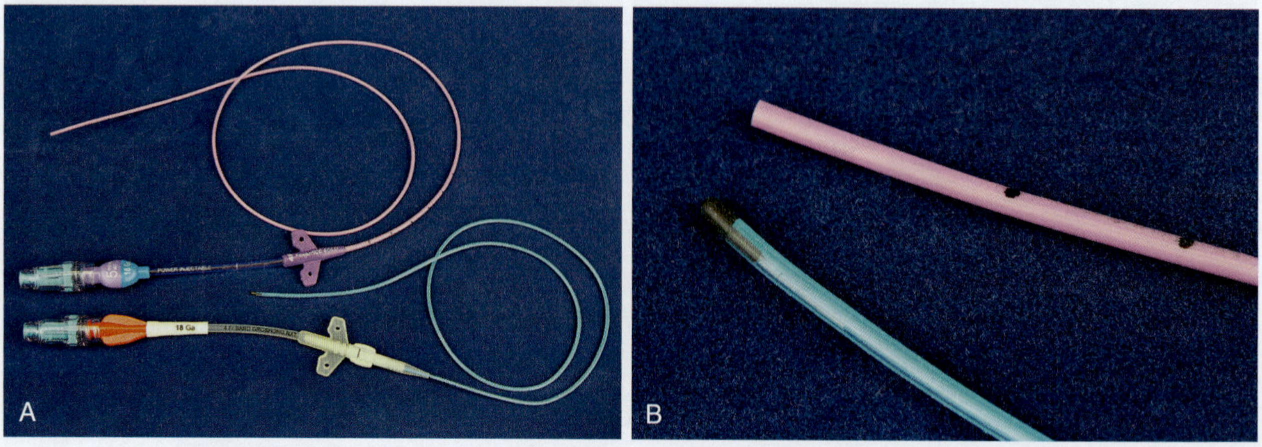

FIG 29.4 **A, Peripherally inserted central catheters (PICCs). B, PICC tips.** *(Courtesy Burl Jantzen.)*

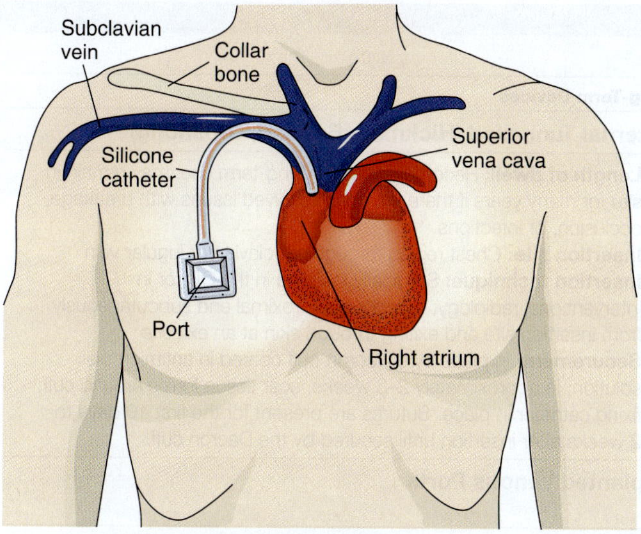

FIG 29.6 Implanted port body and catheter.

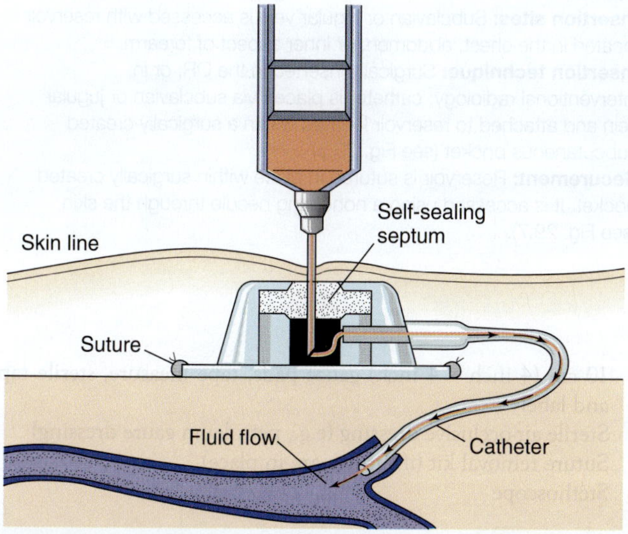

FIG 29.7 Cross-section of implanted vascular access device (VAD) showing access with noncoring needle.

angle through the skin and into the port septum until it hits the back of the port body (Fig. 29.7). IVADs may be valved or nonvalved. To maintain patency when not required for infusion therapy, an IVAD requires a monthly flushing with 0.9% NS. Alternative locking solutions may be indicated according to patient condition, employer policy, and manufacturer instructions for use.

Complications associated with CVADs include intraluminal or extraluminal infections. A local infection can develop around the catheter insertion site or in the pocket of the implanted reservoir. A more serious infection of the bloodstream may be caused by contamination during insertion of the catheter (e.g., from the patient's skin or health care provider's hands), migration of microbes during catheter dwell time, manipulation of the hub, contaminated solutions, or the presence of endogenous microbes. Contamination during care and maintenance is of particular concern and can be influenced by preventive approaches (Gorski et al., 2021). CABSIs are very serious; therefore, bundling of prevention activities (e.g., CVAD insertion bundle) is recommended because it decreases this preventable complication (Gorski et al., 2021; Moureau, 2019).

The key components of a CVAD insertion bundle are as follows:

- Hand hygiene before providing any vascular access and device care.
- Maximal sterile barrier precautions with insertion. (Inserter wears a cap, mask, and sterile gloves and gown, and a large, sterile drape is placed over the patient during insertion.)
- Skin antisepsis with 2% CHG and 70% alcohol.
- Optimal catheter site selection, with avoidance of the femoral vein for central vascular access in adult patients.
- Daily assessment of the CVAD catheter and insertion site, with prompt removal when no longer required for patient plan of care.

Nurses must have evidence-informed knowledge of all CVADs (Table 29.6) to provide the most appropriate care and maintenance techniques, to prevent complications, and to provide safe and effective infusion therapy. Nurses need to use interprofessional collaboration when caring for patients with a CVAD to optimize patient safety.

Delegation and Collaboration

The skill of managing a CVAD cannot be delegated to a UCP. The nurse instructs the UCP about the following:

- Reporting the following to the nurse immediately: bleeding or drainage at CVAD insertion site; patient indications of pain or discomfort at the site or catheter pathway; loose, wet, or soiled dressings; signs and symptoms of shortness of breath or fever; and catheter migration
- Informing the nurse if the EID alarm is triggered or if the container has a low fluid level or is empty
- Assisting with positioning of patient during CVAD insertion and care

Equipment

Site Assessment

- Nonsterile gloves
- Measuring tape (if applicable)

Flushing, Patency, and Locking

- Single-use antiseptic swab or wipe(s)
- Commercially prepared 10-mL barrel prefilled 0.9% NS syringe(s)
- Nonsterile gloves

Site Care and Dressing Change

- CVAD dressing change kit, if available, or the following supplies:
  - Sterile dressing tray
  - Single-use antiseptic applicator (2% CHG in 70% alcohol preferred); alternatives may include CHG in aqueous solution, alcohol, or povidine–iodine (for patients with sensitivities).
  - Sterile gloves
  - Nonsterile gloves
  - Single-use commercially prepared 10-mL barrel syringe prefilled 0.9% NS (one per lumen)
  - Sterile transparent securement dressing; additional ESD, if required; or alternative dressing if required for patient sensitivities
  - Skin barrier swab (for sensitive skin)

Needle-Free Connector Change

- Clean gloves
- Single-use antiseptic swab or wipe(s)
- Needle-free connector(s)
- Commercially prepared 10-mL barrel prefilled 0.9% NS syringe(s)
- Alternative lock solution if required by employer policy or manufacturer instructions.

TABLE 29.6

Central Vascular Access Devices

Short-Term Devices	Long-Term Devices
Nontunnelled Percutaneous	**External Tunnelled (Hickman, Broviac, Groshong)**
• **Length of dwell:** Days to several weeks • **Insertion sites:** Subclavian, external/internal jugular, and femoral veins • **Insertion technique:** Should be placed using ultrasound and maximum barrier precautions maintaining sterile technique; may be placed in the OR for surgical procedures, at the patient's bedside, or in the interventional radiology department • **Securement:** Sutures or an engineered subcutaneous securement device. Sutureless securement is recommended (e.g., using an integrated securement device, subcutaneous securement system, tissue adhesive, or adhesive securement device) along with dressing.	• **Length of dwell:** Recommended for long-term use; may remain in situ for many years if there are no unresolved issues with breakage, occlusion, or infections • **Insertion site:** Chest region through subclavian or jugular vein • **Insertion technique:** Surgically inserted in the OR, or in interventional radiology; tunnelling of proximal end subcutaneously from insertion site and exiting through skin at an exit site • **Securement:** In place by a Dacron cuff coated in antimicrobial solution; in approximately 2–3 weeks, scar tissue forms around cuff, fixing catheter in place. Sutures are present for the first 10 days to 2 weeks after insertion until secured by the Dacron cuff.
Peripherally Inserted Central Catheters (PICCs) (see Fig. 29.4)	**Implanted Venous Ports**
• **Length of dwell:** Recommended for up to 1 year but can remain in situ if no evidence of malfunction (e.g., occlusion, infection, or damage) • **Insertion site:** Upper arm, via basilic, cephalic, or brachial veins • **Insertion technique:** At the patient's bedside by an appropriately trained health care provider • **Securement:** Sutureless securement is recommended (e.g., using an integrated securement device, subcutaneous securement system, tissue adhesive, or adhesive securement device) along with dressing.	• **Length of dwell:** Recommended for long-term use; may remain in situ for many years if there are no unresolved issues with breakage, occlusion, or infections • **Insertion sites:** Subclavian or jugular vein is accessed with reservoir located in the chest, abdomen, or inner aspect of forearm • **Insertion technique:** Surgically inserted in the OR, or in interventional radiology; catheter is placed via subclavian or jugular vein and attached to reservoir located within a surgically created subcutaneous pocket (see Fig. 29.5) • **Securement:** Reservoir is sutured in place within surgically created pocket. It is accessed using a noncoring needle through the skin (see Fig. 29.7).

OR, Operating room.

Short-Term Removal of Central Vascular Access Device (Nontunnelled and PICC)

- Personal protective equipment (PPE) as indicated (goggles, gown, mask, and clean gloves)
- CVAD dressing change kit, which includes sterile gloves, mask, antiseptic swabs for skin disinfection, TSM dressing, 10 cm × 10 cm (4 inch × 4 inch) gauze pads, tape measure, sterile tape, and label
- Sterile air-occlusive dressing (e.g., petroleum gauze dressing)
- Suture removal kit (if sutures are in place)
- Stethoscope

STEP	RATIONALE
ASSESSMENT	
1. Identify patient using at least two person-specific identifiers (e.g., name and date of birth, or name and medical record number) according to employer policy.	Ensures correct patient. Complies with Accreditation Canada's standards and improves patient safety (Accreditation Canada, 2020).
2. Throughout the procedure, the 4 moments for hand hygiene are to be implemented; hand hygiene should occur before initial patient (or patient environment) contact, before an aseptic procedure, after body fluid exposure risk, and after patient (or patient environment) contact. Additional hand hygiene should be performed when hands are visibly soiled.	Proper hand hygiene helps prevent spread of infectious agents to health care providers.
3. Review patient chart to confirm type of CVAD, number of lumens, and previous documentation (e.g., external segment on insertion). Assess patient care needs: times for administration of IV solutions, medications, dressing change, needle-free connector change, and blood sampling (see Skill 9.8). Follow the 10 rights of medication administration (see Chapters 20 and 22).	Care and management depend on type and size of catheter or port, number of lumens, and purpose of therapy. Comparing CVAD external segment measurements facilitates early recognition of migration of displacement (CVAA, 2019).
4. Assess patient for allergies (e.g., povidone–iodine, latex, CHG, and alcohol).	Medications, solutions used during catheter insertion, and use of gloves and tape can cause serious allergic reactions.

ASSESSMENT

STEP	RATIONALE
5. Assess for proper functioning of existing CVAD before initiating therapy: check integrity of catheter, dressing, and catheter patency (ability to flush or infuse solution, and ability to aspirate blood).	Blood return should be obtained and patency confirmed before infusion of solutions or medications (Gorski et al., 2021).
6. Assess patient's knowledge of procedures and signs and symptoms of complications to report.	Provides person-centred care by determining level of instruction needed.

NURSING DIAGNOSES

- Insufficient fluid volume
- Excessive fluid volume
- Insufficient knowledge regarding care of CVAD
- Reduced skin integrity
- Potential for infection
- Potential for injury

Related factors and risk factors are individualized on the basis of patient's condition or needs.

PLANNING

STEP	RATIONALE
1. Expected outcomes following completion of procedure:	
• CVAD will remain free of signs and symptoms of complications (redness, swelling, bleeding, or discomfort at insertion site), and suture or stabilization device will remain intact to prevent catheter migration.	Catheter is patent, properly placed, and without evidence of complications.
• Solutions and medications infuse as prescribed.	Catheter remains patent.
• Patient's CVAD will have ongoing assessment, care, and maintenance according to employer policies, procedures, and guidelines.	Care and maintenance of CVAD includes assessment, site care, dressing changes, needle-free connector changes, and flushing. ANTT must be maintained for all procedures (Gorski et al., 2021).
• Blood draws for diagnostics will be obtained following employer policy to prevent erroneous laboratory results and catheter occlusion.	Catheter remains patent after blood draws.
• Patient and caregiver are able to explain purpose of CVAD and benefits to patient. Patient remains still during procedure. Patient and caregiver are able to explain IV line therapy, care, and maintenance.	Demonstrates patient's and caregiver's understanding of and competency in caring for CVAD.

IMPLEMENTATION

STEP	RATIONALE
1. Collect and organize equipment on clean, clutter-free surface.	
2. Site assessment:	
a. Apply clean gloves.	Reduces transmission of microorganisms.
b. Inspect skin integrity at CVAD insertion site and around dressing.	Identifies complications that may compromise integrity and functionality of CVAD.
c. Palpate insertion site and along catheter pathway. Assess for any discomfort, tenderness, pain, tingling, or numbness.	Identifies complications such as phlebitis, infiltration, and infection.
d. Inspect integrity of securement dressing. Dressing should be dry and intact. If applicable, measure external catheter length under dressing (e.g., PICC) (CVAA, 2019).	There is increased risk of infection or catheter migration if dressing is compromised (e.g., wet, loose). Dressings with securement properties or the addition of an ESD decreases risk of catheter dislodgement, movement, or mechanical phlebitis (Gorski et al., 2021). Comparing CVAD external segment measurements facilitates early recognition of dislodgement or migration (CVAA, 2019).
e. If nonvalved, ensure clamps are engaged when CVAD lumen(s) are not in use.	Reduces the risk of occlusion and infection.
f. Verify that needle-free connector(s) are secure and free of visible debris or blood.	Prevent inadvertent disconnection and/or leaks, infection, and occlusion (Gorski et al., 2021).
3. Patency, flushing, and locking:	CVAD patency (flushing and aspiration of blood return) is assessed prior to each infusion and per employer policy if not in use. CVAD lumens are flushed and locked post medication administration, blood sampling, and discontinuing infusion.

STEP	RATIONALE
IMPLEMENTATION	
a. Prepare and purge air from commercially prepared 10-mL barrel prefilled 0.9% NS syringe(s). CVAD lumens need to be flushed with a minimum of 10 mL of 0.9% NS per CVAD lumen or as per employer policy. Flush volumes may be higher post medication administration (see Chapter 22) and blood sampling (see Skill 9.8). Prepare alternative locking solution if required (e.g., heparin). Maintain ANTT.	Air removed from all devices prior to connection to prevent air embolism (Gorski et al., 2021, p. S160). Commercially prepared prefilled syringes are designed to minimize blood reflux into catheter when disconnecting post flushing compared with a traditional syringe (Gorski et al., 2021).
Critical Decision Point *Always use a single-use commercially prepared 10-mL barrel syringe prefilled with preservative-free 0.9% sodium chloride (NS) when flushing and checking catheter patency* (Gorski et al., 2021).	
b. Vigorously scrub the needle-free connector with antiseptic swab and allow to dry. Use a new antiseptic swab before each entry.	Disinfection prior to each entry reduces intraluminal microbes and risk of infection. Scrub with alcohol swab for a minimum of 5–15 seconds and allow to dry, or use antiseptic solution according to employer policy.
c. Attach commercially prepared 10-mL barrel prefilled 0.9% NS syringe to needle-free connector, maintaining ANTT. Disengage clamp if present.	
d. Flush with 1–2 mL and then gently aspirate for free-flowing blood return. Blood return should be the colour and consistency of whole blood. Avoid aspirating into the needle-free connector and/or flush syringe.	Patency is confirmed by the ability to flush and aspirate blood return without resistance (CVAA, 2019). Assessing for blood return is not required after medication administration or discontinuing an infusion.
e. Using the same attached syringe, flush catheter with entire 10 mL using push–pause or pulsatile technique. Do not forcibly flush against resistance.	Patency is confirmed by the ability to flush and aspirate blood return without resistance (CVAA, 2019). Flushing with appropriate volume using pulsatile technique reduces the risk of catheter occlusion (Gorski et al., 2021).
(1) If using a traditional syringe for flushing (not a commercially prepared 10-mL barrel prefilled), leave 0.5–1 mL at the end before disconnecting.	Leaving 0.5–1 mL when using traditional syringe reduces risk of blood reflux and occlusions.
(2) Flush with appropriate volume according to employer policy.	
f. While flushing, assess CVAD for swelling or leaking at insertion site, signs of pain or discomfort, or for changes in patient's sense of taste or smell.	Identifies signs or symptoms of complications that require further investigation. Commercially prepared NS syringes can cause brief changes in taste and smell while flushing (CVAA, 2019).
g. Engage clamp on catheter if present (or use proper clamping sequence according to needle-free connector) and disconnect flush syringe.	Using the proper clamping sequence ensures positive pressure, minimizing risk of occlusion.
h. If more than one flush syringe required, repeat steps, omitting aspiration of blood return. OPTIONAL: Instill catheter with alternative locking solution (e.g., heparin).	
i. Repeat Steps 3b–3h for all other lumens in order to assess patency.	
j. Discard used supplies and remove gloves.	
4. Insertion site care and dressing change:	
a. Position patient in comfortable position with head slightly elevated. Have patient's arm extended for PICC or midline device.	Enables access to CVAD for providing care.
b. Prepare dressing materials. *TSM dressing:* Change at least every 5–7 days. *Nontransparent dressing:* Change at least every 2 days if unable to assess insertion site. *Nontransparent dressing under TSM:* Change at least every 2 days if unable to assess insertion site.	TSM dressings are preferred because they allow visualization of insertion site.
c. Apply clean gloves. Apply mask if required. Instruct patient to turn head away from site during dressing change or provide mask for patient.	Reduces transmission of microorganisms. Prevents spread of airborne microorganisms over CVAD insertion site.
d. Remove old TSM dressing by peeling the dressing low (close to skin) and slowly toward the insertion site. Stabilize the catheter with disposable forceps from dressing tray or with antiseptic applicator while removing the dressing.	Prevents unintentional catheter dislodgement and MARSI.

STEP	RATIONALE
IMPLEMENTATION	
e. If an additional adhesive stabilization device is present, remove catheter from adhesive stabilization device, then remove stabilization device from the skin. Lift the edge and wet with alcohol while removing. Adhesive devices are to be changed at least every 7 days. If other stabilization devices are used, check manufacturer instructions for use.	Allows for appropriate skin antisepsis; applying alcohol helps reduce the risk of MARSI; and catheter dislodgement. Subcutaneous anchor devices and tissue adhesives may require additional information (Gorski et al., 2021).

Critical Decision Point *If sutures are used for initial catheter stabilization and become loosened or are no longer intact, alternative stabilization measures should be used. Use of an ESD is recommended because sutures are associated with increased risk of infection* (Gorski et al., 2021).

STEP	RATIONALE
f. Assess catheter insertion site and surrounding skin for signs and symptoms of complications (e.g., drainage, swelling, redness, patient report of discomfort). Measure external length using a consistent method and compare to baseline. For PICC, consider measuring arm circumference at a consistent location each time (CVAA, 2019).	Detection of complications for early intervention is critical. Changes in external segment indicate terminal tip of catheter has migrated and may not be in optimal position, requiring reassessment. Increasing arm circumference could indicate thrombosis (Gorski et al., 2021).
g. Remove gloves and discard. Using ANTT, open CVAD dressing kit and other supplies on a clutter-free surface.	ANTT is required to apply new dressing.
h. Perform skin antisepsis with 2% CHG and 70% alcohol (or alternative antiseptic solution based on patient allergies or employer policy). Apply solution using a back-and-forth and up-and-down motion for a minimum of 30 seconds. Allow solution to dry completely without fanning, blotting, or blowing on skin (CVAA, 2019).	Using 2% CHG and 70% alcohol is recommended because it is a broad-spectrum antimicrobial that has an immediate and residual effect. Solution must be completely dry for safety and efficacy and to prevent chemical reactions, itching, and skin breakdown.
i. Apply skin barrier solution and allow to dry completely.	Protects irritated or fragile skin from dressing and stabilization device, if used, and minimizes risk of MARSI.
j. Apply sterile securement dressing or ESD with TSM dressing. CHG-impregnated dressings are recommended for nontunnelled CVADs.	Use of ESDs that enable visual inspection of insertion site can reduce risk of VAD complications (e.g., phlebitis, infection, migration) and unintentional loss of access (Gorski et al., 2021). Use with caution in patients with fragile skin or complicated skin pathologies and in newborns and infants (Gorski et al., 2021).
k. Apply label to dressing with date, initials, and external segment measurement (refer to employer policy).	Indicates when next dressing change is due and whether catheter dislodgement or migration has occurred.
l. Dispose of soiled supplies. Remove gloves and discard.	Reduces transmission of microorganisms.
5. Needle-free connector change:	
a. Assess whether needle-free connector change is required; inspect for any visible blood or disconnection. Determine connector style/type (neutral, negative, or positive displacement).	Needle-free connectors should be changed every 4–7 days if removed for any reason or cannot be flushed clear or if contamination is suspected (CVAA, 2019). Use the appropriate clamping and disconnect sequence for the style/type of needle-free connector (according to manufacturer instructions). Using the correct sequence reduces risk of blood reflux at tip of catheter. Reflux of blood may lead to complications of occlusion and infection.
b. Apply clean gloves.	Reduces transmission of microorganisms.
c. Prepare new sterile needle-free connector(s). Attach commercially prepared 10-mL barrel prefilled 0.9% NS syringe, and prime connector to remove air. Maintain ANTT. Leave prefilled syringe attached.	Priming needle-free connector beforehand prevents air from entering the circulatory system. Maintaining ANTT during preparation is important to reduce risk of infection.
d. Ensure clamps are closed if using a nonvalved catheter. Scrub the connection between the connector and hub of the catheter for a minimum of 15 seconds using an antiseptic swab. Remove connector and repeat the process, scrubbing the hub of the catheter including the treads. Allow to completely air dry. Hold the hub of the catheter and maintain ANTT.	Reduces risk of infection from skin contaminants and other sources.

STEP	RATIONALE
IMPLEMENTATION	
e. Attach new primed, sterile, needle-free connector to catheter hub, ensuring a finger-tight connection. Open the clamp if required and assess patency. Flush a small amount of 0.9% NS from the flush syringe, then aspirate for free-flowing blood return that is the colour and consistency of whole blood. Avoid aspirating into the needle-free connector and/or flush syringe. Then flush the catheter using a push–pause technique. Assess for any resistance: the catheter should flush easily, and the blood return should be the colour and consistency of whole blood. Disconnect the syringe according to the correct clamp disconnection sequence.	Using the appropriate flush–clamp–disconnect sequence decreases risk of catheter occlusion by preventing reflux of blood into catheter tip. If an alternative locking solution is required, scrub needle-free connector with antiseptic swab before attaching syringe, then instill.
f. Observe for any residual blood in the connector or catheter. If present, scrub the connector to disinfect and repeat flush with 10 mL of 0.9% NS using the same technique. Always flush until needle-free connector and catheter are clear of any visible blood.	
g. Repeat steps for all other lumens if present.	
h. Discard used supplies and remove gloves.	
6. Short-term CVAD removal (nontunnelled catheter and PICC) (see Table 29.6):	
a. Collaborate daily with interprofessional team to assess continued need for CVAD. Confirm and review prescription for CVAD removal.	CVADs should be removed promptly if no longer required for plan of care, or if clinically indicated on assessment of signs and symptoms of complications (e.g., dysfunction that cannot be resolved). Review employer policy and procedure for scope of practice responsibilities for CVAD removal (CVAA, 2019).
b. Review patient allergies or skin sensitivity related to supplies (e.g., latex, antiseptic, dressings).	Prevents complications and discomfort.
c. Position patient so the CVAD is below the level of the heart. For nontunnelled CVADs, position patient in supine or Trendelenburg position. Place a moisture-proof pad under arm in appropriate position.	Patient position decreases risk of air embolus upon catheter removal. Moisture-proof pad helps maintain a clean working environment.
d. Prepare supplies using ANTT on a clean, clutter-free surface.	
e. Apply appropriate PPE as indicated by employer policy (e.g., clean gloves and eye protection).	Decreases risk of bloodborne pathogen exposure to health care provider.
f. Gently remove CVAD dressing by stabilizing the catheter and pulling the dressing low (close to skin) and slowly toward the insertion site to prevent accidental removal. If removing a CHG-impregnated dressing, apply moisture from the antiseptic applicator to the gel pad to ease removal. Remove ESD or sutures according to manufacturer instructions for use and according to type of device.	Prevents unintentional catheter dislodgement and MARSI. Prevents skin tears. Allows for inspection of CVAD insertion site before removal.
g. Assess insertion site for sign and symptoms of complications (i.e., redness, drainage, swelling, infection, and skin irritation).	
h. Perform skin antisepsis with 2% CHG and 70% alcohol with a single-use applicator. Apply solution using a friction scrub in a side-to-side and up-and-down motion for a minimum of 30 seconds. Allow to air dry completely without fanning, blotting, or blowing on skin.	Using 2% CHG and 70% alcohol is the preferred antiseptic because it is a broad-spectrum antimicrobial that has an immediate as well as residual effect. Must be left to air dry for safety and efficacy. Consider alternatives for patient sensitivities or according to employer policy.
i. Remove gloves and discard. Apply sterile gloves.	Decreases risk of transmission of microorganisms.
j. Fold sterile air-occlusive dressing (e.g., petroleum gauze) and sterile gauze pad. Place at insertion site with air-occlusive dressing against skin and gauze on top; apply digital pressure.	Application of a petroleum-based dressing against the skin helps seal the skin-to-vein tract and decreases risk of air embolus.
k. Instruct patient to take a deep breath and perform Valsalva's manoeuvre *or* to hold breath while catheter is removed.	Having patient perform the Valsalva's manoeuvre or hold their breath helps prevent air from entering the circulatory system through the skin-to-vein tract (CVAA, 2019; Gorski et al., 2021).

STEP	RATIONALE

IMPLEMENTATION

Critical Decision Point *It is often necessary to apply pressure longer if patient is receiving anticoagulation therapy or has prolonged clotting times.*

STEP	RATIONALE
l. Slowly remove catheter while maintaining digital pressure. Do not pull against resistance; the catheter should be removed easily. After removal, instruct patient to breathe normally. Continue to hold until hemostasis has occurred. Assess for signs and symptoms of complications.	Slow removal helps prevent vasoconstriction, which may result in difficult removal. Pulling against resistance may cause catheter stretching and breakage, resulting in catheter or air embolus. Direct digital pressure is required to prevent bleeding, hematoma formation, and risk of air embolus (CVAA, 2019). Complications may include sudden shortness of breath, coughing, chest pain, hypotension, altered level of consciousness, arrhythmias, and thoracic pain (CVAA, 2019).
m. Leave petroleum-based dressing and sterile gauze in place and cover with a TSM dressing. Instruct patient that dressing must remain in place for at least 24 hours. Label dressing with date and initials. Ask patient to remain in supine or reclining position for 30 minutes after removal of catheter.	Decreases risk of air entering the circulatory system and protects the site from infection.
n. Inspect catheter to ensure it is intact without defect; measure to compare length to insertion length if available.	Ensures entire catheter has been removed with no risk of catheter embolus.
o. Dispose of soiled supplies; remove and dispose of gloves and PPE.	Decreases risk of transmission of microorganisms.

EVALUATION

STEP	RATIONALE
1. CVAD tip confirmation is required postinsertion to confirm preferred location (in the distal superior vena cava or at the cavoatrial junction), prior to initiating infusion therapy. Using electrocardiogram (ECG) technology is preferred because it eliminates patient exposure to radiation, decreases delays in therapy, is cost effective, and increases accuracy of tip location. Alternative methods of tip confirmation include postprocedural chest X-ray or, when CVAD is still in place, fluoroscopy (CVAA, 2019).	Catheter performance is directly related to the position of the terminal tip of the catheter. Using the most accurate method of tip confirmation helps prevent risk of complications such as vein erosion, occlusion, and infection (CVAA, 2019).
2. Daily assessment is required to determine need for CVAD.	CVADs should be removed promptly if no longer required owing to risk of catheter-related infection or catheter-related blood stream infections (CVAA, 2019).
3. Assess and monitor for immediate postinsertion complications.	Postinsertion complications may include, but are not limited to, pneumothorax, cardiac arrhythmias, bleeding, hematoma, and nerve injury (Gorski et al., 2021).
a. Auscultate breath sounds and evaluate for shortness of breath, chest pain, and absent breath sounds.	Signs and symptoms of pneumothorax develop if CVAD pierces intrathoracic space.
b. Monitor vital signs, including heart rate and rhythm.	Assesses for signs of cardiac arrhythmias. Signs and symptoms of arrhythmias may include anxiety, fatigue, fluttering in the chest, tachycardia, bradycardia, lightheadedness, dizziness, sweating and fainting.
c. Monitor patient indications of pain, numbness, tingling, or weakness.	These are signs of nerve injury from catheter insertion; other signs may include paresthesia (burning or prickling sensation) and radiating electric pain (CVAA, 2019).
d. Monitor for hematoma and bleeding.	Signs and symptoms may include persistent external bleeding, increased heart rate, low blood pressure, shortness of breath, bruising or raised dark area around insertion site, and pain or tenderness.
4. Assess patient to determine response to infusion therapy (e.g., laboratory values, I&O, weight, vital signs, postprocedure assessments).	Infusion therapy solutions and medications maintain or restore fluid and electrolyte balance. Early recognition of complications leads to prompt treatment.
5. Assess patient at established intervals for signs and symptoms of CVAD- and infusion therapy–related complications (Table 29.7) according to employer policy.	Complications may include site or systemic infection, inaccurate infusion rates, infiltration, extravasation, and occlusion. Frequently scheduled observation and assessment allow for early detection and treatment of potential complications.
6. Inspect administration set and needle-free connectors to ensure that connections are secure.	Disconnections have potential complications of air embolus, infection, leakage of medication or solutions, or errors in medication delivery (CVAA, 2019).

TABLE 29.7

Complications of Vascular Access Devices

Complication	Assessment	Prevention	Intervention
Catheter damage, breakage	At least once per shift or when flushing: • Check for leaks or holes • Observe insertion site for excess of fluid • Check for kinks at insertion site	Move position of clamps every shift (if present). When dressing is applied, ensure that catheter is positioned with gentle curve upward or in a straight pathway. Use only 10-mL barrel syringes when performing a patency check or flushing. Do not flush against resistance. Do not use sharp objects or scissors during care and maintenance.	If catheter is damaged, stop all infusions and apply a clamp between the break in the catheter and the insertion site. Determine whether catheter can be repaired; repair kits are specific to manufacturer and type of CVAD. Power-rated catheters cannot be repaired and must be removed as soon as possible if damaged.
Occlusion types: • Thrombotic • Nonthrombotic (medication precipitate) • Mechanical (kinks in the catheter internally or externally)	Check for kinks at insertion site or catheter pathway. Check whether dressing and securement are intact. Check for presence of blood in needle-free connector or catheter extension legs. Perform a patency check; should flush without resistance and have brisk blood return. Ask if patient is having any pain or discomfort. Assess patient for swelling in the hand, arm, or chest area. Consultation with health care team may be required. Chest X-ray should be used if all other causes of occlusion have been assessed. IVADs: Check only if noncoring needle is in correct placement.	When applying dressing and securement, check for kinks prior to application. Perform an NS flush before and after administering medication, using a push–pause technique. Always flush until connector and catheter are clear. Do not rely on turning up the EID to flush catheter clear. If a change in catheter patency is observed, it must be investigated and treated appropriately as soon as possible. Thrombotic occlusion will require intervention; discuss with health care provider. Do not leave an unresolved occlusion in any catheter lumen.	*Mechanical occlusions:* • Reposition patient, ask patient to take a deep breath and cough, repeat patency check; often may resolve occlusion. • Perform a dressing and needle-free connector change. • Consult with interprofessional team if unresolved; may require a venogram or chest X-ray to visually confirm cause of occlusion. Discuss treatment plan or need for catheter removal and replacement if required for plan of care. *Thrombotic occlusions:* • Consult with interprofessional team and obtain a prescription for an antithrombotic medication; follow manufacturer instructions for use.
Infection	Assess insertion site for signs and symptoms of local infection: • Redness, drainage, edema, pain or discomfort, erythema Assess patient for signs and symptoms of systemic infection: • Fever, chills, rigors • Monitor laboratory results (elevated white blood cells) • Hypotension • Pain flushing • Edema	Perform hand hygiene prior to providing any vascular access care. Maintain strict aseptic non-touch technique (ANTT®) when providing care and maintenance. Use recommended antiseptics and use according to manufacturer instructions. Ensure dressing is not loose, wet, or soiled; change dressing immediately if compromised.	Consult with interprofessional team to discuss plan of care (e.g., antibiotics, catheter salvage, or catheter removal). Obtain blood cultures if required. Follow employer policy and procedure for suspected catheter-related infections.
Dislodgement or tip migration	Measure external length of catheter every shift and compare to length postinsertion (using a consistent measurement method each time). Observe for signs and symptoms of infiltration or extravasation (e.g., leaking from site, swelling, pain). Ask if patient hears a swishing sound in the ear on side of CVAD (flushing). Assess for changes in pulse rate or rhythm. Observe for visible cuff for tunnelled catheters.	Always maintain dry and occlusive securement and dressings. Use appropriate securement devices for patient's activity level, and use additional stabilization if required (e.g., diaphoretic, restless, or confused patient). Maintain stabilization of catheter when changing dressings. Educate patient to prevent dislodgement during ADLs.	If the catheter has migrated outward and has exceeded the acceptable range noted in employer policy and procedures, follow appropriate guidelines to reconfirm tip placement and discuss with interprofessional team whether catheter can be used or must be replaced, if still required for plan of care. Do not readvance a catheter that has migrated outward. If it has migrated inward, the catheter should be pulled back to its external length at time of insertion to maintain confirmed tip placement.

TABLE 29.7

Complications of Vascular Access Devices—cont'd

Complication	Assessment	Prevention	Intervention
Skin impairment	Assess insertion site daily through TSM dressing or during dressing change for signs and symptoms of impairment such as redness, swelling, rash, skin tears or erosion, pruritis, or blisters. Ask if patient is experiencing itching or discomfort.	Assess nutritional status and consult with interprofessional team if required. Be sure to let skin antiseptics dry completely before applying dressing. Use skin barrier solutions to prevent irritation from adhesive devices or dressings. Remove dressing slowly and gently to avoid skin damage. Do not stretch TSM dressing during application. Do not reinforce loose, wet, or soiled dressing, as this can inhibit the dressing's semipermeable quality and trap moisture. Moisture increases risk of microbial colonization and subsequent risk of extraluminal infection and skin breakdown.	Change soiled or wet dressings immediately. Consider alternative antiseptic or dressing if patient experiences sensitivity. Improve patient's nutritional intake.
Infiltration, extravasation	Assess for erythema, edema, local swelling at the insertion site, malposition of the catheter tip location, patient shortness of breath, lack of blood return, pain during infusion therapy (e.g., burning, stinging).	Perform ongoing assessment of insertion site, surrounding area, and patient reports of discomfort during infusion therapy. Select correct type of VAD for prescribed infusion therapy and patient's vascular access. Assess at least once per shift for migration and potential changes in tip location. Do not rely on EID alarm or alert for infiltration or extravasation.	Consult with interprofessional team and administer antidote if applicable according to employer policy. Remove CVAD as soon as possible. Apply warm or cold compresses if applicable. Administer analgesics if required as prescribed for pain or discomfort. Outline affected area using a skin marker to provide baseline for ongoing skin assessment. Assess area at regular intervals to track progression until resolved. Use photos to track progress when possible. Use a standardized infiltration scale. Complete an adverse reaction report as required by employer policy.
Pneumothorax, hemothorax, air emboli, hydrothorax	Observe for signs of subcutaneous emphysema by palpating skin around insertion site (e.g., crackling, crinkling paper sensation). Assess for patient discomfort, dyspnea, apnea, hypoxia, tachycardia, hypotension, nausea, or confusion.	Always engage clamps on external segment of catheter (if present) when removing needle-free connector or opening the catheter system. Valved CVADs do not require a clamp because the valve remains closed unless aspirating or flushing. Purge all flush syringes, needle-free connectors, and administration sets of air before connecting to VAD.	Administer oxygen as required. Report adverse signs and symptoms to health care provider immediately. If air emboli are suspected, place patient on left side with head down. Remove catheter as prescribed.

ADLs, Activities of daily living; *CLABSI*, central line–associated bloodstream infection; *CVAD*, central vascular access device; *EID*, electronic infusion device; *IV*, intravenous; *IVAD*, intravenous access device; *MARSI*, medical adhesive–related skin injury; *PICC*, peripherally inserted central catheter; *TSM*, transparent semipermeable membrane; *VAD*, vascular access device.

STEP	RATIONALE
EVALUATION	
7. **Use teach-back:** Educate patient and caregiver about plan of care. This may include expected outcomes of treatment, expected duration of therapy, care and maintenance of CVAD, risks associated with CVAD and infusion therapy, and ANTT. For long-term use, ask patient or caregiver to discuss steps in care and to perform procedure (e.g., catheter site cleaning or dressing change). Instruct patient regarding when to report signs and symptoms of complications: "I want to be sure you understand when you need to report signs and symptoms of complications. Can you tell me when you should contact a health care provider?" Develop a revised teaching plan if patient or caregiver is unable to teach back correctly.	Determines patient's and caregiver's level of understanding of instructional topic. Promotes safe, person-centred care.

Unexpected Outcomes	Related Interventions
1. For CVAD complications, see Table 29.7.	• See Table 29.7.
2. Patient or caregiver is unable to explain or perform CVAD care.	• Indicates need for community care referral or additional instruction.

Communication and Documentation

- Immediately notify health care provider of signs and symptoms of any complications.
- Document catheter site care in progress notes in EHR or chart, including catheter location; size of catheter; number of lumens; condition of catheter insertion site or port site, including skin integrity, external catheter length, and midarm circumference for PICC; condition and type of securement device; date and time of dressing change; change of needle-free connectors; flushes used; patency of catheter, including presence or absence of blood return; and patient's tolerance of the procedure.
- Document patient's and caregiver's ability to explain instructions.
- Document catheter removal: patient position, appearance of site, length of catheter removed, integrity of catheter after removal, dressing applied, patient's tolerance of procedure, presence or absence of bleeding from site every 15 minutes for 1 hour, and any problems with removal.
- Document the blood draw: date, time, sample drawn, waste volume, and flushes used.
- Document unexpected outcomes and CVAD complications, health care provider notification, interventions, and patient response to treatment.

Special Considerations

Teaching

- Instruct patient to report discomfort around the site; discomfort in arms, shoulders, or side of the neck; and any shortness of breath.
- Discuss and provide written emergency measures and telephone numbers of health care personnel to be used in case of catheter damage, dislodgement, swelling, redness, or leakage at insertion site; occlusion of catheter; patient temperature above 38°C (100.4°F) (see employer policy); and shivering chills.
- Provide written instructions for dressing changes, inspection of insertion site, flushing, and tubing changes.
- Arrange for instruction and return demonstration of skills by patient or caregiver.
- Have patient or caregiver maintain a list of caregivers and telephone numbers (e.g., health care provider, nurse, social worker, pharmacist, dietitian).

Pediatric

- Central vein catheters that are of a smaller diameter and shorter length are available for children and infants.
- Take care to secure infant catheters in a manner that does not allow them to twist. Small-diameter catheters are fragile; twisting them causes them to tear.
- The amount and dosage of flush solution (heparin or NS) vary with age, size, and catheter diameter and length.
- Record volume of blood draws on I&O record.

Gerontological

- Some older persons have difficulty lying flat in bed, and a modification of the totally supine position during CVAD insertion is often necessary.
- PICC insertion may provide an alternative route of administration that reduces the risk of complications associated with subclavian or jugular insertion.

Care in the Community: Home Management

- Initiate early referral for discharge planning to social services, counsellor, or community care coordinator for assessment of resources.
- Provide patient with written list of providers for supplies and equipment.
- Provide patient with Kelly clamp *without* teeth (bulldog clamp) that can be used in the event of catheter rupture to prevent air embolism, and instruct patient in its use.
- Instruct patient or caregiver in flushing technique, site care, and dressing change, and observe as they perform the procedures.
- Instruct patient and caregiver in adaptations of hospital procedures that they can make at home (e.g., proper hand hygiene instead of sterile gloves).
- Provide education to patient and caregiver about how to recognize signs and symptoms of IV-related complications, actions to take, how to report them, and methods for preservation of CVADs.
- Assess home environment and determine suitable area for dressing changes, avoiding areas where contaminants are potential hazards.
- Provide appropriate information about home disposal of soiled dressings and equipment.

✦ REVIEW QUESTIONS

An 88-year-old patient (she/her) with a history of heart failure and gastric cancer was admitted to the hospital 24 hours ago for dehydration with mild confusion, decreased urine output, postural hypotension, and poor oral intake after receiving chemotherapy. She has been receiving D_5LR at 100 mL/hr by gravity through a peripheral intravenous catheter (PIVC) infusion since admission. Today, her daughter tells the nurse that her mother is having difficulty breathing and is asking for another pillow for her bed.

Review Questions 1 to 3 relate to the case study presented here.

1. On the basis of the daughter's information, which clinical markers should the nurse assess, and which additional signs and symptoms would the nurse expect to find?
2. At morning rounds, the health care team sees the patient and writes changes to the intravenous (IV) solution prescriptions. In addition, a prescription is received to administer furosemide 10 mg by slow direct IV daily for 3 days. Based on the patient's signs and symptoms, which prescriptions can the nurse anticipate? How would the nurse calculate the minute flow rate of an infusion set with a drop factor of 15 gtt/mL, and how would the nurse ensure an accurate flow rate?
3. The following morning, the patient indicates tenderness at her PIVC site. However, the patient no longer has dyspnea or other signs of fluid volume excess (FVE). Her past 24-hour intake was 1 600 mL, and her output was 1 700 mL. Serum electrolyte levels drawn this morning were within normal limits. She reported that she put some tape on her IV dressing last night because it was falling off. There is marked swelling around the IV site with purulent drainage. Her temperature is 38.2°C (100.8°F). Using SBAR (situation–background–assessment–recommendation), show how you would communicate with the health care team about this patient.
4. A patient has a tunnelled central vascular access device (CVAD) placed, and the nurse will be performing catheter care and maintenance, including insertion site assessment, dressing change, needle-free connector change, and flushing with normal saline. Place the following steps in the correct order:
   1. Attach needle-free connector to the catheter hub, flush with 0.9% sodium chloride, remove gloves, perform hand hygiene.
   2. Apply new stabilization device, transparent semipermeable membrane (TSM) dressing, label dressing.
   3. Perform hand hygiene, apply appropriate personal protective equipment (PPE), remove old dressing.
   4. Perform skin antisepsis with 2% CHG and 70% alcohol solution and allow to dry completely.
   5. Remove needle-free connector, scrub exposed catheter hub with antiseptic swab, let dry completely.
   6. Remove and discard clean gloves, perform hand hygiene, apply sterile gloves.
5. Which of the following steps are necessary when inserting a PIVC? (*Select all that apply.*)
   1. Apply tourniquet to arm 10 to 15 cm (4 to 6 inches) above the intended insertion site.
   2. Clean skin using an antiseptic agent (e.g., CHG/alcohol) and allow to dry thoroughly.
   3. Stabilize the vein by placing the thumb proximal to the insertion site, stretching the skin in the direction of insertion.
   4. Use the smallest-gauge, shortest-length catheter suitable for the plan of care and vein size.
   5. Observe for blood in the catheter, lower catheter angle parallel to skin, and advance catheter of the needle into the vein.
   6. Release the tourniquet once the catheter has been secured and the dressing has been applied.

Visit the Evolve site for a complete list of answers to the Review Questions.

✦ NEXT GENERATION NCLEX® (NGN)

For practice with answering exam questions related to unfolding NGN case studies, please consult the Next Generation NCLEX® (NGN)-Style Case Studies for Skills and Techniques on the Evolve website: http://evolve.elsevier.com/Canada/Perry/clinicalskills/

REFERENCES

Accreditation Canada. (2020). *Required organizational practices–2020 handbook.* https://physicians.nshealth.ca/resources/required-organizational-practices-2020-handbook

Arai, S. R., Butzlaff, A., Stotts, N. A., et al. (2014). Quench the thirst: Lessons from clinical thirst trials. *Biological Research For Nursing, 16*(4), 456–466. https://doi.org/10.1177/1099800413505900. [Seminal Reference].

Aseptic Non Touch Technique. (2018). *ANTT core clinical guidelines, 2018.* http://antt.org/ANTT_Site/core_guidelines.html

Canadian Vascular Access Association. (2019). *Occlusion management guideline for central venous access* (2nd ed.). http://cvaa.info/publications/occlusion-management-guideline-omg

El-Sharkawy, A. M., Devonald, M. A. J., Humes, D. J., et al. (2020). Hyperosmolar dehydration: A predictor of kidney injury and outcome in hospitalised older adults. *Clinical Nutrition, 39*(8), 2593–2599. https://doi.org/10.1016/j.clnu.2019.11.030

Fiorini, J., Venturini, G., Conti, F., et al. (2019). Vessel health and preservation: An integrative review. *Journal of Clinical Nursing, 28*(7–8), 1039–1049. https://doi.org/10.1111/jocn.14707

Foster, J., Idossa, L., Mau, L.-W., et al. (2016). Applying health literacy principles: Strategies and tools to develop easy-to-read patient education resources. *Clinical Journal of Oncology Nursing, 20*(4), 433–436. https://doi.org/10.1188/16.CJON.433-436. [Seminal Reference].

Gorski, L. A., Hadaway, L., Hagle, M. E., et al. (2021). Infusion Therapy Standards of practice, 8th edition. *Journal of Infusion Nursing, 44*(1S), S1–S224. https://www.aspirus.org/Uploads/Public/Documents/Library/Infusion_Therapy_Standards_of_Practice,_8th.1.pdf

Hallam, C., Denton, A., Weston, V., et al. (2021). UK vessel health and preservation (VHP) framework: A commentary on the updated VHP 2020. *Journal of Infection Prevention, 22*(4), 147–155. https://doi.org/10.1177/1757177420976806

Holroyd, S. (2020). Frequency volume charts and fluid balance monitoring: Getting it right. *Journal of Community Nursing, 34*(1), 55–58.

Jantzen, D., & Hebig, S. (2024). Fluid, electrolyte, and acid–base balances. In B. Astle, & W. Duggleby (Eds.), *Potter and Perry's Canadian fundamentals of nursing (7th ed., Chapter 41).* Elsevier.

Keenan-Lindsay, L., Sams, C. A., & O'Connor, C. L. (2022). *Perry's maternal child nursing care in Canada* (3rd ed.). Elsevier.

Morata, L., & Bowers, M. (2020). Ultrasound-guided peripheral intravenous catheter insertion: The nurse's manual. *Critical Care Nurse, 40*(5), 38–46. https://doi.org/10.4037/ccn2020240

Moureau, N.L. (Ed.). (2019). *Vessel health and preservation: The right approach for vascular access.* Springer. https://doi.org/10.1007/978-3-030-03149-7

Piredda, M., Bagioli, V., Barrella, B., et al. (2017). Factors affecting difficult peripheral intravenous cannulation in adults: a prospective observational study. *Journal of Clinical Nursing, 26*(7–8), 1074–1084. https://doi.org/10.1111/jocn.13444

Public Health Agency of Canada. (2016). *Routine practices and additional precautions for preventing the transmission of infection in healthcare settings.* https://www.canada.ca/en/public-health/services/publications/diseases-conditions/routine-practices-precautions-healthcare-associated-infections.html. [Seminal Reference].

Voor in 't holt, A. F., Helder, O. K., Vos, M. C., et al. (2017). Antiseptic barrier cap effective in reducing central line-associated bloodstream infections: A systematic review and meta-analysis. *International Journal of Nursing Studies, 69*, 34–40. https://doi.org/10.1016/j.ijnurstu.2017.01.007. [Seminal Reference].

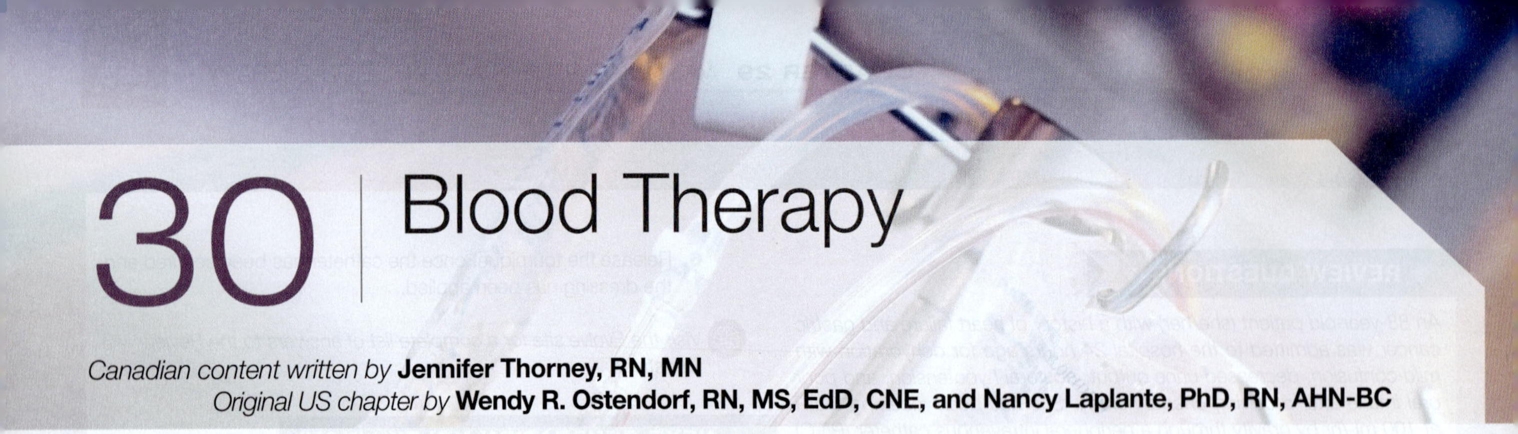

30 Blood Therapy

Canadian content written by **Jennifer Thorney, RN, MN**
Original US chapter by **Wendy R. Ostendorf, RN, MS, EdD, CNE, and Nancy Laplante, PhD, RN, AHN-BC**

SKILLS AND PROCEDURES

OBJECTIVES

Mastery of content in this chapter will enable the nurse to:

- Discuss indications for blood therapy.
- Demonstrate the following skills on selected patients: initiating blood therapy and monitoring for adverse transfusion reactions.
- Describe various transfusion reactions.
- Explain techniques for managing symptoms of adverse transfusion reactions.

MEDIA RESOURCES

- http://evolve.elsevier.com/Canada/Perry/clinicalskills/

PURPOSE

The transfusion of blood and blood components restores and maintains quality of life for patients with hematological disorders, cancer, injury, or surgical intervention. To ensure patient safety, a competent nurse must know the complexities of the ABO and Rh blood group system, the numerous components of blood that can be transfused, and the serious negative outcomes that can occur following transfusion. Never view the transfusion of blood products as routine; overlooking a minor detail is dangerous and can be life threatening to a patient (Gorski, 2019).

STANDARDS OF CARE

- Accreditation Canada (2020)—*Required Organizational Practices–2020 Handbook* (https://physicians.nshealth.ca/resources/required-organizational-practices-2020-handbook)
- Canadian Blood Services (2017–2023)—*Clinical Guide to Transfusion* (https://professionaleducation.blood.ca/en/transfusion/clinical-guide-transfusion)
- Canadian Society for Transfusion Medicine (2021)—*CSTM Standards for Hospital Transfusion Services* (Version 5) (https://www.transfusion.ca/Resources/Standards)
- Health Canada (2023)—*Guidance Document: Blood Regulations* (https://www.canada.ca/en/health-canada/services/drugs-health-products/biologics-radiopharmaceuticals-genetic-therapies/applications-submissions/guidance-documents/blood-regulations/guidance-document-blood-regulations-1.html)
- Healthcare Excellence Canada (2020)—*Hospital Harm Improvement Resource: Infusion, Transfusion, and Injection Complications* (https://www.patientsafetyinstitute.ca/en/toolsResources/Hospital-Harm-Measure/Improvement-Resources/Infusion-Transfusion-Injection-Complications/Documents/HHIR-Infusion-Transfusion-Injectibles-Complications-A11.pdf)
- National Advisory Committee on Blood and Blood Products (2014)—*NAC Companion Document to "Red Blood Cell Transfusion: A Clinical Practice Guideline from the AABB"* (https://nacblood.ca/en/resource/nac-companion-document-red-blood-cell-transfusion-clinical-practice-guideline-aabb)
- Public Health Agency of Canada (2016)—*Transfusion Transmitted Injuries Surveillance System (TTISS): 2009–2013 Summary Results* (https://publications.gc.ca/collections/collection_2016/aspc-phac/HP40-168-2016-eng.pdf)

PRINCIPLES FOR PRACTICE

- Blood product transfusion therapy is the intravenous (IV) administration of red blood cells (Fig. 30.1), blood components (Fig. 30.2), or a plasma protein product (Fig. 30.3) for therapeutic purposes. Transfusions are used to treat hemorrhage, treat symptomatic anemia, and improve oxygen delivery to tissues.
- The most common method of blood transfusion is *allogeneic* blood (blood donated from someone else).
- *Autologous transfusion* (or *autotransfusion*) is a method in which a patient's own blood is collected and reinfused for intravascular volume replacement (Gorski, 2019). Since the late 1990s, preoperative autologous donation (PAD) has been an option for patients concerned with transfusion-related reactions or transmission of disease. PAD may be beneficial for patients undergoing vascular and cardiothoracic surgeries where blood loss may be substantial. Using this process, patients can donate several units of their own blood via phlebotomy, which is performed weekly, approximately 4 to 6 weeks before surgery. The last donation must occur more than 72 hours before surgery.
- To decrease transfusion-related adverse events, blood and its components are treated and stored in controlled environments. Blood is a living tissue; once obtained via the donor, it must

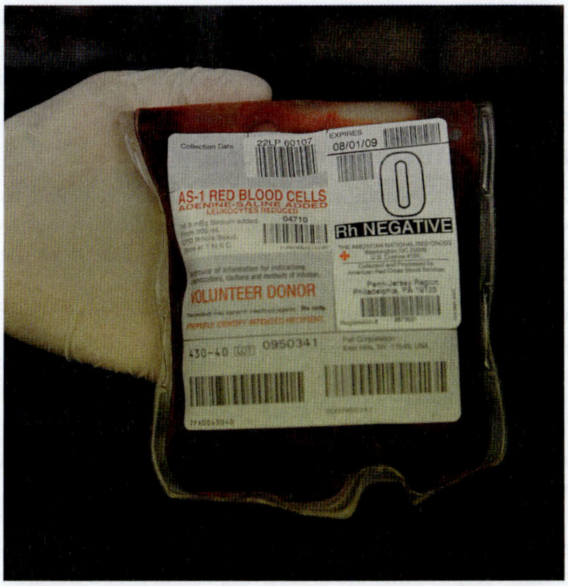

FIG 30.1 Unit of blood. *(Image courtesy of American Red Cross.)*

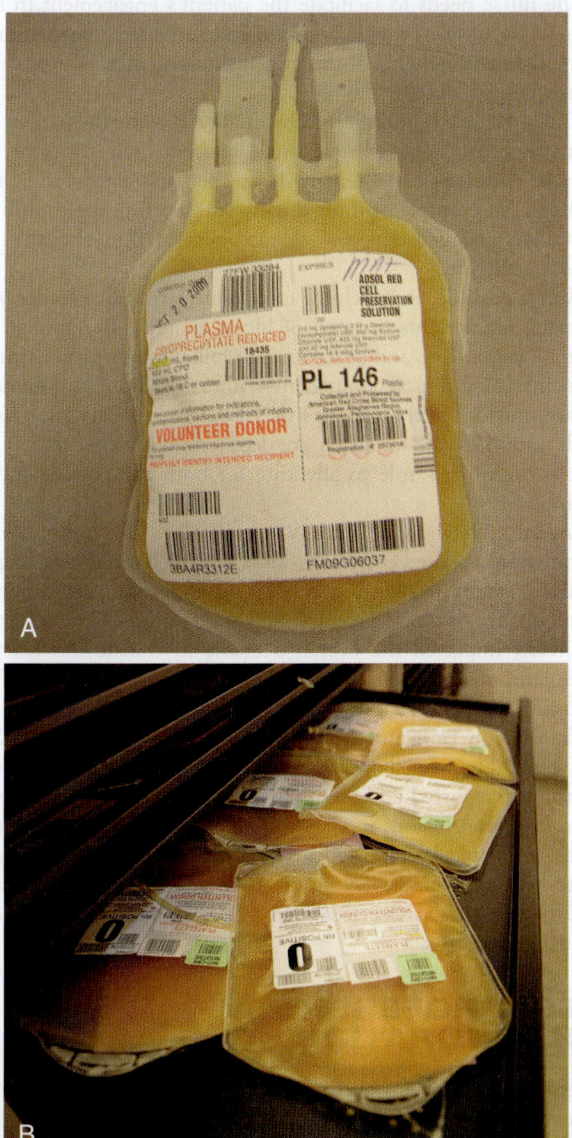

FIG 30.2 A, Bag of apheresis platelets. B, Bags of pooled platelets. *(Images courtesy American Red Cross.)*

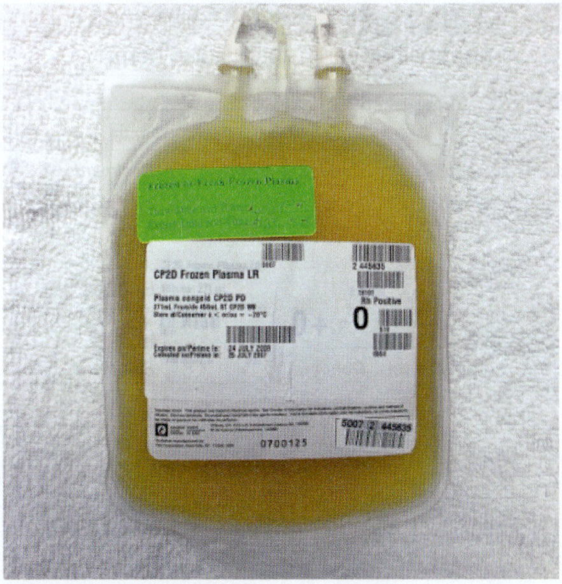

FIG 30.3 Bag of plasma. *(Image courtesy Queen's University School of Medicine. © qscalpel, photo by Adam Szulewski.)*

remain healthy before transfusion. Various anticoagulants and preservatives are used internationally to maintain the shelf life of donated blood.

- Caution is required when infusing multiple units of blood or a unit of blood nearing its expiration. When blood is stored, red blood cells are destroyed continually, which releases potassium (K) from the cells into the plasma. Often, a laboratory test of a patient's K level is prescribed before administering a unit of blood.
- As a nurse, your role during a blood transfusion is to use the principles of interprofessional collaboration to carry out the health care provider's prescription by clearly and respectfully communicating with the blood bank personnel and the prescribing health care provider; safely administering the blood or blood products; assessing a patient before, during, and after the transfusion; and promptly identifying and reporting any transfusion reactions.

ABO System

There are three blood-typing systems: ABO, Rh, and human leukocyte antigen (HLA). These systems ensure a close match between transfused products and a recipient's blood. The ABO system uses the presence or absence of specific antigens on the surface of red blood cells to identify blood groups. When the type A antigen is present, the blood group is type A. When the type B antigen is present, the blood group is type B. When both A and B antigens are present, the blood group is type AB. When blood cells lack both A and B antigens, the blood group is type O. These four blood types are distributed unequally among populations, with type O being the most common in all populations (Lausten et al., 2018) (Table 30.1).

Antibodies that react against the A and B antigens are naturally present in the plasma of people whose red blood cells do not carry the antigen. These antibodies (agglutinins) react against the foreign antigens (*agglutinogens*). Incompatible red blood cells agglutinate (clump together), causing a life-threatening hemolytic transfusion reaction. People with type A blood have anti-B antibodies; people with type B blood have anti-A antibodies. People with type AB blood have neither antibody and can receive all blood types. People with type O blood have both A and B antibodies and can receive only type O blood (Duncan, 2020). The most common transfusion reaction, acute hemolytic transfusion reaction (AHTR), results in 1 death for

TABLE 30.1

ABO Compatibilities for Transfusion Therapy

Component	Compatibilities	
Whole blood	Give type-specific blood only	
Packed red cells (stored, washed, or frozen/washed)	***Donor***	***Recipient***
	O	O, A, B, AB
	A	A, AB
	B	B, AB
	AB	AB
Fresh-frozen plasma	***Donor***	***Recipient***
	O	O
	A	A, O
	B	B, O
	AB	AB, B, A, O
Platelets	RBC: ABO and Rh compatible preferred	
	Donor	***Recipient***
	O	O, A, B, AB
	A	A, AB
	B	B, AB
	AB	AB

Data from Alexander, M., Corrigan, A. M., Gorski, L. A., et al. (2014). *Core curriculum for infusion nursing* (4th ed.). Lippincott.

every 30 incidents of AHTR. It is caused by ABO incompatibility, when a patient receives a transfusion with blood that is not compatible with their ABO blood type (Bahri et al., 2018).

Rh System

The Rh factor is considered when matching blood components for transfusion. The Rh factor is another antigen in red blood cell membranes. Although nearly 50 types of Rh antigen may be present on the surface of red blood cells, the type D antigen is most prevalent and most likely to elicit an immune response. It is the presence or absence of the D antigen that determines a person's Rh type. A person is Rh positive with the D antigen and Rh negative without it (Astle & Duggleby, 2024; Duncan, 2020). Unlike the ABO antigens, naturally occurring antibodies to the Rh(D) antigen do not occur. A person with Rh-negative blood must first be exposed to Rh-positive blood before any Rh antibodies are formed. A person with Rh-negative blood who is exposed to Rh-positive blood will develop enough antibodies to cause a severe transfusion reaction with repeated exposure (Duncan, 2020). Generally, a person with Rh-negative blood receives Rh-negative blood, whereas a person with Rh-positive blood can receive Rh-positive or Rh-negative blood (Astle & Duggleby, 2024).

An Rh-negative mother previously exposed to Rh antigen can transfer Rh antibodies across the placenta to an Rh-positive fetus. This can result in severe fetal hemolysis (i.e., the breakdown of red blood cells, with resultant anemia and jaundice), which is often fatal to the infant. To prevent current or future fetal hemolysis, Rh(D) immunoglobulin (e.g., WinRho) is given by intramuscular injection to the mother at 28 weeks' gestation and again within 72 hours of birth. WinRho significantly reduces alloimmunization by suppressing the immune response and antibody formation in the Rh-negative person who has been in contact with Rh-positive red blood cells (Clarke & Hannon, 2018). Since WinRho is made from human blood, there is a risk of pathogen transmission. To reduce the risk of future fetal hemolysis, it is recommended that in urgent situations, persons under the age of 45 receive O-negative red blood cells (Duncan, 2020).

Acute Transfusion Reactions

- Clinical manifestations range from mild to severe and usually develop in the initial 15 minutes of the transfusion, and therefore best practice is for the nurse to stay with the patient for the first 15 minutes of the transfusion.
- Severe hemolytic reaction is rare (Tyerman & Cobbett, 2023).
- Acute transfusion reactions are detailed in Table 30.2.

PERSON-CENTRED CARE

When administering blood products, the nurse needs to consider a patient's values and cultural and religious beliefs about blood therapy. It is important to seek to understand the patient's health values and goals. A person's perception of their disease or health condition affects how receptive they are to receiving blood. Blood transfusion is often equated to severity of illness.

- The nurse needs to facilitate the patient's engagement in treatment decisions. Provide accurate and unbiased information on the risks and benefits of the transfusion and allay patient anxieties when possible.
- The nurse needs to respect individuality. Provide the patient with an opportunity to ask questions, address their concerns, and make decisions consistent with the person's needs and preferences. An example of individuality is respecting the prohibition of blood transfusions among members of the Jehovah's Witnesses religion.
- When possible, it is helpful to consult a religious leader when caring for patients in need of blood therapy. Be familiar with employer policies and procedures to follow when patients choose an informed refusal. Immediately inform the prescribing health care provider of the patient's decision. Parents have the primary obligation to care for and make decisions about their minor, and it is the nurse's role to advocate for both the patient and the family.
- Patient safety is a priority—specifically the prevention of transfusion-related complications. Over the last decades, ongoing advancement in collection, processing, and testing have improved the quality of blood products and transfusion safety, which has directly impacted the overall decrease in transfusion reactions (Bojanić et al., 2022). To ensure safe patient outcomes, the Transfusion Medicine Laboratory, Canada Vigilance Program, and Transfusion Transmitted Injuries Surveillance System (TTISS) (le système d'hémovigilance du Québec in the province of Quebec) monitor reported adverse reactions related to blood and blood product transfusions in Canada. All adverse reactions to a transfusion should be reported to Transfusion Medicine Laboratory for investigation. TTISS monitors more severe reactions, while Canadian Blood Services/Héma-Québec investigates product-quality concerns.

INTERPROFESSIONAL COLLABORATION

In general, working collaboratively with all health care providers improves clinical outcomes and enhances workplace satisfaction. Interprofessional collaboration has played an essential role in decreasing adverse events and medical errors by fostering communication, role clarification, and mutual respect among health care providers

TABLE 30.2
Transfusion Reactions

Reaction	Etiology	Onset	Signs and Symptoms	Prevention	Nursing Intervention
Acute Immediate (<24 Hours)					
Febrile, nonhemolytic	Most common type of transfusion reaction; caused by WBC antigen–antibody reaction	May begin early in transfusion or as many as several hours after completion	Temperature increase of >1°C (2°F) or more above baseline, chills, headache, vomiting	Premedicate as ordered with antipyretics if prior history of reaction. Use leukocyte-reduced blood products.	**Stop the transfusion.** Change administration set and administer 0.9% sodium chloride at rate to maintain patent IV access. Institute transfusion reaction protocol. Administer antipyretics as ordered to treat fever. Document clinical symptoms, when transfusion was stopped, notification of health care provider and blood bank, nursing interventions and response to interventions, and patient teaching.
Acute hemolytic transfusion reaction (AHTR)	Transfusion of ABO-incompatible RBCs; usually caused by misidentification or improper labelling	Within minutes of transfusion initiation	Fever, with or without chills; tachycardia; hypotension; abdominal, chest, back, and flank pain; dyspnea; red/dark urine; shock	Use extreme care during the entire patient identification process; proper labelling of blood sample; and meticulous verification of ABO/Rh compatibility between donor and recipient before administration. Start transfusion slowly, and monitor carefully for the first 15 minutes.	**Stop the transfusion.** Get help immediately. Change administration set and administer 0.9% sodium chloride at rate to maintain patent IV access. Notify health care provider and blood bank. Treat shock. Maintain blood pressure and renal perfusion. Insert Foley catheter. Monitor intake and output hourly. Dialysis may be required. Obtain blood and urine samples and send to laboratory with unused part of unit of blood. Document reaction according to employer policy.
Allergic reaction (mild to moderate)	Caused by recipient sensitivity to allergens in the blood components	Within minutes of transfusion initiation	Urticaria, pruritus, facial flushing, mild wheezing	May administer antihistamines 30 minutes before transfusion if prescribed.	**Stop the transfusion.** Change administration set and administer 0.9% sodium chloride at rate to maintain patent IV access. Notify health care provider and blood bank. Administer antihistamines as ordered. Monitor and document vital signs every 15 minutes. Transfusion may be restarted if fever, dyspnea, and wheezing are not present.
Severe allergic reaction (anaphylaxis)	Caused by recipient allergy to a donor antigen (usually IgA) Agglutination of RBCs obstructing capillaries and blocking blood flow, causing symptoms in all major organ systems	Within minutes of transfusion initiation	Hypotension, tachycardia, urticaria, bronchospasm, anxiety, shock, nausea, vomiting, diarrhea, abdominal pain	Use autologous blood or blood from donors who are IgA deficient. Transfusion of saline-washed or leukocyte-depleted RBCs.	**Stop the transfusion.** Change administration set and administer 0.9% sodium chloride at rate to maintain patent IV access. Notify health care provider and blood bank. Administer antihistamines, corticosteroids, epinephrine, and antipyretics as ordered. Monitor and document vital signs until stable. Initiate cardiopulmonary resuscitation if necessary.
Transfusion-related acute lung injury (TRALI)	Presence of WBC antibodies from donor who has a WBC-activating agent in blood Leading cause of transfusion-related death	During or within 6 hours of infusion	Fever, respiratory failure, hypoxemia, hypotension, pulmonary edema	Currently there is no method to identify patients at risk.	**Stop the transfusion.** Provide respiratory support, administer oxygen, frequently requires mechanical ventilation, administer vasopressor agents.
Transfusion-associated circulatory overload (TACO)	Related to volume overload; patients older than 70 years and infants are at highest risk	Usually occurs during or within 6 hours of transfusion	Dyspnea, orthopnea, cyanosis, tachycardia, JVD, hypertension, cough	Requires frequent patient monitoring for those at high risk, including slowing infusion rate.	**Stop the transfusion.** Place patient in high Fowler position, notify health care provider, administer oxygen and diuretics.

Continued

TABLE 30.2
Transfusion Reactions—cont'd

Reaction	Etiology	Onset	Signs and Symptoms	Prevention	Nursing Intervention
Delayed Transfusion Reactions					
Transfusion-associated graft-versus-host disease (TA-GVHD)	Usually rare but fatal Donor lymphocytes destroyed by recipient's immune system In immunocompromised patients, the donor lymphocytes are identified as foreign; however, patient's immune system is not capable of destroying, and in turn, patient's lymphocytes are destroyed	8–10 days after transfusion	Maculopapular rash, watery diarrhea, fever, jaundice caused by liver dysfunction, bone marrow suppression (pancytopenia)	Administration of irradiated blood and leukocyte-depleted RBC products as prescribed.	No effective therapy. Treatment of symptoms.
Iron overload	Iron from donated blood binds to protein and is not eliminated	Usually occurs when multiple units (>100 units of PRBCs) are transfused	Cardiac dysfunction, organ failure, arrhythmias, heart failure symptoms, increased serum transferrin, increased liver enzymes, jaundice	Iron chelation, phlebotomy, monitoring of serum iron levels.	No effective therapy. Iron chelation therapy. Monitor patient for heart failure, cardiac disorder, liver disorder, serum transferrin.
Infection-Related Complications					
Bacterial contamination	Microorganism contamination of infused product during donation or in preparing component for infusion Highest risk when administering platelets	Occurs at time of donation Symptoms may appear during transfusion or within 4 hours of completion	High fever, severe chills, hypotension, flushed skin, shock, hemoglobinuria, renal failure, DIC	Use good skin antisepsis prior to venipuncture. Inspect blood unit carefully; do not administer if clots, bubbles, bag leaks, or discoloration of unit is noted.	**Stop the transfusion.** Treat shock and administer ordered steroids and antibiotics. Culture patient's blood, blood components, and all IV solutions.

DIC, Disseminated intravascular coagulation; *IgA,* immunoglobulin A; *IV,* intravenous; *JVD,* jugular vein distension; *PRBCs,* packed red blood cells; *RBC,* red blood cell; *WBC,* white blood cell.

Data adapted from the Association for the Advancement of Blood and Biotherapies. (2020). *Technical manual* (19th ed.); Gorski, L. (2019). *Phillips's manual of IV therapeutics: Evidence-based practice for infusion therapy* (7th ed.). F. A. Davis.

(Goulding et al., 2020). The nurse must understand interprofessional collaboration in order to safely perform the blood transfusion—the nurse needs to understand the role of the laboratory personnel (and how to collaborate with each role) to retrieve the blood product. The nurse should have a comprehensive understanding of the testing and preparation process that was completed prior to retrieval. The nurse must clearly communicate with the prescriber, the laboratory, and the patient for timely and safe patient care. Mutual respect can be demonstrated when all members of the health care team understand the patient's needs and undertake the skill of performing the transfusion through a patient-centred, collaborative approach.

EVIDENCE-INFORMED PRACTICE

Compliance with standards and policies and ongoing education are crucial for maintaining patient safety and reducing potential errors. Safety and risk management are key factors in transfusion therapy. Transfusion-associated circulatory overload (TACO) is the leading cause of transfusion-related death in Canada (Public Health Agency of Canada, 2019). Between 2011 and 2015, the Public Health Agency of Canada (2019) reported a slight increase in the incidence of TACO, emphasizing the need for diligent skill and evidence-informed practice in understanding the implementation of blood transfusions to prevent human error. A human error most often involves misidentification of the patient or of the unit of blood or mislabelling of the pretransfusion blood sample. Advances in technology have helped to decrease transfusion-related errors:

- Electronic bar-code technology helps prevent errors in the identification process between a patient and the compatible blood unit.
- International standard for labelling of blood components (ISBT 128) provides unique numbering of blood components (Fig. 30.4).
- Radiofrequency identification (RFID) is used to standardize and document key steps in the blood collection process as well as verify that the blood unit matches the recipient at the patient's bedside.
- Advanced technological laboratory screening procedures help to ensure safe transfusions in terms of bloodborne pathogens.
- Better assessment of blood and plasma cell integrity is available to avoid loss of blood component function.
- Blood alternative therapies with pharmacological developments such as colloids, crystalloids, erythropoietin, antifibrinolytics, and hematinics reduce the risks associated with transfusing human blood.

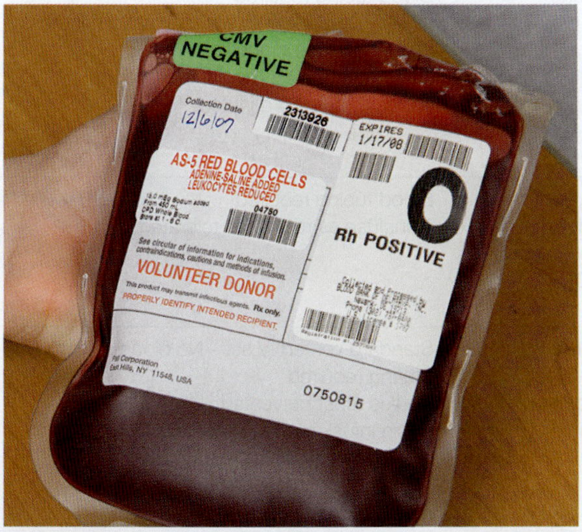

FIG 30.4 Red blood cells (unit of blood with a label). *(Image courtesy American Red Cross.)*

- Choosing Wisely, an Internet site and mobile app, provides rapid access to evidence-informed transfusion recommendations (Canadian Society for Transfusion Medicine, 2021).

SAFETY GUIDELINES

- Administration of blood and blood components requires meticulous attention to detail (e.g., preparation, administration, and monitoring) to prevent life-threatening transfusion reactions (see Table 30.2) and is usually administered via an electronic infusion device.
- Accurate labelling of the pretransfusion sample is important. The nurse needs to follow the employer policy for blood draws and clearly label blood tubes when at the patient's bedside.
- Appropriate pretransfusion blood work ensures safety and provides better red blood cell management in the blood bank. Crossmatch is prescribed to determine compatibility of red blood cells for the patient's blood type when the patient requires a transfusion. When a patient is likely to require blood products, the "type and screen" is prescribed to determine a patient's ABO and Rh type and to perform an antibody screen. This test allows a quick crossmatch should blood be required (Duncan, 2020).
- Restrictive transfusion thresholds limit use of blood products until the hemoglobin level is 70 g/L (80 g/L in certain situations), thus reducing unnecessary transfusions (Canadian Society for Transfusion Medicine, 2021).
- Multiple checks of the blood unit for correct labelling and verification of the correct patient are intended to reduce errors. The nurse follows the 10 rights of medication administration (see Chapter 20) during a transfusion: right medication, right dose, right patient, right route, right time, right documentation, right reason, right patient education, right evaluation, and right to refuse. The patient may sign a right to refuse treatment form.
- The nurse is required to complete several safety checks with another nurse prior to administration of blood or blood products (Box 30.1). Always follow employer policy.
- The nurse reviews employer policy and procedures regarding administration of blood or blood products.
- Two nurses must verify, sign, and document the right blood unit and right patient immediately before administration.
- The patient must be wearing an identification band.

Despite precautions, transfusion therapy carries risks. Infectious diseases such as viruses, bacteria, and parasites can be transmitted through blood transfusion. Canadian Blood Services (2017–2023) suggests that

BOX 30.1

Nurse-to-Nurse Safety Checks Prior to Blood Administration

- Patient's full name
- Unique patient identifier (defined by employer)
- Type of product to be administered
- Volume or amount to be administered
- Rate of infusion or duration (check employer policy for standard administration rate)
- Date and time of transfusion
- Sequence in which products are to be transfused (when multiple products are prescribed together)
- Use of pressure infusion devices when indicated
- Use of blood warmers when indicated
- Modifications, if any, to blood components
- Special transfusion requirements, if any
- Medications related to the transfusion, if required, including dosage, route, and when to administer the medication (i.e., pre-, intra- or post-transfusion)

the risk of viral transmission is greatest when a person donates in the "window period," the interval of time between infectivity and detectability. The majority of noninfectious risks are immune related and are the most common complications. Delayed hemolytic transfusion reaction (DHTR), transfusion-associated graft-versus-host disease (TA-GVHD), and post-transfusion purpura (PTP) may also occur. Nonimmune reactions (e.g., hemoglobinuria, hyperkalemia, hypocalcemia, hypothermia, or iron overload) can be life threatening. Ensuring compatibility between the patient and donor is essential. Human-related errors (e.g., improper labelling, inadequate hand-off between the nurse and the person transporting the blood, or mistakes in completing a blood requisition) that may lead to the administration of incompatible transfusions can occur at every step of the transfusion process.

! SAFETY ALERT When a transfusion reaction occurs, IMMEDIATELY STOP the transfusion while maintaining IV access, check vital signs, and contact the health care provider and the blood bank/laboratory personnel.

✦ SKILL 30.1 Initiating Blood Therapy

Video Clip *NSO Nursing Skills Online Blood Therapy Module 15 / Lesson 2*

Blood is administered for different clinical indications (Table 30.3). A patient's medical condition determines which blood component is required. A health care provider's prescription is required for the administration of a blood product. The nurse is responsible for understanding which blood components are appropriate in various situations. In addition, the nurse must ensure that informed consent has been obtained and that a blood sample has been collected and sent to the laboratory within 72 hours for typing and compatibility screening.

Blood is stored in a refrigerated environment. The refrigeration unit is regulated by the blood bank; blood is never stored in refrigerators on the hospital unit. The blood transfusion must be started soon after the blood has been received. If it cannot be started, contact the blood bank. Blood that has been out of refrigeration for more than 60 minutes must be discarded (Canadian Blood Services, 2017–2023). Always consult employer policy regarding how long blood is allowed to be unrefrigerated before it has to be discarded. In emergency situations, rapid transfusion of cold blood may lead to dysrhythmias and reduction of a patient's core temperature. A blood-warming machine may be used for large transfusions of greater than 50 mL/kg/hr or for patients with cold agglutinins (Fig. 30.5). Special

TABLE 30.3

Blood and Blood Component Products

Blood Product	Major Uses	Storage and Expiration	Administration
Red blood cells (RBC)	Bleeding or anemic nonbleeding patients with signs and symptoms of impaired tissue oxygen delivery: • Tachycardia • Shortness of breath • Dizziness	2–6°C in approved refrigerator only Up to 42 days	• Blood tubing required • Initiate transfusion slowly for first 15 minutes unless massive blood loss • Transfuse over no more than 4 hours • Typically, over 1.5–2 hours, with slower rates for patients at risk for transfusion-associated circulatory overload (TACO)
Plasma	• Liver disease coagulopathy • Massive transfusion • Plasma exchange procedures for thrombotic thrombocytopenic purpura/hemolytic uremic syndrome (TTP/HUS)	Frozen for 1 year Once thawed, expires after 5 days stored at 1–6°C	• Blood tubing required • Initiate transfusion slowly for first 15 minutes unless massive blood loss • Transfuse over no more than 4 hours • Typically, over 30 minutes to 2 hours
Platelets	Control or prevent bleeding in patients with: • Low platelet counts (thrombocytopenia) • Congenital platelet dysfunction • Platelets not functioning because of medications (acetylsalicylic acid [ASA], clopidogrel) • Platelet dysfunction following cardiopulmonary bypass	20–24°C on an agitator to prevent clumping 5 days	• Blood tubing required • Initiate transfusion slowly for first 15 minutes unless massive blood loss • Transfuse over no more than 4 hours • Typically, over 60 minutes
Cryoprecipitate	To replace: • Fibrinogen in patients who are actively bleeding and have a low fibrinogen level • Specific coagulation factors when the specific factor concentrates are not available	Frozen for 1 year Once thawed, expires after 4 hours; stored at 20–24°C	• Blood tubing required • Transfuse as rapidly as tolerated

Albumin (5% and 25%)	• Ascites patients undergoing large-volume paracentesis >5 L
	• Spontaneous bacterial peritonitis (SBP)
	• Hepatorenal syndrome
	• Plasma exchange procedures
		Room temperature lower than 30°C
		Expires as indicated on packaging
			• Standard vented IV set—No blood tubing or filtering required
			• Bottles must be vented
			• Begin infusion slowly, then as tolerated
			• Maximum rate:
			  • Albumin 5%—300 mL/hr
			  • Albumin 25%—120 mL/hr

Continued

TABLE 30.3

Blood and Blood Component Products—cont'd

Blood Product	Major Uses	Storage and Expiration	Administration
Intravenous immune globulin (IVIG)	• Replacement of immunoglobulins • Control of some infections and autoimmune diseases	Storage variable by brand Expires as indicated on packaging	• Standard vented IV set—No blood tubing or filtering required • Bottles must be vented • Infusion pump required • Begin infusion slowly, then as tolerated; maximum rate as indicated on package • Frequent vital sign monitoring
Prothrombin complex concentrate (Octaplex)	Reversal of warfarin or vitamin K deficiency in bleeding patients and those requiring emergency surgery	2–25°C Expires as indicated on packaging Use immediately once reconstituted	• Standard IV set—No blood tubing or filtering required • Infuse over 15–30 minutes • May be given via slow direct IV (usually by a physician) • Dosage based on weight and INR value; usually 2–4 vials • Effect is immediate and lasts 6–12 hours • For complete reversal, vitamin K at 10 mg IV must also be given

INR, International normalized ratio; *IV*, intravenous.

Data from Berta, D. (2020). *Bloody easy—Blood administration: A handbook for health care professionals (version 3).* Ontario Regional Blood Coordinating Network. https://transfusionontario.org/wp-content/uploads/2021/08/Bloody-Easy-Version-3-Interactive-English-Final-Page-Spreads.pdf; Callum, J., Pinkerton, P. H., Lima, A., et al. (2016). *Bloody easy 4—Blood transfusions, blood alternatives, and transfusion reactions: A guide to transfusion medicine* (4th ed.). Ontario Regional Blood Coordinating Network. https://transfusionontario.org/wp-content/uploads/2020/06/EN_BE4-JULY11_FINAL.pdf

tubing is required. Professional blood-warming devices with specialized blood-warming tubing are often used to prevent hemolysis and severe reactions (Canadian Blood Services, 2017–2023). Blood warmers have a safety alarm to prevent the blood from overheating.

Delegation and Collaboration

The skill of initiating transfusion therapy cannot be delegated to an unregulated care provider (UCP). The skill of initiating transfusion therapy by a registered practical nurse (RPN) or licensed practical nurse (LPN) varies by province and territory. Best practice continues to require the registered nurse (RN) to stay with the patient for the first 15 minutes of a transfusion of blood products. After the transfusion has been started and the patient is stable, assistance with monitoring of a patient by a UCP does not relieve an RN of the responsibility to continue assessing the patient during the transfusion. The nurse instructs the UCP about the following:

- What to observe, such as patient indication of shortness of breath, hives, or chills, and reporting this information to the nurse

Equipment

- Y-type blood administration set with a 170- to 260-micron in-line filter (NOTE: Depending on the blood product, special tubing and filter are necessary.)
- Prescribed blood product
- 250-mL bag of 0.9% sodium chloride (normal saline [NS]) for IV use
- 5- to 10-mL prefilled syringe with preservative-free 0.9% NS
- Antiseptic swabs (chlorhexidine gluconate [CHG] solution [preferred], povidone–iodine, or 70% alcohol)
- Clean gloves
- Tape
- Vital signs equipment: thermometer, blood pressure cuff, stethoscope, and pulse oximeter
- Signed transfusion consent form as required by employer policy. (Some employers may require consent for blood products on admission, while others require a separate consent.)

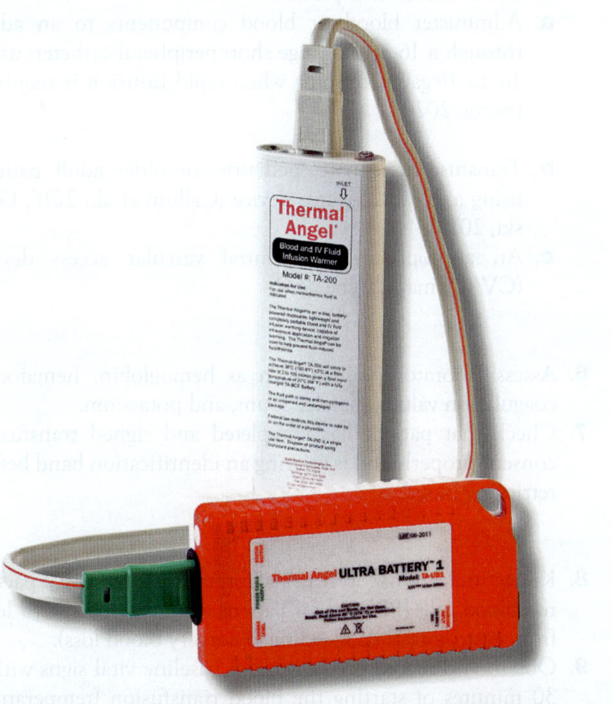

FIG 30.5 Blood-warming system. *(Used with permission of Estill Medical Technologies, Inc. All rights reserved.)*

Optional Equipment

- Rapid infusion pump
- Electronic infusion device (Verify that the pump can be used to deliver blood and blood products.)
- Blood warmer (Used mainly when large-volume or rapid transfusion is needed.)
- Pressure bag
- Cardiac monitor for emergencies

STEP	RATIONALE
ASSESSMENT	
1. Two nurses must identify patient using at least two person-specific identifiers (e.g., name and date of birth, or name and medical record number) according to employer policy.	Ensures correct patient. Complies with Accreditation Canada's standards and improves patient safety (Accreditation Canada, 2020).
2. Throughout the procedure, the 4 moments for hand hygiene are to be implemented; hand hygiene should occur before initial patient (or patient environment) contact, before an aseptic procedure, after body fluid exposure risk, and after patient (or patient environment) contact. Additional hand hygiene should be performed when hands are visibly soiled.	Proper hand hygiene helps prevent the spread of infectious agents to health care providers.
3. Verify health care provider's prescription for specific blood or blood product with appropriate date, time to begin transfusion, special instructions (i.e., irradiated, leukocyte depleted), duration, and any pretransfusion or post-transfusion medications to administer.	A health care provider's prescription must be present before transfusing a blood product. Verifying the prescription helps ensure that the appropriate blood component will be administered (Berta, 2020). Premedications such as an antihistamine or antipyretic may be prescribed, especially if patient demonstrated previous transfusion sensitivity. However, all other scheduled medications should be given at least 30 minutes prior to starting transfusion.
4. Obtain patient's transfusion history and note known allergies and previous transfusion reactions. Verify that type and crossmatch have been completed within the time frame outlined in employer policy. This may vary depending on jurisdiction.	Identifies patient's prior response(s) to transfusion of blood components. If patient has experienced a reaction in the past, anticipate a similar reaction and be prepared to rapidly intervene.
5. Verify that IV cannula is patent and without complications such as infiltration or phlebitis.	Patent IV ensures that transfusion will be infused within established time guidelines.
a. Administer blood or blood components to an adult through a 16- to 22-gauge short-peripheral catheter; use a 16- to 18-gauge cannula when rapid infusion is required (Berta, 2020).	The gauge of the IV cannula should be appropriate for accommodating the infusion of blood or blood components (Berta, 2020). Large-gauge cannulas promote rapid flow of blood components. Rapid transfusion through a cannula that is too small can cause hemolysis of red blood cells (Callum et al., 2016).
b. Transfuse a neonate, pediatric, or older adult patient using a 22- to 25-gauge device (Callum et al., 2016; Gorski, 2019).	Use of smaller cannula gauges, such as 25 gauge, often requires a blood bank to divide the unit so that each half can be infused within the allotted time or with pressure-assisted devices.
c. An appropriate-gauge central vascular access device (CVAD) may also be used.	Use of CVAD for administration of blood depends on catheter gauge and manufacturer recommendations for use. CVADs with multiple lumens allow medications to be administered through a different lumen while blood is infusing (Berta, 2020).
6. Assess laboratory values such as hemoglobin, hematocrit, coagulation values, platelet count, and potassium.	Provides baseline for later evaluation of patient response to transfusion (Astle & Duggleby, 2024; Infusion Nurses Society [INS], 2016).
7. Check that patient has completed and signed transfusion consent properly and is wearing an identification band before retrieving blood.	Informed consent is required before transfusion. The consent form should include risks, benefits, and treatment alternatives; right to accept or refuse transfusion; and opportunity to ask questions. Administration of albumin does not require informed consent. Identification band ensures proper patient identification.
8. Know indications or reasons for transfusion (e.g., packed red blood cells [PRBCs] for patient with low hematocrit level from gastrointestinal bleeding or surgery blood loss).	Allows you to anticipate patient's response to therapy.
9. Obtain and record pretransfusion baseline vital signs within 30 minutes of starting the blood transfusion (temperature, pulse, respirations, and blood pressure). If patient is febrile (temperature >37.8°C [100°F]), notify health care provider before initiating transfusion.	Change from baseline vital signs during infusion alerts you to potential transfusion reaction or adverse effect of therapy (Tyerman & Cobbett, 2023).
10. Assess patient's need for IV fluids or medications while transfusion is infusing.	If IV medications need to be administered during transfusion, second IV site is necessary. No other infusions are to be administered through same IV site as blood transfusion. Administer blood or blood components only with 0.9% sodium chloride (NS) (Callum et al., 2016).
11. Assess patient's understanding of procedure and rationale.	Alleviates some of the anxiety patient may have.

STEP	RATIONALE

NURSING DIAGNOSES

- Decreased cardiac output
- Excessive fluid volume
- Inadequate fluid volume
- Inadequate peripheral tissue perfusion
- Potential for infection
- Reduced stamina
- Insufficient knowledge regarding transfusion

Related factors and risk factors are individualized on the basis of patient's condition or needs.

PLANNING

STEP	RATIONALE
1. Expected outcomes following completion of the procedure:	
• Patient verbalizes understanding of rationale for therapy.	Indicates patient's understanding and ability to make informed decision for consent.
• Patient experiences improved activity tolerance.	Oxygenation is improved.
• Mucous membranes are pink, and patient has brisk capillary refill.	Tissue perfusion is improved.
• Patient's cardiac output returns to baseline.	Intravascular volume is restored.
• Patient's systolic blood pressure improves, and urine output is 0.5–1 mL/kg/hr.	Parameters reflect optimal fluid status and adequate renal blood flow.
• Patient's laboratory values improve in targeted areas (e.g., hemoglobin, hematocrit, coagulation values, platelet count).	Indicates that patient has responded appropriately to blood or blood component infusion.

IMPLEMENTATION

STEP	RATIONALE
1. Perform preadministration protocol:	
a. Obtain blood component from blood bank following employer protocol (see Step 2a illustration). Check the unit of blood and patient documentation with lab personnel.	Timely acquisition ensures that the product is safe to administer. Employer protocol usually encompasses safeguards to ensure quality control throughout transfusion process.

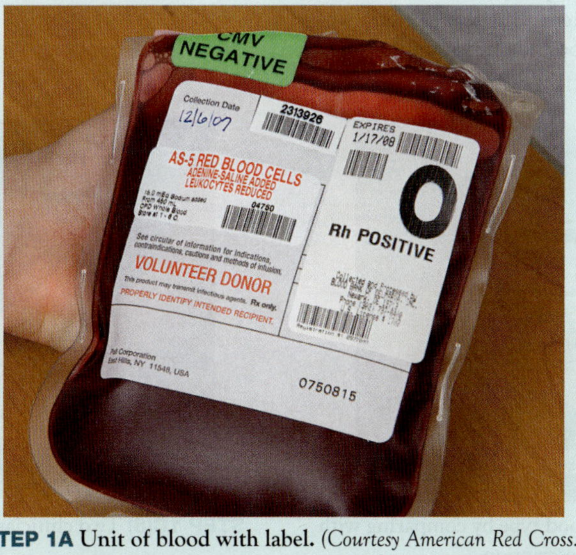

STEP 1A Unit of blood with label. *(Courtesy American Red Cross.)*

STEP	RATIONALE
b. Check blood bag for any signs of contamination (i.e., clumping or clots, gas bubbles, purplish colour) and presence of leaks.	Blood should not be infused if integrity is compromised. Air bubbles, clumping, clots, and discoloration can be an indication of bacterial contamination or inadequate anticoagulation of stored component and are contraindications for transfusion of that product (Berta, 2020). Blood serves as medium for bacterial growth.
c. Verbally compare and correctly verify patient, blood product, and type with another person considered qualified by your employer (e.g., RN or LPN) before initiating transfusion. The following verification process must be used:	Strict adherence to verification procedures before administration of blood or blood components reduces risk of administering wrong blood to patient. Approximately half of all transfusion reactions are related to the wrong patient receiving properly labelled blood (Healthcare Excellence Canada, 2020).

STEP	RATIONALE

IMPLEMENTATION

(1) Recheck patient identity using at least two person-specific identifiers (e.g., name and date of birth, or name and medical record number) according to employer policy. Compare identifiers with information on patient's medication administration record (MAR) or medical record.	Ensures correct patient. Complies with Accreditation Canada's standards and improves patient safety (Accreditation Canada, 2020).
(2) Confirm that transfusion record number and patient's identification number match.	Prevents accidental administration of wrong blood component.

Critical Decision Point *If you notice a discrepancy during the verification procedure, do not administer the product. Notify the blood bank and appropriate personnel as indicated by employer policy. The product should be returned to the blood bank until the discrepancy is resolved* (Gorski, 2019; INS, 2016).

(3) Verify that patient's name is correct on all documents. Check patient identification number and date of birth on identification band and patient record.	
(4) Compare unit number on blood bag with blood bank form to ensure that they are the same.	
(5) Verify that blood type matches on transfusion record and blood bag. Verify that component received from blood bank is the same component that health care provider prescribed (e.g., PRBCs, platelets) (see Step 2c[5] illustration).	Ensures that patient receives correct therapy. Misidentification and improper labelling result in transfusing blood component with wrong ABO group.
(6) Check that patient's blood type and Rh type are compatible with donor blood type and Rh type (e.g., Patient A+: Donor A+ or O+).	Verifies accurate donor blood type and compatibility.
(7) Check expiration date and time on unit of blood.	Never use expired blood because the efficacy of its cell components deteriorates over time and bacterial contamination may occur.
(8) Just before initiating transfusion, two nurses are to check patient identification information with blood unit label information (see Step 1c[8] illustration). Do not administer blood to patient who does not have an identification bracelet or blood identification bracelet (see employer policy).	Serves as last point of patient and blood confirmation (Gorski, 2019).

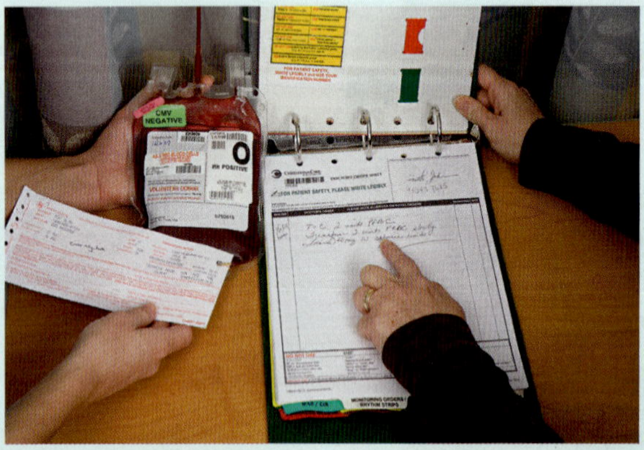

STEP 1C(5) Two clinicians verifying blood type by comparing with health care provider prescription.

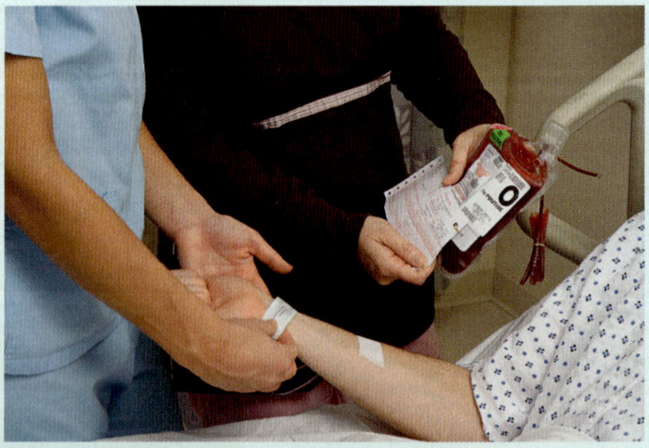

STEP 1C(8) Two clinicians verifying identification of patient and blood product.

(9) Both individuals verify patient and unit identification record process as directed by employer policy.	Documentation is legal medical record.
d. Review purpose of transfusion and ask patient to report any changes that they may feel during the transfusion.	Signs and symptoms of transfusion reactions include chills, low back pain, shortness of breath, rash, hives, or itching (Tyerman & Cobbett, 2023). Prompt notification aids in early intervention.

Critical Decision Point *The blood component should be transfused within 30 minutes of its release from the blood bank. If this cannot be completed because of an elevated patient temperature or other factors, immediately return the blood to the blood bank and retrieve it when you can administer it* (Tyerman & Cobbett, 2023). *DO NOT spike the blood bag until you ensure that no factors exist that would prevent transfusion.*

STEP	RATIONALE

IMPLEMENTATION

STEP	RATIONALE
2. Administer blood component(s):	
a. Apply clean gloves. Reinspect blood product for signs of leakage or unusual appearance.	Using routine practices reduces transmission of microorganisms. Provides ongoing verification of blood product.
b. Open Y-tubing blood administration set for single unit. Use multi-set if multiple units are to be transfused.	Y-tubing facilitates maintenance of IV line access with NS in case patient will need more than 1 unit of blood.
c. Set all clamp(s) to "off" position.	Setting clamps to "off" position prevents accidental spillage and waste of product.
d. Use aseptic technique and spike bag of 0.9% sodium chloride (NS) IV bag with one of the Y-tubing spikes. Hang bag on IV pole and prime tubing. Open upper clamp on NS side of tubing and squeeze drip chamber until fluid covers filter and one-third to one-half of drip chamber (see Step 2d illustration).	Primes tubing with fluid to eliminate air in Y-tubing. Closing clamp prevents spillage and waste of fluid.

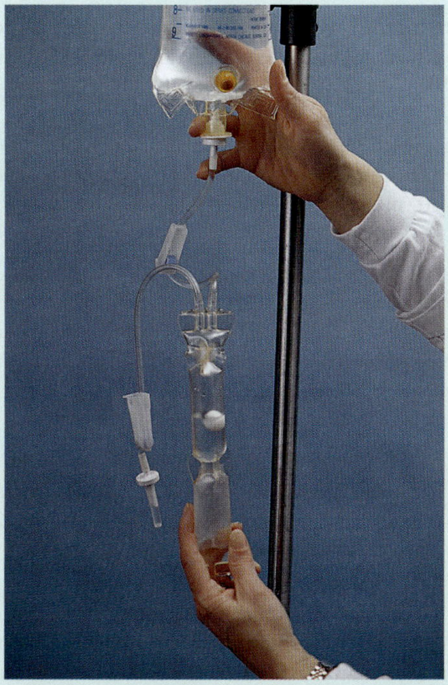

STEP 2D Blood administration set primed with normal saline.

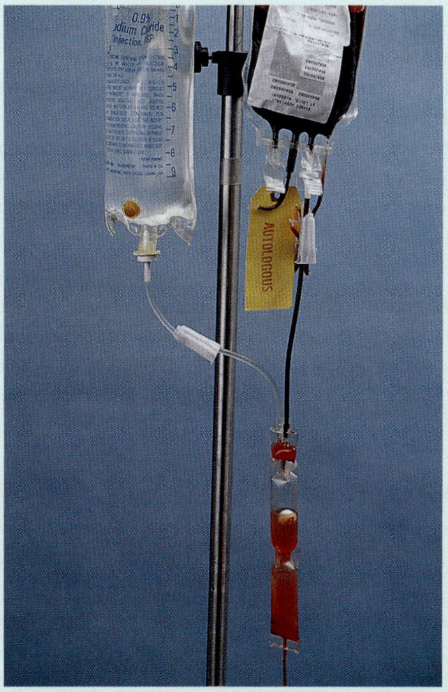

STEP 2F Unit of blood connected to Y-tubing setup.

STEP	RATIONALE
e. Maintain clamp on blood product side of Y-tubing in "off" position. Open common tubing clamp to finish priming tubing to distal end of tubing connector. Close tubing clamp when tubing is filled with NS. All three tubing clamps should be closed. Maintain protective sterile cap on tubing connector.	This step completely primes tubing with NS. IV line is ready to be connected to patient's vascular access device (VAD).
f. Prepare blood component for administration. Gently invert bag two or three times, turning bag back and forth. Remove protective covering from access port. Spike blood component unit with other Y-connection. Close NS clamp above filter, open clamp above filter to blood unit, and prime tubing with blood. Blood will flow into drip chamber (see Step 2f illustration). Tap filter chamber to ensure removal of residual air.	Gentle agitation suspends red blood cells in anticoagulant. A protective barrier drape may be used to catch any potential blood spillage. Tubing is primed with blood unit and ready for transfusion into patient.

Critical Decision Point *NS is compatible with blood products, unlike solutions that contain dextrose, which cause coagulation of blood. Only use 0.9% sodium chloride (NS) to administer blood. No other solutions are to be administered with blood ("piggybacked")* (Callum et al., 2016; Canadian Society for Transfusion Medicine, 2021).

STEP	RATIONALE

IMPLEMENTATION

STEP	RATIONALE
g. Maintaining asepsis, attach primed tubing to patient's VAD by first cleansing the catheter hub with an antiseptic swab. Then, quickly connect NS-primed blood administration tubing directly to patient's VAD.	Reduces transmission of microorganisms from catheter hub. Initiates infusion of blood product into patient's vein.
h. Open common tubing clamp and regulate blood infusion to allow only 2 mL/min to infuse in initial 15 minutes. Remain with patient during first 15 minutes of transfusion. Initial flow rate during this time should be 1–2 mL/min or 10–20 gtt/min (drop factor: 10 gtt/mL).	Many transfusion reactions occur within the first 15 minutes of transfusion. Infusing a small amount of blood component at the beginning minimizes volume of blood to which patient is exposed, thereby minimizing severity of reaction (Tyerman & Cobbett, 2023).

Critical Decision Point *If signs of a transfusion reaction occur,* ***immediately stop the transfusion,*** *start 0.9% sodium chloride (NS) with a new primed tubing attached directly to the VAD hub, and notify the health care provider immediately* (see Skill 30.2). *Do not discard the blood product or tubing because they need to be returned to the blood bank. Do not infuse NS through existing tubing because it will cause blood in tubing to enter patient.*

STEP	RATIONALE
i. Monitor patient's vital signs within 15 minutes of initiating transfusion, at prescribed intervals according to employer policy, at completion of transfusion, and post-transfusion (Tyerman & Cobbett, 2023).	Frequently monitoring patient helps to quickly alert you to transfusion reaction (Canadian Society for Transfusion Medicine, 2021; Gorski, 2019).
j. If there is no transfusion reaction, regulate rate of transfusion according to health care provider's prescription based on drop factor (gtt/mL) for blood administration tubing (see Chapter 29).	Maintaining prescribed rate of flow decreases risk of fluid volume excess while restoring vascular volume. Drop factor for most blood tubing is 10 gtt/mL.

Critical Decision Point *Do not let a unit of blood hang for more than 4 hours because of the danger of bacterial growth. When a longer transfusion time is indicated clinically, the unit may be divided by the blood bank, and the part not being transfused can be properly refrigerated (refer to employer policy). Administration sets should be changed at the completion of each unit or every 4 hours (check employer policy) to reduce bacterial contamination* (INS, 2016). *Blood should only be stored in a refrigerator specifically for blood or blood products to maintain appropriate temperature controls* (Tyerman & Cobbett, 2023).

Critical Decision Point *Medications and solutions should not be infused into the same IV line with a blood component because of the possibility of incompatibility, unless the medication or solution has been approved by Health Canada for use with blood administration. Maintain a separate IV access if patient requires IV solutions or medications* (Gorski, 2019). *Always check employer policy.*

STEP	RATIONALE
k. After blood has infused, clear IV line with 0.9% sodium chloride (NS) and discard blood bag according to employer policy. When consecutive units are prescribed, ensure IV line patency with 0.9% sodium chloride (NS) at keep vein open (KVO) rate as prescribed by health care provider and retrieve subsequent unit for administration.	Infusing IV NS allows remainder of blood in IV tubing to infuse and keeps IV line patent for supportive measures in case of transfusion reaction (Tyerman & Cobbett, 2023). KVO rate must specify infusion rate as required by 10 rights of medication administration.
3. Appropriately dispose of all supplies. Remove gloves and discard.	Routine practices during transfusion reduce transmission of microorganisms.

EVALUATION

STEP	RATIONALE
1. Observe IV site and status of infusion each time vital signs are taken.	Detects presence of IV-related complications (e.g., infiltration, occlusion, phlebitis) and verifies continuous and safe infusion of blood product.
2. Observe for any signs of transfusion reactions such as chills, flushing, itching, dyspnea, or rash during and for 6 hours after transfusion (check employer policy).	Compares presenting signs and symptoms to baseline assessment of patient before transfusion. These are early signs of transfusion reaction or late transfusion reaction (see Table 30.2).

STEP	RATIONALE
EVALUATION	
3. Observe patient and assess laboratory values to determine response to administration of blood component.	Aids in determining whether goals of therapy have been reached or if further blood component therapy will be required. Laboratory results may not reflect transfusion reaction for several hours.
4. Use **teach-back:** "I want to be sure that I explained the reason for your blood transfusion. How can this transfusion help you?" Develop a revised teaching plan if patient or caregiver is unable to teach back correctly.	Determines patient's and caregiver's level of understanding of instructional topic.

Unexpected Outcomes	Related Interventions
1. Patient displays signs and symptoms of transfusion reaction such as chills, flushing, itching, dyspnea, or rash.	• Stop transfusion immediately. • Disconnect blood tubing at VAD hub and cap distal end with sterile connector to maintain sterile system. • Connect new NS solution and primed tubing directly to VAD hub to prevent any subsequent blood from infusing into patient from tubing. • Keep vein open with slow infusion of NS at 1–2 mL/min to ensure venous patency and maintain venous access for medication or to resume transfusion. • Notify health care provider. • See Table 30.2 for interventions.
2. Patient develops infiltration or phlebitis at venipuncture site.	• Transfusion should be stopped at first sign of infiltration, and IV line removed (see Procedural Guideline 29.1). • Insert new VAD in area above previous location or opposite arm. • Restart product if remainder can be infused within 4 hours of initiation of transfusion. • Institute nursing measures to reduce discomfort at infiltrated or phlebotic area.
3. Fluid volume overload occurs, and/or patient exhibits difficulty breathing or has crackles on auscultation of lungs.	• Slow or stop transfusion, elevate head of bed, and inform health care provider of physical findings. • Administer diuretics, morphine, and/or oxygen as prescribed by health care provider. • Continue frequent assessments and closely monitor vital signs and intake and output.

Communication and Documentation

- Before transfusion, document pretransfusion medications, vital signs, location and condition of IV site, and patient education in progress notes in electronic health record (EHR) or chart.
- Document the type and volume of blood component; blood unit number, donor, and recipient identification; compatibility; and expiration date according to employer policy. Document on the transfusion record in progress notes in EHR or chart, MAR, flow sheet, and/or intake and output sheet, depending on employer policy.
- Document volume of NS and blood component infused.
- Document amount of blood received and patient's response to therapy.
- Document vital signs before, shortly after initiation, during, and after transfusion per employer policy.
- Document evaluation of patient and caregiver learning.
- Report signs and symptoms of a transfusion reaction immediately to the health care provider and blood bank. Document in the patient record.
- Report to health care provider any intra-transfusion or post-transfusion deterioration in cardiac, pulmonary, or renal status. Document in the patient record.

DOCUMENTATION EXAMPLE

Patient's hemoglobin was 65 g/L and the primary nurse notified the health care provider of the result. The health care provider prescribed 1 unit of packed red blood cells to be transfused once ready, over 3 hours and followed by a laboratory study of a complete blood count in the evening. Consent for transfusion was signed by the patient and the procedure was explained to the patient. The primary nurse obtained the blood from the blood bank and double-checked the blood and patient identifications with another registered nurse. The primary nurse explained the signs and symptoms of a transfusion reaction to the patient and that they should call for help if experiencing these at any time. Pretransfusion vitals were obtained and documented, and the blood was started at 50 mL/hr per the employer policy. The primary nurse monitored the patient closely for the first 15 minutes, per the employer policy, before increasing the infusion rate. Vitals and infusion rate adjustments were documented in the EMR, and the patient finished receiving the blood transfusion in 3 hours with close observation. The patient did not display any signs of transfusion reaction, and they will have follow-up blood work completed this evening.

Special Considerations

Teaching

- Educate patient and caregiver regarding rationale for transfusion and anticipated amount of time for completion of transfusion.
- Discuss with patient and caregiver the rationale for patient monitoring throughout the transfusion.
- Instruct patient and caregiver to notify the nurse if patient experiences itching, swelling, dizziness, dyspnea, low back pain, chest pain or if feeling generally more unwell than before the infusion because these signs may indicate a transfusion reaction.
- Instruct patient to inform the nurse if redness, pain, tenderness, swelling, bleeding, drainage, or leakage from under the dressing occurs at the IV site.

Pediatric

- Transfuse pediatric patients slowly (1 mL/kg/hr, up to 50 mL/kg/hr) for the first 15 minutes. Then, increase the rate to 5 mL/kg/hr, up to 150 mL/hr. The nurse should stay with the child during this time (Hockenberry et al., 2024).
- Transfusion is not usually required in pediatric patients, unless the hemoglobin level is less than 70 g/L. Neonates under 28 days old may require transfusion sooner (Hockenberry et al., 2024).
- Umbilical catheters may be used in preterm and term infants just after birth (Gorski, 2019).

Gerontological

- Some older persons have decreased cardiac function, thus requiring a slower infusion time. Half units may be obtained if a patient is unable to tolerate the volume of a whole unit of blood or blood component.
- In older persons at risk for TACO, regulate flow rate at 1 mL/kg/hr.

Care in the Community: Home Management

- Patients who have had prior transfusion reactions, acute angina, or heart failure are not appropriate candidates for home transfusion.
- Nursing personnel must be present during the entire transfusion process and for 30 to 60 minutes after transfusion.
- Blood and blood products must be transported in a container with appropriate coolant. Verify and record the temperature at time of delivery.
- Initiate transfusion as soon as possible after the component is obtained from the blood bank.
- When the blood sample is obtained for blood typing and cross-matching, attach the identification band to the patient with their full name and the identification number used by the laboratory. This step ensures that the patient has been correctly identified when blood component transfusion is initiated.
- Instruct patient and caregiver in signs and symptoms of a delayed hemolytic transfusion reaction (i.e., unexplained fever, decrease in hemoglobin and hematocrit levels 2 to 14 days after transfusion) so they can report them and receive treatment, if necessary.
- Return the container, empty bags, and tubing to the community care employer after completion of the transfusion.

✦ SKILL 30.2 Monitoring for Adverse Transfusion Reactions

NSO Nursing Skills Online Blood Therapy Module 15 / Lesson 3

Adverse transfusion reactions may occur any time during a transfusion of blood products and up to 6 hours after a transfusion. Life-threatening reactions usually occur within the first 15 minutes of transfusion. The nurse must remain with the patient during this time to monitor physiological responses.

Several types of adverse reactions may result from a blood transfusion (see Table 30.2). A *hemolytic reaction* is a systemic response to the administration of a blood product that is incompatible with the recipient's blood type. The product either contains allergens to which the recipient is sensitive or allergic, or it is contaminated with pathogens. Some patients who have a history of frequent transfusion may receive premedication with diphenhydramine to combat acquired sensitivities.

Before a transfusion, each blood unit undergoes extensive serological testing to reduce the risk of patients' acquiring a bloodborne disease. Symptoms that indicate an adverse reaction range from fever, chills, and skin rash to hypotension and cardiac arrest. Some patients also experience a delayed transfusion reaction, which sometimes does not occur for days or weeks after the transfusion (Gorski, 2019; Tyerman & Cobbett, 2023). Other possible adverse outcomes that result from transfusion therapy include transmission of diseases, TACO reaction, sepsis reaction, and transfusion-related acute lung injury (TRALI) (Tyerman & Cobbett, 2023). Facilities must report reactions and fatalities that occur as the result of a transfusion reaction to the Canada Vigilance Program, Canadian Blood Services or Héma-Québec, and TTISS.

Delegation and Collaboration

The skill of administering and monitoring blood transfusions cannot be delegated to a UCP. The skill of administering and monitoring blood transfusion by an RPN or LPN varies by provincial and territorial standards of practice as well as employer policy.

After the transfusion has been started and the patient is stable, a UCP can monitor a patient in collaboration with a nurse. This does not relieve an RN of the responsibility to continue to assess the patient during the transfusion. The nurse instructs the UCP about the following:

- The signs and symptoms of a transfusion reaction that the patient may exhibit and immediately reporting these to the nurse

STEP	RATIONALE
ASSESSMENT	
1. Identify patient using at least two person-specific identifiers (e.g., name and date of birth, or name and medical record number) according to employer policy.	Ensures correct patient. Complies with Accreditation Canada's standards and improves patient safety (Accreditation Canada, 2020).

STEP	RATIONALE
ASSESSMENT	
2. Throughout the procedure, the 4 moments for hand hygiene are to be implemented; hand hygiene should occur before initial patient (or patient environment) contact, before an aseptic procedure, after body fluid exposure risk, and after patient (or patient environment) contact. Additional hand hygiene should be performed when hands are visibly soiled.	Proper hand hygiene helps prevent the spread of infectious agents to health care providers.
3. With initiation of a transfusion, observe patient for fever, with or without chills.	Fever indicates onset of AHTR, febrile nonhemolytic reaction, or bacterial sepsis.
4. Assess patient for tachycardia and/or tachypnea and dyspnea.	Indicates AHTR or TACO. In case of TACO, cough may accompany these symptoms.
5. Observe patient for drop in blood pressure.	Hypotension indicates infectious disease transmission, AHTR, or anaphylaxis.
6. Observe patient for hives or skin rash, including on trunk and back.	These signs are early indications of an allergic reaction, anaphylaxis, or TA-GVHD.
7. Observe patient for flushing.	This sign is an early indication of AHTR or febrile nonhemolytic reaction. Sometimes, localized flushing presents with an allergic reaction.
8. Observe patient for gastrointestinal symptoms.	Nausea and vomiting are present in AHTRs, anaphylactic reactions, and infectious disease transmission.
9. Observe patient for wheezing, chest pain, and possible cardiac arrest.	These are all indications of anaphylactic reaction.
10. Be alert to patient reports of headache or muscle pain in presence of fever.	Both indicate febrile nonhemolytic reaction.
11. Monitor patient for *disseminated intravascular coagulation (DIC)* (presence of blood in urine; easily bruises; bleeding from eyes, nose, ears, and mouth; headache; shortness of breath; chest pain; heavier-than-normal periods; signs of a DVT; and neurological decline such as confusion), renal failure, anemia, and hemoglobinemia/hemoglobinuria by reviewing laboratory test results (complete blood count [CBC] with differential, hemoglobin [Hgb], and hematocrit [Hct]).	All are late signs of an AHTR.
12. Auscultate patient's lungs before and during transfusion and monitor central venous pressure (CVP), if possible.	Crackles in base of lungs and rising CVP are indications of TACO.
13. Observe patient for jaundice and increased liver enzyme levels (indicating liver damage) and decreased red blood cells (RBCs), white blood cells (WBCs), and platelets (indicating bone marrow suppression).	These signs indicate TA-GVHD and would occur following transfusion.
14. In patients receiving massive transfusions, observe for mild hypothermia, cardiac dysrhythmias, hypotension, hypocalcemia, and hemochromatosis (iron overload).	Cold blood products affect the cardiac conduction system, resulting in ventricular dysrhythmias. Other cardiac dysrhythmias, hypotension, and tingling indicate hypocalcemia, which occurs when citrate (used as a preservative for some blood products) combines with patient's calcium. Iron overload may occur after 10 transfusions (see Table 30.2). It usually occurs in patients who require chronic transfusions.

NURSING DIAGNOSES

- Inadequate gas exchange
- Excessive fluid volume
- Reduced cardiac output
- Hyperthermia
- Acute pain
- Potential for infection
- Anxiety
- Hypothermia

Related factors and risk factors are individualized on the basis of patient's condition or needs.

PLANNING

STEP	RATIONALE
1. Expected outcomes following completion of procedure:	
• Patient's cardiac parameters (heart rate, blood pressure, CVP) return to baseline.	Intravascular volume is restored, reaction reversed.
• Patient maintains core body temperature of 36–37.2°C (97–99°F).	Helps confirm absence of transfusion reaction, infection, and sepsis.
• Patient has urine output of 0.5–1 mL/kg/hr.	Reflects optimal fluid status.
• Patient maintains oxygen saturation >95%.	Improved tissue perfusion.

STEP	RATIONALE
PLANNING	
• Patient is comfortable.	Absence of transfusion reaction. Appropriate nursing measures keep patient at ease.
2. Patient can explain signs and symptoms of a transfusion reaction.	Reduces anxiety and helps patient and caregiver anticipate nurse's actions.
IMPLEMENTATION	
1. If transfusion reaction is suspected:	
a. Immediately stop transfusion.	Severity of reaction is related to the amount of blood component infused and cause of the reaction. It is critical to prevent any more blood from infusing into patient.
b. Remove blood component and tubing containing blood product. Replace them with new bag of 0.9% sodium chloride (NS) and tubing (see Chapter 29). Connect tubing directly to hub of VAD. Exception: If patient symptoms suggest mild allergic reaction, stop transfusion, administer antihistamine, and restart or discontinue transfusion per health care provider's prescription.	Prevents additional blood in tubing from being infused.
c. Maintain patent VAD using 0.9% sodium chloride (NS) at rate prescribed by health care provider.	NS keeps IV patent and provides route for emergency medications and fluids.
d. Obtain vital signs. Remain with patient for continuous monitoring and assessment. Do not leave patient alone.	Vital signs are objective measures of patient's condition, which can deteriorate rapidly.
e. Notify health care provider.	Transfusion reactions require immediate medical intervention. Follow protocol for emergency interventions for anaphylactic reactions.
f. Notify blood bank.	Blood bank has procedure to follow when notified of transfusion reaction.
g. Obtain blood samples (if needed) from the extremity opposite the extremity receiving transfusion. Check employer policy regarding number and type of tubes to be used.	Typically, one tube of blood will be crossmatched to pretransfusion sample to ensure that correct blood was given to recipient. Blood will be checked for antibodies to determine type of reaction. Second sample will be checked for free hemoglobin in serum, indicating hemolysis, and bilirubin level should be obtained.
h. Return remainder of blood component and attached blood tubing to blood bank according to employer policy.	Sample of this blood will be crossmatched to patient's pretransfusion and post-transfusion samples to determine whether error in crossmatching occurred.
i. Monitor patient's vital signs every 15 minutes (or per employer policy).	Maintains ongoing assessment of patient's cardiopulmonary status and response to treatment.
j. Administer prescribed medications according to type and severity of transfusion reaction:	Follow employer protocol or health care provider's prescription.
(1) Epinephrine	Stimulates sympathetic nervous system to relieve respiratory distress and combat vasodilation in anaphylaxis.
(2) Antihistamine	Diminishes some aspects of allergic response by blocking histamine receptors.
(3) Antibiotics	Administered when bacterial contamination or sepsis is suspected.
(4) Antipyretics/analgesics	Administered to relieve fever and discomfort in AHTRs, febrile nonhemolytic reactions, TA-GVHD, and bacterial sepsis.
(5) Diuretics/morphine	Treats TACO by reducing intravascular volume (diuresis) and decreasing vascular tone (opioid effect).
(6) Corticosteroids	Stabilizes cell membranes, decreasing histamine release. Administered in severe allergic reactions.
(7) IV fluids	Rapid administration of IV fluids counteracts some symptoms of anaphylactic shock.
k. In event of cardiac arrest, initiate cardiopulmonary resuscitation (CPR) (see Chapter 28).	Anaphylaxis can quickly lead to cardiopulmonary arrest. Prompt resuscitation may prevent further complications.
l. Obtain first voided urine sample and send to laboratory; Foley catheter may need to be inserted to obtain urine (see Chapter 34).	Hemoglobinuria occurs with AHTRs. Degree of damage to kidneys is influenced by pH of urine and rate of urinary excretion. Attempts will be made to initiate diuresis and alkalinize urine. If kidney damage is severe, dialysis may be required.
2. Help patient to a comfortable position.	Promotes comfort and safety.
3. Dispose of equipment in appropriate receptacle; remove gloves and discard.	Reduces transmission of microorganisms.

STEP	RATIONALE
EVALUATION	
1. Continue monitoring patient for signs and symptoms of transfusion reactions.	Continued monitoring of patient's cardiopulmonary status and physiological response will indicate whether reaction has been reversed.
2. **Use teach-back:** "I want to be sure that I explained the reactions that can occur when you are getting a blood transfusion. What signs and symptoms would you report?" Develop a revised teaching plan if patient or caregiver is unable to teach back correctly.	Determines patient's and caregiver's level of understanding of instructional topic.

Unexpected Outcomes	Related Interventions
1. Patient's physiological status worsens.	• Appropriate interventions depend on type of transfusion reaction. See Table 30.2 for general guidelines.

Communication and Documentation

- Document the exact time the transfusion reaction was first noted, all vital signs and other physiological assessments, treatments instituted, and patient response in progress notes in EHR or chart. Complete transfusion reaction report (according to employer policy).
- Document your evaluation of patient and caregiver learning.
- Immediately report presence of transfusion reaction and patient's physical assessment findings to health care provider.

Special Considerations

Teaching

- Teach patient and caregiver signs and symptoms of transfusion reactions and steps to take if they occur.

Pediatric

- Irradiated red blood cells and platelets are preferable in children under 6 years of age because of their immature immune systems and to avoid TA-GVHD.

Gerontological

- Administer blood components cautiously to older persons, considering both the rate and amount of infusion, because they are at risk of developing TACO.

Care in the Community: Home Management

- Certain adverse outcomes (development of hepatitis) or transfusion reactions (delayed hemolysis) occur days to weeks after patient has received transfusion and may become evident in the home setting.
- It is important that patients and caregivers be aware of signs and symptoms of adverse occurrences and steps to take should they occur.

✦ REVIEW QUESTIONS

A 72-year-old patient (he/him) is admitted for a hip replacement and has donated 1 unit of autologous blood in case he needs transfusion therapy after surgery. Three weeks earlier, the surgery had been postponed because the patient had a case of pneumonia that required treatment with antibiotics. While awaiting hip surgery, he developed bleeding hemorrhoids, which were surgically repaired yesterday. Today, he tells the nurse that he is very tired, and he passed a great deal of blood with several bowel movements during the night and earlier this morning. His colouring is pale, and his skin is cool to the touch. His blood pressure has dropped since admission, from 130/80 to 100/66 mm Hg. His health care provider told him that he may need a blood transfusion. He had blood drawn this morning, and his hemoglobin has dropped from 100 to 90 g/L. The patient states that he is very concerned about being transfused, and he thinks that the blood he donated will not be good since it was taken over a month ago.

Review Questions 1 to 3 relate to the case study presented here.

1. Based on the patient's concerns, which items would be assessed in preparation for a blood transfusion?

2. After the nurse obtains the unit of packed red blood cells (PRBCs) from the blood bank, the patient is taken to the operating room (OR) for a procedure to stop the rectal bleeding, which will last 1 to 2 hours before starting the blood transfusion. Which actions would the nurse take while waiting for the patient to return?

3. The patient has had no bleeding since his return to the unit from the operating room (OR), and the nurse begins the blood transfusion as prescribed. About 30 minutes after initiating the first unit of packed red blood cells (PRBCs), he reports that he is itchy all over his body and presents with a rash and hives. His vital signs are as follows: temperature, 37°C; pulse, 112 beats/min; respiration, 24 breaths/min; and blood pressure, 126/80 mm Hg. Using SBAR (situation–background–assessment–recommendation), show how the nurse would communicate with the health care team about this patient.

4. Which of the following steps are necessary for initiating a transfusion of packed red blood cells (PRBCs)? (*Select all that apply.*)

1. Infuse blood component with 5% dextrose in water (D_5W).
2. Follow employer policy to verify correct patient and blood product.
3. Check appearance of blood for leaks, bubbles, clots, or purplish colour.
4. Infuse blood component over 4 to 6 hours to prevent fluid volume overload.
5. Obtain vital signs before infusion, after 5 to 15 minutes of initiating infusion, and at its completion.
6. Clear intravenous (IV) line with 0.9% sodium chloride (normal saline) after transfusion.

5. The patient is experiencing an acute hemolytic transfusion reaction (AHTR) while receiving packed red blood cells (PRBCs). Place the following steps in the correct order:

1. Obtain vital signs and remain with the patient.
2. Stop the infusion.
3. Obtain blood and urine samples.
4. Replace the blood component and tubing with a new bag of 0.9% sodium chloride (normal saline [NS]) and new tubing.
5. Notify the blood bank.
6. Notify the health care provider.

6. Which of the following items must be verified to ensure that the correct blood component is transfused to the correct patient? (*Select all that apply.*)

1. Verbally compare and correctly identify the patient's identity using two patient identifiers.
2. Verify that the transfusion record number matches the patient's identification number.
3. Check that the expiration date has not passed.
4. Confirm that the blood collection date is within 72 hours of the transfusion.
5. Have two qualified individuals perform verifications before initiation of transfusion.
6. Verify that the blood component and type to be infused match the patient's.

Visit the Evolve site for a complete list of answers to the Review Questions.

NEXT GENERATION NCLEX® (NGN)

For practice with answering exam questions related to unfolding NGN case studies, please consult the Next Generation NCLEX® (NGN)-Style Case Studies for Skills and Techniques on the Evolve website: http://evolve.elsevier.com/Canada/Perry/clinicalskills/

REFERENCES

Accreditation Canada. (2020). *Required organizational practices–2020 handbook.* https://physicians.nshealth.ca/resources/required-organizational-practices-2020-handbook

Astle, B. J., & Duggleby, W. (2024). *Potter and Perry's Canadian fundamentals of nursing* (7th ed.). Elsevier.

Bahri, T., de Bruyn, K., Leys, R., et al. (2018). Fatal acute hemolytic transfusion reaction due to anti-Wra. *Transfusion Medicine and Hemotherapy, 45*(6), 438–441. https://doi.org/10.1159/000488863

Berta, D. (2020). *Bloody easy–blood administration: A handbook for health care professionals (version 3).* Ontario Regional Blood Coordinating Network. https://transfusionontario.org/wp-content/uploads/2021/08/Bloody-Easy-Version-3-Interactive-English-Final-Page-Spreads.pdf

Bojanić, I., Lukić, M., Plenković, F., et al. (2022). Changes in the incidence of transfusion reactions in hematological patients over the past 30 years. *Transfusion, 62*(3), 600–611. https://doi.org/10.1111/trf.16816

Callum, J., Pinkerton, P. H., Lima, A., et al. (2016). *Bloody easy 4–Blood transfusions, blood alternatives, and transfusion reactions: A guide to transfusion medicine* (4th ed.). Ontario Regional Blood Coordinating Network. https://transfusionontario.org/wp-content/uploads/2020/06/EN_BE4-JULY11_FINAL.pdf [Seminal Reference]

Canadian Blood Services. (2017–2023). *Clinical guide to transfusion.* https://professionaleducation.blood.ca/en/transfusion/clinical-guide-transfusion

Canadian Society for Transfusion Medicine. (2021). *Standards for hospital transfusion services (version 5).* https://cstm.wildapricot.org/CSTM-Blood-Transfusion-Standards

Clarke, G., & Hannon, J. (2018). Hemolytic disease of the fetus and newborn and perinatal immune thrombocytopenia. In G. Clarke & S. Chargé (Eds.), *Clinical guide to transfusion* (Chapter 12). https://professionaleducation.blood.ca/en/transfusion/clinical-guide-transfusion

Duncan, J. (2020). Pre-transfusion testing. In G. Clarke & S. Chargé (Eds.), *Clinical guide to transfusion* (Chapter 8). https://professionaleducation.blood.ca/en/transfusion/clinical-guide-transfusion

Gorski, L. (2019). *Phillips's manual of IV therapeutics: Evidence-based practice for infusion therapy* (7th ed.). F. A. Davis.

Goulding, M., Graham, L., Chorney, D., et al. (2020). The use of interprofessional simulation to improve collaboration and problem solving among undergraduate BHSc medical laboratory science and BScN nursing students. *Canadian Journal of Medical Laboratory Science, 82*(2), 25–33.

Health Canada. (2023). Guidance document: Blood regulations. https://www.canada.ca/en/health-canada/services/drugs-health-products/biologics-radiopharmaceuticals-genetic-therapies/applications-submissions/guidance-documents/blood-regulations/guidance-document-blood-regulations-1.html

Healthcare Excellence Canada. (2020). *Hospital harm improvement resource: Infusion, transfusion, and injection complications.* https://www.patientsafetyinstitute.ca/en/toolsResources/Hospital-Harm-Measure/Improvement-Resources/Infusion-Transfusion-Injection-Complications/Documents/HHIR-Infusion-Transfusion-Injectibles-Complications-A11.pdf

Hockenberry, M., Duffy, E. A., & Gibbs, K. (2024). *Wong's nursing care of infants and children* (12th ed.). Elsevier.

Infusion Nurses Society (INS). (2016). Infusion therapy standards of practice. *Journal of Intravenous Nursing, 39*(Suppl. 1), S1–S161. http://source.yiboshi.com/20170417/1492425631944540325.pdf [Seminal Reference]

Lausten, M. B., Rasmussen, S., & Gazerani, P. (2018). Association between the ABO blood types and post-operative pain. *European Neurological Review, 13*(1), 38–43. https://doi.org/10.17925/ENR.2018.13.1.38

National Advisory Committee on Blood and Blood Products. (2014). *NAC companion document to "red blood cell transfusion: A clinical practice guideline from the AABB."* https://nacblood.ca/en/resource/nac-companion-document-red-blood-cell-transfusion-clinical-practice-guideline-aabb [Seminal Reference]

Public Health Agency of Canada. (2016). *Transfusion Transmitted Injuries Surveillance system (TTISS): 2009–2013 summary results.* https://publications.gc.ca/collections/collection_2016/aspc-phac/HP40-168-2016-eng.pdf [Seminal Reference]

Public Health Agency of Canada. (2019). *Transfusion Transmitted Injuries Surveillance system 2011–2015 summary report.* https://www.canada.ca/en/public-health/services/publications/drugs-health-products/transfusion-transmitted-injuries-surveillance-system-ttiss-2011-2015-summary-results.html

Tyerman, J., & Cobbett, S. (Eds.). (2023). *Lewis's medical–surgical nursing in Canada: Assessment and management of clinical problems* (5th ed.). Elsevier Inc.

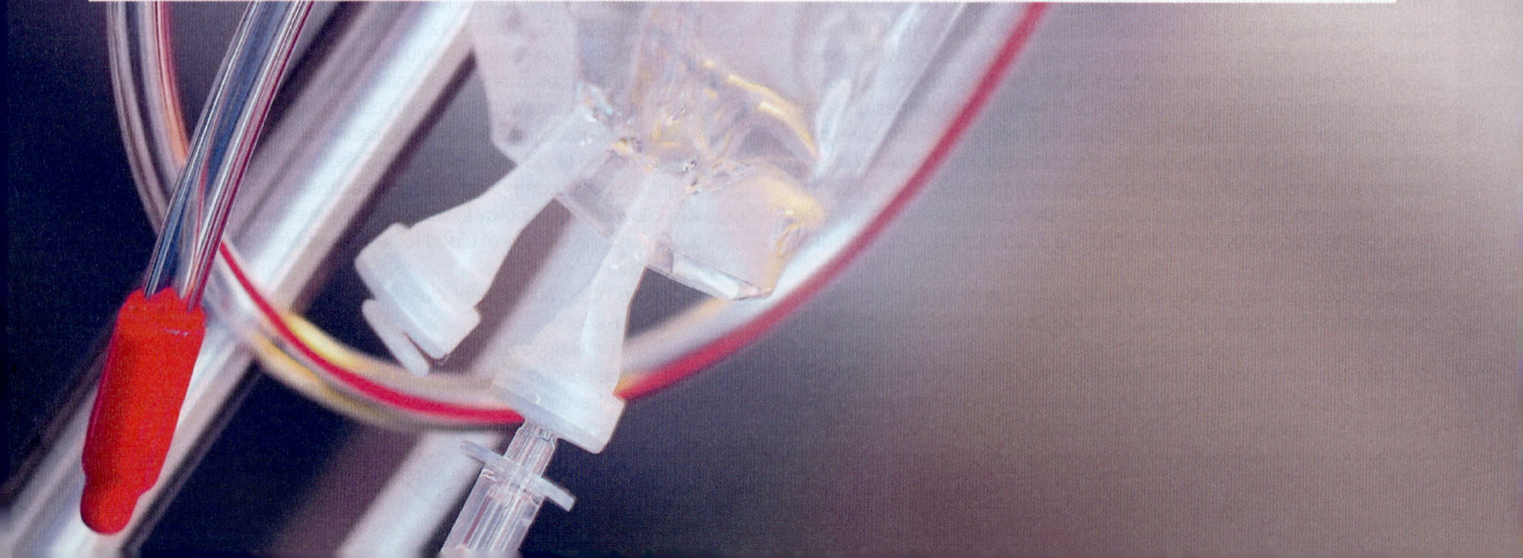

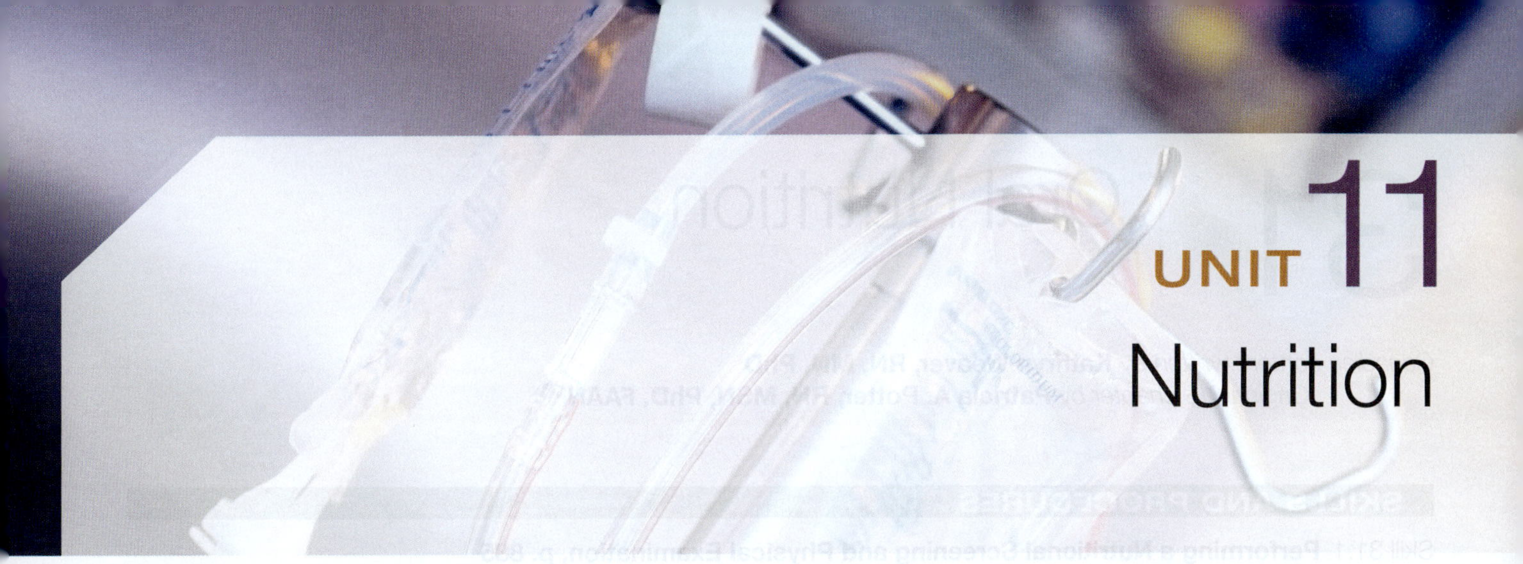

UNIT 11 Nutrition

Providing patients with adequate nutrition requires application of knowledge about normal nutritional needs, the nutritional deficiencies caused by various health conditions, and patients' physical ability to take in nutrients. In addition, knowledge is needed regarding patients' risk for deficiencies and patients' values and cultural beliefs about food and eating habits. Because there are patients who are unable to swallow easily or who require nutritional elements to be delivered by routes other than oral intake, knowledge of the risks involved must be considered to prevent complications such as aspiration and infection. Nutritional standards such as *Canada's Food Guide* provide direction for determining a patient's dietary requirements so that you can compare what is recommended with a patient's actual dietary deficits.

A thorough patient assessment is necessary for you to be able to make dietary recommendations and educate patients and families about nutrition and the role it plays in maintaining health. In outpatient and home health settings, nurses are in an ideal position to better understand a patient's food preferences, meal patterns, and eating habits so that any recommendations are more individualized and likely to be accepted. In acute care, nurses often must focus on assessing whether patients are physically able to self-feed or swallow safely. Patient-centred nutritional care requires patients to partner with you in making decisions about ways to improve their nutritional intake. These decisions also affect how you can support patients who need assistance with self-feeding.

A patient who is on aspiration precautions is at risk of aspirating mucous secretions or food from the oral cavity into the tracheobronchial tree. Aspiration often leads to pneumonia, a serious complication. Your knowledge of patient conditions that pose risks for dysphagia (e.g., stroke, Parkinson's disease, head and neck surgery), the signs of dysphagia, and the presence of cognitive changes allows you to critically anticipate the need for precautions to take during oral feeding. You apply the same knowledge along with therapeutic communication skills and teaching principles to educate caregivers who assist patients with feeding. Often, the expertise of a speech-language pathologist is needed to ensure that foods of the right consistency are offered to patients with dysphagia.

A patient who requires enteral nutrition has serious health problems that prevent the oral intake of nutrients. The safe administration of enteral nutrition requires critical thinking in your assessment of the integrity and function of a feeding tube and whether the patient is at risk for tube displacement and aspiration. Standards for enteral nutrition practices offer the framework for how to identify patient risks, maintain function of a feeding tube, and prevent complications. For example, while preparing to administer a tube feeding, you check the pH of aspirate taken from the tube and find it to be highly alkaline, above what is normally expected. You apply critical thinking to problem solve and determine whether the abnormal pH is due to medications the patient is receiving or possible tube displacement. Similarly, once you have administered a feeding, you critically apply appropriate assessment skills to evaluate whether the patient is tolerating the feeding. Adaptations to a skill are sometimes needed when administering tube feedings. For example, a standard exists for keeping the head of the bed elevated during administration of a tube feeding to prevent aspiration. But what if a patient has a stage 4 pressure injury? Is an upright position safe? Assessment of the patient's condition and priority needs along with collaboration with dietitians and health care providers guides you in the best action to take.

Parenteral nutrition poses significant risks to patients because it is delivered intravenously at a high nutrient concentration. A patient's database must include continuous measurements of intake and output, serum blood tests, vital signs, and body weight. You use these data for ongoing monitoring to detect complications as early as possible. The high concentration of glucose in parenteral solutions predisposes patients to infection, both at the site of intravenous insertion and systemically. You must apply knowledge of the infectious process to anticipate clinical signs. Also, you apply standards of the Infusion Nurses Society (INS) in providing meticulous site care and sterile aseptic dressing changes. You also apply INS standards to correctly monitor parenteral solution infusion rates and know when to act if metabolic or electrolyte imbalances develop.

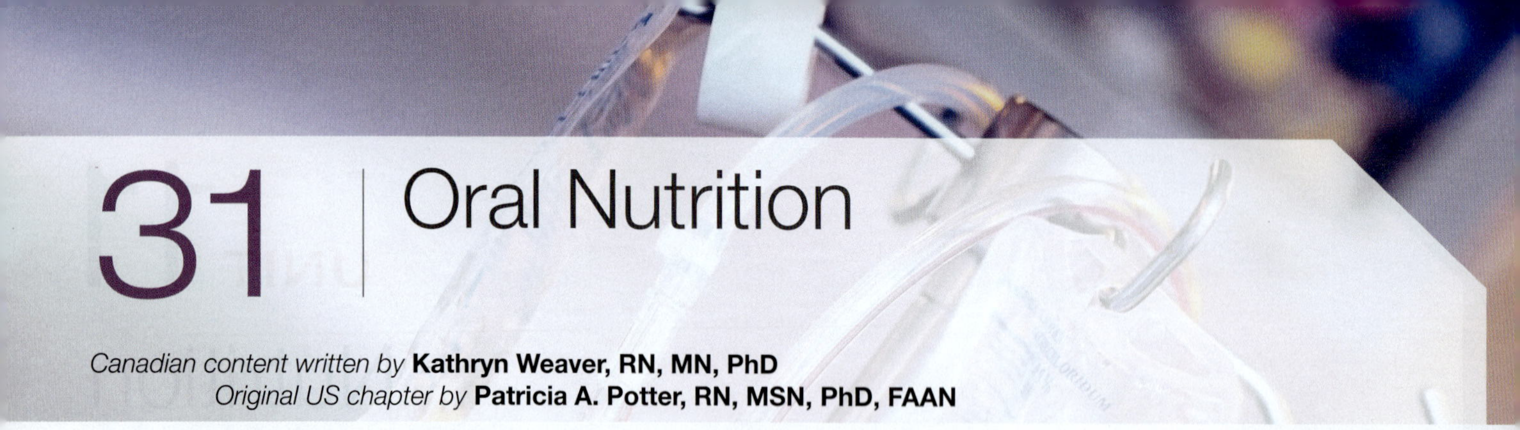

31 Oral Nutrition

Canadian content written by **Kathryn Weaver, RN, MN, PhD**
Original US chapter by **Patricia A. Potter, RN, MSN, PhD, FAAN**

SKILLS AND PROCEDURES

OBJECTIVES

Mastery of content in this chapter will enable the nurse to:

- Perform an accurate nutritional screening.
- Identify the need for a nutritional assessment and collaborate with a dietitian accordingly.
- Assess a patient's ability to swallow.
- Identify risk factors for aspiration.
- Evaluate a patient's tolerance of oral nutrition.
- Identify appropriate techniques to use to prevent a patient from aspirating.
- Demonstrate how to properly feed a patient who cannot self-feed.

MEDIA RESOURCES

- http://evolve.elsevier.com/Canada/Perry/clinicalskills/

PURPOSE

Nutrition is a basic component of health that affects a patient's rate of recovery from illness, surgery, and injury. Malnutrition develops as a result of deficiency in dietary intake, increased requirements associated with disease, complications of an underlying illness such as poor absorption, and excessive nutrient losses, or a combination of these factors (NHS Inform, 2023). Young children, adolescents, and individuals who are pregnant or breastfeeding are the most vulnerable to malnutrition from undernutrition (World Vision, 2021) because their bodies have a greater need for nutrients, such as vitamins and minerals. For example, adolescents with female genitalia are at high risk for iron-deficiency anemia owing to accelerated growth rate and menstruation-related iron loss, while children are at the highest risk of dying from starvation. Nutritional compromise may further result when people lack control over decisions that affect their health and nutrition. In Canada, children 14 years old and under are outnumbered by persons aged 65 plus (Canadian Frailty Network, 2019). Estimates suggest that 30 to 45% of medical patients at an average age of 65 years are malnourished upon admission to hospital. Malnutrition contributes to many conditions, including frailty, a condition estimated to occur in 22% of older Canadians, with an additional 32% considered to be prefrail (Gilmour & Ramage-Morin, 2021). Both categories of frailty are associated with higher risk of mortality from neoplasms, circulatory diseases, and respiratory diseases among community-dwelling older persons.

Every organ system is affected by malnutrition. Complications include alterations in muscle, cardiorespiratory, and gastrointestinal function; immunity and wound healing; and psychosocial effects. As a nurse, you will provide nutritional screening and use interprofessional collaboration (e.g., dietitian, nutritionist, health care provider) to determine the best approaches for supporting patients' nutritional health.

STANDARDS OF CARE

- Accreditation Canada (2020)—*Required Organizational Practices–2020 Handbook* (https://physicians.nshealth.ca/resources/required-organizational-practices-2020-handbook)
- Alberta Health Services (2019)—*Nutrition Guideline: Seniors Health Overview (65 Years and Older)* (https://www.albertahealthservices.ca/assets/info/nutrition/if-nfs-ng-seniors-health-overview.pdf)
- Health Canada (2022a)—*Food and Nutrition* (https://www.canada.ca/en/health-canada/services/food-nutrition.html)
- Health Canada (2023a)—*Canada's Dietary Guidelines for Health Professionals and Policy Makers* (https://food-guide.canada.ca/en/guidelines/)
- Health Canada (2023b)—*Health Canada's Healthy Eating Strategy* (https://www.canada.ca/en/services/health/campaigns/vision-healthy-canada/healthy-eating.html)
- Health Canada (2023c)—*Regulations and Compliance: Nutrition Labelling* (https://www.canada.ca/en/health-canada/services/food-nutrition/food-labelling/nutrition-labelling/regulations-compliance.html)

PRINCIPLES FOR PRACTICE

The Integrated Nutrition Pathway for Acute Care (INPAC) was developed by the Canadian Malnutrition Task Force (Keller, Laur, et al., 2018). The aim of INPAC is to triage all patients to ensure that they receive appropriate nutrition care in health care settings. INPAC encourages all hospital staff to be involved in nutrition care for all patients.

For hospitalized patients, nutritional screening is completed during patient admission. One aim of nutritional screening is to identify common risk factors for nutritional problems (Box 31.1). Nutritional assessment should be completed within 24 hours of screening (Keller, Lengyel, et al., 2018). Food intake, weight history, functional status, and body composition are assessed; the assessment takes approximately 10 minutes.

Recommendations for nutritional care are based on the assessment. If the patient is at risk for malnutrition, optimal oral intake is provided and monitored. Barriers to food intake are assessed in determining a change in nutrition care. Patients who are assessed as being at severe risk of malnutrition may be seen by a dietitian for specialized dietary treatment (Keller, Lengyel, et al., 2018).

- The updated INPAC emphasizes the need for accurate and regular weights, with admission weight and weekly weights considered a minimum for best practice (Keller, Laur, et al., 2018).
- Ensuring the accuracy of food intake estimations and promoting intervention when food intake is defined as low (i.e., ≤50%) are key areas for education and training.
- If a patient is malnourished at admission or during hospitalization, nutrition is flagged in the discharge summary note (completed by the dietitian, health care provider, or nurse). Education is provided to the patient and caregiver. Transfer of care recommendations include dietitian referral if nutrition rehabilitation is ongoing.
- Nothing by mouth (NPO) status should be monitored daily. Being NPO for 3 days may necessitate a comprehensive nutrition assessment because during the first 3 days of NPO, the body loses about 10 g of nitrogen (equivalent to 62.5 g of protein or 169 g of muscle) per day; and although fat loss is minimal, the major losses are a depleted liver store of glycogen (energy), sodium with water, and approximately 500 g of muscle (Canadian Malnutrition Task Force as cited in Canadian Nurses Association, 2018).
- Patients who are malnourished have a longer hospital stay and may experience more complications (e.g., infection rates, mortality) during their period of hospitalization than patients who are in a well-nourished state (Oleynick et al., 2021).
- As a nurse, you are responsible for assisting patients who are on an oral diet to successfully eat an adequate amount of food at a safe and comfortable pace.

The intent of *Canada's Food Guide* (Health Canada, 2023a) is to promote health; reduce the risk of chronic diseases; and provide the basis for federal, provincial, and territorial food and nutrition policy and education initiatives. These guidelines are based on the best available scientific evidence and apply to Canadians aged 2 years and older. The recommended diet consists mainly of plant foods (e.g., fruit, vegetables, whole grains, and plant-based protein such as nuts, seeds, beans, lentils, and soy), whole foods, and minimal use of processed foods and beverages with added sodium, free sugars, or saturated fat. Because sugary drinks such as soda pop, juice, and sports drinks are the main source of total sugars in the Canadian diet, and excess sugar is linked to obesity and heart disease, the guidelines recommend that Canadians make water the beverage of choice to reduce intake of sugary drinks. Canadians are also encouraged to cook more often, eat meals with others, be mindful of eating habits, enjoy food, and be aware of food marketing, which can often be misleading.

Food insecurity occurs whenever the availability of nutritionally adequate and safe food or the ability to acquire food in socially accepted ways is inadequate. Food insecurity is more prevalent in households with children; those led by lone parents who identify as female; those with social assistance, worker's compensation, or employment insurance as the main source of income; those led by an adult with less than a high school diploma; those located in urban areas; and those who rent rather than own their place of residence. Food insecurity is higher in off-reserve Indigenous and recent immigrant households. In 2019, Nova Scotia and Alberta had food insecurity rates significantly above the national average, while only Quebec had a rate that was lower than average (Caron & Plunkett-Latimer, 2022).

In fall 2020, 6 to 9 months into the COVID-19 pandemic, about 1 in 10 Canadians (9.6%) aged 12 and older living in the 10 provinces reported experiencing food insecurity in their household within the past 12 months (Polsky & Garriguet, 2022). This proportion was lower than the approximately 1 in 8 Canadians (12.6%) who had reported household food insecurity in 2019. Emerging reports suggested that the temporary pandemic relief benefits (e.g., the Canada Emergency Response Benefit, available to people who had lost their jobs or were working reduced hours; the Canada Emergency Student Benefit; and supplements to the Canada Child Benefit) helped mitigate the impact of job and income losses for many Canadian households, particularly those with middle and lower incomes. Reduced overall consumer spending as a result of economic shutdowns and slowdowns during the pandemic may also have boosted disposable income for some households. The evidence concerning the prevalence of household food insecurity during the COVID-19 pandemic is still uncertain and suggests that total household food insecurity in Canada may have slightly increased during the pandemic, especially

BOX 31.1

Risk Factors for Potential Nutritional Problems

- Clear- or full-liquid diets for more than 3 days with inappropriate or insufficient nutrient supplementation
- Intravenous feeding (dextrose and saline or saline alone)
- NPO (nothing by mouth) for more than 3 days without nutrient supplementation
- Low intake (<50%) of prescribed diet or tube feedings
- Weight (accounting for edema) 20% above or 10% below a healthy body weight
- Pregnancy weight gain deviating from the normal pattern of gaining 0.45 kg/week during the last 20 weeks of pregnancy; higher-than-normal maternal weight gain is associated with preeclampsia (high blood pressure and organ system damage during pregnancy), low birth weight, and perinatal death
- Diagnoses that increase nutritional needs or decrease nutrient intake: cancer, malabsorption, diarrhea, hyperthyroidism, excessive inflammation, postoperative status, hemorrhage, infected or draining wounds, burns, infection, major trauma
- Chronic use of drugs, especially alcohol, which affects nutritional intake
- Alterations in chewing, swallowing, appetite, taste, and smell
- Body temperature consistently higher than 37°C (98.6°F) for more than 2 days, as fever increases both energy and micronutrient requirements
- Hematocrit: <41% (male reference range), <36% (female reference range) (Moawad, 2021); hemoglobin <140 g/L (male reference range), <120 g/L (female reference range) can signal anemia, which may compromise tissue oxygen delivery ("Hemoglobin level," 2020)
- Decrease in absolute lymphocyte count is a predictor of nutritional risk (1.2–2 × 10^9/L labelled as mild, 0.8–1.19× 10^9/L as moderately malnourished, and <0.8 × 10^9/L as severely malnourished) and surgical complications (Akula & Doctor, 2021)
- Elevated (>5 mmol/L) or decreased (<1.5 mmol/L) total plasma cholesterol, as this is associated with cardiovascular disease risk
- Serum albumin <35 g/L in patients without renal or liver disease, generalized dermatitis, or overhydration, as this is a predictor of nutritional risk and surgical site infection complications (Moman et al., 2022)

Adapted from Grodner, M., Escott-Stump, S., & Dorner, S. (2023). *Foundations and clinical applications of nutrition: A nursing approach* (8th ed.). Elsevier.

in populations that were already vulnerable to food insecurity. There is a need to continue monitoring food insecurity in Canada (Idzerda et al., 2022). Nurses need to maintain awareness of any ongoing disruption in the financial resources of many households, especially low-income households, those with young children, and those in tenuous work environments, particularly as government relief benefits related to COVID-19 have been eliminated.

PERSON-CENTRED CARE

- An understanding of patients' values, beliefs, and attitudes about food and how these values affect food purchase, preparation, and intake enables nurses to support patients in making healthy food choices.
- Interprofessional collaboration has positive effects on patient health outcomes by increasing patient access to nutrition education, self-management training, and nutritional support.
- Individuals follow special patterns of food intake that are based on religion, cultural background, ethics, health beliefs, or concern about the environment. Such special diets (e.g., vegetarian, ovolactovegetarian) do not necessarily provide more or less nutritional benefit than diets based on *Canada's Food Guide* or other nutritional guidelines (Health Canada, 2021c).
- *Canada's Food Guide* was developed by Health Canada (2023a) (Fig. 31.1) as a visual aid to encourage Canadians to fill half of their plates with vegetables and fruits at every meal. Most Canadians need to improve some aspect of their diet. Nurses should use interprofessional collaboration (e.g., dietitian) in considering social factors that influence a person's diet. These factors include personal factors that affect choice of food (e.g., physiological state, food preferences, nutritional knowledge, perceptions of healthy eating and psychological factors); the economic ecosystem (e.g., prices of food, food security, income, and employment); the social environment (e.g., people with whom an individual interacts on a daily basis, including culture, family, acquaintances, friends, and social media); and the physical environment (i.e., infrastructures that affect food availability such as food outlets in their environment, including work sites, schools, restaurants, and supermarkets) (Marcone et al., 2020).
- Some cultures believe in a hot-and-cold theory of health and illness based on the ancient Taoist concept of an essential life force, or qi, present in all objects and aspects of life. For a balanced diet, the yin (cold, dark, passive) and the yang (heat, light, active) are combined in the form of food to create harmony within the body (Dashtdar et al., 2022). Foods are classified as hot or cold on the basis of their effect on the metabolism after consumption, independent of the temperature at which they are served (Xie et al., 2020). Hotness in the body occurs after eating yang-type (hot) foods such as chicken, venison, and low-fibre foods such as coconut water, coffee, honey, alcohol, and milk. Coldness in the body follows consumption of yin-type (cold) foods such as vegetables, fruit, and grains; these yin-type (cold) foods dispel energy and body heat to help balance hot foods. In accordance with their temperature properties, different foods are believed to directly influence health. For example, warming foods such as garlic can help alleviate pain in a person living with rheumatism. An exploration of the dietary choices made by Chinese Canadian patients living with breast cancer to some degree reflected their

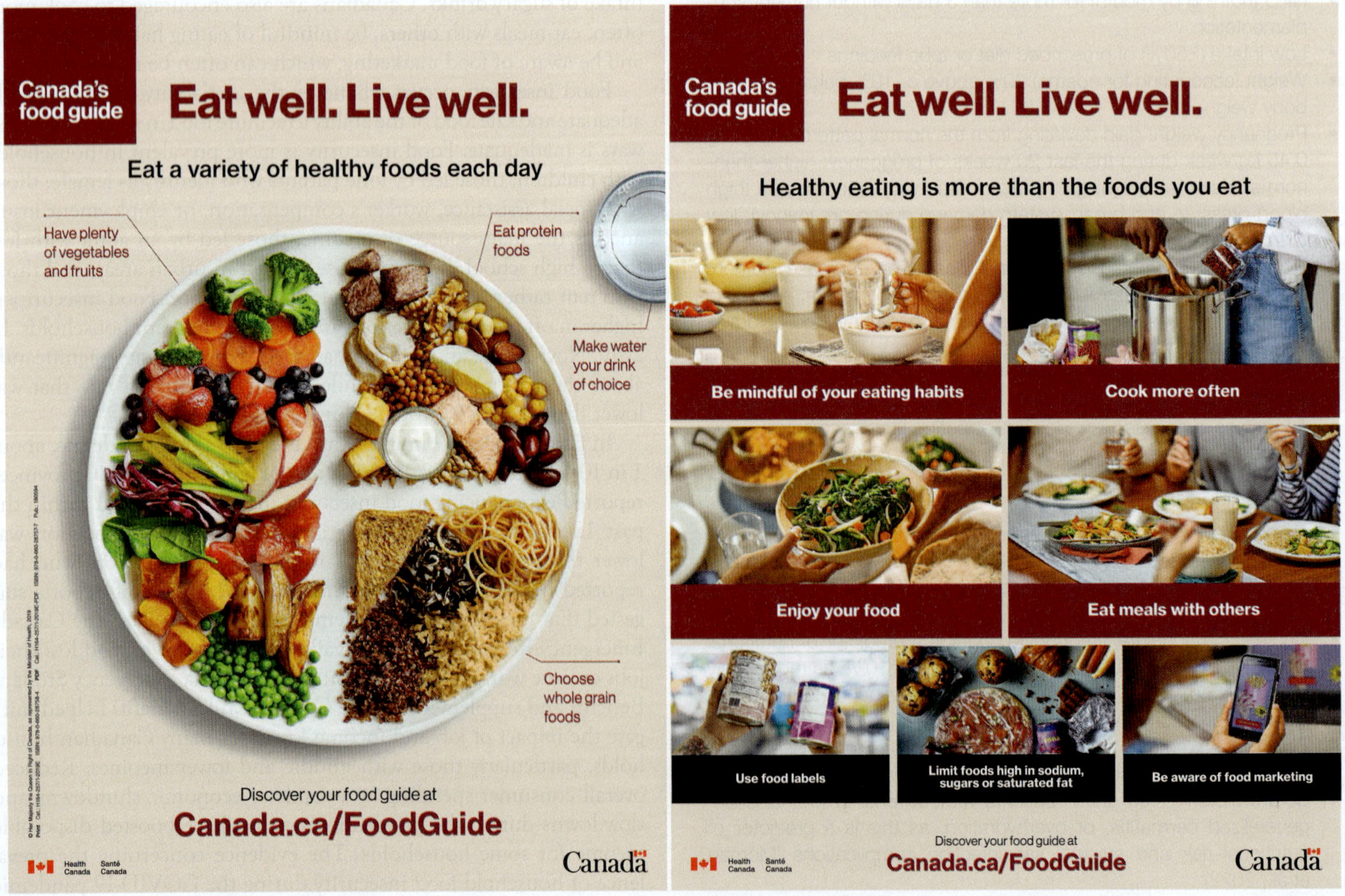
Canada's food guide
Eat well. Live well.
Eat a variety of healthy foods each day
Have plenty of vegetables and fruits
Eat protein foods
Make water your drink of choice
Choose whole grain foods
Discover your food guide at
Canada.ca/FoodGuide
Health Canada Santé Canada
Canada
Canada's food guide
Eat well. Live well.
Healthy eating is more than the foods you eat
Be mindful of your eating habits
Cook more often
Enjoy your food
Eat meals with others
Use food labels
Limit foods high in sodium, sugars or saturated fat
Be aware of food marketing
Discover your food guide at
Canada.ca/FoodGuide
Health Canada Santé Canada
Canada

FIG 31.1 **Canada's Food Guide.** (*© All rights reserved. Canada's Food Guide: Snapshot. Health Canada, 2019. Reproduced with permission from the Minister of Health, 2023.*)

understanding of traditional concepts of yin–yang and hot–cold. To illustrate, one person described adding ginger to cold-natured foods to help balance the coldness (Ng et al., 2021). Eating according to the energetic properties of food and balancing yin and yang foods is a holistic approach that takes into account the whole person, in contrast to the reductionist way the Western diet focuses on calories and eliminating entire categories of nutrients, such as carbohydrates and/or fat (Sweeney, 2020). Awareness of the relationship between culture and food can help nurses learn from their patients and better understand their own basic beliefs about self and others.

EVIDENCE-INFORMED PRACTICE

Safe nutritional support of adult patients living with obesity is an important priority of care. Obesity is a prevalent, complex, progressive, and relapsing chronic disease characterized by abnormal or excess body fat (adiposity) that impairs health. Following an extensive review of published research on obesity conducted worldwide, Obesity Canada and the Canadian Association of Bariatric Physicians and Surgeons developed the *Canadian Adult Obesity Clinical Practice Guidelines* for health care providers, patients, and policymakers (Wharton et al., 2020). Key points from the full guidelines (available at https://obesitycanada.ca/guidelines/) include the following:

- Health care providers should recognize obesity as a chronic disease and the need to ask patients for permission to discuss obesity. If the patient permits, the health care provider may then offer advice and help treat this disease in an unbiased manner. Health care providers also need to be aware of their own attitudes and behaviours toward individuals living with obesity, and should not assume that all patients living with obesity are ready to initiate obesity management.
- A patient with obesity should be assessed using appropriate measurements and in a holistic manner that identifies the root causes, complications, and barriers to obesity treatment. Direct measurement of height, weight and waist circumference, and calculation of body mass index (BMI) may be part of routine physical examination for adults. BMI is an estimate of body fat based on height and weight. For persons with a higher BMI (between 25 and 34.9 kg/m^2), waist circumference can help identify individuals who have increased visceral adiposity and adiposity-related health risks (Health Canada, 2021a). However, the Edmonton Obesity Staging System, a five-stage system of obesity classification, better predicts all-cause mortality when compared with BMI or waist circumference measurements alone and determines the optimal obesity management (Wharton et al., 2020).
- Importantly, these guidelines call upon the obesity research community to shift the focus away from BMI and weight and toward health outcomes. Assessment should include a comprehensive history to identify root causes of weight gain, such as biological factors (e.g., genetics, neurohormonal mechanisms, associated chronic diseases, and obesogenic medications), sociocultural practices and beliefs, social determinants of health, built environment, and individual life experiences (e.g., adverse childhood experiences and psychological factors such as mood, anxiety, binge-eating disorder, attention-deficit/hyperactivity disorder, self-worth, and identity). Working with patients to understand their context and culture and to integrate the root causes of obesity allows for the development of personalized treatment plans.
- Health care providers should discuss the core treatment options (medical nutrition therapy and physical activity) and adjunctive therapies (psychological, pharmacological, and surgical interventions). Adults living with obesity should be encouraged to adopt a healthy, well-balanced eating pattern and engage in regular physical activity (i.e., 30 to 60 minutes of aerobic activity on most days of the week). Nutrition therapy should not be used in isolation because weight loss may be difficult to sustain long term owing to compensatory mechanisms in the brain that promote positive caloric intake by increasing hunger and ultimately causing weight gain. Adjunctive pharmacotherapy is recommended for individuals with a BMI ≥30 kg/m^2, or a BMI ≥27 kg/m^2 and adiposity-related complications, to support medical nutrition therapy, physical activity, and psychological interventions. Bariatric surgery may be considered for people with a BMI ≥40 kg/m^2 or those with a BMI ≥35 kg/m^2 and at least one obesity-related disease.
- Goals of therapy should mainly align with the value that the person living with obesity derives from health-based interventions. Helpful actions include explicitly acknowledging the multiple stereotypes of personal failure or success attached to body composition; enacting behavioural interventions to improve overall health; and redefining success as healthy behaviour change regardless of body size or weight.
- Health care providers are encouraged to engage the person living with obesity, including through family meetings or conferences, in order to make decisions as part of continued follow-up and reassessment. Health care providers also need to advocate for improved care for this chronic disease by addressing barriers affecting access to obesity care in Canada. These barriers include a lack of interdisciplinary obesity management programs, inadequate access to health care providers with expertise in obesity, long wait times for referrals and surgery, and the high costs of some treatments. Canadians affected by obesity are left to navigate the complex landscape of weight-loss products and services, many of which lack scientific rationale and promote unrealistic and unsustainable weight-loss goals.
- Obesity care must be based on evidence-informed principles of chronic disease management that move beyond simplistic approaches of "eat less, move more" and instead address the complex interplay of the multiple genetic, metabolic, behavioural, and environmental drivers of obesity.
- Health care providers must provide person-centred care that validates patients' lived experiences.

Because weight bias and stigma contribute to increased morbidity and mortality independently of weight or BMI, the *Canadian Adult Obesity Clinical Practice Guidelines* (Wharton et al., 2020) refer interprofessional health care team members to the 5As of obesity management:

- *Ask* for permission to discuss weight and explore readiness.
- *Assess* obesity-related risks and "root causes" of weight gain.
- *Advise* on health risks and treatment options.
- *Agree* on health outcomes and behavioural goals.
- *Assist* in accessing appropriate resources and providers.

Using the 5As, health care practitioners can discuss relevant epidemiology and causes of obesity with patients who experience obesity or are at risk for the condition. These patients can be counselled on the complications of obesity and on the risk, benefits, and options available for management of obesity, including behavioural, pharmacological, and bariatric surgery management options.

Regarding older persons living in long-term care homes, Dietitians of Canada (2019a) has established best practices for nutrition, food service, and dining to improve residents' oral intake. Strategies include the following:

- Residents, family members, designated others, and appropriate team members collaborate in the menu planning process to ensure that residents' social, ethnic, cultural, and religious practices, needs, and preferences are assessed. All menus are evaluated and approved by the dietitian.

BOX 31.2

Food Safety Tips

- Wash hands, food preparation surfaces, and utensils with warm, soapy water before touching food.
- For safe internal cooking temperatures for meat, poultry, fish, and eggs, consult Health Canada's website (https://www.canada.ca/en/health-canada/services/general-food-safety-tips/safe-internal-cooking-temperatures.html).
- Wash all fresh fruits and vegetables thoroughly.
- Do not drink unpasteurized milk or juice. Meats and fish that will be eaten raw must be carefully acquired, handled, and stored safely to prevent foodborne illness. Fish intended to be used as sushi should always be bought frozen and delivered at −18°C or below, stored upon arrival in the freezer at −20°C for 7 days or longer, or stored in a blast freezer at −35°C or below for at least 15 hours (Canadian Institute of Food Safety, 2022). Defrost the fish in a refrigerator on the lowest shelf.
- Do not use food past the *expiration date* on a package. Expiration dates indicate the last day a product is safe to consume. These dates are required on certain foods that have specific nutritional compositions that could falter after the determined expiration date. If a food has passed its expiration date, it should be discarded and not used (Canadian Institute of Food Safety, 2020).
- The *best before date*, on the other hand, is the anticipated amount of time that an unopened food product, when stored under appropriate conditions, will retain its freshness, taste, nutritional value, or any other qualities claimed by the manufacturer. After that date, the food is no longer in its ideal state, but this does not necessarily mean that the food is no longer safe to eat.
- Pay attention to food recalls and advisories.
- Refrigerate or freeze all leftover foods within 2 hours to minimize the chance of bacterial growth.
- Thaw frozen foods in the refrigerator.
- Discard food that you suspect is spoiled. Indicate date that food was first refrigerated.
- After food preparation is complete, sanitize countertops, cutting boards, and utensils using a kitchen sanitizer (as directed) or a bleach solution (5 mL bleach to 750 mL of water). Rinse all items carefully with water.
- Clean the inside of the refrigerator, microwave, and other surfaces that come into contact with food regularly with bleach or soap.
- Wash reusable grocery bags frequently.

Adapted from Health Canada. (2021b). *Food safety and you*. https://www.canada.ca/en/health-canada/services/general-food-safety-tips/food-safety-you.html

- Dining rooms must have adequate light, temperature, and good flow for pathways (e.g., walkers placed out of the way and any clutter from walking paths cleared away to ensure a safe route for residents and team members). Help patients with any sensory aids such as hearing aids, glasses, and dentures before their food is served. Use contrasting colours for table coverings/placemats and dishes to help residents with poor vision to identify what is being served. Keep noise level as low as possible. Wheelchairs should fit under tables appropriately. Rotate the order of the "table by table" service regularly to allow all residents the opportunity to be served first.
- Medications are not to be added to food or fluid that is part of the meal without prior documented approval. Whenever possible, medications are provided as residents arrive and leave the dining room to avoid interrupting the dining experience with medications; this approach also allows for more nursing supervision and assistance during dining.
- Each resident's intake of food and fluids is observed and documented throughout the day (i.e., all meals, beverages, snacks, and anything consumed during social activities).
- Residents are given ample time to complete one course before the next is offered, and dirty dishes are removed before providing the next course.
- Regular tables are assigned to team members to allow them to become familiar with the residents and their personal needs, therapeutic diets, fluid consistencies, and dining preferences. These team members are to listen to residents and offer support when appropriate individual requests are made, such as gravy on the side or extra condiments. Team members are seated (never standing) and make appropriate eye contact when helping residents who require assistance.
- The registered dietitian and/or appropriate team members will perform an assessment on residents' ability to swallow solids and liquids. This assessment includes identifying, analyzing, and evaluating potential risks related to feeding and swallowing, as well as proper body positioning and the risk for malnutrition.
- An approved, standardized dysphagia screening tool that includes International Dysphagia Diet Standardisation Initiative (IDDSI) terminology is recommended to identify and determine resident risk for dysphagia. Staff and families are taught to recognize signs of dysphagia to be able to safely assist residents whenever they are eating and drinking. One interdisciplinary care team member who is competent to handle risks such as choking, illness, and other response protocols is assigned to be present at all times while residents are in the dining room.
- As part of person-centred care, nutritious snacks and beverages are provided at times suitable to individual needs.

SAFETY GUIDELINES

- Improper handling, preparation, and storage practices may result in cases of foodborne illness (Health Canada, 2021d). Children younger than 5 years, pregnant women, adults over 65 years, and people with weak immune systems are more likely to become ill from contaminated food (Health Canada, 2019). There are four principles for patients to follow in the home when preparing food: cook food to the right temperature; wash hands and all surfaces (cutting boards, utensils, countertops) often; refrigerate food promptly (within 2 hours); and separate raw meats from other foods to prevent contamination (Box 31.2).
- Identify patients at risk for dysphagia (Wolf et al., 2021), and use interprofessional collaboration (e.g., speech-language pathologist [SLP]) when available to minimize complications such as aspiration pneumonia (Seedat & Strime, 2021). The role of an SLP is to evaluate the patient's ability to swallow and make recommendations to other interprofessional team members; there is a need for ongoing explicit sharing of information between nurses and SLPs about patients' communication support needs (Barnard et al., 2022).
- Ensure that patients receive the correct therapeutic diet. Common dietary errors include wrong diet, meals meant for other patients, allergy conflicts, and meals delivered to a patient when they are NPO (Computrition, 2018).
- Assess a patient's level of consciousness before attempting any oral feeding. Hold oral nutrition if the patient's status has changed such that it has potentially altered their ability to eat (e.g., decrease in level of consciousness), and consult with appropriate health care team members.

✦ SKILL 31.1 Performing a Nutritional Screening and Physical Examination

Nurses screen for patients' actual and potential nutritional alterations by focusing on the effects of an illness, disease, or lifestyle on a patient's nutritional status, such as recent weight loss and decreased oral intake. *Nutritional risk screening* refers to the use of a validated set of usually two or three simple questions to rapidly predict whether a patient is malnourished or at risk for malnutrition; the results of the screening help determine whether a detailed nutritional assessment is indicated. Because malnutrition seen at hospital admission often starts in the community, malnutrition as a comorbidity at hospital admission will continue to be prevalent until nutritional screening in the community is improved (Donnelly et al., 2022). The nutritional screening tools most frequently used in Canadian care settings are shown in Box 31.3.

Nutritional screening involves the application of physical examination findings (including height and weight). A nurse conducts a complete or focused physical examination at the time of a patient's admission to a health care facility. The extent of the examination is determined by patient condition. During an examination, the nurse needs to recognize the physical signs that indicate a nutritional alteration (Table 31.1) and review laboratory results that further support a patient's nutritional status. The most commonly studied blood biomarker for malnutrition is albumin, followed by hemoglobin, total cholesterol, total lymphocyte counts, prealbumin, C-reactive protein, total protein, and transferrin (Keller, 2019). The role of

BOX 31.3

Nutritional Screening Tools

- The Malnutrition Screening Tool (MST), a three-question tool used to assess recent weight and appetite loss, has been validated for use with general medical, surgical, and oncology patients. Designed for use by non–nutrition-trained staff, the MST uses a scoring system to identify patients at high nutrition risk, which can then provide a basis for dietetic referrals and intervention. The MST is available at https://static.abbottnutrition.com/cms-prod/abbottnutrition-2016.com/img/Malnutrition%20Screening%20Tool_FINAL_tcm1226-57900.pdf.
- The Mini Nutritional Assessment (MNA) was developed for patients who are at least 65 years of age. With its short six-question format, the MNA is easy to implement and has been validated in hospitals, long-term care facilities, and community care settings. The MNA is available at https://www.nestle.com/asset-library/documents/library/events/2010-malnutrition-in-older-people/mna_mini_english.pdf.
- The Canadian Nutrition Screening Tool (CNST) consists of two questions developed by the Canadian Task Force on Malnutrition and tested for reliability in Canadian hospitals. Following a positive screening using the CNST, the Subjective Global Assessment (SGA) (see https://subjectiveglobalassessment.com/) is used to assess nutritional status and help prioritize cases. The CNST is available at https://nutritioncareincanada.ca/sites/default/uploads/files/CNST.pdf.
- The SGA requires completion of a questionnaire that includes data on weight change, dietary intake change, gastrointestinal symptoms, changes in functional capacity in relation to malnutrition, and assessment of fat and muscle stores and the presence of edema and ascites. This tool allows for malnutrition diagnosis and classifies patients as follows: A—well nourished; B—mildly/moderately malnourished; or C—severely malnourished.

Adapted from Bachand, M.-P., & Hulst, J. (2020). *Assessing nutritional status* [PowerPoint slides]. Canadian Digestive Diseases Week 2020, Montreal, Quebec. https://www.cag-acg.org/images/cddw/Satsgs_AssessNutrition_Hulst_Bachand.pdf; Steel, C., & Wile, H. (2018). Nutrition screening practices across care settings: Results of a Canadian survey. *Canadian Journal of Clinical Nutrition, 6*(1), 7–19. https://doi.org/10.14206/canad.j.clin.nutr.2018.01.02; Xu, Y. C., & Vincent, J. I. (2020). Clinical measurement properties of malnutrition assessment tools for use with patients in hospitals: A systematic review. *Nutrition Journal, 19*, 106. https://doi.org/10.1186/s12937-020-00613-0

TABLE 31.1

Physical Signs of Nutritional Status Alteration

Body Area	Indicators of Malnutrition
General appearance	Wasting, listless, apathetic, cachectic
Posture	Sagging shoulders, sunken chest, humped back
Hair	Stringy, dull, brittle, dry, thin and sparse, depigmented, easily plucked
Face and neck	Greasy, discoloured, scaly, swollen, dark skin over cheeks and under eyes, lumpiness or flakiness of skin around nose and mouth
Skin	Rough, dry, scaly, pale, pigmented, irritated; bruises and petechiae
Lips	Dry, scaly, swollen, redness and swelling (cheilosis), angular lesions at corner of mouth or fissures or scars
Mouth, oral mucous membranes	Swollen, deep red or magenta mucous membranes, oral lesions
Gums	Spongy, bleed easily, marginal redness, inflamed, receding
Tongue	Swollen, scarlet and raw, magenta colour, beefy (glossitis), hyperemic and hypertrophic or atrophic papillae
Teeth	Missing, broken teeth
Eyes	Conjunctiva pale, redness of conjunctiva, dryness or infection, redness and fissuring of eyelid corners (angular palpebritis), Bitot's spots (dry-appearing patches on the conjunctiva), impaired night vision
Neck (glands)	Thyroid or lymph nodes enlarged
Nails	Spoon-shaped (koilonychias), brittle, ridged
Legs and feet	Edema, tender calf, tingling, weakness, lesions
Musculoskeletal	Flaccid, poor tone, undeveloped, tender, impaired ability to walk, bone deformities (e.g., bowlegs, knocked knees, curved spine), joint pain or swelling
Nerve conduction and mental status	Inattentive, irritable, confused, burning and tingling of hands and feet, loss of position and vibratory sense, cognitive and sensory deficits
Gastrointestinal	Diarrhea; dysgeusia (taste disorder); dysphagia or odynophagia (painful swallowing) due to Plummer-Vinson syndrome, a disorder marked by anemia resulting from iron deficiency, and a web-like growth of membranes in the throat
Endocrine	Thyromegaly

Adapted from Hood, A. (2020). Nutritional status assessment in adults technique. *Medscape*. https://emedicine.medscape.com/article/2141861-technique; Nix McIntosh, S. (2022). *Williams' basic nutrition and diet therapy* (16th ed.). Mosby.

serum biomarkers in diagnosing or monitoring malnutrition is controversial, given their relatively low specificity, the long half-life of albumin (approximately 20 days), and the fact that underlying diseases such as inflammation exert a major influence on these serum visceral proteins. Biomarkers such as prealbumin are, however, valid prognostic indicators of disease outcome and mortality in patients at risk for malnutrition.

The nurse also collects a patient history at the time of admission. Dietary information from the history provides information that will help identify the adequacy of a patient's current diet, appetite changes, type of assistance needed to eat, and food preferences. Findings from a nutritional screening determine whether there is a need for interprofessional collaboration to complete a more detailed assessment of a patient's nutritional status. If a patient is malnourished, an in-depth nutritional assessment, along with treatment, is required by a registered dietitian (Keller, Laur, et al., 2018). In addition, assessment findings can lead to a referral for an SLP if the patient has swallowing difficulties (Heart and Stroke Foundation of Canada, 2021).

Dietitians are considered the best-qualified care providers to assess, design, and implement patients' nutritional treatment plans in collaboration with the health care team (Hewko et al., 2021). Dietitians use a problem-solving method–the nutrition care process–to think critically and make decisions regarding nutrition therapy (Gillis et al., 2021). The nutrition care process has four interrelated steps that are similar to those in the nursing process: nutritional assessment, nutritional diagnosis, nutritional intervention, and nutritional monitoring and evaluation. The dietitian first comprehensively assesses a patient's nutritional status, including medical, social, nutritional, and medication history; physical examination findings; anthropometric measurements; and laboratory data. The goal of the assessment is to develop a nutritional plan of care that effectively addresses a patient's nutritional problems. Using clinical judgement that relies on clinical experience, the dietitian synthesizes various types of information and knowledge with respect to planning context-relevant care (Vo et al., 2021). The dietitian then makes a nutritional diagnosis describing alterations in a patient's nutritional status that the dietitian can treat independently or as part of the health care team. The nutritional intervention is a purposely planned activity intended to resolve nutritional diagnoses. Nutritional monitoring and evaluation are used to identify patient progress, including patient understanding of and adherence to treatment.

Delegation and Collaboration

The skill of performing and interpreting a nutritional screening and physical examination cannot be delegated to an unregulated care provider (UCP). However, measurement of a patient's height and weight can be delegated. The nurse directs the UCP to do the following:

- Measure the patient's weight after voiding, at the same time of day and when wearing the same clothing
- Use the internal bed scale according to employer policy (if applicable)
- To measure the height of a patient who is nonambulatory:
  - *Supine length measurement:* Lower the head of the bed so that the patient is lying down supine. Make a mark at the vertex of the head and the bottom of the heel. Measure the distance between the two marks. This is the patient's height (CNA Training Help, n.d.). Record this number on the patient's chart. This measure may be unreliable in patients with joint contractures.
  - *Four-point method of measurement:* Take serial measurements from vertex of head to medial end of clavicle, lateral aspect of shoulder to anterior superior iliac spine, anterior superior iliac spine to lateral aspect of knee joint, and lateral aspect of knee joint to sole of foot. Add these measurements together to obtain the patient's height. Although this method can potentially lead to errors, it is not altered by joint contractures.
  - *Demi-span or knee height measurement:* Height may be accurately calculated using conversion formulas for women's demi-span (measured from the midsternal notch to the web between the middle and ring fingers along an outstretched arm) and for men's knee height (measured with a knee height caliper) (Cirillo et al., 2018).
- Ensure that measurements take place in a private location to protect the patient's dignity.

Equipment

- Scale (beam, electronic, bed with scale, wheelchair, or chair)
- Nutritional screening form (data sheet and pen or computerized assessment form)
- Tongue blade
- Clean gloves
- Pen light for physical examination

STEP	RATIONALE
ASSESSMENT	
1. Identify patient using at least two person-specific identifiers (e.g., name and date of birth, or name and medical record number) according to employer policy.	Ensures correct patient. Complies with Accreditation Canada's standards and improves patient safety (Accreditation Canada, 2020).
2. Throughout the procedure, the 4 moments for hand hygiene are to be implemented; hand hygiene should occur before initial patient (or patient environment) contact, before an aseptic procedure, after body fluid exposure risk, and after patient (or patient environment) contact. Additional hand hygiene should be performed when hands are visibly soiled.	Proper hand hygiene helps prevent the spread of infectious agents to health care providers.
3. Explain to patient how you intend to apply nutritional assessment information in patient care.	Allows time for patient to ask questions about assessment and improve understanding.
4. Ask patient to report usual body weight (UBW), noting recent changes in weight. Ask whether weight loss was intentional or unintentional.	In adults, weight is usually stable. A weight loss >5% within 1 month is an indicator for further assessment, especially in an adult older than 65 years (Table 31.2).
5. Measure actual body weight (ABW):	Heavier individuals tend to underreport weight to a greater extent than lower-weight individuals (Hodge et al., 2020).

STEP	RATIONALE

ASSESSMENT

STEP	RATIONALE
a. Have patient void. Be sure patient is wearing underwear or hospital gown. Weigh patient either barefoot or with same shoes. Weigh at same time of day.	Improves accuracy of ABW for comparison over time.
b. Make sure that any scale used has been calibrated. If patient is ambulatory, help them stand still on scale with weight evenly distributed over both feet.	Accurate measurement requires use of regularly calibrated and maintained scales. Standing still with equal weight distribution helps in obtaining accurate weight (Grodner et al., 2023).
c. If patient is unable to stand, use wheelchair or bed scale.	Decreases risk of falling. To obtain the patient's weight, weigh the wheelchair separately and subtract wheelchair weight.
d. Record weight to nearest 0.1 kg (0.25 lb).	Provides precise measurement of weight.
6. Measure actual height:	Many individuals say they are slightly taller than they actually are (Hodge et al., 2020).
a. If patient is ambulatory, assist to standing position. If taking height with beam scale, have patient stand erect with weight equally distributed over both feet.	Ensures accurate height measurement (Grodner et al., 2023).
b. Instruct patient to let arms hang free at sides with palms facing thighs.	Prevents movement of shoulders, which will result in inaccurate measurement.
c. Have patient look straight ahead, take a deep breath, and hold position while you bring horizontal bar firmly on top of head. Measure to nearest 0.1 cm (0.04 inches). Make sure your eyes are level with bar to read measurement.	Steady position ensures accurate measurement. Provides precise measurement of height.
d. If patient is nonambulatory, measure height via one of the following methods: • Supine length measurement • Four-point method of measurement • Demi-span or knee height measurement	Currently the most reliable methods to measure nonambulatory patient height.
7. Calculate ideal body weight (IBW):	
a. Calculate via standard height and weight chart. IBW range for normal is 10% above and 10% below IBW.	Use IBW to compare with patient's actual weight to determine whether patient is at risk for nutritional alteration.
b. Use the following formulas: *Males:* 48.1 kg (106 lb) for first 152 cm (5 feet); add 2.7 kg (6 lb) per additional 2.5 cm (1 in). *Females:* 45.4 kg (100 lb) for first 152 cm (5 feet); add 2.25 kg (5 lb) per additional 2.5 cm (inch).	
8. Calculate BMI (see Step 8 illustration): $$BMI = \frac{\text{Actual body weight (kg)}}{\text{Height (m)}^2}$$	BMI is a measure of body fat based on adult height and weight that is widely used to assess health risk associated with underweight and overweight (however, it should not be used as the sole measure for determining healthy weight). Use the following link for an automatic calculation: https://www.diabetes.ca/diabetes-and-you/healthy-living-resources/weight-management/body-mass-index-bmi-calculator
a. Divide weight in kilograms by the square of height in metres (m^2).	Computes BMI kg/m^2 (Table 31.3).
b. Optional formula for BMI: weight (lb)/ [height (inches)]^2 × 703	

TABLE 31.2

Weight Change as an Indicator of Nutritional Status

Weight Loss (% of Body Weight)	Time Period	Nutritional Status
1–2	1 week	Moderate weight loss
>2	1 week	Severe weight loss
5	1 month	Moderate weight loss
>5	1 month	Severe weight loss

Adapted from Grodner, M., Escott-Stump, S., & Dorner, S. (2023). *Foundations and clinical applications of nutrition: A nursing approach* (7th ed.). Elsevier.

TABLE 31.3

Classification of Body Mass Index (BMI) in Adults

Degree of Adiposity	BMI
Underweight	Less than 18.5 kg/m^2
Normal weight	18.5–24.9 kg/m^2
Overweight	25–29.9 kg/m^2
Obesity (class I)	30–34.9 kg/m^2
Obesity (class II)	35–39.9 kg/m^2
Extreme obesity (class III)	Greater than or equal to 40 kg/m^2

STEP	RATIONALE

ASSESSMENT

BMI Table (Metric)

	Underweight			Normal						Overweight					Obese					
BMI	**16**	**17**	**18**	**19**	**20**	**21**	**22**	**23**	**24**	**25**	**26**	**27**	**28**	**29**	**30**	**31**	**32**	**33**	**34**	**35**
Height (cm)	**Body Weight (Kg)**																			
145	34	36	38	40	42	44	46	48	50	53	55	57	59	61	63	65	67	69	71	74
150	36	38	41	43	45	47	50	52	54	56	59	61	63	65	68	70	72	74	77	79
155	38	41	43	46	48	50	53	55	58	60	62	65	67	70	72	74	77	79	82	84
160	41	44	46	49	51	54	56	59	61	64	67	69	72	74	77	79	82	84	87	90
165	44	46	49	52	54	57	60	63	65	68	71	74	76	79	82	84	87	90	93	95
170	46	49	52	55	58	61	64	66	69	72	75	78	81	84	87	90	92	95	98	101
175	49	52	55	58	61	64	67	70	74	77	80	83	86	89	92	95	98	101	104	107
180	52	55	58	62	65	68	71	75	78	81	84	87	91	94	97	100	104	107	110	113
185	55	58	62	65	68	72	75	79	82	86	89	92	96	99	103	106	110	113	116	120
190	58	61	65	69	72	76	79	83	87	90	94	97	101	105	108	112	116	119	123	126
195	61	65	68	72	76	80	84	87	91	95	99	103	106	110	114	118	122	125	129	133
200	64	68	72	76	80	84	88	92	96	100	104	108	112	116	120	124	128	132	136	140

STEP 8 Body mass index for BMI 35 and under. *(From http://bmisite.net/bmi-chart.php.)*

STEP	RATIONALE
9. Obtain dietary information as you complete the nursing history (see Chapter 8):	
a. Assess patient's dietary history, including current diet, food choices and preferences, appetite, food allergies (include on patient identification [ID] band), and food intolerances. NOTE: In outpatient settings, have patient bring 7-day food diary report in electronic or paper format.	Assesses factors affecting dietary adequacy and appetite, including income, food prices, individual preferences and beliefs, cultural traditions, and geographical and environmental aspects (World Health Organization [WHO], 2020). Web-based dietary assessment methods may be more appealing and engaging than paper-based methods, enhance the accuracy of dietary intake reporting (such as the use of digital images to improve memory and portion size estimates), provide rapid feedback to users, and offer potential cost savings for researchers (Eldridge et al., 2018).
b. Assess for any cultural and religious preferences and restrictions in diet. Ask patient whether caregiver believes that certain foods influence health changes to determine level of shared decision making and areas for ongoing education.	Knowing patient preferences demonstrates person-centred care and will improve ability to plan a diet that patient will accept. As a resource, the Food and Agriculture Organization of the United Nations (FAO) provides advice on food, food groups, and dietary patterns for different cultures (FAO, n.d.).
c. Determine medications and other dietary or herbal supplements that patient is taking (over-the-counter and prescribed). Be aware of common drug–drug and drug–nutrient interactions (use interprofessional collaboration [e.g., pharmacist] as required).	Certain medications inhibit or increase action of other medications. Some nutrients interact with medications. For example, vitamin K–rich foods (green leafy vegetables) interfere with action of warfarin (anticoagulant). Medications such as mineral oil laxatives impair nutrient use.
10. Perform physical assessment (see Chapter 8) (see Table 31.1), noting any physical changes reflecting nutritional deficiencies, patient's level of consciousness, responsiveness, and ability to swallow.	The most obvious signs of malnutrition on physical examination are apparent in the skin, mouth, muscles, and central nervous system. Difficulty swallowing predisposes patient to aspiration when eating.
11. Review results of relevant laboratory tests (e.g., albumin, complete blood count [CBC], electrolytes).	Laboratory results can provide clues about nutritional status (refer to Box 31.1).
12. During first meal, determine patient's ability to set up food on plate, manipulate eating utensils, and self-feed.	Independence of feeding was correlated with less malnutrition risk for residents of assisted living (Pakai et al., 2021).
13. Complete a nutritional screening tool if required by employer (see Box 31.3).	Valid tools include key elements for detecting patient's nutritional risk.

NURSING DIAGNOSES

- Reduced ability to swallow
- Inadequate nutrition
- Insufficient knowledge regarding nutritional needs/recommendations
- Obesity
- Overweight
- Potential for weight gain

Related factors and risk factors are individualized on the basis of patient's condition or needs.

STEP	RATIONALE
IMPLEMENTATION	
1. Provide patient help with feeding based on assessment findings (see Skill 31.2).	Level of assistance required depends on patient's motor skills, ability to attend, and ability to swallow and chew normally.
2. Institute aspiration precautions (see Skill 31.3) if needed.	Precautions lessen chance of patient aspirating food or liquid into tracheobronchial tree.
EVALUATION	
1. Review history and physical findings. Note abnormal findings or areas of concern.	Permits prompt identification of risk for malnutrition and need for nutritional interventions.
2. If a BMI measurement was done, compare patient's BMI with recommended BMI for height/weight.	Although BMI can help indicate nutritional risk factors, BMI should not be the only assessment used to inform treatment for individual patients. It has to be used in context with other information, such as laboratory values (e.g., fasting insulin and glucose levels), blood pressure, as well as family history of metabolic disease (Yeo, 2021).
3. Check with the plan of care to determine whether patient's intake and output (I&O) totals should be monitored. If so, monitor and document patient's I&O.	Accurate measurement and documentation of I&O totals are important because medications, intravenous (IV) and fluid administration, dietary decisions, and physician orders for tube feeding are based on the patient's I&O totals.
4. Compare normal laboratory test levels with patient's levels.	When considered with other nutritional parameters, abnormal values can indicate malnutrition (Grodner et al., 2023; Keller, 2019).
5. Compute any score on nutritional screening tool.	Valid tools use a scoring system to identify patients at high nutrition risk.
6. **Use teach-back:** "I want to be sure I explained why we need to do a nutritional screening for you. Tell me what the screening tells us. How will we use that information?" Develop a revised teaching plan if patient or caregiver is unable to teach back correctly.	Determines patient's and caregiver's level of understanding of instructional topic.

Unexpected Outcomes	Related Interventions
1. Patient is gaining or losing a significant amount of weight as evidenced by regular serial measurements.	• Ensure patient is receiving correct caloric diet. • Check that patient is being weighed on same scale, with same type of clothing and shoes, and at same time of day. • Use interprofessional collaboration (e.g., dietitian) to conduct a nutritional assessment and calculate patient's caloric and protein intake and route of nutrition (enteral versus parenteral) (see Chapters 32 and 33). • Implement measures to improve patient's appetite: food appearance, room comfort, providing comfort measures before meal. • Practise person-centred care and include patient and caregiver in meal plan development.
2. Nutritional screening tool score reflects high nutrition risk.	• Refer patient to a dietitian.

Communication and Documentation

- Document assessment results and your evaluation of patient and caregiver learning on progress notes, flow sheet, and nutritional screening form in electronic health record (EHR) or chart.
- Notify health care provider of abnormal findings.
- Make referral to dietitian as indicated.

Special Considerations

Teaching

- To increase patient's and caregiver's awareness of healthy nutrition, provide education about a case-specific nutritional diet.
- Teach families and caregivers not to give fluids by mouth without staff guidance owing to choking risk.
- Provide patient and caregiver with resources to promote healthy eating (e.g., *Canada's Food Guide Plate*) (Health Canada, 2021c) (Box 31.4). Nutrition-focused mobile apps and websites promote patient engagement with their dietary plan.

Cultural

- The act of eating together in community is the basic foundation of all societies. Food gives structure to daily life and ritualistically marks the passage of life stages (e.g., eating cake at a wedding).
- Biological and geographical conditions, as well as cultural norms, determine changes in the food eaten within a certain community. Westerners' rejection of eating raw fish until recent years is one example of this: as Westerners were more exposed to Japanese cuisine, they began to eat more raw fish (Wilson, 2022).
- Food creates bonds between people, and communities may exist whereby food differentiates "us" from "them." Inviting a friend for lunch is an example of the social role of food.

BOX 31.4

Building Healthy Eating Habits

Following *Canada's Food Guide Plate* guidelines will result in healthier eating habits (Health Canada, 2021c):

- When selecting food and beverages, focus on variety, amount, and nutrition. Include all food groups: fruits and vegetables, grain products, meat and alternatives, milk and alternatives, and oils and fats. Also include water intake.
- Eat the right amount for you based on your age, gender, height, weight, and physical activity level.
- Healthier eating habits will help you avoid overweight and obesity and reduce your risk of diseases such as heart disease, diabetes mellitus, and cancer.
- Choose an eating style low in saturated fat, sodium, and added sugars.
- Read nutrition fact labels and ingredient lists carefully for the amounts of saturated fat, sodium, and added sugars when choosing foods and beverages.
- Eating foods with less sodium can reduce your risk of high blood pressure.
- Start with making a few small changes to create healthier eating habits. Think of each change as a personal "win" on your path to healthier living.
- Make half your plate fruits and vegetables.
- Focus on whole fruits, which are more nutritious than fruit juice.
- Vary your vegetables. Dark green and orange vegetables are packed with nutrients.
- Eat a variety of whole grains.
- Choose skim, 1%, or 2% milk or unsweetened fortified soy beverage.
- Choose meat alternatives such as split peas, chickpeas, kidney beans, black beans, lentils, or tofu. Eat heart-healthy fish such as char, herring, mackerel, salmon, sardines, and trout, as these fish are high in omega-3 fats.
- Make calorie-free water your drink of choice.
- Create settings where healthy choices are available and affordable to you and others in your community.
- Professionals, policymakers, partners, industry, families, and individuals can help others make healthy eating a part of their lives.

See more at https://food-guide.canada.ca/en/tips-for-healthy-eating/make-healthy-meals-with-the-eat-well-plate/.

- Food also represents power. A person who does not have enough to eat is powerless, whereas a person who controls another person's food intake holds a certain power over them.
- Food is an important part of gender relations. The traditional role of women in feeding the family has been a factor in the exclusion of individuals who identify as women from public power; however, there is a dimension of power in the act of cooking and determining what other members of the family should eat. The person who controls food intake not only affects bodily functions and health but also may imprint values and virtues, especially on children.
- Culture and society shape a person's diet. Up to 84% of fast-food restaurants serve unhealthy food; 9.78% of businesses use social media to share awareness about their locations, and 8.9% of Canadians visit a fast-food business based on what they saw on social media (Pandurov, 2021).
- There is a negative association between income and obesity. The cost of healthy food, such as fresh fruits and vegetables, has been found to be higher than that of less nutritious, energy-dense food (Bukambu et al., 2020).
- Traditional diets consumed by Indigenous peoples (i.e., before European colonization) were high in animal protein, rich in nutrients, lower in simple sugars (which predispose to obesity and diabetes mellitus), and low in fat or high in marine sources of fat. In addition, good sources of vitamin C, such as rose hips, have been consumed by many Indigenous peoples in a variety of medicinal and food preparations. Not only are traditional foods valued from cultural, spiritual, and health perspectives, but the activities involved in their acquisition and distribution also give Indigenous peoples the opportunity to practise their culture, enact their ancestral responsibilities to the land and live in harmony with creation, contribute to greater physical activity, and may even serve as a political act of resistance and resurgence within the structures of settler colonialism (Robin et al., 2021). *Traditional food* is the term preferred by First Nations and Métis, while *country food* is the term preferred by Inuit (Health Canada, 2023a).
- There is convincing evidence that the omega-3 fatty acids DHA and EHA found in fish and fish oils decrease the risk of cardiovascular disease. Traditional diets, rich in sources of omega-3 fatty acids, beneficially affect the profile of fats consumed, such that greater amounts of DHA and EHA are obtained, and a smaller percentage of the total fat in the diet comes from saturated fats.
- Given the benefits associated with traditional diets, a return to traditional dietary practices seems advisable. However, there are challenges in making this shift. Many Indigenous communities face unique food security challenges related to the consumption of traditional food. Almost half of Indigenous households located on reserve are food insecure owing to low income (Batal, Chan, Fediuk, et al., 2021). Moreover, the willingness to consume traditional or country foods is affected by concerns over contaminants (e.g., cadmium, mercury, PCBs, and pesticides).
- In the first cross-Canada study of First Nations adults below the 60th parallel, low intakes of folate, calcium, magnesium, and vitamins A, D, and C were identified; intake of vitamin B_6 below the recommended level was found among adults aged 51 to 70 years (Batal, Chan, Ing, et al., 2021). As well, intakes were below the recommended average daily intake level for fibre, potassium, and linoleic acid; however, those aged 19 to 70 years had adequate intake of linoleic acid. Sadly, the diets of many Indigenous children are energy dense and low in nutrient-dense foods like fruits and vegetables, an eating pattern that contributes to nutrition-related chronic diseases such as obesity, diabetes, and cardiovascular disease (Gillies et al., 2020).
- Despite challenges such as food insecurity and biocontamination, traditional foods remain important for prevention of chronic diseases; these foods can be successfully promoted in Indigenous communities.
- In 2010, a national food guide was created to reflect the values, traditions, and food choices of First Nations, Inuit, and Métis. This food guide includes both traditional (or country) foods and store-bought foods that are generally available, affordable, and accessible across Canada and provides unique images and content. In 2022, Health Canada provided additional information about the food guide and food safety tips, including being aware that wild game may contain chemical contaminants or natural toxins, parasites, and bacteria; advising the use of steel shots to reduce lead contamination; ensuring that all game is gutted and refrigerated within a few hours of the hunt to avoid spoilage; and cooking to internal temperatures of 74°C for pieces or 82°C for whole game items (Health Canada, 2022b).
- In Canada's North, people are largely unable to grow and produce food for themselves owing to the climate. They struggle to afford the high costs of food and may experience serious mental and physical health consequences from living with food insecurity—malnutrition, chronic diseases, social exclusion,

depression, and suicidal ideation (Robinson, 2021). Nutrition North Canada (NNC), launched in 2011, is a federal government program that helps make perishable and nutritious food and some essential items more affordable and accessible (Health Canada, 2022d). A retail subsidy is applied against the total cost of an eligible product shipped to the eligible community. NNC also subsidizes commercially inspected country foods and traditional foods such as Arctic char, caribou, goose, and muktuk when purchased from a local store or processing plant recognized by the program. The federal government evaluated NNC as successful in improving food access and affordability because there was an increase in the volume of perishable, nutritious foods shipped and a decrease in the cost of a standardized food basket after NNC was launched. However, research findings report a worsening of food insecurity in Nunavut communities (St-Germain et al., 2019) since the introduction of NNC. One interpretation is that NNC led to greater consumption of subsidized foods among the most affluent households while compromising food access among economically vulnerable households because of the removal of the subsidy for common nonperishable foods and essential items. Critics additionally argue that NNC's subsidization of specific foods, but not hunting and fishing equipment—which local people could use to find more food for themselves—makes residents of NNC's eligible communities dependent on the program (Robinson, 2021). More research is needed to better understand the program's impact on food insecurity.

Pregnancy

Health Canada's (2022c) key recommendations for pregnant persons include the following:

- Observe *Canada's Food Guide* by eating the amount and type of food appropriate for a pregnant person.
- Choose foods with healthy fats rather than saturated fat. (e.g., nuts, seeds, fish containing omega-3, and vegetable oils).
- Limit the amount of fresh or frozen tuna, shark, swordfish, escolar, marlin, and orange roughy because of mercury levels—consume no more than 150 g per month.
- Take a multivitamin containing 0.4 mg of folic acid and 16 to 20 mg of iron every day.
- Follow food safety advice (see Box 31.2).
- Eat at least one dark-green and one orange vegetable each day.
- Choose vegetables and fruits prepared with little or no added fat, sugar, or salt.
- Have vegetables and fruits more often than juice.
- Make at least half of the daily grain products whole grain, and choose grain products that are lower in fat, sugar, or salt.
- Drink skim, 1%, or 2% milk each day.
- Select lower-fat alternatives.
- Have meat alternatives such as beans, lentils, and tofu often.
- Select lean meat and alternatives prepared with little or no added fat or salt.
- Satisfy thirst with water as the beverage of choice.
- Limit foods and beverages high in calories, fat, sugar, or salt.
- Be active regularly as part of a healthy pregnancy.

Gerontological

- A systematic review of the contemporary literature on frameworks of healthy aging identified diet as one of 10 determinants of successful healthy aging (Abud et al., 2022). The other determinants identified were physical activity, self-awareness, outlook/attitude, lifelong learning, faith, social support, financial security, community engagement, and independence. Healthy aging appears to result when all these determinants are optimized.

Pediatric

- Anthropometric data include measurement of length, weight, and head circumference in children. These measurements should be compared with standard growth charts to determine percentiles. The WHO growth charts were redeveloped in 2019 through a collaboration between the Dietitians of Canada, the Canadian Paediatric Society, the College of Family Physicians of Canada, Community Health Nurses of Canada, and the Canadian Pediatric Endocrine Group (Dietitians of Canada, n.d.-b).
- The WHO charts (Dietitians of Canada, n.d.-b) include BMI for age and weight for stature percentiles.

Care in the Community: Home Management

- Instruct patient and caregiver about strategies for safe handling, preparation, and storage of food.
- Use interprofessional collaboration (e.g., occupational therapist) to assess the home environment to determine whether the patient or caregiver can prepare a meal safely (see Chapter 42).

✦ SKILL 31.2 Assisting an Adult Patient With Oral Nutrition

Some patients are unable to feed themselves adequately because of the severity of their illness, which may cause musculoskeletal weakness, fatigue, or pain. For example, a patient who loses fine motor skills will have difficulty getting food from their plate and into their mouth. Helping adults with feeding requires time, patience, knowledge of a patient's limitations and nutritional needs, and understanding of a patient's preferences for foods and how to eat a meal. The nurse can improve a patient's nutritional intake by helping with feedings directly or by teaching caregivers how to do so safely. To maintain a patient's dignity during feeding, encourage them to make decisions about food choices, times for eating, and correct use of assistive devices (when needed).

Hospitalized patients receive various therapeutic oral diets that require a health care provider's prescription. A therapeutic diet treats many illness and disease states (Table 31.4). Refer to your employer's dietary manual or consult a dietitian for specific information about therapeutic diets. There are two ways to modify a regular diet: quantitatively or qualitatively (Grodner et al., 2023). *Quantitative modifications* include changes to the number or size of meals served or the amounts of specific nutrients, such as six small feedings or calorie-reduced diet. *Qualitative modifications* involve changes to the consistency, texture, or nutrients, such as clear- or full-liquid diets. The nurse can supplement any diet with oral nutritional supplements. A prescription for a calorie count requires the nurse to record the percentage of each food a patient eats next to the food choice directly on the meal menu. The dietitian calculates caloric intake and determines the need for nutritional supplements or dietary changes.

Altered dentition, improperly fitted dentures, oral lesions or infections, or diseases causing impaired digestion may limit the types and consistencies of foods tolerated. Hemiplegia, a fractured arm, quadriplegia, debilitating illness, or generalized weakness limits self-feeding ability. The presence of IV catheters or tubing, dressings, and bandages also limits the mobility needed for self-feeding. Use interprofessional collaboration (e.g., occupational therapist) to assess a patient's ability to self-feed, and recommend adaptive equipment and supplies for self-feeding. Practise person-centred care when feeding an adult—use compassion, understanding, and common sense to provide a socially meaningful mealtime experience.

TABLE 31.4

Progressive and Therapeutic Diets

Diet	Description
Clear liquid	Foods that are clear and liquid at room or body temperature (e.g., water, apple or cranberry juice, gelatin, popsicles), leave little residue, and are easily absorbed; commonly prescribed for short-term use (24–48 hours) after surgery, before diagnostic tests, and after episodes of diarrhea and vomiting
Full liquid	Includes foods on clear-liquid diet plus addition of smooth-textured dairy products (e.g., milk and ice cream), strained soups and custard, refined cooked cereals, vegetable juice, and pureed vegetables; commonly prescribed before or after surgery for patients who are acutely ill from infection or cannot chew or tolerate solid foods. Verify that patients can tolerate lactose before providing dairy products.
Pureed	Includes foods on full-liquid diet plus easily swallowed foods that do not require chewing (e.g., scrambled eggs; pureed meats, vegetables, and fruits; mashed potatoes). Prescribed for patients with head and neck abnormalities or those who have had oral surgery. Can be modified to be low sodium or low fat.
Mechanical or dental soft	Comprises all previous diets plus addition of ground or finely diced meats, flaked fish, cottage cheese, cheese, rice, potatoes, pancakes, light breads, cooked vegetables, cooked or canned fruit, bananas, and peanut butter; avoid tough meats, nuts, bacon, and fruits with tough skins or membranes; prescribed for patients who have chewing problems or mild gastrointestinal problems; used as a transition diet from liquids to regular
Soft/low residue/low fibre	Addition of low-fibre, easily digested foods such as pastas, moist tender meats, and canned cooked fruits and vegetables; includes easy-to-chew and simply cooked foods; does not permit fatty, rich, and fried foods
High fibre	Addition of fresh uncooked fruits, steamed vegetables, bran, oatmeal, and dried fruits; includes indigestible carbohydrates to relieve constipation, increase gastrointestinal motility, and increase stool weight
Regular or diet as tolerated	No restrictions; permits patient preferences
Sample Therapeutic Diets	
Restricted fluids	Required in severe heart or kidney failure
Sodium restricted	Low levels of sodium: may include a 4-g (no added salt), 2-g (moderate), 1-g (strict), or 500-mg (very strict) diet; often prescribed for patients with heart failure, renal failure, cirrhosis, or hypertension
Fat modified	Cholesterol intake limited to <300 mg daily and fat intake to 30–35%; fatty foods reduced for hypercholesterolemia, malabsorption disorders, and diarrhea
Diabetic	Provides patients with an essential diet treatment for diabetes mellitus; recommended by Diabetes Canada; allows patients to select set amount of food from basic food groups

Adapted from Grodner, M., Escott-Stump, S., & Dorner, S. (2023). *Foundations and clinical applications of nutrition: A nursing approach* (7th ed.). Mosby.

Delegation and Collaboration

The skill of assisting a patient with oral nutrition can be delegated to a UCP. However, the nurse is responsible for determining whether a patient can receive oral nutrition based on their swallowing ability and dietary restrictions. The nurse educates the UCP about the following:

- Explaining any adaptive equipment needed, and proper positioning for patient during and after feeding.
- Explaining any specific swallowing strategies or techniques unique to the patient.
- Reviewing when to stop feeding and reporting immediately to the nurse instances of coughing, gagging, pocketing of food in the mouth, or difficulty swallowing.
- Cautioning not to rush the patient during eating.

Equipment

- Stethoscope
- Washcloths and towels
- Tongue blade
- Adaptive utensils as needed for self-feeding
- Straw
- Oral hygiene supplies (*option*: solution for stomatitis care)
- Clean gloves

STEP	RATIONALE
ASSESSMENT	
1. Identify patient using at least two person-specific identifiers (e.g., name and date of birth, or name and medical record number) according to employer policy.	Ensures correct patient. Complies with Accreditation Canada's standards and improves patient safety (Accreditation Canada, 2020).
2. Throughout the procedure, the 4 moments for hand hygiene are to be implemented; hand hygiene should occur before initial patient (or patient environment) contact, before an aseptic procedure, after body fluid exposure risk, and after patient (or patient environment) contact. Additional hand hygiene should be performed when hands are visibly soiled.	Proper hand hygiene helps prevent the spread of infectious agents to health care providers.

STEP	RATIONALE
ASSESSMENT	
3. Review prescribed diet for type of diet and supplements.	Helps ensure that patient will receive proper diet.
4. Assess presence and condition of teeth. (Apply gloves if there is risk of exposure to saliva.) Determine whether dentures are poorly fitted. Assess severity of mouth discomfort using an appropriate pain rating scale.	Absence of teeth and ill-fitting dentures inhibit normal chewing and influence preparation of food for safe swallowing (Farpour et al., 2020) (see Skill 31.3). Pain can reduce appetite and ability to chew or swallow. These factors increase risk of dysphagia.
5. Have patient speak and swallow: **a.** Watch for laryngeal movement. Ask patient to say "Ah" while using tongue blade and penlight. Check for midline uvula and symmetrical rise of uvula and soft palate. **b.** Use tongue blade to elicit gag reflex (see Chapter 8). Check employer policy before assessing swallowing, as not all jurisdictions allow nurses to assess swallowing ability and gag reflex. In this context, referral to health care provider, SLP, or occupational therapist is indicated.	Patients with damage to cranial nerve IX may experience impaired swallowing; with damage to cranial nerve X, they may exhibit loss of gag reflex, hoarseness, and nasal voice (Gill, 2020).
6. Determine to what extent patient can self-feed. Assess physical motor skills (e.g., ability to grasp utensils, hold cup, and move utensil to mouth). Assess level of consciousness or ability to attend to feeding, visual acuity, and peripheral vision.	Patients with any level of independence should be encouraged to feed themselves. Understanding the patient's physical and cognitive limitations alerts you to the type of help the patient needs. Visual impairments make it difficult to see food and utensils.
7. Assess patient's appetite, recent food and fluid intake, cultural and religious preferences for participating in mealtime, and food likes and dislikes.	Determines type of foods and size of meals that can potentially improve oral intake. Individualizing the assisted-feeding process fosters feelings of patient autonomy (Shune, 2020).
8. Assess for presence of generalized fatigue, pain, or shortness of breath.	Symptoms affect appetite and ability to participate in feeding. Patients eat better when rested.
9. Assess nausea and recent bowel pattern. Is patient passing flatus? Auscultate for bowel sounds.	Determines baseline assessment of gastrointestinal function.
10. Assess need for elimination, hand hygiene, and oral care (including dentures) before feeding.	Reduces interruptions and improves patient's appetite.
11. Review nursing history (see Skill 31.1) for patient's most recent weight and laboratory values.	Provides ongoing monitoring of patient's nutritional status.

NURSING DIAGNOSIS

- Inadequate swallowing
- Acute pain
- Reduced feeding ability
- Reduced stamina
- Potential for insufficient fluid volume
- Potential for aspiration
- Potential for weight loss

Related factors and risk factors are individualized on the basis of patient's condition or needs.

PLANNING

STEP	RATIONALE
1. Expected outcomes following completion of procedure:	
• Patient's weight is maintained or trends toward desired level.	Nutritional intake meets daily needs.
• Patient's nutrition-related laboratory values trend toward normal.	Biochemical markers along with nutritional assessment may indicate nutritional status.
• Patient demonstrates increased ability to self-feed or open items on tray as appropriate.	Indicates increased strength, improved mental status, and increased well-being.
• Patient coughs with no indication of respiratory compromise.	Ineffective cough and respiratory compromise may indicate dysphagia and aspiration.
• Patient has normal vital signs and skin colour while eating.	Indicates tolerance to complete meal.
• Patient is able to describe foods allowed within prescribed diet.	Demonstrates learning.
2. After assessment, allow patient to rest for 30 minutes before mealtime.	Short rest improves patient's energy level and ability to participate in feeding.
3. Administer prescribed analgesic 30 minutes before meal if patient has discomfort.	Analgesic reaches peak level during meal, improving patient's ability to self-feed.
4. Explain to patient how you could set up and help with meal. Allow time for questions.	Minimizes anxiety and engages patient in mealtime.

STEP	RATIONALE
IMPLEMENTATION	
1. Prepare patient's room for mealtime:	
a. Clear over-bed table and arrange any needed supplies.	Reduces transmission of microorganisms and prepares room for food tray.
b. Help patient to comfortable sitting position in chair or place bed in high Fowler's position. If patient is unable to sit, turn patient on side with head of bed (HOB) elevated and chin tucked in position (see Step 1b illustration).	Upright position facilitates swallowing, reducing aspiration risk. Conditions such as pressure injury, traction, or spinal surgery prevent positioning with head elevated. Chin-tuck position decreases the space between the base of the tongue and the posterior pharyngeal wall, creating increased pharyngeal pressure to move the bolus through the pharyngeal region (Paik, 2022) (see Skill 31.3).

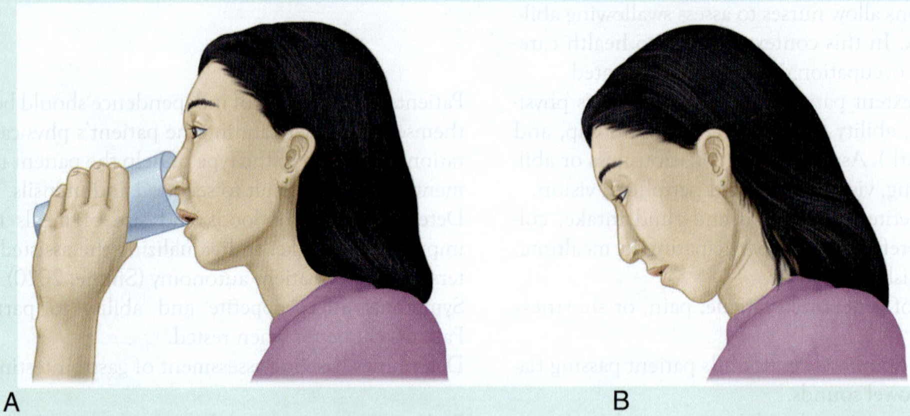

STEP 1B Chin-tuck position.

STEP	RATIONALE
2. Prepare patient for meal:	
a. Help patient with elimination needs and to perform hand hygiene.	Increases patient's comfort, enjoyment of meal, and nutritional intake.
b. Apply clean gloves and offer oral hygiene. If patient has dentures, remove and rinse thoroughly and reinsert. Remove gloves.	Reduces transmission of microorganisms. Moist, clean oral mucosa and teeth improve taste and appetite.
c. Patients with oral mucositis (inflammation of mucous membranes) benefit from rinsing with solutions such as saline, saline–sodium bicarbonate mouthwash, sodium bicarbonate solution, or topical anaesthetics or using mucosal coating agents (Brown & Gupta, 2020). Use interprofessional collaboration to determine best therapy.	Pain of stomatitis causes patients to avoid eating.
d. Help patient put on eyeglasses or insert contact lenses, if used (see Chapter 19).	Enhances patient's ability to self-feed and makes meal more visually appealing.
3. Check environment for distractions. Reduce noise level if possible. *Option:* If patient enjoys music, play a selection of their choice or soothing, low-volume music.	Pleasant environment enhances mealtime experience. Music intervention may reduce agitation in persons with dementia (Soufineyestani et al., 2021).
4. Obtain special assistive devices as needed and instruct on use. Examples include: • Two-handled cup with spout in lid makes it easier to handle cup and drink. Avoids spills. Cup's wide base prevents it from tipping over. • Plate with plate guard (see Step 4 illustration) and nonskid bottom helps person with limited flexibility of hands or poor motor coordination or person who uses only one hand. • Knife, fork, and spoon with large handles or attached splints help with limited hand function or a weak grip.	Devices improve ability to grasp, pick up foods with utensils, and drink liquids.

STEP	RATIONALE

IMPLEMENTATION

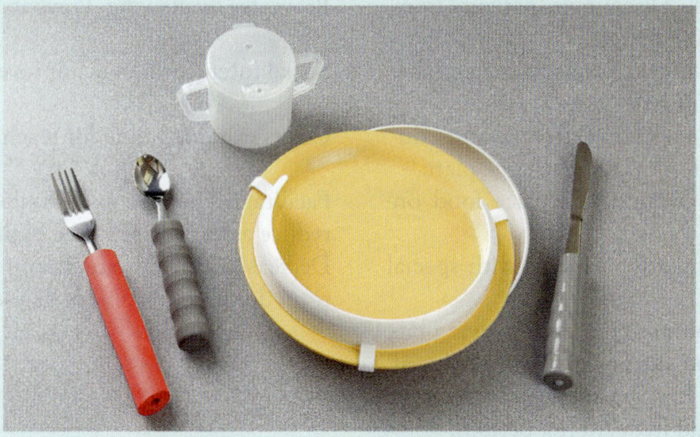

STEP 4 **Mealtime adaptive equipment.** *Clockwise from upper left:* **Two-handled cup with lid, plate with plate guard, utensils with splints, and utensils with enlarged handles.**

STEP	RATIONALE
5. Assess meal tray for completeness and correct diet. Instruct patient about diet, rationale for diet, food options, and dysphagia risks.	Prevents intake of incomplete or incorrect diet. Instruction is more meaningful when applied during real-time activity.
6. Help set up meal tray if patient is unable to do so: open packages, cut up food, apply seasonings or condiments, place napkin.	Allows patient more independence and control. Small pieces are easier to chew and minimize risk of aspiration.
7. Watch patient successfully swallow first bites of food and drink. If patient is able to eat independently, stop here. Return after 15 or 20 minutes, or stay nearby for communication and additional teaching.	Allows patient to be as self-sufficient as possible.

Critical Decision Point *If patient is at risk for aspiration, stay at their side during feeding.*

STEP	RATIONALE
8. Assist patient who cannot eat independently:	
a. Assume comfortable position.	Prevents you from rushing patient through meal.
b. If patient is visually impaired, identify food location on plate as if it were a clock (e.g., vegetables at 3 o'clock, meat at 12 o'clock) (see Step 8b illustration).	Helps patient locate food items and to feed self if given adequate information about food placement on tray.

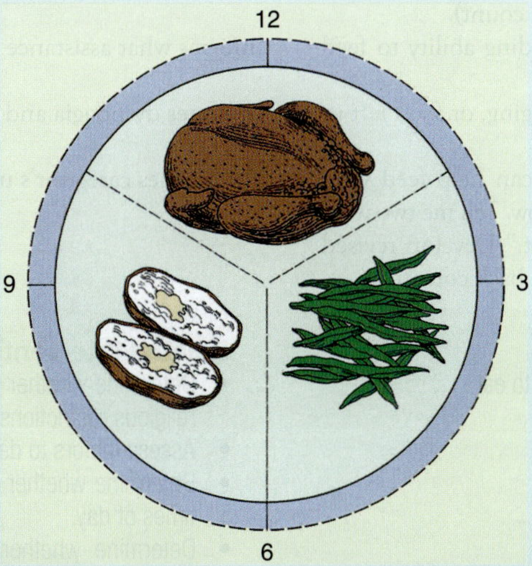

STEP 8B **Clock setup to prepare food on a plate for the visually impaired patient.**

STEP	RATIONALE
c. Ask in which order patient would like to eat and cut food into bite-sized pieces.	Gives patient more independence and control. Small bites reduce risk of aspiration (see Skill 31.3).

STEP	RATIONALE
IMPLEMENTATION	
d. Provide fluids as requested. Discourage patient from drinking all fluids at beginning of meal.	Promotes swallowing. Prevents patient from filling up on fluids.
e. Pace feeding to avoid patient fatigue. Interact with patient, verbally encouraging self-feeding attempts.	Social interaction may improve appetite.
f. Use meal as opportunity to communicate with and educate patient about nutrition topics and discharge plan.	Offers extended time for teaching.
g. Have patient use chin-tuck position and place food on stronger side of mouth.	Facilitates chewing and swallowing. Chin-tuck position may help reduce aspiration risk (see Skill 31.3).
9. Use appropriate feeding techniques for patients with special needs:	Decreased saliva production impairs swallowing. Aspiration results from decreased or absent gag reflex.
a. *Older persons:* Feed small amounts at a time, observing biting, chewing, ability to manipulate tongue to form bolus of food, swallowing, and fatigue. Ensure patient has swallowed food. Offer variety of foods and frequent rest periods.	

Critical Decision Point *If you suspect that patient is aspirating, stop feeding immediately and suction the airway* (see Skill 31.3).

STEP	RATIONALE
b. *Patients living with neurological impairments:* Feed small amounts at a time, observing ability to chew, manipulate tongue to form bolus, and swallow. Have patient open mouth and check for food left inside cheeks (pocketing). Give small amount of thin liquid between bites.	Some patients with limited tongue strength and control are unable to move food to back of mouth for swallowing. Checking for "pocketed" food prevents aspiration (Wayne, 2023).
c. *Patients living with cancer:* Check for food aversions before and during meal. Monitor for fatigue.	Strong, abnormal sense of taste and smell and fatigue are adverse effects of chemotherapy.
10. Help patient with hand hygiene and mouth care after meal is completed. (Apply gloves as needed.)	Maintains comfort.
11. Help patient to resting position, leaving head elevated at least 45 degrees for 30–60 minutes after meal.	Reduces risk of aspiration from regurgitation.
12. Remove and discard gloves.	Reduces transmission of microorganisms.

EVALUATION

STEP	RATIONALE
1. Monitor body weight at least weekly.	Determines ongoing nutritional status.
2. Monitor laboratory values as indicated.	Biochemical markers may help identify changes in nutritional status.
3. Monitor and record I&O (see Chapter 8). Complete intake measurement (e.g., observed intake, calorie count).	
4. Observe patient's ability to self-feed, including ability to feed self, certain items, and part or all of meal.	Informs what assistance patient needs with feeding.
5. Observe patient for choking, coughing, gagging, or food left in mouth during eating.	Indicates dysphagia and possible aspiration.
6. Use teach-back: "We discussed ways you can help feed your spouse that make it easier for them to swallow. Tell me two ways to help feed them and why it is important." Develop revised teaching plan if caregiver is unable to teach back correctly.	Determines caregiver's understanding of instructional topic.

Unexpected Outcomes	Related Interventions
1. Patient is unable to eat entire meal or refuses to eat.	• Determine whether patient has other food preferences and cultural or religious restrictions. • Assess factors to determine what is affecting patient's ability to eat. • Determine whether patient's ability or desire to eat is better at other times of day. • Determine whether patient is in pain, nauseated, or constipated. Implement appropriate interventions (e.g., administering analgesic, antiemetic, or cathartic; providing food or liquid at a temperature patient prefers; offering small, frequent meals). • Provide more frequent oral care. • If inability to eat meal continues, use interprofessional collaboration to develop strategies to assist patient in meeting nutritional requirements.

Unexpected Outcomes	Related Interventions
2. Patient chokes on food.	• Stop feeding immediately; place patient on side with head forward and pointing down; suction mouth and airway. • Contact health care provider if choking occurs repeatedly. • Use interprofessional collaboration as required (e.g., SLP, dietitian) (see Skill 31.3).

Communication and Documentation

- Document in progress notes in EHR or chart the patient's type of diet, amount of feeding assistance needed, tolerance of diet, and percentage of meal eaten (e.g., 25% of food consumed at breakfast).
- If evaluating I&O, document fluid intake on appropriate form (see Chapter 8).
- If patient is receiving oral nutritional supplements to fill or replace meals (e.g., Ensure, Boost), document the amount taken and patient's tolerance.
- Document any swallowing difficulties, food dislikes, or refusal to eat and report to health care provider and dietitian.
- Document your evaluation of caregiver learning.

Special Considerations

Teaching

- See Skill 31.1, Special Considerations, Teaching.

Pediatric

- Human breast milk is the most desirable complete diet for infants during the first 6 months. Infants who are breastfed or bottle-fed do not require additional fluids, especially water or juice, during the first 4 months of life. Excessive intake of water causes water intoxication, failure to thrive, and hyponatremia.
- Babies who are breastfed should receive daily vitamin D supplementation of 10 micrograms (mcg) or 400 international units (IU) (Dietitians of Canada, 2019b).
- Typically, infants do not consume solid foods until 6 months of age. Start with foods that contain iron, and offer them a few times each day to support baby's growth and development (Unger et al., 2019). Iron-fortified infant cereal is usually the first solid food to offer. Iron-rich foods include meats such as beef, lamb, game, poultry, and fish. Meat alternatives include eggs, tofu, and legumes such as beans and lentils.
- Solid foods should not be mixed in a bottle, as this could increase baby's risk of choking; they should be fed with a soft spoon (Centers for Disease Control and Prevention, 2021).

Adolescence

- Developmentally, weight gain is triggered by the release of gonadotropin-releasing hormone, which sends a signal to the adolescent's body to get ready for reproduction.
- Weight gain is also necessary to support height growth in adolescence. The increase in weight and height does not always happen at the same time, and thus the adolescent may seem heavier at times and leaner at others.
- Weight gain is further expected from less physical activity. While primary school students typically run around and play during breaks, high school students tend to sit and socialize.
- Adolescents may have the means to buy the food of their choice and prepare their own meals; they may therefore make poor food choices. Convey recognition of the complex etiology of obesity to help prevent stereotyping of persons who are living with overweight or obesity.

Gerontological

- Some older persons have diminished appetite because of a decline in the olfactory nerve fibres in the nose and number of taste buds, which may limit taste and smell (Sachdev, 2022).
- Interactions between nutrients and medications affect taste of foods or metabolism, absorption, digestion, or excretion of medications. Look at complete medication history to make decisions.
- Being physically active can help individuals stay strong and independent as they grow older. If a patient is overweight or obese, weight loss can improve quality of life and reduce the risk of disease and disability.
- Older persons may refuse to eat certain foods, even if they can feed themselves, because of the way the food looks and smells or because it conflicts with their culture or personal history. Be culturally sensitive when assisting with food selection.

Care in the Community: Home Management

- Assess financial resources of patient and caregiver to determine their ability to purchase nutritionally complete foods for patient.
- Help patient and caregiver identify ways to make meals in the home pleasant and enjoyable experiences.

✦ SKILL 31.3 Aspiration Precautions

Video Clip

The ability to swallow effectively is necessary for the safe transport of food and fluid through the mouth, pharynx, and esophagus into the stomach. It requires the coordination of cranial nerves and the muscles of the tongue, pharynx, larynx, and jaw. Difficulties with feeding, chewing, and swallowing can increase the risk of food getting stuck in the upper airway (causing choking) and/or entering the lungs (causing aspiration). Aspiration is the misdirection of oropharyngeal secretions or gastric contents into the larynx and lower respiratory tract. It often occurs when secretions in the oral pharynx or reflux of gastric content enter the throat and go down the trachea. Patients at risk for aspiration include those with dysphagia (difficulty swallowing).

Some conditions that increase the risk of dysphagia include aging, frailty, cancer of the neck and esophagus, and neurological diseases such as stroke, dementia, and Parkinson's disease (Chen et al., 2021). Medical interventions such as mechanical ventilation and nasotracheal suctioning compromise the gag reflex (Zuercher et al., 2019). Structural obstructions and the adverse effects medications can also cause difficulty swallowing (Krishnan & Pandolfino, 2018) (Box 31.5). Factors that increase the risk of aspiration are decreased level of consciousness; impaired swallowing; nausea or vomiting; reduced gastrointestinal motility; ineffectiveness of patients' endotracheal or tracheostomy tube cuffs; displaced feeding tubes; and large gastric residual volumes, which indicate delayed gastric emptying and may cause distension of the stomach, leading to reflux emesis (Wayne, 2023). Symptoms of dysphagia vary, depending on the swallowing alteration. The nurse should suspect dysphagia if a patient has difficult or painful chewing or swallowing, frequent drooling, loss of food from the mouth during eating, pocketing food in the cheek, and spitting pieces of food out. In addition, a patient might experience choking or coughing when swallowing, a gurgling or wet-sounding voice quality, hoarseness, chest infection, frequent throat clearing, and having the sensation of food getting stuck in the throat after multiple attempts to swallow (Mayo Clinic, 2022).

Inability to coordinate the complex, sequential swallowing mechanism slows eating, results in food being left in the mouth, and may lead to aspiration (Panara et al., 2022). Aspiration of gastric acid causes a chemical pneumonitis (injury caused by the inhalation of sterile gastric contents). Aspiration of bacteria from oral and pharyngeal areas causes aspiration pneumonia (infectious process caused by the inhalation of oropharyngeal secretions that are colonized by pathogenic bacteria), which can be a fatal complication of dysphagia, especially in older persons. *Tachypnea* (>26 respirations/min in adults) is an early sign of aspiration. Other signs include cough; *dyspnea* (difficult breathing); decreased breath sounds; and abnormal breath sounds such as wheezing, rales, and rhonchi (see Chapter 8).

A third type of aspiration, aspiration of a foreign body, may cause an acute respiratory emergency and, in some cases, may predispose the patient to bacterial pneumonia. Both adults and children may inhale foreign bodies. Children have a tendency to swallow a variety of objects such as coins, parts of toys, seeds, and nuts. When the child moves around with their mouth full, the foreign body can enter their airway during deep inspiration. The most common early signs of foreign body aspiration are tachypnea, wheezing, and a wet cough (Goyal et al., 2020); for cases that presented over a week later, fever and dry cough were usually present.

Silent or *asymptomatic aspiration* refers to passage of food or liquid into the trachea and lungs without the development of a protective cough or other signs consistent with aspiration. Lack of outward signs such as coughing reduces awareness by the patient, caregiver, and health team members that aspiration is occurring. This can result in longer periods of ingestion of food and liquid into the lungs, placing the patient at higher risk of developing pneumonia. Nakashima et al. (2018) found silent aspiration to be an independent predictor for mortality in older patients hospitalized for pneumonia. Poor oral hygiene and physical inactivity were important factors related to silent aspiration in these older persons. Yet, children are more likely to silently aspirate than adults, which may be due to immature neurological development or the increased survival rate of premature infants and children with complex medical histories of airway disorders, congenital heart disease, and neurological impairments, including epilepsy/seizures, developmental delay, and cerebral palsy (Velayutham et al., 2018). The subtle signs associated with silent aspiration are easy to miss and include lack of speech, decreased alertness, wet quality to voice, drooling, difficulty controlling secretions, and absence of gag reflex. Because there may be no obvious signs of distress, silent aspiration may go undetected for long periods of time and eventually result in chronic airway disease. Report any noticed aspiration to the health care provider and document this information in the progress notes. Refer the patient for a swallowing assessment if indicated.

Dysphagia Evaluation

As a nurse, you are in a key position to identify your patients' swallowing difficulties and use interprofessional collaboration as required. Conduct your initial nutritional screening (see Skill 31.1) to determine the potential for both aspiration and safe oral intake. When you detect risk factors, use interprofessional collaboration (e.g., SLP) for dysphagia screening (Box 31.6). Dysphagia screening is a minimally

BOX 31.5

Causes of Dysphagia

Neurogenic

- Stroke
- Cerebral palsy
- Guillain-Barré syndrome
- Multiple sclerosis
- Amyotrophic lateral sclerosis (Lou Gehrig's disease)
- Diabetic neuropathy
- Parkinson's disease

Myogenic

- Myasthenia gravis
- Aging
- Muscular dystrophy
- Polymyositis

Obstructive

- Benign peptic stricture
- Lower esophageal ring
- Candidiasis
- Head and neck cancer
- Inflammatory masses
- Trauma or surgical resection
- Anterior mediastinal masses
- Cervical spondylosis

Other

- Gastrointestinal or esophageal resection
- Rheumatological disorders
- Connective tissue disorders
- Vagotomy

BOX 31.6

Criteria for Dysphagia Referral

Before Referral:

If the answer is yes to either of the following two questions, referral at this time is ***not appropriate.***

- Is patient unconscious or drowsy?
- Is patient unable to sit in an upright position for a reasonable length of time?

Also Consider the Next Two Questions Before Making a Referral:

- Is the patient near the end of life?
- Does the patient have an esophageal problem that requires surgical intervention?

When Observing a Patient or Giving Mouth Care, Look for the Following:

- Open mouth (weak lip closure)
- Drooling liquids or solids
- Facial or tongue weakness
- Difficulty moving or swallowing secretions in the mouth
- Slurred, indistinct speech
- Hoarseness
- Poor posture or head control
- Weak, involuntary cough
- Delayed cough (up to 2 minutes after swallow)
- General frailty, confusion, or dementia
- No spontaneous swallowing movements

If the patient has any of the aforementioned symptoms, they may have swallowing problems and need referral to a speech-language pathologist.

invasive procedure that documents the likelihood that dysphagia is present, the need for further swallowing assessment, and the safety of patient intake. The single most important measure to prevent aspiration is to place the patient on NPO until a dysphagia evaluation by an SLP is performed; then a safe diet can resume. A functional oral assessment by an SLP includes observing liquid and food acceptance, bolus formation, lip seal, mastication, dentition, salivation, pocketing, tongue mobility, mandibular movements, propulsion of bolus along palatal vault, and impulsivity or reduced attention (Garand et al., 2020). If the SLP finds serious abnormalities, then videofluoroscopy, the gold standard for dysphagia diagnosis, is indicated.

Dysphagia Management

Dysphagia management includes qualitative dietary modification (i.e., altering the consistency of food and liquids) and is most effective when implemented using an interprofessional approach recommended by the SLP (McGinnis et al., 2019). The SLP's treatment recommendations may include texture modifications for food and liquids (Hill et al., 2021). The dietitian ensures that dietary recommendations are balanced with the nutritional and caloric needs of patients. The nurse assists patients with their mealtime feeding. Thus, interprofessional collaboration (e.g., SLP, dietitian) ensures that appropriate food choices and consistency of liquids are individualized and based on which phase of swallowing is dysfunctional.

In 2019, the Dietitians of Canada supported the IDDSI to standardize terminology and descriptors for texture of foods and liquids that would meet the needs of individuals with dysphagia across all ages and care settings (Dietitians of Canada, n.d.-a). The diet comprises eight levels: thin, slightly thick, mildly thick, liquidized/moderately thick, pureed/extremely thick, minced and moist, soft and bite-sized, and regular (Table 31.5). There is also a category of transitional foods that change texture when moisture (e.g., water, saliva) is applied or temperature is changed—for example, ice chips, ice cream, and certain wafers (IDDSI, 2019).

TABLE 31.5
International Dysphagia Diet Levels

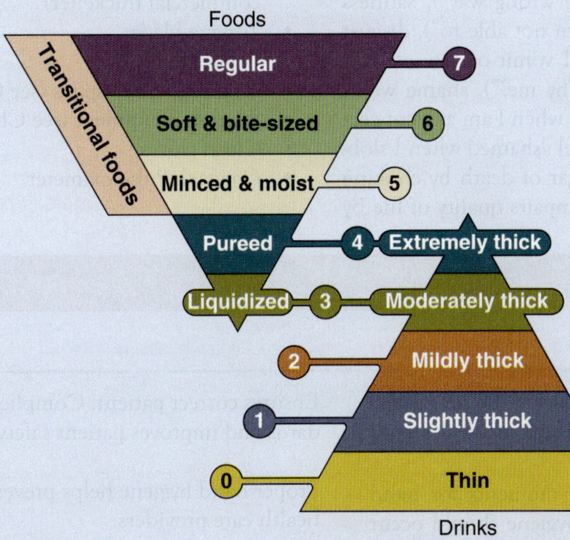

Level	Description/Indications
0: Thin	Flows fast like water; can drink through any nipple, cup, or straw; requires functional ability to safely manage liquids of any type
1: Slightly thick	Thicker than water; requires more effort to drink than thin liquids; reduces speed of flow
2: Mildly thick	Sippable; pours quickly from a spoon, but slower than thin drinks; effort required to drink through standard-bore (5.3-mm) straw; suitable if tongue control is slightly reduced
3: Liquidized/moderately thick	Smooth texture with no lumps; can be drunk from a cup; some effort required to drink through a standard or wide-bore (6.9-mm) straw; allows more time for oral control if pain on swallowing; needs some tongue propulsion effort
4: Pureed/extremely thick	Cannot be drunk from a cup or sucked through a straw; does not require chewing; can be layered or moulded; suitable if pain on chewing or swallowing, missing teeth, poorly fitting dentures
5: Minced and moist	Can be scooped, shaped, and eaten with a spoon or fork; biting is not required; contains small lumps easy to squash with tongue. Suitable if pain or fatigue on chewing, missing teeth, poorly fitting dentures; tongue force needed to move bolus.
6: Soft and bite-sized	Can be eaten with a spoon, fork, or chopsticks; chewing required before swallowing; bite-sized pieces no larger than 8 mm (child) or 15 mm (adult). Suitable if pain or fatigue as above; tongue force and control needed to move food for chewing and move bolus for swallowing.
7: Regular	Normal, everyday foods that are developmentally and age appropriate; includes seeds, bones, and mixed consistencies. Requires ability to bite and chew for long enough to form a swallow-ready bolus and ability to remove bone or gristle from the mouth (i.e., parts that cannot be swallowed safely).

Adapted from International Dysphagia Diet Standardisation Initiative. (2019). *Complete IDDSI framework: Detailed definitions 2.0.* https://iddsi.org/framework/

Thickened liquids are commonly prescribed to prevent aspiration pneumonia. A thickening agent alters flavour and texture qualities. The desired thickness of a liquid depends on a patient's swallowing deficit. It is important to always read the label directions when modifying liquids to prepare the desired thickness correctly. Although there is evidence that thickened liquids can stop immediate aspiration, Hill and colleagues (2021) found low adherence to SLP-prescribed texture-modified diets and fluids, and others reported only limited evidence to indicate that the use of thickened fluids prevents aspiration pneumonia in chronic dysphagia (Bice & Van-Sickle, 2019). More research on this topic is needed.

Consequences of Dysphagia

The physiological consequences of dysphagia include decreased appetite, weight loss, dehydration, malnutrition, and pneumonia (Azer, 2023). A patient's normal nutritional intake is altered when they are unable to consume oral nutrition or must make dietary modifications to swallow without risk of aspiration. Malnutrition may occur secondary to insufficient protein, calorie, and micronutrient intake. Losing the ability to eat and drink safely may affect quality of life. Emotional responses include anger ("I get angry at myself when I am not careful and end up swallowing the wrong way"), sadness ("I feel sad when I see others eating and I am not able to"), disgust ("Meals are disgusting," "I feel disgusted if I vomit or lose control over the food in my mouth"), self-pity ("Why me?"), shame when eating in public spaces ("If people stare at me when I am at a concert or a restaurant, I feel shamed by them," "I feel ashamed when I slobber"), anxiety that therapies may fail, and fear of death by choking (Bushuven et al., 2022). Dysphasia further impairs quality of life by minimizing people's ability to participate in religious rituals (e.g., eating altar bread) and social activities such as going to restaurants with friends.

Delegation and Collaboration

The skill of following aspiration precautions while feeding a patient can be delegated to a UCP. However, the nurse is responsible for the ongoing assessment of a patient's risk for aspiration and determination of positioning and any special feeding techniques. The nurse directs the UCP to do the following:

- Position patient upright (45 to 90 degrees preferred) or according to medical restrictions during and after feeding
- Use aspiration precautions while feeding patients who need help and explain feeding techniques that are successful for specific patients
- Immediately report to the nurse any onset of coughing, gagging, "wet" voice, or pocketing of food

Equipment

- Chair or bed that allows patient to sit upright
- Thickening agents as prescribed (rice, cereal, yogourt, gelatin, commercial thickener)
- Tongue blade
- Penlight
- Oral hygiene supplies (see Chapter 18)
- Suction equipment (see Chapter 25)
- Clean gloves
- *Optional:* Pulse oximeter

STEP	RATIONALE
ASSESSMENT	
1. Identify patient using at least two person-specific identifiers (e.g., name and date of birth, or name and medical record number) according to employer policy.	Ensures correct patient. Complies with Accreditation Canada's standards and improves patient safety (Accreditation Canada, 2020).
2. Throughout the procedure, the 4 moments for hand hygiene are to be implemented; hand hygiene should occur before initial patient (or patient environment) contact, before an aseptic procedure, after body fluid exposure risk, and after patient (or patient environment) contact. Additional hand hygiene should be performed when hands are visibly soiled.	Proper hand hygiene helps prevent the spread of infectious agents to health care providers.
3. Review results of nutritional screening in medical record (see Skill 31.1).	Reveals risk patterns (e.g., patients with dysphagia often alter their eating patterns or choose foods that provide inadequate nutrition).
4. Ask patient or caregiver if patient has difficulties chewing or swallowing various food textures.	Patients are likely to aspirate certain foods more than others.
5. Assess for conditions that cause dysphagia and present risk for aspiration (see Box 31.5). Also assess signs and symptoms of dysphagia (e.g., drooling, hoarseness, food pocketing). Use dysphagia screening tool if available.	Patients with neurological or neuromuscular disease and those with trauma to or surgery of oral cavity or throat are at risk.
6. Assess alertness, orientation, and ability to follow simple commands (e.g., open your mouth; stick out your tongue).	Disorientation and inability to follow commands lead to higher risk of dysphagia.
7. Assess patient's oral cavity, level of dental hygiene, missing teeth, or poorly fitting dentures. (Apply clean gloves if needed.)	Decayed teeth, plaque, and periodontal disease can cause growth of bacteria in the mouth, which creates risk for aspiration of bacteria (Gaeckle et al., 2020).
8. Observe patient during mealtime for signs of dysphagia such as coughing, dyspnea, or drooling. Observe patient's attempt to feed self; note type of food consistencies and liquids they are able to swallow. Note whether patient tires during and by end of meal.	Detects abnormal eating patterns such as frequent clearing of throat or prolonged eating time. Chewing and sitting up for feeding bring on fatigue because the entire swallowing process over the course of a meal—including chewing the food and transporting it from the oral cavity into the pharynx, past a closed larynx, and into the esophagus—requires sustained attention and continuous action of many muscles (Brates et al., 2021).

STEP	RATIONALE

ASSESSMENT

STEP	RATIONALE
9. *Option:* Obtain baseline assessment oxygen saturation.	Research findings differ as to whether oximetry can reliably detect aspiration (Malcom & Baird, 2019).
10. Indicate on patient's EHR, chart, or Kardex that dysphagia/aspiration risk is present. *Option:* Some facilities use different-coloured meal trays to signify patients at risk for aspiration.	Identifying patient as dysphagic reduces risk of improperly prepared oral nutrition without and inadequate supervision.

NURSING DIAGNOSES

- Reduced ability to swallow
- Potential for aspiration

Related factors and risk factors are individualized on the basis of patient's condition or needs.

PLANNING

STEP	RATIONALE
1. Expected outcomes following completion of procedure:	
• Patient does not exhibit signs or symptoms of aspiration.	Interventions for preventing aspiration are successful.
• Patient maintains stable weight.	Patient maintains adequate oral nutrition.
2. Provide patient with 30 minutes of rest.	Fatigue increases risk of aspiration.
3. Explain why you are observing patient while they eat.	Indicators associated with aspiration require further swallowing evaluation such as fluoroscopic examination.
4. Explain to patient and caregiver what you are going to do and why.	Increases patient cooperation and prepares caregiver to assist.

IMPLEMENTATION

STEP	RATIONALE
1. Have patient or caregiver (if helping with feeding) perform hand hygiene.	Educates about and prevents transmission of microorganisms.
2. Apply clean gloves. Provide oral hygiene, including brushing tongue, before meal.	Reduces transmission of microorganisms. Risk for aspiration pneumonia has been associated with poor oral hygiene (Gaeckle et al., 2020).
3. Position patient upright (90 degrees) in chair or elevate HOB to a 45- to 90-degree angle or to highest position allowed by medical condition during meal. For those unable to get out of bed, it is important to raise HOB by at least 30 degrees if possible. Then, have patient tuck chin toward the chest (chin tuck), and, if they are paralyzed on one side, instruct them to turn their head toward the paralyzed side and tilt the body to the nonparalyzed side during the meal.	Appropriate postures or manoeuvres could prevent aspiration during eating or drinking. These actions (chin tuck, head turn, body tilt) direct the food or fluid bolus downward, allowing food and fluid to bypass the weaker side (Chen et al., 2021).
4. *Option:* Apply pulse oximeter to patient's finger; monitor during feeding.	Pulse oximetry is noninvasive, requires little patient cooperation, and is easy to obtain and repeatable. The association between aspiration and oxygen desaturation is inconclusive; therefore, episodes of desaturation during feeding should be interpreted as unspecific "alarm" signals that prompt further thorough assessments (Marian et al., 2017).
5. Use penlight and tongue blade to gently inspect mouth for pockets of food.	Pockets of food found inside cheeks occur when patient has difficulty moving food from mouth into pharynx; may lead to aspiration (Wayne, 2023). Patient is usually unaware of pocketing, particularly persons living with dementia, who lose ability to recognize objects and know when and how to chew or swallow (Jung et al., 2021).
6. Add thickener to thin liquids to create desired consistency according to prescription. Encourage patient to feed self.	Thicker liquids enhance the safety of swallowing and decrease the incidence of aspiration (Teasell et al., 2018).
7. Have patient assume chin-tuck position. Remind patient to not tilt head backward when eating or drinking.	Chin-tuck position is usually effective, as hyperextension of neck makes it easier for food to enter airway. Severe cases of dysphagia may require a more aggressive approach, including enteral feeding. Risk of pneumonia was significantly lower in patients who used percutaneous endoscopic gastrostomy (PEG) feeding than in those with nasogastric (NG) tube, because the NG tube passes through the upper esophageal sphincter (Lin et al., 2022).

IMPLEMENTATION

STEP	RATIONALE
8. If patient is unable to feed self, place 0.5 to 1 teaspoon of food on unaffected side of mouth, allowing utensil to touch mouth or tongue.	Small bites help patient swallow and reduce choking risk (IDDSI, 2019). Provides tactile cue to food; avoids pocketing of food on weaker side.
9. Provide verbal coaching, reminding patient to chew and think about swallowing: "Open your mouth. Feel the food in your mouth. Chew and taste the food. Raise your tongue to the roof of your mouth. Think about swallowing. Close your mouth and swallow. Swallow again. Cough to clear your airway."	Verbal cueing keeps patient focused on normal swallowing. Positive reinforcement enhances patient's confidence in ability to swallow. Double- or repeat-swallowing helps clear any remaining food from unprotected airway (Chen et al., 2021).
10. Avoid mixing food of different textures in same mouthful. Alternate liquids and bites of food. Refer to dietitian for next meal if patient has difficulty with particular consistency.	Single textures are easier to swallow than multiple textures. Alternating solids with liquids removes food residue in mouth and facilitates better transfer to the esophagus (Ellis & Allen, 2018).
11. Monitor swallowing and observe for throat clearing, coughing, choking, gagging, and drooling of food; suction airway as needed (see Chapter 25).	These indications suggest dysphagia and risk for aspiration (Chen et al., 2021).
12. Minimize distractions, do not talk, and do not rush patient. Allow time for adequate chewing and swallowing. Provide rest period as needed during meal.	Environmental distractions during mealtime increase risk of aspiration (Chen et al., 2021). Avoiding fatigue reduces aspiration risk.
13. Use sauces, condiments, and gravies to facilitate cohesive food bolus formation.	Cohesive food bolus helps prevent pocketing and prevents small food particles from entering the airway (van Eck et al., 2020).
14. Ask patient to remain upright for at least 30–60 minutes after meal.	Remaining upright reduces chance of aspiration by allowing food particles remaining in pharynx to clear.
15. Provide thorough oral hygiene after meal (see Chapter 18).	Reduces plaque and secretions containing bacteria that can cause aspiration pneumonia, especially in patients with decreased immunity (Teasell et al., 2018).
16. Remove gloves if worn.	

EVALUATION

STEP	RATIONALE
1. Throughout meal, carefully observe patient's ability to swallow food and fluids of various textures and thickness without choking.	Identifies effort with swallowing and absence of signs related to aspiration. Demonstrating sensitivity to how patient may feel about being watched while they eat or drink enhances trust (Guthrie & Stansfield, 2017).
2. Monitor pulse oximetry readings for high-risk patients while they eat.	Deteriorating oxygen saturation levels indicate aspiration.
3. Monitor patient's I&O, calorie count, and food intake.	Helps detect malnutrition and dehydration.
4. Weigh patient daily or weekly.	Determines whether weight is stable and reflects nutritional status.
5. Observe patient's oral cavity after meal.	Determines presence of food pockets that could be aspirated.
6. Use teach-back: "We talked about why your spouse is at risk of aspirating their food. Tell me the things to observe for that will tell you they are having trouble swallowing. What should you do if these things happen during a meal?" Develop a revised teaching plan if caregiver is unable to teach back correctly.	Determines caregiver's level of understanding of instructional topic.

Unexpected Outcomes	Related Interventions
1. Patient coughs, gags, indicates food "stuck in throat," and has wet quality to voice when eating.	• Stop feeding immediately and place patient on NPO. • Notify health care provider and suction as needed. • Use interprofessional collaboration (e.g., SLP) for swallowing exercises and techniques to improve swallowing.
2. Patient experiences weight loss over next several days or weeks.	• Discuss findings with interprofessional team (e.g., health care provider, dietitian, SLP). Determine whether nutritional supplementation or increasing frequency or quality of foods is needed.

Communication and Documentation

- Document in progress notes in EHR or chart the assessment findings, patient's tolerance of liquid and food textures, amount of help required, position during meal, absence or presence of symptoms of dysphagia during feeding, fluid intake, and amount eaten.
- Report any coughing, gagging, choking, or other swallowing difficulties to health care provider.
- Communicate that patient has dysphagia during hand-off communication at change of shift.
- Document your evaluation of caregiver learning.

DOCUMENTATION EXAMPLE

Patient was sitting upright in bed with over-bed table to eat lunch. Consumed all liquids and semisoft diet as prescribed with no dysphagia, choking, or gagging noted. After setting patient up and orientating them to their plate, no further assistance was required. Remained with patient throughout meal to observe and support independent feeding.

Special Considerations

Pediatric

- Long-term effects for a child diagnosed with pediatric dysphagia include aspiration pneumonia, malnutrition, dehydration, and increased risk of mortality and infectious complications (Lawlor & Choi, 2020).
- The primary goals of oral sensorimotor therapy for children are as follows (Gosa, 2018):
  - Improve safe swallowing and the function of the structures involved in the skills of eating.
  - Achieve maximal functional capacity for feeding and speech by targeting oral muscle tone and strength.
  - Improve range of movement of oral structures, precision of oral movements, oral reflexes, and functional oral movement patterns by using skills appropriate to child's level of development/physical capacity.
  - Ensure collaboration between SLP and caregiver to incorporate dietary preferences and maximize child's quality of life.

Adolescence

- According to adolescents, the concept of weight is not simply a number on the scale; rather, it is a number that evokes feelings of negativity about themselves and is visibly seen by others (Yerges et al., 2021).
- Because weight labelling can initiate the processes of stigma, be sensitive when discussing weight and appearance with adolescents. Begin with general questions about the adolescent to allow for rapport to develop. Use open-ended questions regarding the meaning of health, the meaning of weight, and the adolescent's experiences within their social settings. It may be appropriate to consider asking adolescents and parents about their preferred terms when discussing weight owing to variations in the terms preferred among different cultures and genders. Praise adolescents for any efforts that they are making to eat a healthy diet, get the right amount of sleep, and be active every day. Remind them that every person has an aspect of their body that they feel sensitive about. In addition, adolescents should know that supermodels and other celebrities that they admire have professionals who help them look the way they do, including people who airbrush their photos before they appear on social media.
- Listen well and be available so that the adolescent realizes that their feelings and thoughts matter and that support will be there for them. Help them appreciate what their body does every day. It is important to use nonbiased language, open-ended questions, and a respectful tone when discussing weight. Include adolescents in the conversation and express interest in their lives. Adolescents are highly sensitive to weight-related communication, which often leaves them feeling insecure and upset. They prefer a gentle, encouraging approach that focuses on health management instead of weight management (Auckburally et al., 2021).

Gerontological

- Minimize the use of sedatives and hypnotics, which impair the cough reflex and swallowing (Boscart et al., 2023).

Patients With Physical or Cognitive Challenges

- Patients living with dementia are at high risk for eating and feeding difficulties and inadequate food and fluid intake. Depending on the severity of their cognitive impairment, they may forget to eat, forget they have eaten, fail to recognize food, or eat things that are not food.
- Eating difficulties are likely to worsen in a care facility because people living with dementia often become more confused in an unfamiliar place. Different mealtime routines and foods add to the problem.
- Patients living with dementia may not be able to tell anyone that they are hungry, need help eating, or need more time to chew and swallow.

Care in the Community: Home Management

- Educate the patient and caregiver about aspiration precautions and the most effective techniques for preventing development of aspiration pneumonia.
- Explain to caregiver that older persons with pneumonia often express fewer symptoms than younger adults; therefore, aspiration pneumonia is underdiagnosed. Delirium may be the only manifestation of pneumonia in older persons.
- Dysphagia in the community setting is best managed with an interprofessional person-centred approach that includes the patient, caregiver, health care provider, nurse, occupational therapist, dietitian, and SLP.

✦ REVIEW QUESTIONS

A 73-year-old patient (he/him) with Alzheimer's disease is receiving medication that leaves him with a dry mouth. The results of a nutritional screening indicate he has difficulty swallowing. Symptoms include frequent coughing during mealtime. The patient's respiratory rate is 18 breaths/min and heart rate is 90 beats/min. The speech-language pathologist has recommended a dysphagia mechanically altered diet with liquids thickened to the mildly thick level. The patient currently weighs 62.6 kg (138 lb) and is 177.8 cm (5′10″) tall. His daughter visits frequently at the assisted living facility. Although the patient can feed himself, his daughter usually feeds him during scheduled mealtimes in the busy dining room. She frequently gives him sips of her coffee and bites of his favourite oatmeal cookies. The daughter encourages him to bend his head backward to make sure that he drinks all of the liquid in his cup or glass.

Review Questions 1 to 3 relate to the case study presented here.

1. Determine the patient's body mass index (BMI) and rate his nutritional status.
2. Identify three ways you should teach the daughter to help him swallow and decrease his aspiration risk. Include rationales for your actions.
3. The patient is in the dining area where an unregulated care provider (UCP) is feeding him. The UCP gives the patient some moist ground meat and then cooked fruit. The nurse walks up to the patient's table and notices the patient coughing and beginning to gag. The nurse instructs the UCP to stop feeding. The patient has a respiratory rate of 30 breaths/min and shows that effort is needed to breathe. Document a progress note for this situation.
4. A nurse may delegate the following care to an unregulated care provider (UCP). (*Select all that apply.*)
   1. Nutritional screening
   2. Aspiration precautions
   3. Feeding a patient
   4. Interpreting pulse oximetry readings
   5. Measuring a patient's weight
5. A patient is unable to eat more than 25% of any meal because of pain and nausea. Which of the following interventions are most important for the nurse to perform? (*Select all that apply.*)
   1. Encourage the patient to eat small amounts several times throughout the day.
   2. Ask the patient which foods and beverages cause the least amount of nausea.
   3. Record a chronology of what the patient has been eating for the past 2 days.
   4. Provide the patient with an analgesic 30 minutes before a meal.
   5. Administer an antiemetic to the patient 30 to 60 minutes before a meal.
6. A nurse is examining a patient just admitted to an acute care unit in the hospital.

   List three assessment findings of the skin that would indicate a possible nutritional problem:

   1. ____________
   2. ____________
   3. ____________

Visit the Evolve site for a complete list of answers to the Review Questions.

✦ NEXT GENERATION NCLEX® (NGN)

For practice with answering exam questions related to unfolding NGN case studies, please consult the Next Generation NCLEX® (NGN)-Style Case Studies for Skills and Techniques on the Evolve website: http://evolve.elsevier.com/Canada/Perry/clinicalskills/

REFERENCES

Abud, T., Kounidas, G., Martin, K. R., et al. (2022). Determinants of healthy ageing: A systematic review of contemporary literature. *Aging Clinical and Experimental Research, 34*, 1215–1223. https://doi.org/10.1007/s40520-021-02049-w

Accreditation Canada. (2020). *Required organizational practices–2020 handbook*. https://physicians.nshealth.ca/resources/required-organizational-practices-2020-handbook

Akula, B., & Doctor, N. (2021). A prospective review of preoperative nutritional status and its influence on the outcome of abdominal surgery. *Cureus, 13*(11), e19948. https://doi.org/10.7759/cureus.19948

Alberta Health Services. (2019). *Nutrition guideline: Seniors health overview (65 years and older)*. https://www.albertahealthservices.ca/assets/info/nutrition/if-nfs-ng-seniors-health-overview.pdf

Auckburally, S., Davies, E., & Logue, J. (2021). The use of effective language and communication in the management of obesity: The challenge for healthcare professionals. *Current Obesity Reports, 10*, 274–281. https://doi.org/10.1007/s13679-021-00441-1

Azer, S. A. (2023). *Dysphagia*. StatPearls. https://www.statpearls.com/ArticleLibrary/viewarticle/20803

Bachand, M.-P., & Hulst, J. (2020). *Assessing nutritional status* [PowerPoint slides]. Canadian Digestive Diseases Week 2020, Montreal, Quebec. https://www.cag-acg.org/images/cddw/Satsgs_AssessNutrition_Hulst_Ba chand.pdf

Barnard, R., Jones, J., & Cruice, M. (2022). Addressing patients' communication support needs through speech-language pathologist–nurse information-sharing: Employing ethnography to understand the acute stroke context. *International Journal of Speech Language Pathology, 24*(5), 504–514. https://doi.org/10.1080/17549507.2022.2034944

Batal, M., Chan, H. M., Fediuk, K., et al. (2021). First Nations households living on-reserve experience food insecurity: Prevalence and predictors among ninety-two First Nations communities across Canada. *Canadian Journal of Public Health, 112*(Suppl. 1), 52–63. https://doi.org/10.17269/s41997-021-00491-x

Batal, M., Chan, H. M., Ing, A., et al. (2021). Nutrient adequacy and nutrient sources of adults among ninety-two First Nations communities across Canada. *Canadian Journal of Public Health, 112*(Suppl. 1), 29–40. https://doi.org/10.17269/s41997-021-00490-y

Bice, E., & Van-Sickle, A. (2019). *Modifying more than diets: Rethinking a common practice*. https://dysphagiacafe.com/2019/09/01/modifying-more-than-diets-rethinking-a-common-practice/

Boscart, V., McCleary, L., Sheiban Taucar, L., et al. (2023). *Ebersole and Hess' gerontological nursing and healthy aging in Canada* (3rd ed.). Elsevier.

Brates, D., Troche, M. S., & Molfenter, S. M. (2021). The role of fatigue in the aging swallow: A review. *OBM Geriatrics, 5*(2), 22. https://doi.org/10.21926/obm.geriatr.2102166

Brown, T. J., & Gupta, A. (2020). Management of cancer therapy–associated oral mucositis. *JCO Oncology Practice, 16*(3), 103–109. https://doi.org/10.1200/JOP.19.00652

Bukambu, E., Lieffers, J. R. L., Ekwaru, J. P., et al. (2020). The association between the cost and quality of diets of children in Canada. *Canadian Journal of Public Health, 111*(2), 269–277. https://doi.org/10.17269/s41997-019-00264-7

Bushuven, S., Niebel, I., Huber, J., et al. (2022). Emotional and psychological effects of dysphagia: Validation of the Jugendwerk Dysphagia Emotion and Family Assessment (JDEFA). *Dysphagia, 37*(2), 375–391. https://doi.org/10.1007/s00455-021-10289-1

Canadian Frailty Network. (2019). *Frailty matters*. https://www.cfn-nce.ca/wp-content/uploads/2019/04/CFN-Frailty-Backgrounder-2019-04-29.pdf

Canadian Institute of Food Safety. (2020, August 31). *The difference between best before and expiry dates*. https://www.foodsafety.ca/blog/difference-between-best-and-expiry-dates

Canadian Institute of Food Safety. (2022, February 23). *Your guide to safe sushi service*. https://www.foodsafety.ca/blog/your-guide-to-safe-sushi-service

Canadian Nurses Association. (2018, December 4). *Malnutrition in hospitalized patients: A serious problem calling for interdisciplinary engagement [video]. Canadian nurses association webinar series: Progress in practice*. YouTube. https://www.youtube.com/watch?v=imbmI9LF7VE

Caron, N., & Plunkett-Latimer, J. (2022). *Canadian Income Survey: Food insecurity and unmet health care needs, 2018 and 2019*. Statistics Canada. https://www150.statcan.gc.ca/n1/pub/75f0002m/75f0002m2021009-eng.htm

Centers for Disease Control and Prevention. (2021). *Feeding from a bottle*. https://www.cdc.gov/nutrition/infantandtoddlernutrition/bottle-feeding/index.html

Chen, S., Kent, B., & Cui, Y. (2021). Interventions to prevent aspiration in older adults with dysphagia living in nursing homes: A scoping review. *BMC Geriatrics, 21*, 429. https://doi.org/10.1186/s12877-021-02366-9

Cirillo, D. M., Hart, S. K., Reich, R. R., et al. (2018). Height measures: Evaluating alternatives to standing height in the ambulatory setting. *Clinical Journal of Oncology Nursing, 22*(5), 529–533. https://doi.org/10.1188/18.CJON.529-533

CNA Training Help. (n.d.). *CNA skill: Measuring height and weight for a supine patient*. https://cnatraininghelp.com/cna-skills/measuring-height-and-weight-for-a-supine-patient/

Computrition. (2018). This isn't what I ordered: The severity of hospital tray delivery inaccuracy: What can be done to keep patients safe and satisfied. *During Their Stay [Ebook].* https://www.computrition.com/wp-content/uploads/2020/07/tray-error.pdf

Dashtdar, M., Dashtdar, M. R., Dashtdar, F., et al. (2022). The perspectives of traditional and modern medicine on the nature of hot and cold foods. *Medical Research Journal*, 7(1), 82–93. https://doi.org/10.5603/MRJ.a2022.0001

Dietitians of Canada. (n.d.-a). *Dysphagia.* https://www.dietitians.ca/Advocacy/Interprofessional-Collaborations-(1)/Dysphagia

Dietitians of Canada. (n.d.-b). *WHO growth charts for Canada.* https://www.dietitians.ca/growthcharttraining

Dietitians of Canada. (2019a). *Best practices for nutrition, food service and dining in long term care homes: A working paper of the ontario LTC action group 2019.* https://www.dietitians.ca/DietitiansOfCanada/media/Documents/Resources/2019-Best-Practices-for-Nutrition,-Food-Service-and-Dining-in-Long-Term-Care-LTC-Homes.pdf

Dietitians of Canada. (2019b). *What you need to know about vitamin D.* https://www.unlockfood.ca/en/Articles/Vitamins-and-Minerals/What-you-need-to-know-about-Vitamin-D.aspx

Donnelly, R., Devlin, K., & Keller, H. (2022). Dietitian perspectives: Are we ready for nutrition risk screening in community and primary care? *The Journal of Nutrition, Health & Aging*, 26, 211–212. https://doi.org/10.1007/s12603-022-1735-6

Eldridge, A. L., Piernas, C., Illner, A.-K., et al. (2018). Evaluation of new technology-based tools for dietary intake assessment—an ILSI Europe Dietary Intake and Exposure Task Force evaluation. *Nutrients*, *11*(1), 55. https://doi.org/10.3390/nu11010055

Ellis, P., & Allen, J. (2018). Swallowing difficulties. In R. MacLeod, & L. van den Block (Eds.), *Textbook of palliative care*. Springer. https://doi.org/10.1007/978-3-319-31738-0_19-1

Farpour, S., Smithard, D., & Farpour, H. R. (2020). Dysphagia and oral health in older people. *OBM Geriatrics*, *4*(1), 109. https://doi.org/10.21926/obm.geriatr.2001109

Food and Agriculture Organization of the United Nations. (n.d.). *Food-based dietary guidelines.* https://www.fao.org/nutrition/education/food-dietary-guidelines/home/en/

Gaeckle, N. T., Pragman, A. A., Pendleton, K. M., et al. (2020). The oral–lung axis: The impact of oral health on lung health. *Respiratory Care*, *65*(8), 1211–1220. https://doi.org/10.4187/respcare.07332

Garand, K. L., McCullough, G., Crary, M., et al. (2020). Assessment across the life span: The clinical swallow evaluation. *American Journal of Speech-Language Pathology*, *29*(2S), 919–933. https://doi.org/10.1044/2020_AJSLP-19-00063

Gill, J. (2020, May 20). *Glossopharyngeal and vagus nerve explained—guide to cranial nerves IX and X [Video].* YouTube. https://www.youtube.com/watch?v=f_hCm_vSOPE

Gillies, C., Blanchet, R., Gokiert, R., et al. (2020). School-based nutrition interventions for Indigenous children in Canada: A scoping review. *BMC Public Health*, *20*, 11. https://doi.org/10.1186/s12889-019-8120-3

Gillis, C., Hasil, L., Kasvis, P., et al. (2021). Nutrition care process model approach to surgical prehabilitation in oncology. *Frontiers in Nutrition*, *8*. https://doi.org/10.3389/fnut.2021.644706

Gilmour, H., & Ramage-Morin, P. L. (2021). *Association of frailty and pre-frailty with increased risk of mortality among older Canadians.* Statistics Canada Health Reports. Catalogue No. 82-003-X https://www.doi.org/10.25318/82-003-x202100400002-eng

Gosa, M. M. (2018, September 21). *Pediatric dysphagia treatment: The how and why* [PowerPoint slides]. University of Montevallo. https://www.montevallo.edu/wp-content/uploads/2018/09/Handout-PedDysphagiaTxHowandWhy-2018.pdf

Goyal, S., Jain, S., Rai, G., et al. (2020). Clinical variables responsible for early and late diagnosis of foreign body aspiration in pediatrics age group. *Journal of Cardiothoracic Surgery*, *15*(1), 271. https://doi.org/10.1186/s13019-020-01314-9

Grodner, M., Escott-Stump, S., & Dorner, S. (2023). *Foundations and clinical applications of nutrition: A nursing approach* (8th ed.). Elsevier.

Guthrie, S., & Stansfield, J. (2017). Teatime threats. Choking incidents at the evening meal. *Journal of Applied Research in Intellectual Disabilities*, 30(1), 47–60. https://doi.org/10.1111/jar.12218

Health Canada. (2019). *Food safety for vulnerable populations.* https://www.canada.ca/en/health-canada/services/food-safety-vulnerable-populations/food-safety-vulnerable-populations.html

Health Canada. (2021a). *Body mass index (BMI) nomogram.* https://www.canada.ca/en/health-canada/services/food-nutrition/healthy-eating/healthy-weights/canadian-guidelines-body-weight-classification-adults/body-mass-index-nomogram.html

Health Canada. (2021b). *Food safety and you.* https://www.canada.ca/en/health-canada/services/general-food-safety-tips/food-safety-you.html

Health Canada. (2021c). *Make healthy meals with Canada's food guide plate.* https://food-guide.canada.ca/en/tips-for-healthy-eating/make-healthy-meals-with-the-eat-well-plate/

Health Canada. (2021d). *Safe food storage.* https://www.canada.ca/en/health-canada/services/general-food-safety-tips/safe-food-storage.html

Health Canada. (2022a). *Food and nutrition.* https://www.canada.ca/en/health-canada/services/food-nutrition.html

Health Canada. (2022b). *Food safety for hunting.* https://www.sac-isc.gc.ca/eng/1581553052942/1582645518250

Health Canada. (2022c). *Healthy eating when pregnant and breastfeeding.* https://food-guide.canada.ca/en/tips-for-healthy-eating/pregnant-breastfeeding/

Health Canada. (2022d). *Nutrition North Canada.* https://www.nutritionnorthcanada.gc.ca/eng/1415385762263/1415385790537

Health Canada. (2023a). *Canada's dietary guidelines for health professionals and policy makers.* https://food-guide.canada.ca/en/guidelines/

Health Canada. (2023b). *Health Canada's healthy eating strategy.* https://www.canada.ca/en/services/health/campaigns/vision-healthy-canada/healthy-eating.html

Health Canada. (2023c). *Regulations and compliance: Nutrition labelling.* https://www.canada.ca/en/health-canada/services/ food-nutrition/food-labelling/nutrition-labelling/regulations-compliance.html

Heart and Stroke Foundation of Canada. (2021, January 11). *Taking action for optimal community and long-term stroke care: A resource for healthcare providers—Chapter 3: Body function (physical), section 3.3—nutrition and swallowing* [PowerPoint slides]. https://www.heartandstroke.ca/-/media/1-stroke-best-practices/tacls/tacls-swallowingnutrition-april20

Hemoglobin level. (2020). *Nursing Critical Care*, Vol. 15(4), 34–35. https://doi.org/10.1097/01.CCN.0000660408.76985.53

Hewko, S., Oyesegun, A., Clow, S., et al. (2021). High turnover in clinical dietetics: A qualitative analysis. *BMC Health Services Research*, *21*, 25. https://doi.org/10.1186/s12913-020-06008-5

Hill, C., Clapham, R. P., Buccheri, A., et al. (2021). Assessing adherence and exploring barriers to provision of prescribed texture modifications for dysphagia in a residential aged care facility in rural Australia. *International Journal of Speech Language Pathology*, *24*(1), 67–76. https://doi.org/10.1080/17549507.2021.1953144

Hodge, J. M., Shah, R., McCullough, M. L., et al. (2020). Validation of self-reported height and weight in a large, nationwide cohort of U.S. adults. *PLoS One*, *15*(4), e0231229. https://doi.org/10.1371/journal.pone.0231229

Hood, A. (2020). Nutritional status assessment in adults technique. *Medscape.* https://emedicine.medscape.com/article/2141861-technique

Idzerda, L., Gariépy, G., Corrin, T., et al. (2022). What is known about the prevalence of household food insecurity in Canada during the COVID-19 pandemic: A systematic review. *Health Promotion and Chronic Disease Prevention in Canada*, *42*(5), 177–187. https://doi.org/10.24095/hpcdp.42.5.01

International Dysphagia Diet Standardisation Initiative. (2019). *Complete IDDSI framework: Detailed definitions 2.0.* https://iddsi.org/framework/

Jung, D., Lee, K., De Gagne, J. C., et al. (2021). Eating difficulties among older adults with dementia in long-term care facilities: A scoping review. *International Journal of Environmental Research and Public Health*, *18*(19), 10109. https://doi.org/10.3390/ijerph181910109

Keller, H., Laur, C., Atkins, M., et al. (2018). Update on the Integrated Nutrition Pathway for Acute Care (INPAC): Post implementation tailoring and toolkit to support practice improvements. *Nutrition Journal*, *17*, 2. https://doi.org/10.1186/s12937-017-0310-1

Keller, H., Lengyel, C., Carrier, N., et al. (2018). Prevalence of inadequate micronutrient intakes of Canadian long-term care residents. *British Journal of Nutrition*, *119*(9), 1047–1056. https://doi.org/10.1017/S0007114518000107

Keller, U. (2019). Nutritional laboratory markers in malnutrition. *Journal of Clinical Medicine*, 8(6), 775. https://doi.org/10.3390/jcm8060775

Krishnan, K., & Pandolfino, J. E. (2018). Dysphagia and esophageal obstruction. In R. D. Kellerman, & E. T. Bope (Eds.), *Conn's current therapy 2018* (pp. 199–204). Elsevier.

Lawlor, C. M., & Choi, S. (2020). Diagnosis and management of pediatric dysphagia: A review. *JAMA Otolaryngology–Head & Neck Surgery*, *146*(2), 183–191. https://doi.org/10.1001/jamaoto.2019.3622

Lin, T.-H., Yang, C.-W., & Chang, W.-K. (2022). Evaluation of oropharyngeal dysphagia in older patients for risk stratification of pneumonia. *Frontiers in Immunology*, *12*. https://doi.org/10.3389/fimmu.2021.800029

Malcom, E., & Baird, J. (2019). Pulse oximetry and the enduring neglect of respiratory rate assessment: A commentary on patient surveillance. *British Journal of Nursing*, *28*(19), 1256–1259. https://doi.org/10.12968/bjon.2019.28.19.1256

Marcone, M. F., Madan, P., & Grodzinski, B. (2020). An overview of the sociological and environmental factors influencing eating food behavior in Canada. *Frontiers in Nutrition*, 7. https://doi.org/10.3389/fnut.2020.00077

Marian, T., Schröder, J., Muhle, P., et al. (2017). Measurement of oxygen desaturation is not useful for the detection of aspiration in dysphagic stroke patients. *Cerebrovascular Diseases Extra*, 7(1), 44–50. https://doi.org/10.1159/000453083. [Seminal Reference].

Mayo Clinic. (2022, September 20). *Dysphagia*. https://www.mayoclinic.org/diseases-conditions/dysphagia/symptoms-causes/syc-20372028

McGinnis, C. M., Homan, K., Solomon, M., et al. (2019). Dysphagia: Interprofessional management, impact, and patient-centered care. *Nutrition in Clinical Practice, 34*(1), 80–95. https://doi.org/10.1002/ncp.10239

Moawad, H. (2021). The difference between hemoglobin and hematocrit: Two types of red blood cell measurements. *Very Well Health*. https://www.verywellhealth.com/hematocrit-vs-hemoglobin-5211503

Moman, R. J., Gupta, N., & Varacallo, M. (2022). *Physiology, albumin*. StatPearls. https://www.ncbi.nlm.nih.gov/books/NBK459198/

Nakashima, T., Maeda, K., Tahira, K., et al. (2018). Silent aspiration predicts mortality in older adults with aspiration pneumonia admitted to acute hospitals. *Geriatrics and Gerontology International, 18*(6), 828–832. https://doi.org/10.1111/ggi.13250

Ng, B., Chapman, G. E., Levy-Milne, R., et al. (2021). Exploring the dietary choices of Chinese women living with breast cancer in Vancouver, Canada. *Supportive Care in Cancer, 29*, 1675–1681. https://doi.org/10.1007/s00520-020-05666-9

NHS Inform. (2023, March 10). *Malnutrition*. https://www.nhsinform.scot/illnesses-and-conditions/nutritional/malnutrition

Nix McIntosh, S. (2022). *Williams' basic nutrition and diet therapy* (16th ed.). Mosby.

Oleynick, C., Chiu, E., Pomreinke, H., et al. (2021). What internists should know about malnutrition in hospitalized patients. *Canadian Journal of General Internal Medicine, 16*(4), 32–38. https://doi.org/10.22374/cjgim.v16i4.570

Paik, N.-J. (2022). *Dysphagia treatment and management*. Medscape. https://emedicine.medscape.com/article/2212409-treatment

Pakai, A., Havasi-Sántha, E., Mák, E., et al. (2021). Influence of cognitive function and nurse support on malnutrition risk in nursing home residents. *Nursing Open, 8*(4), 1805–1811. https://doi.org/10.1002/nop2.824

Panara, K., Ramezanpour Ahangar, E., & Padalia, D. (2022). *Physiology, swallowing*. StatPearls. https://www.ncbi.nlm.nih.gov/books/NBK541071/

Pandurov, M. (2021). *20 tasty Canadian fast food industry statistics for 2021*. https://revi ewlution.ca/resources/canadian-fast-food-industry-statistics/

Polsky, J. Y., & Garriguet, D. (2022). *Household food insecurity in Canada early in the COVID-19 pandemic*. Statistics Canada Health Reports. Catalogue No. 82-003-X https://www.doi.org/10.25318/82-003-x202200200002-eng

Robin, T., et al. (2021). Safe food, dangerous lands? Traditional foods and Indigenous peoples in Canada. *Frontiers in Communication, 6*. https://doi.org/10.3389/fcomm.2021.749944

Robinson, T. (2021). *Nutrition North Canada and the fight against food insecurity*. McGill Journal of Political Studies. https://mjps.ssmu.ca/2021/02/15/nutrition-north-canada-and-the-fight-against-food-insecurity/

Sachdev, P. (2022). *What's causing my loss of smell and taste?* WebMD. https://www.webmd.com/brain/ss/slideshow-causes-of-loss-of-smell-and-taste

Seedat, J., & Strime, N. (2021). "Finishing that plate of food . . ." the role of the nurse caring for the patient with dysphagia. *South African Journal of Clinical Nutrition, 35*(2), 39–43. https://doi.org/10.1080/16070658.2021.1940717

Shune, S. E. (2020). An altered eating experience: Attitudes toward feeding assistance among younger and older adults. *Rehabilitation Nursing, 45*(2), 97–105. https://doi.org/10.1097/rnj.0000000000000147

Soufineyestani, M., Khan, A., & Sufineyestani, M. (2021). Impacts of music intervention on dementia: A review using meta-narrative method and agenda for future research. *Neurology International, 13*(1), 1–17. https://doi.org/10.3390/neurolint13010001

Steel, C., & Wile, H. (2018). Nutrition screening practices across care settings: Results of a Canadian survey. *Canadian Journal of Clinical Nutrition, 6*(1), 7–19. https://doi.org/10.14206/canad.j.clin.nutr.2018.01.02

St-Germain, A.-A. F., Galloway, T., & Tarasuk, V. (2019). Food insecurity in nunavut following the introduction of nutrition north Canada. *Canadian Medical Association Journal, 191*(20), E552–E558. https://doi.org/10.1503/cmaj.181617

Sweeney, E. (2020, January 17). *How balancing "warming" and "cooling" foods could benefit your health*. HuffPost. https://www.huffpost.com/entry/warming-cooling-foods_l_5e15f675c5b687c7eb5ebb55

Teasell, R., Foley, N., Martino, R., et al. (2018). *Dysphagia and aspiration following stroke*. http://www.ebrsr.com/sites/default/files/v18-SREBR-CH15-NET.pdf

Unger, S. L., Fenton, T. R., Jetty, R., et al. (2019). Iron requirements in the first 2 years of life. *Paediatric Child Health, 24*(8), 555. https://cps.ca/documents/position/iron-requirements

van Eck, A., Franks, E., Vinyard, C. J., et al. (2020). Sauce it up: Influence of condiment properties on oral processing behavior, bolus formation and sensory perception of solid foods. *Food & Function, 11*(7), 6186–6201. https://doi.org/10.1039/D0FO00821D

Velayutham, P., Irace, A. L., Kawai, K., et al. (2018). Silent aspiration: Who is at risk? *The Laryngoscope, 128*(8), 1952–1957. https://doi.org/10.1002/lary.27070

Vo, R., Smith, M., & Patton, N. (2021). The role of dietitian clinical judgement in the nutrition care process within the acute care setting: A qualitative study. *Journal of Human Nutrition and Dietetics, 34*, 124–133. https://doi.org/10.1111/jhn.12820

Wayne, G. (2023, April 20). *Impaired swallowing (dysphagia) nursing care plan*. Nurseslabs. https://nurseslabs.com/impaired-swallowing/

Wharton, S., Lau, D. C. W., Vallis, M., et al. (2020). Obesity in adults: A clinical practice guideline. *Canadian Medical Association Journal, 192*(31), E875–E891. https://doi.org/10.1503/cmaj.191707

Wilson, B. (2022, February 12). The raw and the cooked. *The Wall Street Journal*. https://www.wsj.com/articles/the-raw-and-the-cooked-11644642060

Wolf, U., Eckert, S., Walter, G., et al. (2021). Prevalence of oropharyngeal dysphagia in geriatric patients and real-life associations with diseases and drugs. *Scientific Reports, 11*, 21955. https://doi.org/10.1038/s41598-021-99858-w

World Health Organization. (2020, April 29). *Healthy diet*. https://www.who.int/news-room/fact-sheets/detail/healthy-diet

World Vision. (2021, August 16). *Malnutrition: How it hurts people, societies and the world*. https://www.worldvision.ca/stories/health/malnutrition-facts-causes-and-effects.

Xie, A., Huang, H., & Kong, F. (2020). Relationship between food composition and its cold/hot properties: A statistical study. *Journal of Agriculture and Food Research, 2*, 100043. https://doi.org/10.1016/j.jafr.2020.100043

Xu, Y. C., & Vincent, J. I. (2020). Clinical measurement properties of malnutrition assessment tools for use with patients in hospitals: A systematic review. *Nutrition Journal*, 19, 106. https://doi.org/10.1186/s12937-020-00613-0

Yeo, G. (2021, July 6). BMI: We know it's flawed, so why do we still use it? *BBC Science Focus*. https://www.sciencefocus.com/comment/bmi-we-know-its-flawed-so-why-do-we-still-use-it/

Yerges, A. L., Snethen, J. A., & Carrel, A. L. (2021). *Adolescent girls with overweight and obesity feel physically healthy and highlight the importance of mental health*. SAGE Open Nursing. https://doi.org/10.1177/23779608211018523

Zuercher, P., Moret, C. S., Dziewas, R., & Schefold, J. C. (2019). Dysphagia in the intensive care unit: Epidemiology, mechanisms, and clinical management. *Critical Care, 23*, 103. https://doi.org/10.1186/s13054-019-2400-2

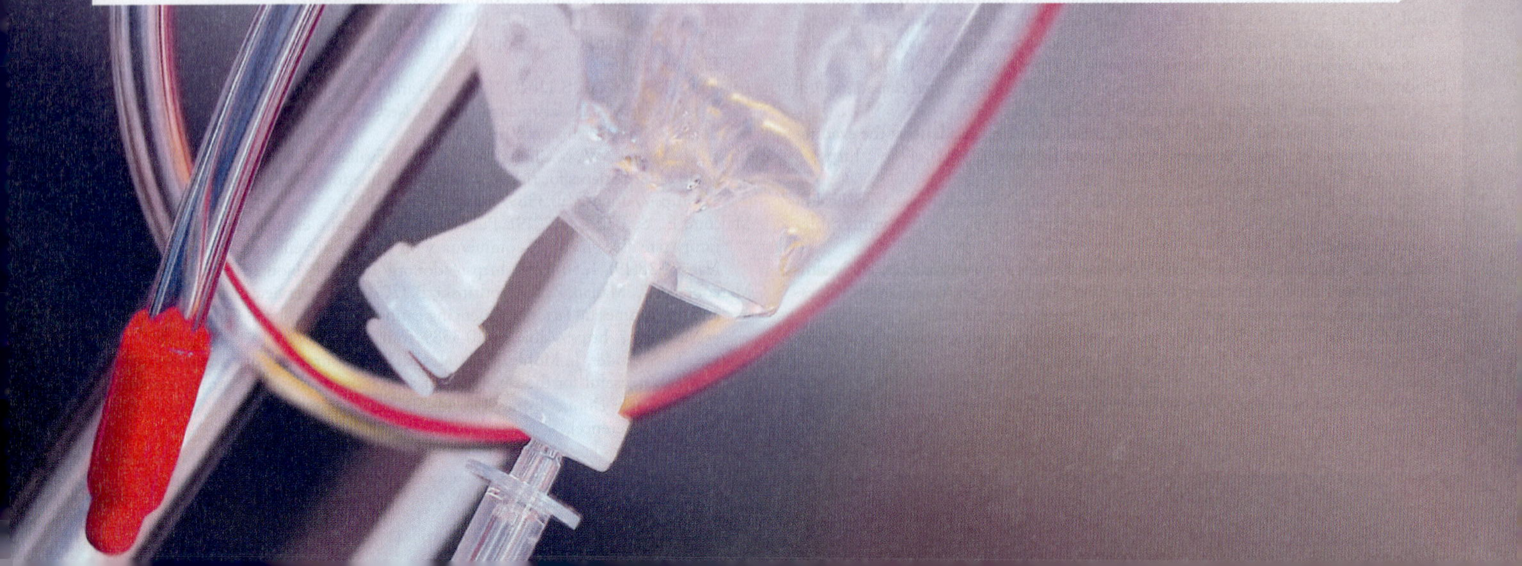

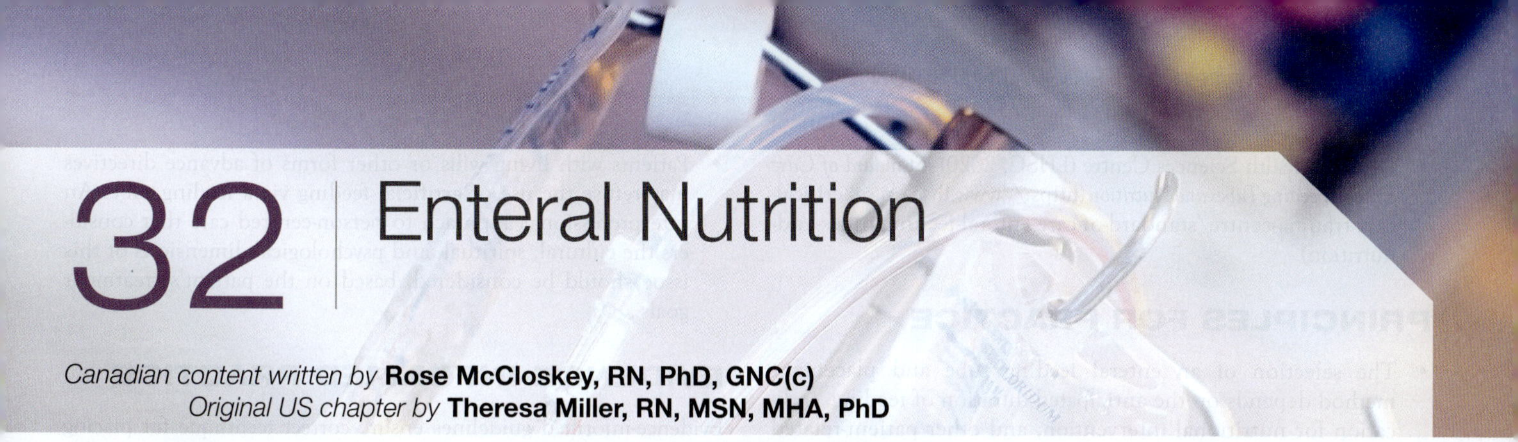

32 Enteral Nutrition

Canadian content written by **Rose McCloskey, RN, PhD, GNC(c)**
Original US chapter by **Theresa Miller, RN, MSN, MHA, PhD**

SKILLS AND PROCEDURES

OBJECTIVES

Mastery of content in this chapter will enable the nurse to:

- Assess patients who are to have enteral tubes inserted.
- Assess patients who are to receive enteral tube feedings.
- Demonstrate the ability to insert a small-bore feeding tube correctly.
- Explain the rationale for the methods used to determine the placement of nasogastric or nasoenteric feeding tubes.
- Explain how to minimize the risk of pulmonary complications during the insertion and maintenance of a feeding tube.
- Demonstrate the appropriate technique for irrigating a feeding tube.
- Demonstrate three appropriate techniques for administering enteral formulas.
- Evaluate a patient's tolerance of enteral feeding.
- Implement and evaluate evidence-informed learning strategies that support patients' ability to care for themselves with a feeding tube in the home setting.

MEDIA RESOURCES

- http://evolve.elsevier.com/Canada/Perry/clinicalskills/

PURPOSE

Enteral nutrition refers to the delivery of nutritional formulas through a tube that has been inserted into the gastrointestinal (GI) tract. Nasogastric (NG) feedings are delivered through a feeding tube introduced through the nose into the stomach. These gastric feedings can be administered as continuous, intermittent, or bolus and delivered via gravity, syringe, or pump method, depending on the patient's needs and tolerance. Nasointestinal (NI) feedings are delivered through a feeding tube introduced through the nose into the small intestine. Intestinal (or small-bowel) feedings are continuous in nature and are therefore delivered via a pump (London Health Sciences Centre [LHSC], 2018). Tubes are placed orally if a patient has trauma to the nose, cranial injury or surgery, facial surgery, or esophageal varices. Candidates for tube feeding include patients who have adequate digestion and absorption but cannot ingest, chew, or swallow food safely or in adequate amounts.

STANDARDS OF CARE

- Accreditation Canada (2020)—*Required Organizational Practices–2020 Handbook* (https://physicians.nshealth.ca/resources/required-organizational-practices-2020-handbook)
- Boullata et al. (2017)—ASPEN safe practices for enteral nutrition therapy (https://doi.org/10.1177/0148607116673053)
- Healthcare Excellence Canada (2009)—*The Safety Competencies: Enhancing Patient Safety Across the Health Professions* (https://www.patientsafetyinstitute.ca/en/toolsResources/safetyCompetencies/Documents/CPSI-SafetyCompetencies_EN_Digital.pdf)
- Institute for Safe Medication Practices Canada (2013)—*Safety Bulletin: Some Liquid Medications May Be Unsuitable for Administration by Enteral Tube* (https://ismpcanada.ca/wp-content/uploads/ISMPCSB2013-05_LiquidMedicationsEnteralTube.pdf)

- London Health Sciences Centre (LHSC, 2020)—*Standard of Care Enteral Feeding Tubes and Nutrition* (https://www.lhsc.on.ca/critical-care-trauma-centre/standard-of-care-enteral-feeding-tubes-and-nutrition)

PRINCIPLES FOR PRACTICE

- The selection of an enteral feeding tube and placement method depends on the anticipated duration of feeding, indication for nutritional intervention, and other patient-related factors such as gastric emptying, GI anatomy, and risk for gastric reflux.
- Nasal tubes are associated with the development of sinusitis, otitis, vocal cord paralysis, and pressure injuries to the nose and sinuses.
- The reflux of tube-feeding formula into the oropharynx can lead to aspiration into the lung.
- It is recommended that the liquid form of medication be used for patients with feeding tubes. If a liquid form is not available, check with a pharmacist prior to crushing pills and tablets (Bandy et al., 2019) and employer policy pertaining to the administration of medications via feeding tubes.
- Radiographic film verification is recommended to confirm correct placement of any bedside-inserted enteral tube before its initial use for feedings or medication administration (Boullata et al., 2017).
- Marking and documenting the exit site of an enteral tube at the time of radiographic confirmation of correct placement enables subsequent monitoring of the location of the tube during feedings (Powers et al., 2021).

PERSON-CENTRED CARE

- The insertion and use of a feeding tube often raises emotional and psychological concerns for patients. The patient and caregiver need reassurance and encouragement throughout the insertion procedure and once the tube feeding is in place. If tube feeding is being considered by a patient's health care provider in the context of advanced illness, the Canadian Virtual Hospice website offers insightful information for health care providers, patients, and family members on navigating this controversial topic (see https://www.virtualhospice.ca/en_US/Main+Site+Navigation/Home/Support/Support/Asked+and+Answered/Nutrition.aspx).
- Nursing interventions such as oral hygiene and care of the nasal passage or tube insertion site promote patient comfort during tube feeding and can reduce complications.
- Although tube feedings offer life-sustaining treatment, artificial nutrition can never replace the social and symbolic benefits of sharing meals. Social, religious, and cultural events involve food; patients requiring long-term tube feeding may feel a sense of loss regarding their ability to participate in life activities.
- Interprofessional collaboration among health care providers can help patients and caregivers use nutritional strategies to preserve or enhance quality of life. For example, a speech-language pathologist (SLP) can evaluate the ability of a patient to swallow safely, and a dietitian can perform advanced nutritional assessments.
- Encourage patients who require long-term tube feedings to use the resources available to them, or initiate a referral to their provincial/territorial home nutrition program, which can provide them with education, supplies, outreach, and networking.
- Patients with living wills or other forms of advance directives may refuse the use of artificial feeding via a feeding tube. An interprofessional approach to person-centred care that considers the cultural, spiritual, and psychological dimensions of this issue should be considered, based on the patient's treatment goals.

EVIDENCE-INFORMED PRACTICE

Evidence-informed guidelines ensure correct technique for placing enteral feeding tubes, initiating and maintaining enteral nutrition, and reducing the risk of feeding tube complications.

- Obtain radiographic confirmation of correct placement of any blindly inserted tube before its initial use for feeding or medication administration (Powers et al., 2021). The most common complication of blindly inserted feeding tubes is improper placement in the esophagus or pulmonary system (Powers et al., 2021).
- Feeding tubes are positioned into the small bowel to reduce the incidence of pulmonary aspiration of stomach contents. Research has not demonstrated this benefit consistently, but newer techniques for detecting aspiration provide some evidence that small-intestine feeding does reduce the incidence of pneumonia (Northington et al., 2022; Powers et al., 2021).
- Tube placement can be examined by testing the pH of aspirate. Gastric pH ≤5 likely indicates a gastric placement (Metheny et al., 2019).
- Maintaining and monitoring tube location during enteral feeding and keeping the head of bed elevated at a minimum of 30 degrees (preferably 45 degrees) effectively reduce aspiration and subsequent pneumonia (LHSC, 2021; VanBlarcom & McCoy, 2018).
- Assessing gastric residual volumes (GRVs) involves withdrawing and measuring stomach contents at regular intervals during tube feeding. Feeding is stopped when GRVs exceed a specified level; however, studies have failed to demonstrate a consistent relationship between GRV and risk for pulmonary aspiration, regurgitation, or pneumonia (Yasuda et al., 2021). Recommendations for stopping tube feeding for elevated GRVs range from 250 to 500 mL, but automatic cessation of feeding should not occur for GRV less than 500 mL in the absence of other signs of intolerance (Boullata et al., 2017; VanBlarcom & McCoy, 2018).
- GRVs are measured every 12 hours until the patient has tolerated the final feeding rate for 24 hours. Some agencies recommend returning the aspirated GRV to the patient through the feeding tube if it is 300 mL or less. After it is determined that the patient can tolerate the feeding rate, GRVs need to be rechecked only if indicated by clinical findings such as abdominal distension, nausea, or vomiting (LHSC, 2020).

SAFETY GUIDELINES

- Be aware of factors that increase a patient's risk of complications related to feeding tube insertion: altered level of consciousness, abnormal clotting, or impaired gag or cough reflex.
- Know the purpose of the feeding and the intended location of the tip of the feeding tube.
- Take precautions to prevent microbial contamination of enteral formulas.
- Be aware of safety measures to prevent pulmonary aspiration of gastric contents and accidental tube displacement by patients.
- Ensure suction equipment is in working order at the bedside.

- Consult with a pharmacist regarding a patient's medications and their route of delivery to determine whether administration via feeding tube is appropriate.
- Use an ENFit connector for all enteral nutrition sets, syringes, and feeding tubes to improve patient safety. The ENFit design features a reverse Luer-Lok connector–with twist-in functionality rather than a friction-held connector–and is incompatible with nonenteral delivery systems (Medline, n.d.), preventing misadministration of an enteral feeding or medication by the wrong route (Guenter & Lyman, 2020).
- A medical device–related pressure injury (MDRPI) is a localized injury to the skin or underlying tissue that forms as a result of sustained pressure from a device. Choose the correct size of medical device(s) to fit the individual, cushion and protect the skin with dressings in high-risk areas (e.g., nasal bridge), and remove or move the device daily to assess the skin (LHSC, 2020).

✦ SKILL 32.1 Inserting and Removing a Small-Bore Feeding Tube

NSO Nursing Skills Online Enteral Nutrition Module 16 / Lessons 1 and 2

Throughout this chapter, nasally placed feeding tubes (8–12 French [Fr]) are referred to as NG *tubes*. However, certain types of NG tubes that are larger and more rigid are used for gastric decompression instead of feeding (see Chapter 35). Small-bore feeding tubes placed by means of either the nasal (via the nose) or the oral (via the mouth) route may be used to deliver enteral nutrition directly into the stomach (NG tube) or small intestine (NI tube; nasojejunal [NJ] tube). Feeding tubes are soft and flexible; some use a removable guidewire or stylet to provide stiffness during tube insertion. Although these wires facilitate placement of a tube, they also add to the risk of pulmonary or esophageal injury during insertion. Insertion of tubes with guidewires or stylets is restricted to interprofessional health team members who are specifically educated/certified to complete this procedure. Nurses working in critical care areas may be certified to complete this advanced skill because they may be required to pass feeding tubes through the mouth (oral gastric tube), especially when a patient is also intubated or when contraindications to nasal placement such as a basilar skull fracture or facial trauma exist.

Placement of a feeding tube requires a health care provider's prescription. All candidates for NG or NI tube placement require an assessment of their coagulation status. Anticoagulation and bleeding disorders pose a risk for epistaxis during nasal tube placement; the health care provider may prescribe platelet transfusion or other corrective measures before tube insertion.

Confirmation of the correct position of a newly inserted tube is mandatory before any feeding or medication is administered. Radiographic confirmation remains the gold standard in confirming tube placement (Boullata et al., 2017).

Delegation and Collaboration

The skill of inserting a feeding tube cannot be delegated to an unregulated care provider (UCP). However, UCPs may help with patient positioning and comfort measures during tube insertion.

Equipment

Tube Insertion

- Small-bore feeding tube (select the smallest diameter possible to enhance patient comfort) (Fig. 32.1)
- 60-mL ENFit syringe
- Stethoscope, pulse oximeter, capnography *(optional)*
- Hypoallergenic tape, semipermeable (transparent) dressing, or tube fixation device
- Skin barrier protectant
- pH indicator strip (scale 1.0–11.0)
- Cup of water and straw or ice chips (for patients who are able to swallow)
- Water-soluble lubricant
- Emesis basin
- Towel or disposable pad
- Facial tissues
- Tape measure
- Clean gloves
- Suction equipment in case of aspiration
- Penlight to check placement in nasopharynx
- Tongue blade
- Oral hygiene supplies
- Gloves

Tube Removal

- Disposable pad
- Tissues
- Clean gloves
- Disposable plastic bag
- Towel
- 60-mL ENFit syringe

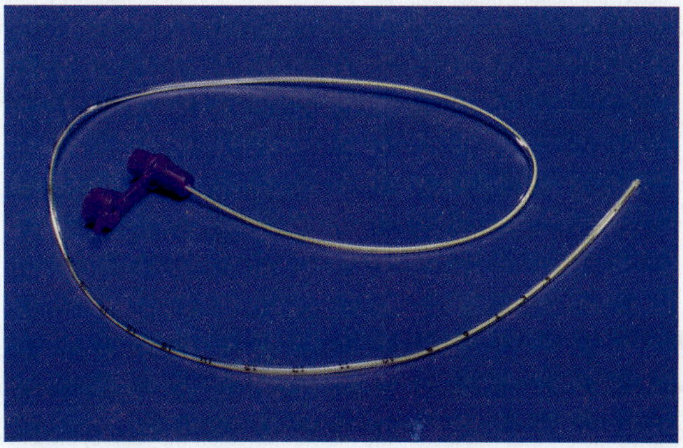

FIG 32.1 Small-bore feeding tube. *(Courtesy Kendall Brands, Mansfield, MA.)*

STEP	RATIONALE

ASSESSMENT

STEP	RATIONALE
1. Identify patient using at least two person-specific identifiers (e.g., name and date of birth, or name and medical record number) according to employer policy.	Ensures correct patient. Complies with Accreditation Canada's standards and improves patient safety (Accreditation Canada, 2020).
2. Throughout the procedure, the 4 moments for hand hygiene are to be implemented; hand hygiene should occur before initial patient (or patient environment) contact, before an aseptic procedure, after body fluid exposure risk, and after patient (or patient environment) contact. Additional hand hygiene should be performed when hands are visibly soiled.	Proper hand hygiene helps prevent the spread of infectious agents to health care providers.
3. Verify health care provider's prescription for type of tube and enteric feeding schedule. Also check prescription to determine whether health care provider wants prokinetic medications (e.g., metoclopramide) given before tube placement. Refer to scope of practice and employer policy before performing the steps.	Health care provider's prescription is needed to insert feeding tube. Prokinetic medications given before tube placement may help advance tube into intestine.
4. Assess patient's knowledge of procedure.	Encourages cooperation, reduces anxiety, and minimizes risks. Identifies teaching needs.
5. Have patient close each nostril alternately and breathe. Examine each naris for patency and skin breakdown (apply clean gloves if drainage present).	Reduces transmission of microorganisms. Sometimes nares are obstructed or irritated, or septal defect is present. Place tube in most patent naris.
6. Review patient's medical history (e.g., for basilar skull fracture, nasal problems, nosebleeds, facial trauma, nasal–facial surgery, deviated septum, anticoagulant therapy, coagulopathy).	History of these problems may require consultation with health care provider to change route of nutritional support. Risk for intracranial tube passage, causing neurological injury, exists for patients with basilar skull fractures and facial trauma.

Critical Decision Point *If a patient is at risk for intracranial passage of the tube, avoid the nasal route. Oral placement or placement under medical supervision using fluoroscopic direct visualization is preferable. Insertion of a gastrostomy or jejunostomy tube is another alternative.*

STEP	RATIONALE
7. Assess patient's height, weight, hydration status, electrolyte balance, and intake and output (I&O).	Provides baseline information to measure nutritional improvement after enteral feedings.
8. Assess patient's mental status (ability to cooperate with procedure, sedation), presence of cough and gag reflex, ability to swallow, critical illness, and presence of artificial airway.	Altered mental status or absence of gag or cough reflex increases risk of transbronchial placement (Caramia, 2018).

Critical Decision Point *Recognize situations in which blind placement of a feeding tube poses an unacceptable risk for placement. Use of devices designed to detect pulmonary intubation such as CO_2 sensors or electromagnetic tracking devices enhances patient safety. While capnography has been found to be a valid verification tool, especially in mechanically ventilated patients, it is not commonly used on nursing units because of lack of availability, inadequate clinical research, and incompatible fitting onto an NG tube* (Judd, 2020).

Alternatively, to avoid insertion complications from blind placement in high-risk situations, such as in critical care, clinicians trained in the use of visualization or imaging techniques should place tubes (Bischoff et al., 2022; Judd, 2020).

STEP	RATIONALE
9. Perform physical assessment of abdomen (see Chapter 8). Remove and dispose of gloves (if worn).	Absent bowel sounds or presence of abdominal pain, tenderness, or distension may indicate a medical problem that contraindicates feedings.

NURSING DIAGNOSES

- Potential for aspiration
- Inadequate nutrition
- Reduced comfort

Related factors and risk factors are individualized on the basis of patient's condition or needs.

PLANNING

STEP	RATIONALE
1. Expected outcomes following completion of procedure:	
• Tube is successfully placed in stomach or small intestine.	Proper position is essential before initiating use of feeding tube.
• Feeding tube remains patent.	Proper irrigation clears tube of formula residue (Bloom & Seckel, 2022).
• Patient has no respiratory distress (e.g., increased respiratory rate, coughing, poor colour) or signs of discomfort or nasal trauma.	Correctly placed tube causes no interference with airway.

STEP	RATIONALE
PLANNING	
2. Explain procedure to patient, including sensations (e.g., burning in nasal passages) that will be felt during insertion.	Increases patient's cooperation with intubation procedure and helps lessen anxiety (Bloom & Seckel, 2022).
3. Explain to patient that they may communicate during intubation by raising an index finger to indicate gagging or discomfort.	Patient must have a way of communicating to alleviate stress and enhance cooperation.
IMPLEMENTATION	
1. Prepare supplies at bedside.	Ensures organized procedure.
2. Stand on same side of bed as naris chosen for insertion and position patient upright in high Fowler's position (unless contraindicated). If patient is comatose, raise head of bed as tolerated in semi-Fowler's position, with head tipped forward (i.e., chin to chest) and a pillow placed behind the head and shoulders. If necessary, have a UCP help with positioning a confused or comatose patient. If patient is forced to lie supine, place in reverse Trendelenburg position.	Allows for easier manipulation of tube. Fowler's position reduces risk of aspiration and promotes effective swallowing. Forward head position helps with closure of airway and passage of tube into esophagus.
3. Apply pulse oximeter and measure vital signs.	Provides baseline for objective assessment of respiratory status during tube insertion.
a. If patient has decrease in oxygen saturation, tube should not be inserted until you determine patient stability.	
4. Place towel over patient's chest. Keep facial tissues within reach.	Prevents soiling of gown. Insertion of tube frequently produces tearing.
5. Determine length of tube to be inserted and mark location with indelible ink.	
a. Measure distance from tip of nose to earlobe to xiphoid process of sternum (see Step 5a illustration). Mark this distance on tube with indelible ink.	Length approximates distance from nose to stomach. Tape is not to be used to mark distance because it can block the nares, be inhaled, collect mucus, and be difficult to remove once placement is confirmed.
b. Measure distance from tip of nose to earlobe to mid-umbilicus for pediatric patient.	
c. Add 20–30 cm (8–12 inches) for NJ tubes.	Length approximates distance from nose to jejunum.

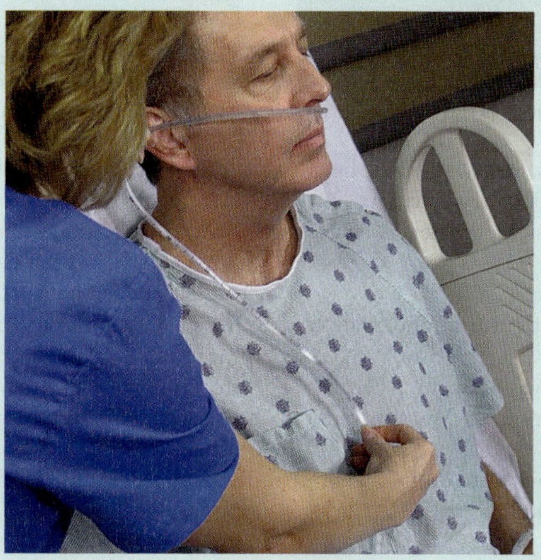

STEP 5A Measure to determine length of tube to insert.

Critical Decision Point *Tip of feeding tube must reach the stomach to avoid the risk of pulmonary aspiration, which can occur when tubes terminate in the esophagus.*

STEP	RATIONALE

IMPLEMENTATION

STEP	RATIONALE
6. Prepare feeding tube for intubation. NOTE: Do not ice or freeze tubes.	Iced tube becomes stiff and inflexible, causing trauma to nasal mucosa.
a. Check employer policy on the training and environment required for the use of stylet or guided tubes.	Most employers permit nurses to insert enteral feeding tubes in targeted practice settings and with advanced education.
7. Prepare tube fixation materials. Cut hypoallergenic tape 10-cm (4-inches) long or prepare membrane dressing or other tube fixation device.	Used to secure tubing after insertion. Fixation devices allow tube to float free of nares, thus reducing pressure on nares and preventing MDRPI (see Step 7 illustration).
8. Apply clean gloves.	Reduces transmission of microorganisms.
9. *Option:* Dip tube with surface lubricant into glass of room-temperature water or apply water-soluble lubricant (see manufacturer instructions).	Activates lubricant to facilitate passage of tube into naris and GI tract.
10. Provide alert patient with a cup of water and straw (if able to swallow). If patient is unable to swallow, assist patient in tucking chin toward their chest.	Patient is asked to swallow water to facilitate tube passage. Closes off glottis and reduces risk of tube entering trachea.
11. Explain next steps to patient and gently insert tube through nostril to back of throat (posterior nasopharynx). This may cause the patient to gag. Aim back and down toward the ear (see Step 11 illustration).	Natural contours facilitate passage of tube into GI tract.

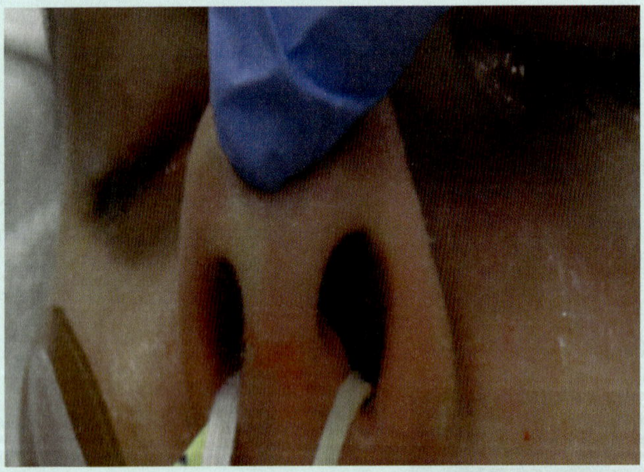

STEP 7 Medical device–related pressure injury (MDRPI) under nose.

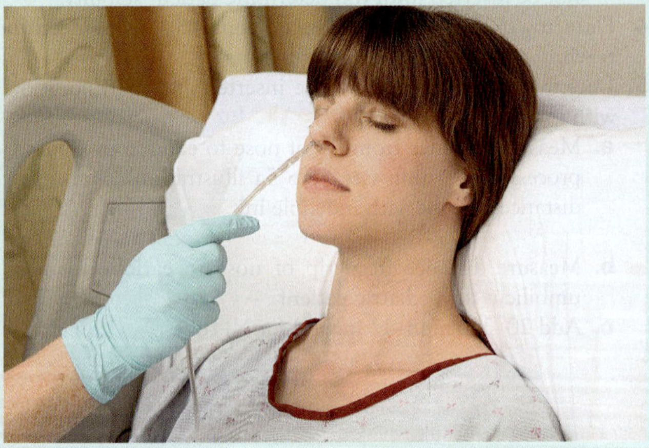

STEP 11 Insert tube through nostril to back of throat.

STEP	RATIONALE
12. Instruct patient to take deep breaths, relax, and flex head toward chest after tube has passed through nasopharynx.	Closes off glottis and reduces risk of tube entering trachea.
13. Encourage patient to swallow small sips of water. Advance tube as patient swallows.	Swallowing facilitates passage of tube past oropharynx. A distinct tug may be felt as the patient swallows, indicating that tube is following expected path.
14. Emphasize to patient the need to mouth breathe and swallow during insertion.	Helps facilitate passage of tube and alleviates patient's fears during procedure.
15. Do not advance tube during inspiration or coughing because it is more likely to enter the respiratory tract. Monitor pulse oximetry and respiratory symptoms.	Can cause tube to inadvertently enter patient's airway, which will be reflected in changes in oxygen saturation and ability to speak.
16. Advance tube each time patient swallows until desired length has been reached (see Step 16 illustration).	Reduces discomfort and trauma to patient. Helps facilitate tube passage.

STEP	RATIONALE

IMPLEMENTATION

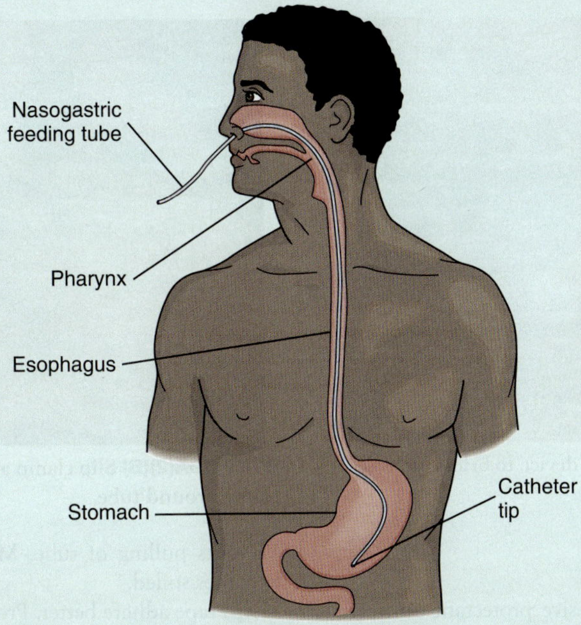

STEP 16 NG tube inserted through nasopharynx and esophagus into stomach.

Critical Decision Point *Do not force the tube or push against resistance. If the patient starts to cough, experiences a drop in oxygen saturation, or shows other signs of respiratory distress, withdraw the tube into the posterior nasopharynx until normal breathing resumes.*

STEP	RATIONALE
17. Check for position of tube in back of throat using penlight and tongue blade.	Tube may be coiled, kinked, or entering trachea.
18. Temporarily anchor tube to nose with a small piece of tape.	Movement of tube stimulates gagging. Assesses general position before anchoring tube more securely.
19. Keep tube secure and check its placement by aspirating stomach contents to measure gastric pH (see Skill 32.2). Also measure amount, colour, and quality of return.	Proper tube position is essential before initiating feeding.

Critical Decision Point *Insufflation of air into the tube while auscultating the abdomen is not a reliable means to determine the position of the feeding tube tip because air movement sounds can be heard when the NG tube is in the esophagus, stomach, or lung* (Judd, 2020).

STEP	RATIONALE
20. Carefully remove temporary tape and re-anchor tube to patient's nose, avoiding placing pressure on nares. Mark exit site on tube with indelible ink; measure and record external length of the tube (i.e., from naris to the end or tip of the NG tube). Select one of the following options for anchoring:	Marking and measuring the tube can alert nurses to possible displacement. A properly secured tube allows patient more mobility and prevents trauma to nasal mucosa. Noting the external length helps determine possible tube dislodgement (Lord, 2018).
a. Apply membrane dressing or tube fixation device:	Permits longer securement without need to change dressing.
(1) *Membrane dressing:*	
(a) Apply skin barrier or adhesive protectant ointment or spray to patient's cheek and area of tube to be secured.	Allows membrane to adhere to skin.
(b) Place tube against patient's cheek and secure tube with membrane dressing, out of patient's line of vision.	Eliminates application of tape around naris. Decreases risk of inadvertent extubation by patient.
(2) *Tube fixation device:*	Secures tube and reduces friction on naris.
(a) Apply wide end of patch to bridge of nose (see Step 20a[2][a] illustration).	
(b) Slip clamp around feeding tube as it exits naris (see Step 20a[2][b] illustration).	

STEP	RATIONALE

IMPLEMENTATION

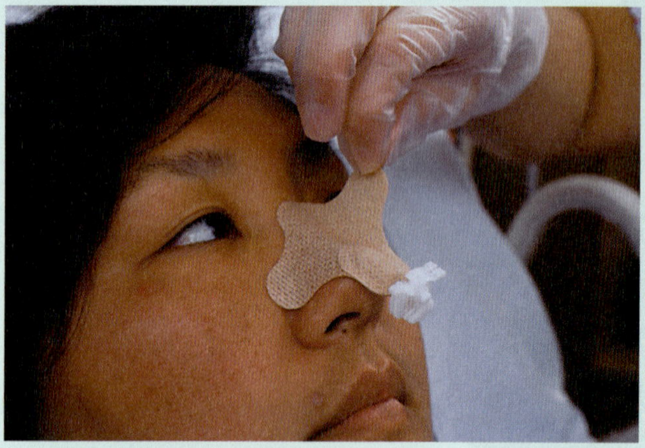

STEP 20A(2)(A) Apply tube fixation device to bridge of nose.

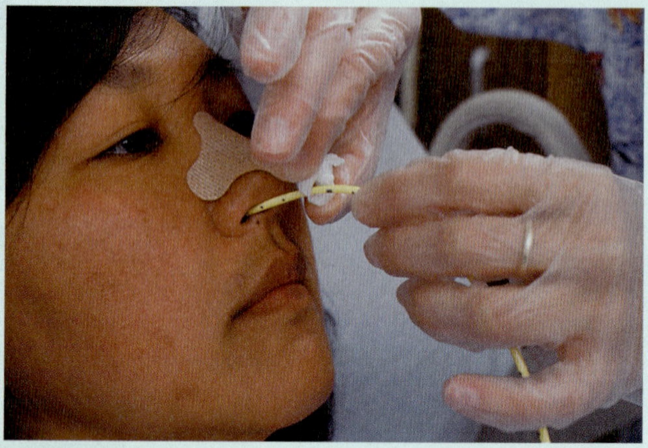

STEP 20A(2)(B) Slip clamp around feeding tube and gently close clamp around tube.

STEP	RATIONALE
b. Apply tape:	Prevents pulling of tube. May require frequent changing if tape becomes soiled.
(1) Apply skin barrier or adhesive protectant ointment on tip of patient's nose and allow it to become "tacky."	Helps tape adhere better. Protects skin.
(2) Remove gloves and tear a horizontal slit up the centre of the tape (see Step 20b[2] illustration).	
(3) Place intact end of tape over bridge of patient's nose. Wrap each strip around tube as it exits (see Step 20b[3] illustration).	Tube is free-floating in the naris with this taping method, resulting in movement of tube in pharynx. Securing tape to naris in this method reduces pressure on naris and risk of MDRPI (Zakaria et al., 2018).
21. Fasten end of tube to patient's gown using clip (see Step 21 illustration). Do not use safety pins to secure tube to gown.	Reduces traction on naris if tube moves. Safety pins can become unfastened and cause injury to patients.

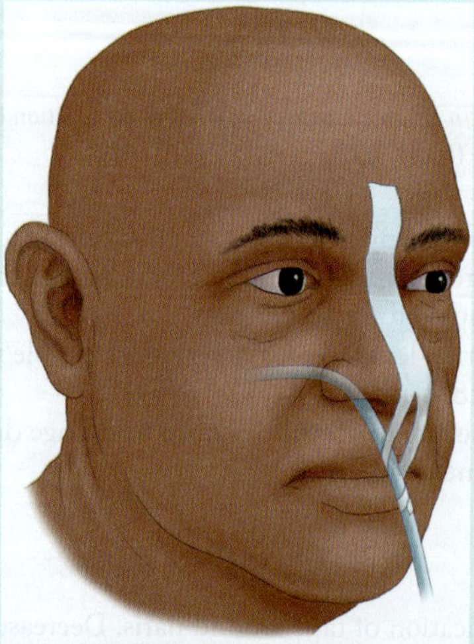

STEP 20B(2) Tear a horizontal slit up the centre of the tape.

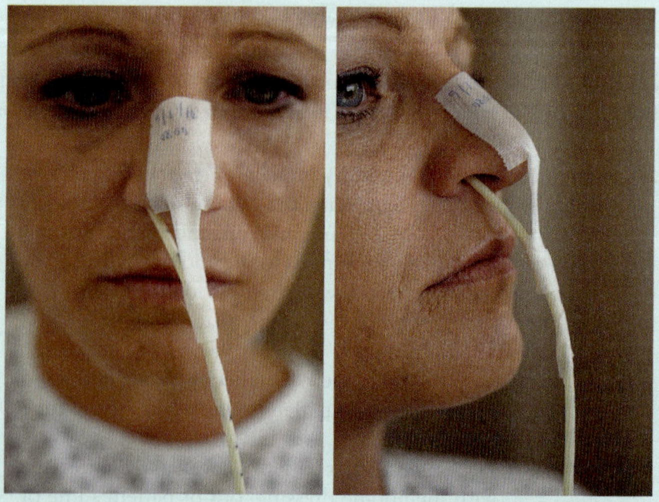

STEP 20B(3) A, Apply tape to anchor nasoenteral tube. B, Naris is free of pressure from tape and tube.

STEP	RATIONALE

IMPLEMENTATION

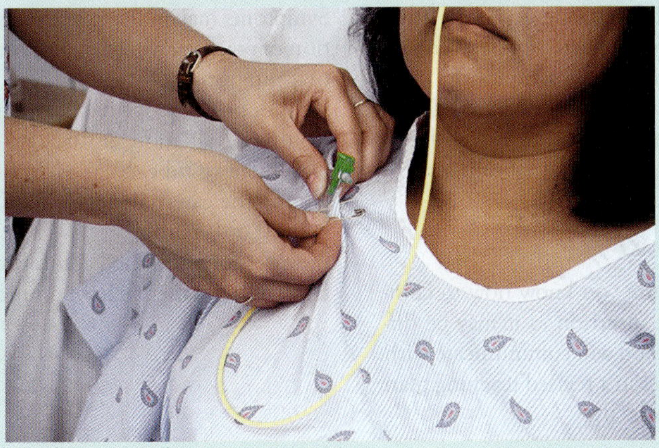

STEP 21 Fasten feeding tube to patient's gown.

STEP	RATIONALE
22. Help patient to a comfortable position; maintain head of bed elevated at least 30 degrees (preferably 45 degrees) unless contraindicated (LHSC, 2021). For intestinal tube placement, place patient on right side, when possible, until radiographic confirmation of correct placement is made.	Promotes patient comfort while patient awaits radiographic (X-ray) confirmation of tube placement. Placing patient on right side promotes passage of NI tube into small intestine.
23. Remove gloves and discard.	Reduces transmission of microorganisms.

Critical Decision Point *Always verify correct placement of feeding tube prior to beginning enteral nutrition.*

STEP	RATIONALE
24. Contact radiology to obtain radiographic film of chest or abdomen.	Radiographic film examination remains the gold standard of practice and is the most accurate method to determine correct placement of feeding tube (Walldorf et al., 2020).
25. Apply clean gloves and administer oral hygiene (see Chapter 18). Clean tubing at nostril with dampened washcloth.	Reduces transmission of microorganisms. Promotes patient comfort and integrity of oral mucous membranes.
26. Remove gloves and dispose of equipment.	Reduces transmission of microorganisms.
27. Tube removal:	
a. Verify health care provider's prescription for tube removal.	Health care provider's prescription is needed to remove feeding tube.
b. Gather equipment.	Ensures organized procedure.
c. Explain procedure to patient.	Encourages cooperation, reduces anxiety, and minimizes risks. Identifies teaching needs.
d. Apply clean gloves.	Reduces transmission of microorganisms.
e. Position patient in high Fowler's position unless contraindicated.	Reduces risk of pulmonary aspiration in event patient should vomit.
f. Place disposable pad or towel over patient's chest.	Prevents mucus and gastric secretions from soiling patient's clothing.
g. Disconnect tube from feeding administration set (if present) and instill 10–20 mL of air into the tube clamp or cap end.	Clears the tube and prevents formula from spilling from tube as it is removed.
h. Remove tape or tube fixation device from patient's nose. Unclip tube from patient's gown.	Allows tube to be removed easily.
i. Instruct patient to take a deep breath and hold it. As you kink the end of the tube securely, completely withdraw the tube by pulling it out steadily and smoothly onto the towel. Inspect intactness of tube, then dispose of in appropriate receptacle.	Prevents inadvertent aspiration of gastric contents while tube is removed. Kinking prevents leakage of fluid from tube. Promotes patient comfort. Reduces transmission of microorganisms.
j. Offer tissues to patient to blow nose.	Clears nasal passages of remaining secretions.
k. Offer mouth care.	Promotes patient's comfort.
l. Remove and dispose of gloves.	Reduces transmission of microorganisms.

STEP	RATIONALE

EVALUATION

1. Observe patient's response to tube placement. Assess lung sounds; have patient speak; check vital signs; note any coughing, dyspnea, cyanosis, or decrease in oxygen saturation	Symptoms may indicate placement in the respiratory tract. Auscultation of crackles, wheezes, dyspnea, or fever may be a delayed response to aspiration.
2. Confirm radiographic film results with health care provider.	Verifies position of tube before initiating enteral feeding.
3. Routinely check condition of nares, location of external exit site marking on tube, measurement of the external tube length, and colour and pH of fluid aspirated from tube.	Routine evaluation ensures no formation of MDRPI and correct placement of tube. Noting the external length helps in detecting possible tube dislodgement (Lord, 2018).
4. Assess patient's level of comfort.	Provides for continued comfort of patient.
5. Use teach-back: "I want to make sure you know how to communicate with me during the tube insertion as it may be difficult for you to speak. Tell me how you will communicate with me during the tube insertion." Develop a revised teaching plan if patient is unable to teach back correctly.	Determines patient's level of understanding of instructional topic.

Unexpected Outcomes	Related Interventions
1. Aspiration of stomach contents into respiratory tract (delayed response or small-volume aspiration) occurs, as evidenced by auscultation of crackles or wheezes, dyspnea, or fever.	• Report change in patient condition to health care provider; if there has not been a recent chest radiographic film, suggest prescribing one. • Position patient on side to protect airway. • Suction nasotracheally and orotracheally. • Prepare for possible initiation of antibiotics.
2. Displacement of feeding tube to another site (e.g., from duodenum to stomach) possibly occurs when patient coughs or vomits.	• Aspirate GI contents and measure pH. • Remeasure external tube length and compare with records. • Request a prescription for radiographic imaging to determine tube placement. • If above verification methods confirm displacement of tube, discuss with health care provider the following options: a. Advancing current tube and reimaging to confirm, or b. Removing current displaced tube completely and reinserting new tube (see Skill 32.1). • If there is question of aspiration, obtain chest radiographic film.

Communication and Documentation

- Document type and size of tube placed, external measurement of tube, patient's tolerance of procedure, condition of naris, and confirmation of tube position by radiographic film examination in progress notes in electronic health record (EHR) or chart.
- Document removal of tube, condition of naris, tube intactness, and patient's tolerance.
- Report any unexpected outcomes and the interventions performed.
- Document your evaluation of patient learning.

Special Considerations

Teaching

- Instruct patient or caregiver on the importance of frequent oral hygiene.
- Instruct patient or caregiver to report tension on feeding tube or displacement of tape or tube fixation device; instruct patient or caregiver to stabilize the tube and call for help.

Pediatric

- The distance from nose to ear to mid-umbilicus better predicts the insertion length for gastric tube placement in neonates and children than the traditional nose-to-ear-to-xiphoid measurements (Northington et al., 2022).
- Radiographic film confirmation is the most accurate assessment of proper tube placement. The best bedside assessment of tube placement is to aspirate gastric contents for colour and pH (Northington et al., 2022). When inserting a feeding tube in an infant, the heart rate and blood pressure may change in response to vagal stimulation.

Gerontological

- Ensure adequate lubrication of tube to decrease discomfort for older persons because of the potential for decreased oral or nasopharyngeal secretions.

Care in the Community: Home Management

- Assess patient's or caregiver's ability to maintain a tube for a feeding program.
- Assess the environmental safety (e.g., adequate space and electricity to operate and maintain needed equipment and supplies) and sanitation of the patient's home to determine potential for infection or injury.
- Teach patient or caregiver how to assess tube placement (see Skill 32.2).
- Teach caregiver correct method for securing a feeding tube and the routine care necessary to reduce pressure injuries.
- Assess patient's and caregiver's understanding of storage and management of equipment and supplies, as well as where and how to obtain supplies and the need for working safety equipment, such as suctioning.

✦ SKILL 32.2 Verifying Feeding Tube Placement

NSO *Nursing Skills Online Enteral Nutrition Module 16 / Lesson 3*

Nurses insert small-bore feeding tubes nasally for intermittent or continuous feeding. It is possible for the tip of a feeding tube to move or migrate into a different location (e.g., from the stomach into the intestine or esophagus, or from the intestine into the stomach). Although all tubes should be marked to document the correct position, tube dislocation can sometimes occur without any external evidence that the tube has moved. The risk of aspirating regurgitated gastric contents into the respiratory tract increases when the tip of the tube accidently dislocates upward into the esophagus.

Following initial radiographic film verification of correct feeding tube position, the nurse must monitor the tube to ensure that the tube tip remains in the intended site. Based on a patient's clinical condition and employer policy, the nurse checks the feeding tube position at regular intervals (often every 4 to 6 hours) and before administering formula or medications through the tube. Radiographic verification is impractical to perform every 4 to 6 hours as well as costly, but the reports of the routine chest and abdominal films should be monitored for reference to the feeding tube location. No single bedside method of monitoring tube position during feeding is completely reliable; there are several techniques to use in combination to detect feeding tube dislocation:

- Monitor the external length of the tube and observe the appearance, volume, and pH of fluid aspirated through it. The colour of the fluid can help differentiate gastric from intestinal placement. Because most intestinal aspirates are stained by bile to a distinct yellow colour and most gastric aspirates are not, the difference in colour can often distinguish the sites (Table 32.1).
- Testing the pH of the aspirate at the bedside and the use of radiographic film are methods that have been suggested for verifying tube placement (Northington et al., 2022). Results should be used in combination with other indicators with careful assessment of a patient in the clinical setting.
- Obtain repeat radiographic film confirmation if bedside methods raise any doubt regarding the location of a tube.

Delegation and Collaboration

The verification of tube placement is the responsibility of the nurse and cannot be delegated to a UCP. The nurse directs the UCP to immediately inform the nurse about the following:

- Patient's respirations change or patient indicates shortness of breath, coughing, or choking.
- Patient vomits or the UCP notices vomitus in the patient's mouth during oral hygiene.
- Bleeding is noted in the nasal or oral cavity.
- Nasal skin irritation or excoriation is present.
- Change in the external length of the tube occurs.

Equipment

- 60-mL ENFit syringe
- Clean gloves
- pH indicator strip (scale 1.0–11.0)
- Small medication cup
- Tape measure

TABLE 32.1
Typical Colour of Gastric Aspirates

Gastric Appearance	Description
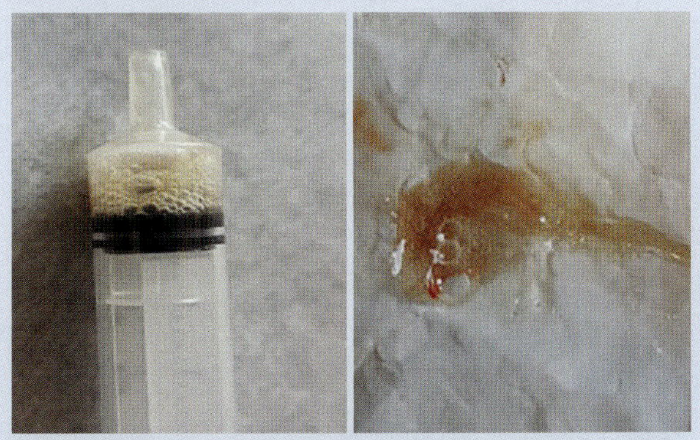	Clear, brown-tinged, mucousy
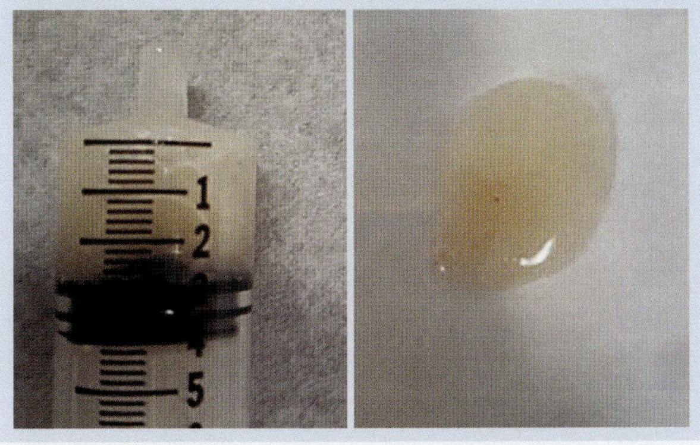	Cloudy, mucousy, white tan

Continued

TABLE 32.1

Typical Colour of Gastric Aspirates—cont'd

Gastric Appearance	Description
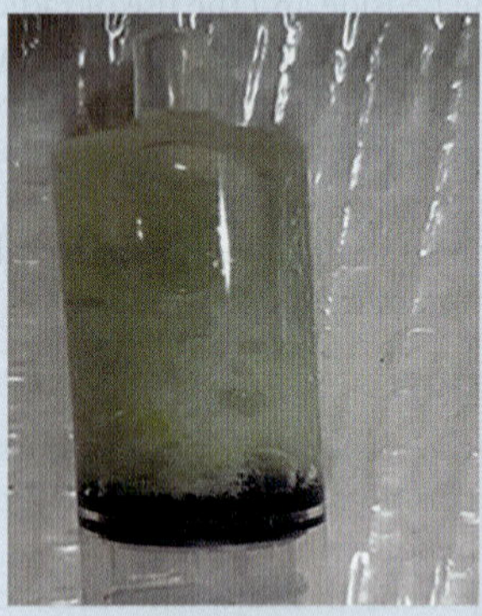 	Clear, light grassy green with sediments
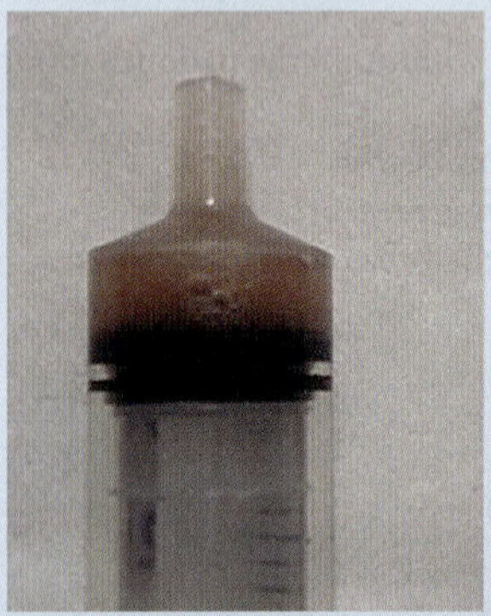 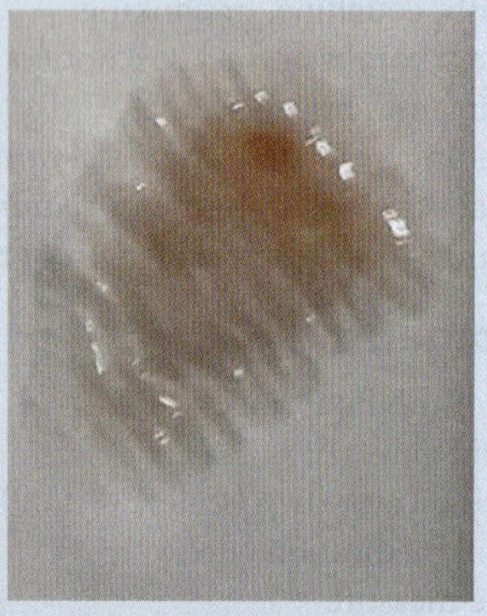	Light brown, mucousy
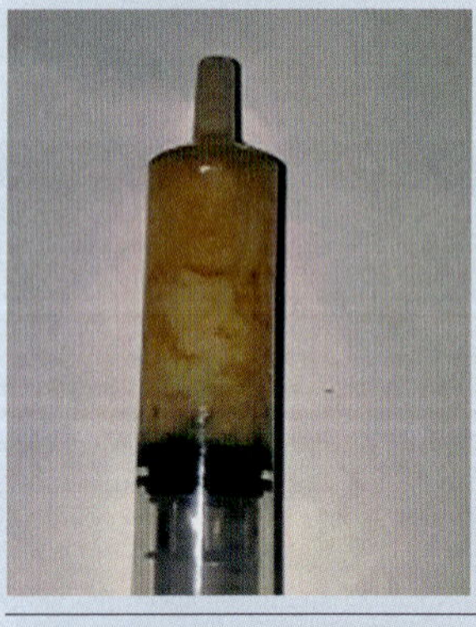 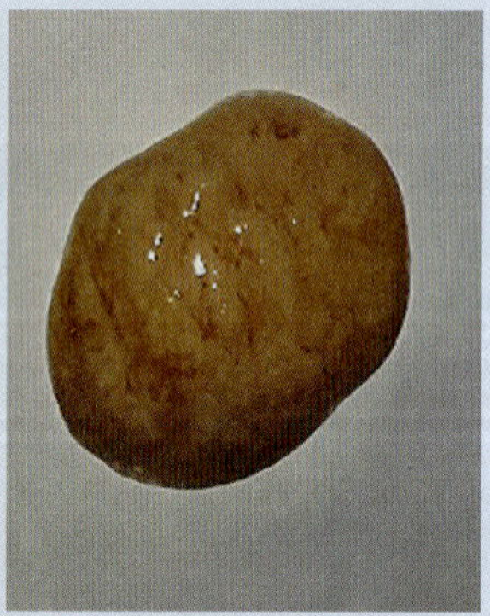	Partially digested formula
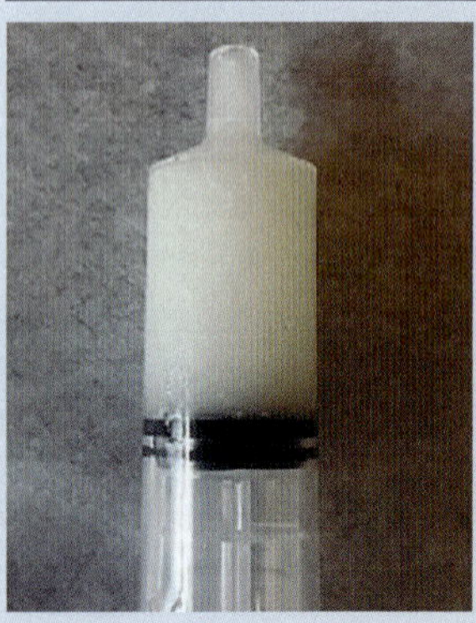 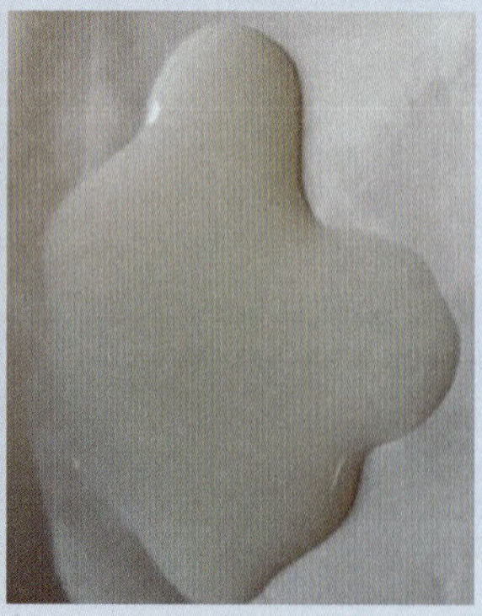	Undigested formula

TABLE 32.1

Typical Colour of Gastric Aspirates—cont'd

Gastric Appearance	Description
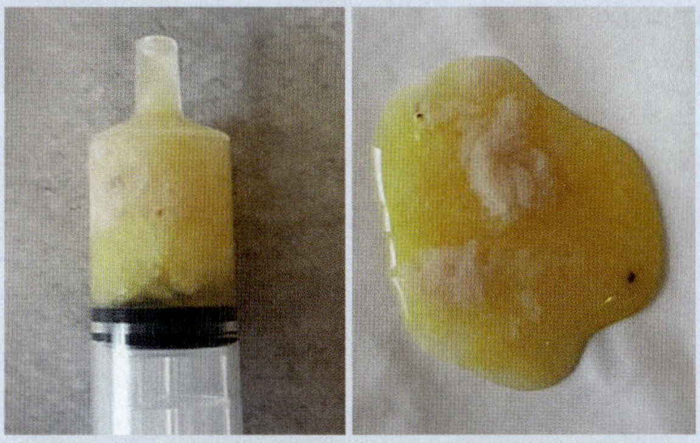	Yellow, partially digested food
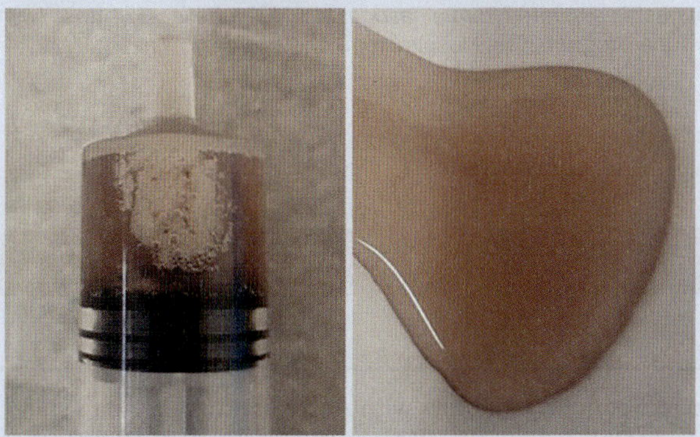	Clear, brown
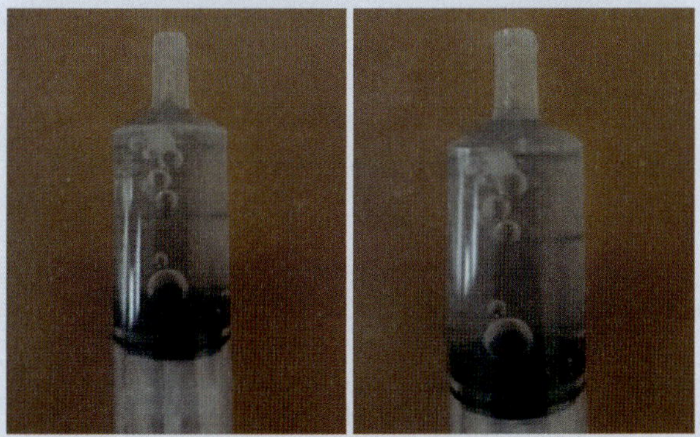	Clear, mucousy
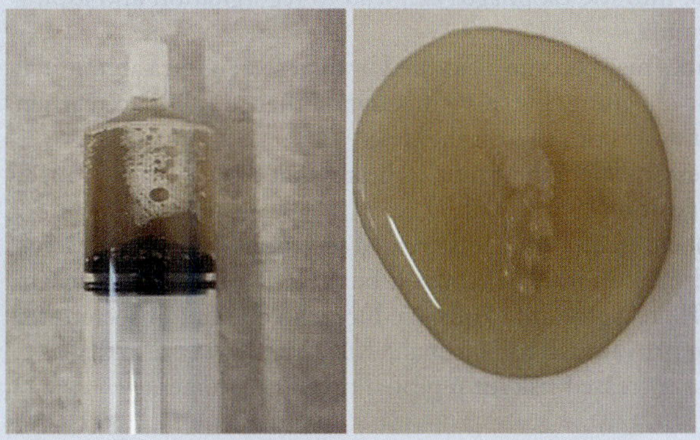	Clear, cloudy, light brown

Continued

TABLE 32.1
Typical Colour of Gastric Aspirates—cont'd

Gastric Appearance	Description
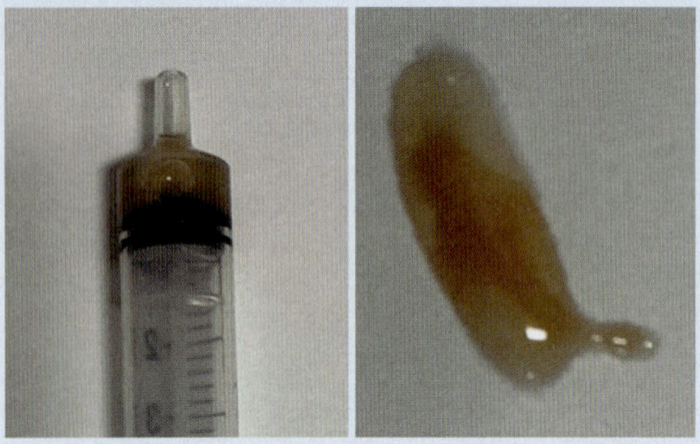	Brown, blood-tinged, mucousy

From The Hospital for Sick Children. (2021, April 8). *HINT: What to consider when the pH of gastric aspirates from a nasogastric (NG) tube is >6?* https://www.connectedcare.sickkids.ca/quick-hits/gastric-ph. Reproduced with permission of the G Tube Program, The Hospital for Sick Children.

STEP	RATIONALE
ASSESSMENT	
1. Identify patient using at least two person-specific identifiers (e.g., name and date of birth, or name and medical record number) according to employer policy.	Ensures correct patient. Complies with Accreditation Canada's standards and improves patient safety (Accreditation Canada, 2020).
2. Throughout the procedure, the 4 moments for hand hygiene are to be implemented; hand hygiene should occur before initial patient (or patient environment) contact, before an aseptic procedure, after body fluid exposure risk, and after patient (or patient environment) contact. Additional hand hygiene should be performed when hands are visibly soiled.	Proper hand hygiene helps prevent the spread of infectious agents to health care providers.
3. Review employer policy for frequency and method of checking tube placement. ***Do not insufflate air into tube to check placement.***	Maintains quality of patient care. Listening for air instilled through the tube is unreliable (Judd, 2020).
4. Observe for signs and symptoms of respiratory distress during feeding: coughing, choking, or reduced oxygen saturation.	Once tube has been correctly placed into the GI tract, its movement into the pulmonary system is unlikely. However, a tube that has been pulled back into the esophagus can lead to regurgitation and aspiration of formula.
5. Identify conditions that increase risk of spontaneous tube migration or dislocation: altered level of consciousness, agitation; retching, vomiting; nasotracheal suction.	Feeding tubes may become dislocated by increases in intra-abdominal pressure or coughing, but most frequently they are displaced when the patient moves or pulls on the tube.
6. Observe and measure the external part of tube for movement of ink mark away from mouth or naris (see Skill 32.1).	Increased external length of tube indicates that distal tip is no longer in correct position (Lord, 2018).
7. Review patient's chart for prescriptions for continuous feeding. Review patient's medication record for a gastric acid inhibitor (e.g., ranitidine) or a proton pump inhibitor (e.g., omeprazole).	Presence of enteral formula in aspirated secretions diminishes usefulness of pH measurements because it buffers the pH of the stomach. Similarly, H_2 receptor antagonists reduce acid content of secretions, also raising pH value (Boullata et al., 2017; Metheny et al., 2019).
8. Review patient's medical record for history of prior tube displacement.	Patient is at increased risk for repeated tube displacement.

NURSING DIAGNOSES

- Inadequate gas exchange
- Potential for aspiration

Related factors and risk factors are individualized on the basis of patient's condition or needs.

STEP	RATIONALE
PLANNING	
1. Expected outcomes following completion of procedure:	
• Colour, pH, and appearance of gastric aspirate are consistent with initial tube placement.	Indicates that tube has likely remained in correct location, initially confirmed by radiographic film (Judd, 2020).
2. Explain procedure to patient.	Demonstrates person-centred care because patient has the right to be informed regarding all procedures. Relieves anxiety.
IMPLEMENTATION	
1. Prepare equipment at bedside and apply clean gloves.	Reduces transmission of microorganisms. Ensures organized procedure.
2. Verify tube placement at the following times:	
a. For patients who are intermittently tube fed, test placement before each feeding (usually a period of at least 4 hours will have elapsed since previous feeding) and before medications.	Each administration of feeding or medication can lead to pulmonary aspiration if the tube is displaced.
b. Follow employer policy regarding when to test pH for patients receiving continuous tube feeding.	Feedings should not be stopped only for the purpose of pH testing. pH testing may be helpful when feedings are interrupted for procedures or diagnostic studies (Judd, 2020). pH testing helps determine likelihood that the tube is in desired location in stomach (i.e., gastric secretions typically have pH <5). However, tube-feeding formula alters the pH of gastric content; therefore, pH testing during continuous feeds may not be reliable (Lord, 2018).
c. Wait for at least 1 hour after administering medication via tube before aspirating gastric contents.	Premature withdrawal of contents will remove unabsorbed medication, reducing dose delivered to patient.
3. If tube feeding is infusing, turn off or place feeding on hold. Clamp or kink feeding tube and disconnect from feeding bag; for intermittent feedings, remove plug at end of tube. Draw up 30 mL of air into a 60-mL ENFit syringe. Flush tube with 30 mL of air before attempting to aspirate fluid. Repositioning patient from side to side is helpful. In some cases, more than one bolus of air is necessary.	A burst of air helps to aspirate fluid more easily. Smaller syringes generate unnecessarily high pressures inside tube. A 60-mL syringe reduces pressure when flushing tube with air (Boullata et al., 2017).
4. Draw back on syringe slowly and obtain 5–10 mL of gastric aspirate (see Step 4 illustration). Observe appearance of aspirate. In patients who are continuously tube fed, aspirates from NG tubes often look like curdled enteral formula. In patients who are intermittently tube fed, gastric aspirates are typically not bile stained (unless intestinal fluid has refluxed into stomach) (Metheny et al., 2019).	Drawing back quickly or using a smaller syringe may cause the tube to collapse. Quantity is sufficient for pH testing. Appearance of aspirate helps to assess position of the tube.

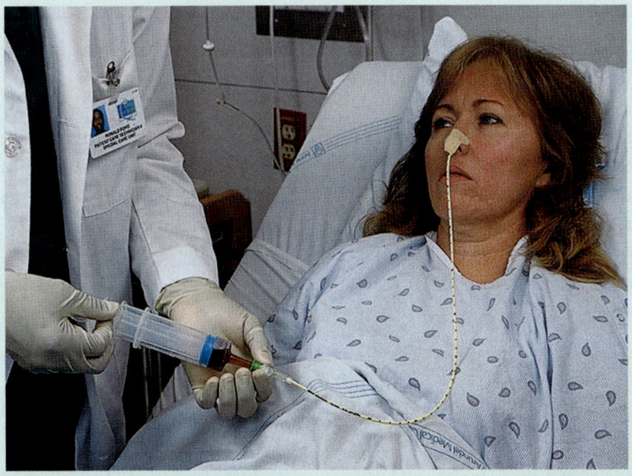

STEP 4 Obtain gastric aspirate.

STEP	RATIONALE

IMPLEMENTATION

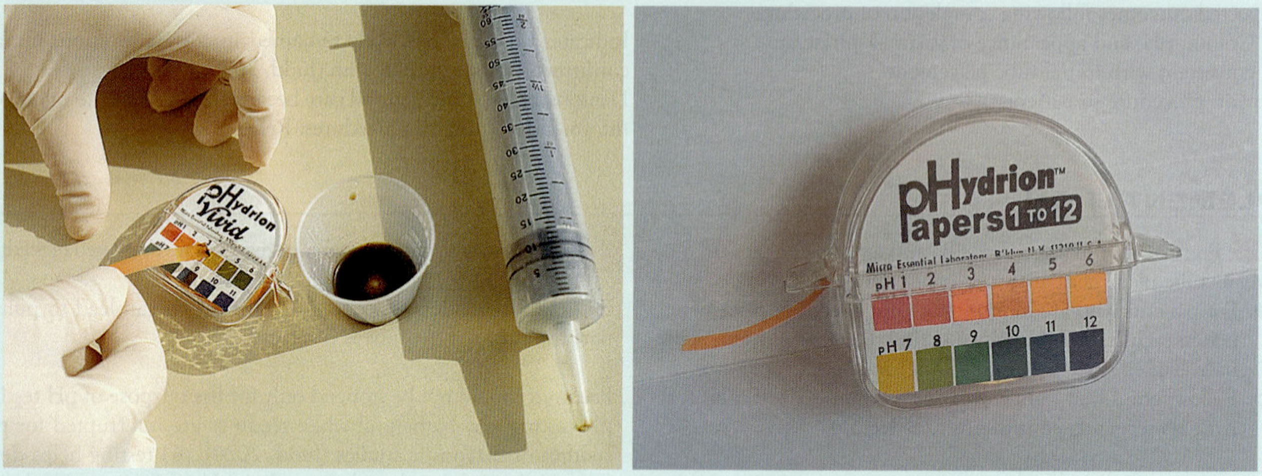

STEP 5 A, Compare colour on test strip with colour on pH chart. B, Test strips. (*B, Courtesy Alia Lagace, University of Manitoba.*)

Step	Rationale
5. Gently mix aspirate in syringe. Expel a few drops into a clean medicine cup. Measure pH of aspirated GI contents by dipping pH strip into fluid or applying a few drops of fluid to strip. Compare colour of strip with colour on chart (see Step 5 illustration) provided by manufacturer.	Mixing ensures equal distribution of contents for testing. The most accurate readings of gastric pH levels are provided by pH paper covering a range of 1.0–11.0 at a minimum.
a. Gastric fluid from a patient who has fasted for at least 4 hours usually has a pH <5.0.	Using pH of 5.0 as the upper cut-off is the safest method for verification of tube location (Judd, 2020).
b. Fluid from a tube in the small intestine of a fasting patient usually has a pH ≥5 (Metheny et al., 2019).	Intestinal contents are more basic than stomach contents. A pH ≥7 indicates intestinal or pulmonary placement (Metheny et al., 2019).
6. If after repeated attempts it is not possible to aspirate fluid from a tube that was confirmed by radiographic film and if (1) there are no risk factors for tube dislocation, (2) the tube has remained in the original taped position, and (3) the patient is not in respiratory distress, continue with irrigation (American Association of Critical-Care Nurses [AACN], 2016; Boullata et al., 2017).	Reports of routine chest or abdominal radiographic films can be used to monitor tube location. Repeat radiographic confirmation of tube position is indicated if external length of tube changes, tape holding the tube comes loose, or patient coughs forcefully or vomits (AACN, 2016).
7. Irrigate tube (see Skill 32.3).	Keeps tube patent.
8. Remove and dispose of gloves and supplies appropriately.	Reduces transmission of microorganisms.

EVALUATION

Step	Rationale
1. Observe patient for respiratory distress: persistent gagging, coughing, drop in oxygen saturation, or changes in respiratory patterns (e.g., rate and depth).	Indicates that tube may be displaced in respiratory tract.
2. Verify that external length of tube, pH, and appearance of aspirate are consistent with initial tube placement.	Indicates that tip of tube is likely to be positioned in same place as it was following radiographic film confirmation.
3. **Use teach-back:** "I want to go over what I explained earlier. Tell me why it is important for me to test and assess the colour and acidity of your stomach contents before feedings." Develop a revised teaching plan if patient or caregiver is unable to teach back correctly.	Determines patient's and caregiver's level of understanding of instructional topic.

Unexpected Outcomes	Related Interventions
1. Red or brown colouring (similar to coffee grounds) of fluid aspirated from feeding tube indicates new or old blood, respectively, in GI tract.	• If colour is not related to medications recently administered, notify health care provider.
2. Patient develops respiratory distress (e.g., dyspnea, decreased oxygen saturation, increased pulse rate) as a result of aspiration or tube displacement into lung.	• Stop any enteral feedings. • Elevate the head of bed. • Perform a respiratory assessment and apply oxygen as needed. • Notify health care provider. • Obtain chest radiographic film as prescribed.

Unexpected Outcomes	Related Interventions
3. Tube cannot be irrigated after testing.	• Reattempt to irrigate tube. Do not force fluid. If unsuccessful, notify health care provider. • Prepare for unclogging procedure based on employer policy.

Communication and Documentation

- Document and report pH value and appearance of aspirate in progress notes in EHR or chart.
- Document your evaluation of patient and caregiver learning.

DOCUMENTATION EXAMPLE

Correct tube placement confirmed with gastric aspirate. 10 mL cloudy, mucousy, light tan fluid aspirated via syringe, pH = 3. Patient tolerated procedure well and is resting in bed at present. Will reassess in 6 hours.

Special Considerations

Teaching

- Have caregiver or patient demonstrate how to check tube placement while patient is still in health care setting.
- Instruct patient not to pull or alter position of enteral tube.

Pediatric

- Decrease the amount of air insufflated according to patient's size (e.g., an infant may only need 1 mL of air; a small child, 5 mL) before withdrawal of gastric secretions.

Care in the Community: Home Management

- See Skill 32.1, Special Considerations, Care in the Community.
- See Skill 32.5, Managing Feeding Tubes in the Home.
- Instruct patient or caregiver not to proceed with feedings or medication administration via the tube if there is any doubt as to its placement.

✦ SKILL 32.3 Irrigating a Feeding Tube

NSO Nursing Skills Online Enteral Nutrition Module 16 / Lesson 4

Feeding tubes must remain patent to ensure that liquid nutritional formulas can pass through easily. All types of feeding tubes require routine irrigation to keep a tube patent. Inability to instill air or fluid suggests that a tube is occluded. Curdled enteral formula and improperly crushed medications are the most common causes of feeding tube occlusion.

Delegation and Collaboration

The skill of irrigating a feeding tube cannot be delegated to a UCP. The nurse directs the UCP to do the following:

- Report when a tube feeding stops infusing

Equipment

- 60-mL ENFit syringe
- Water (tap water or sterile water [see employer policy]; dated and initialled container at patient's bedside)
- Towel
- Clean gloves
- Stethoscope

STEP	RATIONALE
ASSESSMENT	
1. Identify patient using at least two person-specific identifiers (e.g., name and date of birth, or name and medical record number) according to employer policy.	Ensures correct patient. Complies with Accreditation Canada's standards and improves patient safety (Accreditation Canada, 2020).
2. Throughout the procedure, the 4 moments for hand hygiene are to be implemented; hand hygiene should occur before initial patient (or patient environment) contact, before an aseptic procedure, after body fluid exposure risk, and after patient (or patient environment) contact. Additional hand hygiene should be performed when hands are visibly soiled.	Proper hand hygiene helps prevent the spread of infectious agents to health care providers.
3. Apply clean gloves. Inspect volume, colour, and character of gastric aspirates (if obtainable) (see Skill 32.2). Remove and dispose of gloves.	Reduces transmission of microorganisms. Determines correct tube placement.
4. Note ease with which tube feeding infuses through tubing.	Failure of formula to infuse as desired may indicate development of obstruction.
5. Monitor volume of continuous enteral formula administered during shift and compare with prescribed amount.	Indicates whether sufficient volume of feeding is infusing. Serves as baseline to determine tube patency.
6. Refer to employer policy regarding routine irrigation parameters or health care provider's prescription for individual patient needs.	Determines frequency of irrigations.

STEP	RATIONALE

NURSING DIAGNOSES

- Reduced fluid volume
- Excessive fluid volume
- Inadequate nutrition: less than body requirements

Related factors and risk factors are individualized on the basis of patient's condition or needs.

PLANNING

STEP	RATIONALE
1. Expected outcomes following completion of procedure:	
• Feeding tube remains patent.	Irrigation fluid clears solids and secretions from inner lumen of feeding tube.
• Patient receives prescribed caloric intake.	Feeding infuses without interruption.
2. Explain procedure to patient; stress that you are not removing tube.	Decreases patient anxiety.
3. Position patient in high Fowler's (if tolerated) or semi-Fowler's position.	Reduces reflux and risk of pulmonary aspiration during irrigation.

IMPLEMENTATION

STEP	RATIONALE
1. Prepare equipment at patient's bedside and apply clean gloves.	Reduces transmission of microorganisms. Ensures organized procedure.
2. Verify tube placement (see Skill 32.2) if fluid can be aspirated for pH testing and by verifying external tube length.	With tip of tube correctly placed in stomach or intestine, irrigation will not increase risk of pulmonary aspiration.
3. Irrigate routinely before, between, and after medication administration and before an intermittent feeding is administered.	Certain formulas have properties that predispose to tube clogging. Irrigation prevents mixing of medications in tube, which may cause clogging.
4. Draw up 30 mL of water in ENFit syringe. Patient should have individual bottle of solution.	This amount of solution will flush the length of the tube. Water is the most effective agent for preventing tube clogging.

Critical Decision Point *Do not use carbonated beverages or fruit juices to flush tubing.*

STEP	RATIONALE
5. Change irrigation container every 24 hours (according to employer policy).	Ensures clean equipment and solution. Sterile water is required for neonates and patients who are immune suppressed or critically ill (Boullata et al., 2017; The Hospital for Sick Children [SickKids], 2021). Tap water is appropriate in many clinical settings and in home care if municipal water supply is safe (SickKids, 2021).
6. Kink feeding tube while disconnecting it from administration tubing or while removing plug at end of tube.	Prevents leakage of gastric secretions.
7. Insert tip of ENFit syringe into end of feeding tube. Release kink and slowly instill irrigation solution.	Infusion of fluid clears tubing.
8. If unable to instill fluid, reposition patient on left side and try again.	Tip of tube may be against stomach wall. Changing patient's position may move tip away from stomach wall.
9. When water has been instilled, remove syringe. Reinstitute tube feeding or administer medication as prescribed. Flush each medication completely through tube.	Tubing is clear and patent. Ensures that full dose reaches stomach and medications do not mix with formula.
10. Remove and discard gloves; dispose of supplies in appropriate receptacle.	Reduces transmission of microorganisms.

EVALUATION

STEP	RATIONALE
1. Observe ease with which tube feeding instills through tubing.	Irrigated tube is patent, allowing for free flow of solution.
2. Monitor patient's caloric intake.	Total enteral nutrition infuses without difficulty.
3. **Use teach-back:** "I want to be sure that I explained why you need to flush your tube when you return home. Tell me why it is important to flush your tube." Develop a revised teaching plan if patient or caregiver is unable to teach back correctly.	Determines patient's and caregiver's level of understanding of instructional topic.

Unexpected Outcomes	Related Interventions
1. Tube cannot be irrigated and remains obstructed.	• Repeat irrigation; if unsuccessful, notify health care provider. • Several methods can be prescribed to aid in unclogging an obstructed tube—for example, actuated devices, enzymatic mixtures, and warm water (SickKids, 2021). • Tube may need to be removed and a new tube placed.
2. Fluid and electrolyte imbalances occur. Insufficient irrigation can cause water deficiency; excessive irrigations can cause fluid volume excess.	• Notify health care provider of abnormal electrolyte levels or imbalanced I&O.

Communication and Documentation

- Document time of irrigation and amount and type of fluid instilled in progress notes in EHR or chart.
- Report if tubing has become clogged.
- Document your evaluation of patient and caregiver learning.

Special Considerations

Pediatric

- Irrigation of a tube requires a smaller volume of solution in children: 1 to 2 mL for smaller tubes and 5 to 15 mL for larger tubes (Hockenberry et al., 2024).

✦ SKILL 32.4 Administering Enteral Nutrition: Nasogastric, Nasointestinal, Gastrostomy, or Jejunostomy Tube

NSO Nursing Skills Online Enteral Nutrition Module 16 / Lesson 5

Enteral nutrition, or tube feeding, is a method for providing nutrients to patients who are unable to meet their nutritional requirements orally. As a rule, candidates for enteral nutrition must have a sufficiently functional GI tract to absorb nutrients. Examples of indications for enteral feeding include the following:

- Situations in which normal eating is unsafe because of high risk for aspiration: altered mental status, swallowing disorders, impaired gag reflex, dependence on mechanical ventilation, esophageal conditions (e.g., strictures or dysmotility), and delayed gastric emptying.
- Clinical conditions that interfere with normal ingestion or absorption of nutrients or create hypermetabolic states: surgical resection of oropharynx, proximal intestinal obstruction or fistula, pancreatitis, burns, and severe pressure injuries.
- Conditions in which disease- or treatment-related symptoms reduce oral intake: anorexia, nausea, pain, fatigue, shortness of breath, and depression.

Gastric feedings are the most common type of enteral nutrition, allowing tube-feeding formulas to enter the stomach and then pass gradually through the intestinal tract to ensure absorption. In contrast, small-bowel feeding occurs beyond the pyloric sphincter of the stomach, which reduces the risk of pulmonary aspiration (Lord, 2018). General guidelines for the timing of delivery of enteral nutrition are as follows: continuous feeding (typically 25–150 mL delivered continuously anywhere from 12 to 24 hours), intermittent feeding (200–500 mL delivered over 30 to 90 minutes several times during the day), and bolus feeding (50–100 mL delivered over less than 15 minutes several times a day). Feedings are also delivered by a predetermined method: pump, gravity, or bolus. Pump feedings run through an enteral infusion pump that controls the rate. Pump feedings are used in situations where continuous feeding is prescribed and in cases of feeding via a small-bowel feeding tube. The gravity method is used for gastric feeds that are administered intermittently, where the tube feed formula bag is connected to the feeding tube port and the rate is controlled via a roller clamp along the tubing. Patients who receive gravity feeds have typically demonstrated tolerance of receiving their feed within 30 to 90 minutes. Bolus feeds, delivered by syringe method, are the least common, as they are instilled more quickly and thus present a higher risk for abdominal distension. The decision of what type and how much of a given formula is typically determined by the dietitian, based on the patient's fluid, electrolyte, and caloric needs, in collaboration with the interprofessional team. The general rule for initiating a new feed is start low and go slow. The rate and amount will often start low (e.g., 20 mL/hr) for the first 4 hours, with instructions to increase the rate based on tolerance until the desired amount is being delivered to the patient.

Aspiration of enteral nutrition is a serious complication and is a concern for all patients who receive enteral nutrition. Aspiration is the inhalation of oropharyngeal or gastric contents into the larynx and lower respiratory tract (Metheny et al., 2019). Efforts should be made to prevent or minimize aspiration. The AACN (2016) recommends several practices to minimize the risk of aspiration in tube-fed patients:

- Maintain head-of-bed elevation at an angle of 30 to 45 degrees unless contraindicated.
- For patients receiving tube feedings, assess tube placement and GI tolerance at 4-hour intervals.
- Avoid bolus feeding in patients deemed high risk for aspiration.

Delegation and Collaboration

The decision to delegate the skill of administering a nasoenteric tube feeding to a UCP should be made in accordance with employer policy. A nurse must first verify tube placement and patency. The nurse directs the UCP to do the following:

- Elevate the head of the bed to 30 to 45 degrees, or sit the patient up in bed or in a chair unless contraindicated.
- Not to adjust the feeding rate; infuse the feeding as prescribed.
- Report any problems noted while infusing the feeding or any discomfort voiced by the patient.
- Report any gagging, coughing, or choking.
- Provide frequent oral hygiene.

Equipment

- Disposable feeding bag, tubing, or ready-to-hang system
- 60-mL or larger ENFit syringe
- Stethoscope
- Enteral infusion pump for continuous feedings
- pH indicator strip (scale 1.0–11.0)
- Prescribed enteral formula
- Clean gloves
- ENFit connector

STEP	RATIONALE

ASSESSMENT

STEP	RATIONALE
1. Identify patient using at least two person-specific identifiers (e.g., name and date of birth, or name and medical record number) according to employer policy.	Ensures correct patient. Complies with Accreditation Canada's standards and improves patient safety (Accreditation Canada, 2020).
2. Throughout the procedure, the 4 moments for hand hygiene are to be implemented; hand hygiene should occur before initial patient (or patient environment) contact, before an aseptic procedure, after body fluid exposure risk, and after patient (or patient environment) contact. Additional hand hygiene should be performed when hands are visibly soiled.	Proper hand hygiene helps prevent the spread of infectious agents to health care providers.
3. Assess patient's clinical status to determine potential need for tube feedings: decreased level of consciousness, nutritional deficits, head or neck surgery, facial trauma, or impaired swallowing. Use interprofessional collaboration (e.g., dietitian) to consult with nutrition support team and health care provider.	Identify candidates for enteral nutrition before they become nutritionally depleted. A health care provider's prescription is necessary for feedings. Some institutions in Canada have adopted prescription-writing privileges for registered dietitians.
4. Assess patient for food allergies.	Prevents patient from developing allergic responses to feeding.
5. Perform physical assessment of abdomen, including auscultation for bowel sounds, before feeding (see Chapter 8).	Objective measures for assessing tolerance include changes in bowel sounds, expanding girth, tenderness and firmness on palpation, increasing GRV, and vomiting (Tatsumi, 2019). Report findings to health care provider to determine whether tube feeding can proceed safely.
6. Obtain baseline weight and review serum electrolytes and blood glucose level. Assess patient for fluid volume excess or deficit and metabolic abnormalities.	Enteral feedings should restore or maintain a patient's nutritional status. Measures provide objective data and baseline to determine selection of formula and measure effectiveness of feedings.
7. Verify health care provider's prescription for type of formula, rate, route, and frequency.	Ensures that correct formula will be administered in appropriate volume. Enteral formulas are not interchangeable.

NURSING DIAGNOSES

- Inadequate nutrition: less than body requirements
- Reduced swallowing
- Readiness for enhanced nutrition
- Potential for aspiration

Related factors and risk factors are individualized on the basis of patient's condition or needs.

PLANNING

STEP	RATIONALE
1. Expected outcomes following completion of procedure:	
• Patient achieves established target for body weight and fluid/electrolyte balance over time.	Indicates that patient's nutritional status is maintained or improved.
• Patient has no sign of respiratory distress.	Feeding tube does not enter airway, and patient does not aspirate feeding.
• Patient is free of abdominal cramping.	Feeding administered without abdominal distension. Demonstrates tolerance of tube feeding.
2. Explain procedure to patient.	Decreases patient anxiety.

IMPLEMENTATION

STEP	RATIONALE
1. Apply clean gloves.	Reduces transmission of microorganisms and potential contamination of enteral formula.
2. Verify correct formula and check expiration date; note integrity of container.	Ensures that correct therapy is administered and confirms integrity of formula.
3. Prepare formula for administration, following manufacturer guidelines:	
a. Have formula at room temperature.	Cold formula causes gastric cramping and discomfort because liquid is not warmed by mouth and esophagus.
b. Use aseptic technique to connect tubing to container as needed. Use proper ENFit connecter and avoid handling feeding system or touching can tops, container openings, spike, and spike port.	Bag, connections, and tubing must be free of contamination to prevent bacterial growth (Tatsumi, 2019).

STEP	RATIONALE

IMPLEMENTATION

STEP	RATIONALE
c. Shake formula container well. Clean top of canned formula with alcohol swab before opening it.	Ensures integrity of formula. Prevents transmission of microorganisms.
d. For a closed system, connect administration tubing to container. If using an open system, pour formula from Tetra Pak or can into administration bag (see Step 3d illustration).	Formulas are available in closed-system containers (containing a 24- to 48-hour supply of formula) or in an open system (formula must be transferred from Tetra Paks or cans to a bag before administration).

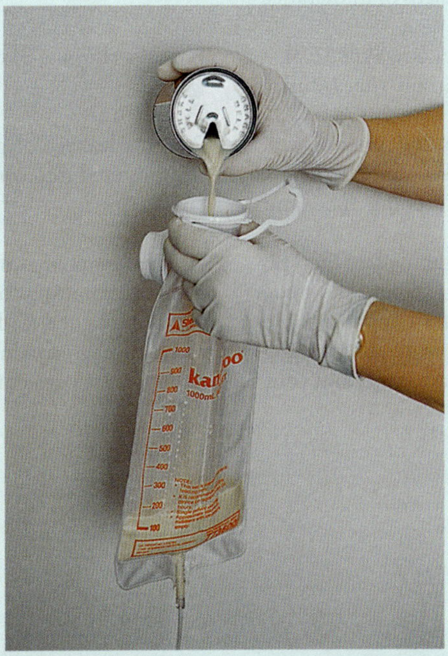

STEP 3D Pour formula into open feeding container.

STEP	RATIONALE
4. Prime the tubing set by opening the roller clamp and allowing administration tubing to fill with formula. Clamp off tubing with roller clamp. Hang container on intravenous (IV) pole.	Prevents introduction of air into stomach once feeding begins.
5. Place patient in high Fowler's position or elevate head of bed at least 30 degrees (preferably 45 degrees). For a patient required to remain supine, place in reverse Trendelenburg position, which raises their head.	Elevated head helps prevent pulmonary aspiration.
6. Verify tube placement (see Skill 32.2):	Verifies whether tip of tube is in stomach or intestine.
a. *Nasoenteric tube:* Attach ENFit syringe and aspirate gastric contents. Observe appearance of aspirate and note pH. Measure external tube length and compare with patient record.	Gastric fluid for patient who has fasted for at least 4 hours usually has pH of 1.0–4.0 (especially when patient is not receiving gastric acid inhibitor).
b. *Gastrostomy tube:* Attach ENFit syringe and aspirate gastric contents. Observe appearance of aspirate and note pH.	Continuous administration of tube feeding elevates pH (Bear et al., 2018). Noting the external length helps determine possible tube dislodgement (Lord, 2018).
c. *Jejunostomy tube:* Attach syringe and aspirate intestinal secretions. Observe appearance; if significant amounts are returned or resemble gastric secretions, check pH. Note the tube position by measuring external length or noting whether the outer measurement markings on the tube are consistent with the patient's medical record.	Presence of intestinal fluid indicates that end of the tube is in the small intestine. If fluid tests acidic on pH test or looks like gastric fluid, tube may be displaced into the stomach. Noting the external length helps determine possible tube dislodgement (Lord, 2018).
7. Check GRV according to employer policy.	GRV determines whether gastric emptying is delayed. Intestinal residual is usually very small. If intestinal feeding residual volume is greater than 10 mL, displacement of tube into stomach may have occurred.
a. Draw up 10–30 mL air into ENFit syringe and connect to end of feeding tube. Inject air slowly into tube. Pull back slowly and aspirate total amount of gastric contents that can be aspirated.	GRV may not be easy to obtain from small-bore feeding tube. A 60-mL syringe should be used to aspirate.

STEP	RATIONALE

IMPLEMENTATION

STEP	RATIONALE
b. Return aspirated contents to stomach slowly unless volume exceeds 250 mL (see employer policy).	Prevents loss of nutrients and electrolytes in discarded fluid. Some questions exist regarding safety of returning high volumes of fluid to stomach (LHSC, 2021).
c. GRVs in range of 200–500 mL should raise concern and lead to implementation of measures to reduce risk of aspiration. Automatic cessation of feeding should not occur for GRV <500 mL in absence of other signs of intolerance (Wen et al., 2019).	Elevated GRV should raise concern and lead to additional measures to reduce risk of aspiration (e.g., elevating head of bed, regular oral hygiene care, use of prokinetic medications) (Lord, 2018).
d. Flush feeding tube with 30 mL of water (see Skill 32.3).	Prevents clogging of tubing.
8. Intermittent feeding (administered at certain times during the day):	
a. Pinch proximal end of feeding tube and remove cap. Connect distal end of administration set tubing to ENFit device (see Step 8a illustration) on feeding tube and release tubing.	Prevents leakage of gastric contents. Ensures that feeding will be administered into correct tubing.
b. Set rate by adjusting roller clamp on tubing (see Step 8b illustration) or attach tubing to feeding pump. Allow bag to empty gradually over 30–45 minutes (length of time to eat a comfortable meal). Label bag with tube-feeding type, strength, and amount. Include date, time, and your initials.	Gradual emptying of tube feeding reduces risk of abdominal discomfort, vomiting, or diarrhea induced by bolus or overly rapid infusion of tube feedings. Labelling provides means to determine when to change administration set and confirms that patient is receiving the correct feeding.

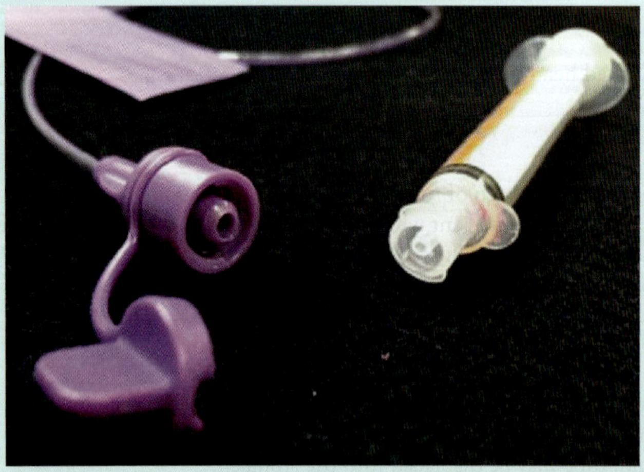

STEP 8A ENFit device.

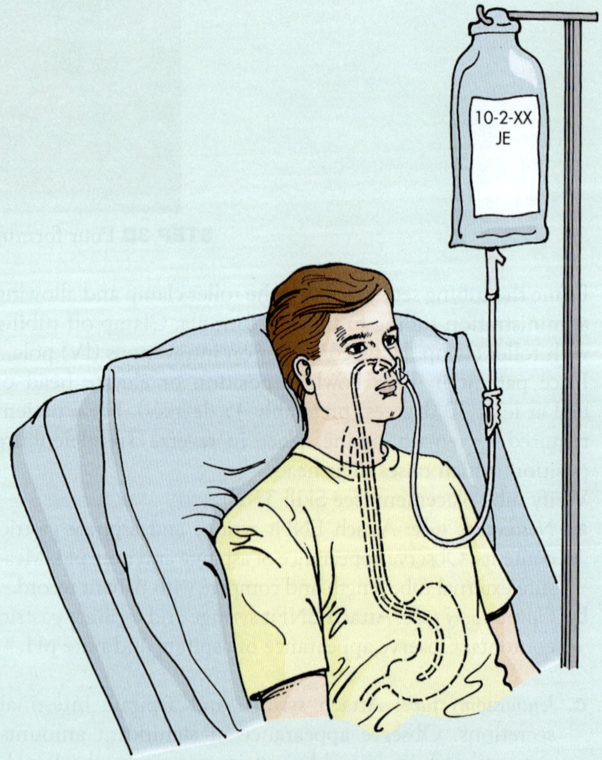

STEP 8B Administer intermittent feeding.

Critical Decision Point *Use pumps designated for tube feeding, rather than those intended for IV fluids.*

STEP	RATIONALE
c. Immediately follow feeding with water (per health care provider's prescriptions and employer policy). Cover end of feeding tube with cap when not in use. Keep bag as clean as possible. Change administration set every 24 hours or according to employer policy.	Prevents tube from clogging. Limits microbial contamination of system.

STEP	RATIONALE

IMPLEMENTATION

STEP	RATIONALE
9. Continuous infusion method:	Method delivers prescribed hourly rate of feeding and reduces risk of abdominal discomfort.
a. Remove cap on tubing and connect distal end of administration set tubing to feeding tube using ENFit connector (see Step 8a illustration).	Prevents leakage of gastric contents.
b. Thread tubing through feeding pump; set rate on pump and turn on (see Step 9b illustration).	Delivers continuous feeding at steady rate and pressure. Feeding pump sounds alarm for increased resistance.

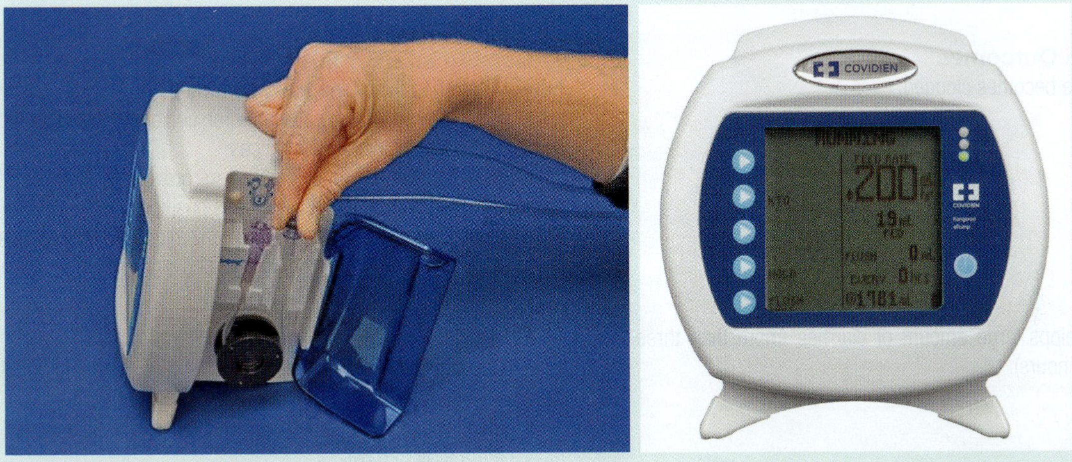

STEP 9B A, Connect tubing through infusion pump. B, Set pump as ordered. *(Images used with permission of Covidien. All rights reserved.)*

STEP	RATIONALE
c. Advance rate of tube feeding (and concentration of feeding) gradually, as prescribed.	Tube feeding can usually begin with full-strength formula. Conservative initiation and advancement of enteral nutrition depend on factors such as patient's age, medical condition, nutritional status, and expected patient tolerance (Bukhari et al., 2020).

Critical Decision Point *Maximum hang time for formula is 12 hours in an open system and 24–48 hours in a closed, ready-to-hang system (if it remains closed). Refer to manufacturer guidelines and employer policy for specific guidelines on hang times* (Lakananurak et al., 2020).

STEP	RATIONALE
10. After feeding, flush tubing with 30 mL water every 4 hours during continuous feeding (see employer policy) or before and after an intermittent feeding. Have dietitian prescribe total free-water requirement per day and obtain health care provider's prescription (see Skill 32.3).	Provides patient with source of water to help maintain fluid and electrolyte balance. Clears tubing of formula.
11. Rinse bag and tubing with warm water whenever feedings are interrupted.	Rinsing bag and tubing with warm water clears old tube feedings and reduces bacterial growth.
12. Dispose of supplies.	Reduces transmission of microorganisms.

EVALUATION

STEP	RATIONALE
1. Measure GRV per employer policy, usually every 4–6 hours, and ask patient whether nausea or abdominal cramping is present.	GI tolerance of tube feedings must be monitored closely to avoid complications.
2. Monitor I&O at least every 8 hours and calculate daily totals every 24 hours.	I&O totals are indications of fluid balance, which can indicate fluid volume excess or deficit.
3. Weigh patient daily until maximum administration rate is reached and maintained for 24 hours; then weigh patient three times per week.	Slow weight gain is indicator of improved nutritional status; however, sudden gain of more than 0.9 kg (2 lb) in 24 hours usually indicates fluid retention.
4. Monitor laboratory values as prescribed by health care provider.	Determines correct administration of formula rate and strength.
5. Observe patient's respiratory status.	Change in respiratory status may indicate aspiration of tube feeding into respiratory tract. Symptoms may include coughing, dyspnea, tachypnea, change in oxygen saturation, crackles, and hoarseness.
6. Examine abdomen and auscultate bowel sounds.	Evaluates status of gastric emptying and peristalsis.
7. For gastrostomy tubes, inspect site for signs of impaired skin integrity and symptoms of infection, injury, or tightness of tube (see Procedural Guideline 32.1).	Enteral tubes can cause pressure and excoriation at insertion site.

STEP	RATIONALE

EVALUATION

8. Observe nasoenteral tube insertion site at least daily (see employer policy). Note skin integrity and look for edema under device, excoriation, or presence of injury.	Allows for early detection of excoriation that can progress to MDRPI.
9. **Use teach-back:** "I want to be sure that I explained to you what you need to look for that means you're not tolerating your tube feeding. Tell me two signs you can look for that may mean you are not tolerating your tube feedings well." Develop a revised teaching plan if patient or caregiver is unable to teach back correctly.	Determines patient's or caregiver's level of understanding of instructional topic.

Unexpected Outcomes	Related Interventions
1. Feeding tube becomes clogged.	• Attempt to flush tube with warm water. • Special products are available for unclogging feeding tubes; do not use carbonated beverages or juices. • Hold feeding and notify health care provider. • Maintain patient in semi-Fowler's position. • Contact pharmacist to change medications to liquid form, and flush before and after intermittent feedings and administering medications (Bandy et al., 2019).
2. Patient develops large amount of diarrhea (more than three loose stools in 24 hours).	• Notify health care provider. • Use interprofessional collaboration (e.g., dietitian) to discuss need to change formula to prevent malabsorption. • Identify and treat underlying medical or surgical issues and infections (Pitta et al., 2019). • Provide perianal skin care after each stool. • Determine other causes of diarrhea (e.g., *Clostridioides difficile* infection, contaminated tube feeding, medications containing sorbitol).
3. Patient develops nausea and vomiting.	• Administer antiemetic as prescribed. • Use prescribed medications to increase gastric motility. • Withhold tube feeding and notify health care provider. • Aspirate for residual.
4. Patient aspirates formula (auscultation of crackles or wheezes, dyspnea, or fever).	• Report change in condition to health care provider. • Position patient on side. • Suction nasotracheally or orotracheally.

Communication and Documentation

- Document amount and type of feeding, infusion rate, method of infusion, patient's response to tube feeding (e.g., GRV, cramping, bowel sounds, patency of tube, condition of skin at tube site) in progress notes in EHR or chart.
- Document volume of formula and any additional water given on I&O form.
- Report type of feeding, status of feeding tube, patient's tolerance, and adverse outcomes.
- Document your evaluation of patient and caregiver learning.

DOCUMENTATION EXAMPLE

Jevity Plus continues to infuse at 65 mL/hr via infusion pump through NG tube with 185 mL infused. Patient states feeling nauseated and "full." Abdomen soft and nondistended, and bowel sounds are present in all four quadrants. Placement of tube verified with measurements of tube at nares at 55 cm and gastric aspirate with a pH of 4. Tube feeding infusion stopped and the head of the bed maintained at a 45-degree angle. Will reassess gastric volume residual in 1 hour and determine whether tube feeding will be resumed.

Special Considerations

Teaching

- Instruct patients and caregivers not to reconnect lines that have separated but to seek clinical assistance.
- Teach patient and caregiver that, if tolerated, patient should remain upright for 1 hour after feedings.
- Instruct patient or caregiver that patient may express feelings of fullness, increased gas, belching, or diarrhea.
- Teach patient or caregiver how to determine correct placement of feeding tube (see Skill 32.2).

Pediatric

- Preterm infants who are at risk for necrotizing enterocolitis frequently receive minimal enteral feeding (MEF) to limit stress on the GI tract. Use of breast milk for the MEF in premature infants reduces sepsis and necrotizing enterocolitis and improves patient outcomes (Cortez et al., 2018).
- Infants who require MEF are sometimes fed using the syringe method while the parent or caregiver holds them to normalize the process and aid in bonding. The syringe can be held lower or higher to achieve the desired rate of instillation that can be tolerated by the baby (Fig. 32.2).

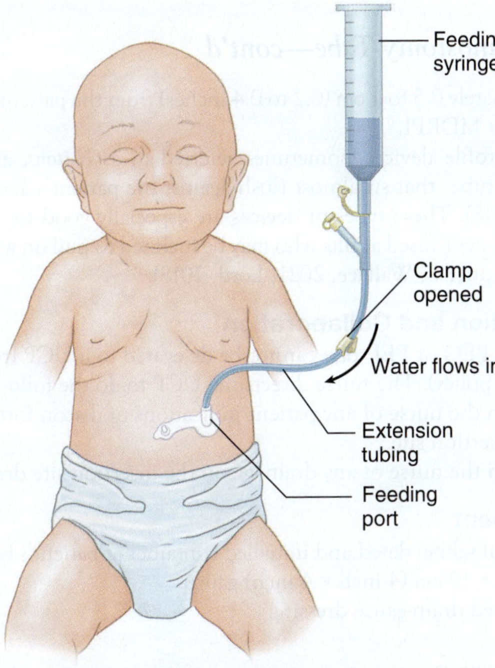

FIG 32.2 Infant being syringe fed.

Gerontological

- Some older persons have decreased gastric emptying; therefore, formula remains in the stomach longer than for younger patients.

Patients With Physical or Cognitive Challenges

- GRV checks are especially important in patients with impaired cognition in order to decrease the risk of pulmonary aspiration.

Care in the Community: Home Management

- See Skill 32.1, Special Considerations, Skill 32.1.
- Instruct patient or caregiver on technique for administering feedings in the home and proper storage and refrigeration of supplies (see Skill 32.5).
- Instruct patient or caregiver about any symptoms or discomfort that may occur during enteral feedings. Reinforce instruction to contact health care provider if symptoms of discomfort occur.
- Teach patient or caregiver how to perform skin care around the gastrostomy or jejunostomy tube and signs and symptoms of infection at insertion site (see Procedural Guideline 32.1).

Procedural Guideline 32.1 *Care of a Gastrostomy or Jejunostomy Tube*

Feeding tubes can be placed directly into the GI tract through the abdominal wall in patients who cannot tolerate nasoenteric feeding tubes or those who require long-term (greater than 4 to 6 weeks) enteral nutrition. The stomach (gastrostomy tube) and jejunum (jejunostomy tube) are the most common sites for long-term feeding tubes. Long-term tubes require endoscopic, radiological, or surgical placement (Lord, 2018). The insertion method used to place tubes may call for specific nursing interventions in the postinsertion period; but otherwise these tubes are used in a similar way to other feeding tubes. Feedings delivered via a gastrostomy tube are relatively safe to administer, provided the patient has normal gastric emptying. Gastrostomy tubes are often called G *tubes*; but they are also commonly referred to as *percutaneous endoscopic gastrostomy (PEG) tubes*, a term used to describe tubes placed endoscopically. Gastrostomy tubes range in size from 12 to 30 Fr (Lord, 2018) and exit through an incision/stoma in the upper left quadrant of the abdomen, where an internal bumper or balloon and an external bumper or disc hold the tube in place (Fig. 32.3).

Once the stoma tract is well formed, balloon gastrostomy tubes are replaced every 6 months by specially trained nurses on the unit (or as needed owing to leaking, damage, or breakage of device).

Jejunostomy tubes are indicated when the risk for regurgitation and aspiration is especially high, as in cases of severely delayed gastric emptying or conditions such as pancreatitis, which limit use of the stomach for feeding. They tend to be smaller in diameter, at 5 to 16 Fr (Lord, 2018). They can be placed directly into the small intestine in a surgical procedure or threaded through the stomach into the jejunum under fluoroscopy. Some jejunal tubes inserted through this transgastric approach are dual-channel devices that have openings in both the stomach and the small-intestine part of the tube. These *combination tubes*, as they are called, allow simultaneous gastric decompression and intestinal feeding for patients with impaired gastric emptying or upper-GI cancers. Each lumen

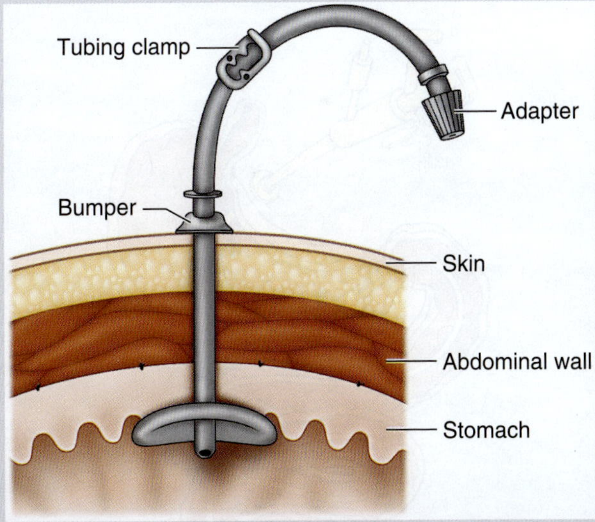

FIG 32.3 Placement of percutaneous endoscopic gastrostomy (PEG) tube into stomach.

of a combination tube is clearly labelled to distinguish between the gastric and jejunal ports (Fig. 32.4).

Sometimes a jejunostomy tube is placed through an existing PEG tube. The percutaneous endoscopic jejunostomy (PEJ) tube is passed through the PEG tube and advanced into the jejunum (Fig. 32.5). The PEJ tube occupies the lumen of the PEG tube; this tube-through-a-tube design does not allow drainage of the stomach during small-intestine feeding. In the case of both combination tubes and PEJ tubes, the nurse must know whether the intended site for formula delivery is gastric or jejunal to ensure safe and effective nutritional care.

Continued

Procedural Guideline 32.1 *Care of a Gastrostomy or Jejunostomy Tube—cont'd*

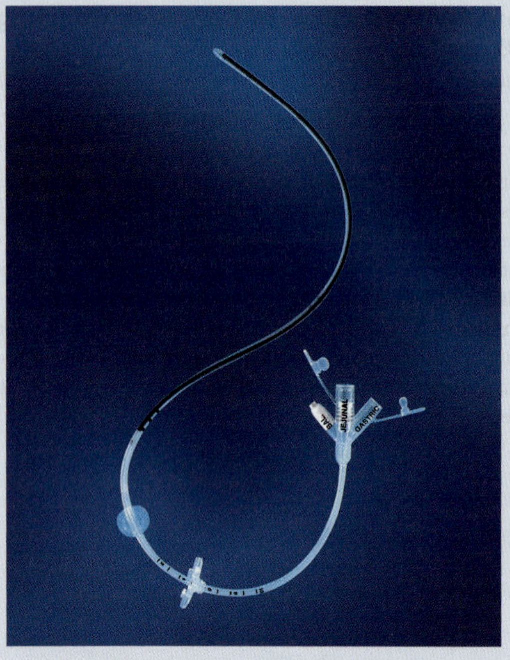

FIG 32.4 **Dual-lumen "combination tube" to allow jejunal feeding and gastric decompression.** *(Image used with permission of Kimberly-Clark Health Care. All rights reserved.)*

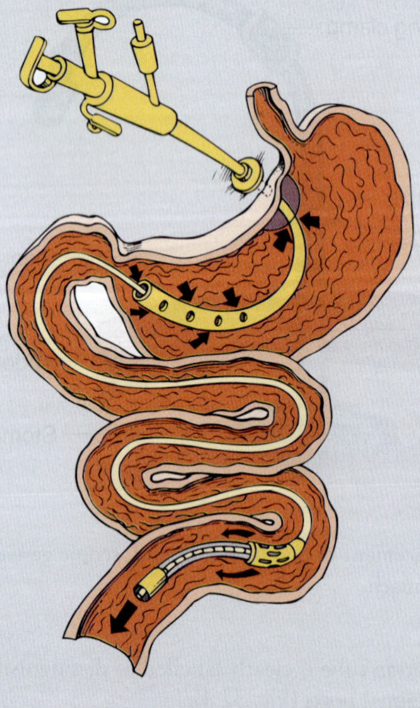

FIG 32.5 **Endoscopic insertion of jejunostomy tube.**

For the first 48 to 72 hours after a new gastrostomy or jejunostomy tube is placed, the stoma tract is considered a surgical wound and is therefore to be cleaned using sterile technique. Postplacement (48 to 72 hours), with a noninfected stoma, clean technique of warm soap and water can be practised daily, and the stoma may be left open to air.

For the first 4 weeks following stoma creation and tube insertion, the external bolster remains fairly tight against the abdomen and should generally not be adjusted. After 4 weeks, the external bolster on a gastrostomy or jejunostomy tube should be positioned approximately 0.5 to 1 cm (0.2 to 0.4 inches) from the patient's skin to prevent MDRPI.

Low-profile devices, sometimes referred to as *buttons*, are gastrostomy tubes that sit almost flush against the patient's abdomen (Lord, 2018). These types of devices are especially good for use in children or confused adults who may be inclined to pull on a longer tube (Gardner & Wallace, 2021; Lord, 2018).

Delegation and Collaboration

Care of a PEG or PEJ tube cannot be delegated to a UCP (refer to employer policy). The nurse directs the UCP to do the following:

- Inform the nurse of any patient indications of discomfort at the insertion site.
- Inform the nurse of any drainage on the insertion site dressing.

Equipment

- Normal saline, dated and initialled container at patient's bedside
- 10 cm × 10 cm (4 inch × 4 inch) gauze
- Prepared drain-gauze dressing
- Tape
- Clean gloves

Procedural Steps

1. Determine whether the exit site is left open to air or if a dressing is indicated. Check health care provider's prescription or verify employer policy.
2. Identify patient using at least two person-specific identifiers (e.g., name and date of birth, or name and medical record number) according to employer policy.
3. Throughout the procedure, the 4 moments for hand hygiene are to be implemented; hand hygiene should occur before initial patient (or patient environment) contact, before an aseptic procedure, after body fluid exposure risk, and after patient (or patient environment) contact. Additional hand hygiene should be performed when hands are visibly soiled. Apply clean gloves.
4. Remove old dressing. Fold dressing with drainage contained inside; remove gloves inside out over dressing. Discard in appropriate container.
5. Assess exit site for evidence of tenderness, leakage, swelling, excoriation, infection, bleeding, redness, or excessive movement (>6 mm [0.25 inches]) of the tube in or out of the stomach.
6. Clean skin around stoma site with warm water and mild soap or saline (according to employer policy) with 10 cm × 10 cm (4 inch × 4 inch) gauze. (If drainage is present, apply clean gloves.) Clean, starting next to the stoma site, and work outward using circular strokes. Carefully clean under external bolster.
7. Rinse and dry site completely.
8. Apply a thin layer of protective skin barrier to exit site, if indicated (e.g., site excoriated).
9. If dressing is prescribed, place a drain-gauze dressing over external bar or disc. **Note:** Do not place dressing under external bar; this can cause gastric tissue erosion or internal abdominal wall pressure.
10. Secure dressing with tape.
11. Place date, time, and your initials on new dressing.
12. Remove gloves and dispose of supplies in appropriate receptacle.
13. Evaluate condition of site routinely (see employer policy).
14. Document appearance of the exit site, drainage noted, and dressing application in progress notes in EHR or chart.
15. Report to health care provider any exit site complications.

✦ SKILL 32.5 Managing Feeding Tubes in the Home

Patients benefit from being able to see tube-feeding equipment and devices up close when learning how to administer home enteral nutrition. Nurses need to provide hands-on experience and ensure patient involvement with decision making about home enteral nutrition whenever possible. Enteral nutrition therapy in the home setting is usually effective when a patient tolerates at least 70% of feeding intake without complications and is medically stable; the patient or caregiver can administer feedings; and there is sufficient time in a controlled environment to learn the skill.

Most patients who receive enteral nutrition in the home have either gastrostomy or jejunostomy tubes. This skill focuses on teaching the patient or caregiver how to administer such feedings in the home. In the home setting, the nurse is often responsible for reinsertion of gastrostomy feeding tubes, and the health care provider is responsible for reinsertion of jejunostomy tubes.

Delegation and Collaboration

The skill of teaching patients and caregivers how to manage feeding tubes in the home cannot be delegated to a UCP. The nurse directs the UCP to do the following:

- Report when the patient has difficulty with feeding, coughing, gagging, respiratory distress, discomfort, or vomiting.

Equipment

- See Skills 32.1 through 32.4 and Procedural Guideline 32.1 for lists of equipment.
- Log in which to record daily weights, I&O, temperature, and feeding residuals

STEP	RATIONALE
ASSESSMENT	
1. Identify patient using at least two person-specific identifiers during first home visit. Facial recognition can be used as one of two identifiers for ongoing subsequent home visits.	Ensures correct patient. Complies with Accreditation Canada's standards and improves patient safety (Accreditation Canada, 2020).
2. Throughout the procedure, the 4 moments for hand hygiene are to be implemented; hand hygiene should occur before initial patient (or patient environment) contact, before an aseptic procedure, after body fluid exposure risk, and after patient (or patient environment) contact. Additional hand hygiene should be performed when hands are visibly soiled.	Proper hand hygiene helps prevent the spread of infectious agents to health care providers.
3. Assess patient's current health status and tolerance of enteral feedings (if already being administered).	Determines whether any changes are needed in feeding schedule.
4. Assess patient's and caregiver's physical function (i.e., vision, fine motor skills). Also assess emotional, financial, and community resources.	Determines patient's and caregiver's ability to manipulate equipment. Availability of resources increases ability to manage self-care at home.
5. Assess environmental conditions of home (sanitation, storage of equipment, work area, supplies, and power source).	Determines whether home environment is safe for enteral feeding, with minimal risks for infection and complications.
6. Assess patient's and caregiver's understanding of the purpose of enteral feedings and positive expected outcomes.	Understanding the rationale of treatment is critical to enhancing participation and cooperation in care.
7. Assess patient's and caregiver's understanding of storage and management of equipment and supplies and where and how to obtain supplies.	Ensures safe home management and decreases risk of complications. Home care delivery companies usually deliver a month's supply at a time. If the patient stores feeding containers in the garage, the containers must be brought into the house a couple hours before use in colder months to be warmed to room temperature (Canadian Cancer Society, 2019). The garage is not a good storage place during hot weather; the basement should be used, if possible.
8. Assess patient's learning readiness and ability to concentrate (consider presence of pain, nausea, or fatigue and patient interest in instruction) and learning style preference.	Presence of significant illness, frailty, or confusion affects a patient's ability to attend to a teaching plan. Indicates need to rely on caregiver for learning and implementation (if available) on a short- or long-term basis. Learning style affects the choice of teaching resources.
9. Observe patient or caregiver administer an enteral feeding (when already prescribed).	Determines which specific components of skill the patient or caregiver can complete easily and which ones are more difficult and require reinforcement.

NURSING DIAGNOSES

- Anxiety
- Insufficient knowledge regarding tube-feeding self-administration
- Reduced ability to self-feeding
- Inadequate nutrition
- Inadequate health maintenance
- Potential for aspiration

Related factors and risk factors are individualized on the basis of patient's condition or needs.

STEP	RATIONALE
PLANNING	
1. Expected outcomes following completion of procedure:	
• Patient or caregiver verbalizes purpose of enteral feedings and enhanced nutritional health.	Provides measurable criteria to determine level of cognitive understanding.
• Patient or caregiver demonstrates proper use of equipment and handling of formulas.	Provides demonstration of skills needed to manage home enteral nutrition.
• Patient or caregiver demonstrates accurate administration of enteral feedings and medications.	Provides demonstration of skills needed to administer home enteral nutrition and medications.
• Patient or caregiver verbalizes understanding of signs, symptoms, and management of complications of feeding.	Confirms that patient or caregiver has knowledge needed to respond when problems with feedings develop.
2. Prepare environment for teaching session: • Select a room that is well lit and has comfortable seating. • Be sure that the patient is close and can see the nurse clearly. • Control sources of noise and distractions.	Improves likelihood that patient and caregiver will be attentive to instruction. Room environment needs to minimize existing sensory alterations. A comfortable environment free of distractions increases a patient's attention.
IMPLEMENTATION	
1. Have patient or caregiver perform hand hygiene with you and explain the importance of skill.	Reduces transmission of microorganisms. Reinforces importance of infection control.
2. Discuss with patient or caregiver the purpose of enteral feeding and enhanced nutritional health.	Reinforces importance of regular feedings.
3. Help patient or caregiver determine a feeding schedule that will maintain nutritional requirements, fit within the patient's or caregiver's schedule, and fit the health care provider's prescription.	Promotes adherence to enteral nutrition therapy. A person-centred approach increases patient confidence in managing their own feedings.
Critical Decision Point *Explain that the caregiver needs to communicate with home health or the health care provider if any changes in feeding schedules are made to fit the daily routine.*	
4. Have patient or caregiver apply clean gloves with you. If a patient has a nasoenteral tube, demonstrate how to identify placement of feeding tube: aspirating gastric fluid, checking pH of gastric fluid, and acceptable pH range (see Skill 32.2).	Reduces transmission of microorganisms. Some nasally placed tubes are inadvertently placed in the respiratory system and migrate to the esophagus or into the respiratory tract. In these cases, check pH periodically. Aspirated secretions with low pH are a strong indicator of gastric placement. However, high pH cannot be used to differentiate between aspirated secretions obtained from respiratory and intestinal tube placements.
Critical Decision Point *Instruct patient or caregiver to avoid administration of all feedings, flushes, or medications if there is any doubt as to placement of the enteral feeding tube.*	
5. Observe how patient or caregiver demonstrate the placement of nasally placed tube.	Return demonstration identifies any areas for further teaching.
6. When the patient has a gastrostomy or jejunostomy tube, observe how patient or caregiver checks for GRV by having them aspirate gastric contents (Tatsumi, 2019). Have patient return aspirated contents to the stomach unless the volume exceeds 250 mL (see employer policy).	Checking gastric residual in a small-bore NG tube can easily lead to occlusion or displacement. GRV in the range of 200–500 mL should raise concern and lead to implementation of measures to reduce the risk of aspiration, such as changing from intermittent to continuous feedings, evaluating the possibility of decreasing opioid analgesics, and starting medication that enhances gastric motility (e.g., metoclopramide). Automatic cessation of feeding should not occur for GRV <500 mL in the absence of other signs of intolerance (Wen et al., 2019).
7. Discuss use of medical asepsis in setting up and changing administration sets, mixing formulas (do not add formula to hanging bag), refrigerating unused formula, limiting amount of formula "hung" at one time to the amount that can be infused in a 4- to 6-hour period (less time in warmer weather), and maintaining and caring for the bag.	Medical aseptic technique minimizes risk of microorganism contamination. Refrigeration and limiting "hang" time reduce growth of microorganisms. Changing administration sets every 24 hours reduces microorganism growth.

STEP	RATIONALE
IMPLEMENTATION	
8. Instruct patient or caregiver that the patient needs to sit up in a chair or have head of bed elevated at least 30 degrees, preferably 45 degrees, while receiving feedings or medications or when tube is flushed.	Decreases risk of aspiration. Aspiration is indicated by increased coughing, difficulty breathing, or increased sputum (Canadian Cancer Society, 2019).
9. Observe how the patient or caregiver mixes, administers, and stores formulas. Discuss flushing of tube after administration of feedings or medications.	Identifies competence and need for further teaching. Regular flushing of tube prevents clogging.
10. Observe how the patient or caregiver changes administration sets and clean bags. Have them dispose of supplies, remove gloves, and perform hand hygiene.	Reduces transmission of infection.
11. Observe how patient or caregiver administer medications and flush tube (see Skill 21.2).	Ensures that medications are given correctly.

Critical Decision Point *Verify that medications do not include any sublingual, enteric-coated, or sustained-release medications. These medications cannot be crushed for administration.*

STEP	RATIONALE
12. Discuss and observe use of infusion pump if patient is receiving continuous feeding.	Use of tube-feeding infusion pumps is complex and requires reinforcement.
13. Discuss measures to stabilize feeding tube in patients with abdominal tubes and how to clean and protect skin insertion site.	Prevents tube from dislodging and skin breakdown.
14. Provide contact information for ordering equipment and supplies or who to call in case of equipment failure.	Ensures that caregiver can respond in an emergency.
15. Discuss emergency plan and actions to take for signs and symptoms of aspiration, such as elevating head of bed, oral suctioning, and calling the health care provider.	Ensures understanding of management of equipment, supplies, emergency plan, and collaboration.
16. Provide patient with written summary of steps or a skills checklist in how to care for enteral nutrition to ensure understanding.	
17. Discuss who to contact and when for signs of diarrhea, constipation, or weight loss.	Provides support to patient or caregiver.

EVALUATION

1. Ask patient or caregiver to state the purpose of home enteral nutrition therapy.	Demonstrates cognitive learning.
2. Observe how patient or caregiver performs medical asepsis techniques, checks tube placement, aspirates residuals, administers medications and feedings, and uses and cleans equipment.	Demonstrates psychomotor learning.
3. Ask patient or caregiver to state the measures used to prevent complications (e.g., verification of tube position before each feeding, elevation of patient's head during feeding, stabilization and flushing of tubing).	Ensures safe home management and identification of areas for teaching.
4. Ask patient or caregiver how to care for cans of open formula.	Ensures safe home management of enteral nutrition and prevention of foodborne illness.
5. Use teach-back: "I want to be sure I explained how to manage problems that can occur with your tube feedings. Tell me how to manage nausea, stomach fullness, and diarrhea." Develop a revised teaching plan if patient or caregiver is unable to teach back correctly.	Determines patient's and caregiver's level of understanding of instructional topic.

Unexpected Outcomes	Related Interventions
1. Feeding tube becomes displaced.	• Instruct patient or caregiver to stop feeding, note the time feeding was stopped, and notify the home care nurse. • The nurse or health care provider will reposition feeding tube and verify placement before initiating any enteral feeding.
2. Signs and symptoms of aspiration are present.	• Stop feeding. Raise head of bed. • Verify tube position. • Notify health care provider.

Unexpected Outcomes	Related Interventions
3. Patient develops diarrhea.	• Notify health care provider. • Use interprofessional collaboration (e.g., dietitian, health care provider) to consider a change in strength, type, or rate of enteral feeding or addition of soluble fibre; review medications; or use antidiarrheal medications.
4. Skin surrounding stoma breaks down, or drainage around insertion site develops.	• Clean stoma area more frequently. • Apply antibiotic ointment around stoma as prescribed. • Contact health care provider.

Communication and Documentation

- Document instructions given to patient and caregiver and their response in the home care record.
- Document specifics of enteral feeding plan, including type and size of tube in the home, formula, and amounts to be administered in specific time frames.
- Patient or caregivers need to document I&O, daily weights, amount of gastric fluid aspirated before each feeding (or every 4 hours if receiving continuous feeding), date and time of feedings, amount and type of formula, any additives, and date and time that administration sets are changed. Provide patient and caregiver with forms for recording details of feedings, weights, and quality and quantity of aspirates.

Special Considerations

Teaching

- Be aware of any cultural considerations that need to be incorporated into the teaching plan. A professional interpreter should be present for patients who have language barriers. All written materials (e.g., checklists and instructions) should be available in patient's preferred language.
- Performing a skill without a nurse in attendance provokes anxiety. Always leave a phone number and instructions on how to reach a home care nurse if needed.
- Teach patient and caregiver the maximum hang time for any enteral feeding. After a can of formula has been opened, it should remain at room temperature for no longer than 8 to 12 hours.
- If the patient has a nasoenteral tube, encourage frequent mouth care to prevent dryness of oral mucous membranes.

Pediatric

- Children are at risk for aspiration and fluid and electrolyte imbalance; thus, teach parents to monitor their child carefully (Hockenberry et al., 2024).
- Children who receive long-term home enteral feedings often experience developmental and growth delays. Other common problems include sleep disturbance, tube blockages, problems with delivery of equipment, and equipment malfunction. Therefore, these children require close follow-up and frequent nutritional monitoring.
- If a child is unable to sit up during or after a tube feeding, teach caregiver how to position the child on their right side during the tube feeding and for approximately 1 hour afterward (Hockenberry et al., 2024).

Gerontological

- Assess for changes and limitations in sensory function, mobility, or dexterity that indicate a need to teach a caregiver how to administer feedings.

✦ REVIEW QUESTIONS

A 72-year-old patient (he/him) was admitted to the acute stroke unit following a cerebral hemorrhage. As a result of the stroke, he has left-sided paralysis and is sometimes not responsive to verbal commands. He recognizes his family and at times has spoken a few words. The patient has been placed on nothing by mouth (NPO) status. The nutrition support team has recommended that he have a small-bore nasogastric (NG) feeding tube inserted for nutritional support. A continuous tube feeding of Isosource HN has been prescribed to run at 55 mL/hr.

Review Questions 1 to 4 relate to the case study presented here.

1. The patient is now ready for his NG tube insertion. Place the following steps in the correct order:
   1. Have patient swallow sips of water while advancing tube past nasopharynx.
   2. Perform hand hygiene.
   3. Tape or clip tube to gown to prevent pulling.
   4. Secure tube to nose.
   5. Measure to determine length of tube to be inserted.
   6. Apply pulse oximeter and measure vital signs.
   7. Obtain radiographic film to determine proper tube placement.
2. Before the patient's first feeding, the nurse aspirates a gastric residual volume of 150 mL. What is the correct nursing action? (*Select all that apply.*)
   1. Consult the registered dietitian.
   2. Stop the feeding immediately.
   3. Continue tube feeding as prescribed.
   4. Discard the gastric aspirate withdrawn through the tube.
   5. Continue to assess for feeding tolerance.
3. The nurse has just inserted an NG tube in the patient's left naris to be used for the purpose of receiving enteral feedings. Identify the appropriate documentation by the nurse for this procedure.
   1. 18 Fr NG tube inserted into the left naris, tube, patient tolerated well, feeding infusing.
   2. 18 Fr NG tube inserted as prescribed, radiographic film obtained and tip is positioned in stomach, both nares are in good condition and intact, and feeding infusing.
   3. 18 Fr NG tube inserted into the left naris, patient tolerated procedure with minimal discomfort, the left naris is intact with no skin breakdown or redness noted, X-ray called and confirmed that the tip of the tube is located in the stomach.

4. 18 Fr NG tube inserted for the first time by the nurse, patient tolerated procedure well, gastric pH was noted to be 5.0, NG tube secured to gown, and feeding infusing.

4. The patient has received feedings for about 12 hours. Four hours ago, the gastric residual volume (GRV) was 200 mL. The nurse is conducting rounds and learns that the patient feels nauseated. Approximately 60 mL of vomitus is in the patient's emesis basin at the bedside. The nurse assesses the patient's abdomen to find that it is tender to touch and distended. Bowel sounds are decreased. The nurse aspirates 300 mL of gastric contents that have the appearance of formula. How does the nurse communicate this situation using SBAR (situation–background–assessment–recommendation)?

5. Which of the following is the most reliable method of verifying the location of blindly inserted feeding tubes?

1. pH testing of fluid withdrawn through the tube
2. Auscultating over the epigastrium while instilling air through the tube
3. Observing the colour and appearance of fluid aspirated through the tube
4. Obtaining radiographic confirmation of tube placement

6. A patient is receiving an enteral feeding. What interventions should the nurse include in the plan of care? (*Select all that apply.*)

1. Ensuring that the central line dressing is occlusive
2. Making sure the total parenteral nutrition (TPN) formula is at room temperature before beginning the infusion
3. Elevating the head of the bed to at least 30 degrees
4. Assessing the capillary blood glucose level prior to the infusion
5. Flushing the feeding tube with sterile water before and after each feeding

7. Which responsibilities can a nurse delegate to an unregulated care provider (UCP)? (*Select all that apply.*)

1. Checking respirations or patient symptoms of shortness of breath, coughing, or choking
2. Verifying tube placement
3. Performing oral hygiene
4. Inspecting skin around the insertion site for irritation or excoriation

Visit the Evolve site for a complete list of answers to the Review Questions.

NEXT GENERATION NCLEX® (NGN)

For practice with answering exam questions related to unfolding NGN case studies, please consult the Next Generation NCLEX® (NGN)-Style Case Studies for Skills and Techniques on the Evolve website: http://evolve.elsevier.com/Canada/Perry/clinicalskills/

REFERENCES

Accreditation Canada. (2020). *Required organizational practices–2020 handbook*. https://physicians.nshealth.ca/resources/required-organizational-practices-2020-handbook.

American Association of Critical-Care Nurses. (2016). *Feeding tube placement*. [Seminal Reference]. https://www.aacn.org/newsroom/feeding-tube-placement

Bandy, K. S., Albrecht, S., Parag, B., et al. (2019). Practices involved in the enteral delivery of drugs. *Current Nutrition Reports*, *8*(4), 356–362. https://doi.org/10.1007/s13668-019-00290-4

Bear, D. E., Hart, N., & Puthucheary, Z. (2018). Continuous or intermittent feeding: Pros and cons. *Current Opinion in Critical Care*, *24*(4), 256–261. https://doi.org/10.1097/MCC.0000000000000513

Bischoff, S. C., Austin, P., Boeykens, K., et al. (2022). ESPEN practical guideline: Home enteral nutrition. *Clinical Nutrition*, *41*(2), 468–488. https://doi.org/10.1016/j.clnu.2021.10.018

Bloom, L., & Seckel, M. A. (2022). Placement of nasogastric feeding tube and postinsertion care review. *AACN Advanced Critical Care*, *33*(1), 68–84. https://doi.org/10.4037/aacnacc2022306

Boullata, J. I., Harvey, L., Mays, A., et al. (2017). ASPEN safe practices for enteral nutrition therapy. *Journal of Parenteral and Enteral Nutrition*, *41*(1), 15–103. https://doi.org/10.1177/0148607116673053

Bukhari, A., Taslim, N. A., As'ad, S., et al. (2020). Comparison of different early enteral feeding formulas on critically ill patients. *Journal of Nutritional Science and Vitaminology*, *66*(Suppl. 1), S2–S10. https://doi.org/10.3177/jnsv.66.S2

Canadian Cancer Society. (2019). *Tube feeding and intravenous (IV) nutrition*. https://cancer.ca/en/treatments/tests-and-procedures/tube-feeding-and-intravenous-iv-nutrition

Caramia, R. (2018). Commentary on intracranial placement of a nasogastric tube in a non-trauma patient. *Journal of Intensive and Critical Care*, *4*(1), 5. https://doi.org/10.21767/2471-8505.100108

Cortez, A., Makker, K., Kramer, D. F., et al. (2018). Maternal milk feedings reduce sepsis, necrotizing enterocolitis and improve outcomes of premature infants. *Journal of Perinatology*, *38*(1), 71–74. https://doi.org/10.1038/jp.2017.149

Gardner, L. A., & Wallace, S. (2021). Nasogastric tube placement: A cross-comparison of verification methods used in Pennsylvania hospitals and how they align with guidelines. *Patient Safety*, *3*(3), 37–45. https://doi.org/10.33940/med/2021.9.4

Guenter, P., & Lyman, B. (2020). Safer enteral nutrition syringes. *Patient Safety*, *2*(4), 58–61. https://doi.org/10.33940/med/2020.12.4

Healthcare Excellence Canada. (2009). *The safety competencies: Enhancing patient safety across the health professions*. https://www.patientsafetyinstitute.ca/en/toolsResources/safetyCompetencies/Documents/CPSI-SafetyCompetencies_EN_Digital.pdf

Hockenberry, M. J., Duffy, E. A., & Gibbs, K. (2024). *Wong's nursing care of infants and children* (12th ed.). Elsevier.

The Hospital for Sick Children. (2021). *HINT: How often do enteral feed bags need to be changed?* https://www.connectedcare.sickkids.ca/quick-hits/2020/02/07/how-often-do-enteral-feed-bags-need-to-be-changed

Institute for Safe Medication Practices Canada. (2013). *Safety bulletin: Some liquid medications may be unsuitable for administration by enteral tube*. https://ismpcanada.ca/wp-content/uploads/ISMPCSB2013-05_LiquidMedicationsEnteralTube.pdf

Judd, M. (2020). Confirming nasogastric tube placement in adults. *Nursing*, *50*(4), 43–46. https://doi.org/10.1097/01.NURSE.0000654032.78679.f1

Lakananurak, N., Nalinthassanai, N., Suansawang, W., et al. (2020). Optimal hang time of enteral formula at standard room temperature and high temperature. *World Journal of Clinical Cases*, *8*(19), 4410–4415. http://dx.doi.org/10.12998/wjcc.v8.i19.4410

London Health Sciences Centre. (2018). *Enteral feeding*. https://www.lhsc.on.ca/critical-care-trauma-centre/enteral-feeding

London Health Sciences Centre. (2020). *Standard of care enteral feeding tubes and nutrition*. https://www.lhsc.on.ca/critical-care-trauma-centre/standard-of-care-enteral-feeding-tubes-and-nutrition

London Health Sciences Centre. (2021). *Procedure: Insertion of an oral/nasal small bowel feeding tube*. https://www.lhsc.on.ca/critical-care-trauma-centre/procedure-insertion-of-an-oral/nasal-small-bowel-feeding-tube

Lord, L. M. (2018). Enteral access devices: Types, function, care, and challenges. *Nutrition in Clinical Practice*, *33*(1), 16–38. https://doi.org/10.1002/ncp.10019

Medline. (n.d.). *ENFit® enteral feeding connectors*. https://www.medline.com/capabilities/clinical-nutrition/enteral-feeding-connectors/

Metheny, N. A., Krieger, M. M., Healey, F., et al. (2019). A review of guidelines to distinguish between gastric and pulmonary placement of nasogastric tubes. *Heart & Lung*, *48*(3), 226–235. https://doi.org/10.1016/j.hrtlng.2019.01.003

Northington, L., Kemper, C., Rempel, G., et al. (2022). Evaluation of methods used to verify nasogastric feeding tube placement in hospitalized infants and children—A follow-up study. *Journal of Pediatric Nursing*, *63*, 72–77. https://doi.org/10.1016/j.pedn.2021.10.018

Pitta, M. R., Campos, F. M., Monteiro, A. G., et al. (2019). Tutorial on diarrhea and enteral nutrition: A comprehensive step-by-step approach. *Journal of Parenteral and Enteral Nutrition*, *43*(8), 1008–1019. https://doi.org/10.1002/jpen.1674

Powers, J., Brown, B., Lyman, B., et al. (2021). Development of a competency model for placement and verification of nasogastric and nasoenteric feeding tubes for adult hospitalized patients. *Nutrition in Clinical Practice*, *36*(3), 517–533. https://doi.org/10.1002/ncp.10671

Tatsumi, H. (2019). Enteral tolerance in critically ill patients. *Journal of Intensive Care*, *7*, 30. https://doi.org/10.1186/s40560-019-0378-0

VanBlarcom, A., & McCoy, M. A. (2018). New nutrition guidelines: Promoting enteral nutrition via a nutrition bundle. *Critical Care Nurse*, *38*(3), 46–52. https://doi.org/10.4037/ccn2018617

Walldorf, J., Michl, P., & Krug, S. (2020). The nasogastric tube is stuck—and causes coughing and dyspnoea: A rare complication. *Intensive and Critical Care Nursing*, *57*, 102786. https://doi.org/10.1016/j.iccn.2019.102786

Wen, Z., Xie, A., Peng, M., et al. (2019). Is discard better than return gastric residual aspirates? A systematic review and meta-analysis. *BMC Gastroenterology*, *19*, 113. https://doi.org/10.1186/s12876-019-1028-7

Yasuda, H., Kondo, N., Yamamoto, R., et al. (2021). Monitoring of gastric residual volume during enteral nutrition. *Cochrane Database of Systematic Reviews*, *2021*(9), Article No. CD013335. https://doi.org/10.1002/14651858.cd013335.pub2

Zakaria, A., Taema, K. M., Ismael, M. S., et al. (2018). Impact of a suggested nursing protocol on the occurrence of medical device-related pressure ulcers in critically ill patients. *Journal of Nursing and Midwifery*, *9*(4), 924–931. https://doi.org/10.15452/CEJNM.2018.09.0025

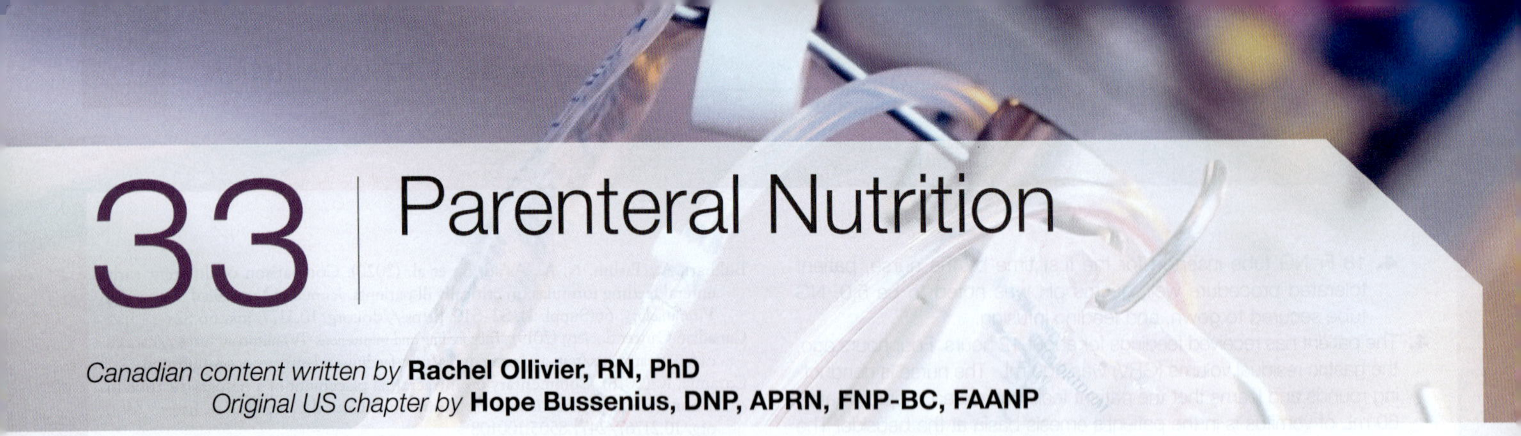

33 | Parenteral Nutrition

Canadian content written by **Rachel Ollivier, RN, PhD**
Original US chapter by **Hope Bussenius, DNP, APRN, FNP-BC, FAANP**

SKILLS AND PROCEDURES

OBJECTIVES

Mastery of content in this chapter will enable the nurse to:

- Describe the purpose and components of parenteral nutrition (PN).
- Identify patients who are candidates for PN.
- Describe the risks associated with PN.
- List the monitoring procedures used for patients receiving PN.
- Identify measures used to prevent complications of PN.
- Demonstrate appropriate nursing care and use of safe precautions when caring for a patient receiving PN.
- Implement and evaluate evidence-informed learning strategies that support patients' abilities to care for themselves when administering PN in the home setting.

MEDIA RESOURCES

- http://evolve.elsevier.com/Canada/Perry/clinicalskills/

PURPOSE

Parenteral nutrition (PN) is a specialized form of nutritional support that is administered intravenously via an infusion pump to patients who are unable to receive nutrients by mouth or through the digestive system. For example, PN may be appropriate for patients recovering from bowel surgery, a bowel obstruction, or severe malnutrition (refer to Box 33.1 for a complete list of indications). PN may be referred to as total parenteral nutrition (TPN) or total nutrient admixture (TNA). In addition, in the community setting, PN meets long-term nutritional needs through infusions if gastrointestinal (GI) issues are expected to be long term (months to years) (Box 33.1).

STANDARDS OF CARE

- Infusion Nurses Society (Gorski et al., 2021)—*Infusion Therapy Standards of Practice*, 8th edition (https://doi.org/10.1097/NAN.0000000000000396)
- Institute for Safe Medication Practices (2015)—*Safe Practice Guidelines for Adult IV Push Medications* (https://www.ismp.org/guidelines/iv-push)
- O'Grady et al. (2002)—*Guidelines for the Prevention of Intravascular Catheter-Related Infections* (https://www.cdc.gov/mmwr/preview/mmwrhtml/rr5110a1.htm)

PRINCIPLES FOR PRACTICE

- PN is used when the GI tract is not sufficiently functional. PN is delivered through a catheter placed in a central venous line in a vein in the arm, neck, or chest. The tip lies within the proximal third of the superior vena cava, the inferior vena cava, or the right atrium, allowing delivery of fluids directly into the bloodstream. Central venous catheters can also be used for the delivery of medication. TPN means that all daily nutritional requirements are received intravenously.
- Peripheral parenteral nutrition (PPN) is delivered through a vein other than the superior vena cava (e.g., cephalic vein). PPN can be used on a short-term basis for up to 2 weeks in circumstances where central venous access is not safe or possible (Worthington et al., 2017). PPN solutions must have an osmolarity of no greater than 900 mOsm/L (Worthington et al., 2017).
- For patients with short-term GI dysfunction, the goal is to provide nutritional requirements while minimizing PN-related complications until patients can resume full oral diets or meet their needs with enteral tube feedings. PN is not intended for the purpose of meeting hydration or fluid needs (Guenter et al., 2018).
- The type of catheter to use for administration of PN depends on patient factors and the expected length of PN therapy. The location of the catheter is defined on the basis of where the distal tip of the catheter lies. Concentrated PN solutions are diluted quickly when infused into a large-diameter central vein (Fig. 33.1).
- Patients who self-administer their PN solutions in the community (see Skill 33.3) will require a central catheter, which may be an implanted subcutaneous port, a peripherally inserted central catheter (PICC), or a tunnelled central access device (Fig. 33.2; see Chapter 29).
- Patients who require PN infusions do so for medical or surgical conditions that are often associated with GI losses (e.g., obstruction, diarrhea, fistula) and organ dysfunction; therefore, electrolyte monitoring is paramount. PN-associated liver disease is a potential complication of nutritional therapy in critically ill

BOX 33.1

Indications for Parenteral Nutrition

Nonfunctional GI Tract
- Small bowel resection
- Small bowel surgery or GI bleed
- Paralytic ileus
- Intestinal obstruction
- Trauma to abdomen, head, or neck
- Severe malabsorption
- Intolerance to slow rates of enteral tube feeding
- Chemotherapy, radiation therapy, bone marrow transplantation
- Severely catabolic patients when GI tract is not functioning for more than 7 days

Gastrointestinal Tract Malfunctional Status
- Enterocutaneous fistula
- Inflammatory bowel disease
- Severe diarrhea
- Moderate-to-severe pancreatitis

Preoperative Parenteral Nutrition
- Preoperative bowel rest
- Severe malnutrition before surgery

GI, Gastrointestinal tract.

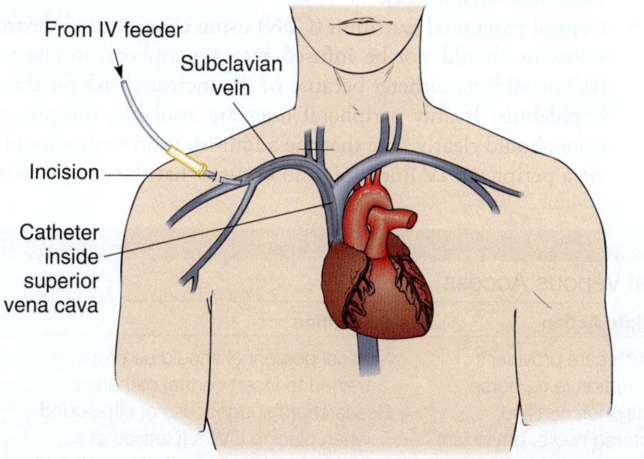

FIG 33.1 Placement of central venous catheter inserted into subclavian vein. ***IV,*** **Intravenous.** (*Courtesy Rolin Graphics.*)

patients, with some patients experiencing liver function deterioration so severe that they may require a liver transplant (Żalikowska-Gardocka & Przybyłkowski, 2020). Thus, a typical laboratory panel ordered for patients receiving PN infusions would include a baseline assessment of electrolytes, serum proteins, complete blood count, triglyceride level, and liver function (Box 33.2).

- The components of the PN solution are amino acids, glucose, and lipids as energy sources, with the addition of electrolytes, minerals, trace elements, vitamins, and water. The addition of a lipid emulsion to the PN solution results in a preparation called a *3:1, 3-in-1,* or *total nutrient admixture (TNA).*
- Because hyperglycemia has been linked to increased infection rates, monitoring blood glucose levels during a PN infusion is important. If possible, PN should not be interrupted to perform routine care or to transport the patient for diagnostic studies (Guenter et al., 2018).
- When the goal is to prepare a patient for a cyclic infusion of PN in the community, glucose levels should be monitored approximately 2 hours after an infusion begins (peak level) and 2 hours after it ends (trough level) to evaluate the need for adding regular human insulin to the infusion bag.

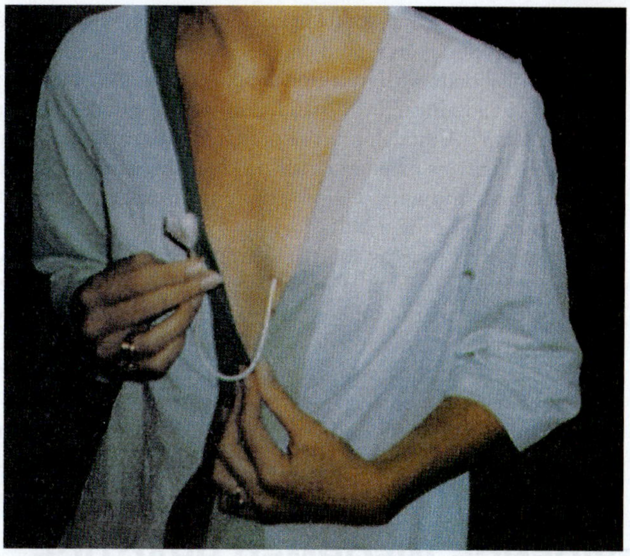

FIG 33.2 Tunnelled catheter used for home central parenteral nutrition. (*From Morgan, S. L., & Weinsier, R. L. [1998]. Fundamentals of clinical nutrition [2nd ed.]. Mosby.*)

BOX 33.2

Typical Monitoring and Laboratory Prescriptions for Patients With Parenteral Nutrition

Monitor
- Fluid intake, urine and gastrointestinal output every 8 hours
- Vital signs every 4 hours
- Glucose level every 6 hours for the first 48 hours of therapy
- Body weight at least three times weekly

Initial and Repeated Weekly
- Complete metabolic panel with sodium (Na), potassium (K), chloride (Cl), carbon dioxide (CO_2), glucose, calcium (Ca), phosphate (PO_4), magnesium (Mg), triglycerides, transaminases, liver function
- Complete blood count (CBC) with hemoglobin, hematocrit, white blood count (WBC), red blood cells (RBCs), lymphocyte count
- Serum proteins, often including albumin, transferrin, C-reactive protein, and/or prealbumin

Daily/Weekly
- Electrolyte panel daily until stable, then weekly
- If glucose levels have been stable for at least 48 hours since initiating parenteral nutrition (PN), glucose testing may then occur daily
- Glucose in preparation for cyclical PN in the community; monitor 2 hours after PN begins and 2 hours after PN ends; adjust insulin per prescriptions

Monthly or Biannually
- Trace elements such as zinc, copper, manganese, selenium (depending on underlying condition such as gastrointestinal issue or malabsorption) and for long-term community PN
- Selected vitamins for long-term community PN patients

- Since a PN solution is typically provided in response to GI issues and to support nutritional needs, it is important to monitor data that describe patient progress (see Box 33.2). Measurement and documentation of intake and output (I&O) enable the nurse to determine when a patient's GI function is changing and the adequacy of fluid intake from the PN solution.

PERSON-CENTRED CARE

- Promote person-centred care by including the patient and caregiver in discussions and decisions about patient autonomy, activities of daily living, individualized care planning, and socialization with friends and loved ones.

- Nurses collaborate with nutrition support teams and health care providers in administering PN and monitoring patients' response to PN therapy. Although practice patterns vary across employers, typically, dietitians or pharmacists provide advice on nutritional support goals and write PN prescriptions in collaboration with other members of the health care team.
- PN may pose concerns for self-identified members of ethnic groups or people with philosophical, religious, or spiritual beliefs that include restriction of animal products. The components of PN are largely synthetic and do not contain pork. The lipid emulsion contains egg phospholipid, a product that may not be appropriate for vegan patients.
- It is important to be mindful of the sense of loss that a patient may experience when unable to consume food, which may be culturally, socially, or religiously connected for some patients.

EVIDENCE-INFORMED PRACTICE

When critically ill patients cannot tolerate enteral nutrition, PN provides an alternative route for nutritional delivery. PN has a decreased infection rate when it is initiated early rather than later in a patient's care (Worthington et al., 2017). Key evidence-informed practice guidelines for the management of critically ill patients in critical care units (CCUs) include the following (Guenter et al., 2018):

- Enteral nutrition is preferred over PN for nutritional support (see Chapter 32).
- If the patient was healthy before the critical illness, with no evidence of protein calorie malnutrition, use of PN should be reserved and initiated only after the first 7 to 10 days of hospitalization, when enteral nutrition is not available.
- PN should be initiated only if the duration of administration is anticipated to be greater than or equal to 7 days.
- In patients stabilized on PN, efforts should be made to reintroduce oral or enteral nutrition.
- PN should not be terminated until at least 60% of energy and protein requirements are being met by the oral or enteral route.
- Initiating supplemental PN prior to this 7- to 10-day period in critically ill patients on some enteral nutrition does not improve outcomes and may be detrimental to patients.

SAFETY GUIDELINES

- Although the use of PN is an important technological advance that has led to improved care for patients with GI issues, a number of complications are associated with the therapy. The most frequent complication is catheter-related bloodstream infection (CRBSI), a risk that exists for both hospitalized patients and those with PN in the community (Table 33.1). It is essential to provide appropriate care of the vascular access device, dressing, and site to minimize CRBSI, including by avoiding blood draws and interruption of the infusions (Gorski, 2018; Gorski et al., 2021) (see Chapter 29).
- Central parenteral nutrition (CPN) using concentrated dextrose solutions should not be infused into a peripheral intravenous (IV) or midline catheter because of the increased risk for thrombophlebitis. If only peripheral lines are available, the prescriptions should clearly state that the administration route should be via a peripheral IV line; doing so ensures that the compounding

TABLE 33.1

Complications of Parenteral Nutrition and Associated Central Venous Access

Problem	Cause	Symptoms	Immediate Action	Prevention
Pneumothorax	Tip of catheter enters pleural space during insertion, causing lung to collapse	Sudden chest pain, difficulty breathing, decreased breath sounds, cessation of normal chest movement on affected side, tachycardia	Per health care provider's prescription (e.g., nurse practitioner, certified registered nurse, physician) may remove the central catheter. Administer oxygen. Insert chest tube to remove air under water-seal drainage or dry one-way valve system.	Medical personnel should be properly trained to insert central catheters. Researchers suggest use of ultrasound when placing CVCs (Gottlieb et al., 2017; Gorski, 2018). Catheter should be secured properly to prevent migration and movement.
Air embolism	IV tubing disconnected; part of catheter system open or removed without being clamped	Sudden respiratory distress: decreased oxygen saturation levels, shortness of breath, coughing, chest pain, decreased blood pressure	Clamp catheter; position patient in left Trendelenburg's position; call health care provider; administer oxygen as needed (Gorski, 2018; Gorski et al., 2021).	Make sure that all catheter connections are secure; clamp catheter when not in use. Never use a stopcock with a CVC. Unless contraindicated, instruct patient in Valsalva manoeuvre for tubing changes (Gorski, 2018; Gorski et al., 2021).
Localized infection (exit site or tunnel)	Poor aseptic technique in removal of skin flora during site preparation and dressing care	*Exit site:* Erythema, tenderness, induration, or purulent drainage within 2 cm (0.8 inches) of skin at exit site *Tunnel:* Same as above but extends beyond 2 cm (0.8 inches) from exit site	Call health care provider. *Exit:* Apply warm compress, provide daily care of site, give oral antibiotics. *Infection:* Collaborate with health care provider regarding removal of catheter (Gorski, 2018; Gorski et al., 2021). *Tunnel:* Remove catheter.	Provide catheter site care using aseptic technique, visually inspect site (including cleaning site), applying new stabilization device, and applying sterile dressing. Change transparent dressings at least every 5–7 days and gauze dressings every 48 hours. Change dressing if damp, loosened, or soiled or when inspection of site is necessary. Use chlorhexidine wipes to cleanse site (Gorski, 2018; Gorski et al., 2021).

TABLE 33.1

Complications of Parenteral Nutrition and Associated Central Venous Access—cont'd

Problem	Cause	Symptoms	Immediate Action	Prevention
Catheter-related sepsis or bacteremia	Catheter hub contamination; contamination of infusate; spread of bacteria through bloodstream from distant site	*Systemic:* Isolation of same microorganism from blood culture and catheter segment, with patient showing fever, chills, malaise, elevated white blood cell count	*Systemic:* Do not exceed hang time of 24 hours for PN that contains dextrose and amino acids, either alone or with fat emulsion added as a 3-in-1 formulation (Gorski, 2018;Gorski et al., 2021). Administer antibiotics intravenously; remove catheter per prescription.	Use full sterile-barrier precautions during catheter insertion and dressing change (Gorski, 2018; Gorski et al., 2021). Do not disconnect tubing unnecessarily. Replace IV tubing and filter every 24 hours. In certain situations, it is necessary to change administration sets with each new PN container (Gorski, 2018; Gorski et al., 2021).
Hyperglycemia	Possible blood-draw error, confirm with bedside glucose device; patient receiving too little insulin (if it is included) in PN solution; receiving steroids; new-onset infection	Excessive thirst, urination, blood glucose >8.9 mmol/L, confusion	Call health care provider for prescription; may need to slow infusion rate.	Review medical history for blood drawn through central line with PN infusing (repeat peripheral blood draw or obtain reading using finger lancet device), glucose intolerance or diabetes, new infection, new medication such as steroids; keep rate as prescribed; never increase PN to "catch up." Maintain blood glucose in range prescribed by health care provider. Use aseptic technique and routine blood glucose monitoring.
Hypoglycemia	PN abruptly discontinued; too much insulin (if it is included in the solution)	Patient is shaky, dizzy, nervous, anxious, hungry; blood glucose <4.4 mmol/L	Call health care provider; if PN discontinued abruptly, may need to restart $D_{10}W$ at previous PN rate (check employer policy). Perform blood glucose monitoring; retest in 15–30 minutes.	Decrease PN, "tapering" gradually until discontinued; blood glucose monitoring is used to ensure adequate insulin.

CVC, Central venous catheter; *$D_{10}W$*, 10% dextrose in water; *IV*, intravenous; *PN*, parenteral nutrition.

TABLE 33.2

Comparison of Central Versus Peripheral Parenteral Nutrition Prescriptions

	Central Parenteral Nutrition	Peripheral Parenteral Nutrition
Osmolality	>600 mOsm/L	<900 mOsm/L (Worthington et al., 2017)
Route of administration	Central venous catheter	Small peripheral vein
Usual daily caloric intake	20–35 calories/kg/day	5–10 calories/kg/day
Usual daily volume (mL)	1 000–2 000	2 000–3 000
Fat emulsion	Minor caloric source	Major caloric source

pharmacy can prepare PPN with a lower osmolarity (Table 33.2), which requires the addition of fluid.

- PPN is used only for short-term situations (maximum of 10 to 14 days) or when there is the need for very low caloric requirements (Worthington et al., 2017). It is difficult to meet total nutrient requirements with PPN because of the limitation in the dextrose concentration that can be delivered peripherally and the inability to meet caloric goals without large volumes of solution.
- Many hospitals use PICCs, termed *PICC lines* (Fig. 33.3), which are typically placed by specially trained advanced vascular access teams or radiologists.

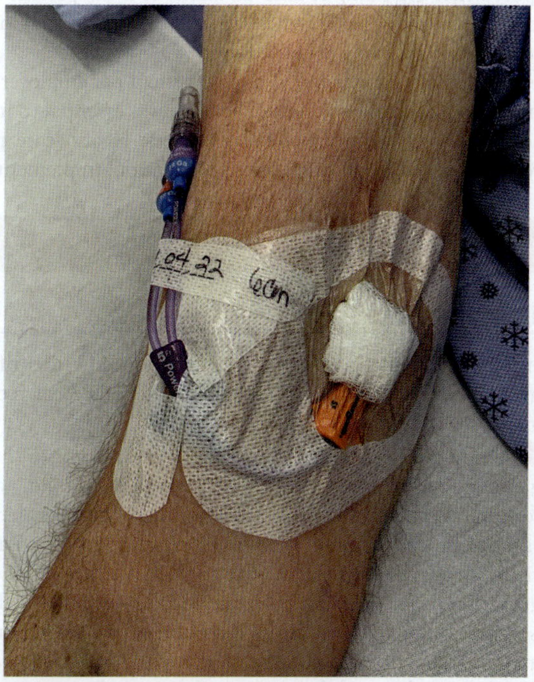

FIG 33.3 **Peripherally inserted central catheter (PICC). Note that the patient's skin appears reddened owing to the chlorhexidine solution applied during insertion.** (*Photo courtesy Rachel Ollivier, RN, PhD, Penticton Regional Hospital.*)

- Following central venous catheter insertion, PN should not be initiated until placement of a venous catheter tip is confirmed through a radiograph or the use of electrocardiographic (ECG) tip verification technology (Gorski, 2018; Gorski et al., 2021).

- Appropriate aseptic technique is needed when handling the central venous catheter (CVC) (or central line), dressings, tubing, and the needleless end-cap PN port (see Skill 29.6).
- PN without lipids can be infused using tubing with a 0.20- or 0.22-micron filter, and lipid-containing emulsions (3-in-1) can be infused using a larger 1.2-micron filter (Gorski, 2018; Gorski et al., 2021). Without a filter in place, particulate matter or large lipid droplets may enter a patient's bloodstream, potentially leading to a pulmonary embolism. The filter should be placed as close to the patient as possible to reduce the risk of patient harm due to particulates, microparticulates, microorganisms, and air emboli (Guenter et al., 2018).
- Malnourished patients receiving PN are at risk for *refeeding syndrome*, a condition in which some electrolytes (e.g., potassium [K], magnesium [Mg], and phosphorus [P]) may shift intracellularly in response to the glucose provided through PN, potentially resulting in low serum levels and risk for arrhythmias and muscle weakness. Adequate electrolyte repletion should occur before initiation of PN. There is also an increased risk of pulmonary edema and heart failure when initiating feeding in malnourished patients.
- Since there is a risk for bloodstream infection in patients with catheters, regular monitoring of temperature and the catheter insertion site is important.

✦ SKILL 33.1 Administering Central Parenteral Nutrition

Administration of CPN through a CVC (or central line) requires the use of strict aseptic technique and application of critical thinking. Because of the composition of PN fluids, patients can experience metabolic and fluid balance changes quickly. In addition, the clinical condition of patients receiving CPN may be poor, especially when they have compromised immunity, have severe underlying illnesses, and are either very young or very old. Nurses need to anticipate changes in a patient's condition that signal the development of complications. Similarly, nurses need to use good judgement to maintain the IV system and ensure that it is functioning properly.

Delegation and Collaboration

The skill of administering PN to a hospitalized patient cannot be delegated to an unregulated care provider (UCP). The nurse directs the UCP to do the following:

- Report when the pump sounds an alarm or if the patient experiences shortness of breath or headaches, weakness or shakiness, or discomfort or bleeding at the IV site
- Measure urinary output and weigh the patient per employer policy

In addition, interprofessional collaboration is essential to improving and promoting positive patient outcomes. Health care providers involved in assessment, diagnosis, consultation, implementation, procedures, monitoring, and evaluation may include registered nurses, licensed (registered) practical nurses, nurse practitioners, dietitians, social workers, physicians, surgeons, and pharmacists, to name a few. Members of these professions may be part of the nutrition support team. Dietitians and pharmacists are often directly involved with deciding the composition of the PN.

Equipment

- Medication administration record (MAR) or computer printout
- PN solution (IV)
- Electronic infusion device (EID) with anti–free-flow control and alarms (Gorski, 2018; Gorski et al., 2021)
- IV infusion tubing with Luer-Lok tip
- Appropriate IV filter (1.2-micron filter for 3-in-1 solutions or lipids containing a membrane that is particulate retentive and air eliminating; 0.20-micron filter for solutions that do not contain lipids) (Gorski, 2018; Gorski et al., 2021)
- 5- to 10-mL syringe with sterile saline flush
- Bedside glucose monitoring kit
- Adhesive tape or tubing label
- Antimicrobial swab
- Clean gloves
- Stethoscope

STEP	RATIONALE
ASSESSMENT	
1. Identify patient using at least two person-specific identifiers (e.g., name and date of birth, or name and medical record number) according to employer policy.	Ensures correct patient. Complies with Accreditation Canada's standards and improves patient safety (Accreditation Canada, 2020).
2. Throughout the procedure, the 4 moments for hand hygiene are to be implemented; hand hygiene should occur before initial patient (or patient environment) contact, before an aseptic procedure, after body fluid exposure risk, and after patient (or patient environment) contact. Additional hand hygiene should be performed when hands are visibly soiled.	Proper hand hygiene helps prevent the spread of infectious agents to health care providers.
3. Assess indications of and risks for protein/calorie malnutrition: weight loss from baseline or ideal, muscle atrophy or weakness, edema, lethargy, failure to wean from ventilatory support, chronic illness, and nothing by mouth (NPO) for more than 7 days. Confer with members of interprofessional team, such as the dietitian or health care provider.	These are clinical indications for PN. These baseline details provide a baseline from which change can be noted (Worthington et al., 2017).

STEP	RATIONALE
ASSESSMENT	
4. Assess vital signs, auscultate patient's lung sounds, inspect for edema of extremities, and measure patient's weight.	Provides baseline for monitoring patient's response to fluid infusion and nutrients. Crackles in lungs are early indication of fluid volume excess.
5. Assess medical record for levels of serum albumin, total protein, transferrin, prealbumin, and triglycerides, and check blood glucose level by finger lancet. Remove gloves and discard.	Provides baseline for measuring patient's nutritional status. In addition, nutritional baseline identifies patient's unique requirements, and PN admixture is tailored to patient's specific needs (Worthington et al., 2017). Serum glucose determines patient's baseline and tolerance of high levels of glucose in PN solution. Reduces transmission of microorganisms.
6. Assess patient's medical history for factors influenced by PN administration (electrolyte levels; renal, cardiac, and hepatic function). Assess for history of allergies.	Some patients require that CPN therapy be adapted by composition or volume (requires health care provider prescription), based on medical history. PN includes constituents (e.g., medications) to which patient may be allergic.
7. Consult with primary health care provider or nurse practitioner, pharmacist, and dietitian on calculation of calorie, protein, and fluid requirements for patient. Physicians and dietitians often work together to form specific prescriptions, although it is essential that interprofessional collaboration is implemented in patient care.	Provides interdisciplinary plan for patient's nutritional support.
8. Verify prescription for nutrients, minerals, vitamins, trace elements, electrolytes, added medications, and infusion rate. Check for compatibility of added medications.	CPN is often prescribed daily in a hospital setting after review of laboratory values. In a community setting, prescriptions may be obtained less frequently (e.g., weekly). Pharmacist that prepare parenteral solutions will check medication compatibility.
9. Assess patient's and caregiver's knowledge of PN, including any previous experience with community management.	Determines level and extent of instruction required.

NURSING DIAGNOSES

- Inadequate nutrition
- Insufficient fluid volume
- Excessive fluid volume
- Potential for unstable blood glucose level
- Potential for infection
- Insufficient knowledge regarding PN purpose and home management

Related factors and risk factors are individualized on the basis of patient's condition or needs.

STEP	RATIONALE
PLANNING	
1. Expected outcomes following completion of procedure:	
• Patient's ideal weight gain is between 0.5 and 1.5 kg (1–3 lb) per week.	Weight indicates patient's nutritional status and determines fluid volume. Weight gain >0.5 kg (1 lb) per day indicates fluid retention.
• Blood glucose levels are maintained per health care provider's prescription for desired glucose range.	Glucose levels needed for specific populations vary according to degree of illness; therefore, a specific prescription from the health care provider is required.
• Central venous access device (CVAD) is patent, and site is free of pain, swelling, redness, purulent drainage, and inflammation.	Ensures that PN is infusing into vein rather than into surrounding tissues and that there are no signs of an access device infection.
• Patient is afebrile.	Shows absence of systemic infection.
• Patient and caregiver are able to discuss purpose and steps for care of PN.	Proper instruction informs patient and caregiver and prepares them for community care if needed.
2. Explain purpose of PN to patient. Ensure that patient and caregiver have opportunity to ask questions or seek further information or clarification.	Promotes person-centred care through patient's understanding of and involvement in their care plan and treatment.
3. If PN solution is refrigerated, remove and let stand at room temperature 1 hour before infusion.	Ensures that solution is administered at room temperature.

STEP	RATIONALE

IMPLEMENTATION

STEP	RATIONALE
1. Check label on PN bag with health care provider's prescription on MAR or computer printout and patient's name. Also check any additives and note solution expiration date. Steps 2–6 may require an independent double-check by another registered nurse, depending on employer policy.	Prevents medication error. *This is the first check for accuracy.*
2. Inspect 2:1 PN solution for particulate matter. Inspect 3:1 PN solution for separation of fat into layer.	Presence of particulate matter or fat emulsion separation requires that solution be discarded.
3. Before leaving medication room, check IV solution a second time using the 10 rights of medication administration (see Chapter 20), including route and rate of delivery. Check label of PN bag against MAR or computer printout.	*This is the second check for accuracy.*
4. Take PN solution to patient in advance of previous solution's emptying. Compare names of solution and additives with MAR at bedside.	*This is the third check for accuracy.*
5. Apply clean gloves. Prepare IV tubing for PN solution:	Reduces transmission of microorganisms.
a. Attach appropriate filter to IV tubing.	Maintains sterility of solution. Air introduced into central circulation could result in air embolus, a fatal IV complication.
b. Prime tubing with PN solution, making sure that no air bubbles remain, and turn off flow with roller clamp (see Step 5b illustration; see Chapter 29). Some infusion pumps and IV tubing require that priming be done on the pump rather than by gravity.	
6. Wipe end port of CVAD (see Step 6 illustration) with alcohol swab and allow to dry. Then attach syringe of 0.9% sodium chloride (normal saline [NS]) solution to needleless port, aspirate for blood return, and flush saline per employer policy.	Scrubbing hub decreases number of microorganisms (Gorski, 2018; Gorski et al., 2021). Determines patency of IV device before infusing PN.
7. Remove syringe. Trace tubing to the body before making the connection (Guenter et al., 2018). Connect Luer-Lok end of PN IV tubing to end port of CVAD; for lines with multiple lumens, label tubing used for PN.	Ensures that tubing is securely connected to IV line. A dedicated line should be used for devices with multiple lumens. Labelling of high-risk catheters prevents connection with inappropriate tube or catheter.

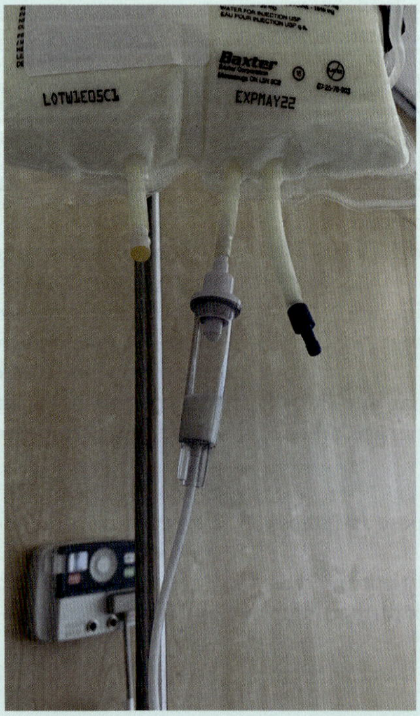

STEP 5B Primed tubing with 3:1 solution. (*Photo courtesy Rachel Ollivier, RN, PhD, Penticton Regional Hospital.*)

IMPLEMENTATION

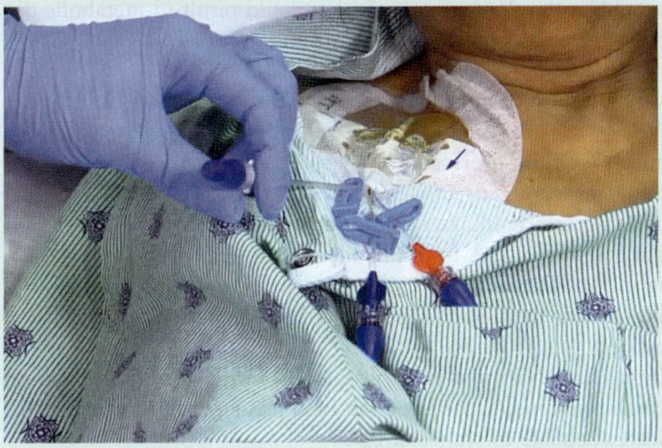

STEP 6 End port of central vascular access device (CVAD). *(From Elsevier. [2021]. Clinical skills: Essentials collection. Mosby.)*

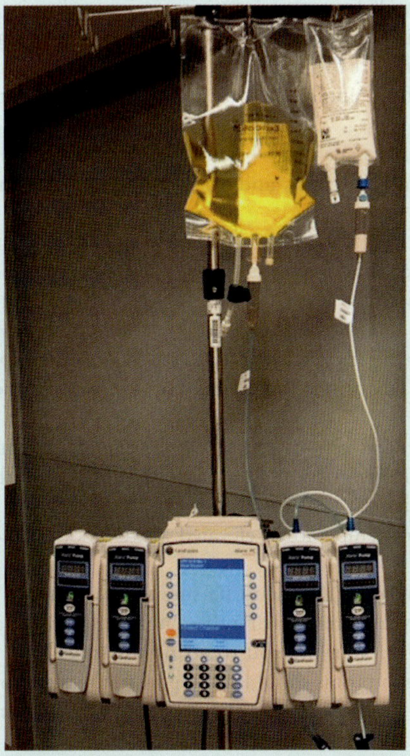

STEP 8 Parenteral nutrition solution infusing via infusion pump. *(Photo by Russell Flores, Vancouver General Hospital.)*

STEP	RATIONALE
8. Place IV tubing in EID. Open roller clamp. Set and regulate infusion rate as prescribed (see Step 8 illustration). Depending on employer policy, the infusion rate (per the prescription) may need to be double-checked by another nurse.	PN infusion rates are prescribed to meet patient's metabolic and electrolyte needs. Maintaining rates prevents electrolyte imbalances.
a. *Continuous infusion (optional):* Infusion rate is immediately set at prescribed rate and given over 24-hour period.	Ensures that blood glucose levels are maintained to prevent hypoglycemia or hyperglycemia (Guenter et al., 2018).
b. *Cycle infusion (optional):* Infusion rate is initiated at about 40–60 mL/hr, and the rate is gradually increased until patient's nutritional needs are met. Before completion of infusion, rate is decreased at about the same rate (mL/hour) until CPN is completed. The infusion is usually given over a shorter time frame (12–18 hours).	Infusion rates are usually increased and decreased to prevent hypoglycemia or hyperglycemia, respectively (Guenter et al., 2018).
9. Infuse all IV medications or blood through alternative IV site or multiple-lumen device. Do not obtain blood samples or central venous pressure readings through same lumen used for CPN.	Prevents drug incompatibility and IV device occlusion (Gorski, 2018).
10. Do not interrupt CPN infusion (e.g., with showers, transport to procedure, blood transfusion), and be sure that rate does not exceed prescribed rate (Guenter et al., 2018).	Prevents development of catheter-related bacteremia (Gorski, 2018; Gorski et al., 2021).
11. PN containing dextrose and amino acids alone or with fat emulsion added as a 3:1 formulation should have a hang time not to exceed 24 hours. Fat emulsions alone should have a hang time not to exceed 12 hours.	Prevents bacterial infection and deterioration of emulsion (Gorski, 2018; Gorski et al., 2021).
12. Change IV administration sets for PN every 24 hours and immediately on suspected contamination. Discard used supplies remove gloves.	Reduces transmission of infection.

STEP	RATIONALE
EVALUATION	
1. Monitor and document infusion rate according to employer policy. If infusion is not running on time, do not attempt to catch up; report this to the health care provider.	Too-rapid or too-slow rate of infusion could result in metabolic disturbances such as hyperglycemia and fluid overload.
2. Monitor fluid intake and urine and GI fluid output every 8 hours.	Prevents fluid imbalance from too-slow or too-rapid rate of infusion.
3. Measure vital signs every 4 hours or per employer policy.	Monitors for fluid overload response.
4. Obtain initial weight, and then weigh at least three times weekly.	Routine measurement of weights will reflect a gain/loss resulting from either caloric intake or fluid retention. Gradual weight gain, if weight gain is the goal, indicates adequate tolerance.
5. Evaluate for fluid retention; palpate skin of extremities; auscultate lung sounds.	Weight gain >0.5 kg (1 lb)/day, dependent edema, lung crackles, and intake greater than output per each 24-hour period indicate fluid retention.
6. Monitor patient's glucose levels every 6 hours (or as prescribed) and other laboratory parameters daily (or as prescribed).	Maintenance of normal electrolyte levels, satisfactory fluid balance, acceptable serum glucose levels, and improvement in serum proteins indicate adequate tolerance of PN.
7. Inspect central venous access site for signs and symptoms of swelling, inflammation, drainage, redness, warmth, tenderness, or edema.	Determines IV patency and absence of infection, infiltration, or phlebitis.
8. Monitor for temperature, elevated white blood cell count, and malaise.	Signs of systemic infection.
9. **Use teach-back:** "I want to be sure that I properly explained to you why you are receiving these nutrients and what signs to look out for. Why are you receiving this nutrition, and what signs and symptoms should you report to the nurse or doctor?" Develop a revised teaching plan if patient or caregiver is unable to teach back correctly.	Determines patient's or caregiver's level of understanding of instructional topic.

Unexpected Outcomes	Related Interventions
1. Redness, swelling, and tenderness are visible around the central venous access site, indicating possible exit site infection.	• Notify health care provider. • Apply a warm compress and initiate daily site care as prescribed. • Systemic antibiotic therapy may be started.
2. Patient develops fever, malaise, and chills, indicating systemic infection.	• Check exit site for signs of infection. • Notify health care provider and consult about need to obtain cultures of exit site or blood. • Systemic antibiotic therapy may be started.
3. Serum glucose level is >8.3 mmol/L or target set by health care provider.	• Notify health care provider. • Indicates intolerance of glucose load in PN solution. • May indicate new-onset infection. • Verify that blood draw was not contaminated by PN, or that proper procedures to interrupt PN and discard first blood draw were followed. • Indicates possible need for addition of insulin to PN, modification of PN solution, or sliding-scale insulin coverage.

Communication and Documentation

- Document condition of CVAD, rate and type of infusion, catheter lumen used for infusion, I&O, blood glucose levels, vital signs, and weights in progress notes in electronic health record (EHR) or chart.

DOCUMENTATION EXAMPLE

2-lumen PICC line to right arm is in situ at 7 cm from insertion site, dressing dry and intact, and patency confirmed per unit policy. No signs of infection noted to site. Infusion of 3:1 solution initiated per institutional policy at a rate of 48 cc/hr with access via purple lumen. I&O, blood glucose, and vital signs recorded on flow sheet.

- If signs of infection, occlusion, fluid retention, or infiltration occur, notify the health care provider.
- Document your evaluation of patient and caregiver learning.

DOCUMENTATION EXAMPLE

Patient teaching regarding indication for infusion was performed and verbal confirmation of understanding was received by writer using teach-back method.

Special Considerations

Teaching

- Provide patient and caregiver instruction on the purpose and goals of CPN. Keep them informed about daily care of the CVC and progress with treatment.
- Inform patient of signs of CVC infection to report to the nurse.

Pediatric

- Consider children's developmental needs when they are on long-term CPN. Perform regular assessments of development to determine child's progress. Implement interventions to encourage expected milestones (Hockenberry et al., 2024).

Gerontological

- Some older persons have impaired ability to tolerate higher fluid volumes because of cardiac or renal impairment.

Care in the Community: Home Management

- See Skill 33.3, Managing Parenteral Nutrition in the Home.

✦ SKILL 33.2 Administering Peripheral Parenteral Nutrition With Lipid (Fat) Emulsion

Video Clip

The administration of PPN requires a lower dextrose content and is intended for short-term use of 2 weeks or less, until central access can be achieved or the patient can be fed orally or enterally. Contraindications to the use of PPN include cardiac failure, severe liver disease, disorders of fat metabolism, uncontrolled diabetes mellitus, shock, and severe blood dyscrasias (Singh, 2023.). The PPN solution has lower concentrations of dextrose and amino acids to reduce osmolality (see Table 33.2) and the risk of phlebitis. Adding a lipid emulsion provides a source of calories with minimal impact on osmolality. A lipid emulsion must be administered through vented IV tubing as a primary IV infusion or a piggyback.

This skill describes piggyback administration of PPN. Administration sets (including piggybacks) used for fat emulsions are changed every 24 hours and immediately on suspected contamination (Guenter et al., 2018). The administration set must have a Luer-Lok design. Indications for PPN include the following:

- *Adequate peripheral access:* Despite its lower osmolality, PPN tends to cause phlebitis and often requires frequent changes in the access location. A midline catheter may be an alternative to the typical short peripheral catheter.
- *Ability to tolerate larger volumes of fluid:* Because of the lower concentration of dextrose in PPN, a larger volume of fluid is required to obtain adequate calories. Some patients with impaired renal or cardiac function do not tolerate PPN.
- *Ability to tolerate lipid emulsions:* Lipid is the most calorically dense nutrient. A 1-L volume of 10% dextrose without lipid provides only 340 calories. A 250-mL volume of 20% lipid solution provides 500 calories.

Delegation and Collaboration

The skill of administering PPN for a hospitalized patient cannot be delegated to a UCP. The nurse directs the UCP to report to the nurse the following:

- Patient indication of burning, pain, or redness at peripheral IV site.
- Infusion pump alarms or a moist IV site dressing.
- Patient complaints of shortness of breath.

Equipment

- MAR or computer printout
- PPN solution
- Lipid emulsion in a glass container or in a separate chamber, such as a prepared PN bag
- IV tubing for PPN with 0.20-micron filter for amino acid-dextrose solution
- IV tubing with a 1.2-micron filter for fat emulsion
- Bedside glucose monitoring kit
- Antimicrobial swab
- Electronic infusion pump with anti-free-flow control and alarms (Gorski, 2018; Gorski et al., 2021)
- Clean gloves
- Stethoscope

STEP	RATIONALE
ASSESSMENT	
1. Identify patient using at least two person-specific identifiers (e.g., name and date of birth, or name and medical record number) according to employer policy.	Ensures correct patient. Complies with Accreditation Canada's standards and improves patient safety (Accreditation Canada, 2020).
2. Throughout the procedure, the 4 moments for hand hygiene are to be implemented; hand hygiene should occur before initial patient (or patient environment) contact, before an aseptic procedure, after body fluid exposure risk, and after patient (or patient environment) contact. Additional hand hygiene should be performed when hands are visibly soiled.	Proper hand hygiene helps prevent the spread of infectious agents to health care providers.
3. Review medical record and assess patient for hypertriglyceridemia. Obtain prescriptions for serum triglyceride level before initiation of PPN and weekly.	Determines patient's ability to metabolize lipid.
4. Apply clean gloves. Select or initiate appropriate functional IV site to administer PPN and lipid emulsion. Assess its patency and function (see Chapter 29).	Reduces transmission of microorganisms. PPN may cause phlebitis; therefore, appropriate vein selection is important.
5. Determine patient's blood glucose level using a finger lancet device.	Provides baseline to determine patient's tolerance of glucose infusion.
6. Assess patient's fluid status by monitoring for edema in extremities, lung sounds, or fluid intake greater than fluid output.	Fluid intake given with PPN may cause fluid overload in older patients or those who have impaired renal or cardiac function.
7. Obtain patient's weight and vital signs. Remove gloves and discard.	Provides baseline information to determine effectiveness and tolerance of PPN solution. Reduces transmission of microorganisms.

STEP	RATIONALE
ASSESSMENT	
8. Check health care provider's prescription against MAR for volume of fat emulsion, PPN solution, and administration time for fat emulsion. Then check name of solution on label against MAR.	The health care provider must prescribe fat emulsions and PPN. Fat emulsions may cause adverse symptoms if infused too rapidly as a separate infusion. Infusion time is normally at least 8 hours. Fat emulsions should hang no longer than 12 hours as a separate infusion from original container. *This is the first check for accuracy.*
9. Read label of fat emulsion solution.	Lipid emulsions are white and opaque; thus, be sure to avoid confusing enteral tube-feeding formula with parenteral lipids.
10. Assess patient's and caregiver's knowledge of PPN.	Determines level and extent of instruction required.

NURSING DIAGNOSES

- Inadequate nutrition
- Excessive fluid volume
- Potential for unstable blood glucose level
- Potential for infection

Related factors and risk factors are individualized on the basis of patient's condition or needs.

STEP	RATIONALE
PLANNING	
1. Expected outcomes following completion of procedure:	
• Triglyceride level is <13.9 mmol/L in most patients.	Indicates adequate clearance of lipid.
• Blood glucose levels are maintained per health care provider's prescription for desired glucose range.	Glucose levels needed for specific populations vary according to degree of illness; therefore, a specific prescription from the health care provider is required.
• Venipuncture site is free of phlebitis, pain, swelling, redness, and inflammation.	Ensures proper administration and monitoring of PPN with lipids.
• Patient does not show signs of systemic infection (e.g., elevated temperature).	Temperature is indication of possible systemic infection related to PPN.
• Patient does not show signs of allergy to lipids.	Monitoring infusion requires observation for allergic response to infusion.
• Patient and caregiver are able to explain purpose of PPN and complications to watch for.	Proper instruction informs patient and caregiver.
2. Explain purposes of PPN and fat emulsion.	Promotes understanding and allows for clarification or questions.
3. Place patient in comfortable position for insertion of IV line or initiation of infusion. Explain associated procedures.	When patients are comfortable, they tolerate procedures more readily.
4. If PPN solution is refrigerated, remove and let stand at room temperature 1 hour before infusion.	Ensures that solution is administered at room temperature (Gorski, 2018).
IMPLEMENTATION	
1. Compare label of PN bag and lipid emulsion bottle with MAR or computer printout; check for correct additives and solution expiration date. Steps 2–5 may require an independent double-check by another nurse, depending on employer policy.	Prevents medication error. *This is the second check for accuracy.*
2. Examine lipid solution for separation of emulsion into layers or fat globules or presence of froth.	Do not administer if these elements appear, as procedure may result in development of a fat embolism.
3. Compare identifiers with information on solution bag label and patient's MAR or medical record at the bedside.	Ensures patient receives correct infusion. *This is the third check for accuracy.*
4. Measure patient's vital signs.	Provides baseline assessment. An immediate allergic reaction can develop once infusion begins.
5. Apply clean gloves. Prepare IV tubing for PPN solution; run solution through tubing to remove excess air. Turn roller clamp to "off" (clamped) position. Some infusion pumps and tubing require priming through the infusion pump. Add sterile capped needle or place sterile cap on end of tubing. Follow same procedure with separate infusion set for lipid infusion.	Reduces transmission of microorganisms. To prevent air from entering vascular system, clear all tubing.

STEP	RATIONALE
IMPLEMENTATION	
6. Wipe end port of peripheral IV infusion tubing with antimicrobial swab and allow to dry. Connect needleless connector at end of PPN tubing to end port of patient's functional peripheral IV line. Gently disconnect old PPN tubing from IV site and insert adapter of new PPN infusion tubing. Open roller clamp on new tubing. Allow solution to run to ensure that tubing is patent; regulate IV drip rate using electronic infusion pump.	Prevents disruption of existing IV infusion and ensures patent infusion. Pump will deliver infusion at prescribed rate.
7. Clean injection cap on needleless peripheral line tubing with antimicrobial swab.	Removes surface organisms at injection site and prevents organisms from entering blood system.
8. Attach fat emulsion infusion tubing to injection cap of IV line; Y-connector may be used if patient is receiving separate PPN and lipid infusions. Label tubing.	Fat emulsions cannot infuse through a 0.20-micron IV filter. Refer to employer policy; if larger 1.2-micron filter is used, lipids may be infused using a Y-connector (Gorski, 2018; Gorski et al., 2021). Labelling high-risk catheters prevents connection with an inappropriate tube or catheter.
9. Open roller clamp completely on fat emulsion infusion and check infusion rate on pump. This step may require an independent double-check by another nurse, depending on employer policy.	Initial slow infusion allows you to observe patient for an allergic response.
10. Infuse lipids initially at 1 mL/min for adults and 0.1 mL/min for a child for the first 15–30 minutes; increase rate as prescribed.	Up to 2.5 g fat/kg per day may be infused, but current practice is generally to give <1 g fat/kg body weight per day in adults.
11. Begin PPN at prescribed rate: 20% lipid solutions are infused over at least 8 hours. All lipids can hang for 12 hours as a separate infusion.	Rate of PPN administration does not need to be increased gradually. A lower concentration of dextrose allows most patients to tolerate a full administration rate without difficulty.
12. Remove and discard gloves and supplies.	Reduces transmission of microorganisms.
EVALUATION	
1. Monitor infusion rate routinely (hourly or more frequently if necessary).	Too-rapid or too-slow rate of infusion could result in metabolic disturbances such as hyperglycemia.
2. Measure vital signs and patient's general comfort level every 10 minutes for the first 30 minutes, then vital signs every 4 hours (or per employer policy).	Monitors patient for lipid allergy.
3. Monitor patient's laboratory values (e.g., triglycerides, liver function) daily and perform blood glucose monitoring as prescribed. Measure serum lipids 4 hours after discontinuing infusion.	Provides objective data to measure response to therapy (e.g., ability of liver to metabolize lipids). Measurement of lipids too soon after infusion will yield incorrect blood values.
4. Monitor temperature every 4 hours and regularly inspect venipuncture site for signs of phlebitis or infiltration.	Onset of fever is a sign of patient's intolerance to fat emulsion or sepsis. Determines integrity of IV system.
5. Evaluate patient's weight, I&O, condition of peripheral extremities (for edema), and breath sounds.	Weight gain, I&O imbalance, peripheral edema, and crackles in lungs indicate fluid retention.
6. Use **teach-back:** "I want to be sure that I properly explained the reasons for your nutrition fluid. Why are you receiving this type of nutrition?" Develop a revised teaching plan if patient or caregiver is unable to teach back correctly.	Determines patient's or caregiver's level of understanding of instructional topic.

Unexpected Outcomes	Related Interventions
1. Patient develops intolerance to fat emulsion, as evidenced by increased triglyceride levels, increased temperature, chills, flushing, headache, nausea and vomiting, diaphoresis, muscle ache, chest and back pain, dyspnea, pressure over eyes, or vertigo.	• Turn PPN infusion off. • Inform health care provider. • Prepare to treat anaphylactic reaction according to health care provider's prescriptions. • Record lipid allergy in patient's medical record.
2. See Unexpected Outcomes and Related Interventions for Skill 33.1.	

Communication and Documentation

- Document condition of IV site, type of solutions, rate and status of infusion, catheter lumen used for infusion, I&O, blood glucose levels, vital signs, weights, and other assessment findings in progress notes in EHR or chart on the appropriate flow sheets.

DOCUMENTATION EXAMPLE

18-gauge IV site to right cephalic vein (lower right arm) in situ, dressing dry and intact with no signs of infection or infiltration. Lipid solution is currently infusing at a rate of 60 cc/hr and the solution appears normal. The patient is tolerating the infusion well. I&O, blood glucose, and vital signs recorded on flow sheet.

- Document any adverse reactions in progress notes in EHR or chart.

DOCUMENTATION EXAMPLE

Upon assessment, patient reported headache, nausea, and chills. Oral temperature measured at 38.4°C. PPN infusion was immediately stopped, and Dr. Reynolds was notified.

- If signs of fat intolerance, infection, occlusion, fluid retention, or infiltration occur, notify the health care provider.
- Document your evaluation of patient and caregiver learning.

Special Considerations

Teaching

- PPN administration does not typically occur in the community unless the patient is in need of long-term nutritional support.

Pediatric

- See pediatric considerations for Skill 33.1.

Gerontological

- Some older persons may have fragile peripheral veins or poor fluid tolerance because of cardiac or renal dysfunction, making PPN an undesirable option.

Care in the Community: Home Management

- See Skill 33.3, Managing Parenteral Nutrition in the Home.

✦ SKILL 33.3 Managing Parenteral Nutrition in the Home

PN in the home is indicated for patients who cannot take adequate nutrition by mouth and when enteral feedings are contraindicated (e.g., cancer, chronic respiratory conditions, or GI disorders). Nurses who manage PN in the home collaborate frequently with dietitians to ensure that patients receive sufficient calories, protein, and fluid. Administering PN in the home requires an interprofessional approach and a patient and caregiver who demonstrate competency in its preparation and administration.

Usually, administration of PN in the home takes about 12 hours; thus, many patients choose to receive their PN during the night. Because of the risks involved with PN and because management in the home is complex, patients receive their first infusion in an acute care setting. After discharge, a home care nurse visits frequently. The home care nurse will need to carefully assess the reaction of the patient or caregiver to the use of the technology needed to administer PN at home and provide emotional support. Although administering PN in the home increases patients' autonomy, it often interferes with their ability to maintain their normal routines. Nurses need to work with the patient or caregiver in a person-centred manner to stress the benefits and offer support in dealing with related issues.

Delegation and Collaboration

The skill of managing PN in the home cannot be delegated to a UCP. The nurse instructs the UCP to do the following:

- Report findings of blood glucose monitoring
- Report vital signs outside of normal range
- Report if patient experiences shortness of breath, headache, weakness, or discomfort
- Report if the catheter dressings are wet or bleeding at the site

Equipment

- IV solution of PN
- IV tubing with optional filter
- Electronic IV infusion pump with anti–free-flow control and alarms
- Home blood glucose monitoring equipment
- Alcohol swabs
- Clean gloves
- Log

STEP	RATIONALE
ASSESSMENT	
1. Identify patient using at least two person-specific identifiers (e.g., name and date of birth, or name and medical record number) according to employer policy.	Ensures correct patient. Complies with Accreditation Canada's standards and improves patient safety (Accreditation Canada, 2020).
2. Throughout the procedure, the 4 moments for hand hygiene are to be implemented; hand hygiene should occur before initial patient (or patient environment) contact, before an aseptic procedure, after body fluid exposure risk, and after patient (or patient environment) contact. Additional hand hygiene should be performed when hands are visibly soiled.	Proper hand hygiene helps prevent the spread of infectious agents to health care providers.
3. Assess patient's ongoing nutritional status and risk for malnutrition by using a nutrition screening tool (see Chapter 31) and performing a physical examination. Identify signs and symptoms of malnutrition (e.g., weight loss or weight below ideal level; muscle atrophy, wasting, or weakness; lethargy; unable to eat for more than 6 days). Include measurement of vital signs.	Nutritional assessment helps in identifying a patient's baseline to determine their response to PN therapy.

STEP	RATIONALE

ASSESSMENT

STEP	RATIONALE
4. Assess patient's fluid status and electrolyte, serum albumin, total protein, transferrin, prealbumin, triglyceride, and glucose levels.	Provides additional baseline assessment data.
5. Assess patient's venous access device for edema, drainage, tenderness, and signs of inflammation (see Chapter 29). Measure circumference of the upper arm if the patient has a PICC; mark place on the arm where measurement was taken.	Infection is a common complication when a patient has a venous access device. Measurement of the arm helps to detect infiltration of the PICC. The mark on the arm ensures consistent measurements over time.
6. Verify health care provider's prescription for PN, including amino acids, dextrose, fat emulsions, vitamins, minerals, trace elements, electrolytes, and flow rate.	Ensures safe and accurate PN administration.
7. Assess patient's learning readiness, anxiety, and ability to concentrate (consider presence of pain, nausea, or fatigue and patient interest in instruction) and learning style preference.	Presence of significant illness, frailty, or confusion affects a patient's ability to attend to a teaching plan. Indicates need to rely on caregiver for learning and implementation (if available) on a short- or long-term basis. Learning style affects the choice of teaching resources.
8. Assess patient's or caregiver's previous knowledge and experience in managing PN in the home. Have patient or caregiver perform return demonstration if they are able to perform the skill.	Determines level of understanding before beginning teaching session.

NURSING DIAGNOSES

- Inadequate nutrition (less than body requirements)
- Anxiety
- Insufficient knowledge regarding PN
- Fatigue
- Readiness for improved nutrition
- Caregiver role strain
- Potential for infection
- Potential for social isolation

Related factors and risk factors are individualized on the basis of patient's condition or needs.

PLANNING

STEP	RATIONALE
1. Expected outcomes following completion of procedure:	
• Patient or caregiver can administer PN correctly.	Indicates that skills have been learned effectively.
• Patient or caregiver demonstrates proper care of the CVC.	Prevents infection and ensures patency of venous access device.
• Patient or caregiver explains how to properly store and maintain formulas for feeding.	Knowledge of infection control principles prevents foodborne illness.
• Patient or caregiver states signs and symptoms that need to be reported to health care provider.	Ensures safe administration of PN at home.
• Patient or caregiver demonstrates correct measurement of blood glucose.	Enables safe monitoring of patient's response to PN therapy.
2. Select setting in the home where patient is most likely to administer PN and that is conducive to a teaching session:	Practising in the same environment where the skill is routinely performed facilitates comprehension and learning.
• Select a room that is well lit with comfortable seating.	
• Be sure that the patient is close and can see the nurse clearly.	
• Eliminate sources of noise and distractions.	Room environment needs to minimize existing sensory alterations. A comfortable environment free of distractions increases patient's attention.

IMPLEMENTATION

STEP	RATIONALE
1. Provide the name and phone number of people or resources available 24 hours a day, 7 days a week, in case problems arise.	Provides assurance and allows patient or caregiver to troubleshoot problems and answer questions.
2. Explain the type and name of infusion, volume and infusion rate, expected outcomes, and components of PN. Explain that PN needs to be stored in refrigerator.	Allows patient or caregiver to verify that correct PN is infused and that patient or caregiver understands expected outcomes of care. Refrigeration maintains integrity of PN.
3. Have patient or caregiver perform each of the following steps with guidance from nurse. Do not rush them.	Allows you to correct errors in technique as they occur and discuss implications.

STEP	RATIONALE

IMPLEMENTATION

STEP	RATIONALE
4. Instruct patient or caregiver to inspect the IV solution bag label, ensure that patient's name is on the label, ensure that solution has not expired, and check bag for leaks.	Ensures that patient or caregiver knows how to check pharmacy-prepared solution to ensure the right patient receives right PN. Bag needs to be intact to maintain a closed system and to ensure that patient receives all prescribed nutrients.
5. Suggest taking PN solution out of the refrigerator for 30–60 minutes before scheduled infusion time.	Chilled solution often causes discomfort; allowing solution to come to room temperature enhances comfort during infusion.
6. Explain the need to inspect fluid in the bag for colour and precipitates.	Changes in colour or precipitates in bag indicate disruption in PN.

Critical Decision Point *Explain to patient that if they observe precipitate, separation of components of mixture, or colour changes, solution needs to be discarded.*

STEP	RATIONALE
7. Have patient or caregiver perform hand hygiene and apply clean gloves with you. Demonstrate how to attach IV tubing to bag, how to attach filter to IV tubing *(optional)*, how to prime IV tubing, and how to load IV tubing into the electronic infusion pump (see Chapter 29).	Reduces transmission of microorganisms. Prepares PN solution for IV administration.
8. Wipe CVC port with alcohol and show how to flush CVC and connect IV tubing to port (see Chapter 29). Use needleless system whenever possible.	CVC needs to be patent, and IV tubing needs to connect to CVC to allow PN to be administered. Needleless systems prevent needlestick injuries.
9. Explain how to determine the appropriate rate of infusion and program the infusion pump (see Skill 29.2). Caution patient and caregiver against changing rate to "catch up."	Ensures that PN is administered at the appropriate rate.
10. Have patient and caregiver remove and dispose of gloves; direct them to perform hand hygiene.	Prevents spread of microorganisms.
11. When infusion is completed, explain and demonstrate how to disconnect IV tubing and flush CVC (see Chapter 29). Ensure that patient or caregiver performs hand hygiene before and after disconnecting CVC.	Flushing CVC following infusion maintains patency of vascular access device. Meticulous hand hygiene prevents infection.
12. Describe appropriate use and storage of infusion pump and supplies. Explain appropriate tubing replacement schedules (e.g., every 24 hours for TNA, 72 hours for 3-in-1 solutions).	Maintains integrity of equipment; appropriate timing of tubing changes prevents infection.
13. Help patient develop a plan for appropriate disposal of supplies, including needles, syringes, and unused medications or solutions, using routine practices for preventing transmission of infection.	Implementation of routine practices is necessary to prevent transmission of communicable diseases and needle-stick injuries.
14. Demonstrate appropriate care of CVC site; discuss how to change dressings, frequency of dressing changes, and signs of infection (see Skill 29.6).	Prevents infection at CVC insertion site.
15. Teach patient and caregiver about signs and symptoms that indicate potential complications from PN therapy (e.g., infection and phlebitis at CVC site, refeeding syndrome, hyperglycemia, hypernatremia, hypophosphatemia, hypokalemia, hypomagnesemia) and when to call for help.	Knowledge of complications of PN therapy allows for early detection and appropriate action.
16. Demonstrate self-monitoring of blood glucose levels. Explain frequency of testing, normal glucose values, and what to do if values fall outside of the expected range (see Chapter 9).	PN increases blood glucose levels, which negatively affects patient outcomes. Frequent monitoring of glucose level helps detect problems early. Expect testing frequency to decrease as patient's condition and response to PN therapy stabilizes.
17. Provide patient with log for recording administration of PN, weights, I&O, and blood glucose levels.	Enables health care provider and patient to evaluate outcomes and detect adverse effects of nutritional therapy.
18. Help patient develop a plan to reorder supplies, PN fluid, and prescribed additives; a plan for emergencies (e.g., what to do if power goes out); and a home safety plan (e.g., how to get to bathroom without tripping over IV tubing).	Plans allow for continuous, safe, and effective administration of PN.

STEP	RATIONALE

EVALUATION

STEP	RATIONALE
1. Have patient or caregiver independently demonstrate initiation, infusion, and discontinuation of PN infusion and CVC site care.	Feedback through return demonstration of psychomotor skill is the best means of evaluating mastery of skill.
2. Watch patient or caregiver clean and store PN, equipment, and supplies.	Proper cleaning and storage help prevent bacterial growth.
3. Ask patient or caregiver to identify expected outcomes of nutritional therapy.	Measures patient's and caregiver's learning and confirms understanding of information.
4. Have patient or caregiver independently demonstrate blood glucose monitoring and recording.	Ensures mastery of skill needed for effective evaluation of patient status.
5. Watch patient or caregiver record information in log. Review patient's or caregiver's log periodically to ensure that information is being recorded correctly.	Health care providers make changes in patient care based on information provided by patient. To ensure that changes are made appropriately, the patient or caregiver needs to record accurate information.
6. Use teach-back: "I want to be sure I explained the common signs and symptoms of infection and other potential complications of PN. Tell me the signs and symptoms of infection to watch out for." Develop a revised teaching plan if patient or caregiver is unable to teach back correctly.	Determines patient's and caregiver's level of understanding of instructional topic.

Unexpected Outcomes	Related Interventions
1. Patient or caregiver is unable to manage home PN therapy or verbalize information that was taught.	• Ask patient or caregiver to describe difficulties experienced while performing skill. • Use a different teaching strategy. • Provide further teaching to caregiver and evaluate need to increase frequency of home visits to ensure safe administration of PN at home.
2. Patient or caregiver reports signs and symptoms of complications from PN or CVC.	• Inform health care provider. • Tell patient or caregiver to call emergency medical services (EMS) if signs and symptoms are severe.

Communication and Documentation

- Document information taught, patient's and caregiver's response, and outcomes of PN therapy (e.g., weight, electrolyte and glucose levels, physical assessment findings) in the home care log.

DOCUMENTATION EXAMPLE

Information regarding signs and symptoms of infection was shared with the patient and their caregiver, Nathan. Both were able to confirm their understanding to this writer using the teach-back method. The patient appears to be tolerating the infusion well, as evidenced by a weight increase of 1.2 kg since last home visit on August 17, 2024. Glucose levels appear stable as per flow sheet.

- Document appearance of CVC site, infusions, glucose monitoring results, and patient's weight in the home care log.

DOCUMENTATION EXAMPLE

Tunnelled triple-lumen CVC site to right chest appears in situ with no signs or symptoms of infection. TPN solution appears normal. Latest blood glucose level is 5.8 mmol/L and current weight is 52.1 kg.

Special Considerations

Teaching

- Assess patient's psychosocial status while providing information. Many patients experience a decrease in quality of life when PN feedings are started in the home, which often increases anxiety and decreases comprehension of information.
- Eating is often a social event. When patients do not eat, they tend to feel socially isolated. Teach patients and caregivers the importance of maintaining social relationships and enhancing social support during PN therapy.
- Always leave a phone number and instructions on how to reach a home care nurse if needed.

Pediatric

- The risk for displacement of the CVC increases as the child grows. Ensure that the placement of the venous access device is confirmed with radiographic film examination as the child grows.
- Teach the caregiver to socialize the child with other children to enhance development (Hockenberry et al., 2024).

Gerontological

- Frail older persons are at high risk of experiencing electrolyte disturbances. Frequently assess and monitor their response to PN therapy and their laboratory values.
- Carefully assess the patient's ability to perform skill. Management of PN at home is complex and requires manual dexterity, visual acuity, and high-level critical thinking and decision-making skills. Include the caregiver in the teaching plan to help with management of home PN.

✦ REVIEW QUESTIONS

A 43-year-old patient (he/him) is admitted to the hospital with a severe exacerbation of Crohn's disease. He has lost 4.5 kg (10 lb) over the last 3 weeks and has recurrent abdominal pain, cramping, and loose stools. He is unable to tolerate food orally and is becoming easily nauseated. He is to receive bowel rest and nutritional support with central parenteral nutrition (CPN) via a central vascular access device (CVAD). The health care provider has inserted a central venous catheter (CVC) (i.e., central line) for 3:1 PN therapy.

Review Questions 1 to 5 relate to the case study presented here.

1. Which of the following physical parameters can change quickly when a patient is receiving CPN and should be part of the nurse's baseline assessment before PN is initiated through a central line? (*Select all that apply.*)
   1. Body temperature
   2. Vital signs
   3. Level of consciousness
   4. Weight loss
   5. Lung sounds
   6. Blood glucose level

2. On the third day after insertion of the central line (CVC), the patient develops a fever and fatigue, preferring to stay in bed. What might the fever indicate, and what could be its source?

3. Two days after beginning CPN infusion, the patient experiences a 2-kg (5-lb) weight gain. He comments, "I'm gaining back some of the weight I lost." What should be the nurse's response? What should the nurse include in a nursing assessment? (*Select all that apply.*)
   1. Reflex responses
   2. Palpation of the skin around the lower extremities
   3. Serum protein levels
   4. Auscultation of lungs
   5. Fluid input and output

4. The nurse takes the patient's vital signs: heart rate 100 beats/min; respirations, 20 breaths/min with bilateral rales; blood pressure, 130/86 mm Hg. The patient denies shortness of breath on exertion. Using SBAR (situation–background–assessment–recommendation), indicate how the nurse would communicate with the health care team about this patient.

5. Place the following steps for administration of central parenteral nutrition (CPN) in the correct order:
   1. Scrub the end port of CVAD with alcohol swab.
   2. Place IV tubing in electronic infusion device (EID). Set and regulate flow rate as prescribed.
   3. Apply clean gloves.
   4. Prime tubing with CPN solution, making sure that no air bubbles remain.
   5. Connect Luer-Lok end of CPN IV tubing to end port of CVAD.
   6. Attach appropriate filter to IV tubing.
   7. Attach syringe of 0.9% normal saline solution to needleless port and flush saline.

6. A patient is being switched from a standard intravenous (IV) solution to peripheral parenteral nutrition (PPN). Which reason(s) should the nurse give the patient about why a large-diameter vein needs to be used for the infusion? (*Select all that apply.*)
   1. The fluid to be administered is very hyperosmolar.
   2. The fluid cannot flow through smaller veins.
   3. Peripheral veins become very irritated because of the content of the fluid.
   4. The patient will have the infusion for an extended amount of time, which will allow for the use of both hands without an IV line in them.
   5. Large veins allow the solution to infuse at the increased rate needed for PPN.

7. A patient with which of the following conditions is a good candidate for short-term PPN? (*Select all that apply.*)
   1. Anastomotic leak
   2. Intestinal obstruction
   3. Severe mucositis
   4. Severe malnutrition before surgery
   5. Pneumonia

8. Place the three checks for accuracy before administering central parenteral nutrition (CPN) in the correct order.
   1. Before leaving the medication room, check intravenous (IV) solution a second time using the 10 rights of medication administration (see Chapter 20). Check label of parenteral nutrition (PN) bag against medication administration record (MAR) or computer printout.
   2. Identify patient using at least two person-specific identifiers (e.g., name and date of birth) according to employer policy. Compare contents of PN solution and additives on label of bag with information on patient's MAR or medical record at bedside.
   3. When preparing PN solution, check label on PN bag by comparing with health care provider's prescription on MAR or computer printout and patient's name.

Visit the Evolve site for a complete list of answers to the Review Questions.

✦ NEXT GENERATION NCLEX® (NGN)

For practice with answering exam questions related to unfolding NGN case studies, please consult the Next Generation NCLEX® (NGN)-Style Case Studies for Skills and Techniques on the Evolve website: http://evolve.elsevier.com/Canada/Perry/clinicalskills/

REFERENCES

Accreditation Canada. (2020). *Required organizational practices handbook*. https://physicians.nshealth.ca/resources/required-organizational-practices-2020-handbook

Gorski, L. A. (2018). *Phillips's manual of IV therapeutics: Evidence-based practice for infusion therapy* (7th ed.). F. A. Davis.

Gorski, L. A., Hadaway, L., Hagle, M. E., et al. (2021). Infusion Therapy Standards of Practice, 8th edition. *Journal of Infusion Nursing, 44*(Suppl. 1), S1–S224. https://doi.org/10.1097/NAN.0000000000000396

Gottlieb, M., Sundaram, T., Holladay, D., et al. (2017). Ultrasound-guided peripheral intravenous line placement: A narrative review of evidence-based best practices. *Western Journal of Emergency Medicine, 18*(6), 1047–1054. https://doi.org/10.5811/westjem.2017.7.34610

Guenter, P., Worthington, P., Ayers, P., et al. (2018). Standardized competencies for parenteral nutrition administration: The ASPEN model. *Nutrition in Clinical Practice, 33*(2), 295–304. https://doi.org/10.1002/ncp.10055

Hockenberry, M. J., Duffy, E. A., & Gibbs, K. (2024). *Wong's nursing care of infants and children* (12th ed.). Elsevier.

Institute for Safe Medication Practices. (2015). *Safe practice guidelines for adult IV push medications*. https://www.ismp.org/guidelines/iv-push

Singh, A. (2023). Parenteral nutrition indications and complications. *MedCare Tips*. https://medcaretips.com/parenteral-nutrition/

Worthington, P., Balint, J., Bingham, A., et al. (2017). When is parenteral nutrition appropriate? *Journal of Parenteral and Enteral Nutrition, 41*(3), 324–377. https://doi.org/10.1177/0148607117695251

Żalikowska-Gardocka, M., & Przybyłkowski, A. (2020). Review of parenteral nutrition-associated liver disease. *Clinical and Experimental Hepatology, 6*(2), 65–73. https://doi.org/10.5114/ceh.2019.95528

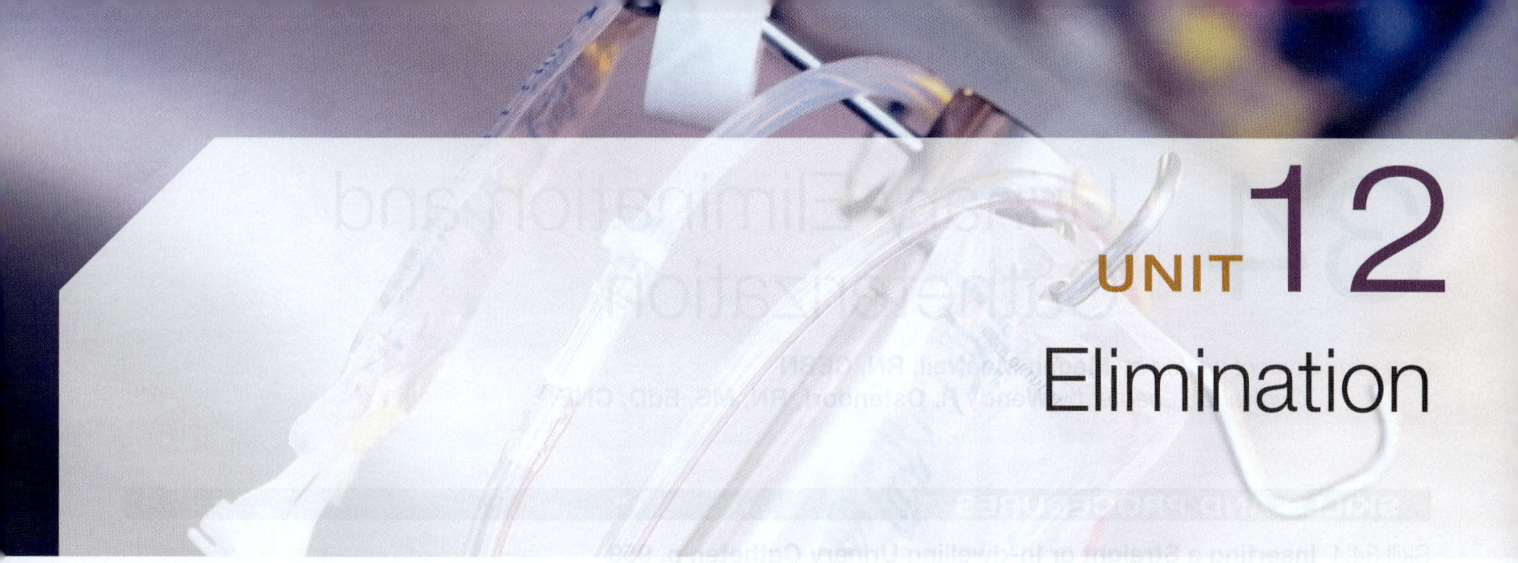

UNIT 12 Elimination

The skills used to support normal urinary elimination apply the principles of preventing infection, promoting patient comfort, protecting skin integrity, and maintaining patient dignity and privacy. Your knowledge base regarding these aims will direct your assessments, identification of patient problems, and clinical decisions about administering the skills correctly. For example, when offering a bedpan to a cisgender female or nonoperative transgender male patient who is overweight, you consider the patient's weight and how to more comfortably position the bedpan. To avoid skin breakdown, you make sure the perineal and anal areas within skinfolds are cleansed thoroughly afterward. Your attention to perineal cleansing may be less stringent for a patient of normal weight. Any skill involving urinary elimination means that a patient needs assistance with a basic need. Thus, your clinical judgement must include consideration of the patient's feelings and perceptions about being unable to provide self-hygiene.

When it is necessary to perform invasive procedures such as urinary catheter insertion or suprapubic catheter care, you rely on your knowledge base about surgical and medical aseptic principles to ensure that infectious microorganisms are not transmitted to patients. Infection control measures based on clinical guidelines for preventing catheter-associated urinary tract infection (CAUTI) are required to prevent microorganisms from entering an existing catheter. Clinical judgement is key when making assessments to inform clinical decision making regarding when an in-dwelling catheter can be removed safely and in a timely manner.

Delivering skills to support normal bowel elimination also involves the application of principles to promote patient comfort, protect skin integrity, and maintain patient dignity and privacy. The administration of an enema is uncomfortable and embarrassing and can make a patient feel helpless. Monitoring a patient's response to your approach and slowly instilling the enema solution reduces cramping, makes it easier for the patient to relax, and allows you to instill more solution for better results. Critical thinking comes into play when you have to adapt a skill such as enema administration—for example, adjusting patient positioning when they cannot turn to the left side.

The insertion, maintenance, and removal of nasogastric tubes used for gastric decompression require you to apply knowledge regarding the nature of a patient's gastrointestinal disease or condition. This knowledge guides what you monitor (e.g., type and amount of drainage and condition of abdomen) to determine patient response. The procedure for nasogastric tube insertion is very uncomfortable. You assess how much a patient either knows or desires to know so that you can effectively partner and make certain that each step causes the least amount of discomfort possible. For example, knowing what is involved in nasogastric tube insertion, a patient can prepare for swallowing and head positioning to assist in making insertion easier. A nasogastric tube creates a high risk for skin irritation and development of a medical device–related pressure injury (MDRPI). You are responsible for conducting ongoing assessments of the condition of a patient's nares and for applying critical thinking regarding frequency of assessment, especially if the patient has other problems contributing to skin breakdown such as diaphoresis and malnutrition.

Surgically placed ostomies for urinary or fecal drainage pose potential problems that require you to apply knowledge of pathological conditions, normal elimination, and how ostomies are designed to function. The existence of an ostomy creates risk for skin breakdown, resultant pain, and difficulty in ostomy pouch placement if skin breakdown is severe. Ostomy care can be complicated, requiring you to rely on an important assessment data resource: a wound, ostomy, and continence (WOC) nurse specialist. Collaboratively you can identify the best strategies for managing patients' ostomies and supporting the patient. The psychological impact of an ostomy can never go unnoticed. Apply principles of therapeutic communication, cultural sensitivity, and grief and loss to better understand the meaning an ostomy has for a patient and the patient-centred approaches to best educate and support the patient.

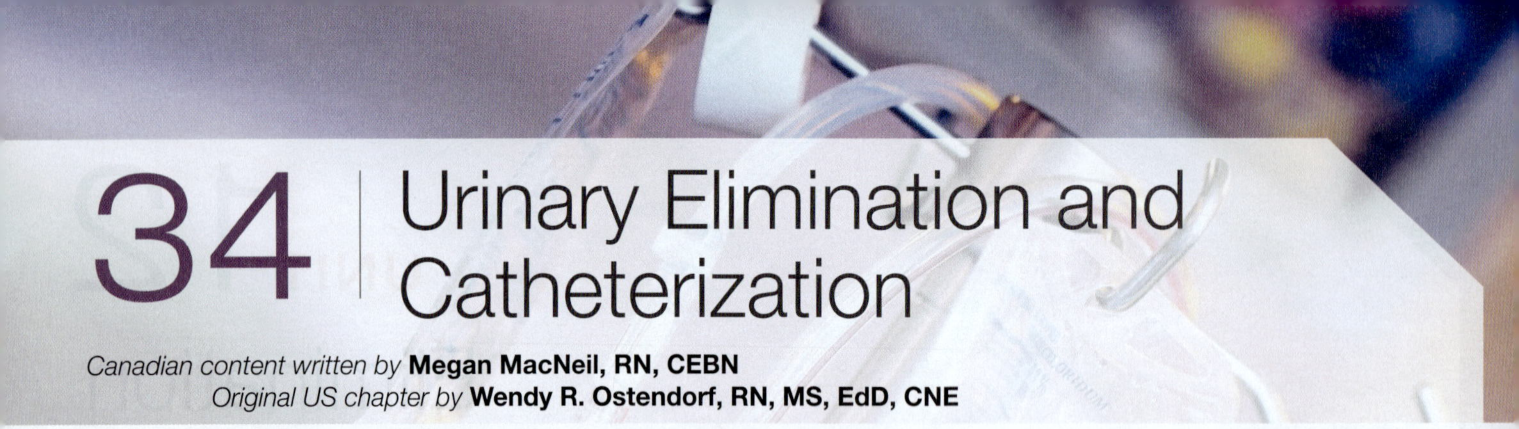

34 Urinary Elimination and Catheterization

Canadian content written by **Megan MacNeil, RN, CEBN**
Original US chapter by **Wendy R. Ostendorf, RN, MS, EdD, CNE**

SKILLS AND PROCEDURES

OBJECTIVES

Mastery of content in this chapter will enable the nurse to:

- Describe nursing interventions that promote normal micturition when toilet access is compromised or after removal of a catheter.
- Explain the relationship between fluid balance and urinary elimination.
- Describe how to use person-centred care principles when caring for patients with urinary elimination alterations.
- Describe ways to provide for patient safety when managing urinary elimination needs.
- Describe ways to stimulate and facilitate urinary elimination.
- Identify factors that increase the risk of catheter-associated urinary tract infection.
- Perform the following skills: place and remove a urinal, insert a urinary catheter, care for an in-dwelling urinary catheter, measure postvoid residual with catheterization and a bladder scan, irrigate a catheter, remove an in-dwelling catheter, apply a condom catheter, and care for a suprapubic catheter.
- Implement and evaluate evidence-informed learning strategies that support patients' ability to care for themselves with intermittent self-catheterization in the home setting.

MEDIA RESOURCES

- http://evolve.elsevier.com/Canada/Perry/clinicalskills/

PURPOSE

A basic human function is urinary elimination, a function that can be compromised by a wide variety of illnesses and conditions. It is the nurse's role to support bladder emptying as needed by helping the patient in toileting, a process that may include use of a commode, urinal, or bedpan. During acute illness, a patient may require urinary catheterization for close monitoring of urinary output or to facilitate bladder emptying when bladder function is compromised. Some patients require long-term in-dwelling catheters, urethral or suprapubic, when the bladder fails to empty effectively. The nurse also implements measures to minimize risk of infection when bladder function is impaired or urinary drainage tubes are required.

STANDARDS OF CARE

- Healthcare Excellence Canada (HEC, n.d.)—*Hospital Harm Improvement Resource: Urinary Tract Infection* (https://www.healthcareexcellence.ca/en/what-we-do/all-programs/hospital-harm-is-everyones-concern/hospital-harm-improvement-resource/)
- Nurses Specialized in Wound, Ostomy, and Continence Canada (NSWOCC), Canadian Nurse Continence Advisors, Urology Nurses of Canada, and Infection Prevention and Control Canada (2020)—*Clean Intermittent Urethral Catheterization in Adults—Canadian Best Practice Recommendations for Nurses* (https://cnca.ca/wp-content/uploads/Clean-Intermittent-Urethral-Catheterization-Adults-for-Nurses-BPR-May2020.pdf)
- Wound, Ostomy, and Continence Nurses Society (WOCN, 2016)—*Care and Management of Patients With Urinary Catheters: A Clinical Resource Guide* (https://cdn.ymaws.com/member.wocn.org/resource/resmgr/document_library/Care_&_Mgmt_Pts_w_Urinary_Ca.pdf)

TABLE 34.1

Signs of Fluid Volume Deficit and Fluid Volume Excess

	Fluid Volume Deficit	Fluid Volume Excess
Eyes	Sunken eyes, dry conjunctivae, decreased or absence of tearing	Periorbital edema, blurred vision, papilledema
Mouth	Sticky, dry mucous membrane; dry, cracked lips; decreased saliva; increased viscosity of saliva; furrowed, shrunken tongue	Excessive salivation
Skin	Increased skin temperature; dry, scaly skin; poor turgor	Edema, anasarca
Cardiovascular	Increased pulse rate, weak pulse, hypotension, decreased pulse volume/pressure, decreased capillary filling, increased hematocrit, flat neck veins	Bounding pulse rate, blood pressure normal with or without orthostatic changes, third heart sound (S_3), distended neck veins
Gastrointestinal	Sunken abdomen, vomiting, diarrhea, abdominal cramps	Vomiting, diarrhea, abdominal cramps
Renal	Oliguria or anuria, increased urine specific gravity (normal = 1.010–1.030)	Decreased urine specific gravity, diuresis (if kidneys are normal)

PRINCIPLES FOR PRACTICE

- Adequate oral intake is essential for bladder health, especially if a patient has an in-dwelling urinary catheter. Some patients with urinary problems limit fluid intake because of their fear of incontinence or increased urinary frequency. The nurse must explain the importance of fluid intake in maintaining urinary health.
- The nurse must know the average output range for a patient. Adult urinary output averages 1 to 2 L in 24 hours, or approximately 0.5 to 1.0 mL/kg/hr (Tyerman & Cobbett, 2023). An hourly output of less than 30 mL/hr for 2 consecutive hours shows the need for further assessment.
- It is important to know the signs of dehydration and fluid overload (Table 34.1). Start measurement of intake and output (I&O) when there is an actual or anticipated change in fluid balance.
- Excessive urination and extreme thirst can occur as a result of inadequate output of the pituitary hormone antidiuretic hormone (ADH) or the lack of normal response by the kidney to ADH. Note that some patients (e.g., with brain tumour or brain surgery) often void very large amounts of urine (e.g., 20 L/day).
- The nurse must assess a patient's most recent serum electrolyte measurements. Abnormal values reflect alterations in fluid balance that can lead to deterioration in a patient's health.
- Weigh a patient to determine fluid status. Ask them to empty their bladder. The patient must be weighed using the same scale, at the same time of day, and wearing comparable articles of clothing, including bed linen if bed weights are necessary.

PERSON-CENTRED CARE

- The personal level of touch needed when helping patients who have problems with urinary elimination requires you as a nurse to understand the patient's values and preferences.
- Determine how patients feel about having to undergo procedures such as catheterization. Try to adapt procedures to minimize the invasive nature of catheterization, and use a person-centred approach to maintain the patient's dignity and communicate respect.
- When caring for patients from diverse cultures, it is important to incorporate into the plan of care sensitivity and awareness of factors that may affect how you manage urinary elimination problems.
- Variations within a cultural group are common. Assess each patient and practise culturally sensitive care. Many cultures have specific beliefs and practices related to elimination, privacy, and gender-specific care. For example:
  - Some cultures emphasize female modesty and prohibit non-related males and females from touching; a same-gender caregiver needs to be provided.
  - Some cultures emphasize interdependence over independence; thus, family presence at the bedside for important decision making is common.
  - Privacy is important in many cultures; thus, careful attention to draping is crucial.

EVIDENCE-INFORMED PRACTICE

- Key recommendations in evidence-informed guidelines to reduce catheter-related problems and infection include reducing inappropriate catheter use and removing catheters as soon as possible (Fekete, 2022; HEC, n.d.; Lawrence et al., 2019; Schaeffer, 2023).
- Studies have shown that bacteriuria can occur within 4 days when open catheters are used, and within approximately 30 days with closed systems. With each catheterization, the risk of acquiring bacteriuria is estimated to be 1 to 3% and is much more prevalent in patients with an in-dwelling catheter than in those experiencing intermittent catheterization (NSWOCC et al., 2020). Complications of long-term catheterization include chronic renal inflammation, chronic pyelonephritis, nephrolithiasis, cystolithiasis, and symptomatic urinary tract.
- Evidence-informed interventions for the prevention of catheter-associated urinary tract infection (CAUTI) include the following:
  - Use aseptic catheter insertion with sterile equipment (Fekete, 2022).
  - Use only trained, dedicated personnel to insert and maintain urinary catheters (HEC, n.d.).
  - Use the smallest catheter possible.
  - Remove catheter as soon as possible (HEC, n.d.; Schaeffer, 2021).
  - Secure in-dwelling catheters to prevent movement and pulling on the catheter.
  - Maintain a sterile, closed urinary drainage system (Schaeffer, 2023).
  - Maintain an unobstructed flow of urine through the catheter, drainage tubing, and drainage bag.
  - Keep the urinary drainage bag below the level of the bladder at all times.

- When emptying the urinary drainage bag, use a separate measuring receptacle for each patient. Do not let the drainage spigot touch the receptacle.
- Perform routine perineal hygiene daily and after soiling.
- Facilities should implement quality improvement and surveillance programs that identify all patients with catheters; these programs include regular educational programming about catheter care.

SAFETY GUIDELINES

- Regularly assess and determine a patient's functional status, such as their ability to safely stand and transfer to a toilet or commode, their ability to follow and understand directions, and their motivation to help in performing self-care activities such as using a toilet, commode, or urinal.
- Evaluate a patient's normal pattern of micturition. Patients taking diuretic medications should have a toilet, commode, or urinal close to their bed or chair. Respond to any request for toileting assistance in a prompt manner to lessen a patient's risk of falling as they try to reach a toilet.
- Consider a patient's age when assessing voiding habits. Toilet training and enuresis are concerns for toddlers and preschoolers. Frail older persons are at higher risk of incontinence because of multiple health care problems and associated physiological changes.
- Patients who need help with elimination should have a call bell within easy reach and be offered assistance at regular intervals, especially in the morning after awakening, after meals, and before bedtime.
- Maintain aseptic technique when catheterizing a patient to prevent CAUTI (Fekete, 2022; HEC, n.d.).

Procedural Guideline 34.1 *Assisting With Use of a Urinal*

Video Clip

A *urinal* is a container that collects and holds urine when a patient's access to a toilet is restricted. Patients who may need a urinal include those who have compromised mobility, severe dyspnea, or other illnesses that make walking to a bathroom impossible or excessively painful. In some instances, a patient with male genitalia may be able to stand at the bedside and use a urinal. Urinals made for female genitalia have a larger opening at the top with a defined rim, which helps position the urinal close against the genitalia (Fig. 34.1). Although these devices are available, most individuals with female genitalia will use a bedpan to void rather than a urinal.

Delegation and Collaboration

The skill of assisting a patient with a urinal can be delegated to an unregulated care provider (UCP). The nurse directs the UCP to do the following:

- Help the patient with special needs or adaptations, such as holding a urinal for the patient
- Provide personal hygiene after urination as necessary
- Measure and record amount of urinary output
- Report immediately any changes in urine colour, clarity, and odour; development of incontinence (involuntary loss of urine); patient reports of dysuria, which could indicate an infection; and any changes in the frequency and amount of urine

Equipment

- Urinal
- Clean gloves
- Graduated cylinder (used for measuring volume if on I&O)
- Supplies for diagnostic urine tests and specimen collection (see Chapter 9)
- Wash basin, washcloths, towels, and soap
- Toilet tissue

Procedural Steps

1. Identify patient using at least two person-specific identifiers (e.g., name and date of birth, or name and medical record number) according to employer policy (Accreditation Canada, 2020).
2. Throughout the procedure, the 4 moments for hand hygiene are to be implemented; hand hygiene should occur before initial patient (or patient environment) contact, before an aseptic procedure, after body fluid exposure risk, and after patient (or patient environment) contact. Additional hand hygiene should be performed when hands are visibly soiled.
3. Assess patient's normal urinary elimination habits, including any episodes of incontinence.

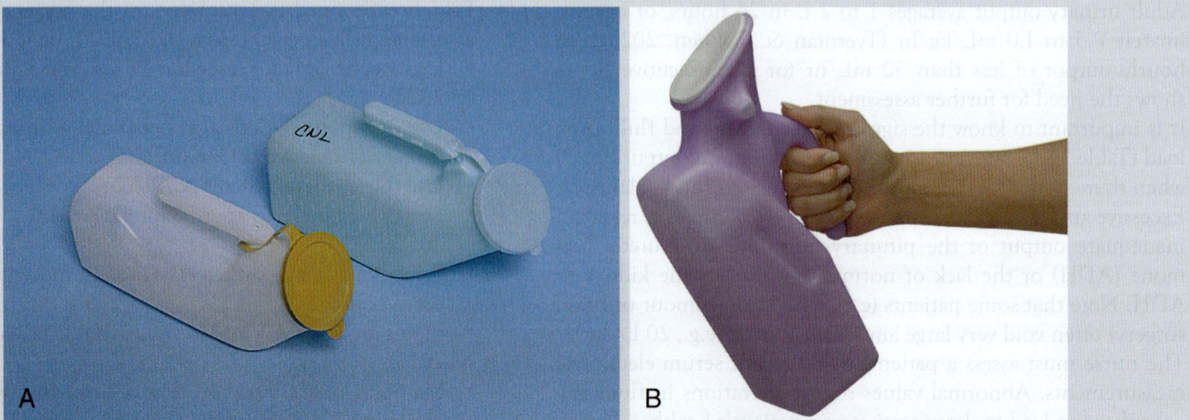

FIG 34.1 **A, Urinals for use with male genitalia. B, Urinals for use with female genitalia.** *(B, Courtesy Briggs Medical Service Co.)*

Procedural Guideline 34.1 *Assisting With Use of a Urinal—cont'd*

4. Determine how much help is needed to place and remove the urinal. (Ask the patient or observe previous use.)
5. Review health care provider prescriptions to determine whether a urine specimen is to be collected.
6. Explain procedure to patient.
7. Provide privacy by closing bedside curtain and room door.
8. Apply clean gloves. Assess for a distended bladder by inspecting the lower one-third of the abdomen or by palpating gently above symphysis pubis.
9. Help patient into appropriate position: for a patient with male genitalia—on side, back, sitting with head of bed elevated, or in standing position; for a patient with female genitalia—lying supine. If needed, place an absorbent pad under patient's buttocks to protect bed linens from accidental spills.

Critical Decision Point *Before having a patient stand to void, assess lower-extremity strength and mobility and assess blood pressure for orthostatic hypotension* (Chapter 7), *especially if there has been a period of prolonged bed rest.*

10. If possible, the patient should hold urinal and position penis in urinal. If needed, help patient by positioning penis completely in urinal and holding urinal in place or by helping to hold urinal. Ensure that urinal is placed dependent of flow of urine.
11. Help a patient on a bedpan into proper position, and stabilize bedpan to keep it in position and dependent of urine flow.
12. Cover patient with bed linens and place the call bell within reach. If possible, give patient further privacy by leaving the bedside after ensuring that they are in a safe and comfortable position. Remove gloves.
13. After patient has finished voiding, remove urinal, and assess characteristics of urine for colour, clarity, odour, and amount. Help patient wash and dry genitalia.
14. Measure urine and record output on I&O record, if needed (see Chapter 8).
15. Empty and clean urinal. Return urinal to patient for future use.
16. Help patient perform hand hygiene as needed.
17. Remove and dispose of gloves.

✦ SKILL 34.1 Inserting a Straight or In-dwelling Urinary Catheter

NSO *Nursing Skills Online Urinary Catheterization Module 17 / Lessons 1 and 2*

Urinary catheterization is the placement of a tube through the urethra into the bladder to remove urine. This is an invasive procedure that requires a health care provider's prescription and strict sterile technique (HEC, n.d.). Urinary catheterization may be short term (usually 2 weeks or less, but sources vary in terms of the exact time frame) or long term (more than 2 weeks) (Fekete, 2022). Short-term catheterization is often used in patients who have acute urinary retention, in those who have had urological and contiguous surgery, and in critically ill patients requiring accurate measurement of urinary output. Examples of patients requiring long-term catheterization include those who have a bladder outlet obstruction that is not medically or surgically correctable and some patients with neurogenic bladder and retention.

Neurogenic bladder is a term used for bladder dysfunction due to neurological damage caused by internal or external trauma, disease, or injury (Gill, 2022) and can be an indication for catheterization. Symptoms can include overflow or urge incontinence, frequency, urgency, incomplete bladder emptying, and urinary retention. Complications of neurogenic bladder may include continuous urine leakage, leading to reduced skin integrity; kidney damage; and urinary tract infection (UTI) (Shelat, 2022).

Conditions that require use of urinary catheters include the need to monitor urinary output, relief of urinary obstruction, postoperative care, or a bladder that empties inadequately as a result of a neurological condition. Excessive accumulation of urine in the bladder increases the risk of a UTI and can cause backward flow of urine up the ureters to the kidneys, causing kidney infection (pyelonephritis), damage, or both. *Urinary incontinence*, an involuntary leakage of urine, may require in-dwelling catheterization if the leaking urine interferes with wound healing. It is important to understand that patients living with urinary incontinence may experience serious impairment in quality of life, with social, psychological, and hygienic consequences (Gascón et al., 2018). Intermittent catheterization is used to measure postvoid residual (PVR) when a bladder scanner is not available or as a way to manage chronic urinary retention. Nurses should attempt to encourage voiding by ensuring that the patient is given privacy when trying to void. Additionally, nurses may encourage voiding by running water, placing the patient's hand in warm water, completing percussion on the suprapubic area, massaging the inner thigh, or having the patient perform the Valsalva's manoeuvre.

A patient with the diagnosis of overactive bladder (OAB) has urinary urgency, incontinence, frequency, and nocturia, with no UTI or obvious pathology (Higuera, 2019). Treatment of OAB includes bladder training and pelvic floor muscle therapy, medications, nerve stimulation, lifestyle changes (e.g., fluid and caffeine restriction, weight loss), and patient education (Higuera, 2019). Bladder training can be carried out using different strategies, all of which share the goal of restoring normal bladder function. Most bladder training programs include a voiding schedule, use of a diary or log to record voiding, and techniques for urgency control and suppression.

The steps for inserting an in-dwelling and a single-use or in-and-out straight catheter are the same. The difference lies in the inflation of a balloon to keep the in-dwelling catheter in place and the presence of a closed drainage system. Urinary catheters are made with one to three lumens (Fig. 34.2). Single-lumen catheters (see Fig. 34.2, A) are used for intermittent catheterization (i.e., the insertion of a catheter for one-time bladder emptying). Double-lumen catheters, designed for in-dwelling catheters, provide one lumen for urinary drainage and

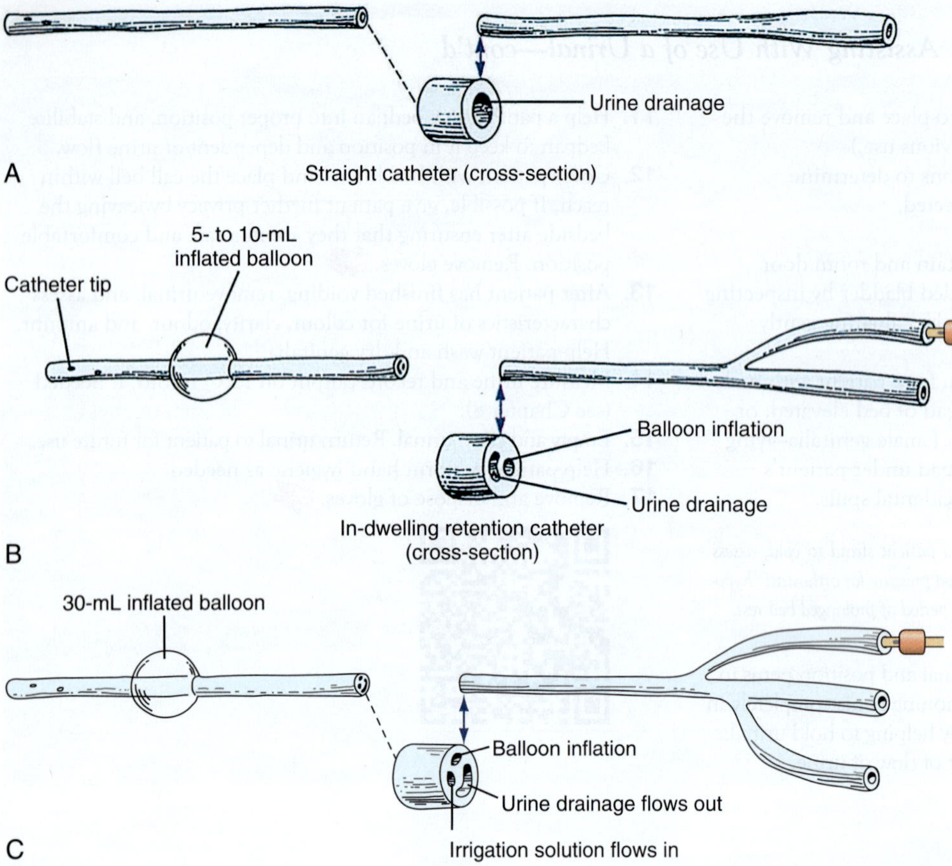

FIG 34.2 A, Single-lumen or straight catheter (cross-section). B, Double-lumen or in-dwelling retention catheter (cross-section). C, Triple-lumen catheter for continuous closed irrigation (cross-section).

a second lumen to inflate a balloon that keeps the catheter in place (see Fig. 34.2, *B*). Triple-lumen catheters (see Fig. 34.2, C) are used for continuous bladder irrigation (CBI) or when it becomes necessary to instill medications into the bladder. One lumen drains the bladder, a second lumen is used to inflate the balloon, and a third lumen delivers irrigation fluid into the bladder.

A health care provider chooses a catheter on the basis of factors such as latex allergy, history of catheter encrustation, previous urological surgeries or catheter insertions, and susceptibility to infection. In-dwelling catheters are made of latex or silicone. Some have special coatings that reduce urethral irritation and encrustation. Silver-coated catheters have been used as a measure to reduce infection, but efficacy data have been inconsistent, with some studies reporting no benefit for prevention of CAUTI (NSWOCC et al., 2020). Straight or intermittent catheters are made of rubber (softer and more flexible) or polyvinyl chloride. Patients who self-catheterize have a large selection of catheters: some have special coatings that do not require lubrication, and others are self-contained systems consisting of a lubricated catheter and packaged with a connected drainage bag.

The size of a urinary catheter is based on the French (Fr) scale, which reflects the internal diameter of the catheter. Most adults with an in-dwelling catheter should have a size 14 to 16 Fr to minimize trauma and risk for infection. Older persons or patients with an enlarged prostate may need a smaller size (12 to 14 Fr). A coudé catheter is also available for patients who have an enlarged prostate with a urinary obstruction; it has a slightly bent tip designed to navigate past the obstruction. Larger catheter diameters increase the risk of trauma to the bladder neck and urethra (Newman et al., 2017). However, larger sizes such as a 20 or 22 Fr are needed in special circumstances, including after urological surgery or in the presence of gross hematuria. Smaller sizes are needed for infants (5 to 6 Fr) and children (8 to 10 Fr).

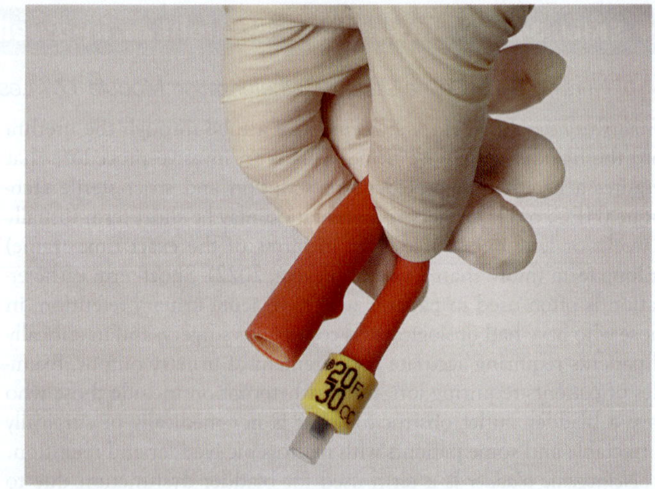

FIG 34.3 Size of catheter and balloon printed on catheter inflation valve.

In-dwelling catheters come in a variety of balloon sizes, from 3 mL for a child to 30 mL for CBI. The size of the balloon is usually printed on the catheter port (Fig. 34.3). The recommended balloon size for an adult is a 5-mL balloon (filled with 10 mL of sterile water). Long-term use of larger balloons (30 mL) has been associated with increased patient discomfort, irritation, and trauma; increased risk of catheter expulsion; and incomplete emptying of the bladder because of urine that pools below the level of the catheter drainage lumen (Newman et al., 2017).

For patients requiring long-term catheterization, catheter changes should be individualized, rather than being implemented at arbitrary times or specific intervals (HEC, n.d.). Catheters should be changed for leaking or blockage if disconnection of the system occurs and before obtaining a sterile specimen for urine culture (HEC, n.d.). Long-term catheterization should be avoided because of its association with UTIs. Best practice involves removal of the catheter as soon as the patient can void (WOCN, 2016).

An in-dwelling catheter is attached to a urinary drainage bag to collect the continuous flow of urine. The bag should always hang below the level of the bladder on the bedframe or a chair to ensure that urine drains down, out of the bladder. The bag should never touch the floor. Never hang the urinary drainage bag on movable parts such as bedrails. When the patient is being transported in a wheelchair, ensure that the tubing and urinary drainage bag do not get caught in the wheels. When a patient ambulates, the bag is carried below the level of the patient's bladder. The only exception to this rule is when a catheter is attached to a specially designed drainage bag (belly bag) that is worn across the abdomen. A one-way valve prevents the backflow of urine into the bladder.

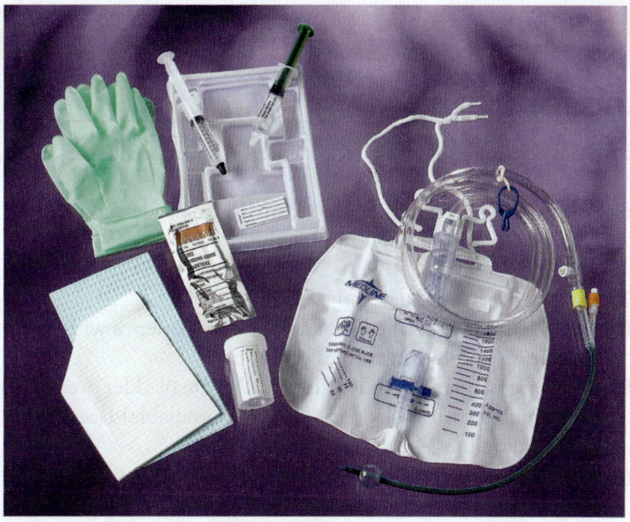

FIG 34.4 **In-dwelling catheterization kit includes drainage device, specimen cup, sterile drapes, sterile gloves, in-dwelling catheter, cleaning solution, sterile saline, sterile cotton balls, forceps, and lubricant.** *(Image used with permission of Medline Industries. All rights reserved.)*

Delegation and Collaboration

The skill of inserting a catheter is usually not delegated to a UCP. However, in some settings, employer policy may permit this skill to be delegated to UCPs who have been properly instructed. UCPs routinely assist with positioning the patient and maintaining patient privacy and comfort, emptying urine from the collection bag, and providing perineal care. The nurse directs the UCP to do the following:

- Assist the nurse with patient positioning, focusing lighting for the procedure, maintaining patient privacy, emptying urine from the collection bag, and assisting with perineal care.
- Report postprocedure patient discomfort or increased temperature to the nurse.
- Report abnormal colour, odour, or amount of urine in the drainage bag and if the catheter is leaking or causes pain.

Equipment

- Catheter kit (Fig. 34.4) containing sterile items (NOTE: Catheter kits vary):
  - *Straight catheterization kit:* Single-lumen catheter, drapes (one fenestrated–with opening in the centre), sterile gloves, lubricant, cleaning solution incorporated in an applicator or to be added to cotton balls, and specimen container
  - *In-dwelling catheterization kit:* Drapes (one fenestrated–with opening in the centre), gloves, lubricant, antiseptic cleaning solution incorporated in an applicator or to be added to cotton balls, specimen container, and a prefilled syringe with sterile water (to inflate balloon). Some kits contain a catheter with an attached drainage bag; others contain only a catheter; others have no catheter.
- Sterile drainage tubing and bag (if not included in in-dwelling catheter insertion kit)
- Device to secure catheter (catheter strap or other device)
- Extra sterile gloves and catheter *(optional)*
- Clean gloves
- Basin with warm water, washcloth, towel, and soap for perineal care
- Flashlight or other additional light source
- Bath blanket, waterproof absorbent pad
- Measuring container for urine

STEP	RATIONALE
ASSESSMENT	
1. Identify patient using at least two person-specific identifiers (e.g., name and date of birth, or name and medical record number) according to employer policy.	Ensures correct patient. Complies with Accreditation Canada's standards and improves patient safety (Accreditation Canada, 2020).
2. Throughout the procedure, the 4 moments for hand hygiene are to be implemented; hand hygiene should occur before initial patient (or patient environment) contact, before an aseptic procedure, after body fluid exposure risk, and after patient (or patient environment) contact. Additional hand hygiene should be performed when hands are visibly soiled.	Proper hand hygiene helps prevent the spread of infectious agents to health care providers.
3. Review patient's medical record, including health care provider's prescription and progress notes. Note previous catheterization, including catheter size, patient's response, and time of catheterization.	Identifies purpose of inserting catheter (such as for measurement of PVR, preparation for surgery, or specimen collection) and potential difficulty with catheter insertion.
4. Review medical record for any pathological condition that may impair passage of catheter (e.g., enlarged prostate gland in men, urethral strictures).	Obstruction of urethra may prevent passage of catheter into bladder.

STEP	RATIONALE
ASSESSMENT	
5. Ask patient about and check medical record for allergies.	Reduces transmission of microorganisms. Identifies allergy to antiseptic, tape, latex, and lubricant.
6. Assess patient's weight, level of consciousness, developmental level, ability to cooperate, and mobility.	Determines positioning for catheterization; indicates how much help is needed to properly position patient, ability of patient to cooperate during procedure, and level of explanation needed.
7. Assess patient's gender and age.	Determines catheter size.
8. Assess patient's knowledge of and prior experience with catheterization and feelings about procedure.	Reveals need for patient instruction, support, or both.
9. Assess for pain and bladder fullness. Palpate bladder over symphysis pubis or use bladder scanner (if available) (see Procedural Guideline 34.2).	Palpation of full bladder causes pain or urge to void, indicating full or overfull bladder.
10. Apply clean gloves. Inspect perineal region, observing for perineal anatomical landmarks, erythema, drainage or discharge, and odour. Remove gloves and discard.	Reduces transmission of microorganisms. Assessment of female perineal landmarks improves accuracy and speed of catheter insertion.

NURSING DIAGNOSES

- Urinary retention
- Acute pain
- Reduced urinary elimination
- Anxiety
- Fear
- Insufficient knowledge regarding catheterization procedure
- Potential for infection

Related factors and risk factors are individualized on the basis of patient's condition or needs.

STEP	RATIONALE
PLANNING	
1. Expected outcomes following completion of procedure:	
• Patient's bladder is not palpable.	Bladder successfully emptied.
• Patient verbalizes absence of abdominal discomfort or bladder pressure or fullness.	Catheterization and free flow of urine through catheter relieve bladder distension and discomfort.
• Patient has urinary output of at least 30 mL/hr as measured in urinary drainage bag.	Verifies presence of catheter in bladder, catheter patency, and adequate kidney function.
• Patient explains purpose of procedure and what to expect.	Reflects patient understanding of procedure.
2. Explain procedure to patient.	Promotes cooperation.
3. Arrange for extra personnel to help as necessary. Organize supplies at bedside.	Some patients are unable to independently assume positioning for procedure. Ensures more efficient procedure.
IMPLEMENTATION	
1. Check patient's plan of care for size and type of catheter (if this is a reinsertion). Use smallest catheter size possible.	Ensures that patient receives correct size and type of catheter. Larger catheter diameters increase the risk of urethral trauma. A small catheter allows for adequate drainage of periurethral glands.
2. Provide privacy by closing room door and bedside curtain.	Promotes person-centred care and protects patient confidentiality.
3. Raise bed to appropriate working height. If side rails are in use, raise side rail on opposite side of bed and lower side rail on working side.	Promotes good body mechanics and patient safety.
4. Place waterproof pad under patient.	Prevents soiling of bed linen.
5. Apply clean gloves. Clean perineal area with soap and water, rinse, and dry (see Chapter 18). Use gloves to examine patient and identify urinary meatus. Remove and discard gloves.	Reduces transmission of microorganisms. Performing hygiene before initiating aseptic catheter insertion removes secretions, urine, and feces that could contaminate sterile field and increase the risk of CAUTI.

Critical Decision Point *Obtain help to position and support patients who have mobility restrictions or are weak, frail, obese, or confused.*

STEP	RATIONALE
6. Position patient:	
a. *Patient with female genitalia:*	
(1) Help patient to dorsal recumbent position (on back with knees flexed). Ask patient to relax thighs so you can rotate their hips.	Exposes perineum and allows hip joints to be externally rotated.

STEP	RATIONALE
IMPLEMENTATION	
(2) Alternate position for patient with female genitalia: Position patient in side-lying position with upper leg flexed at knee and hip. Support patient with pillows if necessary to maintain position.	Alternate position is more comfortable if patient cannot abduct leg at hip joint (e.g., patient has arthritic joints or contractures).
b. *Patient with male genitalia:*	
(1) Position patient supine with legs extended and thighs slightly abducted.	Comfortable position for patient aids in visualization of penis.
7. Drape patient:	Protects patient dignity by avoiding unnecessary exposure of body.
a. *Patient with female genitalia:*	
(1) Drape with bath blanket or use existing bed sheets; pull the bedspread up one side and the top sheet up the other side. Place blanket diamond fashion over patient, with one corner at patient's midsection, side corners over each thigh and abdomen, and last corner over perineum (see Step 7a[1] illustration).	
b. *Patient with male genitalia:*	
(1) Drape patient by covering upper part of body with small sheet or towel; drape with separate sheet or bath blanket so only perineum is exposed (see Step 7b[1] illustration).	

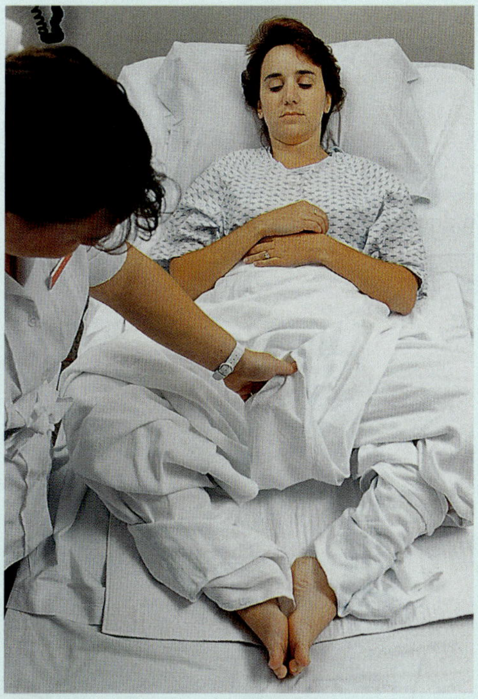

STEP 7A(1) Patient with female genitalia draped and in dorsal recumbent position.

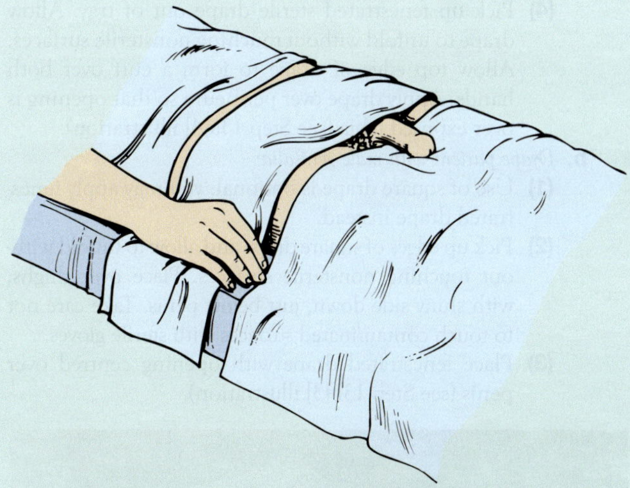

STEP 7B(1) Drape blanket over patient with male genitalia.

STEP	RATIONALE
8. Position light to illuminate genitals or have assistant available to hold light source to visualize urinary meatus.	Adequate visualization of urinary meatus helps with speed and accuracy of catheter insertion.
9. Open outer wrapping of catheterization kit. Place inner wrapped catheter kit tray on clean, accessible surface such as bedside. Patient size and positioning dictate exact placement.	Provides easy access to supplies during catheter insertion.
10. Using sterile technique (see Chapter 6), open inner sterile wrap covering tray containing catheterization supplies. Fold back each flap of sterile covering one at a time, with last flap opened toward the nurse.	Sterile wrap serves as sterile field.

STEP	RATIONALE

IMPLEMENTATION

STEP	RATIONALE
a. *In-dwelling catheterization open system:* Open separate package containing drainage bag, check to make sure that clamp on drainage port is closed, and place drainage bag and tubing in easily accessible location. Open outer package of sterile catheter, maintaining sterility of inner wrapper (see Chapter 6).	Open drainage bag systems have separate sterile packaging for sterile catheter, drainage bag and tubing, and insertion kit.
b. *In-dwelling catheterization closed system:* All supplies are in sterile tray and arranged in sequence of use.	Closed drainage bag systems have catheter preattached to drainage tubing and bag.
c. *Straight catheterization:* All needed supplies are in sterile tray that contains supplies and can be used for urine collection.	
11. Apply sterile gloves.	Maintains surgical asepsis.
12. *Option:* Apply sterile drape with ungloved hands when drape is packed as first item. Touch only edges of drape. Then apply sterile gloves.	Maintains surgical asepsis.
13. Drape perineum, keeping gloves and working surface of drape sterile.	Sterile drapes provide sterile field over which you will work during catheterization.
a. *Drape patient with female genitalia:*	
(1) Pick up square sterile drape, touching only the edges (2.5 cm [1 inch]).	
(2) Allow drape to unfold without touching nonsterile surfaces. Allow top edge of drape (2.5–5 cm [1–2 inches]) to form a cuff over both hands.	When creating cuff over sterile gloved hands, sterility of gloves and workspace is maintained.
(3) Place drape with shiny side down on bed between patient's thighs. Slip cuffed edge just under buttocks as you ask patient to lift hips. Take care not to touch contaminated surfaces with sterile gloves. If gloves are contaminated, remove and apply new pair.	
(4) Pick up fenestrated sterile drape out of tray. Allow drape to unfold without touching nonsterile surfaces. Allow top edge of drape to form a cuff over both hands. Apply drape over perineum so that opening is over exposed labia (see Step 13a[4] illustration).	Opening in drape creates sterile field around labia.
b. *Drape patient with male genitalia:*	
(1) Use of square drape is optional; you may apply fenestrated drape instead.	
(2) Pick up edges of square drape and allow to unfold without touching nonsterile surfaces. Place over thighs, with shiny side down, just below penis. Take care not to touch contaminated surfaces with sterile gloves.	
(3) Place fenestrated drape with opening centred over penis (see Step 13b[3] illustration).	

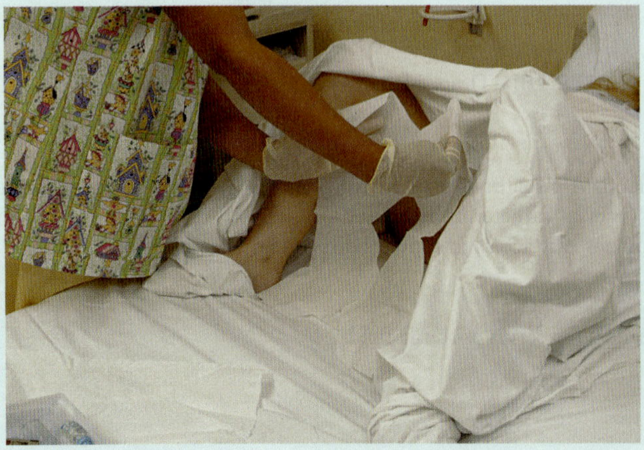

STEP 13A(4) Place sterile fenestrated drape (with opening in centre) over perineum of patient with female genitalia.

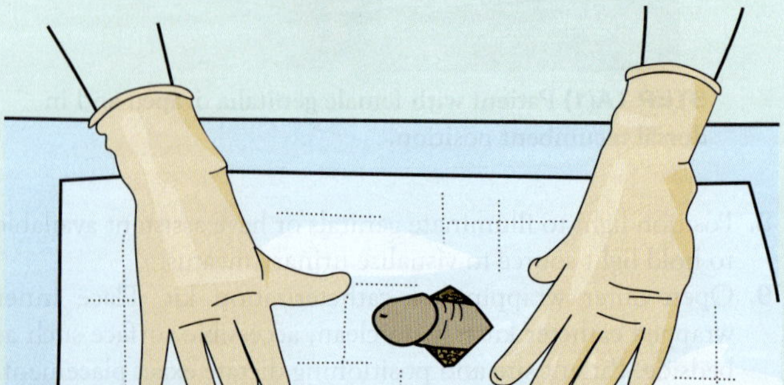

STEP 13B(3) Drape fenestrated drape over patient with male genitalia.

STEP	RATIONALE

IMPLEMENTATION

14. Arrange remaining supplies on sterile field, maintaining sterility of gloves. Place sterile tray with cleaning solution (premoistened swab sticks or cotton balls, forceps, and solution), lubricant, sterile catheter, and prefilled syringe for inflating balloon (in-dwelling catheterization only) on sterile drape between the patient's legs.	Provides easy access to supplies during catheter insertion and helps maintain aseptic technique. Appropriate placement is determined by size of patient and position during catheterization.
a. If kit contains sterile cotton balls, open package of sterile antiseptic solution and pour over cotton balls. Some kits contain package of premoistened swab sticks. Open end of package for easy access (see Step 14a illustration and Fig. 34.4).	Use of sterile supplies and antiseptic solution reduces the risk of CAUTI (HEC, n.d.).
b. Open sterile specimen container if specimen is to be obtained (see Chapter 9).	Makes container accessible to receive urine from catheter if specimen is needed.
c. For in-dwelling catheterization, open sterile wrapper of catheter and leave catheter on sterile field. If part of closed-system kit, remove tray with catheter and preattached drainage bag and place on sterile drape. Make sure that clamp on drainage port of bag is closed. If needed and if part of sterile tray, attach catheter to drainage tubing.	In-dwelling catheterization trays vary. Some have preattached catheters; others need to be attached but are part of the sterile tray; others do not have catheter or drainage system as part of tray.
d. Attach a prefilled water syringe into the balloon port on the catheter. Balloon should be inflated with distilled water only.	Enables preparation for inflation of balloon once catheter is in place: nondominant hand stabilizes catheter while dominant hand inflates balloon using syringe.
e. Open packet of lubricant and squeeze out on sterile field. Lubricate catheter tip by dipping it 2.5–5 cm (1–2 inches) into water-soluble gel for individuals with female genitalia and 12.5–17.5 cm (5–7 inches) for individuals with male genitalia (see Step 14e illustration).	Lubrication minimizes trauma to urethra and discomfort during catheter insertion. Male catheter needs enough lubricant to cover length of catheter inserted.

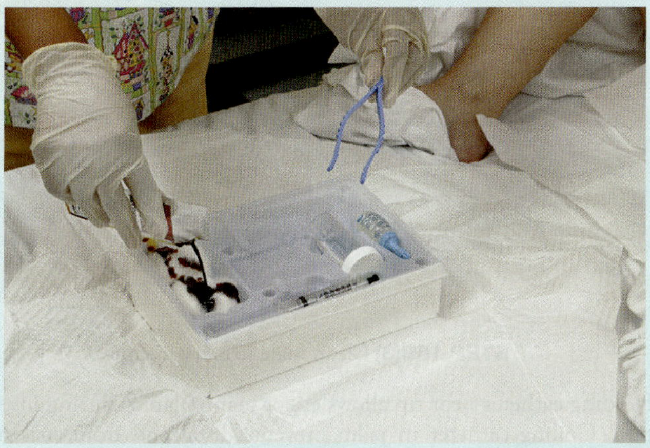

STEP 14A Sterile kit includes antiseptic swabs.

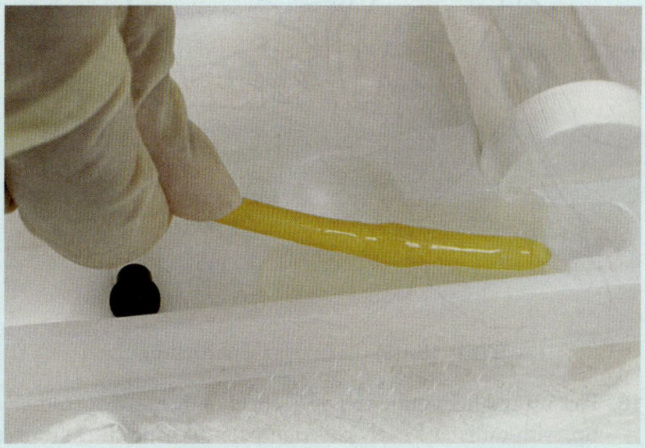

STEP 14E Lubricate catheter.

Critical Decision Point ***It is no longer recommended*** *to pretest a balloon on an in-dwelling catheter by injecting fluid from the prefilled sterile water syringe into the balloon port. Testing the balloon may distort and stretch it and lead to damage, causing increased trauma on insertion.*

15. Clean urethral meatus:	
a. *Patient with female genitalia:*	
(1) Separate labia with fingers of nondominant hand (now contaminated) to fully expose urethral meatus.	Optimal visualization of urethral meatus is possible.
(2) Maintain position of nondominant hand throughout procedure.	Closure of labia during cleaning means that area is contaminated and requires cleaning procedure to be repeated.

IMPLEMENTATION

STEP	RATIONALE
(3) Holding forceps in dominant hand, pick up one moistened cotton ball or pick up one swab stick at a time. Clean labia and urinary meatus from clitoris toward anus, starting with each side followed by the centre. Use new cotton ball or swab for each area that you clean. Clean by wiping far labial fold, near labial fold, and directly over centre of urethral meatus (see Step 15a[3] illustration).	Front-to-back cleaning moves from area of least contamination toward highly contaminated area. Follows principles of medical asepsis (see Chapter 5). Dominant gloved hand remains sterile.
b. *Patient with male genitalia:*	
(1) With nondominant hand (now contaminated) retract foreskin (if uncircumcised) and gently grasp penis at shaft just below glans. Hold shaft of penis at right angle to body. This hand remains in this position for remainder of procedure.	When grasping shaft of penis, avoid pressure on dorsal surface to prevent compression of urethra. Losing grasp during cleaning means that area is contaminated and requires cleaning procedure to be repeated.
(2) Using uncontaminated dominant hand, clean meatus with cotton balls or swab sticks, using circular strokes, cleaning from meatus toward glans in a spiral motion.	Circular cleaning pattern follows principles of medical asepsis (see Chapter 5).
(3) Repeat cleaning three times, using clean cotton ball or swab stick each time (see Step 15b[3] illustration).	

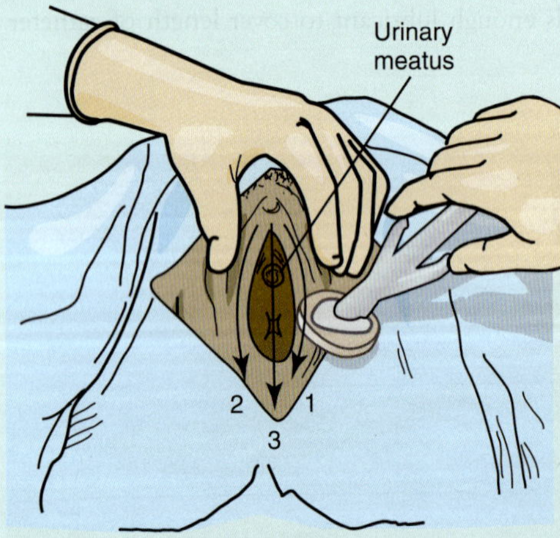

STEP 15A(3) Clean female perineum.

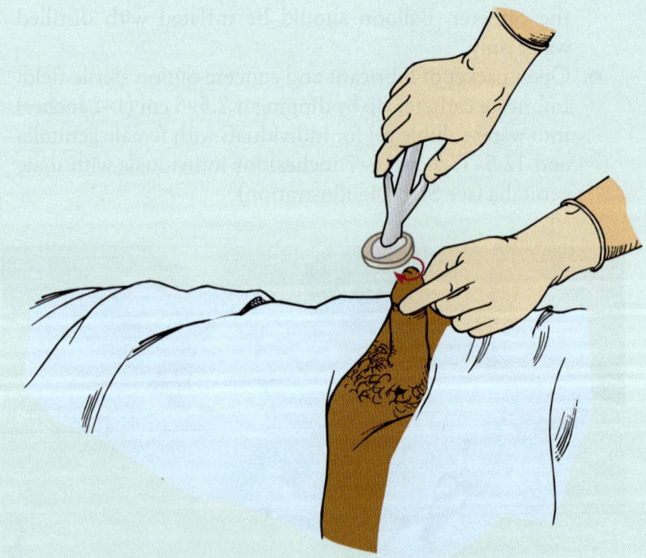

STEP 15B(3) Clean male urinary meatus.

STEP	RATIONALE
16. Pick up and hold catheter 7.5–10 cm (3–4 inches) from catheter tip, with catheter loosely coiled in palm of hand. If catheter is not attached to drainage bag, make sure to position urine tray so end of catheter can be placed there once insertion begins.	Holding catheter near tip allows easier manipulation during insertion. Coiling catheter in palm prevents distal end from striking nonsterile surface.
17. Insert catheter. Explain to patient that a feeling of burning, pinching, or pressure may be experienced as catheter is inserted into urethra. This sensation is normal and will go away quickly.	Helps minimize patient anxiety.
a. *Patient with female genitalia:*	
(1) Ask patient to bear down gently, and slowly insert catheter through urethral meatus (see Step 17a[1] illustration).	Bearing down may help you visualize urinary meatus and promotes relaxation of external urinary sphincter, aiding in catheter insertion.
(2) Advance catheter a total of 5–7.5 cm (2–3 inches) or until urine flows out of catheter. When urine appears, advance catheter another 2.5–5 cm (1–2 inches). Do not use force to insert catheter.	Urine flow indicates that catheter tip is in the bladder or lower urethra. Additional advancement prevents damage to urethra with balloon insertion.

STEP	RATIONALE

IMPLEMENTATION

STEP	RATIONALE
(3) Release labia and hold catheter securely with non-dominant hand.	Prevents accidental expulsion of catheter from the patient's bladder.
b. *Patient with male genitalia:*	
(1) Lift penis to position perpendicular (90 degrees) to patient's body and apply gentle upward traction (see Step 17b[1] illustration).	Straightens urethra to ease catheter insertion.

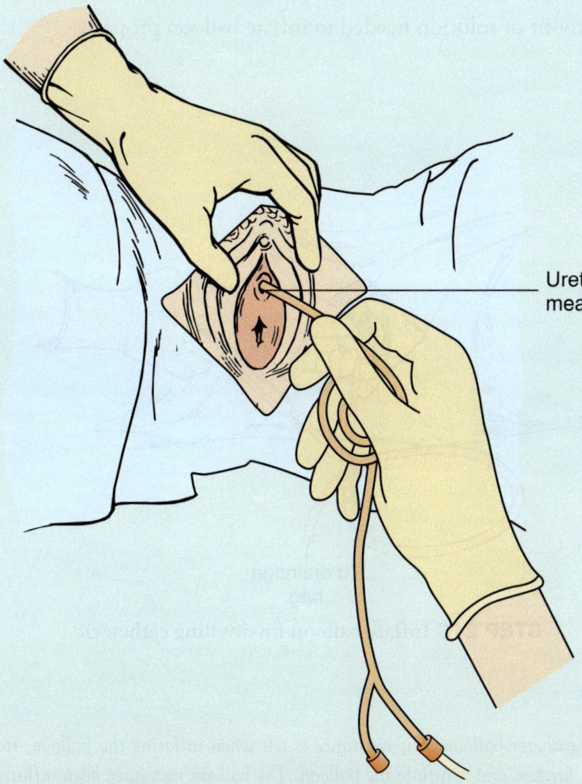

STEP 17A(1) Insert catheter into female urinary meatus.

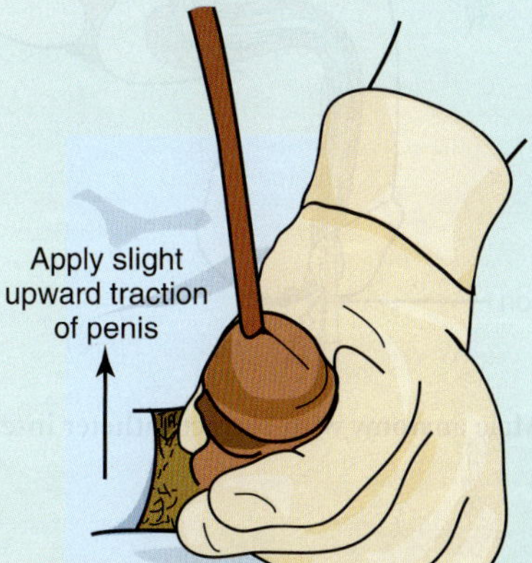

STEP 17B(1) Insert catheter into male urinary meatus.

STEP	RATIONALE
(2) Ask patient to bear down as if to void, then slowly insert catheter through urethral meatus.	Relaxation of external sphincter aids in insertion of catheter.
(3) Advance catheter 17–22.5 cm (7–9 inches) or until urine flows out end of catheter.	Length of male urethra varies. Flow of urine indicates that tip of catheter is in the bladder or urethra but not necessarily that balloon part of in-dwelling catheter is in bladder.
(4) Stop advancing with straight catheter. When urine appears in in-dwelling catheter, advance it to bifurcation (inflation and deflation ports exposed) (see Step 17b[4] illustration).	Further advancement of catheter to bifurcation of drainage and balloon inflation port ensures that it is sufficiently inserted into the bladder (WOCN, 2016).
(5) Lower penis and hold catheter securely in nondominant hand.	Prevents accidental expulsion of catheter from patient's bladder.
18. Allow bladder to empty completely unless employer policy restricts maximum volume of urine drained.	There is no definitive evidence regarding whether there is benefit in limiting maximal volume drained; however, ***draining too much volume at once can cause a large fluid shift in the patient (e.g., fluid volumes >1 L), resulting in dizziness and hypotension.***
19. Collect urine specimen as needed (see Chapter 9). Fill specimen container to 20–30 mL by holding end of catheter over cup.	Sterile specimen for culture analysis can be obtained.
a. Label and bag specimen according to employer policy. Label specimen in front of patient. Send to laboratory as soon as possible.	A fresh urine specimen ensures more accurate findings. Labelling ensures that diagnostic results will be connected to the correct patient.
20. Straight catheterization: When urine stops flowing, withdraw catheter slowly and smoothly until removed.	Minimizes trauma to urethra.

STEP	RATIONALE

IMPLEMENTATION

21. Inflate catheter balloon with amount of distilled water designated by manufacturer.	Improper balloon inflation can result in an asymmetrical balloon, which may cause the catheter tip to bend, resulting in improper drainage, bladder spasms, or leakage (WOCN, 2016).
a. Continue to hold catheter with nondominant hand.	Holding on to catheter before inflating balloon prevents expulsion of catheter from urethra.
b. With free dominant hand, pick up prefilled syringe that is connected to the balloon port at end of catheter.	
c. Slowly inject total amount of solution (see Step 21c illustration).	Full amount of solution needed to inflate balloon properly.

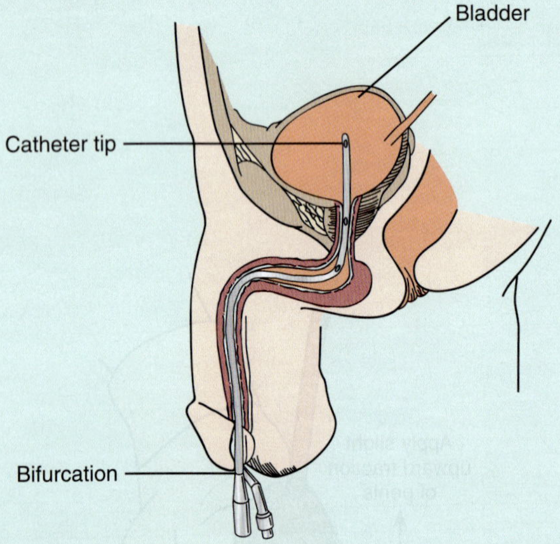

STEP 17B(4) Male anatomy with correct catheter insertion to bifurcation.

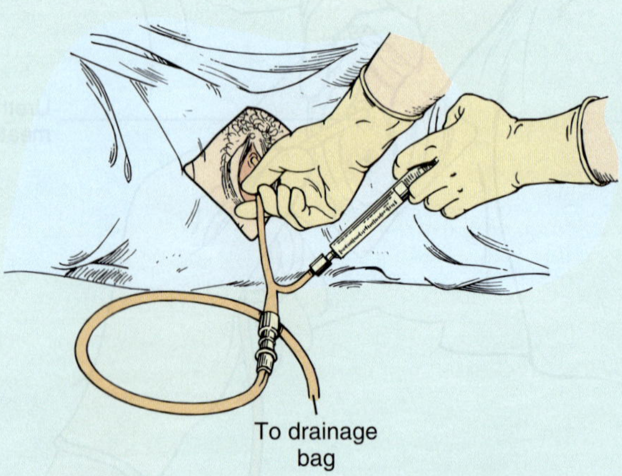

STEP 21C Inflate balloon (in-dwelling catheter).

Critical Decision Point *If the patient indicates sudden pain during inflation of a catheter balloon or if resistance is felt when inflating the balloon, stop inflation, allow the fluid from the balloon to flow back into the syringe, advance the catheter farther, and re-inflate the balloon. The balloon may have been inflating in the urethra. If pain continues, remove the catheter and notify the health care provider.*

d. After inflating catheter balloon, release catheter from nondominant hand. Gently pull catheter until resistance is felt. Then advance catheter slightly.	By moving catheter slightly back into bladder, pressure on bladder neck is avoided.
e. Connect drainage tubing to catheter if it is not already preconnected.	
22. Secure catheter with catheter strap or another securement device attached to the drainage bag tubing and the patient's leg. Leave enough slack to allow leg movement.	Securing catheter reduces the risk of catheter migration, inflammation, necrosis, CAUTI, or accidental catheter removal (Yates, 2018). Leaving enough slack allows for leg movement and penile erection without causing urethral trauma.
a. *Patient with female genitalia:*	
(1) Secure catheter tubing to inner thigh, allowing enough slack to prevent tension (see Step 22a[1] illustration).	
b. *Patient with male genitalia:*	
(1) Secure catheter tubing to upper thigh (see Step 22b[1] illustration) or lower abdomen (with penis directed toward chest). Allow slack in catheter so movement does not create tension on catheter.	Anchoring catheter reduces traction on urethra and minimizes urethral injury (Yates, 2018).

STEP	RATIONALE

IMPLEMENTATION

(2) If retracted, replace foreskin over glans penis. — Leaving foreskin retracted can cause discomfort and dangerous edema.

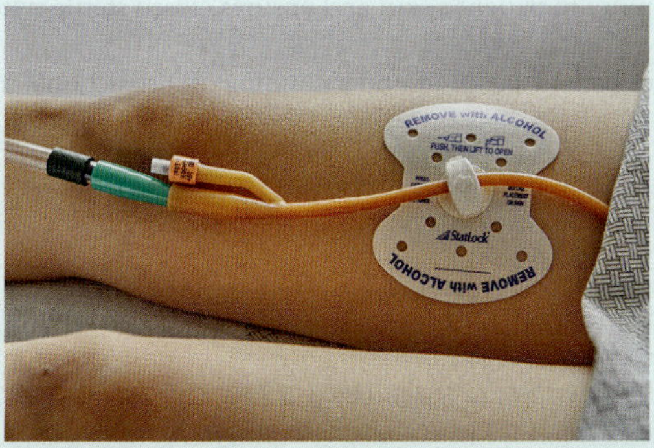

STEP 22A(1) Secure in-dwelling catheter on patient with female genitalia using adhesive securement device.

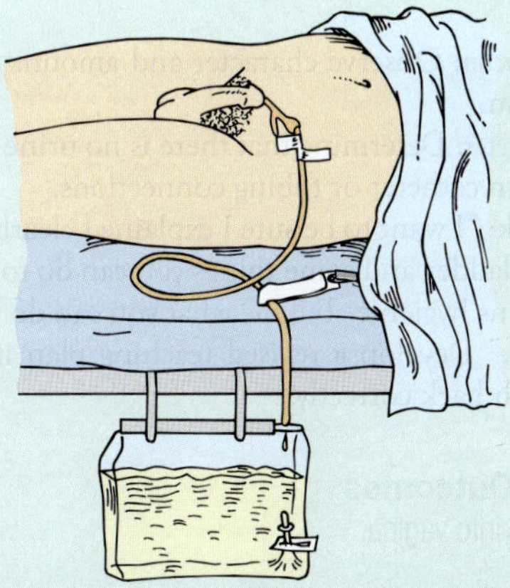

STEP 22B(1) Secure in-dwelling catheter on patient with male genitalia using tape. (*From Sorrentino, S. A., Remmert, L. N., & Wilk, M. J. [2018]. Mosby's Canadian textbook for the support worker [4th ed., Fig. 31.11B]. Elsevier.*)

23. Clip drainage tubing to edge of mattress. Position drainage bag lower than bladder by attaching bag to bedframe. Do not attach bag to side rails of bed (see Step 23 illustration). — Drainage bags that are below level of bladder ensure free flow of urine, thus decreasing the risk of CAUTI (WOCN, 2016). Bags attached to movable objects such as side rail increase the risk of urethral trauma because of pulling or accidental dislodgement.

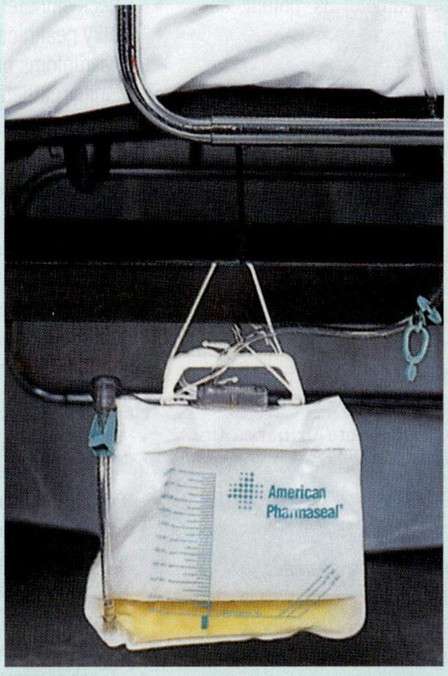

STEP 23 Drainage bag below level of bladder.

24. Check to ensure that there is no obstruction to urine flow. Coil excess tubing on bed and fasten to bottom sheet with clip or another securement device. — Obstruction to flow of urine increases the risk of CAUTI (WOCN, 2016).

25. Help patient to comfortable position.

26. Dispose of supplies in appropriate receptacles.

27. Measure urine and record volume. — Provides baseline for urinary output.

28. Remove gloves and discard. — Reduces transmission of infection.

STEP	RATIONALE
EVALUATION	
1. Palpate bladder for distension or use bladder scan (see Procedural Guideline 34.2) per employer policy.	Determines whether distension is relieved.
2. Ask patient to describe level of comfort.	Determines whether patient's sensation of discomfort or fullness has been relieved.
3. *In-dwelling catheter:* Observe character and amount of urine in drainage system.	Determines whether urine is flowing adequately.
4. *In-dwelling catheter:* Determine that there is no urine leaking (or bypassing) from catheter or tubing connections.	Prevents injury to patient's skin and ensures closed sterile system.
5. Use teach-back: "I want to be sure I explained clearly about the tube in your bladder and some things you can do to ensure the catheter remains hygienic. Tell me what you can do to keep the catheter clean." Develop a revised teaching plan if patient is unable to teach back correctly.	Determines patient's level of understanding of instructional topic.

Unexpected Outcomes	Related Interventions
1. Catheter goes into vagina.	• Leave catheter in vagina. • Clean urinary meatus again. Using a new catheter kit, insert sterile catheter into meatus (check employer policy). **Note:** If gloves become contaminated, start procedure again. • Remove catheter in vagina after successful insertion of second catheter.
2. Sterility is broken during catheterization by nurse or patient.	• Replace gloves if contaminated and start over. • If patient touches sterile field but equipment and supplies remain sterile, avoid touching that part of sterile field. • If equipment or supplies become contaminated, replace with sterile items or start over with new sterile kit.
3. Patient indicates bladder discomfort, and catheter is patent as evidenced by adequate urine flow.	• Check catheter to ensure that there is no traction on it. • Notify health care provider. Patient may be experiencing bladder spasms or symptoms of a UTI. • Monitor catheter output for colour, clarity, odour, and amount.

Communication and Documentation

- Document and report the reason for catheterization, type and size of catheter inserted, amount of fluid used to inflate balloon, specimen collection (if applicable), characteristics and amount of urine, patient's response to procedure, and any education in progress notes in electronic health record (EHR) or chart.
- Document amount of urine on I&O flow sheet record in EHR or chart.
- Report persistent catheter-related pain, inadequate urinary output, and discomfort to health care provider.
- Document your evaluation of patient learning.

DOCUMENTATION EXAMPLE

Inserted a 16 French two-way Foley catheter using sterile technique to manage urinary retention. Balloon inflated with 10 mL of sterile water, patient denied pain with insertion and balloon inflation. Immediately following insertion, 300 mL of clear, amber urine drained, a sample was obtained and sent for lab analysis. Catheter secured to leg with StatLock and urinary drainage bag attached to bed frame. Patient instructed to notify nurse if discomfort develops and verbalized understanding of same.

Special Considerations

Teaching

- Discuss with patient the steps involved in routine care of the catheter and drainage system, which includes avoiding any kinking in the drainage tubing, keeping the drainage bag dependent, avoiding pulling on the catheter, and performing daily hygiene.
- Explain that adequate fluid intake helps prevent catheter blockage.
- Teach patients and family caregivers appropriate assessments, such as signs and symptoms of a UTI, how to prevent a UTI, and signs of skin irritation.

Pediatric

- When caring for an infant or a young child, explain procedures to parents. Describe procedure to a child at a level the child is able to understand (Hockenberry et al., 2024).
- Children and adolescents will experience some discomfort during catheterization. Assistance and gentle holding may be necessary, especially with younger children. Most children prefer to have the parents remain with them during the procedure. Ask adolescents whether they would like a parent to remain with them.
- Catheterization in infants and children may be made easier by use of an adequate amount of catheter lubricant containing 2% lidocaine (Hockenberry et al., 2024).
- Teaching young children to blow into a straw or pinwheel can help to relax pelvic muscles during catheter insertion (Hockenberry et al., 2024).

Gerontological

- The urethral meatus of an older person with female genitalia may be difficult to identify because of urogenital atrophy.

- Symptoms of a UTI in an older person may be difficult to recognize and may be indicated by cognitive changes, lethargy, anorexia, weakness, tachycardia, hypotension, and increased respiratory rate (WOCN, 2016).
- Older persons have an increased risk of contracting UTIs owing to increased prevalence of chronic diseases such as diabetes mellitus and prostatic hypertrophy and a higher prevalence of incontinence.
- The presence of a urinary catheter and its drainage tubing and bag can interfere with the already compromised mobility of the older person.

Patients With Physical or Cognitive Challenges

- Insertion of an in-dwelling catheter may elicit different reactions from a person with cognitive challenges. It is important to carefully consider the needs of the individual and provide care in a sensitive and respectful manner (Tremayne & Pawlyn, 2019).

Care in the Community: Home Management

- Patients who are at home may use a leg bag during the day and switch to a larger-volume bag at night. If a patient changes from a large-volume bag to a leg bag, instruct them on the importance of hand hygiene and cleaning the connection ports with alcohol before changing bags.
- Teach patients and caregivers how to properly position the drainage bag; empty the urinary drainage bag; and observe urine colour, clarity, odour, and amount.
- Educate patients and caregivers about the signs of a UTI and troubleshooting techniques for a leaking catheter.
- Arrange for home delivery of catheter supplies, always ensuring that there is at least one extra catheter, insertion kit, and drainage bag in the home.

✦ SKILL 34.2 Care and Removal of an in-dwelling Catheter

NSO Nursing Skills Online Urinary Catheterization Module 17 / Lesson 5

In patients with an in-dwelling catheter, providing regular perineal hygiene, preventing catheter-related trauma, and removing in-dwelling catheters as soon as possible are important interventions to reduce the risk of CAUTI (HEC, n.d.; Schaeffer, 2021). Prolonged in-dwelling catheterization is a major risk factor for CAUTI. When removing an in-dwelling catheter, the nurse must ensure that the catheter balloon is fully deflated to minimize trauma to the urethra. Clinicians often clamp the catheter tubing before removal, believing that this practice allows the bladder to fill and obtain bladder tone; however, evidence is inconclusive as to whether this practice improves bladder function after catheter removal (WOCN, 2016).

All patients should have their voiding monitored in a voiding record or bladder diary for at least 24 to 48 hours after catheter removal. The nurse records the time and amount of each voiding, including any incontinence, in the patient record to ensure that the patient is able to urinate and empty their bladder properly. On specialty units or under specific circumstances, a bladder scan (see Procedural Guideline 34.2) or ultrasound may be used to monitor bladder functioning by measuring PVR. Abdominal pain and distension, a sensation of incomplete emptying, incontinence, constant dribbling of urine, and voiding in very small amounts can indicate inadequate bladder emptying, requiring intervention.

The risk of a UTI increases with the use of an in-dwelling catheter. Symptoms of infection can develop 2 or more days after catheter removal. Nurses need to inform patients of the risk for infection, prevention measures (e.g., perineal hygiene), and signs and symptoms that need to be reported to the health care provider.

Delegation and Collaboration

The skill of performing routine catheter care can be delegated to a UCP. The skill of removing an in-dwelling catheter can be delegated to a UCP (see employer policy); however, the nurse must first assess a patient's status and verify the health care provider's prescription. The nurse directs the UCP to do the following:

- Report characteristics of the urine (colour, clarity, odour, and amount) before and after catheter removal
- Report the condition of the patient's genital area (e.g., colour, rashes, open areas, odour, soiling from bowel incontinence, trauma to tissues around urinary meatus)
- If permitted by employer policy to remove catheter, check size of balloon and syringe needed to deflate balloon and report if balloon does not deflate and if there is bleeding after removal
- Report time and amount of first voiding after catheter is removed
- Report patient indications of fever, chills, burning, flank pain, back pain, and blood in the urine
- Report patient indications of dysuria, hematuria, urgency, frequency, lower abdominal pain, change in mental status, and lethargy

Collaborate with interprofessional health team members (e.g., wound/ostomy nurse) for specific skin care measures if the patient has perineal skin irritation from the catheter, from adhesive of the catheter stabilization device, or from drainage around catheter insertion site.

Equipment

Catheter Care

- Clean gloves
- Waterproof pad
- Bath blanket
- Soap, washcloth, towel, and basin filled with warm water
- 2% chlorhexidine gluconate (CHG) cloth *(optional)*

Removing a Catheter

- 10-mL or larger syringe without needle (Information on balloon size [mL] is printed directly on balloon inflation valve [see Fig. 34.3].)
- Graduated cylinder to measure urine
- Toilet, bedside commode, urine "hat," urinal, or bedpan
- Bladder scanner (if indicated)

STEP	RATIONALE
ASSESSMENT	
1. Identify patient using at least two person-specific identifiers (e.g., name and date of birth, or name and medical record number) according to employer policy.	Ensures correct patient. Complies with Accreditation Canada's standards and improves patient safety (Accreditation Canada, 2020).
2. Throughout the procedure, the 4 moments for hand hygiene are to be implemented; hand hygiene should occur before initial patient (or patient environment) contact, before an aseptic procedure, after body fluid exposure risk, and after patient (or patient environment) contact. Additional hand hygiene should be performed when hands are visibly soiled.	Proper hand hygiene helps prevent the spread of infectious agents to health care providers.
3. Assess need for catheter care:	
a. Observe urinary output and urine characteristics.	Reduces transmission of microorganisms. A sudden decrease in urinary output may indicate occlusion of catheter. Cloudy, foul-smelling urine associated with other systemic symptoms may indicate CAUTI.
b. Assess for history or presence of bowel incontinence.	The most common bacteria to cause CAUTI are *Escherichia coli*, a major colonizer of the bowel; thus, bowel incontinence increases the risk of CAUTI (Fekete, 2022).
c. Observe for any discharge, redness, bleeding, or presence of tissue trauma around urethral meatus (this may be deferred until catheter care).	Indicates inflammatory process, possible infection, or erosion of catheter through urethra.
d. Assess patient's knowledge of catheter care.	Determines need for patient education related to catheter care.
4. Assess need for catheter removal:	
a. Review patient's medical record, including health care provider's prescription and progress notes. Note length of time catheter has been in place.	Catheters in place for more than a few days cause higher risk for catheter encrustation and UTI.
b. Assess patient's knowledge of and prior experience with catheter removal.	Reveals need for patient instruction and support.
c. Assess urine colour, clarity, odour, and amount. Note any urethral discharge, irritation of genital region, or trauma to urinary meatus (this may be deferred until just before catheter removal).	May be indicator of inflammation or a UTI and source of discomfort during catheter removal.
d. Determine size of catheter inflation balloon by looking at balloon inflation valve.	Determines size of syringe needed to deflate balloon and amount of fluid expected in syringe after deflation.

NURSING DIAGNOSES

- Reduced urinary elimination
- Insufficient knowledge regarding catheter care
- Potential for infection

Related factors and risk factors are individualized on the basis of patient's condition or needs.

PLANNING

STEP	RATIONALE
1. Expected outcomes following catheter care:	
• Genital area is free of secretions, fecal matter, and irritation.	Basic hygiene, especially after bowel movements, reduces the risk of CAUTI (Schaeffer, 2023).
• Patient verbalizes feeling of comfort.	Cleaning relieves local discomfort from irritation of catheter.
2. Expected outcomes after catheter removal:	
• Patient voids at least 150 mL with each voiding no more than 6–8 hours after removal.	Indicates return of voluntary bladder function without urinary retention.
• Patient verbalizes feeling of complete bladder emptying and absence of discomfort.	
• Patient identifies signs and symptoms of a UTI.	Indicates patient learning.
3. Explain procedure to patient. Discuss signs and symptoms of a UTI. If applicable, teach patient how to perform catheter hygiene.	Reduces anxiety and promotes cooperation. Self-care supports patient's sense of autonomy.

STEP	RATIONALE
IMPLEMENTATION	
1. Close room door and bedside curtain.	Provides patient privacy.
2. Raise bed to appropriate working height. If side rails are raised, lower side rail on working side.	Promotes use of proper body mechanics.
3. Organize equipment for perineal care and/or removal of catheter.	Increases efficiency of procedure.
4. Position patient in dorsal recumbent position with waterproof pad under buttocks. Cover patient with bath blanket, exposing only genital area and catheter (see Skill 34.1).	Demonstrates person-centred care and respect for patient dignity by only exposing necessary part of body.
5. Apply clean gloves.	Reduces transmission of microorganisms.
6. Remove catheter securement device while maintaining connection with drainage tubing.	Provides ability to easily clean around catheter and to remove it.
7. Catheter care:	
a. *Patient with female genitalia:* Use nondominant hand to gently separate labia to fully expose urethral meatus and catheter. Maintain position of hand throughout procedure.	Provides full visualization of urethral meatus. Full separation of labia prevents contamination of meatus during cleaning.
b. *Patient with male genitalia:* Use nondominant hand to retract foreskin of penis if not circumcised and hold penis at shaft just below glans. Maintain hand position throughout procedure.	Retraction of foreskin provides full visualization of urethral meatus.

Critical Decision Point *Accidently closing labia or dropping penis during cleaning requires procedure to be repeated.*

STEP	RATIONALE
c. Grasp catheter with two fingers to stabilize it.	Prevents unnecessary traction on catheter. Pulling on catheter is a cause of discomfort for patient and can damage urethra and bladder neck.
d. Assess urethral meatus and surrounding tissues for inflammation, swelling, discharge, or tissue trauma and ask patient whether burning or discomfort is present.	Determines frequency and type of ongoing care required. Indicates possibility of CAUTI or catheter erosion through urethra.
e. Provide perineal hygiene using mild soap and warm water (see Chapter 18). Use solution identified by employer policy.	Antiseptic cleaners have not been proven conclusively to decrease the risk of CAUTI. CHG use has not been supported with sufficient evidence, and there have been rare cases of anaphylaxis due to use of CHG gel (WOCN, 2016).
f. Using clean washcloth, clean catheter.	
(1) Starting close to urinary meatus, clean catheter in circular motion along its length for about 10 cm (4 inches), moving away from body (see Step 7f[1] illustration). Remove all traces of soap. *For patients with male genitalia:* Reduce or reposition foreskin after care.	Reduces presence of secretions or drainage on outside surface of catheter.

STEP	RATIONALE

IMPLEMENTATION

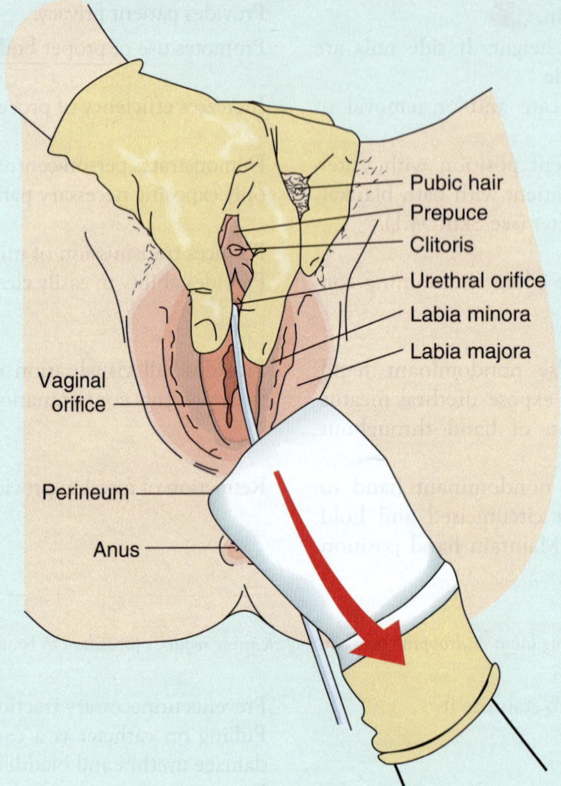

STEP 7F(1) Clean catheter starting at meatus and moving downward while holding it securely.

STEP	RATIONALE
g. Reapply catheter securement device. Allow slack in catheter to ensure movement does not create tension on it.	Securing in-dwelling catheter reduces the risk of urethral trauma, urethral erosion, CAUTI, and accidental removal (HEC, n.d.; Yates, 2018).
8. Routinely check drainage tubing and bag:	
a. Catheter is secured to upper thigh (for patients with female genitalia) or abdomen (for patients with male genitalia).	Maintains unobstructed flow of urine out of bladder (HEC, n.d.; Yates, 2018).
b. Tubing is coiled and secured onto bed linen.	
c. Tubing is not looped or positioned above level of bladder.	
d. Tubing is not kinked or clamped.	
e. Drainage bag is positioned below level of bladder, with urine flowing freely into bag.	
f. Drainage bag is not overfull. Empty drainage bag when half full.	Overfull drainage bag creates tension and pulls on catheter, resulting in trauma to urethra and/or urinary meatus (Yates, 2018).
9. Catheter removal: (Follow Step 7, in this skill, before catheter removal.)	
a. Move syringe plunger up and down to loosen it, and then pull it back to 0.5 mL. Insert hub of syringe into inflation valve (balloon port). Allow balloon fluid to drain into syringe by gravity. The syringe should fill. Make sure that entire amount of fluid is removed by comparing removed amount to volume needed for inflation.	A partially inflated balloon can traumatize the urethral wall during removal. Passive drainage of catheter balloon prevents formation of ridges in balloon. These ridges can cause discomfort or trauma during removal.
b. Pull catheter out smoothly and slowly. Examine it to ensure that it is whole and that tip is intact. The catheter should slide out easily. Do not use force. If you note any resistance, repeat Step 10a to remove remaining water.	A nonwhole (not intact) catheter means that pieces of catheter may still be in the bladder. Notify health care provider immediately.

STEP	RATIONALE
IMPLEMENTATION	
c. Wrap contaminated catheter in waterproof pad. Unhook collection bag and drainage tubing from bed.	Promotes patient comfort and safety.
d. Empty, measure, and record urine present in drainage bag (see Chapter 8).	Documents urinary output.
e. Encourage patient to maintain or increase fluid intake (unless contraindicated).	Maintains normal urinary output.
f. Initiate voiding record or bladder diary. Instruct patient to tell you when the need to empty bladder occurs and that all urine needs to be measured. Make sure that patient understands how to use collection container.	Evaluates bladder function.
g. Explain that many patients experience mild burning, discomfort, or small-volume voiding with first voiding, which are symptoms that soon subside.	Burning results from urethral irritation.
h. Instruct patient to report any signs of a UTI.	
i. Ensure easy access to toilet, commode, bedpan, or urinal. Place urine "hat" on toilet seat if patient is using toilet. Place call bell within easy reach.	Reduces incidence of falls during toileting. Urine hat collects first voided urine.
10. Reposition patient as necessary. Provide hygiene as needed. Lower level of bed and position side rails accordingly.	Promotes patient comfort and safety.
11. Dispose of all contaminated supplies in appropriate receptacle. Remove gloves and discard.	Reduces transmission of microorganisms.
EVALUATION	
1. Inspect catheter and genital area for soiling, irritation, and skin breakdown. Ask patient about discomfort.	Determines whether area has been cleaned properly and whether patient has any irritation.
2. Record time and amount of first voiding after catheter removal.	Indicates return of bladder function after catheter removal.
3. Evaluate patient for signs and symptoms of a UTI.	Any patient who has a catheter or has had a catheter removed recently is at risk for a UTI.
4. **Use teach-back:** "I want to be sure I explained clearly the signs of a urinary tract infection. In your own words, tell me what signs indicate a urinary tract infection." Develop a revised teaching plan if patient is unable to teach back correctly.	Determines patient's level of understanding of instructional topic.

Unexpected Outcomes	Related Interventions
1. Water from inflation balloon does not return into syringe.	• Reposition patient; ensure that catheter is not pinched or kinked. • Remove syringe. Attach new syringe and allow enough time for passive emptying. • Attempt to empty balloon by gently pulling back on syringe plunger. • If catheter balloon does not deflate, *do not* cut balloon inflation valve to drain water. Notify health care provider.
2. Patient has cloudy urine, foul urine odour, fever, chills, dysuria, flank pain, back pain, hematuria, urgency, frequency, lower abdominal pain, change in mental status, and lethargy (Fekete, 2022; MedlinePlus, 2022).	• Assess for bladder distension and tenderness. • Monitor vital signs and urinary output and any changes in level of consciousness. • Report findings to health care provider; signs and symptoms may indicate a UTI. • Consult with health care provider for prescription to remove catheter.
3. Patient is unable to void after catheter removal, has sensation of not emptying, strains to void, or experiences small voiding amounts with increasing frequency.	• Assess for bladder distension. • Help patient into normal position for voiding and provide privacy. • Perform bladder ultrasound or scan (see Procedural Guideline 34.2) to assess for excessive urine volume in bladder. • If patient is unable to void within 6–8 hours of catheter removal or experiences abdominal pain, notify health care provider.

Communication and Documentation

- Document time for catheter care, appearance of urine, and condition of meatus and catheter in progress notes in EHR or chart.
- Document and report time of catheter removal; amount of water removed from balloon; condition of urethral meatus and catheter; and the time, amount, and characteristics of first voided urine in progress notes in EHR or chart.
- Document teaching related to catheter care, catheter removal, and fluid intake in progress notes in EHR or chart.
- Report hematuria, fever, dysuria, inability or difficulty voiding, and any new incontinence after catheter removal to health care provider.
- For patient continuing to have a catheter in place, report signs of a UTI to health care provider.

DOCUMENTATION EXAMPLE

0730 hours verified prescription to remove Foley catheter after patient's recovery from surgical procedure. Catheter care performed and urethral meatus found to be free from tissue trauma, bleeding, or discharge. Passively removed 10 mL of sterile water from balloon. Slowly removed catheter ensuring patient comfort. Catheter inspected upon removal; tip of catheter remains intact. Patient instructed to increase fluid intake to promote voiding and to report any hematuria, difficulty voiding, or incontinence and verbalized understanding of same.

Special Considerations

Cultural Considerations

- Patients from some cultures may prefer a same-gender caregiver to provide care for urinary elimination tasks. Respect for patients' privacy and modesty concerns should be provided.

Teaching

- Unless contraindicated, patients with a catheter should drink at least 2 L of fluid per day to promote continuous flushing of the bladder and to prevent sediment from collecting in the catheter tubing.
- Instruct patient to hold collection bag below the level of the bladder when ambulating.
- Instruct patient not to disconnect the catheter from the collection tubing and bag.

Pediatric

- During catheter removal, do not force catheter out of bladder if you encounter resistance. When excessive tubing has been inserted in the bladder, there have been occurrences of knotting of the tube (Hockenberry et al., 2024).

Gerontological

- Older persons may exhibit atypical signs and symptoms of CAUTI, such as a change in mental status attributed to delirium. A change in mental status may include confusion, agitation, and lethargy.
- In contrast to a UTI, asymptomatic bacteriuria (ASB) is more common in older persons than in younger adults (Fekete, 2022). Residents of long-term care often suffer from significant cognitive deficits, impairing their ability to communicate, and from chronic genitourinary symptoms (e.g., incontinence, urgency, and frequency), making it particularly challenging to diagnose a symptomatic UTI in this group. Furthermore, when infected, residents in long-term care are more likely to present with nonspecific symptoms of a UTI, such as lack of appetite, confusion, and a decline in functional status; fever may be absent or diminished (WOCN, 2016).

Care in the Community: Home Management

- Assess the patient and caregiver for ability and motivation to participate in routine catheter care.
- Collaborate with patients to adapt the home so that those with urinary frequency, urgency, nocturia, and urinary incontinence can reach toileting facilities quickly and safely.

Procedural Guideline 34.2 *Bladder Scan and Catheterization to Determine Residual Urine*

A bladder scanner (Fig. 34.5) is a noninvasive device that creates an ultrasound image of the bladder for measuring the volume of urine in the bladder. The device makes calculations to report accurate urine volumes, especially lower volumes. A bladder scanner is used to assess bladder volume whenever inadequate bladder emptying is suspected, such as after the removal of in-dwelling urinary catheters, in the evaluation of new-onset incontinence, and after urological surgery. The most common use of the bladder scanner is measurement of PVR (i.e., the volume of urine in the bladder after a normal voiding). To obtain the most reliable reading, measure PVR within 5 to 15 minutes of voiding (Power-Kean et al., 2023). A volume less than 50 mL is considered normal. Two or more PVR measurements greater than 100 mL require further investigation. If a bladder scanner is not available, obtain a PVR by measuring urine emptied from the bladder after a straight catheterization.

Delegation and Collaboration

The skill of measuring bladder volume by bladder scan can be delegated to a UCP. The nurse must first determine the timing and frequency of the bladder scan measurement and interpret the measurements obtained. The nurse also assesses the patient's ability to toilet before measuring PVR and the abdomen for distension if urinary retention is suspected. The nurse directs the UCP to do the following:

- Follow manufacturer recommendations for use of the device
- Measure PVR volumes within 5 to 15 minutes after helping the patient to void
- Report and document bladder scan volumes

Equipment

- Bladder scanner (follow manufacturer instructions for use)
- Ultrasound gel
- Cleaning agent for scanner head such as an alcohol pad
- Urethral catheterization tray with single-use catheter for straight/intermittent catheterization (see Skill 34.1)
- Paper towel or washcloth

Procedural Steps

1. Identify patient using at least two person-specific identifiers (e.g., name and date of birth, or name and medical record number) according to employer policy (Accreditation Canada, 2020).
2. Throughout the procedure, the 4 moments for hand hygiene are to be implemented; hand hygiene should occur before initial patient (or patient environment) contact, before an aseptic procedure, after body fluid exposure risk, and after patient (or patient environment) contact. Additional hand hygiene should be performed when hands are visibly soiled.

Procedural Guideline 34.2 *Bladder Scan and Catheterization to Determine Residual Urine—cont'd*

3. Assess I&O record to determine urinary output trends, and check the plan of care to verify correct timing of the bladder scan measurement.
4. Apply clean gloves.
5. Provide privacy by closing the room door and bedside curtain.
6. Discuss procedure with patient. If measurement is for PVR, ask patient to void, then measure voided urine volume. Measurement should be within 5 to 15 minutes of voiding.
7. Measure PVR with the bladder scanner:
   a. Help patient to a supine position with head slightly elevated. Raise bed to appropriate working height. If side rails are raised, lower side rail on working side.
   b. Expose patient's lower abdomen.
   c. Turn on scanner per manufacturer guidelines.
   d. Set gender designation per manufacturer guidelines. Patients with female genitalia who have had a hysterectomy should be designated as male.
   e. Wipe scanner head with alcohol pad or other cleaner and allow to air dry.
   f. Palpate patient's symphysis pubis (pubic bone). Apply generous amount of ultrasound gel (or, if available, a bladder scan gel pad) to midline abdomen 2.5–4 cm (1–1.5 inches) above symphysis pubis.
   g. Place scanner head on gel, ensuring that scanner head is oriented per manufacturer guidelines.
   h. Apply light pressure, keep scanner head steady, and point it slightly downward toward bladder. Press and release the scan button (see Step 7h illustration).
   i. Verify accurate aim (refer to manufacturer guidelines). Complete scan and print image (if needed).
8. Remove ultrasound gel from patient's abdomen with paper towel or moist cloth.
9. Remove ultrasound gel from scanner head and wipe with alcohol pad or other cleaner; allow to air dry.
10. Help patient to comfortable position. Lower bed and replace side rails accordingly.
11. Remove gloves and discard.
12. Measure PVR after using straight/intermittent catheterization (see Skill 34.1). Compare results with prevoiding scan; urine volume should be less.
13. Review health care provider's prescription to determine how often to assess residual urine.
14. Review I&O record to determine urinary output trends.

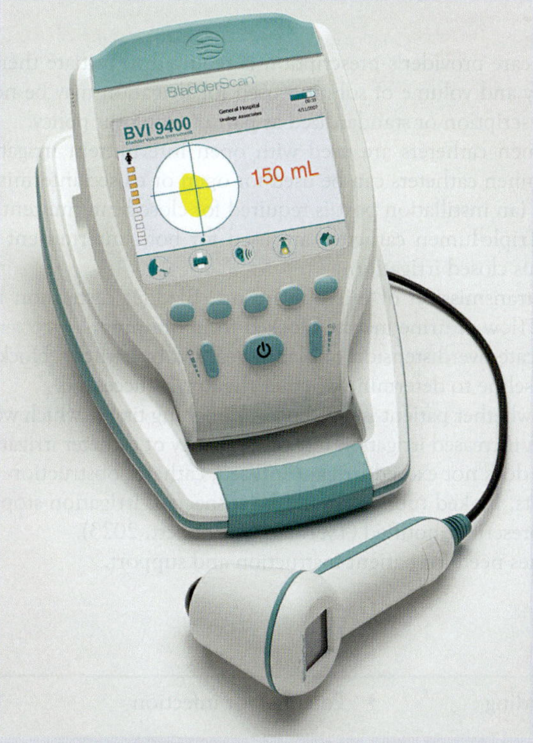

FIG 34.5 Bladder scanner with image.

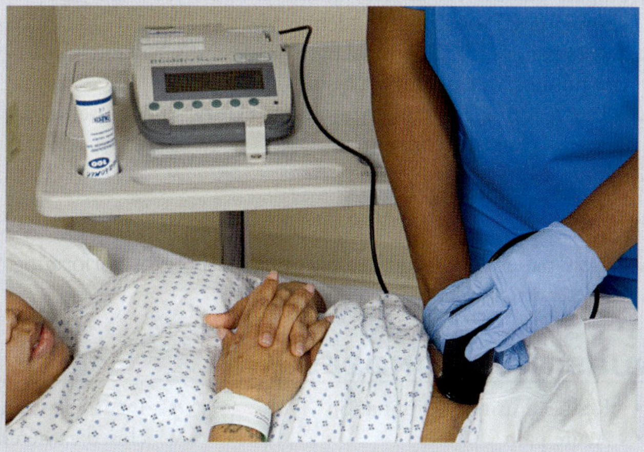

STEP 7H Placement of bladder scan head.

✦ SKILL 34.3 Performing Closed Intermittent Urinary Catheter Irrigation

To maintain the patency of in-dwelling catheters, it is sometimes necessary to irrigate or flush a catheter with sterile solution. However, irrigation is a risk factor for UTIs and thus must be done in a way that maintains a closed urinary drainage system. In some instances, the health care provider will determine that irrigations are needed to keep a catheter patent, such as after genitourinary surgery, when there is a high risk for catheter occlusion from blood clots.

Closed intermittent catheter irrigation provides irrigation of a urinary catheter without disrupting the sterile connection between the catheter and the drainage system.

Delegation and Collaboration

The skill of performing closed intermittent catheter irrigation cannot be delegated to a UCP. The nurse directs the UCP to do the following:

- Report to the nurse if patient indicates pain, discomfort, or leakage of fluid around the catheter
- Monitor and document I&O; report immediately any decrease in urinary output
- Report any change in urine colour, especially the presence of blood clots

Equipment

- Sterile irrigation solution at room temperature (as prescribed)
- Antiseptic swabs
- Clean gloves
- Sterile container
- Syringe to access system: Luer-Lok syringe for needleless access port (per manufacturer instructions)
- Screw clamp or rubber band (used to temporarily occlude catheter as irrigant is instilled)

STEP	RATIONALE
ASSESSMENT	
1. Identify patient using at least two person-specific identifiers (e.g., name and date of birth, or name and medical record number) according to employer policy.	Ensures correct patient. Complies with Accreditation Canada's standards and improves patient safety (Accreditation Canada, 2020).
2. Throughout the procedure, the 4 moments for hand hygiene are to be implemented; hand hygiene should occur before initial patient (or patient environment) contact, before an aseptic procedure, after body fluid exposure risk, and after patient (or patient environment) contact. Additional hand hygiene should be performed when hands are visibly soiled.	Proper hand hygiene helps prevent the spread of infectious agents to health care providers.
3. Verify information in medical record:	
a. Prescription for irrigation method (continuous or intermittent), type of irrigant (sterile saline or medicated solution), and amount of irrigant.	A health care provider's prescription is required to initiate therapy. Frequency and volume of solution used for irrigation may be noted in the prescription or standardized as part of employer policy.
b. Type of catheter in place (see Fig. 34.2).	Single-lumen catheters are used with open intermittent irrigation. Double-lumen catheters can be used for open or closed intermittent irrigation (an instillation port is required for closed intermittent irrigation). Triple-lumen catheters are used for both intermittent and continuous closed irrigation.
4. Palpate bladder for distension and tenderness or use bladder scanner (see Procedural Guideline 34.2).	Reduces transmission of microorganisms. Bladder distension indicates that flow of urine may be blocked from draining.
5. Assess patient for abdominal pain or spasms, sensation of bladder fullness, or catheter bypassing (leaking).	May indicate overdistension of bladder caused by catheter blockage. Offers baseline to determine whether therapy is successful.
6. Observe urine for colour, amount, clarity, and presence of mucous, clots, or sediment.	Indicates whether patient is bleeding or sloughing tissue, which would require an increased irrigation rate or frequency of catheter irrigation.
7. Monitor I&O.	If output does not exceed irrigant infused, catheter obstruction (i.e., blood clots, kinked tubing) should be suspected, irrigation stopped, and the prescriber notified (Tyerman & Cobbett, 2023).
8. Assess patient's knowledge regarding purpose of performing catheter irrigation.	Determines need for patient instruction and support.

NURSING DIAGNOSES

- Reduced urinary elimination
- Acute pain
- Insufficient knowledge regarding closed catheter irrigation
- Potential for infection

Related factors and risk factors are individualized on the basis of patient's condition or needs.

PLANNING

STEP	RATIONALE
1. Expected outcomes following completion of this procedure:	
• Patient reports relief of bladder pain or spasms.	Indicates bladder emptying.
• Urinary output has decreased with an absence of blood clots and sediment. (NOTE: Urine will be bloody following bladder or urethral surgery, gradually becoming lighter and blood tinged in 2–3 days.)	Indicates that catheter is at decreased risk of occlusion with blood clots.
• Absence of fever, lower abdominal pain, and cloudy or foul-smelling urine.	Signs of a UTI are not present.
• Patient explains purpose of procedure and what to expect.	Demonstrates learning.
2. Explain procedure to patient.	Reduces anxiety and promotes cooperation.

STEP	RATIONALE
IMPLEMENTATION	
1. Provide privacy by closing room door and bedside curtain.	Demonstrates person-centred care by promoting patient comfort and dignity.
2. Raise bed to appropriate working height. If side rails are raised, lower side rail on working side.	Promotes use of good body mechanics. Position provides access to the catheter and promotes patient dignity as much as possible.
3. Position patient supine and expose catheter junctions (catheter and drainage tubing).	Position provides access to the catheter and promotes patient dignity as much as possible.
4. Remove catheter securement device.	Eases access to catheter parts.
5. Organize supplies and apply clean gloves.	Ensures an efficient procedure. Reduces transmission of microorganisms.
6. Perform closed intermittent irrigation:	Fluid is instilled through catheter in a bolus, flushing the system. Fluid drains out after irrigation is complete.
a. Pour prescribed sterile irrigation solution into sterile container.	
b. Draw prescribed volume of irrigant (usually 30–50 mL) into sterile syringe using aseptic technique. Place sterile cap on tip of needleless syringe.	Ensures sterility of irrigating fluid.
c. Clamp catheter tubing below soft injection port with screw clamp (or fold catheter tubing onto itself and secure with rubber band).	Occluding catheter tubing below point of injection allows irrigating solution to enter catheter and flow into bladder.
d. Using circular motion, clean catheter port (specimen port) with an antiseptic swab.	Reduces transmission of microorganisms.
e. Insert tip of needleless syringe using twisting motion into port.	Ensures that catheter tip enters lumen of catheter.
f. Inject solution using slow, even pressure.	Gentle instillation of solution minimizes trauma to bladder mucosa.
g. Remove syringe and clamp (or rubber band), allowing solution to drain into urinary drainage bag. (NOTE: Some medicated irrigants may need to dwell in the bladder for a prescribed period, requiring the catheter to be clamped temporarily before being allowed to drain.)	Allows drainage to flow out by gravity. Medications must be instilled long enough to be absorbed by lining of bladder. Clamped drainage tubing and bag should not be left unattended.
7. Anchor catheter with a catheter securement device (see Skill 34.1).	Prevents trauma to urethral tissue caused by pulling catheter.
8. Help patient to a safe and comfortable position. Lower bed and place side rails accordingly.	Promotes patient comfort and safety.
9. Dispose of all contaminated supplies in an appropriate receptacle. Remove gloves and discard.	Reduces transmission of microorganisms.
EVALUATION	
1. Measure actual urinary output by subtracting total amount of irrigation fluid infused from total volume drained into basin.	Determines accurate urinary output.
2. Review I&O flow sheet to verify that hourly output into drainage bag is in appropriate proportion to irrigating solution entering bladder. Expect more output than fluid instilled because of urine production.	Determines urinary output in relation to irrigation.
3. Inspect urine for blood clots and sediment, and ensure that tubing is not kinked or occluded.	Decrease in blood clots means that therapy is successful in maintaining catheter patency. System is patent.
4. Evaluate patient's comfort level.	Indicates catheter patency by absence of symptoms of bladder distension.
5. Monitor for signs and symptoms of infection.	Patients with in-dwelling catheters remain at risk for infection.
6. **Use teach-back:** "I want to be sure I explained clearly about the flushing of your catheter. Tell me in your own words the reason we are flushing your catheter." Develop a revised teaching plan if patient is unable to teach back correctly.	Determines patient's level of understanding of instructional topic.

Unexpected Outcomes	Related Interventions
1. Irrigating solution does not return.	• Examine tubing for clots, sediment, and kinks. • Notify health care provider if irrigant does not flow freely from bladder, patient indicates pain, or bladder distension occurs.
2. Drainage output is less than the amount of irrigation solution infused.	• Examine drainage tubing for clots, sediment, or kinks. • Inspect urine for presence of or an increase in blood clots and sediment. • Evaluate patient for pain and distended bladder. • Notify health care provider.
3. Patient experiences pain with irrigation.	• Examine drainage tubing for clots, sediment, or kinks. • Evaluate urine for presence of or increase in blood clots and sediment. • Evaluate for distended bladder. • Notify health care provider.

Communication and Documentation

- Document irrigation method, amount and type of irrigation solution, amount returned as drainage, characteristics of output, urinary output, and patient tolerance of procedure in progress notes in EHR or chart.
- Report catheter occlusion, sudden bleeding, infection, or increased pain to health care provider.
- Document I&O on the appropriate flow sheet.
- Document your evaluation of patient learning.

Special Considerations

Teaching

- Instruct patient and caregiver to observe urine daily for changes in colour, presence of mucous or blood, and odour.
- Inform patients that bleeding is common after many urological procedures and to expect bright red–tinged urine during the first 48 hours after surgery, followed by a change in colour ranging from pink tinged to clear.
- Instruct patient to maintain adequate oral intake of at least 2 L/day (unless contraindicated).

Care in the Community: Home Management

- Patients and caregivers can be taught to perform catheter irrigations with adequate support, demonstration and return demonstration, and written instructions.
- Teach patients and caregivers to regularly observe urine colour, clarity, odour, and amount.
- Arrange for home delivery and storage of catheter and irrigation supplies.
- Teach patients and caregivers signs of catheter obstruction or a UTI.

✦ SKILL 34.4 Performing Closed Continuous Urinary Catheter Irrigation

Continuous bladder irrigation (CBI) is an example of a continuous infusion of a sterile solution into the bladder, usually using a three-way irrigation closed system with a triple-lumen catheter (Fig. 34.6). CBI is frequently used following genitourinary surgery to keep the bladder clear and free of blood clots or sediment.

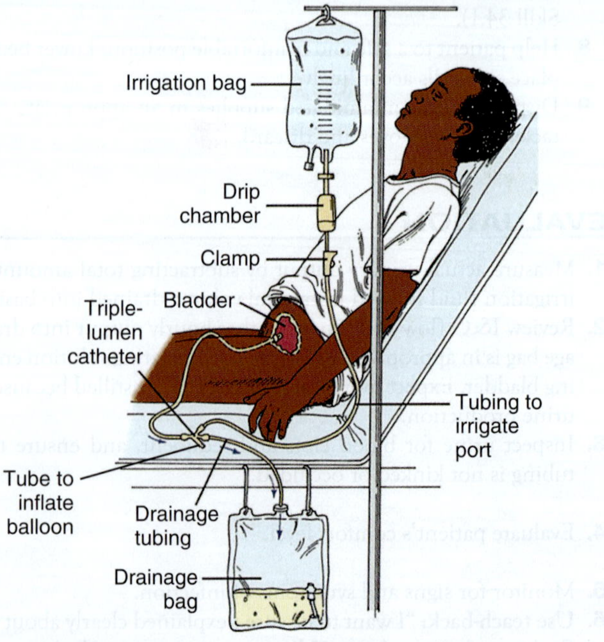

FIG 34.6 Closed continuous bladder irrigation.

Delegation and Collaboration

The skill of performing closed catheter irrigation cannot be delegated to a UCP. The nurse directs the UCP to do the following:

- Report to the nurse if patient indicates pain, discomfort, or leakage of fluid around catheter.
- Monitor and document I&O; report immediately any decrease in urinary output.
- Report any change in urine colour, especially the presence of blood clots.

Equipment

- Sterile irrigation solution at room temperature (as prescribed)
- Antiseptic swabs
- Clean gloves
- Irrigation tubing with clamp to regulate irrigation flow rate
- Y-connector (*optional*) to connect irrigation tubing to double-lumen catheter
- Intravenous (IV) pole (closed continuous or intermittent)

STEP	RATIONALE

ASSESSMENT

STEP	RATIONALE
1. Identify patient using at least two person-specific identifiers (e.g., name and date of birth, or name and medical record number) according to employer policy.	Ensures correct patient. Complies with Accreditation Canada's standards and improves patient safety (Accreditation Canada, 2020).
2. Throughout the procedure, the 4 moments for hand hygiene are to be implemented; hand hygiene should occur before initial patient (or patient environment) contact, before an aseptic procedure, after body fluid exposure risk, and after patient (or patient environment) contact. Additional hand hygiene should be performed when hands are visibly soiled.	Proper hand hygiene helps prevent the spread of infectious agents to health care providers.
3. Verify information in medical record:	
a. Prescription for irrigation method (continuous), type of irrigant (sterile saline or medicated solution), and amount of irrigant.	A health care provider's prescription is required to initiate therapy. Frequency and volume of solution used for irrigation may be noted in the prescription or standardized as part of employer policy.
b. Type of catheter in place (see Fig. 34.2).	Triple-lumen catheters are used for both intermittent and continuous closed irrigation.
4. Palpate bladder for distension and tenderness or use bladder scanner (see Procedural Guideline 34.2).	Reduces transmission of microorganisms. Bladder distension indicates that flow of urine may be blocked from draining.
5. Assess patient for abdominal pain or spasms, sensation of bladder fullness, or catheter bypassing (leaking).	May indicate overdistension of bladder caused by catheter blockage. Provides baseline to determine whether therapy is successful.
6. Observe urine for colour, amount, clarity, and presence of mucous, clots, or sediment.	Indicates whether patient is bleeding or sloughing tissue, which would require an increased irrigation rate or frequency of catheter irrigation.
7. Monitor I&O. When CBI is being used, the amount of fluid draining from the bladder should exceed the amount of fluid infused into the bladder.	If output does not exceed irrigant infused, catheter obstruction (i.e., blood clots, kinked tubing) should be suspected, irrigation stopped, and the prescriber notified (Tyerman & Cobbett, 2023).
8. Assess patient's knowledge regarding purpose of performing catheter irrigation.	Determines need for patient instruction and support.

NURSING DIAGNOSES

- Reduced urinary elimination
- Acute pain
- Insufficient knowledge regarding closed catheter irrigation
- Potential for infection

Related factors and risk factors are individualized on the basis of patient's condition or needs.

PLANNING

STEP	RATIONALE
1. Expected outcomes following completion of this procedure:	
a. Catheter fluid return is greater than volume of irrigating solution instilled.	Indicates patency of drainage system, allowing for drainage of urine and irrigating solution.
b. Patient reports relief of bladder pain or spasms.	Indicates bladder emptying.
c. Urinary output has decreased with an absence of blood clots and sediment. (NOTE: Urine will be bloody following bladder or urethral surgery, gradually becoming lighter and blood tinged in 2–3 days.)	Indicates that catheter is at decreased risk of occlusion with blood clots.
d. Absence of fever, lower abdominal pain, and cloudy or foul-smelling urine.	Signs of a UTI are not present.
e. Patient can explain purpose of the procedure and what to expect.	Demonstrates learning.
2. Explain procedure to patient.	Reduces anxiety and promotes cooperation.

STEP	RATIONALE
IMPLEMENTATION	
1. Provide privacy by closing room door and bedside curtain.	Demonstrates person-centred care by promoting patient comfort and dignity.
2. Raise bed to appropriate working height. If side rails are raised, lower side rail on working side.	Promotes use of good body mechanics. Position provides access to the catheter and promotes patient dignity as much as possible.
3. Position patient supine and expose catheter junctions (catheter and drainage tubing).	Position provides access to the catheter and promotes patient dignity as much as possible.
4. Remove catheter securement device.	Eases access to catheter parts.
5. Organize supplies according to type of irrigation prescribed. Apply clean gloves.	Ensures an efficient procedure. Reduces transmission of microorganisms.
6. Close clamp on new irrigation tubing and hang bag of irrigating solution on IV pole. Insert (spike) tip of sterile irrigation tubing into designated port of irrigation solution bag using aseptic technique (see Step 6a illustration).	Prevents air from entering tubing. Air can cause bladder spasms. Technique prevents transmission of microorganisms.

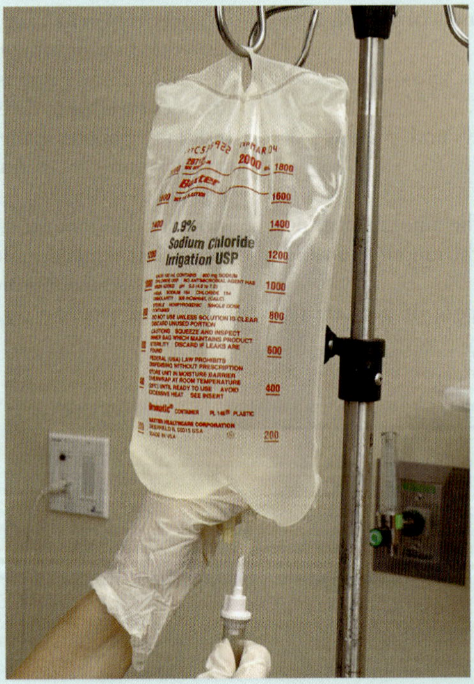

STEP 6A Spiking bag of sterile irrigation solution for continuous bladder irrigation.

STEP	RATIONALE
7. Fill drip chamber half full by squeezing chamber. Remove cap at end of tubing, then open clamp and allow solution to flow (prime) through tubing, keeping end of tubing sterile. Once fluid has completely filled tubing, close clamp and recap end of tubing.	Priming tubing with fluid prevents introduction of air into the bladder.
8. Using aseptic technique, remove cap and connect end of tubing securely to port for infusing irrigation fluid into double- or triple-lumen catheter.	Reduces transmission of microorganisms.
9. Adjust clamp on irrigation tubing to begin flow of solution into bladder. If set volume rate is prescribed, calculate drip rate and adjust rate at roller clamp. If urine is bright red or has clots, increase irrigation rate until drainage appears pink (according to prescribed rate or employer policy).	Continuous drainage is expected. It helps prevent clotting in the presence of active bleeding in the bladder and flushes clots out of the bladder.

Critical Decision Point *Some medicated irrigants may need to dwell in the bladder for a prescribed period, requiring the catheter to be clamped temporarily before being allowed to drain.*

STEP	RATIONALE
IMPLEMENTATION	
10. Observe for outflow of fluid into drainage bag. Empty catheter drainage bag as needed.	Discomfort, bladder distension, and possible injury can occur from overdistension of the bladder when bladder irrigant cannot adequately flow from the bladder. The bag will fill rapidly and may need to be emptied every 1–2 hours.
11. Anchor catheter with a catheter securement device (see Skill 34.1).	Prevents trauma to urethral tissue caused by pulling of catheter.
12. Help patient to a safe and comfortable position. Lower bed and place side rails accordingly.	Promotes patient comfort and safety.
13. Dispose of all contaminated supplies in an appropriate receptacle. Remove gloves and discard.	Reduces transmission of microorganisms.
EVALUATION	
1. Measure actual urinary output by subtracting total amount of irrigation fluid infused from total volume drained into basin.	Determines accurate urinary output.
2. Review I&O flow sheet to verify that hourly output into drainage bag is in appropriate proportion to irrigating solution entering bladder. Expect more output than fluid instilled because of urine production.	Determines urinary output in relation to irrigation.
3. Inspect urine for blood clots and sediment, and ensure that tubing is not kinked or occluded.	Decrease in blood clots means that therapy is successful in maintaining catheter patency. System is patent.
4. Evaluate patient's comfort level.	Absence of symptoms of bladder distension indicate catheter patency.
5. Monitor for signs and symptoms of infection.	Patients with in-dwelling catheters remain at risk for infection.
6. Use **teach-back:** "I want to be sure I explained clearly about the flushing of your catheter. Tell me in your own words the reason we are flushing your catheter." Develop a revised teaching plan if patient is unable to teach back correctly.	Determines patient's level of understanding of instructional topic.

Unexpected Outcomes	Related Interventions
1. Irrigating solution is not flowing at prescribed rate (CBI).	• Examine tubing for clots, sediment, and kinks. • Notify health care provider if irrigant does not flow freely from bladder, patient indicates pain, or bladder distension occurs.
2. Drainage output is less than the amount of irrigation solution infused.	• Examine drainage tubing for clots, sediment, or kinks. • Check bed for wetness due to bypassing of catheter. • Inspect urine for presence of or an increase in blood clots and sediment. • Evaluate patient for pain and distended bladder. • Notify health care provider.
3. Bright-red bleeding with the irrigation (CBI) infusion wide open.	• Assess for hypovolemic shock (vital signs, skin colour and moisture, anxiety level). • Leave irrigation infusion wide open and notify health care provider.
4. Patient experiences pain with irrigation.	• Examine drainage tubing for clots, sediment, or kinks. • Evaluate urine for presence of or increase in blood clots and sediment. • Evaluate for distended bladder. • Notify health care provider.

Communication and Documentation

- Document irrigation method, amount and type of irrigation solution, amount returned as drainage, characteristics of output, urinary output, and patient tolerance of procedure in progress notes in EHR or chart.
- Report catheter occlusion, sudden bleeding, infection, or increased pain to the health care provider.
- Document I&O on the appropriate flow sheet.
- Document your evaluation of patient learning.

DOCUMENTATION EXAMPLE

3000 mL bag of sterile saline infused through intake port of triple-lumen catheter for continuous bladder irrigation. 3500 mL of light pink output free from clots emptied from catheter bag, accounting for 500 mL of urinary output. New 3000 mL sterile saline CBI initiated and maintained at current rate as prescribed. Patient tolerating bladder irrigation well, verbalized no discomfort, and verbalized understanding of need to notify nurse if discomfort occurs.

Special Considerations

Teaching

- See Skill 34.3, Teaching, Special Considerations.

Care in the Community: Home Management

- See Skill 34.3, Care in the Community, Special Considerations.

SKILL 34.5 Applying a Condom-Type External Catheter

NSO *Nursing Skills Online Urinary Catheterization Module 17 / Lesson 3*

The external urinary catheter, also called a *condom catheter* or *penile sheath*, is a soft, pliable, condom-like sheath that fits over the penis, providing a safe and noninvasive way to contain urine. Most external catheters are made of soft silicone to reduce friction. The silicone is clear, allowing for easy visualization of the skin under the catheter. Latex catheters are still available and used by some patients. It is important to verify that a patient does not have a latex allergy before applying this type of catheter.

Condom-type external catheters are held in place by an adhesive coating of the internal lining of the sheath, a double-sided self-adhesive strip, brush-on adhesive applied to the penile shaft, or, in rare cases, an external strap. ***Never use tape to secure a condom catheter.*** The catheter may be attached to a small-volume (leg) drainage bag or a large-volume (bedside) urinary drainage bag, both of which need to be kept lower than the level of the bladder. The condom-type external catheter is suitable for incontinent patients who have complete and spontaneous bladder emptying. The catheters come in a variety of styles and sizes. For the best fit and correct application, it is important to refer to manufacturer guidelines. Condom-type external catheters are associated with reduced risk of UTIs than in-dwelling catheters; thus, they are an excellent option for patients with male genitalia who have urinary incontinence. Other externally applied catheters are available for patients who cannot be fitted for a condom-type external catheter.

An alternative option to the condom catheter is an incontinence device made of a 100% latex-free, hydrocolloid material. The device fits onto the tip of the penis rather than over the penile shaft. It reduces the occurrence of soiling of skin by urine. This device is helpful for patients with retracted anatomy or a small penile tip, which can cause a traditional condom catheter to dislodge (Schaeffer, 2023). Another option is a reusable condom-like device that is held in place by specially designed underwear.

Delegation and Collaboration

Assessment of the skin of a patient's penile shaft and determination of a latex allergy are done by a nurse before catheter application. The skill of applying a condom catheter can be delegated to a UCP, depending on employer policy. The nurse directs the UCP to do the following:

- Follow manufacturer directions for applying the condom catheter and securing device
- Monitor urine I&O and record them, if applicable
- Immediately report any redness, swelling, or skin irritation or breakdown of the glans penis or penile shaft

Equipment

- Condom catheter kit (condom sheath of appropriate size, securement device [internal adhesive or strap], skin preparation solution [per manufacturer directions])
- Urinary collection bag with drainage tubing or leg bag and straps
- Basin with warm water and soap
- Towels and washcloth(s)
- Bath blanket
- Clean gloves
- Scissors, hair guard, or paper towel

STEP	RATIONALE
ASSESSMENT	
1. Identify patient using at least two person-specific identifiers (e.g., name and date of birth, or name and medical record number) according to employer policy.	Ensures correct patient. Complies with Accreditation Canada's standards and improves patient safety (Accreditation Canada, 2020).
2. Throughout the procedure, the 4 moments for hand hygiene are to be implemented; hand hygiene should occur before initial patient (or patient environment) contact, before an aseptic procedure, after body fluid exposure risk, and after patient (or patient environment) contact. Additional hand hygiene should be performed when hands are visibly soiled.	Proper hand hygiene helps prevent the spread of infectious agents to health care providers.
3. Review medical record and assess urinary pattern, ability to empty bladder effectively, and degree of urinary continence.	Incontinent patients are at risk for skin breakdown and thus are candidates for using a condom catheter.
4. Review medical record for history of allergy to rubber or latex. Check patient's allergy wristband.	Condoms are made of latex and can cause serious skin reaction.
5. Apply clean gloves. Assess skin of penis for rashes, erythema, and open areas. (This may be deferred until just before catheter application.) Remove gloves and discard.	Reduces transmission of microorganisms. Provides baseline for comparing changes in condition of the skin after application of the condom catheter.

Critical Decision Point *Apply condom catheters only when the skin on the penile surface is intact.*

STEP	RATIONALE
6. Assess patient's mental status, knowledge of the purpose of using a condom-type catheter, and ability to apply the device. It may be appropriate to include the caregiver in this assessment.	Identifies patient learning needs and whether patient can perform self-application or caregiver needs to be included in instruction.

STEP	RATIONALE

ASSESSMENT

STEP	RATIONALE
7. Verify patient's size and type of condom catheter from plan of care or use manufacturer measuring guide to measure length and diameter of penis in flaccid state (apply gloves for measurement).	Identifies proper size of catheter needed. Penile shaft should be at least 2 cm (0.8 inches) in length to ensure successful application. If it is too small, the condom catheter may fall off and compress the urethra, stopping urine flow or causing local tissue trauma; if it is too big, the catheter may leak or fall off.

NURSING DIAGNOSES

- Urinary incontinence
- Insufficient knowledge regarding catheter application and care
- Potential for impaired skin integrity

Related factors and risk factors are individualized on the basis of patient's condition or needs.

PLANNING

STEP	RATIONALE
1. Expected outcomes following completion of procedure:	
• Patient's skin is free from urine wetness.	Catheter is applied correctly.
• Glans and penile shaft are free of skin irritation or breakdown.	Catheter is secure and not too tight.
• Patient explains purpose of procedure and what to expect.	Reduces anxiety and promotes cooperation.
2. Explain procedure to patient.	Reduces anxiety and promotes cooperation.

IMPLEMENTATION

STEP	RATIONALE
1. Provide privacy by closing room door and bedside curtain.	Promotes patient comfort and dignity.
2. Raise bed to appropriate working height. Lower side rail on working side.	Promotes use of good body mechanics.
3. Prepare urinary drainage collection bag and tubing (large-volume drainage bag or leg bag). Clamp off drainage bag port. Place nearby, ready to attach to condom after application.	Provides easy access to drainage equipment after applying condom catheter.
4. Help patient to a supine or sitting position. Place bath blanket over upper torso. Fold sheets so only penis is exposed.	Respects patient dignity; draping prevents unnecessary exposure of body.
5. Apply clean gloves. Provide perineal care (see Chapter 18). Dry thoroughly before applying device. In an uncircumcised male, ensure that foreskin has been replaced to normal position before applying condom catheter. Do not apply barrier cream.	Reduces transmission of microorganisms. Prevents skin breakdown from exposure to secretions. Removes any residual adhesives. Perineal care minimizes skin irritation and promotes adhesion of new external catheter. Barrier creams prevent sheath from adhering to penile shaft.
6. Clip hair at base of penis as necessary before application of condom sheath. Some manufacturers provide a hair guard that is placed over penis before applying device. Remove hair guard after applying catheter. An alternative to hair guard is to tear a hole in a paper towel, place it over penis, and remove it after application of device.	Hair adheres to the condom and is pulled during condom removal or may get caught in adhesive as the external catheter is applied.

Critical Decision Point *The pubic area should not be shaved because it may increase the risk of skin irritation.*

STEP	RATIONALE
7. Apply condom catheter. With nondominant hand, grasp penis along the shaft. With dominant hand, hold rolled condom sheath at tip of penis with head of penis in cone. Smoothly roll sheath onto penis. Allow 2.5–5 cm (1 to 2 inches) of space between tip of glans penis and end of condom catheter (see Step 7 illustration).	Excessive wrinkles or creases in external catheter sheath after application may mean that patient needs a smaller size.

STEP	RATIONALE

IMPLEMENTATION

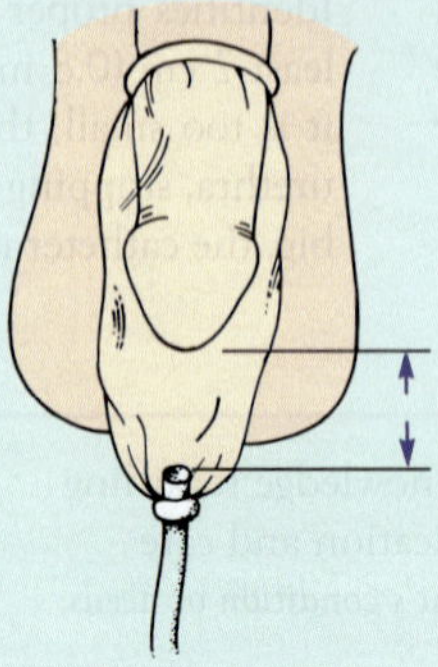

STEP 7 Condom catheter.

8. Apply appropriate securement device as indicated in manufacturer guidelines.
Rationale: The condom must be secured firmly so it is snug and stays on but not tight enough to cause constriction of blood flow. Application of gentle pressure ensures adherence of adhesive with penile skin.

- **a.** Self-adhesive condom catheters: After application, apply gentle pressure on the penile shaft for 10–15 seconds to secure catheter.
- **b.** Outer securing strip-type condom catheters: Spiral wrap penile shaft with strip of supplied elastic adhesive. Strip should not overlap itself. Elastic strip should be snug, not tight (see Step 8b illustration).
  Rationale: Using the spiral-wrap technique allows supplied elastic adhesive to expand so blood flow to penis is not compromised.

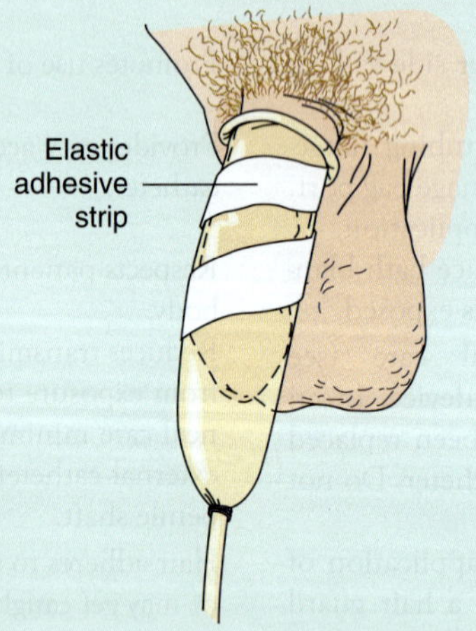

STEP 8B Spiral application of adhesive strip.

Critical Decision Point *Never use regular adhesive tape to secure a condom catheter. Constriction from tape can reduce blood flow to tissues.*

9. Remove hair guard if used. Connect drainage tubing to end of condom catheter. Be sure that condom is not twisted. If using a large drainage bag, secure tubing to thigh to prevent tension on condom.
Rationale: Allows urine to be collected and measured. Keeps patient dry. A twisted condom obstructs urine flow, causing urine pooling, skin irritation, and weakening and deterioration of adhesive, causing catheter to come off.

10. Help patient to a safe, comfortable position. Lower bed and place side rails accordingly.
Rationale: Promotes safety and comfort.

11. Dispose of contaminated supplies in an appropriate receptacle. Remove gloves and discard.
Rationale: Reduces spread of microorganisms.

12. Remove and reapply daily after Steps 7–9 unless an extended-wear device is used. To remove condom, wash the penis with warm, soapy water and gently roll the sheath and adhesive off penile shaft.
Rationale: Prevents trauma and irritation to penile sheath.

STEP	RATIONALE
EVALUATION	
1. Observe urinary drainage.	A twisted condom prevents urine from draining into collection bag.
2. Inspect penis with condom catheter in place within 15–30 minutes after application. Assess for swelling and discoloration and ask patient whether they feel any discomfort.	Determines whether condom is applied too tightly, impeding circulation to penis.
3. Inspect skin on penile shaft for signs of breakdown or irritation at least daily, when performing hygiene, and before reapplying condom.	Changing external catheter reduces risk of infection.
4. Use **teach-back:** "I want to be sure I clearly explained the use of your external condom catheter and some things you can do to prevent it from slipping off. Tell me how you can help keep the catheter on." Develop a revised teaching plan if patient or caregiver is unable to teach back correctly.	Determines patient's and caregiver's level of understanding of instructional topic.

Unexpected Outcomes	Related Interventions
1. Skin around penis is erythematous, ulcerated, or denuded.	• Check for latex allergy or allergy to skin preparation or adhesive device. • Remove condom and notify health care provider. • Do not reapply until penis and surrounding tissue are free from irritation. • Ensure that condom is not twisted and that urine flow is unobstructed after application.
2. Penile swelling or discoloration occurs.	• Remove external catheter. • Notify health care provider. • Reassess current condom size. See manufacturer size chart.
3. Condom catheter does not stay on.	• Ensure that catheter tubing is anchored and that patient understands not to pull or tug on catheter. • Reassess condom catheter size. Refer to manufacturer guidelines for sizing. • Observe whether condom catheter outlet is kinked and urine is pooling at tip of condom, bathing penis in urine; reapply as necessary and avoid catheter obstruction. • Assess need for another brand of external catheter (i.e., one that is self-adhesive).

Communication and Documentation

- Document condom application; condition of penis, skin, and scrotum; urinary output; and voiding pattern in progress notes in EHR or chart.
- Report penile erythema, rashes, or skin breakdown to health care provider.
- Document your evaluation of patient and caregiver learning.

DOCUMENTATION EXAMPLE

Patient experiencing urinary incontinence deemed appropriate for condom catheter. Penis examined and found to be free of rash, erythema, or skin breakdown prior to application of condom catheter. Pericare completed, and condom catheter applied and secured with self-adhesive. Patient displays understanding of teaching by properly explaining how to prevent condom catheter from slipping off.

Special Considerations

Teaching

- Teach patient about signs of skin breakdown or trauma.
- Teach patient to keep condom and catheter kink-free and positioned below level of bladder.
- Teach patient with a leg bag to assess leg straps periodically for tightness and loosen them as necessary.

Pediatric

- Use of condom catheters is uncommon in children. When used in adolescents, take precautions to minimize embarrassment.

Gerontological

- Evaluate patients with neuropathy carefully before applying a condom catheter. The patient may not feel the sensation of pressure from a condom device. Assess penile skin at more frequent intervals, at least twice daily.
- Condom catheters are not recommended in patients with prostatic obstruction.

Patients With Physical or Cognitive Challenges

- Use of male incontinence devices in patients with paraplegia requires routine special assessments because the patient may not be able to identify pain from improper placement. Improper placement can cause pressure and result in a medical device-related pressure injury (MDRPI) (see Chapter 39).

Care in the Community: Home Management

- Teach patient and caregiver appropriate assessments such as signs and symptoms of a UTI, signs of skin irritation, or signs of a poor-fitting catheter sheath.
- Loose-fitting clothing may be needed to accommodate the catheter and drainage system.
- Ensure that patient and caregiver understand correct steps in applying the condom catheter. Manufacturers often supply patient educational materials.
- Teach patient and caregiver to empty drainage bag frequently when half full to avoid placing unnecessary tension on the catheter, as it can lead to problems keeping the catheter intact.

✦ SKILL 34.6 Suprapubic Catheter Care

A *suprapubic catheter* is a urinary drainage tube inserted surgically into the bladder through the abdominal wall above the symphysis pubis (Fig. 34.7). The catheter may be sutured to the skin, secured with an adhesive material, or retained in the bladder with a fluid-filled balloon similar to the one used in an in-dwelling catheter.

Suprapubic catheters are placed when there is blockage of the urethra (e.g., enlarged prostate, urethral stricture, after urological surgery) and when a long-term urethral catheter causes irritation or discomfort or interferes with sexual functioning. Current evidence suggests that when placed correctly, there are rarely any complications from the use of suprapubic catheters (Schaeffer, 2021).

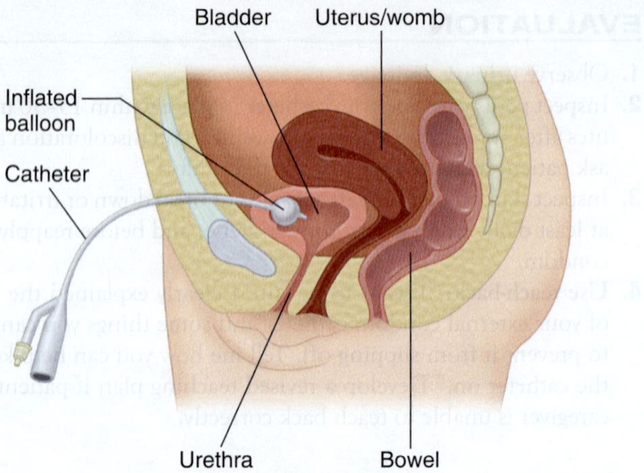

FIG 34.7 Suprapubic catheter.

Delegation and Collaboration

The skill of caring for a newly established suprapubic catheter cannot be delegated to a UCP; however, care of an established suprapubic catheter may be delegated (refer to employer policy). The nurse directs the UCP to do the following:

- Report the patient's discomfort (bladder fullness, abdominal pain, skin irritation) related to the suprapubic catheter.
- Empty the drainage bag and document urinary output in the I&O record.
- Report any change in the amount and character of the urine.
- Report any signs of redness, foul odour, or drainage around the catheter insertion site.

Equipment

- Clean gloves (sterile may be needed in some cases; see employer policy)
- Cleaning agent (sterile normal saline)
- Sterile cotton-tipped applicators
- Sterile surgical drainage gauze (split gauze)
- Sterile gauze dressing
- Washcloth, towel, soap, and water
- Tape
- Velcro tube holder or tube stabilizer *(optional)*

STEP	RATIONALE
ASSESSMENT	
1. Identify patient using at least two person-specific identifiers (e.g., name and date of birth, or name and medical record number) according to employer policy.	Ensures correct patient. Complies with Accreditation Canada's standards and improves patient safety (Accreditation Canada, 2020).
2. Throughout the procedure, the 4 moments for hand hygiene are to be implemented; hand hygiene should occur before initial patient (or patient environment) contact, before an aseptic procedure, after body fluid exposure risk, and after patient (or patient environment) contact. Additional hand hygiene should be performed when hands are visibly soiled.	Proper hand hygiene helps prevent the spread of infectious agents to health care providers.
3. Assess urine in tubing for amount, clarity, colour, odour, and sediment.	Abnormal findings indicate potential complications such as a UTI, decreased urinary output, and catheter occlusion.
4. Apply clean gloves. Observe dressing for drainage and intactness.	Reduces transmission of microorganisms. Drainage indicates a potential complication such as infection. Dressing may become non-occlusive because of tape choice or drainage.
5. Assess catheter insertion site (may be deferred until you clean site) for signs of inflammation (i.e., pain, erythema, edema, and drainage) and for growth of granulation tissue. Ask patient whether they feel any pain at the site; if so, assess for pain using an appropriate pain assessment tool. Remove gloves and discard.	If insertion is new, slight inflammation may be expected as part of normal wound healing but can also indicate infection. Hypergranulation tissue can develop at insertion site as a reaction to catheter. In some instances, intervention may be needed (WOCN, 2016). Reduces transmission of microorganisms.
6. Assess for elevated temperature and chills.	Increased temperature may indicate a UTI or skin site infection.
7. Assess patient's knowledge of purpose of catheter and its care.	Determines level of instruction and support required.
8. Check for allergies.	Patient may be sensitive to tape, latex, or antiseptic solution.

STEP	RATIONALE

NURSING DIAGNOSES

- Reduced urinary elimination
- Acute pain
- Insufficient knowledge regarding catheter care
- Inadequate skin integrity
- Potential for infection

Related factors and risk factors are individualized on the basis of patient's condition or needs.

PLANNING

STEP	RATIONALE
1. Expected outcomes following completion of procedure:	
• Patient indicates no pain or discomfort at insertion site and over bladder.	A patent catheter system keeps bladder empty and maintains patient comfort.
• Urinary output ≥30 mL/hr.	Indicates that catheter is patent.
• Urine remains clear without foul odour, and patient is afebrile.	Indicates that patient is free of CAUTI.
• Catheter exit site is free of infection (i.e., erythema, edema, drainage, tenderness).	Indicates absence of infection and irritation of skin.
• Patient and caregiver can explain purpose of and methods for catheter care.	Evaluates learning.
2. Explain procedure to patient and caregiver.	Reduces anxiety and promotes cooperation. Patients with a suprapubic catheter frequently rely on caregivers for support.

IMPLEMENTATION

STEP	RATIONALE
1. Provide privacy by closing room door and bedside curtain.	Demonstrates person-centred care by promoting comfort and patient's dignity.
2. Raise bed to appropriate working height. If side rails are raised, lower side rail on working side.	Promotes use of good body mechanics.
3. Prepare supplies and open gauze packets in same manner as for applying dry dressing (see Chapter 40).	Keeps dressing sterile until application.
4. Apply clean gloves. Loosen tape and remove existing dressing. Note type and presence of drainage. Remove gloves and discard.	Provides baseline for condition of suprapubic wound. Reduces transmission of microorganisms.
5. Clean insertion site using sterile aseptic technique for newly established catheter: This option is used less frequently; review employer policy or consider individual patient needs. In some facilities, clean gloves are appropriate.	The catheter site is made surgically and thus treated similarly to other incisions, as designated by employer policy. Confirm whether using either medical aseptic or sterile technique is recommended.
a. Apply sterile or clean gloves (see employer policy).	
b. Without creating tension, hold catheter up with nondominant hand while cleaning. Use sterile gauze moistened in saline and clean skin around insertion site in a circular motion, starting near the insertion site and continuing outward in widening circles for approximately 5 cm (2 inches) (see Step 5b illustration).	Moves from area of least contamination to area of most contamination. Tension on the catheter may cause discomfort or damage to the wall of the bladder or cause catheter to slip out of place.
c. With fresh, moistened gauze, gently clean base of catheter, moving up and away from site of insertion (proximal to distal).	Removes microorganisms residing on any drainage that adheres to tubing.
d. Once insertion site is dry, use a sterile gloved hand to apply drain dressing (split gauze) around catheter (see Step 5d illustration). Tape in place.	Collects drainage that develops around catheter insertion site.

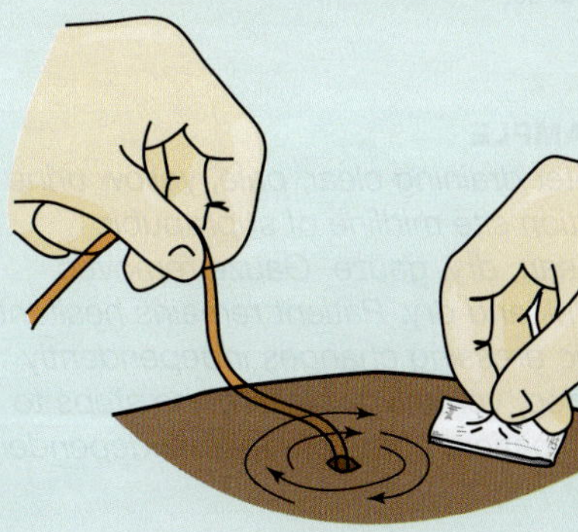

STEP 5B Clean around suprapubic catheter in a circular pattern.

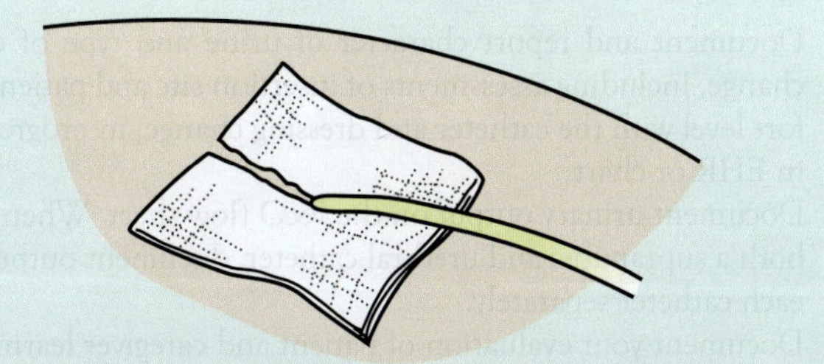

STEP 5D Split drain dressing for suprapubic catheter.

STEP	RATIONALE
IMPLEMENTATION	
6. Clean long-term/established catheter:	
a. Apply clean gloves.	Reduces transmission of microorganisms.
b. Without creating tension, hold catheter erect with nondominant hand while cleaning. Clean with soap and water in a circular motion, starting near catheter insertion site and continuing outward in widening circles for approximately 5 cm (2 inches).	Cleaning and drying suprapubic insertion site requires general hygienic measures; dressing is an option if drainage is not present.
c. With a fresh washcloth or gauze, gently clean base of the catheter, moving up and away from site of insertion (proximal to distal).	Removes microorganisms residing on any drainage that adheres to tubing.
d. *Option:* Apply drain dressing (split gauze) around catheter and tape in place.	
7. Secure catheter to lateral abdomen with tape or Velcro multipurpose tube holder.	Secures catheter and reduces the risk of excessive tension on suture and catheter.
8. Coil excess tubing on bed. Keep drainage bag below level of bladder at all times.	Maintains free flow of urine and decreases the risk of CAUTI (Fekete, 2022; HEC, n.d.).
9. Dispose of all contaminated supplies in an appropriate receptacle. Remove gloves and discard.	Reduces transmission of microorganisms.
EVALUATION	
1. Ask patient to rate pain or discomfort from suprapubic catheter using an appropriate pain assessment tool.	Determines whether bladder is draining and patient is free of infection.
2. Monitor for signs of infection (e.g., fever, elevated white blood cell [WBC] count), and observe urine for clarity, sediment, unusual colour, or odour.	Suprapubic catheters increase the risk of UTIs.
3. Observe catheter insertion site for erythema, edema, discharge, and tenderness. Check dressing every 8 hours at a minimum.	Indicators of an insertion site infection.
4. Use teach-back: "I want to be sure I explained clearly about the care of your suprapubic catheter. Tell me about some of the things you need to do to care for it at home." Develop a revised teaching plan if patient or caregiver is unable to teach back correctly.	Determines patient's and caregiver's level of understanding of instructional topic.

Unexpected Outcomes	Related Interventions
1. Patient develops symptoms of a UTI or catheter site infection.	• Increase fluid intake to at least 2 L in 24 hours (unless contraindicated). • Monitor vital signs and I&O; observe amount, colour, and consistency of urine; assess site. • Notify health care provider.
2. Suprapubic catheter becomes dislodged.	• Cover site with sterile dressing. • Notify health care provider. If this is a newly established catheter, it will need to be reinserted immediately.
3. Skin surrounding catheter exit site becomes red or irritated or develops open areas.	• Notify health care provider. • Change dressing (if used) more frequently to keep site dry. • Consult with wound care nurse.

Communication and Documentation

- Document and report character of urine and type of dressing change, including assessments of insertion site and patient's comfort level with the catheter and dressing change, in progress notes in EHR or chart.
- Document urinary output on the I&O flow sheet. When there is both a suprapubic and urethral catheter, document outputs from each catheter separately.
- Document your evaluation of patient and caregiver learning.
- Report any signs of a UTI or insertion site infection to the health care provider.

DOCUMENTATION EXAMPLE

New suprapubic catheter draining clear, pale, yellow urine free of sediment. Insertion site midline of suprapubic border covered with clean, dry, gauze. Gauze removed and site found to be pink and dry. Patient remains hesitant to complete suprapubic dressing changes independently. Further teaching provided, verbally explained the steps to the patient and had the patient complete them independently with supervision.

Special Considerations

Teaching

- If not contraindicated, encourage patients to consume a minimum of 2 L of fluids daily.
- Teach patient to keep the drainage bag lower than the bladder and to keep tubing free of kinks.
- Patients who have suprapubic catheters may shower. Caution patients against the use of creams, powders, or sprays near the catheter insertion site.

Care in the Community: Home Management

- Teach patient and caregiver how to clean and apply a dressing (if applicable) using clean technique.
- Teach patient and caregiver how to properly position the drainage bag; empty the urinary drainage bag; and observe urine colour, clarity, odour, and amount.
- Arrange for home delivery of catheter supplies, always ensuring that there is at least one extra catheter and drainage bag in the home.
- Teach patient and caregiver the signs of catheter obstruction, UTI, and wound infection.

✦ SKILL 34.7 Teaching Intermittent Self-Catheterization

Most people urinate and empty their bladder four to five times a day (Society of Urologic Nurses and Associates [SUNA], 2019). However, some patients are not able to empty their bladders. Infections in the bladder or kidneys and damage to the kidneys sometimes result from incomplete emptying of the bladder. Clean intermittent self-catheterization (CISC) is a safe and effective way to empty the bladder. The patient performs self-catheterization using clean technique, eliminating the need to wear gloves. Patients who use CISC have a variety of health problems that affect the neuromuscular control of the bladder (Leach, 2018). Current practice supports CISC for use in the home to provide a means to completely empty the bladder, prevent UTIs, and prevent further bladder and kidney damage (NSWOCC et al., 2020). Inadequate or excessive fluid intake, poor catheterization technique and catheter care, and traumatic catheterization can cause UTIs. Teaching proper self-catheterization technique is crucial in preventing infections (SUNA, 2019).

Use of CISC helps patients feel a greater sense of control over their ability to meet their daily needs, which enhances their quality of life. It helps some patients become continent, maintain a positive body image, and experience less anxiety and embarrassment. In addition, CISC allows patients to express their sexuality and sustain satisfying relationships with significant others. However, the skill requires physical and manual dexterity, and patients must adhere to a regular schedule for it to be successful (NSWOCC et al., 2020). When the patient is unable to perform CISC independently, a caregiver may be taught how to perform the skill.

Delegation and Collaboration

The skill of teaching CISC cannot be delegated to a UCP. The nurse instructs the UCP to do the following:

- Document the amount of urine in the paper or digital log if the patient is unable to do so.
- Report to the nurse changes in the colour, odour, or amount of urine.

Equipment

- Soap, water, and clean washcloth
- Mirror *(optional)*
- Urethral catheter (smallest size that can pass easily into the bladder and completely drain patient's urine)
- Lubricant (e.g., water-soluble jelly) if catheter is uncoated
- Container for collection of urine (e.g., urinal)—not needed for patients emptying urine directly into toilet
- Mild soap (e.g., Ivory)
- Catheter storage item or container (e.g., brown paper bag, clean towel)
- Disposable clean gloves (for caregiver)
- Paper or digital log *(optional)*

STEP	RATIONALE
ASSESSMENT	
1. Identify patient using at least two person-specific identifiers during first visit. Facial recognition can be used as one of two identifiers for ongoing subsequent visits.	Ensures correct patient. Complies with Accreditation Canada's standards and improves patient safety (Accreditation Canada, 2020).
2. Review patient's medical record, including prescription for CISC and progress notes. Gather information about voiding history, existing medical and surgical history, patient's usual daily fluid intake, PVR amounts, and daily voiding routine.	Determines reason for CISC, frequency of catheterization, and previous responses to patient education.
3. Assess patient's ability to perform CISC, including developmental level, level of consciousness, motor function, and psychosocial status.	Patient must be physically able to reach urethra and move equipment as needed. Patient who cannot see urethra can be taught to feel for proper location of urethral opening (Wilson, 2015).
4. Assess patient's and caregiver's knowledge about CISC and observe performance of CISC if patient has performed previously.	Effective patient and caregiver education builds on previous knowledge; observation is effective way to assess performance of psychomotor skills.

STEP	RATIONALE

NURSING DIAGNOSES

- Reduced urinary elimination
- Reflex urinary incontinence
- Urinary retention
- Insufficient knowledge regarding self-catheterization
- Readiness for enhanced urinary elimination

Related factors and risk factors are individualized on the basis of on patient's condition or needs.

PLANNING

STEP	RATIONALE
1. Expected outcomes following completion of procedure:	
• Patient or caregiver states signs and symptoms that indicate need for CISC.	Indicates ability to identify appropriate times to use CISC.
• Patient or caregiver correctly demonstrates how to perform CISC and clean and store equipment.	Return demonstration of skill indicates learning.
• Patient or caregiver verbalizes signs and symptoms of complications of CISC (e.g., UTI, urethral bleeding, urethritis, stricture, creation of false passage) and when to contact health care provider.	Urinary complications such as UTIs can occur in patients who use CISC (NSWOCC et al., 2020). Verbalization of signs and symptoms of complications helps patients and caregivers identify potential problems early and seek appropriate care.
2. Select setting in the home that patient or caregiver will most likely use when performing CISC.	Respecting patient's needs, values, and choices is key in person-centred care.
3. Help patient or caregiver select catheter that is easiest to use, causes the least amount of trauma, and is most comfortable.	A variety of single-use and reusable catheters is available.

IMPLEMENTATION

STEP	RATIONALE
1. Teach patient and caregiver how to perform appropriate hand hygiene using soap and water. If caregiver is performing skill, have them apply a pair of clean disposable gloves.	Reduces risk of UTI and trauma, which can lead to urethral strictures. Prevents transmission of infection.
2. Help patient get into a comfortable position. Some patients with male genitalia prefer to stand, whereas others prefer to sit. Patients with female genitalia often need to try different positions to determine which position is most comfortable. Position patient in a place that has adequate lighting.	Patient needs adequate lighting to see meatus and equipment.
3. Teach patient or caregiver how to clean urethral meatus:	
a. *For patients with female genitalia:* Have patient spread labia with one hand and use the other hand to clean urethral opening with a washcloth containing warm, soapy water, and then use a clean, moist washcloth to rinse. Have patient clean in the direction from urethral meatus toward rectum.	Retraction of labia allows for female urethral meatus to be cleaned, reducing risk of infection. Reduces transmission of infection from rectal area to meatus.
b. *For patients with male genitalia:* If patient has not been circumcised, teach them to retract foreskin to expose urethral meatus. Teach patient to hold the penis perpendicular to the body with one hand, use the other hand to clean urethral opening with a washcloth containing warm, soapy water, and then use a clean, moist washcloth to rinse. Have patient clean in a circular motion from meatus outward.	Ensures cleaning of meatus and reduces risk of infection (Wilson, 2015).
4. Teach patient with female genitalia or caregiver how to insert catheter:	
a. Catheter selection depends on patient preference and includes single-use or reusable catheter.	Single-use catheter is disposed of after one use, decreasing the risk of UTIs. Reusable catheter is cleaned and stored between uses.
b. Using a mirror, help patient locate meatus. Explain that it is located just below the clitoris and just above the vaginal opening.	Mirror helps patient with female genitalia visualize anatomy (SUNA, 2019).

STEP	RATIONALE

IMPLEMENTATION

Critical Decision Point *If patient wants to learn how to find the meatus while in a sitting position, teach touch technique by helping them use their fingers to find the urethral opening. Teach the patient to put one finger over the clitoris and another finger over the vaginal opening. Then help them use these two fingers to find the urethral opening. Another method is the tunnel technique. When patient sits with their hips flexed forward, the labia create a "tunnel" that leads to the urethral opening. Teach the patient to slightly separate labia near the clitoris and angle the catheter backward into the urethral opening while placing a finger over the vaginal opening.*

STEP	RATIONALE
c. If an uncoated catheter is selected, have patient lubricate tip of catheter with water-soluble jelly by rotating tip to spread lubricant around bottom 2.5–5 cm (1–2 inches) of catheter. Coated catheters do not require use of separate lubrication.	Lubrication reduces urethral trauma (SUNA, 2019). Coated catheter uses hydrophilic or other coatings that do not require use of separate lubricant.
d. Place outflow end of catheter into urine collection container or let hang over toilet bowl. Slowly and gently insert tip of catheter 5–10 cm (2–4 inches) into meatus until urine begins to flow.	Appearance of urine indicates that catheter tip is in bladder.

Critical Decision Point *If the patient feels resistance at the internal sphincter, teach them to apply firm, gentle, steady pressure until muscles relax and allow the catheter to pass* (SUNA, 2019).

STEP	RATIONALE
5. Teach patient with male genitalia or caregiver how to insert catheter:	
a. Catheter selection depends on patient preference and includes single-use or reusable catheter.	Patient preference is important for adherence to CISC. Single-use catheter is disposed of after one use. Reusable catheter is cleaned and stored between uses.
b. Lubricate tip of uncoated catheter with water-soluble jelly by rotating tip to spread lubricant around bottom 13–18 cm (5–7 inches) of catheter. Coated catheters do not require use of separate lubrication.	Lubrication reduces urethral trauma in uncoated catheters. Dry catheters may cause excoriations in the urethra, which can lead to an entry point for bacterial contamination.
c. Place outflow end of catheter into urine collection container or let hang over toilet bowl. Slowly and gently insert tip of catheter 15–20 cm (6–8 inches) into meatus until urine begins to flow. For an uncircumcised patient, retract foreskin before inserting the catheter. Tell patient that catheter often needs to be inserted all the way for urine to begin to flow.	The male urethra is longer than the female urethra. Flow of urine indicates that catheter tip is in bladder.

Critical Decision Point *Patients may experience some resistance when the catheter reaches the prostatic urethra or the neck of the bladder. If the patient feels resistance, do not pull the catheter in and out. Teach them to apply firm, gentle, steady pressure to fatigue the external sphincter and cause muscle relaxation* (SUNA, 2019).

STEP	RATIONALE
6. Instruct patient or caregiver to hold catheter in place while urine flows into container or toilet.	Release of catheter during procedure often causes catheter to accidently come out before bladder is completely emptied.
7. When urine flow stops, teach patient to slowly and gently remove catheter. For an uncircumcised patient, bring foreskin back over glans penis. Then teach patient to perform hand hygiene.	Removing catheter slowly allows pockets of urine that can accumulate at base of bladder to drain (SUNA, 2019).
8. Give patient log to record amount of urine if needed.	Some patients need to keep track of their urinary output.
9. Single-use catheters are discarded after self-catheterization is complete. Instruct patient to clean reusable catheter with mild soap (e.g., Ivory) and water immediately after use. Rinse catheter completely, allow to air dry, and store in clean, dry towel or brown paper bag.	Minimizes risk of UTIs.
10. Teach patient or caregiver to replace reusable catheters as directed by their health care provider.	Appropriate disposal and replacement of equipment prevent complications associated with CISC.
11. Have caregiver remove and discard gloves (if used).	

STEP	RATIONALE
EVALUATION	
1. Observe patient or caregiver independently demonstrate technique for CISC.	Feedback through return demonstration of psychomotor skill is the best means of evaluating learning of skill.
2. Ask patient to identify plan for timing of CISC and steps to take when problems arise.	Measures patient's cognitive learning and ability to problem solve.
3. Review patient's log and observe patient enter information about urinary output if indicated.	Confirms that patient understands record keeping and the importance of tracking urinary output.
4. **Use teach-back:** "I want to be sure I explained the steps clearly for how to clean and store your catheter. Explain to me how to clean and store your reusable catheter." Develop a revised teaching plan if patient or caregiver is unable to teach back correctly.	Determines patient's and caregiver's level of understanding of instructional topic.

Unexpected Outcomes	Related Interventions
1. Patient is unable to easily pass catheter into the bladder.	• Teach patient not to force catheter into the bladder. • Tell patient to go to the nearest urgent care centre or emergency department if the bladder is full and patient is unable to insert catheter. • Use interprofessional collaboration (e.g., urologist) when appropriate.
2. Patient states that they are having symptoms of a UTI (e.g., intense urge to urinate; flank or abdominal pain; malaise, fever, chills).	• Inform patient's health care provider of symptoms and anticipate treatment with antibiotic.

Communication and Documentation

- Document teaching, patient and caregiver responses, and demonstration in the home care record.
- Document urinary output in home care record and home documentation system (e.g., log).
- Report signs and symptoms of UTIs and difficulty performing CISC to health care provider.

DOCUMENTATION EXAMPLE

Explained clean intermittent self-catheterization to patient and caregiver. Had patient and caregiver demonstrate proper technique, and supported patient when necessary. Patient verbalized signs and symptoms of urinary tract infections and understands when to contact health care provider.

Special Considerations

Teaching

- It is common for patients who perform CISC routinely to have an abnormal urinalysis. Patients should be treated for a UTI only if they have symptoms of an infection (e.g., back pain, pelvic tenderness, malaise, confusion, foul-smelling urine, urgency) (NSWOCC et al., 2020).
- Always leave a phone number and instructions on how to reach the home care nurse if needed.

Pediatric

- Children who are motivated and physiologically and developmentally ready are encouraged to learn how to catheterize themselves. Consult a pediatric urologist; children need special assessment (Hockenberry et al., 2024).
- When teaching children to perform CISC, use developmentally appropriate teaching strategies. Urinary diversion requires special care (see Chapter 36).
- Concerns of children and adolescents who use CISC include leakage and being wet. They also are often concerned about their peers knowing about their condition. Allow children to voice their concerns and help them problem solve what they will do in a variety of situations.

Gerontological

- CISC is highly effective in older persons because it helps restore continence, decreases urinary urge and nocturia, and improves quality of life.
- Older persons may have difficulty performing CISC because of limited manual dexterity. Individualize care for a patient's needs and functional abilities. Educate the patient or caregiver (Boscart et al., 2023).

✦ REVIEW QUESTIONS

The nurse is caring for an 80-year-old patient (she/her) with a history of a stroke, type 2 diabetes mellitus, urinary retention, urinary incontinence, and recurrent urinary tract infections (UTIs). The health care provider has prescribed measurement of postvoid residual (PVR) by either straight catheterization or bladder scan. There is also a prescription for an in-dwelling catheter if the PVR exceeds 400 mL. The patient's spouse will not allow anyone to insert a catheter except her family.

Review Questions 1 to 5 relate to the case study presented here.

1. Which assessments would be pertinent for this patient?
2. Explain why an assessment of PVR is important for this patient.
3. When measuring PVR, should the nurse use a bladder scanner or should a straight catheterization be performed? Give the rationale for your answer.

4. Explain the teaching that would be appropriate when assessing PVR urine.
5. Using SBAR (situation–background–assessment–recommendation), show how you would communicate with the health care team about this patient.
6. Place the following steps for insertion of an in-dwelling catheter in a patient with female genitalia in the appropriate order (not all steps of the procedure are listed here):
   1. Insert and advance catheter.
   2. Lubricate catheter.
   3. Inflate catheter balloon.
   4. Clean urethral meatus with antiseptic.
   5. Drape patient with the sterile square and fenestrated drapes.
   6. When urine appears, advance catheter another 2.5 to 5 cm (1 to 2 inches).
   7. Prepare sterile field and supplies.
   8. Gently pull catheter until resistance is felt.
   9. Attach drainage tubing.
7. The nurse is preparing to remove an in-dwelling urinary catheter. Which nursing interventions should the nurse implement? (*Select all that apply.*)
   1. Attaching a 3-mL syringe to the inflation port
   2. Allowing the balloon to drain into the syringe by gravity
   3. Initiating a voiding record or bladder diary
   4. Pulling catheter quickly
   5. Clamping the catheter before removal
8. Which nursing interventions are appropriate in the care of a patient with a newly inserted suprapubic catheter? (*Select all that apply.*)
   1. Using sterile technique, clean the skin close to the catheter with a circular motion.
   2. Wipe away any drainage on the catheter by wiping down the catheter toward the insertion site.
   3. Inspect the insertion site for erythema, edema, discharge, or tenderness.
   4. Secure the catheter to the abdomen with tape or a tube holder.
   5. Apply upward tension to the catheter when cleaning the site and tubing.

Visit the Evolve site for a complete list of answers to the Review Questions.

✦ NEXT GENERATION NCLEX® (NGN)

For practice with answering exam questions related to unfolding NGN case studies, please consult the Next Generation NCLEX® (NGN)-Style Case Studies for Skills and Techniques on the Evolve website: http://evolve.elsevier.com/Canada/Perry/clinicalskills/

REFERENCES

Accreditation Canada. (2020). *Required organizational practices–2020 handbook.* https://physicians.nshealth.ca/resources/required-organizational-practices-2020-handbook

Boscart, V., McCleary, L., Sheiban Taucar, L., et al. (2023). *Ebersole and Hess' gerontological nursing and healthy aging in Canada* (3rd ed.). Elsevier.

Fekete, T. (2022). Catheter-associated urinary tract infections in adults. *UpToDate.* https://www.uptodate.com/contents/catheter-associated-urinary-tract-infection-in-adults

Gascón, M., Mellão, M. A., Mello, S. H., et al. (2018). The impact of urinary incontinence on the quality of life and on the sexuality of patients with HAM/TSP. *Brazilian Journal of Infectious Diseases, 22*(4), 288–293. https://doi.org/10.1016/j.bjid.2018.07.003

Gill, B. C. (2022). Neurogenic bladder. *Medscape.* https://emedicine.medscape.com/article/453539-overview.

Healthcare Excellence Canada. (HEC) (n.d.). *Hospital harm improvement resource: Urinary tract infection.* https://www.healthcareexcellence.ca/en/what-we-do/all-programs/hospital-harm-is-everyones-concern/hospital-harm-improvement-resource/

Higuera, V. (2019). *Everything you need to know about overactive bladder.* Healthline. https://www.healthline.com/health/overactive-bladder

Hockenberry, M. J., Duffy, E. A., & Gibbs, K. (2024). *Wong's nursing care of infants and children* (12th ed.). Elsevier.

Lawrence, K., Bliss, D. Z., Dailey, M., et al. (2019). The CAUTI prevention tool kit: A professional and collaborative project of the wound, ostomy, and continence nurses society. *The Journal of Wound, Ostomy and Continence Nursing, 46*(2), 154–157. https://doi.org/10.1097/WON.0000000000000505

Leach, D. (2018). Teaching patients a clean intermittent self-catheterisation technique. *British Journal of Nursing, 27*(6), 296–298. https://doi.org/10.12968/bjon.2018.27.6.296

MedlinePlus. (2022). *Catheter-related UTI.* US National Library of Medicine. https://medlineplus.gov/ency/article/000483.htm.

Newman, D., Rovner, E. S., & Wein, A. J. (2017). *Clinical application of urological catheters, devices and products.* Springer. [Seminal Reference]

Nurses Specialized in Wound, Ostomy, and Continence Canada (NSWOCC), Canadian Nurse Continence Advisors, Urology Nurses of Canada, and Infection Prevention and Control Canada. (2020). *Clean intermittent urethral catheterization in adults–Canadian best practice recommendations for nurses.* https://cnca.ca/wp-content/uploads/Clean-Intermittent-Urethral-Catheterization-Adults-for-Nurses-BPR-May2020.pdf

Power-Kean, K., Zettel, S., El-Hussein, M. T., et al. (2023). *Huether and McCance's understanding pathophysiology* (2nd ed.). Elsevier.

Schaeffer, A. (2021). Complications of urinary bladder catheters and preventive strategies. *UpToDate.* https://www.uptodate.com/contents/complications-of-urinary-bladder-catheters-and-preventive-strategies

Schaeffer, A. (2023). Placement and management of urinary bladder catheters in adults. *UpToDate.* https://www.uptodate.com/contents/placement-and-management-of-urinary-bladder-catheters-in-adults

Shelat, A. (2022). Neurogenic bladder. *MedlinePlus.* https://medlineplus.gov/ency/article/000754.htm

Society of Urologic Nurses and Associates (SUNA). (2019). *Adult intermittent self-catheterization: Patient fact sheet.* https://www.suna.org/sites/default/files/download/resources/SUNA_intermittentSelfCathFactSheet.pdf

Tremayne, P., & Pawlyn, J. (2019). Management of in-dwelling urinary catheters for people with learning disabilities. *Learning Disability Practice, 22*(4). https://doi.org/10.7748/LDP.2019.E1949

Tyerman, J., & Cobbett, S. (Eds.). (2023). *Lewis's medical-surgical nursing in Canada: Assessment and management of clinical problems* (5th ed.) Elsevier

Wilson, M. (2015). Clean intermittent self-catheterisation: Working with patients. *British Journal of Nursing, 24*(2), 76–80. https://doi.org/10.12968/bjon.2015.24.2.76 [Seminal Reference]

Wound, Ostomy, and Continence Nurses Society (WOCN). (2016). *Care and management of patients with urinary catheters: A clinical resource guide.* https://cdn.ymaws.com/member.wocn.org/resource/resmgr/document_library/Care_&_Mgmt_Pts_w_Urinary_Ca.pdf [Seminal Reference]

Yates, A. (2018). Catheter securing and fixation devices: Their role in preventing complications. *British Journal of Nursing, 27*(6), 290–294. https://doi.org/10.12968/bjon.2018.27.6.290

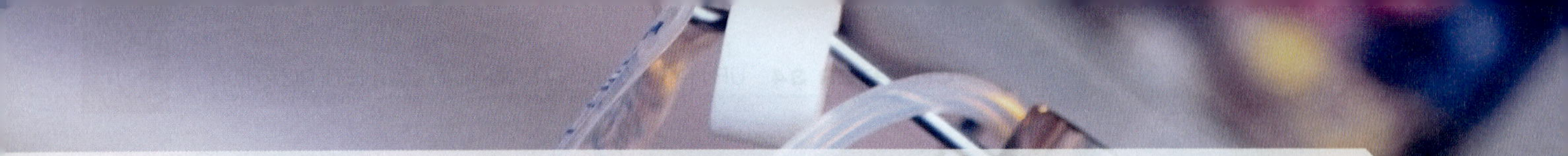

35 Bowel Elimination and Gastric Intubation

Canadian content written by **Maureen Loft, NP-Adult, MScN, PhD**
Original US chapter by **Jane Fellows, MSN, CWOCN**

SKILLS AND PROCEDURES

OBJECTIVES

Mastery of content in this chapter will enable the nurse to:

- Describe factors that promote and impede normal bowel elimination.
- Describe methods to relieve constipation or impaction.
- Describe precautions to follow when administering an enema.
- Describe approaches to managing a patient's comfort during nasogastric tube insertion.
- Perform the following skills: helping a patient use a bedpan, digitally removing stool, administering an enema, and inserting and removing a nasogastric tube.

MEDIA RESOURCES

- http://evolve.elsevier.com/Canada/Perry/clinicalskills/

PURPOSE

Regular elimination of bowel waste products is essential for normal body functioning. Alterations in bowel elimination often indicate early signs, symptoms, or problems in the gastrointestinal (GI) system across the lifespan, particularly in older persons and children (Dumic et al., 2019; Hockenberry et al., 2024). A patient's overall lifestyle patterns, food and fluid intake, medications, functional status, and chronic conditions influence bowel function. Foods may induce symptoms that have a range of effects on bowel elimination (R. Singh et al., 2018). To manage a patient's bowel elimination problems, nurses need to understand factors that promote, impede, or alter normal bowel elimination.

Patients may require the nurse's help to meet bowel elimination needs (e.g., using a bedpan). If a patient is constipated, the nurse will likely administer enemas or digitally remove impacted stool. If severe diarrhea exists, a fecal management system (FMS) protects a patient's perianal skin and collects contaminated fecal waste (R. Singh et al., 2018). When patients undergo abdominal surgery or experience an alteration in GI peristalsis, a nasogastric (NG) tube is inserted for gastric decompression (Sigmon & An, 2022).

STANDARDS OF CARE

- Accreditation Canada (2020)—*Required Organizational Practices—2020 Handbook* (https://physicians.nshealth.ca/resources/required-organizational-practices-2020-handbook)
- Registered Nurses' Association of Ontario (RNAO, 2020)—*A Proactive Approach to Bladder and Bowel Management in Adults*, 4th edition (https://rnao.ca/bpg/guidelines/proactive-approach-bladder-and-bowel-management-adults)
- Rowan-Legg & Canadian Paediatric Society (2011; reaffirmed 2018)—*Managing Functional Constipation in Children* (https://papers.ucalgary.ca/paediatrics/assets/cps-functional-constipation.pdf)
- Wounds Canada (Norton et al., 2021)—*Best Practice Recommendations for the Prevention and Management of Pressure Injuries* (https://www.woundscanada.ca/docman/public/health-care-professional/bpr-workshop/172-bpr-prevention-and-management-of-pressure-injuries-2/file)

PRINCIPLES FOR PRACTICE

- Chronic constipation is a functional GI disorder and a condition frequently encountered in clinical practice (Box 35.1). Approximately 30% of people experience constipation during their lifetime, with older persons being most affected (Dumic et al., 2019).
- Opioid-induced constipation occurs frequently in the palliative care population. Opioids stimulate mu-opioid receptors, which induce analgesia. However, activation of these receptors reduces gastric emptying; increases pyloric, anal, and biliary sphincter tone; reduces biliary track secretions; and increases water absorption from the bowel. All of these factors reduce delayed intestinal transit time, and constipation occurs (Argoff, 2020).

BOX 35.1

Common Causes of Constipation

- Chronic bowel dysfunction (e.g., colonic inertia, irritable bowel syndrome)
- Diseases/conditions (e.g., Parkinson's disease, multiple sclerosis, rheumatoid arthritis, colon cancer, dehydration, diabetes mellitus, stress, depression and eating disorders)
- Low-fibre diet that is high in animal fats (e.g., meats, dairy products, eggs), refined sugars (rich desserts), high-carbohydrate diet, and low fluid intake, all of which slow peristalsis
- Infants/toddlers: Improper formula reconstitution with insufficient water
- Changes in life or routine such as pregnancy, aging, and travel
- Neurological conditions that block nerve impulses to the colon (e.g., stroke, spinal cord injury, tumour)
- Colonic action slowed by medications such as anticholinergics, antispasmodics, anticonvulsants, antidepressants, antihistamines, antihypertensives, antiparkinsonian medications, bile acid sequestrants, diuretics, antacids, iron supplements, calcium supplements, opioids, and chemotherapy medications

- Patients with severe diarrhea may often require an FMS to protect the perianal skin from breakdown, pressure injury formation, and fecal containment (Norton et al., 2021).
- Postoperative ileus and severe abdominal distension, with or without nausea or vomiting, is an indication of failure in the return of adequate bowel function. This causes patient discomfort, increases recovery time, and increases length of hospital stay. When a postoperative ileus occurs, often an NG tube may need to be inserted (Sigmon & An, 2022).

PERSON-CENTRED CARE

- Nurses need to show respect for a person's privacy, provide necessary comfort and hygiene measures, and attend to the patient's emotional needs when performing required skills.
- When caring for patients from diverse cultural and ethnic groups, nurses need to modify nursing interventions to meet their patients' elimination needs and provide for culturally sensitive hygiene needs. For example, hand hygiene can be practised for hygienic reasons, for ritual reasons during religious ceremonies, and for symbolic reasons in specific everyday life situations.
- It is important to determine a patient's normal pattern of bowel elimination and accommodate that pattern while they are in a health care setting. The amount of help needed can be established according to the time of day a patient normally has a bowel movement.
- Nurses should consider developmental changes that affect bowel functioning throughout the lifespan. For example, an older person who becomes less active and has decreased muscle tone and changes in eating patterns is at higher risk of experiencing constipation (Power-Kean et al., 2023).

EVIDENCE-INFORMED PRACTICE

- Nurses assess constipation by obtaining a thorough patient history (e.g., diet, exercise, bowel pattern history, medications). Nurses also need to review medications to identify those associated with an increased risk of developing constipation (e.g., chronic laxative use). Daily dietary fibre intake should be between 25 and 30 g per day (RNAO, 2020).
- Research studies continue to investigate methods of correctly verifying NG tube placement, which is crucial to avoid tube position complications. Radiographic verification of placement of an NG tube immediately following insertion is the gold standard and provides a clear and measurable placement of the tube. Likewise, aspiration of gastric contents and pH values ≤5 are used in subsequent verifications of tube placement (Judd, 2020).
- Pressure applied to the mucous membranes lining the GI tract can cause ischemia and medical device–related pressure injuries (MDRPIs). The resultant pressure injury generally conforms to the pattern or shape of the device.
    - NG and nasoenteral tubes can cause tissue necrosis, skin breakdown, and pressure on the intubated nares. NG tube fixation methods that remove pressure from the nares help reduce the risk of MDRPIs (Gilmour et al., 2023; Wound, Ostomy, and Continence Nurses Society [WOCN], 2016).
    - In-dwelling FMSs are effective in protecting perianal skin from fecal enzyme irritation and subsequent breakdown. However, there is a risk for rectal mucosa necrosis and tearing secondary to the cuff, which is placed internally (S. Singh et al., 2018).
- Methods to reduce MDRPI related to bowel elimination and gastric decompression include the following:
    - Conducting routine and ongoing assessment of nares and secondary pressure sites underlying the medical devices and implementing skin-care practices such as the taping method to reduce the risk of MDRPI (Brophy et al., 2021)
    - Frequently removing tape or the fixation device to inspect underlying skin and provide skin care (Gilmour et al., 2023)
    - Placing thin foam or breathable dressings under medical devices (Gilmour et al., 2023)
    - Positioning NG drainage tubing so as not to cause secondary pressure on the nares from the weight of the drainage tubing itself (Gilmour et al., 2023)
    - Verifying that the patient is not lying on drainage tubing
    - For patients who have an FMS, routinely assessing anal and perianal areas for redness, blistering, edema, and breaks in skin integrity (S. Singh et al., 2018)

SAFETY GUIDELINES

- Promote comfort when a patient uses a bedpan. Encourage the patient to use the bathroom when able.
- Answer the call light promptly to prevent a patient from attempting to get out of bed without help. This is a common factor related to patient falls.
- Patients with neurological, sensory, or motor deficits are prone to constipation. They should be placed on an individualized bowel training schedule (WOCN, 2016).
- Autonomic dysreflexia, which occurs in individuals with spinal injuries at T6 or above, is exhibited as marked hypertension and headache. Assess these patients for flushing, sweating, chills, nasal congestion, blurred vision, and headache (Allen & Leslie, 2022).

! SAFETY ALERT Infants and toddlers, because of their small size, must be closely monitored for dehydration when they are experiencing diarrhea (Hockenberry et al., 2024).

- When digital removal of impacted fecal material is prescribed, obtain patient baseline vital signs and periodically monitor heart rate during the procedure. Observe the patient for signs of distress, pain, discomfort, bleeding, and collapse (WOCN, 2016).
- Follow employer policy to verify correct placement of NG tubes; this process includes radiographic verification after tube insertion and subsequent verification of pH ≤5 (Judd, 2020).
- When a patient with an NG tube indicates nausea or vomits, assess both placement and patency of the tube. Reposition and irrigate the tube as needed.
- When handling fecal matter, always use personal protective equipment (PPE) based on routine practices and additional precautions as required.

✦ SKILL 35.1 Providing a Bedpan

Encouraging patients to use a toilet or commode best supports optimal bowel hygiene. For patients who are on bed rest or unable to ambulate, the use of a bedpan may be required. Two types of bedpans are available (Fig. 35.1). The regular and most commonly used bedpan has a curved, smooth upper end and a tapered lower end. The upper end (wide end) of the regular pan fits under a patient's buttocks toward the sacrum, with the lower end (tapered end) fitting just under the upper thighs toward the foot of the bed. A fracture pan, designed for patients with body or leg casts or those who are restricted from raising their hips (e.g., following total hip joint replacement), slips easily under a patient. The shallow upper end of the pan with a flat, wide rim fits under a patient's buttocks toward the sacrum, with the deep, lower open end toward the foot of the bed.

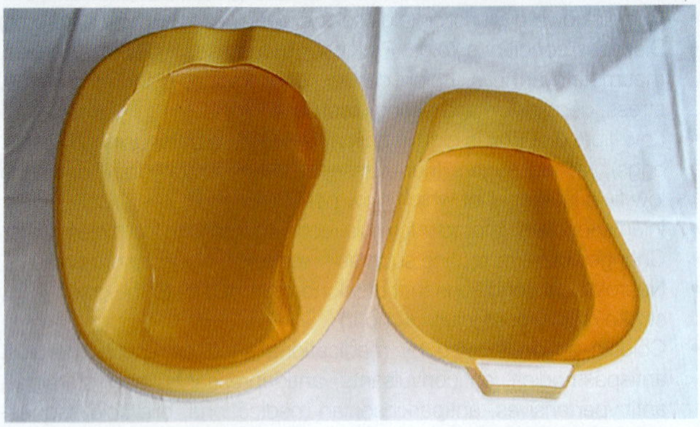

FIG 35.1 Types of bedpans. *Left*, Regular bedpan. *Right*, Fracture bedpan.

Delegation and Collaboration

The skill of providing a bedpan can be delegated to an unregulated care provider (UCP); however, providing or removing a bedpan is more readily facilitated with the assistance of two people. The nurse needs to use interprofessional collaboration to provide optimal patient care and education and to complete patient care in a timely manner. The nurse instructs the UCP to do the following:

- Correctly position patients who have mobility restrictions or therapeutic equipment such as wound drains, intravenous (IV) catheters, or traction
- Provide perineal and hand hygiene for the patient as necessary after use of a bedpan

Equipment

- PPE for transmission-based precautions (e.g., contact)
- Bedpan (regular or fracture) (see Fig. 35.1)
- Bedpan cover
- Toilet tissue
- Specimen container (if necessary); plastic bag clearly labelled with date, patient's name, and identification number
- Basin, washcloths, towels, and soap
- Waterproof absorbent pads (if necessary)
- Clean drawsheet (if necessary)
- Stethoscope

STEP	RATIONALE
ASSESSMENT	
1. Identify patient using at least two person-specific identifiers (e.g., name and date of birth, or name and medical record number) according to employer policy.	Ensures correct patient. Complies with Accreditation Canada's standards and improves patient safety (Accreditation Canada, 2020).
2. Throughout the procedure, the 4 moments for hand hygiene are to be implemented; hand hygiene should occur before initial patient (or patient environment) contact, before an aseptic procedure, after body fluid exposure risk, and after patient (or patient environment) contact. Additional hand hygiene should be performed when hands are visibly soiled.	Proper hand hygiene helps prevent the spread of infectious agents to health care providers.
3. Assess patient's normal bowel elimination habits: routine pattern, character of stool, effect of certain foods or fluids and eating habits on bowel elimination, effect of stress and level of activity on normal bowel elimination patterns, current medications, and normal fluid intake.	Managing a patient's elimination problems depends on thorough understanding of normal elimination and factors that create alterations. Peristalsis is strongest during the hour after the first meal of the day. Anticipate when to offer bedpan.
4. Auscultate abdomen for bowel sounds and palpate lower abdomen for distension.	Normal bowel sounds occur irregularly at a rate of 5–35 per minute. Presence of feces in the colon, often mistaken for an abdominal mass, can be felt as a soft, rounded, boggy mass in the cecum and ascending, descending, or sigmoid colon (Ball et al., 2023).
5. Assess patient to determine level of mobility, including ability to sit upright and lift hips or turn.	Determines whether patient can help position themselves on bedpan or whether assistance will be needed. Determines whether to use regular or fracture bedpan. Older persons, patients living with obesity, patients who have had hip or knee surgery or spinal injury, and debilitated patients often require the assistance of two or more nurses to help them onto or off bedpan.
6. Assess patient's level of comfort. Ask about presence of rectal or abdominal pain, presence of hemorrhoids, or irritation of skin surrounding anus.	Pain limits a patient's ability to help with positioning. Rectal or abdominal pain reduces a patient's ability to bear down during defecation.

STEP	RATIONALE
ASSESSMENT	
7. Apply clean gloves. Inspect condition of perianal and perineal skin. Remove gloves and discard.	Reduces transmission of microorganisms. Repeated diarrhea can cause perineal and perianal skin irritation and skin breakdown.
8. Determine need for stool specimen. This may have been prescribed by the health care provider, or the assessment findings may indicate that a sample is required (e.g., patient is oozing stool, foul odour).	Provides opportunity to obtain specimen container before placing patient on bedpan.

NURSING DIAGNOSES

- Acute pain
- Bowel incontinence
- Diarrhea
- Chronic pain
- Reduced physical mobility
- Chronic functional constipation
- Reduced self-toileting abilities
- Potential for constipation

Related factors and risk factors are individualized on the basis of patient's condition or needs.

PLANNING

STEP	RATIONALE
1. Expected outcomes following completion of procedure:	
• Perianal skin is clean and intact.	Hygiene technique after defecation keeps perianal skin clear of fecal secretions.
• Patient eliminates without pain or discomfort.	Patient is positioned comfortably on bedpan.
2. Explain procedure to patient, including self-help tips (e.g., how to use a trapeze, how to move hips).	Promotes independence, reduces anxiety, and helps patient to assist during procedure.
3. Obtain help from additional nursing personnel as warranted.	Adequate personnel resources minimize muscle strain for you and patient. Reduces patient's discomfort.

IMPLEMENTATION

STEP	RATIONALE
1. Apply clean gloves.	Reduces transmission of microorganisms.

Critical Decision Point *Use a fracture pan if the patient has had a total hip replacement. An abduction pillow may be placed between the legs when turning to decrease the risk of possible dislocation of the new joint (refer to employer policy).*

STEP	RATIONALE
2. Provide privacy by closing curtains around bed or door of room.	Demonstrates person-centred care by reducing embarrassment and promotes bowel elimination.
3. Raise side rail on opposite side of bed.	Protects patient from falling out of bed. Patient can grasp side rail to move about in bed and onto bedpan.
4. Raise bed horizontally according to your height.	Promotes use of good body mechanics and minimizes muscle strain for you and patient.
5. Have patient assume supine position.	Position eases eventual pan placement.

Critical Decision Point *Observe for the presence of drains, dressings, IV fluids, and traction. These devices make it difficult for a patient to help with positioning, and as the nurse you will likely need more personnel to help place the patient on a bedpan.*

STEP	RATIONALE
6. Place patient on bedpan:	
a. *For patients who can help themselves:*	
(1) Apply clean gloves. Raise head of patient's bed 30–60 degrees.	Reduces transmission of microorganisms. Prevents hyperextension of back and provides support to upper torso when patient raises hips. Sitting position promotes defecation.
(2) Remove upper bed linens so they are out of the way but do not expose patient.	Prevents embarrassment to patient; maintains person's dignity and demonstrates respect as part of person-centred care.
(3) Have patient flex knees and lift hips upward.	If legs, upper torso, and arms are supporting body weight, little effort should be required of the patient.

STEP	RATIONALE
IMPLEMENTATION	
(4) Place hand that is closest to the patient's head palm up under the patient's sacrum to help lift. Ask patient to bend knees and raise hips. As patient raises hips, use the other hand to slip the bedpan under them (see Step 6a[4] illustrations). Be sure that open rim of the bedpan is facing toward foot of bed. Do not force pan under patient's hips. *Optional:* Have patient use overhead trapeze frame to raise hips.	Positions bedpan high under buttocks so feces enters pan. Incorrect placement of bedpan causes discomfort for patient and spillage of contents. If legs, upper torso, and arms are supporting body weight, little effort should be required of patient. Forcing bedpan under patient increases risk of friction injury to underlying skin and tissues.
(5) *Optional:* If using a fracture pan, slip it under patient as hips are raised (see Step 6a[5] illustration). Be sure that deep, open, lower end of bedpan is facing toward foot of bed.	Patient requires less manoeuvring and does not have to lift hips.
b. *For patients who are immobile or have mobility restrictions on bedpan:*	
(1) Apply clean gloves. Lower head of bed so that bed is flat or raise head slightly (if tolerated by medical condition).	Helps patient who cannot lift hips, must remain flat, or medically is not permitted to lift hips to roll onto bedpan.
(2) Remove top linens as necessary to turn patient while minimizing exposure.	Prevents embarrassment to patient; demonstrates respect for patient's sense of dignity.
(3) Help patient roll onto side with their back toward you. Place bedpan firmly against patient's buttocks and down into mattress. Be sure that open rim of bedpan is facing toward foot of bed (see Step 6b[3] illustrations).	Incorrect placement causes discomfort to patient and spillage of contents.

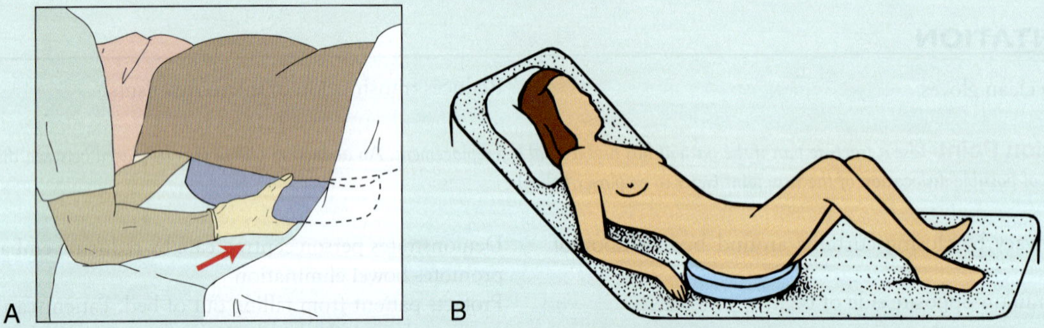

STEP 6A(4) A, Placing bedpan under patient's hips. B, Correct positioning for placing mobile patient on bedpan.

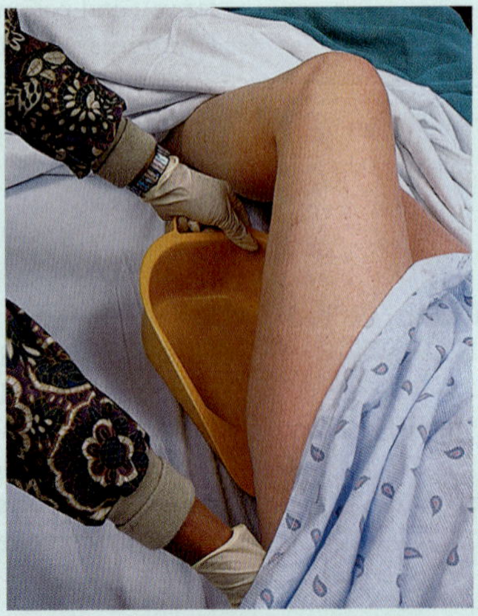

STEP 6A(5) Patient lifts hips as fracture pan is positioned.

STEP	RATIONALE

IMPLEMENTATION

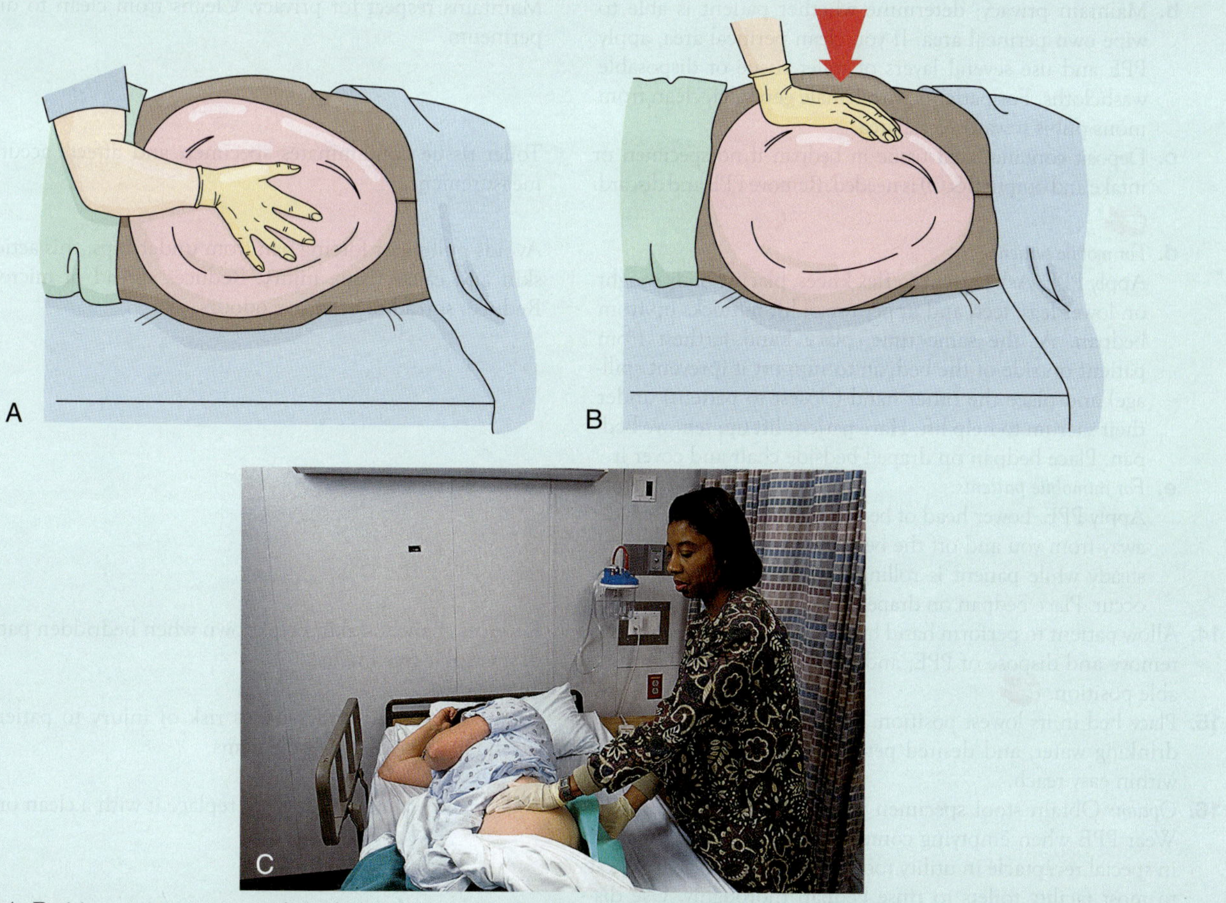

STEP 6B(3) A, Position patient on one side and place bedpan firmly against buttocks. B, Push down on bedpan and toward patient. C, Nurse places bedpan in position. *(A and B from Sorrentino, S. A. [2009]. Mosby's textbook for nursing assistants [7th ed.]. Mosby.)*

Critical Decision Point *If the patient has had total hip replacement, use a fracture pan; an abduction pillow may be used between the patient's legs while they are positioning themselves onto the fracture pan.*

STEP	RATIONALE
(4) Keep one hand against bedpan; place the other around far hip of patient. Ask patient to roll back onto the bedpan, flat in bed. Do not force pan under patient.	Using minimal exertion, this places patient squarely on the pan. Avoid forcing the bedpan under patient, to decrease risk for friction injury to underlying skin and tissues.
(5) Raise patient's head 30 degrees or to a comfortable level (unless contraindicated).	Patient assumes sitting position unless condition necessitates maintaining a flat position.
(6) Have patient bend knees (unless contraindicated).	Relieves stress on back.
7. Maintain patient's comfort, privacy, and safety. Cover patient for warmth. Place a small pillow or rolled towel under lumbar curve of their back. Leave room but stay close by.	Provides added comfort. Pain reduces or eliminates urge to defecate, which will result in bowel elimination problems.
8. Have call bell and toilet tissue within reach of patient.	Promotes safety by preventing patient from reaching over edge of bed for objects out of reach.
9. Ensure that bed is in lowest position and raise upper side rails.	Promotes patient safety and enables patient to reposition pan as needed.
10. Remove PPE and discard.	Reduces transmission of microorganisms.
11. Allow patient to be alone but monitor status and respond promptly once patient signals they are finished using the bedpan.	Reassures patient. Removing the bedpan in a timely manner prevents pressure injuries.
12. Reapply PPE if PPE was removed to perform other activities in the room (e.g., tidy bedside, chart).	Reduces transmission of microorganisms.
13. Remove bedpan:	
a. It is optimal to have assistance of a team member to assist with removal of bedpan. If working alone, place bedpan on floor on a protective barrier.	Working with a team member allows one to immediately empty bedpan contents while the nurse finishes cleaning the patient. Provides area to place bedpan and contents on floor after removal from patient to prevent accidental spilling of full bedpan on bed surface.

STEP	RATIONALE
IMPLEMENTATION	
b. Maintain privacy; determine whether patient is able to wipe own perineal area. If you clean perineal area, apply PPE and use several layers of toilet tissue or disposable washcloths. For patients with female genitalia, clean from mons pubis toward rectal area.	Maintains respect for privacy. Cleans from clean to dirty area of perineum.
c. Deposit contaminated tissue in bedpan if no specimen or intake and output (I&O) is needed. Remove PPE and discard.	Toilet tissue contaminates specimen and affects accurate output measurement.
d. *For mobile patients:* Apply PPE. Ask patient to flex knees, placing body weight on lower legs, feet, and upper torso; lift buttocks up from bedpan. At the same time, place hand farthest from patient on side of the bedpan to support it (prevent spillage) and place the other hand (closest to patient) under their sacrum to help lift. Have patient lift up; remove bedpan. Place bedpan on draped bedside chair and cover it.	Avoids pulling or forcing pan from under hips; this action can pull skin and cause tissue injury. Reduces spread of microorganisms. Reduces spread of offensive odours.
e. *For immobile patients:* Apply PPE. Lower head of bed. Help patient roll onto side away from you and off the bedpan. Hold bedpan flat and steady while patient is rolling off, otherwise spillage will occur. Place bedpan on draped bedside chair and cover it.	
14. Allow patient to perform hand hygiene. Change soiled linens, remove and dispose of PPE, and return patient to a comfortable position.	Reduces chance of skin breakdown when bedridden patient lies on dry, wrinkle-free linens.
15. Place bed in its lowest position. Ensure that call bell, phone, drinking water, and desired personal items (e.g., books) are within easy reach.	Promotes comfort and reduces risk of injury to patient. Patients often fall when reaching for items.
16. *Option:* Obtain stool specimen as prescribed (see Skill 9.2). Wear PPE when emptying contents of bedpan into toilet or in special receptacle in utility room. Use spray faucet attached to most facility toilets to rinse bedpan thoroughly. Use disinfectant if required by employer; store pan. Remove PPE.	If bedpan becomes very soiled, replace it with a clean one.
EVALUATION	
1. Assess characteristics of stool. Note colour, odour, consistency, frequency, amount, shape (see Fig. 35.2), and constituents. Assess characteristics of urine if patient voided in bedpan.	Helps identify significant changes or findings.
2. Evaluate patient's ability to use bedpan.	Provides continual assessment of patient's self-toileting ability.
3. Inspect patient's perianal area and surrounding skin while removing bedpan.	Liquid stool predisposes patients to skin breakdown.
4. **Use teach-back:** "I want to make sure you're comfortable getting off and on the bedpan by using the trapeze to pull your body off the bed. Show me how you will use the trapeze." Develop a revised teaching plan if patient is unable to teach back correctly.	Determines patient's level of understanding of instructional topic.

Unexpected Outcomes	Related Interventions
1. Patient is unable to successfully use bedpan.	• If patient's mobility allows, obtain prescription for use of bedside commode.
2. Patient is incontinent of stool. Avoid use of adult briefs for bedridden patient.	• Establish a regular schedule of offering a bedpan. Adult briefs mask toileting needs and may potentiate skin breakdown called *incontinence-associated dermatitis (IAD)* (McNichol et al., 2018). • Discuss with staff the need to answer the patient's request for toileting help promptly and to use a toileting schedule.
3. Patient develops irritation and breakdown of skin around perianal area.	• Administer perianal skin care using moisture barrier. • Reassess perianal skin with each bowel movement and each position change.

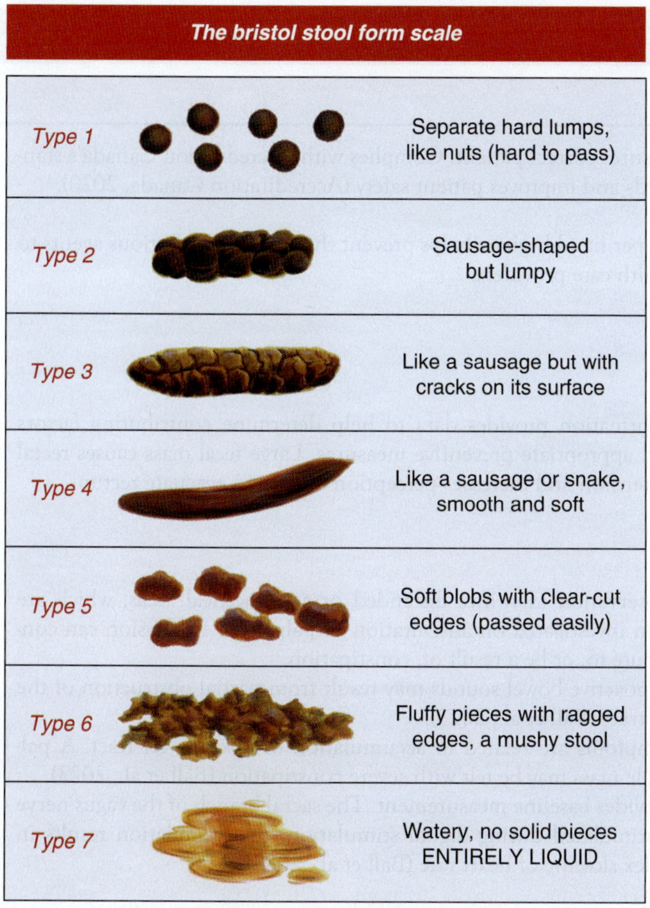

FIG 35.2 Bristol Stool Form Scale. *(From O'Donnell, L. J., Virjee, J., & Heaton, K. W. [1990]. Detection of pseudodiarrhoea by simple clinical assessment of intestinal transit rate. British Medical Journal, 300[6722], 439. © 1990. Reprinted with permission of the BMJ Publishing Group.)*

Communication and Documentation

- Document the type of help needed and whether the patient tolerates getting on and off the bedpan, the character and amount of stool, and urine output (if patient also voids) on flow sheet or in progress notes in electronic health record (EHR) or chart.
- Document your evaluation of patient learning.
- Complete laboratory requisition if you collected a stool or urine specimen and send it to the laboratory. Document the type of specimen sent.

DOCUMENTATION EXAMPLE

Pt assisted onto bedpan with help of one person. Sm. amount soft formed light brown stool noted in bedpan with approx. 100 mL amber urine discarded in pt bathroom. Pt offered washcloth and towel to freshen up. Resting comfortably in bed at present with no voiced concerns.

Special Considerations

Pediatric

- Constipation in early childhood results from environmental changes such as hospitalization, which may lead to reluctance to use a bedpan. Toilet-trained children often regress during hospitalization (Hockenberry et al., 2024).
- Repeated withholding of stool leads to stretching or dilating of the rectum and decreases the sensation or "urge" to defecate (Hockenberry et al., 2024).
- In children over the age of 4 years, encopresis (involuntary discharge of feces) is often the result of chronic constipation (Sood, 2022).

Gerontological

- Older persons have some loss of sphincter control and often require a quick response when requesting a bedpan (Ball et al., 2023; Boscart et al., 2023).
- The use of continence aids such as pads or briefs is more common in older persons. Timely continence care and assessment of skin integrity are critical to prevent skin impairment (Francis, 2018).
- The incidence of constipation is greater among older persons because of impaired rectal sensation to defecate. As a result, older persons do not perceive the need to defecate.
- With increased age, transit time through the bowel increases, causing a normal increase in the time between bowel movements (Lucak et al., 2021).

✦ SKILL 35.2 Removing Fecal Impaction Digitally

Fecal impaction is the inability to pass a collection of hard stool. This condition occurs in all age groups. Physically and mentally incapacitated individuals and institutionalized older persons are at the greatest risk. Patients with acute stroke and spinal cord injuries are also at greater risk for fecal impaction (RNAO, 2020).

Functional constipation is defined by a patient's meeting two or more of the following criteria for at least 3 months: (1) straining with defecation, (2) three or fewer bowel movements in a week, (3) lumpy or hard stools (or both) one-fourth of the time (see Fig. 35.2), (4) sensation of anorectal obstruction or incomplete evacuation, (5) loose stools rarely present without the use of laxatives, or (5) use of digital manoeuvres (Lucak et al., 2021).

Symptoms of fecal impaction include constipation, rectal discomfort, anorexia, nausea, vomiting, abdominal pain, abdominal bloating, diarrhea (leaking around the impacted stool), and urinary frequency. Prevention is the key to managing fecal impaction. With newer bowel management techniques such as transanal irrigation and pharmacological agents, digital removal of fecal material may not be needed.

Delegation and Collaboration

The skill of removing a fecal impaction digitally cannot be delegated to a UCP. The nurse instructs the UCP to do the following:

- Help the nurse position the patient for the procedure
- Monitor heart rate as the nurse removes the impacted fecal material
- Observe the stool for colour and consistency, and immediately report rectal bleeding or bloody mucus to the nurse
- Provide perineal care following each bowel movement

Equipment

- PPE
- Water-soluble local anaesthetic lubricant (Note: Some employers require use of water-soluble lubricant without anaesthetic.)
- Waterproof, absorbent pads
- Bedpan
- Bedpan cover (optional)
- Bath blanket
- Basin, washcloths, towels, and soap
- Vital sign equipment
- Stethoscope

ASSESSMENT

STEP	RATIONALE
1. Identify patient using at least two person-specific identifiers (e.g., name and date of birth, or name and medical record number) according to employer policy.	Ensures correct patient. Complies with Accreditation Canada's standards and improves patient safety (Accreditation Canada, 2020).
2. Throughout the procedure, the 4 moments for hand hygiene are to be implemented; hand hygiene should occur before initial patient (or patient environment) contact, before an aseptic procedure, after body fluid exposure risk, and after patient (or patient environment) contact. Additional hand hygiene should be performed when hands are visibly soiled.	Proper hand hygiene helps prevent the spread of infectious agents to health care providers.
3. Ask patient about normal and current bowel elimination pattern, including frequency and characteristics of stool; use of laxatives, enemas, and other medications; level of exercise; urge to defecate but inability to do so; feelings of incomplete emptying; and sensations of bloating, cramping, and excessive gas.	Information provides data to help determine contributing factors and appropriate preventive measures. Large fecal mass causes rectal distension and increases perception of urge to evacuate rectum.
4. Inspect patient's abdomen for distension.	Observation identifies distended or asymmetrical areas, which are then investigated on auscultation or palpation. Distension can contribute to, or be a result of, constipation.
5. Auscultate all four quadrants for presence of bowel sounds.	Hypoactive bowel sounds may result from partial obstruction of the GI tract (Ball et al., 2023).
6. Palpate patient's abdomen for distension, discomfort, or masses.	Symptoms are related to accumulation of stool in GI tract. A palpable mass may be felt with severe constipation (Ball et al., 2023).
7. Measure patient's current vital signs, including pain level using a validated pain assessment score.	Provides baseline measurement. The sacral branch of the vagus nerve is stimulated during digital stimulation; this stimulation results in reflex slowing of heart rate (Ball et al., 2023).

Critical Decision Point *Because of the potential to stimulate the sacral branch of the vagus nerve, patients with a history of dysrhythmias or heart disease have a greater risk for changes in heart rhythm. Monitor patient's pulse before and during the procedure. This procedure is often contraindicated in cardiac patients; if in doubt, verify with the health care provider.*

STEP	RATIONALE
8. If patient has a spinal cord injury (SCI), review their routine for digital removal of stool; if this step is part of the patient's routine bowel care, it is essential not to interrupt the routine.	The level of SCI and severity of injury affect the pattern of constipation. Injuries to cervicothoracic vertebrae increase the frequency of constipation. Patients with SCI are at risk for autonomic dysreflexia before and after the procedure, which may cause a sudden elevated blood pressure. In these patients, digital removal of stool is a routine intervention for bowel health and should not be interrupted (Allen & Leslie, 2022).
9. Apply clean gloves. Observe consistency of stool (see Fig. 35.2), seepage of liquid stool, or continued passage of small amounts of hard stool. Observe anal area for signs of irritation or hemorrhoids. Remove gloves and discard.	Reduces transmission of microorganisms. Seepage of stool is symptomatic of an impaction high in the colon. Patient may be able to pass small pieces of hard stool or liquid fecal material around the impacted mass. Leakage of fecal contents causes skin irritation and increases risk of pressure injury formation (Fletcher, 2020).
10. Determine whether patient is receiving anticoagulant therapy or has a past history of rectal surgery.	This procedure may be contraindicated. Manipulation of the rectum can cause bleeding, which is prolonged with anticoagulants.
11. Check patient's record for health care provider's prescription for digital removal of impaction and use of anaesthetic lubricant.	Written prescription required before performing procedure because it involves excessive stimulation of the vagus nerve.

NURSING DIAGNOSES

- Acute pain
- Chronic functional constipation
- Diarrhea

Related factors and risk factors are individualized on the basis of patient's condition or needs.

STEP	RATIONALE
PLANNING	
1. Expected outcomes following completion of procedure:	
• Impacted stool is removed successfully.	Indicates that rectum is clear of stool.
• Patient is free of abdominal or rectal discomfort.	Fecal impaction causes direct pain to rectum and indirect abdominal discomfort through abdominal distension.
• Vital signs remain within patient's baseline.	Indicates absence of vagal stimulation.
2. Explain procedure to patient.	Information reduces anxiety and encourages patient participation in therapeutic elimination protocol.
3. Arrange supplies at bedside.	Ensures access to supplies during procedure.
IMPLEMENTATION	
1. Obtain help to change patient's position if necessary. Raise bed horizontally to a comfortable working height.	Promotes patient safety and use of good body mechanics.
2. Pull curtains around bed or close door to room.	Maintains patient's privacy and prevents unnecessary exposure of body.
3. Lower side rail on patient's right side. Keeping far side rail raised, help patient to a left side-lying position with the knees flexed and back (Fig. 35.3).	Promotes patient safety. Provides access to rectum. The left side-lying position promotes rectal sphincter relaxation; mimics the squatting position, which aids in defecation (RNAO, 2020); and promotes an anatomical approach for insertion of the index finger.
4. Drape patient's trunk and lower extremities with a bath blanket and place a waterproof pad under the patient's buttocks.	Maintains patient's privacy and prevents unnecessary exposure of body.
5. Apply clean gloves and place bedpan next to patient.	Reduces transmission of microorganisms.
6. Lubricate gloved index finger and middle finger of dominant hand with anaesthetic lubricant.	Prevents transmission of microorganisms. Reduces discomfort and permits smooth insertion of finger into anus and rectum.
7. Instruct patient to take slow, deep breaths during the procedure. Gradually and gently insert gloved index finger and feel anus relax around finger. Insert middle finger (Fig. 35.4).	Slow, deep breaths help to relax the patient. Gradual insertion of the index finger helps to dilate the anal sphincter.
8. Gradually advance fingers slowly along rectal wall toward umbilicus.	Guiding finger toward rectal wall follows the natural direction of the colon, allowing for access to impacted stool high in the rectum.
9. Gently loosen fecal mass by moving fingers in scissors motion to fragment fecal mass. Work fingers into hardened mass.	Loosening and penetrating of mass allows for removal of stool in small pieces, resulting in less discomfort to patient.
10. Work stool downward toward end of rectum. Remove small sections of feces and discard into bedpan.	Prevents need to force finger into rectum and minimizes trauma to mucosa.
11. Observe patient's response, and periodically assess heart rate and look for signs of fatigue.	Vagal stimulation slows the heart rate and causes dysrhythmias. This procedure often exhausts a patient.

Critical Decision Point *Stop the procedure if the heart rate drops or rhythm changes from the patient's baseline or if the patient has dyspnea or indicates palpitations.*

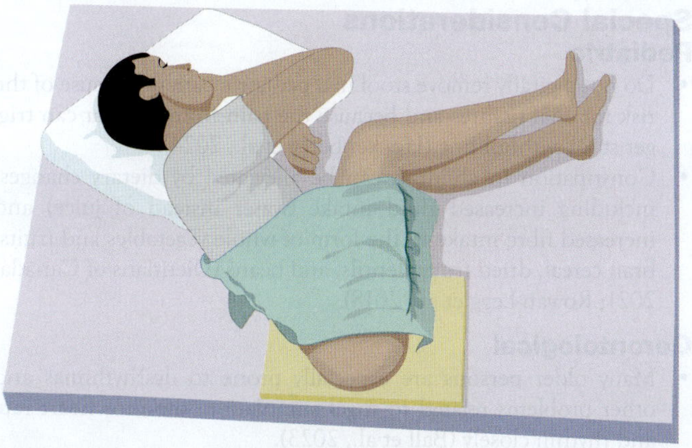

FIG 35.3 Patient in left side-lying position for digital removal of feces. *(Redrawn from Peate, I. [2016]. How to perform digital removal of faeces. Nursing Standard, 30[40], 36–39, Figure 2.)*

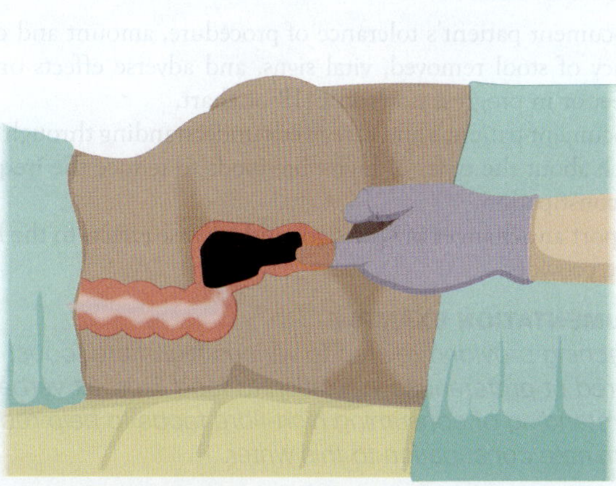

FIG 35.4 Patient in left side-lying position for digital removal of feces (cross-section shown). *(Redrawn from Peate, I. [2016]. How to perform digital removal of faeces. Nursing Standard, 30[40], 36–39, Figure 3.)*

STEP	RATIONALE
IMPLEMENTATION	
12. Continue to clear rectum of feces and allow patient to rest at intervals.	Rest improves patient's tolerance of procedure, allowing heart rate to return to normal.
13. After removal of impaction, perform perineal hygiene (see Procedural Guideline 18.1).	Promotes patient's sense of comfort and cleanliness.
14. Remove bedpan and inspect feces for colour and consistency. Dispose of feces in toilet.	Reduces transmission of microorganisms.
15. If needed, help patient to toilet or clean and store bedpan. (Procedure may be followed by enema or cathartic.)	Removal of impaction stimulates defecation reflex.
16. Remove PPE. Remove gloves by turning them inside out and discarding in a proper receptacle.	Reduces transmission of microorganisms.
EVALUATION	
1. Apply clean gloves, perform rectal examination for stool, and observe anal and perianal area for irritation or skin breakdown following the disimpaction. Remove and dispose of gloves.	Reduces transmission of microorganisms. Determines whether rectum is clear. Fecal material, especially diarrhea, causes irritation to perianal tissues (Fletcher, 2020).
2. Reassess vital signs and compare to baseline value. Continue to monitor patient for 1 hour for bradycardia.	Determines extent of vagal stimulation.
3. Auscultate bowel sounds.	Determines presence of peristaltic activity.
4. Palpate abdomen to determine whether it is soft and nontender.	Discomfort is relieved.
5. **Use teach-back:** "I want to make sure you start consuming the high-fibre foods and fluids that we recommended to help prevent constipation. Tell me which foods you will eat regularly." Develop a revised teaching plan if patient or caregiver is unable to teach back correctly.	Determines patient's and caregiver's level of understanding of instructional topic.

Unexpected Outcomes	Related Interventions
1. Patient experiences trauma to rectal mucosa as evidenced by rectal bleeding.	• Assess anal and perianal region for source of bleeding. • Stop procedure if bleeding is excessive and notify health care provider.
2. Patient experiences bradycardia (heart rate <60 beats/min), decrease in blood pressure, and decrease in level of consciousness as a result of vagus nerve stimulation.	• Stop procedure and measure vital signs. • Notify health care provider and remain with patient.
3. Patient has seepage of liquid stool after procedure is complete.	• Assess patient for continuing impaction. • Notify health care provider for possible rectal suppository (see Chapter 20) or enema. • Increase patient's fluid intake and dietary fibre.

Communication and Documentation

- Document patient's tolerance of procedure, amount and consistency of stool removed, vital signs, and adverse effects on flow sheet or in progress notes in EHR or chart.
- Document patient's and caregiver's understanding through teach-back about the types of high-fibre foods to reduce the frequency of constipation.
- Report any changes in vital signs and adverse effects to the health care provider.

DOCUMENTATION EXAMPLE

Pt teaching provided related to various high-fibre foods; explored pt preferences in relation to food likes. Pt verbalized understanding of consuming high-fibre foods to help reduce or eliminate constipation to this writer.

Special Considerations

Pediatric

- Do not digitally remove stool in a pediatric patient because of the risk for anal fissures and because the pain from the tear can trigger stool withholding (Hockenberry et al., 2024).
- Constipation in children can be alleviated by dietary changes, including increased fluid intake (water instead of juice) and increased fibre intake in the form of whole vegetables and fruits, bran cereal, dried fruits, lentils, and beans (Dietitians of Canada, 2021; Rowan-Legg et al., 2018).

Gerontological

- Many older persons are especially prone to dysrhythmias and other problems related to vagal stimulation; monitor heart rate and rhythm closely (Ball et al., 2023).

- For older persons, a diet with adequate dietary fibre adds bulk, weight, and form to the stool and improves defecation (Zheng & Yao, 2018). The recommended daily fibre intake is 25 to 30 g daily (RNAO, 2020).
- Laxative use for chronic constipation in older persons must be individualized to the patient's cardiac and renal comorbidities, medication interactions, and adverse effects (Zheng & Yao, 2018).

✦ SKILL 35.3 Administering an Enema

Video Clip NSO Nursing Skills Online Bowel Elimination/Ostomy Care Module 18 / Lesson 2

An *enema* is the instillation of a solution into the rectum and sigmoid colon to promote defecation through stimulation of peristalsis. Typically, enemas treat constipation or empty the bowel before diagnostic procedures or certain types of abdominal surgery. The volume or type of fluid that breaks up the fecal mass stretches the rectal wall and initiates the defecation reflex. Table 35.1 summarizes common types of enemas.

Cleansing enemas promote complete evacuation of feces from the colon. They act by stimulating peristalsis through infusion of large volumes of solution. Oil-retention enemas act by lubricating the rectum and colon, allowing feces to absorb oil and become softer and easier to pass.

Medicated enemas contain pharmacological therapeutic agents. Some are prescribed to reduce dangerously high serum potassium levels (e.g., sodium polystyrene sulfonate enema) or to reduce bacteria in the colon before bowel surgery (e.g., neomycin enema).

Delegation and Collaboration

The skill of administering an enema can be delegated to a UCP. (NOTE: If a medicated enema is prescribed, then it cannot be delegated to a UCP.) The nurse instructs the UCP to do the following:

- Properly position patients who have mobility restrictions or therapeutic equipment such as drains, IV catheters, or traction
- Inform the nurse immediately if patient has rectal bleeding or new abdominal pain (EXCEPTION: patient reports cramping, a normal side-effect of enemas) or rectal bleeding
- Inform the nurse immediately if there is blood in the stool or around the rectal area or any change in vital signs.

Equipment

- PPE
- Water-soluble lubricant
- Waterproof, absorbent pads
- Toilet tissue
- Bedpan, bedside commode, or access to toilet
- Bath blanket
- Basin, washcloths, towel, and soap
- Stethoscope

Enema Bag Administration

- Enema container with tubing and clamp (Fig. 35.5)
- IV pole
- Appropriately sized rectal tube (adult: 22 to 30 Fr; child: 12 to 18 Fr)
- Correct volume of warmed (tepid) solution
  - Adult: 750 to 1 000 mL
  - Adolescent: 500 to 700 mL
  - Pediatric: The weight of the child usually determines the volume for the enema. For example, with a phosphate enema, calculate 6 mL/kg (up to 135 mL) for total volume. Enemas are not recommended for children under 2 years of age (Rowan-Legg et al., 2018).

Prepackaged Enema

- Prepackaged enema container with lubricated rectal tip (Fig. 35.6)

TABLE 35.1

Types of Enemas

Type of Enema	Description and Implications
Tap-water (hypotonic) enema	Do not repeat after first installation because water toxicity or circulatory overload can develop.
Physiological normal saline	Safest enema to administer. Infants and children can tolerate only this type because of their predisposition to fluid imbalance.
Hypertonic solution (e.g., commercially prepared Fleet enema)	Useful for patients who cannot tolerate large volumes of fluid.
Harris flush enema	A return-flow enema that helps expel intestinal gas. Administer a small amount (100–200 mL) of enema solution into the patient's rectum and colon. Lower the enema container to allow the total volume of solution to flow back. The repeated back-and-forth administration and return of the fluid reduces flatus and promotes the return of peristalsis.
Soapsuds enema (SSE)	Pure castile soap is added to either tap water or normal saline. Use only pure castile soap. The recommended ratio of pure soap to solution is 5 mL (1 teaspoon) to 1 000 mL (1 quart) warm water or saline. Add soap to the enema bag after water is in place to reduce excessive suds.
Oil-retention enema	Oil-based solution. The colon absorbs a small volume, which softens stool for easier evacuation.
Carminative solution	Relieves gaseous distension. Example: MGW solution, which contains 30 mL of magnesium, 60 mL of glycerin, and 90 mL of water.

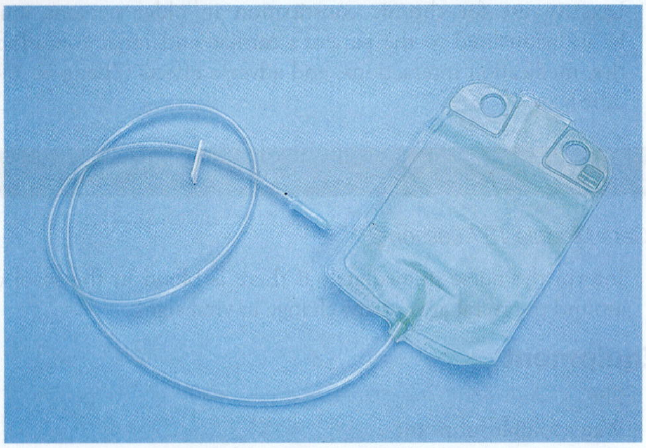

FIG 35.5 Enema bag with tubing.

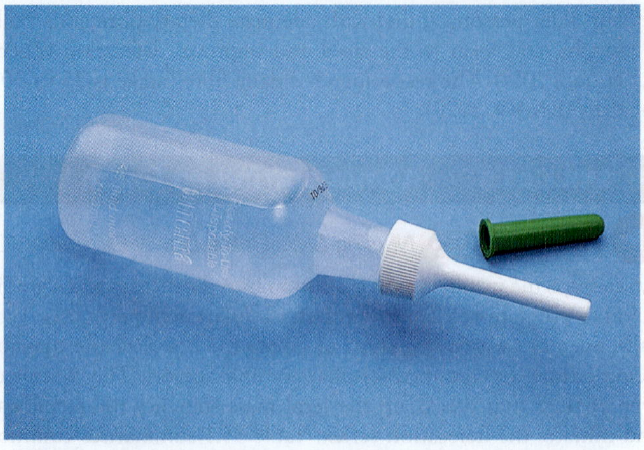

FIG 35.6 Prepackaged enema container with rectal tip and cap.

STEP	RATIONALE
ASSESSMENT	
1. Identify patient using at least two person-specific identifiers (e.g., name and date of birth, or name and medical record number) according to employer policy.	Ensures correct patient. Complies with Accreditation Canada's standards and improves patient safety (Accreditation Canada, 2020).
2. Throughout the procedure, the 4 moments for hand hygiene are to be implemented; hand hygiene should occur before initial patient (or patient environment) contact, before an aseptic procedure, after body fluid exposure risk, and after patient (or patient environment) contact. Additional hand hygiene should be performed when hands are visibly soiled.	Proper hand hygiene helps prevent the spread of infectious agents to health care providers.
3. Review health care provider's prescription for an enema and clarify reason for administration.	A prescription from a health care provider is usually required for a hospitalized patient. The prescription states which type of enema the patient will receive.
4. Assess last bowel movement, normal versus most recent bowel pattern, presence of hemorrhoids, and presence of abdominal pain or cramping.	Determines need for enema and type of enema used. Also establishes baseline for bowel function. Hemorrhoids may obscure rectal opening and cause discomfort or bleeding during evacuation.
5. Assess patient's mobility and their ability to turn and position on their side.	Determines whether assistance is needed for positioning patient.
6. Inspect abdomen for presence of distension and auscultate for bowel sounds.	Establishes baseline for determining effectiveness of enema.
7. Assess patient for allergy to any active ingredients of Fleet enema.	Reduces risk of allergic reaction.
8. Determine patient's level of understanding of purpose of enema.	Allows for planning appropriate teaching measures.

Critical Decision Point *"Enemas until clear" prescription means that enemas are repeated until the patient passes fluid that is clear of fecal matter. The fluid the patient passes may also be tinted and have small flecks of fecal matter. Check employer policy, but usually the patient should receive only three consecutive enemas to avoid disruption of fluid and electrolyte balance. It is essential to observe the contents of the solution passed.*

NURSING DIAGNOSES

- Acute pain
- Constipation
- Chronic functional constipation
- Potential for constipation

Related factors and risk factors are individualized on the basis of patient's condition or needs.

STEP	RATIONALE
PLANNING	
1. Expected outcomes following completion of procedure:	
• Stool is evacuated.	Solution clears rectum and lower colon of stool.
• Enema return is clear.	Indicates that all solid fecal material in colon has passed.
• Abdomen is flat, nontender, and not distended.	Gas and feces are expelled.
2. Arrange supplies at bedside.	Ensures access to supplies during procedure.
IMPLEMENTATION	
1. If enema is medicated, the skill is usually not delegated to a UCP (see employer policy). Check accuracy and completeness of each medication administration record (MAR) by comparing with the health care provider's written prescription. Check patient's name, type of enema, and time for administration. Compare MAR with label of enema solution.	The prescription is the most reliable source and only legal record of medications or procedure that a patient is to receive. Ensures that patient receives correct enema.
2. Pull curtain around bed or close room door.	Maintains privacy and reduces embarrassment for patient.
3. Place bedpan or bedside commode in easily accessible position. If patient will be expelling contents in toilet, ensure that toilet is available; place patient's nonskid slippers and bathrobe in an easily accessible position.	A bedpan is used if patient is unable to get out of bed. Nonskid slippers help prevent a patient who may be rushing to the bathroom from falling. An extra gown provides modesty for patient.
4. With side rail raised on patient's right side and bed raised to an appropriate working height, help patient turn to a left side-lying position with the right knee flexed. Encourage patient to remain in this position until the procedure is complete. Place a child in the dorsal recumbent position.	Allows enema solution to flow downward by gravity along the natural curve of the sigmoid colon and rectum, thus improving retention of solution.

Critical Decision Point *Patients with poor sphincter control require placement of a bedpan under the buttocks. Administering an enema with the patient sitting on the toilet is unsafe because the curved rectal tubing can abrade the rectal wall.*

STEP	RATIONALE
5. Apply clean gloves and place waterproof pad, absorbent side up, under hips and buttocks. Cover patient with a bath blanket, exposing only the rectal area, with the anus clearly visible.	Reduces transmission of microorganisms. Pad prevents soiling of linen. Blanket provides warmth, reduces exposure of body, and allows patient to feel more relaxed and comfortable.
6. Separate buttocks and examine perianal region for abnormalities, including hemorrhoids, anal fissure, and rectal prolapse.	Findings influence approach for inserting enema tip. Prolapse contraindicates enema.
7. Administer enema.	
a. *Administering prepackaged disposable enema:*	
(1) Remove plastic cap from tip of container. Tip may already be lubricated. Apply more water-soluble lubricant as needed.	Lubrication provides for smooth insertion of rectal tube without causing rectal irritation or trauma. With presence of hemorrhoids, extra lubricant provides added comfort.
(2) Gently separate buttocks and locate anus. Instruct patient to relax by breathing out slowly through the mouth.	Breathing out promotes relaxation of external rectal sphincter.
(3) Expel any air from enema container.	Introducing air into the colon causes further distension and discomfort.
(4) Insert lubricated tip of container gently into anal canal toward umbilicus (see Step 7a[4] illustration): • Adult and adolescent: 7.5–10 cm (3–4 inches) • Child: 5–7.5 cm (2–3 inches) • Infant: 2.5–3.75 cm (1–1.5 inches)	Gentle insertion prevents trauma to rectal mucosa.

STEP	RATIONALE

IMPLEMENTATION

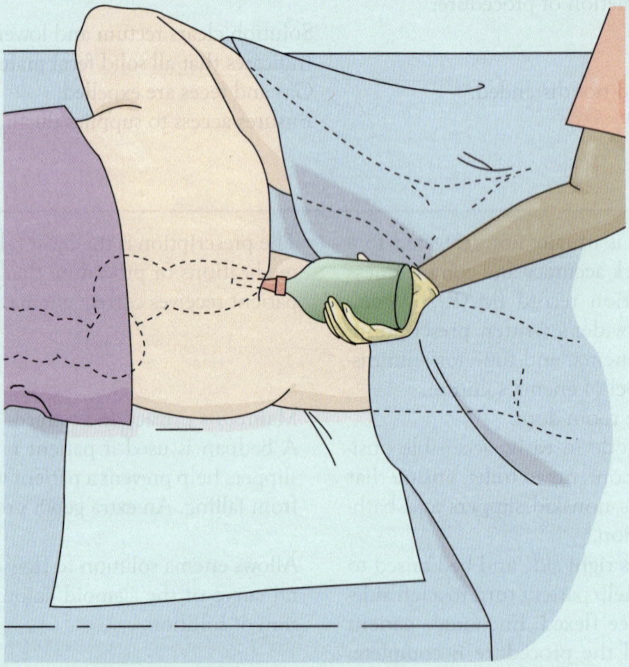

STEP 7A(4) **With patient in left side-lying position, insert tip of commercial enema into rectum.** *(From Wilk, M. J. [2022]. Sorrentino's Canadian textbook for the support worker [5th ed.]. Elsevier Inc.)*

Critical Decision Point *If pain occurs or you feel resistance at any time during the procedure, stop and discuss this with the health care provider. Do not force insertion.*

STEP	RATIONALE
(5) Roll plastic bottle from bottom to tip until entire solution has entered rectum and colon. Instruct patient to retain solution until the urge to defecate occurs, usually 2–5 minutes.	Prevents instillation of air into the colon and ensures that entire solution enters the rectum. Hypertonic solutions require only small volumes to stimulate defecation.
b. *Administering enema in standard enema bag:*	
(1) Add warmed solution to enema bag according to health care provider's prescription (i.e., solution type and volume). Adjust faucet so that tap water is warm, then fill basin with water. Place saline container in basin of warm water before adding saline to the enema bag. Check temperature of solution by pouring small amount of solution over inner wrist.	Hot water burns intestinal mucosa. Cold water causes abdominal cramping and is difficult to retain.
(2) If soapsuds enema (SSE) is prescribed, add castile soap after water.	Reduces suds in enema bag.
(3) Raise container, release clamp, and allow solution to flow long enough to fill tubing.	Removes air from tubing.
(4) Reclamp tubing.	Prevents further loss of solution.
(5) Lubricate 6–8 cm (2.5–3 inches) of tip of rectal tube with lubricant.	Allows smooth insertion of rectal tube without risk of causing irritation or trauma to mucosa.
(6) Gently separate buttocks and locate anus. Instruct patient to relax by breathing out slowly through the mouth. Touch patient's skin next to the anus with tip of the rectal tube.	Patient's breathing out and feeling skin being touched with tube promotes relaxation of external anal sphincter.
(7) Insert tip of rectal tube slowly by pointing it in the direction of the patient's umbilicus. Length of insertion varies (see Step 7a[4]).	Careful insertion prevents trauma to rectal mucosa from accidental lodging of tube against the rectal wall. Insertion beyond the proper limit can cause bowel perforation.

STEP	RATIONALE

IMPLEMENTATION

Critical Decision Point *If the tube does not pass easily, do not force it. Consider allowing a small amount of fluid to infuse and then try to reinsert the tube slowly. The instillation of fluid relaxes the sphincter and provides additional lubrication. If impaction is present, remove it* (see Skill 35.2) *before administering the enema.*

STEP	RATIONALE
(8) Hold tubing in the rectum continuously until the end of fluid instillation.	Prevents expulsion of rectal tube during bowel contractions.
(9) Open regulating clamp and allow solution to enter slowly, with container at patient's hip level.	Rapid infusion stimulates evacuation of tubing and can cause cramping.
(10) Raise height of enema container slowly to an appropriate level above the anus: 30–45 cm (12–18 inches) for high enema; 30 cm (12 inches) for regular enema (see Step 7b[10] illustration); 7.5 cm (3 inches) for low enema. Instillation time varies with volume of solution administered (e.g., 1 L may take 10 minutes). An IV pole may be used to hold an enema bag once you establish a slow flow of fluid (see Step 7b[10] illustration).	Allows for continuous, slow instillation of solution. Raising the container too high causes rapid instillation and possible painful distension of colon. High pressure causes rupture of the bowel in an infant.

Critical Decision Point *Temporary cessation of infusion minimizes cramping and promotes the ability to retain solution. Lower the container or clamp tubing if the patient indicates they are experiencing cramping or if fluid escapes around the rectal tube.*

STEP	RATIONALE
(11) Instill all solution and clamp tubing. Tell patient that the procedure is completed and that you will remove the tubing.	Prevents entrance of air into rectum. Patients may misinterpret sensation of removing tube as loss of control.
8. Place layers of toilet tissue around tube at anus and gently withdraw rectal tube and tip.	Provides for patient's comfort and cleanliness.
9. Explain to patient that some distension and abdominal cramping are normal. Ask patient to retain solution as long as possible until the urge to defecate occurs. This usually takes a few minutes. Stay at the bedside. Have patient lie quietly in bed, if possible. (For an infant or a young child, gently hold buttocks together for few minutes.)	Solution distends the bowel. Length of retention varies with type of enema and patient's ability to contract rectal sphincter. Longer retention promotes stimulation of peristalsis and defecation.

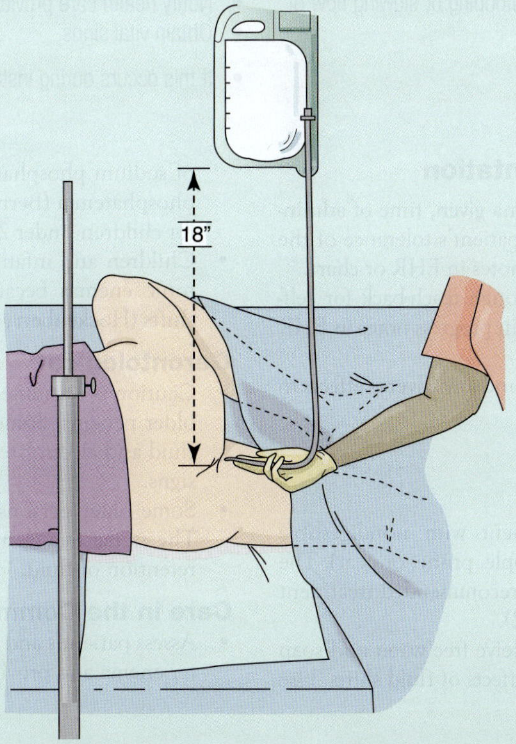

STEP 7B(10) IV pole is positioned so that bottom of enema bag is located 45 cm (18 inches) above anus. *(From Sorrentino, S. A. [2009]. Mosby's textbook for nursing assistants [7th ed.]. Mosby.)*

STEP	RATIONALE
IMPLEMENTATION	
10. Discard enema container or disposable bag and tubing in proper receptacle. Remove PPE and discard.	Reduces transmission and growth of microorganisms.
11. Help patient to the bathroom or commode, if possible. If using a bedpan, apply clean gloves and help patient to as near a normal position for evacuation as possible (see Skill 35.1).	Normal squatting position promotes defecation. Reduces transmission of microorganisms.
12. Observe character of stool and solution (caution patient against flushing toilet before inspection).	Determines whether enema was effective.
13. Help patient as needed to wash anal area with warm soap and water (use gloves for perineal care).	Fecal contents irritate the skin. Hygiene promotes patient's comfort.
14. Remove and discard gloves.	Reduces transmission of microorganisms.
EVALUATION	
1. Inspect colour, consistency, and amount of stool; odour; and fluid passed.	Determines whether stool is evacuated or fluid is retained. Note abnormalities such as presence of blood or mucus.
2. Assess for abdominal distension.	Determines whether distension is relieved.
3. **Use teach-back:** "I want to be sure I explained clearly how to position yourself in bed if you need to give yourself an enema. Tell me how you would position yourself." Develop a revised teaching plan if patient is unable to teach back correctly.	Determines patient's level of understanding of instructional topic.

Unexpected Outcomes	Related Interventions
1. Severe abdominal cramping, bleeding, or sudden abdominal pain develops and is unrelieved by temporarily stopping or slowing flow of solution.	• Stop enema. • Notify health care provider. • Obtain vital signs.
2. Patient is unable to hold enema solution.	• If this occurs during installation, slow the rate of infusion.

Communication and Documentation

- Document the type and volume of enema given, time of administration, characteristics of results, and patient's tolerance of the procedure on flow sheet or in progress notes in EHR or chart.
- Document patient's understanding through teach-back for self-administration of a prepackaged enema in progress notes in EHR or chart.
- Report the failure of patient to defecate and any adverse effects to the health care provider.

Special Considerations

Pediatric

- Infants frequently respond to treatment with nondigestible osmotically active carbohydrates (e.g., apple, prune, or pear). The use of oral stool softeners is the initial recommended treatment for constipation in children (Sood, 2022).
- Children and infants usually do not receive free water and soap enemas because of the serious adverse effects of fluid shifts. Use of sodium phosphate enemas should be limited to avoid hyperphosphatemia (Bernal et al., 2018); these are not recommended for children under 2 years of age (Sood, 2022).
- Children and infants usually do not receive prepackaged hypertonic enemas because hypertonic solutions cause rapid fluid shifts (Hockenberry et al., 2024).

Gerontological

- Caution is warranted when administering enemas prescribed for older persons. Some older persons become tired, are at risk for fluid and electrolyte imbalances, and experience changes in vital signs.
- Some older persons may have difficulty retaining enema fluid. The nurse may gently hold the buttocks together to help with retention of fluid.

Care in the Community

- Assess patient's and caregiver's ability and motivation to administer enema and provide instruction as needed.

PROCEDURAL GUIDELINE 35.1 *Applying a Fecal Management System*

A fecal management system (FMS) protects the perineum from exposure to fecal enzymes and prevents feces from spreading to wounds. In addition, the FMS is useful for patients with severe fecal incontinence, such as those with *Clostridioides difficile*–associated diarrhea. FMS systems are latex-free, in-dwelling rectal catheters with a low-pressure balloon that holds the catheter in place in the rectum and soft, flexible drainage tubing attached to a containment device. These systems have an irrigation port to maintain patency of the catheter and promote fecal drainage. Risks associated with use of this in-dwelling device include rectal necrosis, loss of rectal tone, pressure injury, and fistula formation (S. Singh et al., 2018). Nurses must use interprofessional collaboration to discuss options for patients; certain situations contraindicate the use of an FMS (Box 35.2).

Delegation and Collaboration

The skill of applying a topical (external) fecal containment device cannot be delegated to a UCP. The UCP can assist the nurse by helping to position a patient during device application. The nurse instructs the UCP to do the following:

- Report to the nurse any instances of leakage or change in appearance of skin around the device noted during routine care
- Report to the nurse immediately any increase in patient's rectal pain or sensation of pressure or rectal bleeding

Equipment

- FMS, also called fecal containment device (FCD) kit (Fig. 35.7)
- PPE
- Protective bed pad
- Bath basin

Procedural Steps

1. Identify patient using at least two person-specific identifiers (e.g., name and date of birth, or name and medical record number) according to employer policy (Accreditation Canada, 2020).
2. Review medical record for contraindications for use of an FMS (see Box 35.2).
3. Assess for frequency and amount of diarrhea over the last 24–48 hours.
4. Assess patient for allergy to silicone. Note that these devices are latex-free.
5. Apply PPE. Perform perineal hygiene, and observe patient's anal region for swelling, hemorrhoids, redness, irritation, or drainage. Presence of these findings may contraindicate placement of the device or may indicate need for other interventions to protect the perianal skin.
6. Change gloves and perform digital rectal examination to ensure the absence of rectal impaction. Remove and discard gloves.
7. Apply new clean gloves.
8. Apply the FMS:
   a. Prepare system by connecting the collection bag to catheter tube assembly.
   b. Deflate cuff, usually done with 60-mL syringe supplied in the kit.
   c. Fill 60-mL syringe with quantity of tap water recommended by manufacturer and attach syringe to inflation port. DO NOT inflate at this time. Inflation port is colour coded.
   d. Position patient in left knee–chest position. This position helps maximize sphincter relaxation.
   e. Place protective bed pad under patient's dependent hip.
   f. Fold cuff according to manufacturer instructions and lubricate cuff. Note that a folded cuff should be the size of your index finger.
   g. Generously lubricate anal sphincter.
   h. Gently separate patient's buttocks (UCP can assist), exposing perianal area for entire procedure. Make sure that the perianal area is clean and dry. It may be necessary to perform perineal hygiene again.
   i. Insert cuff using your index finger as a guide. Once the cuff is in the rectal vault, it will open to its original shape.
      (1) Inflate cuff with quantity of water recommended by manufacturer by slowly depressing the syringe plunger; the cuff will inflate. Use the pilot balloon as a guide: If the balloon indicates overinflation or underinflation, withdraw all fluid from the cuff, reposition it in the rectal vault, and reinflate it.

BOX 35.2

Contraindications for Use of Fecal Management Systems

- Suspected or confirmed anal pathology
- Pediatric population
- Existing weak anal sphincter
- Anorectal stricture or stenosis
- Anorectal surgery
- Colorectal surgery in the preceding 12 months
- Severe hemorrhoids
- Rectal tumour
- Fecal impaction
- Allergy or sensitivity to silicone
- Inflammatory processes of the rectum (e.g., Crohn's disease, radiation proctitis)
- Anticoagulated patients

From Whiteley, I., & Sinclair, G. (2014). Faecal management systems for disabling incontinence or wounds: Literature review. *British Journal of Nursing, 23*(16), 881. [Seminal Reference].

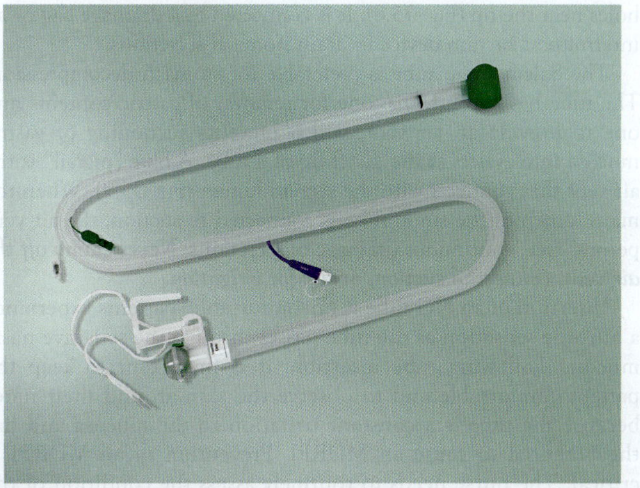

FIG 35.7 DIGNICARE® stool management system. *(Copyright © 2016 C. R. Bard, Inc. Used with permission.)*

PROCEDURAL GUIDELINE 35.1 *Applying a Fecal Management System—cont'd*

(2) Remove syringe from injection port and gently pull on the catheter to ensure that cuff sits against the rectal floor.

j. Note position of indicator line in relation to patient's anus. Changes in indicator line position may indicate need for cuff to be repositioned. Remove gloves and discard.

9. Irrigate cuff as needed: Fill syringe with 45 mL of tap water and attach to clear irrigation port. Observe flow; if leakage occurs, the cuff may need repositioning (see manufacturer instructions).

Critical Decision Point *If the catheter tubing is obstructed with fecal contents, irrigate the catheter. Attach a filled syringe to the FLUSH port and irrigate. Ensure that the flush port remains parallel to the catheter to prevent kinking.*

10. If stool sampling is needed, use sample port (see Fig. 35.7). Apply clean gloves, open sample port, and either tilt or milk the catheter tubing to collect a sample or insert a slip-tip catheter to withdraw fecal material. Close sample port when finished. Remove gloves and discard.

11. Replace collection bag as needed:
   a. Apply clean gloves.
   b. Disconnect drainage tubing from the collection bag.
   c. If necessary, attach bag plug into the collection bag hub.
   d. Connect new bag to tubing.
   e. Dispose of fecal contents per employer policy. Remove PPE and discard.
12. Remove the FMS:
   a. Apply PPE.
   b. Attached depressed 60-mL syringe to cuff infusion port and slowly withdraw all water.
   c. Once cuff is deflated, grasp the catheter as close to the patient as possible and slowly slide it out of the anus.
   d. Dispose of the FMS according to employer policy. Remove PPE and discard.
13. Position patient in a comfortable position and perform any hygiene needed.
14. Monitor patient for diarrhea and record amounts on I&O record every shift.
15. Record application of device and appearance of skin in progress notes in EHR or chart.

✦ SKILL 35.4 Inserting, Maintaining, and Removing a Nasogastric Tube for Gastric Decompression

There are times when normal peristalsis may be altered temporarily, such as after major surgery or with conditions that affect the GI tract. When peristalsis is slowed or absent, a patient cannot eat or drink fluids without experiencing abdominal distension. The temporary insertion of an NG tube into the stomach serves to decompress the stomach, keeping it empty until normal peristalsis returns.

An NG tube is a hollow, pliable tube inserted through a patient's nasopharynx into the stomach. It allows for the removal of gastric secretions and the introduction of solutions into the stomach. Sometimes an NG tube is used for enteral feedings, but a softer, small-bore feeding tube is preferred for feeding purposes (see Chapter 32). The Levin and Salem sump tubes are the most common ones used for stomach decompression. The Levin tube is a single-lumen tube with holes near the tip (Fig. 35.8). It is connected to a drainage bag or an intermittent suction device to drain stomach secretions.

The Salem sump tube is preferable for stomach decompression. The tube has two lumens: one for removal of gastric contents and one to provide an air vent, which prevents suctioning of gastric mucosa into eyelets at the distal tip of a tube. A blue "pigtail" is the air vent that connects with the second lumen (Fig. 35.9). When the main lumen of the sump tube is connected to suction, the air vent permits free, continuous drainage of secretions. ***Never clamp off the air vent, connect to suction, or use for irrigation.***

Insertion of an NG tube is uncomfortable; patients experience a burning sensation as the tube passes through the sensitive nasal mucosa. Following tube insertion, it is important to keep the patient comfortable and to observe the skin around their nares because the tube is a constant irritation to the mucosa and has the potential to cause an MDRPI. Prevention of an MDRPI is critical. The nurse needs to routinely assess the condition of the nares and mucosa for inflammation, blistering, and excoriation (Gilmour et al., 2023).

Delegation and Collaboration

The skill of inserting and maintaining an NG tube cannot be delegated to a UCP. The nurse instructs the UCP to do the following:

- Measure and record the drainage from an NG tube
- Provide oral and nasal hygiene measures
- Perform selected comfort measures, such as positioning or offering ice chips, if allowed
- Anchor the tube to the patient's gown during routine care to prevent accidental displacement
- Immediately report to the nurse any signs of redness or irritation to the nares

Equipment

- 14- or 16-Fr NG tube (Smaller-lumen catheters are not used for decompression in adults because they are unable to remove thick secretions.) (*Option:* A dual-purpose tube, one that is used for both gastric decompression and enteral feedings, may be prescribed for selected patients.)
- Water-soluble lubricant
- pH test strips (measure gastric aspirate acidity); use paper with a range of at least 1.0–11.0 or higher
- Tongue blade
- Flashlight
- Emesis basin
- Bulb or catheter-tipped syringe
- 2.5-cm (1-inch) wide hypoallergenic tape or commercial fixation device
- Safety pin and rubber band
- Clamp, drainage bag, or suction machine with pressure gauge if wall suction is to be used
- Towel
- Glass of water with straw

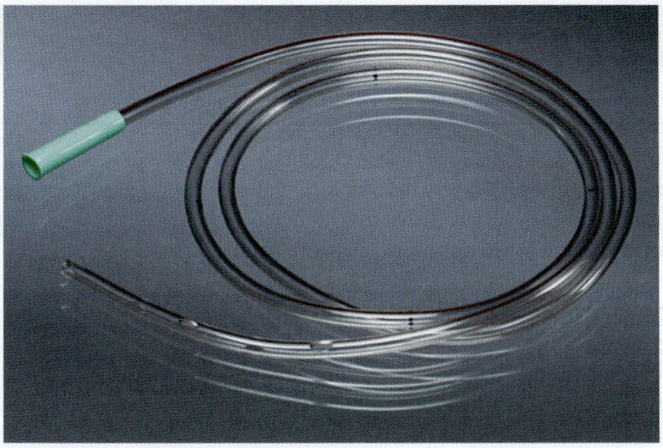

FIG 35.8 Levin tube. *(Courtesy Bard Medical, Covington, GA.)*

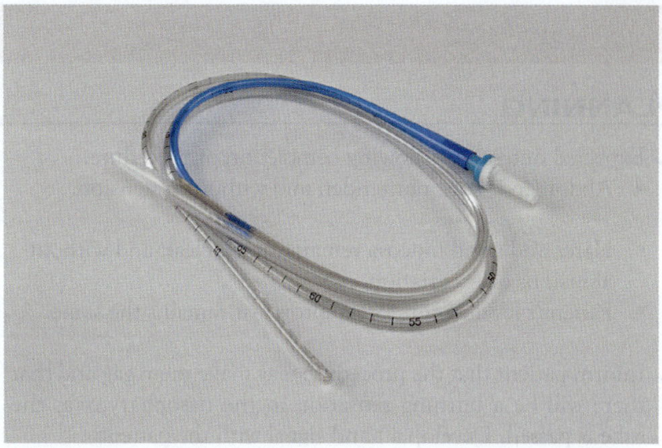

FIG 35.9 Salem sump tube. *(Courtesy Covidien, Mansfield, MA.)*

- Facial tissues
- Normal saline
- Tincture of benzoin *(optional)*
- Suction equipment
- Stethoscope
- PPE

STEP	RATIONALE
ASSESSMENT	
1. Identify patient using at least two person-specific identifiers (e.g., name and date of birth, or name and medical record number) according to employer policy.	Ensures correct patient. Complies with Accreditation Canada's standards and improves patient safety (Accreditation Canada, 2020).
2. Throughout the procedure, the 4 moments for hand hygiene are to be implemented; hand hygiene should occur before initial patient (or patient environment) contact, before an aseptic procedure, after body fluid exposure risk, and after patient (or patient environment) contact. Additional hand hygiene should be performed when hands are visibly soiled.	Proper hand hygiene helps prevent the spread of infectious agents to health care providers.
3. Apply appropriate PPE. Inspect condition of patient's nares and nasal and oral cavity.	Documents whether skin on nares is intact or irritated before NG tube insertion. Determines need for special nursing hygiene measures after tube placement.
4. Ask if patient has a history of nasal surgery or congestion and allergies, and note whether a deviated nasal septum is present.	Alerts nurse to potential obstruction. Insert tube into *uninvolved* nasal passage. Procedure may be contraindicated if surgery is recent.
5. Auscultate for bowel sounds. Palpate patient's abdomen for distension, pain, and rigidity. Remove and discard gloves if applied.	In the presence of diminished or absent bowel sounds, auscultate abdomen for at least 1 minute in each quadrant (Ball et al., 2023). Documents baseline for any abdominal distension, GI ileus, and general GI function, which later serves as baseline for comparison once the tube is inserted.
6. Assess patient's level of consciousness and ability to follow instructions.	Determines patient's ability to help during the procedure.

Critical Decision Point *If the patient is confused, disoriented, or unable to follow commands, get help from another staff member to insert the tube.*

7. Determine whether patient has had a previous NG tube and, if so, which naris was used.	Patient's previous experience complements any explanations and prepares patient for NG tube placement.
8. Verify health care provider's prescription for type of NG tube to be placed and whether tube is to be attached to suction or a drainage bag.	Requires prescription from health care provider. Adequate decompression depends on NG suction.

NURSING DIAGNOSES

- Acute pain
- Inadequate GI motility
- Insufficient knowledge regarding purpose of gastric decompression
- Inadequate oral mucous membrane
- Potential for impaired skin integrity

Related factors and risk factors are individualized on the basis of patient's condition or needs.

STEP	RATIONALE
PLANNING	
1. Expected outcomes following completion of procedure:	
• Abdomen is soft, nontender, and without distension.	Correctly positioned NG tube remains patent, drains gastric secretions, and relieves gastric distension.
• Nares and nasal mucosa remain intact, clear, and without abrasions or excoriation.	Ensures absence of irritation or pressure injury formation from NG tube.
• Patient's level of comfort improves or remains the same.	A correctly inserted NG tube prevents abdominal discomfort from progressing.
2. Inform patient that the procedure may make them gag and that there will be a burning sensation in the nasopharynx as the tube is passed. Develop a hand signal with the patient.	Increases patient's cooperation and ability to anticipate nurse's action. If patient is unable to tolerate the procedure, use of a hand signal will alert the nurse.
3. Arrange supplies at bedside.	Ensures efficient access to supplies during procedure.
IMPLEMENTATION	
1. Position patient upright in high Fowler's position unless contraindicated. If patient is comatose, raise head of the bed as tolerated in semi-Fowler's position with the head tipped forward, chin to chest.	Promotes patient's ability to swallow during procedure. Good body mechanics prevent injury to nurse and patient.
2. Place bath towel over patient's chest. Give facial tissues to patient and allow them to blow their nose, if necessary. Place an emesis basin within reach.	Prevents soiling of patient's gown. Tube insertion through nasal passages may cause tearing and coughing with increased salivation.
3. Pull curtain around bed or close room door.	Provides privacy and preserves dignity as part of person-centred care.
4. Wash bridge of nose with soap and water or alcohol swab. Dry thoroughly.	Removes oils from nose to allow fixation devices to adhere completely.
5. Stand on patient's right side if right-handed or on left side if left-handed. Lower side rail.	Allows easier manipulation of tubing.
6. Instruct patient to relax and breathe normally while you are occluding one naris. Then repeat this action for the other naris. Select the nostril with greater airflow.	Tube passes more easily through naris that is more patent.
7. Measure distance from tip of patient's nose to earlobe to xiphoid process of sternum (see Step 7 illustration).	This length approximates distance from nose to stomach. The NEX (nose–earlobe–xiphoid) method is commonly used in clinical settings with adult patients.
8. Use indelible ink to mark the length of tube that will be inserted.	Indicates length of tube to be inserted.
9. Prepare tube fixation materials. Cut hypoallergenic tape 10 cm (4 inches) long, or prepare membrane dressing or another tube fixation device (see Step 21a[2]).	Fixation devices allow the tube to float free of the nares, thus reducing pressure on the nares and preventing MDRPI (Fumarola et al., 2020).
10. Apply clean gloves.	Reduces transmission of microorganisms.
11. Apply pulse oximetry/capnography device and measure vital signs. Monitor oximetry/capnography during insertion.	Provides objective assessment of respiratory status before and during tube insertion.
12. *Option:* Dip tube with surface lubricant into a glass of room-temperature water or lubricate 7.5–10 cm (3–4 inches) end of tube with water-soluble lubricant (see manufacturer instructions).	Water activates lubricant, minimizes friction against nasal mucosa, and aids in insertion of the tube. Water-soluble lubricant is less toxic than oil-based lubricant if aspirated.

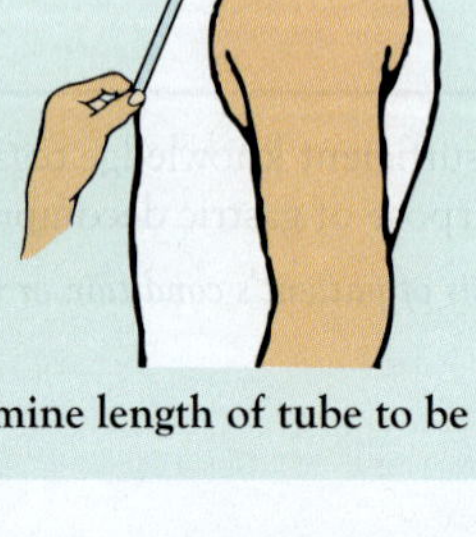

STEP 7 Determine length of tube to be inserted.

STEP	RATIONALE
IMPLEMENTATION	
13. Hand an alert patient a cup of water if they are able to hold the cup and swallow, unless contraindicated. Check employer policy related to use of a straw when drinking. If patient is unconscious, do not use water. Watch for patient coughing. Explain to patient that you are about to insert NG tube and how you will do so (see Step 14).	Swallowing water facilitates tube passage. The use of a straw may cause the patient to swallow additional air and worsen gastric distension. Coughing may indicate that tube is inadvertently entering the lungs. Explanation decreases patient anxiety and increases patient cooperation.
14. Insert tube gently and slowly through the naris to back of the throat (posterior nasopharynx). Aim back and down, toward patient's ear.	Natural contour facilitates passage of tube into GI tract and reduces gagging.
15. Have patient relax and flex head toward their chest after tube is passed through nasopharynx.	Closes off glottis and reduces risk of tube entering the trachea.
16. Inserting tube using swallow or no-swallow technique:	
a. Encourage patient to swallow by having them take small sips of water when possible. Advance tube as the patient swallows, rotating tube gently 180 degrees while inserting. Advance tube each time the patient swallows until you reach the desired length.	Swallowing facilitates passage of past the oropharynx. A tug may be felt as patient swallows, indicating that tube is following desired path.
b. If using no-swallow technique, ask patient to take a deep breath and hold it when tube reaches pharynx (Shlamovitz, 2022). Once tube is inserted 15–20 cm, have patient perform abdominal breathing.	In a recent randomized controlled trial, researchers found that no-swallow technique of NG tube insertion decreased patient discomfort; increased success rate at first intubation; and reduced nausea, tearing, mucosal injury, and changes in vital signs (Shlamovitz, 2022).
17. Do not advance tube during inspiration or coughing because it will likely enter respiratory tract. Monitor oximetry/capnography.	When tube inadvertently enters airway, changes in oxygen saturation or end-tidal carbon dioxide (CO_2) (capnography) occur.

Critical Decision Point *Do not force the NG tube. If the patient starts to cough or has a drop in oxygen saturation or increased CO_2, withdraw the tube into the posterior nasopharynx until normal breathing resumes.*

STEP	RATIONALE
18. Using a penlight and tongue blade, verify that tube is not positioned in back of throat.	Tube could become coiled or kinked or enter trachea.
19. Temporarily anchor tube to patient's nose with a small piece of tape.	Securing NG tube prevents movement of tube and subsequent gagging. Allows for verification of tube placement.
20. Verify tube placement. Check employer policy for recommended methods of checking tube placement:	
a. Follow prescription for bedside X-ray and notify radiology for examination of chest and abdomen.	Radiography is the gold standard for verifying initial NG tube placement; this step must be completed before any medication or liquid is administered (Judd, 2020).
b. While waiting for radiography, follow these procedures: Attach a bulb or catheter-tipped syringe to end of NG tube. Aspirate gently back on syringe to obtain gastric contents, observing amount, colour, and quality of return (see Step 20b illustration).	Observation of gastric contents is useful to verify initial tube placement. Gastric contents are usually green but can sometimes be off-white, tan, bloody, or brown in colour. Other common aspirate colours include yellow or bile stained (duodenal placement); pale watery yellow (esophageal placement); and tan/off-white, with aspirate having consistency of mucous (tracheobronchial placement) (Lord, 2018).
c. Use pH test paper to measure aspirate for pH with colour-coded pH paper. Be sure that paper range of pH is at least 1.0–11.0 (see Step 20c illustration).	Evidence supports pH testing for use as an indicator of tube placement: pH ≤5 likely indicates gastric placement; intestinal or respiratory pH is usually ≥7 (Judd, 2020).
21. Anchor tube with a fixation device, avoiding application of pressure on nares. Select one of the following fixation methods:	Proper anchoring and marking of tube helps prevent migration of tube and formation of MDRPI.
a. *Applying tape.*	
(1) Apply tincture of benzoin or other skin adhesive to bridge of patient's nose and allow it to become "tacky."	Helps tape adhere better. Protects underlying skin.

STEP	RATIONALE

IMPLEMENTATION

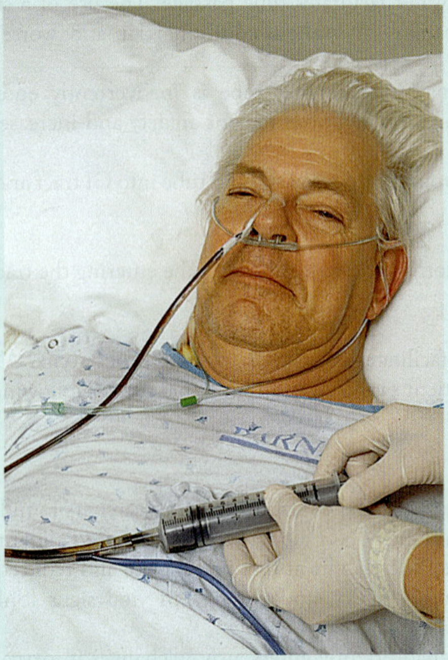

STEP 20B Aspiration of gastric contents.

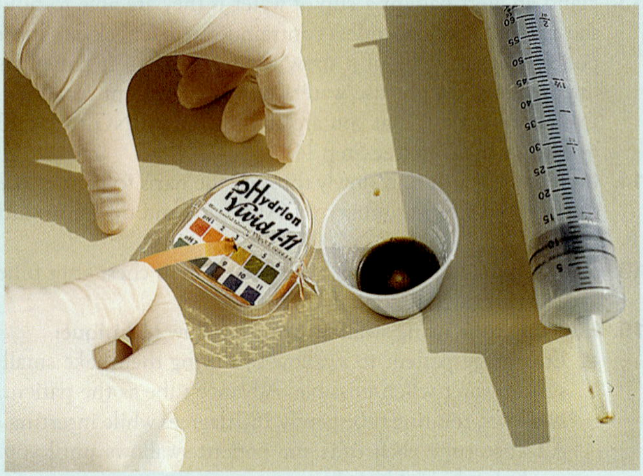

STEP 20C Checking pH of gastric aspirate.

STEP	RATIONALE
(2) Tear small horizontal slits at one-third and two-thirds of length of tape without splitting tape (see Step 21a[2] illustration). Fold middle sections toward one another to form a closed strip.	Tape strip holds tubing to lessen rubbing against soft palate and naris.
(3) Print date and time on tape and place top end of tape over bridge of patient's nose.	
(4) Wrap bottom end of tape around tube as it exits patient's nose (see Step 21a[4] illustration).	
b. *Applying tube fixation device using shaped adhesive patch (see manufacturer instructions).*	Secures tube and reduces friction on nares.
(1) Apply wide end of patch to bridge of nose (see Step 21b[1] illustration).	
(2) Slip connector around tube as it exits the nose (see Step 21b[2] illustration).	
22. Fasten end of NG tube to patient's gown with a piece of tape (see Step 22 illustration). Do not use safety pins to fasten tube to gown.	Anchors tubing to prevent pulling on nose.
23. Keep head of bed elevated at least 30 degrees (preferably 45 degrees) unless contraindicated or patient is upright in semi-sitting position (WOCN, 2016).	Reduces patient's risk of aspirating stomach contents.

Critical Decision Point *If inserting a Salem sump tube, keep the pigtail of the tube above the level of the stomach to prevent a siphoning action that will clog the tube.*

STEP	RATIONALE
24. Assist radiology as needed in obtaining prescribed X-ray of the chest and abdomen.	Radiography is the gold standard for verifying NG tube placement (Judd, 2020).
25. Remove gloves and help patient to comfortable position.	Reduces transmission of microorganisms.
26. Once tube placement is confirmed, measure amount of tube that is external, then use indelible marker to mark exit of tube at nares as a guide for any tube displacement. Record this information in progress notes in EHR or chart.	The mark alerts nurses and other health care providers to possible tube displacement, which will require confirmation of tube placement.

Critical Decision Point *Never reposition the NG tube in a patient who has had gastric surgery, as positioning can rupture the suture line.*

STEP	RATIONALE

IMPLEMENTATION

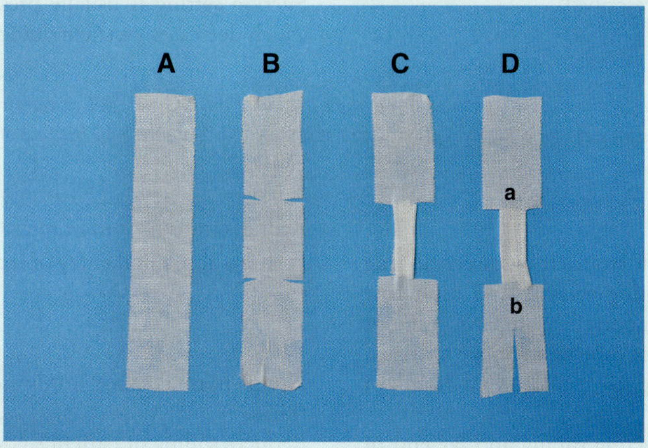

STEP 21A(2) Taping method. A, Start with a piece of tape. B, Make two slits on both sides of the tape. C, Fold the middle section inward. D, Tear a new slit in bottom of tape. Top part (a) should attach to patient's nose; bottom part (b) should be wrapped around the tube.

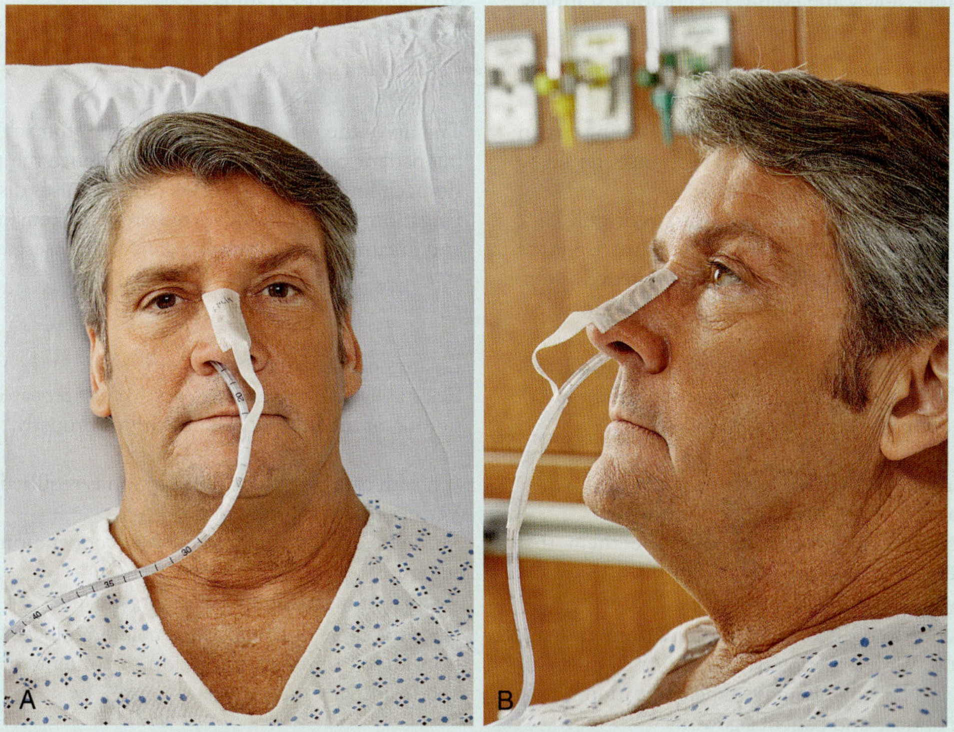

STEP 21A(4) A, Tape applied to anchor nasogastric tube. B, Nares are free of pressure from tape and tube.

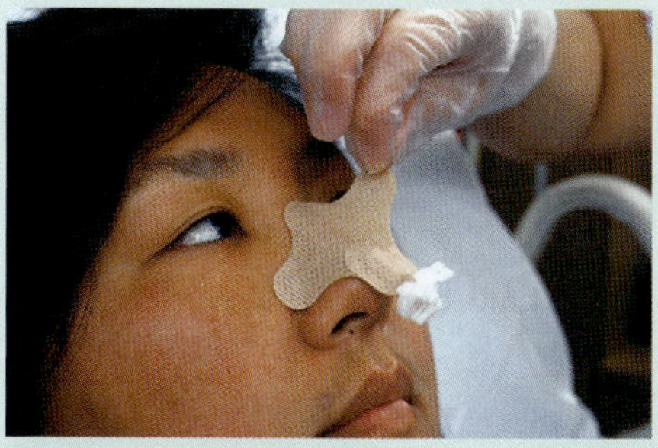

STEP 21B(1) Apply patch to bridge of nose.

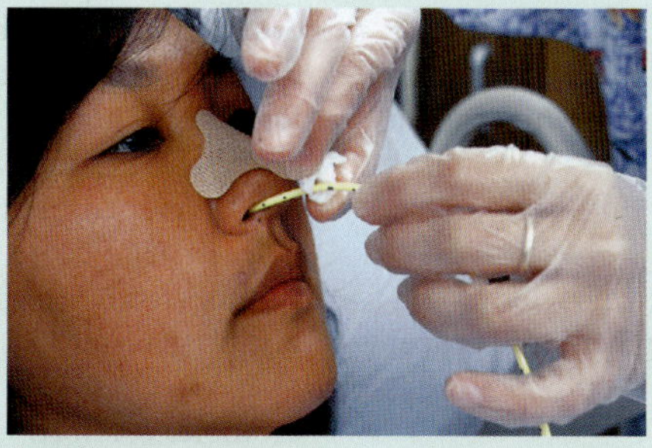

STEP 21B(2) Slip connector around nasogastric tube.

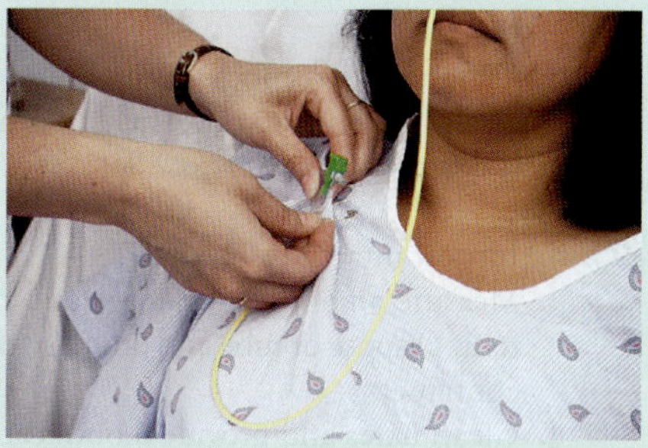

STEP 22 Fasten nasogastric tube to patient gown.

IMPLEMENTATION

STEP	RATIONALE
27. Attach NG tube to suction as prescribed.	Suction setting is usually prescribed to be low and intermittent, which decreases gastric irritation from NG tube.

Critical Decision Point *If the lumen of the tube is narrow and secretions are thick, the NG tube will not drain as desired. Irrigate the tube* (see Step 30). *Use interprofessional collaboration to discuss the need for a higher suction setting if unable to irrigate the tube because of thick secretions.*

STEP	RATIONALE
28. Irrigating NG tube:	
a. Apply clean gloves.	Reduces transmission of microorganisms.
b. Check for tube placement in stomach by disconnecting NG tube, connecting irrigating syringe, and aspirating contents (see Step 20b). Temporarily clamp NG tube or reconnect it to the connecting tube and remove syringe.	Prevents accidental entry of irrigating solution into lungs.
c. Empty syringe of aspirate and use it to draw up 30 mL of normal saline.	Use of normal saline minimizes loss of electrolytes from stomach fluids.
d. Disconnect NG from connecting tubing and lay end of connection tubing on towel.	Reduces soiling of patient's gown and bed linen.
e. Insert tip of irrigating syringe into end of NG tube. Remove clamp. Hold syringe with tip pointed at the floor and inject saline slowly and evenly. Do not force solution.	Position of syringe prevents introduction of air into vent tubing, which causes gastric distension. Solution introduced under pressure causes gastric trauma.

Critical Decision Point *Do not introduce saline through blue pigtail air vent of the Salem sump tube.*

STEP	RATIONALE
f. If resistance occurs, check for kinks in tubing. Turn patient onto their left side. Repeated resistance should be reported to the health care provider.	The tip of the tube may lie against the stomach lining. Repositioning patient on their left side may dislodge the tube away from the stomach lining. Buildup of secretions causes distension.
g. After instilling saline, immediately aspirate or pull back slowly on syringe to withdraw fluid. If amount aspirated is greater than amount instilled, record difference as output. If amount aspirated is less than amount instilled, record difference as intake.	Irrigation clears tubing so the stomach remains empty. Measure and document amount of irrigant fluid inserted in tube as intake.
h. Use a bulb syringe to place 10 mL of air into blue pigtail.	Ensures patency of air vent.
i. Reconnect NG tube to drainage or suction. (Repeat irrigation if solution does not return.)	Re-establishes drainage collection; may repeat irrigation or repositioning of tube until NG tube drains properly.
29. Removing NG tube:	
a. Verify prescription to remove NG tube.	A health care provider's prescription is required for this procedure.
b. Auscultate abdomen for presence of bowel sounds.	Verifies return of peristalsis.
c. Explain procedure to patient and reassure them that removal is less distressing than insertion.	Minimizes anxiety and increases cooperation. Tube passes out smoothly.
d. Apply clean gloves.	Reduces transmission of microorganisms.
e. Turn off suction and disconnect NG tube from drainage bag or suction. With irrigating syringe, insert 20 mL of air into lumen of NG tube. Remove tape or fixation device from bridge of nose and patient's gown.	Have tube free of connections before removal. Clears gastric fluids from tube to prevent aspiration of contents or soiling of clothing and bedding.
f. Hand patient facial tissue; place a clean towel across their chest. Instruct patient to take and hold breath as tube is removed.	Some patients wish to blow their nose after the tube is removed. The towel keeps the gown from getting soiled. Temporary airway obstruction occurs during tube removal.
g. Clamp or kink tubing securely and pull tube out steadily and smoothly into towel held in other hand while patient holds their breath.	Clamping prevents tube contents from draining into oropharynx. Reduces trauma to mucosa and minimizes patient's discomfort. Towel covers tube, which is an unpleasant sight. Holding breath helps prevent aspiration.
h. Inspect intactness of tube.	
i. Measure amount of drainage and note character of content. Dispose of tube and drainage equipment into proper container.	Provides accurate measure of fluid output. Reduces transfer of microorganisms.
j. Clean nares and provide mouth care.	Promotes comfort.

STEP	RATIONALE
IMPLEMENTATION	
k. Position patient comfortably and explain procedure for drinking fluids if not contraindicated. Instruct patient to notify you if nausea occurs.	Sometimes patients are not allowed anything by mouth (NPO) for up to 24 hours. When fluids are allowed, prescriptions usually begin by allowing patient a small amount of ice chips each hour and increase as patient is able to tolerate more.
30. For all procedures, clean equipment and return to their proper place. Place soiled linen in utility room or proper receptacle.	Proper disposal of equipment prevents spread of microorganisms and ensures proper exchange procedures.
31. Remove and discard gloves.	Reduces transmission of microorganisms.
EVALUATION	
1. Observe amount and character of contents draining from NG tube. Ask if patient feels nauseated.	Determines whether tube is decompressing stomach of contents.
2. Auscultate for presence of bowel sounds. Turn off suction while auscultating.	Sound of the suction apparatus is sometimes misinterpreted as bowel sounds.
3. Palpate patient's abdomen periodically. Note any distension, pain, or rigidity.	Determines success of abdominal decompression and return of peristalsis.
4. Inspect condition of nares and nose.	Evaluates onset of skin and tissue irritation.
5. Observe position of tubing.	Prevents tension applied to nasal structures.
6. Explain that it is normal for patient to have sore throat or irritation in pharynx.	Tissue in pharynx is tender and thus irritated by NG tube.
7. **Use teach-back:** "I need to be sure I explained why you need the NG tube and the importance of letting me know if you feel nauseated. Tell me why it is important for me to know if you feel nauseated." Develop a revised teaching plan if patient or caregiver is unable to teach back correctly.	Determines patient's and caregiver's level of understanding of instructional topic.

Unexpected Outcomes	Related Interventions
1. Patient indicates nausea or has distended and painful abdomen.	• Assess patency of tube. NG tube may be occluded or no longer in the stomach. • Irrigate tube. • Verify that suction is on as prescribed. • Notify health care provider if distension is unrelieved.
2. Patient develops irritation or erosion of skin around naris.	• Provide frequent skin care to area. • Use taping method designed to reduce MDRPI (see taping methods in Steps 21a and 21b). • Consider switching tube to other naris.
3. Patient develops signs and symptoms of pulmonary aspiration (fever, shortness of breath, or pulmonary congestion).	• Perform complete respiratory assessment. • Notify health care provider. • Obtain chest X-ray examination as prescribed.

Communication and Documentation

- Document length, size, and type of NG tube inserted and in which naris it was inserted. In addition, record patient's tolerance of procedure, confirmation of tube placement, location of distal tip of tube, character of gastric contents, pH value, results of radiography, whether the tube is clamped or connected to a drainage bag or to suction, and amount of suction supplied on flow sheet or in progress notes in EHR or chart.

DOCUMENTATION EXAMPLE

Insertion of NG tube prescribed for gastric decompression for small bowel obstruction explained to patient, patient questions answered, and consent obtained by health care provider. 16F NG tube inserted after patient placed in high Fowler's position. Skin around nares inspected and found intact. NG inserted through right naris and advanced to 52 cm and secured there with secure fit adhesive. Patient tolerated procedure well. Abdominal X-ray confirmed placement in stomach and NG attached to low, intermittent wall suction. Immediately after suction initiated, 500 mL of green liquid with small blood clots from gastric contents observed. Surgical team notified of blood within gastric contents.

- Document patient's and caregiver's understanding through teach-back of what to report to the nurse and the purpose of the NG tube in progress notes in EHR or chart.
- Document difference between amount of normal saline instilled and amount of gastric aspirate removed on I&O sheet. Record the amount and character of contents draining from the NG tube during every shift.
- Document removal of the tube "intact," patient's tolerance of procedure, and final amount and character of drainage.

Special Considerations

Pediatric

- Children usually have an NG tube for feeding, and often the tube is removed between feedings and reinserted as needed. If a tube is to be left in place for a young child, the child will need some type of hand restraint to keep them from pulling the tube out.

Gerontological

- Check for ill-fitting dentures, and remove them for the patient's safety and comfort during the insertion.
- Oral and nasal mucosal drying is sometimes present. Adequately lubricate the tube for insertion.

✦ REVIEW QUESTIONS

An older adult patient with mild dementia was admitted to the hospital with a fractured hip 3 days earlier. Surgical repair of the hip was done, and the patient took opioid medication for pain for 2 days after surgery. A stool softener was also prescribed to be administered once a day. In reviewing the patient's record, the nurse finds that the patient had two small liquid incontinent bowel movements the previous evening. The patient is unable to remember the last time their bowels moved, but the patient states that they feel "pressure in my bottom." The patient's family does not know when the patient's last bowel movement was because the patient is independent in toileting at home. However, a family member recalls that the patient had reported being constipated several days prior to surgery.

Review Questions 1 to 5 relate to the case study presented here.

1. The health care provider orders a soapsuds enema (SSE) to be given. The nurse positions the patient on their side and inserts the enema tubing. When the clamp is released to allow the fluid to be instilled, the fluid does not flow into the patient. What is the likely cause?
2. The nurse assesses that the patient may have a fecal impaction, so the nurse requests an order from the physician for which of the following priority actions?
   1. Laxatives to supplement the stool softeners that the patient is taking
   2. Digital removal of the stool mass present in the patient's rectum
   3. Changes to the patient's diet to increase fibre and fluids
   4. Wait until the next day and try the enema again
3. The patient develops nausea and vomiting, and the health care provider orders a nasogastric (NG) tube to be inserted. Place the following steps in the correct order:
   1. Verify order for NG tube.
   2. Tape tube to nose.
   3. Apply clean gloves.
   4. Identify patient using at least two identifiers (e.g., name and date of birth, or name and medical record number) according to agency policy.
   5. Pass the tube along the floor of the nasal passage, then just past the nasopharynx.
   6. Instruct the patient to flex their head forward and swallow while the tube is advanced.
   7. Measure distance to insert tube as length from tip of nose to earlobe to xiphoid process.
4. Before the patient is discharged from the hospital, which instructions would the nurse include when educating the patient and the patient's caregiver about management of chronic constipation? (*Select all that apply.*)
   1. Increase fibre and fluid intake.
   2. Use a low-volume enema daily.
   3. Avoid gluten.
   4. Take laxatives twice a day.
   5. Exercise for 30 minutes every day.
   6. Schedule time to use the toilet at the same time every day.
   7. Take probiotics 5 times a week.
5. Given that the patient has dementia and is now less mobile until their hip heals, what methods should the nurse use to remind the patient about managing their health at home after discharge?

Visit the Evolve site for a complete list of answers to the Review Questions.

✦ NEXT GENERATION NCLEX® (NGN)

For practice with answering exam questions related to unfolding NGN case studies, please consult the Next Generation NCLEX® (NGN)-Style Case Studies for Skills and Techniques on the Evolve website: http://evolve.elsevier.com/Canada/Perry/clinicalskills/

REFERENCES

Accreditation Canada. (2020). *Required organizational practices–2020 handbook*. https://physicians.nshealth.ca/resources/required-organizational-practices-2020-handbook

Allen, K., & Leslie, S. (2022). *Autonomic dysreflexia*. StatPearls. https://www.ncbi.nlm.nih.gov/books/NBK482434/

Argoff, C. (2020). Opioid-induced constipation: A review of health-related quality of life, patient burden, practical clinical considerations, and the impact of peripherally acting μ-opioid receptor antagonists. *The Clinical Journal of Pain*, *36*(9), 716–722. https://doi.org/10.1097/AJP.0000000000000852

Ball, J. W., Dains, J. E., Flynn, J. A., et al. (2023). *Seidel's guide to physical examination* (10th ed.). Elsevier.

Bernal, C. J., Dole, M., & Thame, K. (2018). The role of bowel management in children with bladder and bowel dysfunction. *Current Bladder Dysfunction Reports*, *13*, 46–55. https://doi.org/10.1007/s11884-018-0458-3

Borowitz, S. (2017). *Encopresis*. Medscape. https://emedicine.medscape.com/article/928795-overview#a3s

Boscart, V., McCleary, L., Sheiban Taucar, L., et al. (2023). *Ebersole and Hess' gerontological nursing and healthy aging in Canada* (3rd ed.). Elsevier.

Brophy, S., Moore, Z., Patton, D., et al. (2021). What is the incidence of medical device-related pressure injuries in adults with the acute hospital setting? A systematic review. *Journal of Tissue Viability*, *30*(4), 489–498. https://doi.org/10.1016/j.jtv.2021.03.002

Dietitians of Canada. (2021). *Constipation in children*. UnlockFood.ca. http://www.unlockfood.ca/en/Articles/Childrens-Nutrition/Health-Conditions/Constipation-in-Children.aspx

Dumic, I., Nordin, T., Jecmenica, M., et al. (2019). Gastrointestinal tract disorders in older age. *Canadian Journal of Gastroenterology and Hepatology, 2019*, Article ID 6757524. https://doi.org/10.1155/2019/6757524

Fletcher, J. (2020). Pressure ulcer education 6: Incontinence assessment and Care. *Nursing Times, 116*(3), 42–44. https://www.nursingtimes.net/clinical-archive/tissue-viability/pressure-ulcer-education-6-incontinence-assessment-and-care-10-02-2020/

Francis, K. (2018). Damage control: Differentiating incontinence-associated dermatitis from pressure injury. *Nursing, 48*(6), 18–25. https://doi.org/10.1097/01.nurse.0000532739.93967.20

Fumarola, S., et al. (2020). Overlooked and underestimated: Medical adhesive–related skin injuries [Best practice consensus document on prevention]. *Journal of Wound Care, 29*(Suppl. 3c), S1–S24. https://doi.org/10.12968/jowc.2020.29.Sup3c.S1

Gilmour, N., Froese, M., Gray, L. J., et al. (2023). *Preventing medical treatment related skin and tissue injuries in adults and children. evidence informed practice tools.* Winnipeg Regional Health Authority. https://professionals.wrha.mb.ca/evidence-informed-practice-tools/.

Hockenberry, M. J., Duffy, E. A., & Gibbs, K. (2024). *Wong's nursing care of infants and children* (12th ed.). Elsevier

Judd, M. (2020). Confirming nasogastric tube placement in adults. *Nursing, 50*(4), 43–46. https://doi.org/10.1097/01.nurse.0000654032.78679.f1

Lord, L. M. (2018). Enteral access devices: Types, function, care, and challenges. *Nutrition in Clinical Practice, 33*(1), 16–38. https://doi.org/10.1002/ncp.10019

Lucak, S., Lunsford, T. N., & Harris, L. A. (2021). Evaluation and treatment of constipation in the geriatric population. *Clinics in Geriatric Medicine, 37*, 85–102. https://doi.org/10.1016/j.cger.2020.08.007

McNichol, L. L., Ayello, E. A., Phearman, L. A., et al. (2018). Incontinence-associated dermatitis: State of the science and knowledge translation. *Advances in Skin & Wound Care, 31*(11), 502–513. https://doi.org/10.1097/01.ASW.0000546234.12260.61

Norton, L., Parslow, N., Johnston, D., et al. (2021). Best practice recommendations for the prevention and management of pressure injuries. In *Foundations of best practice for skin and wound management: A supplement of wound care Canada. Wounds Canada.* https://www.woundscanada.ca/docman/public/health-care-professional/bpr-workshop/172-bpr-prevention-and-management-of-pressure-injuries-2/file

Power-Kean, K., Zettel, S., El-Hussein, M. T., et al. (2023). *Huether and McCance's understanding pathophysiology* (2nd Cdn. ed.). Elsevier.

Registered Nurses' Association of Ontario. (2020). *A proactive approach to bladder and bowel management in adults,* 4th edition. https://rnao.ca/bpg/guidelines/proactive-approach-bladder-and-bowel-management-adults

Rowan-Legg, A., & Canadian Paediatric Society. (2011; reaffirmed 2018). *Managing functional constipation in children.* https://papers.ucalgary.ca/paediatrics/assets/cps-functional-constipation.pdf

Shlamovitz, G. Z. (2022). *Nasogastric intubation technique.* Medscape. https://emedicine.medscape.com/article/80925-technique

Sigmon, D., & An, J. (2022). *Nasogastric tube.* StatPearls. https://www.ncbi.nlm.nih.gov/books/NBK556063/

Singh, R., Salem, A., Nanavati, J., & Mullin, G. E. (2018). The role of diet in the treatment of irritable bowel syndrome: A systematic review. *Gastroenterology Clinics of North America, 47*(1), 107–137. https://doi.org/10.1016/j.gtc.2017.10.003

Singh, S., Bhargava, B., Vasantha, P., et al. (2018). Clinical evaluation of a novel intrarectal device for management of fecal incontinence in bedridden patients. *The Journal of Wound, Ostomy and Continence Nursing, 45*(2), 156–162. https://doi.org/10.1097/WON.0000000000000408

Sood, M. R. (2022). *Chronic functional constipation and fecal incontinence in infants, children, and adolescents: Treatment.* UpToDate. https://www.uptodate.com/contents/chronic-functional-constipation-and-fecal-incontinence-in-infants-children-and-adolescents-treatment

Whiteley, I., & Sinclair, G. (2014). Faecal management systems for disabling incontinence or wounds: Literature review. *British Journal of Nursing, 23*(16), 881. [Seminal Reference].

Wound, Ostomy, and Continence Nurses Society. (2016). *Guideline for prevention and management of pressure ulcers (injuries)* (2nd ed.). [Seminal Reference].

Zheng, S., & Yao, J. (2018). Expert consensus on the assessment and treatment of chronic constipation in the elderly. *Aging Medicine, 1*(1), 8–17. https://doi.org/10.1002/agm2.12013

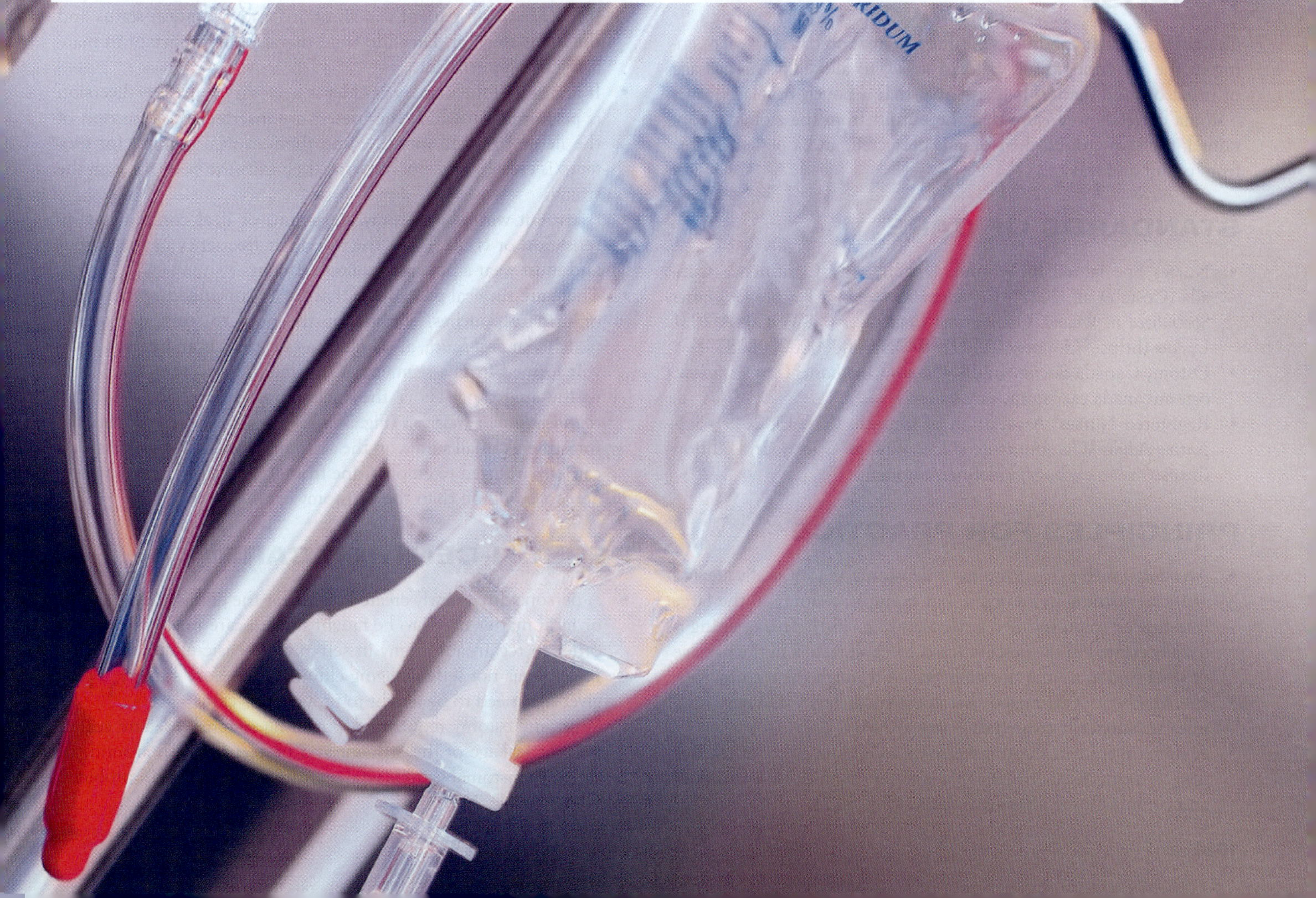

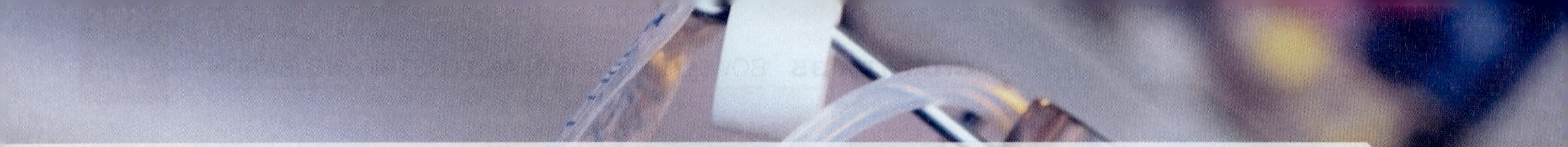

36 | Ostomy Care

Canadian content written by **Sayedeh Haddis Razeghi, RN, BScN**
Original US chapter by **Jane Fellows, MSN, CWOCN**

SKILLS AND PROCEDURES

OBJECTIVES

Mastery of content in this chapter will enable the nurse to:

- Identify the types of fecal and urinary diversions.
- Explain the differences in consistency of effluent based on the type of ostomy.
- Pouch a fecal or urinary diversion.
- Describe methods used to maintain integrity of the peristomal skin.
- Catheterize a urinary diversion.

MEDIA RESOURCES

- http://evolve.elsevier.com/Canada/Perry/clinicalskills/

PURPOSE

Certain diseases or conditions require the creation of a surgical opening in the abdominal wall, called a *stoma*, to allow for the passage of urine or fecal matter. It is essential that a pouch be placed over a stoma correctly to ensure that the output from the stoma is contained, the skin around the stoma is protected, and a patient is free from odour and leakage.

STANDARDS OF CARE

- Nurses Specialized in Wound, Ostomy, and Continence Canada (Costa et al., 2022)—*Canadian Standards of Practice for Nurses Specialized in Wound, Ostomy, and Continence (NSWOCs): A 2021 Update* (https://doi.org/10.1097/WON.0000000000000839)
- Ostomy Canada Society (n.d.)—*Ostomy Care Basics* (https://www.ostomycanada.ca/ostomy-care-basics/)
- Registered Nurses' Association of Ontario (RNAO, 2019)—*Supporting Adults Who Anticipate or Live With an Ostomy*, 2nd edition (https://rnao.ca/bpg/guidelines/ostomy)

PRINCIPLES FOR PRACTICE

- An *ostomy*, such as a colostomy or ileostomy, is a surgically created artificial opening in an organ. For example, a stoma in the large intestine or colon is called a *colostomy* (Fig. 36.1). This opening is usually created in the descending colon and results in the passage of stool similar to that normally passed through the rectum.
- In Canada, it is estimated that approximately 13 000 new ostomies are surgically created each year (RNAO, 2019).
- A stoma placed in the transverse or ascending colon is an *ileostomy*. It drains fecal effluent that is watery to thick in consistency and contains some digestive enzymes (Fig. 36.2).
- The character of the output of a bowel stoma (called *effluent*) is influenced by a patient's medications and hydration status and the foods they eat. Diet and fluid therapy are important in managing ostomy effluent.
- If removal of the urinary bladder is necessary, a urinary diversion is performed in which the ureters are inserted into a section of the ileum or small intestine and then an ileal conduit (or *urostomy*) is created (Fig. 36.3). Urine then exits the body through the stoma.
- A patient with a colostomy, ileostomy, or ileal conduit has no sensation or control over the timing or frequency of the output and must wear a pouch to collect effluent.
- There are surgical procedures that create continent internal fecal or urinary pouches, eliminating the need to wear an external pouch. An *ileal pouch*, also known as a *J-pouch*, is an internal reservoir formed from a segment of the ileum that is then connected to the anal canal above the anal sphincter (Fig. 36.4, *A–B*). A *continent urinary reservoir* (Fig. 36.5) is a reservoir created from the intestine. A small stoma on the abdominal wall allows access via a catheter inserted to empty urine from the pouch. These surgeries are less common than the ileostomy or urostomy.

PERSON-CENTRED CARE

- A person with a newly created stoma for the elimination of urine or fecal matter needs to be taught how to care for the ostomy in order to regain autonomy in self-care for basic elimination. If a patient was not self-managing elimination before surgery, a caregiver may need to be taught to provide this care.
- With any ostomy requiring a pouching system, a secure seal to prevent leakage of the effluent and protect the skin around the stoma (peristomal skin) is vital to avoid peristomal skin problems (Taneja et al., 2019).

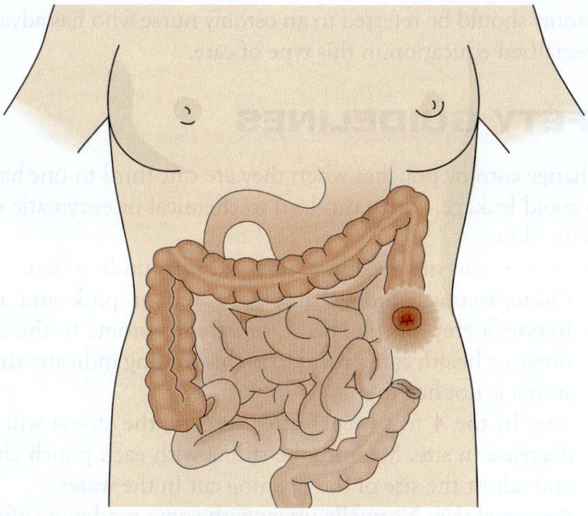

FIG 36.1 Sigmoid colostomy.

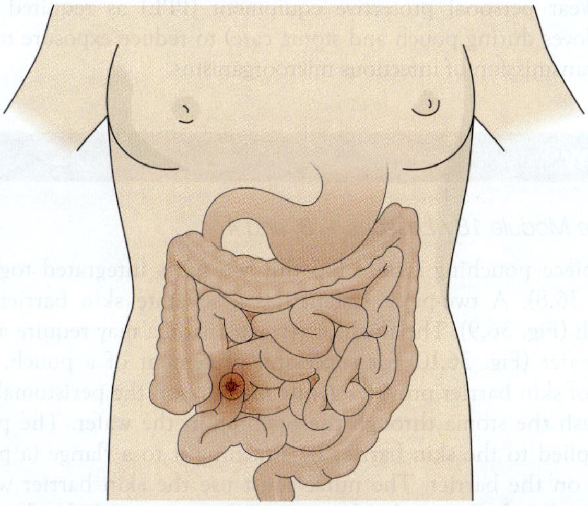

FIG 36.2 Ileostomy.

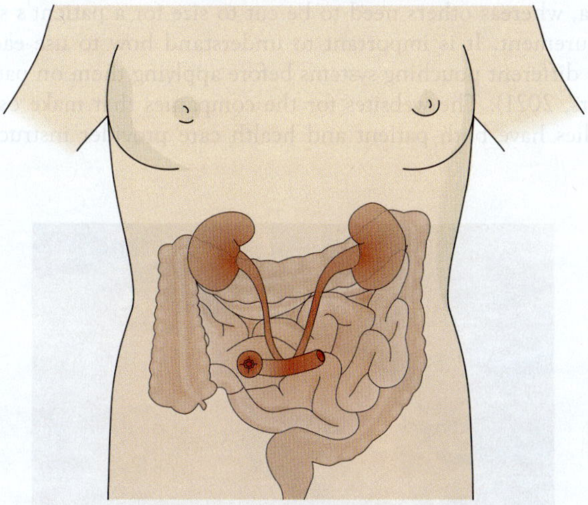

FIG 36.3 Urostomy (ileal conduit).

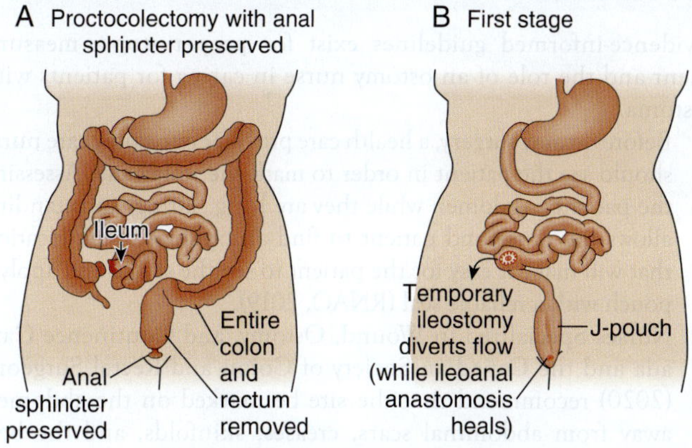

FIG 36.4 Ileal pouch anal anastomosis.

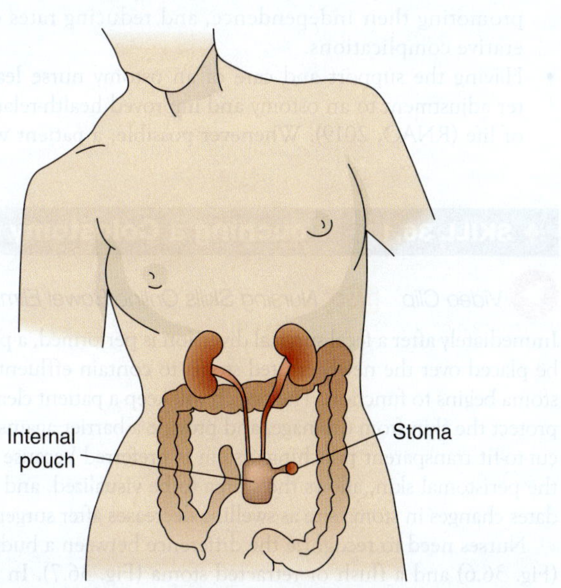

FIG 36.5 Continent urinary diversion.

- A reliable and effective pouching system is an essential factor in facilitating a patient's emotional adjustment to an ostomy (Carmel et al., 2021).
- In addition to the stress of illness and surgical recovery, patients with ostomies face the fear of social rejection, concern about sexual function and intimacy, and the need to receive help with personal care (Medina-Rico et al., 2019).
- Having an ostomy can significantly impact a patient's quality of life, leading to a range of physical, psychological, and social restrictions. Some patients also face significant changes in their perceived body image, lifestyle, and intimate relationships (Medina-Rico et al., 2019). Always practise person-centred care with these patients and encourage them to express their feelings about their ostomy.
- In communicating with a patient during ostomy care, it is important to be sensitive and avoid conveying anything that the patient may interpret as disrespect or disgust. Practise person-centred care, prepare adequately for the procedure, arrange interprofessional collaboration when necessary, and maintain a calm, professional demeanour. Do not act offended by the odour or appearance of the effluent in the pouch or the appearance of the stoma. A negative reaction from caregivers only reinforces a patient's feelings that this alteration in bodily function makes them personally and socially unacceptable.
- When patients come to a hospital with an ostomy, encourage them to be able to resume self-care as soon as possible. Respect a patient's routine of care even if it differs from usual care in the facility. Offer educational materials to support the patient's development of ostomy self-care (Abdelmohsen, 2020).

EVIDENCE-INFORMED PRACTICE

Evidence-informed guidelines exist for proper stoma measurement and the role of an ostomy nurse in caring for patients with a stoma.

- Before ostomy surgery, a health care provider or ostomy care nurse should see the patient in order to mark the stoma site. Assessing the patient's abdomen while they are lying, sitting, and standing allows the nurse and patient to find an optimal stoma location that will make it easy for the patient to see the stoma and apply a pouch with a reliable seal (RNAO, 2019).
- Nurses Specialized in Wound, Ostomy, and Continence Canada and the Canadian Society of Colon and Rectal Surgeons (2020) recommend that the site be marked on the abdomen away from abdominal scars, creases, skinfolds, and the belt line. Studies show that preoperative stoma site marking is crucial for improving patients' postoperative quality of life, promoting their independence, and reducing rates of postoperative complications.
- Having the support and care of an ostomy nurse leads to better adjustment to an ostomy and improved health-related quality of life (RNAO, 2019). Whenever possible, a patient with a new ostomy should be referred to an ostomy nurse who has advanced, specialized education in this type of care.

SAFETY GUIDELINES

- Change ostomy pouches when they are one-third to one-half full to avoid leakage, which can lead to chemical or enzymatic injury to the skin.
- Know the signs of a healthy stoma and surrounding skin:
  - *Colour/moisture:* Stoma should be red or pink and moist. Report a grey, purple, black, or very dry stoma to the charge nurse or health care provider, as this finding indicates that the stoma is not healthy.
  - *Size:* In the 4 to 6 weeks after surgery, the stoma will likely decrease in size. Measure the stoma with each pouch change, and adjust the size of the opening cut in the wafer.
  - *Peristomal skin:* Normally intact with some reddening after the adhesive wafer is removed. Presence of blisters, a rash, or excoriated skin is abnormal.
- Wear personal protective equipment (PPE) as required (e.g., gloves during pouch and stoma care) to reduce exposure to and transmission of infectious microorganisms.

SKILL 36.1 Pouching a Colostomy or an Ileostomy

Video Clip *NSO Nursing Skills Online Bowel Elimination/Ostomy Care Module 18 / Lessons 1, 3, and 4*

Immediately after a fecal surgical diversion is performed, a pouch must be placed over the newly created stoma to contain effluent when the stoma begins to function. The pouch will keep a patient clean and dry, protect the skin from drainage, and provide a barrier against odour. A cut-to-fit transparent pouching system is preferred because it protects the peristomal skin, allows the stoma to be visualized, and accommodates changes in stoma size as swelling decreases after surgery.

Nurses need to recognize the difference between a budded stoma (Fig. 36.6) and a flush or retracted stoma (Fig. 36.7). In the immediate postoperative period, the stoma may be edematous and the abdomen distended. These symptoms will resolve over a 4- to 6-week period after surgery, but during this time it will be necessary to revise the pouching system to meet the changing size of the stoma and the changes in body contours (Carmel et al., 2021).

There are many types of pouching systems. All have a protective layer that adheres to the skin, called a *skin barrier*, and a pouch. A one-piece pouching system has the two parts integrated together (Fig. 36.8). A two-piece system has a separate skin barrier and pouch (Fig. 36.9). The flush or retracted stoma may require a convex wafer (Fig. 36.10) for successful placement of a pouch. This type of skin barrier provides gentle pressure on the peristomal skin to push the stoma through the opening in the wafer. The pouch is applied to the skin barrier by attaching it to a flange (a plastic ring) on the barrier. The nurse must use the skin barrier with a flange that fits a pouch of corresponding size made by the same manufacturer to avoid leakage between the skin barrier and pouch. Some pouching systems have precut openings in the barrier for the stoma, whereas others need to be cut to size for a patient's stoma measurement. It is important to understand how to use each of these different pouching systems before applying them on patients (Myers, 2021). The websites for the companies that make ostomy supplies have both patient and health care provider instructions

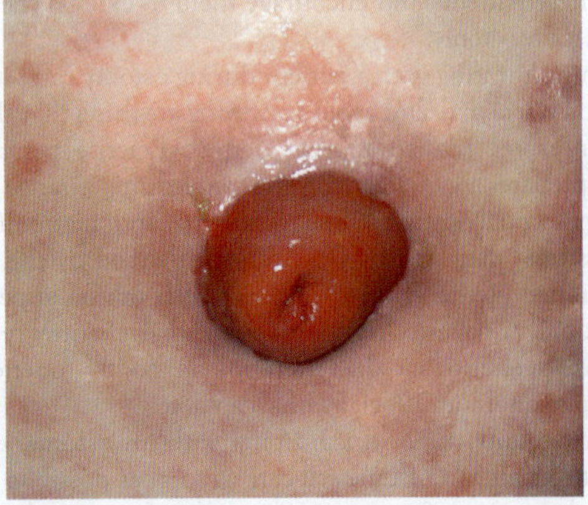

FIG 36.6 Budded stoma. *(Courtesy Jane Fellows.)*

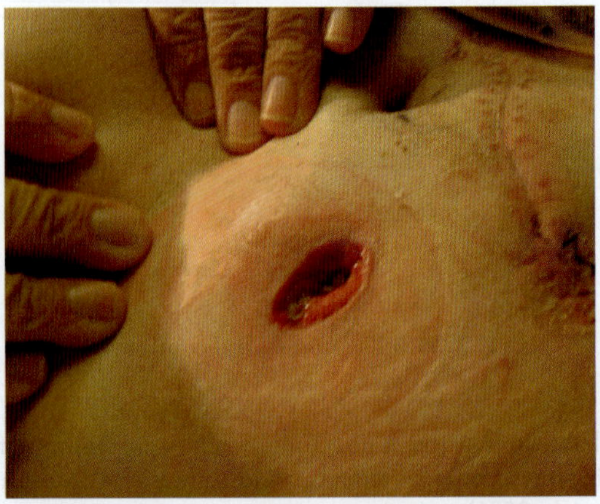

FIG 36.7 Retracted stoma. *(Courtesy Jane Fellows.)*

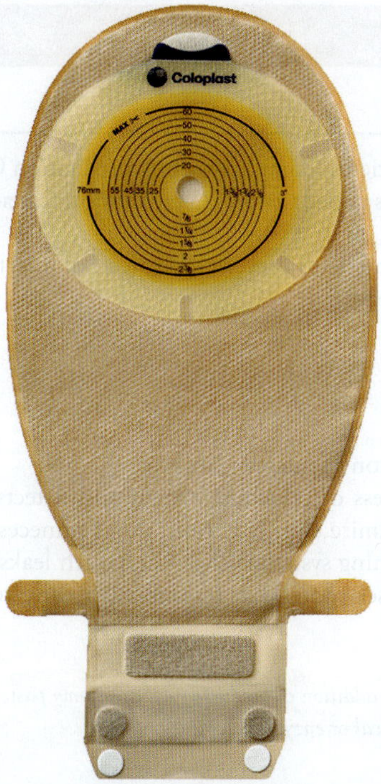

FIG 36.8 One-piece pouch with Velcro closure. *(Courtesy Coloplast, Minneapolis, MN.)*

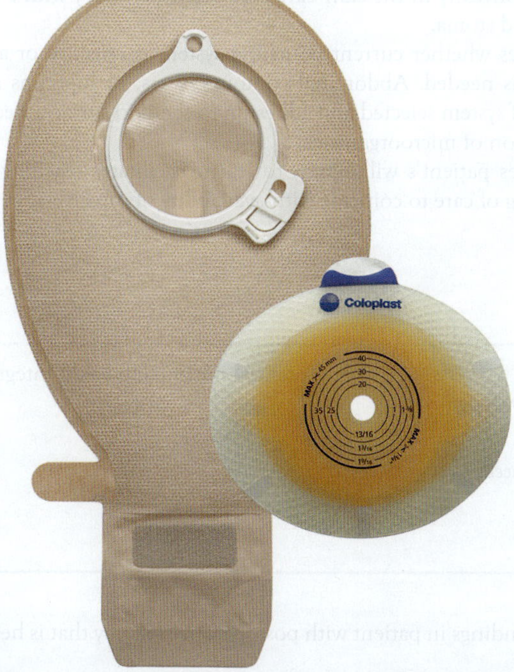

FIG 36.9 Two-piece pouching system with separate skin barrier and attachable pouch. *(Courtesy Coloplast, Minneapolis, MN.)*

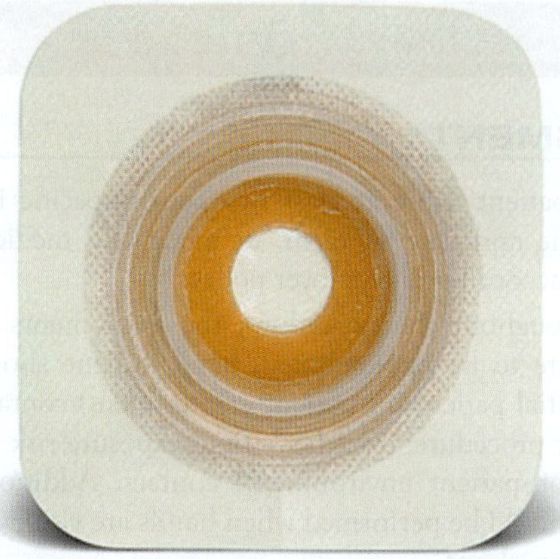

FIG 36.10 Convex skin barrier wafer. *(Used with permission of Convatec, Inc. All rights reserved.)*

that are helpful in understanding how to use the pouching systems (e.g., https://www.coloplast.ca; https://www.convatec.ca/; https://www.hollister.ca/en-ca/).

Delegation and Collaboration

The skill of pouching a new ostomy should not be delegated to an unregulated care provider (UCP). In some facilities, care of an established ostomy (4 to 6 weeks or more after surgery) can be delegated to UCPs. The nurse directs the UCP about the following:

- The expected amount, colour, and consistency of drainage from an ostomy
- The expected appearance of the stoma
- Special equipment needed to complete a particular patient's pouching
- The changes in a patient's stoma and surrounding skin integrity that should be reported

Collaborate with the interprofessional health care team (e.g., wound, ostomy, and continence [WOC] nurse), when available, for postsurgical assessment, selection of proper barrier and pouch, and patient education on self-care.

Equipment

- Skin barrier/pouch–clear, drainable one-piece or two-piece system, cut-to-fit or precut size
- Pouch closure device such as a clip, if needed
- Ostomy measuring guide
- Adhesive remover *(optional)*
- Clean gloves
- Washcloth
- Towel or disposable waterproof barrier
- Basin with warm tap water
- Scissors
- Waterproof bag for disposal of pouch
- PPE (e.g., gown and goggles if there is any risk of splashing when emptying pouch)

STEP	RATIONALE
ASSESSMENT	
1. Identify patient using at least two person-specific identifiers (e.g., name and date of birth, or name and medical record number) according to employer policy.	Ensures correct patient. Complies with Accreditation Canada's standards and improves patient safety (Accreditation Canada, 2020).
2. Throughout the procedure, the 4 moments for hand hygiene are to be implemented; hand hygiene should occur before initial patient (or patient environment) contact, before an aseptic procedure, after body fluid exposure risk, and after patient (or patient environment) contact. Additional hand hygiene should be performed when hands are visibly soiled.	Proper hand hygiene helps prevent the spread of infectious agents to health care providers.
3. Apply clean gloves.	Reduces transmission of microorganisms.
4. Observe existing skin barrier and pouch for leakage and length of time in place. Pouch should be changed every 3–7 days, not daily (Carmel et al., 2021). If an opaque pouch is being used, remove it to fully observe stoma. Dispose of this type of pouch in proper receptacle.	Assesses effectiveness of pouching system and detects potential for problems. To minimize skin irritation, avoid unnecessary changing of the entire pouching system. When the pouch leaks, skin damage from effluent causes more skin trauma than early removal of the wafer.

Critical Decision Point *Repeated leakage may indicate the need for a different type of pouch or addition of products such as ostomy paste or barrier rings. If the pouch is leaking, change it. Taping or patching it to contain effluent leaves the skin exposed to chemical or enzymatic irritation.*

STEP	RATIONALE
5. Observe amount of effluent in pouch and empty it if it is more than one-third to one-half full by opening pouch and draining it into a container for measurement of output. Note consistency of effluent and record intake and output (I&O).	Weight of the pouch may disrupt the seal of adhesive on the skin. Monitor fluid balance and bowel function after surgery. Normal colostomy effluent is soft or formed stool, whereas normal ileostomy effluent is liquid.
6. Observe stoma for type, location, colour, swelling, presence of sutures, trauma, and healing or irritation of peristomal skin.	Stoma characteristics influence selection of an appropriate pouching system. Convexity in the skin barrier is often necessary with a flush or retracted stoma.
7. Observe placement of stoma in relation to abdominal contours and presence of scars or incisions. Remove and dispose of gloves.	Determines whether current pouching system is effective or a new selection is needed. Abdominal contours, scars, or incisions affect the type of system selected and adhesion to the skin surface. Reduces transmission of microorganisms.
8. Explore patient's attitudes, perceptions, knowledge, and acceptance of their stoma. Discuss patient's interest in learning self-care. Identify others who will be helping patient after they leave hospital.	Determines patient's willingness to learn. Facilitates teaching plan and timing of care to coincide with availability of caregivers.

NURSING DIAGNOSES

- Reduced skin integrity
- Insufficient knowledge regarding pouching of an ostomy
- Alteration in body image
- Willingness to enhance knowledge
- Potential for impaired skin integrity

Related factors and risk factors are individualized on the basis of patient's condition or needs.

STEP	RATIONALE
PLANNING	
1. Expected outcomes following completion of procedure:	
• Stoma is red and moist; peristomal skin is intact and free of irritation; sutures are intact.	Normal findings in patient with postoperative ostomy that is healing.
• Stoma drains a moderate amount of liquid or soft stool, and flatus is in pouch, which can be seen with bulging of pouch. (Flatus may not be observable if pouch has a gas filter.)	Stoma is functioning normally. A snug seal around the stoma has been attained. Flatus indicates return of peristalsis after surgery.
• Patient and/or caregiver observe stoma and steps of procedure.	Reveals acceptance of alteration in body image and interest in self-care.
• Patient asks questions about the procedure and attempts to help with pouch change.	Indicates readiness to learn and begin self-care.
2. Explain procedure to patient; encourage patient's interaction and questions.	Lessens patient's anxiety and promotes person-centred care.
3. Assemble equipment and close room curtains or door.	Optimizes use of time; provides privacy.

STEP	RATIONALE

IMPLEMENTATION

STEP	RATIONALE
1. Have patient assume semireclining or supine position (same position assumed during assessment and pouching). (**Note:** Some patients with established ostomies prefer to stand.) If possible, provide patient with a mirror for observation.	When patient is semireclining, there are fewer skinfolds, allowing for ease of application of pouching system.
2. Apply clean gloves.	Reduces transmission of microorganisms.
3. Place towel or disposable waterproof barrier under patient and across patient's lower abdomen.	Protects bed linen; maintains patient's dignity.
4. If not done during assessment, remove the used pouch and skin barrier gently by pushing skin away from barrier. Use adhesive remover to facilitate removal of skin barrier. Empty pouch and dispose of it in appropriate receptacle. Measure output if needed. **Note:** There may be no output at the time of first pouch change.	Reduces skin trauma. Improper removal of pouch and barrier can cause peristomal skin irritation or breakdown.
5. Clean peristomal skin gently with warm tap water using a washcloth; do not scrub the skin. If you touch the stoma, minor bleeding is normal. Pat skin dry. Have washcloth handy for additional cleaning if there is output from the stoma while preparing the pouch.	Soap leaves residue on skin, which may irritate the skin. The pouch does not adhere to wet skin. Avoid the use of creams or oils because they prevent the ostomy appliance from sealing around the stoma. If excess hair is noted on the skin around the stoma, clip the area using scissors to help the appliance better adhere to the skin (RNAO, 2019). Ileostomies have frequent output, especially after eating.
6. Measure stoma (see Step 6 illustration). Expect size of stoma to change in the first 4–6 weeks after surgery.	Allows for proper fit of pouch that will protect peristomal skin.
7. Trace pattern of stoma measurement on pouch backing or skin barrier (see Step 7 illustration).	Prepares for cutting of opening in pouch.
8. Cut opening on backing or skin barrier wafer (see Step 8 illustration). If using mouldable or shape-to-fit barrier, use your fingers to mould shape-to-fit stoma.	Customizes pouch to provide appropriate fit over stoma.
9. Remove protective backing from adhesive backing or wafer (see Step 9 illustration).	Prepares skin barrier for placement.
10. Apply pouch over stoma (see Step 10 illustration). Press firmly into place around stoma and outside edges. Have patient hold their hand over the pouch to apply heat to secure seal.	Pouch adhesives are heat and pressure sensitive and hold more securely at body temperature.
11. Close end of pouch with clip or integrated closure. Remove drape from patient. Help patient to assume a comfortable position.	Ensures that pouch is secure. Contains effluent.
12. Remove and dispose of gloves and other PPE.	Reduces transmission of microorganisms.

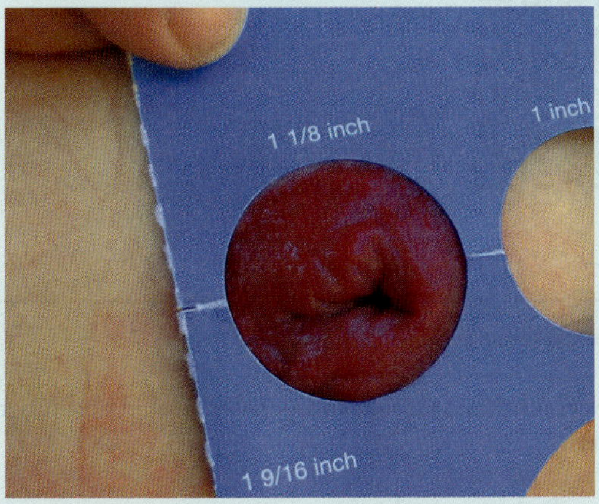

STEP 6 Measure stoma. *(Courtesy Coloplast, Minneapolis, MN.)*

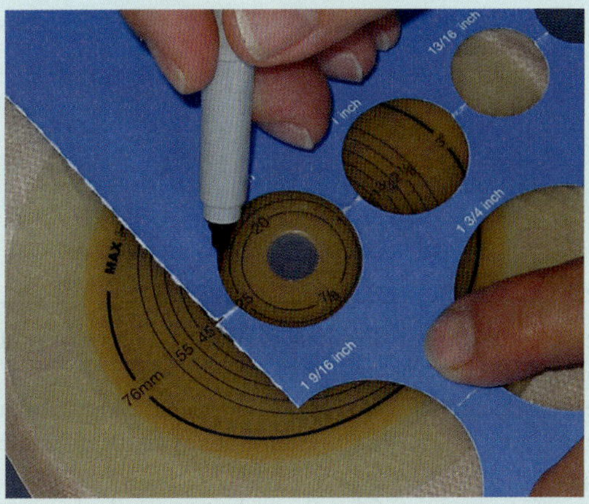

STEP 7 Trace measurement on skin barrier. *(Courtesy Coloplast, Minneapolis, MN.)*

STEP	RATIONALE

IMPLEMENTATION

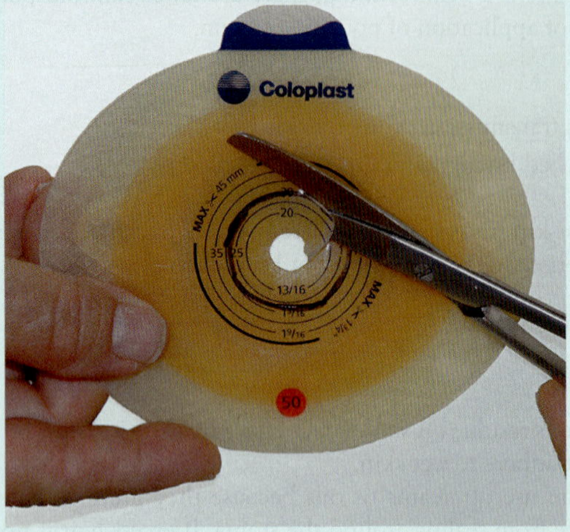

STEP 8 Cut opening in wafer. *(Courtesy Coloplast, Minneapolis, MN.)*

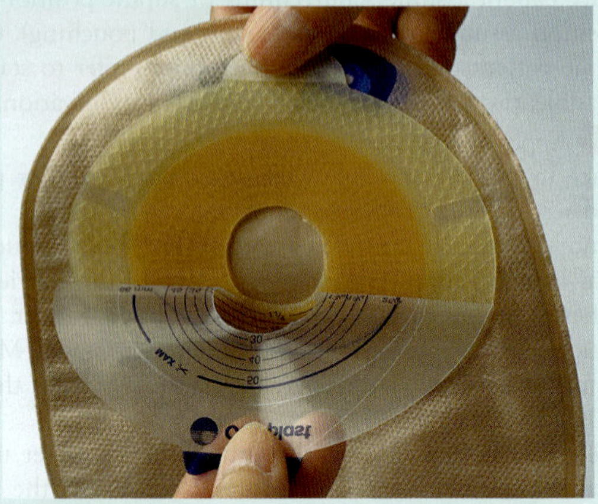

STEP 9 Remove protective backing. *(Courtesy Coloplast, Minneapolis, MN.)*

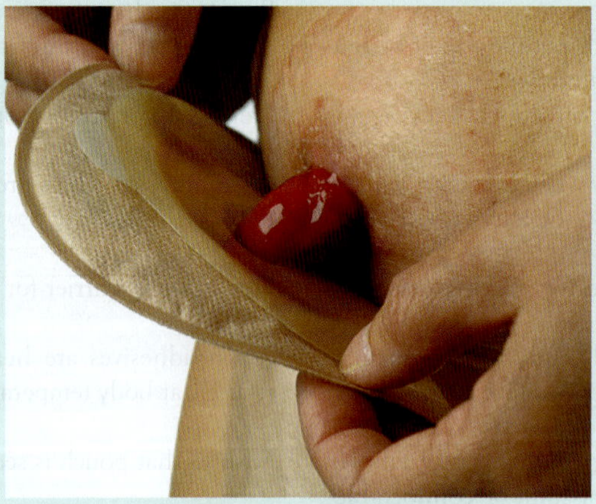

STEP 10 Apply pouch over stoma. *(Courtesy Coloplast, Minneapolis, MN.)*

EVALUATION

STEP	RATIONALE
1. Observe condition of skin barrier and adherence of pouch to abdominal surface.	Determines presence of leaks.
2. Observe appearance of stoma, peristomal skin, abdominal contours, suture line, and presence of any flatus during pouch change.	Determines condition of stoma and peristomal skin and progress of wound healing.
3. Observe for presence of any flatus during pouch change	Determines whether peristalsis is returning.
4. Observe patient's and caregiver's willingness to view stoma and ask questions about procedure.	Determines level of adjustment to and understanding of stoma care and pouch application. Allows planning for future education needs and progress toward acceptance of altered body image.

STEP	RATIONALE
EVALUATION	
5. Use **teach-back:** "I want to be sure you understand what is involved in changing your ostomy pouch. Tell me how often you should empty your pouch and things you can do to stop the skin around your stoma from becoming sore." Develop a revised teaching plan if patient or caregiver is unable to teach back correctly.	Determines patient's and caregiver's level of understanding of instructional topic.

Unexpected Outcomes	Related Interventions
1. Skin around stoma is irritated, blistered, or bleeding, or a rash is noted. This may be caused by undermining of pouch seal by fecal contents, causing irritant dermatitis, or by adhesive removal, causing skin stripping or fungal or other skin eruption.	• Remove pouch more carefully. • Change pouch more frequently or use a different type of pouching system. • Avoid use of acetone-based products. • Arrange for interprofessional collaboration, including an ostomy care nurse.
2. Necrotic stoma is manifested by purple or black colour, dry instead of moist texture, failure to bleed when washed gently, or tissue sloughing.	• Report to nurse in charge or health care provider. • Document appearance.
3. Patient refuses to view stoma or participate in care.	• Obtain referral for ostomy care nurse. • Allow patient to express feelings. • Encourage caregiver support.

Communication and Documentation

- Document type of pouch and skin barrier applied; time of procedure; amount and appearance of effluent in the pouch; location, size, and appearance of stoma; and condition of peristomal skin in the electronic health record (EHR) or chart.
- Document patient's and caregiver's level of participation, teaching that was done, and response to teaching.
- Report any of the following to the health care provider: abnormal appearance of stoma, suture line, peristomal skin, or character of output.

DOCUMENTATION EXAMPLE

Patient's right lower quadrant end-ileostomy was changed at 1600 hours. Stoma is budded and measures 35 mm and appears moist, pink, and warm. Peristomal skin is intact, with no erythema or ecchymosis noted. Flatus present and effluent emptied for 125 mL of brown, liquid stool. Stoma cleansed with warm water. Barrier ointment applied, along with a two-piece flat Coloplast appliance, which is intact and well-sealed. Patient tolerated procedure well. Patient looks at stoma and actively participates in care. Patient demonstrated good understanding of appliance change by cleansing and measuring stoma and cutting appliance appropriately.

Special Considerations

Teaching

- Teach changing of a pouch whenever doing a pouch change, even if the patient does not appear interested. Do not insist that the patient look at the stoma; allow time for adjustment.
- Include the caregiver in teaching to facilitate the patient's readiness to learn.
- Some patients accept a stoma with minimal emotional difficulty; some may never completely adjust to it. Practise person-centred care–individualize care according to the patient's situation and circumstances (Giordano et al., 2020).
- Give the patient plain-language teaching materials that clearly state each step for a pouch change. Audio, video, and online instructions are also available. Consider using materials that have illustrations for each step. For patients who do not speak English, provide a professional interpreter.
- Give patients a list of equipment and the name, address, phone number, and website of the supplier.

Pediatric

- Pediatric stoma surgery is usually done because the neonate has necrotizing enterocolitis (NEC), Hirschsprung's disease, or a congenital disorder (Sena et al., 2020). These stomas are often temporary, with closure of the ostomy occurring when the surgical repair has healed and the neonate is medically ready for surgery. Children and adolescents may have ostomy surgery for conditions such as Gardner syndrome, typhlitis, inflammatory bowel disease, and trauma (Minkes, 2022).
- To prevent parastomal hernias, stomas should be brought through the rectus abdominis in older children and adolescents (Minkes, 2022).
- The most common complications with pediatric stomas are skin irritation and infection (e.g., *Candida* infection, dermatitis). It is important to teach caregivers appropriate wound care (Minkes, 2022).
- The skin of a preterm infant is not fully developed and is more absorbent than that of a full-term infant. Avoid use of skin sealants and adhesive removers on these infants (Kenner & Boykova, 2021).
- Select pediatric pouches designed especially for neonates, infants, and children. The pouches are smaller and have a more skin-sensitive adhesive on the barrier.
- Adolescents requiring an ostomy benefit from presurgical contact with other adolescents who have an ostomy. Practise person-centred care by facilitating conversations with adolescent patients about their care issues and concerns, as well as about their life in general (e.g., school, family, and spirituality) (Lataillade & Chabal, 2021).

Gerontological

- Evaluate an older person's cognitive status for understanding ostomy self-care instructions. Include a caregiver in the care plan (if appropriate).
- Adapt care approaches for older persons who have impaired manual dexterity or limited vision. If a patient is unable to custom-cut the size of the skin barrier, consider having barriers precut by an ostomy equipment supplier or using a precut pouching system.
- Costs of ostomy supplies and reimbursement are an issue for patients on a fixed income if not covered by insurance.

Care in the Community: Home Management

- Evaluate home toileting facilities and patients' ability to empty the pouch directly into a toilet.
- A patient may shower without covering a pouch. A patient may take the pouch off in the shower to clean the peristomal skin if they wish to do so and if cleared by health care provider.
- If a pouching system has a clamp to close the pouch, have patients carry an extra clamp with them in case that one breaks or gets lost.
- Patients should avoid storing pouches in extremely hot or cold locations. Temperature affects barrier and adhesive materials.

✦ SKILL 36.2 Pouching a Urostomy

Because urine flows continuously from an incontinent urinary diversion, placement of a pouch is more challenging than with a fecal diversion. In the immediate postoperative period, urinary stents extend out from a stoma (Fig. 36.11). A surgeon places the stents to prevent stenosis of the ureters at the site where the ureters are attached to the conduit. The stents will be removed during the hospital stay or at the first postoperative visit with the surgeon.

The stoma is normally red and moist. It is made from part of the intestinal tract, usually the ileum. A normal stoma protrudes above the skin. An ileal conduit is usually located in the right lower quadrant of a patient's abdomen. While the patient is in bed, the pouch may be connected to a bedside drainage bag to decrease the need for frequent emptying. When the patient goes home, a bedside drainage bag may be used at night to avoid having to get up to empty the pouch. Each type of urostomy pouch comes with a connector for the bedside drainage bag (Fig. 36.12). Incorrect pouch placement, large volumes of urine in the pouch, or a urinary pouch without an antireflux valve promotes reflux of urine back into the urostomy and ureters, increasing risk of infection. The risk of reflux is reduced by attaching a urinary pouch to straight drainage when high urinary output is expected. A patient must understand the importance of draining the pouch frequently and using clean technique during stomal and skin care. If the pouch does not contain an integrated gas (flatus) filter, the patient needs to be taught how to release built-up gas from the pouch.

Delegation and Collaboration

The skill of pouching a new incontinent urinary diversion cannot be delegated a UCP. In some facilities, care of an established urostomy (4 to 6 weeks or more after surgery) can be delegated to UCPs. The nurse directs the UCP about the following:

- Expected appearance of the stoma
- Expected amount and character of the output and when to report changes
- Change in the patient's stoma and surrounding skin integrity that should be reported
- Special equipment needed to complete the procedure for a particular patient

Equipment

- Urinary pouch (with antireflux flap) and skin barrier; clear, drainable one- or two-piece system, cut-to-fit or precut size
- Appropriate adapter for connection to bedside drainage bag
- Measuring guide
- Bedside urinary drainage bag
- Clean gloves
- Washcloth
- Towel or disposable waterproof barrier
- Basin with warm tap water
- Scissors
- Adhesive remover
- Absorbent wick made from gauze rolled tightly in the shape of a tampon
- Waterproof bag for disposal of pouch
- Mirror for patient to observe ostomy
- PPE as required (e.g., gown and goggles if there is any risk of splashing when emptying pouch)

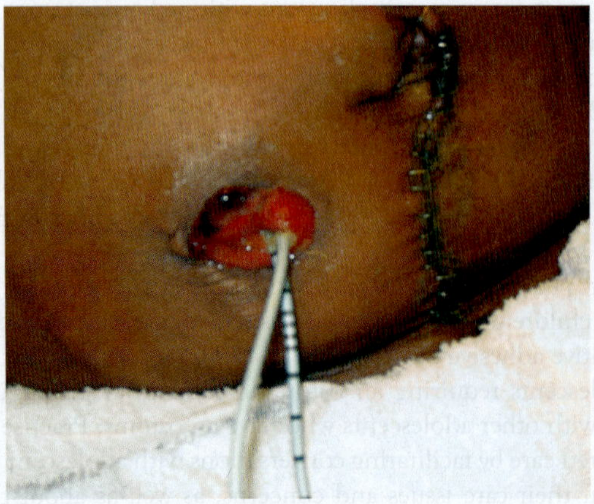

FIG 36.11 Urostomy stoma with stents in place. *(Courtesy Jane Fellows.)*

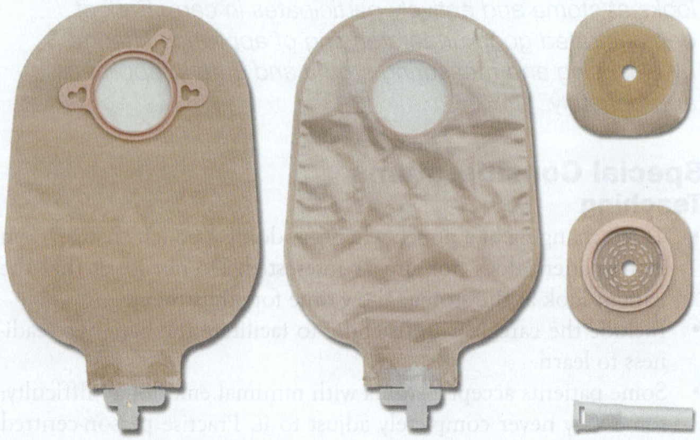

FIG 36.12 Urostomy pouching system with adapter to connect pouch to bedside drainage bag. *(Courtesy Hollister Inc., Libertyville, IL.)*

STEP	RATIONALE
ASSESSMENT	
1. Identify patient using at least two person-specific identifiers (e.g., name and date of birth, or name and medical record number) according to employer policy.	Ensures correct patient. Complies with Accreditation Canada's standards and improves patient safety (Accreditation Canada, 2020).
2. Throughout the procedure, the 4 moments for hand hygiene are to be implemented; hand hygiene should occur before initial patient (or patient environment) contact, before an aseptic procedure, after body fluid exposure risk, and after patient (or patient environment) contact. Additional hand hygiene should be performed when hands are visibly soiled.	Proper hand hygiene helps prevent the spread of infectious agents to health care providers.
3. Apply clean gloves.	Reduces transmission of microorganisms.
4. Observe existing skin barrier and pouch for leakage and length of time in place. Pouch should be changed every 3–7 days, not daily (Carmel et al., 2021). If urine is leaking under the wafer, change the pouch.	Assesses effectiveness of pouching system and allows for early detection of potential problems. To minimize skin irritation, avoid changing the entire pouching system unnecessarily. Repeated leakage may indicate need for a different type of pouch to provide a reliable seal.
5. Observe characteristics of urine in pouch or bedside drainage bag. Empty pouch if it is more than one-third to one-half full by opening valve and draining it into a container for measurement.	There may be blood or large amounts of mucus in urine after surgery, but this should resolve in the first 1–2 weeks after surgery. Weight of pouch can disrupt seal. Urine from ileal conduit will contain mucus because of flow through intestinal segment.
6. Observe stoma for colour, swelling, presence of sutures, trauma, and healing of peristomal skin. Assess type of stoma. Remove and dispose of gloves.	Consider stoma characteristics in selecting appropriate pouching system. Convexity in skin barrier is often necessary with a flush or retracted stoma.
7. Explore patient's perceptions, acceptance, and knowledge of stoma and interest in learning self-care. Identify others who will be helping patient after leaving hospital.	Facilitates teaching plan and timing of care to coincide with availability of caregivers.

NURSING DIAGNOSES

- Reduced skin integrity
- Insufficient knowledge regarding care of urostomy
- Alteration in body image
- Willingness for enhanced knowledge
- Potential for impaired skin integrity

Related factors and risk factors are individualized on the basis of patient's condition or needs.

STEP	RATIONALE
PLANNING	
1. Expected outcomes following completion of procedure:	
• Stoma is red and moist with stents protruding from it. Peristomal skin is free of irritation and intact. Sutures are intact.	These are normal findings for postoperative urinary diversion.
• Urine drains freely from stents or stoma.	These are normal findings after surgery.
• Urine is yellow with some mucus shreds and is without foul odour. Urine may be pink or contain small blood clots after surgery.	It is normal for most individuals to have some mucus shreds in their urine when the bowel is being used to make the ileal conduit; however, if the number of shreds increases or the urine has a foul odour, the patient should be screened for a urinary tract infection (UTI).
• Volume of output is within acceptable limits (≥30 mL/hr).	Normal output reveals ureters draining without obstruction.
• Patient and caregiver observe stoma and procedural steps.	Shows adjustment to change in body image and a willingness to learn self-care.
• Patient asks questions about procedure and may help with pouch change.	Indicates readiness to learn and begin self-care.
2. Explain procedure to patient; encourage their interaction and questions.	Lessens patient's anxiety and promotes person-centred care.
3. Assemble equipment and close room curtains or door.	Optimizes use of time; provides privacy.
IMPLEMENTATION	
1. Position patient in semireclining or supine position. If possible, provide patient with a mirror for observation.	When patient is semireclining, there are fewer skin wrinkles, allowing for ease of pouch application.
2. Apply clean gloves.	Reduces transmission of microorganisms.
3. Place towel or disposable waterproof barrier under patient and across patient's lower abdomen.	Protects bed linen; maintains patient's dignity.

STEP	RATIONALE
IMPLEMENTATION	
4. If not done during assessment, remove the used pouch and skin barrier gently by pushing skin away from the barrier. If stents are present, pull pouch gently around them and lay towel underneath. Empty pouch and measure output. Dispose of pouch in an appropriate receptacle.	Reduces risk of trauma to skin and of dislodging stents. Keeps urine from leaking onto skin. Urine output provides information about renal status and whether volume is within acceptable limits (≥30 mL/hr).
5. Place rolled gauze at stoma opening. Maintain gauze at stoma opening continuously during pouch measurement and change.	Using wick at stoma opening prevents peristomal skin from becoming wet with urine during pouch change.
6. While keeping rolled gauze in contact with stoma, clean peristomal skin gently with warm tap water and washcloth; do not scrub skin. If you touch the stoma, minor bleeding is normal. Pat skin dry.	Avoid using soap. It leaves residue on the skin, which can irritate it. The pouch does not adhere to wet skin.
7. Measure stoma (see illustration, Skill 36.1, Step 6). Expect size of stoma to change during the first 4–6 weeks after surgery.	Allows for proper fit of pouch that will protect peristomal skin.
8. Trace pattern on pouch backing or skin barrier (see illustration in Skill 36.1, Step 7).	Prepares for cutting of opening in pouch.
9. Cut opening in pouch (see illustration in Skill 36.1, Step 8). If using mouldable or shape-to-fit barrier, use your fingers to mould shape-to-fit stoma.	Customizes pouch to provide appropriate fit over stoma.
10. Remove protective backing from adhesive backing or wafer surface (see illustration in Skill 36.1, Step 9). Remove rolled gauze from stoma.	Prepares pouch for application to skin.
11. Apply pouch (see illustration in Skill 36.1, Step 10). Press adhesive barrier firmly into place around stoma and outside edges. Have patient hold their hand over the pouch for 1–2 minutes to secure seal.	Pouch adhesives are heat and pressure sensitive and will hold more securely at body temperature.
12. Use adapter provided with pouches to connect pouch to the bedside urinary bag. Keep tubing below level of the bag.	Allows patient to rest without having to empty pouch frequently. Tubing position allows for collection and measurement of urine and prevents backflow of urine into stoma.
13. Remove drape from patient. Help patient to assume a comfortable position. Remove and dispose of gloves and other disposables.	Reduces transmission of microorganisms.
EVALUATION	
1. Observe appearance of stoma, peristomal skin, and suture line during pouch change.	Determines condition of stoma and peristomal skin and progress of wound healing.
2. Evaluate character and volume of urinary drainage.	Determines whether stoma and/or stents are patent. Character of urine reveals degree of concentration and whether there is a possible UTI.
3. Observe patient's and caregiver's willingness to view stoma and ask questions about procedure.	Determines level of adjustment to and understanding of stoma care and pouch application.
4. **Use teach-back:** "I want to be sure you understand what is involved in changing your ostomy pouch. Let's review what we discussed. Tell me how often you should empty your pouch and how often you should change it." Develop a revised teaching plan if patient or caregiver is unable to teach back correctly.	Determines patient's and caregiver's level of understanding of instructional topic.

Unexpected Outcomes	Related Interventions
1. Skin around stoma is irritated, blistered, or bleeding, or maceration is noted as result of chronic exposure to urine.	• Check stoma size and opening in skin barrier. • Resize skin barrier opening, if necessary. • Remove pouch more carefully. • Consult ostomy care nurse.
2. No urine output for several hours or output is <30 mL/hr. Urine has foul odour.	• Increase fluid intake (if allowed). • Notify health care provider. • Obtain urine specimen for culture and sensitivity if prescribed.
3. Patient and caregiver are unable to observe stoma, ask questions, or participate in care.	• Consult ostomy care nurse. • Allow patient to express feelings. • Encourage caregiver support.

Communication and Documentation

- Document type of pouch, time of change, condition and appearance of stoma and stents and peristomal skin, and character of urine in EHR or chart.
- Document urinary output on I&O form.
- Document patient's and caregiver's reaction to stoma and level of participation.
- Document your evaluation of patient and caregiver learning.
- Report abnormalities in stoma or peristomal skin and absence of urinary output to nurse in charge or health care provider.

DOCUMENTATION EXAMPLE

Patient's left-lower quadrant urostomy appliance was changed at 1430 hours. Stoma is round and appears red and moist and measures 25 mm. Stents ×2 present and protruding from stoma. Sutures around stoma are present and intact. Peristomal skin is intact with no signs of irritation present. Urine in pouch emptied of 325 mL of clear, yellow urine with small amounts of mucus shreds. Stoma cleansed with warm water. Skin barrier ointment and two-piece flat Coloplast appliance applied. Appliance is well-sealed and intact. Patient looks at stoma and participates in care. Patient asked appropriate questions and demonstrated understanding of appliance change by measuring and fitting appliance. Patient correctly verbalized abnormal findings to assess for to this writer and knows to seek a health care provider if any abnormal signs identified.

Special Considerations

Teaching

- Follow teaching considerations in Skill 36.1.
- Teach patients the significance and importance of drinking about 2 L (2 quarts) of fluid daily to decrease risk of developing a UTI (Carmel et al., 2021). Explain that some mucus in the urine is expected but that patients should report any blood in their urine, excessively cloudy urine, chills, fever (38.3°C [101°F] or higher), or back (flank) pain to their health care provider.

Pediatric

- In neonates, urinary diversions are less common than fecal ostomies.
- Select pediatric pouches designed especially for neonates, infants, and children; these pouches are smaller and have a more skin-sensitive adhesive on the barrier.

Gerontological

- Follow gerontological considerations in Skill 36.1.
- Older persons have decreased thirst and may not normally consume adequate fluids. Explain the importance of fluid intake to promote healthy renal function and decrease risk of developing a UTI.

Care in the Community: Home Management

- Follow care-in-the-community considerations described in Skill 36.1.
- Instruct patient that pouch can be connected to straight drainage at night. Make sure that patient understands that the adapter will be needed to connect the pouch to the bedside drainage bag (see Fig. 36.12).
- Urinary drainage bag should be rinsed with tap water after use.

✦ SKILL 36.3 Catheterizing a Urinary Diversion

Catheterization of a urinary diversion is the only method to obtain an accurate culture and sensitivity specimen to screen a patient for infection. Check employer policy to identify the appropriate health care team member to collect this specimen. When it is necessary to obtain a urine specimen from a urinary diversion, the best method is to insert a sterile catheter into the stoma. Obtaining a specimen of urine in a pouch does not provide an accurate finding because of the likely risk for contamination by microorganisms growing in the stagnant urine. With the use of strict aseptic technique, catheterization is relatively safe and easy. If a patient uses a two-piece system, remove the pouch from the skin barrier and replace it after catheterization without disturbing the skin barrier. If a patient uses a one-piece system, remove the pouch to obtain the specimen and replace it with a new pouch after the procedure. To prevent trauma to the tissues, one needs to understand how the stoma and implanted ureters are constructed for a patient (see Fig. 36.3).

Delegation and Collaboration

The skill of catheterizing a urinary diversion cannot be delegated a UCP. The nurse directs the UCP to do the following:

- Inform the nurse if the patient has peristomal or flank pain (sign of kidney infection)
- Inform the nurse if there is a change in colour, odour, or amount of urine or if there is blood in the urine

Equipment

- Urinary catheterization supplies (contained in prepackaged sterile catheter kit or gathered separately):
  - 14- to 16-Fr sterile catheter
  - Water-soluble lubricant
  - Antiseptic swabs (e.g., povidone–iodine or chlorhexidine gluconate [CHG])
  - Sterile gloves
  - Sterile specimen container
  - Absorbent gauze wick
  - Bed protection barrier
  - Towels
  - Urinary pouch, if needed
  - Clean gloves

STEP	RATIONALE
ASSESSMENT	
1. Identify patient using at least two person-specific identifiers (e.g., name and date of birth, or name and medical record number) according to employer policy.	Ensures correct patient. Complies with Accreditation Canada's standards and improves patient safety (Accreditation Canada, 2020).

STEP	RATIONALE

ASSESSMENT

STEP	RATIONALE
2. Throughout the procedure, the 4 moments for hand hygiene are to be implemented; hand hygiene should occur before initial patient (or patient environment) contact, before an aseptic procedure, after body fluid exposure risk, and after patient (or patient environment) contact. Additional hand hygiene should be performed when hands are visibly soiled.	Proper hand hygiene helps prevent the spread of infectious agents to health care providers.
3. Obtain health care provider's prescription for catheterization.	This invasive procedure requires a health care provider's prescription.
4. Observe for signs and symptoms of a UTI: elevated temperature, chills, foul-smelling urine, and elevated white blood cell (WBC) count.	Determines need to perform catheterization to obtain sterile specimen from urinary diversion. Having a urinary diversion poses a risk for reflux of urine back to the kidneys, resulting in infection.
5. Assess patient's understanding of need for the procedure and how it is done.	Determines willingness to cooperate and reduces patient's anxiety.

NURSING DIAGNOSES

- Insufficient knowledge regarding catheterization procedure
- Potential for infection
- Potential for injury: urinary tract

Related factors and risk factors are individualized on the basis of patient's condition or needs.

PLANNING

STEP	RATIONALE
1. Expected outcomes following completion of procedure:	
• Urine specimen is not contaminated with bacteria during procedure.	Urine is obtained correctly. Laboratory results are accurate.
• Patient describes risks for infection and techniques to prevent infection.	Demonstrates patient's learning.
2. Assemble equipment and close room curtain or door.	Optimizes use of time and provides privacy.
3. Explain procedure to patient, including sensations that will be felt. If possible, obtain specimen when the patient is due for a pouch change (if using one-piece system).	Lessens anxiety and promotes patient's cooperation. Cleaning the stoma and surrounding skin may cause a cool sensation. Insertion of the catheter may cause a sensation of mild pressure, or it may not be felt at all. Changing the pouch too frequently could result in skin trauma.

IMPLEMENTATION

STEP	RATIONALE
1. If possible, help patient into sitting position, and drape towel across their lower abdomen.	Gravity facilitates flow of urine. Maintains patient's dignity. Towel absorbs urine.
2. Apply clean gloves.	Reduces transmission of microorganisms.
3. Remove pouch. If patient uses a two-piece system, remove the pouch but leave barrier attached to the skin.	Allows access to stoma.
4. Remove gloves and discard.	Avoids contamination.
5. Open sterile catheterization kit according to instructions or open needed equipment and place on sterile barrier using aseptic technique (see Chapter 5). If not using a catheterization kit, place gauze pad on sterile field and squeeze a small amount of lubricant onto the gauze. Apply sterile gloves.	Prepares sterile work field.
6. If needed, have patient hold absorbent gauze wick on the stoma while you prepare catheterization supplies.	Prevents leakage of urine onto peristomal skin, linens, and clothing.
7. Clean surface of stoma with antiseptic swabs using a circular motion from centre outward. Use a new swab each time; repeat process twice. Allow CHG antiseptic to dry or wipe off excess antiseptic with dry sterile gauze or cotton ball.	Removes surface bacteria. CHG must dry to achieve antibacterial effect.

Critical Decision Point *If the patient has stents in place, use an antiseptic swab to clean the ends of the stents and place the stents in the sterile cup. Allow urine to drip into the cup until you obtain an adequate amount for a specimen. Then proceed directly to Step 13.*

STEP	RATIONALE
8. Remove lid from sterile specimen container.	Sterile container collects a small volume of urine.

STEP	RATIONALE
IMPLEMENTATION	
9. Lubricate tip of catheter with water-soluble lubricant, keeping catheter sterile.	Facilitates passage of catheter through the stoma.
10. With your dominant hand, gently insert catheter tip into the stoma. Do not force the catheter; redirect course as needed. Place distal end of the catheter into the specimen container. Have patient cough; massage their abdomen near the stoma or turn patient on their side.	Use care to avoid trauma to conduit. Movement and coughing may facilitate flow of urine from conduit.
11. Hold container below level of the stoma. If needed, wait several minutes to get an adequate amount of urine.	Culture and sensitivity studies require only 3–5 mL of urine (check employer policy).
12. Withdraw catheter slowly; place an absorbent pad over the stoma.	Keeps skin dry.
13. Apply lid to specimen container.	Prevents accidental spillage.
14. Reapply a new pouch or reattach pouch if patient uses a two-piece system (see Skill 36.2).	The pouch is necessary to contain urine.
15. Dispose of used pouch and equipment properly.	Avoids unpleasant odour in room.
16. Label specimen in presence of the patient, place it in a biohazard bag, and send it to the laboratory at once. Remove gloves and discard.	Ensures that laboratory results are assigned to correct patient. Labelling ensures acceptance and processing of specimen by laboratory. Leaving urine to sit for a long period at room temperature will adversely affect laboratory results.
EVALUATION	
1. Compare results of culture and sensitivity with expected findings. Mucus is a normal finding if patient has an ileal conduit.	Determines presence of infection. If contamination appears likely, a second specimen will be needed.
2. **Use teach-back:** "I want to be sure you understand the reason we needed to collect the urine. Tell me in your own words why we did this procedure to get urine from your stoma. What are the signs of a urinary tract infection when you have a urostomy?" Develop a revised teaching plan if patient or caregiver is unable to teach back correctly.	Determines patient's and caregiver's level of understanding of instructional topic.

Unexpected Outcomes	Related Interventions
1. Unable to obtain urine specimen.	• Reposition patient. • If there is still no urine, push fluids and try again later. • Inform health care provider if unable to obtain specimen on second attempt.
2. Skin or stoma reveals complications.	• Notify health care provider. • Consult with ostomy care nurse about pouching system or skin barrier to use.

Communication and Documentation

- Document time the specimen was collected; patient's tolerance of the procedure; and appearance of urine, skin, and stoma in EHR or chart.
- Document your evaluation of patient and caregiver learning.
- Report results of laboratory test to the nurse in charge or health care provider.

DOCUMENTATION EXAMPLE

Patient's stoma was catheterized at 1530 hours for culture and sensitivity. Previous pouch removed. Stoma is red, moist, and intact. Peristomal skin is intact and free from signs of irritation. Stoma cleansed with chlorhexidine swabs. Catheter inserted into stoma with no resistance. Patient tolerated procedure well. Specimen successfully obtained and sent to lab. Patient able to verbalize why the procedure was done and understands to report signs of a UTI.

Special Considerations

Teaching

- Explain common symptoms of a UTI: flank pain, dark or bloody urine, foul-smelling urine, fever (38.3°C [101°F] or higher), confusion.
- Encourage patient to notify a health care provider if symptoms of infection develop.
- Reinforce the importance of fluid intake of 2 L/day, or as tolerated.

✦ REVIEW QUESTIONS

A young adult (she/her) with Crohn's disease had surgery this week to resect a portion of her large intestine and now has an ileostomy. She understands that this surgery was necessary to treat her abdominal pain and chronic infection from abscesses in her intestine, but she is having trouble coping with the change in her body image with an ileostomy. The patient is reluctant to learn how to empty or change her pouch.

Review Questions 1 to 4 relate to the case study presented here.

1. Because the patient's pouch has overfilled and there has been leakage under the ostomy wafer, the patient has burning pain. The nurse changing her pouch notes a raw, weeping area of the skin around the stoma. Which actions are most appropriate in this situation? (*Select all that apply.*)
   1. Cleaning the area with alcohol to help dry the raw skin
   2. Consulting a wound, ostomy, and continence (WOC) nurse
   3. Reviewing the importance of emptying the pouch before it is one-half full
   4. Cutting the opening in the skin barrier larger than before so that the skin barrier is not covering the raw skin
   5. Recommending that the patient measure the stoma again and cut a new pattern because the stoma may have changed size since surgery

2. Place the following steps for changing an ostomy pouch in the correct order:
   1. Close the end of the pouch.
   2. Measure the stoma.
   3. Cut the hole in the wafer.
   4. Press the pouch into place over the stoma.
   5. Remove the old pouch.
   6. Trace the correct measurement onto the back of the wafer.
   7. Observe the stoma and the skin around it.
   8. Cleanse and dry the peristomal skin.

3. In documenting the patient's response to receiving instruction about ostomy care, which statement would be most appropriate to include in the medical record? Why?
   1. "Patient refuses to participate in care and will not look at her stoma. Family members and health care provider notified of her refusal."
   2. "Patient is tearful and appears frightened by her stoma and the ostomy care required. Explained the steps needed to empty and change her pouch while performing pouch change and encouraged patient that she will have another opportunity to participate and learn self-care."

4. When would the nurse refer this patient to a WOC nurse or ostomy care specialist?
   1. At the time of discharge from the hospital
   2. As soon as possible after surgery
   3. When the health care provider requests that the nurse make a referral
   4. When the patient requests to see the WOC nurse

5. A nurse is caring for a patient with a urostomy. Which of the following assessments are necessary to rule out the presence of a urinary tract infection (UTI)? (*Select all that apply.*)
   1. Fluid intake
   2. Appearance of urine
   3. Condition of peristomal skin
   4. Body temperature
   5. Patient self-report of comfort level
   6. Blood pressure

Visit the Evolve site for a complete list of answers to the Review Questions.

✦ NEXT GENERATION NCLEX® (NGN)

For practice with answering exam questions related to unfolding NGN case studies, please consult the Next Generation NCLEX® (NGN)-Style Case Studies for Skills and Techniques on the Evolve website: http://evolve.elsevier.com/Canada/Perry/clinicalskills/

REFERENCES

Abdelmohsen, S. A. (2020). Effectiveness of structured education on patient's knowledge and practice regarding colostomy care. *Asia-Pacific Journal of Oncology Nursing, 7*(4), 370–374. https://doi.org/10.4103/apjon.apjon_24_20

Accreditation Canada. (2020). *Required organizational practices–2020 handbook*. https://physicians.nshealth.ca/resources/required-organizational-practices-2020-handbook

Carmel, J. E., Colwell, J. C., & Goldberg, M. T. (2021). *Wound, ostomy, and continence nurses society core curriculum: Ostomy management* (2nd ed.). Wolters Kluwer.

Costa, I., LeBlanc, K., & Rajhathy, E. M. (2022). Canadian standards of practice for nurses specialized in wound, ostomy and continence (NSWOCs): A 2021 update. *Journal of Wound, Ostomy and Continence Nursing, 49*(1), 100–101.

Giordano, V., Nicolotti, M., Corvese, F., et al. (2020). Describing self-care and its associated variables in ostomy patients. *Journal of Advanced Nursing, 76*(11), 2982–2992. https://doi.org/10.1111/jan.14499

Kenner, C., & Boykova, M. V. (2021). *Neonatal nursing care handbook: An evidence-based approach to conditions and procedures* (3rd ed.). Springer.

Lataillade, L., & Chabal, L. (2021). Therapeutic patient education: A multifaceted approach to ostomy care. *Advances in Skin & Wound Care, 34*(1), 36–42. https://doi.org/10.1097/01.ASW.0000722756.35017.02

Medina-Rico, M., Zárate-Velasco, A. M., Quiñonez, A., et al. (2019). Sexuality in people with ostomies: A literature review. *Sexuality and Disability, 37*(4), 571–586. https://doi.org/10.1007/s11195-019-09604-4

Minkes, R. (2022). Stomas of the small and large intestine in children–Treatment and management. *Medscape*. https://emedicine.medscape.com/article/939455-treatment

Myers, T. M. (2021). *Fast facts for wound care nursing: Practical wound management* (2nd ed.). Springer.

Nurses Specialized in Wound, Ostomy, and Continence Canada & Canadian Society of Colon and Rectal Surgeons. (2020). *Canadian practice enabler from the position statement on preoperative stoma site marking for fecal diversions–ileostomy and colostomy*. https://cscrs.ca/wp-content/uploads/2020/03/Preoperative-stoma-site-marking-enabler-2020-final-highres.pdf

Ostomy Canada Society. (n.d.). *Ostomy care basics*. https://www.ostomycanada.ca/ostomy-care-basics/

Registered Nurses' Association of Ontario (RNAO). (2019). *Supporting adults who anticipate or live with an ostomy* (2nd ed.). https://rnao.ca/bpg/guidelines/ostomy

Sena, J. F., da Silva, P. I., Lucena, S. K. P., et al. (2020). Validation of educational material for the care of people with intestinal stoma. *Revista Latino-Americana de Enfermagem, 28*, e3269–e3269. https://doi.org/10.1590/1518-8345.3179.3269

Taneja, C., Netsch, D., Rolstad, B. S., et al. (2019). Risk and economic burden of peristomal skin complications following ostomy surgery. *The Journal of Wound, Ostomy and Continence Nursing, 46*(2), 143–149. https://doi.org/10.1097/won.0000000000000509

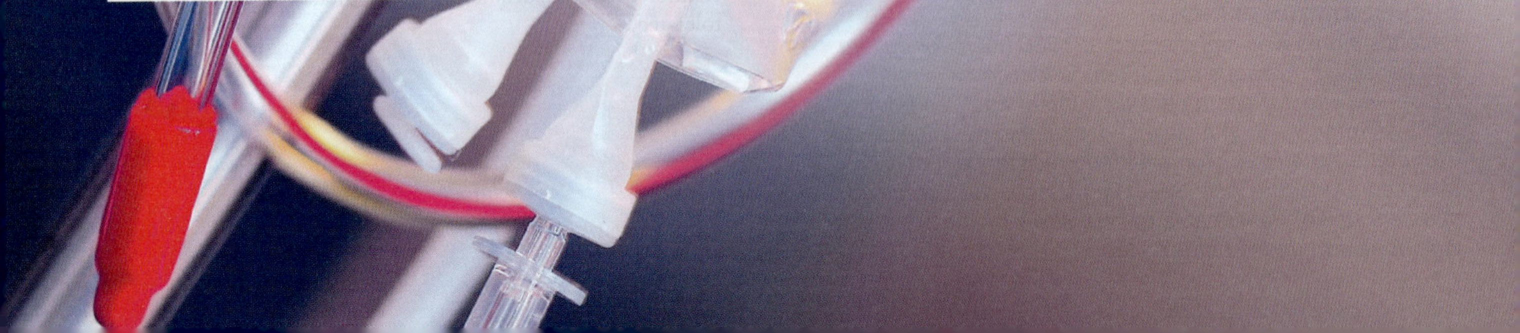

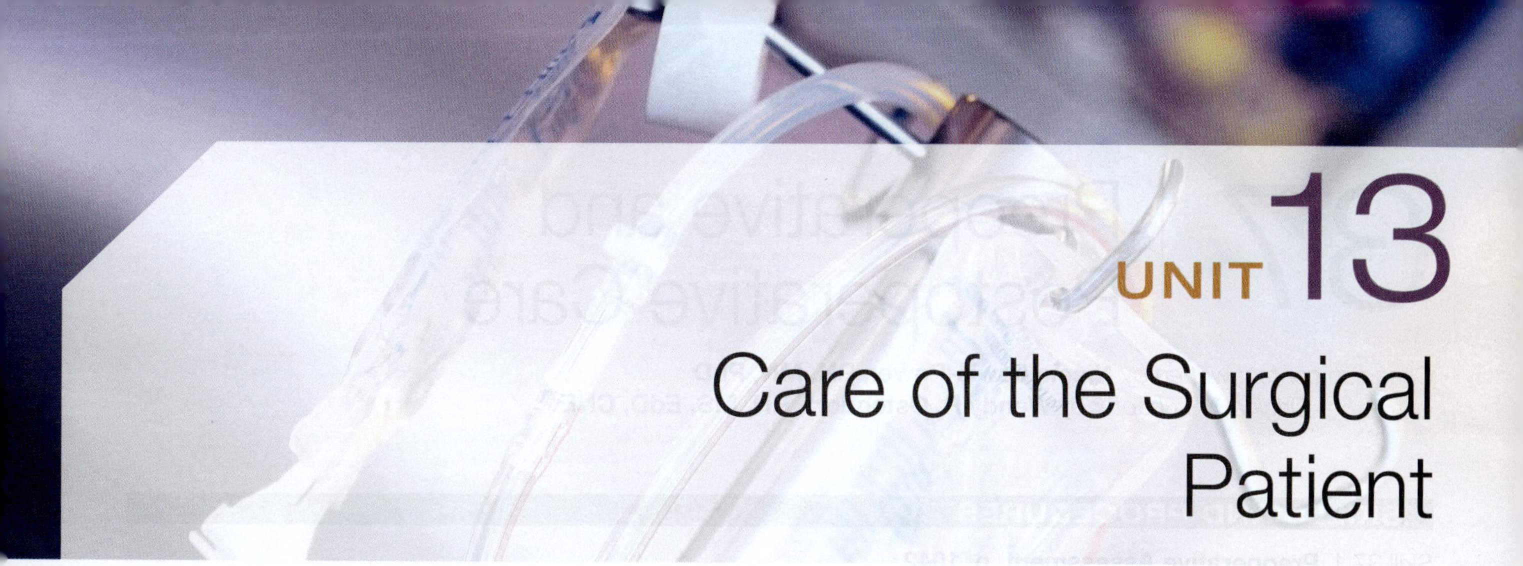

UNIT 13 Care of the Surgical Patient

The care of a surgical patient involves a number of routines: educational topics to cover during preoperative preparation, the procedures used for physical preparation, the type of monitoring to conduct during surgical recovery, and the bodily responses to support during recovery. However, the manner in which you perform these routines is highly individualized. Patient education, in particular, must be patient-centred to ensure that a patient is properly informed and prepared to participate in the surgical experience and to then follow necessary postoperative guidelines. For example, a young adult with limited health literacy and visual challenges requires you to adapt an instructional approach that differs greatly from that used to teach an older person with no known health problems. Because surgery often invokes anxiety and fear, your application of therapeutic communication techniques and knowledge of the stress response is key in identifying potential problems and then adapting teaching strategies accordingly. Also, critical assessment of a patient's resources in the home or community care setting allows you to anticipate how to adjust routine explanations so that recommended guidelines fit the patient's home environment.

Critical thinking must be employed when you conduct a preoperative assessment. A comprehensive patient database must include the patient's current health status, physical risks for undergoing surgery, and knowledge of the impending procedure. A caregiver or close friend who will assist with postoperative care after discharge should be included. You will apply critical thinking attitudes and intellectual standards to ensure that the data you collect are thorough and relevant to the patient. Each category of a preoperative assessment will trigger various questions leading to clarity and relevance. For example, consider the process of assessing a patient for a chronic health condition; if one exists, you must explore the effects the condition has on the physical systems most affected by surgery. If a patient has a history of bronchitis, then your knowledge of its impact on lung function will prompt you to assess whether the patient is able to cough effectively, the amount of mucous production normally expressed, and the status of lung sounds. Such information guides you to which interventions to deliver (e.g., coughing, incentive spirometry, hydration for mucous clearing) and provides a database for evaluating the patient response after interventions are performed.

The physical preparation of a patient for surgery is usually standardized, but there are variations depending on the type of surgery scheduled. For example, a patient undergoing surgery involving the intestines will have to follow a preoperative bowel preparation protocol. A patient undergoing a hip replacement may be required to do more physical exercise and even visit a physiotherapist before entering the hospital. As a nurse, you are responsible for anticipating the standard and individualized forms of preparation required and educating patients about the rationale for the therapies. Standard physical preparation just before surgery involves inserting an intravenous line for fluid administration, verifying allergies and blood type, placing antiembolic devices on the lower extremities, and gathering a patient's personal items. During this process, the ongoing provision of psychological support and educational instruction informs the patient and potentially minimizes anxiety.

Knowledge of the anticipated effects of surgery, a patient's preoperative health status, and the standard postoperative assessments of airway, breathing, and circulation place you in a position to critically judge how a patient initially recovers from surgery. Always be alert. Let the patient's ongoing responses guide you in choosing the frequency and type of assessments needed. Then, allow those assessments to direct your interventions. For example, when working in a recovery room, if a patient seems slow to awaken from anaesthesia, focus on monitoring vital signs and level of consciousness, and if breathing is shallow, turn the patient to one side with the head elevated. If a patient awakens quickly with stable vital signs, focus on pain management and preventive therapies such as coughing and incentive spirometry.

As a patient recovers from the initial postoperative phase of recovery, your assessment and scope of interventions broaden to include all body systems. Airway, breathing, and circulation remain priorities. Pain becomes a priority as well, because if it is left uncontrolled, patient recovery will be slowed. For example, acute pain will limit the ability of a patient to be mobile and initiate self-care. Postoperative assessment and corresponding supportive care include all bodily systems most likely to be affected by a particular surgery. Skin integrity will apply to all surgeries, requiring you to document a precise and accurate description of a surgical wound to monitor healing. Patients forced to be more immobile after surgery, such as after knee or hip replacement and spinal surgery, require close examination of circulatory status to monitor for deep vein thrombosis. Patients placed on early ambulation protocols will require monitoring of tolerance to exercise and the effects of ambulation on comfort.

Critical thinking during postoperative recovery of a patient requires knowledge of surgical conditions, use of evidence-informed knowledge for prevention of complications, and application of what you assess about each patient to make patient-centred adaptations needed for recovery.

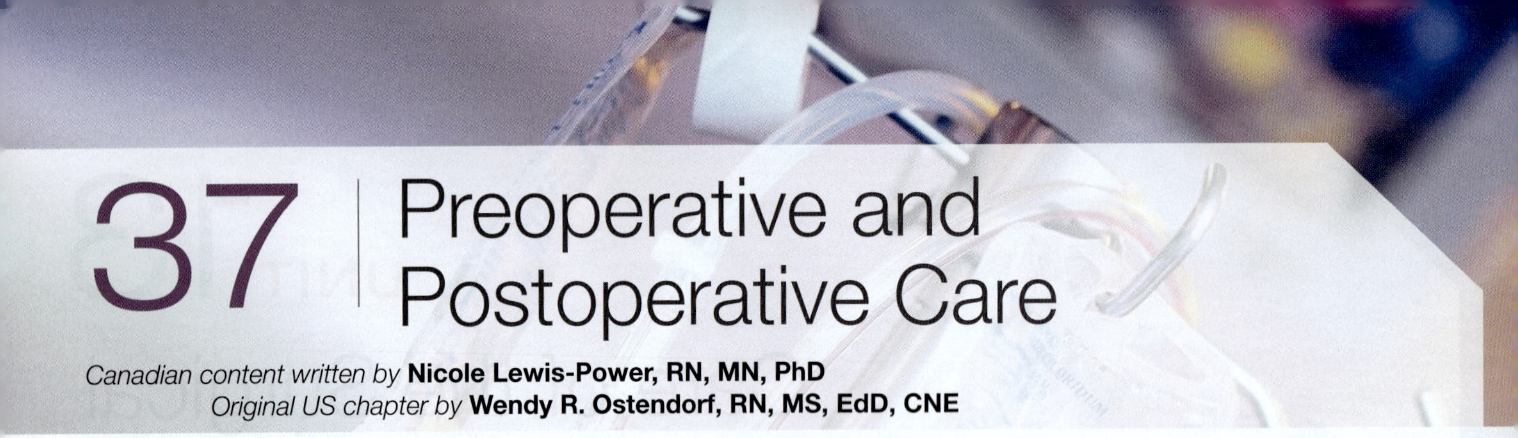

37 Preoperative and Postoperative Care

Canadian content written by **Nicole Lewis-Power, RN, MN, PhD**
Original US chapter by **Wendy R. Ostendorf, RN, MS, EdD, CNE**

SKILLS AND PROCEDURES

OBJECTIVES

Mastery of content in this chapter will enable the nurse to:

- Explain how to integrate person-centred care into preoperative and postoperative care.
- Describe the physical preparations needed for a patient facing surgery.
- Identify risk factors that have the potential to affect a patient's clinical outcomes postoperatively.
- Describe cultural differences that might affect the implementation of preoperative and postoperative procedures.
- Describe the benefits of structured preoperative teaching.
- Explain the rationale for each postoperative exercise.
- Successfully teach a patient to perform postoperative exercises.
- Describe the differences in nursing assessment performed during the immediate postoperative period versus the convalescent phase of recovery.
- Conduct an assessment of a preoperative and a postoperative patient.

MEDIA RESOURCES

- http://evolve.elsevier.com/Canada/Perry/clinicalskills/

PURPOSE

Surgical care of patients is in a continuous state of technological advancement. As a result, patients have shortened lengths of stay because of less invasive surgery and less time spent in a hospital. During the preoperative phase, the nursing role focuses on physical, psychological, sociocultural, and spiritual preparation while also validating existing information, reinforcing patient education, and providing nursing care to prepare the patient and family for the surgical experience (American Society of PeriAnesthesia Nurses [ASPAN], 2023). During the postoperative phase, when a patient returns from the operating room (OR), the nurse initially is responsible for completing a thorough assessment of the patient's physical and mental status while also providing continuous monitoring of their condition and ongoing education during the recovery process.

STANDARDS OF CARE

- Accreditation Canada (2020)—*Required Organizational Practices—2020 Handbook* (https://physicians.nshealth.ca/resources/required-organizational-practices-2020-handbook)
- National Association of PeriAnesthesia Nurses of Canada (NAPANc, 2023)—*Standards for Practice*, 5th edition (http://napanc.ca/index.php/standards)
- Operating Room Nurses Association of Canada (2023)—*ORNAC Standards, Guidelines, and Position Statements for Perioperative Registered Nurses*, 16th edition (https://www.ornac.ca/en/standards)

PRINCIPLES FOR PRACTICE

- A variety of diagnostic tests are coordinated before surgery to ensure that the surgeon and anaesthesia care providers have the information needed to determine a patient's risks during surgery and the postoperative period.
- The National Association of PeriAnesthesia Nurses of Canada (NAPANc, 2023) identifies patient assessment, data collection, and management as critical to all phases of the perianaesthesia environment and has provided specific guidelines for care of the pediatric and older person populations.
- The speed of a patient's recovery depends on how effectively the nurse anticipates potential complications, initiates necessary supportive and preventive therapies, and actively involves the patient and caregiver in the recovery process.

- Preoperative and postoperative patient education improves outcomes after surgery. The shift in how surgical services are now provided poses special challenges to meeting patients' educational needs within a reduced time frame. Because most patients undergo surgery in an ambulatory setting and thus avoid a hospital stay, it is essential that they receive adequate information to ensure that they or their caregivers can manage postoperative care activities in the home setting.
- NAPANc (2023) advocates that the registered nurse take part in the preanaesthesia phase—allowing the nurse to anticipate patient outcomes from surgery and anaesthesia—and that the nurse use critical thinking and clinical judgement to interpret and analyze preoperative data and assessments. This analysis enables recognition of the need for further testing, interprofessional collaboration, or additional interventions to prevent intraoperative and postoperative complications.

PERSON-CENTRED CARE

- Engaging and involving patients and caregivers in patient care results in safer and more patient-centred care (Bombard et al., 2018).
- To provide culturally competent care to a surgical patient, the nurse should begin by assessing the family to determine not only who should be involved but also who is legally responsible for making decisions and giving consent for surgery.
- To better understand the culture and needs of the patient, the nurse may be required to request specific information from the patient, their family, or a religious leader.
- When providing preoperative teaching, include caregivers. The use of professional interpreters for patients who do not speak English is necessary to provide competent informed patient care.
- Before surgery, it is important to accommodate a patient's religious and cultural needs and adapt the patient's care to encompass their practices and beliefs whenever possible. Identify cultural and religious beliefs and practices that may affect patients' and caregivers' reactions to the surgical experience, such as diet, pain, blood transfusions, and disposal of body parts, including hair.
- Both before and after surgery, assess patient preferences for pain medication. Many patients believe that pain medication leads to addiction, and they will therefore attempt to endure the pain without medication. Patients who come from cultures that value men's ability to control their emotions may be unwilling to verbalize their pain.
- Persons from certain religious or cultural backgrounds may request to wear articles such as jewellery, medallions, or undergarments. To accommodate these needs and deliver person-centred care, nurses may need to allow such articles (e.g., medals, underclothing) to be worn until just before surgery. If articles are removed, the nurse must ensure that they are returned promptly after surgery.

EVIDENCE-INFORMED PRACTICE

Approximately 8 000 people in Canada die from health care–associated infections (HAIs) annually. Approximately 200 000 people contract an HAI every year. The cost of treating *Clostridioides difficile* infections alone in 2012 was estimated to be $281 million (Public Health Agency of Canada, 2018). Surgical site infection (SSI) is the most common HAI among surgical patients, with 77% of patient deaths reported to be related to an SSI (Healthcare Excellence Canada, 2016).

The following evidence-informed guidelines have been identified to reduce the incidence of SSIs (Healthcare Excellence Canada, 2016):

- Adequate perioperative antimicrobial coverage
- Appropriate hair removal
- Maintenance of perioperative glucose control
- Perioperative normothermia

There are also strict guidelines for use of antibiotics (McCubbin et al., 2021). The goal of prophylactic antibiotic therapy is to select the most effective antibiotics for maximum coverage and administer them when they are most beneficial for protecting patients from infection with as little risk as possible:

- Overall, it is recommended that prophylactic antibiotics be given as close to the time of incision as possible (within 60 minutes) and not for longer than 24 hours after surgery.
- Vancomycin and fluoroquinolones (i.e., ciprofloxacin, levofloxacin) may be given up to 2 hours before incision because of their longer infusion times. Antibiotic use after incision closure does not reduce infection rates, and when the antibiotics are continued, infections are more likely to be caused by a resistant organism (Centers for Disease Control and Prevention, 2019).
- Prophylactic antibiotics should be discontinued within 24 hours after the end of surgery in most cases.

SAFETY GUIDELINES

- Know the type and nature of any previous surgery. Anatomical and physiological alterations affect a patient's risk for operative problems.
- Identify the factors and conditions that increase a patient's risks during surgery. Preoperative preparation and postoperative care depend on knowledge of these risk factors.
- Know the rationale for and extent of the impending surgery. Each type of surgical procedure requires a different type of nursing care and allows nurses to anticipate potential complications correctly.
- Ensure that the patient has signed the informed consent. A nurse may witness a patient's signature, but in most facilities this practice is discouraged, as it is the health care provider's (e.g., surgeon) responsibility to ensure informed consent has been obtained. Witnessing a signature is not a declaration that the witness provided information about risks and alternatives. Should the patient or family not be fully informed about the surgical procedure, it is the nurse's responsibility to advocate for the patient and inform the health care provider of this lack of knowledge. Informed consent is required by law to help protect patients' rights, autonomy, and privacy. Failure to obtain consent can result in professional sanctions, civil liability, and/or criminal charges. The surgeon should provide the information and obtain consent for medical or surgical interventions. They should give the patient information about the extent and type of surgery; alternative therapies; and usual risks, benefits, and consequences of not having surgery. See employer policy regarding consent (Table 37.1) (Canadian Nurses Protective Society, 2018).
- Complete the preoperative checklist according to employer policy.
- Administer pain relief therapies according to a patient's perioperative needs. Pain can slow a patient's recovery following surgery.
- Restrict patient activity after administration of preoperative and postoperative sedatives to minimize the risk of patient falls.

TABLE 37.1

Information Needed for Informed Consent

Parameter	Example
Name of procedure/surgery	Abdominal hysterectomy under general anaesthesia
Description of procedure/surgery	Removal of uterus only through an incision in the abdominal wall at the top of the pubic hairline; done while unconscious
Person performing procedure/surgery	Dr. Rachel Jones, assisted by Dr. William Smith
Benefits of procedure/surgery	To remove uterus with fibroids and stop excessive bleeding Abdominal route necessary because of anticipated adhesions from prior abdominal surgery
Potential risks and adverse effects of procedure/surgery	Risk of hemorrhage and infection from surgery; risk of excessive sedation and allergic reaction to medications used with general anaesthesia; accidental damage to bladder, intestines, and/or nerves controlling these organs
Approximate length of time for procedure/surgery	About 1 hour; 1–2 hours in postanaesthesia care unit (PACU)
Approximate length of time needed for recovery	3–4 days on surgical unit; 4–6 weeks before resuming physically stressful work
Alternative treatments	Removal of uterus vaginally; radiation to shrink fibroids
Consequences of refusing treatment	Continuation of pain and vaginal bleeding, risk of developing anemia; after menopause, fibroids should regress

✦ SKILL 37.1 Preoperative Assessment

A thorough preoperative nursing assessment of a patient's physiological and psychological condition allows a nurse to identify patient risks and plan for care during and after surgery. The assessment documents baseline data for future comparisons to determine the effect of instruction and whether complications have developed during the perioperative period. Many health care facilities have a designated department devoted to completing thorough preoperative screening and testing. Laboratory tests, electrocardiograms (ECGs), chest X-ray films, and other tests are often obtained 1 to 2 weeks in advance of the scheduled surgical procedure. Perioperative staff perform a thorough assessment and review the test results to identify any potential abnormalities that may need further evaluation and treatment before surgery.

The nurse assesses the patient again 1 to 2 hours before the scheduled time of surgery to ensure that there are no changes in the patient's physical condition. Advanced planning gives nurses time to follow up on any unexpected outcomes. Before beginning this assessment, the nurse needs to establish a trusting relationship with the patient. It is not unusual for the patient to remember and report at this time facts that were not previously told to the surgeon. The nurse should speak with the patient in a private environment free of interruptions to encourage open communication. The nurse initiates a preprocedure checklist, beginning with the decision to perform a procedure, maintained with ongoing data collection and assessment, and verified immediately before moving the patient to the procedure room (Accreditation Canada, 2020). Typically, the surgeon, anaesthetist, or nurse completes an assessment, and the patient signs a consent form after receiving an explanation of the procedure from the surgeon. Current test results and notices of any special considerations during the procedure, such as a need for blood products or special equipment, should be available.

Delegation and Collaboration

The skill of performing a preoperative assessment cannot be delegated to an unregulated care provider (UCP). The nurse instructs the UCP to do the following:

- Obtain vital signs and weight and height measurements

Equipment

- Stethoscope
- Blood pressure (BP) monitoring equipment
- Pulse oximetry
- Thermometer
- Watch or clock with a second hand
- Method to measure height and weight
- Access to laboratory, ECG, X-ray films, and other diagnostic equipment as needed
- Preprocedure checklist
- Preoperative assessment form

STEP	RATIONALE
ASSESSMENT	
1. Identify patient using at least two person-specific identifiers (e.g., name and date of birth, or name and medical record number) according to employer policy.	Ensures correct patient. Complies with Accreditation Canada's standards and improves patient safety (Accreditation Canada, 2020).
2. Throughout the procedure, the 4 moments for hand hygiene are to be implemented; hand hygiene should occur before initial patient (or patient environment) contact, before an aseptic procedure, after body fluid exposure risk, and after patient (or patient environment) contact. Additional hand hygiene should be performed when hands are visibly soiled.	Proper hand hygiene helps prevent the spread of infectious agents to health care providers.

STEP	RATIONALE

ASSESSMENT

STEP	RATIONALE
3. Prepare equipment and room for assessment. Don clean gloves if required by employer policy.	Reduces transmission of infection. Makes assessment more efficient.
4. Determine whether patient has any communication impairment (e.g., blindness, hearing loss), can read and understand English, and is mentally competent. For example, give patient an informational brochure and have them explain part of the contents. Obtain a professional interpreter if needed.	Without effective communication, the patient may not fully comprehend a diagnosis, understand the proposed treatment, or effectively consider the alternatives presented. Relying on a caregiver as an interpreter cannot guarantee the accuracy of explanations.
5. Assess patient's understanding of the intended surgery and anaesthesia. Ask patient to offer a description rather than asking a simple yes-or-no question (e.g., "Tell me in your own words what your surgery will involve"). Ask about the patient's and caregiver's expectations of surgery and care. Include questions concerning fears, cultural practices, and religious beliefs, if applicable.	Patient may have misconceptions and incomplete knowledge. Asking about fears, cultural practices, and religious beliefs allows patient's and caregiver's priorities to be anticipated and the plan to be adapted so that appropriate instruction and support are provided to patient and caregiver.
6. Ask if patient has an advance care plan (see Chapter 17).	Advance care plans protect patient's rights by communicating patient's treatment preferences if patient is unable to communicate.
7. Collect nursing history and identify surgical risk factors:	Allows for anticipation of possible complications and planning for interventions to reduce patient risks.

Critical Decision Point *If patient is having emergency surgery, focus on assessment of primary body system affected.*

STEP	RATIONALE
a. Condition requiring surgery.	Allows anticipation of postoperative needs and possible complications.
b. Chronic illnesses and associated risks (e.g., hypertension: bleeding, stroke; postoperative respiratory depression and arrest; asthma: impaired ventilation; hiatal hernia: aspiration; diabetes mellitus: impaired wound healing; methicillin-resistant *Staphylococcus aureus*: impaired wound healing and sepsis).	Some chronic conditions increase the risk of complications from surgery and anaesthesia.
c. Determine whether patient has obstructive sleep apnea (OSA). Many facilities use the STOP-Bang assessment tool (http://www.stopbang.ca/): STOP* • Do you SNORE loudly (louder than talking or loud enough to be heard through closed doors)? • Do you often feel TIRED, fatigued, or sleepy during the daytime? • Has anyone OBSERVED you stop breathing during your sleep? • Do you have or are you being treated for high blood PRESSURE? BANG • BMI >35 kg/m^2 • AGE >50 years old • NECK circumference >40 cm (16 inches) • GENDER: Male *Any question answered *Yes* is a risk factor.	In the surgical population, a STOP-Bang score of 5–8 identifies patients with high probability of moderate/severe OSA. The STOP-Bang score helps the health care team to stratify patients for unrecognized OSA, practise perioperative precautions, or triage patients for diagnosis and treatment (Gumidyala & Selzer, 2022). Patients with OSA will require special anaesthesia precautions. Patients with OSA are often sensitive to sedative medications, especially if the OSA is untreated. Even minimal sedation can cause airway obstruction and ventilatory arrest, thus requiring close monitoring of patient postoperatively (Gumidyala & Selzer, 2022).
d. Last menstrual period (for patients with female genitalia in childbearing years).	Anaesthetic medications and other medications could injure the fetus.
e. Previous hospitalizations.	Determines whether patient is familiar with hospital procedures.
f. Full medication history, including prescription, over-the-counter (OTC), medical cannabis and herbal remedies, and date and time of last doses.	Patient may not report OTC medications and herbal remedies unless specifically asked. All such remedies may interact with anaesthetic medications or other medications given during surgery. Patient may be instructed to take any routine BP, cardiac, or seizure medications. Changes in dosages of oral diabetic medications or insulin may be prescribed.
g. Previous experience with surgery and anaesthesia; have patient clarify whether any undesirable outcomes occurred.	Information helps prevent recurrent problems with planned surgery.
h. Family history of complications from surgery or anaesthesia.	Family history of reactions to anaesthetic medications may indicate familial condition such as malignant hyperthermia, which is life threatening.
i. Allergies to medications, food, or tape, including specific questions about natural rubber latex. Ask patients whether they have had any problem with medication or anything placed on their skin.	Allergies to medications or latex can be life threatening. Prevention of latex allergy in sensitized patients requires specific precautions. Often, patients with latex allergies are scheduled as the first case of the day. In addition, many patients do not understand that rubber and latex are the same. Using both words helps to obtain accurate information.

STEP	RATIONALE
ASSESSMENT	
j. Physical impairment (e.g., paralysis, reduced range of motion [ROM] of extremity).	Physical impairments may cause limited mobility and situations that could lead to problems with positioning and risk for pressure injury formation. Communicate this information to the OR nurse because these patients may need special positioning or OR bed surfaces.
k. Prostheses and implants (e.g., implantable medication-delivery pump, dentures, hearing aid, pacemaker, internal defibrillator, hip prosthesis).	These devices are often removed prior to surgery (see employer policy) because they could become damaged or malfunction from electrical equipment used during surgery. Report this information to the OR nurse.
l. Smoking, alcohol, and drug use.	Preoperative alcohol consumption is associated with an increased risk of general postoperative morbidity, general infections, wound complications, pulmonary complications, prolonged hospital stay, and admission to a critical care unit (Egholm et al., 2018). Preoperative use of illicit medications can lead to pulmonary complications, poor pain control, and withdrawal symptoms. Smoking can lead to cardiopulmonary complications.
m. Occupation.	Anticipates how postoperative restrictions will affect the patient's return to work.
8. Obtain patient's weight, height, and vital signs (see Chapters 7 and 8).	Height and weight are used to calculate medication dosages. Vital signs provide a baseline for postoperative comparison.

Critical Decision Point *Many patients with OSA are morbidly obese, placing them at increased risk for aspiration of acidic gastric fluid at the time of induction of anaesthesia. For this reason, many of these patients receive medications to suppress gastric acid production, neutralize the acid, or stimulate emptying of the stomach. Use interprofessional collaboration (e.g., health care provider) to discuss possible prescription for acid-suppressing medication.*

STEP	RATIONALE
9. Assess patient's respiratory status, including auscultation of lungs, adventitious sounds, character and rate of respirations, oxygen saturation, ability to breathe lying flat, use of oxygen or continuous positive airway pressure (CPAP) at home, and chest X-ray film report.	Poor respiratory condition can affect the patient's response to general anaesthesia. Use of CPAP may indicate that the patient has OSA, a condition that poses risks after surgery.
10. Auscultate heart sounds and evaluate patient's circulatory status, including apical pulse, ECG report, and peripheral pulses (see Chapter 8).	Screens for possible cardiac problems that may contraindicate surgery. Circulation may be a factor in positioning patient on the OR table.
11. Assess patient's risk for postoperative thrombus formation (e.g., older persons, immobilized patients, patients with personal or family history of blood clots, use of birth control pills, hormones). Ask patient about any leg pain. Observe calves for swelling, warmth, and redness; observe calves for symmetry; and palpate pedal pulses.	Circulation slows after general anaesthesia, increasing tendency for blood clot formation. Immobilization during surgical procedure promotes venous stasis. Manipulation and positioning can cause accidental trauma to leg veins.

Critical Decision Point *Homans' sign is not always present when a deep vein thrombosis (DVT) exists* (Schwartsmann et al., 2019). *If you suspect a thrombus, notify the surgeon and refrain from manipulating the extremity any further. Surgery will usually need to be postponed. Antiembolism stockings or a venous flexus foot pump* (Fig. 37.1) *may be prescribed for patients at risk for thrombus formation* (see Chapter 12).

STEP	RATIONALE
12. Complete a gastrointestinal (GI) assessment; identify time of patient's last intake of food or drink (see Chapter 8).	With patient under general anaesthesia, the esophageal sphincter relaxes, and the stomach contents can be aspirated.

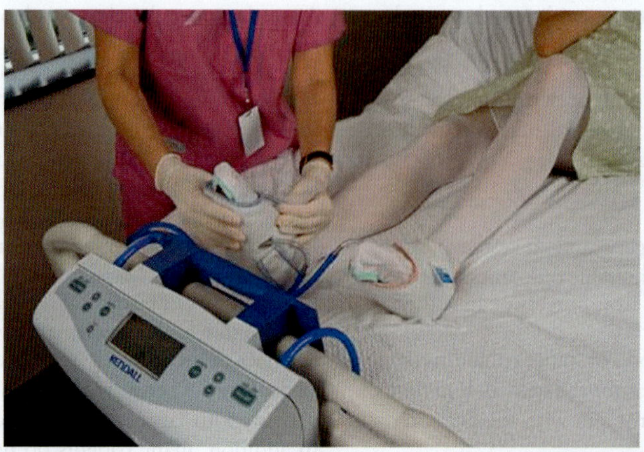

FIG 37.1 Venous plexus foot pump with bedside controls. *(Courtesy Tyco Healthcare Group LP.)*

STEP	RATIONALE
ASSESSMENT	
13. Complete neurological assessment; determine patient's neurological status, including level of consciousness (LOC), cognitive function, and sensation, and note neurological deficits (see Chapter 8).	Patient's neurological status affects attentiveness to instruction. Offers important baseline for postoperative evaluation.
14. Assess patient's musculoskeletal system, including ROM of joints (see Chapter 8).	If ROM is limited, extra care is needed to prevent injury related to positioning in surgery.
15. Examine patient's skin; identify any breaks in skin integrity and determine level of hydration (see Chapter 8). Pay particular attention to area of body on which patient will be positioned.	If skin is thin, broken, or bruised, extra padding is needed during surgery. Hydration may affect skin integrity.
16. Assess patient's emotional status, including level of anxiety, coping ability, and caregiver support. Assess potential for abuse from a partner or caregiver.	If patient has a high level of anxiety or fear, use interprofessional collaboration (e.g., social worker, pastoral care, advanced practice nurse) as required. Any suspected or reported abuse requires follow-up, according to provincial/territorial regulations.
17. Review results of laboratory tests, including complete blood count, electrolytes, urinalysis, and other diagnostic tests.	Laboratory work provides an assessment of major body systems.
18. Remove gloves and discard, if donned.	

NURSING DIAGNOSES

- Inadequate knowledge regarding preoperative plan of care
- Potential for perioperative positioning injury
- Potential for impaired skin integrity
- Potential for infection

Related factors and risk factors are individualized on the basis of patient's condition or needs.

STEP	RATIONALE
PLANNING	
1. Expected outcomes following completion of procedure:	
• Patient provides appropriate preoperative information required to establish plan of care.	Identifies patient's knowledge of preoperative plan of care.
• Patient remains alert and appropriately responsive to assessment questions.	Identifies patient readiness to learn.
• Patient does not incur any injury during preoperative preparation in OR.	Precautions taken because of assessment findings prevent positional and skin injury.
IMPLEMENTATION	
1. Communicate to preoperative team the risk factors that increase patient's vulnerability to intraoperative complications.	Limitations in mobility and sensation should affect how patient is positioned for surgery. Presence of OSA and any cardiopulmonary abnormalities can influence anaesthesia approach.

Critical Decision Point *Even though the surgeon and anaesthesia provider will conduct a separate assessment, your findings may reveal surgical risk factors not previously identified.*

STEP	RATIONALE
2. Based on patient's cognitive status, experience, and nature of the planned surgery, present preoperative instructions to patient and caregiver (see Skill 37.2).	Assessment findings influence the approach to instructions and topics to discuss.
EVALUATION	
1. Determine whether patient information is complete so that plan of care can be established. Validate unclear information with patient and caregiver.	Provides preoperative baseline of assessment data.
2. Evaluate patient's ability to cooperate (e.g., makes eye contact, answers appropriately).	Establishes patient's ability to participate in assessment.
3. **Use teach-back:** "I want to be sure I explained what you need to know about your intended surgery and anaesthesia. Tell me why you are having surgery and when your surgery is scheduled." Develop a revised teaching plan if patient is unable to teach back correctly.	Determines patient's level of understanding of instructional topic.

STEP	RATIONALE
Unexpected Outcomes	**Related Interventions**
1. Patient does not understand what surgery will be performed.	• Notify surgeon.
2. Patient reports allergy to latex.	• Remove all supplies containing latex from patient's room. • Post latex precautions sign on door or stretcher. • Notify surgeon, anaesthesia provider, and OR nurse.

Communication and Documentation

- Document findings in the preoperative section of the progress notes or other designated employer form in the electronic health record (EHR) or chart.
- Report abnormal laboratory values or other concerns to the health care provider (surgeon or anaesthesiologist).
- Document your evaluation of patient and caregiver learning.

DOCUMENTATION EXAMPLE

Patient is ready for surgery with preoperative checks and assessment complete. Patient accurately able to explain purpose of their surgery to writer, has no allergies, and has no acute concerns.

Special Considerations

Teaching

- Whenever you provide printed educational materials to a patient about their surgery or recovery process, ensure that the materials are age appropriate and at the patient's literacy level.
- It is important that any preoperative educational strategy focus on improving a patient's sense of empowerment.

Pediatric

- Involve the parent or guardian in the preoperative preparation to decrease the child's anxiety.
- Consider a child's developmental level when performing preoperative assessment and preoperative preparation (e.g., use stories, films, books, tours, toys, and games) (Keenan-Lindsay et al., 2022).
- Encourage parent or guardian to accompany the child to the surgery holding area.

Gerontological

- Age-related changes may result in diminished short-term memory. Additional assessment and teaching may be necessary.
- An older person may have some limitation in ROM. If this limitation is significant, notify the OR nurse so that the surgical position can be modified.

SKILL 37.2 Preoperative Teaching

Video Clip

With hospital stays becoming shorter and growth in ambulatory surgical procedures, there is a greater demand for patient preparation and support. Patient education must go beyond simply providing information because patients and families must be prepared to assume more preoperative and postoperative responsibilities. Preoperative patient teaching involves helping a patient understand and prepare mentally for the surgical experience. Effective education focuses on each patient's individual needs. Patients feel empowered when they have received knowledge that meets their needs, expectations, and/or preferences.

In the past, patients received preoperative teaching the day or evening before surgery—when patients are feeling most anxious. Health care cost reduction practices now have most patients arrive at the hospital or ambulatory care centre the morning of surgery. Preoperative teaching is not effective at this time because of patient anxiety and stress related to surgical preparation (Wongkietkachorn et al., 2018). Many health care facilities now provide outpatient education programs to prepare patients and their caregivers for a specific surgery. For example, patients who require a total knee replacement go to preoperative preparation classes with other patients requiring the same surgery. Effective preoperative teaching increases patient satisfaction, promotes psychological well-being, and may decrease complications that lead to a longer hospital stay (Tyerman & Cobbett, 2023).

As a nurse, plan your teaching based on the preoperative assessment. Make every attempt to ensure the patient's privacy. Select the best learning method for the patient. In many settings, video, written, and online materials are available to help you. Whenever possible, have the caregivers who will be responsible for the patient's care after surgery present during teaching. Later, the caregivers serve as coaches and help the patient perform postoperative exercises. Plan to have the patient demonstrate expected postoperative skills to allow for practice and facilitate understanding.

Patients and their families are often anxious about impending surgery, which hinders learning. Speak in a clear, slow voice to reduce the patient's anxiety and promote understanding. You may need extra time for teaching and reinforcement to ensure patient understanding. After surgery, high anxiety can lead to negative psychological and physiological outcomes. Preoperative information about expected perioperative sensations decreases the distress associated with surgery. By teaching and setting expectations before surgery (pain level, average length of surgery), the patient and the nurse can make a significant contribution to success in the postoperative recovery phase.

Delegation and Collaboration

The skills of preoperative teaching cannot be delegated to a UCP. The UCP can reinforce and help patients perform postoperative exercises. The nurse instructs the UCP about the following:

- Any precautions or safety issues unique to the patient (e.g., fall precautions, mobility limitations, bleeding precautions, weight-bearing issues, dietary concerns)
- Informing the nurse of any identified concerns (e.g., patient is unable to perform the exercises correctly)

Equipment

- Stretcher or bed
- Pillow
- Incentive spirometer
- Preoperative education flow sheet
- Positive expiratory pressure (PEP) device
- Stethoscope

STEP	RATIONALE

ASSESSMENT

STEP	RATIONALE
1. Identify patient using at least two person-specific identifiers (e.g., name and date of birth, or name and medical record number) according to employer policy.	Ensures correct patient. Complies with Accreditation Canada's standards and improves patient safety (Accreditation Canada, 2020).
2. Throughout the procedure, the 4 moments for hand hygiene are to be implemented; hand hygiene should occur before initial patient (or patient environment) contact, before an aseptic procedure, after body fluid exposure risk, and after patient (or patient environment) contact. Additional hand hygiene should be performed when hands are visibly soiled.	Proper hand hygiene helps prevent the spread of infectious agents to health care providers.
3. Ask about patient's previous experiences with surgery and anaesthesia.	Allows you to individualize teaching and address specific patient concerns.
4. Determine whether patient and caregiver understand the surgery.	Determines whether correction of misunderstanding is necessary.
5. Identify patient's cognitive level, language, and culture. If patient does not speak English, have a professional interpreter present to assist you.	These factors may alter the patient's ability to understand the meaning of the surgery and can affect the postoperative healing course if there are mixed messages or misunderstandings.
6. Assess patient's risk for postoperative respiratory complications (see Skill 37.1). Check nursing history for patient's height and age.	General anaesthesia predisposes a patient to respiratory problems (see Chapters 23 and 25). The presence of underlying respiratory conditions or patient's inability to perform postoperative respiratory exercises increases the patient's risk of pulmonary complications. Height and age are used to set incentive spirometer parameters.
7. Assess patient's anxiety related to surgery.	If patient's anxiety is still high, directs you to provide additional emotional support. Indicates patient's readiness to learn.
8. Assess caregiver's willingness to learn and support patient following surgery.	Caregiver's presence after surgery can be a potential motivating factor for patient recovery. In addition, the caregiver can coach the patient through postoperative exercise and observe for any postoperative problems.
9. Assess patient's medical prescriptions.	Preoperative and postoperative prescriptions often require adaptations in the way patient performs exercises.

NURSING DIAGNOSES

- Anxiety
- Inadequate knowledge regarding postoperative exercises

Related factors and risk factors are individualized on the basis of patient's condition or needs.

PLANNING

STEP	RATIONALE
1. Expected outcomes following completion of procedure:	
• Patient demonstrates culturally appropriate eye contact, asks and answers questions appropriately.	Identifies patient's readiness to learn.
• Patient correctly performs splinting, turning and sitting, breathing exercises, and leg exercises.	Patient will be prepared to participate in postoperative exercises following surgery.
• Family identifies location of waiting room and time frame when they can expect status on their family member.	Family anxiety may be reduced with preoperative expectations clearly provided.
• Caregivers verbalize ability to help prepare patient at home before surgery.	Caregivers can assist patient with necessary preparations before surgery at home.
• Caregivers provide emotional support for patient before surgery.	Both patient and caregiver have support for surgery.

IMPLEMENTATION

STEP	RATIONALE
1. Inform patient and caregiver of date, time, and location of surgery; anticipated length of surgery; additional time in postanaesthesia recovery area; and where to wait.	Reduces transmission of infection. Accurate information helps reduce stress associated with surgery.
2. Answer questions that patient and caregiver ask.	Responding to patient and caregiver questions helps decrease their anxiety and demonstrates your concern for them.

STEP	RATIONALE
IMPLEMENTATION	
3. Instruct patient about preoperative bowel or skin preparations, as needed. Check medical prescriptions and employer policy regarding number of preoperative showers and medications to be used for each shower (2% chlorhexidine gluconate [CHG] is used most often). Following each preoperative shower, instruct patient to rinse the skin thoroughly and dry with a fresh, clean, dry towel. Patient should don clean clothing.	Proper skin preparation is a critical element in preventing SSIs. Rinsing skin removes residual antiseptic preparation that may cause skin irritation. After use, towels contain microorganisms that can grow in the presence of moisture. Using fresh towel after each shower and donning clean clothing minimizes risk of reintroducing microorganisms to clean skin (Association of periOperative Registered Nurses, 2023).
4. Instruct patient about extent and purpose of food and fluid restrictions for period specified before surgery (e.g., no clear liquids at least 2 hours before surgery, no light meal [e.g., toast and a clear liquid] 6 hours or more before surgery, no meat or fried foods 8 hours before surgery, unless otherwise specified by surgeon or anaesthesiologist) (Dobson et al., 2023).	During general anaesthesia muscles relax; and gastric contents can reflux into esophagus, leading to aspiration. Anaesthetic eliminates patient's ability to gag.
5. Describe perioperative routines (e.g., time-out, site marking, intravenous [IV] therapy, urinary catheterization, enema, hair clipping or removal, laboratory tests, transport to OR).	Allows patient to anticipate and recognize routine procedures, reducing anxiety.
6. Describe planned effect of preoperative medications.	Provides information about what to expect, decreasing patient anxiety.
7. Review which routine medications patient needs to discontinue before surgery.	Some medications are discontinued before surgery to minimize effects that can cause surgical risks. For example, anticoagulants may increase bleeding and are usually discontinued several days before surgery. Insulin dosages are usually adjusted because of reduced intake of food before surgery.
8. Describe perioperative sensations (e.g., BP cuff tightening, ECG leads, cool room, and beep of monitor).	Misconceptions and concerns about anaesthesia have been ranked high among preoperative patients.
9. Describe pain control methods to be used after surgery. Many patients have a patient-controlled analgesia (PCA) pump (see Chapter 16).	Patients are fearful of postoperative pain. Explaining pain management techniques reduces this fear. Establishes what pain is acceptable; patients will know they will not be pain-free, but their pain will be managed.
10. Describe what patient will experience after surgery (e.g., where patient will be on awakening, frequent vital signs, catheters, drains, tubes, alternating pressure from sequential compression device, intermittent pneumatic compression devices, postoperative exercises).	Provides concrete description of what patient can expect after surgery to ensure patient is prepared.
11. Teach turning:	
a. Instruct patient on turning and sitting up (especially suited for abdominal and thoracic surgery):	Promotes circulation and ventilation.
(1) Turn onto right side: Have patient assume supine position and move to side of bed (in this case, left side) if permitted by surgery. Instruct patient to move by bending knees and pressing heels against mattress to raise and move buttocks (see Step 11a[1] illustration). The top side rails on both sides of the bed should be in up position.	Positioning begins on side of bed so that turning to other side does not cause patient to roll toward edge of bed. Buttocks lifting prevents shearing force against sheets. If patient's bed has a turn-assist feature, use it to help position them.
(2) Have patient splint incision with right hand; or, with right hand, have patient hold pillow over incisional area. Patient should keep right leg straight and flex their left knee up (see Step 11a[2] illustration). Have patient grab right side rail with their left hand, pull toward right, and roll onto their right side. Reverse process to turn to left side.	Supports incision and decreases discomfort while turning.

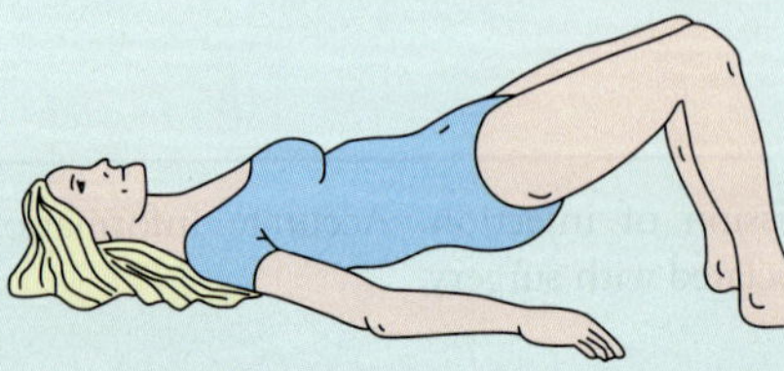

STEP 11A(1) Buttocks lift for moving to side of bed.

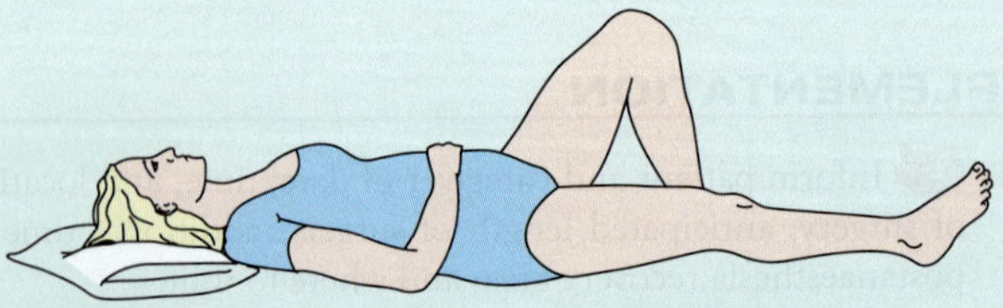

STEP 11A(2) Leg position when turning to right.

STEP	RATIONALE
IMPLEMENTATION	
(3) Instruct patient to turn every 2 hours from side to side while awake. Often, patient requires assistance with turning after surgery. If patient is unable to turn, assist or turn patient every 2 hours unless contraindicated by operative procedure.	Reduces risk of vascular, pulmonary, and pressure injury complications.

Critical Decision Point *Some patients, such as those who have had back surgery or vascular repair, are restricted from flexing their legs after surgery. Some patients are restricted from turning or may need help for positioning* (see Chapter 11).

STEP	RATIONALE
(4) Have patient sit up on right side of bed. Elevate head of bed and have patient turn onto their right side. While lying on right side, patient pushes on mattress with left arm and swings feet over edge of bed with nurse's help. For patient to sit up on left side of bed, reverse this process.	Sitting position lowers diaphragm to permit fuller lung expansion.

Critical Decision Point *Caution patient to always ask for assistance, particularly the first time sitting up on the side of the bed, to reduce risk of a fall.*

STEP	RATIONALE
12. Teach coughing and deep breathing: If patient has an abdominal or thoracic incision, teach patient to place a pillow over the incision area and their hands over the pillow in order to splint the incision.	Patient may be unable or reluctant to deep breathe because of weakness or pain, resulting in secretions remaining in base of the lungs. Collection of secretions increases risk of pulmonary atelectasis and pneumonia. Deep breathing and coughing exercises place a strain and stress on the suture line, causing discomfort. Splinting provides a firm support and reduces incisional pulling and pain.
a. Help patient to high Fowler's position in bed with their knees flexed, or have patient sit on side of bed or chair in an upright position.	Sitting position facilitates diaphragmatic expansion.
b. Instruct patient to place palms of their hands across from one another lightly along lower border of rib cage or upper abdomen (see Step 12b illustration).	This allows patient to feel the rise and fall of their abdomen during deep breathing.
c. Have patient take slow, deep breaths, inhaling through the nose. Explain that patient will feel normal downward movement of the diaphragm during inspiration. Demonstrate as needed.	Helps prevent hyperventilation or panting. Slow, deep breathing allows for more complete lung expansion.
d. Have patient avoid using chest and shoulder muscles while inhaling.	Increases unnecessary energy expenditure and does not promote full lung expansion.
e. Have patient take slow, deep breath; hold for count of 3 seconds; and slowly exhale through the mouth as if blowing out a candle (pursed lips).	Resistance during exhalation helps prevent alveolar collapse.
f. Have patient repeat breathing exercise three to five times.	Repetition reinforces learning.
g. Have patient take two slow, deep breaths, inhaling through the nose and exhaling through pursed lips.	Deep breaths expand lungs fully, so air moves behind mucus to facilitate coughing.
h. Have patient inhale deeply a third time and hold breath to count of 3. Have patient cough fully for two or three consecutive coughs without inhaling between coughs.	Deep breathing moves up secretions in the respiratory tract to stimulate cough reflex without voluntary effort on the part of the patient (Tyerman & Cobbett, 2023).
i. Caution patient against clearing their throat.	Clearing the throat does not remove mucus from deeper airways.
j. Have patient practise several times. Instruct patient to perform turning, coughing, and deep breathing every 2 hours. Have caregiver coach patient to exercise.	Ensures mastery of technique. Frequent pulmonary exercises and movement decrease risk of postoperative pneumonia (Tyerman & Cobbett, 2023).

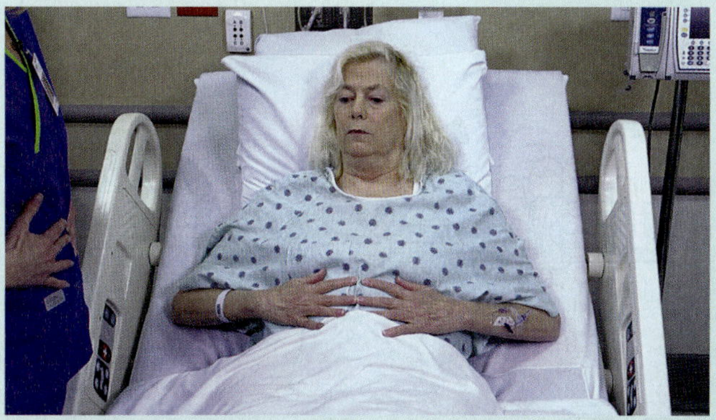

STEP 12B Deep-breathing exercise—placement of hands on upper abdomen during inhalation.

IMPLEMENTATION

STEP	RATIONALE
13. Teach use of an incentive spirometer (see also Skill 25.3):	Provides visual aid of respiratory effort. Encourages deep breathing to loosen secretions in lung bases.
a. Position patient in sitting position in chair or in reclining position in bed, with head of bed elevated at least 45 degrees.	Facilitates diaphragm lowering and lung expansion.
b. Either set or indicate to patient on the incentive spirometer device scale the volume level to be reached with each breath (targeted tidal volume). Use manufacturer directions to set volume.	Establishes goal of volume level necessary for adequate lung expansion. Manufacturers determine target on basis of patient height and age.
c. Explain to patient how to place mouthpiece of incentive spirometer so lips completely cover the mouthpiece (see Step 13c illustration). Have patient demonstrate until position is correct.	Validates patient's understanding of instructions, evaluates psychomotor skills, and lets patient ask questions.
d. Instruct patient to exhale completely, then position mouthpiece so lips completely cover it, and inhale slowly, maintaining constant flow through unit until reaching goal volume (see Step 13d illustration).	Promotes complete inflation of lungs and minimizes atelectasis.
e. Once maximum inspiration is reached, have patient hold breath for 2–3 seconds and then exhale slowly.	Promotes alveolar inflation.
f. Instruct patient to breathe normally for a short period between each of the 10 breaths taken on incentive spirometer. Have patient repeat this every hour while awake.	Prevents hyperventilation and fatigue.
14. Teach PEP therapy and "huff" coughing:	
a. Set PEP device for setting prescribed.	Higher settings require more effort.
b. Instruct patient to assume semi-Fowler's or high Fowler's position in bed or to sit in a chair, and place nose clip on patient's nose (see Step 14b illustration).	Promotes optimum lung expansion and expectoration of mucus.

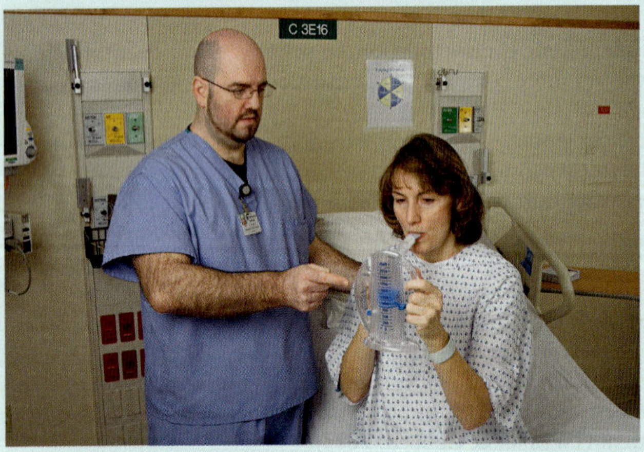

STEP 13C Patient demonstrates incentive spirometry.

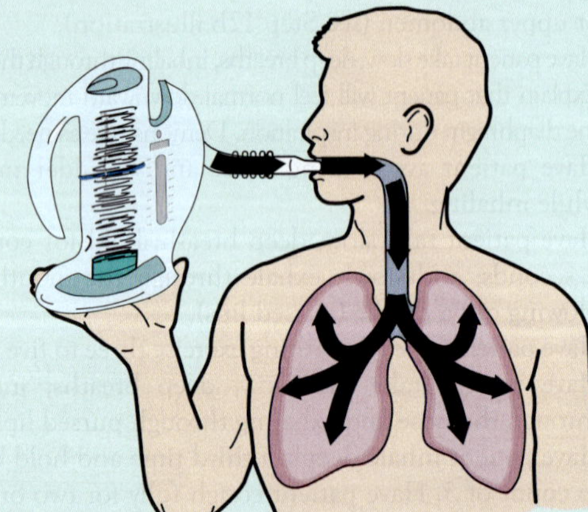

STEP 13D Diagram of use of incentive spirometer.

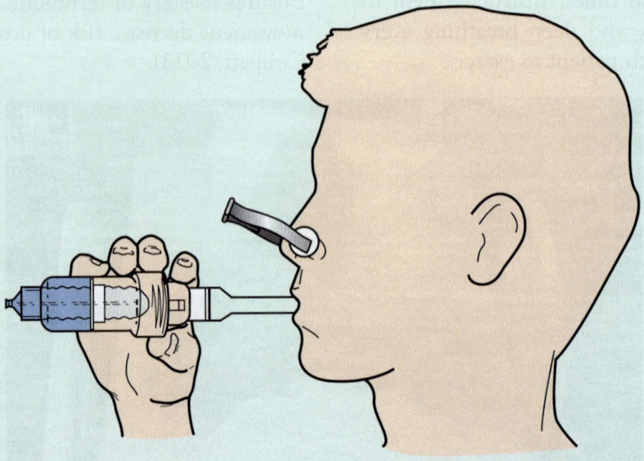

STEP 14B Diagram of use of positive expiratory pressure device.

STEP	RATIONALE
IMPLEMENTATION	
c. Have patient place lips around the mouthpiece. Instruct patient to take a full breath and exhale two or three times longer than length of inhalation. Repeat pattern for 10 to 20 breaths.	Ensures that patient does all breathing through the mouth. Ensures that patient uses device properly.
d. Remove device from mouth and have patient take a slow, deep breath and hold it for 3 seconds.	Promotes lung expansion before coughing.
e. Instruct patient to exhale in quick, short, forced "huffs." Repeat exercise every 2 hours while patient is awake.	"Huff" coughing, or forced expiratory technique, promotes bronchial hygiene by increasing expectoration of secretions.
15. Teach controlled coughing:	Deep breaths expand lungs fully so air moves behind mucus and facilitates effective coughing.
a. Explain importance of maintaining an upright position.	Position facilitates diaphragm excursion and enhances thorax and abdominal expansion.
b. Demonstrate coughing. Have patient take two slow, deep breaths, inhaling through the nose and exhaling through (pursed lips) mouth.	Consecutive coughs help remove mucus more effectively and completely than one forceful cough.
c. Have patient inhale deeply a third time and hold breath to count of 3. Patient should cough fully for two or three consecutive coughs without inhaling between coughs (see Step 15c illustration). (Tell patient to push all air out of lungs.)	Clearing the throat does not remove mucus from deeper airways. A dull, forceful cough is most effective in removing mucus.
d. Caution patient against clearing their throat instead of coughing deeply.	Clearing the throat does not remove mucus from deeper airways.
e. If surgical incision is either thoracic or abdominal, teach patient to place either hands or pillow over incisional area and place hands over pillow to splint the incision (see Step 15e illustration). During breathing and coughing exercises, patient should press gently against incisional area for splinting and support.	Surgical incision cuts through muscles, tissues, and nerve endings. Deep-breathing and coughing exercises place additional stress on the suture line and cause discomfort. Splinting the incision with hands or a pillow provides firm support and reduces incisional pulling and pain.
f. Patient continues to practise coughing exercises, splinting imaginary incision (see Step 15f illustration). Instruct patient to cough two or three times every 2 hours while awake.	Deep coughing with splinting effectively expectorates mucus with minimal discomfort.

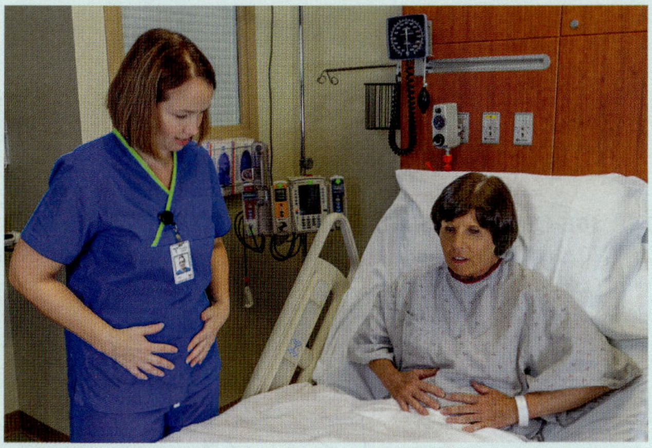

STEP 15C Controlled coughing with placement of hands on upper abdomen.

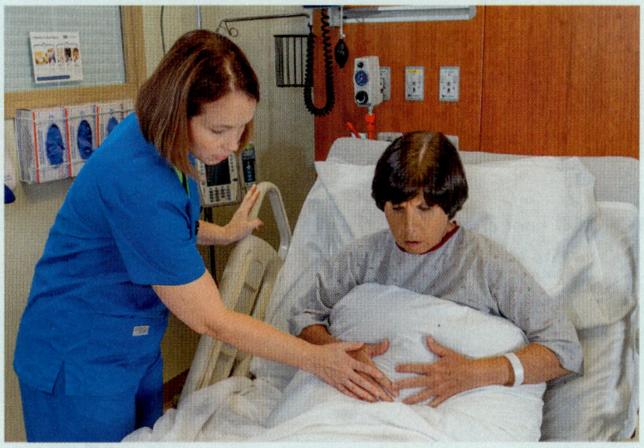

STEP 15E Patient splinting abdomen with pillow.

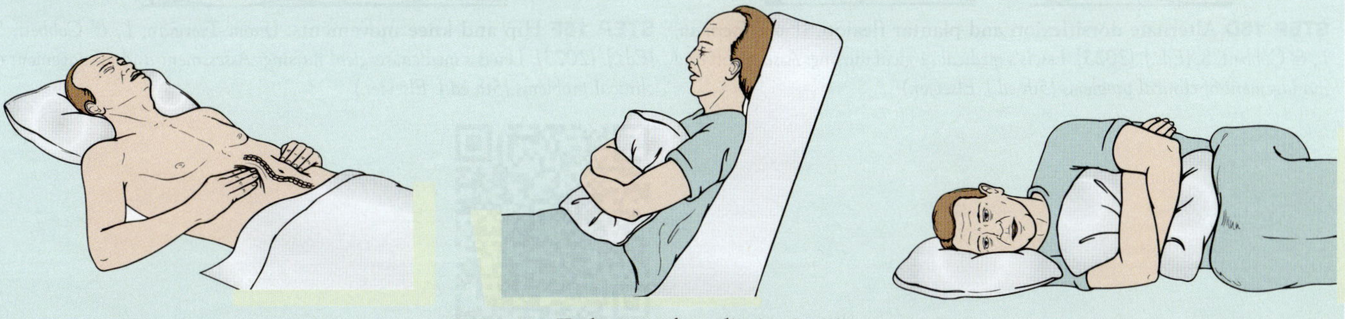

STEP 15F Techniques for splinting incisions.

STEP	RATIONALE
IMPLEMENTATION	
g. Instruct patient to examine sputum for consistency, odour, amount, and colour changes and to notify a nurse if any changes are noted.	Sputum consistency, odour, amount, and colour changes indicate presence of a pulmonary complication such as pneumonia.
16. Teach leg exercises:	
a. Instruct patient in performing leg exercises. Encourage them to perform the following exercises every 1–2 hours while patient is awake: ankle rotation, dorsiflexion and plantar flexion, leg extension and flexion, and straight-leg raises.	Leg exercises facilitate venous return from lower extremities and reduce risk of circulatory complications such as venous thrombus.
b. Position patient supine.	
c. Instruct patient to rotate each ankle in a complete circle and draw imaginary circles with the big toe five times (see Step 16c illustration).	Promotes joint mobility and venous return.
d. Have patient alternate dorsiflexion and plantar flexion and instruct patient to feel calf muscles tighten and relax. Repeat five times (see Step 16d illustration).	Helps maintain joint mobility and promote venous return to prevent thrombus formation.
e. Have patient perform quadriceps setting by tightening thigh and bringing knee down toward mattress and relaxing. Repeat five times (see Step 16e illustration).	Quadriceps-setting exercises contract muscles of upper legs, maintain knee mobility, and improve venous return to the heart.
f. Instruct patient to alternate raising legs straight up from bed surface. Leg should be kept straight. Repeat five times (see Step 16f illustration).	Causes quadriceps muscle contraction and relaxation, which help promote venous return (Tyerman & Cobbett, 2023).
17. Have patient continue to practise exercises before surgery at least every 2 hours while awake. Teach patient to coordinate turning and leg exercises with diaphragmatic breathing and use of incentive spirometer.	Leg exercises stimulate circulation, which prevents venous stasis and thus helps prevent formation of DVT (Tyerman & Cobbett, 2023).
18. Verify that patient's expectations of surgery are realistic. Correct expectations as needed.	May prevent postoperative anxiety or anger.
19. Reinforce therapeutic coping strategies. If ineffective, encourage alternatives.	Therapeutic coping strategies promote postoperative adherence and recovery.

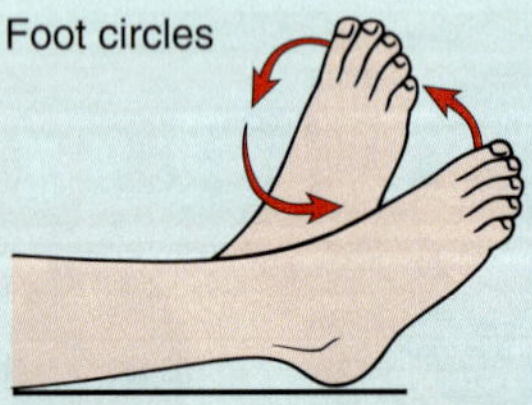

STEP 16C Foot circles. *(From Tyerman, J., & Cobbett, S. [Eds.]. [2023]. Lewis's medical-surgical nursing: Assessment and management of clinical problems [5th ed.]. Elsevier.)*

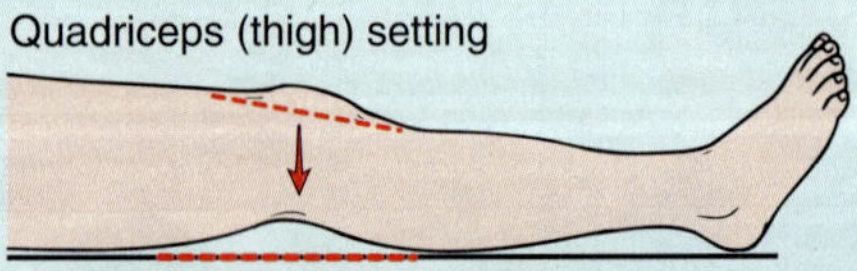

STEP 16E Quadriceps (thigh) setting. *(From Tyerman, J., & Cobbett, S. [Eds.]. [2023]. Lewis's medical-surgical nursing: Assessment and management of clinical problems [5th ed.]. Elsevier.)*

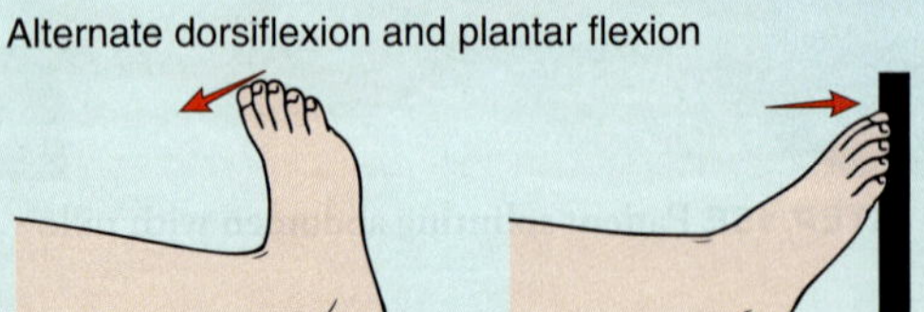

STEP 16D Alternate dorsiflexion and plantar flexion. *(From Tyerman, J., & Cobbett, S. [Eds.]. [2023]. Lewis's medical-surgical nursing: Assessment and management of clinical problems [5th ed.]. Elsevier.)*

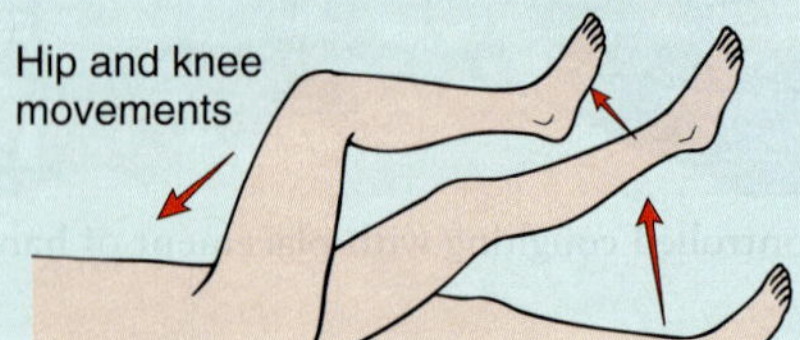

STEP 16F Hip and knee movements. *(From Tyerman, J., & Cobbett, S. [Eds.]. [2023]. Lewis's medical-surgical nursing: Assessment and management of clinical problems [5th ed.]. Elsevier.)*

STEP	RATIONALE

EVALUATION

Step	Rationale
1. Observe patient's demonstration of splinting, turning and sitting, deep breathing, use of incentive spirometer, PEP therapy, and leg exercises.	Validates patient's ability to perform postoperative exercises and use devices.
2. Ask family to identify location of waiting room and validate if correct.	Establishes family's knowledge of where they can wait for patient information.
3. Ask caregiver if they are able to help prepare patient at home before surgery.	Establishes that postoperative care in the community is in place for patient on discharge.
4. Observe level of emotional support caregiver provides patient.	Identifies preoperative emotional support for patient.
5. **Use teach-back:** "I want to be sure I explained what you need to know about getting ready for surgery. Tell me which medications you should not take before surgery." Develop a revised teaching plan if patient or caregiver is unable to teach back correctly.	Determines patient's and caregiver's level of understanding of instructional topic.

Unexpected Outcomes	Related Interventions
1. Patient identifies incorrect procedure, site, date, or time of surgery.	• Provide correct information verbally and in writing for patient and caregiver.
2. Patient incorrectly performs one of the postoperative exercises. Anxiety and fatigue can alter a patient's performance.	• Explain and demonstrate correct exercise technique. • Explain importance of the postoperative exercise as it pertains to patient recovery. • Instruct patient to repeat demonstration.

Communication and Documentation

- Document all preoperative patient and caregiver teaching in the progress notes in EHR or chart.
- Document your evaluation of patient and caregiver learning.

DOCUMENTATION EXAMPLE

Preoperative teaching completed. Patient can correctly perform splinting of their abdomen, breathing exercises, and leg exercises. Patient accurately able to explain the purpose of these techniques and is willing to perform them postop.

Special Considerations

Teaching

- Nurses are responsible for ensuring that patient education materials are clear, concise, in plain language, person centred, and based on the patient's needs and abilities. In addition, the nurse must evaluate the effectiveness of the teaching (Arnold & Boggs, 2019).

Pediatric

- Use an age-appropriate level of communication and provide simple explanations using familiar terms.
- The use of pictures, models, equipment, and play, rather than verbal explanations, increases learning in preschool and school-age children.
- Teaching coughing, deep breathing, and leg exercises is not usually necessary for young children. The normal responses of crying and moving extremities will maintain lung expansion and peripheral circulation.
- Adolescents need to receive the same preoperative instructions and teaching as adults to support their developmental level.

Gerontological

- Physiological changes that occur with aging may require admission to hospital before surgery for additional diagnostic tests and stabilization of the condition (Table 37.2).
- Age-related changes in the central nervous system may diminish short-term memory. Additional time and reinforcement may be necessary for older persons to learn and comprehend information (Boscart et al., 2023). The greater the number of different exposures to new material, the higher the probability that the material will be learned.
- Reinforce teaching with verbal explanations, audiovisual resources, pamphlets, and demonstrations. Consider sight and hearing deficits when providing both written and verbal instructions (Boscart et al., 2023).

Care in the Community: Home Management

- Review coughing, deep breathing, abdominal splinting, relaxation, leg exercises, and ambulation before patient admission and after discharge.

TABLE 37.2

Physiological Factors That Place Older Persons at Risk for Complications During Surgery

Alteration	Surgery Risk	Nursing Implications
Cardiovascular		
Degenerative change in myocardium and valves	Reduced cardiac reserve	Assess baseline vital signs.
Rigidity of arterial walls and reduction in sympathetic and parasympathetic innervation to the heart	Predisposes patient to postoperative hemorrhage and rise in systolic and diastolic blood pressure	Maintain adequate fluid balance to minimize stress to heart. Ensure that blood pressure is adequate to meet circulatory demands.
Increase in calcium and cholesterol deposits within small arteries; arterial walls thickened	Predisposes patient to clot formation in lower extremities	Teach patient techniques for performing leg exercises and proper turning. Apply bilateral antiembolism stockings, sequential compression devices (SCDs) (see Chapter 12).
Integumentary		
Decreased subcutaneous tissue and increased fragility of skin	Prone to pressure injuries and skin tears	Assess skin every 4 hours; pad all bony prominences during surgery. Turn or reposition (see Chapter 39).
Pulmonary		
Rib cage stiffens and enlarges	Reduced vital capacity	Teach patient proper technique for coughing and deep-breathing exercises and use of incentive spirometer.
Reduced diaphragm excursion	Greater residual capacity or volume of air left in lung after normal breath increases, reducing amount of new air brought into lungs with each inspiration	Encourage deep breathing. Use incentive spirometer to enhance exhalation.
Lung tissue is less distensible; alveoli enlarged	Reduced blood oxygenation	Assess oxygen saturation via pulse oximetry (SpO_2).
Renal		
Reduced blood flow to kidneys	Blood loss that causes decrease in circulation to the kidney	Monitor urinary output and laboratory data (i.e., blood urea nitrogen [BUN], creatinine).
Reduced glomerular filtration rate and excretory times	Limits ability to remove medications or toxic substances	Assess for adverse effects of medications.
Reduced bladder capacity	Increase in voiding frequency; larger amount of urine stays in the bladder after voiding	Instruct patient to notify nurse immediately when sensation of bladder fullness develops.
	Sensation of need to void may not occur until bladder is filled	Keep call light or bedpan within easy reach.
Neurological		
Sensory losses, including reduced tactile sense, increased pain tolerance	Patient is less able to respond to early warning signs of surgical complications	Inspect bony prominences for signs of pressure.
Decreased reaction time	Patient becomes confused easily after anaesthesia	Orient patient to surrounding environment. Observe for nonverbal signs of pain. Maintain a safe environment. Institute fall precautions.
Metabolic		
Lower basal metabolic rate	Reduced total oxygen consumption and nutritional needs	Ensure adequate nutritional intake once diet is resumed.
Reduced number of red blood cells and hemoglobin levels	Reduces ability to carry adequate oxygen to tissues	Administer necessary blood products. Assess for adequacy of oxygenation, fatigue, and infection.
Change in total amounts of body potassium and water volume	Greater risk of fluid or electrolyte imbalance	Monitor electrolyte levels.

✦ SKILL 37.3 Physical Preparation for Surgery

Video Clip

Preparing a patient for surgery involves activities and procedures that help decrease anxiety, ensure patient safety, and decrease the risk of perioperative complications. The type of surgery determines the preparation required before surgery (e.g., low-residue and clear-liquid diets, enemas, cathartics, and oral antibiotics for patients who will undergo bowel surgery). Smoking cessation should be encouraged, and patients should be offered nicotine substitutes. Nicotine delays wound healing, increases the risk of infection, and increases the risk of venous thromboembolism (VTE) (Al-Nasser, 2020; Mitri et al., 2021). Patients whose blood work indicates a low hemoglobin level and/or abnormal electrolyte levels or coagulopathies often require inpatient therapy before surgery.

Because many patients are admitted on the day of surgery, much of the preoperative preparation is often the responsibility of the patient or the primary caregiver. Therefore, it is important that a preadmission nurse or nurse in the surgeon's practice provide adequate instructions. Patient teaching should include any food and fluid restrictions; which medications, if any, are permitted on the morning of surgery; and the need for surgical site preparation the evening before surgery (see Skill 37.2). It is also important to include action that a patient will need to take if they omit any of these procedures by mistake. Written instructions are a useful adjunct to teaching because a patient and caregiver can refer to them for any points that are unclear or forgotten. Videos and pamphlets are also useful adjuncts in preparing patients and their families.

The revised Joint Commission standards, which are incorporated into the National Patient Safety Goals, include the Universal Protocol for Preventing Wrong Site, Wrong Procedure, Wrong Person Surgery (The Joint Commission, 2023). The Universal Protocol was implemented as an added safety measure to ensure that the correct person, procedure, and surgical site are verified at the time of scheduling the procedure, on admission or entry into the facility, and each time the responsibility for care of the patient is transferred to another caregiver. A final verification check involving the entire surgical team occurs immediately before the start of the procedure. If the case involves laterality (right versus left), multiple structures (e.g., fingers, toes, lesions), or multiple levels (e.g., spine), the final verification should include a site marking by the person performing the procedure. The site markings need to be visible after the patient has been prepared and draped. Patients should be involved in this process when they are awake and aware. Immediately before starting the procedure a "time-out" is called. The entire operative team, using active communication, verifies correct patient identity, correct side and site, agreement on the procedure to be done, correct patient position, and availability of correct implants and any special equipment or special requirements. This final verification process should be documented.

Delegation and Collaboration

The skill of coordinating the patient's preparation for surgery cannot be delegated to a UCP. Depending on employer policy, the UCP may administer an enema; obtain vital signs in stable patients; apply antiembolism stockings; and help patients remove clothing, jewellery, and prostheses. The nurse instructs the UCP about the following:

- Using routine practices and additional precautions (infection control) when preparing a patient for surgery
- Observing and using precautions if the patient has an IV catheter or other invasive devices in place

Equipment

NOTE: Equipment varies by procedure prescribed.

- Vital sign equipment: stethoscope, BP cuff, thermometer, pulse oximeter
- Oxygen equipment
- Suction equipment as prescribed
- Hospital gown
- IV solution and administration set (see Chapter 29)
- Skin-cleaning solution
- Compression (antiembolism) stockings (see Chapter 12)
- Intermittent compression devices (ICDs)
- Venous foot pump
- Urinary catheterization kit (see Chapter 34)
- Preoperative checklist
- Medications (e.g., sedative)
- Clean gloves

STEP	RATIONALE
ASSESSMENT	
1. Identify patient using at least two person-specific identifiers (e.g., name and date of birth, or name and medical record number) according to employer policy.	Ensures correct patient. Complies with Accreditation Canada's standards and improves patient safety (Accreditation Canada, 2020).
2. Throughout the procedure, the 4 moments for hand hygiene are to be implemented; hand hygiene should occur before initial patient (or patient environment) contact, before an aseptic procedure, after body fluid exposure risk, and after patient (or patient environment) contact. Additional hand hygiene should be performed when hands are visibly soiled.	Proper hand hygiene helps prevent the spread of infectious agents to health care providers.
3. Complete the preoperative assessment (see Skill 37.1).	Provides all baseline assessment data for surgical team.
4. Assess and record patient's heart rate, BP, respiratory rate, oxygen saturation, and temperature.	Provides baseline for patient's preoperative status.
5. If patient is same-day admission or an ambulatory patient, validate that admission preparations were completed as prescribed. Specific preparations to review include NPO (nothing by mouth) status, administration of medications, skin preparation, and bowel preparation, if applicable.	Failure to complete preparation could lead to perioperative or postoperative complications and may necessitate postponement or cancellation of surgery.
6. Ask if patient has advance care plan. If so, place it in their medical record.	Document conveys patient's wishes if life support measures are necessary.

STEP	RATIONALE

NURSING DIAGNOSES

- Inadequate knowledge regarding the surgical experience
- Fear
- Anxiety
- Acute pain
- Reduced oral mucous membrane
- Reduced physical mobility
- Potential for impaired skin integrity
- Potential for delayed surgical recovery
- Potential for infection
- Potential for perioperative positioning injury
- Potential for disturbed body image

Related factors and risk factors are individualized on the basis of patient's condition or needs.

PLANNING

STEP	RATIONALE
1. Expected outcomes following completion of procedure:	
• Patient can state which surgical procedure is being performed and the risks and benefits of surgery.	Identifies preparation for informed consent.
• Patient states that anxiety is decreased.	Decreased anxiety increases participation.

IMPLEMENTATION

STEP	RATIONALE
1. Help patient put on hospital gown and remove personal items. Patients are often anxious before surgery. Before any procedure, decrease patient's anxiety by explaining how equipment or preparation will feel (e.g., cold, tight) before touching patient.	Reduces transmission of infection. Allows patient to orient to surroundings and understand presurgical procedures.
2. Instruct patient to remove makeup, nail polish, hairpins, and jewellery.	Hair appliances and jewellery anywhere on the body may become dislodged and cause injury during positioning and intubation. Rings decrease circulation in fingers. Makeup, nail polish, and false nails impede assessment of skin and oxygenation. In addition, acrylic nails harbour pathogenic organisms (Hewlett et al., 2018).
3. Ensure that money and valuables have been locked up or given to a caregiver.	Patient might not return to the same location after surgery. Prevents valuables from being misplaced or lost.
4. Ensure that patient has followed appropriate fluid and food restrictions per surgeon or anaesthesiologist prescription (see Skill 37.2).	Extent and type of restriction vary by employer policy and health care provider. Under general anaesthesia, sphincters in the stomach relax, and stomach contents may reflux into esophagus and trachea.
5. Verify presence of allergies and ensure that allergy/sensitivity band or other safety armbands are present.	Alerts surgeons and health care team to potential allergies and risk of falls.
6. Verify that patient has followed instructions about omission or ingestion of medications as instructed.	Missed or inaccurate dosage could precipitate complications.
7. Verify that bowel preparation (e.g., laxative, cathartic, enema) has been completed by patient or caregiver at home, if prescribed.	Proper bowel evacuation is needed for surgery to be performed.

Critical Decision Point *In some situations, additional enemas and/or cathartics are prescribed. Emptying the bowel is necessary for bowel surgery and decreases the risk of postoperative ileus. Enemas are used when surgery is near the lower intestine.*

STEP	RATIONALE
8. Ensure that medical history and physical examination results are in the patient's record.	Ensures that pertinent laboratory and diagnostic test results are available and that all preoperative preparations have been completed (Canadian Medical Protective Association, n.d.).
9. Verify that surgical consent, anaesthesia consent, and consent for blood transfusion are complete. In addition, all of the following should be present: name of procedure; name of surgeon(s); date; name of person authorized to obtain surgical consent; signature of surgeon (or authorized person) obtaining consent, anaesthesia provider delivering anaesthesia, and witness to the patient signature; and patient's signature.	Ensures patient's agreement to undergo intended procedure. In most settings, the surgeon obtains consent, and the nurse verifies that consent is complete and consistent with patient's understanding (refer to employer policy).
10. Ensure that necessary laboratory work, ECG, and chest X-ray film studies have been completed and results recorded on chart.	Diagnostic test results may indicate a medical problem and provide data for postoperative comparison.
11. Verify that blood type and crossmatch are completed, if prescribed, by surgeon and that blood transfusions are available as needed.	In many cases, surgery cannot begin without availability of blood units.

STEP	RATIONALE
IMPLEMENTATION	
12. Instruct patient to void.	Prevents risk of bladder distension or rupture during surgery.
13. Initiate IV therapy; refer to employer policy or surgeon's prescriptions (see Chapter 29).	An IV line provides access for fluids and medications to be administered to patient when in OR.
14. Administer preoperative medications as prescribed (e.g., preoperative antibiotics, prophylactic medications).	Preoperative medications are used for various reasons and should be administered as prescribed for maximum effectiveness.
15. Apply compression stockings, if prescribed (see Chapter 12).	Compression stockings promote circulation during periods of immobilization, reducing risk of embolism.
16. Apply ICDs, if prescribed. Note: ICDs may or may not be used in combination with compression stockings. Verify prescription.	ICDs push blood from superficial veins into deep veins, decreasing venous stasis.

Critical Decision Point *ICDs do not provide effective DVT prophylaxis if the device is not applied correctly or if the patient does not wear the device continuously except during bathing, skin assessment, and ambulation. ICDs are not to be worn when a patient has an active DVT because of the risk for pulmonary embolism.*

STEP	RATIONALE
17. Apply clean gloves. Clean and prepare surgical site, if prescribed. Remove and discard gloves.	Reduces transmission of microorganisms. Cleaning with antimicrobial soap decreases bacterial flora on skin.
18. Insert urinary catheter, if prescribed (see Chapter 34). Note: There are times when a urinary catheter is placed while patient is in OR.	Maintains bladder decompression and provides for monitoring of urinary output during surgery.
19. Allow patient to wear eyeglasses or a hearing aid as long as possible before surgery so that patient is able to sign consents and read materials. Remove contact lenses, eyeglasses, hairpieces, and dentures just before surgery (see checklist completed before surgery noting that all items are removed before proceeding to OR).	These aids facilitate patient cooperation by ensuring that patient has clear vision and maximal auditory perception throughout the preoperative phase.
20. Place cap over patient's head and hair.	Cap contains hair and minimizes OR contamination during surgery. Plastic or reflective caps reduce heat loss during surgery.
21. Place patient on bed rest with call light within reach and inform them not to get out of bed without help. Allow family members to remain at bedside until patient is transferred to surgical area. Maintain a quiet and relaxing environment.	There is an increased chance of injury when patient tries to ambulate to void when sedated and unattended.
22. Help patient onto stretcher for transport to OR.	Some ambulatory surgery patients walk to OR.

STEP	RATIONALE
EVALUATION	
1. Have patient describe surgical procedure and its benefits and risks.	Confirms level of knowledge needed to sign informed consent.
2. Have patient repeat preoperative instructions.	Provides evidence that patient understands instructions.
3. Monitor patient for signs and symptoms of anxiety, and ask how patient and family are feeling.	Increased heart rate and BP, dilated pupils, dry mouth, increased sweating, and muscle rigidity or shaking are responses to stress and anxiety. Asking patient about their feelings gives them permission to express concerns, which can be further explored.
4. Use teach-back: "I want to be sure you understand what will happen after your surgery. Tell me what you expect to happen once you get to the recovery room." Develop a revised teaching plan if patient is unable to teach back correctly.	Determines patient's level of understanding of instructional topic.

STEP	RATIONALE
Unexpected Outcomes	**Related Interventions**
1. Patient is unable to give consent, and family member is unavailable.	• In emergencies, obtain telephone consent from next of kin. Two people must witness oral consent (see employer policy). • Document explanation of situation and fact that oral consent was obtained and witnessed. • At earliest opportunity, person giving oral consent must sign written consent. A signed telegram or signed fax may also be considered oral consent. Follow employer policy.
2. Patient did not remain NPO, which may place them at risk for aspiration and may indicate that they did not understand instructions or forgot.	• Use interprofessional collaboration (e.g., surgeon, anaesthesiologist) to discuss food and fluid intake. Surgery may be postponed or cancelled.
3. Informed consent has not been signed and witnessed. Surgeon and anaesthesiologist did not provide information or ensure that consent forms were signed.	• Patient is not ready for surgery. Patient must sign consent before administration of preoperative medications or any medication that alters the central nervous system. Notify health care provider, surgeon, and anaesthesiologist.
4. Vital signs are above or below the patient's baseline or expected range.	• May indicate infection, pain, anxiety, or cardiovascular dysfunction. Notify surgeon and anaesthesiologist.
5. Patient did not void.	• Patient did not need to void or was unable to void. Assess for bladder distension.

Communication and Documentation

- Document preoperative physical preparation on preoperative checklist in EHR or chart.
- Document disposition of patient valuables and belongings (i.e., whether locked up according to employer policy or given to caregiver) in EHR or chart.
- Report lack of signed and witnessed consent form or failure of patient to maintain NPO status and action taken.
- Document your evaluation of patient and caregiver learning.

DOCUMENTATION EXAMPLE

Patient's preop checklist completed per employer policy. Preoperative medications given as prescribed by health care provider with no concerns noted by the patient. Patient is ready for the OR, vital signs stable and within normal limits, patient resting quietly while waiting to be brought to the OR at 1030 hours.

Special Considerations

Pediatric

- Give the child as many choices related to procedures as possible.
- Keep parent–child separation to the minimum time possible. When a parent or guardian cannot be present, it is important to leave a favourite possession with the child.
- Allow the parent or guardian to accompany their child to the surgery holding area.

Gerontological

- Some older persons may have cognitive, sensory, or physical impairments, and it may take an older person more time to dress for surgery and complete the needed physical preparation.

✦ SKILL 37.4 Providing Immediate Anaesthesia Recovery in the Postanaesthesia Care Unit

The first phase of postoperative care takes place during the immediate recovery period. This phase extends from the time the patient leaves the OR to the time the patient is stabilized in the postanaesthesia care unit (PACU), meets the discharge criteria, and is transferred to the nursing unit.

The first 1 to 2 hours are the most critical period for assessing the aftereffects of anaesthesia, including airway clearance, cardiovascular complications, temperature control, and neurological function (Table 37.3). A patient's condition can change rapidly; assessments must be timely, knowledgeable, and accurate. Nurses need to be aware of the common complications and problems associated with each type of anaesthesia (Table 37.4). Quick judgement regarding the most appropriate interventions is essential. A patient is usually ready for discharge to the general unit when specific standardized criteria are met. The Aldrete score is one of several scoring systems for assessment (Table 37.5). It uses parameters of activity, respiration, circulation, consciousness, and oxygen saturation. A score of 8 or less indicates that additional monitoring is required. A score of 10 indicates full recovery of the patient.

Recovery from ambulatory surgery requires the same assessments. However, the depth of general anaesthesia may be less because the surgery is less involved and of shorter duration. Some patients have only IV conscious sedation, and intensive monitoring is required for a shorter time period. As soon as the patient is stable and alert, the nurse needs to give instructions for care in the community to the patient and caregiver, including demonstrations and written instructions.

Delegation and Collaboration

The skill of initiating immediate anaesthesia recovery of a patient cannot be delegated to a UCP. The UCP may provide basic comfort and hygiene measures. The nurse instructs the UCP by doing the following:

- Explaining any restrictions for how to provide comfort measures (e.g., repositioning, turning, applying warming blanket)

TABLE 37.3

Postanaesthesia Monitoring and Management of Complications

Condition	Interventions
Airway	
Mechanical obstruction: Decreased LOC and muscle relaxants, resulting in flaccid muscles and tongue blocking airway	Hyperextend neck; pull mandible forward; use nasal or oral airway; encourage deep breathing.
Retained thick secretions: Irritation from anaesthesia; anticholinergic medications; history of smoking	Suction; encourage coughing.
Laryngospasm: Stridor from excessive secretions or airway irritation	Encourage patient to relax and breathe through the mouth. If extreme, it may require positive-pressure ventilation with oxygen, a small dose of muscle relaxant (prescribed by anaesthesiologist), and intubation.
Laryngeal edema: Allergic reaction, irritation from ET tube, fluid overload	Administer humidified oxygen, antihistamines, steroids, sedatives; in some cases, perform reintubation.
Bronchospasm: Pre-existing asthma, anaesthetic irritation (expiratory wheeze)	Administer bronchodilators as prescribed.
Aspiration: Vomiting from hypotension, accumulated gastric secretions and delayed gastric emptying, pain, fear, position changes	Position patient on side; suction airway; administer antiemetic as prescribed.
Breathing: Hypoventilation/Hypoxemia	
CNS depression: Anaesthesia, analgesics, muscle relaxants (respiratory rate shallow)	Encourage patient to cough and deep breathe; use mechanical ventilator; administer narcotic antagonist and muscle-relaxant reversal medication.
Mechanical restriction: Obesity, pain, tight cast or dressings, abdominal distension	Reposition patient; give analgesic; loosen cast or dressings; implement measures to reduce gastric distension (e.g., NG intubation, NG suction).
Circulation	
Hypovolemia: Blood loss, dehydration	Administer IV fluids or blood replacement.
Hypotension: Anaesthesia/medication effects, vasodilation (possibly from spinal anaesthesia), narcotics	Elevate patient's legs; give oxygen, IV fluids, or blood replacement; administer vasopressors; monitor I&O, stimulation, hemoglobin, and hematocrit.
Cardiac failure: Pre-existing cardiac disease; circulatory overload; excessive/too-rapid fluid replacement	Provide digitalization and diuretics; monitor ECG.
Cardiac arrhythmias: Hypoxemia; MI; hypothermia; imbalance of potassium, calcium, magnesium	Provide IV fluid replacement; monitor ECG and urine output; identify and treat cause.
Hypertension: Pain, distended bladder, pre-existing hypertension, vasopressor medications	Compare with preoperative baseline; identify and determine cause.
Compartment syndrome: Pressure from edema causing enough compression to obstruct arterial and venous circulation, resulting in ischemia, permanent numbness, loss of function; forearm and lower leg are most common sites	Obtain compartment pressures to diagnose, and elevate extremity no higher than heart level; remove or loosen bandage or cast to relieve compression; if left untreated, amputation may be required. Do not apply ice.

CNS, Central nervous system; *ECG,* electrocardiogram; *ET,* endotracheal; *I&O,* intake and output; *IV,* intravenous; *LOC,* level of consciousness; *MI,* myocardial infarction; *NG,* nasogastric.

TABLE 37.4

Focused Assessment of Patient Problems Related to Anaesthesia Type

Anaesthesia Type	Focused Assessment
General	Hypotension; changes in heart rate or rhythm; lowered body temperature; respiratory depression; emergence delirium in the form of shivering, trembling, confusion, or hallucinations
Spinal	Headache, hypotension, decreased cardiac output, cyanosis, difficulty breathing
Local	Skin rash; allergic reaction with edema of the face, lips, mouth, or throat; restlessness; bradycardia; hypotension; ischemic necrosis at injection site
Moderate sedation	Respiratory depression, bradycardia, hypotension, nausea and vomiting
Epidural	Cyanosis, breathing difficulties, decreased heart rate, irregular heart rate, pale skin colour, nausea and vomiting

Data from Lilley, L. L., Collins, S. R., & Snyder, J. S. (2020). *Pharmacology and the nursing process* (9th ed.). Mosby; Rothrock, J. C. (2019). *Alexander's care of the patient in surgery* (16th ed.). Mosby.

TABLE 37.5
Aldrete Score for Postanaesthesia Monitoring

Parameter	Description of Patient's Condition	Score
Respirations	Able to breathe deeply and cough freely	2
	Dyspnea or limited breathing	1
	Apneic	0
Oxygen saturation	Able to maintain O_2 saturation >92% on room air	2
	Requires supplemental O_2 to maintain SpO_2 >90%	1
	O_2 saturation <90% even with supplemental O_2	0
Circulation	BP ±20% of preoperative level	2
	BP ±20–50% of preoperative level	1
	BP ±50% of preoperative level	0
Consciousness	Awake and oriented	2
	Wakens with stimulation	1
	Not responding	0
Movement	Moves four limbs on own	2
	Moves two limbs on own	1
	Moves no limbs on own	0

BP, Blood pressure; *O_2,* oxygen; *SpO_2,* pulse oximetry.

From College of Physicians and Surgeons of British Columbia. (2018). *Accreditation standards patient care: Post-anesthesia care (Appendix D)*. https://www.cpsbc.ca/files/pdf/NHMSFAP-AS-Post-anesthesia-Care.pdf

- Offering instruction in providing needed supplies

NOTE: Other appropriate personnel may be allowed to do more in ambulatory surgery recovery, such as provide initial by-mouth (PO) liquids—always refer to employer policy.

Equipment

- Equipment for physical assessment
- Various types and sizes of artificial airways
- Constant and intermittent suction
- Oxygen equipment (e.g., mask, oxygen regulator, oxygen tubing, and positive-pressure delivery system)
- Pulse oximeter
- End-tidal carbon dioxide (CO_2) monitor
- BP monitoring equipment
- Adjustable lighting
- ECG monitor
- Arterial blood gas supplies
- Bladder scanner
- Bedside portable ultrasound to assess pulses
- Thermoregulation equipment, including thermometers, blanket warmers, and cooling blankets
- IV supplies (if prescribed) (see Chapter 29)
- Adult and pediatric emergency cart with defibrillator
- Stock supplies (e.g., facial tissues, dressings, bedpans, urinals, emesis basins)
- Personal protective equipment
- Latex-free supplies and equipment

STEP	RATIONALE

ASSESSMENT

Step	Rationale
1. Identify patient using at least two person-specific identifiers (e.g., name and date of birth, or name and medical record number) according to employer policy.	Ensures correct patient. Complies with Accreditation Canada's standards and improves patient safety (Accreditation Canada, 2020).
2. Throughout the procedure, the 4 moments for hand hygiene are to be implemented; hand hygiene should occur before initial patient (or patient environment) contact, before an aseptic procedure, after body fluid exposure risk, and after patient (or patient environment) contact. Additional hand hygiene should be performed when hands are visibly soiled.	Proper hand hygiene helps prevent the spread of infectious agents to health care providers.
3. Receive hand-off report from circulating nurse and anaesthesia provider, including procedure performed, range of vital signs, any complications, estimated blood loss (EBL), other fluid loss, fluid replacement during surgery, type of anaesthesia, medications given, type of airway and size, extent of surgical wound, restrictions to movement of position during surgery, and any preoperative medical and nursing diagnoses.	Determines patient's general status and allows nurse to anticipate type of assessment needed, the need for special equipment, potential treatment measures, and nursing care interventions in PACU.
4. On patient's arrival in PACU, review surgeon's prescriptions.	Allows nurse to focus on priority interventions; assists nurse in organizing care.
5. Consider type of surgical procedure, restrictions to movement, and type of anaesthesia used.	Influences type of assessments necessary, type of complications for which to observe, and specific nursing interventions needed.
6. Perform thorough patient assessment, including vital signs; pulse oximetry; pain; assessment of body systems to include (e.g., respiratory, cardiac, neurological, GI, genitourinary, and metabolic); and fluid status. Assess patient's surgical site and drains, skin integrity, safety, and anxiety level.	Reduces transmission of infection. Provides baseline for ongoing postoperative evaluations. Identifies priority nursing interventions.

STEP	RATIONALE

ASSESSMENT

STEP	RATIONALE
7. Take vital signs and monitor pulse oximetry during initial stabilization (ASPAN, 2023).	Monitors patient stability.
8. Discharge from phase I level of care is based on specific criteria, not a time limit. Criteria should address assessment of airway patency, oxygenation, hemodynamic stability, thermoregulation, neurological stability, intake and output (I&O), tube patency, dressings, pain and comfort management, and postanaesthesia scoring system, if used. See employer policy for required frequency of assessment.	Discharge instructions are developed in consultation with anaesthesia department.

Critical Decision Point *Be sure to turn patient on side (when possible) to observe underlying skin and accumulation of blood or serous drainage not otherwise visible.*

NURSING DIAGNOSES

- Inadequate airway clearance
- Inadequate breathing pattern
- Inadequate spontaneous ventilation
- Inadequate tissue perfusion
- Acute pain
- Inadequate gas exchange
- Inadequate swallowing
- Inadequate fluid volume
- Excessive fluid overload
- Inadequate thermoregulation
- Acute confusion
- Inadequate skin integrity
- Inadequate physical mobility
- Reduced verbal communication
- Inadequate protection
- Potential for aspiration
- Potential for urinary retention

Related factors and risk factors are individualized on the basis of patient's condition or needs.

PLANNING

STEP	RATIONALE
1. Expected outcomes following completion of procedure:	
• Patient's airway remains clear; respirations are deep, regular, and within normal limits by time of transfer. Oxygen saturation remains >95%.	No occurrence of pulmonary changes except those expected from effects of anaesthetic or analgesic.
• Patient's BP, pulse, and temperature remain within previous baseline or expected range by time of transfer.	No occurrence of cardiovascular, pulmonary, or thermoregulatory changes except those expected from effects of anaesthetic or analgesic.
• Dressings are clean, dry, and intact by time of discharge from recovery.	Indicates wound stabilization without signs of bleeding or infection.
• I&O is within expected parameters by time of discharge from recovery.	Adequate urinary elimination is maintained. Fluid intake (IV and/or PO) is adequately maintained.
• Patient reports relief of discomfort after receiving analgesia or other pain relief measures by time of transfer from immediate recovery area (usually 1–2 hours).	Pain relief measures effectively alter patient's reception or perception of pain.
• Patient's postoperative assessments are within expected normal postoperative parameters.	Patient is stable and may be prepared for the next phase of postoperative recovery.
2. Prepare equipment for continued monitoring and care activities.	Reduces transmission of infection.

IMPLEMENTATION

STEP	RATIONALE
1. While receiving hand-off report as patient enters PACU on stretcher or bed, immediately attach oxygen tubing to regulator, hang IV fluids, and check IV flow rates. Connect any drainage tubes to gravity drainage or continuous or intermittent suction as prescribed. Attach cardiac monitor. Ensure that in-dwelling catheter and bag are in drainage position and patent.	Maintaining oxygenation and circulation are two priorities. Inhaled oxygen improves the percentage of oxygen delivered to alveoli. IV fluids maintain circulatory volume and provide a route for emergency medications. Drainage tubes must remain patent and in proper position to allow fluid to drain.

STEP	RATIONALE

IMPLEMENTATION

STEP	RATIONALE
2. Continue ongoing assessment of all vital signs every 5–15 minutes until patient stabilizes or more frequently if clinically indicated (see employer protocol). Compare findings with patient's baseline. Provide warm blankets as needed for patient comfort.	Vital signs reveal onset of postoperative complications from surgery or anaesthesia (e.g., respiratory depression, hypothermia or hyperthermia, pulse irregularity, or hypotension). Acute blood loss may lead to hypovolemic shock; signs include reduced BP, elevated heart and respiratory rates, pale skin, and restlessness. General anaesthetic may affect the temperature-regulating centre, and a lower metabolic rate causes hypothermia. Malignant hyperthermia is a rare inherited condition that develops after patient receives an anaesthetic and is a medical emergency (Ebbitt et al., 2020).

Critical Decision Point *If the patient underwent a short procedure under procedural sedation, check employer policy for sedation recovery guidelines. The perianaesthesia registered nurse monitoring a patient who receives procedural sedation/analgesia should have no other responsibilities that compromise continuous patient monitoring. The nurse should monitor oxygenation until the patient is no longer at risk for hypoxemia. Ventilation and circulation are monitored at regular intervals until patients are suitable for discharge* (NAPANc, 2023).

STEP	RATIONALE
3. Maintain patent airway after general anaesthesia:	Ensures appropriate oxygenation.
a. Position patient on their side with head facing down and neck slightly extended (see Step 3a illustration). Never position a patient with hands over chest (reduces chest expansion).	Extension prevents occlusion of airway at the pharynx. Downward position of head moves the tongue forward, and mucus or vomitus can drain out of the mouth, preventing aspiration.

Critical Decision Point *Always stay with a sedated patient until respirations are well established. Patients with an artificial airway may gag and vomit, become restless, or stop breathing. Closely monitor patients with a history of OSA.*

STEP	RATIONALE
b. Place a small, folded towel or small pillow under the patient's head. If patient is restricted to a supine position, elevate head of bed approximately 10 to 15 degrees, extend patient's neck, and turn their head to the side. Have emesis basin available if patient becomes nauseated.	Supports head in extended position. Prevents aspiration if patient should vomit.

Critical Decision Point *If the patient is unable to extend their neck, turn their head to the side, if possible; suction the oropharynx* (see Chapter 23) *frequently.*

STEP	RATIONALE
c. Encourage patient to cough and deep breathe on awakening and every 15 minutes.	Promotes lung expansion and expectoration of mucous secretions.
d. Suction artificial airway and oral cavity as secretions accumulate.	Clears airway of secretions.
e. Once gag reflex returns, have patient spit out oral airway (see Step 3e illustration). Do not tape oral airway.	Indicates that patient can clear airway independently. If airway is taped, patient will gag and oral airway may obstruct airway.

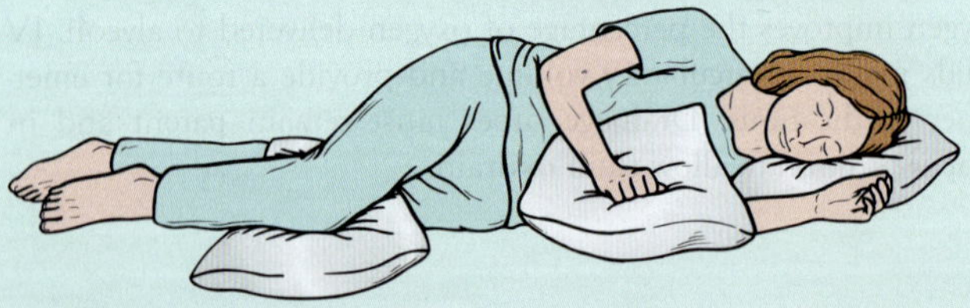

STEP 3A Position of patient during recovery from general anaesthesia.

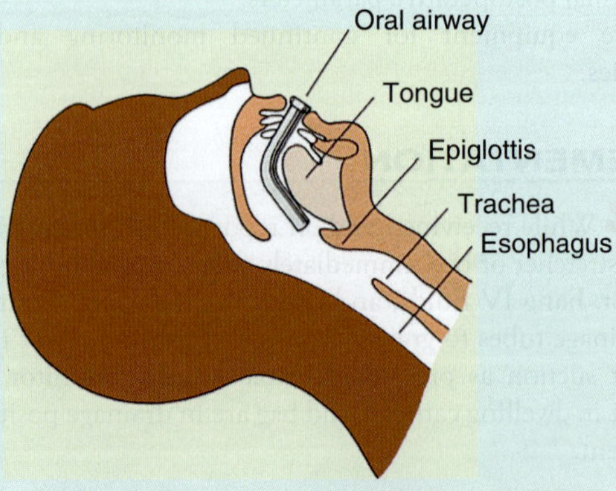

STEP 3E Oral airway position before removal.

STEP	RATIONALE
IMPLEMENTATION	
f. Avoid rapid position changes in patients who had spinal anaesthesia, as this may cause changes in patient's BP. Good body alignment is needed. Maintain IV infusion. Encourage fluid intake (only if patient can take fluids, such as with ambulatory surgery).	Rapid movements are avoided so as not to cause spinal headache from loss of cerebrospinal fluid. Increased IV or PO fluids help the body replace cerebrospinal fluid.

Critical Decision Point *Because of the shorter half-life of medications used today, many patients have the oral airway removed before leaving the OR. PACU nurse must assess that respiratory effort is adequate; otherwise, the airway may need to be replaced, and the patient may need a ventilator.*

STEP	RATIONALE
4. Call patient by name in a normal tone of voice. If there is no response, attempt to arouse patient by touching or gently moving a body part. Explain that surgery is over and that the patient is in the recovery area.	Determines patient's LOC and ability to follow commands.
5. Assess circulatory perfusion by inspecting colour of nail beds, mucous membranes, and skin. Palpate for skin temperature. Test for capillary refill (see Chapter 8).	Pink or normal colour of skin, nail beds, and mucous membranes and brisk (≤3 seconds) capillary refill indicate adequate perfusion. Warm extremities indicate adequate circulation.
6. Inspect colour of nail beds and skin. Palpate for skin temperature.	Indicators of peripheral tissue perfusion.
7. Assess closely for any behavioural or clinical changes reflecting potential cardiovascular and pulmonary complications of general anaesthesia (see Table 37.3). Monitor laboratory findings.	Postoperative patients who are sedated often become hypoxic.
8. *If patient had general anaesthesia:* As patient arouses, introduce yourself and orient them to surroundings.	
9. Monitor sensory, circulatory, pulmonary, and neurological responses after spinal or epidural anaesthesia:	Reflects return of spinal function.
a. Monitor for hypotension, bradycardia, and nausea and vomiting.	Blockage of the sympathetic nervous system results in vasodilation of major vessels and systemic hypotension.
b. Maintain adequate IV infusion.	Maintains BP by increasing fluid volume and fills temporarily expanded vascular space.
c. Keep patient supine or with head slightly elevated and maintain position.	Minimizes risk of postspinal anaesthesia headache from leakage of spinal fluid at injection site, with increased pressures caused by elevation of upper body. Headache is more common with spinal than epidural anaesthesia (Tyerman & Cobbett, 2023).
d. Observe patients in PACU until they regain movement in extremities.	Patients fear permanent loss of function.
e. Assess respiratory status, level of spinal sensation, and mobility in lower extremities. Drowsiness will be apparent after IV sedation. Level of anaesthesia depends on location of sensation change. Have patient close eyes and use alcohol wipe to test sensation along sensory dermatomes. Have patient identify whether warm or cold. *If patient had spinal anaesthesia:* Remind them that loss of extremity sensation and movement is normal and will return in several hours.	Spinal block is set within 20 minutes of onset. However, if level of anaesthesia moves above sixth thoracic vertebra (T6), respiratory muscles are affected. Patients often feel short of breath and may require mechanical ventilation if respiratory muscles are severely affected.
10. Monitor source of I&O.	
a. Observe dressing and drains for any evidence of bright red blood. Inspect surgical incision for swelling or discoloration. Note condition of surgical dressing, including amount, colour, odour, and consistency of drainage. Mark dressing with circle around drainage using a black pen. Place time of marking and check area every 10–15 minutes, marking any changes and noting vital signs.	Determines extent of fluid loss and condition of underlying wound. Size, location, and depth of wound influence amount of drainage.
b. Reinforce pressure dressing or change simple dressing, if prescribed (see Chapter 40). Continue to monitor condition of incision, surrounding tissue, and amount and colour of any drainage if incision is exposed or covered with transparent dressing.	Pressure dressing should not be removed because it helps maintain hemostasis (termination of bleeding) and absorb drainage. Changing dressings immediately after surgery can disrupt wound edges and aggravate drainage. The first dressing changes most often occur 24 hours after surgery and are usually done by the surgeon. Minor surgical wounds may not have dressings but simply skin closure; or wounds may be covered with a transparent dressing, which allows for observation of the incision and surrounding tissue (Lei et al., 2019).

STEP	RATIONALE

IMPLEMENTATION

STEP	RATIONALE
c. Inform surgeon of unexpected bloody drainage and reinforce dressing as indicated. Apply direct pressure. Also look underneath patient for any pooling of bloody drainage. Monitor for decreased BP and increased pulse.	Progressive increase or changes in characteristics of drainage warrant a call to the surgeon because they could indicate hemorrhage (Tyerman & Cobbett, 2023). Hemorrhage from a surgical wound is most likely within the first few hours, indicating inadequate hemostasis during surgery. As the dressing becomes saturated, blood often oozes down the patient's side and collects underneath them.
d. Inspect condition and contents of any drainage tubes and collecting devices. Note character and volume of drainage.	Determines patency of drainage tube and extent of wound drainage.
e. Observe amount, colour, and appearance of urine from in-dwelling Foley catheter (if present).	Urine output <30 mL/hr is a sign of decreased renal perfusion or altered renal function.
f. If a nasogastric (NG) tube is present, assess drainage. If NG tube is not draining, check placement and irrigate if necessary with normal saline (see Chapter 35).	Maintains patency of tube to ensure gastric decompression. Expected drainage is dark or pale, yellow, or green and 100–200 mL/hr. Bloody drainage occurs after some surgeries.
g. Monitor and maintain IV fluid rates. Observe IV site for signs of infiltration (see Chapter 29).	Provides adequate hydration and circulatory function.
11. Promote comfort:	
a. Provide mouth care by placing a moistened washcloth on lips, swabbing oral mucosa with a dampened swab or soft toothbrush, or applying petrolatum to lips.	The mouth is dry from NPO status and preoperative anticholinergics such as atropine.
b. Provide a warm blanket or active rewarming therapy to promote warmth and minimize shivering.	General anaesthesia impairs thermoregulation, OR environment is cold, and exposure of body cavity results in internal heat loss. Shivering increases oxygen consumption, predisposes patient to arrhythmias and hypertension, impairs platelet function, alters medication metabolism, impairs wound healing, and increases hospitalization costs because of cumulative adverse outcomes (NAPANc, 2023).
c. Help patient with position changes and provide supportive pillows.	Improves ventilation and circulation.
12. Continue monitoring pain (including quality, severity, and location) as patient awakens and until transfer to the surgical unit or discharge (see Chapter 16). Do not assume that all postoperative pain is incisional pain.	Pain is often not directly related to the surgical procedure (e.g., chest pain [myocardial infarction or pulmonary embolism] or muscle pain [trauma from positioning]). Referred pain (in shoulder) often occurs after laparoscopy. Systematic assessment of pain helps patients achieve functional status.
a. Provide pain medication as prescribed and when vital signs have stabilized.	Promotes patient comfort.
13. Explain patient's condition to patient, and inform them of plans for transfer to nursing unit or discharge.	Decreases anxiety, which can interfere with recovery process.
14. When patient's condition stabilizes, contact anaesthesiologist to approve care transition (i.e., transfer to nursing unit or discharge to home).	Surgeon is responsible for authorizing transfer or discharge.
15. Before discharge to home from an ambulatory surgery unit, provide verbal and written instructions (Box 37.1).	Patient and caregiver must be aware of potential complications and follow-up care.

Critical Decision Point *If the patient is to be discharged to home, ensure that the patient has someone to drive them home and observe them for signs and symptoms of complications. Review with the patient and driver reportable signs and symptoms and emergency care needed.*

BOX 37.1

Postanaesthesia and Ambulatory Surgery Discharge Criteria

Postanaesthesia Discharge Criteria

- Patient awake (or has returned to baseline)
- Vital signs stable
- No excess bleeding or drainage
- No respiratory depression
- Oxygen saturation (SaO_2) >90%
- Pain controlled
- Report given

Ambulatory Surgery Discharge Criteria

- All postanaesthesia care unit (PACU) discharge criteria met
- No intravenous (IV) narcotics for last 30 minutes
- Minimal nausea and vomiting
- Pain controlled
- Voided (if appropriate to surgical procedure/prescriptions)
- Able to ambulate if age appropriate and not contraindicated
- Responsible adult present to accompany patient
- Discharge instructions given and understood

STEP	RATIONALE
EVALUATION	
1. Compare all vital sign assessment measurements with patient's baseline and expected normal levels.	Evaluates patient's respiratory, cardiovascular, and thermoregulatory status throughout recovery.
2. Inspect surgical wound and dressings for drainage. Be sure to assess for wound drainage under patient.	Provides data to measure progress of wound healing.
3. Measure I&O. Urine output should be at least 30–50 mL/hr.	Indicates onset of fluid imbalances.
4. Auscultate bowel sounds and ask if patient has passed flatus.	Allows evaluation of return of peristalsis and diet tolerance.
5. Measure patient's perception of pain after implementing pain relief measures such as positioning and use of analgesics.	Determines level of comfort achieved and effectiveness of pain relief measures.
6. Complete system-specific physical assessments, as appropriate, according to patient's unique type of surgery (e.g., craniotomy: neurological assessment; neck surgery: airway status; vascular surgery: circulation and bleeding; orthopedic surgery: neurovascular status and immobility or positioning).	Allows monitoring of patient's course of recovery.
7. **Use teach-back:** "I want to be sure you know what to expect when you go home. Tell me the signs and symptoms to expect if you were to get an infection." Develop a revised teaching plan if patient or caregiver is unable to teach back correctly.	Determines patient's and caregiver's level of understanding of instructional topic.

Unexpected Outcomes	Related Interventions
1. Patient exhibits respiratory depression (pulse oximetry <95%, respiratory rate <10 breaths/min or shallow).	• Promptly report to surgeon. • Administer oxygen as prescribed by nasal cannula. Give patients with chronic obstructive pulmonary disease (COPD) ≤2 L/min of oxygen. • Encourage deep breathing every 5–15 minutes. • Position patient to promote chest expansion (on side or in semi-Fowler's). • Administer prescribed medications (e.g., epinephrine, muscle relaxant, narcotic reversal medication).

2. Patient exhibits signs of hypovolemia related to internal or incisional hemorrhage.	• Elevate patient's legs enough to maintain downward slope toward trunk of body. Do not lower head past flat position because this position increases respiratory effort and potentially decreases cerebral perfusion.
	• Promptly report patient's present status to surgeon.
	• Administer oxygen at 6–10 L/min by mask per prescription.
	• Increase rate of IV fluid or administer blood products as prescribed.
	• Monitor BP and pulse every 5–15 minutes.
	• Apply pressure dressings as follows, per prescription:
	  • *Abdominal dressing:* Cover bleeding area with several thicknesses of gauze compresses, and place tape 7–10 cm (3–4 inches) beyond width of dressing with firm, applying even pressure on both sides close to the bleeding source. Maintain pressure as you tape the entire dressing to maximize pressure at source of bleeding.
	  • *Dressing on extremity:* Apply rolled gauze, pressing gauze compress over bleeding site. Do not continue tape around entire extremity, only covering the bleeding site.
	  • *Dressing in neck region:* Cover with several thicknesses of gauze, and place tape 7–10 cm (3–4 inches) beyond width of dressing. Apply with pressure, but do not occlude carotid artery or airway. Assess every 5–15 minutes for carotid pulse and evidence of airway obstruction.
	• Patient remains NPO because it is often necessary to return to surgery to control bleeding.

STEP	RATIONALE
Unexpected Outcomes	**Related Interventions**
3. Patient indicates severe incisional pain; analgesic dosage may be insufficient.	• Administer analgesics; reassess and provide analgesia before pain becomes severe. • Pain sometimes lowers BP; analgesia may restore vital signs to normal. Monitor vital signs carefully. • For patients with PCA, be sure that patient is using device correctly. Teach caregiver not to manipulate PCA. • *Orthopedic surgery:* The earliest symptom of compartment syndrome in an extremity is pain unrelieved by analgesics. Other symptoms include numbness, tingling, pallor, coolness, and absent peripheral pulses. The surgeon must be notified. Do not elevate extremity above level of the heart because this increases venous pressure. Application of ice is contraindicated because vasoconstriction will occur (Tyerman & Cobbett, 2023).
4. Vital signs are above or below the patient's baseline or expected range.	• Alterations may result from anaesthetic effects. Ensure patient is fully awake. • Medicate for pain as indicated. • Notify health care provider.
5. I&O measurements are imbalanced.	• Possible fluid volume excess or deficit. Continue to monitor and notify health care provider.

Communication and Documentation

- Document in progress notes in EHR or chart patient's arrival time at PACU; include vital signs and other physical parameters, LOC, and pain severity. Also include condition of dressings and tubes, character of drainage, and all nursing measures initiated.
- Document vital signs and I&O on appropriate flow sheets.
- Report any abnormal assessment findings and signs of complications to the health care provider and/or surgeon.
- Document your evaluation of patient and caregiver learning.

DOCUMENTATION EXAMPLE

Patient states they have pain; crying and holding their incision. Pain assessment complete, pain ranked as a 7 out of 10 by the patient. PRN morphine IV 5 mg SUBCUT administered as prescribed. Patient reminded of splinting their incision. Patient was helped to change position in the bed and states they are comfortable.

Special Considerations

Teaching

- If patient had spinal or epidural anaesthetic, remind caregiver that loss of extremity movement for several hours is normal.
- Reinforce preoperative teaching regarding coughing, deep breathing, leg exercises, and information concerning ambulation and pain control.
- Patient teaching for ambulatory surgical patients includes the following:
  - Surgeon's office and surgery centre telephone number (or appropriate 24-hour emergency contact)
  - Follow-up appointment date and time
  - Review of prescribed medications
  - Guidelines related to specific surgery
  - Dressing and wound care
  - Pain control
  - Activity restrictions
  - Guidelines related to possible effects of anaesthesia
  - Dietary restrictions
  - Activity restrictions
  - Signs and symptoms of complications

Pediatric

- Maintenance of body temperature in infants and children after surgery is a priority because of their immature temperature-control mechanisms.
- Infants and children normally have higher metabolic rates and other differences in physiological makeup compared with adults, resulting in greater oxygen, fluid, and calorie needs.
- Vomiting is a major concern in young children because of increased risk of fluid and electrolyte imbalances and risk of aspiration. Vomiting is also more likely because surgery in children is often necessitated by accidental injuries without benefit of NPO status.
- Keep parent–child separation to a minimum. If parent or guardian cannot be present, leave a favourite possession with the child.
- Refer to NAPANc (2023), PeriAnesthesia Care of the Pediatric Client.

Gerontological

- The ability of older persons to tolerate surgery depends on the extent of physiological changes that have occurred with aging, the presence of any chronic diseases, and the duration of the surgical procedure.
- When communicating with older persons, be aware of any auditory, visual, or cognitive impairment that may be present.
- Refer to NAPANc (2023): Alterations of Aging Clients and Effect of Anesthesia on Geriatric Response.

Care in the Community: Home Management

- Teach ambulatory surgery patients and caregivers about any postoperative exercises, home modifications, or activity limitations.
- If the patient is discharged with dressing changes, suggest that the bedroom or bathroom is usually ideal for this procedure.
- Be informed as to which supports and services are available in the community where the patient lives, and provide the patient with a list of these services or information on how to access a list of available services in their community.
- Assess need for a community health care referral. Check provincial/territorial regulations to determine who is eligible to receive care in the community and what services community care nurses can provide in the patient's home.

✦ SKILL 37.5 Providing Early Postoperative and Convalescent-Phase Recovery

The second phase of recovery is the postoperative convalescent period. The American Society of PeriAnesthesia Nurses (ASPAN) defines the phase II level of care as the period when nursing roles focus on preparation for care in the home or an extended-care environment. This period extends from the time a patient is discharged from the PACU to the time they are discharged from the inpatient hospital. Outpatient surgical patients undergo convalescence at home. All patients who have undergone surgical procedures have similar postoperative needs. However, nursing care becomes very individualized and depends on the nature of a patient's surgery, pre-existing medical conditions, the onset of complications, and the speed of recovery. Not all surgical patients recover at the same rate. During the convalescent period, the nurse begins preparation for discharge and actively includes the patient and caregivers in the process. The nurse promotes the patient's independence, educates the patient and caregiver about any limitations imposed by surgery, and provides resources needed for the patient to assume an improved state of wellness.

Delegation and Collaboration

The skill of providing early postoperative and convalescent-phase recovery cannot be delegated to a UCP. The UCP may obtain vital signs (if the patient is stable), apply a nasal cannula or oxygen mask (but not adjust oxygen flow), and provide hygiene or repositioning for comfort. The nurse instructs the UCP by doing the following:

- Explaining how often to take vital signs
- Reviewing specific safety concerns and what to observe and report back to the nurse
- Explaining any precautions that affect how to provide basic hygiene and comfort measures

Equipment

- Postoperative bed (recliner for day surgery recovery)
- Stethoscope, sphygmomanometer, thermometer
- IV fluid poles and infusion pumps, as needed
- Emesis basin
- Washcloth and towel
- Waterproof pads
- Equipment for oral hygiene
- Pillows
- Facial tissue
- Oxygen equipment, bag–valve masks, and emergency cart with defibrillator for adults and children
- Suction equipment (to suction airway)
- Dressing supplies
- Intermittent suction (to connect to NG tube or wound drainage tubes)
- Orthopedic appliances (if needed)
- Clean gloves
- Personal protective equipment (PPE) as indicated
- Malignant hyperthermia cart (Ebbitt et al., 2020)
- Latex-free supplies and equipment
- Transport equipment, including wheelchair and cart

STEP	RATIONALE
ASSESSMENT	
1. Identify patient using at least two person-specific identifiers (e.g., name and date of birth, or name and medical record number) according to employer policy.	Ensures correct patient. Complies with Accreditation Canada's standards and improves patient safety (Accreditation Canada, 2020).
2. Throughout the procedure, the 4 moments for hand hygiene are to be implemented; hand hygiene should occur before initial patient (or patient environment) contact, before an aseptic procedure, after body fluid exposure risk, and after patient (or patient environment) contact. Additional hand hygiene should be performed when hands are visibly soiled.	Proper hand hygiene helps prevent the spread of infectious agents to health care providers.
3. Obtain report from PACU nurse summarizing patient's current status.	Allows nurse to prepare hospital room with necessary supplies and equipment for patient's specific needs.
4. On patient's arrival on nursing unit, collect a more detailed hand-off report from nurse accompanying patient.	Detailed report helps nurse plan appropriate assessment and nursing care measures. Data provide baseline for detecting any change in patient's condition.
5. Review patient's chart for information pertaining to type of surgery; complications; medications administered; preoperative medical risks; baseline vital signs, including PACU vitals; and patient's usual medications given or not given before surgery.	Nature of surgery, intraoperative complications, and presence of medical risks dictate complications to observe for. Vital signs provide means for detecting postoperative changes. The list of patient's usual medications may necessitate a call to the surgeon for prescriptions concerning timing and dose of medications not given before surgery.
6. Review postoperative medical prescriptions.	Offers additional guidelines for type of care to provide.
7. Assess patient's and caregiver's knowledge and expectations of surgical recovery.	Patient will be better prepared to participate in care.

STEP	RATIONALE

NURSING DIAGNOSES

- Reduced airway clearance
- Inadequate breathing pattern
- Reduced gas exchange
- Inadequate tissue perfusion
- Acute confusion
- Acute pain
- Dehydration
- Excessive fluid overload
- Inadequate knowledge regarding postoperative care
- Inadequate nutrition
- Inadequate physical mobility
- Reduced skin integrity
- Reduced verbal communication
- Inadequate protection
- Potential of aspiration
- Potential of urinary retention

Related factors and risk factors are individualized on the basis of patient's condition or needs.

PLANNING

STEP	RATIONALE
1. Expected outcomes following completion of procedure:	
• Patient's breath sounds remain clear bilaterally.	No occurrence of pulmonary changes except those expected from effects of anaesthetic or analgesic.
• Patient's vital signs remain within normal limits, consistent with preoperative baseline.	No occurrence of cardiovascular, pulmonary, or thermoregulatory changes except those expected from effects of anaesthetic or analgesic.
• Incision wound edges are well approximated; no drainage is noted.	Indicates wound healing without signs of bleeding or infection.
• Fluid balance is evident by I&O records.	Adequate urinary elimination is maintained. Fluid intake (IV and/or PO) is adequately maintained.
• Patient describes pain as <4 on a scale of 0 (no pain) to 10 (worst pain ever) while engaged in moderate activity by time of discharge.	Pain relief measures effectively alter patient's reception or perception of pain.
• Normal bowel sounds are present after bowel surgery or general anaesthesia within 48–72 hours after surgery.	Indicates return of GI function.
• Patient or caregiver describes signs indicating complications that need to be reported, dietary modifications, and activity restrictions in the home. Identifies plans for follow-up visit and demonstrates incision care.	Involves patient in plan of care and minimizes anxiety. As recovery progresses, the patient is able to make more choices regarding how procedures should be performed. Caregiver can serve as a coach or provide direct assistance and help the patient remember explanations given.
2. Arrange equipment at bedside.	Reduces transmission of infection. Improves efficiency of care activity.
3. If patient is being transported by stretcher, prepare for transfer with bed in a high position (level with stretcher), with sheet folded to side and room for stretcher to be placed beside bed easily (see Chapter 11).	Arrangement of equipment facilitates safe and smooth transfer process.

IMPLEMENTATION

STEP	RATIONALE
1. Early initial postoperative care:	
a. Help transport staff, using slide board, to move patient from stretcher to bed (see Chapter 11).	Ensures proper body mechanics.
b. Attach any existing oxygen tubing, position IV fluids, verify IV flow-rate settings on infusion pump, and check drainage tubes (e.g., Foley catheter or wound drainage).	Maintains patency of IV and integrity of drainage tubing.
c. Maintain airway. If patient remains sleepy or lethargic, keep their head extended and support it in a side-lying position (see Chapter 23).	Minimizes chances of aspiration and obstruction of airway with tongue.
d. Conduct initial assessment of LOC and vital signs, and compare findings with vital signs in recovery area and patient's baseline values. Continue monitoring as prescribed.	Patient's status may change during transfer. Movement of patient and their pain level influence stability of vital signs. Change in vital signs may reveal onset of postoperative complications.
e. Encourage patient coughing, deep breathing, and use of incentive spirometry and PEP device (see Skill 37.2) to prevent atelectasis.	Anaesthesia, medications, and intubation irritate airways, resulting in secretions and atelectasis. Coughing and use of devices expands chest, aerates lungs, and mobilizes secretions.
f. Assess GI system for return of bowel sounds.	Indicates return of GI function.
g. If NG tube is present, check placement and irrigate (see Chapter 35). Connect to a proper drainage device. Connect all other drainage tubes to an appropriate suction or collection device. Secure tube to prevent tension on tubing.	Transfer and movement may dislodge tubes, which would interfere with drainage.

STEP	RATIONALE
IMPLEMENTATION	
h. Assess patient's surgical dressing for appearance, presence, and character of drainage. Unless contraindicated by surgeon, outline drainage along edges with a pen and reassess in 1 hour for change. If no dressing is present, inspect condition of the wound (see Chapter 40).	The wound can hemorrhage quickly during the early postoperative period. Observations of wound and dressings provide data to measure progress of wound healing.

Critical Decision Point *If unable to change dressing, mark area of drainage and label with time, date, and initials. Record frequency of reinforcement. Never use a felt-tip marker to mark the dressing because ink can bleed into gauze, contaminating the incision site.*

STEP	RATIONALE
i. Palpate abdomen for bladder distension or use bladder ultrasound when available. If a Foley catheter is present, check placement. Ensure that catheter is draining freely and properly secured. Patient may have continuous bladder irrigations or a suprapubic catheter (see Chapter 34).	Anaesthesia often contributes to urinary retention. Urinary stasis increases risk of a urinary tract infection (UTI).
j. If no urinary drainage system is present, explain that voiding within 8 hours after surgery is expected. Male patients may void successfully if allowed to stand.	Anaesthetics and analgesics depress the sensation of bladder fullness. The patient may still have no sensations below the level of spinal or epidural anaesthetic.
k. Measure all sources of fluid I&O (including estimated blood loss during surgery).	Altered fluid and electrolyte balance is a potential complication of major surgery.
l. Describe purpose of equipment and frequent observations to patient and caregiver.	Unfamiliar sights (e.g., equipment, patient's appearance) often provoke anxiety.
m. Position patient for comfort, maintaining correct body alignment. Avoid tension on surgical wound site.	Reduces stress on suture line. Helps patient relax and promotes comfort.
n. Place call light within reach and raise side rails (one of two or three of four). Instruct patient to call for help to get out of bed.	Promotes patient's safety as effects of anaesthesia continue to diminish. Raising all side rails may be considered physical restraint.
o. Assess patient's level of pain on an age-appropriate pain scale. Check last time analgesic was given. PCA may be used for pain control (see Chapter 16). Medicate patient as prescribed, either around the clock or as needed (prn), during the first 24–48 hours. Explain to patient how you plan to assist with pain control; review medications prescribed and their frequency.	Determines level of discomfort. Adequate pain control is needed to enable patient to carry out breathing exercises, coughing, and ambulation.
2. Continued postoperative care:	
a. Assess vital signs at least every 4 hours or as prescribed.	Temperature >38°C (100.4°F) in the first 48 hours may indicate atelectasis, the normal inflammatory response, or dehydration. A temperature >37.8°C (100°F) on the third day or after often indicates wound infection, pneumonia, or phlebitis (Tyerman & Cobbett, 2023). Altered BP or pulse is associated with cardiovascular complications (see Table 37.3).
b. Closely monitor progress of wound healing and change dressings as prescribed.	Wound infection occurs most often within 3–6 days after surgery. Wound dehiscence occurs most often 3–11 days after surgery (see Chapter 40).
c. Monitor drainage (see Step 2c, illustration A) and maintain wound drainage devices such as Jackson-Pratt, Hemovac, or Penrose drains. Jackson-Pratt and Hemovac drainage systems must be emptied when they are half full of drainage or air and recharged (compressed to discharge air) (see Step 2c, illustration B).	Wound drainage devices promote healing from inside to outside and relieve pressure on suture line. Compressing flexible closed container and then plugging drainage hole creates negative suction pressure.

STEP	RATIONALE

IMPLEMENTATION

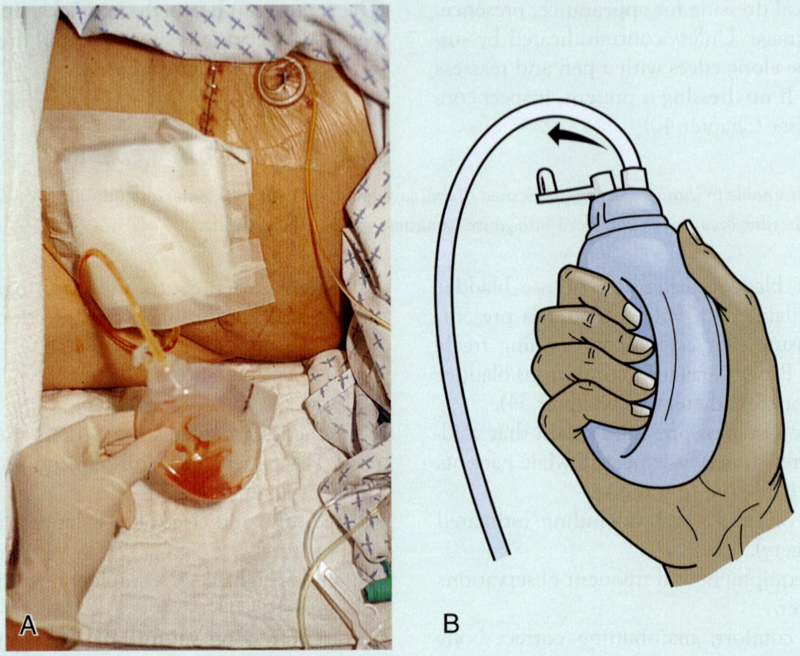

STEP 2C A, Note colour of drainage from device. B, Charging Jackson-Pratt drainage system.

STEP	RATIONALE
d. Provide oral care at least every 2 hours as needed. If permitted, offer ice chips.	Medication such as an anticholinergic given before surgery makes the mouth dry. Oral care and ice chips promote comfort.
e. Encourage patient to turn, cough, deep breathe, and use incentive spirometer and PEP device at least every 2 hours (see Skill 37.2).	Promotes adequate ventilation and minimizes hypoventilation and atelectasis. This is especially necessary for patients with a history of smoking, pneumonia, or COPD or for patients who are confined to bed rest.
f. Monitor function of sequential compression devices. If prescribed, apply elastic stockings to lower extremities (see Chapter 12). Explain to patient that compression device will inflate and deflate intermittently.	Stockings increase venous return (Liu & Cheng, 2021). Explanation decreases anxiety and fosters cooperation.
g. Promote ambulation and activity as prescribed (see Chapter 12). Assess vital signs before and after activity to assess tolerance. Patients often are encouraged to be up in a chair the evening of surgery or the next morning and progress to walking in the room or hallway.	Ambulation is the most significant nursing intervention to prevent postoperative complications. Mobility promotes circulation, lung expansion, and peristalsis. Postural hypotension is caused by sudden position changes.
h. Progress patient's intake from clear liquids to regular diet as tolerated if nausea and vomiting do not occur.	Nausea and vomiting are associated with anaesthesia and surgery. IV fluids are usually discontinued when oral intake is tolerated. Some patients must be NPO for several days until flatus returns or bowel sounds are heard.
i. Include patient and caregiver in decision making; answer questions as they arise.	Promotes patient's sense of control and independence and improves self-esteem.
j. Provide an opportunity for patients who must adjust to change in body appearance or function to verbalize their feelings.	Radical surgery, amputation, or inoperable cancer often results in anxiety and depression. Grief response to loss of a body organ is common and should be expected.

STEP	RATIONALE
IMPLEMENTATION	
3. Convalescent phase:	
a. Assess patient's home environment for safety, cleanliness, and availability of community resources and help for patient. (NOTE: In many settings, this is done by a case manager and not a staff nurse. Use the information to revise any teaching you provide.)	Provides information about patient's need for care in the community. Verifies patient's and caregiver's level of knowledge and any additional teaching needs for discharge. Helps promote uncomplicated discharge and patient's independence and participation in care.
b. Provide instruction on care activities that patient or caregiver will perform at home (e.g., dressing change, medication administration, exercises, IV therapy).	Enables patient to achieve self-care at home.
c. Keep patient and caregiver informed of progress made toward recovery, including when patient can expect to be discharged from hospital. Provide answers to individual patient questions or concerns.	Decreases anxiety and helps patient know what to anticipate. Encourages participation in discharge planning.

EVALUATION

1. Auscultate breath sounds bilaterally.	Determines status of airways.
2. Monitor trends in vital signs.	Provides data to measure progress of postoperative status.
3. Evaluate I&O records. Assess time of patient's first postoperative urination.	Indicates onset of urination.
4. Auscultate bowel sounds.	Evaluates return of peristalsis and diet tolerance.
5. Ask patient to describe pain on a scale of 0 (no pain) to 10 (worst pain ever) after moderate activity.	Determines level of comfort achieved and effectiveness of pain relief measures.
6. Inspect incision (wound edges are well approximated, no drainage noted).	Provides data to measure progress of wound healing.
7. Have patient or caregiver describe incision care, dietary modifications or restrictions, activity restrictions, medication schedule, and plans for follow-up visit.	Identifies need for further teaching.
8. **Use teach-back:** "I want to be sure I explained what you need to know about your activity level after surgery. In your own words, tell me how you will be more active after your surgery." Develop a revised teaching plan if patient is unable to teach back correctly.	Determines patient's level of understanding of instructional topic.

Unexpected Outcomes	Related Interventions
1. Vital signs are above or below patient's baseline or expected range. Initially, this could be related to anaesthesia effects, pain, hypovolemic shock, airway obstruction, fluid and electrolyte imbalance, or hypothermia.	• Identify contributing factors. • Notify surgeon.
2. Patient indicates severe incisional pain.	• Report to surgeon; discuss alternative analgesic option. • Try nonpharmacological pain control measures (see Chapter 16).

Communication and Documentation

- Document patient's arrival at the nursing unit, vital signs, assessment findings, and all nursing measures initiated in progress notes in EHR or chart.
- Continue to document these factors every 4 hours or more frequently as patient's condition warrants.
- Document vital signs and I&O on appropriate flow sheet.
- Report any abnormal assessment findings and signs of complications to surgeon.
- Document your evaluation of patient and caregiver learning.

Special Considerations

Teaching

- Instruct patient and caregiver to identify signs and symptoms and appropriate actions to take for infection, respiratory, circulatory, or GI difficulties and wound disruptions.
- Provide important phone numbers to patient and caregiver for use in emergency and follow-up care on discharge.
- Teach patient about appropriate wound care, dietary recommendations, and activity restrictions.

Pediatric

- Assessment of a child's perceptions of the surgical experience includes reinforcement of positive experiences and clarification of misconceptions. Drawing and storytelling are effective methods that allow children to share their thoughts and feelings (Keenan-Lindsay et al., 2022).
- Infants and children normally have higher metabolic rates and differences in physiological makeup compared with adults, resulting in greater oxygen, fluid, and calorie needs. Vomiting is a concern because of increased risk of fluid and electrolyte imbalances and risk of aspiration.
- Use an appropriate pain assessment tool to determine the child's pain level.

Gerontological

- Older persons often experience a longer and more difficult postoperative recovery. Assess carefully for the development of postoperative complications.
- Assess for postoperative delirium and changes in mental status along with potential causes.
- Older persons may not request pain medication because they believe it should be tolerated as an expected effect of surgery (Tyerman & Cobbett, 2023).

Care in the Community: Home Management

- Teach the patient and caregiver about postoperative exercises, home modifications, activity limitations, wound dressing care, medications, and nutritional needs.
- If the patient is discharged with dressing changes, the bedroom or bathroom is usually ideal for the procedure. Have the patient and caregiver perform return demonstration of dressing change.
- Make referral to community care services if patient and caregiver will have difficulty providing the expected level of care needed.
- If the patient is having surgery in an ambulatory surgery centre, they must be accompanied by another person to allow for discharge after the procedure (see Box 37.1).

✦ REVIEW QUESTIONS

The nurse is assigned to care for a 52-year-old patient (she/her) who is 152 cm (5 feet) tall and weighs 113.4 kg (250 lb). The patient is married with three adult children and is employed as an attorney. The nurse just received the patient from the postanaesthesia care unit (PACU) following an abdominal hysterectomy for fibroid tumours and a bladder neck suspension. Her previous medical history includes 30 years of two-pack-per-day cigarette smoking and type 2 diabetes mellitus, and she has been on birth control pills for 20 years. She has an abdominal dressing that has a small amount of shadowing on it, is on oxygen at 2 L/min via nasal cannula, and has both a Foley catheter and a suprapubic catheter draining pink-tinged urine. She has an intravenous (IV) infusion of D_5 0.5% normal saline (NS) infusing at 125 mL/hr and a morphine patient-controlled analgesia (PCA) device. She received cefazolin IV piggyback approximately 45 minutes before her incision was made and is to receive her second dose 8 hours later.

Review Questions 1 to 3 relate to the case study presented here.

1. Which postoperative complications is this patient at risk of developing, and what are the nursing implications? Provide the rationale.
2. What postoperative teaching should the patient receive, and who should be included in the teaching?
3. On postoperative day 2, the patient appears anxious and has a pulse oxygenation of 82%. On assessment, her left lung sounds are diminished when compared with the right lung. She also indicates that her left leg is painful and swollen. Using SBAR (situation–background–assessment–recommendation), show how the nurse would communicate with the health care team about this patient.
4. Prevention of surgical site infections (SSIs) requires numerous actions by both the surgical team and the patient. Which of the following measures are used to reduce SSIs? (*Select all that apply.*)
   1. Discharge patient from the hospital as soon as possible.
   2. Give prophylactic antibiotic therapy as close to the time of incision as possible.
   3. Shave excess hair with a razor just before the surgery begins.
   4. Control hyperglycemia in patients with and without diabetes.
   5. Give a shower or bath after the preoperative enema is evacuated.
5. There are numerous measures to prevent venous thromboembolism (VTE) during the postoperative period. Which of the following interventions are most appropriate before the surgery begins? (*Select all that apply.*)
   1. Performing an assessment for Homans' sign
   2. Ensuring that bilateral lower-extremity sequential compression devices are on and functioning
   3. Teaching coughing and breathing techniques to patient
   4. Instructing patient how to ambulate after surgery
   5. Teaching patient how to do leg exercises
6. Which assignment would the nurse delegate to an unregulated care provider (UCP)? (*Select all that apply.*)
   1. Managing the postoperative care of the patient
   2. Initial assessments on arrival to the postanaesthesia care unit (PACU)
   3. Emptying the Foley catheter
   4. Caring for the patient by monitoring and providing comfort measures
   5. Assessing the intravenous site

Visit the Evolve site for a complete list of answers to the Review Questions.

✦ NEXT GENERATION NCLEX® (NGN)

For practice with answering exam questions related to unfolding NGN case studies, please consult the Next Generation NCLEX® (NGN)-Style Case Studies for Skills and Techniques on the Evolve website: http://evolve.elsevier.com/Canada/Perry/clinicalskills/

REFERENCES

Accreditation Canada. (2020). *Required organizational practices–2020 handbook*. https://physicians.nshealth.ca/resources/required-organizational-practices-2020-handbook

Al-Nasser, B. (2020). Influence of tobacco smoking on perioperative risk of venous thromboembolism. *Turkish Journal of Anaesthesiology and Reanimation*, 48(1), Article 11. https://doi.org/10.5152/TJAR.2019.08683

American Society of PeriAnesthesia Nurses. (2023). *2023–2024 perianesthesia nursing standards, practice recommendations, and interpretive statements*. https://www.aspan.org/Publications-Resources/ASPAN-Publications/ASPAN-Standards

Arnold, E. C., & Boggs, K. U. (2019). *Interpersonal relationships: Professional communication skills for nurses* (8th ed.). Saunders.

Association of periOperative Registered Nurses. (2023). *Guidelines for perioperative practice*. https://www.aorn.org/guidelines-resources/guidelines-for-perioperative-practice

Bombard, Y., Baker, G. R., Orlando, E., et al. (2018). Engaging patients to improve quality of care: A systematic review. *Implementation Science*, *13*, Article 98. https://doi.org/10.1186/s13012-018-0784-z

Boscart, V., McCleary, L., Sheiban Taucar, L., et al. (2023). *Ebersole and Hess' gerontological nursing and healthy aging in Canada* (3rd ed.). Elsevier.

Canadian Medical Protective Association. (n.d.). *Good practices*. https://www.cmpa-acpm.ca/en/education-events/good-practices

Canadian Nurses Protective Society. (2018). *InfoLAW: Consent to treatment: The role of the nurse*. https://cnps.ca/article/consent-to-treatment/

Centers for Disease Control and Prevention. (2019). *Guidelines for environmental infection control in health care facilities*. https://www.cdc.gov/infectioncontrol/pdf/guidelines/environmental-guidelines-P.pdf

Dobson, G., Chau, A., Denomme, J., et al. (2023). Guidelines to the practice of anesthesia: Revised edition 2023. *Canadian Journal of Anesthesia*, *70*(1), 16–55. https://doi.org/10.1007/s12630-022-02368-0

Ebbitt, L., Johnson, E., Herndon, B., et al. (2020). Suspected malignant hyperthermia and the application of a multidisciplinary response. *Healthcare*, *8*(3), Article 328. https://doi.org/10.3390/healthcare8030328

Egholm, J. W., Pedersen, B., Møller, A. M., et al. (2018). Perioperative alcohol cessation intervention for postoperative complications. *Cochrane Database of Systematic Reviews*, *2018*(11), Article CD008343. https://doi.org/10.1002/14651858.CD008343.pub3

Gumidyala, R., & Selzer, A. (2022). Preoperative optimization of obstructive sleep apnea. *International Anesthesiology Clinics*, *60*(1), 24–32. https://doi.org/10.1097/AIA.0000000000000353

Healthcare Excellence Canada. (2016). *The Canadian surgical site infection prevention audit–results*. https://www.patientsafetyinstitute.ca/en/toolsResources/SSI-Audit-2016/Pages/default.aspx [Seminal Reference]

Hewlett, A. L., Hohenberger, H., Murphy, C. N., et al. (2018). Evaluation of the bacterial burden of gel nails, standard nail polish, and natural nails on the hands of health care workers. *American Journal of Infection Control*, *46*(12), 1356–1359. https://doi.org/10.1016/j.ajic.2018.05.022

The Joint Commission. (2023). *Hospital: 2023 national patient safety goals*. https://www.jointcommission.org/standards/national-patient-safety-goals/hospital-national-patient-safety-goals/

Keenan-Lindsay, L., Sams, C. A., & O'Connor, C. L. (2022). *Perry's maternal child nursing care in Canada* (3rd ed.). Elsevier.

Lei, J., Sun, L., Li, P., et al. (2019). The wound dressings and their applications in wound healing and management. *Health Science Journal*, *13*(4), Article 662. https://www.itmedicalteam.pl/articles/the-wound-dressings-and-their-applications-in-wound-healing-and-management-106117.html

Liu, H., & Cheng, L. (2021). Study on the wearing performance of compression stockings and its influence on the blood flow velocity of lower limbs. *E3S Web of Conferences*, *237*, Article 04037. https://doi.org/10.1051/e3sconf/202123704037

McCubbin, K. D., Anholt, R. M., de Jong, E., et al. (2021). Knowledge gaps in the understanding of antimicrobial resistance in Canada. *Frontiers in Public Health*, *9*, Article 1523. https://doi.org/10.3389/fpubh.2021.726484

Mitri, A., Lin, G., Waldman, R. A., & Grant-Kels, J. M. (2021). Effects of tobacco and vaping on the skin. *Clinics in Dermatology*, *39*(5), 762–771. https://doi.org/10.1016/j.clindermatol.2021.05.004

National Association of PeriAnesthesia Nurses of Canada (NAPANc). (2023). *Standards for practice* (5th ed.). http://napanc.ca/index.php/standards

Operating Room Nurses Association of Canada. (2023). *The ORNAC standards, guidelines, and position statements for perioperative registered nurses* (16th ed.). https://www.ornac.ca/en/standards

Public Health Agency of Canada. (2018). *Evaluation of healthcare-associated infection activities at the public health agency of Canada 2012–13 to 2016–17*. https://www.canada.ca/en/public-health/corporate/transparency/corporate-management-reporting/evaluation/healthcare-associated-infection-activities-2012-2017.html

Schwartsmann, C. R., Binz, M. A. R., Ferreira, M. T., et al. (2019). Clinical, laboratory and echografic evaluation of patients with deep vein thrombosis following total knee arthroplasty. *Open Journal of Orthopedics*, *9*(2), 23–29. https://doi.org/10.4236/ojo.2019.92003

Tyerman, J., & Cobbett, S. (2023). *Lewis's medical-surgical nursing in Canada: Assessment and management of clinical problems* (5th ed.). Elsevier.

Wongkietkachorn, A., Wongkietkachorn, N., & Rhunsiri, P. (2018). Preoperative needs-based education to reduce anxiety, increase satisfaction, and decrease time spent in day surgery: A randomized controlled trial. *World Journal of Surgery*, *42*(3), 666–674. https://doi.org/10.1007/s00268-017-4207-0

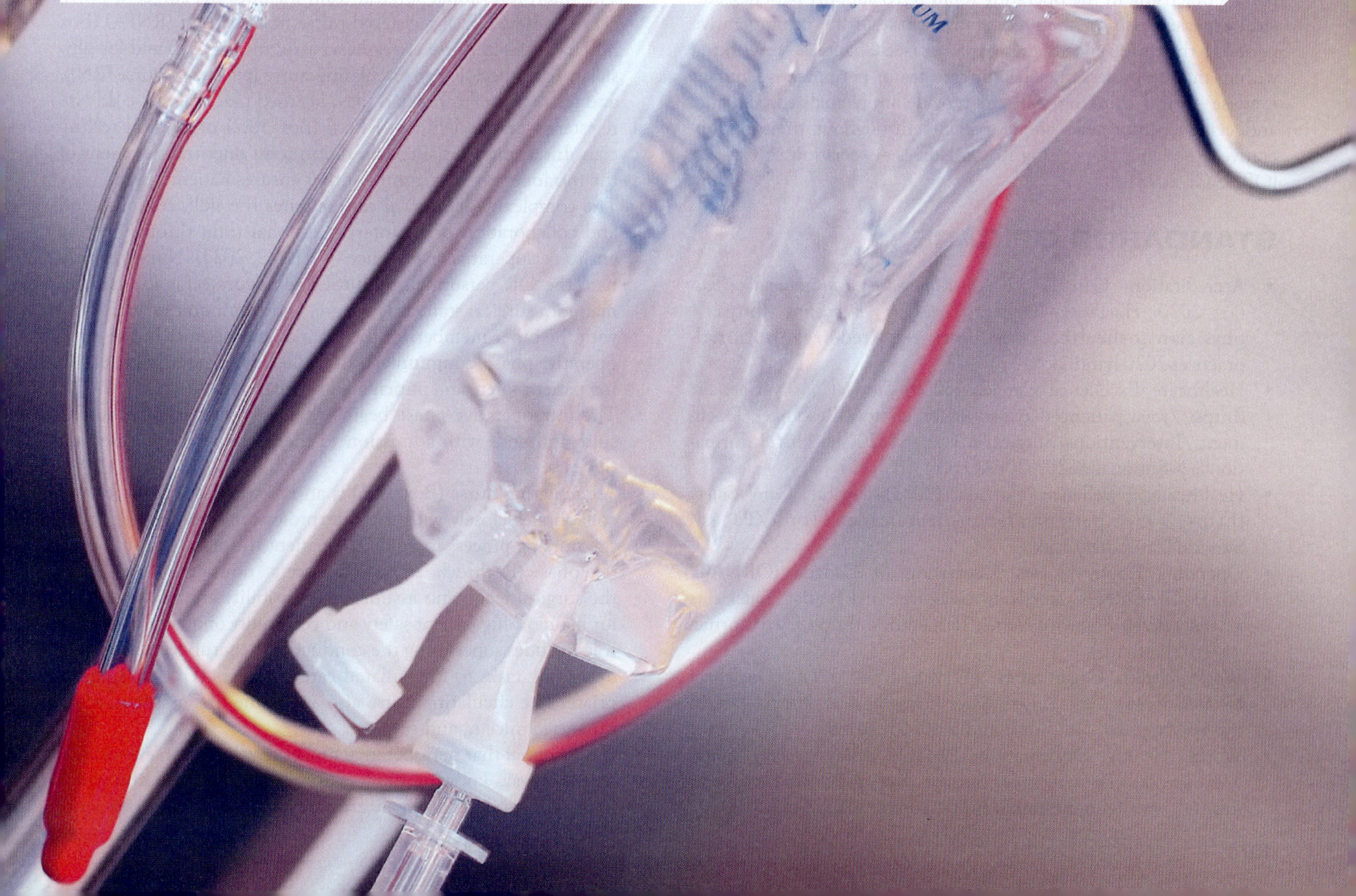

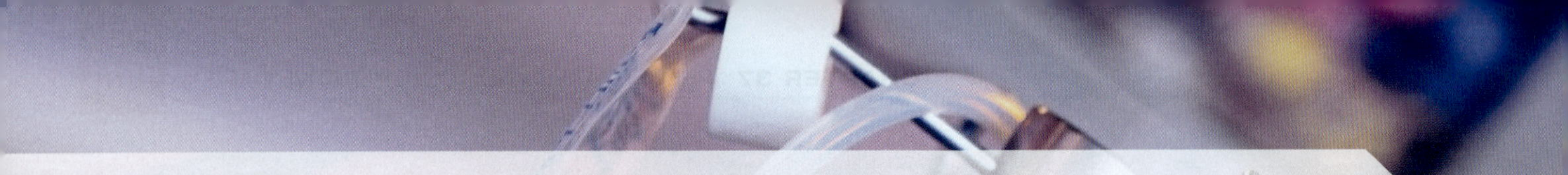

38 | Intraoperative Care

Canadian content written by **Shelley L. Cobbett, RN, GnT, MN, EdD**
Original US chapter by **Nancy Mirarchi, MSN, RN, CNOR**

SKILLS AND PROCEDURES

OBJECTIVES

Mastery of content in this chapter will enable the nurse to:

- Describe the meaning of a sterile conscience.
- Describe the roles of a registered nurse in the operating room.
- Identify guidelines for the use of sterile technique in the operating room.
- Perform surgical hand antisepsis correctly.
- Explain how to correctly don a sterile surgical gown.
- Apply sterile gloves using the closed technique.

MEDIA RESOURCES

- http://evolve.elsevier.com/Canada/Perry/clinicalskills/

PURPOSE

Nurses practising in the operating room (OR) support patients' surgical experiences from the preoperative phase to the intraoperative period to the various postoperative phases (see Chapter 37). Working within an interprofessional health care team, perioperative nurses exercise critical thinking skills to provide individualized, holistic, and evidence-informed care to patients throughout their perioperative experience (Operating Room Nurses Association of Canada [ORNAC], 2023).

STANDARDS OF CARE

- Accreditation Canada (2020)—*Required Organizational Practices–2020 Handbook–Briefing, Time-Out, Debriefing* (https://physicians.nshealth.ca/resources/required-organizational-practices-2020-handbook)
- Healthcare Excellence Canada (2009)—*Surgical Safety Checklist* (https://www.patientsafetyinstitute.ca/en/toolsResources/Documents/Interventions/Surgical%20Safety%20Checklist/Information%20Rationale%20%20FAQ.pdf)
- Healthcare Excellence Canada (2022)—*Surgical Care Safety* (https://www.patientsafetyinstitute.ca/en/Topic/Pages/Surgical-Care-Safety.aspx)
- Operating Room Nurses Association of Canada (ORNAC, 2023)—*The ORNAC Standards, Guidelines, and Position Statements for Perioperative Registered Nurses*, 16th edition (https://www.ornac.ca/en/standards)
- World Health Organization (WHO, 2009)—*WHO Guidelines for Safe Surgery: Safe Surgery Saves Lives—Surgical Safety Checklist* (https://apps.who.int/iris/handle/10665/44185)
- World Health Organization (WHO, 2018)—*Global Guidelines for the Prevention of Surgical Site Infection* (2nd ed.) (https://www.who.int/publications/i/item/9789241550475)

PRINCIPLES FOR PRACTICE

- The interprofessional surgical team includes the surgeon, physician's assistant (PA), registered nurse first assistant (RNFA) (Box 38.1), registered nurse anaesthesia assistant (RNAA) and/or physician anaesthesiologist, circulating nurse (registered nurse [RN]), and scrub nurse/technician (RN, licensed practical nurse [LPN]/registered practical nurse [RPN]) (Box 38.2) or surgical technician. Interprofessional collaboration is an important element of the intraoperative environment that ensures patient safety.
- The complexity of surgical care requires the skill, commitment, and collaboration of an interprofessional team throughout the entire perioperative experience (ORNAC, 2023). Nurses coordinate the OR personnel, monitor and advocate for the patient, maintain surgical standards of care, and communicate effectively with the other members of the team as appropriate. In the intraoperative phase, communication and teamwork are vital to ensuring patient safety and anticipated surgical outcome.
- The intraoperative phase begins when a patient enters the OR suite and ends with admission to the postanaesthesia care unit (PACU).
- A circulating nurse (Box 38.3) is an RN who both manages and collaborates closely with the interprofessional team while using the nursing process to guide the patient through the intraoperative phase (Rothrock, 2019). They are a "nonsterile" member of the surgical team who assumes responsibility and accountability for maintaining patient safety and continuity of quality care. This role includes supervising the conduct of the scrub technician and delegating tasks to unregulated care providers (UCPs) as appropriate. The circulating nurse also assists the first assistant, scrub nurse/technician, and surgeon.
- It is essential that perioperative nurses develop a *sterile conscience*, that is, always knowing the location of a sterile field and which items are sterile and which are nonsterile. A sterile conscience

BOX 38.1

Role and Responsibilities of a Registered Nurse First Assistant

The role of the registered nurse first assistant (RNFA) is an expansion of the traditional perioperative nursing role, and therefore areas of responsibility overlap, including preoperative, intraoperative, and postoperative roles. The intraoperative roles of an RNFA include the following:

- Participating in "time-out" procedure with other surgical team members (safety measure taken to ensure correct patient; signed consent; correct procedure; correct site, side, and level; correct patient position; correct implants/equipment present; and provision of appropriate answers to any questions or concerns)
- Assisting the anaesthesia care provider
- Assisting with patient positioning, skin preparation, and draping
- Providing surgical exposure (assisting in retracting tissues and suctioning surgical field)
- Assessing the patient and monitoring hemostasis and blood loss
- Safe handling and/or cutting of tissue
- Suturing and using surgical instruments and medical devices safely and correctly
- Performing wound closure
- Monitoring and protecting against contamination of the sterile field
- Applying human anatomical and physiological considerations in practice; recognizing structure, function, and location of tissues and organs; manipulating tissues accordingly to avoid injury
- Ensuring preoperative and postoperative patient management in collaboration with other health care providers
- Initiating intraoperative actions according to employer policy if surgeon becomes incapacitated
- Collaborating with the interprofessional health care team to ensure optimal surgical outcome

Adapted from Operating Room Nurses Association of Canada. (2023). *The ORNAC standards, guidelines, and position statements for perioperative registered nurses* (16th ed.). https://www.ornac.ca/en/standards

BOX 38.2

Role of the Scrub Nurse

- Helps circulating nurse prepare the OR and opens supplies
- Performs surgical hand antisepsis and dons sterile gown and gloves
- Prepares sterile field with procedure-appropriate supplies and instruments, verifying that all are in working condition
- Participates in "time-out" procedure with other surgical team members
- Performs sponge, sharps, and instrument counts with circulating nurse before incision is made, at the beginning of wound closure, and at the end of the surgical procedure to ensure that there is no retained foreign body in the patient (Rothrock, 2019)
- Labels all liquids and/or medications on the sterile field with a sterile marking pen when liquid or medication is out of the original container or package
- Gowns and gloves surgeons and assistants as they enter the OR
- Assists surgeons with sterile draping of patient
- Keeps sterile field orderly and monitors progress of procedure and any breaks in aseptic technique
- Passes sterile instruments and supplies to surgeons and assistants during surgery
- Handles surgical specimens per employer policy
- Constantly monitors location of all sponges and sharps in the sterile field

OR, Operating room.

requires knowledge of the principles of aseptic technique; self-discipline; good communication skills to identify, address, and correct any breaks in sterile technique; and the maturity to overcome personal preferences.

BOX 38.3

Role of the Circulating Nurse

- Coordinates care of the patient undergoing surgery and collaborates with interprofessional surgical team using evidence-informed practice and individualized approach for patient care
- Provides appropriate care during admission to the OR and during preinduction, induction, intraoperative, and emergence phases
- Develops, modifies, and documents the individualized plan of care or a clinical pathway to meet the specific needs of the patient
- Organizes and prepares OR before start of surgical procedure; checks that equipment works properly
- Gathers supplies for surgical procedure and opens sterile supplies for scrub nurse/technician
- Performs surgical counts and accurately documents sponges, sharps, and instruments with scrub nurse/technician before incision is made, at the beginning of wound closure, and at the end of surgical procedure
- Ensures that all liquids and/or medications on the sterile field are labelled with a sterile marking pen when liquid or medication is out of the original container or package
- Sends for patient at appropriate time
- Conducts preoperative patient assessment, including the following steps:
  - Explains role and identifies patient
  - Reviews medical record and verifies procedure and consents
  - Confirms that dentures and prostheses are removed
  - Confirms patient's allergies, NPO status, laboratory values, ECG, X-ray film studies, skin condition, and circulatory and pulmonary status
- Safely transfers patient to operating table and positions patient according to surgeon preference and procedure type, and postoperatively, using safety precautions (e.g., safety belt, securing arms, padding bony prominences)
- Participates in "time-out" procedure with other surgical team members
- Applies conductive pad to patient if electrocautery to be used; may prepare patient's skin; may apply ECG electrodes
- Applies antiembolism stockings and sequential compression device per health care provider prescription
- Explains briefly to patient what the circulating nurse and the scrub nurse/technician are doing
- Assists surgical team by tying gowns and arranging equipment
- Assists anaesthesia personnel during induction and extubation
- Uses a surgical conscience to maintain and monitor integrity of the sterile field
- Strives to provide environmental conditions conducive to positive patient outcomes
- Continuously monitors procedure for any breaks in aseptic technique and anticipates needs of health care team; opens additional sterile supplies for scrub nurse/technician
- Continuously monitors patient throughout surgery
- Handles surgical specimens per employer policy
- Documents on perioperative progress notes
- Communicates to family and PACU personnel during surgical procedure

ECG, Electrocardiogram; *NPO*, nothing by mouth; *OR*, operating room; *PACU*, postanaesthesia care unit.

- While a patient is in the OR and the OR team is gowned and gloved, it is recommended that a surgical safety checklist or the WHO checklist be completed (WHO, 2009) (Fig. 38.1). The surgical safety checklist is a tool that is used to promote safety in any perioperative environment (Healthcare Excellence Canada, 2009; ORNAC, 2023). The WHO checklist identifies three phases of an operation, each corresponding to a specific period in the normal flow of work: before the induction of anaesthesia ("sign

Surgical Safety Checklist

World Health Organization | Patient Safety — A World Alliance for Safer Health Care

Before induction of anaesthesia → **Before skin incision** → **Before patient leaves operating room**

Before induction of anaesthesia
(with at least nurse and anaesthetist)

Has the patient confirmed his/her identity, site, procedure, and consent?
- ☐ Yes

Is the site marked?
- ☐ Yes
- ☐ Not applicable

Is the anaesthesia machine and medication check complete?
- ☐ Yes

Is the pulse oximeter on the patient and functioning?
- ☐ Yes

Does the patient have a:

Known allergy?
- ☐ No
- ☐ Yes

Difficult airway or aspiration risk?
- ☐ No
- ☐ Yes, and equipment/assistance available

Risk of >500ml blood loss (7ml/kg in children)?
- ☐ No
- ☐ Yes, and two IVs/central access and fluids planned

Before skin incision
(with nurse, anaesthetist and surgeon)

- ☐ **Confirm all team members have introduced themselves by name and role.**
- ☐ **Confirm the patient's name, procedure, and where the incision will be made.**

Has antibiotic prophylaxis been given within the last 60 minutes?
- ☐ Yes
- ☐ Not applicable

Anticipated Critical Events

To Surgeon:
- ☐ What are the critical or non-routine steps?
- ☐ How long will the case take?
- ☐ What is the anticipated blood loss?

To Anaesthetist:
- ☐ Are there any patient-specific concerns?

To Nursing Team:
- ☐ Has sterility (including indicator results) been confirmed?
- ☐ Are there equipment issues or any concerns?

Is essential imaging displayed?
- ☐ Yes
- ☐ Not applicable

Before patient leaves operating room
(with nurse, anaesthetist and surgeon)

Nurse Verbally Confirms:
- ☐ The name of the procedure
- ☐ Completion of instrument, sponge and needle counts
- ☐ Specimen labelling (read specimen labels aloud, including patient name)
- ☐ Whether there are any equipment problems to be addressed

To Surgeon, Anaesthetist and Nurse:
- ☐ What are the key concerns for recovery and management of this patient?

This checklist is not intended to be comprehensive. Additions and modifications to fit local practice are encouraged.

Revised 1 / 2009

FIG 38.1 The World Health Organization Surgical Safety Checklist. (*Used with permission, World Health Organization.*)

in"), before the incision of the skin ("time-out"), and before the patient leaves the OR ("sign out") (WHO, 2009). In each phase, a checklist coordinator, usually the circulating nurse, must confirm that the surgery team has completed the listed tasks before it proceeds with the operation.

- The surgical safety checklist verifies the patient's identity, ascertains whether the patient has any allergies, confirms that the surgical site is marked and verifies the site marking, asks the patient whether they have any questions, and ensures adherence to safety protocols (ORNAC, 2023; WHO, 2009). The surgical checklist consists of three parts: *briefing*, the period from the patient's transfer to the operating bed to the induction of anaesthesia; *time-out*, the period immediately prior to the incision; and *debriefing*, the period after the surgery is complete but before the patient's transfer to the PACU (Accreditation Canada, 2020; ORNAC, 2023).
- Time-outs are standardized by each facility, initiated by a designated member of the team, and involve all immediate members of the surgical/procedure team who will be participating in the procedure from start to finish. It is during the time-out that the team members agree, at a minimum, that the correct patient and site have been identified and that the correct procedure is scheduled to be done on the correct body part or area. A designated member of the team must document the time-out according to employer policy before the procedure begins (ORNAC, 2023; Rothrock, 2019).

PERSON-CENTRED CARE

- The patient may be unsure of what to expect and have concerns regarding pain, disfigurement, and length of recovery. It is a nurse's responsibility to practise person-centred care and encourage questions.
- The circulating nurse requires specialized knowledge to take care of the surgical patient, a role that includes closely monitoring the patient's intraoperative response to the experience.
- Patient needs vary on the basis of preoperative health, type of surgical procedure, and cultural and religious beliefs. Nurses need to obtain information regarding cultural and religious preferences that may affect the patient's acceptance of education, blood administration, and surgical interventions.
- Information is communicated to the interprofessional team to ensure comprehensive intraoperative care.

EVIDENCE-INFORMED PRACTICE

- Decreased glove perforation results in decreased surgical site infection (SSI) and also protects the health care provider from

exposure to contaminated blood and body fluids and subsequent infection (ORNAC, 2023). Evidence-informed research offers the following gloving guidelines:
- Double-gloving is superior to single-gloving.
- Double-gloving provides an additional barrier; there is a significant reduction in the perforation of the innermost layers when double-gloving is used compared with single-gloving (ORNAC, 2023; Rothrock, 2019; Tlili et al., 2018).
- In addition, double-gloving and using the perforation indicator system (lighter pair of gloves worn over a darker pair) helps a health care provider better identify glove failure (ORNAC, 2023; Tlili et al., 2018).

- Current evidence-informed research links perioperative hypothermia with an increase in morbidity and mortality. Specifically, hypothermia can put patients at additional risk for SSI, cardiac arrhythmias, changes in medication metabolism, and increased incidence of surgical bleeding. Patients at risk for hypothermia include older persons, those with low body weight or metabolic disorders, those in a cold surgical environment or who receive cold infusions, and those undergoing open-cavity surgical procedures and general surgeries (Association of periOperative Registered Nurses [AORN], 2023).
- Interventions effective in preventing hypothermia include forced-air warming. Commencement of active warming preoperatively and monitoring it throughout the intraoperative period is effective. Combined strategies, including preoperative commencement of warming and the use of warmed fluids plus forced-air warming during surgery, are also effective (Spruce, 2018; Steelman et al., 2018).

OR personnel are responsible for adhering to specific infection control practices based on individualized employer guidelines. Basic evidence-informed infection control practices include the following:
- Hand hygiene should be performed (with specific attention given to areas between the thumb and first digit) when OR staff arrive at the health care facility, before and after patient contact, before a procedure, after body fluid exposure, before and after donning gloves and other personal protective equipment (PPE), before and after eating, after contact with contaminated items, when items or hands are visibly soiled, and before leaving the health care facility (ORNAC, 2023; Rothrock, 2019).
- Hand scrub using alcohol-based hand-rub products should be approved by the employer's infection control department, and an established standardized protocol should be followed (ORNAC, 2023). The user must be made aware of and follow the manufacturer's written instructions regarding storage, dispensing, technique, and amount of product required (ORNAC, 2023; Rothrock, 2019).
- OR personnel should use approved brushless, alcohol-based surgical hand-rub products (with added emollients) that limit damage to the user's skin, improve adherence to hand antisepsis protocols, simplify application technique, and reduce material waste (i.e., water, brushes, and packaging) (Rothrock, 2019).
- Fingernails should be clean, short, natural, and look healthy, and nail polish should not be worn. Avoid use of any nail enhancements (artificial nails, acrylics, extenders, and gels) (ORNAC, 2023).
- An addition to the ORNAC (2023) standards, under "Exceptional Clinical Events," is a section related to pandemic planning for surgical suites. The need for urgent surgeries is not diminished by the presence of a pandemic, and emergency preparedness plans that maintain quality patient care should be current in all facilities. Strategies are required to manage organizational resources, including personnel, bed capacity, ORs, equipment, and supplies (ORNAC, 2023). Other considerations identified by ORNAC (2023) include the following:
  - A phased approach may be required during a pandemic, including minimizing or restricting access (e.g., visitors), changed staffing ratios or delegation of duties, decreased elective surgeries, changed surgical-time allotment, decreased admissions, consolidation of services, and an increase in specific supplies/equipment (e.g., PPE, UPP [universal pandemic precautions] supplies).
  - A comprehensive patient screening process using specific pandemic-related questions should be conducted prior to the surgery.
  - Planning for patients who are positive for the specific virus that caused the pandemic (e.g., SARS-CoV-2) should include a designated pandemic clinical pathway, patient flows (e.g., bypassing holding area and directly admitted to the OR; shortest possible transfer routes), masking for nonintubated patients, and consideration of identification with a pandemic-specific patient wristband system.
  - Consideration should be given to continue providing oncological procedures, including palliative treatments.
  - Specific patient discharge teaching instructions need to include pandemic considerations.

SAFETY GUIDELINES

- ORNAC (2023) recommends the following measures to reduce intraoperative errors and promote a culture of safety: using a time-out, decreasing distractions, nonpunitive error reporting, commitment to root cause analysis, and increasing staff education.
- All items used within a sterile field must be sterile.
- Gowns used by scrub people must be sterile before donning. Once in place, gowns are sterile from the front chest and shoulders to table level and on the sleeves to 5 cm (2 inches) above the elbow to the cuff circumferentially.
- Persons who are sterile must keep their hands in view, above waist level and below neckline, to avoid contamination.
- When wearing a sterile gown, one should not fold the arms with hands tucked in the axillary region. This area is not considered sterile once the gown is donned. Perspiration can lead to strike-through, contamination that occurs when moisture permeates a sterile barrier.
- Sterile-draped tables are sterile only at table level. The sides of the drape extending below table level are nonsterile.
- All personnel moving around or within a sterile field must do so in a manner consistent with maintaining the sterility of that field. Scrubbed persons move from sterile areas to other sterile areas, contacting a sterile field only with sterile gowns and gloves. Nonsterile health care team members always stay at least 30 cm (about 1 foot) away from the sterile field while keeping it in constant view; they touch only nonsterile areas.
- All sterile supplies and equipment are grouped around the sterile-draped patient.
- Nonsterile people must avoid reaching over the sterile field.
- Scrubbed team members remain close to the sterile field. When changing position, they need to turn face-to-face or back-to-back.
- Breaks in aseptic technique should be monitored and corrected immediately.

✦ SKILL 38.1 Surgical Hand Antisepsis

In the OR setting, surgical hand antisepsis must be achieved through effective surgical scrub or antiseptic hand rub (ORNAC, 2023; Rothrock, 2019). Use of an antimicrobial preparation for hand antisepsis is an integral part of the presurgical scrubbing procedure for OR personnel that reduces patient risk of acquiring postoperative infections. Although the skin cannot be sterilized, the number of microorganisms can be greatly reduced by chemical, physical, and mechanical means.

Through the use of an antimicrobial agent and sterile brushes or sponges, the surgical hand scrub removes debris and transient microorganisms from the nails, hands, and forearms; reduces the resident microbial count to a minimum; and inhibits rapid and rebound growth of microorganisms (ORNAC, 2023; Rothrock, 2019). Evidence suggests that completing a brushless hand-rub technique using approved hand hygiene products, with or without water, has the same antimicrobial efficacy as performing the traditional hand scrub with a brush (AORN, 2023). Both methods of surgical hand antisepsis are currently used in OR settings.

Surgical hand-scrub procedure for all staff (water-based or waterless) should follow a standardized protocol established and approved by the facility and the manufacturer's recommendations (follow employer policy) (ORNAC, 2023). When using water-facilitated scrub methods, the hands and arms are to be dried with a sterile towel prior to gowning (Rothrock, 2019). Some procedures, described as clean procedures (e.g., laryngoscopy and proctoscopy), require performing hand hygiene but are not necessarily surgical hand antisepsis. At a minimum, the 4 moments of hand hygiene are used throughout the intraoperative period—before initial patient (or patient environment) contact, before aseptic procedure, after body fluid exposure risk, and after patient (or patient environment) contact (Infection Prevention and Control, 2022).

Delegation and Collaboration

The skill of surgical hand antisepsis can be assigned to any member of the interprofessional health care team. The RN routinely observes surgical hand antisepsis to ensure staff adherence.

Equipment

- Deep sink with foot or knee controls for dispensing water and soap
- Antimicrobial agent approved by employer (dispenser with foot controls)
- Surgical scrub brush with plastic nail file
- Paper face mask, cap or hood, surgical shoe covers
- Protective eyewear/face shield
- Sterile towel
- Sterile pack containing sterile gown

STEP	RATIONALE
ASSESSMENT	
1. Determine type and length of time for hand hygiene (follow employer policy).	Guidelines vary regarding ideal time needed for surgical scrub.
2. Remove bracelets, rings, and watches.	Jewellery harbours microorganisms and protects them from removal. Jewellery interferes with hand hygiene and donning of PPE (ORNAC, 2023). Skin under rings has been shown to harbour more pathogens; therefore, rings should not be worn (ORNAC, 2023).
3. Inspect fingernails, which must be short (not extending beyond the fingertips), clean, natural, and healthy. Nail polish should not be worn. Never wear artificial nails, extenders, or enhancers.	Long nails and chipped or old nail polish harbour microorganisms (ORNAC, 2023). Long fingernails can puncture gloves, causing contamination. Artificial nails interfere with hand hygiene and promote the growth of *Staphylococcus aureus*, Gram-negative microorganisms, and fungus (ORNAC, 2023).
4. Inspect condition of cuticles, hands, and forearms for presence of abrasions, cuts, or open lesions.	Cuts, abrasions, exudative lesions, fresh tattoos, or hangnails tend to ooze serum, which may contain pathogens. Individuals with these conditions should not have patient contact until conditions heal (AORN, 2023).
NURSING DIAGNOSIS	
• Potential for infection	
Related factors and risk factors are individualized on the basis of patient's condition or needs.	
PLANNING	
1. Expected outcomes following completion of procedure: • Patient does not develop signs of SSI.	Indicates that microorganisms are not transferred to patient and sterile field.

STEP	RATIONALE
IMPLEMENTATION	
1. Don surgical shoe covers, cap or hood, face mask, and protective eyewear.	Protective eyewear prevents exposure to blood or body fluids that may splash from sterile field, which increases risk of infection (e.g., human immunodeficiency virus [HIV], hepatitis B virus [HBV]).
Critical Decision Point *Laser surgery requires special protective eyewear to prevent eye damage from stray laser energy.*	
2. Perform prescrub wash at beginning of work shift.	Prevents contamination of hands after scrub.
a. Turn water on using foot or knee control and adjust to comfortable temperature.	
b. Wet hands thoroughly with water. Follow manufacturer directions for application of soap.	
c. Rub hands, covering all surfaces with lather, including backs of hands, fingertips, inner webs, and palms, washing for at least 15 seconds.	A short prescrub wash/rinse of at least 15 seconds at the beginning of the work shift removes gross debris and superficial microorganisms (AORN, 2023).
d. Rinse hands well. Dry hands thoroughly with disposable towel and discard towel.	Rinsing removes all soap and remaining debris.
3. Perform surgical hand scrub (with sponge):	
a. Turn water on using foot or knee control. Clean under nails of both hands with disposable nail pick or cleaner (see Step 3a illustration). Rinse hands and forearms under running water, keeping hands and forearms elevated and elbows down.	Removes dirt and organic materials that harbour microorganisms.
b. Dispense antimicrobial scrub agent according to manufacturer instructions, (ORNAC, 2023). Apply agent to wet hands and forearms with soft, nonabrasive sponge.	Ensures removal of resident microorganisms on all surfaces of hands and arms (ORNAC, 2023).
c. Scrub for the length of time recommended (follow manufacturer instructions). Visualize each finger, hand, and arm as having four sides (see Step 3c illustrations). Wash all four sides effectively, keeping hand elevated and elbow down. Repeat for other hand, fingers, and arm.	Times vary by product. Scrubbing all surfaces ensures removal of resident microorganisms on hands and arms (ORNAC, 2023). The direction of the scrubbing procedure is from the hands to the elbows (ORNAC, 2023). Keeping hands elevated and elbows down prevents microorganisms from flowing back onto hands.

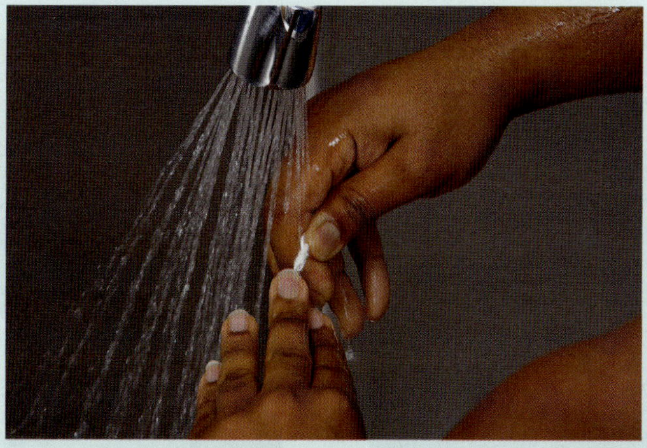

STEP 3A Clean under fingernails.

STEP	RATIONALE

IMPLEMENTATION

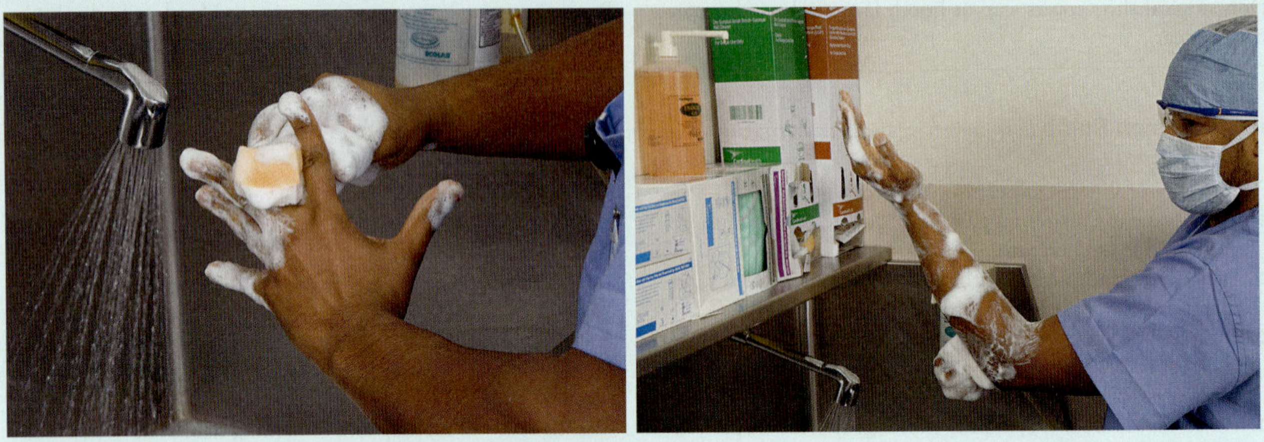

STEP 3C A, Scrub sides of fingers. B, Scrub forearms.

STEP	RATIONALE
d. Avoid splashing surgical attire. Discard sponges in appropriate container.	
e. Rinse hands and arms, running water from fingertips to elbows in one continuous motion, holding hands higher than elbows and away from surgical site (see Step 3e illustration).	Hands remain the cleanest part of the upper extremities.
f. Turn off water using foot or knee controls, and back into the OR holding hands higher than elbows and away from surgical attire.	
g. Approach sterile setup and grasp sterile towel, taking care not to drip water on sterile field (see Step 3g illustration).	Water contaminates field.
h. Keeping hands and arms above the waist and outstretched, carefully grasp one end of sterile towel to dry one hand thoroughly, moving from fingers to elbow in rotating motion (see Step 3h illustration).	Avoids sterile towel from contacting nonsterile scrub attire and transferring contamination to hands. Dries skin from cleanest (hands) to least clean (elbows).

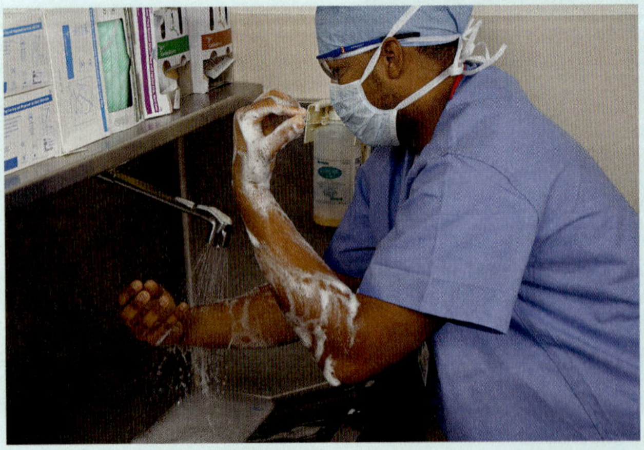

STEP 3E Rinse arms.

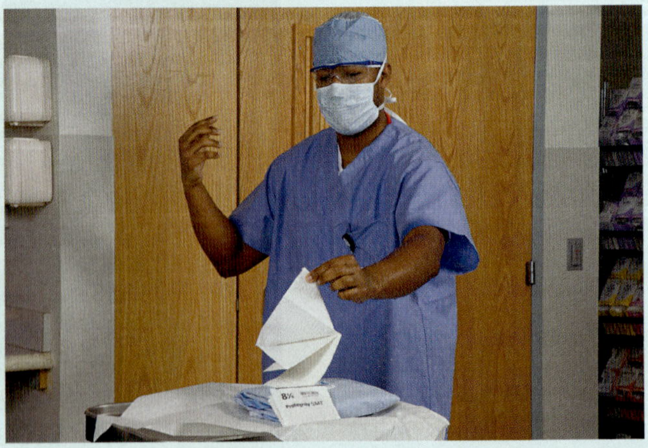

STEP 3G Grasp sterile towel.

STEP	RATIONALE

IMPLEMENTATION

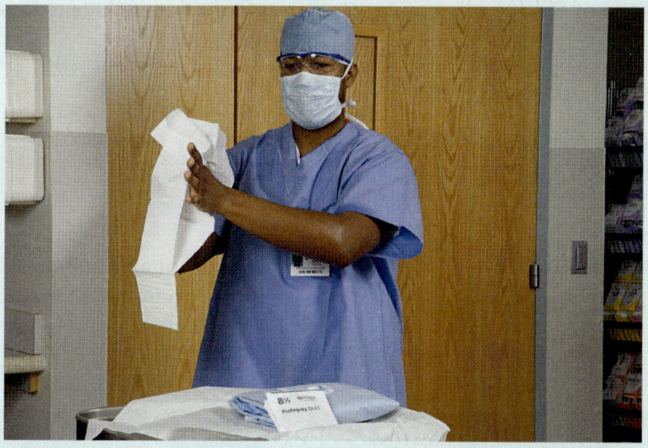

STEP 3H Dry hands thoroughly.

i. Use opposite end of towel to dry other hand. — Avoids transfer of microorganisms from elbow to opposite hand.

j. Drop towel into linen hamper or into circulating nurse's hand, making sure hands do not fall below waist level.

4. Perform spongeless surgical hand scrub with alcohol-based hand-rub product:

a. After prescrub wash (Step 2), turn water on using foot or knee control. Clean under nails of both hands with disposable nail pick or cleaner. Rinse hands and forearms under running water. Dry hands thoroughly with paper towel. Turn off water.

b. Dispense manufacturer-recommended amount of surgical hand antiseptic/scrub agent (see Step 4b illustration). Apply agent to hands and forearms according to manufacturer's written instructions for application, recommended volume, and specified time. — A broad-spectrum hand antiseptic agent has the ability to kill microorganisms when applied, promotes reduction in microorganism regrowth on all surfaces of hands and arms, and has a cumulative effect over time (ORNAC, 2023).

c. Repeat antimicrobial product application if indicated in manufacturer instructions.

d. Rub thoroughly until completely dry (see Step 4d illustration). Proceed to OR to don gloves.

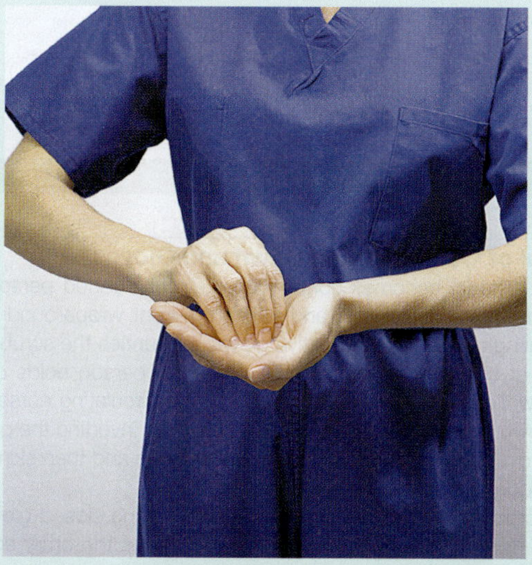

STEP 4B Dispense antimicrobial agent into hands. (*Photo Courtesy 3M Health Care.*)

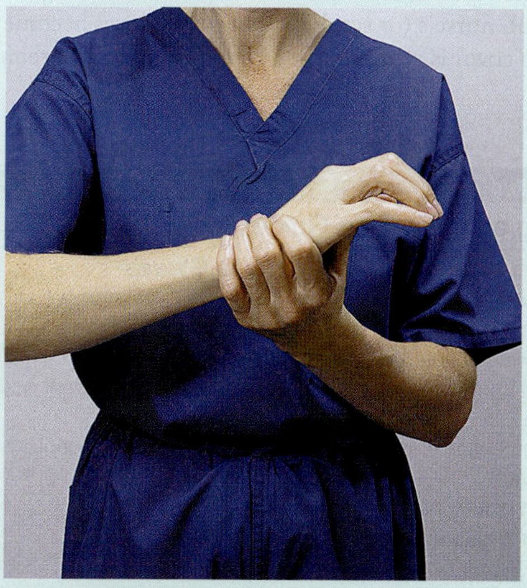

STEP 4D Rub thoroughly until completely dry. (*Photo Courtesy 3M Health Care.*)

STEP	RATIONALE
EVALUATION	
1. Monitor patient after surgery for signs of SSI (usually occurs 2–3 days after surgery).	Signs of infection include redness, heat, swelling, pain, and purulent drainage.

Unexpected Outcomes	Related Interventions
1. Redness, heat, swelling, pain, or purulent drainage may develop at surgical site, which often indicates infection of wound.	• Individualize interventions based on patient's situation (e.g., wound care, antibiotic therapy).

Communication and Documentation

- No documentation is required for surgical hand antisepsis.
- Document area and description of surgical site in progress notes in electronic health record (EHR) or chart after surgery to provide baseline for monitoring wound.

✦ SKILL 38.2 Donning a Sterile Gown and Closed Gloving

Immediately following surgical hand antisepsis, surgical personnel apply a sterile gown and then apply sterile gloves. All members of the surgical team must prepare in this manner before entering the sterile field. Once applied, the surgical gown is considered sterile in the front, from the chest to the waist or table level. The sleeves are considered sterile from 5 cm (2 inches) above the elbow to the level of the cuff (ORNAC, 2023). The neckline, shoulders, under the arms, sleeve cuffs, and back of the gown are considered nonsterile (ORNAC, 2023). Surgical gowns should cover all garments worn underneath. All sterile gowns that are free of tears, punctures, strain, and abrasion provide an effective barrier against microorganisms, particulates, and fluids passing between nonsterile and sterile areas and reduce the risk of contamination (ORNAC, 2023).

All members of the surgical team use the closed-glove method to apply gloves when entering the sterile field. If a glove becomes contaminated during surgery, the circulating nurse, wearing protective nonsterile gloves, grasps the outside of the glove and pulls it off inside out, leaving the stockinette cuff of the gown in place. Another sterile team member assists in regloving. The open method can be used when only one glove has been contaminated. In some settings, the scrub nurse will wear two pairs of sterile gloves. If both of the scrub nurse's (or scrub technician's) gloves become contaminated, the gown is removed first, then the gloves are removed, and then the nurse regowns and regloves using the closed-glove method (Box 38.4).

Delegation and Collaboration

The RN can assign the skills of donning a sterile gown and closed gloving to a surgical technologist or LPN/RPN. The RN routinely observes sterile gown application and closed gloving to ensure staff adherence.

The nurse collaborates with the interprofessional health care team to follow sterile practices, prevent infection, and achieve optimal patient outcomes.

Equipment

- Package of properly sized sterile gloves (latex-free if sensitivity or allergy is present)
- Sterile pack containing sterile gown
- Clean, flat, dry surface (table or Mayo stand) on which to open gown and gloves
- Paper face masks, cap or hood, surgical shoe covers
- Protective eyewear/face shield

BOX 38.4

Gloving and Gowning Guidelines

When to Change Surgical Sterile Gloves

- After each patient contact
- When a defect is noted
- Following suspected or actual contamination
- When perforation from a needle, suture, or other event occurs
- Immediately following use of methyl methacrylate
- If unintentional electric shock from the electrocautery device is received
- When gloves swell or become loose
- According to employer policy

Removal of Contaminated Gown and Gloves

- When a gown becomes contaminated, the scrubbed person steps away from the sterile field and unties the front wraparound tie. The circulating nurse dons protective gloves and unties the scrub nurse's gown at the neck and back. The scrubbed person holds out their arms while facing the circulating nurse. The circulating nurse grasps the gown at the shoulders and pulls it off while inverting the gown.
- The gloves are removed using a glove-to-glove and then skin-to-skin technique and are discarded immediately.
- The scrub nurse regowns and regloves self, using closed-glove technique (from another table) or gowns and gloves the other scrubbed personnel.

From Operating Room Nurses Association of Canada. (2023). *The ORNAC standards, guidelines, and position statements for perioperative registered nurses* (16th ed., pp. 135–137). https://www.ornac.ca/en/standards

STEP	RATIONALE

ASSESSMENT

STEP	RATIONALE
1. Select proper size and type of sterile gloves. Select latex-free gloves if patient or any surgical personnel in OR are sensitive or allergic to latex.	Proper fit ensures ease of handling instruments and supplies. Prevents latex allergic response.

Critical Decision Point *Know your employer's policy because double-gloving may be recommended to reduce the risk of glove perforation during a surgical procedure* (ORNAC, 2023; Tlili, 2018).

STEP	RATIONALE
2. Select proper size and type of sterile surgical gown.	Ill-fitting gown impedes movement of extremities.

NURSING DIAGNOSIS

- Potential for infection

Related factors and risk factors are individualized on the basis of patient's condition or needs.

PLANNING

STEP	RATIONALE
1. Expected outcomes following completion of procedure: • Patient does not develop signs of SSI.	Nurse maintains aseptic technique and does not contaminate gown or gloves.

IMPLEMENTATION

STEP	RATIONALE
1. Donning sterile gown:	
a. Open sterile gown and glove package on clean, dry, flat surface. Scrub nurse (before scrubbing hands) or circulating nurse can do this for you, preferably on a small table, separate from sterile field, containing sterile instruments and supplies.	Provides sterile area for gloving.
b. Perform surgical hand antisepsis (see Skill 38.1). Dry hands thoroughly.	
c. Pick up gown (folded inside out) from sterile package, grasping inside surface at collar.	Hands are not completely sterile. Inside surface of gown will contact surface of skin and thus is considered contaminated.
d. Lift folded gown directly upward and step back, away from table.	Prevents gown from touching nonsterile object.
e. Locate neckband; with both hands grasp inside front of gown just below neckband.	Clean hands may touch inside of gown without contaminating outer surface.
f. Keeping gown at arm's length away from body, allow it to unfold with inside of gown toward body. Do not touch outside of gown or allow it to touch floor.	Outside of gown remains sterile.
g. With hands at shoulder level, slip both arms into armholes simultaneously (see Step 1g illustration). Do not allow hands to move through cuff opening. Have circulating nurse pull gown over your shoulders by reaching inside the arm seams. Pull gown on, leaving sleeves covering hands.	Careful application prevents contamination. Gown covers hands to prepare for closed gloving.
h. Have circulating nurse tie gown at neck and waist (see Step 1h illustration). If gown is wraparound style, do not touch sterile front flap until scrub nurse/technician has gloved (see Step 3b).	Secures gown without contaminating it.

STEP	RATIONALE

IMPLEMENTATION

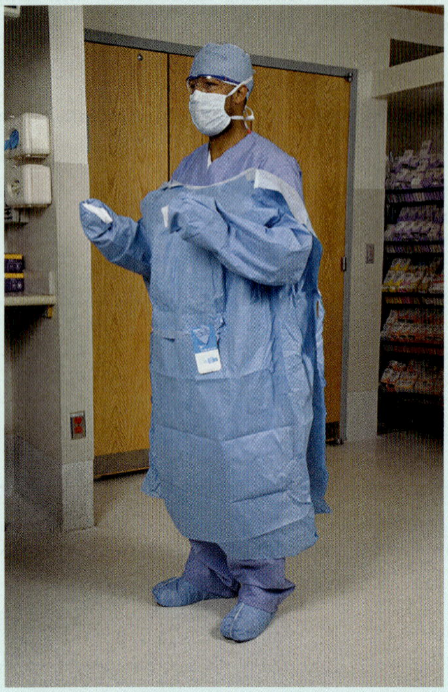

STEP 1G Place arms in sleeves.

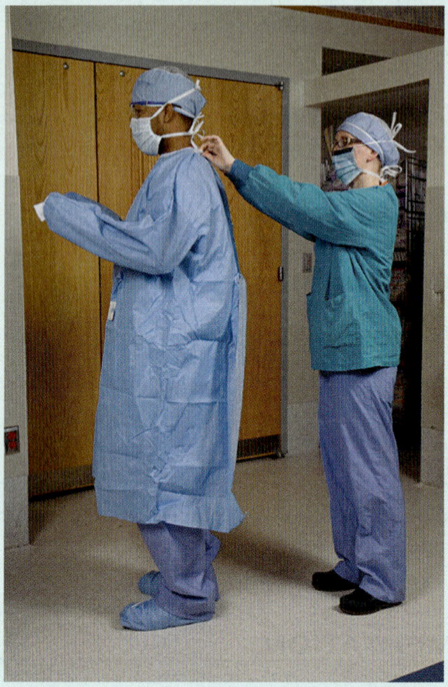

STEP 1H Circulating nurse ties scrub gown.

2. Applying gloves using closed-glove method:

a. With hands covered by gown cuffs and sleeves, open inner sterile glove package (see Step 2a illustration). — Sterile gown cuff touches sterile glove surface.

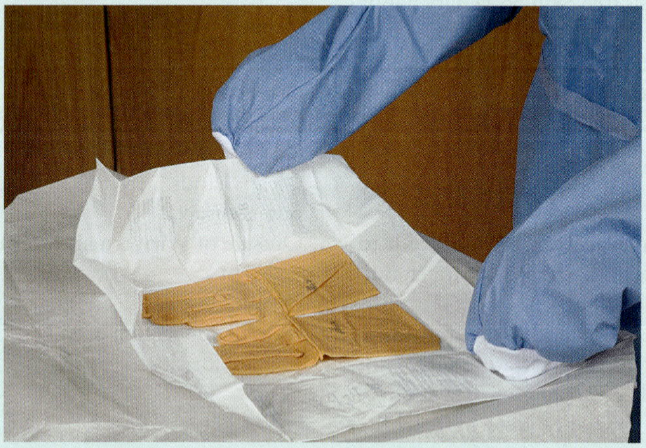

STEP 2A Scrub nurse opens glove package.

b. Grasp folded cuff of glove for dominant hand with nondominant hand. — Sterile gown touches sterile glove.

c. Extend covered dominant hand and forearm forward with palm up and place palm of glove against palm of dominant hand. Glove fingers point toward elbow. — Positions glove for application over cuffed hand, keeping glove sterile.

d. While holding glove cuff through gown with dominant hand on which it was placed, grasp back of glove cuff with nondominant hand and turn glove cuff over end of dominant hand and gown cuff (see Step 2d illustration). — Positions glove over gown for hand insertion.

e. Grasp top of glove and underlying gown sleeve with covered nondominant hand. Carefully extend fingers into glove, being sure that cuff of glove covers cuff of gown.

STEP	RATIONALE

IMPLEMENTATION

f. Glove nondominant hand in same manner with gloved dominant hand (see Step 2f, illustration *A*). Keep hand inside sleeve. Be sure that fingers are fully extended into both gloves (see Step 2f, illustration *B*).	Gloves remain sterile.

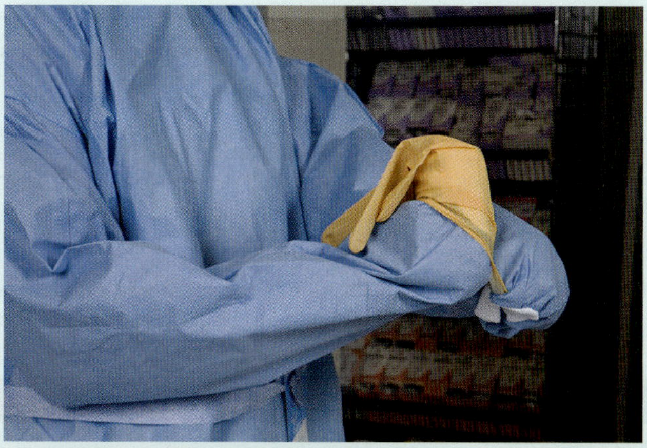

STEP 2D Glove applied as hands remain inside cuffs.

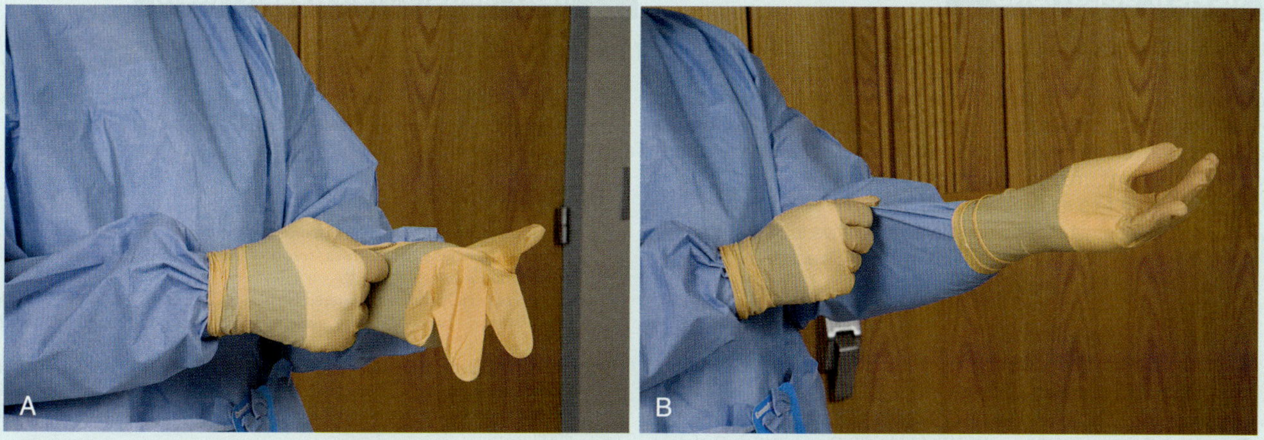

STEP 2F A, Second glove applied. B, Gloved fingers extended.

3. Donning wraparound gown:	
a. Grasp sterile front flap/paper tab with gloved hands and untie.	Front of gown is sterile.
b. Pass sterile paper tab to a member of sterile surgical team or to nonsterile team member (e.g., circulating nurse) (see Step 3b illustration). Keep gown tie in right hand. Circulating nurse stands still as scrub nurse/technician turns.	Nonsterile team member uses caution to avoid touching sterile tie when taking sterile paper tab while scrub nurse/technician turns.

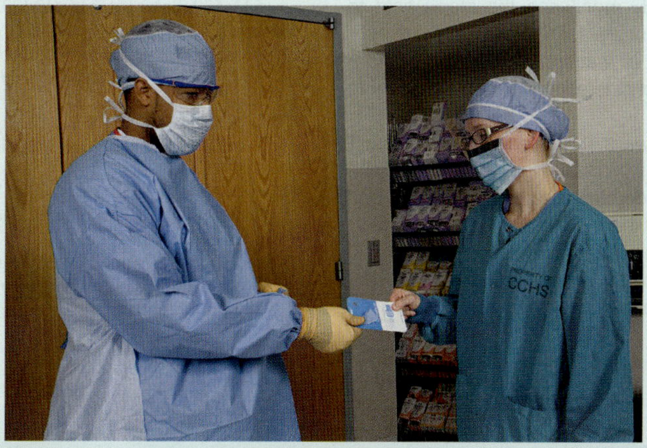

STEP 3B Paper tab on disposable gown is passed to circulating nurse.

STEP	RATIONALE
IMPLEMENTATION	
c. Allowing margin of safety, turn to left one-half turn, covering back with extended gown flap. Retrieve sterile tie only from team member and secure both ties in place.	Manoeuvre covers entire body with gown. Nonsterile team member pulls off paper tab and discards it.
EVALUATION	
1. Monitor patient after surgery for signs of SSI (usually occurs 2–3 days after surgery).	Signs of infection include redness, heat, swelling, pain, and purulent drainage.

Unexpected Outcomes	Related Interventions
1. Redness, heat, swelling, pain, or purulent drainage develops at surgical site, which often indicates infection of wound.	• Individualize interventions based on patient's situation (e.g., wound care, antibiotic therapy).

Communication and Documentation

- No documentation is required for sterile gowning and gloving.
- Document area and description of surgical site in progress notes in EHR or chart after surgery to provide baseline for monitoring wound.

✦ REVIEW QUESTIONS

You are the circulating nurse in the general operating room (OR) where your first case scheduled at 0730 hours is a 78-year-old patient (she/her) weighing 46 kg who is scheduled for a total abdominal hysterectomy. You meet the patient in the surgical waiting area, perform a preoperative assessment, and review their electronic medical record. The patient confirms all necessary information before entry into the OR.

Review Questions 1 to 5 relate to the case study presented here.

1. Choose the circumstances when the perioperative team will practise hand hygiene throughout intraoperative care. (*Select all that apply.*)
  1. Before touching the patient
  2. Before a procedure
  3. After body fluid exposure
  4. After touching the patient
  5. After touching the environment

2. Describe the purpose and types of surgical hand antisepsis.

3. The circulating nurse follows the World Health Organization Surgical Safety Checklist guidelines to reduce intraoperative errors by participating in a time-out with the perioperative team. The time-out procedure: (*Select all that apply.*)
  1. Ensures correct patient, correct procedure, and correct site
  2. Reviews antibiotic prophylaxis
  3. Discusses patient-specific surgical and anaesthesia concerns
  4. Confirms the presence of correct imaging and equipment
  5. Occurs after the patient leaves the OR

4. The circulating nurse is constantly monitoring the sterile field to ensure that sterile technique is maintained. Principles of sterile technique include the following: (*Select all that apply.*)
  1. The front of a sterile gown is considered sterile from the chest to the level of the sterile field.
  2. Unscrubbed team members always stay at least 30 cm (about 1 foot) away from the sterile field while keeping it in constant view.
  3. Surgical gowns should be an adequate size to wrap around and completely cover the scrubbed team member's body.
  4. Sterile-draped tables are sterile only at table level.

5. List the risk factors for hypothermia for this patient. What interventions can be used to prevent unplanned hypothermia?

Visit the Evolve site for a complete list of answers to the Review Questions.

✦ NEXT GENERATION NCLEX® (NGN)

For practice with answering exam questions related to unfolding NGN case studies, please consult the Next Generation NCLEX® (NGN)-Style Case Studies for Skills and Techniques on the Evolve website: http://evolve.elsevier.com/Canada/Perry/clinicalskills/

REFERENCES

Accreditation Canada. (2020). *Required organizational practices–2020 handbook.* https://physicians.nshealth.ca/resources/required-organizational-practices-2020-handbook

Association of periOperative Registered Nurses. (2023). *Guidelines for perioperative practices.* https://www.aorn.org/guidelines-resources/guidelines-for-perioperative-practice

Healthcare Excellence Canada. (2009). *Surgical safety checklist.* https://www.patientsafetyinstitute.ca/en/toolsResources/Documents/Interventions/Surgical%20Safety%20Checklist/Information%20Rationale%20%20FAQ.pdf [Seminal Reference]

Healthcare Excellence Canada. (2022). *Surgical care safety.* https://www.patientsafetyinstitute.ca/en/Topic/Pages/Surgical-Care-Safety.aspx

Infection Prevention and Control. (2022). *IPAC Canada practice recommendations: Hand hygiene in health care settings.* https://ipac-canada.org/photos/custom/Members/pdf/22Nov11_Hand%20Hygiene_Practice%20Recommendation.pdf

Operating Room Nurses Association of Canada. (2023). *The ORNAC standards, guidelines, and position statements for perioperative registered nurses* (16th ed.). https://www.ornac.ca/en/standards

Rothrock, J. (2019). *Alexander's care of the patient in surgery* (16th ed.). Mosby.

Spruce, L. (2018). Back to basics: Unplanned hypothermia. *AORN Journal, 108*(5), 533–539. https://doi.org/10.1002/aorn.12389

Steelman, V. M., Chae, S., Duff, J., et al. (2018). Warming of irrigation fluids for prevention of perioperative hypothermia during arthroscopy: A systematic review and meta-analysis. *Arthroscopy, 34*(3), 930–942.e2. https://doi.org/10.1016/j.arthro.2017.09.024

Tlili, M., Belgacem, A., Sridi, H., et al. (2018). Evaluation of surgical glove integrity and factors associated with glove defect. *American Journal of Infection Control, 46*(1), 30–33.

World Health Organization. (2009). *WHO guidelines for safe surgery: Safe surgery saves lives.* https://www.who.int/publications/i/item/9789241598552 [Seminal Reference]

World Health Organization. (2018). *Global guidelines for the prevention of surgical site infection* (2nd ed.). https://www.who.int/publications/i/item/9789241550475 [Seminal Reference]

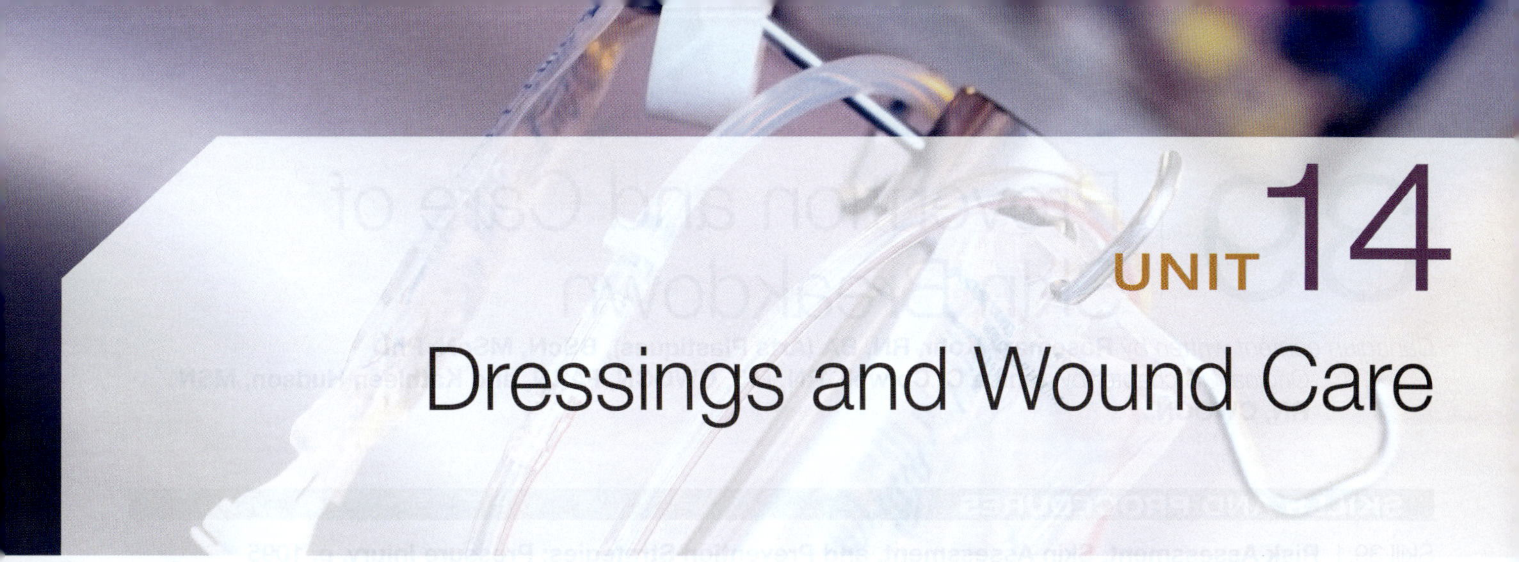

UNIT 14 Dressings and Wound Care

Implementing proper dressing and wound care is essential to patient comfort and safety. When patients have wounds from surgeries, trauma, or pressure injuries, the outermost layer of their skin is no longer intact. That fact alone increases the patient's risk for further infection, tissue damage, and decreased mobility and dependence. It is important that you use your critical thinking skills to continually assess the patient's skin integrity to judge the status of any wounds and wound healing as well as the effectiveness of therapeutic measures, such as specific wound care therapies and irrigations, pressure injury prevention and care, and specialized dressings.

Frequent and thorough wound assessments are essential to determine the status of wound healing. Use your knowledge of wound healing and the nature of any condition causing the wound to critically think about the specific assessment parameters you will use when observing the patient's wound. Also consider a patient's risk factors for poor wound healing. As you collect assessment data, identify cues and use clinical judgement to determine the specific wound care problem. For example, a postoperative patient shows signs of a wound infection, and as a result the surgical incision was opened for twice-a-day wound irrigations. You need to critically assess the status of ongoing wound healing: determine changes in both wound drainage and wound margin, and review results of any wound cultures. Evaluate the patient's response to wound irrigation, and use clinical judgement to evaluate whether the interventions are effective or whether different therapies are needed.

Prevention of pressure injuries is one goal for safe patient care. There are many patients at risk for these injuries, which can begin as a small, blistered area on the skin that may rapidly progress. Frequent skin assessment of high-risk areas, such as pressure points or the skin under medical devices, such as a tracheostomy or orthopedic device, is crucial. Use knowledge of your patient's current activity and mobility status, current and concurrent illnesses, and nutritional status when you perform a physical assessment to identify skin and areas at risk. Your experience in caring for patients allows you to anticipate problems. For example, experience in caring for patients with feeding tubes prompts you to assess for early signs of a medical device–related pressure injury (MDRPI). As you collect the assessment data and identify cues, use clinical judgement to plan and implement appropriate skin care and prevention interventions. Your initial assessments are a baseline that enable you to later clinically judge the patient's response to these interventions. Preventing pressure injuries from starting or progressing is a major nursing responsibility and begins immediately for all patients, especially those at high risk.

The application of dressings prevents some injuries to wounds, as well as being therapeutic in promoting wound healing. Use clinical judgement when assessing the patient's skin and wounds for early indications of tissue damage. Consider a patient's physical condition and care status to anticipate what to assess. For example, you are caring for a patient who is underweight and has limited mobility related to bilateral traction for leg fractures. Because of the immobility, you know to assess dependent areas of the skin and note that there is a reddened, intact, small blister on their right hip. After consulting with a wound care specialist, you choose a transparent film dressing to protect the area while allowing for ongoing assessment of the wound status. In another example, you are caring for a patient with an open abdominal wound that requires irrigation followed by packing with fine mesh gauze. This intervention promotes wound healing within the wound; however, in order to assess wound healing, you must routinely remove the dressing and packing and inspect the wound. In both of these examples, you will use clinical judgement to determine the effectiveness of the dressing for wound healing. In the first example, you need to evaluate the response to the transparent dressing. Was it protective or did the wound progress? In the second example, you need to fully assess the wound bed and critically analyze wound-healing criteria. Is the wound base showing signs of healing?

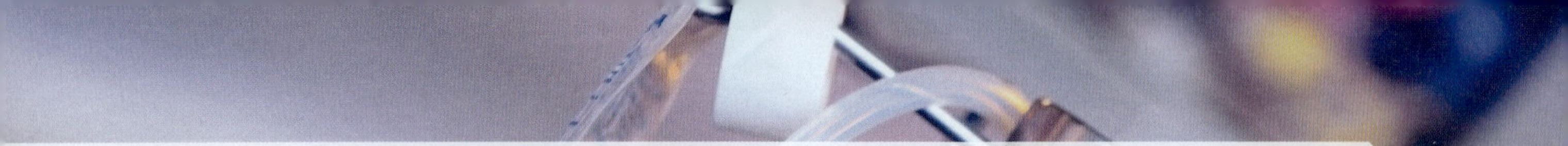

39 Prevention and Care of Skin Breakdown

Canadian content written by **Rosemary Kohr, RN, BA (Arts Plastiques), BScN, MScN, PhD**
Original US chapter by **Janice C. Colwell, RN, MS, CWOCN, FAAN, and Kathleen Hudson, MSN, RN, CWOCN**

SKILLS AND PROCEDURES

OBJECTIVES

Mastery of content in this chapter will enable the nurse to:

- Describe the response of the body during each stage of the wound-healing process.
- Differentiate between primary- and secondary-intention wound healing.
- Explain factors that promote or impair normal wound healing.
- Identify risk factors for the development of skin breakdown (e.g., pressure injury).
- Describe guidelines for the prevention of skin breakdown.
- Perform a skin assessment.
- Describe valid and reliable tools for assessing a patient's risk for pressure injuries.
- Identify outcome criteria for patients at risk for pressure injuries or impaired skin integrity.
- Explain the teaching needs of patients and caregivers regarding the prevention and treatment of skin breakdown (particularly pressure injury).
- Perform a wound irrigation.
- Remove sutures or staples.
- Demonstrate care of a wound drainage system.
- Explain the purpose and use of negative-pressure wound therapy and wound vacuum treatment.

MEDIA RESOURCES

- http://evolve.elsevier.com/Canada/Perry/clinicalskills/

PURPOSE

The skin is the body's largest organ. In its role as sensory protection, the skin defends the body in recognizing pain, touch and pressure, and temperature. The acidic pH of the skin creates an *acid mantle*, which further serves to protect the skin from external bacteria, viruses, and other potential contaminants. It also plays a major role in thermoregulation, metabolism, immunity, and fluid balance regulation (Bryant & Nix, 2024a). Intact skin is the body's first line of defence against invasion by infectious microorganisms. If there is a break in the integrity of the skin, appropriate, evidence-informed wound care is necessary to promote wound closure and restore the skin barrier (Orsted et al., 2017/2021).

Care of a patient's skin is essential for both preventing and managing skin breakdown. Pressure injuries are of particular importance in health care settings: they are one type of skin breakdown that often can be prevented by implementing evidence-informed practices such as pressure off-loading, management of incontinence, adequate nutritional intake, and consistent, regular repositioning schedules. In addition, frequent monitoring of the patient's skin can be done by educating the patient, caregiver, and unregulated care providers (UCPs) about wound assessment and prevention strategies (Orsted et al., 2017/2021).

STANDARDS OF CARE

- Accreditation Canada (2020)—*Required Organizational Practices–2020 Handbook* (https://physicians.nshealth.ca/resources/required-organizational-practices-2020-handbook)
- Edsberg et al. (2016)—*Revised National Pressure Ulcer Advisory Panel Pressure Injury Staging System* (https://doi.org/10.1097/WON.0000000000000281)
- European Pressure Ulcer Advisory Panel (EPUAP), National Pressure Injury Advisory Panel (NPIAP), & Pan Pacific Pressure Injury Alliance (PPPIA) (2019)—*Prevention and Treatment of Pressure Ulcers/Injuries: Quick Reference Guide*, 3rd edition (https://guidelinesales.com/store/ViewProduct.aspx?id=15037164)
- Healthcare Excellence Canada (n.d.)—*Pressure Ulcer: Introduction* (https://www.healthcareexcellence.ca/en/what-we-do/

all-programs/hospital-harm-is-everyones-concern/hospital-harm-improvement-resource/pressure-ulcer-introduction/)

- Norton et al. (2017/2021)—*Best Practice Recommendations for the Prevention and Management of Wounds* (https://www.woundscanada.ca/docman/public/health-care-professional/bpr-workshop/172-bpr-prevention-and-management-of-pressure-injuries-2/file)
- Wound, Ostomy, and Continence Nurses Society (WOCN, 2016)—*Guideline for Prevention and Management of Pressure Ulcers (Injuries)*, 2nd edition (https://www.wocn.org/)

PRINCIPLES FOR PRACTICE

- The skin is the largest external organ. It has two layers: the *epidermis* and the *dermis* (Fig. 39.1). The epidermis has five layers:
  - The *stratum corneum*, the outermost layer, consists of flattened, dead keratinized cells. The stratum corneum prevents dehydration of the underlying cells and is a physical barrier against entry of certain chemicals.

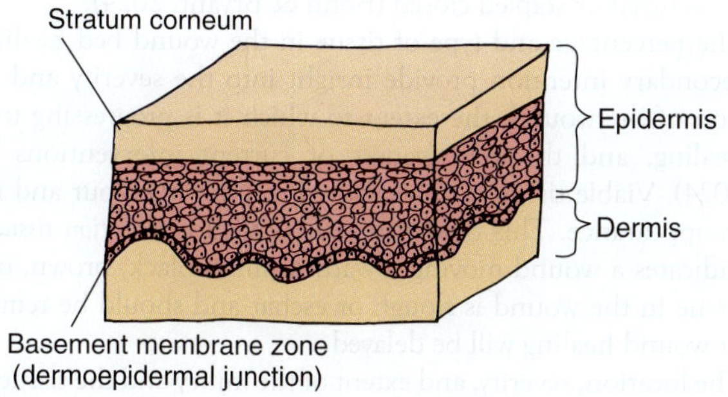

FIG 39.1 Diagram of layers of skin and subcutaneous tissue.

  - The next three layers of the epidermis are the *stratum lucidum*, *stratum granulosum*, and *stratum spinosum*.
  - The *stratum germinativum*, the innermost layer, is sometimes called the *basal layer*. Important features of the stratum germinativum are the epidermal protrusions, or "peaks and valleys," that point downward into the dermis. These provide resiliency and integrity to the skin structure. *Melanocytes*, the cells that give skin its colour, are also found in this layer. As individuals age, this layer flattens out, decreasing the skin's resiliency.
- The area that separates the epidermis from the dermis is called the *dermoepidermal junction*, or *basement membrane zone*.
- Beneath the epidermis is the dermis. Collagen (a tough, fibrous protein layer), blood vessels, and nerves compose the dermal layer. Collagen constitutes about 70% of the dermis and is essential in wound healing. The dermis restores the physical properties of the skin and its structural integrity. Restoration of both the epidermal and dermal layers is necessary to promote healing. Local or systemic infection, impaired circulation, and breakdown of tissue directly impair the wound-healing ability of the skin layers (Bohn & Bryant, 2024).
- Pressure injuries occur from unrelieved, prolonged soft tissue compression, which interferes with blood flow to the tissue; if this compression continues for an extended period of time, the tissue dies from lack of blood flow, or *tissue ischemia*. Ischemia develops when pressure on the skin is greater than vascular pressure inside the vessels, causing the vessels to collapse and decreasing tissue perfusion.
- The most common sites for the development of pressure injuries are over bony prominences such as the sacrum, coccyx, ischial tuberosities, greater trochanters, heels, scapulae, iliac crests, and lateral and medial malleoli (Nix & Bryant, 2024). Figure 39.2

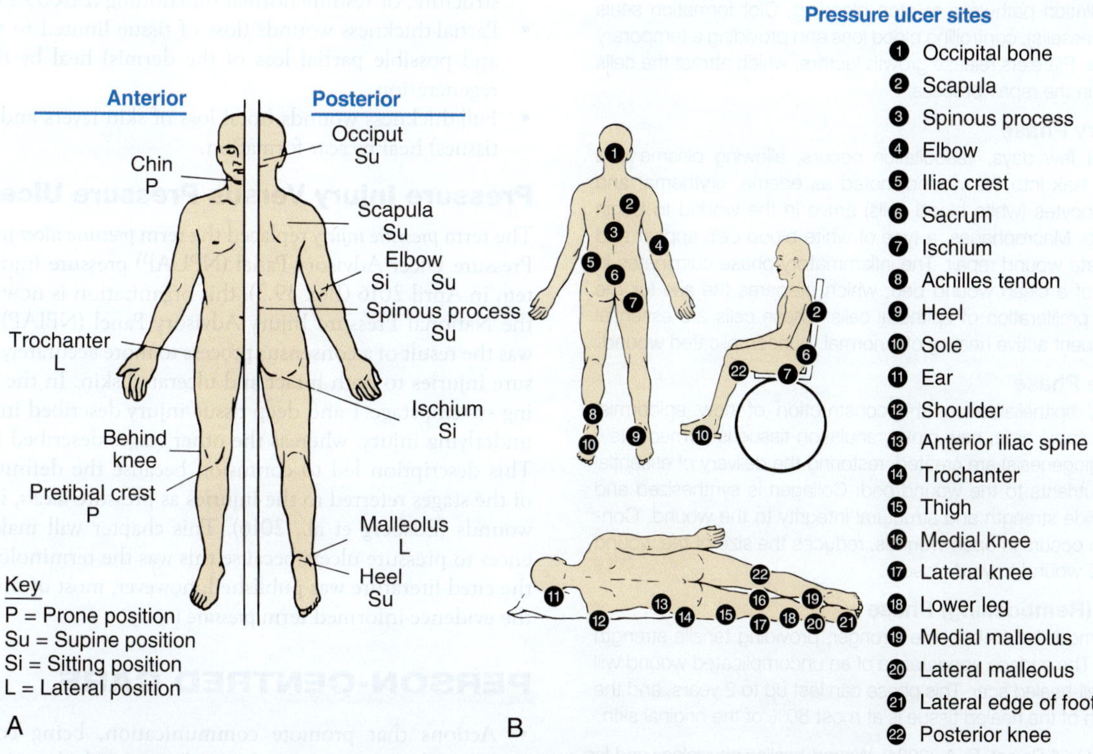

FIG 39.2 A, Bony prominences most frequently underlying pressure injuries. B, Pressure injury sites.
(From Trelease, C. C. [1988]. Developing standards for wound care. Ostomy & Wound Management, 26, 50.)

shows pressure points over bony prominences, where pressure injuries can develop in sitting or lying positions.

- Wounds should be assessed on a scheduled basis. If the assessment indicates that the wound is not healing as expected, the plan of care needs to be changed to support wound healing.
- A thorough wound assessment includes the identification of the type of wound healing (e.g., primary, secondary, or tertiary intention) and the type of tissue and characteristics of the wound base, as well as the condition of the wound edges and periwound skin. All these parameters should be considered when determining treatment options. In the case of a pressure injury, the assessment includes identifying the stage of injury (Kottner et al., 2019), discussed later in this chapter.
- The wound-healing process consists of *phases*, which for explanatory purposes are presented as distinct—but in reality, these phases overlap. In a full-thickness wound, the phases are hemostasis, inflammation, proliferation, and remodelling or maturation (Box 39.1). Every wound or injury, no matter what type, follows the same phases of wound healing. Chronic wounds are those wounds that stall at a particular point in the wound-healing trajectory.
- During the proliferative stage, fibroblasts migrate to the site of injury. Fibroblasts increase the synthesis of collagen, which forms the healing ridge that can be palpated under an intact healing incision by days 5 to 9 (Fig. 39.3) (Bohn & Bryant, 2024).
- Wound healing occurs by primary, secondary, and tertiary intention (Fig. 39.4).
  - Healing by *primary intention* occurs when the edges of a clean surgical incision remain close together. The wound heals quickly, and tissue loss is minimal or absent (Bohn & Bryant, 2024). The skin cells regenerate quickly, and capillary walls stretch across the wound, under the suture line, to form a smooth surface as they join.
  - Wounds that are left open and allowed to heal by scar formation are classified as healing by *secondary intention* (Beitz, 2022). Tissue loss and open wound edges occur. Granulation tissue gradually fills in the area of the wound (Fig. 39.5). This process is typical of severe laceration or massive surgical intervention with skin loss.
    - In secondary intention, there is a gap between the edges. Connective tissue develops, which supports new capillaries. This type of healing results in the formation of scar tissue to close the wound. The slowness of this process places a patient at greater risk for infection because there is no epidermal barrier until later in the healing process.
  - Healing by *tertiary intention* is sometimes called *delayed primary intention* or *closure*. It occurs when surgical wounds are not closed immediately but left open for 3 to 5 days to allow edema or infection to diminish. Then, the wound edges are sutured or stapled closed (Bohn & Bryant, 2024).
- The percentage and type of tissue in the wound bed healing by secondary intention provide insight into the severity and duration of the wound, the extent to which it is progressing toward healing, and the effectiveness of current interventions (Nix, 2024). Viable tissue is normally red to pink in colour and moist in appearance. This type of tissue is called *granulation tissue* and indicates a wound moving toward healing. Black, brown, or tan tissue in the wound is slough or eschar and should be removed, or wound healing will be delayed.
- The location, severity, and extent of the injury and the tissue layer or layers involved all affect the wound-healing process (Bohn & Bryant, 2024). In addition, there are underlying factors that prevent the ability of cells and tissues to regenerate, return to normal structure, or resume normal functioning (Box 39.2).
- Partial-thickness wounds (loss of tissue limited to the epidermis and possible partial loss of the dermis) heal by the process of regeneration.
- Full-thickness wounds (total loss of skin layers and some deeper tissues) heal by scar formation.

BOX 39.1

Phases of Wound Healing (Full-Thickness Wounds)

Hemostasis Phase

Immediately upon injury, blood vessels constrict, and clotting factors activate coagulation pathways to stop bleeding. Clot formation seals the disrupted vessel(s), controlling blood loss and providing a temporary bacterial barrier. Platelets release growth factors, which attract the cells needed to begin the repair process.

Inflammatory Phase

Within the first few days, vasodilation occurs, allowing plasma and blood cells to leak into the wound, noted as edema, erythema, and exudate. Leukocytes (white blood cells) arrive in the wound to begin wound cleanup. Macrophages, a type of white blood cell, appear and begin to regulate wound repair. The inflammatory phase culminates in the formation of a clean wound bed, which prepares the site for the migration and proliferation of epithelial cells. These cells are essential for the subsequent active healing of a normal, noncomplicated wound.

Proliferative Phase

In this phase, epithelialization (the construction of new epidermis) begins. At the same time, new pink granulation tissue is formed. New capillaries (angiogenesis) are created, restoring the delivery of essential oxygen and nutrients to the wound bed. Collagen is synthesized and begins to provide strength and structural integrity to the wound. Contraction, which occurs in open wounds, reduces the size of the wound and moves the wound toward closure.

Maturation (Remodelling) Phase

Collagen is remodelled to become stronger, providing tensile strength to the wound. The surface appearance of an uncomplicated wound will be that of a well-healed scar. This phase can last up to 2 years, and the tensile strength of the healed tissue is at most 80% of the original skin.

Data from Bohn, G., & Bryant, R. A. (2024). Wound-healing physiology and factors that affect the repair process. In R. A. Bryant & D. P. Nix (Eds.), *Acute and chronic wounds: Intraprofessionals from novice to expert* (6th ed., pp. 143–163). Elsevier Inc.

Pressure Injury Versus Pressure Ulcer

The term *pressure injury* replaced the term *pressure ulcer* in the National Pressure Ulcer Advisory Panel (NPUAP) pressure injury staging system in April 2016 (Box 39.3); this organization is now referred to as the National Pressure Injury Advisory Panel (NPIAP). This update was the result of a consensus process to more accurately describe pressure injuries to both intact and ulcerated skin. In the previous staging system, stage 1 and deep tissue injury described intact skin with underlying injury, whereas the other stages described open injuries. This description led to confusion because the definitions for each of the stages referred to the injuries as pressure *ulcers*, implying open wounds (Edsberg et al., 2016). This chapter will make some references to pressure ulcers because this was the terminology used when the cited literature was published; however, most of this text will use the evidence-informed term *pressure injury*.

PERSON-CENTRED CARE

- Actions that promote communication, being conscious of a patient's privacy (e.g., using drapes and sheets), and prompt removal of soiled dressings and bed linens are inherent aspects of care for every patient.

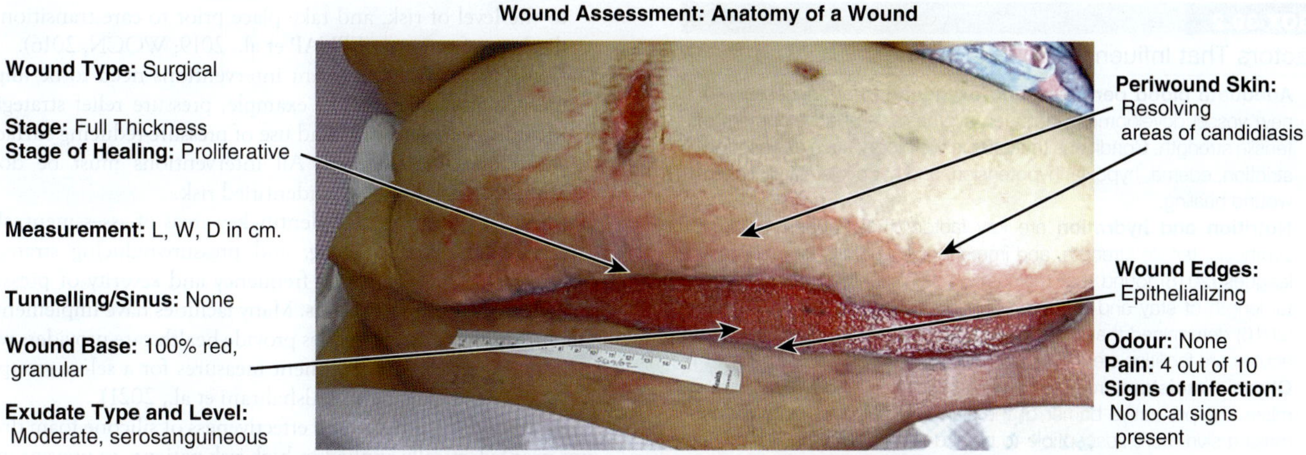

FIG 39.3 Surgical wound with epithelialization occurring. Epithelial healing ridge apparent. *(From Bryant, R. A., & Nix, D. P. [Eds.]. [2024]. Acute and chronic wounds: Intraprofessionals from novice to expert [6th ed.]. Elsevier Inc.)*

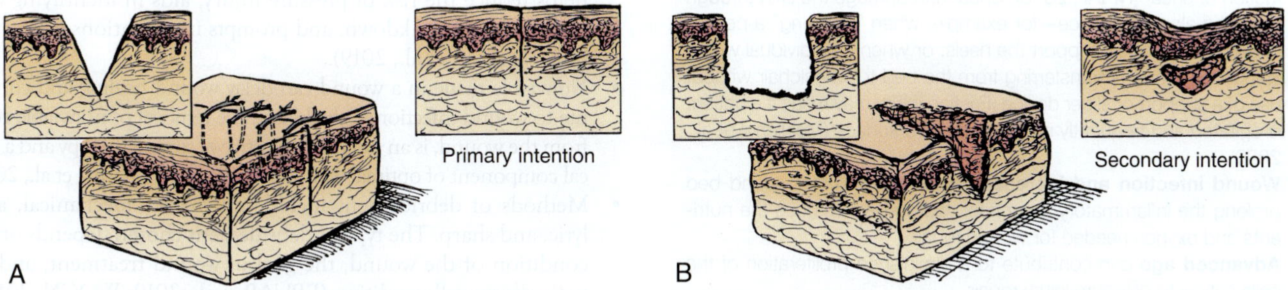

FIG 39.4 Wound healing by primary intention such as with a surgical incision. A, Wound healing edges are pulled together and approximated with sutures, staples, or adhesive tape strips; healing occurs by connective tissue deposition. B, Wound healing by secondary intention. Wound edges are not approximated, and healing occurs by granulation tissue formation and contraction of the wound edges. *(From Bryant, R. A., & Nix, D. P. [Eds.]. [2024]. Acute and chronic wounds: Intraprofessionals from novice to expert [6th ed.]. Elsevier Inc.)*

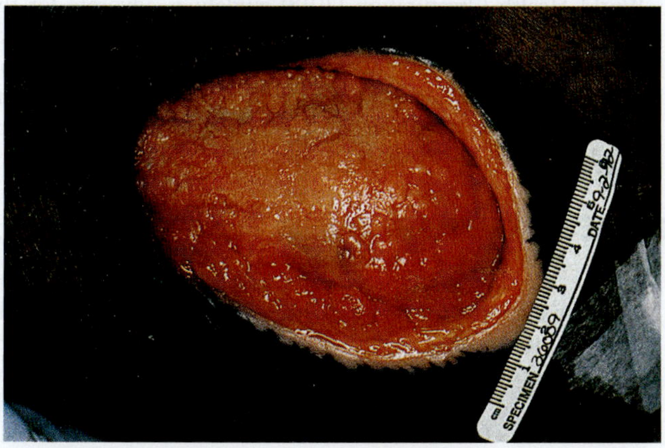

FIG 39.5 Open wound with granulation tissue.

- Sensitivity toward cultural differences is essential. Paying attention to the patient's and family's cultural and religious needs will help to allay anxiety and miscommunication.
- In providing skin care, nurses need to recognize potentially sensitive issues, such as whether care needs to be provided by health care personnel who have the same gender as the patient. In some cultures, it may be inappropriate to expose body parts to a member of the opposite sex (Squitieri et al., 2020). Use of a professional translator may also be required to ensure that communication is clearly understood by the patient, caregiver, and health care provider. Unless unavoidable (e.g., emergency situation), family members or other staff members should not be used as translators.
- When changing dressings or assessing wounds, it is important to recognize that blood and secretions may hold different meanings for some cultures (e.g., bed linens or gowns may be considered "dirty" and should be promptly changed; blood may be seen as a life force, so the presence of it on dressings or sheets should first be explained and then removed as soon as possible).
- Some religious beliefs may prohibit the use of dressings containing any animal-derived products (e.g., some dressings may contain animal-derived collagen) (Chong et al., 2017; Farroha, 2020).
- Encourage patients to talk about any traditional home remedies and practices that they may have used or might use. It is important to respectfully explain to the patient and caregiver when to avoid these practices if they could increase the risk of infection or negatively affect wound healing.

EVIDENCE-INFORMED PRACTICE

- Risk assessment is a central component of clinical practice aimed at identifying individuals susceptible to skin breakdown in order

BOX 39.2

Factors That Influence Wound Healing

- **Adequate blood perfusion and oxygenation** are necessary for new vessel development, collagen synthesis, and development of tensile strength. Conditions that affects the blood, such as vasoconstriction, edema, hypoxia, hypotension, and hypovolemia, will affect wound healing.
- **Nutrition and hydration** are key factors that support collagen synthesis, tensile strength, and immune function. Hudson and colleagues (2018) found that malnutrition significantly impacts hospital length of stay and mortality. Importantly, Allard and colleagues (2016) determined that over 45% of patients admitted to Canadian acute care facilities were clinically malnourished on admission.
- **Chronic moisture** from fecal and urinary incontinence compromises the protective barrier of the skin and may macerate tissue, making skin more susceptible to breakdown. In addition, alteration in the skin's pH (acid mantle) caused by exposure to urine or feces can compromise the barrier effectiveness of the acid mantle (Elias, 2017).
- **Pressure off-loading** is a key element in skin breakdown, occurring either through the unrelieved pressure from immobility or through friction or shear (NPIAP, 2016). Shear can damage the skin through dragging along a surface—for example, when "boosting" a person in bed, forgetting to support the heels, or when an individual with a spinal cord injury is transferring from the bed to wheelchair without use of a support or slider device. Friction injury may result if a patient is agitated and frequently rubbing across a surface (McNichol et al., 2020).
- **Wound infection and increased bioburden** in the wound bed prolong the inflammatory response; microorganisms use the nutrients and oxygen needed for wound repair.
- **Advanced age** can contribute to a diminished proliferation of the cells critical to pressure injury repair.
- A patient with **diabetes mellitus** may have impaired wound healing because of abnormal and prolonged inflammation, reduced collagen synthesis, and impaired epithelial migration. Hyperglycemia is associated with compromised neutrophil function and impaired migration.
- **Corticosteroid therapy or the use of other immunosuppressive agents** such as chemotherapy increases a patient's susceptibility to infection.
- **Medical devices** can cause pressure injury or skin breakdown if the device lies over a bony prominence. In the case of nonbony locations, injury can result from a poorly positioned or ill-fitting device or incorrect device use. These types of skin injuries are called *medical device–related pressure injuries (MDRPIs)*—injuries resulting from devices designed and applied for diagnostic or treatment purposes. The injury generally conforms to the shape of the device (WOCN, 2016).

Adapted from Bohn, G., & Bryant, R. A. (2024). Wound-healing physiology and factors that affect the repair process. In R. A. Bryant & D. P. Nix (Eds.), *Acute and chronic wounds: Intraprofessionals from novice to expert* (6th ed., pp. 143–163). Elsevier Inc.

to target appropriate prevention and treatment interventions (Hajhosseini et al., 2020; WOCN, 2016):

- Ensure that a complete skin assessment is part of the risk assessment screening policy at all health care facilities (EPUAP et al., 2019; WOCN, 2016). Ongoing, regular skin assessment is necessary to detect early signs of skin breakdown, particularly pressure-related damage.
- In individuals at risk for skin breakdown (see factors in Box 39.2), a comprehensive skin assessment should be conducted as soon as possible, within 8 hours of admission (or first visit in a community setting). Ongoing assessment and evaluation should be part of the patient care plan, be related to the level of risk, and take place prior to care transition or discharge from care (EPUAP et al., 2019; WOCN, 2016).
- If risk is identified, relevant interventions need to be implemented immediately. For example, pressure relief strategies, including repositioning and use of pressure-reducing surfaces, should be implemented. All interventions must be documented in relation to the identified risk.

- Skin integrity bundles that identify key areas of assessment, skin care measures, repositioning, and pressure-reducing strategies are effective in reducing the frequency and severity of pressure injuries in critically ill patients. Many facilities have implemented this approach, as these bundles provide health care providers with specific preventive and treatment measures for a select group of at-risk or high-risk patients (Alshahrani et al., 2021).
- There is some evidence of the effectiveness of silicone foam dressings prophylactically applied in high-risk patients to prevent pressure injury development (Fulbrook et al., 2019; Jackson et al., 2019). However, frequent repositioning, visual inspection of the area, and incontinence management are also essential.
- Routine assessment of skin under and around medical devices helps reduce the risk of pressure injury, aids in identifying early stages of skin breakdown, and prompts interventions (Cao et al., 2022; Jackson et al., 2019).
- Nonviable tissue in a wound can delay wound healing and contribute to wound infection. *Debridement,* the removal of nonviable tissue from the wound, is an essential objective of topical therapy and a critical component of optimal wound management (Manna et al., 2023).
- Methods of debridement include enzymatic, mechanical, autolytic, and sharp. The type of debridement chosen depends on the condition of the wound, the goal of wound treatment, and the patient's overall condition (EPUAP et al., 2019; WOCN, 2016).
- Enzymatic debridement is the topical application of enzymes such as collagenase over necrotic tissue. Collagenase can effectively digest the collagen isoforms that are found in necrotic tissue to enhance cell migration (EPUAP et al., 2019). When collagenase is used on a wound, the necrotic tissue is covered with the collagenase, and a moisture-retentive dressing can be used to soften the tissue (Lumbers, 2018).
- World Health Organization (2018) guidelines advocate for the use of triclosan-coated sutures because there is moderate evidence to support their use for reducing the risk of surgical site infection or postoperative wound complications. It is important that the primary repair approximate the wound edges and that the incision be adequately perfused.

SAFETY GUIDELINES

- Patients should be routinely assessed for risk of skin breakdown, especially patients who have any underlying factors that would increase the risk of pressure injury. The Braden Risk Assessment tool (Braden Scale; https://www.bradenscale.com/) and the Norton Scale (WOCN, 2016) are valid and reliable tools that provide guidance for effective interventions to reduce the risk of skin breakdown. However, evidence is inconclusive as to whether the use of risk assessment scales reduces the incidence of pressure injuries (WOCN, 2016). It is the combination of identified risk (based on a risk assessment tool), critical thinking, clinical judgement, and targeted interventions aimed at the specific risk factors that decreases potential pressure injury development.
- Standard risk assessment tools provide instructions for preventive interventions. These interventions include documenting the location of pressure points and establishing a repositioning routine, to be implemented every 1–2 hours as patient condition

BOX 39.3

Staging of Pressure Injuries

Description

Stage 1 Pressure Injury: Nonblanchable Erythema of Intact Skin

Intact skin with a localized area of nonblanchable erythema, which may appear differently in darkly pigmented skin. Presence of blanchable erythema or changes in sensation, temperature, or firmness may precede visual changes. Colour changes do not include purple or maroon discoloration; these may indicate deep tissue pressure injury.

Stage 1 Pressure Injury—Lightly Pigmented

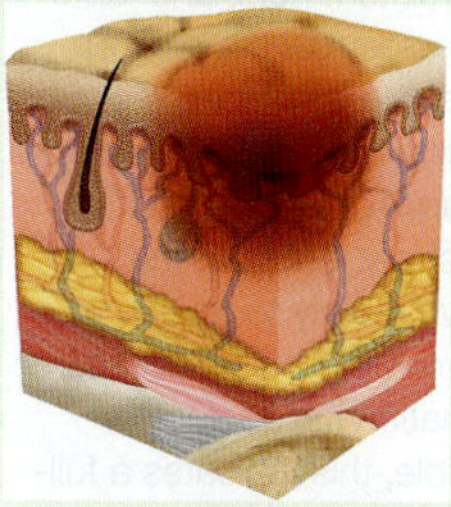

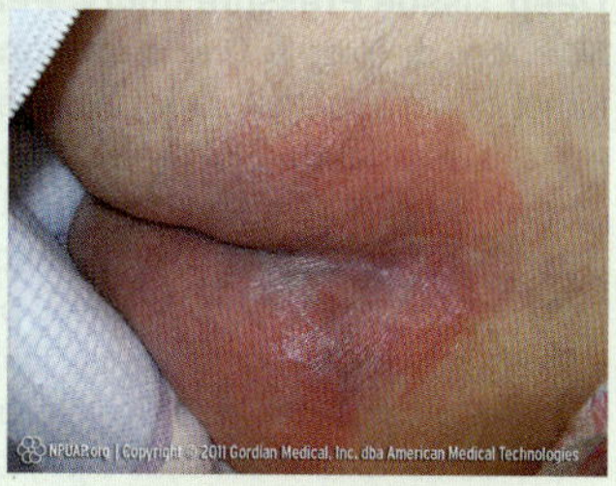

Stage 1 Pressure Injury—Darkly Pigmented

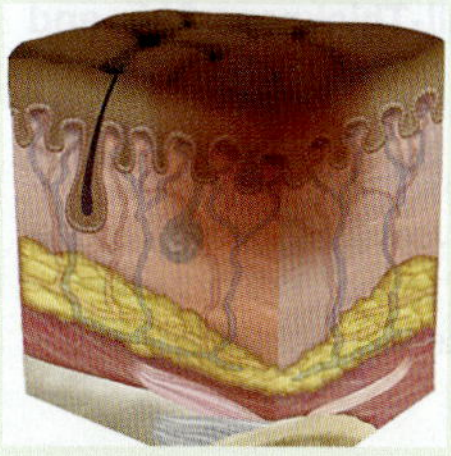

Stage 2 Pressure Injury: Partial-Thickness Skin Loss With Exposed Dermis

Partial-thickness loss of skin with exposed dermis. The wound bed is viable, pink or red, and moist and may also present as an intact or ruptured serum-filled blister. Adipose (fat) and deeper tissues are not visible. Granulation tissue, slough, and eschar are not present. These injuries commonly result from adverse microclimate and shear in the skin over the pelvis and shear in the heel. This stage should not be used to describe moisture-associated skin damage (MASD), including incontinence-associated dermatitis (IAD), intertriginous dermatitis (ITD), medical adhesive–related skin injury (MARSI), or traumatic wounds (skin tears, burns, abrasions).

Stage 2 Pressure Injury

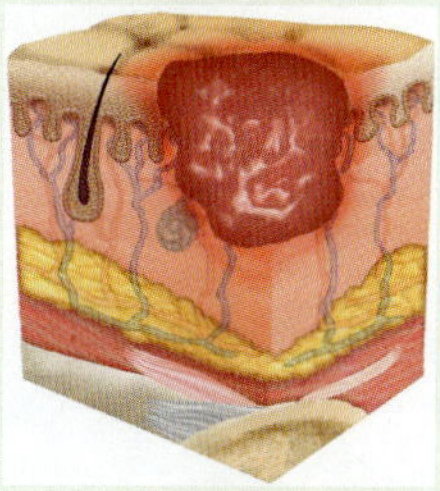

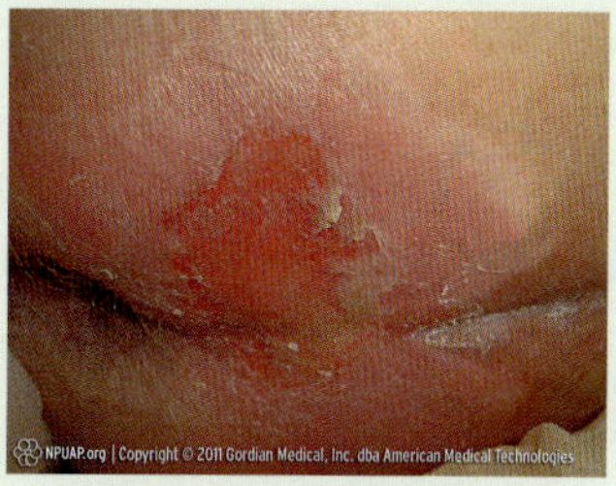

Stage 3 Pressure Injury: Full-Thickness Skin Loss

Full-thickness loss of skin, in which adipose (fat) is visible in the injury and granulation tissue and epibole (rolled wound edges) are often present. Slough and/or eschar may be visible. The depth of tissue damage varies by anatomical location; areas of significant adiposity can develop deep wounds. Undermining and tunnelling may occur. Fascia, muscle, tendon, ligament, cartilage, and/or bone are not exposed. If slough or eschar obscures the extent of tissue loss, this is an *Unstageable Pressure Injury*.

Stage 3 Pressure Injury

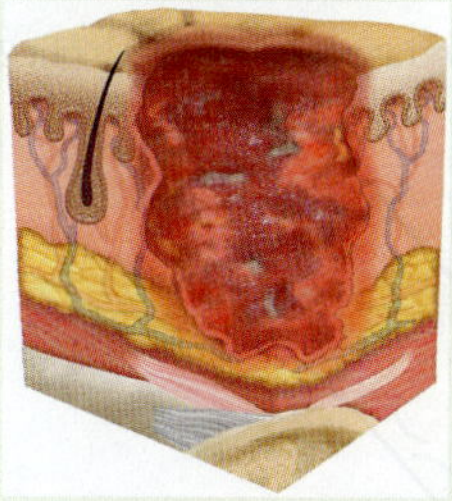

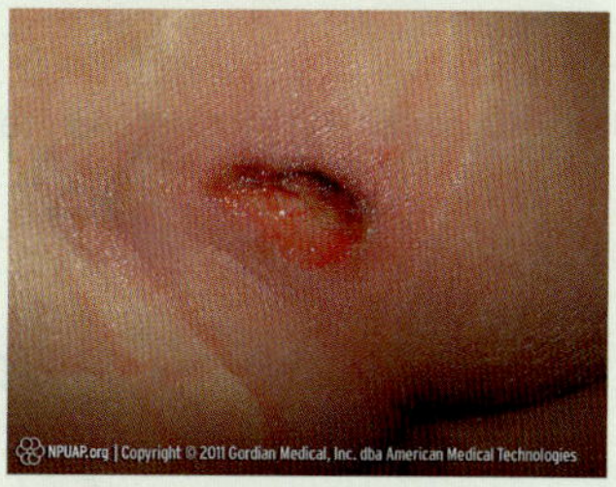

Stage 4 Pressure Injury: Full-Thickness Skin and Tissue Loss

Full-thickness skin and tissue loss with exposed or directly palpable fascia, muscle, tendon, ligament, cartilage, or bone in the injury. Slough and/or eschar may be visible. Epibole (rolled edges), undermining, and/or tunnelling often occur. Depth varies by anatomical location. If slough or eschar obscures the extent of tissue loss, this is an *Unstageable Pressure Injury*.

Stage 4 Pressure Injury

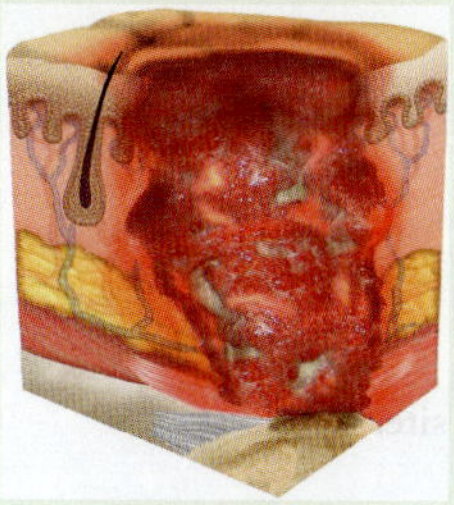

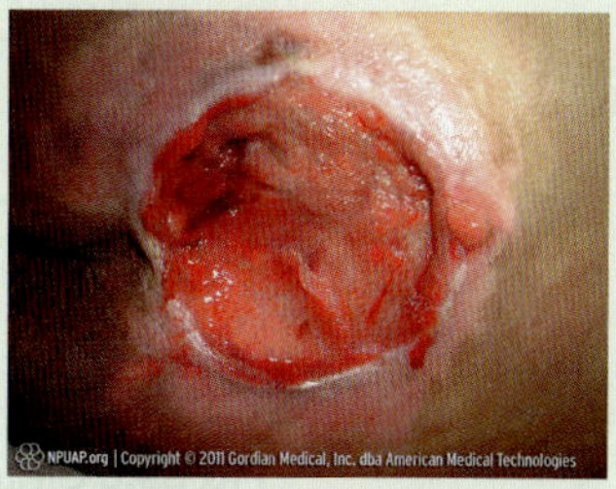

Continued

BOX 39.3

Staging of Pressure Injuries—cont'd

Description

Deep Tissue Pressure Injury: Persistent Nonblanchable Deep Red, Maroon, or Purple Discoloration

Intact or nonintact skin with localized area of persistent nonblanchable deep red, maroon, or purple discoloration or epidermal separation revealing a dark wound bed or blood-filled blister. Pain and temperature change often precede skin colour changes. Discoloration may appear differently in darkly pigmented skin. This injury results from intense and/or prolonged pressure and shear forces at the bone–muscle interface. The wound may evolve rapidly to reveal the actual extent of tissue injury or may resolve without tissue loss. If necrotic tissue, subcutaneous tissue, granulation tissue, fascia, muscle, or other underlying structures are visible, this indicates a full-thickness pressure injury (*Unstageable, Stage 3, or Stage 4*). Do not use *deep tissue pressure injury (DTPI)* to describe vascular, traumatic, neuropathic, or dermatological conditions.

Deep Tissue Pressure Injury

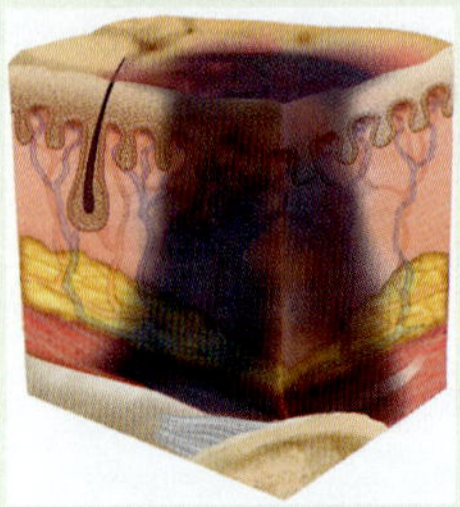

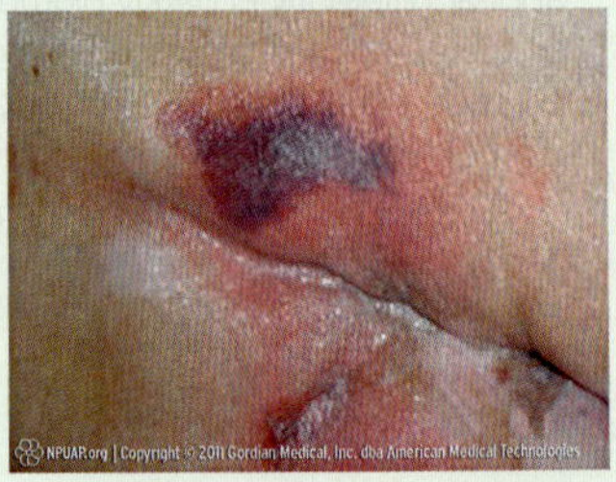

Unstageable Pressure Injury: Obscured Full-Thickness Skin and Tissue Loss

Full-thickness skin and tissue loss in which the extent of tissue damage within the injury cannot be confirmed because it is obscured by slough or eschar. If slough or eschar is removed, a Stage 3 or Stage 4 pressure injury will be revealed. *Stable eschar* (i.e., dry, adherent, intact without erythema or fluctuance) on a heel or ischemic limb *should not be softened or removed*.

Dark Eschar

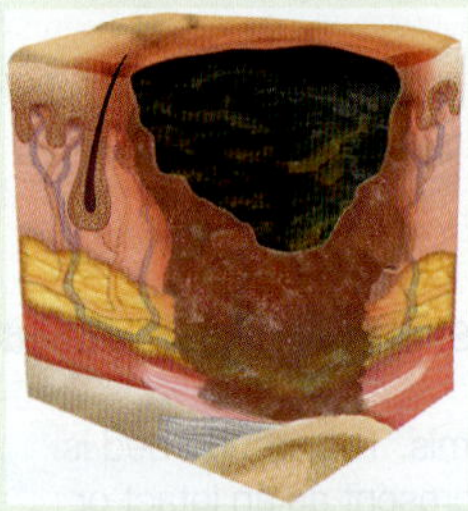

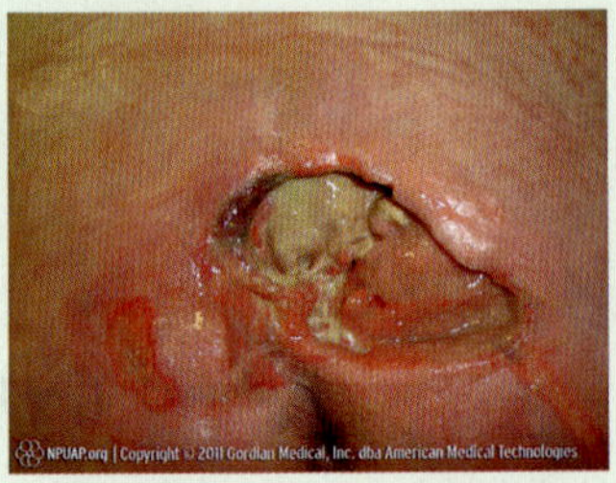

Slough Eschar

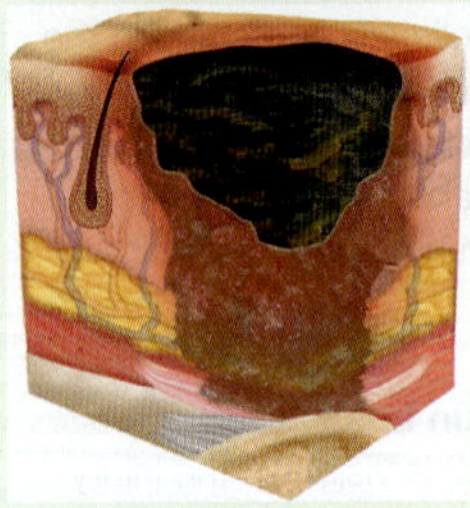

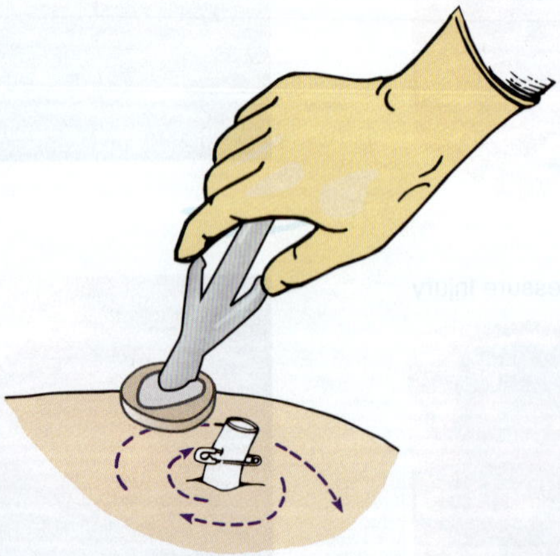

FIG 39.6 Cleaning drain site.

allows—doing so ensures redistribution of pressure from the superficial capillaries and allow tissues to compensate for temporary ischemia. Nurses need to follow appropriate lifting and handling guidelines to avoid friction and shear (see Chapter 11).

- Patients at high risk of sustaining a pressure injury should be placed on specialized beds, overlays, or mattresses (see Chapter 13), which redistribute pressure over the entire body surface to prevent excess pressure over bony prominences. By distributing pressure evenly over a patient's body surface, less pressure is applied to a concentrated area. Similar products to redistribute pressure (e.g., high-density foam, gel, or inflatable air cushion) should be provided for at-risk patients (e.g., those sitting in a wheelchair or geriatric chair).
- Patients who are incontinent of stool or urine must be cleaned as soon as possible. Use gentle cleansing cloths and/or no-rinse perineal cleanser. Prolonged skin moisture from urinary and fecal incontinence creates alteration in skin pH as well as, in the case of fecal incontinence, fecal enzyme action on the skin—all significant risk factors for skin breakdown (Thayer et al., 2022). Areas subjected to repeated episodes of incontinence should be protected with a barrier ointment, cream, or paste, but these products must not interfere with the effectiveness of continence briefs (adult diapers). Avoid the use of cornstarch or baby powder (Yates, 2018). Fecal containment devices are available for difficult-to-manage fecal incontinence (see Chapter 35).

- Minimize friction and shear through the use of lift sheets when repositioning patients to reduce rubbing of skin against sheets. Ensure heels are not dragging when repositioning. Raise the head of the bed no more than 30 degrees (unless medically contraindicated) to prevent sliding and shear injury and to decrease pressure on the coccyx (WOCN, 2016).
- Adequate nutrition helps prevent and treat pressure injuries (WOCN, 2016). A diet high in protein with enough calories, vitamins, and minerals helps maintain normal tissue status and promotes healing. With tissue injury, the body needs more energy (calories) for healing; nutrient deficiencies may result in impaired or delayed healing. Monitoring a patient's nutritional status is part of the nurse's total assessment (WOCN, 2016).
- Use interprofessional collaboration (e.g., wound care nurse, dietitian) to support optimal wound healing.
- Do not remove an initial surgical dressing for direct wound inspection until the health care provider writes a prescription for removal. If drainage has saturated the initial dressing or the patient is experiencing unanticipated or increased pain, contact the health care provider for reassessment of the surgical site.
- If needed, provide analgesia 30 minutes before a dressing change.
- Healed skin from a prior injury or ulceration is weaker than skin that has never had an injury.
- Know a patient's nutritional status. Tissue repair and infection resistance are directly related to adequate nutrition, including proteins, carbohydrates, lipids, vitamins, and minerals. Patients who are malnourished are at increased risk for wound infections and wound infection–related sepsis (Munoz et al., 2020). Recognize that culture and religion may prohibit certain foods and may also affect nutritional intake during designated religious holidays.
- Understand the risks of obesity. Inadequate vascularization decreases delivery of nutrients and cellular elements required for healing. The patient is at greater risk for wound infection and dehiscence or evisceration (Beitz, 2022; Williamson, 2020).
- When a drain is present, clean the drain site using a circular stroke, starting with the area immediately next to the drain (Fig. 39.6). Using sterile gauze, clean immediately next to the drain and attempt to clean a little farther out from the drain.
- Identify factors that decrease oxygenation, such as decreased hemoglobin level, smoking, and underlying cardiopulmonary conditions. Adequate oxygenation at the tissue level is essential for white blood cell activity and phagocytosis, fibroblast proliferation and collagen synthesis, and re-epithelialization (Bohn & Bryant, 2024). Tissue repair is negatively influenced by a hematocrit value below 33% and a hemoglobin value below 10 g/100 mL. Hemoglobin level and oxygen release to tissues are reduced in smokers.
- Know the types of medications prescribed. Steroids reduce the inflammatory response and slow collagen synthesis. Cortisone depresses fibroblast activity and capillary growth. Chemotherapy depresses bone marrow production of white blood cells and impairs immune function.
- Identify the presence of chronic diseases or chronic trauma, such as diabetes mellitus or radiation. Decreased tissue perfusion and failure to release oxygen to tissues result from diabetes mellitus.

✦ SKILL 39.1 Risk Assessment, Skin Assessment, and Prevention Strategies: Pressure Injury

NSO Nursing Skills Online Wound Care Module 19 / Lessons 1 and 4

The key to preventing the development of pressure injuries is the early identification of an at-risk patient and the implementation of prevention strategies. The *Guideline for Prevention and Management of Pressure Ulcers (Injuries)* (WOCN, 2016) is a compilation of international research and expert reviews that address the following:

- Identifying individuals at risk of developing pressure injuries and initiating an early prevention program
- Implementing appropriate strategies and plans to attain and maintain intact skin and preventing skin breakdown and complications
- Promptly identifying and managing complications
- Involving patient and caregiver in patient's self-management of skin care and pressure injury
- Implementing cost-effective strategies and plans that prevent and treat pressure injuries

The current recommendation is to perform a pressure injury risk assessment on patient admission to a health care facility and to repeat this on a regularly scheduled basis or when there is a significant change in a patient's condition (WOCN, 2016). For example, if a patient who was ambulatory on admission becomes confined to bed because of a surgical procedure, this person is potentially at higher risk for skin breakdown than when first admitted. When assessing patients, the nurse needs to use risk assessment tools such as the Braden Scale or the Norton Scale (WOCN, 2016).

The Braden Scale has six subscale parameters: sensory perception, moisture, activity, mobility, nutrition, and risk of friction and shear (Ayello & Braden, 2002; Braden & Bergstrom, 1989, 1994). The maximum score is 23, indicating little to no risk, with scores ranging from "at risk" to "very high risk" (Table 39.1). It is important to understand how to interpret the meaning of a patient's total score and, more importantly, the subscores. The higher the score, the lower the risk. Specific interventions related to the subscore results should be documented and implemented.

As a nurse, you need to inspect a patient's skin and bony prominences at least daily and in good light. Direct (artificial) lighting may be required in order to identify pressure-related skin changes on individuals with a darker skin tone. Remove medical devices or tape securing these devices, shoes, socks, antiembolic stockings, and heel and elbow protectors for skin inspection (Jackson et al., 2019). Inspect all bony prominences, including back of head, shoulders, rib cage, elbows, hips, ischium, sacrum, coccyx, knees, ankles, and heels (see Fig. 39.2). Palpate any reddened or discoloured areas with a gloved finger to determine whether the erythema blanches. Blanching is normal and expected. If you palpate an area that does not blanch (abnormal reactive hyperemia), this area is a site for potential skin breakdown.

TABLE 39.1

Braden Risk Assessment Scale Score Interpretation

Classification	Risk Scores
At risk	15–18
Moderate risk	13–14
High risk	10–12
Very high risk	≤9

Data from British Columbia Provincial Nursing Skin and Wound Committee. (2014). *Braden scale for predicting pressure ulcer risk in adults & children/infants*. https://tiffanycare.com/wp-content/uploads/2017/03/Braden-Risk-Assessment-Scale.pdf

Delegation and Collaboration

While the skill of performing a pressure injury risk assessment cannot be delegated to an unregulated care provider (UCP), the nurse should instruct the UCP to do the following:

- Frequently change the patient's position and help the patient use specific positions that have been individualized for the patient
- Report any redness or break in the patient's skin
- Report any abrasion from medical devices

Equipment

- Risk assessment tool (use employer-approved tool)
- Documentation record
- Pressure-redistribution mattress, bed, and/or chair cushion
- Positioning aids
- Clean gloves

STEP	RATIONALE
ASSESSMENT	
1. Identify patient using at least two person-specific identifiers (e.g., name and date of birth, or name and medical record number) according to employer policy.	Ensures correct patient. Complies with Accreditation Canada standards and improves patient safety (Accreditation Canada, 2020).
2. Throughout the procedure, the 4 moments for hand hygiene are to be implemented; hand hygiene should occur before initial patient (or patient environment) contact, before an aseptic procedure, after body fluid exposure risk, and after patient (or patient environment) contact. Additional hand hygiene should be performed when hands are visibly soiled.	Proper hand hygiene helps prevent the spread of infectious agents to health care providers.
3. Review medical record to assess patient's risk for pressure injury formation:	Determines need to administer preventive care and identifies specific factors that place patient at risk (EPUAP et al., 2019).
a. Paralysis or immobilization caused by restrictive devices	Patient unable to turn or reposition independently or relieve pressure.
b. Presence of a medical device such as a nasogastric (NG) tube, oxygen equipment, artificial airways, drainage tubing, or mechanical devices (Pittman, 2022).	Medical devices have the potential to exert pressure on a patient's nares or ears or on tissue adjacent to devices such as artificial airways and drainage tubes (Jackson et al., 2019).
(1) If not medically contraindicated, remove medical device to observe and palpate skin and tissues under and around each medical device.	Pressure area assumes the same configuration as medical device (Padula et al., 2023; WOCN, 2016).
c. Sensory loss (e.g., hemiplegia, spinal cord injury)	Patient unable to feel discomfort from pressure and does not independently change position.
d. Circulatory disorders (e.g., peripheral vascular diseases, vascular changes from diabetes mellitus, neuropathy)	Impaired circulation reduces tissue perfusion of tissue layers in skin.
e. Increased temperature	Increases metabolic demands of tissues. Accompanying diaphoresis leaves skin moist.
f. Anemia	Decreased hemoglobin level reduces oxygen-carrying capacity of blood and amount of oxygen available to tissues.
g. Malnutrition	Inadequate nutrition leads to weight loss, muscle atrophy, and reduced tissue mass. Nutrient deficiencies result in impaired or delayed healing (Munoz et al., 2020).
h. Fecal or urinary incontinence	Skin becomes exposed to a moist environment that contains bacteria. Excessive moisture macerates skin (Parnham et al., 2020).
i. Heavy sedation and anaesthesia	Patient is not alert and does not turn or change position independently. Sedation alters sensory perception.
j. Age	Neonates and very young children are at high risk for pressure injury, the head being the most common site (WOCN, 2016). There is loss of dermal thickness in older persons, impairing the ability to distribute pressure (Nix & Bryant, 2024).
k. Dehydration	Results in decreased skin elasticity and turgor.
l. Edema	Edematous tissues are less tolerant of pressure, friction, and shear.
m. Existing pressure injuries	Limit surfaces available for position changes, placing available tissues at increased risk.
n. History of pressure injury	Tensile strength of skin from previously healed pressure injury is ≤80%; therefore, this area cannot tolerate pressure as much as undamaged skin can (Bohn & Bryant, 2024).

STEP	RATIONALE
ASSESSMENT	
4. Use an employer-approved risk assessment tool such as the Braden Scale or Norton Scale. Perform risk assessment when patient enters the health care facility and repeat on a regularly scheduled basis or when there is a significant change in patient's condition (WOCN, 2016).	Valid and reliable risk assessment tools help evaluate patient's risk of developing a pressure injury. Identifying risk factors that contribute to the potential for skin breakdown enables targeting of specific interventions that decrease the risk of skin breakdown.
5. Obtain risk score and evaluate its meaning based on patient's unique characteristics. To calculate risk score, use Braden Scale (https://www.bradenscale.com/) and Tables 39.1 and 39.2.	Risk cut-off score depends on the instrument used. Score involves identifying contributing risk factors and minimizing negative outcomes.
6. Assess condition of patient's skin over regions of pressure (see Fig. 39.2). Apply gloves as needed with open and draining wounds.	Body weight against bony prominences places underlying skin at risk of breakdown.
a. Inspect skin for discoloration (see Box 39.2 for patients with darkly pigmented skin) and tissue consistency (firm or boggy) and palpate for abnormal sensations (Nix, 2024).	Indicates that tissue was under pressure; hyperemia is a normal physiological response to hypoxemia in tissues.
b. Palpate discoloured area on skin and under and around medical devices. Release your fingertip and look for blanching.	If, on palpation, an area of redness blanches (lightens in colour), this indicates normal reactive hyperemia–tissue is not at risk of skin breakdown. Tissue that does not blanch when palpated indicates abnormal reactive hyperemia, an indication of possible ischemic injury.
c. Inspect for pallor or mottling.	Persistent hypoxia in tissues that were under pressure is an abnormal physiological response.
d. Inspect for absence of superficial skin layers.	Represents early pressure injury formation; usually a partial-thickness wound that may have resulted from friction, shear, or both.
e. Inspect for changes in skin temperature, edema, and tissue consistency, especially in individuals with darkly pigmented skin.	Localized heat, edema, and induration have been identified as warning signs of pressure injury development. Because it is not always possible to observe changes in skin colour on darkly pigmented skin, these additional signs should be considered in the assessment (EPUAP et al., 2019).
f. Inspect for wound drainage.	Wound drainage increases risk of skin breakdown because drainage is caustic to skin and underlying tissues. Tubing from drainage devices (e.g., Jackson-Pratt, Hemovac) causes pressure under the device and on adjacent skin (Reddy, 2022).
7. Assess skin and tissue around and beneath medical devices every nursing shift for additional areas of potential pressure injury resulting from medical devices (Jackson et al., 2019) (Table 39.3).	Patients at high risk have multiple sites of pressure necrosis from medical devices in areas other than bony prominences (de Assis et al., 2021). Pressure points around medical devices (e.g., oxygen cannula and masks, drainage tubing) can cause pressure injury to underlying tissue and become full-thickness pressure injuries (Cao et al., 2022; Jackson et al., 2019; Padula et al., 2023).

TABLE 39.2

Pressure Injury Risk Assessment

Level of Care	Initial	Reassessment
Acute care	Within 8 hours of admission (EPUAP et al., 2019)	• On a defined schedule (e.g., every 24–72 hours) • Whenever a major change in patient's condition occurs
Critical care	On admission	• Every 24 hours (Lin et al., 2020) (see employer policy)
Long-term care	On admission	• Weekly for first 4 weeks after admission • Routinely on quarterly basis • Whenever resident's condition changes or deteriorates
Community care	On admission	• Per employer policy

STEP	RATIONALE

ASSESSMENT

8. Observe patient for preferred positions when in bed or chair. Note and care for contractures; provide pressure relief with, for example, foam wedges.	Preferred positions result in weight of body being placed on certain bony prominences. Presence of contractures may lead to pressure being exerted in unexpected places.
9. Observe ability of patient to initiate and help with position changes.	Potential for friction and shear injuries increases when patient is dependent on others for position changes.

TABLE 39.3

Strategies to Prevent Medical and Immobilization Device–Related Pressure Injuries

Device	Pressure Areas	Prevention Strategies*
Nasogastric tubes	Nares Skin on nasal bridge	Secure tube using pressure-relieving techniques, which direct pressure from tube away from the nares (see Chapters 32 and 35). Reposition tube.
Endotracheal tubes	Lips Tongue	Remove securing device daily and inspect for pressure injury (Jackson et al., 2019). Rotate tube every shift or more often.
Nasotracheal tube	Nose/nasal bridge Nares	Remove securing device daily and inspect for pressure injury (Jackson et al., 2019). Reposition.
Tracheostomy tubes	Front of neck and stoma site Back of neck	Remove securing device daily. Increase stoma care. Apply pressure reduction dressing to back of neck.
Oxygen and cannula and tubing	Ears Nose	Apply pressure reduction dressing to external ear. Periodically remove cannula to relieve pressure and inspect for pressure injury (Padula et al., 2023).
Noninvasive positive-pressure ventilation (NIPPV)/bilevel positive airway pressure (BiPAP)	Forehead Nose/nasal bridge	Pretreat bridge of nose with pressure reduction dressing before application of mask. If possible, remove mask for a few minutes.
Drainage tubing	Area immediately next to drainage tube Adjacent area during patient position changes	Apply appropriate dressing around drainage tube. Check tubing placement with each position change. Instruct patient not to lie on tubing (Jackson et al., 2019).
In-dwelling catheter	Thighs Female: Urethra, labia Male: Tip of penis	Provide meticulous perineal care. Anchor and secure catheter to reduce pressure.
Orthopedic devices	All areas where device comes in contact with patient's skin and tissues	When possible and not contraindicated, inspect area under the device.
Neck collar	Neck and occipital region Scalp	Remove hard collars as soon as possible and replace with softer collar (Jackson et al., 2019). Inspect scalp daily.
TED (thromboembolic deterrent) hose or stockings (*not the same as compression stockings*)	Calf Behind knee Heel Toes	Verify proper fit. Remove stockings for observation of pressure points. These are worn only by nonambulatory patients. *Compression stockings* must be fitted after circulation has been assessed (ankle-brachial pressure index or vascular flow studies), which should be documented in patient's history. Compression stockings are designed for ambulatory individuals and generally are applied on arising and removed at bedtime.
Immobilization devices	Wrists Ankles	Apply dressing between patient's skin and immobilizer (Jackson et al., 2019). Verify space between immobilizer and patient's skin. Ensure assistance from person (e.g., unregulated care provider), and remove restraints one at a time to inspect skin.

*In addition to routine inspection and cleansing of skin under and around medical device.

STEP	RATIONALE
ASSESSMENT	
10. Assess patient's and caregiver's understanding of what a pressure injury is and the individual risks for patient to develop pressure injuries.	Gaps in understanding of the significance of a pressure injury and thus its prevention may lead to exacerbation of skin breakdown.

NURSING DIAGNOSES

- Inadequate peripheral tissue perfusion
- Insufficient knowledge regarding pressure injury prevention
- Inadequate nutrition
- Reduced mobility
- Reduced skin integrity
- Potential for impaired skin integrity

Related factors and risk factors are individualized on the basis of patient's condition or needs.

STEP	RATIONALE
PLANNING	
1. Expected outcomes following identification/assessment and intervention plan:	
• Risk factors are identified.	Establishes approach to patient needs and baseline for future assessment.
• Patient experiences no change from baseline skin assessment.	Prevention interventions diminish occurrence or worsening of pressure injury.
• Skin is intact with no evidence of erythema or signs of breakdown.	Prevention strategies reduce risk factors.
• Patient and caregiver are able to articulate and respond to patient's individual risk factors for pressure injury.	Demonstrates knowledge transfer.
2. Explain procedure(s) and purpose to patient and caregiver.	Relieves anxiety and provides opportunity for education.
IMPLEMENTATION	
1. Implement prevention guidelines adapted from WOCN (2016) *Guideline for Prevention and Management of Pressure Ulcers (Injuries).*	Reduces patient's risk of developing pressure injury.
2. Close room door or bedside curtain.	Demonstrates person-centred care by maintaining patient privacy.
3. If patient has open, draining wounds, wear sterile surgical gloves.	Use of routine practices and additional precautions prevents accidental exposure to body fluids.
4. Following initial assessment, continue to inspect skin at least once a day.	
a. Observe patient's skin; pay particular attention to bony prominences and areas around and under medical devices and tubes. If you find a reddened area, gently press area with a gloved finger to check for blanching. If area does not blanch, ensure pressure off-loading; suspect tissue injury and recheck in 1 hour. Discoloration may vary from pink to deep red.	Routine skin inspection is fundamental to risk assessment and in selecting interventions to reduce risk of injury (WOCN, 2016). Persistent redness when lightly pigmented skin is pressed can indicate tissue injury. If the area of redness blanches (pales in colour), it indicates that the skin is likely not at risk of breakdown.

Critical Decision Point *Do not massage reddened areas because doing so may cause additional tissue trauma. Reddened areas indicate blood vessel damage, and massaging can further damage the vessel* (Nix & Brant, 2024).

STEP	RATIONALE
b. If patient has darkly pigmented skin, look for colour changes that differ from their normal skin colour.	Darkly pigmented skin may not blanch. A change in colour may occur at the site of pressure; this change in colour *differs* from patient's usual skin colour (EPUAP et al., 2019) (see Box 39.2).
5. Each shift, check all treatment and assistive devices (e.g., catheters, feeding tubes, casts, braces) for potential pressure points (see Table 39.3).	Pressure from these devices increases risk of injury to bony prominences and other areas.
a. Verify that device is correctly sized, positioned, and secured.	Incorrect size, placement, and securing of medical device can cause excessive pressure and rubbing by device on underlying skin (de Assis et al., 2021).

STEP	RATIONALE

IMPLEMENTATION

STEP	RATIONALE
b. Consider shielding underlying skin with protective dressing (low-profile nonadherent [silicone] foam, hydrocolloid or dimethicone barrier, applied as a wipe).	Silicone foam dressing provides moisture-vapour transfer, wicking moisture away from the body. Hydrocolloid is occlusive but can provide protection from friction and shear. Dimethicone barrier functions as "second skin" barrier (de Assis et al., 2021; Jackson et al., 2019).

Critical Decision Point *Inspect skin around and beneath orthopedic devices (e.g., cervical collar, braces, or cast). Note any abrasions or warmth in areas where devices can rub against the skin* (Jackson et al., 2019; Padula et al., 2023).

STEP	RATIONALE
6. Remove and dispose of gloves.	
7. Review patient's pressure injury risk assessment score, paying attention to subscores.	Risk scores aid in identifying interventions to lessen or eliminate current risk factors.
8. If immobility, inactivity, or poor sensory perception is a risk factor(s) for patient, consider one of the following interventions:	Immobility and inactivity reduce a patient's ability or desire to independently change position. Poor sensory perception decreases a patient's ability to feel sensation or pressure discomfort.
a. Identify appropriate schedule to reposition patient (in consultation with patient). Plan regular assessment of skin condition to identify early signs of pressure damage. If skin changes occur, re-evaluate the plan.	Reduces duration and intensity of pressure. Some patients may require more frequent repositioning (EPUAP et al., 2019; WOCN, 2016).
b. When patient is in side-lying position in bed, use 30-degree lateral position (see Step 8b illustration). Avoid using 90-degree lateral position.	Reduces contact between trochanter and support surface.
c. When needed, use pillow bridging (see Step 8c illustration).	Use of pillows prevents direct contact between bony prominences.

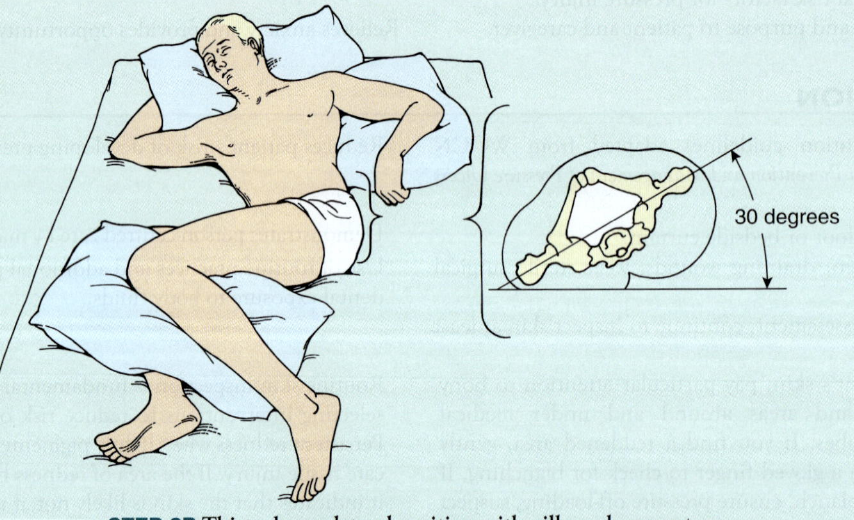

STEP 8B Thirty-degree lateral position with pillow placement.

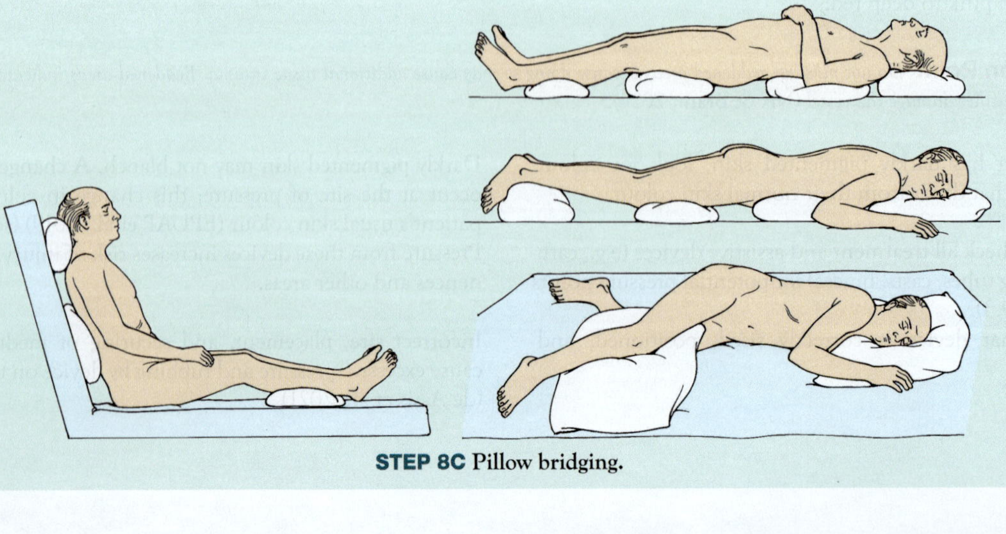

STEP 8C Pillow bridging.

STEP	RATIONALE
IMPLEMENTATION	
d. *In bed:* Ensure pressure-redistribution surface is in place for patient lying in bed. Make sure pressure on heels is reduced.	Reduces amount of pressure exerted on tissues.
e. *In chair:* Use pressure-redistribution device, and shift points under pressure at least every hour (WOCN, 2016). Make sure heels are also provided with pressure off-loading.	Reduces amount of pressure on body areas (e.g., sacrum, ischium, heels).
9. If friction and shear are identified as risk factors, consider the following interventions:	Friction and shear damage tissue from the epidermis to below the dermis through repeated action.
a. Use safe patient handling guidelines to reposition patient (see Chapter 11). For example, use slide board or transfer sheets to move patient from bed to stretcher.	Proper repositioning of patient prevents creating shear from dragging patient along sheets. Slide board provides slippery surface to reduce friction. Use of "lift team," when appropriate, keeps patient's skin, including heels, off sheets.
b. Ensure that heels are free from surface of bed by using a pillow under calves to elevate heels or use a heel-suspension device; knees should be in 5- to 10-degree flexion (Delmore et al., 2019; WOCN, 2016).	"Floating" heels from bed surface offload the heel completely and redistribute weight of the leg along the calf without applying pressure on the Achilles tendon (Delmore et al., 2019).
c. Maintain head of bed at 30 degrees or lower or at the lowest degree of elevation consistent with patient's condition (do not lower head of bed if patient is at risk for aspiration (WOCN, 2016).	Decreases potential for patient to slide toward foot of bed and incur shear injury.
10. If patient receives *low score* on moisture subscale (e.g., Braden Scale), consider one of the following interventions:	Continual exposure of patient's skin to body fluids increases risk of skin breakdown and pressure injury development.
a. Apply clean gloves. Cleanse and pat skin dry after each incontinent episode (WOCN, 2016). Apply moisture barrier protectant (e.g., cream, ointment) to perineum and surrounding skin according to manufacturer instructions.	Reduces transmission of microorganisms. Friction and shear are increased in the presence of moisture. Barrier protects skin from fecal or urinary incontinence. Some barrier products only require once per day application. Overuse leads to occlusion of skin.
b. If skin is denuded, use protective barrier cream or ointment (e.g., dimethicone or petroleum jelly) after each incontinent episode, depending on manufacturer instructions (Smart & Sibbald, 2020).	Provides barrier between skin and stool or urine, allowing for healing. Ensure barrier cream or ointment does not affect absorption of the continence brief.
c. If moisture source is from wound drainage, consider appropriate dressing. Ensure protective barrier to protect skin is in place. Use interprofessional collaboration to discuss collection device if indicated.	Avoids frequent exposure of skin to wound drainage, which can lead to maceration and skin breakdown.
11. If friction and shear are risk factors and patient is confined to a wheelchair:	If sitting is prolonged, relief of pressure by changing from lying to sitting position is insufficient. Patients should be encouraged to reposition; if pressure injury risk factors are present, provide pressure relief cushion (e.g., ROHO, EHOB, or gel cushion) (WOCN, 2016).
a. Tilt patient's chair seat to prevent them from sliding forward; support arms, legs, and feet to maintain proper posture (EPUAP et al., 2019).	
b. Limit amount of time patient spends in a chair without pressure relief (EPUAP et al., 2019).	
c. For patients who can reposition themselves while sitting, encourage pressure relief every 15 minutes using chair push-ups, forward lean, or side-to-side movement (WOCN, 2016).	Assess ability of patient to comply. Continue to use pressure-reduction cushion for chair, since most patients have difficulty managing repositioning on their own.
12. Educate patient and caregiver regarding pressure injury risk and prevention (WOCN, 2016).	Improves adherence to interventions that reduce pressure injury risk.
13. Remove gloves and discard in appropriate receptacle.	Reduces transmission of microorganisms.
EVALUATION	
1. Observe patient's skin for areas at risk for tissue damage, noting change in colour, appearance, or texture (Table 39.4).	Enables evaluation of effectiveness of prevention techniques.

STEP	RATIONALE
EVALUATION	
2. Observe patient's tolerance of position change by measuring level of comfort on appropriate pain rating scale.	Position changes sometimes interfere with patient's sleep and rest pattern.
3. Compare subsequent risk assessment scores and skin assessments.	Provides ongoing comparison of patient's risk level to facilitate appropriateness of plan of care.
4. Use teach-back: "I just want to make sure I explained why your skin needs to be checked regularly. Tell me in your own words why we will be checking your skin on a regular basis." Develop a revised teaching plan if patient or caregiver is unable to teach back correctly.	Determines patient's and caregiver's level of understanding of instructional topic.

Unexpected Outcomes	Related Interventions
1. Skin becomes mottled, reddened, purplish, or bluish.	• Notify health care provider; use interprofessional collaboration (e.g., wound care specialist, dietitian, physiotherapist) as necessary. Re-evaluate patient's circulation and oxygen saturation, immobility and position changes, and bed surface.
2. Areas under pressure develop persistent discoloration, induration, or temperature changes.	• Notify health care provider. • Modify patient's positioning and turning schedule. • Perform more frequent reassessment of condition.

Communication and Documentation

- Document any skin changes, patient's risk score and subscores, and skin assessment on flow sheet in progress notes in electronic health record (EHR) or chart. Describe positions, turning intervals, pressure-redistribution devices, and other prevention measures. Note patient's response to the interventions.
- Document your evaluation of patient's and caregiver's understanding of the need for frequent skin and pressure injury assessment education.
- Report to health care provider the need for additional interprofessional collaboration for the high-risk patient and the time frame for consultation.

DOCUMENTATION EXAMPLE

Full-body assessment conducted. Braden Risk Assessment subscale scores: Sensory 4; Moisture, Activity, Mobility: all 3 out of 4. Nutrition: 2; Potential risk for friction and shear. Nonblanchable erythema located on left heel (approx. 2 cm × 3 cm) and coccyx (approx. 3 cm × 4.5 cm). Otherwise, patient's skin is intact, clean, and dry. Reviewed with patient the need to off-load pressure by repositioning every 2 hours as well as ensuring wheelchair gel cushion is in place/used. Patient able to demonstrate how to reposition self. Reviewed need for patient to inform caregivers to pay attention to repositioning/use of gel cushion. Patient aware of Braden Risk Assessment and importance of improving nutrition. Able to describe ways to increase food intake (e.g., using high-protein drink). Patient and caregiver aware of effective moisture management with use of scant amount of barrier cream to sacral area daily and frequent toileting/change of adult brief. Care when repositioning patient in bed/chair to avoid friction/shear (lift, don't drag). Reassess daily. Consult dietitian to review nutritional status with patient.

TABLE 39.4
Wound Colour/Tissue

Wound Colour	Description
Black or brown wounds/ eschar	Black or brown tissue is eschar, which represents full-thickness tissue destruction. Black is used to describe necrotic tissue or desiccated tissue such as tendon. It is also related to gangrenous lesions secondary to peripheral vascular disease.
Yellow wounds/slough	Yellow tissue represents nonviable tissue and in some cases the presence of an infection. Sloughy tissue, which can be yellow, cream coloured, or grey slough, is often accompanied by purulent drainage.
Red wounds/granulation	Red tissue represents the presence of granulation tissue. The red colour is the result of an increasing amount of new blood vessels in the wound and is considered healthy.

Special Considerations

Teaching

- Help patient and caregiver understand the multiple factors involved in preventing and treating pressure injuries.
- Explain and demonstrate positioning options to achieve pressure redistribution.
- Explain the purpose and maintenance of pressure-redistribution devices (see Chapter 13).
- When teaching patients to change position for pressure redistribution, suggest using television programming and commercial intervals or a clock or phone with an alarm as reminders.

Pediatric

- Infants and young children in diapers are at risk of skin breakdown; also assess occipital area and ensure child has a pressure-reduction pillow or mattress.

Gerontological

- Re-evaluate sitting posture and position because body weight and muscle tone change with age.
- In older persons, thinning skin leads to a decrease in padding protection over bony prominences, and the time for epidermal regeneration is diminished, leading to slower healing (Wysocki, 2024).
- When interpreting the Braden Scale score, consider a score of ≤18 as an indication that the older person is at risk (Huang et al., 2021).

Care in the Community: Home Management

- Identify community resources such as relatives, neighbours, or community (e.g., church) members who may be able to provide safe assistance (e.g., meals, transfer from bed or chair). Review available professional health care services and resources the patient and caregiver may wish to access (e.g., home care services).
- Closely monitor patients at home with the following risk factors: poor nutrition, dementia, wheelchair or bed dependence, incontinence, anemia, fracture, obesity, or skin drainage.
- Remind patient and caregiver that repositioning needs to occur while a patient is sitting in a chair. Suggest that patient considers shifting position every 15 minutes. Small shifts, such as moving or repositioning the legs, redistribute pressure over bony prominences. Patients who sit for long periods in a wheelchair or a chair should have an appropriate and functional pressure-reduction cushion (WOCN, 2016). Ensure that the wheelchair and the cushion are assessed for ongoing functionality.

Procedural Guideline 39.1 *Performing a Wound Assessment*

Video Clip **NSO** *Nursing Skills Online Wound Care Module 19 / Lesson 1*

Normal wound healing occurs in an organized fashion. Evaluation of wound status provides an ongoing assessment of wound healing and helps determine wound treatments. The frequency of wound assessment depends on the patient's overall condition, employer policy, the type of dressings used, and overall patient goals (Nix, 2024). Check employer policy for frequency of wound assessment and specific wound assessment tool.

Routine wound assessment, including documentation of wound measurement, provides valuable information regarding the status of the wound. For example, is wound healing progressing as expected or is it delayed? Is there new drainage? Wound size may be affected by debridement. An expected finding is an increase in the size of the wound when necrotic tissue is removed. An increase in the amount and consistency of the drainage and new presence of odour may indicate a wound infection; a wound culture may be necessary if systemic antibiotics are prescribed.

Assessment of the wound occurs before, during, and after the wound is cleaned and irrigated. The following parameters are included when performing a wound assessment:

- *Location:* Note the anatomical position of the wound.
- *Type of wound:* If known, identify the etiology of the wound (i.e., surgical, pressure, trauma).
- *Extent of tissue involvement:* A full-thickness wound involves both the dermis and epidermis. A partial-thickness wound involves only the epidermal layer. If the wound is a pressure injury, use the staging system of the EPUAP et al. (2019) (see Box 39.3).
- *Type and percentage of tissue in wound base:* Describe the type of tissue (i.e., granulation, slough, eschar) and the approximate percentage of each type.
- *Wound size:* Follow employer policy to measure wound dimensions, which include width, length, and depth.
- *Wound exudate:* Describe the amount, colour, and consistency. Serous drainage is clear like plasma; sanguineous or bright red drainage indicates fresh bleeding; serosanguinous drainage is pink; and purulent drainage is thick and yellow, pale green, or white.
- *Presence of odour:* Note the presence or absence of odour, which may indicate infection.
- *Wound edge:* Determine whether the wound edges are rolled, jagged, or smooth and either pink (healing) or white (maceration) in colour.
- *Periwound area:* Assess the colour, temperature, and integrity of surrounding skin. Note any indication of reaction to dressing (e.g., redness from adhesive tape).
- *Pain:* Use a validated pain assessment scale to evaluate pain.

Delegation and Collaboration

The skill of wound assessment cannot be delegated to a UCP. It is the nurse's responsibility to assess and document wound characteristics. The nurse directs the UCP to report the following to the nurse:

- Drainage from the wound that is present on sheets or as strike-through from the dressing
- Presence of odour in the area of the wound
- Patient indicating increasing pain at the wound site
- Any dressing that is no longer adherent

Equipment

- Personal protective equipment (PPE) (e.g., clean gloves, gown, and goggles if splash or spray risk exists)
- Employer tool to document assessment, including measuring guide
- Cotton-tipped applicator
- Dressing supplies, as prescribed
- Disposable waterproof biohazard bag

Procedural Steps

1. Identify patient using at least two person-specific identifiers (e.g., name and date of birth, or name and medical record number) according to employer policy.
2. Throughout the procedure, the 4 moments for hand hygiene are to be implemented; hand hygiene should occur before initial patient (or patient environment) contact, before an aseptic procedure, after body fluid exposure risk, and after patient (or patient environment) contact. Additional hand hygiene should be performed when hands are visibly soiled.
3. Examine patient record, locating the last wound assessment for comparison with current wound assessment. Review record to determine etiology of the wound, interventions to treat the underlying cause, past dressing protocol, and wound characteristics from the last wound assessment.
4. Assess comfort level or pain on an appropriate pain rating scale and identify symptoms of anxiety. Offer pain medication prior to assessment, if indicated.
5. Close room door or bed curtains and position patient.
   a. Position patient comfortably to permit observation of wound in well-lit room.
   b. Expose area of the wound only, and maintain patient privacy.
6. Explain procedure of wound assessment to patient and caregiver (if caregiver wishes to remain during the assessment, then ensure patient permission).

Continued

Procedural Guideline 39.1 *Performing a Wound Assessment—cont'd*

7. Form a cuff on waterproof biohazard bag and place near bed.
8. Apply clean gloves and remove soiled dressings.
9. Examine dressings for quality of drainage (colour, consistency), presence or absence of odour, and quantity of drainage (note whether dressings were saturated, slightly moist, or had no drainage). Discard dressings in waterproof biohazard bag. Discard gloves.
10. Apply clean gloves.
11. Inspect wound and determine type of wound healing (e.g., primary or secondary intention).
12. Use employer-approved assessment tool and assess the following:
    a. Wound healing by primary intention (surgical wound):
        (1) Assess anatomical location of wound on body.
        (2) Note whether incisional wound margins are approximated or closed together. The wound edges should be together with no gaps.
        (3) Observe for presence of drainage. A closed incision should not have any drainage.
        (4) Look for evidence of infection (presence of erythema, odour, or wound drainage).
        (5) Lightly palpate along incision to feel a healing ridge (see Fig. 39.3). The ridge will appear as an accumulation of new tissue, presenting as firmness beneath the skin and extending to about 1 cm (0.5 inches) on each side of the wound between 5 and 9 days after the incision was created. This is an expected, positive sign (Bohn & Bryant, 2024).
    b. Wound healing by secondary intention (e.g., pressure injury or contaminated surgical or traumatic wound:
        (1) Assess anatomical location of wound.
        (2) Assess wound dimensions: Measure size of wound (including length, width, and depth). If using a ruler, use disposable centimetre measuring guide. Measure length by placing a ruler above wound at the point of greatest length (or head to foot). Measure width from side to side (Nix, 2024) (see Step 12b[2] illustration). Measure depth by inserting cotton-tipped applicator in area of greatest depth and placing a mark on applicator at skin level. Discard measuring guide and cotton-tipped applicator in a biohazard bag. If using an e-documentation system with automatic photo measurement, follow employer instructions for use.

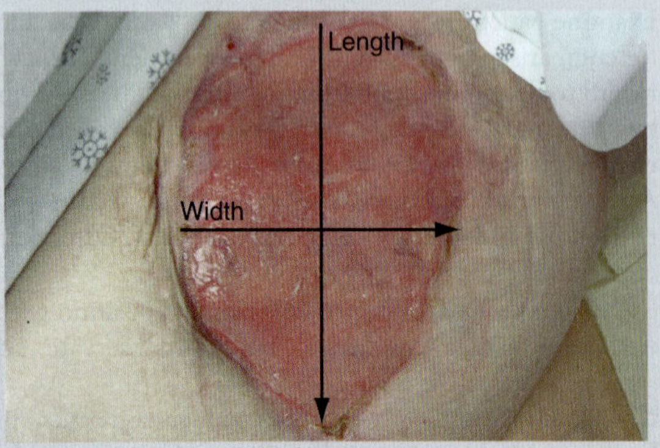

STEP 12B(2) Measuring wound length and width.

        (3) Assess for *undermining* (i.e., the destruction of tissue under intact skin around the wound perimeter): Use cotton-tipped applicator to gently probe wound edges. Measure depth and note location using the face of a clock as a guide. The 12 o'clock position (top of wound) would be toward the head of the patient, and the 6 o'clock position would be the bottom of the wound, toward the patient's feet. Document the number of centimetres that the area extends from the wound edge (e.g., underneath intact skin).
        (4) Assess extent of tissue loss: If the wound is a pressure injury, determine deepest viable tissue layer in wound bed and its stage. If necrotic tissue does not allow visualization of base of the wound, then the stage cannot be determined. If the wound is not a pressure injury, determine whether there is partial-thickness loss (epidermis and part of the dermis) or full-thickness loss (loss of both the epidermis and the dermis). If it is a pressure injury, use the staging system of the EPUAP et al. (2019) (see Box 39.3).
        (5) Observe tissue type, including percentage of granulation, slough, and necrotic tissue.
        (6) Note presence of exudate: amount, colour, consistency, and odour. Indicate amount of exudate by using part of dressing saturated (completely or partially saturated) or in terms of quantity (e.g., scant, moderate, or copious).
        (7) Note whether wound edges are rounded toward wound bed, macerated (white in colour), or jagged—any of these features may indicate delayed wound healing. Describe presence of epithelialization at wound edges (if present) because this indicates movement toward healing.

Critical Decision Point *Compare the wound assessment to previous assessments and determine progress toward healing. If there is no movement toward healing or if you notice deterioration or increased drainage, consider a wound care consultation. Lack of wound healing is often related to infection. Notify the health care provider and use interprofessional collaboration (wound care nurse) as indicated.*

13. Inspect the periwound skin, including colour, texture, and temperature, and describe skin integrity (e.g., open, macerated areas; blistering). Periwound assessment provides clues about the effectiveness of wound treatment and possible wound deterioration (Nix, 2024).
14. Determine whether previous dressing is still appropriate based on wound characteristics. If it is, apply dressings as prescribed. If not, use interprofessional collaboration to discuss a change in treatment plan, or if the prescription states "according to best practice," decide which dressing is most appropriate and apply it. Use an indelible (waterproof) marker to label the new dressing with the time, date, and nurse's initials.
15. Reassess patient's pain and level of comfort, including pain at wound site, using an appropriate pain rating scale after dressing is applied.

Procedural Guideline 39.1 *Performing a Wound Assessment—cont'd*

16. Discard biohazard bag, soiled supplies, and gloves per employer policy.
17. Document wound assessment findings and dressing details, including when the next dressing change should be completed. Confirm comparison of assessment with previous wound assessments to monitor wound healing (see previous Critical Decision Point).

✦ SKILL 39.2 Performing a Wound Irrigation

Video Clip

Wound irrigation is used to clean open surgical or chronic wounds such as pressure injuries. Typically, the irrigation of an open wound involves the use of clean gloves. Review the health care provider's prescription to determine whether a sterile solution is required. The use of sterile solutions may be necessary with new traumatic wounds (Atwood et al., 2024). Irrigation involves introducing the cleaning solution directly into the wound with a syringe, syringe and catheter, pulsed lavage device, or a handheld shower. A proper wound-cleaning solution is one that does not harm the tissue and uses adequate force to agitate and wash away surface debris and devitalized tissue containing bacteria (Table 39.5) (Jaszarowski & Murphree, 2022).

When using a syringe, the tip remains 2.5 cm (1 inch) above the wound. If a patient has a deep wound with a narrow opening, attach a soft catheter to the syringe to allow the fluid to enter the wound. Pulsed lavage delivers kinetic and mechanical energy and suction (a form of subatmospheric pressure). When pulsed lavage is used, normal saline may be delivered at between 4 and 15 psi (pressurized irrigation) through a mechanical apparatus. Suction (subatmospheric pressure) may be used to aspirate wound debris and remove microorganisms. The use of mechanical energy through a pressurized spray also aids the removal of wound debris. Ambulatory patients often benefit from the use of a handheld shower for wound cleaning; the shower spray should be held approximately 30 cm (12 inches) from the wound.

Delegation and Collaboration

The skill of wound irrigation cannot be delegated to a UCP unless it is an established chronic wound and is permitted by employer policy. It is the nurse's responsibility to assess and document wound characteristics. If relevant, the nurse directs the UCP to do the following:

- Notify the nurse when the wound is exposed so an assessment can be completed
- Report to the nurse the patient's pain, presence of blood, and drainage

TABLE 39.5

Wound-Cleaning Considerations

	Mechanical Force	
	High Pressure	**Low Pressure**
Wound base characteristics	Presence of necrotic tissue (eschar, fibrin slough), debris, or other particulate matter	Presence of granulation tissue or new epithelial cells
	Significant bacterial burden	No/Minimal serous or serosanguinous exudate
	Moderate/large amount of exudate	
Clinical outcome(s)	Loosen, soften, and remove devitalized tissue from wound	Prevent trauma to viable wound tissue
	Separate eschar from fibrotic tissue, or separate fibrotic tissue from granulating base	Remove wound care product residue
Solution	Normal saline or potable municipal tap water (warmed, if possible)	Normal saline or potable municipal tap water (warmed, if possible)
	Volume of solution depends on size of wound	Volume of solution depends on size of wound
Delivery systems	35-mL syringe/19-gauge angiocatheter	Pouring saline directly from bottle
		Bulb syringe
		Piston syringe

Adapted from Spear, M. (2011). Wound cleansing: Solutions and techniques. *Plastic Surgical Nursing, 31*(1), 29–31.

Equipment

- Irrigant/cleaning solution (volume 1.5 to 2 times the estimated wound volume)
- Irrigation delivery system (as prescribed), depending on amount of pressure desired
- 35-mL syringe with a 19-gauge angiocatheter to facilitate optimum pressure for cleaning with minimal risk of tissue injury (Bryant & Nix, 2024b)
- PPE (e.g., clean gloves, gown, and goggles if splash or spray risk exists)
- Waterproof underpad, if needed
- Dressing supplies (see Tables 39.2 and 40.1)
- Disposable waterproof biohazard bag
- Extra towels and padding (to protect bed)
- Wound assessment supplies (see Procedural Guideline 39.1)

STEP	RATIONALE
ASSESSMENT	
1. Identify patient using at least two person-specific identifiers (e.g., name and date of birth, or name and medical record number) according to employer policy.	Ensures correct patient. Complies with Accreditation Canada's standards and improves patient safety (Accreditation Canada, 2020).
2. Throughout the procedure, the 4 moments for hand hygiene are to be implemented; hand hygiene should occur before initial patient (or patient environment) contact, before an aseptic procedure, after body fluid exposure risk, and after patient (or patient environment) contact. Additional hand hygiene should be performed when hands are visibly soiled.	Proper hand hygiene helps prevent the spread of infectious agents to health care providers.
3. Review health care provider's prescription to ensure best practice for irrigation of open wound and type of solution to be used.	Open-wound irrigation requires a medical prescription, including type of solution(s) to use.
4. Assess patient's level of comfort using an appropriate pain rating scale.	Provides baseline to determine tolerance of procedure.
5. Review patient's chart for signs and symptoms related to patient's open wound.	Provides ongoing data to indicate change in wound status (Nix, 2024).
a. Extent of impairment of skin integrity, including size of wound	
b. Verify number of drains present (if any)	Awareness of drain position facilitates safe dressing removal and determines need for special dressings.
c. Drainage, including amount, colour, consistency, and any odour noted	Ongoing data; drainage should decrease in a healing wound. When drainage increases, it is often related to infection (Bohn & Bryant, 2024).
d. Wound tissue colour	Colour represents balance between necrotic and new scar tissue. Proper selection of wound care products on the basis of wound colour facilitates removal of necrotic tissue and promotes new tissue growth (Nix, 2024).
e. Culture reports and/or use of antimicrobial dressings	An infected wound has an increase in bioburden and critical colonization of bacteria. Culture reports identify the type of bacteria and selection of appropriate systemic antibiotics. Wound cultures are relevant if systemic antibiotic treatment is required (Hurlow & Kalan, 2024). Antimicrobial dressings may be used.
6. Assess patient for history of allergies to antiseptics, solutions, medications, tapes, or dressing material.	If patient has known allergies, it is recommended to apply a sample of prescribed wound treatment as a skin test before flushing wound with a large volume of solution or selecting different tape or dressing material.
7. Assess patient's and caregiver's understanding of need for irrigation and signs of wound infection.	Determines extent of instruction required.

NURSING DIAGNOSES

- Acute pain
- Insufficient knowledge related to purpose of irrigation
- Reduced skin integrity
- Reduced tissue integrity
- Potential for infection
- Potential for injury

Related factors and risk factors are individualized on the basis of patient's condition or needs.

STEP	RATIONALE

PLANNING

STEP	RATIONALE
1. Expected outcomes following completion of procedure:	
• Patient states acceptable level of comfort and pain on a validated pain rating scale after wound irrigation.	Patient's comfort ensured by premedication, appropriately administered irrigation, application of clean dressing, and repositioning.
• Wound begins to demonstrate signs of healing; wound is free of excessive drainage, exudate, and inflammation.	Wound closure and healing progress in absence of debris and in presence of protective dressing.
• Skin integrity is maintained; no redness, edema, or inflammation is noted in surrounding tissue.	No further skin and tissue damage has resulted from wound irrigation.
• Patient is able to describe signs of wound healing and infection.	Demonstrates learning.
2. Administer analgesic at least 30 minutes before starting wound irrigation procedure.	Promotes pain control and enables patient to move more easily and be positioned to facilitate wound irrigation (Leren et al., 2020).
3. Explain procedure to patient and caregiver. Describe signs of healing and infection during irrigation.	Promotes cooperation and reduces anxiety.
4. Gather appropriate supplies for wound irrigation and dressing.	Ensures an organized procedure.
5. Close room door or bed curtains, and position patient.	Maintains privacy.
a. Position patient comfortably to permit gravitational flow of irrigating solution over wound and into collection receptacle (see Step 5a illustration).	Directing solution from top to bottom of wound and from clean to contaminated area prevents further infection. Position patient during planning stage, keeping in mind bed surfaces needed for later preparation of equipment.

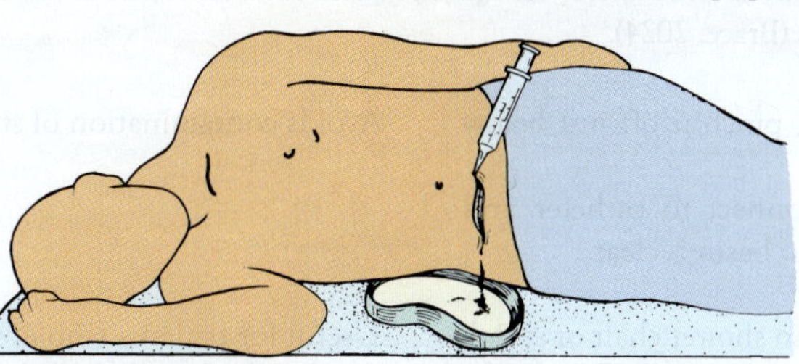

STEP 5A Patient position for wound irrigation.

STEP	RATIONALE
b. Position patient so wound is vertical to collection basin. Irrigant should be at room temperature.	Room-temperature solution increases comfort and reduces vascular constriction response in tissues.
c. Place padding or extra towel on bed under area where irrigation will take place.	Protects bedding from becoming wet.

IMPLEMENTATION

STEP	RATIONALE
1. Form a cuff on waterproof biohazard bag and place near bed.	Cuffing helps to maintain a large opening, thereby enabling placement of contaminated dressings without touching bag itself.
2. Apply PPE (gown, mask, goggles as indicated); apply clean gloves and remove old dressing.	Reduces transmission of microorganisms. Protects nurse from splashes or sprays of body fluid.
3. Discard old dressing and gloves in biohazard bag.	Reduces transmission of microorganisms.
4. Apply clean or sterile gloves (see employer policy). Perform wound assessment and examine recent charted assessment of patient's open wound (see Procedural Guideline 39.1).	Provides ongoing data on wound healing. Use sterile precautions when sterile gloves are needed.
5. Expose area near wound only.	Provides privacy and prevents chilling of patient.
6. Irrigate wound with wide opening:	
a. Fill a 35-mL syringe with warmed irrigation solution.	Irrigating a wound involves mechanical force, which helps with separation and removal of necrotic debris and surface bacteria (Jaszarowski & Murphree, 2022). Flushing a wound helps remove debris and facilitates healing by secondary intention. Warmed (body temperature) irrigant promotes wound healing.
b. Attach 19-gauge angiocatheter.	Catheter lumen delivers ideal pressure for cleaning and removing debris (Lumbers, 2018). Mechanical debridement may include irrigation, which can be done using a 35-mL syringe attached to 19-gauge angiocatheter, with irrigation pressures delivered at between 4 and 15 psi (WOCN, 2016).

IMPLEMENTATION

STEP	RATIONALE
c. Hold syringe tip 2.5 cm (1 inch) above upper end of wound and over area being cleaned.	Prevents syringe contamination. Careful placement of syringe prevents unsafe pressure of flowing solution.
d. Using continuous pressure, flush wound; repeat Steps 6a-6c until solution draining into basin is clear.	Flushing the wound helps remove debris; clear solution indicates removal of all debris.
7. Irrigate deep wound with very small opening:	
a. Attach soft catheter to filled irrigation syringe.	Catheter permits direct flow of irrigant into wound. Expect wound to take longer to empty when opening is small.
b. Gently insert tip of catheter into opening about 1.3 cm (0.5 inches).	Prevents tip from touching fragile inner wall of wound.

Critical Decision Point *Do not force the catheter into the wound because this will cause tissue damage. Ensure that irrigant solution will be flushed out of the wound; avoid irrigating when the wound base will not permit effective flushing out of solution.*

STEP	RATIONALE
c. Using slow, continuous pressure, flush wound.	Administering stream of solution using slow mechanical force loosens particulate matter on wound surface and promotes healing (Brace, 2024).

Critical Decision Point *Pulsatile high-pressure lavage is often the irrigation method of choice for necrotic wounds. Pressure settings should be set per provider prescription, usually between 4 and 15 psi, and should not be used on skin grafts, exposed blood vessels, muscle, tendon, or bone. Use with caution if the patient has a coagulation disorder or is taking anticoagulants* (Brace, 2024).

STEP	RATIONALE
d. While keeping catheter in place, pinch it off just below syringe.	Avoids contamination of sterile solution.
e. Remove and refill syringe. Reconnect to catheter and repeat until solution draining into basin is clear.	
8. Clean wound with handheld shower:	
a. With patient seated comfortably in shower chair or standing if condition allows, adjust spray to gentle flow; make sure that water is warm.	Useful for patients who are able to shower with help or independently. May be accomplished at home.
b. Shower for 5–10 minutes with shower head 30 cm (12 inches) from wound.	Ensures that wound is cleaned thoroughly.
9. When indicated (e.g., determining appropriate systemic antibiotic), obtain cultures (see Chapter 9) after cleaning with nonbacteriostatic saline.	The WOCN (2016) recommends using quantitative bacterial cultures (tissue biopsy or swab cultures). The most common types of wound culture are swab technique, aspirated wound fluid, or tissue biopsy (Hurlow & Kalan, 2024).

Critical Decision Point *Obtain a wound culture for systemic antibiotic use if there is inflammation around the wound, purulent odour or drainage, or new drainage; when the patient is febrile and systemic infection is suspected; or when antimicrobial topical treatments are not effective.*

STEP	RATIONALE
10. Dry wound edges with gauze; dry patient after shower. Remove and dispose of gloves.	Prevents maceration of surrounding tissue from excess moisture.
11. Apply clean or sterile gloves (see employer policy). Apply appropriate dressing and label with time, date, and nurse's initials.	Reduces transmission of microorganisms. Maintains protective barrier and healing environment for wound.
12. Remove mask, goggles, and gown.	Reduces transfer of microorganisms.
13. Dispose of equipment and soiled supplies. Remove and dispose of gloves.	Reduces transmission of microorganisms.
14. Help patient to a comfortable position.	

STEP	RATIONALE
EVALUATION	
1. Have patient rate level of comfort and pain using an appropriate pain rating scale.	Patient's pain should not increase as result of wound irrigation.
2. Monitor type of tissue in wound bed.	Identifies wound-healing progress and determines type of wound cleaning and dressing needed.
3. Inspect dressing periodically (see employer policy).	Determines patient's response to wound irrigation and need to modify plan of care.
4. Evaluate periwound skin integrity.	Determines whether extension of wound has occurred or signs of infection are present (warm, red periwound skin).
5. Observe for presence of retained irrigant.	Retained irrigant is medium for bacterial growth and subsequent infection.
6. **Use teach-back:** "I want to be sure that I explained why your wound was cleaned (irrigated) today. Tell me why it is important to clean (irrigate) your wound." Develop a revised teaching plan if patient or caregiver is unable to teach back correctly.	Determines patient's and caregiver's level of understanding of instructional topic.

Unexpected Outcomes	Related Interventions
1. Bleeding or serosanguinous drainage appears.	• Review medications (e.g., anticoagulant therapy). • Notify health care provider of bleeding. • Flush wound during next irrigation using less pressure.
2. Increased pain or discomfort occurs.	• Decrease pressure during wound irrigation. • Assess patient's need for additional analgesia before wound care.
3. Suture line opening extends.	• Notify health care provider. • Re-evaluate amount of pressure to use for next wound irrigation.

Communication and Documentation

- Document wound assessment before and after irrigation; amount, colour, and odour of drainage on dressing removed; amount and type of solution used; irrigation device used; patient's tolerance of the procedure; and type of dressing applied after irrigation on flow sheet in progress notes in EHR or chart.
- Document patient's and caregiver's understanding through teach-back of reasons for wound irrigation.
- Immediately report to the health care provider any evidence of fresh bleeding, sharp increase in pain, retention of irrigant, or signs of shock.

Special Considerations

Teaching

- Instruct patient and caregiver regarding wound care technique, observe their return demonstration of the technique, and provide written instructions.
- Explain the need for specialized supplies such as irrigating solutions and dressings and the need to maintain asepsis when performing care.
- Teach patient and caregiver the signs of a healing wound, improper wound healing, and wound infection.

Pediatric

- Some pediatric patients are very frightened. They might verbally and physically try to prevent the nurse from cleaning the wound. Having the child take active part in the procedure or supporting the child to work out their feelings about wound irrigation through play therapy on a doll with a wound helps the child to be more cooperative.
- Neonatal skin is immature and easily damaged from pressure and wound care products. Check that products are approved for use with this population. Remember that in neonates, the skin readily absorbs products.

Gerontological

- Wound irrigations are traumatic, frightening, and painful to some older persons. Assess patient's cooperation before irrigating the wound. Be aware of patient's cognitive level of understanding when performing wound irrigation.

Care in the Community: Home Management

- Assess patient's home environment to determine adequacy of resources for performing wound care; check especially for adequate lighting, safe (treated) water supply (municipal water that undergoes standard government testing), and storage of supplies.
- Plan wound care in conjunction with patient's total rehabilitation goals. The objective of wound care management in a subacute care setting is to return the patient to their home environment.
- Provide encouragement to address underlying factors (e.g., nutrition, continence management, pressure off-loading), including education for patient and caregiver about wound-healing expectations of chronic wounds (Bohn & Bryant, 2024).
- If ambulatory, patients will often be appropriate for wound care management in an outpatient clinic. Be sure that the patient has directions to the clinic and knows where to park and where to obtain dressing supplies in advance (if necessary).
- Solutions to use for irrigation in the home include potable tap water, distilled water, cooled boiled water, and normal saline (WOCN, 2016). Normal saline can be made in the home (dissolve 8 teaspoons of salt in 3.5 L of distilled water; keep refrigerated for up to 1 month). The saline solution should be allowed to reach room temperature before use.

✦ SKILL 39.3 Removing Sutures and Staples

Nurses need to have the skills and equipment to remove sutures and staples. Generally, staple and suture removal is prescribed by the health care provider. The prescription will state whether to remove the staples or sutures all at once, or to remove every other suture or staple in the first phase, with the remainder removed in the second phase.

Sutures and staples generally are removed within 7 to 14 days after surgery if healing is adequate (Oropallo, 2024). Retention sutures usually remain in place for 14 to 21 days. Timing the removal of sutures and staples is important. They must remain in place long enough to ensure initial wound closure with enough strength to support internal tissues and organs. Sutures left in longer than 14 days generally leave suture marks (Oropallo, 2024).

Sutures are threads of wire or other materials used to sew body tissues together. They come in different sizes and are absorbent or nonabsorbent. They are placed within tissue layers in deep wounds and superficially as the final means of wound closure. The choice of suture technique depends on the type and anatomical location of the wound, thickness of the skin, degree of tension, and desired cosmetic effect (Fig. 39.7) (Oropallo, 2024). A patient's history of wound healing, the site of the wound, the tissues involved, and the purpose of the sutures determine the suture material selected. For example, a patient with repeated abdominal surgeries might require wire sutures for greater strength to promote wound closure.

Staples are stainless-steel wires, are quick to use, and provide strength. The location of the incision sometimes restricts their use because there must be adequate distance between the skin and the structures that lie below the skin, including bone and vascular structures. They are used for skin closure of abdominal incisions and orthopedic surgery when appearance of the incision is not critical. Removal requires a sterile staple extractor and aseptic technique.

If there is any sign of suture line separation during the removal process, the remaining sutures or staples are left in place and a description is documented and reported to the health care provider. In some cases, these are removed several days to 1 week later. After sutures or staples are removed, the nurse applies Steri-Strips over the incision to provide support. The strips loosen over time (5 to 7 days) and can be removed when half of the strip is no longer attached to the skin.

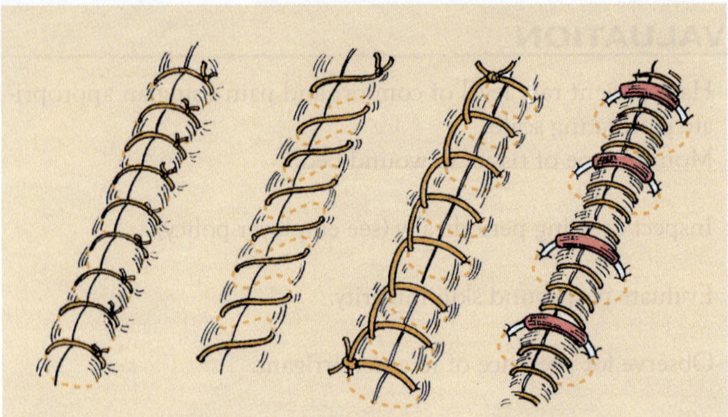

FIG 39.7 Types of sutures. A, Intermittent. B and C, Continuous. D, Blanket.

Delegation and Collaboration

The skill of staple and suture removal cannot be delegated to a UCP. The nurse directs the UCP to report any of the following to the nurse:

- Drainage, bleeding, or swelling at the incision site or an elevation in the patient's temperature
- Patient's indication of pain
- Any dehiscence of the closed wound (following suture removal)

Equipment

- Disposable waterproof biohazard bag
- Sterile suture removal set (forceps and scissors) or sterile staple extractor
- Sterile antiseptic swabs
- Gauze pads
- Steri-Strips or butterfly adhesive strips
- Clean gloves (sterile gloves optional)

STEP	RATIONALE
ASSESSMENT	
1. Identify patient using at least two person-specific identifiers (e.g., name and date of birth, or name and medical record number) according to employer policy.	Ensures correct patient. Complies with Accreditation Canada's standards and improves patient safety (Accreditation Canada, 2020).
2. Throughout the procedure, the 4 moments for hand hygiene are to be implemented; hand hygiene should occur before initial patient (or patient environment) contact, before an aseptic procedure, after body fluid exposure risk, and after patient (or patient environment) contact. Additional hand hygiene should be performed when hands are visibly soiled.	Proper hand hygiene helps prevent the spread of infectious agents to health care providers.
3. Review patient's chart for the following information:	
a. Check health care provider's prescription.	Health care provider's prescription is required for removal of sutures.
b. Review specific directions related to suture or staple removal.	Indicates specifically which sutures are to be removed (e.g., every other suture).
c. Determine history of conditions that may pose risk for impaired wound healing: advanced age, cardiovascular disease, diabetes, immunosuppression, radiation, obesity, smoking, poor nutrition, infection.	Pre-existing health disorders affect speed of healing and sometimes result in dehiscence.

STEP	RATIONALE

ASSESSMENT

4. Assess patient for history of allergies. Use latex-free gloves.	Determines whether patient is sensitive to antiseptic, latex, or other supplies used (e.g., paper tape).
5. Assess patient's comfort level on an appropriate pain rating scale. Ensure comfort measures are in place prior to removing sutures or staples (e.g., positioning, analgesia if prescribed).	Provides baseline of patient's comfort level to determine response to therapy.
6. Inspect incision for healing ridge and skin integrity of suture line for uniform closure of wound edges, normal colour, and absence of drainage and inflammation. Apply clean gloves, if necessary, to palpate wound. Remove and dispose of gloves after assessment.	Indicates adequate wound healing for support of internal structures without continued need for sutures or staples (Oropallo, 2024). Reduces transmission of microorganisms.
7. Assess patient's or caregiver's knowledge of wound care and what observations the patient needs to make when performing their own wound care.	Determines extent of instruction required.

Critical Decision Point *If wound edges are separated or signs of infection are present, the wound has not healed properly. Notify the health care provider because sutures or staples may need to remain in place or other wound care may need to be initiated.*

NURSING DIAGNOSES

- Acute pain
- Insufficient knowledge regarding incision care
- Reduced skin integrity
- Potential for infection

Related factors and risk factors are individualized on the basis of patient's condition or needs.

PLANNING

1. Expected outcomes following completion of procedure:	
• All suture material or staples are removed.	Removes source of infection or irritation from retained sutures.
• Suture line is intact.	Wound is healing and does not require protective dressings.
• Patient states acceptable level of comfort on an appropriate pain rating scale following removal of sutures or staples.	Some patients require pain medication before suture or staple removal.
• Patient or caregiver can describe wound care following suture removal.	Demonstrates learning.
2. Explain to patient how you will remove staples and that suture removal is usually not a painful procedure, although patient may feel pulling or tugging of skin.	Gains patient cooperation and reduces anxiety.
3. Administer prescribed analgesic, if needed, at least 30 minutes before procedure.	Promotes patient comfort and helps minimize movement during suture removal.

IMPLEMENTATION

1. Close curtains or room door.	Provides privacy.

Critical Decision Point *For a patient who is highly anxious or has an extensive wound, consider administering analgesic 30 minutes before suture removal. Assess patient comfort and pain level to ensure effectiveness of analgesic prior to suture or staple removal. Offer alternative comfort measures, such as squeezing a ball, distraction, or breathing techniques. Talking through the procedure with the patient during suture removal is often helpful in relieving anxiety.*

2. Position patient comfortably while exposing suture line. Ensure that light is directed to suture line.	Aids visibility and correct placement of forceps or extractor during removal process, ultimately reducing soft tissue injury.
3. Place cuffed waterproof disposal bag within easy reach.	Provides for easy disposal of contaminated dressings and prevents the passing of items over sterile work area.
4. Prepare materials needed for suture or staple removal: **a.** Open sterile suture removal kit or staple extractor kit. **b.** Open sterile antiseptic swabs and place on inside surface of kit. **c.** Obtain gloves (sterile gloves, if policy indicates).	Ensures an organized procedure.

STEP	RATIONALE

IMPLEMENTATION

STEP	RATIONALE
5. Apply clean gloves. Carefully remove dressing; discard dressing and gloves in prepared refuse disposal bag.	Reduces transmission of microorganisms.
6. Inspect incision and suture line (see Step 6 illustration).	Determines adequacy of wound healing.

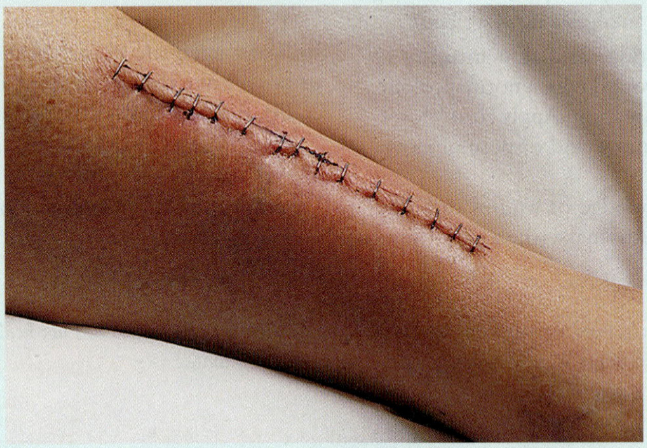

STEP 6 Suture line secured with staples.

STEP	RATIONALE
7. Apply clean or sterile gloves, as required by employer policy.	Reduces transmission of infection.
8. Clean sutures or staples and healed incision with antiseptic swabs or sterile saline, according to employer policy. Start down the incision line and then to each side of the incision line, using a new antiseptic swab or gauze for each swipe.	Removes surface bacteria from incision and sutures or staples.

Critical Decision Point *When removing sutures, remove every **second** suture to help decrease the chance of wound dehiscence. Steri-Strips can be applied to support the incision prior to removal of all sutures (see employer policy).*

STEP	RATIONALE
9. Remove staples:	
a. Place lower tips of staple extractor under the first staple. As you close the handles, the upper tip of the extractor depresses the centre of the staple, causing both ends of the staple to bend upward and simultaneously exit their insertion sites in the dermal layer (see Step 9a illustration).	Avoids placing excessive pressure on suture line and secures smooth removal of each staple.
b. Carefully control staple extractor.	Avoids placing pressure on suture line and minimizes patient discomfort.
c. As soon as both ends of staple are visible, move it away from the skin surface (see Step 9c illustration) and continue until staple is over refuse bag.	Prevents scratching of tender skin surface with sharp, pointed ends of staple. Provides comfort and infection control.

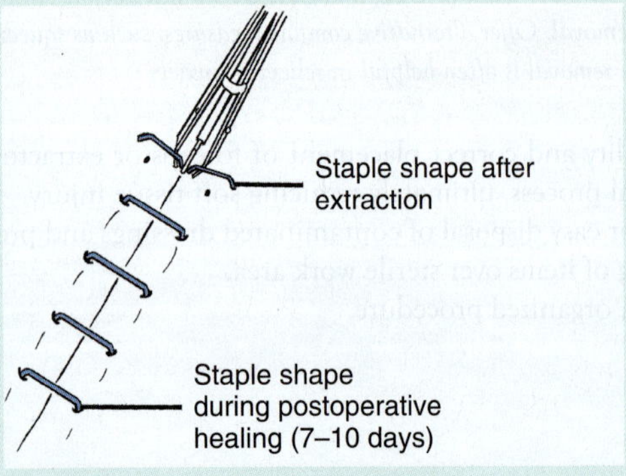

STEP 9A Staple extractor placed under staple.

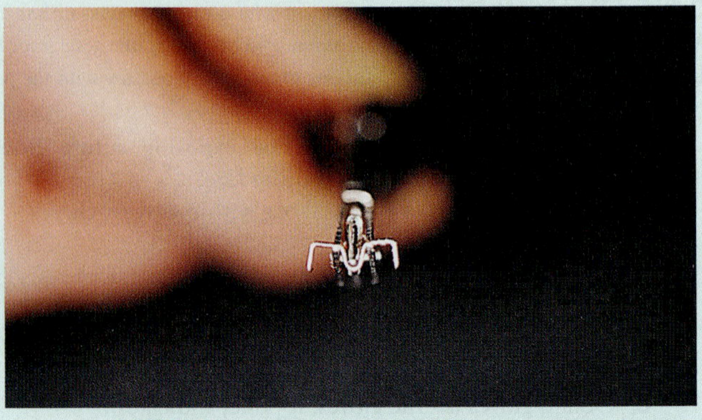

STEP 9C Metal staple removed by extractor.

STEP	RATIONALE

IMPLEMENTATION

STEP	RATIONALE
d. Release handles of staple extractor, allowing staple to drop into refuse bag.	Avoids contamination of sterile field with used staples.
e. Repeat Steps 9a–9d until all staples have been removed.	
10. Remove interrupted sutures:	
a. Place gauze a few centimetres from the suture line. Hold scissors in your dominant hand and forceps (clamp) in your nondominant hand.	Gauze serves as receptacle for removed sutures. Placement of scissors and forceps allows for efficient suture removal.

Critical Decision Point *Placement of scissors and forceps is very important. Avoid pinching the skin around the wound when lifting up the suture. Likewise, avoid cutting the skin around the wound by accident when snipping the suture.*

STEP	RATIONALE
b. Grasp knot of suture with forceps and gently pull up knot while slipping tip of scissors under suture near skin (see Step 10b illustration).	Releases suture.
c. Snip suture as close to the skin as possible at end distal to knot.	

Critical Decision Point *Never snip both ends of the suture; there will be no way to remove the part of the suture situated below the surface.*

STEP	RATIONALE
d. Grasp knotted end with forceps, then in one continuous, smooth motion, pull suture through from the other side (see Step 10d illustration). Place removed suture on gauze.	Smoothly removes suture without placing additional tension on suture line.

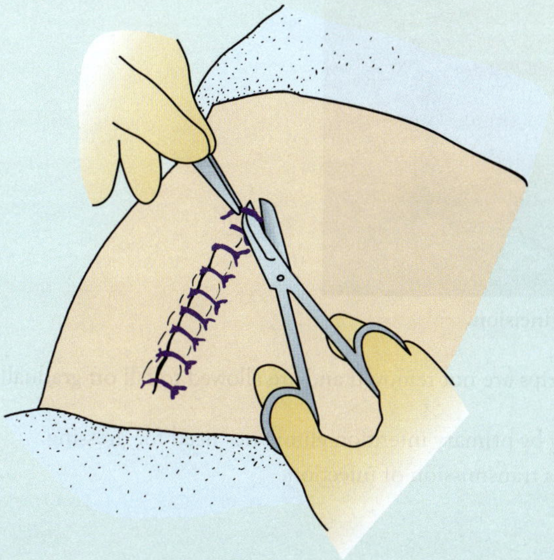

STEP 10B Removal of intermittent suture. Nurse cuts suture as close to the skin as possible, away from knot.

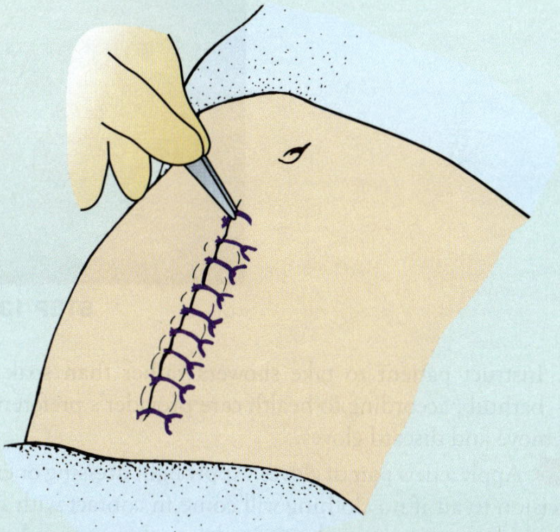

STEP 10D Nurse removes suture, never pulling contaminated stitch through tissues.

Critical Decision Point *Never pull the exposed surface of any suture into tissue below the epidermis. The exposed surface of any suture is considered contaminated.*

STEP	RATIONALE
e. Repeat Steps 10a–10d until you have removed every other suture.	
f. Observe healing level. Based on observations of wound response to suture removal and health care provider's original prescription, determine whether remaining sutures will be removed at this time. If so, repeat Steps 10a–10d until you have removed all sutures.	Determines status of wound healing and whether suture line will remain closed after all sutures have been removed.
g. If there is any doubt about wound healing, immediately stop suture removal and notify health care provider.	

STEP	RATIONALE

IMPLEMENTATION

11. Remove continuous and blanket stitch sutures:

- **a.** Place sterile gauze a few centimetres from suture line. Grasp scissors in dominant hand and forceps in nondominant hand.
  - *Rationale:* Gauze serves as receptacle for removed sutures. Placement of scissors and forceps allows for efficient suture removal.
- **b.** Snip first suture close to skin surface at end distal to knot.
  - *Rationale:* Releases suture.
- **c.** Snip second suture on same side.
  - *Rationale:* Releases interrupted sutures from knot.
- **d.** Grasp knotted end and gently pull in one continuous, smooth motion, removing suture from beneath skin. Place suture on gauze compress.
  - *Rationale:* Smoothly removes sutures without placing additional tension on suture line. Prevents pulling of contaminated part of suture through skin.
- **e.** Repeat Steps 11a–11d in consecutive order until entire line is removed.

12. Inspect incision to ensure that all sutures have been removed and to identify any trouble areas. Gently wipe suture line with antiseptic swab to remove debris and clean incision.
- *Rationale:* Reduces risk of further separation of incision line.

13. Apply Steri-Strips if *any* separation greater than two stitches or two staples in width is apparent, to maintain contact between wound edges.
- *Rationale:* Supports wound by distributing tension across wound and eliminates closure-technique scarring.

- **a.** Cut Steri-Strips to allow strips to extend 4–5 cm (0.5–2 inches) on each side of incision.
- **b.** Remove from backing and apply across incision (see Step 13b illustration).

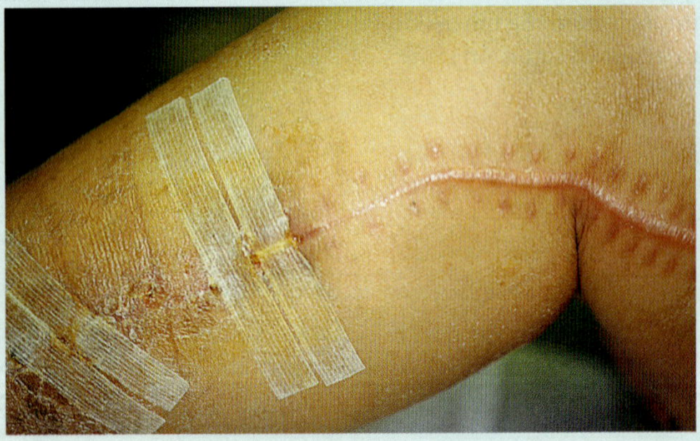

STEP 13B Steri-Strips over incision.

- **c.** Instruct patient to take showers rather than soak in a bathtub, according to health care provider's preference.
  - *Rationale:* Steri-Strips are not removed and are allowed to fall off gradually.

14. Remove and discard gloves.
- *Rationale:* Healing by primary intention eliminates need for dressing.

15. Apply a new pair of gloves. Apply light dressing or expose incision to air if no clothing will come in contact with suture line. Instruct patient about applying their own dressing, if needed, at home.
- *Rationale:* Reduces transmission of infection.

16. Dispose of sharps (disposable staple extractor and/or scissors) in designated sharps disposal bin and discard all contaminated materials. Remove and dispose of gloves.
- *Rationale:* Provides a safe environment because instruments are sharp and contaminated. Reduces transmission of infection.

EVALUATION

1. Assess site where sutures or staples were removed; inspect condition of soft tissues, including skin. Look for any pieces of removed suture left behind.
- *Rationale:* Ensures that sources of infection have been removed.

2. Determine whether patient has pain along incision.
- *Rationale:* Determines comfort level and can indicate whether suture material remains in skin.

3. **Use teach-back:** "I want to be sure that I explained the signs of a wound or incision infection before you are discharged. Tell me what signs of infection you should watch for." Develop a revised teaching plan if patient or caregiver is unable to teach back correctly.
- *Rationale:* Determines patient's and caregiver's level of understanding of instructional topic.

Unexpected Outcomes	Related Interventions
1. Retained suture is present.	• Notify health care provider. • Instruct patient to notify health care provider if signs of suture line infection develop following patient's discharge from facility.
2. Patient experiences wound separation or drainage secondary to healing problems.	• Leave remaining sutures or staples in place. • Place Steri-Strip closures across suture line. • Notify health care provider.

Communication and Documentation

- Document on flow sheet in progress notes in EHR or chart the time at which the sutures or staples were removed and the number of sutures or staples removed; cleaning of the suture line, appearance of the wound, level of healing of the wound, and type of dressing applied; and patient's response to suture or staple removal.
- Document patient's and caregiver's understanding of why the sutures were removed.
- Immediately report to the health care provider any suture line separation, dehiscence, evisceration, bleeding, or purulent drainage.

Special Considerations

Teaching

- Teach patient to observe for any sign of separation of wound edges before removing remaining sutures or staples and inspect incision for continued healing.
- Reinforce instruction about resuming bathing and showering activities, avoiding abdominal strain during defecation, and getting adequate nutrition and ambulation.
- Teach patient to avoid placing additional stress on suture line through activities such as lifting or bending. Patients who have had abdominal surgery or injury need to avoid heavy lifting for several weeks.
- Instruct patient that sometimes there is a small amount of drainage from the wound immediately after suture removal.

Pediatric

- Help is sometimes necessary to keep infants from moving during the suture removal procedure.
- Topical anaesthetic solutions (e.g., lidocaine, eutectic mixture of local anaesthetics [EMLA]) applied to intact skin may provide short-term (20 minutes) anaesthesia (Trottier et al., 2019).

Gerontological

- Some older persons need reassurance about suture or staple removal. Depending on their cognitive status, they may not understand the procedure.
- An older person's skin is often at higher risk for dehiscence after sutures or staples are removed.

✦ SKILL 39.4 Managing Wound Drainage: Emptying, Shortening, and Removing Drains

NSO *Nursing Skills Online Wound Care Module 19 / Lesson 2*

If drainage accumulates in a wound bed, wound healing is delayed. Drainage is facilitated when the surgeon inserts either a closed- or open-drain system, even if the amount of drainage is small. The drain is inserted directly through a small stab wound near the suture line into the area of the wound.

An open-drain system (e.g., a Penrose drain [Fig. 39.8]) is used to remove drainage from the wound and deposit it onto the skin surface. A sterile safety pin is inserted through this drain, outside the skin, to prevent the tubing from moving into the wound.

A closed-drain system, such as a Jackson-Pratt drain (Fig. 39.9) or Hemovac drain, relies on the presence of a vacuum to withdraw accumulated drainage from around the wound bed into the collection device. A Jackson-Pratt drain collects fluid in the range of 100 to 200 mL/24 hours. A Hemovac or ConstaVac drainage system is used for larger amounts of drainage (500 mL/24 hours). The collection

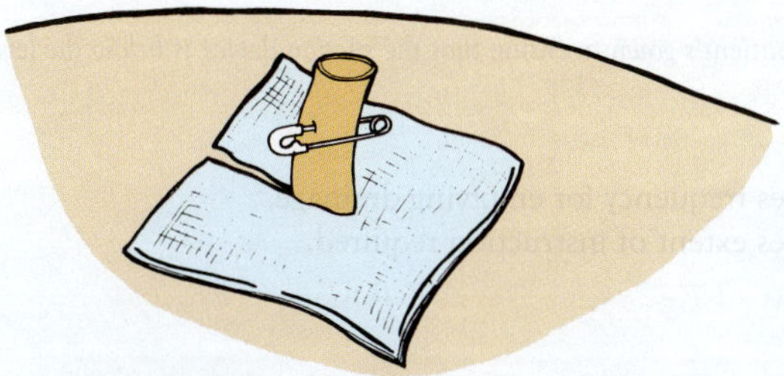

FIG 39.8 Penrose drain with drain-split gauze.

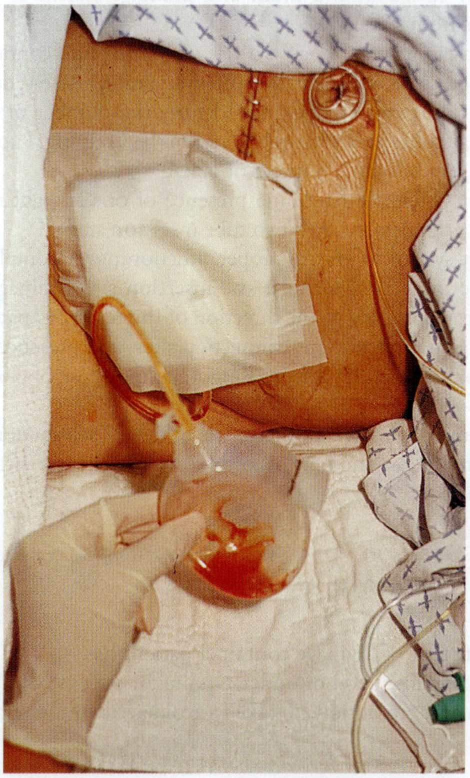

FIG 39.9 Jackson-Pratt wound drainage system.

device is connected to a clear plastic drain with multiple perforations. Drainage collects in a closed reservoir or suction bladder. The closed system collects fluid but operates only if the tubing is patent and a vacuum exists. If the drainage device is half full, empty the chamber and measure the drainage. After measurement, re-establish the vacuum and ensure that all drainage tubes are patent.

Drainage tubes can also be shortened or removed, depending upon the health care provider's prescription. It is important to follow aseptic technique to minimize the risk of infection when shortening or removing drains.

Delegation and Collaboration

The assessment of wound drainage and maintenance of drains and the drainage system cannot be delegated to a UCP. However, the nurse may delegate emptying a closed drainage container or pouch, measuring the amount of drainage, and reporting the amount on the patient's intake and output (I&O) record to a UCP. The nurse instructs the UCP to do the following:

- Report any increase in frequency of emptying the drain other than once a shift
- Report any change in amount, colour, or odour of drainage
- Review with the nurse the I&O procedure

Equipment

- Graduated cylinder or specimen container
- Antiseptic wipes
- Gauze sponges, including split-gauze sponges for drain site
- 10 cm × 10 cm (4 inch × 4 inch) sterile gauze dressings, as needed
- Clean gloves
- Safety pin(s)
- PPE (e.g., goggles, mask, and gown if risk of spray from drain is present)
- Disposable drape or barrier
- *Optional:* Normal saline for cleaning insertion site

STEP	RATIONALE
ASSESSMENT	
1. Identify patient using at least two person-specific identifiers (e.g., name and date of birth, or name and medical record number) according to employer policy.	Ensures correct patient. Complies with Accreditation Canada's standards and improves patient safety (Accreditation Canada, 2020).
2. Throughout the procedure, the 4 moments for hand hygiene are to be implemented; hand hygiene should occur before initial patient (or patient environment) contact, before an aseptic procedure, after body fluid exposure risk, and after patient (or patient environment) contact. Additional hand hygiene should be performed when hands are visibly soiled.	Proper hand hygiene helps prevent the spread of infectious agents to health care providers.
3. Review medical record to identify presence, location, and purpose of closed wound drain and drainage system as patient returns from surgery.	Drainage tubing is usually placed near the wound through a small surgical incision.
4. Wear clean gloves if there is a risk of coming into contact with drainage or if indicated by employer policy. Assess drainage present on patient's dressing. Identify the number of wound drainage tubes and what each one will be draining. Label each drainage tube with a number or label.	Assigning a labelling system to each drain helps with consistent documentation when the patient has multiple drainage tubes.
5. Inspect system to determine presence of one straight tube or Y-tube arrangement with two tube insertion sites.	Allows nurse to plan skin care and identify quantity of sterile dressing supplies needed.
6. Inspect system to ensure proper functioning. A complete systematic inspection includes the insertion site, drainage moving through tubing in the direction of the reservoir, patency of drainage tubing, airtight connection sites, and presence of any leaks or kinks in the system. Remove and dispose of gloves.	A properly functioning system maintains suction until the reservoir is filled or drainage is no longer being produced or accumulated. Tension on drainage tubing increases injury to skin and underlying muscle.
7. Determine whether drainage tube needs self-suction, wall suction, or no suction, according to health care provider's prescription.	Some drainage tubes, such as Hemovac, can be used with self-suction or wall suction.

Critical Decision Point *Attach tape and a safety pin to drainage tubing and pin to patient's gown to ensure that the suction device is below the level of the wound and does not pull on the insertion site.*

STEP	RATIONALE
8. Identify type of drainage container patient has.	Determines frequency for emptying drainage.
9. Assess patient's level of understanding of purpose of drainage system and precautions to take to avoid accidental removal.	Determines extent of instruction required.

STEP	RATIONALE

NURSING DIAGNOSES

- Insufficient knowledge regarding wound drain function
- Reduced skin integrity
- Potential for infection
- Potential for injury

Related factors and risk factors are individualized on the basis of patient's condition or needs.

PLANNING

STEP	RATIONALE
1. Expected outcomes following completion of procedure:	
• Wound healing continues.	Patient is comfortable and wound drainage is collected.
• Vacuum is re-established.	Suction system is intact.
• Tubing is patent.	Fluid is draining away from wound area.
• Patient describes precautions to prevent accidental drain removal.	Demonstrates learning.
2. Explain procedure to patient.	Promotes patient's cooperation and reduces anxiety.

IMPLEMENTATION

STEP	RATIONALE
1. Close room door or bedside curtains.	Provides privacy.
2. Apply clean gloves.	Reduces transmission of microorganisms.
3. Place open specimen container or graduated container (for measuring output) on bed between you and the patient.	Permits measuring and discarding of wound drainage.
4. Empty Hemovac or ConstaVac:	Prevents entry of pathogens.
a. Maintain asepsis while opening the plug on the port indicated for emptying drainage reservoir.	Vacuum will be broken, and reservoir will pull air in until chamber is fully expanded.
(1) Tilt suction container in direction of plug.	Drains fluid toward plug.
(2) Slowly squeeze two flat surfaces together, tilting toward measuring container.	Prevents splashing of contaminated drainage. Squeezing empties reservoir of drainage.
b. Drain contents into measuring container (see Step 4b illustration).	Contents counted as fluid output (see Chapter 8).
c. Hold uncovered antiseptic swab in dominant hand. Place suction device on a flat surface, with open outlet facing upward; continue pressing downward until bottom and top are in contact (see Step 4c illustration).	Cleaning plug reduces transmission of microorganisms into drainage evacuation.

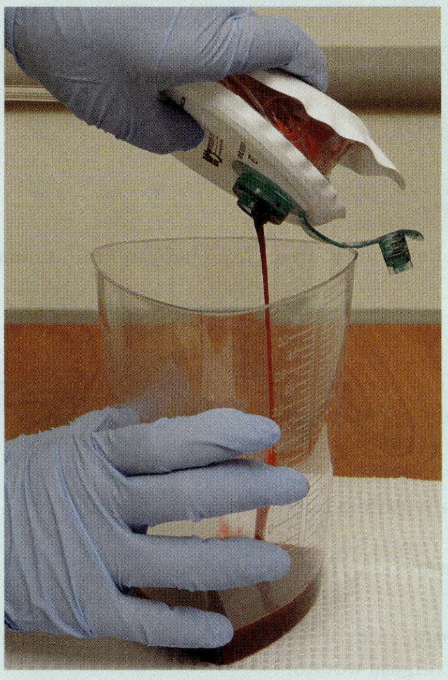

STEP 4B Hemovac contents drained into measuring container.

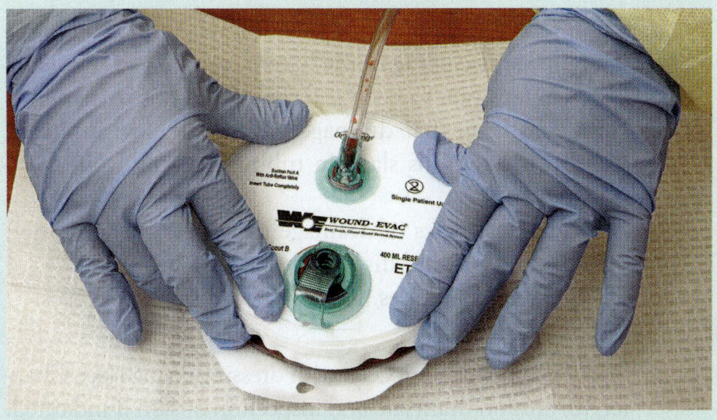

STEP 4C Hemovac compressed to create suction.

STEP	RATIONALE
IMPLEMENTATION	
d. Holding surfaces together with one hand and using an antiseptic swab, quickly clean opening, plug with other hand, and immediately replace plug; secure suction device on patient's bed.	Compression of surface of Hemovac creates vacuum.
e. Check device for re-establishment of vacuum, patency of drainage tubing, and absence of stress on tubing.	Facilitates wound drainage and prevents tension on drainage tubing.
5. Empty Hemovac with wall suction:	Empties drainage and re-establishes suction to wound bed.
a. Turn off suction.	
b. Disconnect suction tubing from Hemovac port.	
c. Empty Hemovac as described in Step 4.	
d. Use an antiseptic swab to clean port opening and the end of suction tubing. Reconnect tubing to port.	Cleaning plug reduces transmission of microorganisms.
e. Set suction level as prescribed or on low if health care provider does not specify suction level.	Re-establishes wound suction.
6. Empty Jackson-Pratt suction drain:	
a. Open port on top of bulb-shaped reservoir (see Step 6a illustration).	Breaks vacuum on drain.
b. Tilt bulb in direction of port and drain toward opening. Empty drainage from device into measuring container (see Step 6b illustration). Clean end of emptying port and plug with antiseptic wipe.	Reduces transmission of microorganisms.

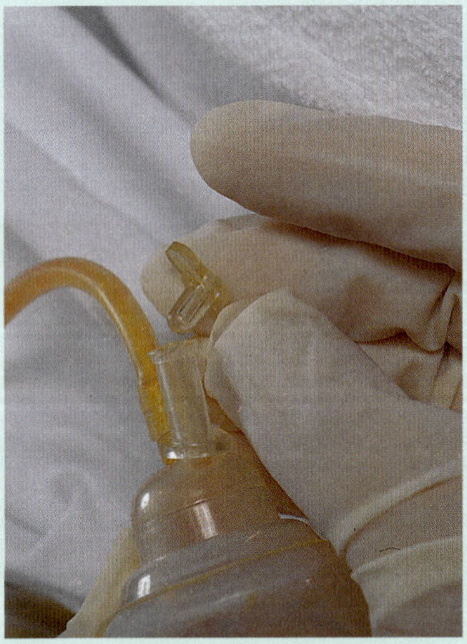

STEP 6A Opening port of Jackson-Pratt device.

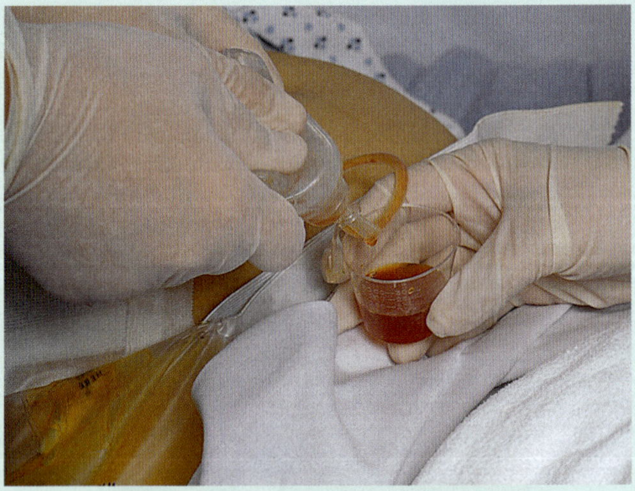

STEP 6B Emptying contents from Jackson-Pratt drainage device.

STEP	RATIONALE
c. Compress bulb over drainage container. While compressing bulb, replace plug immediately.	Re-establishes vacuum.
d. Use a safety pin to secure drainage tubing to patient's gown, ensuring that drainage system is below insertion site. Ensure there is slack in tubing running from reservoir to wound.	Pinning drainage tubing to patient's gown prevents tension or pulling on tubing and insertion site.
e. Note characteristics of drainage in measuring container; measure volume and discard by flushing in commode.	Contents count as fluid output.
f. Discard soiled supplies. Remove and dispose of gloves.	Reduces transmission of microorganisms.
g. Apply clean gloves. Proceed with dressing change (see Chapter 40) around drain site and inspection of skin if indicated. Split-drain sponge dressings are often used around drainage tubes (see Step 6g illustration) and taped in place.	Reduces transmission of microorganisms. Prevents entrance of bacteria into surgical wound.

STEP	RATIONALE

IMPLEMENTATION

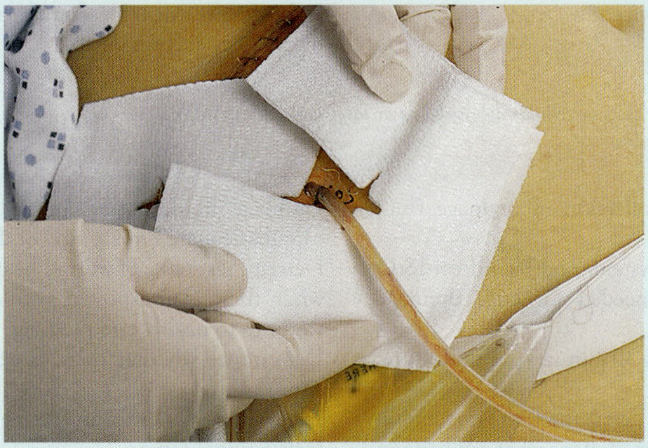

STEP 6G Applying split-gauze dressing around a Jackson-Pratt drainage tube.

STEP	RATIONALE
7. Discard contaminated materials. Remove and dispose of gloves.	Reduces transmission of microorganisms.
8. Shortening a drain:	Drains can be shortened by withdrawing them gradually (typically by 2 cm/day), which allows the site to heal gradually. Drains that protect postoperative sites from leakage form a tract and are usually kept in place longer (typically for about a week) (Knott, 2021).
a. Check health care provider's prescription for length in centimetres by which the drain is to be shortened.	
b. Check patient chart to assess whether the drain is sutured into place.	
c. Explain procedure to patient.	
d. Put on clean gloves and remove soiled dressing; discard dressing and remove gloves.	Reduces transmission of infection
e. Don sterile gloves; clean incision and drain area.	Reduces transmission of infection
f. If drain is sutured, clamp sterile forceps onto drain and remove suture(s).	To prevent drain from slipping into the wound.
g. Using second sterile forceps, gently pull prescribed amount of drainage tube out.	To prevent transmission of microorganisms.
h. Insert new sterile pin into drain close to the skin, leaving 2 cm of drain above the newly inserted pin; take sterile scissors and cut drain between the two pins.	
9. Discard all equipment. Remove and discard gloves.	
10. Removing a drain:	
a. Confirm health care provider's prescription for drain removal.	
b. Explain procedure to patient and offer analgesia.	When removing a drain, inform patient that there may be some discomfort when drain is pulled out. Offer preprocedure analgesia to minimize patient discomfort (Knott, 2021).
c. Don clean gloves and applicable PPE.	Reduces transmission of infection
d. Ensure reservoir is empty; remove dressing.	
e. Clean the incision and drain.	Removes surface bacteria from incision and drain.
f. Carefully cut and remove the securing suture following aseptic technique.	
g. Holding two 10 cm × 10 cm (4 inch × 4 inch) sterile gauze dressings in nondominant hand, stabilize skin.	
h. Ask patient to take a deep breath and exhale slowly; remove drain as patient exhales.	Minimizes discomfort and promotes relaxation.
i. Firmly grasping drainage tube close to the skin with dominant hand, use swift and steady motion to withdraw drain.	
j. Clean wound and apply sterile dressing.	
11. Discard supplies and remove gloves.	Reduces transmission of microorganisms.

STEP	RATIONALE

EVALUATION

1. Observe for drainage in suction device.	Indicates presence of vacuum, patency of tubing, and functioning of drainage suction device.

Critical Decision Point *Inspect for clots or cellular debris. Clots or large collections of debris may block drainage flow. The Y-site in the drainage tubing is especially prone to clogging.*

2. Inspect wound for drainage or collection of drainage fluid under skin, causing seroma.	Drainage should not be significant under suture line. It may indicate inadequate functioning of drainage suction device.
3. Measure drainage from drainage system, and record on I&O form every 8–12 hours and as needed for large drainage volume.	Determines status of wound healing. Collect diagnostic specimen when there is unexpected purulence or a pungent odour, report findings to health care provider, and record in progress notes.
4. If drain was removed, assess dressing 30 minutes postprocedure.	Determines whether there is excessive drainage from the drain site.
5. **Use teach-back:** "I want to be sure I explained why it is important for you not to pull on your drain. Tell me what can happen if you pull the drain out accidently." Develop a revised teaching plan if patient or caregiver is unable to teach back correctly.	Determines patient's and caregiver's level of understanding of instructional topic.

Unexpected Outcomes	Related Interventions
1. Site where tube exits becomes infected.	• Notify health care provider about presence of signs of infection: purulent drainage, odour, reddened site, increased white blood cell count, and elevated temperature. • Use aseptic technique when changing dressings.
2. Bleeding appears in or around drainage collector.	• Determine amount of bleeding and notify health care provider if it is excessive. • Assess for tension on patient's drainage tubing. • Secure tubing to prevent pulling and pain.
3. Patient experiences pain.	• Assess patient's level of pain. • Medicate patient. • Stabilize drainage tubing to reduce tension and pulling against incision. • Notify health care provider if signs of wound infection are present.
4. Drainage suction device is not accumulating drainage.	• Assess drainage tubing for clots. • Assess drainage system for air leaks or kinks. • Notify health care provider.

Communication and Documentation

- Document emptying the drainage suction device; re-establishing vacuum in the suction device; amount, colour, and odour of drainage; dressing change to drain site; and appearance of drain insertion site on flow sheet in progress notes in EHR or chart.
- Document amount of drainage on I&O record.
- Document drain shortening, amount by which drain length was shortened, appearance of skin at drain site, how drain was resecured, and dressing applied.
- Document drain removal, drain output and characteristics, and dressing applied.
- Document your evaluation of patient and caregiver learning.
- Immediately report a sudden change in amount of drainage, either output or absence of drainage flow, to the health care provider. Also report pungent odour of drainage or new evidence of purulence, severe pain, or dislodgement of the drainage tube to the health care provider.

Special Considerations

Teaching

- Instruct patient about anticipated postoperative drainage, expected progress of wound healing and drainage volume, and estimated date of removal of drain as volume diminishes.
- Teach patient or caregiver how to empty and record amount of drainage. If patient is going home with a drainage device, ask patient or caregiver to record the amount emptied and bring this information to their next outpatient visit.

Pediatric

- Have parent or guardian help pediatric patient keep drainage tube in place and avoid dislodging them.

Gerontological

- Be aware that older persons with large amounts of drainage will need additional fluid intake because they are more likely to become dehydrated.
- Take measures to prevent a confused patient from pulling out a drain collector.

Care in the Community: Home Management

- Assess health literacy and provide appropriate (written) instructions in drain care. Include the importance of measuring and documenting the amount of drainage. The patient should communicate the volume of drainage daily to the health care provider.

✦ SKILL 39.5 Negative-Pressure Wound Therapy

Negative-pressure wound therapy (NPWT), or wound vacuum, is the application of subatmospheric (negative) pressure to a wound through suction to facilitate healing and collect wound fluid (Netsch & Nix, 2024). There are a number of types of NPWT, from the large canister and vacuum that is attached to the bed and connected to a wall plug to small mini-NPWT products that provide the patient with complete mobility. When managing NPWT, you need to know how the product functions. Nurses may require additional training before using the product (see employer policy).

The primary effects of negative pressure at the wound surface (Figs. 39.10 and 39.11) (Netsch, 2022) are as follows:

- Removal of wound exudates
- Maintenance of a moist wound surface
- Reduction of edema with improved perfusion
- Macrodeformation (traction on the sides of the wound), which promotes wound contraction
- Microdeformation and mechanical stretch on cells in the wound bed, which changes cell shape and activates intracellular processes to promote healing.

Indications for NPWT include chronic, acute, traumatic, subacute, and dehisced wounds; partial-thickness burns; injuries (e.g., diabetic and pressure); flaps and grafts once nonviable tissue is removed; and selected high-risk postoperative surgical incisions (e.g., orthopedic, sternal). NPWT is also used in wounds with tunnels (i.e., a channel has formed that extends from any part of the wound through subcutaneous tissue or muscle), undermining, or sinus tracts, as long as the wound filler can fill the dead space and is easily retrieved (Netsch & Nix, 2024). Research also supports the use of an installation of wound-rinsing agents to facilitate healing in some chronic wounds (WOCN, 2016).

Contraindications to NPWT include necrotic tissue with eschar present; untreated osteomyelitis; unexplored fistulas; malignancy in the wound; exposed vasculature; and exposed nerves, anastomotic site, or organs. Safety precautions need to be considered for patients at high risk for bleeding or hemorrhage; patients taking anticoagulants; and patients requiring magnetic resonance imaging (MRI), hyperbaric chamber, or defibrillation (Netsch & Nix, 2024).

There are a number of different NPWT systems. These may be gauze or foam based and designed for either acute care settings or outpatient care (Netsch, 2022). NPWT can be delivered intermittently or continuously. Research and reviews of evidence show improved microvascular blood flow and granulation tissue formation with intermittent versus continuous therapy delivered at 125 mm Hg (WOCN, 2016). However, for patients with severe pain, lower levels of pressure (75–80 mm Hg) can be used to reduce pain and discomfort without compromising effectiveness (EPUAP et al., 2019; Netsch & Nix, 2024).

Delegation and Collaboration

The skill of applying NPWT cannot be delegated to a UCP. The nurse directs the UCP to do the following:

- Use caution in positioning or turning the patient to avoid tubing displacement
- Report to the nurse any change in dressing shape or integrity
- Report to the nurse any change in the patient's temperature or comfort level
- Report any wound fluid leakage around the edges of the adhesive drape

Equipment

- Application of the NPWT unit requires a health care provider's prescription. Vacuum-assisted closure (VAC) products are available in several different systems. The most appropriate approach when using a VAC system is to refer to manufacturer instructions. The following information is relevant to any type of VAC product.

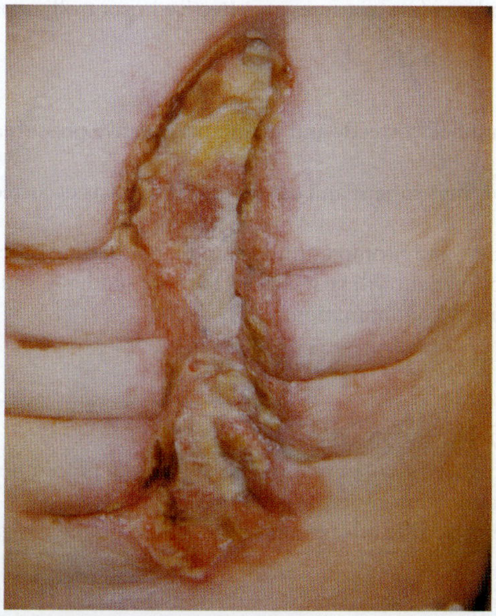

FIG 39.10 Dehisced wound before negative-pressure wound therapy. *(Courtesy KCI Licensing, San Antonio, TX.)*

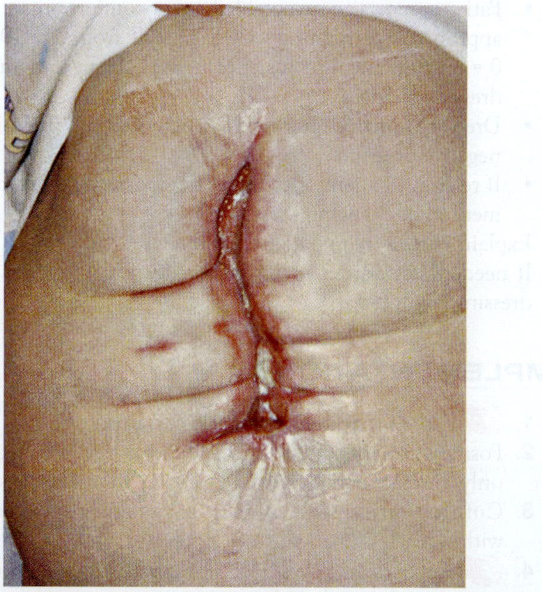

FIG 39.11 Dehisced wound after negative-pressure wound therapy. *(Courtesy KCI Licensing, San Antonio, TX.)*

STEP	RATIONALE
ASSESSMENT	
1. Identify patient using at least two person-specific identifiers (e.g., name and date of birth, or name and medical record number) according to employer policy.	Ensures correct patient. Complies with Accreditation Canada's standards and improves patient safety (Accreditation Canada, 2020).
2. Throughout the procedure, the 4 moments for hand hygiene are to be implemented; hand hygiene should occur before initial patient (or patient environment) contact, before an aseptic procedure, after body fluid exposure risk, and after patient (or patient environment) contact. Additional hand hygiene should be performed when hands are visibly soiled.	Proper hand hygiene helps prevent the spread of infectious agents to health care providers.
3. Review the health care provider's prescriptions for type of VAC as well as frequency of dressing change, amount of negative pressure, type of foam or gauze to use, and pressure cycle (intermittent or continuous), if applicable.	Determines frequency of dressing change, negative-pressure setting, and special instructions.
4. Review medical record for signs and symptoms related to condition of patient's wound.	Provides baseline to compare findings with previous dressing change assessments and reflects wound-healing progress.
5. Assess patient's level of comfort using an appropriate pain rating scale.	Provides baseline to measure response to dressing therapy.
6. Apply clean gloves. Assess location, appearance, and size of wound (see Procedural Guideline 39.1). Remove and dispose of gloves.	Reduces transmission of microorganisms. Provides information regarding status of wound healing, presence of complications, and proper type of supplies and help needed.
7. Assess patient's and caregiver's knowledge of purpose of dressing and whether they will participate in dressing the wound.	Identifies patient's learning needs. Prepares patient and caregiver if dressing will need to be changed at home.

NURSING DIAGNOSES

- Acute pain
- Chronic pain
- Insufficient knowledge regarding purpose of dressing
- Reduced skin integrity
- Potential for infection

Related factors and risk factors are individualized on the basis of patient's condition or needs.

STEP	RATIONALE
PLANNING	
1. Expected outcomes following completion of procedure:	
• Patient's wound shows evidence of healing as wound decreases in size with less drainage, redness, or swelling.	Dressing is effective in promoting healing and preventing infection.
• Patient reports an acceptable level of comfort on an appropriate pain rating scale (e.g., scale from 0 to 10, with 0 = no pain and 10 = worst pain ever) during and after dressing changes.	Analgesic and comfort measures are effective in controlling pain.
• Dressing remains intact with airtight seal and prescribed negative pressure.	Dressing is applied correctly and maintains negative pressure.
• If relevant, patient or caregiver demonstrates correct method of changing dressing.	Demonstrates that patient and caregiver learning has occurred.
2. Explain procedure to patient and caregiver.	Relieves anxiety and promotes understanding of healing process.
3. If needed, administer prescribed analgesic 30 minutes before dressing change.	A comfortable patient will be less likely to move suddenly, causing wound or supply contamination.
IMPLEMENTATION	
1. Close room door or cubicle curtains.	Provides for patient privacy.
2. Position patient comfortably and drape to expose wound site only. Instruct patient not to touch wound or sterile supplies.	Promotes patient's cooperation and organized procedure. Prevents contamination of sterile supplies.
3. Cuff top of disposable waterproof biohazard bag and place within reach of work area.	Cuff prevents accidental contamination of top of outer bag.
4. Apply clean gloves. If risk of spray exists, apply protective gown, goggles, and mask.	Reduces transmission of microorganisms from soiled dressings to nurse's hands.

STEP	RATIONALE

IMPLEMENTATION

STEP	RATIONALE
5. Follow manufacturer instructions for removal and replacement because use of each NPWT unit varies slightly. Turn off NPWT unit by pushing therapy on/off button.	Deactivates therapy and allows for proper drainage of fluid in drainage tubing.
a. Keeping tube connectors attached to NPWT unit, raise tubing connectors; disconnect tubes from one another and drain fluids into drainage collector.	Prevents backflow of any drainage in tubing back into wound.
b. Before lowering tubing connectors, tighten clamp on canister tube and disconnect canister and dressing tubing at connection points.	Prevents drainage from exiting tubing when removed.
6. Remove transparent film by gently stretching it, then slowly pulling it away from the skin.	Prevents injury to wound tissue. Protects periwound skin from potential breakdown caused by removal of transparent adhesive.
7. Remove old dressing one layer at a time and discard in bag. Observe drainage on dressing. Use caution to avoid applying tension on any drains that are present.	Determines type and amount of dressings needed for replacement. Prevents accidental removal of drains.
8. Assess wound. Observe surface area and tissue type, colour, odour, and drainage within the wound. Measure length, width, and depth of wound as prescribed.	Measurement of wound is necessary to assess wound-healing progression and justify continuation of NPWT (Netsch & Nix, 2024). Determines condition of wound and need for replacement of dressing.

Critical Decision Point *At this stage, a wound care nurse or health care provider might debride the wound. Debridement of eschar or slough, if present, should be performed in order to remove devitalized tissue and thus prepare the wound bed* (Netsch & Nix, 2024).

STEP	RATIONALE
9. Remove and discard gloves in waterproof bag. Avoid having patient see old dressing because the sight of wound drainage may be upsetting.	Reduces transmission of microorganisms. Lessens patient anxiety during procedure.
10. Clean wound:	Irrigation removes wound debris and cleans wound bed.
a. Apply sterile or clean gloves, depending on employer policy and wound status.	Prevents transmission of microorganisms.
b. If prescribed, irrigate wound with normal saline or other solution prescribed (see Skill 39.2). Gently blot periwound with gauze to dry thoroughly.	Cleaning periwound is essential for an airtight seal.

Critical Decision Point *If drainage appears purulent or has a foul odour or if there is a change in amount or colour of drainage, notify the health care provider about the potential for increased bioburden. A wound culture may be appropriate, and this may be an indication that NPWT should be discontinued* (Wynn & Freeman, 2019).

STEP	RATIONALE
11. Apply skin protectant, barrier film, solid skin-barrier sheet, or hydrocolloid dressing to periwound skin.	Maintains airtight seal needed for NPWT wound therapy and protects periwound skin from moisture-associated skin damage (Netsch & Nix, 2024).
12. Fill any uneven skin surfaces (e.g., creases, scars, and skinfolds) with skin-barrier product (e.g., paste, strip).	Further helps to maintain airtight seal (Netsch & Nix, 2024).
13. Remove and discard gloves.	Prevents transmission of microorganisms.
14. Depending on type of wound, apply sterile or new clean gloves (see employer policy).	Fresh sterile wounds require sterile gloves. Chronic wounds require clean technique (WOCN, 2016).
15. Apply NPWT:	
a. Prepare NPWT filler dressing. Consult with wound care expert for appropriate type.	Filler dressing depends on NPWT used and can include foam or gauze dressings with or without antimicrobials such as silver. The type of dressing may be adjusted based on undermining, tunnelling, or sinus tracts present (Netsch & Nix, 2024).
(1) Measure wound and select appropriately sized dressing.	Establishes baseline for wound size. Black polyurethane (PU) foam has larger pores and is most effective in stimulating granulation tissue and wound contraction. White soft foam is denser, with smaller pores, and is used when growth of granulation tissue needs to be restricted (Netsch & Nix, 2024).
(2) Using sterile scissors, cut filler dressing foam to wound size, making sure to fit foam to exact size and shape of wound, including tunnels and undermined areas.	Proper size of foam dressing maintains negative pressure on entire wound (Netsch & Nix, 2024).

STEP	RATIONALE

IMPLEMENTATION

Critical Decision Point *In some instances, an antimicrobial product such as a silver-impregnated contact layer or topical antibiotic is required. These products help reduce the bioburden of the wound.*

STEP	RATIONALE
b. Place filler dressing in wound, following manufacturer instructions. Be sure that filler dressing is in contact with entire wound base, margins, and tunnelled and undermined areas. Count number of filler dressings and document in patient's chart. *Dressing must* ***not*** *be placed over intact periwound skin.*	Maintains negative pressure on entire wound. Edges of foam dressing must be in direct contact with patient's skin. Dressing count provides nurse who removes dressing with number of filler dressings that should be removed.
c. Place suction device per manufacturer instructions.	
d. Apply NPWT transparent dressing over foam wound dressing.	
(1) Trim transparent dressing to cover wound and dressing so it will extend onto periwound skin approximately 2.5–5 cm (1–2 inches).	Prepares dressing of appropriate size for wound.
(2) Apply transparent dressing, keeping it wrinkle-free (see Step 15d[2] illustration).	Ensures wound is properly covered and negative-pressure seal can be achieved (Box 39.4). Dressing should be airtight, with no tunnels or gaps, to ensure a good seal when suction is activated.

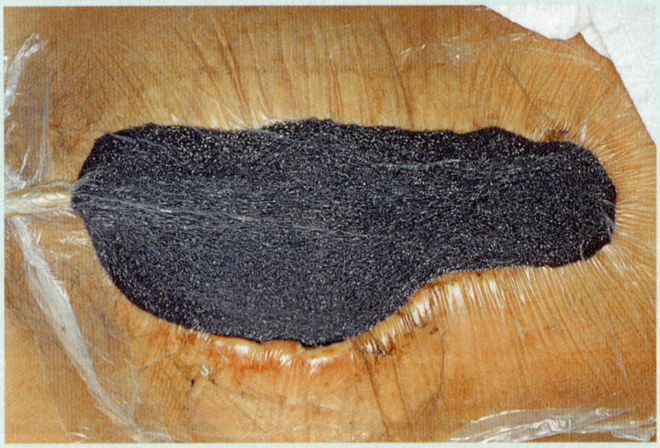

STEP 15D(2) Foam wound filler; transparent dressing over existing wound.

BOX 39.4

Maintaining an Airtight Seal With Negative-Pressure Wound Therapy

To avoid loss of suction (negative pressure), the wound and dressing must stay sealed after therapy is initiated. Problem seal areas include wounds around joints; wounds near skin creases and folds; and wounds exposed to moisture, such as diaphoresis, wound drainage, and urine or stool. The following points may help to maintain an airtight seal:

- Clip hair on skin around wound (check employer policy).
- Fill uneven skin surfaces with a skin-barrier product such as paste or strips.
- Make sure that the periwound skin surface is dry.
- Cut transparent film to extend 2.5–5 cm (1–2 inches) beyond wound perimeter.
- Frame periwound area with skin sealant, solid skin barrier, hydrocolloid, or transparent film dressing.
- Cut or mould transparent dressing to fit wound.
- Avoid wrinkles when applying transparent film.
- Identify any air leaks with a stethoscope and repair them with a sealant dressing (e.g., transparent dressing). Use only one or two additional layers for large leaks. Multiple layers reduce moisture-vapour transmission and cause maceration of the wound.
- Avoid adhesive remover because it leaves a residue that hinders film adherence.

Data from Netsch, D. S. (2022). Refractory wounds: Assessment and management. In L. L. McNichol, C. R. Ratliff, & S. S. Yates (Eds.), *Wound, Ostomy, and Continence Nurses Society core curriculum: Wound management* (2nd ed., pp. 214–233). Wolters Kluwer; Netsch, D. S., & Nix, D. P. (2024). Negative pressure wound therapy. In R. A. Bryant & D. P. Nix (Eds.), *Acute and chronic wounds: Intraprofessionals from novice to expert* (6th ed., pp. 488–500). Elsevier Inc.

STEP	RATIONALE

IMPLEMENTATION

Step	Rationale
(3) Secure tubing to transparent film, aligning drainage holes to ensure occlusive seal. Do not apply tension.	Excessive tension may compress foam dressing and impede wound healing. It also produces shear force on periwound area (Agarwal et al., 2019).
(4) Secure tubing several centimetres away from dressing, avoiding pressure points.	Drainage tubes placed over bony pressure prominences can cause medical device–related pressure injuries (MDRPIs) (Jackson et al., 2019; Netsch & Nix, 2024).
16. After wound is completely covered, connect tubing from dressing to tubing from canister and NPWT unit and set at prescribed suction level:	Intermittent or continuous negative pressure can be administered at 80–125 mm Hg (Netsch & Nix, 2024; WOCN, 2016).
a. Remove canister from sterile packing and push unit until you hear click. NOTE: An alarm sounds if canister is not properly engaged.	
b. Connect dressing tubing to canister tubing. Make sure that both clamps are open.	
c. Place on a level surface or hang from foot of the bed. NOTE: Unit sounds alarm and deactivates therapy if tilted beyond 45 degrees.	
d. Press power button (commonly this is a green-lit button) and set pressure as prescribed.	
17. Inspect NPWT system:	
a. Verify that system is on. This information is displayed differently for each type of NPWT unit. For example, on some units the display screen shows "Therapy On." Check employer policy and procedure for specific information.	
b. Verify that all clamps are open and all tubing is patent.	
c. Examine system to be sure that seal is intact and therapy is working.	Negative pressure is achieved when a tight seal is present (Netsch, 2022).
d. If a leak is present, use strips of transparent film to patch areas around edges of the wound.	
18. Record initials, date, and time on new dressing.	Provides reference for next dressing change.
19. Help patient to a comfortable position. Patient may ambulate with NPWT.	Enhances patient comfort and relaxation.
20. Discard gloves and dispose of any dressing material.	Prevents transmission of microorganisms.

EVALUATION

Step	Rationale
1. Inspect condition of wound on ongoing basis; note drainage (any evidence of bleeding) and odour.	Determines status of wound healing.
2. Ask patient to rate pain using an appropriate pain rating scale.	Determines patient's level of comfort following procedure.
3. Verify airtight dressing seal and correct negative-pressure setting.	Determines effective negative pressure is being applied.
4. Measure wound drainage output in canister on a regular basis.	Monitors fluid balance and wound drainage.
5. **Use teach-back:** "I want to be sure I explained clearly what your wound should look like as it is healing and the signs of infection to watch for before you are discharged. Explain to me what your wound will look like as it begins to heal." Develop a revised teaching plan if patient or caregiver is unable to teach back correctly.	Determines patient's and caregiver's level of understanding of instructional topic.

Unexpected Outcomes	Related Interventions
1. Wound appears inflamed and tender, drainage has increased, and odour is present.	• Notify health care provider. • Obtain wound culture. • Increase frequency of dressing changes.

Unexpected Outcomes	Related Interventions
2. Patient reports increase in pain.	• Patient may need more analgesia. • Instill normal saline to moisten foam and other filler dressings to allow them to loosen from granulation tissue. • If using black foam, switch to polyvinyl alcohol (PVA) white soft foam. • Decrease pressure setting. • Change from intermittent to continuous cycling. • Change type of NPWT system.
3. Negative-pressure seal has broken.	• Take preventive measures (see Box 39.4).
4. Wound hemorrhages.	• Stop NPWT immediately and notify health care provider.
5. Patient discharged to home with NPWT.	• Ensure patient has prescriptions for NPWT products to continue treatment.

Communication and Documentation

- Document appearance of wound, characteristics of drainage, placement of NPWT (type of dressing, pressure mode and setting), and patient response to dressing change on flow sheet in progress notes in EHR or chart.
- Document your evaluation of patient and caregiver learning.
- Report brisk, bright red bleeding, evidence of poor wound healing, evisceration or dehiscence, and possible wound infection to the health care provider immediately.

Special Considerations

Teaching

- Successful NPWT relies on the patient's and caregiver's cooperation with treatment. NPWT can be difficult to use when the patient is unable to consciously cooperate (e.g., dementia) (Netsch & Nix, 2024).
- If relevant, patients and caregivers need to learn how to administer analgesics appropriately. Patient tolerance of and adherence to NPWT are difficult if dressing changes are painful (Netsch & Nix, 2024).
- Educate patients and caregivers about the signs and symptoms that indicate development of an infection and to report this to the health care provider immediately.
- Teach patient and caregiver points to follow to maintain negative-pressure seal.
- Explain how NPWT works and why dressing is not changed daily.

Pediatric

- NPWT therapy is not appropriate for fragile neonatal skin.
- For older pediatric patients, the same approach is used as for adult patients.

Gerontological

- Older persons have fragile skin and decreased healing potential, owing to numerous factors. Assess the patient's suitability for NPWT (e.g., adequate nutrition, perfusion).
- Use skin care practices to protect periwound tissue. Transparent film may be irritating to fragile skin. A skin protectant is one method to reduce the risk of tissue injury.
- Therapy may need to start with lower negative pressures (e.g., 75 mm Hg) and slowly titrate to more negative pressure.

Care in the Community: Home Management

- The patient and caregiver are usually not required to change the larger NPWT treatment methods; however, small units may be managed by a patient or caregiver. Provide support and ongoing follow-up to ensure appropriate use of the NPWT product, including by maintaining the seal, observing for infection, and changing the dressing (if appropriate).
- Provide information to the patient and caregiver regarding proper disposal of contaminated products.

✦ REVIEW QUESTIONS

A patient is 6 days postoperative from a colon resection for a perforated diverticulum and has been readmitted because of excessive drainage from their midline abdominal incision. On admission, half of the staples in the incision were removed by the admitting resident. The wound has been left to heal by secondary intention; saline-moistened gauze dressings are to be applied every 12 hours. On admission, the patient had a computed tomography (CT) scan that showed fluid accumulation. The fluid was drained in interventional radiology, and the drain was left in place and attached to a bulb syringe.

Review Questions 1 to 3 relate to the case study presented here.

1. The abdominal wound will heal by which type of wound healing, and what principle will guide the wound toward healing?
2. Name two types of wound irrigation that may be appropriate for the twice-daily irrigation prescribed by the health care provider.
3. The patient was discharged with an open wound and instructed to use twice-daily irrigation and to apply a saline-moistened nonadherent gauze wound dressing. The patient returns to the wound clinic 1 week after discharge, reporting increased tenderness around the wound and some light-yellow drainage. The nurse takes the patient's vital signs and notes a temperature of 38.7°C (101.6°F). Wound assessment reveals yellow, foul-smelling purulent drainage and red wound edges. Use SBAR (situation–background–assessment–recommendation) documentation to communicate these findings to the health care team.
4. A patient has recently undergone a colon resection and has an abdominal wound healing by secondary intention. For 4 days

following the surgical procedure, the patient has had a moist saline gauze dressing changed twice a day. The unregulated care provider (UCP) calls the nurse to the room because they have noted excessive drainage from under the abdominal wound dressing. Based on this finding, which of the following assessments will the nurse plan to do? (*Select all that apply.*)

1. Ask the UCP to obtain vital signs and note the patient's temperature.
2. Reinforce the dressing and call the surgical team.
3. Remove the dressings and assess how many of the dressings are soaked with drainage; note its colour, consistency, and any presence of odour.
4. Suggest ambulation to help the wound drain additional fluid.
5. Instruct the UCP to change the dressing as needed.
6. Observe the wound tissue for colour and presence of abnormal drainage and the periwound area for redness or warmth.

5. A patient has an extensive abdominal wound and is to have half of the staples removed and the incision cleaned. Place the following steps for preparing and interacting with the patient in the correct order:

1. Assess healing ridge and skin integrity of suture line.
2. Describe to the patient how you will remove the staples.
3. Place upper tip of the staple remover under the staple to ease removal.
4. Assess patient for pain.
5. Lift up on staple when depressing the extractor handles.
6. Clean incision before removing staples, starting at sides next to incision.

6. The nurse notes approximately 60 mL of bright red drainage in the Jackson-Pratt drain 6 hours after surgery. Which two nursing interventions should be included in the care for this patient?

1. Emptying the drain in 24 hours
2. Shaking the bulb to thin the drainage
3. Calling the surgeon to report the finding
4. Securing the drain above the level of the wound
5. Emptying the drain immediately and checking the volume again in 2 hours

Visit the Evolve site for a complete list of answers to the Review Questions.

NEXT GENERATION NCLEX® (NGN)

For practice with answering exam questions related to unfolding NGN case studies, please consult the Next Generation NCLEX® (NGN)-Style Case Studies for Skills and Techniques on the Evolve website: http://evolve.elsevier.com/Canada/Perry/clinicalskills/

REFERENCES

Accreditation Canada. (2020). *Required organizational practices–2020 handbook*. https://physicians.nshealth.ca/resources/required-organizational-practices-2020-handbook

Agarwal, P., Kukrele, R., & Sharma, D. (2019). Vacuum assisted closure (VAC)/negative pressure wound therapy (NPWT) for difficult wounds: A review. *Journal of Clinical Orthopaedics and Trauma, 10*(5), 845–848. https://doi.org/10.1016/j.jcot.2019.06.015

Allard, J. P., Keller, H., Jeejeebhoy, K. N., et al. (2016). Malnutrition at hospital admission—Contributors and effect on length of stay: A prospective cohort study from the Canadian malnutrition task force. *Journal of Parenteral and Enteral Nutrition, 40*(4), 487–497. https://doi.org/10.1177/0148607114567902. [Seminal Reference].

Alshahrani, B., Sim, J., & Middleton, R. (2021). Nursing interventions for pressure injury prevention among critically ill patients: A systematic review. *Journal of Clinical Nursing, 30*(15–16), 2151–2168. https://doi.org/10.1111/jocn.15709

Atwood, R. E., Bradley, M. J., & Elster, E. A. (2024). Traumatic wounds: Bullets, blasts, and vehicle crashes. In R. A. Bryant, & D. P. Nix (Eds.), *Acute and chronic wounds: Intraprofessionals from novice to expert* (6th ed., pp. 620–636). Elsevier Inc.

Ayello, E. A., & Braden, B. (2002). How and why to do pressure ulcer risk assessment. *Advances in Skin & Wound Care, 15*(3), 125–131. https://doi.org/10.1097/00129334-200205000-00008. [Seminal Reference].

Beitz, J. M. (2022). Wound healing. In L. L. McNichol, C. R. Ratliff, & S. S. Yates (Eds.), *Wound, Ostomy, and Continence Nurses Society core curriculum: Wound management* (2nd ed., pp. 39–55). Wolters Kluwer.

Bohn, G., & Bryant, R. A. (2024). Wound-healing physiology and factors that affect the repair process. In R. A. Bryant, & D. P. Nix (Eds.), *Acute and chronic wounds: Intraprofessionals from novice to expert* (6th ed., pp. 143–163). Elsevier Inc.

Brace, J. A. (2024). Wound debridement. In R. A. Bryant, & D. P. Nix (Eds.), *Acute and chronic wounds: Intraprofessionals from novice to expert* (6th ed., pp. 430–440). Elsevier Inc.

Braden, B. J., & Bergstrom, N. (1989). Clinical utility of the Braden Scale for predicting pressure sore risk. *Decubitus, 2*(3), 44–46 [Seminal Reference].

Braden, B. J., & Bergstrom, N. (1994). Predictive validity of the Braden Scale for pressure sore risk in a nursing home population. *Research in Nursing & Health, 17*(6), 459–470. https://doi.org/10.1002/nur.4770170609. [Seminal Reference].

Bryant, R. A., & Nix, D. P. (2024a). Principles for practice development to facilitate outcomes and productivity. In R. A. Bryant, & D. P. Nix (Eds.), *Acute and chronic wounds: Intraprofessionals from novice to expert* (6th ed., pp. 1–17). Elsevier Inc.

Bryant, R. A., & Nix, D. P. (2024b). Principles of wound healing and topical management. In R. A. Bryant, & D. P. Nix (Eds.), *Acute and chronic wounds: Intraprofessionals from novice to expert* (6th ed., pp. 441–457). Elsevier Inc.

Cao, S., Gu, M., Feng, M., et al. (2022). Implementation of evidence in preventing medical device–related pressure injury in ICU patients using the i–PARIHS framework. *Journal of Nursing Management, 30*(1), 318–327. https://doi.org/10.1111/jonm.13458

Chong, S. J., Kok, Y. O., Choke, A., et al. (2017). Comparison of four measures in reducing length of stay in burns: An Asian centre's evolved multimodal burns protocol. *Burns, 43*(6), 1348–1355. https://doi.org/10.1016/j.burns.2017.03.011. [Seminal Reference].

de Assis, I. I. C., dos Santos, J. E., Abib, M. L. V. S., et al. (2021). Medical device-related pressure injury in an intensive care unit: A cross-sectional study. *Wound Management & Prevention, 67*(11), 26–32. https://doi.org/10.25270/wmp.2021.11.2632

Delmore, B., Ayello, E. A., Smith, D., et al. (2019). Refining heel pressure injury risk factors in the hospitalized patient. *Advances in Skin & Wound Care, 32*(11), 512–519. https://doi.org/10.1097/01.asw.0000579704.28027.d2

Edsberg, L. E., Black, J. M., Goldberg, M., et al. (2016). Revised National Pressure Ulcer Advisory Panel pressure injury staging system. *The Journal of Wound, Ostomy and Continence Nursing, 43*(6), 585–597. https://doi.org/10.1097/WON.0000000000000281. [Seminal Reference].

Elias, P. M. (2017). The how, why and clinical importance of stratum corneum acidification. *Experimental Dermatology, 26*(11), 999–1003. https://doi.org/10.1111/exd.13329. [Seminal Reference].

European Pressure Ulcer Advisory Panel, National Pressure Injury Advisory Panel, & Pan Pacific Pressure Injury Alliance. (2019). *Prevention and treatment of pressure ulcers/injuries: Quick reference guide* (3rd ed.). https://guidelinesales.com/store/ViewProduct.aspx?id=15037164

Farroha, A. (2020). Reduction in length of stay of patients admitted to a regional burn centre during COVID-19 pandemic. *Burns, 46*(7). Article 1715. https://doi.org/10.1016/j.burns.2020.05.028

Fulbrook, P., Mbuzi, V., & Miles, S. (2019). Effectiveness of prophylactic sacral protective dressings to prevent pressure injury: A systematic review and meta-analysis. *International Journal of Nursing Studies, 100*. Article 103400. https://doi.org/10.1016/j.ijnurstu.2019.103400

Hajhosseini, B., Longaker, M., & Gurtner, C. (2020). Pressure injury. *Annals of Surgery 271*(4), 671–679. https://doi.org/10.1097/SLA.0000000000003567

Healthcare Excellence Canada. (n.d.). *Pressure ulcer: Introduction*. https://www.healthcareexcellence.ca/en/what-we-do/all-programs/hospital-harm-is-everyones-concern/hospital-harm-improvement-resource/pressure-ulcer-introduction/

Huang, C., Ma, Y., Wang, C., et al. (2021). Predictive validity of the Braden Scale for pressure injury risk assessment in adults: A systematic review and meta-analysis. *Nursing Open, 8*(5), 2194–2207. https://doi.org/10.1002/nop2.792

Hudson, L., Chittams, J., Griffith, C., et al. (2018). Malnutrition identified by academy of nutrition and dietetics/American society for parenteral and enteral nutrition is associated with more 30-day readmissions, greater hospital mortality, and longer hospital stays: A retrospective analysis of nutrition assessment data in a major medical center. *Journal of Parenteral and Enteral Nutrition, 42*(5), 892–897. https://doi.org/10.1002/jpen.1021

Hurlow, J., & Kalan, L. (2024). Wound infection and bioburden: Detection and management. In R. A. Bryant, & D. P. Nix (Eds.), *Acute and chronic wounds: Intraprofessionals from novice to expert* (6th ed., pp. 411–429). Elsevier Inc.

Jackson, D., Sarki, A. M., Betteridge, R., et al. (2019). Medical device–related pressure ulcers: A systematic review and meta-analysis. *International Journal of Nursing Studies, 92*, 109–120. https://doi.org/10.1016/j.ijnurstu.2019.02.006

Jaszarowski, K. A., & Murphree, R. W. (2022). Wound cleansing and dressing selection. In L. L. McNichol, C. R. Ratliff, & S. S. Yates (Eds.), *Wound, Ostomy, and Continence Nurses Society core curriculum: Wound management* (2nd ed., pp. 136–156). Wolters Kluwer.

Knott, L. (2021). Surgical drains: Indications, management and removal. *Patient*. https://patient.info/doctor/surgical-drains-indications-management-and-removal

Kottner, J., Cuddigan, J., Carville, K., et al. (2019). Prevention and treatment of pressure ulcers/injuries: The protocol for the second update of the international Clinical Practice Guideline 2019. *Journal of Tissue Viability, 28*(2), 51–58. https://doi.org/10.1016/j.jtv.2019.01.001

Leren, L., Johansen, E., Eide, H., et al. (2020). Pain in persons with chronic venous leg ulcers: A systematic review and meta-analysis. *International Wound Journal, 17*(2), 466–484. https://doi.org/10.1111/iwj.13296

Lin, F., Zijing, W., Song, B., et al. (2020). The effectiveness of multicomponent pressure injury prevention programs in adult intensive care patients: A systematic review. *International Journal of Nursing Studies, 102*. Article 103483. https://doi.org/10.1016/j.ijnurstu.2019.103483

Lumbers, M. (2018). Wound debridement: Choices and practice. *British Journal of Nursing, 27*(15), S16–S20. https://doi.org/10.12968/bjon.2018.27.15.S16

Manna, B., Nahirniak, P., & Morrison, C. A., (2023). *Wound debridement*. National Library of Medicine. https://www.ncbi.nlm.nih.gov/books/NBK507882/

McNichol, L., Mackey, D., Watts, C., et al. (2020). Choosing a support surface for pressure injury prevention and treatment. *Nursing, 50*(2), 41–44. https://doi.org/10.1097/01.NURSE.0000651620.87023.d5

Munoz, N., Posthauer, M. E., Cereda, E., et al. (2020). The role of nutrition for pressure injury prevention and healing: The 2019 international Clinical Practice Guideline recommendations. *Advances in Skin & Wound Care, 33*(3), 123–136. https://doi.org/10.1097/01.asw.0000653144.90739.ad

National Pressure Injury Advisory Panel. (2016). *NPIAP pressure injury and stages*. https://cdn.ymaws.com/npiap.com/resource/resmgr/NPIAP-Staging-Poster.pdf. [Seminal Reference].

Netsch, D. S. (2022). Refractory wounds: Assessment and management. In L. L. McNichol, C. R. Ratliff, & S. S. Yates (Eds.), *Wound, Ostomy, and Continence Nurses Society core curriculum: Wound management* (2nd ed., pp. 214–233). Wolters Kluwer.

Netsch, D. S., & Nix, D. P. (2024). Negative pressure wound therapy. In R. A. Bryant, & D. P. Nix (Eds.), *Acute and chronic wounds: Intraprofessionals from novice to expert* (6th ed., pp. 488–500). Elsevier Inc.

Nix, D. P. (2024). Skin and wound inspection and assessment. In R. A. Bryant, & D. P. Nix (Eds.), *Acute and chronic wounds: Intraprofessionals from novice to expert* (6th ed., pp. 192–212). Elsevier Inc.

Nix, D. P., & Bryant, R. A. (2024). Pressure ulcers/injuries. In R. A. Bryant, & D. P. Nix (Eds.), *Acute and chronic wounds: Intraprofessionals from novice to expert* (6th ed., pp. 213–257). Elsevier Inc.

Oropallo, A. (2024). Perfusion, oxygenation, and incision care. In R. A. Bryant, & D. P. Nix (Eds.), *Acute and chronic wounds: Intraprofessionals from novice to expert* (6th ed., pp. 581–596). Elsevier Inc.

Orsted, H. L., Keast, D. H., Forest-Lalande, L., et al. (2017/2021). Best practice recommendations for the prevention and management of wounds. In *Foundations of best practice for skin and wound management: A supplement of Wound Care Canada. Wounds Canada*. https://www.woundscanada.ca/doclink/wc-bpr-prevention-and-management-of-wounds/

Padula, W. V., Cuddigan, J., Ruotsi, L., et al. (2023). Best-practices for preventing skin injury beneath personal protective equipment during the COVID-19 pandemic: A position paper from the National Pressure Injury Advisory Panel. *Journal of Clinical Nursing, 32*(3–4), 625–632. https://doi.org/10.1111/jocn.15682

Parnham, A., Copson, D., & Loban, T. (2020). Moisture-associated skin damage: Causes and an overview of assessment, classification and management. *British Journal of Nursing, 29*(12), S30–S37. https://doi.org/10.12968/bjon.2020.29.12.S30

Pittman, J. (2022). General concepts related to skin and soft tissue injury caused by mechanical (external) factors. In L. L. McNichol, C. R. Ratliff, & S. S. Yates (Eds.), *Wound, Ostomy, and Continence Nurses Society core curriculum: Wound management* (2nd ed., pp. 314–322). Wolters Kluwer.

Reddy, M. (2022). Pressure injuries: Prevention and management. In A. J. Sinclair, J. E. Morley, B. Vellas, et al. (Eds.), *Pathy's principles and practice of geriatric medicine* (6th ed., pp. 1403–1405). Wiley. https://doi.org/10.1002/9781119484288.ch111

Smart, H., & Sibbald, R. (2020). Skin care for the protection and treatment of incontinence associated dermatitis (IAD) to minimise susceptibility for pressure injury (PI) development. *World Council of Enterostomal Therapists Journal, 40*(4), 40–44.

Squitieri, L., Tsangaris, E., Klassen, A. F., et al. (2020). Patient-reported experience measures are essential to improving quality of care for chronic wounds: An international qualitative study. *International Wound Journal, 17*(4), 1052–1061. https://doi.org/10.1111/iwj.13374

Thayer, D. M., Rozenboom, B. J., & LeBlanc, K. (2022). Prevention and management of moisture-associated skin damage (MASD), medical adhesive–related skin injury (MARSI), and skin tears. In L. L. McNichol, C. R. Ratliff, & S. S. Yates (Eds.), *Wound, Ostomy, and Continence Nurses Society core curriculum: Wound management* (2nd ed., pp. 323–354). Wolters Kluwer.

Trottier, E. D., Doré-Bergeron, M.-J., Chauvin-Kimoff, L., et al. (2019). Managing pain and distress in children undergoing brief diagnostic and therapeutic procedures. *Paediatrics and Child Health, 24*(8), 509–521. https://doi.org/10.1093/pch/pxz026

Williamson, K. (2020). Nursing people with bariatric care needs: More questions than answers. *Wounds UK, 16*(1), 64–71. https://www.wounds-uk.com/journals/issue/608/article-details/nursing-people-with-bariatric-care-needs-more-questions-than-answers

World Health Organization. (2018). *Global guidelines for the prevention of surgical site infection* (2nd ed.). https://www.who.int/publications/i/item/global-guidelines-for-the-prevention-of-surgical-site-infection-2nd-ed

Wound, Ostomy, and Continence Nurses Society. (2016). *Guideline for prevention and management of pressure ulcers (injuries)* (2nd ed.). https://www.wocn.org/. [Seminal Reference].

Wynn, M., & Freeman, S. (2019). The efficacy of negative pressure wound therapy for diabetic foot ulcers: A systematised review. *Journal of Tissue Viability, 28*(3), 152–160. https://doi.org/10.1016/j.jtv.2019.04.001

Wysocki, A. B. (2024). Anatomy and physiology of skin and soft tissue. In R. A. Bryant, & D. P. Nix (Eds.), *Acute and chronic wounds: Intraprofessionals from novice to expert* (6th ed., pp. 117–142). Elsevier Inc.

Yates, A. (2018). Incontinence-associated dermatitis in older people: Prevention and management. *British Journal of Community Nursing, 23*(5), 218–224. https://doi.org/10.12968/bjcn.2018.23.5.218

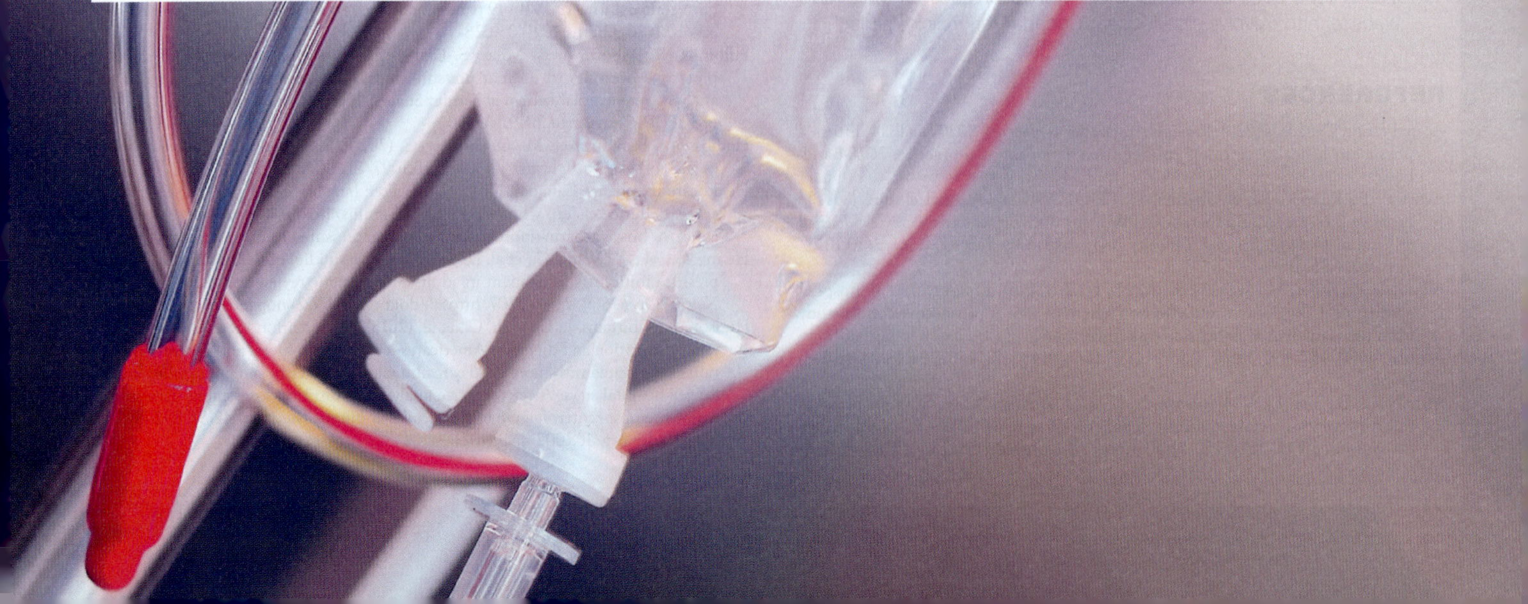

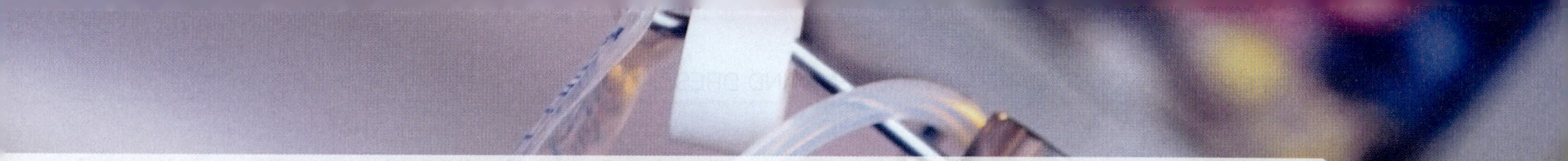

40 Wound Care Management and Dressings

Canadian content written by **Rosemary Kohr, RN, BA (Arts Plastiques), BScN, MScN, PhD**
Original US chapter by **Anne Griffin Perry, RN, MSN, EdD, FAAN; Janice C. Colwell, RN, MS, CWOCN, FAAN; and Kathleen Hudson, MSN, RN, CWOCN**

SKILLS AND PROCEDURES

OBJECTIVES

Mastery of content in this chapter will enable the nurse to:

- Assess a wound correctly.
- Understand the purposes and techniques of applying dressings, bandages, and abdominal binders.
- Understand how to choose the correct dressing for a wound based on its characteristics.
- Apply dressings correctly.
- Apply an abdominal binder correctly.

MEDIA RESOURCES

- http://evolve.elsevier.com/Canada/Perry/clinicalskills/

PURPOSE

The correct use of dressings, bandages, and binders supports underlying tissues and promotes wound healing. Knowledge and application of proper wound dressing techniques are essential nursing practices. Selection of the type of dressing is based on specific characteristics of the wound; the expected outcomes desired; and, for chronic wounds, the practicality and feasibility of having caregivers perform dressing changes in the home setting.

STANDARDS OF CARE

- Accreditation Canada (2020)—*Required Organizational Practices–2020 Handbook* (https://physicians.nshealth.ca/resources/required-organizational-practices-2020-handbook)
- European Pressure Ulcer Advisory Panel (EPUAP), National Pressure Injury Advisory Panel (NPIAP), & Pan Pacific Pressure Injury Alliance (2019)—*Prevention and Treatment of Pressure Ulcers/Injuries: Quick Reference Guide*, 3rd edition (https://guidelinesales.com/store/ViewProduct.aspx?id=15037164)
- Harris et al. (2017/2021)—*Best Practice Recommendations for Prevention and Management of Surgical Wound Complications* (https://www.woundscanada.ca/docman/public/health-care-professional/bpr-workshop/555-bpr-prevention-and-management-of-surgical-wound-complications-v2/file)
- Healthcare Excellence Canada (n.d.)—*Pressure Ulcer: Introduction* (https://www.healthcareexcellence.ca/en/what-we-do/all-programs/hospital-harm-is-everyones-concern/hospital-harm-improvement-resource/pressure-ulcer-introduction/)
- Orsted et al. (2017/2021)—*Best Practice Recommendations for the Prevention and Management of Wounds* (https://www.woundscanada.ca/docman/public/health-care-professional/bpr-workshop/165-wc-bpr-prevention-and-management-of-wounds/file)

PRINCIPLES FOR PRACTICE

- Acute wounds go through a predictable, standard process as they heal. Wound healing consists of the following phases: hemostasis, inflammation, proliferation (repair), and maturation (remodelling). Chronic wounds stall in this trajectory, often remaining in the inflammatory or proliferation phase (Ermer-Seltun & Rolstad, 2022).
- The TIME framework addresses barriers to wound healing and identifies key clinical assessments and treatment options (Ermer-Seltun & Rolstad, 2022; Piemonte et al., 2019; Sibbald et al., 2021):
  - **Tissue management** involves removing nonviable, unhealthy tissue from the wound bed. Wound debridement reduces bioburden of the wound, thus reducing the risk of wound infection and promoting effective wound healing. Tissue management also controls for hypergranulation and hypertrophic scar formation, both of which affect wound healing.
  - **Inflammation and infection** are influenced by the presence of nonviable tissue, high bacterial loads, and impaired

leukocytes. The goal is to identify and treat wound infection and inflammation promptly.
- **Moisture balance** is crucial in wound healing. When a wound surface is too wet or too dry, the repair process is delayed. The goal is to keep a wound surface moist, not wet.
- **Edge** of the wound requires assessment to ensure the integrity of the perimeter of the wound. A closed or compromised wound edge prevents resurfacing and wound repair. The goal is to have a proliferative wound edge.

- The key principles of creating a physiological wound environment are adequate moisture, temperature control, pH balance, and control of bacterial burden.
- Effective dressings control wound moisture and drainage, debride dead tissue, protect the wound, and reduce the spread of infection.
- Primary wound healing occurs when tissue is cut cleanly and margins are reapproximated (i.e., surgical incisions).
- Secondary wound healing occurs when skin is left open, healing through the formation of granulation tissue at the base of the wound combined with epithelialization from the sides.
- Dressing material is selected on the basis of its characteristics, to promote wound healing (Box 40.1).
- There are many types of alternative dressings beyond those covered in this chapter; it is the nurse's responsibility to be familiar with the particular dressing they are applying and to follow employer policies.

PERSON-CENTRED CARE

- Numerous dressings and products are available for the management of acute and chronic wounds; select dressings to achieve individual patient care outcomes (Table 40.1).
- A priority in wound care management is patient comfort:

BOX 40.1

Dressing Characteristics and Outcomes

Characteristics
- Nontraumatic and able to absorb exudate and allow for moisture-vapour transfer*
- Keeps wound bed moist and surrounding periwound tissues dry and intact
- Appropriate for infected wounds*
- Can be removed without trauma, pain, or leaving dressing fragments in the wound
- Conforms to body part for ease of movement
- Maintains stable physiological wound environment
- Easy to apply and remove with easy-to-follow patient and caregiver instructions
- Cost effective

Outcomes
- Reduces volume of exudate and amount of necrotic tissue
- Resolves or prevents periwound erythema or maceration
- Reduces wound dimensions or depth of sinus tract
- Reduces pain intensity during dressing changes

Data from Bryant, R. A., & Nix, D. P. (2024). Principles of wound healing and topical management. In R. A. Bryant & D. P. Nix (Eds.), *Acute and chronic wounds: Intraprofessionals from novice to expert* (6th ed., pp. 441–457). Elsevier Inc.; Orsted, H. L., Keast, D. H., Forest-Lalande, L., et al. (2017/2021). Best practice recommendations for the prevention and management of wounds. In *Foundations of best practice for skin and wound management: A supplement of Wound Care Canada.* Wounds Canada. https://www.woundscanada.ca/docman/public/health-care-professional/bpr-workshop/165-wc-bpr-prevention-and-management-of-wounds/file

*Not including hydrocolloid dressings.

- Select dressings that help reduce pain. For example, nonadherent (e.g., silicone) dressings will generally reduce wound-related pain (Oropallo & Quraishi, 2024).
- If a patient's pain is due to eroded or denuded skin around the margin of a wound, use skin sealants or barriers or a dressing with a silicone-based border (Bryant & Borchert, 2024).
- If required, provide patients with an appropriate analgesic dose 30 minutes before a dressing change to maximize comfort when the dressing and tissues are manipulated.

- Patients may not admit to requiring pain relief related to dressing change. Discuss with the patient in advance the issue of pain relief. Culture may play a role in a patient's approach to pain. As well, individuals sometimes feel the need to experience pain "to know what's going on." However, it is important to explain the benefit of pain management for wound healing. If acceptable and appropriate, recommend pharmacological and nonpharmacological pain relief measures before dressing changes. These measures may include altering sensory stimulus (e.g., providing a squeeze ball), letting the patient remove the dressing or perform the dressing change, and allowing for "time-outs" during painful dressing changes (Oropallo & Quraishi, 2024).
- Provide an opportunity for caregivers to be present during dressing changes if acceptable to the patient. Caregivers can then see the actual dressing change, thus enabling them to give the patient comfort and emotional support. Provide relevant teaching (e.g., phases of wound healing, rationale for dressing selection) and answer questions during this time.
- If a patient has a chronic wound, assess the patient's or caregiver's knowledge about proper wound care. Patients might have preferences regarding the timing of wound dressing changes (e.g., morning versus afternoon or evening, changing the dressing before or after a certain activity). Encouraging the patient or caregiver to perform wound care at these preferred times can improve patient comfort, engagement, and adherence to the wound care regimen.
- If it is likely that the patient will continue to use the same type of dressing while at home, educate them and the caregiver on the proper techniques of changing it and disposing of medical waste. Also instruct them on how to assess for increased bioburden and for infection.
- Person-centred care includes recognizing the influence of an individual's culture on their health beliefs. For instance, the patient may attribute different meanings to wounds and trauma, blood loss, and disposal of soiled dressings and linens. In addition to ensuring privacy, the act of changing a dressing may require gender-congruent caregivers (e.g., female caregiver for female patient). It is important to ensure that culture and religion have been assessed to determine whether there are additional steps to take in caring for the patient and family.

EVIDENCE-INFORMED PRACTICE

- Management of chronic wounds is a challenge. These wounds often have bacterial bioburden and slough. The TIME framework (see Principles for Practice, earlier) provides an organized approach to wound healing (Ermer-Seltun & Rolstad, 2022; Piemonte et al., 2019; Sibbald et al., 2021).
- Wounds change as they move through the healing phases. Pay attention to the wound itself: the absorption requirements to maintain a moist wound environment, bacterial load, and the need to remove slough or eschar and devitalized tissue (Baron et al., 2020).
- Wound cleaning and irrigation using noncytotoxic solutions with surfactants remove loose devitalized tissue, thus reducing

TABLE 40.1

Wound Care Dressing Categories*

Gauze Dressing	
Composition	Cotton or synthetic material; woven or nonwoven. Available as sterile or nonsterile in multiple sizes (square, ribbon) and as sterile/flat (Nu-Gauze) for packing; nonabsorptive.
Use	To protect surgical or minimally draining wounds or for wound packing. Requires a cover dressing to remain intact.
Not Suitable For	Contact layer in granulating wounds or for heavily draining wounds. Gauze do not support moisture-vapour transfer, so has a limited role in absorbing drainage.
Characteristics	Gauze dressings for wounds should be *nonwoven* if touching the wound bed to avoid potential irritation of the wound bed from gauze fibres. Gauze can sometimes be used when first assessing a wound, to provide protection and some absorption of drainage. Gauze dressings are used mostly to clean wounds, occasionally for packing—packing should be *light* to avoid compression of wound edges.
Frequency of Change	Daily or when saturated or soiled.
Examples	Curity Gauze Sponges, Kerlix Super Sponges, KLING Gauze, Curity AMD Packing Strips
Transparent Film	
Composition	A waterproof adhesive membrane, impermeable to fluids and bacteria.
Use	Best for securing intravenous (IV) tubing, etc. A transparent film is generally useful for keeping a dressing intact and occlusive—for example, in negative-pressure wound therapy (NPWT).
Not Suitable For	Because of the limited moisture-vapour transfer effect, transparent film is not suitable for wounds with moderate to large amounts of drainage. Not recommended for wounds with fragile periwound skin (e.g., skin tears) or drainage, since these dressings tend to hold in moisture and thus may macerate periwound skin and inhibit cell migration in the base of the wound. Should not be used on wounds where infection is suspected nor on third-degree burns.
Characteristics	Help visualize wound and skin underneath dressing. Must be removed using lateral pull: Support dressing and begin to remove at transverse edge. Pull and allow adhesive to be lifted through the mechanical pulling action. Go slowly. Avoid using adhesive remover, as it will further dry patient's skin.
Frequency of Change	Every 3–4 days or when drainage or exudate remains on the wound or periwound skin (maceration of the underlying tissue).
Examples	BioClusive Plus, OpSite, POLYSKIN, Suresite
Hydrocolloid Dressing	
Composition	Gel-forming agents that, once in contact with the wound bed, create autolysis of slough in the wound bed. Maintains a moist environment by forming a gelatinous mass as an occlusive dressing. Self-adhesive (or with transparent film borders), moulds to body contours, and occlusive—waterproof and, if intact, resistant to external contaminants.
Use	Autolytic debridement of noninfected wounds with slough or necrotic tissue; most commonly used for pressure injuries (stage II, stage III, or unstageable). Thin hydrocolloid may be used to protect area from friction or shearing.
Not Suitable For	Critically colonized or infected wounds; wound with moderate to significant drainage; third-degree burns, arterial wounds. Also not for patients with fragile skin at risk for further damage from an adhesive dressing. Avoid using on dry eschar (e.g., diabetic heel ulcers) if debridement will not be of benefit.
Characteristics	Available in different shapes and sizes; select one that provides coverage of wound bed and allows 2–3 cm of intact hydrocolloid dressing around wound (i.e., avoid using overly large dressing). Protect periwound skin with barrier wipe or spray prior to application of dressing because there is potential for periwound maceration. Ensure dressing is completely sealed on application to support autolysis. Dressing will begin to wrinkle, and cream-coloured material is visible through the dressing as autolysis occurs. Odour may be noted when dressing is removed—this is characteristic of hydrocolloids and not to be confused with infection.
Frequency of Change	Every 5–7 days or when the autolyzed material is within 1.5 cm of the border (avoid strike-through/leakage). Irrigate and cleanse wound well; apply fresh hydrocolloid if additional autolysis is required. Protect periwound skin.
Examples	Tegaderm, Duoderm, Granuflex, NU-DERM, ULTEC
Hydrogel Dressing	
Composition	Glycerin- or water-based polymers. Designed to provide moisture to a dry wound bed, thus supporting autolytic debridement.

Continued

TABLE 40.1

Wound Care Dressing Categories*—cont'd

Use	Most effective in promoting moisture in a dry wound bed, which supports wound healing. Can be used in partial- or full-thickness wounds and pressure injury; shallow to deep wounds; dry to light exudate; necrotic wounds.
Not Suitable For	Third-degree burns; wounds with existing drainage. Not generally in conjunction with hydrocolloids or other dressings where its addition may macerate the periwound or wound bed.
Characteristics	Can be in sheet or tube format. Apply sparingly to wound bed (approximately 1.5 mm). Can be used to moisten ribbon or gauze dressing to decrease trauma to wound bed. Can also be mixed with Iodosorb (cadexomer iodine) to help with application. Requires a cover dressing.
Frequency of Change	Per wound bed requirement and selected cover dressing. Generally, every 2–4 days to allow time for hydrogel to interact with wound bed tissue.
Examples	IntraSite Gel, Normlgel, Skintegrity Gel, Spenco 2nd Skin (most product names end in *gel*)
Alginate and Hydrofibre Dressings	
Composition	These two types of dressings are similar in use but different in composition. The main difference between them is that when wet, the *hydrofibre* dressing turns into a gel form that is atraumatic and easy to remove from a wound (i.e., retains shape: the needle-bonding threads). *Alginates* are made of highly absorbent, nonwoven material that strengthens or forms a hydrophilic gel when exposed to wound drainage; composed of fibrous product derived from seaweed (contains sodium and calcium). *Hydrofibres* are soft, sterile, nonwoven pad or ribbon dressings composed of sodium carboxymethylcellulose, which is incorporated in the form of a fleece held together by a needle-bonding process.
Use	For moderately to heavily draining wounds; shallow or deep wounds; pressure injury; venous ulcers. Can be used in conjunction with other cover dressings to provide additional absorption of exudate.
Not Suitable For	Dry wounds; third-degree burns; wounds covered with dry eschar; not in combination with hydrogels (which are designed for the opposite purpose).
Characteristics	Come in sheets or ribbon, so can be fluffed into a wound bed or used to provide light packing in a tunnelling wound. These dressings are highly absorbent—they must be removed in one piece from the wound bed (if using ribbon, ensure amount is measured and documented on application and removal). Alginates also have hemostatic properties, so are useful for postsurgical debridement, for example. Determine whether nonwoven gauze or packing ribbon could be used instead, since alginate and hydrofibre dressings are more expensive; however, they are more effective than gauze for absorbing drainage.
Frequency of Change	Per wound requirements. Generally aim for minimum of 2 days (otherwise, gauze may be used if wound requires daily change).
Examples	ALGICELL calcium alginate, AQUACEL, Maxorb II, NU-DERM Alginate, Sorbsan
Foam Dressing	
Composition	Absorbent, nonadherent polyurethane or film-coated layer used to protect wounds and maintain moist healing environment through moisture-vapour transfer from wound bed. Available in adhesive and nonadhesive forms, also "regular" or "lite" versions.
Use	Moderate-to-heavy exudate wounds; partial- and full-thickness wounds; shallow and deep wounds; stage III and stage IV pressure injuries.
Not Suitable For	Dry wounds; ischemic wounds with dry eschar; third-degree burns.
Characteristics	Foam dressings come in many varieties, shapes, and sizes. They may be simple pads or with a border (either adhesive or silicone). Silicone-based foam dressings provide hydrophobic protection for healing tissue and protect the periwound skin (so no skin preparation is required). Foam dressings are designed to absorb drainage and permit rapid moisture-vapour transfer, which decreases maceration to the wound bed and periwound skin and supports an optimally moist wound environment. Soft and conformable, the borderless foam dressing can be used on several areas of the body (e.g., elbows, heels) and secured with gauze wrap (e.g., Kling).
Frequency of Change	Given moisture-vapour transfer and fluid handling capabilities, foam dressings should be changed when drainage appears to fill the dressing (with approximately 1–2 cm [0.4–0.8 inches] of nonsaturated foam dressing at edges). Dressings should be changed as needed—usually every 3–5 days—but generally can be left intact for 7 days if there is no sign of infection or dressing saturation.
Examples	ALLEVYN, Biatain, Mepilex, Restore Foam, Tegaderm Foam

Adapted from Bryant, R. A., & Nix, D. P. (2024). Principles of wound healing and topical management. In R. A. Bryant & D. P. Nix (Eds.), *Acute and chronic wounds: Intraprofessionals from novice to expert* (6th ed., pp. 441–457). Elsevier Inc.

*Please refer to manufacturer monographs for specific dressings.

bioburden in chronic wounds and improving wound healing (Tyldesley et al., 2019).

- Comprehensive wound assessment not only helps to predict pressure injury risk but also aids in identifying hard-to-heal wounds in a timely manner (Mahoney, 2020).
- Some studies have shown that various dressings may be effective in reducing surgical site infection in postoperative wounds (Simon & Hollenbeck, 2022) and preventing pressure injuries (Lichterfeld-Kottner et al., 2021; Sillmon et al., 2021).

SAFETY GUIDELINES

- Know the underlying cause of the wound and its identified type. Wounds related to vascular insufficiency, diabetes mellitus, pressure, trauma, and surgery have specific factors that need to be considered when developing a treatment plan. Health care providers with additional skill and training, such as enterostomal therapists (also called nurses specialized in wound, ostomy, and continence [NSWOC]), may be required to assess and participate in planning for appropriate wound care. Not knowing the cause of a wound can have serious negative effects if treatments are used that are contraindicated for certain types of wounds (Bryant & Nix, 2024).
- Identify appropriate wound-cleaning agents and appropriate concentration. Some products, used at full strength, may be cytotoxic and impede wound healing. Verify the type and frequency of wound-cleaning agents to apply (World Health Organization [WHO], 2018).
- Be aware of the anticipated amount and type of wound exudate or drainage (Box 40.2). Select dressings that provide adequate exudate management. Heavily draining wounds may require more frequent dressing changes or benefit from the use of superabsorbent polymer materials that absorb and wick away drainage from the wound or periwound. Also, increased drainage is an indicator that a wound is potentially tipping into critical bacterial colonization or infection.
- Determine whether wound drainage devices are present in the wound in order to prevent their accidental dislocation when you remove the old dressing (see Skill 40.3).
- Verify that any wound drainage devices do not place pressure on adjacent skin, as this can result in medical device–related pressure injury (MDRPI) (Alshahrani et al., 2021).
- A wound is a break in skin integrity that increases a patient's risk of infection. Hand hygiene is critical in reducing the risk of introducing bacteria into a wound in the postoperative phase (WHO, 2018).
- To protect yourself and the patient, use surgical gloves when changing a dressing.
- In the home setting, assess the patient's and caregiver's knowledge of infection control practices and provide patient education as needed.

BOX 40.2

Types of Wound Drainage

Serous, which is a clear, watery plasma

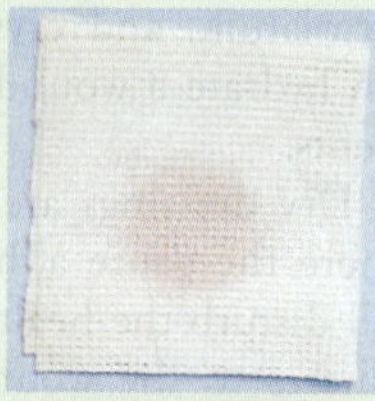

Sanguineous, which indicates fresh bleeding, bright red

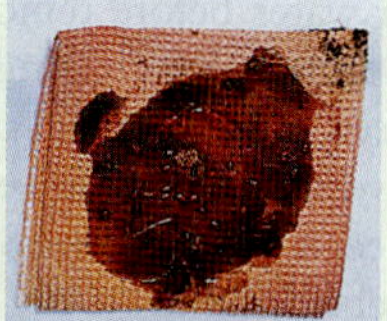

Serosanguineous, which is a pale, red, more watery drainage than sanguineous drainage

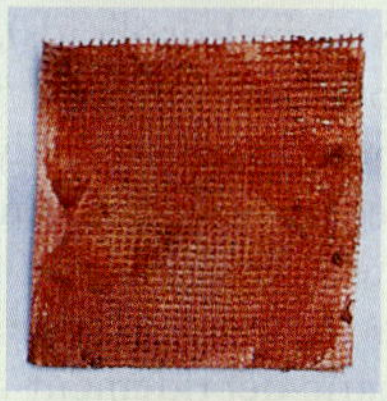

Purulent, which is a thick, yellow, green, tan, or brown drainage

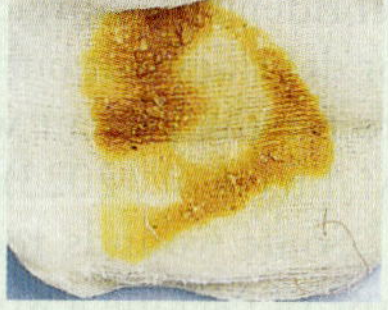

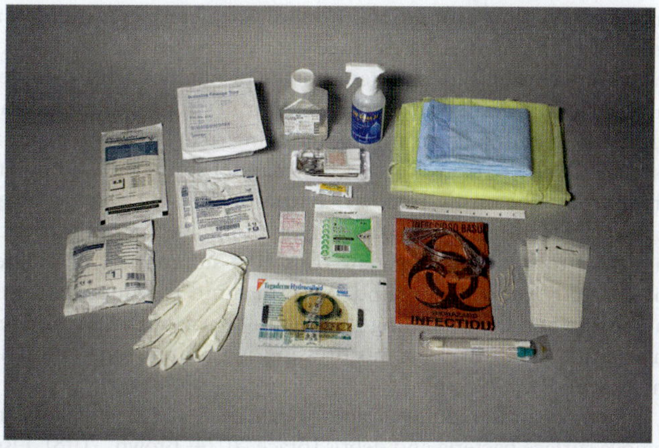

FIG 40.1 Dressing set with personal protective equipment and wound cleaners.

✦ SKILL 40.1 Applying a Dry Dressing

NSO *Nursing Skills Online Wound Care Module 19 / Lesson 3*

Dry, *nonwoven* gauze dressings may be used for a wound healing by primary intention with little drainage (Fig. 40.1). Dry dressings protect the wound from injury, reduce discomfort, and promote healing. Dry gauze dressings do not interact with wound tissues and should cause minimal wound irritation (Bryant & Nix, 2024). These dressings are commonly used for abrasions and nondraining postoperative incisions (see Table 40.1).

Dry dressings have the disadvantage of allowing moisture to evaporate quickly, which can cause a dressing to dry out. As a result, frequent dressing changes are usually needed, and there are increased infection rates when compared with semi-occlusive dressings (Bryant & Nix, 2024). However, dry gauze may come impregnated with a variety of substances, such as zinc oxide paste, iodinated agents, petrolatum, and crystalline sodium chloride. Impregnated gauze can hydrate a wound and absorb exudate or deliver antimicrobial agents.

Dry dressings are not appropriate for actively healing wounds where the gauze adhering to wound drainage or the wound bed will disturb the healthy tissue when the gauze is removed. If gauze adheres to the wound, moisten the dressing with normal saline or water before removing it to minimize wound trauma and pain. Damp-to-dry dressings (also called *wet-to-dry* or *moist-to-dry*) are rarely used as mechanical debridement because this method is not selective for nonviable versus healing tissue and is painful. This practice is no longer considered an appropriate method for wound debridement.

The current options for wound debridement include autolysis (e.g., hydrocolloids), enzymatic, and surgical and maggot therapy. Hydrotherapy is considered mechanical debridement but should be used only when the bath or pool can be thoroughly decontaminated. Enzymatic debriding agents applied directly to the wound bed (or the scored eschar) work by digesting collagen in the necrotic tissue (Brace, 2024; EPUAP et al., 2019). Enzymatic debridement and maggot therapy are less commonly used, but when available, they provide effective and selective tissue debridement. Surgical debridement remains the gold standard for debridement but may not be readily available or not appropriate for the patient with underlying medical or other conditions (Manna et al., 2023).

Some wounds require packing to promote healing. The purpose of packing a wound is to fill dead space and avoid the potential for abscess formation when a wound closes too soon (Bryant & Nix, 2024). Gauze impregnated with simple hydrogel can be used when there is *undermining* (i.e., the destruction of tissue under intact skin around the wound perimeter) or wound *tunnelling* (i.e., a channel has formed that extends from any part of the wound through subcutaneous tissue or muscle). The hydrogel-moistened gauze will prevent the gauze from sticking to the wound edges and potentially harming granulating tissue. Ribbon gauze is used to fill the narrow areas in the channel so that the complete dressing can be easily removed during a dressing change. Alginate or hydrofibre ribbon dressings are optimal for wounds with moderate to significant exudate. Box 40.3 summarizes principles for correctly packing a wound. Keep in mind the importance of measuring and documenting the ribbon or packing dressing used in wounds to ensure that no dressing is unintentionally left in the wound.

Open wounds require cleaning with each dressing change to remove surface bacteria and debris (Brace, 2024; Brown, 2018). Usually, normal saline is the solution of choice, but commercially prepared wound cleaners are also appropriate. Municipal (treated) tap water may also be used. Use an irrigating catheter or syringe for cleaning if a wound is deep (see Chapter 39).

Delegation and Collaboration

The nurse is responsible for wound assessments, care of acute new wounds, wound care requiring sterile technique, and evaluation of wound healing; none of these actions can be delegated to an unregulated care provider (UCP). However, the nurse should instruct the UCP about the following:

- Any unique modifications to the dressing change, such as the need for use of special tape or taping techniques to secure the dressing
- Reporting pain, fever, bleeding, or wound drainage to the nurse immediately

BOX 40.3

Principles for Packing a Wound

- Use the wound characteristics to decide which type of packing is appropriate.
- Make sure that the packing material can be safely used to pack a wound.
- Clean the periwound and wound; apply barrier to the periwound skin.
- Moisten the packing material with a noncytotoxic solution (e.g., normal saline) or a scant amount of hydrogel. Never use full-strength cytotoxic solutions (e.g., povidone–iodine) to pack a healable wound (Alves et al., 2021; Gmur & Karpiński, 2020).
- Use *nonwoven* gauze, if available (woven gauze may leave fibres in the wound bed). Loosen or "fluff" the gauze before packing it into the wound.
- Loosely pack the wound. Tight packing of a wound will result in pressure to the walls of the wound, slowing down the healing process.
- Do not let the packing material drag or touch the surrounding wound tissue before you put it into the wound (avoid contamination).
- Lightly fill all the wound dead space with the packing material.
- When the wound surface has been reached, make sure the packing can be affixed and readily removed; never pack the wound higher than the wound surface.
- Document and measure the amount of packing going into the wound and the amount being removed.

Equipment

- Clean gloves
- Sterile gloves (*optional*)
- Sterile dressing set (scissors, forceps) (*optional*; check employer policy)
- Sterile drape (*optional*)
- Sterile dressings: fine-mesh gauze, 10 cm × 10 cm (4 inch × 4 inch) gauze, absorbent pads
- Sterile basin (*optional*)
- Antiseptic ointment (as prescribed)
- Wound cleaner (as prescribed)
- Sterile normal saline or prescribed solution
  - Debriding gel (as prescribed)
  - Tape, Montgomery ties, hypoallergenic tape (*optional*)
  - Skin barrier (optional if using Montgomery ties or silicone-based dressings)
- Protective waterproof underpad
- Biohazard bag
- Measurement devices (cotton-tipped applicator, measuring guide, camera)
- Personal protective equipment (PPE) (e.g., gown, goggles, mask), as needed
- Additional lighting, if needed (e.g., flashlight, treatment light)

STEP	RATIONALE

ASSESSMENT

STEP	RATIONALE
1. Identify patient using at least two identifiers (e.g., name and date of birth, or name and medical record number) according to employer policy.	Ensures correct patient. Complies with Accreditation Canada's standards and improves patient safety (Accreditation Canada, 2020).
2. Throughout the procedure, the 4 moments for hand hygiene are to be implemented; hand hygiene should occur before initial patient (or patient environment) contact, before an aseptic procedure, after body fluid exposure risk, and after patient (or patient environment) contact. Additional hand hygiene should be performed when hands are visibly soiled.	Proper hand hygiene helps prevent the spread of infectious agents to health care providers.
3. Assess patient for allergies, especially antiseptics, tape, or latex, and acquire specific prescriptions for dressing change.	Reduces risk of localized or systemic allergic reactions to these supplies.
4. Ask patient to rate level of pain using a pain scale of 0–10 (0 = no pain, 10 = worst pain ever)—or use a visual scale, such as the FACES Pain Scale, if the patient is nonverbal or has cognitive deficits—and assess character of pain. If needed, administer prescribed analgesic 30 minutes before dressing change.	Superficial wounds with multiple exposed nerves may be intensely painful, whereas deeper wounds with destruction of dermis should be less painful (Kordestani, 2019; Oropallo & Quraishi, 2024). A comfortable patient is less likely to move suddenly, which could cause wound or supply contamination. Provides baseline to measure response to dressing therapy.
5. Assess size, location, and condition of wound. Review previous progress notes in electronic health record (EHR) or chart.	Helps plan for proper dressing type and securement of supplies needed and determines whether help is needed during dressing procedure.
6. Assess patient's and caregiver's knowledge of purpose of dressing change.	Determines level of support and explanation required.
7. Assess need for and readiness and willingness of patient or caregiver to participate in dressing wound.	Identifies areas for patient education to prepare patient or caregiver if dressing must be changed at home.
8. Review health care provider's prescriptions for type of dressing.	Indicates types of dressing supplies needed.
9. If this is a subsequent dry dressing change, review previous nursing charting regarding dressing change.	Provides baseline information prior to implementing the dressing change.
10. Identify patients at risk for wound healing problems, including older persons; premature infants; those with obesity, diabetes mellitus, circulation disorders, nutritional deficit, immunosuppression, or high levels of stress; those undergoing radiation therapy; and those using steroids.	Physiological changes resulting from aging, chronic illness, obesity, poor nutrition, medications that affect wound healing, and cancer treatments have the potential to affect wound healing (Dilley et al., 2024; Kordestani, 2019).

NURSING DIAGNOSES

- Acute pain
- Chronic pain
- Insufficient knowledge regarding need for specific type of dressing
- Reduced skin integrity
- Potential for infection
- Potential for caregiver role strain (e.g., taking on dressing changes between nurse visits)

Related factors and risk factors are individualized on the basis of patient's condition or needs.

PLANNING

STEP	RATIONALE
1. Expected outcomes following completion of procedure:	
• Patient's wound shows evidence of healing by its decrease in size and reduced drainage, redness, or swelling.	Indicates wound is healing appropriately.
• Patient reports less pain than that experienced at previous assessment after dressing change.	Indicates patient has appropriate analgesia.
• Dressing remains clean, dry, and intact.	Indicates proper application and securement of dressing.
• Patient or caregiver explains purpose of dressing and method of dressing application.	Indicates understanding and that learning has occurred.
2. Explain procedure to patient.	Decreases patient's anxiety.

IMPLEMENTATION

STEP	RATIONALE
1. Close room or cubicle curtains.	Provides for privacy.
2. Position patient comfortably and drape to expose only the wound site. Instruct patient not to touch wound or sterile supplies.	Draping provides access to wound while minimizing exposure. Dressing supplies become contaminated when touched by the patient's hand.
3. Place disposable biohazard bag within reach of work area. Apply clean gloves. Apply gown, goggles, and mask if there is a risk of splashing.	Ensures easy disposal of soiled dressings. Reduces transmission of microorganisms.
4. Gently remove tape, bandages, or ties: Use your nondominant hand to support the dressing and, with your dominant hand, pull tape parallel to skin and toward dressing. If dressing is over a hairy area, remove it in the direction of hair growth. Get patient's permission to clip or shave area (check employer policy). Remove any adhesive from skin.	Pulling tape toward the dressing reduces stress on the suture line or wound edges, irritation, and discomfort.
5. With gloved hand or forceps, remove dressing one layer at a time, observing appearance and drainage of dressing. Carefully remove outer secondary dressing first; then remove inner primary dressing that is in contact with wound bed. If drains are present, slowly and carefully remove dressings (see Step 5 illustration) and avoid putting tension on any drainage devices. Keep soiled undersurface from patient's sight.	Purpose of primary dressing is to remove necrotic tissue and exudate. Appearance of drainage may be upsetting to patient. Avoids accidental removal of drain.
a. If dressing adheres to wound, moisten dressing and remove gently, alerting patient to potential discomfort.	Prevents injury to wound surface and periwound during dressing removal.

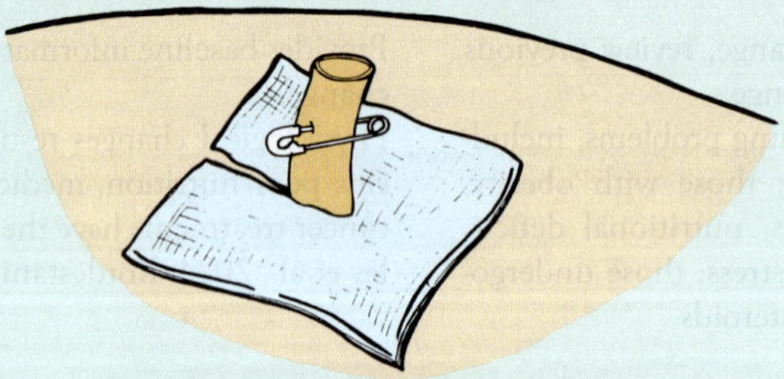

STEP 5 Penrose drain with split gauze.

STEP	RATIONALE
6. Inspect wound and periwound for appearance, colour, size (length, width, and depth), drainage, edema, presence and condition of drains, approximation (wound edges are together), granulation tissue, or odour (see Chapter 39). Use measuring guide or ruler to measure size of wound (see Chapter 39). Gently palpate wound edges for bogginess or patient report of increased pain.	Assesses condition of wound and periwound condition. Indicates status of healing.
7. Fold dressings with drainage contained inside and remove gloves inside out. With small dressings, remove gloves inside out over dressing (see Step 7 illustrations). Dispose of gloves and soiled dressing according to employer policy. Cover wound lightly with sterile gauze pad.	Contains soiled dressings, prevents contact between nurse's hands and drainage, and reduces cross-contamination.

STEP	RATIONALE

IMPLEMENTATION

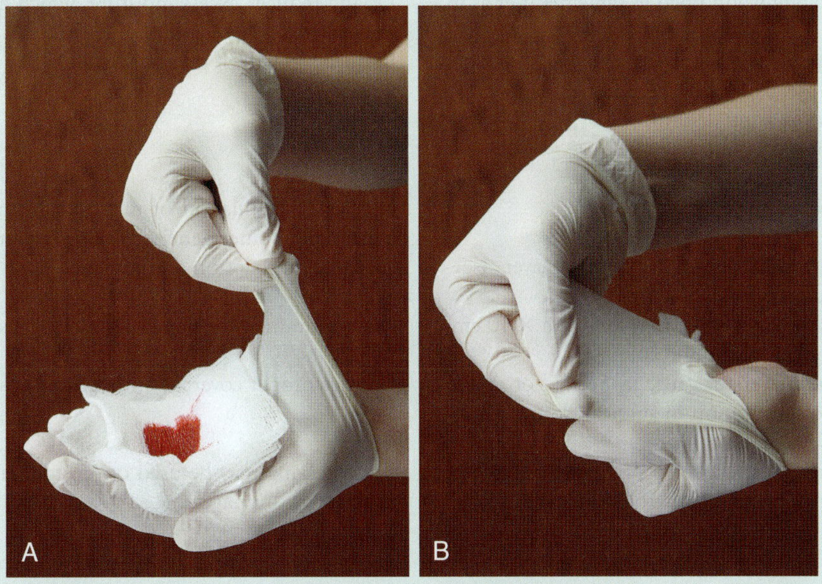

STEP 7 A and B, Dispose of soiled dressings by placing in gloved hand and pulling glove off over dressing and then off hand.

STEP	RATIONALE
8. Describe appearance of wound and any indicators of wound healing to patient.	Wounds may be unsettling and frightening to patients. It helps the patient to know that wound appearance is as expected and whether healing is taking place.
9. If required, use sterile dressing tray or individually wrapped sterile supplies on over-bed table (see Chapter 6). Pour any prescribed solution into sterile basin.	Sterile dressings remain sterile while on or within sterile surface. Preparation of all supplies before dressing change prevents break in technique during dressing change.
10. Clean/irrigate wound (see Chapter 39):	
a. Apply clean gloves. Use normal saline, municipal (treated) tap water, sterile water, or wound cleanser set to "stream" or "spray" as needed (irrigating or cleaning the wound).Gauze pads may be used to gently cleanse surface of the wound and remove any soiled matter.	Removes nonadherent sloughy matter and other loose debris from the wound that may interfere with the healing process. Reduces transmission of microorganisms from previously cleaned area.
b. Clean from least to most contaminated area (see Chapter 39) (see Step 10b illustration).	Cleaning in this direction prevents introduction of microorganisms into wound.
c. Clean around any drain (if present), using circular strokes starting near drain and moving outward and away from insertion site (see Step 10c illustration) (see Chapter 39).	Correct aseptic technique while cleaning helps prevent contamination.

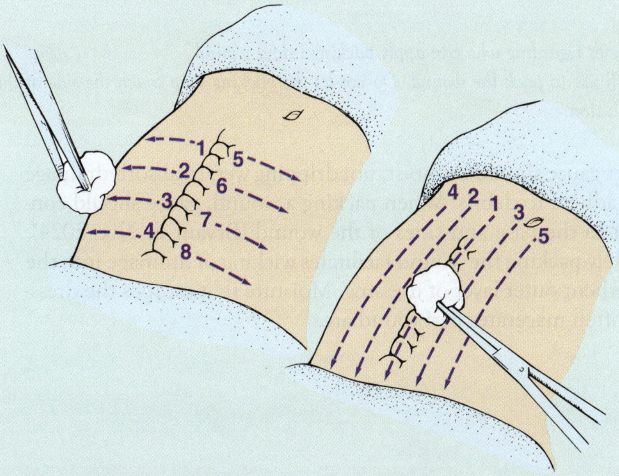

STEP 10B Methods for cleaning a wound; cleaning from least to most contaminated area.

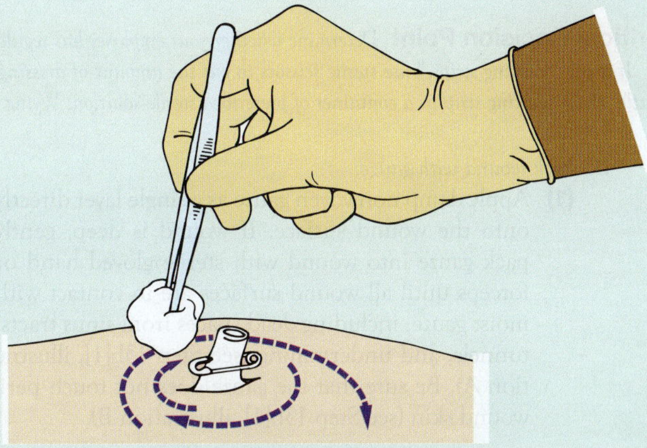

STEP 10C Cleaning around a drain site.

STEP	RATIONALE
IMPLEMENTATION	
11. Use sterile dry gauze to blot wound bed in same manner as in Step 10.	Drying reduces excess moisture, which could eventually harbour microorganisms.
12. Apply antiseptic ointment (if prescribed) with sterile cotton-tipped applicator or gauze, using same technique to apply it as for cleaning. Remove gloves and discard.	Reduces growth of microorganisms.
13. Apply dressing (see employer policy).	
a. *Dry sterile dressing:*	
(1) Apply clean gloves (see employer policy).	Reduces transmission of microorganisms. Sterile gloves may be required by some agencies and for certain wound conditions.
(2) Apply loose, woven gauze as contact layer (see Step 13a[2] illustration).	Promotes absorption of drainage.
(3) If drain is present, apply precut, split 10 cm × 10 cm (4 inch × 4 inch) gauze around drain.	Secures drain and promotes drainage absorption at site.
(4) Apply additional layers of gauze as needed or dressing designed for absorption in surgical wound dressing (e.g., AQUACEL Extra)	Ensures proper coverage and optimal absorption.
(5) If required, apply absorbent pad (e.g., Mesorb) and affix with tape or gauze roll (see Step 13a[5] illustration).	This dressing may be used on postoperative wounds when there is excessive drainage.

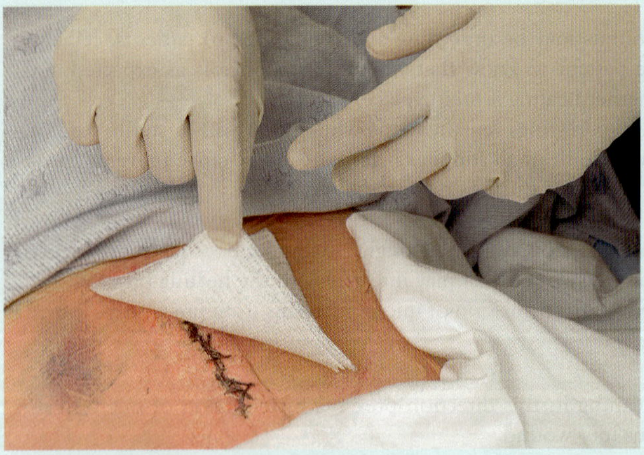

STEP 13A(2) Placing dry gauze dressing over simple wound.

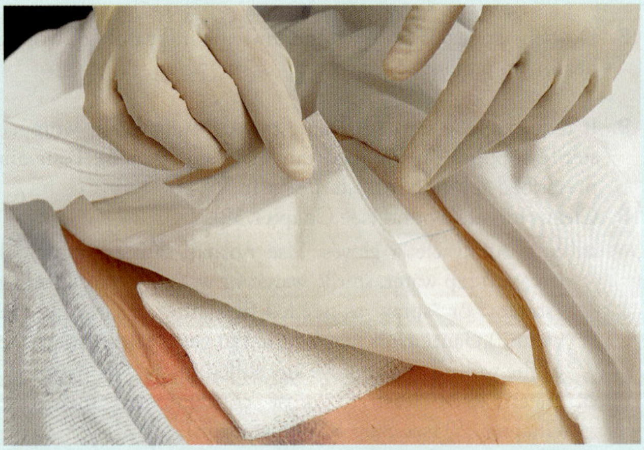

STEP 13A(5) Placing abdominal pad over gauze dressing.

Critical Decision Point *Determine whether your employer has regulations or policies regarding who can apply packing into a wound.*

If using "packing strips," use sterile scissors to cut the amount of dressing that you will use to pack the wound. Do not let the packing strip touch the side of the bottle. Place packing strip in a container of prescribed sterile solution. Wring out excess solution.

STEP	RATIONALE
b. *Pack wound with gauze:*	
(1) Apply damp nonwoven gauze as a single layer directly onto the wound surface. If wound is deep, gently pack gauze into wound with sterile gloved hand or forceps until all wound surfaces are in contact with moist gauze, including dead spaces from sinus tracts, tunnels, and undermining (see Step 13b[1], illustration *A*). Be sure that the gauze does not touch periwound skin (see Step 13b[1], illustration *B*).	Inner gauze should be moist, not dripping wet, to absorb drainage and adhere to debris. When packing a wound, gauze should conform to the base and sides of the wound (Bryant & Nix, 2024). Loosely packing the wound facilitates wicking of drainage into the absorbent outer layer of dressing. Moisture that escapes the dressing often macerates periwound area.

STEP	RATIONALE

IMPLEMENTATION

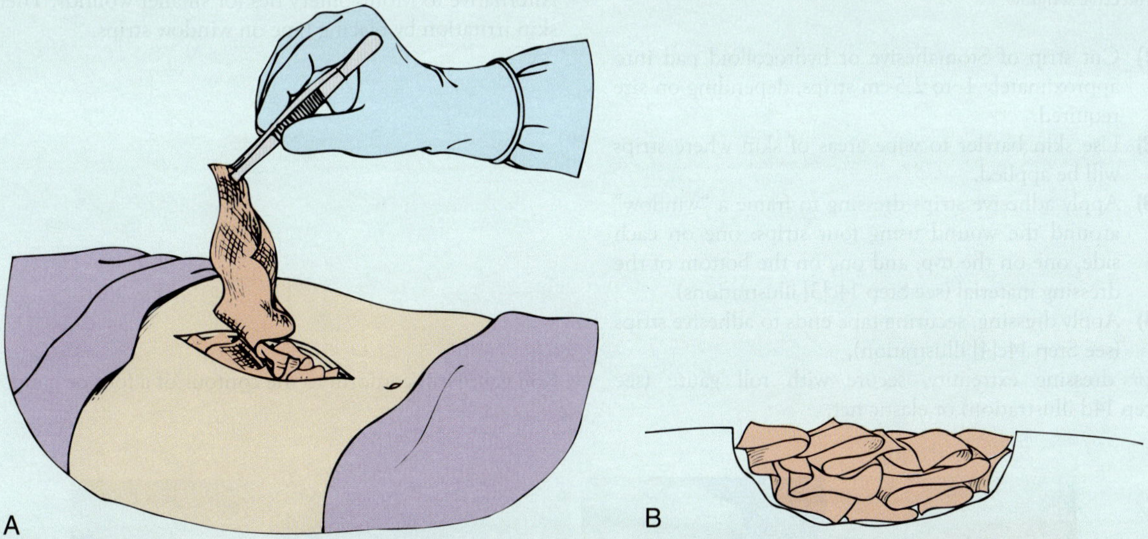

STEP 13B(1) A, Packing wound with fine-mesh gauze. B, Cross-section of deep wound packed loosely with roll gauze.

Critical Decision Point *Be sure to count and document how many pieces of gauze are packed in the wound, especially deep wounds. This practice ensures that all gauze from previous dressing change has been removed from the wound.*

Critical Decision Point *When packing the wound, do not overpack or underpack it* (Bryant & Nix, 2024). *Packing should fill the wound but not be above the level of the skin.*

STEP	RATIONALE
(2) Cover with absorbent pad (e.g., Mesorb) or gauze.	Protects wound from microorganisms.
14. Secure dressing:	
a. *Tape:* Apply tape 2.5–5 cm (1–2 inches) beyond dressing. Use hypoallergenic tape when necessary.	Supports wound and ensures placement and stability of dressing.
b. *Montgomery ties* (see Step 14b illustrations):	Prevents skin irritation. Ties allow for repeated dressing changes without removal of tape.
(1) Be sure that skin is clean. Application of skin barrier is recommended (see Chapter 39).	Skin barrier (e.g., Cavilon wipe) protects intact skin from stretch and tension of adhesive tape.
(2) Expose adhesive surface of tape ends.	
(3) Place ties on opposite sides of dressing over skin or skin barrier.	
(4) Secure dressing by lacing ties across dressing snugly enough to hold it secure but without placing pressure on skin.	

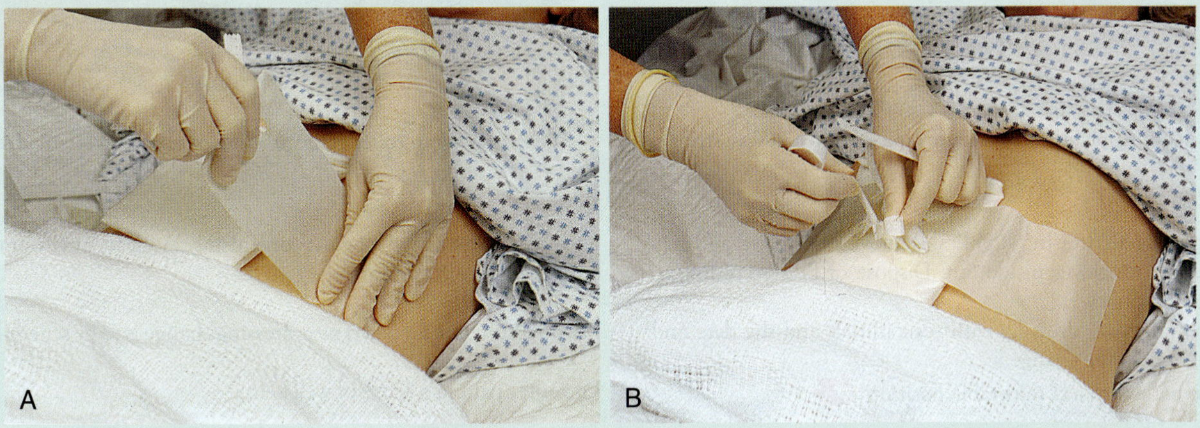

STEP 14B Montgomery ties. A, Each tie is placed at side of gauze dressing. B, Securing ties encloses dressing.

STEP	RATIONALE

IMPLEMENTATION

c. *Protective window:*

Alternative to Montgomery ties for smaller wounds. There is less skin irritation by placing tape on window strips.

(1) Cut strip of Stomahesive or hydrocolloid pad into approximately 1- to 2.5-cm strips, depending on size required.

(2) Use skin barrier to wipe areas of skin where strips will be applied.

(3) Apply adhesive strips dressing to frame a "window" around the wound using four strips: one on each side, one on the top, and one on the bottom of the dressing material (see Step 14c[3] illustrations).

(4) Apply dressing, securing tape ends to adhesive strips (see Step 14c[4] illustration).

d. For dressing extremity, secure with roll gauze (see Step 14d illustration) or elastic net.

Roll gauze can conform to the contour of a foot or hand.

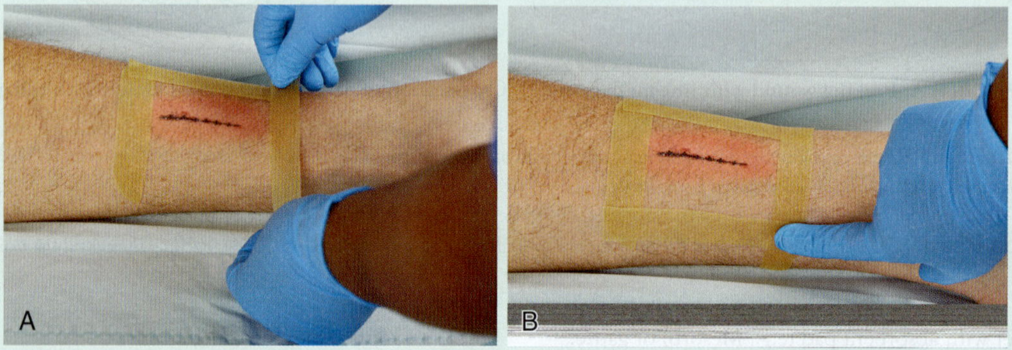

STEP 14C(3) A and B, Apply adhesive strips to frame a "window" around wound using four strips.

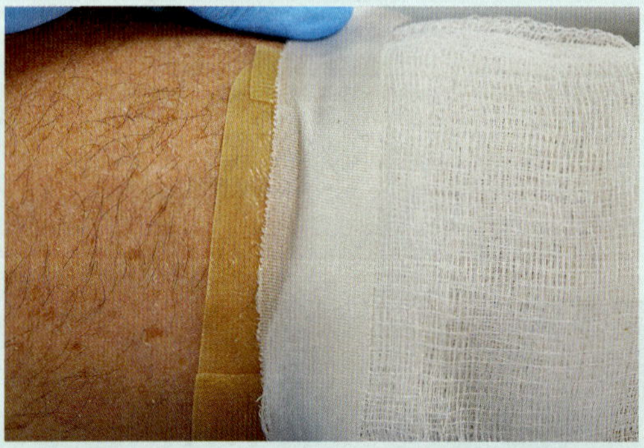

STEP 14C(4) Apply dressing; secure tape ends to adhesive strips.

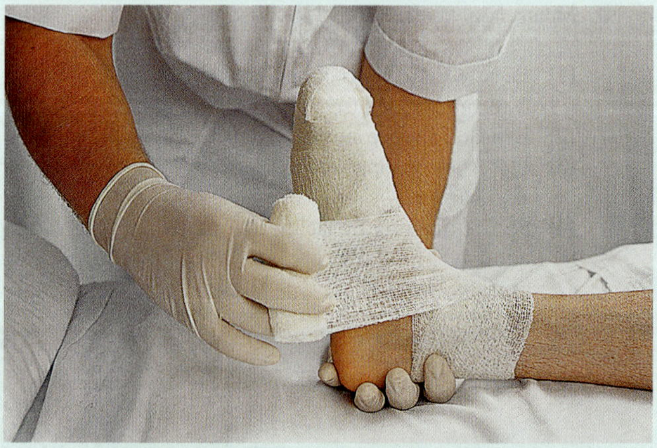

STEP 14D Wrap roller gauze around extremity to secure dressing.

15. Dispose of all dressing supplies. Remove cover gown and goggles; remove gloves inside out. Dispose of PPE according to employer policy.

Reduces transmission of microorganisms. A clean environment enhances patient comfort.

16. Label tape over dressing with your initials and the date and time of dressing change.

Provides timeline for when next dressing change is to be scheduled.

17. Help patient to a comfortable position.

Promotes patient's sense of well-being.

STEP	RATIONALE
EVALUATION	
1. Observe appearance of wound for healing: measure size of wound; observe amount, colour, and type of drainage and periwound erythema or swelling.	Determines rate of healing.
2. Ask patient to rate pain using a pain scale of 0–10 (0 = no pain, 10 = worst pain ever) or a visual scale, such as the FACES Pain Scale, if the patient is nonverbal or has cognitive deficits.	Increased pain often indicates wound complications such as infection or that wound dressing is pulling on tissue.
3. Inspect condition of dressing at least every shift.	Determines status of wound drainage.
4. Use **teach-back:** "I want to be sure I explained why and how often you need to continue these dressing changes in the hospital and at home. Tell me why it is important to change your dressing and how often you will do this." Develop a revised teaching plan if patient or caregiver is unable to teach back correctly.	Determines patient's and caregiver's level of understanding of instructional topic.

Unexpected Outcomes	Related Interventions
1. Wound appears inflamed and painful, drainage is evident, and/or odour is present, periwound skin is warmer than adjacent skin.	• Monitor patient for signs of infection (e.g., fever, increased white blood cell count). • Notify health care provider. • Obtain wound cultures, as prescribed. • If there is yellow, tan, or brown necrotic tissue, use interprofessional collaboration (e.g., wound care specialist, health care provider) to determine need for debridement (Table 40.2).
2. Wound bleeds during dressing change.	• Observe colour and amount of bloody drainage. If excessive, you may need to apply direct-pressure dressing and/or calcium alginate (e.g., Kaltostat). • Inspect area along the dressing and directly underneath patient to determine amount of bleeding. • Obtain vital signs, as needed. • Notify health care provider.
3. Patient reports sensation that "something has given way under the dressing."	• Observe wound for increased drainage or dehiscence (partial or total separation of wound layers) or evisceration (total separation of wound layers and protrusion of viscera through wound opening). • If dehiscence or evisceration occurs, protect the wound. Cover it with a moist sterile dressing. • Instruct patient to lie still. • Stay with patient to monitor vital signs. • Immediately notify health care provider.

Communication and Documentation

- At each dressing change, document the following on the flow sheet and progress notes in EHR or chart: appearance and wound measurement (length × width × depth), characteristics of drainage, presence of necrotic tissue, type of dressing applied, patient's response to dressing change, and patient's level of comfort.
- Document patient's and caregiver's understanding through teach-back of effective dressing change.
- Report any unexpected appearance of wound drainage, accidental removal of a drain, bright red bleeding, or evidence of wound dehiscence or evisceration.

DOCUMENTATION EXAMPLE

Left lower quadrant abdominal abscess, treated by incision and drainage 2 days ago. Dressing: moderate amount serosanguinous drainage; incision site has slight erythema, wound edges clean, smooth, pink. Patient states that pain is localized and "manageable," 3/10 on pain scale (receiving analgesics per health care provider prescription). Reviewed signs/symptoms of infection; patient able to describe signs/symptoms of infection and when to contact health care provider if changes occur.

Wound appearance: L 3 cm × W 2 cm × D 6 cm. No undermining or tunnelling noted. Wound bed pink/moist. No pus, purulence, or odour noted. Irrigated with warmed NS until clear, applied barrier wipe to periwound, applied 6 cm AQUACEL Ag ribbon dressing lightly packed into wound as per prescription, covered with Medipore, and secured with tape. Plan to change q2 days or when external dressing shows drainage.

TABLE 40.2

Problems Associated With Wound Care and Dressings

Problem	Nursing Activities
Solutions or dressings used may be irritating to periwound skin	Protect healthy skin with protective periwound barrier composed of dimethicone (e.g., Cavilon wipes) or petrolatum or zinc oxide. If zinc oxide is used, it should be removed with mineral oil. Avoid scrubbing the skin because doing so can harm the epithelial layer.
Wound becomes excessively dry	Wounds change over time. Consider selecting a dressing that donates moisture to the wound bed (e.g., hydrogel). This can be mixed with nonwoven gauze to lightly fluff into the wound bed. Cover with a simple gauze pad.
Wound is deep, and retention of dressing in cavity is suspected	Irrigate wound copiously with prescribed solution to loosen dressing for removal. Use continuous "ribbon" or strip of gauze to dress deep wounds, and secure to periwound skin if there is danger of the packing slipping into the deep wound.
Wound drainage is damaging healthy tissue	Always protect periwound skin with a barrier product. If drainage is significant and difficult to manage with a superabsorbent dressing, consider a drainage collection device.
Patient's skin is irritated by tape	Use silicone tape. Or, if there are frequent dressing changes, use Montgomery ties or straps (as needed) or fabric tape with multidirectional stretch. Secure dressing with a binder or elastic net, or wrap with roll gauze if on an extremity.

Special Considerations

Teaching

- Explain expected wound appearance and risks of improper wound care. Provide patient and caregiver with a list of signs to report to the health care provider, taking into account your assessment of the literacy level of the patient and caregiver. A written list or illustrations and images may be appropriate.
- Demonstrate wound care and, if appropriate, encourage the patient or caregiver to perform a dressing change with and without supervision. Provide supportive information for reference (e.g., steps to follow, with illustrations).

Pediatric

- Some pediatric patients are fearful of dressing changes. If appropriate, explain the procedure and allow the child to handle and see the dressings (in sterile packaging or sample). Prepare to take time to engage in activities to decrease child's anxiety and fear. If a play therapist is available (or another care provider or family member), plan in advance to have their support to assist in keeping the child cooperative during the dressing change (Boles, 2018).
- Older children may need something to do during dressing changes. Listening to music or watching a video helps relieve some of the boredom or stress they may feel during the procedure (Robertson et al., 2020).

Gerontological

- Normal aging-related changes in skin and tissue and in the inflammatory response may delay wound healing (Boscart et al., 2023).
- Adhesive tape often irritates older persons' skin and causes skin tears. Use paper tape, nonallergenic (e.g., silicone) tape, wraps, or an elastic net to avoid skin trauma.
- Consider risk factors in older persons for impaired skin integrity, such as sensory impairment, dry and dehydrated skin, or impaired nutritional status, that will affect wound healing (Boscart et al., 2023).
- Another option is to create a Stomahesive window. Cut strips of Stomahesive into approximately 1- to 2.5-cm strips. Use a skin barrier to wipe areas of intact skin where you will place the strips. Apply the adhesive strips to two or four sides of the wound, framing it. Apply dressing. Apply tape to the Stomahesive strips.

Care in the Community: Home Management

- While patients at home will initially receive nursing visits for wound care and dressing changes, when possible, patients and caregivers are encouraged to become adept at managing wound care on their own as visits from the community health nurse become less frequent.
- Consider resources within the home, the caregiver's ability, as well as the time required for dressing change when selecting the dressing procedure to be done in the home setting.
- Provide education for the patient and caregiver to increase their confidence and ability to perform independent dressing changes. As the nurse, you will continue to provide support and reassurance and monitor the wound's progress, as required.
- Select dressings that can remain intact longer, if appropriate (to decrease frequency of dressing changes and home visits).
- If the patient or caregiver will be changing the dressing, provide instruction on proper methods of disposing medical waste.

✦ SKILL 40.2 Applying a Pressure Bandage

A pressure bandage is a temporary treatment to control excessive, sudden, unanticipated bleeding. Hemorrhage may occur during surgical intervention (e.g., cardiac catheterization, arterial puncture, organ biopsy) or after surgery or be a life-threatening occurrence related to accidental trauma (e.g., stabbing, suicide attempt). Pressure dressings are essential to stopping the flow of blood and promoting clotting at the site until definitive action can be taken to stop the source of the bleeding.

Given the emergent nature of an acute bleeding episode, the aseptic techniques considered essential in most dressing applications are secondary to halting the bleeding. A pressure dressing applied in an emergency is usually temporary; the wound can be cleaned and the dressing changed once the bleeding has been controlled.

Delegation and Collaboration

The skill of applying a pressure dressing in an emergency situation cannot be delegated to a UCP. However, if the application requires more than one person, a UCP can assist the nurse. The nurse directs the UCP to do the following:

- Assist the nurse as required
- Observe the pressure dressing during care activities to make sure that it remains in place and that there is no visible bleeding from the site
- Check underneath the patient and observe for bleeding after dressing has been applied
- Contact the health care provider if bleeding persists

Equipment

- Necessary dressings: nonadherent gauze and absorbent pads, hemostatic dressings, roller gauze
- Adhesive tape (hypoallergenic, if necessary)
- Adhesive remover *(optional)*
- Clean gloves
- PPE (e.g., gown, goggles, mask), as needed
- Equipment for vital signs

STEP	RATIONALE
ASSESSMENT	
1. If the situation permits, identify patient using two person-specific identifiers (e.g., name and date of birth, or name and medical record number) according to employer policy.	Ensures correct patient. Complies with Accreditation Canada's standards and improves patient safety (Accreditation Canada, 2020).
2. Throughout the procedure, the 4 moments for hand hygiene are to be implemented; hand hygiene should occur before initial patient (or patient environment) contact, before an aseptic procedure, after body fluid exposure risk, and after patient (or patient environment) contact. Additional hand hygiene should be performed when hands are visibly soiled.	Proper hand hygiene helps prevent the spread of infectious agents to health care providers.
3. Anticipate patients at risk for unexpected bleeding–including those with traumatic injury, arterial puncture, donor graft site, postoperative incision, or wounds after surgical debridement–and surgical patients with a history of bleeding disorder.	Familiarity with conditions associated with unexpected bleeding allows rapid response to bleeding.
4. Assess location where hemorrhage has occurred.	Helps identify proper type and amount of supplies needed.
5. Assess patient for allergies to antiseptics, tape, or latex. If patient is nonresponsive and no history is available, use nonlatex or nonallergenic supplies.	Prevents localized or systemic allergic reaction.
6. Quickly assess patient's anxiety level.	Determines need for education and positive reinforcement during procedure.
7. Assess patient's baseline vital signs before onset of hemorrhage.	If data are available, baseline vital signs indicate status of circulatory function.

NURSING DIAGNOSES

- Reduced skin integrity
- Potential for imbalanced fluid volume

Related factors and risk factors are individualized on the basis of patient's condition or needs.

STEP	RATIONALE
PLANNING	
1. Expected outcomes following completion of procedure:	
• Patient shows cessation of bleeding and no evidence of hematoma formation.	Hemostasis is achieved.
• Patient maintains stable blood pressure and heart rate.	Hemodynamic stability is achieved with minimal blood loss.
• Distal circulation is maintained with intact pulses (distal to site of injury).	
IMPLEMENTATION	
Phase I: Immediate Action—First Nurse	
1. Apply clean gloves. Identify external bleeding site. To observe area underneath patients with large absorbent pads, you will need to turn the patient. NOTE: Wounds to the groin area, which are not always visible, can also result in large amounts of blood loss.	Quick identification increases response time to stop bleeding. Maintaining asepsis and privacy is considered only if time and severity of blood loss permit.

Critical Decision Point *If the patient is bleeding from a thoracic or abdominal surgical or traumatic wound, turn the patient over to fully assess the amount of hemorrhage.*

STEP	RATIONALE
2. Apply immediate manual pressure to bleeding site.	Hemostasis is maintained as supplies are prepared.
3. Seek help.	Bandage must be secured quickly. Situation could be life threatening.

STEP	RATIONALE

IMPLEMENTATION

Phase II: Applying Pressure Bandage—Second Nurse

STEP	RATIONALE
4. Apply clean gloves. Quickly identify source of bleeding: • *Arterial bleeding* is bright red and gushes forth in waves, related to the patient's heart rate; if the vessel is very deep, flow is steady. • *Venous bleeding* is dark red and flows smoothly. • *Capillary bleeding* is oozing of dark red blood; self-sealing controls this bleeding.	Determines method of application and supplies to use.
5. Elevate affected body part (e.g., extremity) if possible.	Helps slow rate of bleeding.
6. The first nurse continues to apply direct pressure as the second nurse unwraps a roller bandage and places it within easy reach. The second nurse quickly cuts three to five lengths of adhesive tape and places them within reach; *do not take the time to clean wound until bleeding is controlled.*	Pressure dressing controls bleeding temporarily. Preparation allows for pressure bandage to be secured quickly.
7. *In simultaneous coordinated actions:*	
a. Rapidly cover bleeding area with multiple thicknesses of gauze compresses. The first nurse slips fingers out as the other nurse exerts adequate pressure to continue controlling bleeding (see Step 7a illustrations).	Gauze is absorbent. Layers provide bulk against which local pressure can be applied to bleeding site.

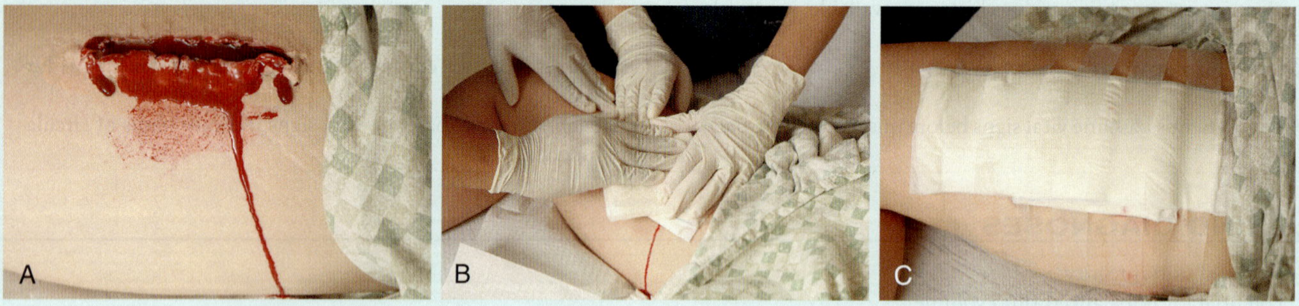

STEP 7A A, Bleeding wound. B, Nurses apply pressure dressing. C, Dressing applied.

STEP	RATIONALE
b. Place adhesive strips 7–10 cm (3–4 inches) beyond width of dressing with even pressure on both sides of fingers as close as possible to central bleeding source. Secure tape on distal end, pull tape across dressing, and keep firm pressure as the proximate end of tape is secured.	Tape exerts downward pressure, promoting hemostasis. To ensure blood flow to distal tissues and prevent a tourniquet effect, adhesive tape must not be continued around the entire extremity.
c. Remove fingers temporarily and quickly cover centre of area with third strip of tape.	Provides pressure to source of bleeding.
d. Continue reinforcing area with tape as each successive strip is overlapped on alternating sides of centre strip. Keep applying pressure.	Prevents tape from loosening.
e. When pressure bandage is on the extremity, apply roller gauze: Apply two circular turns tautly on both sides of fingers that are pressing the gauze. Compress over bleeding site. Simultaneously remove finger pressure and apply roller gauze over centre. Continue with figure-eight turns. Secure end with two circular turns and a strip of adhesive (see Procedural Guideline 40.1).	Roller gauze acts as a pressure bandage, exerting more even pressure over the extremity.
8. Remove gloves and discard.	

Critical Decision Point *Start pressure bandage from distal to proximal, working toward the heart. If bleeding continues, contact the health care provider for immediate assistance.*

STEP	RATIONALE

EVALUATION

1. Observe dressing for control of bleeding.	An effective pressure bandage controls bleeding without blocking distal circulation.
2. Evaluate adequacy of circulation (distal pulse, skin characteristics).	Determines level of perfusion to distal body parts.
3. Estimate volume of blood loss (e.g., count number of dressings used, weigh saturated dressing).	Helps determine blood and fluid replacement needs.
4. Monitor vital signs.	Identifies patient's response to blood loss and early stages of hypovolemic shock.

Unexpected Outcomes	Related Interventions
1. There is continued bleeding. Fluid and electrolyte imbalance, tissue hypoxia, confusion, hypovolemic shock, and cardiac arrest develop.	• Notify health care provider. • Reinforce or adjust pressure dressing. • Initiate intravenous (IV) therapy per prescription. • Place patient in Trendelenburg position; provide covers for warmth. • Monitor vital signs every 5–15 minutes (apical pulse, distal pulses, and blood pressure) (see employer policy).
2. Pressure dressing is too tight and thus occludes circulation.	• Inspect areas distal to pressure dressing to ensure that circulation has not been occluded. • Adjust dressing as needed.

Communication and Documentation

- Immediately report to the health care provider the current status of patient's bleeding control, time the bleeding was discovered, estimated blood loss, nursing interventions (including effectiveness of applied pressure bandage), apical and distal pulses, blood pressure, patient's mental status, signs of restlessness, and need for health care provider to assess the patient without delay.
- Document assessment, application of pressure dressing, and patient response on flow sheet in progress notes in EHR or chart.

Special Considerations

Teaching

- Explain to patient and caregiver (if present) the need to monitor vital signs.
- Explain need for patient to remain quiet and stay in position to reduce bleeding.

Pediatric

- If family members and health care providers can remain calm, child may calm down and be more cooperative (Hockenberry et al., 2024).

Gerontological

- Because of the normal changes associated with aging, the older person has increased risk for vascular and tissue changes distal to the pressure dressing. Perform frequent evaluation of skin and pulse distal to the pressure bandage (Boscart et al., 2023).

Care in the Community: Home Management

- If the patient is at risk for hemorrhage, instruct on the following:
  - How the caregiver or patient should apply pressure with clean towels or linen
  - Immediate activation of emergency system (9-1-1)
  - How to position patient by elevating the affected body part (if extremity)
  - CAUTION: If a puncture wound occurs from a penetrating object (e.g., knife, toy, building materials), instruct caregivers *not to* remove the object. Removal will cause more rapid blood loss and may damage underlying structures.
  - How to position patient to promote elevation of the affected body part (if extremity) and relaxation.

✦ SKILL 40.3 Applying a Transparent Dressing

NSO *Nursing Skills Online Wound Care Module 19 / Lesson 3*

A transparent film dressing is a clear, adherent, nonabsorptive sheet of polyurethane that is impermeable to fluids and bacteria (Bryant & Nix, 2024). Once the transparent film is applied, a moist exudate forms over the wound surface, which prevents tissue dehydration and allows for rapid, effective healing by speeding up epithelial cell growth. However, transparent film dressings may contribute to maceration of the wound or periwound skin because of the occlusive nature of these dressings, which have limited moisture-vapour transfer capabilities.

The most appropriate use of transparent dressings is over an IV catheter insertion site to stabilize the catheter. The synthetic membrane acts as a temporary second skin, adheres to undamaged skin to contain exudate, and minimizes wound contamination from the exterior environment.

Transparent film dressings should not be used on skin tears or fragile skin, since in addition to their occlusive nature, these dressings are difficult to remove without damaging periwound skin—particularly if the lateral pull technique is not used to release the adhesive in a gradual manner.

When applying dressings, including transparent film, hydrocolloid, foam, hydrogel, and other specialty dressings, follow the general principles discussed in this section.

Delegation and Collaboration

The assessment of the wound and care of a new acute wound cannot be delegated to a UCP. However, the nurse directs the UCP to do the following:

- Report any signs of bleeding, drainage, infection, or poor wound healing immediately to the nurse

Equipment

- Sterile gloves *(optional)*
- Dressing set *(optional)*
- Sterile normal saline or other prescribed cleaning agent
- Clean gloves
- Cotton swabs
- Biohazard bag for disposal
- Transparent dressing (size as needed)
- Sterile 10 cm × 10 cm (4 inch × 4 inch) gauze pads
- Skin-preparation materials *(optional)*
- PPE (e.g., gown, goggles, mask), as needed

STEP	RATIONALE
ASSESSMENT	
1. Identify patient using at least two person-specific identifiers (e.g., name and date of birth, or name and medical record number) according to employer policy.	Ensures correct patient. Complies with Accreditation Canada's standards and improves patient safety (Accreditation Canada, 2020).
2. Throughout the procedure, the 4 moments for hand hygiene are to be implemented; hand hygiene should occur before initial patient (or patient environment) contact, before an aseptic procedure, after body fluid exposure risk, and after patient (or patient environment) contact. Additional hand hygiene should be performed when hands are visibly soiled.	Proper hand hygiene helps prevent the spread of infectious agents to health care providers.
3. Assess location, appearance, and size of wound. Determine size of dressing needed. Plan appropriate dressing based on fragility of patient's periwound skin and the amount of drainage or exudate from the wound.Review previous progress notes in EHR or chart.	Determines type of materials needed for dressing change. These dressings are applied over clean, debrided wounds that are not actively bleeding.
4. Review health care provider's prescriptions for frequency and type of dressing change.	Health care provider prescribes frequency of dressing changes and special instructions.
5. Assess patient for allergies, especially antiseptics, tape, or latex.	Prevents local or systemic allergic reaction.
6. Ask patient to rate level of pain using an appropriate pain rating tool. If necessary, administer prescribed analgesic 30 minutes before dressing change.	A comfortable patient will be less likely to move suddenly, which can cause wound or supply contamination. Provides baseline to measure response to dressing therapy.
7. Assess patient's knowledge of purpose of dressing.	Identifies patient's learning needs.
8. Assess patient's risks for impaired wound healing (e.g., aging, poor nutrition).	Physiological changes caused by aging, chronic illness, poor nutrition, medications, and cancer treatments have the potential to affect wound healing (Kordestani, 2019).

NURSING DIAGNOSES

- Acute pain
- Impaired skin integrity
- Risk for infection

Related factors and risk factors are individualized on the basis of patient's condition or needs.

STEP	RATIONALE
PLANNING	
1. Expected outcomes following completion of procedure:	
• Wound heals appropriately.	Dressing is effective in preventing infection and promoting healing.
• Patient experiences minimal discomfort during dressing change.	Adequate pain control is achieved.
2. Explain procedure to patient.	Relieves anxiety and promotes understanding of healing process.
3. Position patient comfortably and to allow for access to dressing site.	Facilitates application of dressing.
IMPLEMENTATION	
1. Close door or room curtains; keep sheet or gown draped over body parts not requiring exposure.	Provides privacy and decreases transfer of microorganisms.
2. Expose wound site, minimizing exposure. Instruct patient not to touch wound or sterile supplies.	Dressing supplies become contaminated when touched by the patient's hand.

IMPLEMENTATION

STEP	RATIONALE
3. Place biohazard bag within reach of work area.	Ensures easy disposal of soiled dressing.
4. Apply clean gloves. Apply PPE (e.g., gown, mask, goggles), as needed.	Reduces transmission of microorganisms from soiled dressings to nurse's hands.
5. Remove old dressing by stretching film in direction parallel to wound rather than pulling it.	Stretching action gently breaks dressing seal (Bryant & Nix, 2024). Reduces excoriation, tearing, or irritation of skin after dressing removal.
6. Dispose of soiled dressing in waterproof bag. Remove gloves by pulling them inside out and dispose of them in waterproof bag.	Reduces transmission of microorganisms.
7. Prepare dressing supplies. Ensure dressings are sterile (package sealed) prior to use.	Reduces risk of break in sterile technique.
8. Pour saline or prescribed solution over 10 cm × 10 cm (4 inch × 4 inch) sterile gauze pads.	Maintains sterility of dressing.
9. Apply clean or sterile gloves (check employer policy).	Allows nurse to handle dressings.
10. Clean wound and periwound area gently with 10 cm × 10 cm (4 inch × 4 inch) sterile gauze pads moistened in sterile normal saline or sprayed with noncytotoxic wound cleaner. Clean from least to most contaminated area (see Skill 40.1).	Reduces introduction of microorganisms into wound.
11. Pat skin around wound. Dry thoroughly with dry 10 cm × 10 cm (4 inch × 4 inch) sterile gauze pads.	Transparent dressing with adhesive backing does not adhere to a damp surface (Bryant & Nix, 2024).
12. Inspect wound for tissue type, colour, odour, and drainage; measure wound, if indicated.	Provides baseline for monitoring wound healing.

Critical Decision Point *If the patient has thin or fragile skin, use a skin barrier on the periwound skin before dressing application to protect patient's skin from further injury* (Bryant & Borchert, 2024).

STEP	RATIONALE
13. Remove gloves and discard.	Reduces transmission of microorganisms.

Critical Decision Point *If the wound has a large amount of drainage, choose another dressing that can absorb drainage and provide effective moisture-vapour transfer.*

STEP	RATIONALE
14. Apply clean gloves and apply transparent dressing according to manufacturer directions. *Do not stretch film during application, and avoid making wrinkles.*	Reduces transmission of microorganisms. Wrinkles provide tunnel for exudate drainage.
a. Remove paper backing, taking care not to allow adhesive areas to touch one another.	
b. Place film smoothly over wound without stretching (see Step 14b illustrations).	Ensures coverage of wound. Prevents shearing of skin from dressing that is too tight. Stretching can also break wound seal.
c. Use your fingers to smooth dressing and help it adhere.	
d. Label dressing with your initials and the date and time of dressing change on outer label of dressing (see Step 14d illustration).	Provides record for determining when to next change dressing.

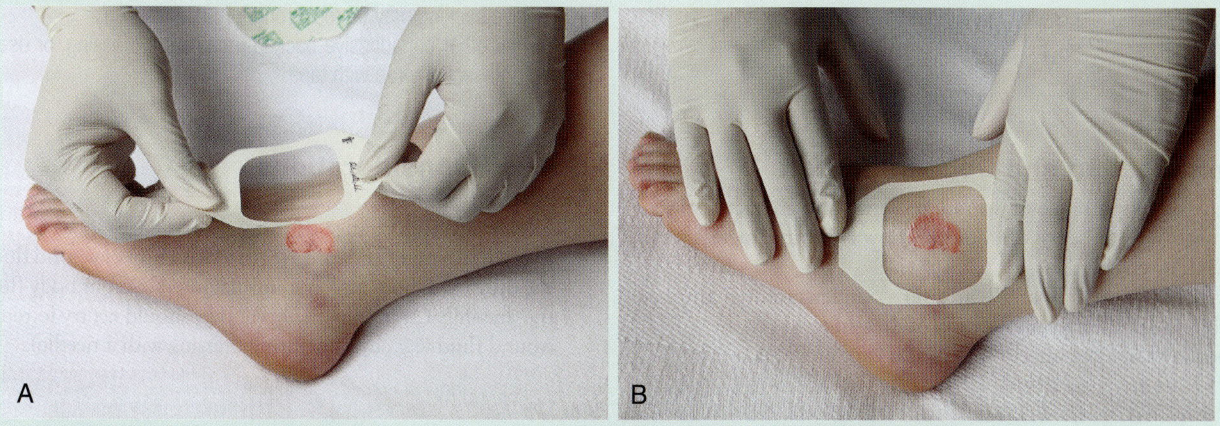

STEP 14B A, Transparent dressing placed over a small wound on ankle. B, Place film smoothly without stretching it.

STEP	RATIONALE

IMPLEMENTATION

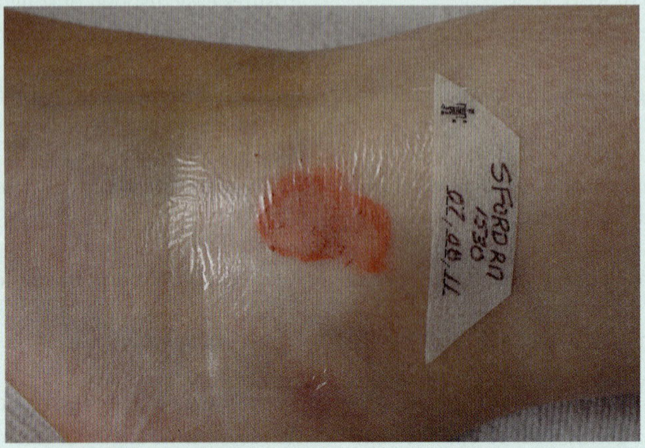

STEP 14D Transparent dressing correctly labelled.

STEP	RATIONALE
15. Discard soiled dressing materials properly. Remove gloves by pulling them inside out and discard in prepared bag.	Reduces transfer of microorganisms.
16. Help patient to a comfortable position.	Enhances patient comfort and relaxation.

EVALUATION

STEP	RATIONALE
1. Inspect appearance of wound and amount of drainage and measure size.	A clear dressing allows observation of wound and status of wound healing.
2. Inspect periwound areas.	Identifies any injury to surrounding skin.
3. Ask patient to rate pain using an appropriate pain rating scale.	Determines any change in pain during procedure.
4. Use teach-back: "I want to be sure you understand how to apply this transparent dressing, since you will be using it at home. Show me how you will apply this dressing." Develop a revised teaching plan if patient or caregiver is unable to teach back correctly.	Determines patient's and caregiver's level of understanding of instructional topic.

Unexpected Outcomes	Related Interventions
1. Wound is inflamed and tender; accumulation of fluid with a white, opaque appearance and erythema of surrounding tissue; increased drainage or change in the colour of drainage; necrosis; and/or odour is present.	• Remove dressing and obtain wound culture according to employer policy. • A different type of dressing may be required. • Notify health care provider.
2. Dressing does not stay in place.	• Evaluate size of dressing used for adequate wound margin (2.5–3.75 cm [1–1.5 inches]). • Assess for increased drainage from wound. • Dry patient's skin thoroughly before reapplication of dressing.
3. Outer layer of patient's skin tears on removal of dressing.	• Adhesive backing may be too strong for patient's skin. • Consider other nonadhesive-backed transparent dressing, or use gauze wrap and secure wrap with tape.

Communication and Documentation

- Document appearance of wound, presence and characteristics of drainage, and presence of odour on flow sheet in progress notes in EHR or chart.
- Document patient's and caregiver's understanding through teach-back of effective application of dressing.
- Report any signs of infection to health care provider.

Special Considerations

Teaching

- Explain need to change dressing should edges loosen.
- Explain to patient and caregiver that collection of wound fluid under the dressing is not "pus" but normal interaction of body fluids with the dressing. Caution patient that they should *not* try to remove this wound fluid (e.g., by puncturing dressing with a needle).

Pediatric

- Adhesive backing may cause skin tears on premature infants' immature skin (Kelly-O'Flynn et al., 2020).
- Children may find this procedure more tolerable if they know that the longer the dressing is left on, the easier it is to remove (Sahyoun et al., 2021).

Gerontological

- Adhesive backing may be too strong for the skin of older persons. Do not use a film dressing that has an adhesive backing with a stronger bond to the epidermis than the epidermis has to the dermis (Boscart et al., 2023).

Care in the Community: Home Management

- The wound may be cleaned in the shower if approved by the health care provider.
- Many types of transparent dressings exist. Some newer options allow for moisture-vapour transfer (to some degree) and can remain in place for several weeks (e.g., absorbent clear acrylic dressings). Ensure that the patient understands how the dressing functions and the ways to keep it intact.

✦ SKILL 40.4 Applying a Hydrocolloid, Hydrogel, Foam, Alginate, or Hydrofibre Dressing

NSO *Nursing Skills Online Wound Care Module 19 / Lesson 3*

Current wound care dressings have several different characteristics and different mechanisms of action, depending on the needs of a particular wound at a particular time in the wound healing process (see Table 40.1).

Hydrocolloid dressings are designed to promote autolytic debridement when there is no evidence of infection (Weller et al., 2020). These dressings can be left intact (5 to 7 days) to work effectively. The periwound skin should be protected with a barrier wipe prior to application of the hydrocolloid. Hydrocolloid dressings are often the choice for sacral pressure injury wounds requiring autolytic debridement when there is no evidence of infection in the wound bed.

Hydrogel dressings promote moist wound healing and autolysis (Bryant & Nix, 2024). The gel dressings are nonadherent and less painful to remove. A dry wound still requires a dressing—and if debridement or enhanced healing is of benefit, a scant amount of hydrogel dressing the thickness of a dime will donate moisture to the wound bed.

Polyurethane foam dressings are sheets of foamed polymers that contain small, open cells capable of holding wound exudate away from a wound bed (Bryant & Nix, 2024). The foam dressings protect the wound surface while maintaining a moist, insulated environment. These dressings are designed to wick moisture away from the wound through moisture-vapour transfer, thus avoiding saturation of the wound bed and periwound skin.

Alginate and hydrofibre dressings, designed primarily to absorb drainage, promote autolysis, granulation, and epithelialization (Bryant & Nix, 2024). The dressing may come as a sheet or rope that can be packed into a wound. The nurse can lightly pack deep tracking wounds with either of these types of absorptive dressings, which provide easy removal with little risk for retention of the dressing deep in the wound cavity (Bryant & Nix, 2024).

Delegation and Collaboration

The skill of applying a hydrocolloid, hydrogel, foam, alginate, or hydrofibre dressing cannot be delegated to a UCP. The nurse directs the UCP to do the following:

- Help position the patient during dressing application
- Immediately report to the nurse any pain, fever, bleeding, wound drainage, or slippage of dressing

Equipment

- Sterile gloves *(optional)*
- Clean gloves

Dressing Set *(optional)*

- Sterile scissors *(optional)*
- Sterile drape *(optional)*
- Necessary primary dressings: gauze, hydrocolloid, hydrogel, foam, alginate, or hydrofibre
- Secondary dressing of choice
- Sterile 10 cm × 10 cm (4 inch × 4 inch) gauze pads
- Irrigating solution if indicated (see Skill 39.2)
  - Debriding gel (as prescribed)
  - Skin barrier wipe
  - Tape (nonallergenic paper or adhesive) or Montgomery ties, as needed
- Measuring guide (tape measure, tracing paper, camera), as needed
- Adhesive remover (generally not required)
- Biohazard bag
- PPE (e.g., gown, goggles, mask), as needed

STEP	RATIONALE
ASSESSMENT	
1. Identify patient using at least two person-specific identifiers (e.g., name and date of birth, or name and medical record number) according to employer policy.	Ensures correct patient. Complies with Accreditation Canada's standards and improves patient safety (Accreditation Canada, 2020).
2. Throughout the procedure, the 4 moments for hand hygiene are to be implemented; hand hygiene should occur before initial patient (or patient environment) contact, before an aseptic procedure, after body fluid exposure risk, and after patient (or patient environment) contact. Additional hand hygiene should be performed when hands are visibly soiled.	Proper hand hygiene helps prevent the spread of infectious agents to health care providers.
3. Assess for presence of allergies, especially antiseptics, tape, or latex.	Prevents localized or systemic reaction to supplies.
4. Inspect location, size, and condition of wound.	Determines supplies and help needed.

STEP	RATIONALE
ASSESSMENT	
5. Ask patient to rate pain using an appropriate pain rating scale. If necessary, administer prescribed analgesic 30 minutes before dressing change.	Patient may require pain medication before dressing change. Allows for peak effect of medication during procedure.
6. Review health care provider's prescriptions for frequency and type of dressing change. *Do not use alginate or absorptive dressings on nonexudative wounds.*	Prescription indicates type of dressing or application to use. Wounds change in their requirements over time. If dressing prescription is no longer appropriate, contact the health care provider to provide an up-to-date wound description for relevant prescription change.
7. Review previous progress notes in EHR or chart. Note possible need to use customized shape or size of dressing to fit body parts that are difficult to size (e.g., sacrum, heels, or elbows).	Customized shapes aid in person-centred dressing selection and better dressing adherence.
8. Assess patient's knowledge of purpose of dressing and determine need to include caregiver in dressing wound.	Identifies patient's and caregiver's learning needs.

NURSING DIAGNOSES

- Acute pain
- Chronic pain
- Insufficient knowledge regarding application of hydrocolloid, hydrogel, foam, alginate, or hydrofibre dressing
- Reduced skin integrity
- Potential for infection

Related factors and risk factors are individualized on the basis of patient's condition or needs.

STEP	RATIONALE
PLANNING	
1. Expected outcomes following completion of procedure:	
• Patient's wound shows evidence of healing as it becomes smaller in size or shallower in depth with less drainage, redness, or swelling.	Dressing is effective in promoting healing.
• Patient reports pain that is less than previously assessed level, using an appropriate pain rating scale during and after dressing change.	Pain control is achieved during dressing removal and reapplication.
• Dressing remains clean, dry, and intact.	Dressing is applied correctly.
• Patient or caregiver explains procedure correctly.	Demonstrates that learning has occurred.
2. Explain procedure to patient or caregiver.	Relieves anxiety and promotes understanding of healing process.
3. Position patient comfortably to allow access to dressing site.	Facilitates application of dressing.
IMPLEMENTATION	
1. Close room door or room curtains.	Provides for patient privacy.
2. Expose wound site and drape patient. Instruct patient not to touch wound or sterile supplies.	Draping provides access to wound while minimizing exposure. Dressing supplies become contaminated when touched by the patient's hand.
3. Place biohazard bag within reach of work area. Fold top of bag to make a cuff.	Ensures easy disposal of soiled dressings. The nurse should not reach across a sterile field.
4. Apply clean gloves. Apply appropriate PPE, as needed, if there is risk of splashing.	Reduces transmission of microorganisms.
5. Using nondominant hand, gently remove tape, bandages, or ties from existing dressing. Pull tape parallel to skin and toward dressing. If dressing is over hairy areas, remove tape in the direction of hair growth and get patient's permission to clip or shave area before applying new dressing (check employer policy). Remove any adhesive from skin.	Pulling tape toward dressing reduces stress on wound edges, irritation, and discomfort.
6. With gloved hand or forceps, remove old dressing one layer at a time. Note amount and character of drainage (see Step 6 illustration). Use caution to avoid placing tension on any drains.	Reduces irritation and possible injury to skin. Prevents accidental removal of drain.

STEP	RATIONALE

IMPLEMENTATION

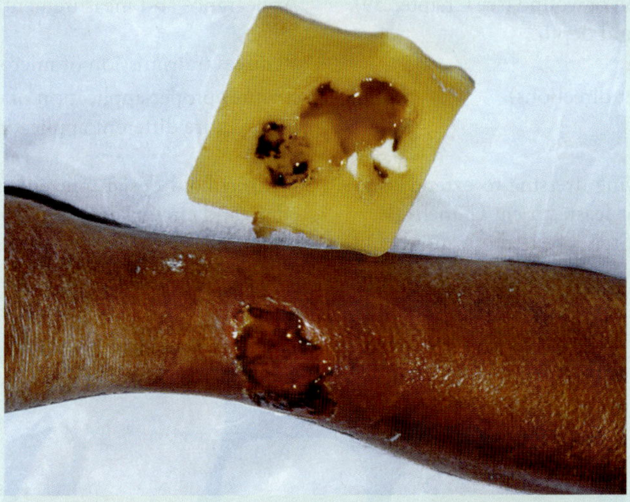

STEP 6 Hydrocolloid dressing after removal from venous injury. Purulent-appearing exudate is present on dressing and wound. This is expected with autolysis under the dressing and is not evidence of infection. *(From Bryant, R. A., & Nix, D. P. [2024]. Acute and chronic wounds: Intraprofessionals from novice to expert [6th ed.]. Elsevier Inc.)*

Critical Decision Point *Check removal directions for the specific brand of dressing used. Some brands require that the old dressing be soaked, irrigated, or moistened for removal. Consider "lateral pull" to gently loosen adhesive from skin. If necessary, use adhesive remover to ease off the dressing, but avoid contact between adhesive remover and the wound.*

STEP	RATIONALE
7. Fold dressings with drainage contained inside and remove gloves inside out. With small dressings, remove gloves inside out to enclose dressing (see Skill 40.1). Dispose of gloves and soiled dressing according to employer policy. Cover wound lightly with a sterile 10 cm × 10 cm (4 inch × 4 inch) gauze pad.	Contains soiled dressings; prevents contact between nurse's hands and drainage; reduces cross-contamination.

Critical Decision Point *Hydrocolloid dressings interact with wound fluids and form a soft, whitish-yellowish gel, which is sometimes hard to remove and may have a faint odour. A residual gel substance occurs in wound beds with some absorption dressings. This is a normal occurrence; do not confuse these findings with pus or purulent exudate, wound infection, or wound deterioration* (Bryant & Nix, 2024). *Foam dressings should have a well-marked area of saturation of wound fluid or exudate (with approximately 1.5 cm of nonsaturated foam at dressing edges).*

STEP	RATIONALE
8. Prepare sterile field with sterile dressing kit or individually wrapped sterile supplies on over-bed table (see Chapter 6). Pour prescribed cleaning solution into sterile bowl.	Creates sterile work area.
9. Remove gauze cover over wound.	
10. Clean wound:	
a. Apply clean gloves. Sterile gloves are optional (see employer policy). Clean wound and periwound area gently with 10 cm × 10 cm (4 inch × 4 inch) sterile gauze pads moistened in sterile normal saline or sprayed with noncytotoxic wound cleanser.	Reduces transmission of microorganisms into wound. Effective cleaning and irrigation remove residual dressing gel or slough without injuring newly formed delicate granulation tissue in healing wound bed.
b. Clean from least contaminated to most contaminated area.	Cleaning in this direction prevents introduction of microorganisms into noncontaminated areas.
c. Clean around any drain, using circular stroke starting near drain and moving outward away from insertion site (see Skill 40.1).	
11. Use dry sterile gauze to blot dry wound bed and on skin around wound.	Dressing will not adhere to damp surface. Periwound maceration can enlarge wound and impede healing.

STEP	RATIONALE

IMPLEMENTATION

12. Inspect appearance and condition of wound (see Chapter 39). Measure wound length, width, and depth.
    - *Rationale:* Appearance and measurement indicate state of wound healing.
13. Remove gloves and discard.
    - *Rationale:* Reduces transmission of microorganisms.
14. Apply dressing (see manufacturer directions).
    - *Rationale:* Ensures proper application of dressing. Different brands of dressings require different application techniques.

    a. *Hydrocolloid dressings:*

    (1) Select proper size, allowing dressing to extend onto intact periwound skin at least 2.5 cm (1 inch) (Bryant & Nix, 2024) (see Step 14a[1] illustration). Do not stretch dressing; avoid producing wrinkles and tenting.
    - *Rationale:* Hydrocolloid design prevents shear and friction from loosening edges and circumvents need for tape along dressing borders (Bryant & Nix, 2024).

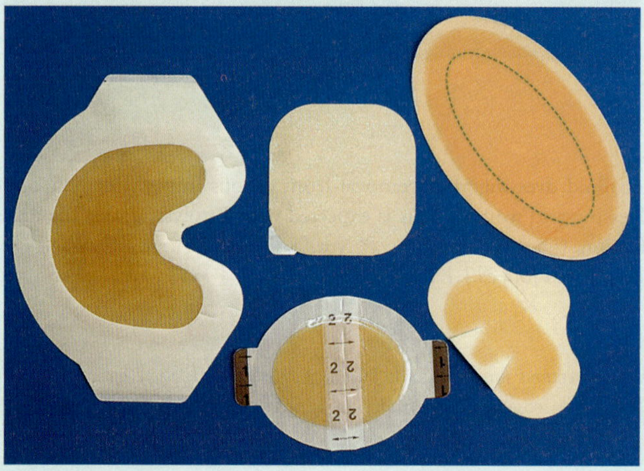

STEP 14A(1) Variety of sizes and shapes of hydrocolloid dressings. *(Courtesy Bonnie Sue Rolstad.)*

    (2) For a deep wound, apply hydrocolloid granules, impregnated gauze, or paste before the wafer.
    - *Rationale:* Functions as filler material to ensure contact with all wound surfaces.

    (3) Remove paper backing from adhesive side and place over wound. Do not stretch, and avoid producing wrinkles or tenting. Hold dressing in place for 30–60 seconds after application.
    - *Rationale:* Moulds dressing at body temperature (Bryant & Nix, 2024). Warmth of nurse's hand over the dressing helps with adherence.

    (4) If dressing is cut from a larger piece, tape edges with nonallergenic tape to avoid rolling or adherence to clothing.

Critical Decision Point *Edges of dressing may be notched to help mould around wound. Consider using custom shapes and sizes to better conform to certain parts of the body, such as heels, elbows, and sacrum.*

    b. *Hydrogel dressings:*

    (1) Apply skin barrier wipe to surrounding skin that will encounter any adhesive or gel.
    - *Rationale:* Protects periwound skin. Because of the high water content of gels, care must be taken to protect periwound skin through use of a skin barrier (Bryant & Nix, 2024).

    (2) Apply gel or gel-impregnated gauze directly into wound, spreading evenly over wound bed (see Step 14b[2] illustration). Apply gel to wound cavity no more than about one-third full or pack gel-impregnated gauze loosely, including any undermined or tunnelled areas. Cover with appropriate moisture-retentive dressing that will still allow for moisture-vapour transfer. *Option:* Hydrogel sheets composed of water should be cut to size of wound only.
    - *Rationale:* Hydrogels donate moisture to the wound bed, thus facilitating autolytic debridement of wounds. Filling the wound cavity partially full allows for expansion with absorption of exudate (Bryant & Nix, 2024).

STEP	RATIONALE

IMPLEMENTATION

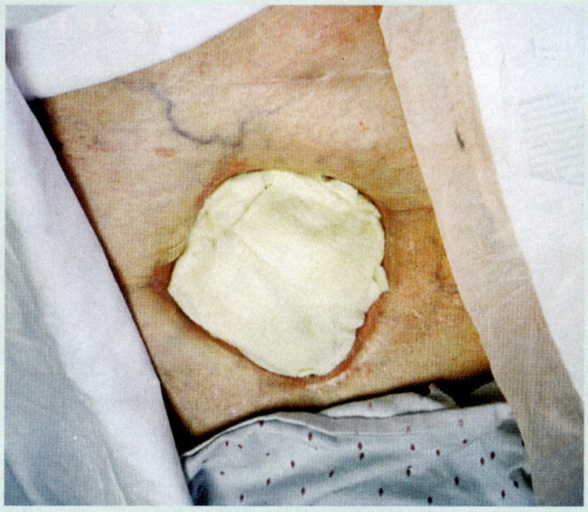

STEP 14B(2) Hydrogel-impregnated gauze used to maintain moist wound bed and fill dead space in this deep abdominal wound with undermining. *(From Bryant, R. A., & Nix, D. P. [2024]. Acute and chronic wounds: Intraprofessionals from novice to expert [6th ed.]. Elsevier Inc.)*

STEP	RATIONALE
(3) Apply skin barrier cream or spray to periwound skin.	Protects skin around wound from maceration.
(4) Secure dressing with nonallergenic tape if secondary dressing is not self-adhering.	
c. *Foam dressings:*	
(1) Know removal and application characteristics of the specific brand of foam dressing.	Some foam dressings have silicone in the dressing itself; some have a silicone dressing border only. With silicone dressings, no skin barrier protectant is required.
(2) If dressing is not silicone foam, a skin barrier wipe is required. Apply to the surrounding skin that will come in contact with dressing adhesive.	Protects periwound skin from maceration or irritation from adhesive.
(3) If using a foam dressing without a border, use an appropriately sized dressing; if required, a nonborder foam dressing can be cut to extend 2.5 cm out onto intact periwound skin. Nonborder foam requires a "window-pane" border created with tape. Do not cover the entire foam dressing, just the borders. Foam dressings with a border should extend approximately 2.5 cm (1 inch) on all sides over intact periwound skin. Verify which side of the foam dressing should be placed toward the wound bed and which side should be facing away from it; check product instructions.	Ensures proper absorption and keeps wound exudate away from wound bed (Bryant & Nix, 2024).
(4) Cut foam to fit around drain or tube.	
d. *Alginate or hydrofibre dressings:*	
(1) Cut sheet or rope to fit size of wound or loosely pack into wound space (see Step 14d[1] illustration), filling one-half to one-third full.	Highly absorptive product expands with absorption of serous fluid or exudate (Bryant & Nix, 2024).

STEP	RATIONALE

IMPLEMENTATION

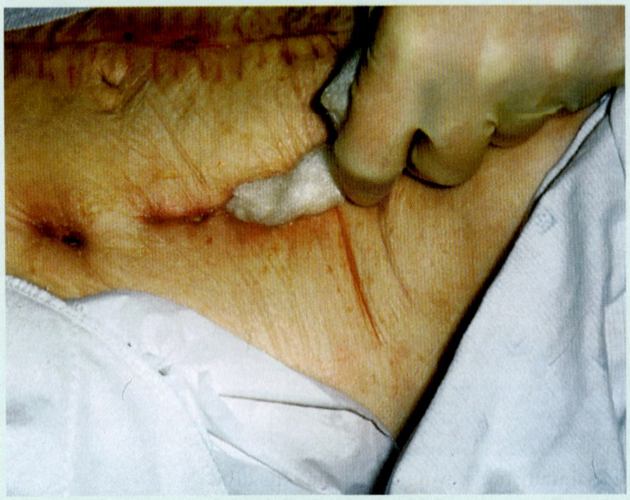

STEP 14D(1) Alginate dressing applied to fill dead space and absorb exudate in full-thickness abdominal wound. *(From Bryant, R. A., & Nix, D. P. [2024]. Acute and chronic wounds: Intraprofessionals from novice to expert [6th ed.]. Elsevier Inc.)*

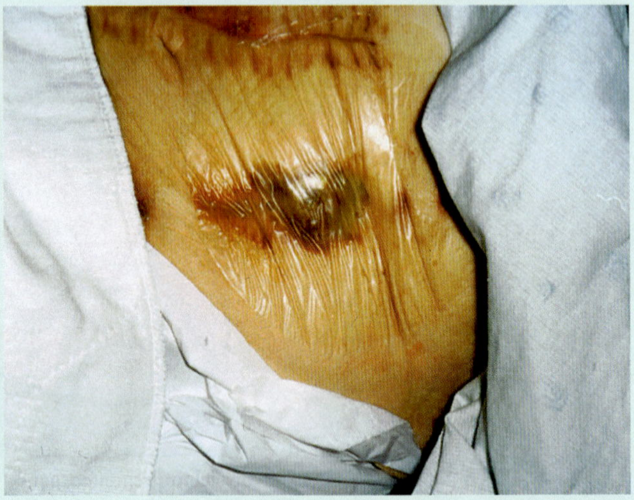

STEP 14D(2) Alginate dressing secured with secondary transparent dressing. *(From Bryant, R. A., & Nix, D. P. [2024]. Acute and chronic wounds: Intraprofessionals from novice to expert [6th ed.]. Elsevier Inc.)*

STEP	RATIONALE
(2) Apply secondary dressing: absorbent pad (e.g., Mesorb) or foam dressing to cover. Select cover dressing according to anticipated frequency of primary dressing change (see Step 14d[2] illustration).	Secondary dressing helps maintain appropriate moisture in the wound bed, supports moisture-vapour transfer, and prevents drainage on bed linens and clothing.
15. Label dressing with your initials and the date and time of dressing change.	Provides timeline for next dressing change.
16. Discard soiled dressing materials properly. Remove gloves by pulling them inside out and discard in prepared bag.	Reduces transfer of microorganisms.
17. Help patient return to a comfortable position.	Enhances patient comfort and relaxation.

EVALUATION

STEP	RATIONALE
1. Inspect appearance of wound: measure length × width × depth of wound; observe amount and colour of drainage; and observe presence of periwound edema or erythema. Palpate around wound for tenderness.	Determines status of wound healing.
2. Evaluate patient's level of comfort.	Documents patient's level of comfort after procedure.
3. Inspect condition of dressing at least every shift or as prescribed.	Determines integrity of wound dressing.
4. **Use teach-back:** "I want to be sure I explained why I need to use this type of dressing for your wound. Tell me why this dressing material is the best option for your wound." Develop revised teaching if patient or caregiver is unable to teach back correctly.	Determines patient's and caregiver's level of understanding of instructional topic.

Unexpected Outcomes	Related Interventions
1. Wound develops more necrotic tissue and increases in size.	• In rare instances, some wounds do not tolerate hypoxia induced by hydrocolloid dressings. In these patients, discontinue use. Notify the health care provider. • Evaluate appropriateness of wound care protocol. • Assess and treat the underlying conditions. Evaluate for other factors impairing wound healing.

Unexpected Outcomes	Related Interventions
2. Dressing does not stay in place.	• Evaluate size of dressing used for adequate margin (2.5–3.5 cm [1–1.4 inches]) • Ensure that periwound skin is not macerated and has an appropriate skin barrier wipe to assist in keeping dressing intact. • If patient is incontinent or diaphoretic, some dressings may be difficult to adhere. Consider alternatives (e.g., using roll gauze or elastic net). • Consider custom shapes for body parts that are difficult to fit. • Dressing may be secured with roll gauze, tape, or transparent dressing (assess for fragile skin).
3. Periwound skin is macerated.	• Assess moisture-control property of dressing or application technique, including skin barrier protectant; incontinence or diaphoresis may also require management.

Communication and Documentation

- Document the following on flow sheet in progress notes in EHR or chart: appearance, colour, and size of wound; characteristics of drainage; response to dressing change; condition of periwound skin; and patient's level of comfort.
- Graph wound surface area (L × W) or volume (L × W × D) if wound is chronic. Wound progress should demonstrate 50% or more wound closure at 4 weeks of standard treatment (Foltynski et al., 2021).
- Document patient's and caregiver's understanding through teach-back of proper wound dressing change.
- Report signs of infection, necrosis, or deteriorating wound status to health care provider immediately.

Special Considerations

Teaching

- Explain expected wound appearance, fluid or gel accumulation in wound bed, and possible odour with use of specific dressing.
- Because application techniques can vary with brand, tell patient and caregiver not to purchase a brand of dressing different from the one for which the nurse gave instructions. If a different brand must be used, the patient and caregiver should check with the nurse for any additional instructions or modifications in application and removal techniques.

Pediatric

- See Pediatric Considerations for Skills 40.1, 40.2, and 40.3.

Gerontological

- See Gerontological Considerations for Skills 40.1, 40.2, and 40.3.
- Avoid early and frequent removal of a hydrocolloid dressing to reduce injury to surrounding intact skin.

Procedural Guideline 40.1 *Applying Gauze and Elastic Bandages*

NSO *Nursing Skills Online Wound Care Module 19 / Lesson 1*

Gauze and elastic bandages secure or wrap hard-to-cover areas of the body such as dressings on extremities and amputation stumps. Bandages act as a secondary dressing, providing protection, pressure, immobilization, and anchoring of underlying dressings or splints. There are numerous types of and applications for bandages. They are available in rolls of various widths and materials, including gauze, elastic, webbing, elasticized knit, and muslin. Gauze bandages are lightweight and inexpensive, mould easily around body contours, and permit air circulation to prevent skin maceration. Elastic bandages apply compression to a body part. Elastic compression to a lower extremity prevents edema by promoting the return of blood from the peripheral to the central circulation.

When applying a bandage, select a type of bandage turn (Table 40.3) and width, depending on the size and shape of the body part to be bandaged. For example, bandages with a width of 7.5 cm (3 inches) are commonly used for the adult leg.

Delegation and Collaboration

The skill of applying an elastic bandage for compression cannot be delegated to a UCP. The nurse assesses the condition of any wound or dressing before applying a bandage. The skill of applying bandages to secure nonsterile dressings can be delegated to a UCP (refer to employer policy). The nurse directs the UCP about the following:

- Modifying the bandage application, such as through the use of special taping
- Reviewing what to observe and report back to the nurse (e.g., patient's indication of pain, numbness, or tingling after application or changes in patient's skin colour or temperature)

Collaborate with the interprofessional health care team (e.g., physiotherapist) to ensure that the patient's extremity has sufficient support and that the elastic bandage is necessary and applied appropriately. Proper use and application is especially important when an elastic bandage is prescribed for an amputated limb (Matthews et al., 2019)

Equipment

- Correct width and number of gauze or elastic bandages
- Clips or adhesive tape
- Clean gloves if wound drainage is present
- Pillow *(optional)*

Continued

Procedural Guideline 40.1 *Applying Gauze and Elastic Bandages—cont'd*

TABLE 40.3

Types of Bandage Turns

Type	Description	Purpose or Use
Circular turn 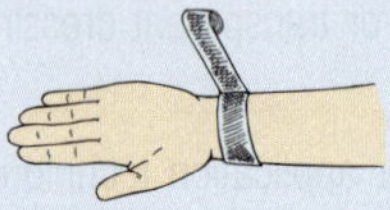	Bandage turn completely overlaps previous turn	Anchors bandage at first and final turn; covers small body part (e.g., finger, toe)
Spiral turn 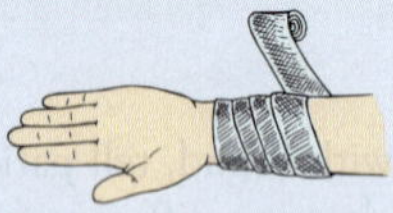	Bandage ascending body part, with each turn overlapping previous one by one-half or two-thirds width of bandage	Covers cylindrical body parts (e.g., wrist, upper arm)
Spiral-reverse turn 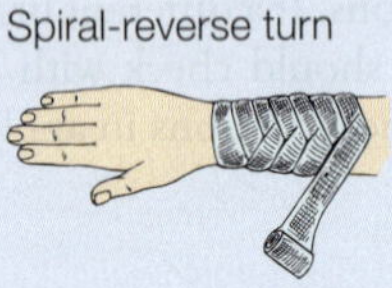	Turn requiring twist (reversal) of bandage halfway through each turn	Covers cone-shaped body parts (e.g., forearm, thigh, calf); useful with nonstretching bandages such as gauze or flannel
Recurrent turn 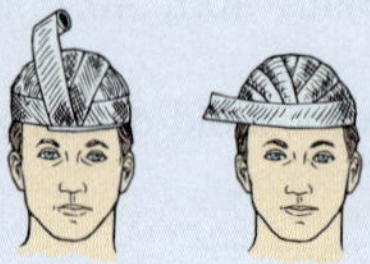	Bandage first secured with two circular turns around proximal end of body part; half turn made perpendicular up from bandage edge; body of bandage brought over distal end of body part to be covered, with each turn folded back over on itself	Covers uneven body parts (e.g., head or stump)

Procedural Steps

1. Identify patient using at least two person-specific identifiers (e.g., name and date of birth, or name and medical record number) according to employer policy.
2. Throughout the procedure, the 4 moments for hand hygiene are to be implemented; hand hygiene should occur before initial patient (or patient environment) contact, before an aseptic procedure, after body fluid exposure risk, and after patient (or patient environment) contact. Additional hand hygiene should be performed when hands are visibly soiled.
3. Review patient's medical record for specific prescriptions related to application of gauze or elastic bandage. Note area to be covered, type of bandage required, frequency of change, and previous response to treatment.
4. Assess patient's level of comfort using an appropriate pain rating scale. If necessary, administer prescribed analgesic 30 minutes before dressing change.
5. Observe adequacy of circulation by palpating temperature of skin and pulses, presence of edema, and sensation (distal to area to be bandaged). Observe skin colour and movement of body part to be wrapped. NOTE: Impaired circulation may result in pain, coolness to touch when compared with the opposite side of the body, cyanosis or pallor of skin, diminished or absent pulses, edema or localized pooling, and numbness and/or tingling of body part.
6. Apply clean gloves (if drainage or a break in skin is present). Inspect skin of area to be bandaged for alterations in integrity as indicated by presence of abrasion, discoloration, or chafing. Pay close attention to areas over bony prominences.
7. Inspect the condition of any wound for appearance, size, and presence and character of drainage, and be sure the wound it is covered with a proper dressing. If not, reapply dressing (check employer policy for type of gloves to use). Remove gloves and discard.
8. Assess for size of bandage:
   a. *Gauze or basic elastic bandage to secure a dressing:* Assess size of area to be covered. Each successive roll of gauze or elastic should overlap the previous layer. Use smaller widths for upper extremities, larger widths for lower extremities.
   b. *Elastic bandage to provide simple compression:* Assess circumference of lower extremity before or shortly after patient gets out of bed in the morning or after patient has been in bed for at least 15 minutes. Select width that will cover and overlap without bulkiness.
9. Identify patient's and caregiver's present knowledge level and their ability to manipulate the bandage if bandaging will be continued at home.
10. Close room door or curtains. Position patient comfortably in an anatomically correct supine position in bed.
11. Apply clean gloves if drainage is present.
12. Apply gauze or elastic bandage to secure dressings:
    a. Elevate dependent extremity for 15 minutes before applying elastic bandage to promote venous return.
    b. Make sure that primary dressing over wound is securely in place.
    c. Begin elastic bandage application at the distal end of the body part. Hold the roll of bandage in your dominant hand and use the other hand to lightly hold the beginning layer.
    d. Apply even tension during application and begin with two circular turns to anchor the bandage. Continue to maintain even tension, and transfer the roll to your dominant hand as you wrap the bandage (see Step 11d illustration).

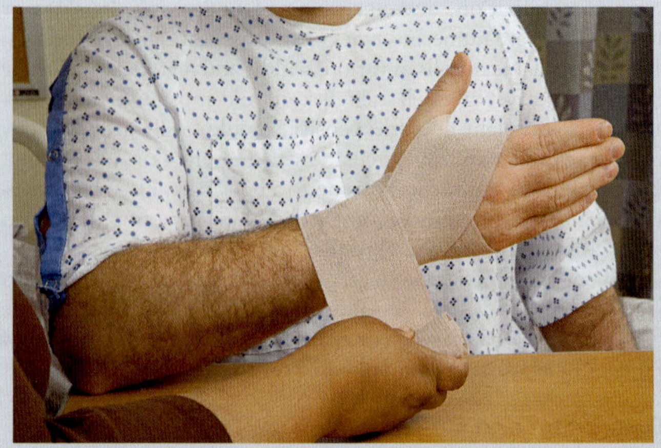

STEP 11D Hold elastic bandage in dominant hand and apply using circular turns.

Procedural Guideline 40.1 *Applying Gauze and Elastic Bandages—cont'd*

e. Apply bandage from distal point toward proximal boundary (see Step 11e illustration), using appropriate turns to cover various shapes of body parts (see Table 40.3). Roll gauze, overlapping each layer by one-half to two-thirds the width of the bandage.

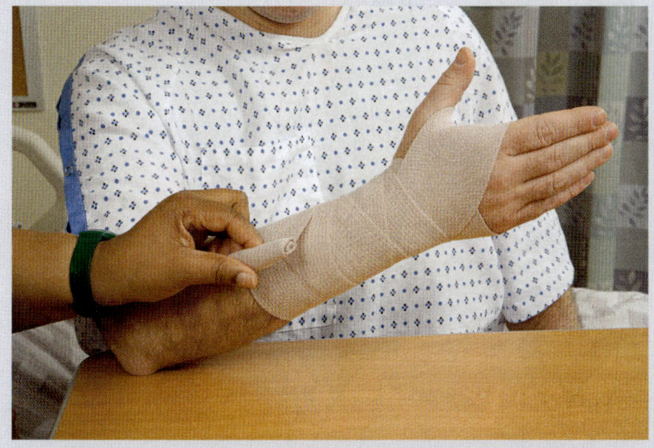

STEP 11E Apply bandage from distal to proximal area.

f. Double check tension and ensure that the bandage is snug but not tight and that the primary dressing or splint is positioned correctly. A tight bandage may cause numbness and tingling from impaired circulation or pressure on peripheral nerves.

g. While unrolling an elastic bandage, stretch the bandage slightly. Explain to the patient that smooth, even pressure will be applied to improve circulation, reduce swelling, immobilize the body part, and provide pressure.

h. End bandage with two circular turns; secure end of gauze or elastic bandage to outside layer of bandage, not skin, with tape or clips (see Step 11h illustration).

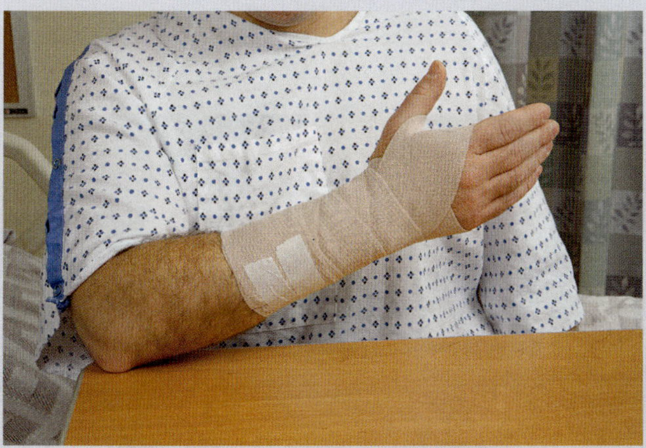

STEP 11H Secure with tape or closure device.

Critical Decision Point *Keep toes or fingertips uncovered and visible for follow-up circulatory assessment, except in cases in which toes or fingers are treated because of wounds.*

13. Apply elastic bandage over stump (see Step 13 illustrations):
    a. Elevate stump with a pillow or support it with the help of another person.
    b. Secure bandage by wrapping it twice around the proximal end of the stump or person's waist (depending on size of stump).
    c. Make a half turn with bandage perpendicular to its edge.
    d. Bring body of bandage over distal end of stump.
    e. Continue to fold bandage over stump, wrapping from distal to proximal points.
    f. Secure with metal clips, Velcro if provided, or tape.
14. Remove gloves, if worn, and discard.
15. Assess degree of tightness of bandage, wrinkles, looseness, and presence of drainage.
16. Evaluate distal circulation when bandage application is complete, at least twice during next 8 hours, and then at least every shift.
    a. Observe skin colour for pallor or cyanosis.
    b. Palpate skin for warmth.
    c. Palpate distal pulses and compare bilaterally.
    d. Ask patient to rate pain using an appropriate pain rating scale and to describe any numbness, tingling, or other discomfort in order to evaluate for neurological and vascular changes.
17. Observe mobility of extremity.
18. **Use teach-back:** "I want to be sure I explained how to apply the elastic roll to your sprained ankle. Show me how you would apply this elastic roll to your ankle." Develop a revised teaching plan if patient or caregiver is unable to teach back correctly.
19. Record patient's level of comfort, circulation status, type of bandage applied, presence of swelling, and range of motion at baseline and after bandage application on flow sheet in progress notes in EHR or chart.
20. Report any changes in neurological or circulatory status to health care provider.

Continued

Procedural Guideline 40.1 *Applying Gauze and Elastic Bandages—cont'd*

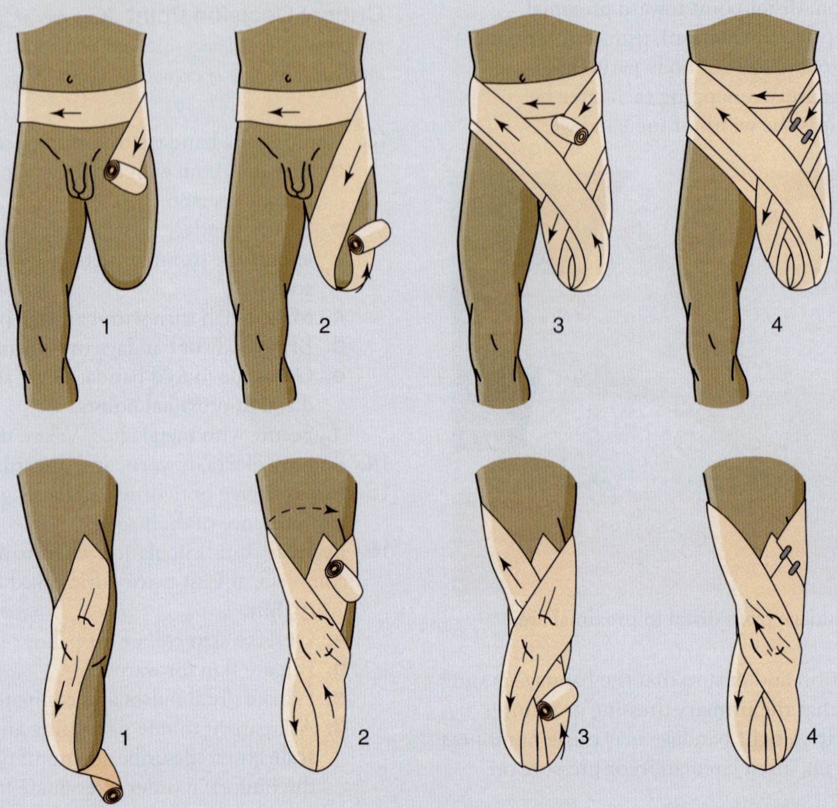

STEP 13 Top, Correct method for bandaging midthigh amputation stump. Note that bandage must be anchored around patient's waist. Bottom, Correct method for bandaging midcalf amputation stump. Note that bandage need not be anchored around waist.

(From Monahan, F., Sands, J. K., Neighbors, M., et al. [Eds.]. [2007]. Phipps' medical-surgical nursing: Health and illness perspectives [8th ed.]. Mosby.)

Procedural Guideline 40.2 *Applying an Abdominal Binder*

Binders are bandages made of large pieces of material specially designed to fit a specific body part. Most binders are made of elastic or cotton. The most common type is the abdominal binder. Breast binders are not used as often in current practice because sports bras are preferred for breast support following certain surgeries.

An abdominal binder supports large abdominal incisions that are vulnerable to tension or stress as a patient moves or coughs (Fig. 40.2). The binder also lessens pain in postoperative patients. In addition, abdominal binders provide a noninvasive intervention for enhancing recovery of walk performance, controlling pain, and improving the patient's experience following major abdominal surgery (Saeed et al., 2019). Binders support underlying muscles and large incisions, lessening muscle stress, which helps a patient move more freely without additional discomfort.

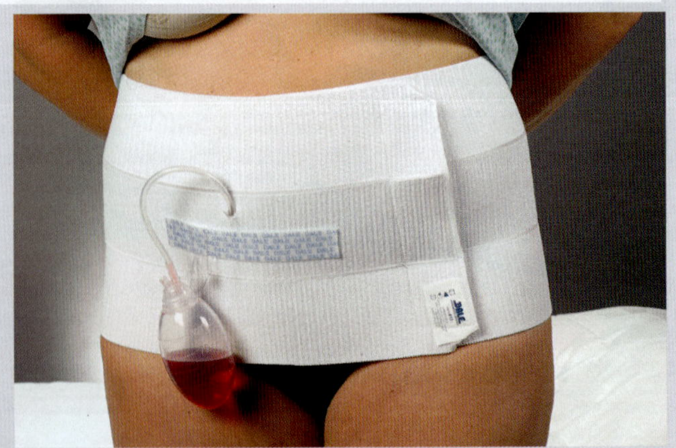

FIG 40.2 **Abdominal binder with Velcro closures.** *(Courtesy Dale Medical Products, Plainville, MA.)*

Procedural Guideline 40.2 *Applying an Abdominal Binder—cont'd*

Delegation and Collaboration

The skill of applying a binder may be delegated to a UCP, depending on employer policy. The nurse is responsible for assessing the condition of any incision, the skin, and the patient's ability to breathe before binder application. The nurse instructs the UCP about the following:

- How to modify the skill, such as using special wrapping or the manner of securing the binder
- Reporting patient's indication of pain, numbness, tingling, or difficulty breathing after the abdominal binder has been applied or any changes in the patient's skin colour or temperature

Equipment

- Clean gloves if wound drainage is present
- Gauze bandage, as needed
- Correct type and size of binder
- Closures for cloth binder

Procedural Steps

1. Identify patient using at least two person-specific identifiers (e.g., name and date of birth, or name and medical record number) according to employer policy.
2. Throughout the procedure, the 4 moments for hand hygiene are to be implemented; hand hygiene should occur before initial patient (or patient environment) contact, before an aseptic procedure, after body fluid exposure risk, and after patient (or patient environment) contact. Additional hand hygiene should be performed when hands are visibly soiled.
3. Review medical record for prescription for binder (check employer policy).
4. Observe patient who needs support of thorax or abdomen; observe their ability to breathe deeply, cough effectively, and turn or move independently.
5. Inspect skin for actual or potential alterations in integrity. Observe for irritation, abrasion, and skin surfaces that rub against one another.
6. Inspect any surgical dressing for intactness, presence of drainage, and coverage of incision. Change any soiled dressing before applying binder (using clean gloves).
7. Determine patient's comfort level. Ask patient to rate pain using an appropriate pain rating scale. Administer prescribed analgesic 30 minutes before dressing change.
8. Gather necessary data regarding size of patient and appropriate binder to use (see manufacturer guidelines) to ensure proper fit.
9. Determine patient's knowledge of the purpose of the binder.
10. Close curtains or room door.
11. Apply clean gloves (if contact with wound drainage is likely).
12. Apply abdominal binder:
    a. Position patient in supine position with head slightly elevated and knees slightly flexed.
    b. Help patient roll on the side away from you toward raised side rail while they firmly support the abdominal incision and dressing with their hands. Fanfold far side of binder toward midline of binder.
    c. Place binder flat on bed, right side up. Fanfold far side of binder toward midline of binder so patient can roll over with minimal effort.
    d. Place fanfolded ends of binder under patient.
    e. Instruct patient (or help them) to roll over folded binder. For overweight patients, consider asking a nurse colleague to help.
    f. Unfold and stretch ends out smoothly on far side of bed. Then stretch out ends on near side of bed.
    g. Instruct patient to roll back into supine position.
    h. Adjust binder so supine patient is centred over binder, using symphysis pubis and costal margins as lower and upper landmarks.
    i. If patient is very thin, pad iliac prominences with gauze bandage.
    j. Close binder. Pull one end of binder over centre of patient's abdomen. While maintaining tension on that end of the binder, pull the opposite end of the binder over the centre and secure with Velcro closure tabs or metal fasteners. This method provides continuous wound support and comfort.

Critical Decision Point *After binder is in place, assess patient's ability to breathe deeply and cough effectively. When applied correctly, an abdominal binder over midline abdominal incisions should not have any effect on the patient's pulmonary function.*

13. Assess patient's comfort level and adjust binder as necessary.
14. Remove gloves and discard.
15. Ask patient to rate pain using an appropriate pain rating scale.
16. Remove binder and surgical dressing to assess skin and wound characteristics at least every 8 hours.
17. Evaluate patient's ability to ventilate properly, including deep breathing and coughing, every 4 hours to determine presence of impaired ventilation and potential pulmonary complications.
18. Document condition of skin, circulation, integrity of underlying dressing, and patient's comfort level at baseline and after application of binder in progress notes in EHR or chart. Also record type of bandage applied.
19. Report any complications (e.g., pain, skin irritation, impaired ventilation) to the nurse in charge.
20. Report reduced ventilation (e.g., pulse oximetry, pulmonary function tests) to health care provider immediately.

✦ REVIEW QUESTIONS

A 75-year-old patient (he/him) is postoperative day 2 after having an exploratory laparotomy with a total gastrectomy for gastric cancer. The patient has developed a fever of 38.5°C (101.3°F). There was purulent drainage coming from his midline incision and surrounding erythema. The patient rates their pain at a 6 out of 10 and has not received any pain medication in the past 4 hours. Temperature is 38.5°C (101.3°F), blood pressure (BP) is 130/80 mm Hg, pulse is 95 beats/min, respirations (RR) are 20 breaths/min, and oxygen saturation (SaO_2) is 96%. Approximately 5 cm (2 inches) of the incision was opened at bedside by the removal of 10 staples.

Review Questions 1 to 3 relate to the case study presented here.

1. Based on the type of wound and amount of wound drainage, which type of dressing would be appropriate for this patient?
2. On assessing the patient on postoperative day 3, you notice a large amount of bright red blood coming from the base of the open wound. How should you proceed, and which type of dressing should be chosen?
3. Using SBAR (situation–background–assessment–recommendation), show how would you communicate with the health care team about this patient.
4. Of the following dressings, which are the most appropriate for a shallow wound with minimal exudate? (*Select all that apply.*)
   1. Nonadherent gauze dressing
   2. Calcium alginate dressing
   3. Hydrogel dressing
   4. Transparent film dressing
   5. Hydrocolloid dressing
5. Match each type of wound drainage (left column) with the correct definition (right column).

Serous	1. Yellow, green, or brown drainage
Serosanguineous	2. Indicates fresh bleeding, bright red
Sanguineous	3. Pale, red, more watery drainage
Purulent	4. Clear, watery plasma

6. Which of the following steps are necessary to prepare the patient for a dressing change on an open abdominal wound? (*Select all that apply.*)
   1. Assessing size, location, and condition of wound
   2. Explaining procedure to the patient
   3. Reviewing all blood results
   4. Asking the patient to rate their pain level
   5. Assessing the patient about allergies

Visit the Evolve site for a complete list of answers to the Review Questions.

✦ NEXT GENERATION NCLEX® (NGN)

For practice with answering exam questions related to unfolding NGN case studies, please consult the Next Generation NCLEX® (NGN)-Style Case Studies for Skills and Techniques on the Evolve website: http://evolve.elsevier.com/Canada/Perry/clinicalskills/

REFERENCES

Accreditation Canada. (2020). *Required organizational practices–2020 handbook*. https://physicians.nshealth.ca/resources/required-organizational-practices-2020-handbook

Alshahrani, B., Sim, J., & Middleton, R. (2021). Nursing interventions for pressure injury prevention among critically ill patients: A systematic review. *Journal of Clinical Nursing*, *30*(15–16), 2151–2168. https://doi.org/10.1111/jocn.15709

Alves, P. J., Barreto, R. T., Barrois, B. M., et al. (2021). Update on the role of antiseptics in the management of chronic wounds with critical colonisation and/or biofilm. *International Wound Journal*, *18*(3), 342–358. https://doi.org/10.1111/iwj.13537

Baron, J. M., Glatz, M., & Proksch, E. (2020). Optimal support of wound healing: New insights. *Dermatology*, *236*(6), 593–600. https://doi.org/10.1159/000505291

Boles, J. (2018). The powerful practice of distraction. *Pediatric Nursing*, *44*(5), 247–251. https://www.pemcrew.com/uploads/1/2/5/9/125977418/the_powerful_practice_of_distraction.pdf

Boscart, V., McCleary, L., Sheiban Taucar, L., et al. (Eds.). (2023). *Ebersole and Hess' gerontological nursing and health aging in Canada* (3rd ed.) Elsevier.

Brace, J. A. (2024). Wound debridement. In R. A. Bryant, & D. P. Nix (Eds.), *Acute and chronic wounds: Intraprofessionals from novice to expert* (6th ed., pp. 430–440). Elsevier Inc.

Brown, A. (2018). When is wound cleansing necessary and what solution should be used? *Nursing Times*, *114*(9), 42–45. https://www.nursingtimes.net/clinical-archive/tissue-viability/when-is-wound-cleansing-necessary-and-what-solution-should-be-used-20-08-2018/

Bryant, R. A., & Borchert, K. (2024). Draining wounds and fistulas. In R. A. Bryant, & D. P. Nix (Eds.), *Acute and chronic wounds: Intraprofessionals from novice to expert* (6th ed., pp. 709–731). Elsevier Inc.

Bryant, R. A., & Nix, D. P. (2024). Principles of wound healing and topical management. In R. A. Bryant, & D. P. Nix (Eds.), *Acute and chronic wounds: Intraprofessionals from novice to expert* (6th ed., pp. 441–457). Elsevier Inc.

David, J. A., & Chiu, E. S. (2018). Surgical debridement. In D. Orgill (Ed.), *Interventional treatment of wounds* (pp. 3–15). Springer International.

Dilley, J. R., Vlad, L. G., & Molnar, J. A. (2024). Skin care needs of the patient with obesity. In R. A. Bryant, & D. P. Nix (Eds.), *Acute and chronic wounds: Intraprofessionals from novice to expert* (6th ed., pp. 665–676). Elsevier Inc.

Ermer-Seltun, J. M., & Rolstad, B. S. (2022). General principles of topical therapy. In D. B. Doughty, & L. L. McNichol (Eds.), *Wound, ostomy, and continence nurses society core curriculum: Wound management* (2nd ed., pp. 136–156). Wolters Kluwer.

European Pressure Ulcer Advisory Panel, National Pressure Injury Advisory Panel, & Pan Pacific Pressure Injury Alliance. (2019). *Treatment of pressure ulcers/injuries: Quick reference guide* (3rd ed.). https://guidelinesales.com/store/ViewProduct.aspx?id=15037164

Foltynski, P., Ciechanowska, A., & Ladyzynski, P. (2021). Wound surface area measurement. *Biocybernetics and Biomedical Engineering*, *41*(4), 1454–1465. https://doi.org/10.1016/j.bbe.2021.04.011

Gmur, M. K., & Karpiński, T. M. (2020). Povidone-iodine in wound healing and prevention of wound infections. *European Journal of Biological Research*, *10*(3), 232–239. https://doi.org/10.5281/ZENODO.3958220

Harris, C. L., Kuhnke, J., Haley, J., et al. (2017/2021). Best practice recommendations for prevention and management of surgical wound complications. In *Foundations of best practice for skin and wound management: A supplement of Wound Care Canada*. Wounds Canada. https://www.woundscanada.ca/docman/public/health-care-professional/bpr-workshop/555-bpr-prevention-and-management-of-surgical-wound-complications-v2/file

Healthcare Excellence Canada. (n.d.). *Pressure ulcer: Introduction*. https://www.healthcareexcellence.ca/en/what-we-do/all-programs/hospital-harm-is-everyones-concern/hospital-harm-improvement-resource/pressure-ulcer-introduction/

Hockenberry, M. J., Duffy, E. A., & Gibbs, K. (2024). *Wong's nursing care of infants and children* (12th ed.). Elsevier.

Kelly-O'Flynn, S., Mohamud, L., & Copson, D. (2020). Medical adhesive-related skin injury. *British Journal of Nursing*, *29*(6), S20–S26. https://doi.org/10.12968/bjon.2020.29.6.S20

Kordestani, S. (2019). *Atlas of wound healing. A tissue regeneration approach*. Elsevier.

Lichterfeld-Kottner, A., Vogt, A., Tomova-Simitchieva, T., et al. (2021). Effects of loading and prophylactic dressings on the sacral and heel skin: An exploratory cross–over trial. *International Wound Journal*, *18*(6), 909–922. https://doi.org/10.1111/iwj.13596

Mahoney, K. (2020). Part 2: Wound cleansing and debridement. *Journal of Community Nursing*, *34*(3).

Manna, B., Nahirniak, P., & Morrison, C.A. (2023). Wound debridement. *StatPearls [Internet]*. https://www.ncbi.nlm.nih.gov/books/NBK507882/

Matthews, C. N., Chen, A. F., Daryoush, T., et al. (2019). Does an elastic compression bandage provide any benefit after primary TKA? *Clinical Orthopaedics and Related Research*, *477*(1), 134–144. https://doi.org/10.1097/CORR.0000000000000459

Oropallo, A., & Quraishi, W. (2024). Wound pain. In R. A. Bryant, & D. P. Nix (Eds.), *Acute and chronic wounds: Intraprofessionals from novice to expert* (6th ed., pp. 536–546). Elsevier Inc.

Orsted, H. L., Keast, D. H., Forest-Lalande, L., et al. (2017/2021). Best practice recommendations for the prevention and management of wounds. In *Foundations of best practice for skin and wound management: A supplement of Wound Care Canada*. Wounds Canada. https://www.woundscanada.ca/docman/public/health-care-professional/bpr-workshop/165-wc-bpr-prevention-and-management-of-wounds/file

Piemonte, G., Benelli, L., Braschi, F., et al. (2019). The local treatment: Methodology, debridement, and wound bed preparation. In M. Matucci-Cerinic, & C. P. Denton (Eds.), *Atlas of ulcers in systemic sclerosis: Diagnosis and management* (pp. 145–159). Springer.

Robertson, E., Treadgold, C., Parker, B., et al. (2020). Positive distraction for children during burn wound care in Australia–An evaluation of the "Captains on Call" pilot. *Journal of Pediatric Nursing*, *54*, 10–17. https://doi.org/10.1016/j.pedn.2020.05.001

Saeed, S., Rage, K. A., Memon, A. S., et al. (2019). Use of abdominal binders after a major abdominal surgery: A randomized controlled trial. *Cureus*, *11*(10). Article e5832. https://doi.org/10.7759/cureus.5832

Sahyoun, C., Cozzi, G., Leroy, P. L. J. M., et al. (2021). Towards integrated procedural comfort care: Redefining and expanding "non-pharmacology. In K. P. Mason (Ed.), *Pediatric sedation outside of the operating room* (pp. 783–795). Springer.

Sibbald, R. G., Elliott, J. A., Persaud-Jaimangal, R., et al. (2021). Wound bed preparation 2021. *Advances in Skin & Wound Care*, *34*(4), 183–195. https://doi.org/10.1097/01.asw.0000733724.87630.d6

Sillmon, K., Moran, C., Shook, L., et al. (2021). The use of prophylactic foam dressings for prevention of hospital-acquired pressure injuries: A systematic review. *The Journal of Wound, Ostomy and Continence Nursing*, *48*(3), 211–218. https://doi.org/10.1097/WON.0000000000000762

Simon, S., & Hollenbeck, B. (2022). Risk factors for surgical site infections in knee and hip arthroplasty patients. *American Journal of Infection Control*, *50*(2), 214–216. https://doi.org/10.1016/j.ajic.2021.11.006

Tyldesley, H. C., Salisbury, A.-M., Chen, R., et al. (2019). Surfactants and their role in biofilm management in chronic wounds. *Wounds International*, *10*(1), 20–24. https://woundsinternational.com/journal-articles/surfactants-and-their-role-biofilm-management-chronic-wounds/

Weller, C. D., Team, V., & Sussman, G. (2020). First-line interactive wound dressing update: A comprehensive review of the evidence. *Frontiers in Pharmacology*, *11*. Article 155. https://doi.org/10.3389/fphar.2020.00155

World Health Organization. (2018). *Global guidelines for the prevention of surgical site infection* (2nd ed.). https://www.who.int/publications/i/item/global-guidelines-for-the-prevention-of-surgical-site-infection-2nd-ed

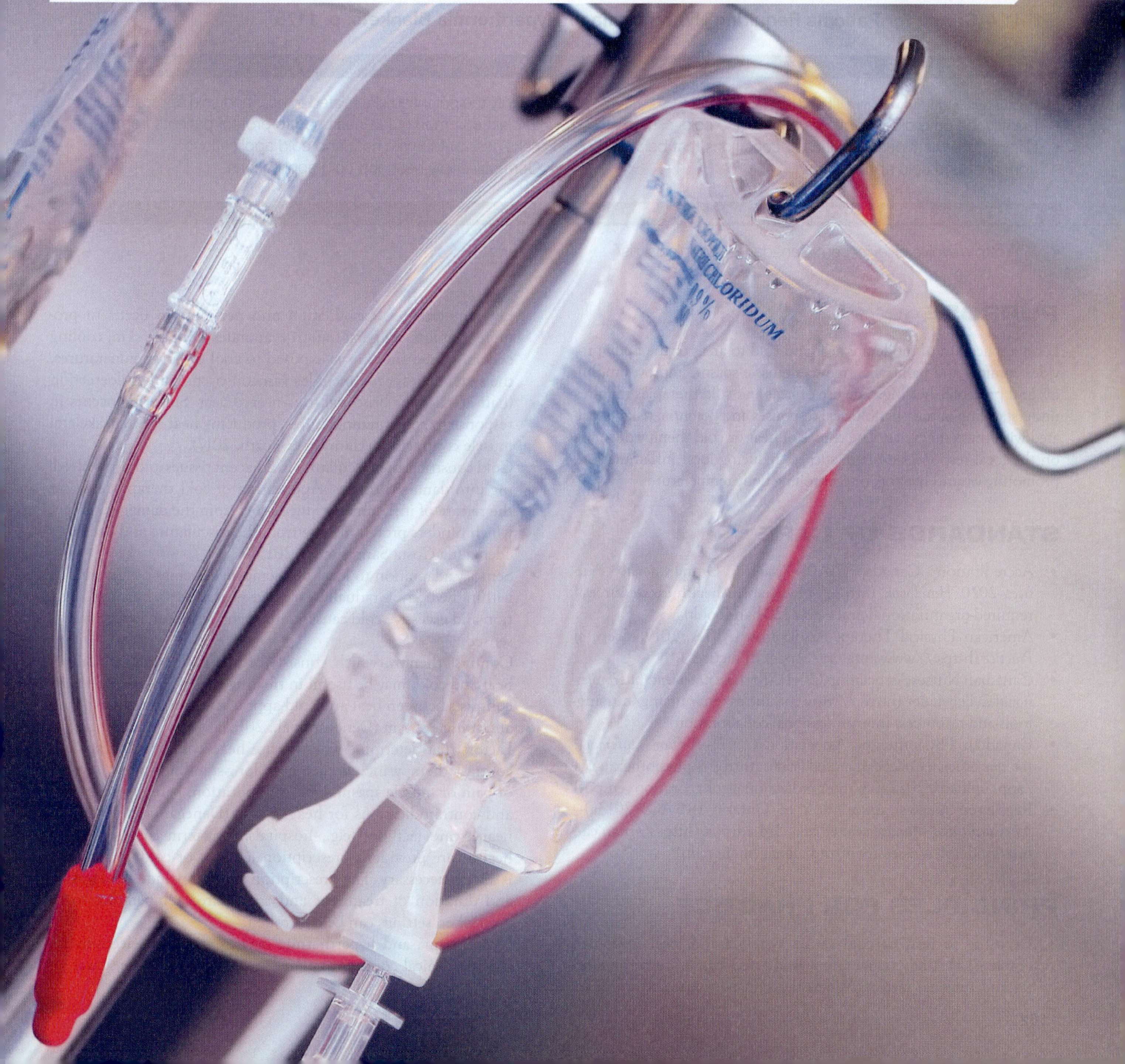

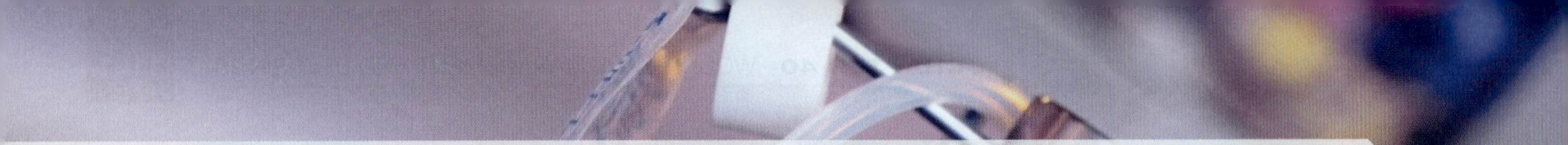

41 Therapeutic Use of Heat and Cold

Canadian content written by **Keri Durocher, RN, MN, PhD(c)**
Original US chapter by **Anne Griffin Perry, RN, MSN, EdD, FAAN**

SKILLS AND PROCEDURES

OBJECTIVES

Mastery of content in this chapter will enable the nurse to:
- Identify the physiological effects of heat and cold.
- Differentiate the types of injuries or conditions that benefit from heat and cold applications.
- Identify the potential risks related to heat and cold applications.
- Explain common guidelines used to protect patients from risks associated with heat and cold applications.
- Correctly apply heat and cold applications.

MEDIA RESOURCES

- http://evolve.elsevier.com/Canada/Perry/clinicalskills/

PURPOSE

Local application of moderate heat and cold to areas of the body provides comfort and pain relief, reduces muscle spasm, improves mobility, and promotes healing. Safe use of heat and cold therapies requires understanding of the physiological responses and potential risks associated with these therapies. The choice of heat or cold therapy depends on the local responses desired, such as reducing local inflammation, promoting wound healing, or controlling body temperature.

STANDARDS OF CARE

- Accreditation Canada (2020)—*Required Organizational Practices—2020 Handbook* (https://physicians.nshealth.ca/resources/required-organizational-practices-2020-handbook)
- American Physical Therapy Association (APTA, 2019)—*Scope of Practice* (https://www.apta.org/ScopeOfPractice/)
- Canadian Nurses Association (2011)—*Position Statement: Interprofessional Collaboration* (https://www.cna-aiic.ca/en/nursing/nursing-tools-and-resources/interprofessional-collaboration)
- Canadian Physiotherapy Association (2012)—*Position Statement: Interprofessional Collaboration and Practice* (https://physiotherapy.ca/app/uploads/2022/08/inter-professional-collaboration_en.pdf)
- Registered Nurses' Association of Ontario (RNAO, 2013a)—*Assessment and Management of Pain*, 3rd edition (https://rnao.ca/bpg/guidelines/assessment-and-management-pain)

PRINCIPLES FOR PRACTICE

- Exposure to heat or cold causes systemic and local responses (Table 41.1). Body temperature is affected by both environmental and internal factors. When the skin is exposed to warm or hot temperatures, vasodilation and perspiration occur to promote heat loss. As perspiration evaporates from the skin, cooling occurs. When the skin is exposed to cool or cold temperatures, the systemic response includes vasoconstriction and piloerection (hair erection or bristling) to conserve heat. Shivering occurs in response to cooler temperatures, producing heat through skeletal muscle contraction (Hannon & Porth, 2017).
- Cold constricts the vasculature in adjacent tissues and slows bleeding into damaged tissues. Application of cold therapy decreases the release of inflammatory mediators from the damaged tissues, which hinders protein release from the vasculature and decreases edema (da Costa Santos et al., 2015).
- Sensory adaptation to local temperature extremes occurs quickly within the body. Gradually, excessive heat causes a burning sensation and excessive cold causes a numbing sensation before pain is sensed.
- Contrast therapy, which consists of alternating applications of heat and cold, may be useful in treating athletic injuries. Sensory contrasts between heat and cold appear effective in reducing pain and muscle spasm (Denegar et al., 2018).
- Factors that determine when to use heat, cold (cryotherapy), or contrast therapy include acute or long-standing injury, severity of pain or muscle spasm, ease of application, patient preference, and contraindications for heat or cold (Denegar et al., 2018). In health care facilities (e.g., hospitals, long-term care settings) a health care provider's prescription for heat or cold applications is always necessary. The prescription should include the location and duration of treatment and the desired temperature to be used when settings can be controlled.
- Hypothermia and hyperthermia devices are used selectively for specific clinical conditions. They are designed to raise, lower, or

TABLE 41.1

Pathophysiological Effects of Heat and Cold Applications

	Cold	Heat
Pain	↓	↓
Spasm	↓	↓
Metabolism	↓	↑
Blood flow	↓	↑
Inflammation	↓	↑
Edema	↓	↑
Joint stiffness	↓	↓

Data from da Costa Santos, V., dos Santos Cardoso, C., Figueiredo, C. P., et al. (2015). Effect of cryotherapy on the ankle temperature in athletes: Ice pack and cold water immersion. *Fisioterapia em Movimento, 28*(1), 23–30; Denegar, C. R., Saliba, E., & Saliba, S. F. (2018). *Therapeutic modalities for musculoskeletal injuries* (4th ed.). Human Kinetics; LeBlanc, K. (2018). Skin integrity and wound care. In B. J. Kozier, G. Erb, A. Berman, et al. (Eds.), *Fundamentals of Canadian nursing: Concepts, process, and practice* (4th Canadian ed., pp. 930–982). Pearson Canada.

maintain body temperature through heat or cold transfer between the device and the patient.

PATIENT-CENTRED CARE

- The meaning and significance of heat and cold therapy may have varied interpretations, depending on a patient's culture (Giger & Haddad, 2020). Therefore, as part of person-centred care, it is important to assess the culture-specific perceptions of heat and cold for each patient and caregiver:
  - Reinforce the purpose of the therapy and identify patient concerns or questions to promote understanding of the purpose and benefits of the therapy.
  - During application of heat or cold therapy, the patient, or their extremities, may be exposed; maintain patient comfort and privacy through the use of additional blankets, privacy curtains, and closed room doors. Some patients may refuse exposure to reduce body temperature.
  - Include family members or professional interpreters to promote acceptance of critical therapies such as hypothermia or ice packs that may contradict a patient's or family's cultural beliefs and practices.
- Inform the patient and caregiver about the rationale for heat and cold as primary or adjuvant therapies. Lack of education about the benefits of heat or cold therapies may contribute to perceptions that pain is being trivialized (RNAO, 2013b).
- Heat or cold may be used with other nonpharmacological measures such as physiotherapy, massage, and other interventions to reduce pain and improve sleep, mood, and general well-being. Nonpharmacological approaches are not intended to replace adequate pharmacological management. Interprofessional collaboration is critical in determining an appropriate treatment plan (RNAO, 2013a).
- Assess the patient's and caregiver's past experiences with heat and cold therapies. Prior experiences will influence preference for heat or cold and willingness to participate in the treatment plan (Denegar et al., 2018; RNAO, 2013a).

EVIDENCE-INFORMED PRACTICE

- The application of ice or cryotherapy is one of the most widely used therapeutic modalities in the management of acute musculoskeletal injuries. Patients who use a numerical rating score for pain have reported decreased pain following application of ice on their neck. Cold therapy reduces the conduction of pain impulses, which occurs when the skin temperature is lowered (da Costa Santos et al., 2015; Denegar et al., 2018).
- Ice compresses applied after scleral buckling eye surgery help reduce swelling and pain in the operative area (Li & Wang, 2016).
- Cold therapy decreases nerve conduction velocity, formation and accumulation of edema, and blood flow to injured tissues. As a result, the physiological effects of cold therapy include reduced inflammation, pain, and edema and better control of bleeding (Benchahong et al., 2021; Hannon & Porth, 2017; Li & Wang, 2016).
- Cold therapy is recommended for treatment of acute injury to reduce inflammation, pain, spasm, and edema. Heat application is recommended for the treatment of long-standing injuries owing to its physiological effects of increased blood flow and tissue temperature (Denegar et al., 2018; Wang et al., 2021).
- Contrast therapy, using an alternating cold-to-heat ratio of 1 minute of cold to 3 (or 4) minutes of heat, effectively treats musculoskeletal injuries by reducing inflammation and edema and improving joint function (Denegar et al., 2018).
- There are varied recommendations about optimal length of time for heat or cold applications (Denegar et al., 2018). Treatment length is determined by the health care provider and adjusted according to individual needs and situation.

SAFETY GUIDELINES

- Use a trauma-informed approach to care when providing heat and cold applications, to improve support of the patient and minimize potential harm.
- Know the patient's risk for injury from heat or cold, as some individuals are more predisposed to injury than others (Table 41.2).
- Exposed layers of skin are more sensitive to temperature variations than intact skin. Therefore, damaged skin should be protected when applying heat or cold therapy.
- Do not microwave towels or medical products used for heat application, as this may provide excessive heat and increase risk of tissue injury.
- Many devices such as heating pads or water-flow pads have thermostats to regulate temperature. Always check the temperature of a heating device or moist compress before applying it directly to the skin.
- Burns and skin injuries sustained from heat or cold therapies are serious reportable events and are preventable. Prompt reporting to the appropriate health team member enables early, appropriate treatment to minimize discomfort and tissue damage.
- It is important to individualize care to meet a patient's needs and preferences. Patient teaching, safety, comfort, and privacy are important when using heat or cold therapies.
- Consider patient age, skin and circulation, vital signs, ability to sense temperature, and ability to communicate before applying heat or cold therapies. Children, older persons, or patients with sensory impairment or peripheral vascular diseases have a greater risk for injury from heat and cold applications (see Table 41.2).
- Heat or cold therapies should be used with caution in patients who have diabetes mellitus, peripheral vascular disease, or any alterations in sensation or pain perceptions. Patients with these conditions also require more frequent skin assessment during treatment. Heat or cold applications should be avoided in areas treated with radiation therapy for at least 5 days after treatment (RNAO, 2013b).

TABLE 41.2

Characteristics of Heat and Cold Application

	Examples of Conditions	Precautions	Adverse Outcomes
Cold application	Immediately after direct trauma such as sprain, strains, fractures, muscle spasms; after superficial lacerations or puncture wounds; minor burns; persistent pain from arthritis, joint trauma; delayed onset muscle soreness; inflammation	Circulatory insufficiency Sensory impairment Radiation therapy Diabetes mellitus	Cardiovascular effects (bradycardia) Nerve and tissue damage Impaired wound healing Frostbite
Heat application	Inflamed or edematous body area; new surgical wound; infected wound; arthritis; degenerative joint disease; localized joint pain, muscle strains; low back pain; menstrual cramps; hemorrhoid, perianal, and vaginal inflammation; local abscess	Pregnancy Laminectomy sites Spinal cord injury Malignancy Vascular insufficiency Radiation therapy Acute injury Extreme caution when using heat or cold therapies with eyes, testes, heart area	Burns Infections Increased pain Increased inflammation Secondary tissue injury

TABLE 41.3

Heat Application: Moist Versus Dry

Type	Advantages	Disadvantages
Moist application	Reduces drying of skin and softens wound exudate	Skin maceration with prolonged exposure
	Conforms well to body area being treated	Cools rapidly because of moisture evaporation
	Penetrates deeply into tissue layers	Increases risk of burns because moisture conducts heat
	Lessens sweating and insensible fluid loss	
Dry application	Less likely to burn skin	Increases insensible fluid loss through sweating
	Does not cause skin maceration	Does not penetrate deep into tissue
	Retains temperature longer because it is not influenced by evaporation	Increases drying of skin

- Cold or contrast therapy cannot be used if patients have Raynaud's phenomenon or cold urticaria (cold allergy) (Denegar et al., 2018; LeBlanc, 2018).
- Heat should not be used for an area that is bleeding, is being treated with products that contain menthol, or has decreased sensation, or within 24 hours after acute injury (LeBlanc, 2018; RNAO, 2013b).
- Dry or moist applications may be used in heat or cold therapies, depending on the expected outcome for the patient. Temperature travels from an external source, such as a compress or a heating pad, to the surface of the skin. A substance that conducts temperatures poorly is a good insulator and thus protects skin and tissues. However, there are distinct advantages to using both dry and moist applications (Table 41.3).
- Extremities or perineal areas have decreased fat and underlying tissue and are more sensitive than other areas to temperature extremes. Modify the intensity of heat and cold when treating sensitive skin areas.
- Check the patient frequently during heat or cold application. The condition of the skin indicates whether tissue injury may be occurring. Observe for signs of excessive redness, maceration, or blistering.
- Inform the patient to not adjust the temperature settings.
- Position the patient so it is possible for them to move away from the temperature source to decrease the risk for injury from temperature exposure. A hospitalized patient should always have a call light within reach.
- Do not leave unattended a patient who is unable to sense temperature changes or move away from the temperature source.
- Be aware of the systemic effects of heat in dilating blood vessels and increasing local blood flow. If vasodilation is significant, the patient's blood pressure may decrease, causing dizziness and increased risk of falls. While heat applications may reduce swelling and transmission of pain impulses, excessive use of heat is a noxious stimulus that may increase pain and tissue damage (Hannon & Porth, 2017).

✦ SKILL 41.1 Application of Moist Heat (Compress and Sitz Bath)

Moist heat is beneficial in increasing muscle and ligament flexibility, promoting relaxation and healing, and relieving muscle spasm. Moist heat applied as a compress may also be beneficial for treating arthritic or sprained joints, strained muscles, back pain, and rheumatoid arthritis and in any treatment where heat is applied to the skin to promote circulation. Factors to consider before application include level of temperature and duration of the heat therapy and the nature of the tissues being treated.

Compresses and commercial packs (Fig. 41.1) are examples of moist heat applications used for a variety of conditions. A warm compress is sterile or clean gauze moistened with a prescribed heated solution (i.e., normal saline or sterile water) that is applied directly to

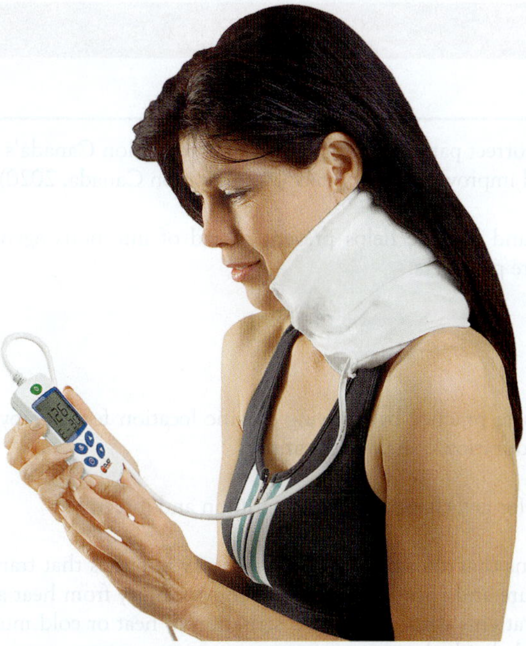

FIG 41.1 **Digital moist heat pack.** *(Image used with permission from Theratherm, Chattanooga, a DJO Company. All rights reserved.)*

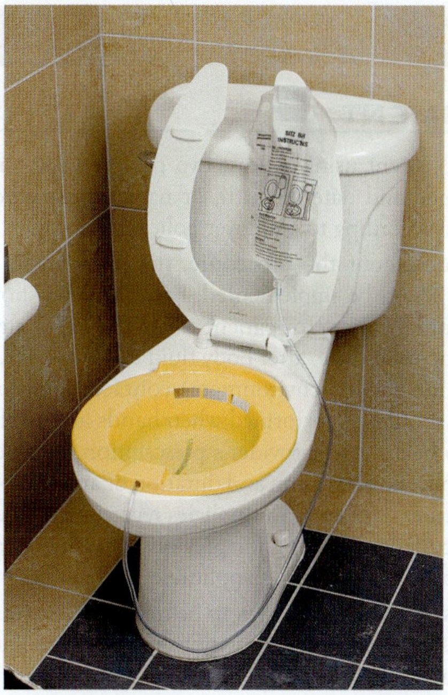

FIG 41.2 **Disposable Sitz bath.** *(Used with permission, Briggs Corporation.)*

an affected area. Commercially packaged sterile, premoistened compresses, available in some facilities, require a special infrared lamp to heat them. Plain sterile or clean gauze is heated by adding the gauze to a container of warmed solution. A commercial heat pack produces its own moisture by drawing moisture from humidity in the air and retaining it in the outer flannel cover of the hot pack.

Moist heat application also includes the use of warm baths, soaks, and Sitz baths. A warm bath or soak involves immersion of a body part in a warmed solution. Warm soaks and Sitz baths promote circulation, reduce edema and inflammation, promote muscle relaxation, debride wounds, and may contain medicated solutions. In particular, a Sitz bath causes localized vasodilation that may result in decreased blood pressure. A body part that is too large to immerse may be soaked by wrapping it in a dressing saturated with the warmed solution.

Sitz baths require a special tub or chair basin that allows a patient to sit in water without immersing the legs, feet, and upper trunk (Fig. 41.2). Sitz basins are disposable and especially easy to use in the home. Portable baths fit easily on top of toilets. Patients who have undergone perineal or rectal surgery, had an episiotomy during childbirth, or have painful hemorrhoids or perineal inflammation benefit from a Sitz bath.

When preparing a soak or bath, remember that the heated solution will be in direct contact with the patient's skin. Assess the patient's skin for excessive redness or blistering after 10 to 15 minutes, and check water temperature frequently to prevent burns. The solution temperature should be kept constant to enhance the therapeutic effects of the moist heat. When adding heated solution to a soak basin or bath, remove the patient's body part and re-immerse it once the solution has mixed and the temperature has been checked.

Delegation and Collaboration

The skill of applying moist heat may be delegated to an unregulated care provider (UCP) (see employer policy). If there are risks or expected complications, the skill cannot be delegated. In most settings, the nurse applies any sterile applications. Explanation of the purpose of the treatment, assessment of the patient's overall condition and the skin and tissues in the area being treated, and evaluation of the patient's response cannot be delegated. Where applicable, the nurse instructs the UCP about the following:

- Proper temperature of the application
- Skin changes to immediately report to the nurse (e.g., burning, blistering, or excessive redness)
- Specific patient concerns and changes in vital signs to immediately report to the nurse (e.g., pain, dizziness or light-headedness, increased or decreased pulse, decreased blood pressure)
- Specific positioning and application time requirements based on employer policy and manufacturer instructions
- Reporting when treatment is completed to allow the nurse to evaluate patient's response

Equipment

All Moist Heat Applications

- Prescribed analgesia (if prescribed)
- Dry bath towel, bath blanket
- Prescribed solution (i.e., heated normal saline) or commercially prepared compresses or commercial heat pack
- Biohazard waste bag
- Clean gloves
- Compress
- Clean basin
- Waterproof pad
- Ties or cloth tape
- Clean gauze or towel
- Moist heat application options according to the health care provider's prescription:
  - Sterile compress: sterile basin, sterile gauze, and sterile gloves
  - Aquathermia pad
  - Disposable Sitz bath: prescribed solution and any topical medication to be applied after the soak

STEP	RATIONALE

ASSESSMENT

STEP	RATIONALE
1. Identify patient using at least two person-specific identifiers (e.g., name and date of birth, or name and medical record number) according to employer policy.	Ensures correct patient. Complies with Accreditation Canada's standards and improves patient safety (Accreditation Canada, 2020).
2. Throughout the procedure, the 4 moments for hand hygiene are to be implemented; hand hygiene should occur before initial patient (or patient environment) contact, before an aseptic procedure, after body fluid exposure risk, and after patient (or patient environment) contact. Additional hand hygiene should be performed when hands are visibly soiled.	Proper hand hygiene helps prevent spread of infectious agents to health care providers.
3. Refer to health care provider's prescription for type of moist heat application, location and duration of application, desired temperature, and employer policies regarding temperature.	Ensures safe practice by verifying specific location for therapy and type and duration of heat application.
4. Check patient's charting for previous assessments and dressing change information as applicable.	To assess for any changes in skin condition and integrity.
5. Assess skin around area to be treated. Perform neurovascular assessments for sensitivity to temperature and pain by measuring light touch, pinprick, and temperature sensation (see Chapter 8).	Conditions that alter conduction of sensory impulses that transmit temperature and pain predispose patients to injury from heat applications. Patients with diminished sensation to heat or cold must be monitored closely during treatment.

Critical Decision Point *Patients living with diabetes mellitus, vascular diseases, paralysis, rheumatoid arthritis, peripheral neuropathy, or other alterations in sensation or pain perceptions, as well as those using certain cardiovascular medications, are at greater risk for thermal injury.*

STEP	RATIONALE
6. Refer to patient's medical record to identify any contraindications to moist heat application: unstable cardiac conditions, active bleeding, therapeutic medicinal patch, acute inflammatory reactions, recent musculoskeletal injury or radiation therapy, and skin conditions such as eczema.	Patients with certain cardiovascular conditions and who exhibit adverse effects of certain medications such as cardiac, hypertensive, and vasoactive medications may be at risk for sudden changes in blood pressure and blood flow caused by vasodilation. Heat causes vasodilation, which aggravates active bleeding and can in turn increase hemorrhage or bleeding into soft tissues adjacent to the musculoskeletal injury (LeBlanc, 2018). Vasodilation increases the rate of medication absorption when direct heat is applied over the medication patch.
7. Assess patient's level of consciousness and responsiveness (e.g., confusion, disorientation, dementia).	Patients with altered level of consciousness are unable to sense or report reduced sensation of discomfort and will require close supervision during therapy.
8. Assess patient's mobility: ability to position self for soak application, position self in bath, and sit up from bath.	Determines level of help needed to position patient for treatment.
9. When applying moist heat, apply clean gloves and assess the wound for size, colour, drainage volume, pain (use a pain assessment method appropriate for the patient's age, culture, or cognitive state) (RNAO, 2013a), and odour (this may be deferred until dressing is removed [see Step 5c in Implementation] and heat is applied). Remove and discard gloves.	Reduces transmission of microorganisms. Provides baseline to determine change in wound following heat application. Provides baseline for patient's comfort level.
10. Assess patient's blood pressure and pulse.	Establishes baseline to determine response to therapy.
11. Assess patient's range of motion of affected area if being treated for muscle sprain.	Provides baseline to determine whether range of motion improves following therapy.
12. Assess patient's and caregiver's understanding of application and related safety factors.	Determines need for health teaching.

NURSING DIAGNOSES

- Acute pain
- Persistent pain
- Inadequate peripheral tissue perfusion
- Insufficient knowledge regarding heat therapy
- Reduced physical mobility
- Reduced skin integrity
- Potential for injury

Related factors and risk factors are individualized on the basis of patient's condition or needs.

STEP	RATIONALE

PLANNING

STEP	RATIONALE
1. Expected outcomes following completion of procedure:	
• Affected area is pink and warm to touch immediately after heat application.	Vasodilation increases blood flow to site.
• After multiple applications, wound shows signs of healing (e.g., tissue granulation; reduced edema, inflammation, drainage).	Moist heat increases blood flow, enhances white blood cell infiltration, and removes waste products from cells (da Costa Santos et al., 2015).
• Patient denies burning sensation.	Indicates temperature applied appropriately.

Critical Decision Point *Once the therapeutic effect time has been exceeded for heat application, vasoconstriction can result* (Karadağ et al., 2019).

STEP	RATIONALE
• Patient reports increased mobility and decreased pain in affected region.	Heat reduces edema and inflammation and relaxes stiff and strained muscles. Heat used in conjunction with physical therapy, exercise, or both improves function and mobility (da Costa Santos et al., 2015; Denegar et al., 2018).
• Blood pressure and pulse are within patient's normal range.	No systemic vascular changes occur. Goal of therapy is to achieve localized vascular response.
• Patient or caregiver demonstrates how to apply therapy safely.	Measures level of understanding necessary for care in the community.
2. Assemble and prepare equipment and supplies.	Organization of supplies prevents unnecessary delays in procedure.
3. Explain steps of procedure and purpose to patient. Describe expected sensations such as warmth and wetness. Explain precautions to prevent burning.	Minimizes anxiety and promotes cooperation during procedure.

IMPLEMENTATION

STEP	RATIONALE
1. Close room door and close bedside curtains.	Decreases drafts, thus decreasing transmission of microorganisms. Provides privacy.
2. Apply clean gloves.	Reduces transmission of microorganisms.
3. Position patient in bed, keeping affected body part in proper alignment. Expose area of body where heat will be applied, and drape patient with bath blanket or towel as needed.	Limited mobility in an uncomfortable position causes muscular stress. Draping prevents cooling and maintains privacy.
4. Place waterproof pad under patient (not required with Sitz bath or commercial heat pad).	Protects bed linen from moisture and soiling.
5. Apply moist clean or sterile compress:	
a. Heat prescribed solution to desired temperature by immersing closed bottle of solution in a basin of warm water.	Prevents burns by ensuring proper temperature of solution.
b. Prepare aquathermia pad if needed. Temperature is usually preset by manufacturer or bioengineering.	Prevents burning by using proper temperature.
c. Remove any existing dressing covering the wound. Inspect the wound and surrounding skin.	Reduces transmission of microorganisms. Provides baseline to measure wound healing.

Critical Decision Point *An inflamed wound appears reddened, but the surrounding skin is less red in colour. If skin surrounding the wound is inflamed or reddened or has active bleeding or drainage, moist heat application may be contraindicated. Verify with health care provider.*

STEP	RATIONALE
d. Dispose of gloves and dressing in appropriate receptacle.	Reduces transmission of microorganisms.
e. Prepare compress with appropriate aseptic or sterile technique.	A sterile compress is needed when applied to open wound.
(1) Pour warmed solution into container. If sterile asepsis is required, use sterile technique to open sterile gauze and add it to warmed sterile solution (see Chapter 6).	A sterile compress is needed when applied to an open wound.
(2) If using a commercially prepared compress, follow manufacturer instructions for warming.	Prevents injury associated with procedure.

Critical Decision Point *To avoid injury to a patient, test the temperature of sterile solution by applying a drop to your forearm (without contaminating solution). It should feel warm to the skin without burning.*

IMPLEMENTATION

STEP	RATIONALE
f. Apply clean gloves, or if sterile asepsis is needed, apply sterile gloves.	Reduces transmission of microorganisms. Allows manipulation of sterile dressing and touching an open wound.
g. Pick up one layer of immersed gauze, wring out excess solution, and apply lightly to wound; avoid surrounding unaffected skin. *Option:* Apply commercial compress or heat pack over wound only; use only with clean wounds.	Excess moisture macerates skin and increases risk of burns and infection. Skin is sensitive to a sudden change in temperature.
h. After a few seconds, lift edge of gauze to assess for redness.	Increased redness indicates burn.
i. If patient tolerates compress, pack gauze snugly against wound. Ensure all wound surfaces are covered with the warm compress.	Packing the compress prevents rapid cooling from ambient air currents.
j. Cover moist compress with dry sterile dressing (Fig. 41.3) and towel. If necessary, pin or tie in place. Remove and dispose of gloves.	Dry sterile dressing prevents transfer of microorganisms to wound via capillary action caused by moist compress. Towel insulates compress to prevent heat loss.
k. *Option:* When using a gauze compress, apply aquathermia (Fig. 41.4), a commercial heat pack, or waterproof heating pad (see Skill 41.2) over the towel. Keep it in place for the desired duration of application.	Provides constant temperature to compress.
l. Leave compress in place for 20 minutes or per health care provider's prescription or employer policy. If aquathermia pad or commercial heat pack is *not* used, change warm compress using sterile technique every 5–10 minutes or as prescribed for duration of therapy.	Maintains constant temperature for best therapeutic benefit. Moist heat promotes transfer of heat to underlying subcutaneous tissues, which helps reduce thermal injury to skin. Rebound phenomenon, in which the opposite effect begins, occurs after maximum therapeutic effect is achieved. Maximum vasodilation from heat occurs in 20–30 minutes (LeBlanc, 2018).
m. After prescribed time, apply clean gloves. Remove pad, towel, and compress. Evaluate wound and skin and replace dry sterile dressing (using sterile gloves) as prescribed.	Continued exposure to moisture macerates skin. Prevents entrance of microorganisms into wound site.
n. Assist patient to preferred position.	Maintains patient's comfort.
o. Dispose of equipment and soiled compress.	Reduces transmission of microorganisms.
6. Prepare Sitz bath or warm soak to intact skin or wound:	
a. Remove any existing dressing covering the wound. Inspect the wound and surrounding skin. Dispose of gloves and dressing in appropriate receptacle.	Provides baseline to determine response to warm soak. Reduces transmission of microorganisms.

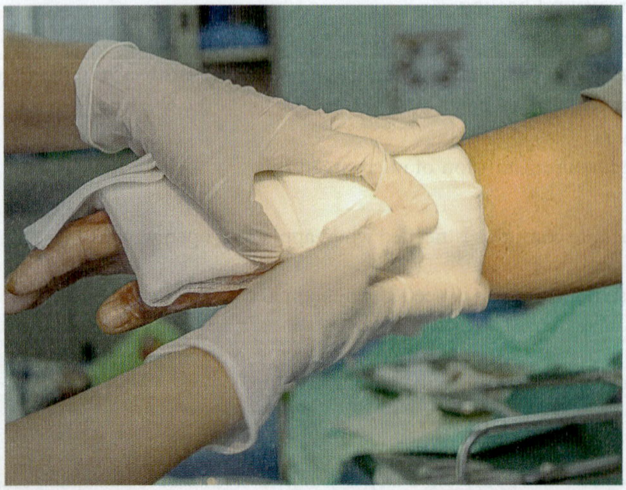

FIG 41.3 Wet to dry dressing. (*From Sonas Home Health Care. [2018]. How to change a wound dressing. https://www.sonashomehealth.com/how-to-change-wound-dressing/*)

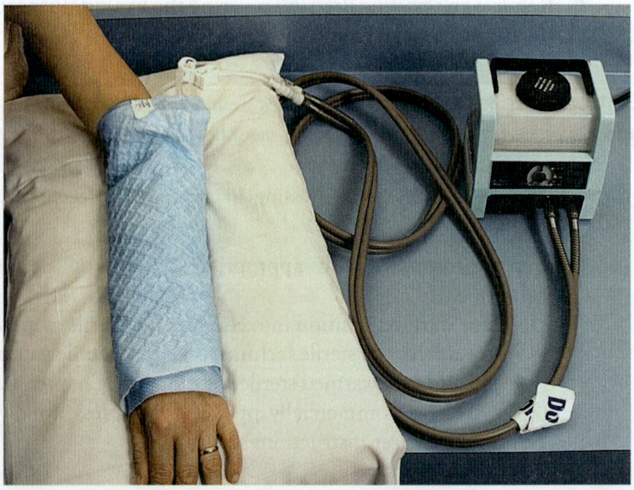

FIG 41.4 Aquathermia heating unit. (*Biology Forums. [2017]. Aquamatic pad and heating unit provide dry heat treatment to a patient's arm. https://biology-forums.com/index.php?action=gallery;sa=view;id=27068. Reprinted with permission.*)

STEP	RATIONALE
IMPLEMENTATION	
b. When exudate or drainage is present, apply new clean gloves and cleanse intact skin around open area with clean cloth and soap and water. Sterile gloves and gauze may be needed to clean an open wound. Remove gloves and discard.	Cleaning removes microorganisms so that bath or soak solution does not spread infection.
c. Fill Sitz bath or bathtub in bathroom with warmed solution. Check temperature. *Option:* If using normal saline, warm per employer policy or health care provider's prescription.	Ensures proper temperature and reduces risk of burns.
d. Assist patient to bathroom to immerse body part in Sitz bath, bathtub, or basin. Cover patient with bath blanket or towel as needed.	Prevents falls. Covering patient prevents heat loss through evaporation and maintains temperature and privacy.
e. Assess heart rate and that the patient does not feel lightheaded or dizzy. Ensure call light is within reach.	Provides baseline to determine whether vascular response to vasodilation occurs during treatment.
f. After 15–20 minutes, remove patient from soak or bath; dry body areas thoroughly. (Wear clean gloves.)	Avoids excess cooling. Enhances patient's comfort.
g. Drain solution from basin or tub. Clean the basin or tub according to employer policy. Dispose of soiled linen and gloves.	Reduces transmission of microorganisms.
EVALUATION	
1. Inspect condition of body part or wound treated for evidence of healing. Assess skin colour, temperature, edema, and sensitivity to touch.	Evaluates effectiveness of treatment and risk for potential injury.
2. Assess patient's comfort level using an appropriate pain assessment method (see employer policy). Consider the patient's age, clinical condition, cognitive or developmental level, literacy, ability to communicate, culture, and ethnicity when using a pain assessment method such as verbal or face picture rating scales or nonverbal indicators of pain (RNAO, 2013a).	Determines whether patient was exposed to temperature extreme that may cause injury. Evaluates patient's subjective response to therapy.
3. Obtain blood pressure and pulse and compare with baseline.	Determines whether systemic vascular response to vasodilation has occurred.
4. Evaluate range of motion of affected body part.	Determines whether edema or muscle spasm is relieved.
5. Use teach-back: "I want to be sure I demonstrated how to apply a moist warm compress so you can do this at home. Show me how you would apply this compress at home." Develop a revised teaching plan if the patient or caregiver is unable to teach back correctly.	Determines patient's and caregiver's level of understanding.

Unexpected Outcomes	Related Interventions
1. Patient's skin is reddened and sensitive to touch, either during treatment or 30 minutes after, or patient reports burning.	• Discontinue moist heat application immediately. • Verify proper temperature or check device for proper functioning. • Notify health care provider and, if there is a burn, complete an incident or adverse event report (see employer policy).
2. Patient describes burning sensation and increased discomfort.	• Reduce temperature of compress. • Assess for skin breakdown. • Notify health care provider.

Communication and Documentation

- Document procedure, noting type, location, and duration of application; solution and temperature; condition of body part, wound, and skin before and after treatment; and patient's response to therapy on flow sheet in progress notes in electronic health record (EHR) or chart.
- Document preprocedure and postprocedure vital signs.
- Document your evaluation of patient and caregiver learning.
- Report any unexpected changes in condition of skin or wound to health care provider.

DOCUMENTATION EXAMPLE

Patient ambulated to washroom at 1000 hours. Writer assisted patient to use Sitz bath. Sitz bath was placed on toilet per package directions, and patient immersed perineum in warm water for 15 minutes, per the health care provider's prescription. Skin remains dry and intact after procedure, with episiotomy sutures well-approximated. Patient reports improved comfort after procedure and verbalizes understanding of instructions for Sitz bath frequency and water temperature.

Special Considerations

Teaching

- If a patient needs to continue heat applications after discharge, have the patient or caregiver give a return demonstration before discharge.
- Caregivers and patients need to learn and demonstrate the assessments required for patients with reduced sensation in order to determine appropriate compress temperature.

Pediatric

- The skin of infants and children is thin and fragile and therefore easily damaged. Use special caution with application of heat in this population (Hockenberry et al., 2024). Remain with children during the procedure for safety.
- It may be helpful to incorporate play into the time a child is required to soak. Place clean bath toys in the basin or bath soak. Adult supervision is necessary.

Gerontological

- Normal aging results in thinning and increased fragility of a patient's skin, which increases risk of skin damage. If an older person is receiving long-term steroid therapy or is malnourished, the skin becomes even more fragile. Skin also becomes less elastic and more prone to tears. Chronic diseases may contribute to impaired circulation to a skin area or impaired sensation for pain or temperature (Boscart et al., 2023).
- Older persons who have lost subcutaneous tissue and fat have lost the insulating effect of these tissues. As a result, they may experience alterations in thermoregulation and have an increased risk of injury from heat applications (Boscart et al., 2023).

Care in the Community: Home Management

- When necessary, assess availability of a caregiver to help patient apply moist heat, the caregiver's understanding of the purpose of the procedure, and the caregiver's willingness to adhere to the procedure.
- Assess physical environment to determine adequacy of facilities for patient's use. The patient may need assistive devices to get in or out of a tub or a commode chair to set up a Sitz bath.
- Assess the patient's health state to determine whether continuous supervision is needed during therapy.

✦ SKILL 41.2 Application of Aquathermia and Dry Heat

A water-flow pad (e.g., an aquathermia pad), electric heating pads, and commercial heat packs (Fig. 41.5) are common forms of dry heat therapy. Air-activated wearable heat wraps that maintain a temperature of 40°C (104°F) can be worn for up to 8 to 10 hours. The aquathermia pad (water-flow pad) consists of a waterproof rubber or plastic pad connected by two hoses to an electrical control unit that has a heating element and motor. Distilled water circulates through hollowed channels in the pad to the control unit where water is heated (or cooled).

Dry heat devices are applied directly to the surface of the skin. For this reason, extra precautions need to be taken to prevent burns and skin and tissue injury. Conventional heating pads use dry heat and are often used in the home. A cotton or flannel cloth must cover the heating pad. The pad has a temperature-regulating unit for setting the heat to high, medium, or low. Instruct patients not to turn the setting higher once they have adapted to the temperature.

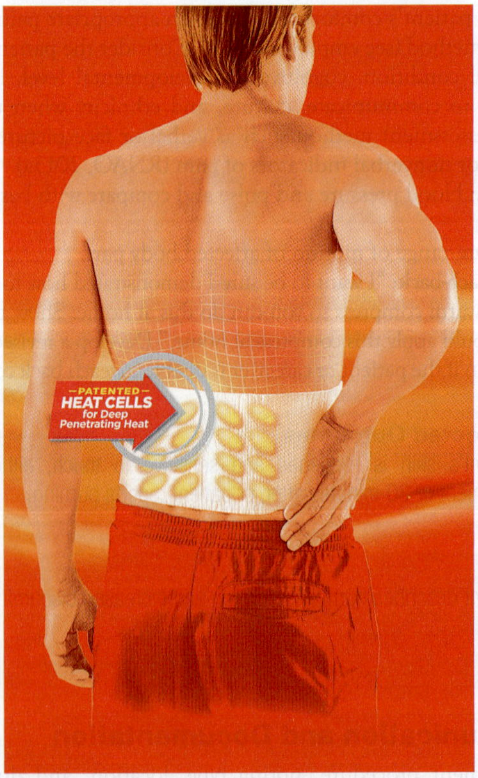

FIG 41.5 **Dry heat wrap.** (*Image used with permission, ThermaWrap, Pfizer Consumer Healthcare. All rights reserved.*)

Delegation and Collaboration

The skill of applying aquathermia and dry heat may be delegated to a UCP (see employer policy). The nurse must assess and evaluate the condition of the skin and tissues in the area being treated and explain the purpose of the treatment. If there are risks or expected complications, this skill cannot be delegated. The nurse instructs the UCP about the following:

- Specific positioning and time requirements to keep the application in place based on the health care provider's prescription or employer policy.
- Immediately reporting excessive redness or pain during application.
- Reporting to the nurse when treatment is completed to allow the nurse to evaluate patient's response.

Equipment

- Aquathermia pad or commercial heat pack
- Distilled water (for aquathermia pad)
- Bath towel or pillowcase
- Tape, ties, or gauze roll

STEP	RATIONALE
ASSESSMENT	
1. Identify patient using at least two identifiers (e.g., name and date of birth, or name and medical record number) according to employer policy.	Ensures correct patient. Complies with Accreditation Canada's standards and improves patient safety (Accreditation Canada, 2020).
2. Throughout the procedure, the 4 moments for hand hygiene are to be implemented; hand hygiene should occur before initial patient (or patient environment) contact, before an aseptic procedure, after body fluid exposure risk, and after patient (or patient environment) contact. Additional hand hygiene should be performed when hands are visibly soiled.	Proper hand hygiene helps prevent spread of infectious agents to health care providers.
3. Refer to health care provider's prescription for location, duration of therapy, and desired temperature. Employer policy usually sets recommended temperature for aquathermia pad.	A prescription is required to help ensure the patient's safety. Preset temperature on the device reduces risk of skin and tissue injury.
4. Check patient's chart for previous assessments and dressing change information as applicable.	Assesses for any changes in skin condition and integrity.
5. Assess skin integrity around the area being treated. Assess skin colour, temperature, sensitivity to touch, blistering, and excessive dryness (see Chapter 8).	Provides baseline to determine change in skin condition after heat application.
6. Assess patient's level of consciousness and responsiveness.	Patients with reduced level of consciousness are unable to sense or report reduced sensation or discomfort.
7. Assess patient's comfort level using a pain assessment method that can be understood by the person or caregiver. Consider the patient's age, clinical condition, cognitive or developmental level, literacy, ability to communicate, culture, and ethnicity when using a pain assessment method such as verbal or face picture rating scales or nonverbal indicators of pain (RNAO, 2013a). Assess range of motion if patient is being treated for muscle sprain.	Provides baseline to determine whether pain relief or improved range of motion is achieved.
8. Check electrical plugs and cords for obvious fraying or cracking.	Prevents injury from accidental electrical shock.
9. Determine patient's or caregiver's knowledge of procedure, including steps for application and safety precautions.	Heating pads are frequently used in the home. Assessment determines extent of health teaching required.

NURSING DIAGNOSES

- Acute pain
- Persistent pain
- Insufficient knowledge regarding heat application
- Reduced physical mobility
- Reduced skin integrity
- Reduced peripheral tissue perfusion
- Potential for injury

Related factors and risk factors are individualized on the basis of patient's condition or needs.

STEP	RATIONALE
PLANNING	
1. Expected outcomes following completion of procedure:	
• Skin is pink and warm to touch after application.	Vasodilation from heat exposure increases blood flow to affected part.
• Patient reports increased range of motion and a decrease in pain of inflamed tissues or strained muscles.	Thermoreceptors are activated by changes in skin temperature. Superficial heat increases joint mobility by increasing connective tissue extensibility, reducing pain, and reduced tissue viscosity; cold increases tissue viscosity whereas heat decreases it. (LeBlanc, 2018).
• Patient or caregiver correctly applies pad.	Measures level of understanding necessary for safe care in the community.
2. Prepare equipment and supplies.	Organization of supplies prevents unnecessary delays in procedure.
3. Explain procedure, purpose, and precautions.	Improves likelihood of patient's adherence to therapy.

STEP	RATIONALE

IMPLEMENTATION

STEP	RATIONALE
1. Close room door and close bedside curtains.	Provides for patient's privacy.
2. Apply clean gloves, and position patient to expose area being treated.	Reduces transmission of microorganisms. Patient must be able to assume position for several minutes during heat application.
3. Apply heat therapy.	
a. Aquathermia heating pad:	
(1) Cover or wrap area to be treated with single layer of bath towel or enclose pad with a pillowcase.	Prevents heated surface from touching patient's skin directly, thus reducing risk of injury to patient's skin.

Critical Decision Point *Do not pin wrap to the heating pad because this may cause a leak in the device.*

STEP	RATIONALE
(2) Place pad over the affected area and secure it with tape, a tie, or gauze as needed (see Step 3a[2] illustration).	Pad delivers dry, warm heat to injured tissues. Pad should not slip onto a different body part.
(3) Turn on aquathermia unit and check temperature setting. Temperature of unit is usually set by employer's bioengineering department.	Prevents exposure of patient to temperature extremes.
b. Apply commercially prepared heat pack (follow manufacturer guidelines to break pouch inside the larger pack).	Activates chemicals within pack to warm outer surface.

Critical Decision Point *Never position the patient in such a way that they are lying directly on the heating device. This position prevents dissipation of heat and increases risk of burns.*

STEP	RATIONALE
4. Remove and dispose of gloves.	Reduces transmission of microorganisms.
5. Monitor skin condition over site every 5 minutes and ask patient about sensation of burning.	Determines whether heat exposure is causing any burn, blistering, or injury to underlying skin.
6. After no more than 20 minutes (or as prescribed by health care provider), apply clean gloves and remove pad and store it.	Reduces transmission of microorganisms. Rebound phenomenon, in which the opposite effect begins, occurs after maximum therapeutic effect is achieved. Maximum vasodilation from heat occurs in 20–30 minutes (LeBlanc, 2018).
7. Assist patient to preferred position and dispose of soiled linen and gloves.	Promotes comfort. Reduces transmission of microorganisms.

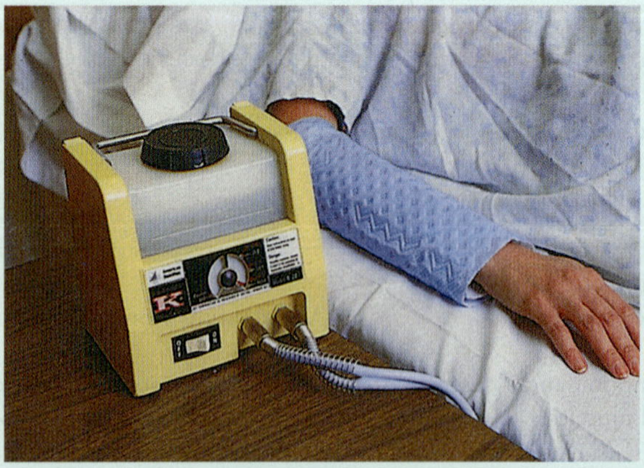

STEP 3A(2) Aquathermia pad.

STEP	RATIONALE
EVALUATION	
1. Inspect condition of skin for integrity, colour, temperature, dryness, and blistering. Evaluate again 30 minutes following treatment.	Evaluates response of skin to heat exposure.
2. Evaluate range of motion. Assess comfort level using a pain assessment method that can be understood by the patient or caregiver. Consider the patient's age, clinical condition, cognitive or developmental level, literacy, ability to communicate, culture, and ethnicity when using a pain assessment method such as verbal or face picture rating scales or nonverbal indicators of pain (RNAO, 2013a).	Heat reduces edema and relieves pain from muscle stiffness and spasm (Denegar et al., 2018).

Critical Decision Point *Instruct the patient not to actively exercise the muscle to evaluate results of therapy. Active exercise can aggravate muscle strain.*

STEP	RATIONALE
3. Use **teach-back:** "I want to be sure I explained how to safely use a heating pad at home. Explain to me why a layer of cloth between the pad and your skin is important." Develop a revised teaching plan if patient or caregiver is unable to teach back correctly.	Determines patient's and caregiver's level of understanding.

Unexpected Outcomes	Related Interventions
1. See Skill 41.1, Unexpected Outcomes.	
2. Patient reports that body part remains painful to move.	• Discontinue aquathermia pad or heat pack use. • Observe for localized swelling. • Notify health care provider.
3. Patient or caregiver applies heat incorrectly or is unable to explain precautions.	• Reinstruct patient or caregiver as necessary. Consider possible home health referral.

Communication and Documentation

- Document appearance and condition of skin, degree of range of motion of affected part, type of application, temperature and duration of therapy, and patient's response on flow sheet in progress notes in EHR or chart.
- Document evaluation of patient and caregiver learning.
- Report increased pain, reduced range of motion, burn, blistering, or other injury to the skin to health care provider.

DOCUMENTATION EXAMPLE

Writer applied aquathermia dry heat wrap to patient's left calf at 1315 hours, per the health care provider's prescription. Prior to the application, patient's skin was dry and intact. Patient had adequate perfusion to bilateral lower extremities with capillary refills of less than 2 seconds, warm to touch, and strong dorsalis pedis pulses were palpated. Two minutes after the application, patient reported "intense" pain, rated as 9/10 and radiating to the left thigh. Writer immediately removed the application. Patient's skin remains intact but reddened, with blanching noted upon palpation. Patient continues to have full range of motion. Writer immediately reported these findings to the health care provider.

Special Considerations

Teaching

- Highlight safety precautions during the procedure so these will be followed by the patient or caregiver.
- Instruct patient and caregiver not to use the highest heat setting and to check frequently for redness or blistering on the skin exposed to the heating device.

Pediatric

- Infants and children have skin that is thin and fragile and therefore easily damaged. Use special caution in this population (Hockenberry et al., 2024) when using dry heat therapy. Remain with children during the procedure for safety and effectiveness.

Gerontological

- Older persons are more at risk for burns because of loss of heat sensation and they have thin, fragile skin that is susceptible to burns.
- Check site frequently during all treatments.

Care in the Community: Home Management

- Assess patient's and caregiver's understanding of and ability and motivation to adhere to procedure.
- Assess home environment for safety of facilities (e.g., condition of electrical outlets and equipment).
- Discourage use of a conventional heating pad. However, if the patient has limited resources and chooses to use this pad at home, instruct them on all safety precautions.

SKILL 41.3 Application of Cold

A variety of cold (cryotherapy) modalities, such as ice packs, moist cold compresses, chemical cold packs, electromechanical or compression devices, or cold-soak immersion of a body part, are available. Cold therapy treats localized inflammatory responses that lead to edema, hemorrhage, muscle spasm, or pain (see Table 41.1). Improvement to joint mobility following cold therapy is related to facilitating mobility, relieving pain, inhibiting muscle spasm, and reducing muscle tension (Denegar et al., 2018).

Cold exerts a profound physiological effect on the body, reducing inflammation caused by injuries to soft tissue and the musculoskeletal system (APTA, 2019). Cold is one step in the PRICE principle (i.e., the acronym used in treating sprains and strains) (Maughan & Jackson, 2023). The overall goal of the PRICE principle is to limit the amount of swelling at the injury site and promote healing:

- P–Protect from further injury
- R–Restrict/Rest activity
- I–Apply Ice
- C–Apply Compression
- E–Elevate injured area

Cold application leads to vasoconstriction, which reduces blood flow to the injured part, thereby reducing the fluid accumulation and slowing the bleeding and hematoma formation associated with trauma. The lower temperature also suppresses muscle spasm and produces a local anaesthetic response (Denegar et al., 2018; Hannon & Porth, 2017). Cold applications produce maximal analgesia, control the inflammatory response, decrease nerve conduction, and improve mobility (da Costa Santos et al., 2015).

A cold compress usually consists of a commercial cold pack or a gauze dressing or washcloth that has been immersed in an iced or chilled solution to achieve the desired temperature. Although a clean compress is most common, open wounds require sterile applications. The size or thickness of gauze depends on the site of injury. For example, a cold compress to the eye requires thicker gauze that fits a small area to maintain a cold temperature. Thin gauze works more effectively for larger areas such as the face.

Ice bags and cold packs come in a variety of sizes to fit different body parts (Fig. 41.6). When a commercial ice bag or cold pack is unavailable, use a plastic bag or glove filled halfway with crushed ice. Squeeze the bag or glove to expel the air, which hampers cold conduction. Wrap all of these items in a towel or cloth before application.

Electrically controlled continuous cold-flow therapy devices simultaneously provide cold and compression (e.g., Cryo/Cuff; Fig. 41.7). Compression acts together with cold to reduce blood flow and edema formation while providing support to the soft tissues. The cooling pad has the advantage of delivering a constant cool temperature. Elevating the extremity during treatment further augments venous return. Treatment with one of these devices provides all components of the PRICE method for managing this type of injury (APTA, 2019).

Delegation and Collaboration

The skill of applying cold applications may be delegated to a UCP (see employer policy). The nurse must assess and evaluate the patient and explain the purpose of the treatment. If there are risks or possible complications, this skill cannot be delegated. The nurse instructs the UCP to do the following:

- Keep the application in place for only the time specified in the health care provider's prescription
- Immediately report to the nurse any excessive redness on the skin, increase in pain, or decrease in sensation
- Report when treatment is completed to allow the nurse to evaluate patient's response

Equipment

All Compresses, Bags, and Packs

- Clean gloves (if blood or body fluids are present)
- Cloth tape or ties or elastic wrap bandage
- Soft cloth cover: towel, pillowcase, or stockinette
- Bath towel or blanket and waterproof pad

Cold Compress

- Absorbent gauze (clean or sterile) folded to desired size
- Basin
- Prescribed solution at desired temperature

Ice Bag or Gel Pack

- Ice bag
- Ice chips and water or
- Reusable or disposable commercial gel pack (cold pack)

Electrically Controlled Cooling Device

- Cool water-flow pad or cooling pad and electrical pump
- Gauze roll or elastic wrap

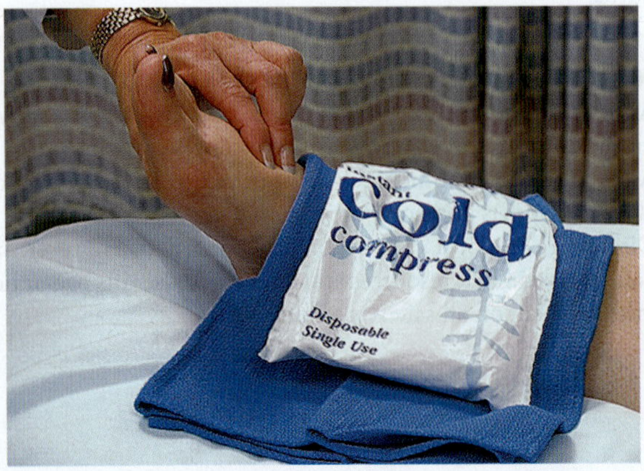

FIG 41.6 Commercial ice pack.

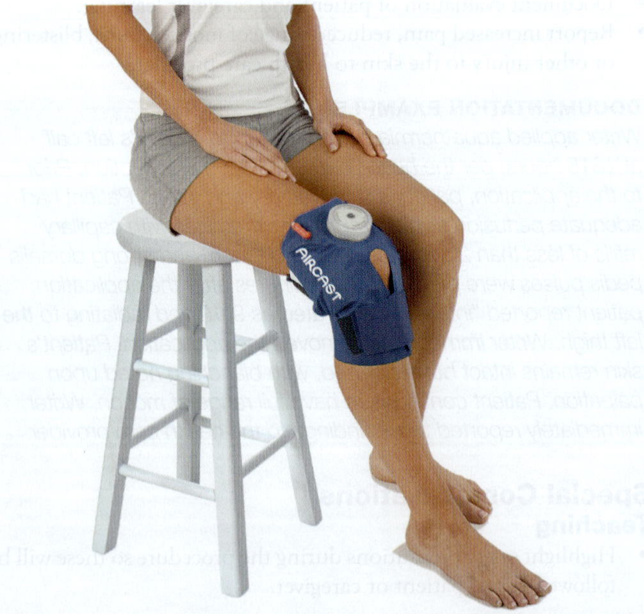

FIG 41.7 Cryo/Cuff includes integrated cooler. (*Image of AirCast Cryo/Cuff used with permission of DJO Global.*)

STEP	RATIONALE

ASSESSMENT

STEP	RATIONALE
1. Identify patient using at least two person-specific identifiers (e.g., name and date of birth, or name and medical record number) according to employer policy.	Ensures correct patient. Complies with Accreditation Canada's standards and improves patient safety (Accreditation Canada, 2020).
2. Throughout the procedure, the 4 moments for hand hygiene are to be implemented; hand hygiene should occur before initial patient (or patient environment) contact, before an aseptic procedure, after body fluid exposure risk, and after patient (or patient environment) contact. Additional hand hygiene should be performed when hands are visibly soiled.	Proper hand hygiene helps prevent spread of infectious agents to health care providers.
3. Refer to health care provider's prescription for type, location, and duration of application. Temperature of the cooling pad will be prescribed or preset.	A health care provider's prescription is required for all cold applications in most facilities (e.g., hospitals, long-term care).
4. Inspect condition of the injured or affected part. Gently palpate area for edema (apply clean gloves if there is risk of exposure to body fluids).	Reduces transmission of microorganisms. Provides baseline to determine change in condition of injured tissues.

Critical Decision Point *Keep injured part in alignment and immobilized. Movement can cause further injury to strains, sprains, or fractures.*

STEP	RATIONALE
5. Perform neurovascular check and inspect surrounding skin for integrity, presence of pulses, colour, temperature, and sensitivity to touch (see Chapter 8).	Determines whether patient is insensitive to cold extremes, which increases risk of injury.
6. Consider time elapsed since injury occurred.	Apply cold therapy as soon as possible after injury to reduce swelling, inflammation, tissue bleeding, and pain (Brooks & Hergenroeder, 2023; Maughan & Jackson, 2023).
7. Assess patient's level of consciousness and responsiveness.	Patients with reduced level of consciousness are unable to sense or report reduced sensation or discomfort.
8. Assess patient's comfort level using an appropriate pain assessment method (see employer policy). Assess range of movement of affected part if muscle sprain is involved.	Provides baseline to determine whether pain relief or improved range of motion is achieved with therapy.
9. Review medical history for conditions that contraindicate cold therapy: peripheral vascular diseases (e.g., Raynaud's phenomenon, diabetic neuropathy, rheumatoid arthritis, frostbite).	These conditions increase risk of skin and tissue injury when exposed to cold.
10. Assess patient's or caregiver's understanding and knowledge of procedure.	Cold applications are frequently used at home. Determines extent of instruction required.

NURSING DIAGNOSES

- Acute pain
- Persistent pain
- Reduced peripheral tissue perfusion
- Insufficient knowledge regarding cold application
- Reduced physical mobility
- Potential for injury

Related factors and risk factors are individualized on the basis of patient's condition or needs.

PLANNING

STEP	RATIONALE
1. Expected outcomes following completion of procedure:	
• Affected area is slightly pale and cool to touch.	Result of vasoconstriction.
• There is decreased edema, bleeding, or both in tissues at site of injury.	Cold reduces blood flow to the affected part by reducing protein extravasation from vasculature and subsequent edema formation (Brooks & Hergenroeder, 2023).
• Patient reports or shows evidence of decreased pain as determined by an appropriate pain assessment method.	Cold creates a localized analgesic effect by decreasing local swelling, reducing the inflammatory response, and decreasing nerve conduction (Brooks & Hergenroeder, 2023).
• Patient's range of motion increases.	Cold reduces swelling.
• Patient or caregiver correctly states how to apply cold and provides return demonstration.	Measures level of understanding necessary for safe care in the community.
2. Prepare equipment and supplies.	Organization prevents unnecessary delays.
3. Explain procedure and precautions.	Improves likelihood of adherence to therapy.

STEP	RATIONALE
IMPLEMENTATION	
1. Close room door and bedside curtain. Apply clean gloves.	Provides privacy for patient. Reduces transmission of microorganisms.
2. Position patient to keep body part in proper alignment and only expose area to be treated; drape patient with bath blankets.	Prevents further injury to body part. Avoids unnecessary exposure of body, maintaining patient's comfort and privacy.
3. Place towel or absorbent pad under area to be treated.	Protects ben linen from moisture and soiling.
4. Apply cold compress:	
a. Place ice and water in basin and test temperature on inner aspect of arm.	Extreme temperature can cause tissue damage.
b. Submerge gauze into basin filled with cold solution; wring out excess moisture.	Excess moisture is uncomfortable to patient.
c. Apply compress to affected area, moulding it gently over site.	Ensures that cold is directed over site of injury.
d. Remove, remoisten, and reapply compress to maintain temperature as needed.	Ensures consistency of treatment.
5. Apply ice pack or bag:	
a. Fill bag with water, secure cap, and invert.	Ensures that there are no leaks.
b. Empty water and fill bag two-thirds full with small ice chips and water.	Partially filled bag is easier to mould over body part.
c. Express excess air from bag, secure bag closure, and wipe bag dry.	Excess air interferes with cold conduction. Allows bag to conform to area and promotes maximum contact.
d. Squeeze or knead commercial ice pack according to manufacturer instructions.	Releases alcohol-based solution to create cold temperature.
e. Wrap pack or bag with single layer of towel, pillowcase, or stockinette. Apply over injury. Secure with tape as needed.	Protects patient's tissue and absorbs condensation. Prevents direct exposure of cold against patient's skin.
6. Apply commercial gel pack:	
a. Remove from freezer.	
b. Wrap pack with a towel, pillowcase, or stockinette. Apply pack directly over injury.	Protects patient's tissue and absorbs condensation. Prevents direct exposure of cold against patient's skin.
c. Secure with gauze, cloth tape, or ties as needed.	

Critical Decision Point *Do not reapply the ice pack to red or bluish areas; continual use of the ice pack increases ischemia.*

STEP	RATIONALE
7. Apply electrically controlled cooling device:	
a. Prepare device according to manufacturer instructions. Some devices are gravity-fed and require manual filling with iced water. Motorized units circulate chilled water.	Ensures safe temperature application.
b. Make sure that all connections are intact and the temperature, if adjustable, is set (see employer policy).	Ensures safe temperature application.
c. Wrap cooling device in a single layer of towel or pillowcase.	Prevents adverse reactions from cold such as burn or frostbite.
d. Wrap cooling device around body part.	Ensures even application of cold temperature.
e. Turn device on and check correct temperature. Temperature is usually preset in health care settings (see employer policy).	Ensures effective therapy. Preset temperature reduces risk of skin and tissue injury.
f. Secure with elastic wrap bandage, gauze roll, or ties.	Ensures cold is distributed to the correct body part.
8. Remove and dispose of gloves in proper container.	Reduces transmission of microorganisms.
9. Check condition of skin every 5 minutes for duration of application.	Determines whether there are adverse reactions to cold (e.g., mottling, redness, burning, blistering, numbness).
a. If area is edematous, sensation may be reduced; use extra caution during cold therapy and assess site more often.	
b. Numbness and tingling are common sensations with cold applications and indicate adverse reactions only when severe and coupled with other symptoms. Stop treatment if the patient experiences a burning sensation or the skin begins to feel numb.	During cold application, patient's skin will initially feel cold, followed by relief of pain. As cryotherapy continues, the patient will feel a burning sensation, pain, and finally numbness.
10. After 20 minutes (or as prescribed), apply clean gloves, remove compress or pad, and gently dry off any moisture.	Reduces transmission of microorganisms. Drying prevents maceration of skin.

STEP	RATIONALE

IMPLEMENTATION

Critical Decision Point *Areas with little body fat (e.g., knee, ankle, and elbow) do not tolerate cold as well as fatty areas (e.g., thigh and buttocks). For bony areas, decrease duration of cold application.*

STEP	RATIONALE
11. Assist patient to a comfortable position.	Maintains comfort.
12. Remove and dispose of supplies. Dispose of soiled linen and gloves.	Reduces transmission of microorganisms.

EVALUATION

STEP	RATIONALE
1. Inspect affected area for integrity, colour, temperature, and sensitivity to touch. Re-evaluate 30 minutes after the procedure.	Determines reaction to cold application.
2. Palpate affected area gently for edema, bruising, and bleeding (apply gloves if there is risk of exposure to body fluids).	Determines effectiveness of treatment and development of skin or tissue injury.
3. Assess the patient's comfort level using an appropriate pain assessment method (see employer policy).	Determines whether pain has been relieved.
4. Measure range of motion of affected body part.	Determines whether edema or muscle spasm is decreased.
5. **Use teach-back:** "I want to be sure I showed you how to apply an ice pack. Show me how to apply an ice pack." Develop a revised teaching plan if patient or caregiver is unable to teach back correctly.	Determines patient's and caregiver's level of understanding.

Unexpected Outcomes	Related Interventions
1. Skin appears mottled, reddened, or bluish after exposure to cold.	• Stop treatment. • Notify health care provider.
2. Patient reports burning pain and numbness.	• Stop therapy. • Notify health care provider.
3. Patient or caregiver is unable to describe or demonstrate therapy.	• Provide further instruction and demonstration.

Communication and Documentation

- Document appearance and condition of the skin and affected body part; procedure, including type, location, and duration of application; and patient's response on flow sheet in progress notes in EHR or chart.
- Document evaluation of patient and caregiver learning.
- Report sensations of burning, numbness, or unrelieved skin colour changes to health care provider.

DOCUMENTATION EXAMPLE

At 2030 hours, writer applied ice bag with appropriate protective cloth layers to patient's inferior jaw postoperatively, per the health care provider's prescription. Prior to application, skin was noted to have mild ecchymosis and 1+ pitting edema to bilateral cheeks. Skin remained dry and intact. Ice bag was removed after 20 minutes. Edema was no longer pitting after removal, and skin temperature was warm to touch. Patient did not report any pain with procedure. Writer to repeat procedure at 2130 hours per health care provider's prescription.

Special Considerations

Teaching

- Injuries requiring this type of therapy usually occur outside of acute care settings. Patients at risk for injury, such as those who participate in sports, should know how to minimize the extent of injury using cold.

Pediatric

- A greater metabolic rate and larger trunk in relation to the rest of the body make children more prone to hypothermia (Hockenberry et al., 2024).
- Infants have an immature temperature control mechanism; thus, mottling of extremities is common and does not always indicate an adverse reaction (Hockenberry et a., 2024).
- Cool soaks decrease itching with some skin lesions.
- The same precautions and play techniques as those used with warm soaks may be useful in cold therapy with children.

Gerontological

- Older persons are more at risk for tissue damage because of altered responses to change in body temperature; therefore, they need frequent skin assessment during treatment (Boscart et al., 2023).

✦ SKILL 41.4 Caring for Patients Requiring Hypothermia or Hyperthermia Blankets

A hypothermia or hyperthermia blanket raises, lowers, or maintains body temperature through conductive heat or cold transfer between the blanket and the patient (Fig. 41.8). Adjusting body temperature using a hypothermia or hyperthermia blanket must be carefully controlled to avoid overwhelming the body's thermoregulatory centre and cardiopulmonary functions. Because oral temperatures are inaccurate in circumstances of vasoconstriction and sluggish blood flow, the patient's temperature is continuously monitored with a special thermistor probe capable of measuring core body temperatures as low as 25°C (77°F) (Hannon & Porth, 2017).

Patients may develop high, prolonged fevers from infectious neurological diseases, as adverse effects of anaesthesia, and following severe brain injury. Induced hypothermia prevents or moderates neurological outcomes following neurosurgery, traumatic brain injury, and acute stroke (Rittenberger & Callaway, 2023). Therapeutic hypothermia decreases cerebral metabolic rate and oxygen demand and has been found to improve neurological outcomes and survival (Kurisu & Yenari, 2019). The recommended temperature range is 33 to 36°C (96.8–104°F) for targeted temperature management of patients following cardiac arrest (Boulé-Laghzali et al., 2019).

Following severe trauma or major surgery such as cardiac surgery, thermoregulation is essential. Hypothermia causes vasoconstriction, shivering, increased oxygen demand, altered coronary blood flow, cardiac dysrhythmias, acid–base imbalances, and impaired coagulation. Rapid rewarming can be life threatening. Interventions to progressively raise body temperature should be directed by an experienced health care provider and focus on heat retention, restoration of normal core body temperature, and tissue preservation (Zieber, 2018).

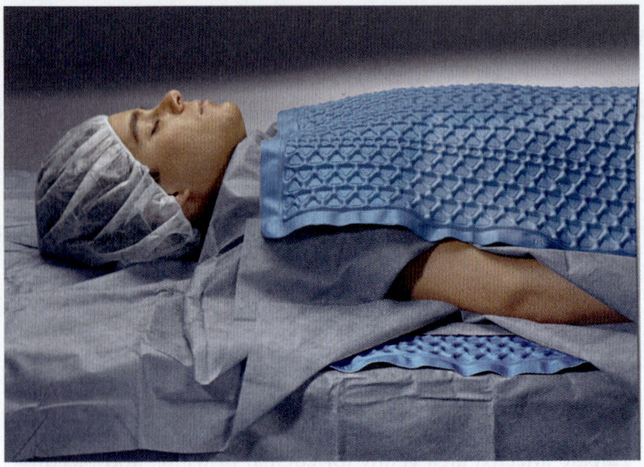

FIG 41.8 **Hypothermia cooling blanket is applied over a paper sheet before additional top sheet is applied to bed.** (*Courtesy Cincinnati Sub-Zero Maxi-Therm Hyper-Hypothermia Blanket.*)

Delegation and Collaboration

The skill of applying a hypothermia or hyperthermia blanket cannot be delegated to a UCP. The nurse is responsible for assessing and evaluating treatment and related patient education. The nurse instructs the UCP to do the following:

- Maintain proper temperature of the blanket throughout the treatment and discontinue the therapy as specified in the health care provider's prescription
- Report any unexpected patient outcomes (e.g., shivering or redness to the skin) to the nurse
- Inform the nurse when treatment is completed to allow the nurse to evaluate patient's response to treatment

Equipment

- Hypothermia or hyperthermia blanket with control panel and rectal probe
- Sheet or thin bath blanket
- Distilled water to fill the unit, if necessary
- Clean gloves
- Rectal thermometer

STEP	RATIONALE
ASSESSMENT	
1. Identify patient using at least two person-specific identifiers (e.g., name and date of birth, or name and medical record number) according to employer policy.	Ensures correct patient. Complies with Accreditation Canada's standards and improves patient safety (Accreditation Canada, 2020).
2. Throughout the procedure, the 4 moments for hand hygiene are to be implemented; hand hygiene should occur before initial patient (or patient environment) contact, before an aseptic procedure, after body fluid exposure risk, and after patient (or patient environment) contact. Additional hand hygiene should be performed when hands are visibly soiled.	Proper hand hygiene helps prevent spread of infectious agents to health care providers.
3. Refer to health care provider's prescription and check that patient's current body temperature indicates use of hypothermia or hyperthermia blanket.	Instituting therapy requires a health care provider's prescription.
4. Obtain patient's vital signs and assess neurological status, mental status, and peripheral circulation.	Establishes baseline data to use for comparison during therapy.

STEP	RATIONALE

ASSESSMENT

5. Verify that other less intensive measures are not able to restore the patient's body temperature to the desired level.	Use of a hypothermia or hyperthermia blanket is not without risk and should be instituted only when other measures are not effective.

Critical Decision Point *Antipyretic therapy may be used in combination with a cooling blanket. Very high fevers (>41°C [105.8°F]) damage parenchymal cells throughout the body, particularly in the brain, which may result in irreversible neuron damage* (Hannon & Porth, 2017; Zieber, 2018).

6. Assess patient's skin on the chest and extremities, paying close attention to bony prominences such as hands and feet.	Areas that are more exposed to the blanket are at greater risk for skin and tissue injury. Establishing baseline data helps determine whether skin injury or development of pressure injury is the result of therapy.

NURSING DIAGNOSES

- Hyperthermia
- Hypothermia
- Reduced peripheral tissue perfusion
- Reduced skin integrity
- Potential for skin injury

Related factors and risk factors are individualized on the basis of patient's condition or needs.

PLANNING

1. Expected outcomes following completion of procedure:	
• Temperature is within normal range.	Indicates that therapy is effective.
• Absence of shivering with hypothermia blanket.	Shivering increases metabolic rate, heat production, and oxygen consumption. Shivering also causes vasoconstriction, which can injure skin of distal body regions (Rittenberger & Callaway, 2023).
• Skin does not show signs of injury or burns.	Indicates that treatment is not causing adverse effects.
2. Explain procedure and precautions to patient or caregiver.	Increases cooperation with treatment and reduces anxiety.
3. Prepare blanket according to employer policy, manufacturer instructions, and prescription. Manufacturer instructions are usually located on the machine.	Facilities have specific policies on maintaining and using equipment. Ensures correct and safe use of equipment.

IMPLEMENTATION

1. Apply clean gloves. Position patient comfortably.	Reduces transmission of microorganisms.
2. Turn on blanket and observe that cool or warm light is on. Set the blanket temperature to desired level.	Verifies that blanket is set correctly for prescribed therapy to reduce or increase patient's body temperature.
3. Verify that blanket temperature limits are set at desired safety ranges.	Safety ranges prevent excessive cooling or warming. Blanket automatically shuts off when preset body temperature is achieved.
4. Cover hypothermia or hyperthermia blanket with thin paper, a cloth sheet, or bath blanket.	A thin covering prevents direct contact with the blanket, thus reducing risk of injury to skin. Covering provides insulation between the patient and appliance and protects skin from contact with plastic blanket.
5. Position hypothermia or hyperthermia blanket following manufacturer instructions.	Provides distribution of blanket against patient's skin.
a. Wrap patient's hands and feet in gauze.	Reduces risk of thermal injury to distal areas of body.
b. Wrap scrotum with towels.	Protects sensitive tissue from direct contact with cold or heat.
6. Continuously monitor patient's temperature using a thermistor probe according to the blanket manufacturer instructions.	Accurate and continuous monitoring of patient's core body temperature is required during warming or cooling to prevent the body's thermoregulation mechanisms and cardiopulmonary functions from being overwhelmed.
7. Turn and position patient regularly to prevent development of pressure injuries and impaired body alignment (see Chapter 11). Keep linens free of perspiration and condensation.	Reduces risk for pressure injury development due to skin moisture created by blanket and patient's body temperature.
8. Double-check fluid thermometer on control panel of blanket before leaving room.	Verifies that blanket temperature is maintained at desired level.
9. Remove gloves and discard.	Reduces transmission of microorganisms.

STEP	RATIONALE
EVALUATION	
1. Monitor patient's temperature and vital signs every 15 minutes during the first hour of therapy. Evaluate automatic temperature control thereafter every 30 minutes visually and every 4 hours by assessing the patient's temperature.	Provides continuous evaluation of patient's response to therapy during initial and continuous therapy. Ensures appropriate discontinuation of treatment when the patient's temperature reaches desired level. Decreases risk of subnormal body temperature. Verifies accuracy of thermistor probe and automatic temperature control device.
2. Observe skin for indications of burns, change in colour, and other injuries.	Hypothermia and hyperthermia blankets have the potential to cause skin injuries.
3. Observe patient for signs of shivering.	Early signs of shivering, which may result in negative outcomes, include electrocardiographic changes, facial muscle twitching, and hyperventilation.
4. Determine patient's level of comfort.	Prompt assessment reduces risk of severe injuries.
5. **Use teach-back:** "I want to be sure I explained why this blanket is important for your loved one's care. Tell me why we are using the blanket." Develop revised teaching if caregiver is unable to teach back correctly.	Determines caregiver's level of understanding.

Unexpected Outcomes	Related Interventions
1. Patient's core body temperature decreases or rises rapidly. This indicates that temperature is extreme, which may result in injury to patient.	• Adjust blanket temperature no more than 0.6°C (1°F) every 15 minutes to avoid complications. • Report temperature changes to health care provider.
2. Patient's core body temperature remains unchanged.	• Patient may need hypothermic or hyperthermic treatment to axilla, groin, and neck in addition to those areas covered by blanket. • Discuss use of antipyretic with health care provider.
3. Patient begins to shiver. Shivering increases metabolic rate and heat production, causing patient's core body temperature to rise, and increases oxygen consumption.	• Adjust temperature range and assess whether shivering decreases. • If shivering continues, stop treatment and notify health care provider.

Communication and Documentation

- Document the following baseline data: vital signs, neurological and mental status, peripheral circulation, and skin integrity when therapy was initiated. Include type of hyperthermia–hypothermia unit; control settings (manual or automatic and temperature settings); temperature monitoring method, date, time, and duration; and patient's response to treatment in progress notes in EHR or chart.
- Document repeated measurements of vital signs on temperature graphic EHR or chart to document response to therapy.
- Document evaluation of caregiver learning.
- Report any unexpected outcome to health care provider.

DOCUMENTATION EXAMPLE

At 0300 hours, writer assisted with the application of a hypothermia blanket, per the health care provider's prescription. The blanket was applied over a paper sheet, and a top sheet was applied over the hypothermia blanket. Prior to the application, patient's skin was warm to touch centrally and peripherally, with no evidence of skin breakdown or abnormalities. At 0315 hours, patient's thermometer probe began signalling a core temperature of 32°C. Writer immediately assisted with the removal of the blanket and reported this finding to the health care provider. After removal, patient's temperature remains stable at 36°C per probe reading.

Special Considerations

Teaching

- Instruct patients and their families not to move the patient off the blanket.

Pediatric

- Infants have an immature temperature control mechanism; thus, mottling of extremities is common and does not always indicate an adverse reaction (Hockenberry et al., 2024).

Gerontological

- Some older persons are more at risk for tissue damage because of loss of cold sensation. Check patient frequently during all treatments (Boscart et al., 2023).

✦ REVIEW QUESTIONS

The nurse is assigned to care for a 58-year-old patient who is postoperative day 1 following total left knee arthroplasty. The patient has type 1 diabetes mellitus that is regulated with insulin. The surgeon has prescribed an electronically controlled cold compression cuff to be applied to the left knee for 2 to 3 hours, followed by a 1- to 2-hour break with compression loosened. The patient is receiving oral pain medication every 4 hours for pain.

Review Questions 1 to 3 relate to the case study presented here.

1. Place in the correct order the following statements describing how the nurse will begin the cold application. Explain your choice(s).
    1. Refer to the health care provider's prescription for location and duration of the application.
    2. Explain the procedure and precautions to the patient to avoid injury to the skin.
    3. Assess the condition of the injured or affected body part.
    4. Assess the patient's current pain level.
2. What is the major risk associated with cold application for this patient and how should the nurse assess for this risk?
3. After 24 hours of intermittent cold therapy using a compression cuff, the patient reports a burning sensation. The nurse observes a reddened 2-cm area and a blister on the skin under the compression cuff. The left leg is warm with normal colour, and pulses are present distal to the compression cuff. The patient denies incisional pain and the incision is clean and intact. Show how the nurse would use SBAR (situation–background–assessment–recommendation) to communicate with the health care team about this patient.

Visit the Evolve site for a complete list of answers to the Review Questions.

✦ NEXT GENERATION NCLEX® (NGN)

For practice with answering exam questions related to unfolding NGN case studies, please consult the Next Generation NCLEX® (NGN)-Style Case Studies for Skills and Techniques on the Evolve website: http://evolve.elsevier.com/Canada/Perry/clinicalskills/

REFERENCES

Accreditation Canada. (2020). *Required organizational practices–2020 handbook.* https://physicians.nshealth.ca/resources/required-organizational-practices-2020-handbook

American Physical Therapy Association. (2019). *Scope of practice.* https://www.apta.org/ScopeOfPractice/

Benchahong, S., Pongrojpaw, D., Chanthasenanont, A., et al. (2021). Cold therapy for pain relief during and after amniocentesis procedure: A randomized controlled trial. *Journal of Obstetrics and Gynaecology Research, 47*(8), 2623–2631. https://doi.org/10.1111/jog.14832

Boscart, V., McCleary, L., Sheiban Taucar, L., et al. (2023). *Ebersole and Hess' gerontological nursing and healthy aging in Canada* (3rd ed.). Elsevier.

Boulé-Laghzali, N., Pérez, L. D., Dyrda, K., et al. (2019). Targeted temperature management after cardiac arrest: The Montreal Heart Institute experience. *CJC Open, 1*(5), 238–244. https://doi.org/10.1016/j.cjco.2019.07.001

Brooks, G. P., & Hergenroeder, A. C. (2023). *Musculoskeletal injury in children and skeletally immature adolescents: Overview of treatment principles for nonoperative injuries.* UpToDate. https://www.uptodate.com/contents/musculoskeletal-injury-in-children-and-skeletally-immature-adolescents-overview-of-treatment-principles-for-nonoperative-injuries

Canadian Nurses Association. (2011). *Position statement: Interprofessional collaboration* https://www.cna-aiic.ca/en/nursing/nursing-tools-and-resources/interprofessional-collaboration. [Seminal Reference].

Canadian Physiotherapy Association. (2012). *Position statement: Interprofessional collaboration and practice* https://physiotherapy.ca/app/uploads/2022/08/inter-professional-collaboration_en.pdf. [Seminal Reference].

da Costa Santos, V., dos Santos Cardoso, C., Figueiredo, C. P., et al. (2015). Effect of cryotherapy on the ankle temperature in athletes: Ice pack and cold water immersion. *Fisioterapia em Movimento, 28*(1), 23–30. https://doi.org/10.1590/0103-5150.028.001.AO02. [Seminal Reference].

Denegar, C. R., Saliba, E., & Saliba, S. F. (2018). *Therapeutic modalities for musculoskeletal injuries* (4th ed.). Human Kinetics.

Giger, J., & Haddad, L. (2020). *Transcultural nursing: Assessment and intervention* (8th ed.). Elsevier.

Hannon, R. A., & Porth, C. M. (2017). *Pathophysiology: Concepts of altered health states* (2nd ed.). Wolters Kluwer. [Seminal Reference].

Hockenberry, M. J., Duffy, E. A., & Gibbs, K. (2024). *Wong's nursing care of infants and children* (12th ed.). Elsevier.

Karadağ, S., Taşci, S., Doğan, N., et al. (2019). Application of heat and a home exercise program for pain and function levels in patients with knee osteoarthritis: A randomized controlled trial. *International Journal of Nursing Practice, 25*(5), e12772. https://doi.org/10.1111/ijn.12772

Kurisu, K., & Yenari, M. A. (2019). Therapeutic hypothermia for ischemic stroke; pathophysiology and future promise. *Neuropharmacology, 134,* 302–309. https://doi.org/10.1016/j.neuropharm.2017.08.025

LeBlanc, K. (2018). Skin integrity and wound care. In B. J. Kozier, G. Erb, A. T. Berman, et al. (Eds.), *Fundamentals of Canadian nursing: Concepts, process, and practice* (4th ed., pp. 930–982). Pearson Canada.

Li, Z., & Wang, Q. (2016). Ice compresses aid the reduction of swelling and pain after scleral buckling surgery. *Journal of Clinical Nursing, 25*(21–22), 3261–3265. https://doi.org/10.1111/jocn.13362. [Seminal Reference].

Maughan, K. L., & Jackson, J. (2023). *Ankle sprain in adults: Evaluation and diagnosis.* UpToDate. https://www.uptodate.com/contents/ankle-sprain-in-adults-evaluation-and-diagnosis

Registered Nurses' Association of Ontario. (2013a). *Assessment and management of pain* (3rd ed.). https://rnao.ca/bpg/guidelines/assessment-and-management-pain. [Seminal Reference].

Registered Nurses' Association of Ontario. (2013b). Non-pharmacological interventions. In *Assessment and management of pain* (3rd ed, pp. 36–37). https://rnao.ca/bpg/guidelines/assessment-and-management-pain

Rittenberger, J., & Callaway, C. (2023). *Post-cardiac arrest management in adults.* UpToDate. https://www.uptodate.com/contents/initial-assessment-and-management-of-the-adult-post-cardiac-arrest-patient

Wang, Y., Li, S., Zhang, Y., et al. (2021). Heat and cold therapy reduce pain in patients with delayed onset muscle soreness: A systematic review and meta-analysis of 32 randomized controlled trials. *Physical Therapy in Sport, 48,* 177–187. https://doi.org/10.1016/j.ptsp.2021.01.004

Zieber, E. M. P. (2018). Vital signs. In B. Kozier, G. Erb, A. Berman, et al. (Eds.), *Fundamentals of Canadian nursing: Concepts, process, and practice* (4th ed., pp. 630–667). Pearson Canada.

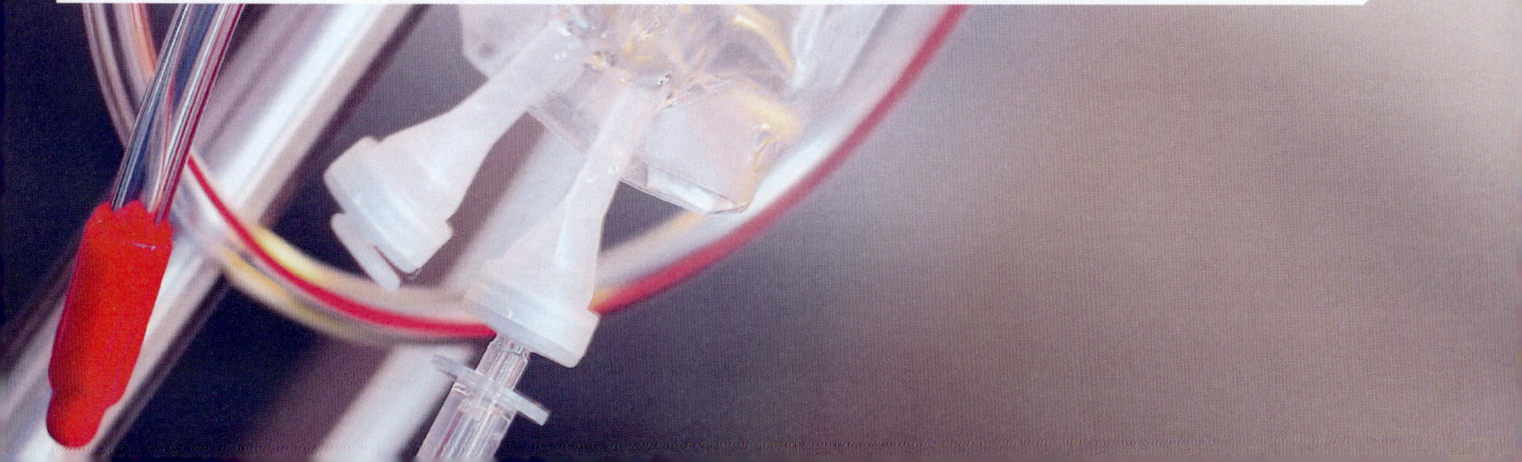

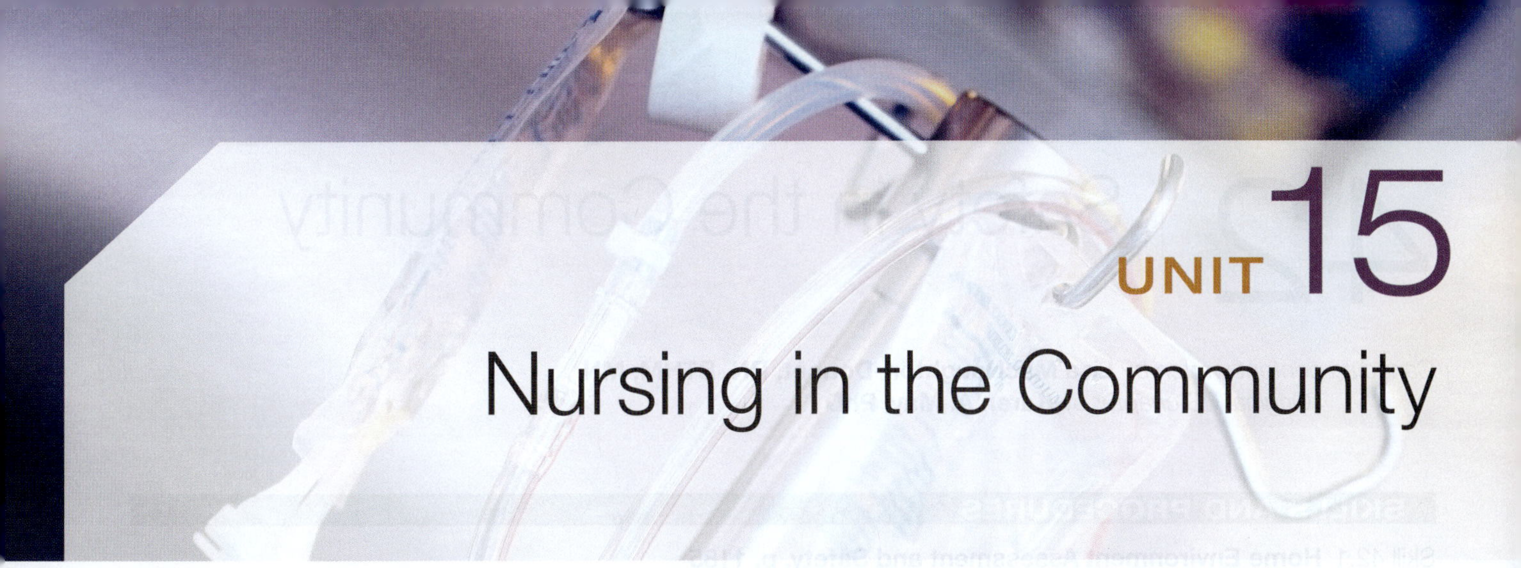

UNIT 15

Nursing in the Community

Patients who require home care are dependent on nurses to critically assess and identify all the factors within the home that could affect their safety and health outcomes. Use a patient-centred, systematic, ongoing process to assess a patient's health status and needs. Home health nurses manage patients' problems, often over several weeks. Establishing an initial database of a patient's health status and home environment is essential in order to monitor for change. Once problems and needs have been identified, a home health nurse discusses them with the patient, family members, and other caregivers. Together, they determine goals and outcomes that reflect the patient's desires, priorities, cultural values, and preferences. The two greatest priorities in home health care are patient safety and education to enable patients to perform self-care.

Patient safety in the home begins with a home environment assessment, which enables you to make adaptations to the home that will minimize the effects of a patient's limitations or deficiencies. It also allows for a patient's strengths to be maximized. If a patient returns home with an unsteady gait or poor balance, an assessment of the condition of stairs and common walkways leads you to recommend alterations such as installing railings along stairs, removing objects or rugs that can cause tripping, and repairing uneven walking surfaces. The same patient will require you to exercise your clinical judgement regarding which strategies are appropriate for fire safety. A recurring principle is to be sure your recommendations are accepted by patients and caregivers and that resources (economic, people, time) are available to make needed changes in the home.

Patients who have cognitive challenges require special consideration to keep them safe in the home. Your assessment focuses on the level of deficit a patient is experiencing, the level of caregiver support available, and any hazards existing in the home. You will critically apply your assessment findings to provide interventions that maximize a patient's abilities by simplifying tasks and providing consistency in daily activities. Often, a caregiver has found ways to manage a patient with cognitive deficits by minimizing anxiety, reducing wandering, and keeping the patient engaged. When successful interventions exist, use them in your plan of care. Your knowledge of cognitive challenges offers guidance in helping caregivers anticipate the progression of the disease.

The list of nursing skills that a patient and/or caregiver may have to perform in the home has become lengthy owing to the trend in early discharge of patients from hospitals. In all cases, patient safety and education are necessary so that patients know not only how to perform skills correctly but also what problems or complications to anticipate and when to contact a health care provider. When you instruct a patient or caregiver on performing a skill, follow the same basic steps that you would use as a nurse. However, adapt the steps of each skill so that the patient can follow infection control and safety principles and use equipment that can be obtained for the home. Also, plan skills at times that are convenient for patients (when possible). Do not use shortcuts but make evidence-informed adaptations. The use of therapeutic communication and education principles will promote trusting relationships with a patient and caregiver, instilling confidence in the patient. A patient needs to be competent in performing a skill and to know when to seek help from a health care provider.

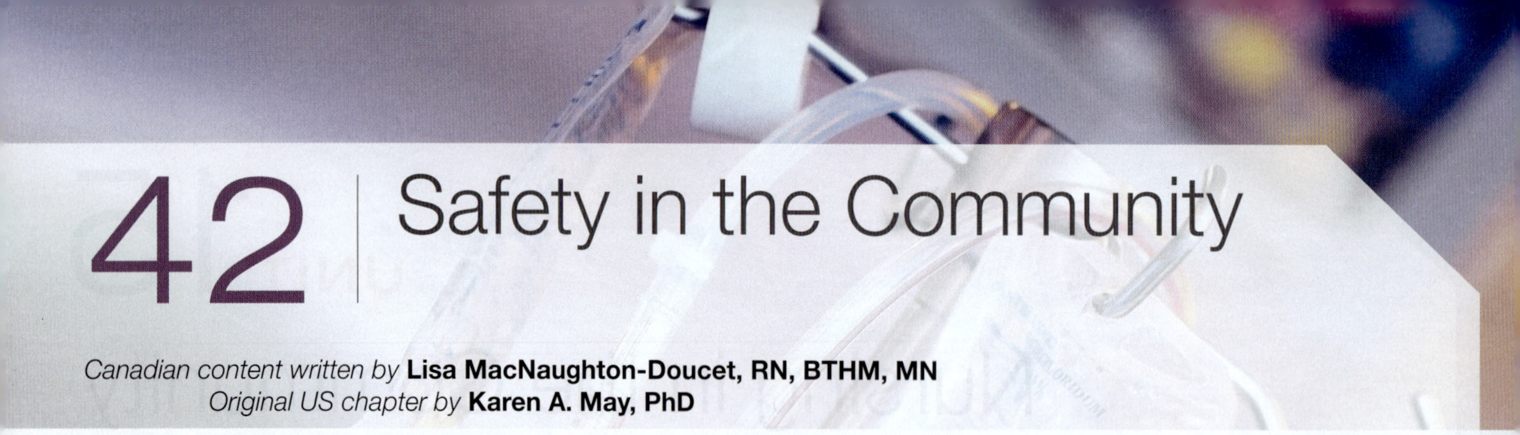

42 Safety in the Community

Canadian content written by **Lisa MacNaughton-Doucet, RN, BTHM, MN**
Original US chapter by **Karen A. May, PhD**

SKILLS AND PROCEDURES

OBJECTIVES

Mastery of content in this chapter will enable the nurse to:

- Identify patients at risk for safety hazards and possible accidents in the home.
- Promote self-care of patients in the home.
- Describe factors within a home environment that create risks for patient injury.
- Perform a home safety risk assessment.
- Identify interventions to improve the physical safety of the home environment.
- Identify interventions to reduce the risk of harm to persons with sensory, cognitive, and/or mental status alterations.
- Recommend strategies to ensure safe medication administration within the home.
- Perform a falls risk assessment.

MEDIA RESOURCES

- http://evolve.elsevier.com/Canada/Perry/clinicalskills/

PURPOSE

In the community setting, nurses improve patient safety through health promotion and injury prevention (Franklin & Sleet, 2018). The home has many safety hazards; the key to preventing home-related injuries is to eliminate risks before any injuries occur (Feist, 2019). Safety in the home begins before a patient is discharged from a health care facility. An interprofessional approach to hospital discharge planning is critical to ensure that patients are returning to a safe environment in which falls and injuries can be prevented. Before discharge, patients may be assessed for the need to have home modifications and/or the home may be assessed for safety hazards to help create a supportive home environment, thereby mitigating the risk for hospital readmission and ensuring good quality of life at home (Kirchner-Heklau et al., 2021).

STANDARDS OF CARE

- Alzheimer Society of Canada (ASC, n.d.)—*Making Your Environment Safe* (https://alzheimer.ca/en/help-support/im-caring-person-living-dementia/ensuring-safety-security/making-your-environment-safe)
- Canadian Paediatric Society (n.d.)—Caring for Kids—*Safety and Injury Prevention at Home* (https://caringforkids.cps.ca/handouts/safety-and-injury-prevention)
- Community Health Nurses of Canada (2019)—*Canadian Community Health Nursing Professional Practice Model and Standards of Practice* (https://www.chnc.ca/en/standards-of-practice)
- Health Excellence Canada (2017)—*Patient/Client Safety in the Home* (https://www.patientsafetyinstitute.ca/en/education/PatientSafetyEducationProgram/PatientSafetyEducationCurriculum/Pages/Module-18-Patient-Client-Safety-in-Home-Care.aspx
- Parachute Canada (n.d.)—*Discover How to Prevent Injuries Before They Happen* (https://www.parachutecanada.org/en/injury-topics/)

PRINCIPLES FOR PRACTICE

- Safety in the home involves communication between a patient, caregiver(s), and interprofessional care providers.
- The goal is to create an environment in which a patient can perform self-care safely and effectively, with or without the assistance of a caregiver.
- Taking a trauma-informed approach to care is essential for supporting the patient. Care workers entering a patient's home need to support an environment of physical, social, and psychological safety and acceptance. Transparent communication, trust, and mutual collaboration help the patient to maintain a sense of control in their environment and diminish the risk of the patient feeling traumatized or threatened (Hatcher, 2020).
- Insurance coverage, including provincial/territorial medicare, can be extremely limited for services offered in the community. Therefore, the time spent in the home with the patient must be well planned and used to the fullest.
- Patients living in socioeconomically disadvantaged areas may be at increased risk for injury because of the possibility of higher exposure to environmental hazards.
- Falls prevention is a critical aspect of care, especially in the community.

- A patient history to assess injury prevention and risk for falls in the home and immediate environment is part of the plan of care.

PERSON-CENTRED CARE

- As a nurse conducting home safety assessments, it is important for you to respect the patient's living space and respect that people live in a wide range of home environments that are influenced by the social determinants of health, including socioeconomic status, informal caregiver support, cultural background, and health care beliefs (Community Health Nurses of Canada, 2019). Take time to listen to the patient's health concerns and apply the knowledge you have about the person to understand which interventions within the home are likely to be accepted by the patient and caregiver.
- Communication is an essential, continuous process between you and the patient. At the first meeting, introduce yourself and ask the patient how you should refer to them. If a language or other communication barrier exists, it may be necessary to seek assistance from assistive technology or the services of a professional interpreter.
- Collaborate with the patient in assessing their home environment. Ask them whether they are willing to give you a tour of their home and explain the purpose of such a tour. Do not focus solely on what is wrong (e.g., barriers or features in disrepair); instead, point out why safety is an issue for the person (based on their health condition) and explain why a change in the immediate environment of the home may make them safer.
- Assess for culture-specific health-related beliefs that may affect a patient's willingness to use home care services. For example, an Indigenous person may have a sense of mistrust and reluctance based on previous experiences with the residential care or foster care systems and authority figures (Leckey et al., 2021). As another example, it is customary in some Muslim families for the male head of the household to speak on behalf of the female members of the household (Attum et al., 2023).
- When assessing the availability of caregivers, recognize that families, neighbours, and friends can have valuable roles in caring for the patient. Caregivers may live with the patient, live in the community, or even live a great distance away. Regardless, all members of the patient's care circle can contribute to their health and safety in the community. With the patient's permission, include these caregivers when performing the home safety assessment.
- Assess and provide support for any caregivers; the presence or absence of a caregiver could be the difference between a person remaining in the home or being readmitted to a facility.

EVIDENCE-INFORMED PRACTICE

Safety in the home is influenced by extrinsic factors, such as the physical environment, and intrinsic factors that can affect the person's ability to remain at home in a safe environment. In-home safety threats are common and may lead to high rates of mortality, morbidity, and incapacity. They often affect persons from lower socioeconomic groups or ethnic or gender minorities. Home safety is a priority across the lifespan and across populations and must be considered based on current knowledge about all ages and stages of the population, from the young child to the older person. Other priority groups at risk for unsafe home environments include persons with physical or cognitive challenges (e.g., persons living with Alzheimer's disease, dementia, or diminished visual or auditory abilities). Living in an unsafe environment can have negative impacts on the health and well-being of patients at home. The nurse must therefore be prepared to assess the home environments of patients representing a wide variety of populations (Davis & Davis, 2022).

Home health services may not be fully publicly funded because these services are funded differently from hospital and physician services. Home health services are not an insured benefit covered within the *Canada Health Act* (Health Canada, 2016). Fee structures and eligibility criteria may vary among provinces/territories for home health services and are contingent upon variables such as patient/family income, living arrangements, number of hours required, and types of services. Patients may be required to pay out of pocket or use private insurance plans, if they have them, to help subsidize the services that enable them to remain at home safely.

The federal government provides home care services to certain populations, including First Nations people living on reserve, Inuit, eligible veterans, federal inmates, and members of the Canadian Armed Forces and Royal Canadian Mounted Police (Health Canada, 2019).

SAFETY GUIDELINES

- Injury prevention begins with making timely and adequate home repairs (e.g., replacing loose floor tile, securing railings on stairwells). When patients do not have the resources to maintain a safe home environment, a nurse's role is to help identify appropriate resources or services in the community.
- The nurse plays a key role in interprofessional collaboration, working within a team of health care providers together with the patient and their caregiver(s) to determine the best approaches for meeting a patient's safety needs.
- The goal is to create a healthy environment in which the patient can optimize self-care safely and effectively.
- When helping a patient alter their home environment, make changes in a way that allow the person to retain as much of their independence and ability to perform self-care as possible. Ask the patient or caregiver whether they have concerns or questions about safety or suggestions to improve safety.
- Modifications to the home environment should be made in collaboration with the interprofessional team (e.g., occupational therapist [OT]) and should match the patient's physical strengths, remaining functional abilities, and resources.

✦ SKILL 42.1 Home Environment Assessment and Safety

The home environment should be a place where a person feels comfortable and safe. They should be able to move about freely within their home, regardless of its size, and have a sense of control over their daily routine. Achieving this level of autonomy requires maintenance of one's personal space and a sense of privacy. Taking a strengths-based approach, you can help a patient maintain independence and reduce risks in the home environment by conducting a home safety assessment.

Patients who require care in the community often experience physical alterations (e.g., progressive physical or sensory changes due to aging) that require modifications in their home environment. For example, if a patient has poor balance but good upper-arm strength, you may need to collaborate with an OT to make modifications (e.g., install handrails on both sides of a staircase and in the bathroom) to enable the person to safely walk or move throughout the house, ascend and descend stairs, and enter and exit a bathtub or shower.

Teaching a patient to safely use assistive devices (e.g., walker or cane) may help them increase their mobility and maintain independence (Fig. 42.1).

Respect the concept of personal space. Making changes too rapidly without a patient's consent leads to more problems than benefits. Appreciate the arrangement of a patient's space within the home, and do not move things or suggest modifications without their permission. Provide a rationale to the patient as to why changes are beneficial or needed. Knowing the rooms that a patient uses most frequently can help in making the adjustments to create a safe environment.

Delegation and Collaboration

The UCP, under the direction of and in collaboration with a regulated health care provider, may contribute to a home safety assessment while maintaining scope-of-practice guidelines and employer regulations.

Equipment

- Home safety checklist

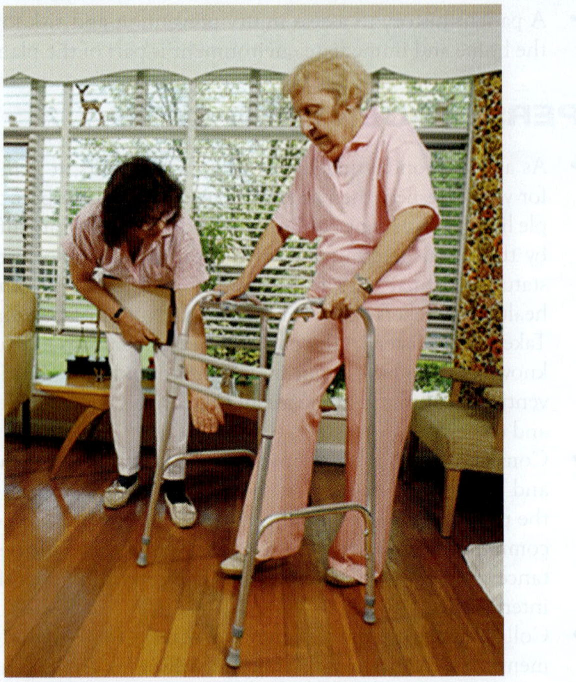

FIG 42.1 Use of a walker may help a patient remain mobile.

STEP	RATIONALE
ASSESSMENT	
1. Identify patient using at least two person-specific identifiers (e.g., name and date of birth, or name and medical record number) according to employer policy.	Ensures correct patient. Complies with Accreditation Canada's standards and improves patient safety (Accreditation Canada, 2020).
2. Throughout the procedure, the 4 moments for hand hygiene are to be implemented; hand hygiene should occur before initial patient (or patient environment) contact, before an aseptic procedure, after body fluid exposure risk, and after patient (or patient environment) contact. Additional hand hygiene should be performed when hands are visibly soiled.	Proper hand hygiene helps prevent the spread of infectious agents to other people.
3. Review risk factors that predispose patients to injuries within the home:	
a. Visual impairment	Reduced visual function alters a patient's balance, depth perception, or adaptation to dark or glaring light.
b. Hearing impairment	Prevents patient from hearing normal environmental sounds (e.g., call-out by caregiver). Prevents clear perception of home-installed alarms (e.g., smoke alarm). Interferes with communication; patient unable to hear clearly and interpret what you are saying (Hirst & Stares, 2020).
c. Neuromuscular alterations (e.g., lower-extremity weakness, unsteady gait, impaired balance, poor ankle dorsiflexion)	Age-related changes in the neurological system include slowing of reaction time (Hirst & Stares, 2020). Gait disorders make patients vulnerable to trips and falls (Schniepp et al., 2021).
d. Reduced energy or fatigue	Predisposes patients to falls.
e. Incontinence or nocturia	Frequent trips to the bathroom may cause a patient with other deficits to accidently trip or fall. Dementia affects the patient's ability to locate the bathroom and recognize the need to void (ASC, 2021).
f. History of stroke, parkinsonism, delirium, seizures, dementia, syncope	These conditions present multiple reasons for falls (Beghi et al., 2018), including impaired gait and coordination, visual changes, diminished cognition, pain, and muscle weakness.
g. Cardiopulmonary conditions: postural hypotension, arrhythmias, palpitations, difficulty breathing, shortness of breath	These conditions present multiple reasons for falls, including dizziness, light-headedness (Manemann et al., 2018), fatigue, and unsteady gait.

STEP	RATIONALE
ASSESSMENT	
h. Medication usage and history, including polypharmacy and use of sedatives, antihypertensives, antidepressants, and diuretics	Polypharmacy (use of five or more medications) and medications increase the risk of drug–drug interaction (Hirst & Stares, 2020) and can alter the patient's sense, balance, and judgement, all of which increase the risk of falls.
i. History of previous fall—obtain detailed description of previous fall	Previous fall increases risk of future fall. Helps identify circumstances that may lead to a fall (Ninomiya et al., 2020).
4. Determine whether patient has had other injuries or near misses within the home (e.g., near falls, slips, and missteps).	Onset, location, and activity associated with a fall provide further details on causative factors and how to prevent future falls (Sharif et al., 2018).
5. Have patient who has had a near fall or actual fall maintain a fall diary (Box 42.1) and teach the patient and caregiver what to do in the event of a fall.	Information in a fall diary is helpful in determining antecedents and consequences of falling.
6. Conduct *"timed up-and-go" (TUG)* test for basic mobility (see Skill 14.1).	This simple screening examination is useful in detecting difficulties with balance or gait. Collaborate with the interprofessional team (e.g., physiotherapist, pharmacist, dietitian, gerontologist, or neurologist) for further assessment (Rohm, 2020). The TUG test is a quick way to assess a patient's balance and gait (Buck, 2018).
7. Determine whether patient has a fear of falling. Indicators while ambulating are apprehension (observed in facial expressions); sweating or trembling; clutching people or objects; reluctance to change position; and wobbly, reduced mobility after fall.	Some patients may restrict mobility and participation in activities of daily living (ADLs) or instrumental activities of daily living (IADLs) because of a fear of falling (Liu et al., 2021).

Critical Decision Point *In addition to the patient, be sure to include caregivers as a resource in assessments because they may witness accident trends or patterns.*

STEP	RATIONALE
8. Partner with patient and caregivers to conduct home safety assessment:	Provides comprehensive review of all areas within the home that pose hazardous situations.
a. Front and back entrances:	
(1) Are walkways to front and back door even and free of holes or cracks?	Uneven pavement and holes may not be seen by patient, causing tripping and falls.
(2) Are home entrances, including walkways, well lit?	Poorly lit areas prevent individuals from seeing variations in walking surface.
(3) Does patient have nonskid strips and safety treads or bright-coloured paint on outdoor steps? Which colours are most easily seen by patient? Are these colours used?	Nonskid surfaces can help prevent slips on stairs. Colour on steps enables patient to see edges, accommodating for any reduced depth perception.
(4) Are doormats in good repair with nonskid backing and tapered edge?	Raised edges pose risk for tripping. Doormats without nonskid backing slide when stepped on, causing patient to lose balance.

BOX 42.1

Fall/Near-Fall Diary

Diary Setup

- In a notebook, write down the following five headings at the top of the long edge of the page: "Date," "Time of Fall," "Activity at Time of Fall," "Symptoms," and "Injury."
- Instruct patient or caregiver to complete the information under each heading as soon as possible after a fall.
- At the bottom of the page, list emergency contact numbers for the patient to call in case a fall results in serious injury.
- Instruct patient to bring the diary to the health care provider's office at the next scheduled visit or to share this information with the community care nurse during the next home visit.

If the Patient Falls

- Stay calm and assess the situation. It can take a few minutes to feel pain from injuries. Do not try to lift them up yourself; you could make things worse.
- A fall may require emergency care. If the patient hit their head or hurt their back, neck, or hip, or if you are unsure whether they are injured, call 9-1-1. While waiting for help, keep them comfortable and warm.
- The patient may need follow-up medical care if they blacked out or were dizzy before they fell, if an injury appears later, if they struggle to recover after the fall, or if they are unsteady on their feet again after the fall.

Adapted from Meiner, S. E., & Yeager, J. J. (Eds.). (2018). *Gerontologic nursing* (6th ed.). Mosby; NHS Inform. (2023). *What to do if someone falls.* https://www.nhsinform.scot/media/2971/what-to-do-if-someone-falls.pdf

STEP	RATIONALE
ASSESSMENT	
(5) Are doors in good repair and do they open and close easily? Can patient open and close all doors easily?	Opening and closing a door is difficult if grasp is weak. Tripping may occur while opening door and cause a fall.
(6) Are there sturdy handrails on both sides of stairs leading to entrance?	Handrails are recommended to be on both sides of the hallway and stairs.
(7) Are steps in good condition with even, flat surfaces?	Uneven surfaces predispose to tripping.
(8) Are doorways and stairs free of clutter?	Reduces risk of tripping or falling.
b. Kitchen:	The kitchen is one of the most hazard-oriented rooms in the home.
(1) Does patient wear clothing with short or close-fitting sleeves when cooking?	Short or close-fitting sleeves are less likely to accidently catch on fire when person works at stove.
(2) Does patient always stay in kitchen when cooking?	Lack of attention when using fire is a risk.
(3) Does patient have a loud timer to signal when food is cooked?	Prevents burning of food and risk for fire.
(4) Does patient keep stovetop and oven clean and grease-free?	Grease is highly flammable.
(5) Are stove control dials easy to see and use?	Patient may accidently use higher flame than is necessary for cooking safely.
(6) Is charged, easy-to-use fire extinguisher close at hand?	Extinguisher should always be ready for use.
(7) Has the expiry date been checked?	Over time, extinguishers lose their pressure, decreasing their effectiveness to extinguish fires (Fire-Alert, n.d.).

Critical Decision Point *Have patient identify the nearest exits and who to call in the event of a fire.*

STEP	RATIONALE
(8) Are emergency numbers for family members, health care providers, police, fire, and poison control posted on or near telephone or listed in contacts on cell phone?	Availability of emergency phone numbers and extinguisher ensures quick response if fire or accident occurs.
(9) Can items in kitchen cabinets and shelves be reached without climbing on a stool or chair?	Climbing on step stools or chairs creates risks for falls.
(10) Is there adequate lighting over the sink, stove, and work areas?	Good lighting makes it easier to see control knobs or dials and increases patient safety when they are using sharp knives or utensils.
(11) Are kitchen throw rugs and mats slip resistant?	Rugs or mats that are not slip resistant can easily slide on tile or wood floors.
(12) Assess food safety: Is the refrigerator stocked with food? Are perishable foods in the refrigerator and nonperishable foods safe to eat? Is food stored appropriately? Are expiration dates past? Is there evidence that food has spoiled? Does patient know how to prepare and store food safely?	Proper food storage and preparation can prevent foodborne illnesses. Heating food to a high enough temperature for a long enough time kills the harmful bacteria that cause foodborne illness (Health Canada, 2021). Eating foods that have spoiled or with expiration dates that have passed puts patient at risk for foodborne illness (e.g., food poisoning).
c. Bathroom:	
(1) Can patient unlock the bathroom door from both sides of the door?	Functional locks prevent person from being trapped in bathroom.
(2) Is tub or shower equipped with nonskid mats, abrasive strips, or surfaces that are not slippery?	Tub or shower bottoms can be very slippery, creating risk for falls (MedlinePlus, 2022).
(3) Does bathroom floor have a nonslip surface or rug with nonskid backing?	Wet floors increase risk of falls.
(4) Does patient avoid using slippery bath oils when bathing?	Use of bath oils makes tub surface slippery and increases risk of falls.
(5) Do bathtub and shower have at least one grab bar or handrail placed where the patient can reach it?	Grab bars provide extra support while manoeuvering into and out of tubs or showers. Grab bars placed correctly where patient can safely reach them help to steady gait and lessen chance of falls (MedlinePlus, 2022).
(6) Is patient careful not to place towels on grab bars?	Some patients accidently grab towel instead of bar when needing support. Towel can slip off bar.
(7) Does shower have stable stool or chair and handheld sprayer? Is shower easy to access (walk-in versus step-in to tub area)?	Shower stool allows patient to sit while showering.
(8) Are cold and hot water faucets clearly marked, and is temperature on water heater 49°C (120.2°F) or lower?	Accidental burns can occur from exposure to hot water.

STEP	RATIONALE
ASSESSMENT	
d. Bedroom:	
(1) Is a night light placed in bedroom or bath?	Older persons have altered night vision.
(2) Is a working smoke detector installed just outside the bedroom door?	Alarm installed just outside bedroom can awaken person early enough to help them escape fire.
(3) Can patient turn on light without having to get out of bed in the dark? Is a flashlight available at the bedside? A flashlight can be attached to a walker or cane.	Getting out of bed without proper lighting or the ability to adjust to light changes and reaching for necessary objects put patient at risk for falls.
(4) Is furniture arranged to provide clear path from bed to bathroom?	Obstructed path creates barrier that causes tripping and falls.
(5) Is phone with emergency numbers within easy reach of bed?	In an emergency, patients need to be able to reach the phone without having to get out of bed.
(6) Are other alarm systems available? Push buttons that call for help? Nursery listening devices for cognitively impaired or non-ambulatory patients?	Alarm systems placed in a readily accessible location can alert caregivers when person requires immediate help. Bedside phone, cell phone, intercom buzzer, or medical alert system can be placed in readily accessible location.
e. Living room and other rooms:	
(1) Are electrical or extension cords removed from under furniture and carpeting? Kept out of the way of traffic?	Patients can easily trip or fall over electrical cords. Hidden cords are tripping and fire hazards.
(2) Can patient turn on light without having to walk into a dark room?	Darkened room can disorient and prevent patient from seeing uneven surfaces.
(3) Are hallways and walkways free from objects and clutter?	Objects and clutter in common walkway can cause patient to trip, leading to a fall.
(4) Are loose area rugs securely attached to floor and not placed over carpeting? (For best safety, consider removing throw rugs.)	Loose edges of rugs are easy for person to trip over.
(5) Is furniture arranged in each room so patient can walk around easily?	Furniture creates obstacles to walking in room.
(6) Is all furniture steady and without sharp edges?	Patients often use edges of furniture for support when standing.
f. Around the house:	
(1) Are all living areas and stairways well lit?	Adequate lighting helps people see any barriers or uneven walking surfaces.
(2) Is flooring or carpeting throughout house in good repair?	Frayed carpet or irregular surfaces can cause tripping and result in fall.
(3) Are all thresholds level with floor or no more than 1.25 cm (0.5 inch) in height?	Uneven thresholds can cause tripping.
(4) Are light switches located at top and bottom of stairs?	Prevents individual from having to walk up or down part of stairs in dark.
(5) Does lighting produce glare or shadows on stairs or floor surfaces?	Older persons are sensitive to glare because their visual pathway becomes distorted.
(6) Do handrails run continuously from top to bottom of flights of stairs?	Handrails provide source of physical support when ascending and descending stairs.
(7) Are handrails securely attached to the wall?	Ensure at least one handrail is installed on stairs. It is recommended that handrails be installed on both sides of hallway or stairwell to reduce fall risk (Canadian Centre for Occupational Health and Safety, 2017).
(8) Are step coverings in good condition?	Loosened covering can cause tripping.
(9) Are guns kept in the house? Are trigger locks installed on all guns? Are guns stored unloaded? Is ammunition in a secure location?	Following gun safety standards decreases risk of injury and death related to gun use (Health Canada, 2019).
g. General fire safety:	
(1) Does patient have properly working smoke detectors with fresh batteries?	Smoke alarms should be properly located, with batteries checked monthly and replaced annually (Health Canada, 2022).

Critical Decision Point *Check to see when the battery in the smoke alarm was last changed; the battery should be changed annually. Instruct patient to change the battery each time they change their house clocks for daylight saving time.*

STEP	RATIONALE
ASSESSMENT	
(2) Does patient have several emergency exit plans, in case of fire?	Exit plan helps people anticipate route of escape when fire does occur. Exit should not have locks that are difficult to open or any physical barriers.
(3) Has patient determined a meeting place in event of emergency, such as at mailbox in front of home?	Use of a common emergency meeting location is an efficient method for determining that all members are safely out of the house.
(4) Does patient use portable electric heaters? Are they kept at least 1 metre away from flammable items?	Portable electric heaters should be a minimum of 1 metre away from other materials (Health Canada, 2020).
(5) Is furnace area free of items that can catch fire?	Heaters, furnaces, and chimneys pose fire risks.
(6) Does a qualified professional check the furnace and chimney annually?	Buildup of creosote within the chimney can catch fire. An overheated motor in the furnace can burn out and possibly cause fire.
(7) Does patient who smokes report smoking in bed?	Smoking was the cause of 9% of all residential fires across Canada (Garis & Biantoro, 2019). Smoking in bed poses additional fire risk, as patient may fall asleep while cigarette is lit.
h. General electrical safety:	
(1) Are electrical cords in good condition (i.e., not frayed, spliced, or cracked)?	Damaged cords can short-circuit and lead to fire (Health Canada, 2020).
(2) Are electrical cords kept away from water?	Use of any appliance or device that is exposed to water creates risk for electrical shock.
(3) Does patient use extension cords or outlet extenders with a built-in circuit breaker or fuse?	Prevents overloading of circuit, which can lead to fire.
(4) Do all wall outlets and switches have cover plates?	Prevents physical contact with wiring (Health Canada, 2020).
(5) Does patient use light bulbs of correct wattage for each fixture?	Use of excessive wattage can lead to fire.
(6) Is main electrical fuse box for home easily accessible and clearly labelled?	In event of emergency, fuse box should be easy to access so that proper circuit can be cut off.
i. Carbon monoxide (CO) safety:	
(1) Are furnace flues checked regularly for patency?	Obstructed flues are a common cause of CO toxicity.
(2) Is there a working CO detector in the home?	CO is a colourless and odourless toxic gas that can be emitted from a furnace and can lead to serious injury or death (Buck, 2018).
9. Assess patient's financial resources; determine monthly income used for ongoing expenses.	Determines potential financial resources available for making repairs to home. Reveals need for low-cost community service support.
10. Assess patient's and caregiver's willingness to make changes. Has patient accepted limitations that pose risk for injury? Determine how important functional independence is for patient.	Some patients perceive attempts to improve safety within the home as intrusive. If you show that necessary revisions to their home environment will preserve independence, the patient will participate more willingly.

NURSING DIAGNOSES

- Reduced physical mobility
- Anxiety
- Reduced memory
- Insufficient home maintenance
- Insufficient knowledge regarding safety risks
- Potential for injury and falls
- Potential for foodborne illness

Related factors and risk factors are individualized on the basis of patient's condition or needs.

PLANNING

STEP	RATIONALE
1. Expected outcomes:	
• Patient and caregiver describe potential environmental risks within home that predispose to accidents.	Demonstrates patient's and caregiver's recognition of safety risks that are of greatest concern.
• Patient and caregiver initiate actions to correct environmental risks, making the home environment safer.	Patient sees value in modifying the living environment.
• Patient remains injury-free.	Environmental barriers are reduced or removed to minimize injuries.
2. Prioritize with patient and caregiver which environmental barriers pose greatest risk.	Patient's physical and/or cognitive deficits make certain environmental risks more hazardous. Prioritization helps patient make best choices.
3. Recommend calling in a reliable contractor if major home repairs are necessary and acceptable to patient.	Ensures that repairs are made safely and correctly.

STEP	RATIONALE

IMPLEMENTATION

STEP	RATIONALE
1. Increase overall home safety:	
a. Ensure there is direct light source in areas where patient reads, cooks, uses tools, or conducts hobby work. High-intensity light on the object or surface that is involved works best.	Visual impairment in older persons usually is a result of cataracts, macular degeneration, glaucoma, or diabetic retinopathy (Hirst & Stares, 2020).

Critical Decision Point *Avoid fluorescent lighting because it creates excessive glare.*

STEP	RATIONALE
b. Consider satin and nonglossy finishes for walls, cabinets, and countertops in kitchen. Have sheer curtains or adjustable shades in other living areas.	Reduces glare for older persons.
c. Consider installing drawers with glide mechanisms in kitchen cabinets. Install C-ring handles in lower cabinets.	Makes access to food and kitchen supplies easier.
d. Install automatic door openers, level doorknob handles, and hook-and-chain locks (Boscart et al., 2023).	Devices may be easier to grasp and use. Remote-controlled door locks can also provide additional security.
e. Turn pot handles toward the centre of the stovetop, and tilt pot lids toward the back of the stove to prevent steam burns.	Reduces risk of injury and falls (Ottawa Public Health, n.d.).
2. Reduce risk of falls:	
a. Install treads with uniform depth of 22.5 cm (9 inches) and 22.5-cm (9-inch) risers (vertical face of steps).	If stairs are of uniform size, person does not have to continually adjust vision or stride.
b. Rearrange furniture to open space through hallways and major rooms.	Creates unobstructed pathway for ambulation.
c. Reduce clutter within living areas (e.g., footstools, flowerpots, extension cords, children's toys, stacked newspapers or magazines).	Mobility hazards resulting from clutter are especially risky at night.
d. Secure all carpeting, mats, and tile; place nonskid backing under small rugs and doormats. Remove throw rugs or mats in nonessential (dry) areas.	Reduces patient's risk of slipping when they step onto rug.
e. Use interprofessional collaboration when appropriate. For example, collaborate with an OT for use of specialized floors that absorb the impact of falls; collaborate with physiotherapist for use of low-rise beds, if not contraindicated.	May cushion patient's fall. Lowers distance to the floor's surface.
f. Ensure there are enough electrical outlets installed to be able to plug light or electronic device (e.g., television, video, stereo) into nearby outlet. Secure electrical cords against baseboards.	Prevents need to run extension cords across walkways.
g. Install nonskid strips on surface of bathtub and in shower stall. Be sure that floor is clean and dry, wipe up spills immediately.	Reduces chances of slipping on tub or shower.
h. Have grab bar installed in studs at tub, toilet, and shower (see Step 2h illustration). Have patient select vertical or horizontal placement if choice is available. If possible, be sure that bar is a different colour from the wall and is easy to see.	Grab bars placed where patient can safely reach them help to steady their gait and reduce chance of falls.
i. Have handrails installed alongside any stairway (see Step 2i illustration). Be sure that stairways are well lit, with switches at top and bottom of steps.	Handrails in stairwell provide greatest stability for patient.

STEP	RATIONALE

IMPLEMENTATION

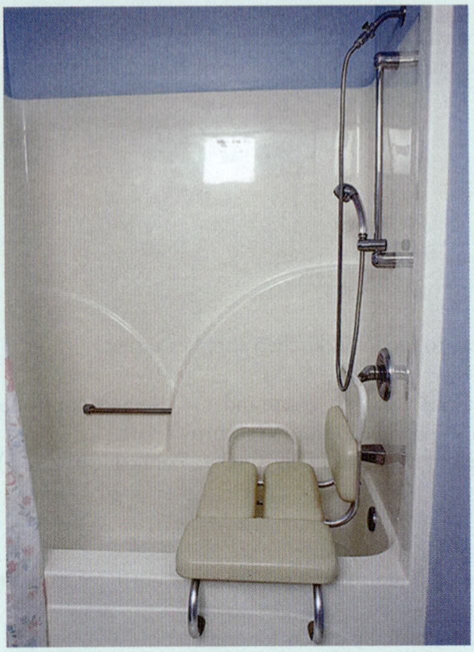

STEP 2H **Grab bars and safety seat installed in shower.**

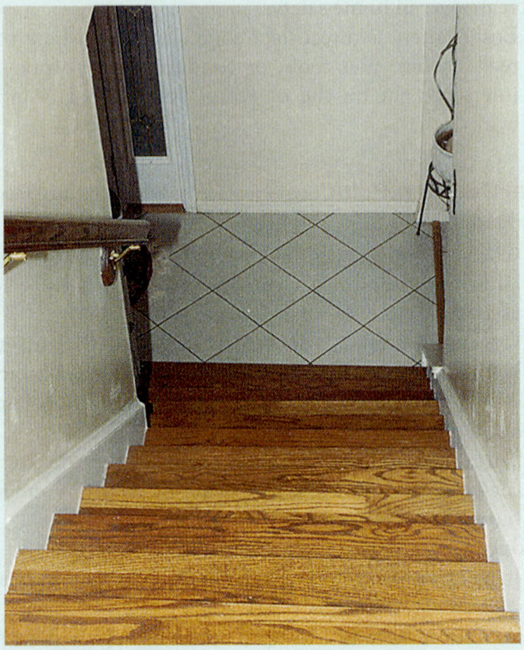

STEP 2I **Handrails installed along stairways provide security for patients with visual, balance, and coordination issues.**

j. Install appropriate broad-beam lighting for outside walkways.	Provides full illumination.
k. Keep lighted phone easily accessible, next to patient's bed.	Prevents patient from having to get up out of bed, often in dark.
l. Install motion-sensor exterior lighting for walkways and driveway.	Reduces risk of patient falls caused by dark surroundings.
m. Use interprofessional collaboration (e.g., OT, physiotherapist) for use of padding or types of clothing that will cushion bony prominences (see Step 2m illustration).	Specially designed hip protectors may be available to help cushion falls.

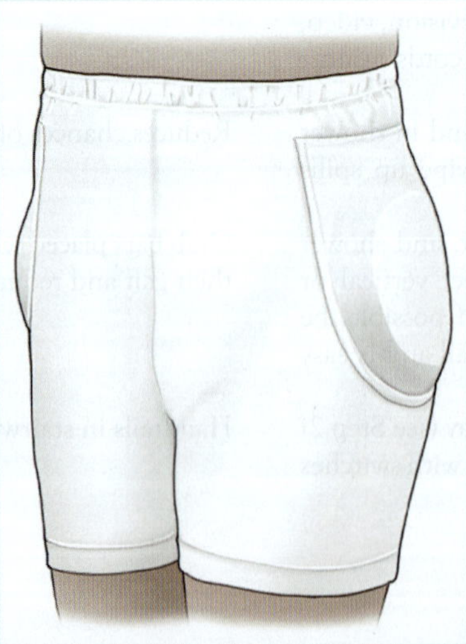

STEP 2M **Padded clothing may reduce risk of pressure injuries.** *(From Sorrentino, S. A., & Remmert, L. N. [2021]. Mosby's textbook for nursing assistants [10th ed.]. Elsevier.)*

STEP	RATIONALE
IMPLEMENTATION	
3. Prevent spread of infection:	
a. Instruct patient and caregiver to wash hands for at least 15 seconds before, during, and after meal preparation.	Clean hands will help reduce the risk of food poisoning (Centers for Disease Control and Prevention, 2022).
b. Teach patient and caregiver cleaning practices to prevent spread of infection.	Cleaning kitchen surfaces and utensils will help eliminate bacteria and reduce the risk of food poisoning (Health Canada, 2021).
c. Instruct patient not to share eating and drinking utensils.	Some infections are spread by saliva.
d. Instruct patient to clean appliances and surfaces daily.	Regular cleaning reduces risk of contamination and spread of infection (Health Canada, 2021).
e. Instruct patient in safe food preparation and storage.	Ensures safe thawing and cooking of foods. Adhering to safe storage times for food in refrigerator and freezer helps prevent foodborne illnesses (Health Canada, 2021).
f. Set refrigerator at 4°C (39.2°F) or lower and freezer to −18°C (−0.4°F) or lower.	Keeps food out of the temperature danger zone for refrigerated foods (between 4°C [39.2°F] and 60°C [140°F]), where bacteria can grow quickly (Health Canada, 2021).
4. Increase fire safety:	
a. Have smoke detectors installed near each bedroom, in kitchen, and in basement. Be sure that a detector is located on each floor of the home. Alarm should be close enough to patient to alert them, especially if they are sleeping.	Fires most frequently start in the basement near the furnace, dryer, or electrical wiring; in the kitchen; or in living areas where there is extensive wiring.
b. Have patient select fire extinguisher that is easy to handle and manipulate (see Step 4b illustration). Ask them to read instructions (if appropriate) and demonstrate its proper use (Health Canada, 2022).	Some older persons or patients with disabilities have difficulty gripping mechanisms on certain extinguishers.

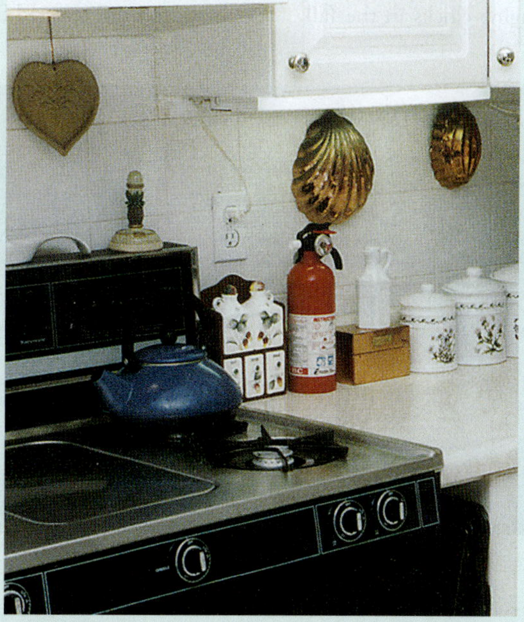

STEP 4B Fire extinguisher accessible in kitchen.

STEP	RATIONALE
c. Have area around furnace cleared of any flammable items.	Reduces risk of fire.
d. Instruct patient to verify that any portable electric heater has emergency shut-off feature and that equipment housing and electrical cords are intact.	Portable electric heaters can be overturned by accident, which can cause fire; the safety mechanism on newer models will turn the unit off immediately (Farrell, 2023).
e. Have patient make appointments for maintenance of furnace and chimney cleaning in appropriate season.	Furnace maintenance prevents short-circuits and fires. Accumulation of creosote on chimney walls can lead to fire.
f. Have patient check light-bulb wattage in all fixtures.	Ensures proper wattage being used; wattage that exceeds recommendation can cause fire.
g. Have patient establish routine for cooking, ensure the stove is clean, and ensure that items such as potholders and towels are kept away from burners.	Food cooking on stove can easily boil over or begin to burn when unattended.

STEP	RATIONALE
IMPLEMENTATION	
h. If patient is a smoker, review need to keep ashtrays clean and emptied. Placing a small amount of water or sand in the bottom of the ashtray is useful if patient is visually impaired.	Patients with reduced vision may be unable to tell whether a cigarette, cigar, or match has extinguished.
i. Strongly discourage smoking in bed or smoking after taking medication that diminishes alertness. Instruct patient and caregiver to put their cigarette out at first sign of feeling drowsy.	Risk factors for burns and fire. Patient's reaction time may be slower when tired.
j. Recommend that patient install power strips or surge protectors for plugging in multiple appliances and devices.	Reduces risk of electrical short, which can cause fire.
5. Increase burn safety:	
a. Have setting on hot water heater adjusted to 49°C (120.2°F) or lower (Buck, 2018).	Prevents scalding.
b. Instruct patient to always turn cold water on first.	Prevents direct exposure to hot water.
c. Install touch pads on lamps.	Light is easy to turn on without risk of touching hot light bulb.
d. Use colour codes (red = hot, blue = cold) on water faucets. If patient has difficulty distinguishing these colours, choose two that are easily distinguished.	Prevents accidental burning from turning on wrong faucet.
6. Increase carbon monoxide safety:	
a. Have condition of furnace venting checked annually just before turning on furnace for colder season.	Improper venting prevents escape of CO, a poisonous gas that alters hemoglobin to prevent formation of oxyhemoglobin and reduces oxygen supply to tissues.
b. Caution patients against using gas stove or barbecue grill for heating inside home.	Both appliances are sources of CO.
c. Have battery-operated CO detector installed in home; check or replace battery when changing clocks in the fall and spring (see Step 6c illustration).	Detector produces alarm when CO reaches unsafe levels. Battery operation is not affected by power outages.

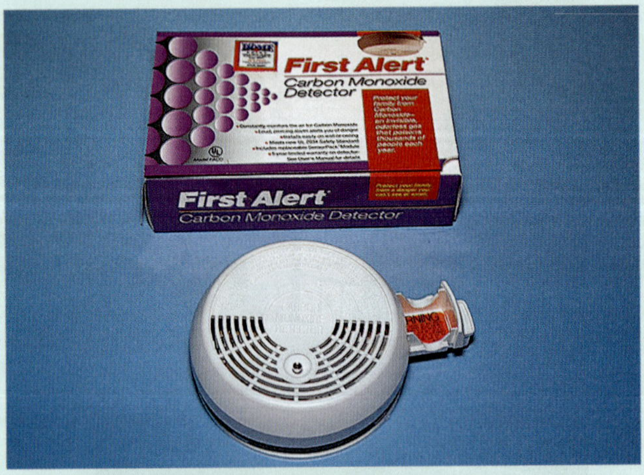

STEP 6C CO detector.

STEP	RATIONALE
7. Increase firearm safety:	
a. Teach patient about dangers associated with keeping guns in home.	Following firearm safety standards decreases risk of injury and death.
b. If guns are kept in home, teach patient to store them unloaded in a locked cabinet. Teach patient to store ammunition in a secured area separate from guns. Store keys in a place inaccessible to children.	Following firearm safety standards decreases risk of injury and death.

STEP	RATIONALE
EVALUATION	
1. Have patient and caregiver(s) identify safety risks revealed in home safety assessment.	Demonstrates patient's understanding of safety risks and the relative importance of modifying each risk to increase home safety.
2. During follow-up visit or call to patient, ask patient to discuss plans for making any modifications and observe changes patient has implemented.	Evaluates extent to which patient sees risks as potentially harmful and carries out suggested changes.
3. During follow-up visits or calls, ask patient whether they have experienced any falls or other injuries at home.	Reveals whether risks have been eliminated, depending on patient's previous history of injury.
4. During subsequent home visits, reassess for progression of dementia.	Evaluates for potential new risks to patient and caregiver.
5. Use teach-back: "I want to be sure I explained why you should make changes to your home to make it safer. Tell me why this is important." Develop a revised teaching plan if patient or caregiver is unable to teach back correctly.	Determines patient's and caregiver's level of understanding of instructional topic.

Unexpected Outcomes	Related Interventions
1. Patient and caregiver do not acknowledge risks identified in home safety assessment.	• Determine reason or reasons patient is reluctant to make changes. Consider limited resources, disbelief concerning need to make changes, fear of loss of autonomy, or other reasons. • Review implications of risks to patient's safety and welfare. • Consider offering videos and/or diagrams to help identify and explain home safety risks to patient.
2. Patient fails to make changes agreed on in previous plan.	• Determine reason for failure to make changes. • Help prioritize greatest risks. • Suggest making a single change and gauge patient's response.
3. Patient suffers fall or burn within home.	• Conduct assessment of contributing factors and conditions in environment at time of injury. • Make revisions based on assessment findings.

Communication and Documentation

- Retain a copy of the home safety assessment in patient's record.
- Document any instruction provided, patient's and caregiver's response, and changes made within the environment in progress notes in the electronic health record (EHR) or chart.

DOCUMENTATION EXAMPLE

During today's home visit, focused assessment was completed on falls prevention while reviewing home safety precautions. Patient encouraged to keep record of falls/near falls in a diary. During assessment, noted a small area rug in both the foyer and bathroom that may increase risk of a fall. Patient encouraged to remove unnecessary area rugs in high-traffic areas and was given rationale for their removal. Patient agreed and will ask caregiver to remove rugs during next home visit.

Special Considerations

Teaching

- Caregivers will benefit from learning how to safely help the patient ambulate or transfer from bed to chair or wheelchair to chair, depending on patient's mobility limitations (see Chapter 11).
- Instruct patient and caregiver about what to do in case the patient falls, including access to emergency help and how to prevent further injury.
- Teach patient and caregiver how to use any emergency assistive devices (e.g., devices that are worn around the patient's neck and a special monitor connected to the patient's telephone).
- Reinforce to caregivers the importance of preserving patient autonomy as much as possible.

Pediatric

- Assess the developmental stage of the child when considering home safety. Major risks include suffocation and strangulation, choking, falls, fire prevention, burns and scalds, poisoning, electrical injuries, drowning, and gun safety. Safety interventions to consider are as follows (Canadian Paediatric Society, 2020):
  - Install child-resistant door handle covers, especially for rooms with hazards and exit doors.
  - Keep all sharps and breakable or heavy objects in a latched drawer, locked cabinet, and out of reach.
  - Anchor top-heavy furniture or objects (televisions, dressers, bookcases) to the wall.
  - Tie up dangling cords, and push small appliances to the back of the counter when not in use.
- Caution caregivers working in the kitchen not to pour hot liquids near an infant or young child.
- When child is being bathed in the tub, an adult must always stay with them.

Gerontological

- Use "aging in place" resources and consider the person's personal health and context, without having to completely redesign the home.
- Offer resources from the National Council on Aging (https://www.ncoa.org/older-adults) and the Canadian Association of Retired Persons (CARP) (https://www.carp.ca).

Patients With Physical and Cognitive Challenges

- Consider safety measures for patients with diminished vision:
    - Have a place for everything.
    - Move fragile items out of traffic paths.
    - Remind visitors to push their chairs under the table, close/open doors fully.
    - Cover sharp corners and ensure furniture is stable.
    - Secure rug edges to prevent slips/trips and avoid clutter.
    - Keep electrical outlets covered, and tape down electrical cords that are lying on the floor.
    - Apply coloured tape or paint to colour-code controls of stove, oven, dryer, toaster, and other appliances and even on stairs.
    - Refer to the Canadian National Institute for the Blind for additional resources (https://www.cnib.ca/).
- Consider safety measures for patients with diminished hearing:
    - Find a quiet location to talk in order to reduce background noise, and face the patient and maintain eye contact while talking (National Institute on Aging [NIA], 2023).
    - When speaking, stand in good lighting and use facial expression or gestures; repeat yourself if necessary, using different words (NIA, 2023).
    - Use baby monitors that can trigger an under-pillow vibrating alarm, or connect a bedside lamp to an alarm that turns on the light when activated (Oshawa Hearing Aid Clinic, 2020).
    - Install smoke detectors and CO detectors with flashing lights or an extra loud alarm. Some display the word "FIRE" in orange (Fitzgerald, 2021).
    - Install a light-activated, vibrating, or loud doorbell with additional receivers located throughout the home (Fitzgerald, 2021).

✦ SKILL 42.2 Adapting the Home Setting for Patients With Cognitive Deficits

Patients with cognitive impairments may have to make adaptations to preserve their ability to function safely within their homes. An important aspect of safety is a person's ability to perform routine ADLs and IADLs. ADLs include a patient's ability to bathe, dress, go to the toilet, transfer, and feed themselves. IADLs include the ability to use a telephone, prepare meals, travel, do housework, take medication, and shop. Caregivers often do not understand changes in a patient's cognition and thus require help to determine whether a patient is competent to stay at home safely. Three common cognitive conditions that affect patients are depression, dementia, and delirium (the "3 Ds"). Signs and symptoms of depression, dementia, and delirium can, at first, appear to be similar, yet they become distinct as the conditions progress. Dementia and depression are progressive illnesses, whereas delirium has a rapid onset within hours to days (Hirst & Stares, 2020). *Depression* may result from social isolation (e.g., an older person becomes homebound and has few visitors and lives alone). Depression is common among older persons receiving care in the community and is characterized by functional impairment, lethargy, and isolation. It is estimated that almost half of people with dementia have also been diagnosed with depression (Heerema, 2021). It is essential to watch for signs and symptoms of depression in a person with dementia. These include apathy and loss of interest, tearfulness, loss of appetite, losing weight, irritability, psychosomatic complaints, and fatigue (Heerema, 2021).

Dementia is a progressive cognitive illness that involves memory loss; difficulties with thinking, problem solving, and language; and changes in mood or behaviour (Hirst & Stares, 2020). Dementia leads to a decline in the ability to perform basic ADLs and IADLs. In 2016, approximately 430 000 Canadians diagnosed with dementia lived at home (Canadian Institute for Health Information [CIHI], 2018). Individuals with dementia have been shown to score worse on behavioural and cognitive scales compared with those without dementia; they were also more likely to live in long-term care or require support to remain safely at home (CIHI, 2018). Some patients with dementia are at risk of wandering. Wandering in a safe environment is not harmful and can be a healthy outlet (ASC, 2022). However, a wandering patient may try to leave their place of residence unattended, necessitating the caregiver's intervention to ensure the patient's safety.

Delirium is an acute cognitive condition. Signs and symptoms of delirium include onset of short-term confusion, excitement, disorganization, disorientation, hallucinations, illusions, being easily distracted, switching from subject to subject, rambling, irrelevant or pressured speech, and disturbance in sleep–wake cycles (Hirst & Stares, 2020). Once the underlying issue is treated, symptoms of delirium diminish. It is important to seek immediate treatment if delirium is suspected.

Delegation and Collaboration

The skill of assessing and adapting the home environment for patients with cognitive deficits cannot be delegated to a UCP. The nurse is responsible for the assessment of cognitive function. The nurse directs the UCP to do the following:

- Inform the nurse when there is a change in the patient's mood, memory, and ability to maintain the home or perform self-care

Equipment

- Use appropriate tools to assess cognitive and functional status (e.g., Mini-Mental State Examination [MMSE] and the Geriatric Depression Scale [GDS]) (Hirst & Stares, 2020). Consider using the following tools:
    - Calendar
    - Paper for making lists
    - Medication organizer *(optional)*
    - Bulletin board or poster board *(optional)*
    - Electronic location device *(optional)*

STEP	RATIONALE
ASSESSMENT	
1. Identify patient using at least two person-specific identifiers (e.g., name and date of birth, or name and medical record number) according to employer policy.	Ensures correct patient. Complies with Accreditation Canada's standards and improves patient safety (Accreditation Canada, 2020).

STEP	RATIONALE
ASSESSMENT	
2. Throughout the procedure, the 4 moments for hand hygiene are to be implemented; hand hygiene should occur before initial patient (or patient environment) contact, before an aseptic procedure, after body fluid exposure risk, and after patient (or patient environment) contact. Additional hand hygiene should be performed when hands are visibly soiled.	Proper hand hygiene helps prevent the spread of infectious agents to other people.
3. Assess patient over several short periods of time. Adapt assessment if patient has sensory disabilities.	Respects dignity of patient. Improves likelihood of gathering relevant data.
4. Ensure the room is well lit with minimal outside noises or interruptions. Listen carefully and speak clearly and in a normal tone of voice.	Optimal environment for assessment of patient's cognitive, functional, and mental status provides a more valid assessment.
5. Ask patient to describe their own level of health and have them describe how it affects their ability to perform ADLs and IADLs. Ask caregivers (if available) to confirm description. Screen for at-risk behaviours (e.g., medication nonadherence, unsupervised use of stove).	Question requires patient to focus on one topic. Allows you to assess attention and concentration. Also determines whether patient is fully perceptive of physical and cognitive capabilities.

Critical Decision Point *Adapt communication to patient's and caregiver's level of understanding and comprehension. Use communication skills that demonstrate to the patient that you are listening to and value their views. The caregiver can supplement answers with the patient's consent, but the patient remains the focus of the interview.*

STEP	RATIONALE
6. Ask patient and caregiver, if appropriate, how they are handling household management responsibilities: "Tell me which bills you pay each month. Can you tell me what each one is for?" Regarding ADLs: "Can you tell me about your normal day? When do you get up, eat meals, and get dressed? Tell me what you do to dress or bathe each morning."	Provides comparison of patient and caregiver perceptions. Interaction helps to measure short-term memory, judgement, and problem solving.
7. Assess patient's adherence to taking medications. Review the number and type of medications being taken, the patient's understanding of each medication's purpose as prescribed (or as chosen for over-the-counter [OTC] medications), time of day taken, and dosages. Conduct pill count over the course of a week (caregivers may need to help). Also assess where the patient stores medications. Give special attention to pain medications, anticonvulsants, antihypertensives (especially beta-adrenergic blockers), diuretics, digoxin, Aspirin, and anticoagulants. Have patient or caregiver keep an updated list of medications that can be brought to the emergency department if needed. Ask to see medications and the list used.	Depression, dementia, and delirium can lead to poor medication adherence. Older persons frequently experience medication interactions from polypharmacy. Some medications or combinations of medications place the patient at risk for adverse effects that increase the chance of injury because of physical or cognitive changes. There can be several barriers to medication adherence: patient-related factors, such as disease-related knowledge, health literacy, and cognitive function; medication-related factors, such as adverse effects and polypharmacy; and other factors, including patient–provider relationship. Keeping a list of medications allows health care providers easy access to medication history.
8. Determine whether patient has caregivers who help with self-care or household management responsibilities. What level of support is provided? How frequently is the caregiver available? Does the patient perceive satisfaction in caregiver's support? What level of satisfaction does the caregiver perceive? Does the caregiver have access to or take advantage of respite care?	Relationship between caregivers and the patient helps define how difficult it is to provide support. The caregiver role is often stressful, particularly if the individual has other responsibilities such as parenting, work, or school. Determines availability of resource to patient and quality of that support.
9. During discussion, observe patient's dress, nonverbal expressions, appearance, and cleanliness.	Conditions such as depression and dementia can result in patient's inability to attend to personal appearance.

Critical Decision Point *Do not confuse behavioural changes with lack of available resources to maintain hygiene. Also be aware of signs and symptoms of abuse or neglect* (see Chapter 8). *Report suspected abuse immediately.*

STEP	RATIONALE
10. Observe immediate home environment.	Behavioural changes associated with cognitive dysfunction are evident in a disorderly home and inappropriate placement of objects (e.g., carton of orange juice placed inside kitchen cabinet instead of in refrigerator).

STEP	RATIONALE

ASSESSMENT

11. If you suspect a cognitive or mental status change:
    a. Complete the MMSE (e.g., Folstein test) for dementia.
    MMSE screens for orientation, attention and calculation, recall, language, and intelligence. The highest possible score is 30. A score of <24 is often considered an indication of impaired cognition (Folstein et al., 1975).
    b. Complete a depression screening, such as the GDS.
    GDS is recommended because it takes 5 minutes to administer and has been tested, validated, and used extensively for depression in older persons (Guse, 2018).
12. If you suspect the patient is at risk of wandering or is wandering, observe for the following behaviours (caregivers might provide information as well):
    - Repeated shadowing or seeking whereabouts of caregiver
    - Revisiting one destination many times
    - Inability to locate landmarks or getting lost in a familiar setting
    - Going into unauthorized or private places
    - Searching for "missing" people or places
    - Walking with no apparent destination or purpose
    - Haphazard or continuous moving, walking, or pacing
    - Walking that cannot easily be redirected

    Alerts caregivers to potential safety risks. When wandering extends outside a safe environment, the patient is at increased risk for injury or death.
13. Assess which current environmental strategies caregivers are using to deal with wandering (e.g., latches and alarms on doors, visual cues such as stop signs, constant supervision, and wearing identification band).
    Helps determine level of intervention necessary. Allows for assessment of how caregiver (who may or may not be a family member) is dealing with issues of wandering and need for additional outside support.
14. Assess caregiver for signs and symptoms of stress.
    Helps determine whether caregiver is feeling burdened or overwhelmed and needs help.

NURSING DIAGNOSES

- Acute confusion
- Reduced self-care (feeding, toileting, bathing, dressing, grooming)
- Caregiver role strain
- Wandering
- Reduced memory
- Reduced role performance
- Insufficient health and/or home maintenance
- Potential for injury

Related factors and risk factors are individualized on the basis of patient's condition or needs.

PLANNING

1. Expected outcomes following completion of procedure:
    - Patient can complete household management responsibilities within existing abilities.
      Modifications are made that help patient apply remaining cognitive functions.
    - Patient receives appropriate combination of medications for diagnosed conditions.
      Assistive devices enable patient to adhere to prescribed medication regimen.
    - Patient is able to safely perform self-care activities or receives appropriate help.
      Interventions preserve patient's autonomy and maximize their functionality.
    - Caregiver describes steps to take to minimize wandering.
      Instruction prepares caregiver to use strategies to manage wandering.
    - Patient experiences fewer episodes of wandering.
      Strategies to manage wandering are effective.
    - Caregiver identifies community resources for support.
      Services available may include respite care, adult day care programs, and support groups.
2. If patient has difficulty with self-care or fine motor skills, use interprofessional collaboration and home care resources to identify the best plan of care.
   OTs can recommend assistive devices and self-care adaptations. Home support services provide added resources for meal preparation and home cleaning. Respite care provides caregiver with temporary rest from continuous responsibilities.
3. Consider patient's level of cognitive impairment. Some patients may require only minor adaptations, while others will depend more on the help of caregivers.
   Retention of patient's independence and autonomy in a safe environment is the goal.
4. Determine best time of day for the patient.
   Some patients are more alert and responsive in the morning than in the afternoon and vice versa.

STEP	RATIONALE
IMPLEMENTATION	
1. If patient has difficulty remembering when to perform tasks (e.g., paying bills, making appointments), help to create a list or post reminder notes in a conspicuous location (e.g., bulletin board, front of refrigerator).	Lists and organizers help patient cope with memory loss and continue to safely perform activities.
2. If patient has difficulty remembering when to take medicines, help to create list or reminder note, provide medication container organized by days of week, or recommend wristwatch with alarm or schedule of text messages to signal medication administration times.	Reminder systems have benefit if the patient or caregiver is motivated and willing to adhere to them.
3. When patient has difficulty completing tasks such as paying bills or bringing groceries into the home from the store, help simplify the task.	Decreases frustration by arranging for assistance to complete tasks (e.g., paying bills through automated bank withdrawals or designating a person to buy and deliver groceries).
4. If patient has difficulty bathing, dressing, writing, and feeding, offer assistive devices (see Step 4 illustrations).	Assistive eating devices have larger handles, cup handles, or plate edges to help with meals. Assistive dressing devices use Velcro, large zippers, and elastic to facilitate independence when dressing.

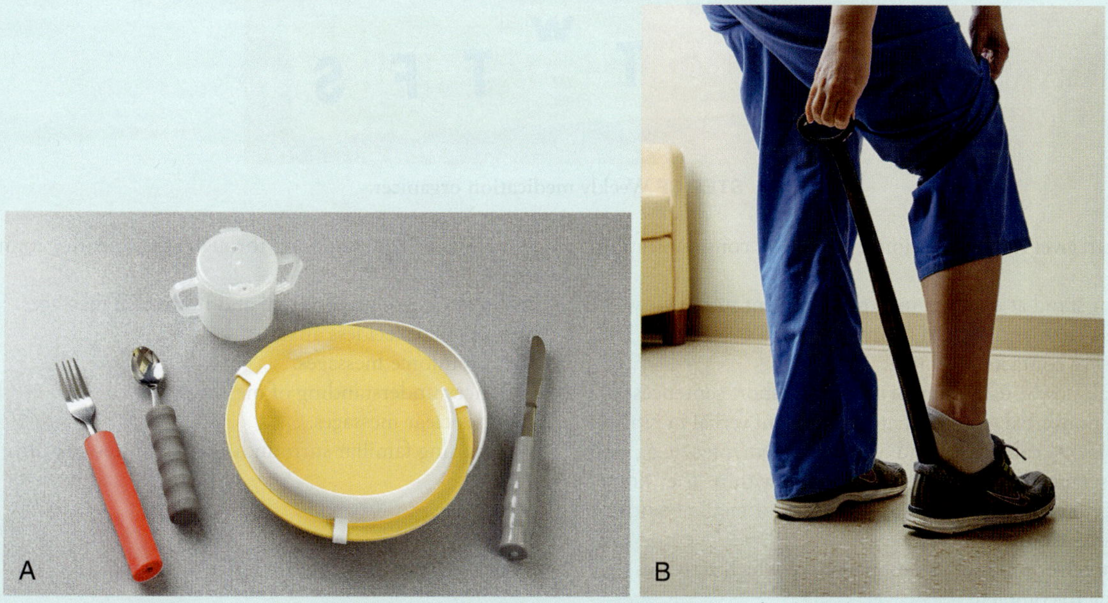

STEP 4 **A, Assistive feeding devices. B, Assistive device to help put on shoes.** *(Image used with permission of ArcMate Manufacturing Corporation. All rights reserved.)*

STEP	RATIONALE
5. Help patient and caregiver determine a routine schedule for ADLs such as eating, bathing, daily exercise, home cleaning, and napping. Have a large calendar posted in a conspicuous area to write in appointments or special planned events.	Consistency creates a sense of security and keeps patient oriented to daily activities. Routines provide security and decrease frustration.
6. Instruct caregiver to focus on patient's strengths rather than disabilities in performing ADLs (e.g., if patient has limited use of right hand, try approaches that maximize use of left hand).	Retains patient's autonomy and sense of self-worth.
7. Have caregiver help set up activities so patient can complete tasks (e.g., chopping vegetables before cooking, placing wash basin on table in bedroom for sponge bath, placing clothes to wear for that day on the bed, unpacking groceries on countertop for eventual storage, arranging food on plate with items in clockwise orientation [e.g., vegetables at 0900 hours, salad at 1500 hours, meat at 1800 hours]).	Helps patient master task even though they are unable either physically or cognitively to perform all the steps.
8. Use interprofessional collaboration, and include patient and caregiver, to generate options for scheduling medications.	Medications sometimes cause physiological changes that create risk for injury.
a. Inquire whether medications that are likely to cause confusion can be prescribed to be administered at bedtime.	Reduces risk of confusion during waking hours; confusion contributes to disorientation and risk of falling.

STEP	RATIONALE

IMPLEMENTATION

Critical Decision Point *Do not recommend bedtime medication administration if patient has nocturia because the patient will be at greater risk of falling.*

STEP	RATIONALE
b. Space antihypertensives and antiarrhythmics at different times to minimize adverse effects.	These medications cause blood pressure changes and dizziness, thus increasing risk of falls.
c. When possible, reduce the number of pain medications used.	These medications create sedative effects, increasing risk of falls.
d. Have diuretics taken early in the day rather than at night.	Diuretic effect occurs during the day while patient is awake and less fatigued.
e. Discuss with health care provider the possibility of prescribing medications for patient to take at the same time.	If safe and appropriate, taking medications at the same time will alleviate the problem of patient needing to remember multiple administration times.
f. Discuss use of medication organizer and dispenser (see Step 8f illustration).	Organizing medications in a dispenser helps patient and caregiver avoid medication errors (e.g., duplicating or missing a dose).

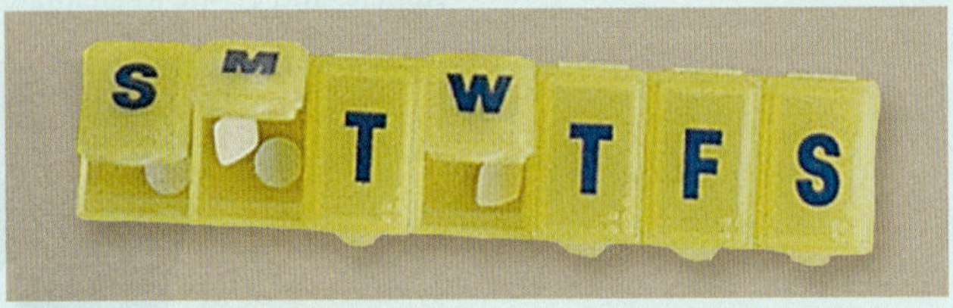

STEP 8F Weekly medication organizer.

STEP	RATIONALE
9. Teach caregiver how to use simple and direct communication:	Relays care and support through therapeutic communication techniques.
a. Sit or stand at eye level in front of patient in full view.	Promotes reception of verbal and nonverbal messages.
b. Use a calm and relaxed approach.	Helps patient feel less anxious.
c. Use eye contact and touch.	Helps reinforce messages.
d. Speak slowly, using simple words and short sentences.	Enhances understanding of messages.
e. Use nonverbal gestures that complement verbal messages.	Provides clear messages.
10. Place clocks, calendars, and personal mementos (e.g., pictures, scrapbooks) throughout rooms within the home. Enhance environment with the addition of tactile boards or three-dimensional art.	Maintaining familiar surroundings maximizes cognitive function.
11. Have caregiver routinely orient patient to which activities they are going to complete.	Supports patients with progressive dementia.
12. Be sure that patient has regular naps or rest periods during the day.	Fatigue adds to any mental status changes. Gives patient energy to perform planned activities.
13. Have caregiver encourage and support frequent visits from family and friends. Teach caregiver how to use humour and reminiscing about favourite stories to promote social interaction.	Participation in social activities prevents boredom and restlessness.
14. Provide a safe place for the person to wander (e.g., large room or fenced yard).	Reduces risk of injury and leaving residence.
15. Recommend installation of door locks or electronic guards if patient wanders.	Reduces chance of patient exiting home unsupervised.
16. Create a calm, safe setting that is appropriate for the patient's abilities.	Decreases agitation and minimizes behavioural symptoms.
17. Teach caregiver to assess for pain using an appropriate pain assessment tool (see employer policy).	Untreated pain can lead to depression, loss of appetite, social withdrawal, restlessness, aggression, and agitation (Achterberg et al., 2019). Untreated pain may lead to unstable balance and increased risk for falls (Cetin & Calik, 2020).
18. Monitor patient for personal comfort (e.g., hunger, thirst, constipation, full bladder, comfortable temperature).	Reduces stimuli that prompt wandering (Hirst & Stares, 2020).
19. Keep a list of places to which patient may wander (e.g., former homes or workplaces).	Patient may seek a familiar place.

STEP	RATIONALE
IMPLEMENTATION	
20. Install motion detector with a portable alarm near front door (i.e., exit) of residence.	Alerts caregiver to patient's attempt to exit residence.
21. Consider having patient wear an electronic locating device.	Alerts caregiver to patient's location (ASC, 2022) and enhances patient safety.
22. Assess need for full-time care.	
EVALUATION	
1. During follow-up visits, ask patient to review household management activities completed the morning of that day and previous day.	Determines patient's ability to recall events and evaluates whether patient completed planned activities.
2. Review with patient and caregiver the revised schedule for medication administration.	Evaluates understanding of regimen.
3. Ask for a medication count since last visit.	Tracking doses confirms whether patient is adhering to regimen.
4. Ask caregiver to describe ways that will increase the patient's success in completing household management and self-care activities.	Measures learning.
5. Ask caregiver to show schedules of ADLs and specific approaches used. Observe environment for presence of reality orientation cues.	Determines caregiver's success in applying information and making environmental changes.
6. Ask caregiver to describe options for minimizing wandering.	Measures learning.
7. Ask caregiver to report number of occurrences of wandering.	Determines whether reduction in wandering has occurred.
8. **Use teach-back:** "I want to be sure I explained how you can help reduce your partner's wandering. Tell me some ways you can do this." Develop revised teaching if caregiver is unable to teach back correctly.	Determines caregiver's level of understanding of instructional topic.

Unexpected Outcomes	Related Interventions
1. Patient is unable to complete ADLs or IADLs as planned.	• Further modifications are sometimes necessary. • Reassess what occurred when task was not completed. • Ask caregiver to offer suggestions.
2. Patient experiences medication interaction from multiple medications.	• Have health care provider evaluate patient's medication regimen. • Recommend feasibility of pharmacy consultation.
3. Caregiver is unable to describe or implement techniques that will improve patient's orientation and ability to complete activities.	• Reinstruction and discussion are necessary. • Support for caregiver is sometimes necessary before caregiver can learn how to support someone else.
4. Caregiver is unable to describe or implement strategies to decrease wandering.	• Consider that caregiver is unable to provide necessary support; analyze other options for support. • Reinstruction and discussion are necessary. • Caregiver may not have resources available to adapt environment.
5. Patient's wandering increases.	• Reassess strategies and precipitating factors prompting wandering.
6. Patient misses medication doses or takes wrong dosage.	• Review method for administering medications (e.g., medication dispenser). • Reconsider strategies to organize and schedule medications. • Assess patient for adverse effects.

Communication and Documentation

- Document assessment of patient's cognitive, functional, and mental status; recommended interventions; and patient's and caregiver's response in progress notes in EHR or chart.
- Report to health care provider any decline in patient's behaviour or health status.

DOCUMENTATION EXAMPLE

Patient has diagnosis of vascular dementia and lives with partner, who is the primary caregiver. Caregiver reported that patient is no longer able to manage meal preparation or brush teeth independently. Collaboratively assisted caregiver and patient to create an organizer to help with meal preparation and shopping, and a daily schedule for brushing teeth by using timer prompts and writing on the calendar in the kitchen. Both patient and caregiver are agreeable to using these tools, which will be reassessed on next home visit. Will send progress note to health care provider about the change in patient's cognitive status.

Special Considerations

Teaching

- Instruct caregiver in signs and symptoms of dementia, depression, and delirium. If delirium is suspected, contact health care provider immediately. If patient's functionality continues to decline, the caregiver may choose to learn more ADL support skills (e.g., how to help with hygiene, dressing, transfer and turning, toileting).

Pediatric

- Children with cognitive impairment are often unaware of inherent dangers during play and other activities. Adult supervision is critical.

Gerontological

- Elder abuse is becoming a growing concern for older persons living at home longer, particularly those with cognitive decline. *Elder abuse* is as any form of intentional physical, emotional, mental, financial, sexual, or spiritual maltreatment by a person in a position of trust and power (Government of Ontario, 2023). Types of abuse include physical abuse (e.g., hitting, rough handling, giving too much or too little medication, use of restraints), sexual abuse (e.g., unwanted sexual activity or sexually suggestive behaviour), emotional abuse (e.g., intimidation, insults, humiliation), financial abuse (e.g., threatening to take, or persuading person to give away, money or possessions), violation of rights and freedoms (e.g., withholding information, denying spiritual practices), and neglect (e.g., failing to provide food, clothing, safe shelter, medical attention, personal care, and necessary supervision) (Government of Ontario, 2023). Assess for signs and symptoms of elder abuse, such as unexplained injuries, changes in financial situation, conflicts between the patient and caregiver, the patient being nervous or afraid of the caregiver, lack of hygiene, and neglected environment. Report abuse immediately if suspected.
- Caregivers may need access to respite programs, which will allow them to have planned time away from their caregiving role.
- Consider that patients may not have caregivers who are able or willing to care for them. Additional help from a paid caregiver may be required if available; ability to afford in-home care may also affect the patient's ability to stay in their home and not be placed in assisted living facility.
- If wandering is an ongoing problem, have the caregiver provide current photographs of the patient to local police. Recommend the national MedicAlert Safe and Found program, which provides 24-hour emergency and wandering response services and support services (ASC, 2022; MedicAlert Foundation Canada, n.d.).

Patients With Physical and Cognitive Challenges

- Ensure a calm and predictable environment to reduce stimuli that may cause agitation and increase the risk of wandering and unintentional injury.
- Approach patients who have diminished vision or hearing calmly, and stand directly in front of them to avoid startling them.
- Face patients who have a hearing impairment while speaking, or speak into the ear from which the patient hears the best.

✦ SKILL 42.3 Medication and Medical Device Safety

On the first visit, review and list all patient's medications and medication bottles. It is important to note medication name, dosage, frequency, and route and compare that list with any previous lists (e.g., known medications ordered by health care provider and any specific instructions). This process is known as *medication reconciliation*; the goal is to ensure that there are no errors or omissions in a patient's medication regimen while also assessing for any need to make changes to the medications prescribed (Buck & Picinbono-Larose, 2018). Community pharmacies are a valuable resource for information on medications.

Patients in the home frequently manage the administration of medications and use of medical devices such as syringes, blood glucose monitoring equipment, dressing supplies, and even intravenous (IV) devices. These tasks include administration, storage, and disposal of medications and medical devices. It is critical that a patient administer medications correctly, use devices properly, clean equipment thoroughly, and remove waste properly. Infection control is just one safety principle that a patient and caregiver must learn for the home setting. Nurses need to make sure that patients know the regulations regarding waste disposal and follow the procedures in accordance with local and provincial/territorial laws (e.g., place soiled dressings in securely fastened plastic bags before adding to regular garbage; use garbage containers with tight lids to avoid attracting animals).

Patients who require special consideration include those with acute sensory or neurological impairment; those with chronic illness such as diabetes mellitus or arthritis; and older persons, who frequently have physical limitations that make manipulating medical devices and dispensing medications difficult. For example, patients with arthritic hands are often unable to open medication containers because of weakness in the hands and the pain created by pressure on the joints.

Delegation and Collaboration

The skill of assessing for and monitoring medication and medical device safety cannot be delegated to a UCP. The nurse directs the UCP to do the following:

- Make suggestions that further ensure patient safety regarding the use of basic infection control practices
- Make suggestions about how to properly dispose of sharps, needles, and contaminated supplies in the home

Equipment

- Coloured marking pens
- Labels
- Puncture-resistant sharps container or 2-L hard plastic bottle with cap
- Duct, masking, or adhesive tape
- Assistive devices (e.g., syringe magnifier)
- Medication organizers

STEP	RATIONALE
ASSESSMENT	
1. Identify patient using at least two person-specific identifiers (e.g., name and date of birth, or name and medical record number) according to employer policy.	Ensures correct patient. Complies with Accreditation Canada's standards and improves patient safety (Accreditation Canada, 2020).
2. Throughout the procedure, the 4 moments for hand hygiene are to be implemented; hand hygiene should occur before initial patient (or patient environment) contact, before an aseptic procedure, after body fluid exposure risk, and after patient (or patient environment) contact. Additional hand hygiene should be performed when hands are visibly soiled.	Proper hand hygiene helps prevent the spread of infectious agents to other people.
3. Assess patient's sensory, musculoskeletal, and neurological function (see Chapter 8), specifically hand strength, ability to read labels on containers, ability to read doses on syringe, and ability to prepare medicine in a syringe.	Reveals any deficits that will affect preparation and use of medications or medical devices. Print size on the label may be too small to read.
4. If caregiver provides routine help, ask caregiver whether they have any concerns about being able to care for patient.	Assesses caregiver's health. Nurses can help educate caregivers on the need for help and provide information to avoid injury.
5. Assess patient's medication regimen and length of time that the patient has been receiving each medication. Ask patient to describe doses and schedule for each medication.	Determines how familiar patient or caregiver is with the regimen and assesses potential misunderstanding of instructions.
6. Assess patient's and caregiver's health literacy level (e.g., ask them to read a medication label out loud to you).	Helps ensure that patient and caregiver can read and understand medication that patient is taking. Helps prevent medication errors.

Critical Decision Point *Be sure that medication labels are not confusing for a patient. For example, the Spanish word for eleven is written as "once." A Spanish-speaking patient could confuse a medication direction that requires them to take a medication 1 time per day as 11 times per day.*

STEP	RATIONALE
7. Ask patient to show you where medications are stored in the home. Look at each container.	Determines condition and labelling of containers.
8. Assess temperature of storage area.	Medication, including insulin, should not be stored in extreme heat or extreme cold (Roedler, 2020) or near food in the refrigerator.
9. If patient self-administers injections, ask to see where they store supplies and what they use to dispose of used syringes and needles.	Determines sterility of equipment and whether method of disposal creates risk for needle-stick injuries to patient, caregiver, or nurse.
10. If patient uses a glucose-monitoring device, ask to see where the monitor, lancets, and glucose strips are stored. Also ask how patient disposes of lancets.	Allows you to examine cleanliness of equipment, sterility of lancets, and condition of glucose strips. Sharps should be disposed of in a puncture-proof container.

NURSING DIAGNOSES

- Insufficient knowledge regarding medication safety
- Insufficient health maintenance
- Nonadherence
- Caregiver role strain
- Potential for injury
- Potential for infection

Related factors and risk factors are individualized on the basis of patient's condition or needs.

PLANNING

STEP	RATIONALE
1. Expected outcomes following completion of procedure:	
• Patient and caregiver discuss principles of medication safety.	Patient education includes information and techniques for safe medication administration.
• Patient and caregiver prepare medications independently.	Adaptations successfully accommodate patient's and caregiver's deficits in handling and manipulating equipment.
• Patient and caregiver identify correct conditions for storing medications, medical devices, and supplies.	Instruction focuses on ensuring infection control measures.
• Patient and caregiver dispose of used medical equipment and supplies correctly.	Appropriate receptacles and methods for disposal are made available and used.

IMPLEMENTATION

STEP	RATIONALE
1. Teach patient and caregiver the following principles to ensure that medications are safe to use:	
a. Always use prescriptions provided by your pharmacy (Pharmacy Association of Nova Scotia [PANS], n.d.).	Medications must be of full strength and used for an appropriate pharmacological reason to have therapeutic benefit.
b. Do not take any expired medicine as noted on the container.	Expired medication is sometimes toxic or no longer effective.
c. Do not place different medicines in the same container.	Prevents accidental "mix-up" of medications and medication error.
d. Do not place medications in pill containers different from their original ones.	Prevents accidental "mix-up" of medications and confusion about expiration dates.
e. Always finish prescribed medication; do not save for future illness.	Prevents underdosing or inappropriate dosing.
f. Wash hands before and after administering or taking medication.	Contaminated hands are source of infection transmission.
2. Recommend approaches to preparing medications:	
a. For patients with weakened grasp or pain in hands and fingers, recommend a screw-top container.	Tops of childproof containers are difficult to remove.

Critical Decision Point *If the patient has children or grandchildren who have easy access to the medication storage area or patient's purse, ensure that medications are stored in a secure place.*

STEP	RATIONALE
b. For patients taking multiple medications, propose the use of a colour-coding system. The same colour is used for medications that need to be taken at the same time. Mark tops of bottle caps with a coloured marking pen.	Technique helps patient take correct medications and doses at correct times of day. Best used when patient is reliable in self-administration.
c. Provide specially designed syringes with large numerals or syringe magnifier for patients with visual alterations (see Step 2c illustration).	Ensures that accurate dose of medication is prepared in syringe.

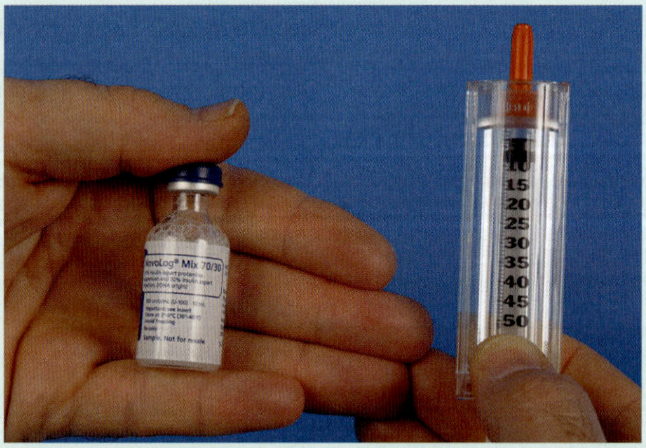

STEP 2C Syringe with magnifier.

STEP	RATIONALE
d. For patients who have difficulty manipulating syringes, offer spring-loaded needle insertion aid.	Delivers injection safely without manipulation of plunger.

Critical Decision Point *Teach caregivers what to do following a needle-stick injury. Wash the affected area thoroughly with soap and water and dry. If the patient has acquired immunodeficiency syndrome (AIDS), hepatitis, or some other communicable disease, caregivers should pursue appropriate laboratory testing.*

STEP	RATIONALE
e. Teach caregivers how to properly draw up prescribed volume of medication into syringe. When necessary, have caregiver prepare extra prefilled syringes for patient's use when the caregiver is absent.	Ensures that caregiver knows proper preparation techniques and that patient has access to injections. Watch patient and caregiver draw up and dispense medications to determine whether more teaching is needed.
3. Recommend approaches to storing medications and supplies:	
a. Store medications in a safe, dry place, preferably in the kitchen, away from the microwave or stove.	Moisture and excessive heat may cause medications to decompose.
b. Keep liquid medications and parenteral medications, especially insulin, in a cool place.	Prevents decomposition of medication.

STEP	RATIONALE

IMPLEMENTATION

Critical Decision Point *Although manufacturers recommend storing insulin in the refrigerator, injecting cold insulin can sometimes make the injection more painful. To avoid this problem, store the bottle of insulin being used at room temperature. Insulin kept at room temperature will last for approximately 1 month. However, remember to store extra bottles in the refrigerator if a patient buys more than one bottle at a time* (Roedler, 2020). *If insulin is stored in the refrigerator, be sure that medication is in a bin or container, away from food.*

STEP	RATIONALE
c. Keep medical supplies such as syringes, dressing supplies, and glucose meter in an airtight container (e.g., plastic storage bin) and store in a cool place, such as a bedroom closet.	Ensures that supplies are not exposed to moisture or other contaminants.
d. Instruct patient and caregiver to use a new needle with each medication administration.	Multiple use of the same needle puts patient at risk for infection.
4. Review with patient and caregiver the proper techniques to dispose of medications, "sharps," and disposable medical supplies:	Proper practices are necessary to prevent patient injury.
a. Return expired and unused prescription medications to the pharmacy for disposal (PANS, n.d.).	Medications can be harmful to the environment when disposed of improperly (Public Safety Canada [PSC], 2022).
(1) DO NOT FLUSH unused medications.	Environmental impact studies report that flushing medications down the toilet could be having an adverse impact on the environment (PSC, 2022).
(2) Return all unused medications to the community pharmacy. Patients are advised against disposing of any medications in the home setting (PSC, 2022).	Medication return programs at local pharmacies will ensure safe and proper disposal of medications (PSC, 2022).
b. Obtain a sharps container from a medical supply store or IV equipment supplier. (If finances are limited, have patient use a small-neck plastic bottle such as a soda bottle.) Dispose of all needles and lancets in container.	A puncture-proof container prevents exposure to contaminated needle. A small-neck container makes it difficult for anyone to easily retrieve a used needle or sharp.
c. Caution against filling a sharps container to the point where needles protrude from the opening. Return container to pharmacy when it is three-fourths full, securing top with duct tape or adhesive tape.	Prevents needle-stick injuries.
d. Dispose of soiled dressings, used glucose testing trips, and IV tubing in a separate, sealed plastic garbage bag. Place in a second plastic bag (double-bagged) and discard appropriately as garbage.	Prevents contamination with other items in the home. Minimizes chances of caregiver's exposure to infectious waste.

EVALUATION

STEP	RATIONALE
1. Have patient and/or caregiver describe steps to take to ensure that medications are safe to use.	Demonstrates learning.
2. Observe how patient and/or caregiver prepare and administer medication dose.	Evaluates ability to physically manipulate medications and necessary equipment.
3. Observe home setting for appropriate storage of medications and supplies.	Evaluates patient's and/or caregiver's adherence to recommendations.
4. Have patient or caregiver describe how sharps or medical equipment is discarded.	Demonstrates learning.
5. Do medication counts (pills remaining in containers) at successive intervals, such as twice a week for 2 weeks.	Verifies that patient is taking correct number of medications over a period of time.
6. **Use teach-back:** "I want to be sure I explained the importance of not throwing needles and sharp objects (e.g., lancets) in the garbage. Tell me how to dispose of these safely and why it is important." Develop a revised teaching plan if patient or caregiver is unable to teach back correctly.	Determines patient's and caregiver's level of understanding of instructional topic.

Unexpected Outcomes	Related Interventions
1. Patient or caregiver is unable to recall principles for safe use of medications.	• Reinstruction is necessary, or patient and caregiver need a chance to ask more questions regarding benefit of precautions. • Offer simple, plain-language, written instructions.

Unexpected Outcomes	Related Interventions
2. Patient or caregiver has difficulty or is unable to prepare and administer medication.	• Offer further help to set up equipment. • Offer assistive aids. • Provide reinstruction on steps used to prepare medication.
3. Medications and medical devices are not stored in a secure or appropriate location.	• Assess whether patient chooses to store items conveniently rather than safely or has limited resources. • Reinstruction and discussion are necessary.
4. Sharps and disposable medical equipment are not disposed of properly.	• Provide reinstruction. • Arrange to provide appropriate containers.
5. Excess or insufficient number of pills found during pill count.	• Review with patient and caregiver daily medications prescribed. • Re-evaluate use of dosage reminders. • Notify health care provider.

Communication and Documentation

- Document instructions and recommendations to patient and caregiver and results of return demonstrations in progress notes in EHR or chart.
- Report to health care provider any unsafe situation.

DOCUMENTATION EXAMPLE

During today's home visit, this writer reviewed medication administration with patient who has several medications dispensed in bottles and who lives alone. Patient successfully identified the purpose of each medication, yet was unable to remember the order in which to take the medication throughout the day. Patient agreed to allow writer to contact the community pharmacy and arrange to have medications dispensed in blister packs for ease of use. The blister packs will be ready for pickup this evening, and the caregiver has agreed to pick them up and deliver them to patient.

Special Considerations

Pediatric

- Store sharps container in an area that is inaccessible to children.
- Store medications in child-resistant container or a locked cabinet or drawer.
- Avoid taking medicines in front of children and do not leave caps loose.
- Never call medicine "candy."

Gerontological

- Changes that naturally occur as individuals age, including reduced gastric acid, delayed gastric emptying, decreased circulatory plasma, impaired peripheral blood flow, increased or decreased body fat, and decreased renal function, may contribute to an altered drug response in older persons (Hirst & Stares, 2020).

Patients With Physical and Cognitive Challenges

- Consider the following for patients with diminished vision:
  - Ask the pharmacy to type larger labels on all medication containers or ask for labels to be written in Braille to ensure readability for patients who are legally blind.
  - Have the patient practise feeling different pills for the size of different medication bottles, until these become familiar (American Printing House for the Blind [APHB], n.d.).
  - Separate medications by location: keep breakfast pills in the kitchen and evening pills on the bedroom nightstand (APHB, n.d.).
  - Arrange to have medications prepackaged in blister packs (APHB, n.d.).
- Consider the following for patients with diminished hearing:
  - Encourage the use of visual reminders for medication, such as a calendar, alarm with a light, or cell phone app.

✦ REVIEW QUESTIONS

A nurse receives a home referral for a patient (she/her) recently hospitalized for heart failure. In preparation for her initial visit, the nurse reviews the referral report. The patient is 79 years old and lives with her 59-year-old sibling in a split-level four-bedroom home that they have owned for over 50 years. The patient has a history of osteoporosis and early-onset Parkinson's disease. The patient has been prescribed both a diuretic and an angiotensin-converting enzyme inhibitor for heart failure. This medication is in addition to the medications she takes for Parkinson's and glaucoma. She has advanced glaucoma and diminished hearing but does not wear hearing aids. The sibling, who is employed as a service worker at a local elementary school, reportedly provides assistance when the patient has difficulty with activities of daily living (ADLs). The home referral is aimed at performing an assessment of the patient's home situation and any health implications.

Review Questions 1 to 5 relate to the case study presented here.

1. After reviewing the referral history, which of the following factors should the nurse assess to determine the patient's fall risk, considering the known effects of the patient's health conditions? (*Select all that apply.*)

1. Fatigue
2. Joint discomfort
3. Cognitive change
4. Reduced depth perception
5. Impaired gait
6. Hearing acuity

2. The nurse assesses the patient's knowledge of the medications they are now prescribed to take. The nurse asks the patient to

describe the medication schedule and whether there are any problems in following that schedule. Which of the following problems might the nurse anticipate the patient to have, based on the nurse's knowledge of Parkinson's disease and glaucoma?
1. Ability to store medications in a dry place
2. Ability to read medication label and warning stickers on bottle
3. Ability to use a medication organizer
4. Health literacy level
5. Ability to open medication bottle
6. Caregiver ability to assist in medication preparation

3. The nurse chooses to assess the patient's ability to follow a medication schedule successfully. What is the best approach for measuring this outcome?
4. The nurse plans an assessment of the patient's home environment for potential hazards. Which of the following hazards is most likely to pose risks because of the patient's glaucoma?
   1. Absence of handrails on both sides of staircase to upper level of home
   2. Presence of throw rugs or mats on floors
   3. Condition of lighting over sink, stove, and work area
   4. Phone with emergency numbers within easy reach at bedside
   5. Condition of furniture in living room
5. The nurse visits the patient again 7 days later. The patient has missed two doses of the diuretic prescribed for heart failure. The patient has difficulty recalling the times the medications are due to be taken. The nurse asks the patient whether the patient's sibling can be involved in a discussion regarding ways to improve medication adherence. The patient agrees. What is the first priority for the nurse to consider before involving the sibling in the plan of care?
   1. Sibling's health literacy
   2. Sibling's concerns about being able to care for the patient
   3. Sibling's willingness to make changes to home environment
   4. Sibling's functional limitations that affect their ability to assist the patient

Visit the Evolve site for a complete list of answers to the Review Questions.

NEXT GENERATION NCLEX® (NGN)

For practice with answering exam questions related to unfolding NGN case studies, please consult the Next Generation NCLEX® (NGN)-Style Case Studies for Skills and Techniques on the Evolve website: http://evolve.elsevier.com/Canada/Perry/clinicalskills/

REFERENCES

Accreditation Canada. (2020). *Required organizational practices–2020 handbook.* https://physicians.nshealth.ca/resources/required-organizational-practices-2020-handbook

Achterberg, W., Lautenbacher, S., Husebo, B., et al. (2019). Pain in dementia. *Pain Reports, 5*(1), e803. https://doi.org/10.1097/PR9.0000000000000803

Alzheimer Society of Canada. (n.d.). *Making your environment safe.* https://alzheimer.ca/en/help-support/im-caring-person-living-dementia/ensuring-safety-security/making-your-environment-safe

Alzheimer Society of Canada. (2021). *Toilet problems, continence, and dementia.* https://www.alzheimers.org.uk/get-support/daily-living/toilet-problems-continence

Alzheimer Society of Canada. (2022). *Tracking devices.* https://alzheimer.ca/en/help-support/im-caring-person-living-dementia/ensuring-safety-security/locating-devices

American Printing House for the Blind. (n.d.) *Organizing your medications.* https://visionaware.org/for-seniors/health-and-aging/managing-your-medication/organizational-systems/

Attum, B., Hafiz, S., Malik, A., et al. (2023). *Cultural competence in the care of Muslim patients and their families.* StatPearls. https://www.ncbi.nlm.nih.gov/books/NBK499933/

Beghi, E., Gervasoni, E., Pupillo, E., et al. (2018). Prediction of falls in subjects suffering from Parkinson disease, multiple sclerosis, and stroke. *Archives of Physical Medicine and Rehabilitation, 99*(4), 641–651. https://doi.org/10.1016/j.apmr.2017.10.009

Boscart, V., McCleary, L., Sheiban Taucar, L., et al. (2023). *Ebersole and Hess' gerontological nursing and health aging in Canada* (3rd ed.). Elsevier.

Buck, M. (2018). Safety. In B. Kozier, G. Erb, A. Berman, et al. (Eds.), *Fundamentals of Canadian nursing: Concepts, process, and practice* (4th ed., pp. 761–791). Pearson Canada.

Buck, M., & Picinbono-Larose, C. (2018). Medications. In B. Kozier, G. Erb, A. Berman, et al. (Eds.), *Fundamentals of Canadian nursing: Concepts, process, and practice* (4th ed., pp. 792–874). Pearson Canada.

Canadian Centre for Occupational Health and Safety. (2017). *Stairways–Falls prevention.* https://www.ccohs.ca/oshanswers/safety_haz/stairs_fallprevention.html. [Seminal Reference].

Canadian Institute for Health Information. (2018). Dementia in home and community care. In *Dementia in Canada [Report].* https://www.cihi.ca/en/dementia-in-canada/dementia-care-across-the-health-system/dementia-in-home-and-community-care

Canadian Paediatric Society. (n.d.). *Caring for kids–Safety and injury prevention at home.* https://caringforkids.cps.ca/handouts/safety-and-injury-prevention

Canadian Paediatric Society. (2020). *Keep your young child safe around the house.* https://caringforkids.cps.ca/handouts/safety-and-injury-prevention/keep_your_young_child_safe

Centers for Disease Control and Prevention. (2022). *Handwashing: A healthy habit in the kitchen.* https://www.cdc.gov/handwashing/handwashing-kitchen.html

Cetin, S. Y., & Calik, B. B. (2020). Investigation of the relationship between activity performance, frequency of fall, and pain in elderly people living at home. *Topics in Geriatric Rehabilitation, 36*(2), 97–102. https://doi.org/10.1097/TGR.0000000000000268

Community Health Nurses of Canada. (2019). *Canadian community health nursing professional practice model and standards of practice.* https://www.chnc.ca/en/standards-of-practice

Davis, K. L., & Davis, D. D. (2022). *Home safety techniques.* StatPearls. https://www.ncbi.nlm.nih.gov/books/NBK560539/

Farrell, M. H. J. (2023). *How to be sure you're using your space heater safely.* https://www.consumerreports.org/space-heater/space-heater-safety-tips-a1096367334/

Feist, H. (2019). Emergency nursing. In M. El Hussein, & J. Osuki (Eds.), *Brunner and Suddarth's Canadian textbook of medical-surgical nursing* (4th ed., pp. 2338–2379). Wolters Kluwer.

Fire-Alert. (n.d.). *Can I use an expired fire extinguisher?* https://fire-alert.ca/expired-fire-extinguisher/

Fitzgerald, R. (2021). *Deaf or hearing loss: Home safety checklist.* https://www.uphomes.com/blog/deaf-or-hearing-loss-home-safety-checklist.html

Folstein, M. F., Folstein, S. E., & McHugh, P. R. (1975). "Mini-mental state": A practical method for grading the cognitive state of patients for the clinician. *Journal of Psychiatric Research, 12*(3), 189–198. https://doi.org/10.1016/0022-3956(75)90026-6. [Seminal Reference].

Franklin, R. C., & Sleet, D. A. (2018). Injury prevention and health promotion: A global perspective. *Health Promotion Journal of Australia: Official journal of Australian Association of Health Promotion Professionals, 29*(2), 113–116. https://doi.org/10.1002/hpja.191

Garis, L., & Biantoro, C. (2019). *Fires in Canada originating from smoking materials: Analysis of Canadian fire incidents.* University of the Fraser Valley, School of Criminology and Criminal Justice & Centre for Public Safety and Criminal Justice Research. https://cjr.ufv.ca/wp-content/uploads/2019/03/Fires-in-Canada-Originating-from-Smoking-Materials-March-2019.pdf

Government of Ontario. (2023). *Information about elder abuse.* https://www.ontario.ca/page/information-about-elder-abuse

Guse, L. (2018). Comprehensive assessment of the older adult. In K. Mauk (Ed.), *Gerontological nursing: Competencies for care* (4th ed., pp. 620–702). Jones & Bartlett Learning.

Hatcher, T. L. (2020). *Integrating trauma informed care in home health: COVID-19 considerations.* https://www.relias.com/blog/integrating-trauma-informed-care-home-health

Health Canada. (2016). *Home and community health care.* https://www.canada.ca/en/health-canada/services/home-continuing-care/home-community-care.html

Health Canada. (2019). *Canada's health care system.* https://www.canada.ca/en/health-canada/services/health-care-system/reports-publications/health-care-system/canada.html

Health Canada. (2020). *Electrical product safety.* https://www.canada.ca/en/health-canada/services/home-safety/electrical-products.html

Health Canada. (2021). *Food safety and you.* https://www.canada.ca/en/health-canada/services/general-food-safety-tips/food-safety-you.html

Health Canada. (2022). *Fire safety in your home.* https://www.canada.ca/en/health-canada/services/home-safety/fire-safety.html

Health Excellence Canada. (2017). *Patient/client safety in the home.* https://www.patientsafetyinstitute.ca/en/education/PatientSafetyEducationProgram/PatientSafetyEducationCurriculum/Pages/Module-18-Patient-Client-Safety-in-Home-Care.aspx

Heerema, E. (2021). How to recognize the symptoms of depression in dementia. https://www.verywellhealth.com/recognizing-the-symptoms-of-depression-in-dementia-98566

Hirst, S., & Stares, R. (2020). Health care of the older adult. In M. El Hussein, & J. Osuki (Eds.), *Brunner and Suddarth's Canadian textbook of medical-surgical nursing* (4th ed., pp. 210–237). Wolters Kluwer.

Kirchner-Heklau, U., Krause, K., & Saal, S. (2021). Effects, barriers and facilitators in predischarge home assessments to improve the transition of care from the inpatient care to home in adult patients: An integrative review. *BMC Health Services Research*, *21*, 540. https://doi.org/10.1186/s12913-021-06386-4

Leckey, R., Schmieder-Gropen, R., Nnebe, C., et al. (2021). Indigenous parents and child welfare: Mistrust, epistemic injustice, and training. *Social & Legal Studies*, *31*(4), 559–579. https://doi.org/10.1177/09646639211041476

Liu, M., Hou, T., Li, Y., et al. (2021). Fear of falling is as important as multiple previous falls in terms of limiting daily activities: A longitudinal study. *BMC Geriatrics*, *21*(350). https://doi.org/10.1186/s12877-021-02305-8

Manemann, S., Chamberlain, A. M., Boyd, C. M., et al. (2018). Fall risk and outcomes among patients hospitalized with cardiovascular disease in the community. *Circulation: Cardiovascular Quality and Outcomes*, *11*(8), e004199. https://doi.org/10.1161/CIRCOUTCOMES.117.004199

MedicAlert Foundation Canada. (n.d.). *Safe and found.* https://www.medicalert.ca/safe-and-found

MedlinePlus. (2022). *Bathroom safety for adults.* US National Library of Medicine. https://medlineplus.gov/ency/patientinstructions/000021.htm

National Institute on Aging. (2023). *Hearing loss: A common problem for older adults.* https://www.nia.nih.gov/health/hearing-loss-common-problem-older-adults

Ninomiya, K., Takahira, N., Ikeda, T., et al. (2020). Predictors of falls in patients during the first year after total hip arthroplasty: A prospective cohort study. *Health Science Reports*, *3*(3), E184. https://doi.org/10.1002/hsr2.184

Oshawa Hearing Aid Clinic. (2020). *Home safety for people with hearing loss.* https://www.oshawahearing.ca/blog/home-safety-tips/

Ottawa Public Health. (n.d.). *Kitchen safety tips.* https://www.ottawapublichealth.ca/en/Public-Health-Topics/resources/Documents/kitchen_safety_tips_en.pdf

Parachute Canada. (n.d.). *Discover how to prevent injuries before they happen.* https://www.parachutecanada.org/en/injury-topics/

Pharmacy Association of Nova Scotia. (n.d.). *Medication storage and disposal.* https://pans.ns.ca/medication-storage-disposal

Public Safety Canada. (2022). *Prescription drug return initiatives in Canada.* https://www.publicsafety.gc.ca/cnt/rsrcs/pblctns/prscptn-drg-rtrn/index-en.aspx

Roedler, R. (2020). Assessment and management of patients with diabetes mellitus. In M. El Hussein, & J. Osuki (Eds.), *Brunner and Suddarth's Canadian textbook of medical-surgical nursing* (4th ed., pp. 1136–1190). Wolters Kluwer.

Rohm, C. D. (2020). Interprofessional collaboration to reduce falls in the acute care setting. *Medsurg Nursing*, *29*(5), 303–307.

Schniepp, R., Huppert, A., Decker, J., et al. (2021). Fall prediction in neurological gait disorders: Differential contributions from clinical assessment, gait analysis, and daily-life mobility monitoring. *Journal of Neurology*, *268*, 3421–3434. https://doi.org/10.1007/s00415-021-10504-x

Sharif, S. I., Al-Harbi, A. B., Al-Shihabi, A. M., et al. (2018). Falls in the elderly: Assessment of prevalence and risk factors. *Pharmacy Practice*, *16*(3), 1206. https://doi.org/10.18549/PharmPract.2018.03.1206

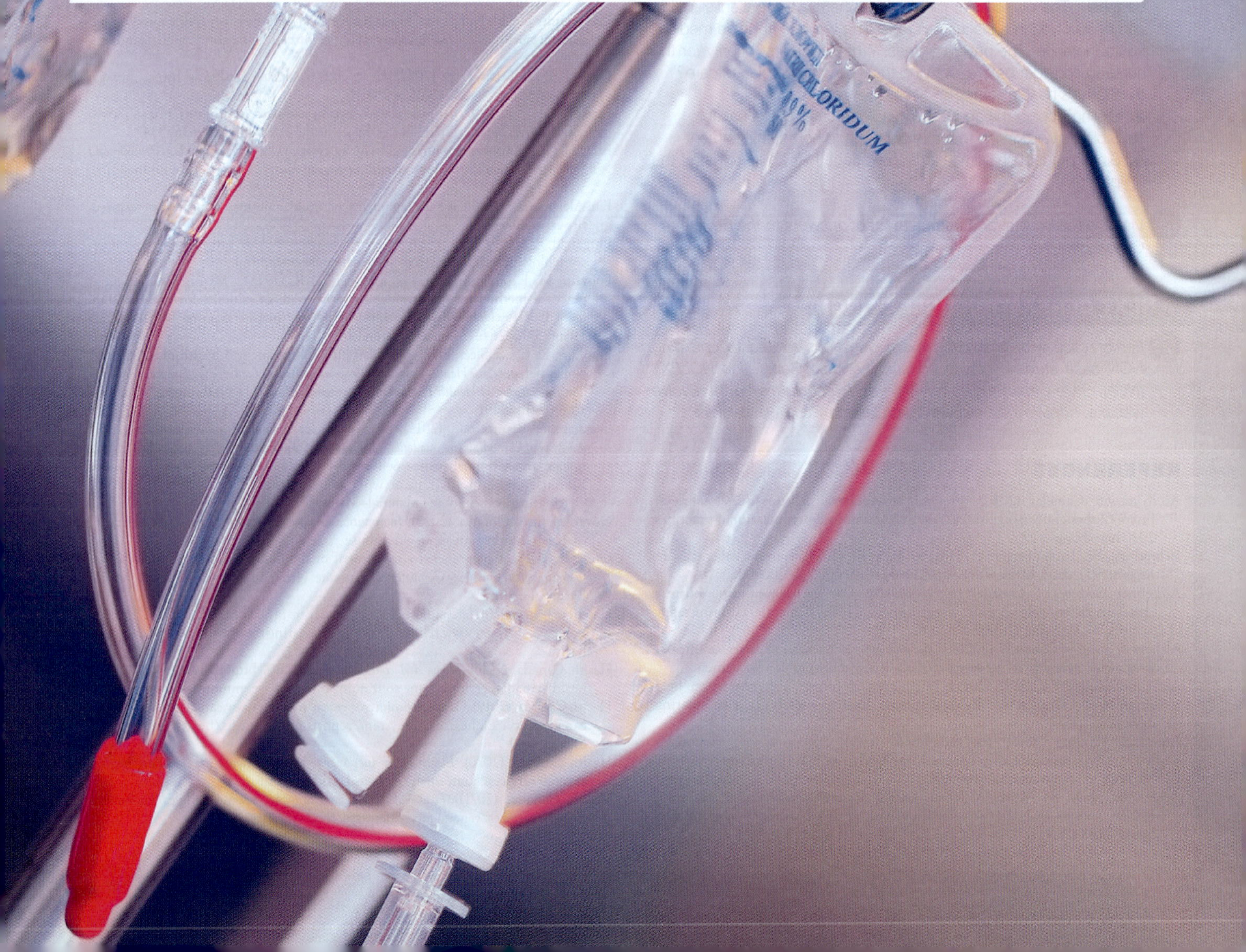

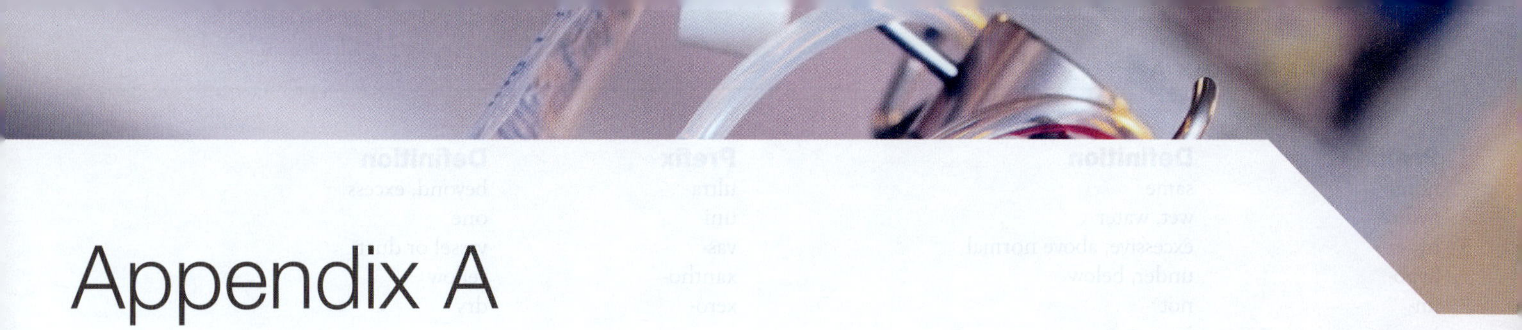

Appendix A

TERMINOLOGY/COMBINING FORMS: PREFIXES AND SUFFIXES

Medical terminology is similar to a foreign language. Many medical terms are derived from Latin and Greek sources. They often consist of two or more simple words or word elements. A word root or *combining form* may be put together with a *prefix* and a *suffix*.

Root—The basis of a word

Example: *nephr*/o/tic (degenerative changes in the kidney)

Root: nephr- (kidney)

Linking vowel—A vowel that joins the combining form to the suffix or another combining form

Example: nephr/*o*/sis (disease of the kidneys)

Linking vowel: o

Prefix—The beginning of a word

Example: *hyper*/active (excessively active)

Prefix: hyper- (excessive)

Suffix—The ending of a word

Example: nephr/*itis* (inflammation of the kidney)

Suffix: -itis (inflammation)

Combining form—The union of a word root with a linking vowel

Example: *hepato*/megaly (enlargement of the liver)

Combining form: hepato- (liver)

The following tables contain some of the most commonly used prefixes and suffixes.

COMMON PREFIXES

Prefix	Definition
a-	without
ab-	away from
abd-	abdominal
acu-	sharp
ad-	toward
adip-	fat
ad lib-	freely, as wanted
aero-	air, gas
al-	toward
ambi-	both
an-	not
ana-	up
ante-	before, in front of
anti-	against
arteri-	artery
arthro-	joint
auto-	self
bi-	two
brady-	slow
cata-	down
chole-	bile
cili-	eyelid
circum-	around
co-	with, together
cogni-	know
colo-	colon
con-	with, together
contra-	against
crani-	skull
cut-	skin
cyt-	cell
de-	from, lack of
demi-	half
dent-	tooth
derm-	skin
dia-	through, across
diplo-	double, two-fold
dis-	to free or undo
dors-	back
dur-	hard
dy-	two
dys-	bad, painful, difficult, abnormal
ec-	out, out from
ecto-	outside
em-	in
embol-	to insert
encephalo-	brain
endo-	in, within
entero-	intestine
epi-	above, on
erythro-	red
eso-	within, inward
et-	and
eu-	good, normal
ex-	out, away from
exo-	outside
extra-	outside
faci-	face
fiss-	split, cleft
fore-	before, in front of
gastro-	stomach
glosso-	relating to the tongue
glyco-	sugar
haplo-	simple, single
heme-	iron-based
hemi-	one half
hepat-	liver
hetero-	different
histo-	tissue

Prefix	Definition
homo-	same
hydro-	wet, water
hyper-	excessive, above normal
hypo-	under, below
im-	not
in-	in, not
infra-	under, below
inter-	between
intra-	in, within
isch-	deficiency
iso-	equal, alike
lapis-	stone
lapra-	loin or flank, sometimes abdomen
latero-	side
macro-	large
mal-	bad
meato-	opening
medi-	middle
melano-	black
mesa-	middle
meso-	middle
meta-	beyond, change
micro-	small
mono-	one
morpho-	form, structure
multi-	many, much
neo-	new
nephro-	kidney
oculo-	eye
onco-	tumour
oro-	mouth
osteo-	bone
pan-	all
para-	beside, beyond
per-	through, by
peri-	around
phago-	eating
poly-	many, much
post-	after, behind
pre-	before, in front of
primi-	first
pro-	before, in front of
pseudo-	false
quadri-	four
re-	again, backward
retro-	backward, behind
rhabdo-	rod-shaped, striated
rhodo-	red
scler-	hardening
semi-	one half
stetho-	chest
sub-	under, below
super-	above, excessive
supra-	above, excessive
sym-	together
syn-	union, together, joined
tachy-	rapid
tetra-	four
therm-	heat
trans-	through, across
tri-	three
ultra-	beyond, excess
uni-	one
vas-	vessel or duct
xantho-	yellow
xero-	dry

COMMON SUFFIXES

Suffix	Definition
-ac	pertaining to
-agra	excessive pain
-al	pertaining to
-algia	painful condition, pain
-apheresis	removal
-ar	pertaining to
-ary	pertaining to
-ase	enzyme
-bi	two, double
-blast	developing cell
-cele	hernia, swelling, sac
-centesis	puncture of a cavity
-clasis	break, fracture
-clysis	irrigation, washing
-coccus	berry shaped
-crit	to separate
-cyte	cell
-desis	fusion, binding, fixation
-drome	to run
-dynia	pain
-ectasis	expansion, dilation
-ectomy	excision, removal of a body part
-emesis	vomiting
-emia	blood
-er	one who
-gen	forming, producing, origin
-genesis	forming, producing, origin
-genic	origin, formation
-grade	to go
-gram	the record made, mark
-graph	instrument for recording, machine
-graphy	the process, process of recording
-ia	condition
-iasis	morbid condition
-iatry	treatment, medicine
-ic/-ical	pertaining to
-icle	small, minute
-ism	condition
-ist	one who specializes in, specialist
-itis	inflammation
-lith	stone, calculus
-logist	specialist in the study of
-logy	process of study
-lysis	dissolution, setting free
-malacia	softening, soft
-megaly	enlargement
-meter	instrument for measuring
-metry	act of measuring
-odynia	pain
-oid	form, shape
-ole	small, minute
-ology	study or science of

Suffix	Definition
-oma	tumour
-opsy	to view
-or	one who
-orrhea	flow, discharge
-osis	condition or state
-ous	pertaining to
-para	to bear (offspring)
-paresis	partial paralysis
-pathy	disease, suffering
-penia	deficiency, lack of, decrease
-pexy	fixation
-phagia	eating, swallowing
-phasia	speech
-philia	attraction for
-phobia	fear
-physis	to grow
-plasia	formation, growth
-plasm	growth, formation
-plasty	mold, shape, repair
-plegia	paralysis
-poiesis	formation, production
-ptosis	downward displacement, falling
-ptysis	spitting
-rrhage	bursting forth, rupture
-rrhaphy	suturing in place
-rrhea	flow, discharge
-rrhexis	rupture
-scope	instrument to visually examine
-scopy	process of examining, visual examination
-sepsis	infection
-sis	state of, condition
-spasm	involuntary spasm
-stalsis	constriction
-stasis	control, constant level, stop
-stenosis	narrowing, stricture
-stomy	creation of an opening
-therapy	treatment
-tic	pertaining to
-tome	instrument for cutting
-tomy	process of cutting, incision
-toxic	poison
-tresia	opening
-tripsy	surgical crushing
-trophy	nourishment
-ula	small, minute
-ule	small, minute
-y	process

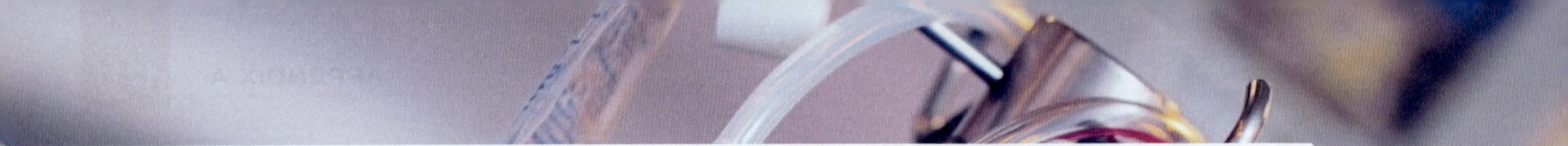

Index

Page numbers followed by "*f*" indicate figures, "*t*" indicate tables, and "*b*" indicate boxes.

Q

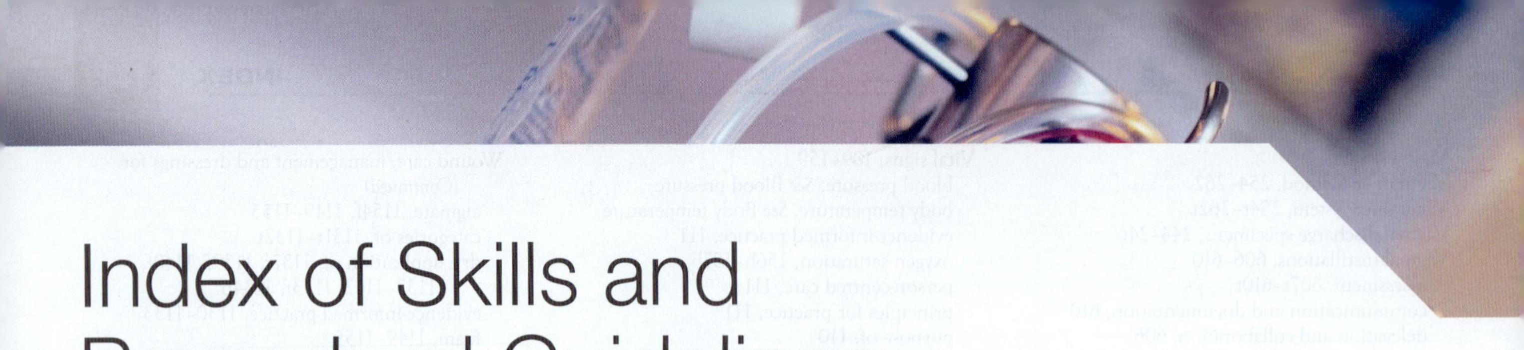

Index of Skills and Procedural Guidelines